D0220567

*Fundamental Principles and Practice of*

# Anaesthesia

To our children

Alison, Jo, David Chris
Charlotte
Lacy, Martha, Frank
Kristin and Matthew

# *Fundamental Principles and Practice of* **Anaesthesia**

*Edited by*

Peter Hutton BSc PhD MB ChB FRCP FRCA
*Henry Hill Hickman Professor of Anaesthesia*
*Featherstone Department of Anaesthesia and Intensive Care,*
*University of Birmingham, UK*

Griselda M Cooper MB ChB FRCA
*Senior Lecturer in Anaesthesia*
*Featherstone Department of Anaesthesia and Intensive Care,*
*University of Birmingham, UK*

Francis M James III MD
*Professor Emeritus, Department of Anesthesiology*
*Wake Forest University School of Medicine,*
*Winston-Salem, North Carolina, USA*

John Butterworth MD
*Professor, Department of Anesthesiology*
*Wake Forest University School of Medicine,*
*Winston-Salem, North Carolina, USA*

*Foreword by*

Leo Strunin MD FRCA FRCPC
*President, Association of Anaesthetists of Great Britain and Ireland;*
*BOC Professor of Anaesthesia, Director of Anaesthetics Unit*
*The Royal London Hospital, University of London, UK*

MARTIN DUNITZ

First published in the United Kingdom in 2002
by Martin Dunitz Ltd, The Livery House, 7–9 Pratt Street, London NW1 0AE

Tel.: +44 (0) 20 74822202
Fax.: +44 (0) 20 72670159
E-mail: info@dunitz.co.uk
Website: http://www.dunitz.co.uk



A CIP record for this book is available from the British Library.

ISBN 1-899066-57-8

Distributed in the USA by
Fulfilment Center
Taylor & Francis
7625 Empire Drive
Florence, KY 41042, USA
Toll Free Tel.: +1 800 634 7064
E-mail: cserve@routledge_ny.com

Distributed in Canada by
Taylor & Francis
74 Rolark Drive
Scarborough, Ontario M1R 4G2, Canada
Toll Free Tel.: +1 877 226 2237
E-mail: tal_fran@istar.ca

Distributed in the rest of the world by
ITPS Limited
Cheriton House
North Way
Andover, Hampshire SP10 5BE, UK
Tel.: +44 (0)1264 332424
E-mail: reception@itps.co.uk

Composition by Creative Associates, Oxford UK
Manufactured in China by Imago

# Contents

## Section 2 Integrated basic sciences

Contents

## Section 3 The presenting patient

Contents

## Section 4 Special subjects: physiology and pharmacology

Contents

# Foreword

Throughout the world the modern anaesthetist may be found practising in many aspects of acute medical care. These include preoperative assessment clinics, the traditional role in the operating theatres for both in-patient and day-stay units, post-anaesthetic recovery, high dependency units, intensive care medicine, emergency and perioperative medicine, and pain management. The training of young doctors to be the anaesthetists of the future is well developed in many countries. The regulatory bodies of this training have a prime responsibility to make sure that the trainee has developed the proper competencies to be a professional anaesthetist, as defined by the necessary knowledge, skills and attitudes, at the completion of the training period. However this is not the end. The whole purpose of training is to produce anaesthetists who will provide, wherever they practice and throughout their careers, safe and competent anaesthesia care for their patients and, in addition, be the teachers of the next generation.

It is therefore crucial, first of all, that we recruit suitable doctors to anaesthesia practice, and, second, that training programmes provide the necessary environment to produce successful professionals. Key to any training is the acquisition of knowledge, which is the bedrock of developing future skills and attitudes. In days gone by, see one, do one — get on with it and teach the next one characterized such acquisition. However, times have changed. Training is now increasingly regulated and only by passing regular assessments can a trainee progress through their training programme. Many programmes have formal examinations as part of their assessment process and the regulatory bodies reasonably expect that at such examinations, particularly if conducted in the early years of training, trainees should be able to demonstrate, usually in written and oral formats, that they possess the necessary knowledge to proceed. Even without formal examination, it seems axiomatic that there must be some form of assessment to determine that trainees have acquired the necessary knowledge before they can practise unsupervised.

How then to acquire the knowledge for the broad range of competencies required of the modern anaesthetist? Of more immediate interest to the trainee just commencing their career with examinations looming, where should they look? The written word, for example in conventional textbooks and journals, has always been an integral part of providing knowledge. However, by their nature these sources may be too complex and detailed for the early years of training and perhaps best left for final specialist training and lifelong continuous professional development.

*Fundamental Principles and Practice of Anaesthesia*, edited by Professor Peter Hutton and his colleagues, is a novel approach to providing written information aimed at the early years of training. When one travels around the world, meeting anaesthetic colleagues and watching their practice, one is struck by the many similarities and relatively uniform approach to problems. Obviously local circumstances dictate some differences. This book rightly takes the view that the information presented in its four sections: Basic anaesthetic practice, Integrated basic science, The presenting patient and Special subjects, has a universality of principles and is appropriate for international use. The authors are all in clinical practice and are involved in postgraduate training and examination. They have used their experience to produce a text that the aspiring anaesthetist should use to get started and can feel confident that the required knowledge for safe practice is included. Getting the principles right at the start is surely the best way to ensure that one can maintain professional attitudes throughout a working lifetime.

Leo Strunin MD FRCA FRCPC
*President, Association of Anaesthetists of Great Britain and Ireland;*
*BOC Professor of Anaesthesia,*
*Barts and The London School of Medicine and Dentistry,*
*Queen Mary s College, University of London UK*

# Preface

This book is a foundation text in anaesthesia, developed to meet the needs of the first two or three years of postgraduate training. It covers the clinical anaesthesia, basic science, and principles of peri-operative medicine that are required for the appropriate examination sections of the UK and Irish Colleges, the American Board of Anesthesiology, the Royal College of Physicians and Surgeons of Canada, the European Diploma of Anaesthesia and Intensive Care, the Australian & New Zealand College, the Hong Kong College, and the National University of Singapore. For the final examinations of these institutions, trainees will need some additional information on aspects of specialized anaesthesia, intensive care and pain management.

The book consists of four sections:

- **Section 1 – Basic anaesthesia practice** – describes the principles of the preoperative visit, general and regional anaesthesia, monitoring, and postoperative care, including intensive care.
- **Section 2 – Integrated basic sciences** – begins with general physiological and pharmacological principles relevant to anaesthesia. This leads on to systematic physiology and pharmacology, more detailed pharmacology of anaesthetics, and concludes with chapters on applied physics, clinical measurement, and statistics.
- **Section 3 – The presenting patient** – describes the peri-operative care of patients with co-existing conditions that have significant implications for the management of anaesthesia.
- **Section 4 – Special subjects: physiology and pharmacology** – covers a variety of topics which, although necessary to practice and understanding, do not conveniently fall into the other parts of the book. These chapters have been subdivided into groupings on physiology and pharmacology, practical procedures and clinical practice.

This book differs in concept, content, arrangement and layout from other texts intended for this period of training. Common clinical problems and their solutions are emphasized whenever possible, and the relevance of basic science to safe practice is an underlying theme. The authors are from both sides of the Atlantic. All are active clinicians involved in postgraduate education and the majority are examiners for their relevant College. This emphasizes the editors' belief that the basic science and clinical knowledge needed to underpin safe practice are essentially universal, even though the style of delivery may depend on local custom. For example, the use of anaesthetic rooms is common in the UK but rare in the US, yet the requirements for a safe induction or establishment of a regional block are the same in both locations. This book, by describing principles rather than local practice, will encourage trainees to think in a similar way – an important consideration for those who broaden their clinical experience by working in another country. Where differences cannot be avoided (e.g. the colour coding of cylinders, or accepted pollution levels), the convention for each country is given.

The selection of material for an integrated text such as this is, on occasion, difficult. We have tried to ensure that the core knowledge necessary for understanding and safe practice is included, and have amplified those sections which, through our knowledge of teaching and examining postgraduate trainees, frequently require reinforcement or are poorly understood. We have also included a few subjects outside the normal curricula (e.g. principles of genetics, ageing) which are likely to become immensely important in the future. The final responsibility for content lies with the editors rather than the individual contributors. Wherever possible, cross referencing between sections has been used to link basic science with clinical practice.

The text is heavily supported with line drawings, clinical photographs, and tables. This is appropriate for what is, in many of its aspects, a visual subject. The diagrams have been selected or specially designed to give a specific message; tables contain group data, comparisons and material requiring specific emphasis.

In comparison with other books covering the same ground, we have deliberately avoided heavy referencing. The role of the textbook is changing, and will continue to change under the influence of electronic publishing. We believe that a modern textbook should be an instructional manual, universally applicable, which describes, in a clear, unambiguous and attractive way, accepted safe practice and the established basic science which underpins it. It should be an integrated whole and not try to contain chapters all of which are an 'up-to-the-minute' monograph. Our preference has been to develop logical principles, rather than referencing the text heavily with 'cutting edge opinion' (which can quickly become out of date). Furthermore, the majority of trainees make little use of the references. Instead, like us, they obtain articles from recent research journals and electronic sources for project work and presentations. We have therefore, in the majority of instances, simply listed *Further reading* at the end of each chapter for those who wish to extend their study. A few of these sources have been chosen for their historical importance. The test of this book will be in its continuing relevance and applicability rather than as a dated reference source.

Finally, our very grateful thanks go to Caroline Denver for her unfailing secretarial support, and to Helen Barham who has been an outstanding freelance editor.

# Contributors

**Lesley Bromley FRCA**
Senior Lecturer in Anaesthetics, Academic Department of Anaesthetics, University College London School of Medicine, The Middlesex Hospital, London UK

**Joanna M Budd MB BS FRCA**
Consultant Anaesthetist, Worcester Royal Infirmary, Worcester UK

**Ken Burchett MB ChB FRCA**
Consultant in Anaesthesia and Critical Care, Queen Elizabeth Hospital, Kings Lynn, Norfolk UK

**John Butterworth IV MD**
Professor and Section Head, Cardiothoracic Anesthesia, Department of Anesthesiology, Wake Forest University School of Medicine, Winston-Salem, North Carolina USA

**Mark A. Cannon MD**
Assistant Professor and Co-Director, Cardiothoracic Intensive Care Unit, Division of Cardiothoracic Anesthesia and Critical Care, Vanderbilt University Medical Center, Nashville, Tennessee USA

**Michael L. Cannon MD**
Assistant Professor, Department of Anesthesiology, Wake Forest University School of Medicine, Winston-Salem, North Carolina USA

**Thomas H. Clutton-Brock MB ChB MRCP FRCA**
Senior Lecturer in Anaesthesia and Intensive Care Medicine, University Department of Anaesthesia and Intensive Care, Queen Elizabeth Hospital, Birmingham UK

**David F. Cochrane MB ChB FRCA**
Consultant Anaesthetist, North Bristol NHS Trust, Frenchay Hospital, Bristol UK

**David M. Colonna MD**
Assistant Professor, Department of Anesthesiology, Wake Forest University School of Medicine, Winston-Salem, North Carolina USA

**Denis Connolly MB FFARCSI**
Consultant Anaesthetist and Medical Director, Musgrave Park Hospital, Stockman s Lane, Belfast Northern Ireland

**Laura S. Dean MD**
Assistant Professor, Department of Anesthesiology, Wake Forest University School of Medicine, Winston-Salem, North Carolina USA

**Chris Dodds MRCGP FRCA**
Consultant Anaesthetist and Director, Department of Anaesthesia, South Cleveland Hospital, Middlesborough UK

**Sylvia Y. Dolinski MD**
Assistant Professor, Department of Anesthesiology, Wake Forest University School of Medicine, Winston-Salem, North Carolina USA

**Robert O. Feneck MB BS FRCA**
Consultant Anaesthetist and Honorary Senior Lecturer, St Thomas Hospital; Guys, King s and St Thomas School of Medicine and Dentistry, London UK

**Jonathan W. Freeman TD FRCA**
Consultant Anaesthetist and Intensivist, Department of Anaesthesia, Queen Elizabeth Hospital, Birmingham UK

**Thomas Gallacher FRCA**
University Department of Anaesthesia, Queen Elizabeth Hospital, Birmingham UK

**Leanne Groban MD**
Assistant Professor, Department of Anesthesiology, Wake Forest University School of Medicine, Winston-Salem, North Carolina USA

**Sandy L. Hack Pharm D BCNSP BS**
Clinical Co-ordinator, Nutrition Support, Department of Pharmacy, Wake Forest University Baptist Medical Center, Winston-Salem, North Carolina USA

**Timothy N. Harwood MD**
Assistant Professor, Department of Anesthesiology, Wake Forest University School of Medicine, Winston-Salem, North Carolina USA

**Nigel J. N. Harper MB ChB FRCA**
Consultant in Anaesthesia and Intensive Care, Manchester Royal Infirmary, Central Manchester and Manchester Children s University Hospitals NHS Trust; Honorary Clinical Lecturer, University of Manchester, Manchester UK

**Jennifer M. Hunter MB ChB PhD FRCA**
Professor of Anaesthesia, University Department of Anaesthesia, The University of Liverpool, Liverpool UK

**Timothy J. Jones FRCS**
Department of Cardiothoracic Surgery, Queen Elizabeth Hospital, Birmingham UK

**Jeffrey S. Kelly MD FACEP**
Associate Professor, Department of Anesthesiology, Wake Forest University School of Medicine, Winston-Salem, North Carolina USA

**Kin-Leong Kong MD MB BS FRCA**
Consultant Anaesthetist, City Hospital NHS Trust, Birmingham; Honorary Senior Clinical Lecturer, University of Birmingham, Birmingham UK

**Kate Leslie MD FANZCA**
Department of Anaesthesia, The Royal Melbourne Hospital, Parkville, Victoria Australia

**Drew A. MacGregor MD**
Associate Professor of Anesthesiology (Critical Care), Associate Professor of Internal Medicine (Pulmonary and Critical Care), Department of Anesthesiology, Wake Forest University School of Medicine, Winston-Salem, North Carolina USA

**Mavji Manji MB BCh MRCP (UK) FRCA**
Consultant, Intensive Care Medicine and Anaesthesia, University Hospital Birmingham NHS Trust, Birmingham UK

**Patrick P. McCaslin MD**
Anesthesiology Department, St Tammany Parish Hospital, Covington, Louisiana USA

**John J. McCloskey MD**
Assistant Professor, Department of Anesthesiology, Wake Forest University School of Medicine, Winston-Salem, North Carolina USA

**S. John Mihic PhD**
Associate Professor, Section of Neurobiology and Waggoner Center for Alcohol and Addiction Research, University of Texas at Austin, Austin, Texas USA

**J. Peter Millns MB BS FRCA**
Consultant Anaesthetist, Department of Anaesthesia, Birmingham Women's Hospital NHS Trust, Birmingham UK

**Samiran Nath BSc MB ChB MRCP (UK)**
Specialist Registrar in Cardiology and General Medicine, Department: Department of Cardiology, North Manchester General Hospital, Manchester UK

**Peter Nightingale FRCA FRCP**
Consultant in Anaesthesia and Intensive Care, Withington Hospital, Manchester UK

**Annette G. Pashayan MD**
Medical Director and Staff Anesthesiologist, HealthSouth Greensboro Specialty Surgical Center, Winston-Salem, North Carolina USA

**Melissa A. Polkinghorne RN**
Assistant Nurse Manager and Operating Room Laser Nurse, Duke University Medical Center, Durham, North Carolina USA

**Richard C. Prielipp MD**
Professor and Section Head, Critical Care Medicine, Department of Anesthesiology, Wake Forest University School of Medicine, Winston-Salem, North Carolina USA

**Charles S. Reilly MD FRCA**
Professor and Head of Anaesthesia, University of Sheffield, Royal Hallamshire Hospital, Sheffield UK

**Douglas G. Ririe MD**
Assistant Professor, Department of Anesthesiology, Wake Forest University School of Medicine, Winston-Salem, North Carolina USA

**Pamela H. Roberts MD**
Associate Professor, Department of Anesthesiology, Wake Forest University School of Medicine, Winston-Salem, North Carolina USA

**Kashemi D. Rorie PhD**
Research Assistant, Department of Anesthesiology, Wake Forest University School of Medicine, Winston-Salem, North Carolina USA

**David J. Rowbotham MB ChB MD MRCP FRCA**
Professor of Anaesthesia and Pain Management, Head of Department, Department of Anaesthesia, Critical Care and Pain Management, Leicester Warwick Medical School, University Hospitals of Leicester, Leicester UK

**David Saunders PhD FRCA**
Department of Anaesthesia, Southampton General Hospital, Southampton UK

**John W. Sear BSc PhD FFARCS FANZCA**
Consultant Anaesthetist, John Radcliffe Hospital, Oxford UK

**Maire P. Shelly MB ChB FRCA**
Consultant in Anaesthesia and Intensive Care, Withington Hospital, Manchester UK

**Robert J. Sherertz MD**
Professor of Internal Medicine (Infectious Diseases), Section head of Infectious Diseases, Department of Internal Medicine, Wake Forest University School of Medicine, Winston-Salem, North Caroline USA

**David A. Stump PhD**
Director, Cerebral Blood Flow Laboratory, Department of Anesthesiology, Wake Forest University School of Medicine, Winston-Salem, North Carolina USA

**Anne J. Sutcliffe BSc MB ChB FRCA**
Consultant in Anaesthesia and Intensive care, Honorary Senior Lecturer, Queen Elizabeth Hospital, Edgbaston, Birmingham UK

**Joseph R. Tobin MD**
Associate Professor and Section Head, Pediatric Anesthesia & Critical Care, Department of Anesthesiology, Wake Forest University School of Medicine, Winston-Salem, North Carolina USA

**Andrew A. Tomlinson MB BS FRCA**
Consultant Anaesthetist, North Staffordshire Hospital, Stoke-on-Trent UK

**Christopher. J. Vallis BSc FRCA FRCPCH DCH**
Consultant Paediatric Anaesthetist, Department of Anaesthesia, Royal Victoria Infirmary, Newcastle upon Tyne UK

**Michael H. Wall MD**
Assistant Professor, Department of Anesthesiology, Wake Forest University School of Medicine, Winston-Salem, North Carolina USA

**Anthony D. Wilkey FRCA**
Consultant Anaesthetist, Featherstone Department of Anaesthesia and Intensive Care, Queen Elizabeth Hospital, Birmingham UK

**Matthew J. Wilson BM ChB BA(Oxon) FRCA**
Consultant Anaesthetist, University Hospital Birmingham, Women's Hospital Birmingham; Honorary Senior Lecturer in Anaesthesia, University of Birmingham, Birmingham UK

ERRATA

Because of problems with software conversion the following items were printed incorrectly.

**Pg. 151, Fig. 11.1**: left hand side

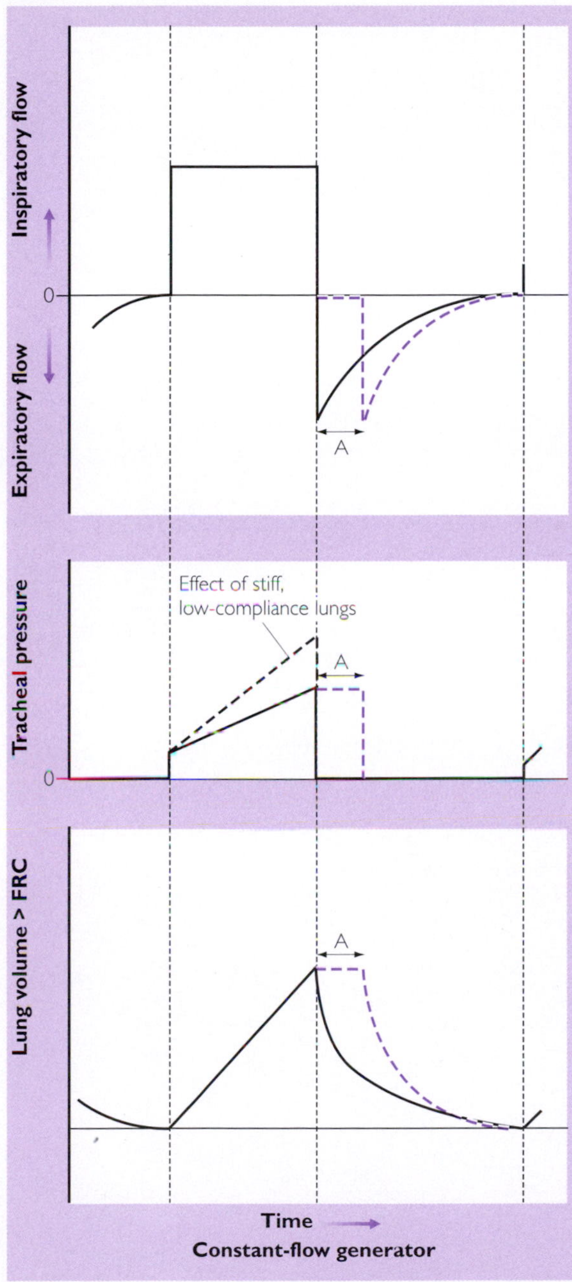


**Pg. 679, Fig. 37.47**

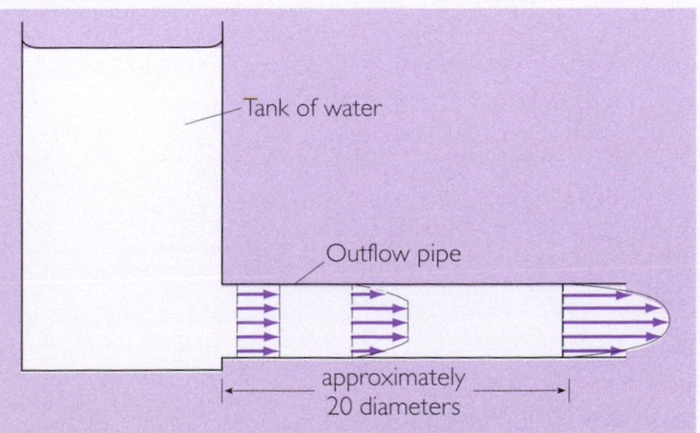


**Pg. 750**, beneath Fig. 40.4

$$y = \frac{1}{\sigma\sqrt{2\pi}} \cdot e^{\frac{-1}{2}\left(\frac{x-\mu}{\sigma}\right)^2}$$

**Pg. 751**

$$\frac{\Sigma|x-\bar{x}|}{n} = \text{Mean absolute deviation} \quad (1)$$

$$\frac{\Sigma\,(x-\bar{x})^2}{n} = S^2 \text{ (variance)} \quad (2)$$

$$\Sigma\,(x-\bar{x})^2 = \Sigma x^2 - \frac{(\Sigma x)^2}{n} = \text{SS (sum of squares)} \quad (3)$$

$$\sqrt{\frac{\Sigma\,(x-\bar{x})^2}{n}} = \text{S (standard deviation)} \quad (4)$$

**Pg. 752**

$$\text{SD }(\bar{x}) = \sqrt{\frac{\sigma^2}{n}} = \frac{\sigma}{\sqrt{n}} \approx \frac{S}{\sqrt{n}} \approx \text{SEM} \quad (6)$$

**Pg. 755**

$$\text{var}\,(\bar{x}_1 - \bar{x}_2) = \text{var}\,(\bar{x}_1 + \bar{x}_2) = \frac{\sigma_1^2}{n_1} + \frac{\sigma_2^2}{n_2} \quad (7)$$

$$\text{SE difference} = \sqrt{\frac{S_1^2}{n_1} + \frac{S_2^2}{n_2}} \quad (8)$$

$$\text{SE difference} = \sqrt{\frac{(10.4)^2}{100} + \frac{(12.4)^2}{100}} \quad (9)$$

$$= 1.61 \text{ mmHg}$$

**Pg. 759**

$$\text{b (slope)} = \frac{\Sigma\,(x-\bar{x})\,(y-\bar{y})}{\Sigma\,(x-\bar{x})^2} \quad (10)$$

$$r = \frac{\Sigma\,(x-\bar{x})\,(y-\bar{y})}{\sqrt{\Sigma\,(x-\bar{x})^2\,\Sigma\,(y-\bar{y})^2}} \quad (11)$$

$$t = \sqrt{\frac{n-2}{1-r^2}} \quad (12)$$

**Pg. 895, Fig. 57.3**: the lower x-ray is the wrong way up

# Section 1

# Basic anaesthesia practice

# Chapter 1 Anaesthesia and the preoperative visit

P. Hutton

## THE SCOPE OF ANAESTHESIA PRACTICE

Anaesthesia makes numerous contributions to hospital practice, some of which are shown in Table 1.1. The expansion of activities from its original role as a provider of intraoperative unconsciousness has developed in response to the clinical needs of patients. Anaesthetists have often 'filled the gap' not provided by others and in doing so have developed a specialty that has a major impact on modern hospital care. The term 'perioperative physician' is being applied to anaesthetists with increasing frequency. Almost two-thirds of all patients attending a hospital will, at some time during their stay, benefit from the skills of an anaesthetist. In the United Kingdom, the cost of employing anaesthetists is approximately 3% of the budget of a hospital but they have an impact on over 60% of its income (Figure 1.1).

In a number of instances, the 'subspecialty' areas shown in Table 1.1 have almost developed sufficiently to constitute disciplines in their own right. The work of one consultant anaesthetist can therefore be completely different to that of another. A trainee entering anaesthesia consequently has a wide spectrum of career opportunities. Despite this diversity of clinical activity, there is nevertheless a common core of theoretical knowledge, practical skills and experience that all doctors describing themselves as anaesthetists require, and that, in part, is what this book is about.

Although the specialty has an excellent clinical record of development, innovation and safety, the same cannot always be said for its public image. Surveys of patients have repeatedly shown that they know little about our activities and most of them have no idea of the training and commitment required to qualify as an anaesthetist. Not long ago a colleague of mine had his pride dented when a patient remarked 'you seem to know quite a lot, you should have gone in for being a doctor!' Even our surgical colleagues, who only see us individually for part of the working week, often have little concept of what we are doing when we are not with them.

Therefore, all anaesthetists, whatever their grade, should make every effort to communicate clearly with

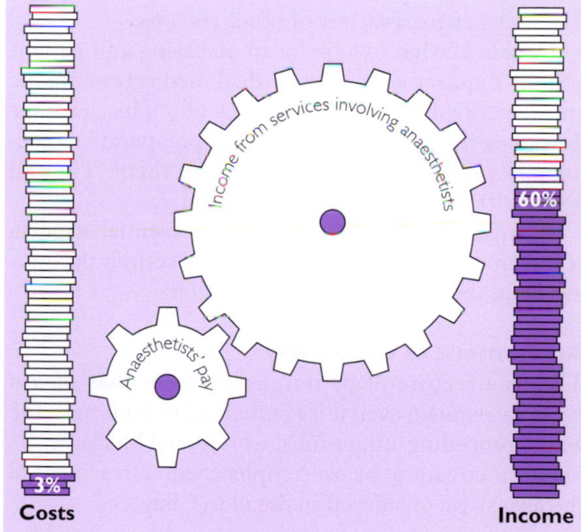


**Figure 1.1.** The cost of anaesthetists and their impact on hospital income. (Audit Commission, *Anaesthesia Under Examination*, 1997.)

**Table 1.1. Some of the ways in which anaesthesia contributes to hospital practice**

| | |
|---|---|
| Preoperative assessment | Accident and emergency services |
| Intraoperative care | Dental surgery |
| Postoperative care | Radiology |
| Acute pain management | Radiotherapy |
| Chronic pain management | Palliative care |
| Intensive care medicine | Sleep studies |
| Resuscitation | Burns, cardiology, psychiatry etc. |
| Obstetric care | Various outpatient activities |

both patients and colleagues. This is particularly so when talking to patients, who often have little knowledge of what to expect and even less of what is possible. Providing patients with good information must be one of our priorities. In addition, it is also a major component of sound risk-management strategy.

## THE PREOPERATIVE VISIT

The preoperative visit is a key part of all anaesthetic procedures, for both the patient and the anaesthetist. Patients like to meet their anaesthetist and it is bad practice if they are not informed about the anaesthetic technique that will be used. The visit gives the patient the opportunity to ask questions, which need to be answered in a manner appropriate to their age and intellect. Whenever possible, the visit should be carried out by the same person who administers the anaesthetic and the visit recorded on the anaesthetic sheet.

In the past, premedicant drugs contributed more to the anaesthetic technique itself than they do now. This is because modern drugs have made the process of induction and recovery so much smoother. The reduction in dependence on the effect of the premedicant has, however, in no way reduced the importance of the preoperative visit and, where appropriate, the prescription of drugs for a variety of other reasons.

Details of what to look for in assessing a fit patient and the requirements of individual medical conditions are described in Chapters 41 – 66. This chapter describes the general objectives of preoperative visiting and comments briefly on each of them. They all begin with A and are listed in Table 1.2.

It is clear that some of these are essential aspects of the process, whereas others apply selectively depending upon the patient and the operation.

### Assessment of the airway

This is a feature of patient assessment that *should never be omitted*, even if it is intended to undertake the whole procedure under local or regional blockade. Its importance cannot be overemphasized. Assessment of the airway is considered in detail in Chapter 7.

### Appraising and answering

As discussed above, all patients deserve to be given an explanation of the process that they are about to undergo in language appropriate to their understanding. Their behaviour will vary from I don t want to know anything Doc to nothing less than demanding a detailed account of every possible complication. Common sense is obviously needed in dealing with different individuals. Although one is often tempted to do so, do not lie, when questioned, to please the patient, especially about the risks of awareness. Quite often, good rapport and a straightforward answering of queries are the best anxiolytic available.

If the patient asks questions about the *surgery* to be performed, it is probably satisfactory to answer simple queries to which there is an unambiguous answer, but *do not* become involved in details of surgical technique. These should be dealt with by the surgical staff whose responsibility it is.

If a local block or the use of suppositories is planned, it is mandatory in current practice that the patient be informed about these before any premedication is given, and agreement to their use noted on the anaesthetic chart.

### Anxiolysis

Often, as described above, all that is required for anxiolysis in the typical patient undergoing minor surgery is the reassurance of the preoperative visit. For those of nervous disposition, and if major surgery (particularly with an uncertain outcome) is planned, pharmacological anxiolysis is usually preferred by both the patient and the anaesthetist. This may also, on occasions, include night sedation before surgery. The most common preparations used in current practice are short-acting benzodiazepines (e.g. temazepam 10 – 30 mg depending on age and weight). If the timing of surgery is uncertain, the longer-acting diazepam is more satisfactory. For the traditional heavy premedication , which may be preferred for some patients, a generous dose of diazepam 2 hours before surgery followed by an intramuscular opioid 1 hour later is, in the opinion of the author, hard to beat. For elderly people or those with ischaemic heart disease, prescribe nasal or facemask oxygen after the opioid.

### Anaesthetic history

All patients must be asked if they, or their relatives, have had any anaesthetics previously and if there were any complications. In addition to possibly revealing rare familial traits (e.g. malignant hyperpyrexia), this

**Table 1.2. The objectives of the preoperative visit**

| | |
|---|---|
| Assessment of the airway | Antiemesis |
| Appraising and answering | Antisialogogue therapy |
| Anxiolysis | Antacid therapy |
| Anaesthetic history | Antibiotic therapy |
| Amnesia | Antiasthma and antiallergy therapy |
| Analgesia | Associated conditions and existing therapies |
| Antithrombosis | Antivagal therapy |
| Assessment of drug response | |

not infrequently allows previous imperfect experiences to be taken into account (e.g. fear of needles) and, whenever possible, the patient s fears allayed or appropriate action taken (e.g. prophylaxis for nausea and vomiting).

Repeat anaesthesia should avoid the use of halothane unless, on balance, it is still the best agent for the proposed procedure and no other acceptable alternative is available. If this is indeed the case, the reasons for using it need to be documented.

There now seems little doubt that, on very rare occasions, repeated halothane anaesthesia can result in severe liver damage. The shorter the exposure time, the stronger the reaction, although in some cases the diagnosis of halothane-related damage has been made with exposures over a year previously. In published series of fulminant hepatic failure, halothane hepatitis has sometimes represented up to 5% of cases. Risk factors are shown in Table 1.3.

The risk of halothane hepatitis has resulted in the Committee on Safety of Medicines (CSM) issuing practice guidelines. These are given in Table 1.4.

Although it is possible to argue with some of these recommendations, they nevertheless represent the published practice guidelines so, unless there are very strong reasons not to do so, they should be adhered to.

### Amnesia

There are some patients who want to remember nothing about the operative procedure that they are about to undergo; there are others who feel cheated if amnesia for induction and recovery occurs. A reasonable approach is to respect the patient s wishes and, if they request no memory of events after leaving the ward, to prescribe a generous dose of lorazepam or use some other heavy premedication.

### Analgesia

As described above, opioids can, on occasion, form part of the premedication and can be commenced preoperatively for postoperative pain relief.

After opioid administration, most patients breathing air have a fall in their oxygen saturation, so those at risk (e.g. with ischaemic heart disease) need to have facemask or nasal oxygen prescribed. Opioids also produce nausea in a proportion of patients and this may require the prescription of an antiemetic.

Non-steroidal anti-inflammatory drugs are increasingly being used for minor and moderate pain control postoperatively and, if the surgical procedure is short, need to be given at an appropriate time preoperatively so that they can be acting properly when the patient wakes up.

The other reason for giving analgesics preoperatively is to control existing pain (e.g. from appendicitis). Once the surgical diagnosis has been made and the operation planned, there is no reason to withhold analgesics. Although analgesia should be initiated by the surgical team, if it has not been, the anaesthetist should make sure that it is when he or she sees the patient.

The preoperative visit should also be used as an opportunity to discuss the various methods of postoperative analgesia available to the patient. The activities of the acute pain service can be outlined and options such as epidural or patient-controlled analgesia explained.

### Antithrombosis

Patients who present for surgery may be on antiplatelet drugs or anticoagulants, or may need them to reduce the incidence of postoperative deep vein thrombosis (DVT) or arterial thromboembolism. Whether a patient should be given anticoagulants depends on the operation and the patient.

**Table 1.3. Risk factors for halothane hepatitis**

| | |
|---|---|
| High | Recent previous exposure |
| | Previous adverse reaction |
| Uncertain but some evidence of association with | Obesity |
| | Female gender |
| | Drug allergy |
| | Lymphocyte sensitivity to phenytoin |
| | Family history of halothane hepatotoxicity |

**Table 1.4. Halothane exposure guidelines (CSM, 1991)**

| | |
|---|---|
| Avoid halothane exposure if | Previous exposure within 3 months |
| | Previous adverse reaction to halothane |
| | Family history of adverse reaction to halothane |
| | Adverse reaction to other halogenated hydrocarbon anaesthetic |
| | Pre-existing liver disease |

Patients who are already established on antiplatelet therapy (e.g. aspirin) can have their therapy continued, unless there are specific reasons to stop it. It is difficult to say exactly what these are at present because they vary from hospital to hospital and doctor to doctor.

Similarly, patients on maintenance anticoagulation should *not* have their clotting status reversed without very strong reasons to do so. The usual practice is to convert patients from warfarin to heparin therapy preoperatively so that, if necessary, the anticoagulation can be reversed quickly and for a limited period. Trainees should follow local guidelines and refer to consultant staff for advice in particular cases. It would not be wise, in the current climate of opinion, to undertake epidural and spinal blocks in the presence of antiplatelet or full anticoagulant therapy. Whether patients at risk of arterial thromboembolism (e.g. with carotid stenosis) should have preoperative aspirin started prophylactically is highly contentious at present. Over the next few years, guidelines on the use of aspirin therapy will undoubtedly become clearer.

The prophylaxis of DVT and pulmonary embolism (PE) using heparin has been studied for many years and there is now more agreement on its management. One problem is the fact that frank PE occurs in only a small percentage of those who acquire a DVT and that anticoagulant therapy itself is not without complications. There is, however, a growing consensus emerging that has been helped by a recent intercollegiate report and several review articles. *A key point is that the only effective treatment is prevention: therefore prophylaxis should be offered to all patients at risk.*

The risk factors for venous thromboembolism are given in Table 1.5.

For the purposes of determining the prophylactic regimen, patients can be stratified into low, medium and high risk. Reasonable definitions of these categories are given in Table 1.6.

Suggested guidelines for the prophylaxis of venous thromboembolism are given in Table 1.7. Since there is still debate about optimal therapy, trainees should always follow local guidelines and protocols.

Low molecular weight heparin has been shown to have been significantly superior to unfractionated heparin only in the prophylaxis of venous thromboembolism in patients undergoing major lower-limb orthopaedic surgery.

It is part of the anaesthetist's responsibilities to draw the attention of the surgical staff to medium- and high-risk cases if appropriate prophylactic measures have not been taken.

### Assessment of drug response

Giving a drug as a premedication (e.g. intramuscular morphine) allows its depressant effect to be seen at approximately peak level when the patient is in the anaesthetic room. This may give a guide to the safe dosage of any postoperative regimen that is subsequently prescribed.

### Antiemesis

Antiemetics are relevant in two ways: first, patients may present for urgent surgery (e.g. after trauma) with the possibility of having a full stomach. Second, postoperative nausea and vomiting (PONV) is a common problem in both elective and urgent patients (see Chapter 5, Table 5.10). There are various drugs that can be given to alleviate PONV, which are described more fully in Chapters 5 and 27.

One important point is that some drugs, for example, metoclopramide, promote gastric emptying whereas others, for example, prochlorperazine, reduce nausea and vomiting but may have little action

**Table 1.5. Risk factors for venous thromboembolism**

| Patient-specific factors | Surgical or disease-related factors |
|---|---|
| Age > 40 years | Trauma or surgery especially of the pelvis, hip and lower limb |
| Severe obesity | Malignancy, especially pelvic or with abdominal metastases |
| Immobility (bed rest over 4 days) | Heart failure |
| Pregnancy | Recent myocardial infarction |
| Puerperium | Paralysis of lower limb(s) |
| Oral contraceptive medication | Severe infection |
| High-dose oestrogens | Inflammatory bowel disease |
| Previous DVT or PE | Nephrotic syndrome |
| Any type of thrombophilia | Polycythaemia |
| Homocystinaemia | Paraproteinaemia |
| | Behçet's disease |
| | Paroxysmal nocturnal haemoglobinuria |

DVT, deep vein thrombosis; PE, pulmonary embolism.
Adapted from Verstraete M. *BMJ* 1997;314:123 and Wheatley T, Veitch PS. *Br J Anaesth* 1997;78:118.

**Table 1.6. Categories of risk of venous thromboembolism**

| Low risk (proximal vein thrombosis 0.4%, fatal PE < 0.2%) | Medium risk (proximal vein thrombosis 2–4%, fatal PE < 0.2–0.5%) | High risk (proximal vein thrombosis 10–20%, fatal PE 1–5%) |
|---|---|---|
| Patients undergoing minor surgery (< 30 min) with no other risk factors | Major general, urological, gynaecological, cardiothoracic, vascular or neurological surgery in patients > 40 years or a patient with one or more other risk factors | Fracture or major orthopaedic surgery of pelvis, hip or leg |
| Patients < 40 years undergoing surgery (> 30 min) with no other risk factors | Major trauma or burns | Major pelvic or abdominal surgery for cancer |
| Patients with minor trauma or minor medical illness | Oral contraceptive medication | Major surgery, trauma or illness in patients with previous DVT, PE, or thrombophilia |
| | Minor trauma, surgery or illness in patients with previous DVT, PE or thrombophilia | Leg paralysis (including stroke) |
| | Plastercast immobilization of the leg in a patient with minor injury | Critical ischaemia or major leg amputation |
| | Major acute medical illness such as myocardial infarction, heart failure, chest infection, cancer or inflammatory bowel disease | |

DVT, deep vein thrombosis; PE, pulmonary embolism.
Adapted from Verstraete M. *BMJ* 1997;314:123 and Wheatley T, Veitch PS. *Br J Anaesth* 1997;78:118.

**Table 1.7. Suggested guidelines for prophylaxis of venous thromboembolism**

| Category of risk | Suggested guidelines |
|---|---|
| Low | Compression stockings<br>No drug therapy |
| Medium | Compression stockings (unless severe leg ischaemia) or intermittent pneumatic compression leggings plus:<br>Subcutaneous heparin (5000 IU 2 hours before surgery and 12-hourly till fully mobile) |
| High | Compression stockings and/or intermittent pneumatic compression leggings plus:<br>Subcutaneous heparin started before surgery (approx. 5000 IU 8-hourly) to keep APTT 1.5–2.5 of control value or<br>Warfarin to INR of 2–3 or<br>Consider formal monitored anticoagulation in very high-risk cases<br>Consider LMWH in major orthopaedic cases |

APTT, activated partial thromboplastin time; INR, international normalized ratio; IU, international units; LMWH, low molecular weight heparin. Adapted from Verstraete M. *BMJ* 1997;314:123.

being prescribed an antiemetic, should have one that promotes gastric emptying, *provided that they do not have intestinal obstruction*. Starved, elective patients who are having the risk of PONV reduced, can be prescribed something that acts more centrally, e.g. ondansetron.

Antiemetics *do not* reduce the need for using appropriate measures in patients at risk of pulmonary aspiration (see Chapter 7).

### Antisialogogue therapy

Antisialogogues used to be prescribed regularly when gas inductions were common, particularly if ether was to be used as part of the technique. From the patient's point of view, they produce an unpleasant, dry mouth which emphasizes the preoperative starve. They are now probably best reserved for those cases in which a gas induction is intended or in which a difficult or awake intubation is anticipated. The drug with the best drying action and least central effect is glycopyrrolate.

Hyoscine (scopolamine) is also effective and its mildly sedative effect may be advantageous.

### Antacid therapy

There are two objectives to antacid therapy: the first is to render the stomach contents less acid to minimize the effects of any pulmonary aspiration, and the second is to reduce the incidence of stress ulceration.

Prophylaxis for aspiration should be used when there is an increased risk, as defined in Chapter 7.

Stress ulceration can occur after any form of major surgery but particularly after major surgery in patients who are debilitated. Prophylaxis for this (as opposed to the effects of aspiration) with $H_2$-receptor blockers can be commenced orally or parenterally at the time of premedication, and continued until the patient is eating and mobilizing normally.

### Antibiotic therapy

Prophylactic antibiotics are given regularly for several types of surgery and in those at high risk of postoperative pulmonary infection. It is negligent to omit them in patients known to be at risk of subacute bacterial endocarditis. Hospitals have set policies for prophylactic antibiotic therapy to minimize the emergence of resistant strains of bacteria. These need to be adhered to. Although the prescription of surgically related antibiotics is, strictly speaking, the surgeon s remit, it does not remove the moral responsibility from the anaesthetist to check that they have been given and to mention it if they have been overlooked. This is particularly so if the antibiotics are not required for the surgical procedure itself but for another reason (e.g. valvular heart disease).

### Antiasthma and antiallergy therapy

All patients with asthma need to be taken seriously and treated as described in Chapter 53. The prescription for other allergies (e.g. hay fever) can be based on the patient s usual dose requirements.

### Associated conditions and administration of existing therapy

Patients who are on maintenance therapy need to have their drug regimens reviewed. In general, cardiovascularly related drugs (β-adrenoceptor antagonists, antihypertensives, etc.) should be continued, whereas others, for example, antidiabetic drugs may have to be stopped. Each should be dealt with on its merits, as described in Chapters 41 – 66.

### Antivagal therapy

The preoperative prescription of drugs for their antivagal action is now rare. If vagolysis is required it can be administered at the time of induction.

## FURTHER READING

Association of Anaesthetists of Great Britain and Ireland. *Anaesthesia and Anaesthetists: Information for patients and their relatives*. London: Association of Anaesthetists of Great Britain and Ireland, 1997.

Audit Commission. *Anaesthesia Under Examination*. London: Audit Commission, 1997.

Kanto J, Watanabe H, Namiki. Pharmacological premedication for anaesthesia. *Acta Anaesthesiol Scand* 1996;**40**:982 – 90.

Neuberger JM. Halothane and the implications of hepatitis. In: Kaufman L, ed. *Anaesthesia Review 8*. London: Churchill Livingstone, 1991: 179 – 94.

Practice guidelines for preoperative fasting and the use of pharmacologic agents to reduce the risk of pulmonary aspiration; application to healthy patients undergoing elective procedures. *Anesthesiology* 1999;**90**:896 – 905.

Royal College of Anaesthetists and the Association of Anaesthetists of Great Britain and Ireland. *Good Practice. A Guide for Departments of Anaesthesia*. London: Royal College of Anaesthetists and Association of Anaesthetists of Great Britain and Ireland, 1998.

Van Aken H, Thomson D, Smith G, Zorab J. 150 years of anaesthesia – a long way to perioperative medicine: the modern role of the anaesthesiologist. *Eur J Anaesthesiol* 1998;**15**:520 – 3.

Verstraete M. Prophylaxis of venous thromboembolism. *BMJ* 1997;**314**:123 – 5.

Wheatley T, Veitch PS. Recent advances in prophylaxis against deep vein thrombosis. *Br J Anaesth* 1997;**78**:118 – 20.

# Chapter 2 Induction of general anaesthesia

P. Hutton

## BASIC PRINCIPLES

This chapter deals with the induction of general anaesthesia in an adult. The induction of children is described in Chapter 42. Variations required because of age and specific medical conditions can be found in the relevant sections of Chapters 43 – 66. From the patient s viewpoint, induction of anaesthesia is a very important time, partly because anxiety is maximal, especially in the unpremedicated person. It is therefore important that the process is purposeful without undue delays and that the environment is peaceful, gives an impression of confidence, and has no distracting noises.

Depending upon the hospital, it will be the normal practice to induce patients in either the anaesthetic room or the operating room. Anaesthetic rooms are common in the UK but rare in the USA. The pattern varies in other countries across the world.

Where anaesthetic rooms are used, they are generally popular with both patients and staff and, if two trained anaesthetists are present, allow the list to proceed more rapidly because one patient can be induced while surgery is finishing on another. If the patient is seriously ill, if there is insufficient monitoring equipment for two locations or if transporting or moving them puts the patient at undue risk, anaesthesia should be induced in the operating room with the patient on the operating table. The basic principle is to induce anaesthesia only in a properly equipped environment with a properly trained assistant. The latter is vital; anaesthesia should never be induced without support. The safe movement of a patient from a trolley to an operating table is described in Chapter 3 (see Figure 3.5).

Before inducing anaesthesia (even though in some instances it is also the responsibility of others) it is the responsibility of the anaesthetist to ensure the following:

- That it is the correct patient who has consented for the correct operation. Check the wrist band or other identity tag.
- That the surgeon is ready and has had the opportunity to check the identity of the patient and the details of the proposed surgery.
- That the correct notes, radiographs, etc. are present.
- That there is a competent anaesthetic assistant and, if the patient is overweight or requires special positioning after induction, that extra people are immediately available.
- That the patient is on a bed or trolley that tips head down.
- That all the equipment in the anaesthetic room and operating room likely to be required is present and checked. Details of this are given elsewhere.
- That resuscitation drugs and a self-inflating bag are available.
- That in particular there is a powerful sucker available and a ready supply of 100% oxygen.
- That the availability of any special intravenous fluids (e.g. blood, fresh frozen plasma [FFP]) has been confirmed.
- That, unless there are any specific, unusual reasons to the contrary, the conditions for minimal monitoring are met. All routine patients should be induced with an ECG, pulse oximeter, and a non-invasive blood pressure cuff in place. Equipment should also be available for checking the position of an endotracheal tube (see Airway management, Chapter 7).
- That there is reliable intravenous access. If a drip or intravenous cannula is *in situ* on arrival, its patency needs checking.
- That appropriate postoperative and recovery facilities are available.

The duration of starvation for elective patients is discussed in Chapter 7. For many years it has been the practice to remove a patient s false teeth on the ward. This not only reduces the self-confidence of the patient, but it is also sometimes easier to maintain an airway on a face mask if the false teeth are left in. Consequently, it is difficult to be rigid in the approach to the removal of teeth except to say that, if they are left in, they should be recognized as a potential airway hazard and, if the anaesthetist subsequently removes them, they must be kept safely and (even worse if it happens) not mixed up with anyone else s.

General anaesthesia can be induced by either intravenous or inhalational agents in both elective and urgent cases. The salient features of these procedures are described below.

## ELECTIVE INTRAVENOUS INDUCTION

Intravenous induction is the most frequently used general-purpose method of producing unconsciousness and has a high degree of patient acceptability. A great advantage to the anaesthetist is the rapid passage from consciousness to the plane of surgical anaesthesia with few excitatory side effects. There are a number of intravenous induction agents available, the properties of which are described in Chapter 32. If there is a specific contraindication to a particular drug (e.g. allergy), it should not be used. The manufacturer's product inserts, journal papers, and textbooks all tend to give a range of induction doses specified on a milligram per kilogram basis. This is because doses are predictable for populations but not for individuals: titration to response is the key to success for individual patients. Intravenous induction of children is described in Chapter 42.

Preoxygenation is often recommended and is mandatory for emergency cases and patients with a difficult airway. It is, however, by no means universally applied to healthy elective cases. Although being the 'counsel of perfection' and recommendable on safety grounds, it is something that a number of patients find raises their anxiety levels (particularly if they don't like facemasks) and it inhibits conversation between the anaesthetist and patient. In practice, some anaesthetists only use preoxygenation if there is a specific indication, others employ it routinely.

The intravenous induction agent should be injected steadily into a well-sited intravenous cannula under direct observation or into a well-running intravenous drip. Pain on injection can occur and is more common in the smaller veins on the back of the hand. If pain is experienced, make sure that the injection is not going subcutaneously or intra-arterially. The management of extra-venous injection is described later.

The greater the dose of drug and the faster the injection rate, the quicker sleep is induced and the more adverse the physiological side effects. Practical experience is the best guide as to how fast to induce anaesthesia in particular patients, the less fit responding best to slow induction. Always allow sufficient time for the induction agent to act in patients with a slow circulation time. Remember that an intravenous induction administers a potent drug to a patient and, from then onwards, the anaesthetist has no control over the subsequent actions and pharmacology of the agent. This contrasts with volatile agents which can be removed by ventilation. Factors that affect the dose of intravenous induction agent required are as follows:

- If a patient is premedicated, less is required.
- The dose is reduced by the simultaneous administration of intravenous opioids.
- Elderly patients require less.
- Malnourished individuals require less.
- Less is required in a poor circulatory state (e.g. shock).

Although minimal monitoring (Chapter 12) is required, nothing replaces the finger on the pulse and clinical observation during the induction process. Apart from when using the sympathomimetic agent ketamine, the most common physiological changes on loss of consciousness are respiratory depression (there may be apnoea for short periods) and a fall in blood pressure (BP). The latter results from a combination of direct myocardial depression, vasodilatation, and obtunding of the baroreceptor response. If the fall in BP is thought to be too great, it can be treated with intravenous fluids or vasoconstrictors. In fit patients an initial fall of 20% in systolic pressure is not uncommon and usually requires no treatment other than observation. The majority of physiological changes seen on intravenous induction are predictable in direction, but vary in magnitude from patient to patient. This is, however, also the time when, very rarely, the first signs of anaphylaxis and malignant hyperpyrexia may be seen (see Chapter 13).

Immediately after loss of consciousness, the subsequent conduct of anaesthesia will be determined by the intended choice of airway and whether neuromuscular blocking drugs are to be used. Airway management and maintenance of anaesthesia are described separately in Chapters 7 and 3, respectively, but there are some important points of general relevance to be made:

- It is bad practice and produces a risk of awareness for relaxants to be given before consciousness is lost.
- It is vital, once consciousness is lost, to achieve immediate control of the airway and to ensure a continued supply of oxygenated gas to the lungs. *This point cannot be emphasized too strongly*, especially in patients who have not been fully preoxygenated.
- If the intravenous induction agent is not to be continued as an infusion, anaesthesia must be maintained by volatile or gaseous agents delivered with the inspired gas. This cannot occur if the anaesthetist does not have control of the airway and there is the risk of awareness in the presence of medium- or long-acting relaxants, particularly during intubation.
- The insertion of an oral airway cannot usually be achieved without trauma, etc. in an unrelaxed patient in a light plane of anaesthesia.
- *Try to recognize as early as possible when you are unable to ensure a safe airway*. Unless experienced help is immediately available, allow the patient to wake up or, if the condition is life threatening, proceed to emergency measures such as cricothyrotomy. Dealing with this situation is described in Chapter 7.

One very unusual but always embarrassing and perplexing situation is when the patient fails to go to sleep within the expected time. The three most obvious reasons for this are as follows:

1. The cannula is not in a vein. This usually causes pain, and, because of its importance, is considered fully later in this chapter.
2. There is venous obstruction (e.g. inflated tourniquet).
3. The wrong drug has been given.

But do not forget a fourth:

4. *The drug is taking an unusually long time to reach its target receptors because the cardiac output is seriously low.*

A number of drugs used at the time of induction (including antibiotics, barbiturates, and relaxants) are reconstituted from powders. This step introduces another potential mistake, especially when the compounds look similar when made up. Cefuroxime is not as effective as thiopentone (thiopental) in producing unconsciousness and vecuronium is a poor substitute for midazolam! The important thing is not to continue inexorably administering the contents of a syringe when the expected outcome is not occurring. If the wrong drug has been given, treat the consequences appropriately and draw all subsequent drugs up again from fresh ampoules.

Remember (as stated in point 4, above) that one very serious reason why no effect is seen after injection is that the patient's cardiac output is very low (myocardial failure, shock). *It is very easy to overdose sick patients by failing to wait long enough for a response.*

Once anaesthesia has been satisfactorily induced, proceed to maintenance as described in Chapter 3.

## ELECTIVE INHALATIONAL INDUCTION

Elective inhalational induction of children is described in Chapter 42.

The indications for elective inhalational induction *in adults* are as follows:

- Airway obstruction or abnormal anatomy – when this is present, have emergency oxygenation devices (e.g. cricothyrotomy kit) to hand and the personnel available to do an emergency tracheostomy (see Chapter 7 on difficult and failed intubation);
- Patient request;
- Needle phobia;
- Difficult peripheral intravenous access;
- Bronchopleural fistula/empyema (rare today);
- Intravenous induction agents are contraindicated.

Paradoxically, both the advantages and disadvantages of inhalational induction derive from its gradual onset. During intravenous induction, the rise in serum level of the agent is controlled totally by the volume, concentration and speed of the injection; during inhalational induction, the rise in partial pressure of the agent is controlled by the solubility of the agent and the uptake from the lungs. Inhalational induction is therefore slower, more controllable, and easier to reverse. This can be a great advantage in cases of airway obstruction or difficult airway, and allows the patient to be woken up independently of the rate of drug metabolism. Cardiovascular changes after inhalational induction in adults are similar to those for intravenous induction. Although implicated as a trigger for malignant hyperpyrexia, there are no recorded cases of anaphylaxis from volatile agents (see Chapter 13), so that serious hypotension and bradycardia, etc. must be assumed to result from an anaesthetic cause (e.g. overdose, hypoxia, etc.) in the first instance.

The gradual change from the awake to the asleep state can, however, be accompanied by adverse events. The detailed stages of inhalational induction were first reported by Snow in 1847, but classically described for ether in a spontaneously breathing patient by Guedel in 1937. For reference, Guedel's classification is shown diagrammatically in Figure 2.1. It can be seen that he described four stages, the third of which he divided into three planes.

### *Stage 1*

The stage of analgesia between the beginning of induction and the onset of unconsciousness, i.e. still awake but markedly reduced response to painful stimuli. This is the state that, on occasion, when paralysed, can result in awareness without severe pain.

### *Stage 2*

The stage of uninhibited response or 'excitement' when there is restlessness, non-cooperation, struggling, breath-holding, coughing, swallowing, and vomiting. It lasts from the loss of consciousness to the onset of regular breathing.

### *Stage 3*

This is the stage of surgical anaesthesia:

- *Plane I:* onset of regular breathing to loss of eyeball movements.

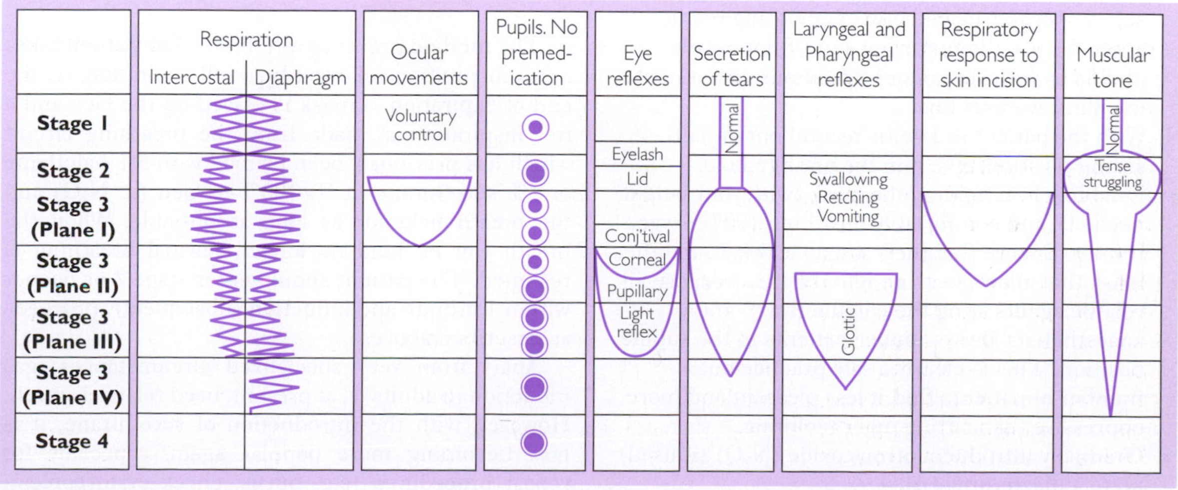

**Figure 2.1.** Diagrammatic representation of Guedel's classification of the signs of ether anaesthesia. (After Guedel AE, modified by Atkinson RS, Rushman GB, Lee JA. *Synopsis of Anaesthesia*, Bristol: Wright, 10th edn, 1987: 166.)

- *Plane II:* cessation of eyeball movement to loss of intercostal action.
- *Plane III:* progressive intercostal paralysis with progressive lack of diaphragmatic power associated with reducing tidal and minute volumes and rising $Pa_{CO_2}$. This is a suitable degree of anaesthesia for maintenance.
- *Plane IV:* from complete intercostal paralysis to diaphragmatic paralysis.

***Stage 4***

Progression from diaphragmatic paralysis to death from apnoea and cardiac depression.

These exact, detailed descriptions have not been published for any inhalational anaesthetic other than ether, although they are often erroneously regarded as universal in their applicability. They do, however, serve as a valuable model for the events occurring during inhalational induction and remind us that, between loss of consciousness and the onset of surgical anaesthesia, there is an interim state accompanied by restlessness where salivation, breath-holding, bronchospasm, laryngospasm, hiccoughs, regurgitation, and vomiting are possible.

Inhalational induction in the adult requires their cooperation, otherwise an inelegant brawl develops between the anaesthetist and patient. Only the experienced assistant will have the necessary restraining skills to deal with restlessness. Uninformed onlookers may carry graphic descriptions back to the wards, despite the patient's lack of recall for events. Properly carried out, gas induction in adults can nevertheless be very acceptable to all concerned and is probably experiencing something of a revival.

## The basic principles of an inhalational induction in an adult

1. Discuss the procedure with the patient beforehand, explain exactly what you will do and, if appropriate, prescribe premedication, not forgetting that a drying agent may be helpful.
2. Ensure that your assistant knows what you are going to do and what he or she is expected to do.
3. When the patient arrives in the prepared and safety checked anaesthetic or operating room, apply the usual monitoring and (if not needle phobic or with very poor intravenous access) put in an intravenous line.
4. With the patient in a semi-recumbent or half-sitting position, give him the mask to hold. Establish him holding the mask (with your help if needed), and comfortably breathing 100% oxygen from it. Ensure that there are no leaks around the mask that allow gas to go into the eyes because all volatile agents sting the conjunctiva. Some anaesthetists always induce patients in the supine position. This is clearly a safe practice but a number of patients find it less pleasant and more oppressive than sitting up or reclining.
5. Gradually introduce nitrous oxide ($N_2O$) (if used) up to a maximum of 50%.
6. Depending on the volatile agent to be used, increase it gradually at a rate compatible with the response to airway irritation. Sevoflurane can be pushed rapidly over a few breaths to 5% or more, whereas halothane, isoflurane, or enflurane need to proceed more slowly at up to 1–1.5% per five breaths or so, depending on the patient. Of the latter three agents, halothane is by far the easiest to use.
7. Once the patient shows the onset of inattention and/or abnormal eye movements and/or restlessness, if not already doing so, take over holding the facemask and gently pull the jaw into the best airway position. Prevent air leaks around the mask. Do not at this stage attempt to insert an oral airway. If dealing with a needle phobic, an assistant could now establish intravenous access to accelerate induction with a reduced dose of intravenous agent.
8. Press on through the episodes of breath-holding relentlessly increasing the concentration of volatile agent. It is often helpful to *very slightly* raise the expiratory pressure in the breathing circuit at this stage by partially screwing down the expiratory valve. If breath-holding becomes a real problem, keep the volatile agent going but return to 100% oxygen as the carrier gas. When regular respiration supervenes and the jaw becomes loose, insert an oral airway. Lower the patient to the horizontal and continue as planned.

As soon as induction is complete, the concentration of volatile agent needs to be reduced to a suitable maintenance value. *If at any time during induction there is a severe bradycardia or marked hypotension, lower the patient to the horizontal and return to 100% oxygen.*

An alternative method of carrying out a gas induction is to use the single-breath technique. For success this requires two important elements:

1. a very cooperative patient who understands what to do;
2. an anaesthetist who demonstrates clearly to the patient on him- or herself using a mask not attached to a breathing circuit, what the patient has to do.

The method proceeds as follows. The patient takes a full inspiration followed by a full expiration. At the end of expiration, a mask is placed on the face and a full inspiration is made from the breathing circuit which has previously been primed with 5% halothane or 8% sevoflurane in 50–100% oxygen (± $N_2O$) and the breath held for as long as possible. When the breath can be held no longer, normal breathing is resumed. The patient should enter stage 2 or deeper within 1 minute and induction subsequently proceeds as described above.

Apart from very specialized circumstances, gas induction in adults is, at present, used relatively rarely. However, with the introduction of sevoflurane, it is now becoming more popular again, especially for repeat procedures (e.g. burns, check cystoscopies), and some patients are even requesting it.

## INDUCTION OF A PATIENT WITH A DIFFICULT AIRWAY OR KNOWN RISK OF ASPIRATION

The guidelines for dealing with these situations are given in Chapter 7.

## MANAGEMENT OF ACCIDENTAL EXTRAVENOUS INJECTION OF INTRAVENOUS INDUCTION AGENT

If pain occurs on intravenous injection of any drug, always make sure that it is not going extravenously.

### Extravascular/subcutaneous injection

Most intravenous induction agents (and especially barbiturates because of their alkalinity) are irritants when injected extravascularly. The extent of pain and damage depend upon the volume and concentration of the injection. These can vary from minor irritation and erythema to severe pain, tissue necrosis, and sloughing.

Once injected, there is relatively little that can be done to reverse the process. Pain can be alleviated by infiltrating the area with 1% lignocaine (lidocaine) (without vasoconstrictor), the penetration of which can be assisted by the addition of hyaluronidase. Vasodilatation and comfort are aided by warm compresses and simple analgesics.

### Intra-arterial injection

This can lead to serious damage to the blood supply of the affected limb, with permanent ischaemic sequelae. Traditionally, the most common occurrence of an intra-arterial injection was that of a barbiturate into an artery in the antecubital fossa. In modern practice it is probably an inadvertent injection into an arterial monitoring line that has a catheter with an unnecessary tap. The consequences of intra-arterial injection of other drugs such as antibiotics can be just as disastrous as those of barbiturates. *If the patient is already anaesthetized, the symptoms described below will be absent and realization of the event may be delayed.*

Although arterial monitoring lines are at risk from all drugs, the inadvertent intra-arterial administration of thiopentone will be described because of its importance. Although the clinical picture varies with the dose and concentration, the classic response is immediate and agonizing pain shooting down the arm into the hand and fingers. The severity is such that it is unlikely to be caused by any other event during induction. The pain may subsequently last for a short time, be persistent or return later, presumably because of attacks of vascular spasm. There have been reports of intra-arterial injection not followed by pain, but these are extremely rare. After the pain, the limb blanches, the pulse disappears, and the limb then becomes mottled and cyanosed. An intense chemical arteritis develops and there may be crystal deposition in small vessels. The arterial distribution will determine the muscles, skin, and other tissues involved.

Management is as follows:

- On suspicion, immediately stop the injection and send for senior assistance. Unless it is life saving, abandon the surgery or at least delay it until the outcome of the event is clear.
- Leave the needle or cannula *in situ*. If it comes out, put a 20-gauge cannula back into the artery, if necessary more proximally, above the site of injury.
- Into the artery inject lignocaine 100 mg and papaverine 40 mg in 10–20 ml saline.
- Give 4000 IU heparin intravenously (unless otherwise contraindicated or unless a sympathetic block is to be done immediately).
- Keep the limb warm to encourage vasodilatation.
- Prescribe analgesia.
- Consider sympathectomy by local anaesthetic (e.g. stellate ganglion block), but remember the effects of heparinization and balance the risks.
- Longer term management depends upon the extent of damage and may involve limb salvage surgery or plastic reconstruction.

## FURTHER READING


Dundee JW, Bryant AM. *Intravenous Anaesthesia*, 2nd edn. Edinburgh: Churchill Livingstone, 1988.

*Guedel AE. *Inhalation Anesthesia*. New York: Macmillan, 1937.

*Guedel AE. *Inhalation Anesthesia*, 2nd edn. New York: Macmillan, 1951.

Hartmannsgruber MWB, Schulte-Steinberg H, Conzen P, Doenicke A. New intravenous induction agents. In: Frink EJ, Brown BR, eds. *New Intravenous Induction Agents. Baillière's Clin Anaesthesiol* 1995;**9**:51–66.

*Macintosh RR, Bannister FB. *Essentials of General Anaesthesia*, 3rd edn. Oxford: Blackwells, 1943.


*These books, available from many department libraries, give a fascinating and graphic account of the practical management of inhalational anaesthesia. Although the monitoring and agents have changed, the basic principles of safe practice have not.

# Chapter 3 Maintenance of anaesthesia

P. Hutton

## BASIC REQUIREMENTS AND OBJECTIVES

Maintenance of anaesthesia is the operative phase of the anaesthesia process between the end of induction (or establishment of a regional block) and arriving in recovery or transferring to a high dependency or intensive care unit. In most patients anaesthesia is maintained under general anaesthesia, but some of those with a regional block are sedated or remain fully conscious during surgery. During the maintenance of anaesthesia, however it is carried out and however short the duration, patients must be properly monitored in a safe environment and a proper record kept. The objectives of maintenance of anaesthesia (whatever form it takes) are:

- to supply oxygen and to remove $CO_2$ from the tissues via the alveoli;
- to observe physiological parameters and to make therapeutic manoeuvres to keep them within safe limits, bearing in mind any coincidental pathologies. Adequate monitoring, as described in Chapter 12, is essential. No matter how short the procedure, it is not optional;
- to detect, treat or prevent any adverse event;
- to pay particular attention to organs at specific risk, e.g. kidneys after an episode of shock, cerebral blood flow in an arteriopath;
- to manage fluid balance;
- to maintain the patient's body temperature;
- to produce good operating conditions;
- to initiate an analgesic regimen so that the patient does not have severe pain postoperatively.

These objectives can be met in a variety of ways as described below. Monitoring, fluid balance, regional anaesthesia and specific specialty requirements are described in other chapters of the book.

## GENERAL ANAESTHESIA

In addition to the above objectives, general anaesthesia should guarantee unconsciousness and lack of recall from induction to recovery, i.e. no sensory awareness of any kind by the patient.

General anaesthesia can be maintained with the patient either breathing spontaneously or being ventilated. Both methods can be supplemented with local or regional anaesthesia. Techniques can be subdivided as shown in Figure 3.1, and each has its advantages and disadvantages. These are summarized in Tables 3.1 and 3.2.

One cornerstone of good practice in maintenance anaesthesia is to note the wide individual variation in pharmacokinetic and pharmacodynamic responses and duration of action to both volatile and intravenous anaesthetics, opioids, and neuromuscular blockers. This makes it necessary to titrate the administration of drugs to an individual patient's response. (There are some specialized situations – for example, induced hypothermia – where, during maintenance, even an individual patient's response changes but these are not considered further here.)

As shown in Figure 3.1, maintenance of general anaesthesia can be achieved either by a single hypnotic drug or combination of drugs, or by employing regional blockade to reduce or abolish the transmission of painful stimuli to the central nervous system (CNS). Single-drug general anaesthesia is now only practised for very short procedures causing little physiological upset, e.g. single shot thiopentone (thiopental) or propofol for manipulation of a fracture or extraction of a loose incisor tooth. The problem of using a single drug for longer procedures is the need for a combination of hypnosis and analgesia with or without muscle relaxation. A volatile or intravenous agent provides excellent hypnosis, but requires a dose that is considerably in excess of that required for loss of consciousness to prevent the response to painful stimuli. Consequently, the unwanted cardiovascular system and respiratory system side effects may be unacceptably high.

The normal method of maintenance anaesthesia is therefore to use a balanced technique that targets hypnosis, analgesia, and relaxation (if required) separately, with the analgesic component continuing into

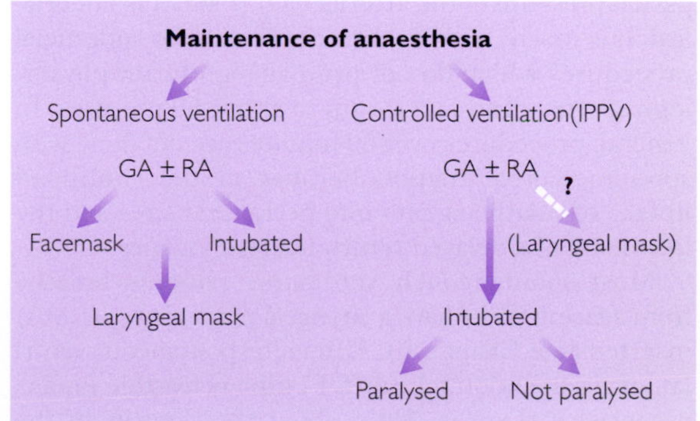


**Figure 3.1.** Methods of maintaining anaesthesia. GA, general anaesthesia; RA, regional anaesthesia; IPPV, intermittent positive-pressure ventilation.

**Table 3.1. Advantages and disadvantages of spontaneous ventilation**

| Advantages | Disadvantages |
|---|---|
| Disconnection does not result in failure of ventilation | Alveolar ventilation falls and $Pa\text{CO}_2$ rises |
| Undetected awareness is less likely to occur because patient is not paralysed and is able to move | Greater depth of anaesthesia may be required to achieve good surgical conditions |
| Light anaesthesia can be detected by increased respiratory rate which itself increases uptake of volatile agents | Depressant effects of volatile and intravenous agents on the cardiovascular and respiratory systems may be marked |
| There are no problems initiating ventilation when surgery ends | May be longer time to recovery of consciousness |

**Table 3.2. Advantages and disadvantages of controlled ventilation**

| Advantages | Disadvantages |
|---|---|
| Can produce the necessary surgical conditions with control over alveolar ventilation and hence $Pa\text{CO}_2$ | If a disconnection occurs, it is likely to result in a serious outcome |
| Allows combinations of drugs to be used which provide rapid reversal and recovery | Higher risk of awareness because patients are unable to move in response to pain |
| Makes some types of surgery possible that otherwise would not be, e.g. thoracic operations | May produce postoperative weakness and poor ventilation |
| | Hyperventilation may result in $CO_2$ wash-out with postoperative underventilation |
| | Introduces all the risks of ventilated patients, e.g. barotrauma, tube down right main bronchus, etc. |

the postoperative phase. Intraoperatively, it is necessary to have an adequate but not excessive depth of anaesthesia. This has to be adjusted to each individual patient's requirements. In practice, this is done by ensuring that the pulse, blood pressure, etc. are within normal physiological limits and that there is an absence of autonomic or emotional responses, e.g. sweating, lacrimation.

### Spontaneous ventilation

This is a suitable form of maintenance for procedures where relaxation is not required and in which the partial pressure of the arterial $CO_2$ ($Pa\text{CO}_2$) is not critical. It is mostly used in current practice for superficial procedures which do not provoke significant physiological stress and last for up to about 60 minutes. In general, procedures over 60 minutes are not done with spontaneous ventilation because of the continued uptake of volatile agents into peripheral sites and the likelihood of a delayed return to consciousness.

Most spontaneously ventilating patients breathe from a facemask or have a laryngeal mask airway (LMA) inserted (see Chapter 6). Although spontaneous ventilation via an endotracheal (ET) tube is feasible (and is essential if there is doubt about the security of the airway), intubation requires either a high concentration of volatile agent for laryngoscopy or the use of a neuromuscular blocking agent to introduce the tube, together with a sufficient depth of anaesthesia to overcome tracheal and laryngeal reflexes during maintenance.

If a patient has had a gas induction, the transfer to spontaneous maintenance is usually straightforward, merely being a continuation of the induction process. It is, however, much more usual to convert from an intravenous induction to volatile/gaseous maintenance. The wash-out curve from a single dose of intravenous induction agent, together with the wash-in curve of a volatile agent, is shown in Figure 3.2. It can be seen that, as the one falls, the other should rise for a steady state of anaesthesia to be maintained. The various breathing systems used to achieve this and their necessary fresh gas flows are described in Chapters 9 and 10.

Assuming that conversion is from an intravenous induction to volatile agent maintenance on a facemask or laryngeal mask, some common problems experienced in establishing and maintaining spontaneous ventilation are as follows:

- Following intravenous induction the patient may not continue to breathe smoothly after the introduction of nitrous oxide ($N_2O$) and/or volatile agents. Such a situation should be dealt with as described in Chapter 2 or a second smaller dose of intravenous agent given to smooth the transition.
- Apnoea occurs. This can be minimized by giving the induction agent slowly but in some patients

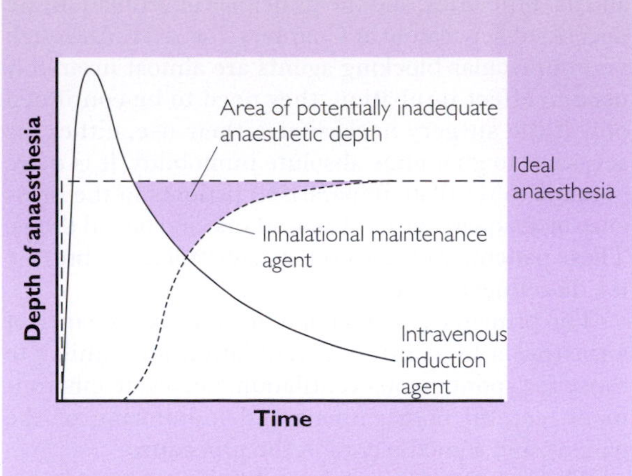


**Figure 3.2.** Diagrammatic representation of the conversion from induction to maintenance. It can be seen that, as the effects of the induction agent on hypnosis reduce, they must be compensated for by a rise in the serum level of the maintenance agent.

seems impossible to prevent. The problem with apnoea is that, while it continues, no gaseous or volatile agent is being taken up. Oxygenation is paramount at all times, so when apnoea occurs, try to hand ventilate the lungs and gradually increase the concentration of volatile agent. Excessive hyperventilation lowers the $Pa\text{CO}_2$ and prolongs the time to spontaneous breathing. Once this has occurred, the fractional inspired concentration of oxygen ($F\text{IO}_2$) needs to be kept high, together with an adequate concentration of volatile agent in combination with a low minute volume. This maintains oxygenation and anaesthesia while the $CO_2$ drifts upwards. During complete apnoea, the $Pa\text{CO}_2$ rises at between 0.4 and 0.8 kPa/min (3–6 mmHg/min).

- Inability to maintain an airway is always a serious problem requiring immediate resolution. It can often be resolved by the use of the adjuncts and techniques described in Chapters 6 and 7. Sometimes anaesthesia has to be deepened by a further dose of intravenous agent to accommodate an oral or nasal airway. If a serious airway problem is not resolved very quickly, the patient should be allowed to wake up, if necessary maintaining oxygenation by emergency methods (see Chapters 6 and 7).
- Breath-holding/coughing/laryngospasm/bronchospasm/hiccough occurs. All these are related to an inadequate depth of anaesthesia associated with a noxious stimulus such as inserting an airway, using too high a concentration of volatile agent too soon, or a response to the start of surgery. The message is the same for all: maintain oxygenation and deepen anaesthesia. An incremental dose of induction agent (especially propofol) is often helpful.
- The response to the start of surgery. This may be nothing, enough to trigger respiration, or an unexpected physiological response with increased breath-holding, tachycardia, hypertension, and movement. The important thing is to observe when surgery is starting (you are not always told!), and be ready for the outcome. If no movement occurs, anaesthesia may be too deep and could possibly be lightened; if movement is very significant it may be necessary to stop surgery and give an additional dose of intravenous agent. Otherwise if, as is usual, the respiration rate increases slightly but with few other adverse responses, deepen anaesthesia by increasing the concentration of volatile agent.
- The concentration of volatile agent required is reduced by the addition of opioids, non-steroidal anti-inflammatory drugs, or other analgesics, which also continue to have an analgesic effect in the postoperative period. It is therefore beneficial for them to be acting at least at the termination of surgery. The practical problem with opioids is that they reduce the drive to ventilation. If given intramuscularly intraoperatively, their take-up is gradual and their effects on respiration are easier to handle. If given intravenously, unless they are given very slowly or by dilute infusion, the frequent result is temporary apnoea during which manual ventilation is required.
- All spontaneously ventilating techniques result in changes in the $Pa\text{CO}_2$. The individual and combined effects of volatile agents and opioids all increase the $Pa\text{CO}_2$ threshold for the triggering of respiration, depress the slope of the $CO_2$ response curve and reduce alveolar ventilation (see Chapters 21, 33 and 34). These effects are opposed by the sympathetic response to surgery, which increases the rate and depth of breathing. During spontaneous ventilation, depending on the balance of the various components, the $Pa\text{CO}_2$ is usually between 5.5 and 8.5 kPa (41–64 mmHg). With insufficient fresh gas flow this can rise to dangerously high levels. The lack of control by the anaesthetist over the $CO_2$ level makes spontaneous ventilation inappropriate for those situations in which the intracranial and intraocular pressures are critical. The reduction in alveolar ventilation and rise in the $Pa\text{CO}_2$ also requires the $F\text{IO}_2$ to be increased to compensate.

Capnography can be very useful during spontaneous ventilation for a variety of reasons. If, for instance, the depth of anaesthesia is too light (see Figure 2.1 and accompanying text), the respiratory rate can be high and irregular, with the end-tidal $CO_2$ varying from breath to breath. This reflects uncoordinated, sometimes shallow, breathing with incomplete alveolar emptying. Consequently, under these conditions, the end-tidal $CO_2$ is not a guide to the $Pa\text{CO}_2$ but indicates inadequate anaesthesia.

As anaesthesia progresses and becomes 'smoother', the breathing becomes regular and, although the end-tidal $CO_2$ is more constant, it may still not be representative of the $Pa\text{CO}_2$. Obtaining a reliable sample of end-tidal gas from which to estimate the $Pa\text{CO}_2$ depends on the presence of a well-defined alveolar plateau. During spontaneous ventilation, the ingress of fresh gas and low tidal volumes can combine to reduce the reliability of capnography other than as an indicator of respiratory rate (Figure 3.3). Exceptions to this are when gas is sampled from within the ET tube or LMA. Capnography during spontaneous ventilation is considered further in Chapter 12.

Spontaneously breathing techniques are almost exclusively used with gaseous and/or volatile agents. Although success is possible with intravenous agents, it is very difficult to produce a smooth anaesthetic with manual administration; it can, however, be done well with pre-programmed infusion pumps. The problems of maintenance with intravenous agents are identical to those listed above.

As the end of surgery is approached, the concentration of anaesthetic agent can be reduced to minimize the time to awakening. The process of recovery is described in Chapter 4.

Related but separate problems of spontaneous ventilation such as pollution, malignant hyperthermia, etc. are described in other chapters of the book.

### Controlled ventilation by intermittent positive pressure ventilation

Maintenance by controlled ventilation requires the patient to be intubated with a correctly sited ET tube. Some anaesthetists ventilate via the laryngeal mask (as described in Chapter 6), but this is not universal and is not considered further here. Methods of intubation and its difficulties, and the principles of ventilation, are described separately in Chapters 7 and 11. Although neuromuscular blocking agents are almost invariably used to effect intubation, they need to be continued only if the surgery necessitates their use, either for access or to guarantee absolute immobility. It is quite possible to ventilate unparalysed patients in the presence of adequate doses of anaesthetic and opioid drugs. These patients will, however, usually still fail to breathe if a disconnection occurs.

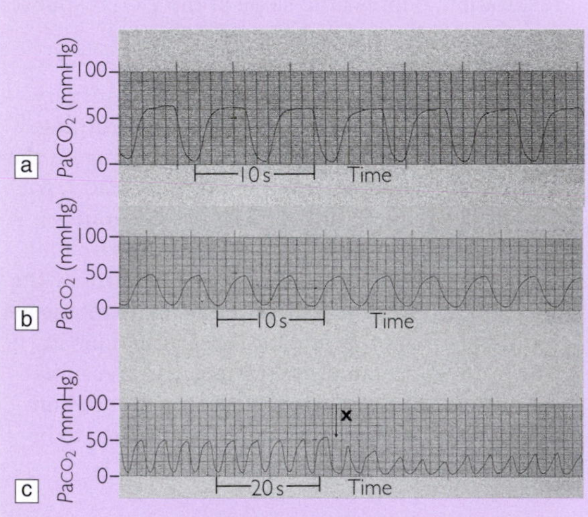


**Figure 3.3.** Capnograms during spontaneous ventilation from a Mapleson A breathing system fed by fresh gas at 4.5L/min. (Breathing systems are described in Chapter 9.) (a) Gas sampled from within an endotracheal tube while breathing spontaneously during anaesthesia. Note the well-defined alveolar plateau and the level of $CO_2$ concentration. (b) Gas sampled from a nasopharyngeal airway while breathing spontaneously during anaesthesia. Note the absence of a proper alveolar plateau and the non-zero inspired level of $CO_2$. This will not give an accurate estimate of $Pa\text{CO}_2$. (c) Gas sampled from an oral airway while breathing spontaneously on a facemask. The first part of the trace is similar to (b). At X the catheter has slipped from the oral airway into the free space between the mask and the face. Note the further deterioration of the capnogram as a result of the effect of mixing between fresh and expired gas.

The principles of good practice for maintenance of anaesthesia by controlled ventilation are similar to those for spontaneous ventilation, i.e. a safe environment, careful management and monitoring of the patient, and a good record of the procedure.

Whilst intubating and establishing intermittent positive-pressure ventilation (IPPV), the concepts of Figure 3.2 still apply and, whether using volatile or intravenous agents to maintain hypnosis, their blood concentrations need to be raised before those of the induction agent fall too low. This can be done by giving a loading dose of intravenous agent followed by an infusion (or a computer-controlled exponentially decreasing infusion, see Chapter 32), or by using overpressure with a volatile agent before reducing it to its maintenance value (Chapter 33). It is usual to administer an opioid (either by bolus or infusion) to provide analgesia that at the same time reduces the necessary dose of intravenous or volatile hypnotic.

The concept of balanced anaesthesia is that an intravenous or volatile agent is given for hypnosis, an opioid or regional block for analgesia, and relaxation to permit ventilation and to provide good operating conditions. In healthy patients, after bolus administration, modern neuromuscular blocking agents (vecuronium, atracurium, pancuronium, rocuronium and mivacurium) have a very dependable duration of action. In our practice, routine monitoring of their effects with a nerve stimulator is not used in healthy adults. We would, however, recommend the use of neuromuscular monitoring if we were using atracurium or mivacurium by infusion, or if the patient had liver, renal, or other metabolic derangement. Neuromuscular monitoring is also obviously recommended in those instances in which patient movement would cause serious problems (e.g. surgery under an operating microscope).

Controlled ventilation maintenance potentially poses a few more serious hazards to patients than spontaneous ventilation. These are listed in Table 3.2 and are described below.

#### *Awareness*

The patient may be awake during surgery but unable to move to indicate his or her distress. Awareness in a paralysed patient can (without very sophisticated cerebral monitoring, not described here) only be recognized by observation of physiological parameters. It should always be considered in the presence of unexplained hypertension and tachycardia, sweating, lacrimation, movement of the superficial temporalis muscle, large pupils and non-specific twitching. The usual cause is a failure to administer the anaesthesia as intended (e.g. empty vaporizer, infusion pump not turned on). If you think awareness may be happening, assume that it is. Check the delivery of anaesthesia and, if in doubt, give a bolus of intravenous induction agent until you are sure all is well. Occasionally, awareness without pain occurs and this may be more difficult to detect from physiological signs.

### *Disconnection*

A paralysed patient will die or suffer serious hypoxic damage if a disconnection is not detected almost immediately. This makes the constant monitoring of ventilation either by clinical (e.g. stethoscope) or electronic methods (e.g. expired $CO_2$, expired flow, or airway pressure) mandatory. Our recommendation would be always to use a disconnection monitor of some type whenever a patient is subject to controlled ventilation. Unnoticed disconnection is a very serious event that will always (correctly) be classed as negligent. Disconnection is discussed in more detail in Chapter 12.

### *Large shifts in $P_{aCO_2}$*

Although for most operations the objective is to ventilate to normocapnia, when the minute volume is no longer under physiological control it is possible inadvertently to:

1. hyperventilate the lungs, driving the $P_{aCO_2}$ down to less than 50% of its normal value and seriously upsetting $CO_2$ homoeostasis;
2. underventilate the lungs or ventilate with $CO_2$-containing gas so that the $P_{aCO_2}$ becomes grossly elevated.

The consequences of hyper- and hypocapnia are given in Table 3.3. For these reasons we would strongly recommend the use of a capnograph when patients are artificially ventilated, and it is essential if a partial rebreathing or circle system is used (see Chapter 10).

### *The conclusion of surgery*

The principles of management as surgery comes to an end are similar to those for spontaneous ventilation. The depth of anaesthesia needs to be lightened in the presence of adequate analgesia at a level of relaxation that can be easily reversed. Common problems at the end of a laparotomy are the tone of the abdominal muscles and diaphragmatic contractions during closure. There is sometimes a warning of spontaneous diaphragmatic efforts on the capnograph trace. These appear as a dip at the end of the alveolar plateau (Figure 3.4) and, when seen, unless the abdomen is already closed, a *small* incremental dose of neuromuscular blocking agent is probably going to be necessary. If a nerve stimulator is being used, and one or two twitches can be felt on the train of four (see Chapters 24 and 35), there is usually no problem in apposing muscle layers and subsequently reversing the patient.

## SEDATION

Sedation means different things to different people, and some medical staff are particularly imprecise with its use. A widely accepted definition of sedation is:

> '. . . a carefully controlled technique in which a single intravenous drug, or a combination of oxygen and nitrous oxide, is used to reinforce hypnotic suggestion and reassurance in a way which allows treatment to be performed with minimal physiological and psychological stress, but which allows verbal contact with the patient to be maintained at all times. The

**Table 3.3. Consequences of not ventilating to normocapnia**

| System/function | Hypercapnia | Hypocapnia |
|---|---|---|
| Heart | Hypertension<br>Increased myocardial work<br>Increased myocardial oxygen consumption<br>Increased cardiac output<br>Onset of arrhythmias | Myocardial depression<br>Reduced cardiac output |
| Peripheral vasculature | Vasodilatation | Vasoconstriction |
| CSF (immediate effects) | $CO_2$ level rises | $CO_2$ level falls |
| Cerebral blood flow | Increases | Decreases |
| Regional blood flow | Some increased, steal effects | Some decreased, steal effects |
| Postoperative breathing | High drive but rapid breathing with increased oxygen consumption | Poor drive, may be difficult to trigger breathing;<br>Underventilation later to compensate for CSF changes and $CO_2$ wash-out |
| Oxyhaemoglobin dissociation curve | Moved to right: aids delivery of oxygen to tissues | Moved to left: hinders delivery of oxygen to tissues |

CSF, cerebrospinal fluid.

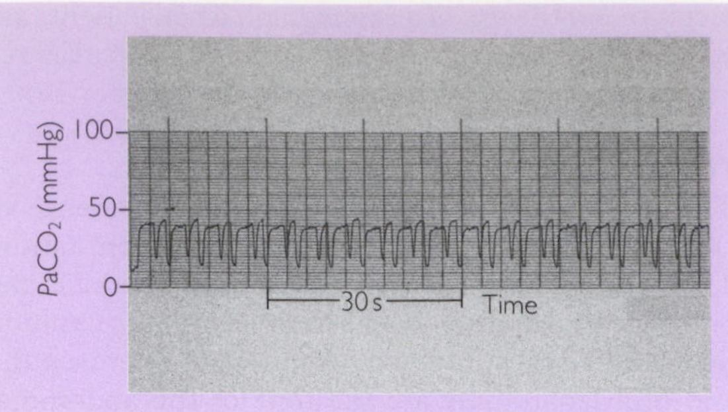


**Figure 3.4.** A capnogram taken from a patient breathing against the ventilator. Note the inspiratory effort causing a dip in the alveolar plateau. There is a non-zero inspiratory $CO_2$ level because a partial rebreathing circuit is being used.

> technique must carry a margin of safety wide enough to render unintended loss of consciousness unlikely.' (From the Standing Dental Advisory Committee [UK], *Sedation and Resuscitation in Dentistry*, March 1990.)

Any state producing a greater obtundation of consciousness should be regarded as general anaesthesia. Two important aspects of this definition are, first, *that drugs are used to augment the reassurance of human contact* and, second, *that verbal contact is possible, thereby confirming a competent larynx*.

Although superficially straightforward, sedation requires considerable practice for it to be done well. The state of anxiolysis without loss of consciousness can be achieved by small doses of midazolam, diazepam or propofol. In some centres, patient-controlled sedation has been a success. Often, particularly with midazolam, the sedated patient becomes disinterested in the surgical activities rather than becoming drowsy. Inhalational sedation with $N_2O$ is practised widely in dentistry but not so commonly in operating rooms. Concentrations of $N_2O$ of up to 30% are usual. The dose required on an individual basis, like that for intravenous sedation, is very variable: above 25% $N_2O$, disorientation and confusion may begin to occur in some patients whereas others will retain verbal contact to much higher levels.

From the anaesthetist's point of view, be wary of the surgical request along these lines: 'We've got a frail old chap for a strangulated hernia. We'll do it under local but could you be there to give a bit of sedation if required.' Translated, this means: 'I'm going to give some local which might not work. If this happens please be there to give the patient a general anaesthetic.' This scenario underlines the lack of understanding of the dangers of sedative techniques in many who request them, and it is salutary to remember that there are more deaths under sedation than under anaesthesia. Consequently, all patients receiving sedation need routine assessment and to be treated in an environment in which everything is immediately available for airway control and resuscitation. They should also receive appropriate non-invasive monitoring.

After sedation, patients need to be cared for in a properly equipped recovery area and meet the normal criteria for ward or street fitness before being discharged.

## POSITIONING

Apart from the small number of awake patients having minor surgery under a local peripheral block, who can position themselves, all other patients are at risk of damage from the position in which they are placed on the operating table. Although there are many positions adopted for specialized surgery, this section will deal only with the supine, prone (on a flat table), and lithotomy positions.

The surgical procedure, and the position necessary to do the operation, are information required for preoperative assessment because, for some patients, the optimal operative position can put them at considerable risk, e.g. thyroidectomy in a patient with rheumatoid arthritis. Cases such as these need to be planned in advance with the surgeon. It is sensible, if the operative position is potentially damaging, to get the patient to adopt it at the time of the preoperative visit (e.g. make sure their hips flex sufficiently for the lithotomy position).

The operating table is made of smooth, non-slip, anti-static rubber which covers foam cushions. For comfort and ease of moving the patient, he or she should be separated from it by a wrinkle-free linen sheet. Once the patient is anaesthetized (or subject to regional blockade that involves a joint), the tone of the muscles around a joint is lost and it is easy to force joints unwittingly into positions that would be intolerable in the awake patient. Furthermore, the position may be maintained without relief for some considerable time. Consequently, once a patient is anaesthetized, great care needs to be taken with all movement, no matter how trivial. In addition, all pressure points need to be well padded, with special attention paid to the elbows, knees, greater trocanters, ischial tuberosities, fibulae, and heels, especially in emaciated and elderly patients. Vital to safety is the presence of sufficient trained staff to help with moving. If a patient normally wears a cervical collar or other surgical joint support, it is sound advice, whenever possible, to leave it on throughout anaesthesia and surgery. Once the patient is safely on the table and anaesthetized, any request to move the table position must be done carefully with anticipation of the problems that it might cause.

*Do not forget to continue monitoring the patient if positioning takes a long time.*

### The supine position

Assuming the patient is anaesthetized, sedated or premedicated, he or she will be brought to the operating table on a trolley. First, if appropriate, connect the patient to the ventilator or other breathing system and confirm ventilation. Then adjust the height of the trolley and/or table to the same level. Ensure that the helpers are in position, supporting the patient on the canvas, together with any sliding aids. Establish control of the situation. Hold the patient's head and neck securely and move the whole patient on a count of three onto the table (Figure 3.5). If used, confirm that the ET tube or laryngeal mask has stayed in the correct position. The helpers should stay until the arms are secured with padded restraints, straps, or towels. Whenever possible, the arms should be by the patient's side or folded across the chest. Check that the ulnar

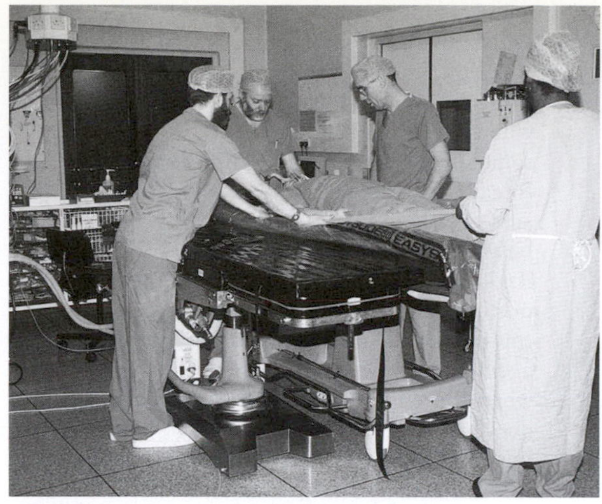

**Figure 3.5.** Moving a patient safely from a trolley to the operating table. Note that the table and trolley have been brought to the same height. A low-friction roller is being used to reduce the effort required by the operating room staff. The anaesthetist, having connected the patient to the breathing system, is carefully supporting the head and the others are waiting for instructions to move. It is important that everybody moves the patient together to maintain the alignment of axial joints and to prevent the inadvertent fall of a limb.

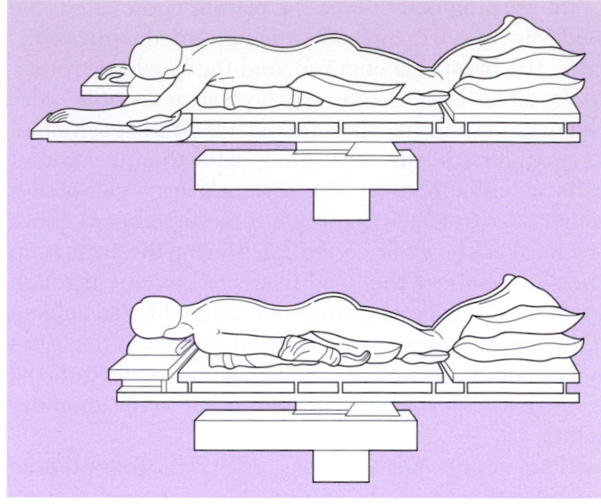

**Figure 3.6.** Two versions of the prone position. Note the chest rolls and hip pillows to free the abdomen and the comfortable support for the head. One pillow would also be adequate for the lower limbs. (Adapted from Martin JT, Warner MA. *Positioning in Anesthesia and Surgery*, 3rd edn. Philadelphia: Saunders, 1997.)

nerve at the elbow is not subject to localized pressure. If necessary, exchange the pillow for a smaller head-rest. Lift the heels onto foam-rubber pads and ensure that the pressure points mentioned above are checked. To prevent electrical and diathermy accidents, make sure that no metal parts are touching the patient.

If the arms have to be moved from the sides (e.g. to be strapped to a transverse bar at chest or neck level), move the joints in their normal way.

Damage to the brachial plexus is described below under 'The prone position'. If in doubt, the safety of limb movements can be checked by moving one's own limbs to similar positions. The basic supine position is well tolerated in normal patients, with no significant adverse cardiovascular or respiratory effects. Very occasionally, a large abdominal tumour can mimic the effects of the pregnant uterus: this can be corrected in the same way as managing a pregnant patient (Chapter 45). In all cases the eyelids need to be closed to prevent corneal damage, and, if used, the catheter mount and/or breathing filter supported so as not to put pressure on nerves or tissues, especially around the orbit.

### The prone position

The prone position carries many more hazards than the supine. The ability of the patient to turn the head to one side and to put their hands above their head should be checked preoperatively. This chapter assumes that the prone position is required for a simple procedure on the sacrum or anus, that the patient will be on a flat table and that the arms will adopt one of the two positions shown in Figure 3.6.

In the prone position, the face is into the pillow, putting the eyes and airway at risk. After induction, it is wise to intubate such a patient with a non-kinking ET tube and to tape and pad the eyes. The tube needs to be fixed securely at a length that ensures that the cuff is safely below the cords, with the tip not likely to slip into the right main bronchus. *A facemask or laryngeal mask is contraindicated for a prone patient because of the difficulty of intubating should problems arise.*

Although many people adopt the prone position for normal sleep, during anaesthesia compression of the abdominal contents hampers diaphragmatic movement and a free abdomen also reduces venous bleeding in the surgical field. This is particularly so in obese people. It is regarded as standard practice to take pressure off the abdomen by supporting the chest and pelvis on pillows, and the majority of prone patients are ventilated rather than being allowed to breathe spontaneously. When finally positioned, the pelvis and chest supports should allow the anaesthetist's hand to pass between the abdomen and the table. This ensures unrestricted diaphragmatic movement.

This account describes pronating the patient from the trolley onto the table (as opposed to turning the patient over when already on the table). The trolley is first moved into position alongside the operating table and the patient cared for initially as described for the supine patient. To effect the transfer, six people are required: two to push the patient over (standing next to the trolley), two to receive the patient (standing on the far side of the table), one at the feet, and the anaesthetist at the head. The patient's arms are put alongside the body as he or she lies supine before transfer. The patient is then disconnected from the ventilator and, on a prearranged count from the anaesthetist, the receivers put their arms across the table and the pushers start to rotate the patient first to the lateral and then completely over into the prone position, the patient now lying on the arms of the receivers with the head turned to one side. Throughout this, the anaesthetist supports the patient's neck and keeps it fixed in position relative to the turning body. Once the patient is pronated, the trolley is removed, the patient reconnected to the ventilator, the breathing checked, and the 'pushers' return to the table. The 'receivers' (whose arms are still under the patient) and the anaesthetist adjust the position of the patient and the others help with the insertion of pillows and supports. The patient's arms can be left down by the sides or put on a transverse board above the head as shown in Figure 3.6. Moving the arms from the side to above the head needs to be done through the normal anatomical range of the shoulder and elbow. The final placement should be in a position that does not strain the shoulders or brachial plexus and puts the arms in a ventral position with respect to the shoulder joints.

The prone position has many more potential complications than the supine. These are as follows:

- Resuscitation after cardiac arrest is virtually impossible in the prone position. If this happens, the patient will almost inevitably have to be turned over into the supine position.
- The patient can be dropped.
- The arm(s) can be trapped between the table and trolley or allowed to fall down.
- The neck can be twisted.
- The eyes can be subject to abrasion and pressure: the periorbital ridges, lips and cheeks, and nerves and tissues over them can be compressed by tubes, catheter mounts, badly placed supports, or folded cloths.
- The ET tube connectors and catheter mount can become disconnected without it being noticed.
- Female breasts need to be positioned medially and not extended laterally because traction of this nature can produce interstitial bleeding at the medial breast edges.
- The brachial plexus is vulnerable during turning and positioning and can be left stretched and compressed in the final position (Figure 3.7). This is also true in the supine position if the arms are dropped or put in unusual positions. Particular dangers exist if the arm is used as a lever to move the patient. The mechanisms of injury are as follows:
  - when the arm is abducted and externally rotated with the elbow extended and the forearm supinated, the plexus is stretched across the humeral head and compressed between the clavicle and first rib. This is worse if: the arm is abducted beyond 90° and pushed posteriorly; the scapula is prevented from rotating by the weight of the patient; the arm accidentally falls posteriorly;
  - when there is extreme abduction of the arms above the head, especially if the forearms are not in a forward position, stretching is inevitable; try putting your hands behind your head and getting somebody to push your elbows backwards!
  - when the neck is extended and flexed to the opposite side;
  - when the patient is put in a steep head-down or head-up position, tension on the wrists or badly positioned shoulder supports can produce problems;
  - although not described in detail here, the lateral position can also put the plexus at risk if the upper arm is strapped to a supporting bar in an abducted position, particularly if the head is not well supported.

Prevention of brachial plexus injuries consists of careful movement and positioning of the arms. Only roll the patient with the arms by the sides. If abduction of the arm is necessary, make sure that there is no backward displacement. If the patient needs to be head up or down, employ a standard non-slip mattress in preference to braces and straps.

### The lithotomy position

The lithotomy position is so called because historically it was used for removal of bladder stones. It is now an

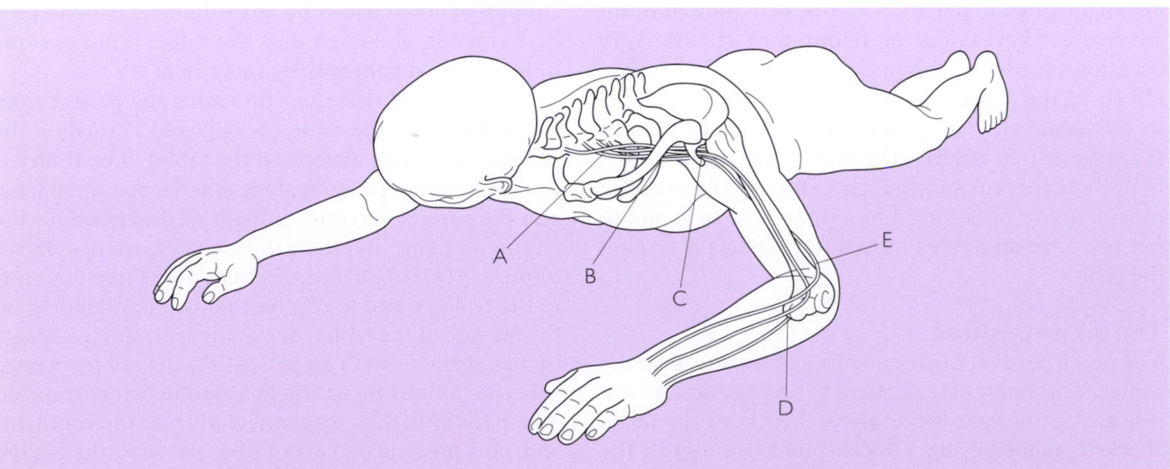


**Figure 3.7.** Sources of injury to the brachial plexus in a pronated patient. A, Head position stretching plexus against its anchors in the shoulder; B, potential closure of retroclavicular space by malpositioned chest supports when arms at side and neurovascular bundle trapped against first rib; C, head of humerus pushed into neurovascular bundle if arm and axilla not relaxed; D, compression of ulnar nerve at elbow; E, radial nerve at risk of external compression. (Adapted from Martin JT, Warner MA. *Positioning in Anesthesia and Surgery*, 3rd edn. Philadelphia: Saunders, 1997.)

inexact term in general use, used to describe the patient lying supine with the thighs abducted and legs raised, for operations on the genitals, urinary tract, anus, rectum, and perineum. Typical positions are shown in Figure 3.8 and each may involve a head-down tilt at some stage. It is important at the preoperative visit to know what position is intended and to ensure that the patient can adopt it. Check on symptoms of regurgitation. Ask specifically about a history of backache, sciatica, and any other neural symptoms in the lower limbs and document them.

When anaesthetized, the patient should first be placed supine as described above, with the sacrum in the correct position for removal of the foot of the table. Put the poles and stirrups into position. The legs must then be lifted simultaneously and the feet secured safely in the stirrups. Stirrups and leg holders come in a variety of designs. When content that the legs are safe, remove or lower the foot of the table. If a head-down tilt is anticipated, intubation and ventilation are strongly recommended in all but short procedures in elective, fit patients. The following are the complications of the lithotomy position:

- As the legs are elevated, the venous capacitance of the legs is reduced and the central blood volume is augmented. If there is significant intraoperative blood loss that has not been replaced, hypotension can occur when the legs are lowered.
- In the head-down position, there is a risk of passive regurgitation, especially in patients with a hiatus hernia.
- In the head-down position, the abdominal contents fall against the diaphragm and hinder respiratory movement. This is a particularly important factor in obese patients.
- The nerves most at risk are the common peroneal and saphenous. Both can be compressed by the supporting poles as shown in Figure 3.9. Damage can be avoided by good positioning and adequate padding. Also, a variety of postoperative neuropathies has been reported, which include the following nerves:
  - the ulnar – pressure from supports;
  - obturator – probably surgical;
  - femoral – compression against the inguinal ligament during excessive abduction and rotation of thigh;
  - sciatic – surgical or compression in the sciatic notch.
- If the feet or calves are bound too tightly in supports, the circulation is reduced and there have been cases of development of the compartment syndrome. This is a condition in which tissue oedema (usually secondary to direct damage, hypoxia, or ischaemia) is limited from volume expansion by inelastic fascial compartments, producing an interstitial tissue pressure that prevents arterial flow.
- Postoperative backache and prolapsed intervertebral disc symptoms have been reported after lithotomy, especially with long procedures. Explanations offered are abnormal flattening of the normal lumbosacral curvature, sacroiliac strain, and rotary stress on the lumbosacral spine (with asymmetrical movement and/or positioning).

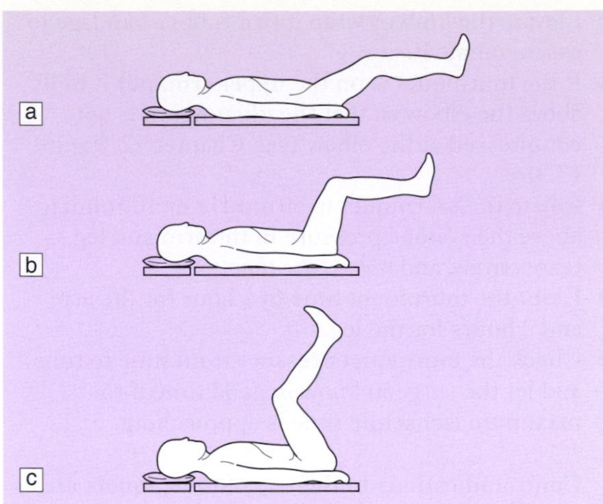


**Figure 3.8.** Examples of the lithotomy position. (a) is described as low lithotomy, (b) as standard and (c) as high.

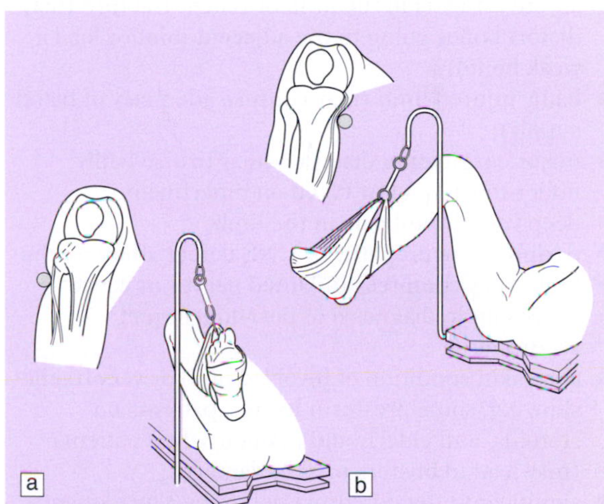


**Figure 3.9.** Nerve damage from lithotomy poles. (a) Lateral pressure compresses the common peroneal nerve just caudal to the head of the fibula, and (b) medial pressure compresses the saphenous nerve in the region of the medial condyle of the tibia. (Adapted from Martin JT, Warner MA. *Positioning in Anesthesia and Surgery*, 3rd edn. Philadelphia: Saunders, 1997.)

## TOURNIQUETS

Tourniquets are used on the arms and legs to produce a bloodless surgical field. As it is impossible to do definitive clinical trials correlating limb damage with cuff pressure and duration of inflation, the recommended cuff pressures and durations of inflation are determined by custom and practice. Although recommendations vary slightly from publication to publication, reasonable guidelines are as follows:

- Pad the upper arm or thigh with cotton wool or towelling and apply the tourniquet firmly, without pinching the skin.

- Elevate the limb or wrap it in a rubber bandage to exsanguinate it.
- If the tourniquet is on the upper arm, put it well above the elbow so that the ulnar nerve is not compressed at the elbow (see Chapter 12, Figure 12.9)
- Inflate the tourniquet to 50 mmHg or 100 mmHg above the systolic pressure in the arm and leg, respectively, and *record the time*.
- Limit the tourniquet time to 1 hour for the arm and 2 hours for the leg.
- Check the tourniquet pressure from time to time and let the surgeon know in good time if the maximum ischaemic time is approaching.

Contraindications to the use of tourniquets are as follows:

- sickle-cell disease (may precipitate sickling);
- severe peripheral vascular disease (may produce permanent ischaemia or damage to 'pipe-stem' arteries);
- severe arthritis in the limb or recent fracture (may distort bones going to the adjacent joint or load a weak bone);
- badly injured limb (may confuse adequacy of blood supply);
- major coagulation disorder (may bruise badly under tourniquet or bleed on reperfusion);
- deep vein thrombosis in the limb;
- peripheral neuropathy or CNS defect affecting the limb (may compress inflamed nerves or cause confusion in diagnosis of post-tourniquet syndrome);
- poor skin condition of involved limb or very fragile skin, e.g. some pre-term babies, patients on steroids, and elderly and malnourished patients (may lead to blisters or skin damage);
- significant infection proximal to the tourniquet (may cause transfer of bacteria into general circulation).

When the tourniquet is released, there is a return of acidotic, hypercapnic, hypoxic blood into the circulation. The limb becomes warm and flushed with reactive erythema, and the return of the blood to the circulation can produce a transient hypotension and tachycardia. These latter effects are more pronounced for a leg than an arm for obvious reasons.

## CONSERVATION OF BODY HEAT

Methods of heat loss and the measurement of temperature are covered in Chapters 38 and 73. Conscious humans are homoeotherms despite wide variations in ambient conditions. Control of body temperature is best in young adults and worst at the extremes of age.

The maintenance of a fixed body temperature represents a balance between heat generated from metabolism and received under unusual conditions (e.g. sunstroke) and heat lost to the surroundings. Heat loss is increased by low environmental temperatures and sweating, and is reduced by peripheral vasoconstriction.

Intraoperatively, apart from unusual situations such as hypothalamic disturbances, malignant hyperthermia, and severe, developing sepsis, the body temperature falls. The core temperature typically falls by 1°C in the first hour of anaesthesia. Thereafter the rate of fall reduces. The reasons for the fall in temperature are:

- ambient temperature is lower than body temperature;
- reduced metabolic rate;
- obtunding of effective thermoregulation by anaesthesia;
- loss of heat from exposed body cavities (especially the abdomen and thorax).

Heat loss and temperature fall can be reduced by:

- maintaining the ambient temperature high;
- covering the skin with a waterproof sheet to prevent evaporation of spilt liquids;
- putting on drapes to keep draughts off the patient and to reduce surface heat loss;
- warming inspired gases;
- warming intravenous fluids;
- using warming mattresses and heating blankets.

The advantages of maintaining body temperature are that:

- drugs and enzyme systems work predictably;
- there is optimal neural and neuromuscular transmission;
- postoperative shivering with its tissue hypoxia is minimized;
- postoperative fluid replacement is more predictable because the patient does not have to be 'filled up peripherally' as they re-warm and reverse their peripheral vasoconstriction.

Although there are no firm guidelines published on which patients should have their temperatures measured intraoperatively, the following are probably reasonable suggestions:

- patients subject to active heat conservation and warming techniques;
- operations on the abdomen or thorax in which there will be wide exposure of the cavity and contents lasting in excess of 1 hour;
- any operation expected to last for over 2.5 hours;
- any operation with an expected blood loss of over 1 litre;
- any patient with Raynaud's disease or autonomic dysfunction;
- patients whose body temperature is known to be abnormal preoperatively;
- patients whose temperature is likely to be altered deliberately intraoperatively (e.g. induced hypothermia);
- any patient with a family history of malignant hyperthermia.

## THE CONCLUSION OF MAINTENANCE ANAESTHESIA

For those patients with only a local block and no sedation or anaesthesia, the block can be allowed to wear off in the presence of adequate analgesia.

For those patients who have received sedation or a general anaesthetic, within a reasonable time of the end of surgery a satisfactory emergence requires the following:

- return of consciousness with intact laryngeal reflexes and mentation;
- return of muscle power and with it the ability to cough and move;
- adequate analgesia, hopefully with no nausea.

Details of the management of reversal and recovery are given in Chapter 4.

## FURTHER READING


Articles in: Peter K, Conzen P, eds. *Inhalation Anaesthesia. Baillière's Clin Anaesthesiol* 1993;**7**:839–1078.

Martin JT, Warner MA. *Positioning in Anesthesia and Surgery*, 3rd edn. Philadelphia: WB Saunders, 1997

White DC. The maintenance of anaesthesia. In: Aitkenhead AR, Jones RM, eds. *Clinical Anaesthesia*. Edinburgh: Churchill Livingstone, 1995: 173–87.

# Chapter 4 Emergence, reversal and recovery from anaesthesia

P. Hutton

## GENERAL PRINCIPLES

Patients can be awakened (after general anaesthesia), extubated (if necessary), and recovered from the effects of regional or general anaesthesia in either the operating room or a designated recovery area. The principles are the same wherever recovery occurs: safe transport and positioning, good oxygenation, appropriate monitoring and equipment, facilities for re-intubation and resuscitation, well-trained staff, and immediate availability of powerful suction. This chapter describes the management of routine patients who would be expected to recover satisfactorily and return to the ward. Patients expected to require care on an intensive care unit (ICU) are described in Chapter 17. Other aspects of postoperative care are described in Chapter 5.

### Regional blockade

Patients who have had a regional block and are fully conscious or have been sedated (i.e. they have remained in verbal contact with intact laryngeal reflexes) can be recovered in a comfortable position, which they adopt for themselves.

### Spontaneous ventilation

If a patient has had general anaesthesia and been breathing spontaneously, as the end of surgery approaches the volatile or intravenous agent can be gradually reduced so as to minimize the time of unconsciousness. When surgery has been completed the volatile or intravenous agent should be discontinued and 100% $O_2$ administered. The time to return of consciousness will depend on the initial concentration of the agent, the duration of surgery, and the level of analgesia. The elimination of volatile agents depends on the minute volume; that of intravenous agents depends on metabolism.

### Controlled ventilation

If neuromuscular blocking agents are used only for intubation at the start of the case, the effect of the agent will have disappeared by the end and the patient can be treated as described above for spontaneous ventilation. If, however, as is more usual, relaxation is maintained until the end of surgery, reversal will be needed with neostigmine, accompanied by either atropine or glycopyrrolate to prevent a serious bradycardia. Patients must not, however, be allowed to regain consciousness in the presence of paralysis; this situation is very distressing.

If surgery finishes unexpectedly soon after giving a dose of long-acting neuromuscular blocking agent (e.g. 'open and shut' laparotomy), be patient and *do not reverse the block too soon*. It does not save time in the long run and in the short term produces a patient with incoordinate twitches who is distressed and barely able or unable to breathe.

Once the reversal drugs have been given, the patient should be ventilated with 100% oxygen and any remaining hypnotic agents stopped (if they are still running). The ideal conclusion to routine surgery after reversal of blockade is that the patient begins to breathe spontaneously and is extubated as he or she wakes up.

Details of monitoring neuromuscular block and its reversal can be found in Chapters 35 and 39.

### Moving the patient from theatre

Whether awake or asleep, extubated or not, the patient should not be moved from the operating table until the anaesthetist is satisfied that:

- the cardiorespiratory status of the patient is stable and satisfactory;
- the bed or trolley has an oxygen cylinder attached, can be tipped head-down, and is correctly positioned;
- suction equipment is available;
- the monitoring equipment that is needed is functioning satisfactorily;
- the necessary breathing system equipment is present;
- there are sufficient trained staff available.

### Transfer to recovery ward staff

On arrival in recovery the handover to recovery staff should include the following information:

- the nature of the surgery that has taken place, including any complications that might affect recovery (e.g. excessive blood loss, recent opioid administration);
- the site of the wound, dressings, and drains;
- important aspects of the patient's general health, e.g. cardiac disease, asthma;
- the type of anaesthetic given, including details of regional blocks;

- unexpected intraoperative events, e.g. serious arrhythmias, bronchospasm, hypotension;
- physiological parameters within an acceptable range;
- prescription of postoperative analgesia, antiemetics, and fluids.

The ideal features of a recovery room, the basic equipment it should contain and the important features of patient trolleys or beds are given in Tables 4.1–4.3. An adequately equipped recovery bay is shown in Figure 4.1.

## THE PATIENT RECOVERING FROM A REGIONAL BLOCK (WITH OR WITHOUT SEDATION OR GENERAL ANAESTHESIA)

After the return of consciousness, as a patient recovers from a regional block two things are mandatory:

1. the observance and documentation of the return of normal sensation and motor function together with monitoring of basic physiological data (pulse, blood pressure, oxygen saturation etc.);
2. the provision of adequate analgesia as the block wears off.

**Table 4.1. Ideal features of a recovery room**

| | |
|---|---|
| Close to operating room | 1.5 bays per operating room |
| Curtains or screens for privacy | Ability to segregate children and very ill patients |
| Adequate space per bay | Adequate space between trolleys or beds |
| Wide doors | Temperature above 21°C |
| Well ventilated | Well lit |
| Reasonable relative humidity (approx. 40%) | Ceiling hooks or stands for drips, etc. |
| Plenty of power sockets for equipment | Easily available telephone(s) |
| Suction, oxygen, and air pipeline outlets | Waste gas scavenging points |

**Table 4.2. Basic equipment for each recovery bay**

| At each bed or trolley space | Also, immediately available should be |
|---|---|
| Properly trained member of staff | Intubation equipment |
| Oxygen facemasks and nasal specula | Emergency airways |
| Self-inflating or other hand ventilation bag | Standard anaesthetic and analgesic drugs |
| Sharps disposal box | Properly equipped resuscitation cart, including emergency drugs and defibrillator |
| Stethoscope | Extra staff in emergencies |
| Emergency bell | Range of intravenous fluids |
| Twin (pipeline) oxygen outlets | |
| Powerful suction and range of suction catheters | |
| Anaesthesia facemasks and airways | |
| Vomit bowl and tissues | |
| Basic monitoring equipment (see text) | |

**Table 4.3. Requirements of trolleys or beds used for the recovery of patients**

| | |
|---|---|
| Oxygen cylinder with sufficient gas | Easy and rapid head-down tilt (from head end) |
| Portable sucker | Sides that are comfortable when in position |
| Adjustable back rest | Large wheels that lock easily |
| Easy to clean | Shelf or tray for notes, etc. |

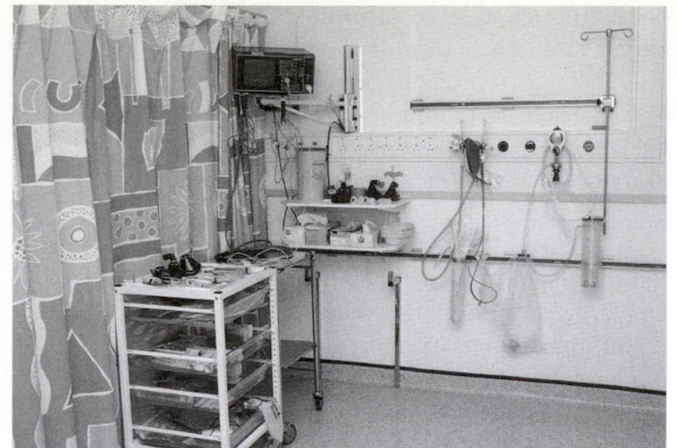

**Figure 4.1.** A properly equipped recovery bay. Note the presence of adequate monitoring equipment, stethoscope, dual wall oxygen supplies, and powerful suction. The equipment trolley in the foreground can be moved from bay to bay and contains emergency airway equipment. The retractable curtain allows privacy for the patient when appropriate. The very important element missing from this picture is the presence of a properly trained member of staff. (Courtesy of University Hospital Birmingham NHS Trust.)

A common cause of patient discomfort in recovery after a spinal or epidural block is a full bladder, which can be relieved by temporary catheterization. Further details of regional blocks and their complications are given in Chapter 15.

## THE PATIENT RECOVERING FROM GENERAL ANAESTHESIA

### Routine care

Unless there is a specific contraindication (e.g. surgical traction), it is good practice to allow patients to emerge from anaesthesia in the left lateral position, to reduce the chance of aspiration from passive regurgitation or vomiting.

All patients require supplemental oxygen and monitoring on arrival and during their stay in recovery. A proper chart must be kept, recording their physiological parameters and general progress. The basic monitoring for each patient should be careful clinical observation, pulse oximeter, non-invasive blood pressure, ECG, and pain score. Additional monitoring to meet clinical need in specific cases (e.g. arterial line after craniotomy) can be individually tailored. *Any patient who was difficult to intubate must be extubated awake*. Aspects of care are as follows.

### Respiratory function

Recovery staff should be given instructions to contact the anaesthetist responsible if the oxygen saturations on any patient are persistently below normal levels (e.g. 95%).

A patient arriving in recovery after facemask anaesthesia needs to have the airway maintained until consciousness returns.

If a laryngeal mask airway (LMA) has been used, the traditional advice is to allow the patient to recover consciousness with the LMA in position and to allow them to pull it out (with the cuff still inflated) when the larynx is competent. Saliva and other secretions that have collected above the mask are brought up on the upper surface of the LMA and expectorated. Occasionally, patients do not tolerate this and as anaesthesia lightens they chew the tube. This not only cuts off their air supply but also damages the tube. It can be prevented by putting a rubber wedge or other form of bite bar between their front teeth.

An alternative approach is to remove the mask at a deep level of anaesthesia. This requires the secretions above the mask to be sucked away before removal and for the patient's airway to be maintained by a suitably trained person until consciousness returns. Often it is necessary to insert an oral airway to do this satisfactorily.

Patients who have been intubated and ventilated will frequently have been extubated in the operating room before transit and will hopefully be conscious on arrival in recovery. They can be given added oxygen from a simple facemask or a fixed performance mask.

If a tracheal tube is still in place (and this is the policy in some units), it should be attached to an appropriate breathing system and removed when there is adequate ventilation and oxygenation and the patient is wakening. Some patients (particularly very obese ones) will breathe adequately only when sitting up. If in doubt, the tube can remain *in situ* until the patient shows signs of self-extubation.

The adequacy of ventilation is usually assessed on clinical grounds as (depending on the age):

- a respiratory rate of 10–20 breaths/min;
- no signs of distress;
- normal colour and oxygen saturation readings.

Some degree of hypoventilation is common in the immediate postoperative period, the reduction in oxygen flux being compensated for by a high inspired fractional $O_2$ from a facemask or nasal speculum. *It is important to remember that, in the presence of alveolar hypoventilation, a high inspired oxygen concentration can compensate for hypoxia while allowing the arterial $CO_2$ to rise to an unacceptably high level* (see Chapter 5, Figure 5.11). It is therefore obligatory to measure respiratory rate and observe the bellows function of the patient's lungs and not to rely on pulse oximeter saturations alone.

### Cardiovascular function

The patient's heart rate and blood pressure should be monitored regularly (initially at 5-min intervals) and the prescribed fluids given. If the recorded parameters fall outside the acceptable range, the anaesthetist needs to investigate. Two important practice points are:

1. the most common cause of hypotension is hypovolaemia;
2. the most common cause of hypertension is pain.

## CLINICAL PROBLEMS IN THE RECOVERY PERIOD

Clinical problems in the recovery period are listed in Table 4.4.

**Table 4.4. Clinical problems in the recovery period**

| |
|---|
| Failure to wake up and make regular and/or coordinated breathing efforts |
| Failure of ventilation in the presence of adequate ventilatory efforts |
| Hypoxaemia |
| Abnormal pulse rate and arrhythmias |
| Blood pressure abnormalities |
| Pain control |
| Fluid balance |
| Postoperative nausea and vomiting |
| Abnormal body temperature |
| Confusion |

### Failure to wake up and make regular and/or coordinated breathing efforts

When intubated, or after extubation, patients sometimes make no effort to breathe. When this occurs, continued oxygenation of the patient by the most appropriate means, and monitoring of vital signs are essential. The following are the causes of this situation.

#### *Common causes*

- Excess residual opioid (of any single or combination of routes and drugs).
- Excess residual volatile or intravenous anaesthetic agent.
- Intraoperative hyperventilation leading to hypocapnia.
- Normocapnia but arterial $CO_2$ partial pressure ($Pa\text{CO}_2$) still too low to trigger respiration in presence of opioids and/or volatiles.

#### *Less common causes*

- Residual neuromuscular blocking agents.
- Residual benzodiazepines.
- Sedative premedication still active.
- Existing preoperative condition, e.g. confusion, liver disease, renal disease, diabetes, existing cerebral pathology, hypothyroidism, occult myopathies, etc., acidosis, or alkalosis.
- Effects of unexpected cerebral migration of epidural and spinal local and opioid agents.
- Unknown self-medication.

#### *Rare causes*

- Very high $Pa\text{CO}_2$.
- Intraoperative cerebrovascular accident (CVA).
- Severe hypothermia.
- Porphyria, the post-ictal state and other small-print oddities.

The common causes can usually be identified by a review of the pupils and the anaesthetic chart, capnography, and assessment of residual neuromuscular block and vapour analyser. If in doubt about the cause, do a dipstick test to eliminate hypoglycaemia: it is simple and easy to do and reassuring to know the result. The $Pa\text{CO}_2$ often has to be 6 kPa (45 mmHg) or above to trigger respiration in the presence of effective opioid analgesia. Opioid overdose can be diagnosed by the use of naloxone, but this can allow breakthrough pain and is short acting.

If failure to breathe is the result of inadequate neuromuscular transmission alone, the patient usually has large pupils, makes discoordinate and ineffective respiratory efforts, accompanied by peripheral twitching and eyebrow raising. This can be very distressing and the kindest and safest thing is to keep the patient ventilated in the presence of a hypnotic until neuromuscular function has recovered. The pharmacology of reversal is described in Chapter 35.

### Failure of ventilation in the presence of adequate ventilatory efforts

This has four main causes and an uncommon fifth. The first three are related to the obstruction of gas flow (upper airway obstruction, laryngeal obstruction, and bronchospasm) and the fourth is inhibition of chest expansion because of pain. The fifth is the presence of a pneumothorax. If the patient is conscious they are always distressed and usually frightened.

#### *Upper airway obstruction*

This can be caused by the tongue, poor pharyngeal tone, blood, secretions, jaw position, and, very importantly, a throat pack that has not been removed. Usually, at least initially, the obstruction is partial and the breathing stertorous. An increasing degree of obstruction is demonstrated by the use of accessory muscles of respiration, tracheal tug and paradoxical movement of the chest and abdominal wall. With total obstruction, there is no sound combined with extreme ventilatory effort.

This situation must be remedied immediately, first by giving 100% oxygen and elevating the chin, turning the patient on to the left lateral position (if appropriate) and suctioning the airway. If this is not successful, then the manoeuvres described in gas induction of anaesthesia (see Chapter 2) and airway management (see Chapter 7) should be used. If the obstruction cannot be rectified very quickly and the patient becomes hypoxic, re-intubation will be necessary. This should be decided upon early and the appropriate hypnotic and neuromuscular blocking agent given while there is still a good pulse and blood pressure. If re-intubation is not possible, the usual emergency oxygenation measures will be required (see Chapters 6 and 7).

#### *Laryngeal obstruction*

Laryngospasm, when it occurs, usually produces partial obstruction of the larynx. It is recognized by a characteristic high-pitched inspiratory stridor in the presence of strenuous breathing efforts. Complete obstruction may present identically to upper airway obstruction as described above. It can be precipitated by:

- blood or secretions on the vocal cords;
- reflex irritation from an oral or nasopharyngeal airway that is too long;
- inadequate reversal of neuromuscular blockade;

- extubation while between deep anaesthesia and the awake state;
- damage to the recurrent laryngeal nerve (thyroid surgery) (see Chapter 7).

The management is (if possible) to open the mouth and suck out any secretions very quickly, then to apply a close-fitting mask supplied with 100% oxygen at positive pressure (partially close the breathing system outlet valve) and pull the jaw into the best position. If the mouth cannot be opened easily, do not waste time, but apply the mask directly. If there is stridor (indicating air movement) and the patient remains a good colour, press on until the spasm improves. If s/he becomes hypoxic, or if there is no gas movement, treat as above for total upper airway obstruction.

Laryngeal oedema causing obstruction is less common but less easily remedied. If it occurs, usually after prolonged intubation or in specific states (e.g. pre-eclampsia, infections), management is by anti-inflammatory drugs (e.g. dexamethasone) combined with antibiotics and nebulized gases. If severe, intubation or re-intubation may be necessary until it resolves. This usually requires one or more days on an ICU.

#### *Bronchospasm*

This can occur in people with asthma or in previously normal people. The causes are:

- a patient known to have asthma;
- the presence of a tracheal tube, especially if touching the carina when anaesthesia is light;
- secretions in the bronchial tree;
- an allergic or anaphylactic reaction;
- aspiration of gastric contents.

The principles of management are essentially as for laryngospasm with the expectation that it will improve. If the patient is conscious and still intubated but making good inspiratory efforts, it is probably best to remove the endotracheal tube. If the bronchospasm does not resolve quickly, sympathomimetic bronchodilators (e.g. nebulized or intravenous salbutamol) or intravenous aminophylline should be given and the episode treated as an asthmatic attack (see Chapter 53). A chest radiograph must be done to look for evidence of aspiration or a pneumothorax.

### Pain

If the patient is unable to make adequate ventilatory efforts because of pain, this clearly needs to be treated in the most appropriate way. This will vary from situation to situation depending upon what analgesic techniques are already bring used. The principles of postoperative pain control are given in Chapter 5.

### Pneumothorax

Although a pneumothorax is rare in recovery, it needs to be remembered. Its presentation and management are described in Chapter 13.

### Hypoxaemia

Hypoxaemia is inadequate carriage of oxygen by the red cells. It is diagnosable from blood gas results, which reveal a low $Pa\text{O}_2$ or from clinical observation or the pulse oximeter, both of which assess the level of oxygen saturation. Clinical observation is highly observer dependent, and also depends on the ambient lighting and it is influenced by the level of haemoglobin (see Chapters 39 and 52).

Hypoxaemia can result from any of the factors listed above that affect ventilatory drive, and the failure of inspired gas to reach the alveoli.

Hypoxaemia in the postoperative period may also be the result of diffusion hypoxia and ventilation–perfusion ($\dot{V}/\dot{Q}$) abnormalities. The exhalation of nitrous oxide after it has been switched off is associated with a reduced uptake of fresh gas into the alveoli (see Chapter 33). When the patient is allowed to breathe room air, this produces diffusion hypoxia, a mild condition that resolves spontaneously in a few hours in fit patients. It can be compensated for by giving a higher percentage of oxygen in the inspired air.

$\dot{V}/\dot{Q}$abnormalities can occur because general anaesthesia also induces a reduced functional residual capacity, the closing volume may change, and the cardiac output may have fallen (see Chapters 5 and 21). They can also result from pulmonary oedema, atelectasis and broncho- or aspiration pneumonia.

Oxygen therapy is described in Chapter 5.

### Abnormal pulse rate and arrhythmias

The most common postoperative arrhythmia is sinus tachycardia, which may be caused by pain, hypovolaemia, hypercapnia, hypoxia, anticholinergics, or sympathetic stimulation. The management is the diagnosis and treatment of the underlying cause. In otherwise fit patients, pain and fluid depletion should be top of the list. Sinus bradycardia is found frequently in young, fit people and is occasionally secondary to neostigmine. It can occur from vagal stimulation (e.g. after vomiting or during suction), but is an end-stage phenomenon in hypoxia. Bradycardia itself only needs treatment if there is symptomatic hypotension.

Patients with existing cardiac disease obviously need a greater degree of surveillance during recovery. Even so, the common abnormalities of rhythm described above are usually the result of the common causes listed. Other arrhythmias, such as multifocal ventricular ectopies, supraventricular tachycardias, or morphological ECG changes could be caused by ischaemia or impending or actual infarction. If this is suspected, immediately do a twelve-lead ECG and take blood samples for cardiac enzymes. Such a patient may need to be re-routed from the ward to a high dependency unit (HDU) or ICU for better observational care.

### Blood pressure abnormalities

Hypertension occurs because of anxiety, pain, or pre-existing hypertension. It is augmented by the physiological response to hypercapnia and hypoxia. After some procedures that affect physiological responses (e.g. carotid surgery, removal of phaeochromocytoma), blood pressure homoeostasis can be lost. The management of hypertension is the management of the cause, with pain right at the top of the list.

Hypotension is most commonly the result of inadequate fluid replacement. It needs rapid correction because, if it persists, vital organs can be damaged and $\dot{V}/\dot{Q}$ mismatches maintained. Other causes are decreased myocardial contractility and peripheral vasodilatation.

First-line management in an average-sized adult should usually be to give a test load of 500 ml colloid and observe the response. It is very easy to underestimate the losses of fluid into body cavities and tissues postoperatively. In the rare event that adequate filling pressures are obtained and the blood pressure remains low, it is time for an arterial line, inotropes, and expert management.

### Pain control

Some of the effects of poor pain management and the adverse consequences of analgesic drugs have been described above. The principles of postoperative pain control are described in Chapter 5.

### Fluid balance

Some problems with fluid balance have been described above. The principles of management are dealt with in Chapter 14.

### Postoperative nausea and vomiting

The factors affecting this and its management are described in Chapter 5.

### Abnormal body temperature

Hyperthermia is rare unless the patient is pyrexial preoperatively; degrees of hypothermia are common.

Hyperthermia can occur *de novo* when anticholinergic drugs (which prevent sweating) are given in the presence of infection. Malignant hyperpyrexia is very rare but should be considered, if only to exclude it.

Hypothermia is multifactorial in cause but usually associated with long operations that have exposed large body cavities. Measures to conserve body heat should have been taken intraoperatively (see Chapters 3 and 73) and these need to be continued in recovery. Hypothermia results in peripheral vasoconstriction, shivering and tissue hypoxia, reduced neuromuscular transmission, and, occasionally, hypertension. It may contribute to slow awakening and, on occasion, requires a period of elective postoperative ventilation while the temperature recovers. The difference between skin and core temperatures is a good guide to the effectiveness of management.

### Confusion

Transient agitation in patients during the early stages of recovery is not uncommon and usually resolves with effective pain management and reassurance. If it continues, or is actually frank confusion, it needs to be taken seriously. There are a large number of causes, some of which have already been described. Others to think about are:

- hypoxaemia and/or hypercapnia;
- hypotension;
- continuing pain;
- hypothermia;
- inadequate reversal of relaxation;
- gastric or bladder distension or irritation from indwelling catheter;
- hallucinations (note alcohol);
- CVA.

Patients with confusion need to be kept in recovery until it abates or discharged to an environment (e.g. an HDU) that can cope with it.

## CRITERIA FOR DISCHARGE FROM RECOVERY

Patients leave recovery to go to the normal ward or to a more specialized unit such as an HDU. The criteria for discharge to specialized units will obviously depend upon the exact situation and local guidelines.

For discharge to a normal ward, patients need to meet the criteria listed in Table 4.5.

When the ward staff arrive to take the patient back, there needs to be a proper handover similar to that described above for when the patient arrives in recovery from the operating room. Transport back to the ward should be on a suitable designed trolley or bed (see Table 4.3).

**Table 4.5. Criteria for discharge from recovery to a normal ward**

| A patient should be fully conscious and lucid and: |
|---|
| Possess a clear and reliable airway |
| Have physiological parameters within the expected range |
| Have pain adequately controlled (to their level of satisfaction) |
| Be well hydrated with good tissue perfusion |
| Be mentally comfortable with their condition and not unduly anxious |

## FURTHER READING


Association of Anaesthetists of Great Britain and Ireland. *Immediate Postanaesthetic Recovery*. London: Association of Anaesthetists of Great Britain and Ireland, 1993.

Cooper GM. Monitoring the recovery from anaesthesia. In: Hutton P, Prys-Roberts C, eds. *Monitoring in Anaesthesia and Intensive Care*. Philadelphia: WB Saunders, 1994: 350–64.

Frost EAM, Thomson DA, eds. *Post-anaesthetic Care*. *Baillière's Clin Anaesthesiol* 1994;**8**:749–910.

Hartley M, Vaughan RS. Problems associated with tracheal extubation. *Br J Anaesth* 1993;**71**:561–8.

Hutton P, Clutton-Brock TH. The benefits and pitfalls of pulse oximetry. *BMJ* 1993;**307**:457–8.

# Chapter 5 Postoperative care

C. Dodds and P. Hutton

Depending on the site and severity, operations can cause tissue damage, activation of stress responses, and local organ damage. The general health and robustness of the patient has a profound effect on the outcome of these responses, but the actions and postoperative care by the anaesthetic and surgical teams play a major role in whether or not there is permanent harm or even death.

The crucial nature of the postoperative period has been recognized for many years. In 1863 in *Notes on Hospitals*, Florence Nightingale stated, 'The most important perhaps of all the elements are the complications occurring after operations.'

The definition used in deciding what is 'postanaesthetic' or 'postoperative' varies from 24 hours (reporting to coroners) to 30 days (for operative mortality data). Therefore the whole of the patient's stay in hospital is, to a greater or lesser degree, the responsibility of the anaesthetist – acting as a 'perioperative physician'. The care of the patient in the immediate postoperative recovery period is described in Chapter 4.

The postoperative management of the patient includes active steps to reduce and control pain, the reduction or elimination of nausea and vomiting, and the preservation of physiological homoeostasis. Frequently, when difficulties arise, they do not occur in isolation; proper management requires careful prioritization of treatments. Some patients will require intensive or high dependency care, and their selection and management is described in Chapter 17.

Any injury (be it trauma, surgery, burns, or haemorrhage) induces a physiological 'stress' response that is proportional to the magnitude of the injury. This results in release of various hormones (ACTH [and hence cortisol], endorphins, growth hormone, vasopressin, prolactin, catecholamines, and aldosterone). There is a period of intense catabolism: fatty acids are mobilized and utilized, amino acids are converted into carbohydrate, and nitrogen is lost from the body as a result of the breakdown of protein. Blood glucose is increased. Sodium and water are retained, although there is increased urinary potassium loss. The metabolic rate, body temperature, oxygen consumption, and carbon dioxide production increase.

The stress response has been suggested to be necessary for survival and recovery but it can be seen that some of its effects are potentially adverse, particularly in the cachectic patient or one with cardiac disease. High-dose opioid anaesthetic techniques and regional blockade can modify the degree of hormonal response but the benefits of this are controversial.

## ACUTE PAIN MANAGEMENT

This section describes the management of pain in the postoperative period. Accompanying relevant information on the pharmacology of analgesic drugs is given in Chapter 34 and on local anaesthetics in Chapter 36. The practical aspects of regional anaesthesia are dealt with in Chapter 15.

### Pain: definition and effects

Pain is usually defined as:

> *as an unpleasant sensory and emotional experience resulting from a stimulus that has already caused, is causing, or is likely to cause tissue damage.*

The fact that it is experienced by the patient alone (the rest of us are just observers of the response) and is affected by subjective emotional factors means that it must be treated on an individual basis. Value judgements from medical and nursing staff that categorize patients as 'tough' or 'soft' are unfair, unhelpful, and counterproductive. An example of the variation in dose requirements of alfentanil between individuals after surgery is shown in Figure 5.1.

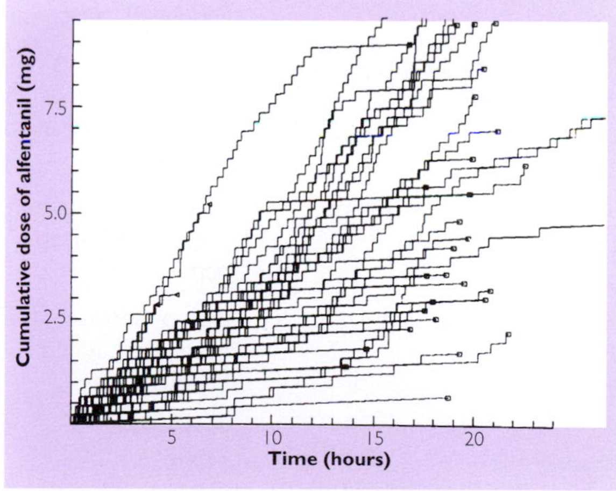


**Figure 5.1.** An example of the variability in postoperative requirements for alfentanil. Each line represents the cumulative dose for an individual patient, each of whom had the same operation and was allowed to self-administer via a patient-controlled analgesia system. (Adapted from Lehman KA. The pharmacology of opioid analgesics – discussion. In: Harmer M, Rosen M, Vickers MD, eds. *Patient-controlled Analgesia*. Oxford: Blackwell Scientific Publications, 1985, 27.)

If patients are experiencing significant pain, they are subject to its adverse effects, as listed in Table 5.1. Effective pain management abolishes or at least minimizes these. The best approach is to treat each patient on their merits because the benefits of pain relief can be attained only if it is successful. Unfortunately, reports from the UK, the USA, and Australia have demonstrated the continuing poor quality of postoperative pain relief in hospitals. Basic humanitarian considerations dictate that postoperative pain management requires our continued attention.

### Management and measurement of pain

Effective pain management starts with the preoperative assessment of the patient, and an understanding of the nature and extent of the proposed surgery. Factors relevant to acute pain management in an individual patient are given in Table 5.2. Patients have differing strategies for coping with pain and there are wide variations in their tolerance to it. Elderly patients often complain much less than young or middle-aged ones. Assessment of the mental state of the patient is important because it may, for instance, determine whether they are capable of using a patient-controlled analgesia (PCA) system, or whether a nurse-administered protocol is safer.

It is clear that the preoperative visit is the time when postoperative pain management should be planned. Most analgesic regimens are started during surgery, but some anaesthetists are of the opinion that analgesia should begin preoperatively. This is termed 'pre-emptive analgesia' and is intended to reduce analgesic

| Table 5.2. Factors relevant to acute pain management in an individual patient |
|---|
| Personality and psychological make-up |
| Site and extent of surgery |
| Patient's tolerance to pain |
| Patient's response to analgesics |
| Reason for surgery and likely outcome |
| Expectations of postoperative pain and its relief |
| Previous experience of postoperative pain |
| Existing pain problems and therapy (e.g. arthritis) |
| Coping responses and family support |
| Attitudes to the use of drugs |

**Table 5.1. The adverse effects of pain**

| Modality | Effects | Consequences |
|---|---|---|
| Psychological | Distress<br>Humiliation | Depression<br>Withdrawal<br>Fear |
| CVS | Hypertension<br>Tachycardia<br>Peripheral vasoconstriction | Myocardial oxygen requirements increased |
| Respiratory system | If breathing hurts:<br>Low tidal volumes<br>Decreased ventilation<br>Poor coughing | Hypoxaemia<br>Atelectasis<br>Pneumonia<br>Hypercapnia if ventilatory depression is severe |
| Central nervous system | Altered sleep pattern, possibly with sleep deprivation | Anxiety state<br>Hypoxaemia during sleep |
| Locomotor system | Lack of normal movement, even when in bed<br>Venous stasis | Increased risk of DVT and PE<br>Muscle wasting<br>Aching joints, etc. |
| Endocrine system | Increases in:<br>ADH<br>Cortisol<br>Aldosterone | Water and sodium retention<br>Hyperglycaemia<br>Oedema |
| Gastrointestinal system | Gastric stasis and dilatation<br>Ileus<br>Poor oral intake | Nausea and vomiting<br>Increased aspiration risk |
| Urological system | Urinary retention | Agitation<br>Discomfort<br>Associated CVS changes |

ADH, antidiuretic hormone; DVT, deep vein thrombosis; PE, pulmonary embolism; CVS, cardiovascular system.

requirements later. Enthusiasts believe that it exerts its beneficial effects by limiting 'immediate early gene' (IEG) expression, which is linked with the 'wind-up' phenomenon. Even a transient noxious stimulation leads to the expression of the IEG c-*fos* within 10 min of stimulation in the superficial layers of the dorsal horn of the spinal cord. This area has a high proportion of connections to higher pain centres. Unfortunately, clear-cut clinical data to support the benefits of the administration of analgesia before tissue injury are limited. Pre-emptive analgesia remains a contraversial subject.

The management of postoperative pain continues to evolve and it is the anaesthetist's responsibility to ensure that it occurs. It is probably managed best in hospitals that run an acute pain control service. The potential benefits of an acute pain service are given in Table 5.3.

| Table 5.3. The potential benefits of an acute pain service |
|---|
| Improved relief of pain |
| Improved patient and staff satisfaction |
| Allows method of pain relief to be tailored to patients' needs |
| Focuses teaching of nursing and medical staff |
| Sets standards for practice |
| Promotes safety standards |
| Can reduce hospital stay |
| Can reduce postoperative complications |
| Cost-effective |
| Improves both the standing and understanding of anaesthesia as a specialty within the hospital and among the public |

Assessment of pain should be done regularly and recorded clearly. The site and nature of the pain, what exacerbates it, and what relieves it should be noted. Postoperative pain is usually characterized by a constant painful ache related to the incisional site and which is exacerbated with tearing sensations during movement such as coughing or as a result of physiotherapy. The pain is normally time limited, subsides over 2 or 3 days, although this can be very variable, and remains localized. New pain in a different site may indicate new pathology (e.g. pulmonary embolus, perforated ulcer).

One of the keys to successful pain control *is the precise definition of what the patient is experiencing and the monitoring of treatment*. This necessitates regular observations of the patient by a trained observer. The assessment of pain can be made by a variety of scoring systems. Examples of two such systems in current adult and paediatric use, which can be filled in by either the patient or the nurse, are shown in Figures 5.2 and 5.3. Another version, which combines cardiovascular and respiratory observations with pain measurement, is shown in Figure 5.4. If treatment is unsuccessful, it is obvious that dosing modifications are necessary. Continued recording of unremitting pain, with no attempt to respond to the clinical findings to try and ameliorate it, is a complete waste of time. It is particularly important to try to assess pain in the confused elderly patient because the pain itself may be the cause of the confusion.

The requirements for the success of an acute pain service are given in Table 5.4. Of particular importance is the establishment of agreed protocols and immediate back-up for nursing staff if difficulties arise. These two factors mean that prescription of a limited range of drugs may be best so that experience is gained rapidly and confidence exists to use effective doses.

## Therapeutic options for pain control

The choice of drug, route, and timing is the key to success. Wherever opioids and local anaesthetics are used, resuscitation equipment and naloxone must be immediately available.

For convenience of reference, the ways in which analgesics can be administered are given in Appendix

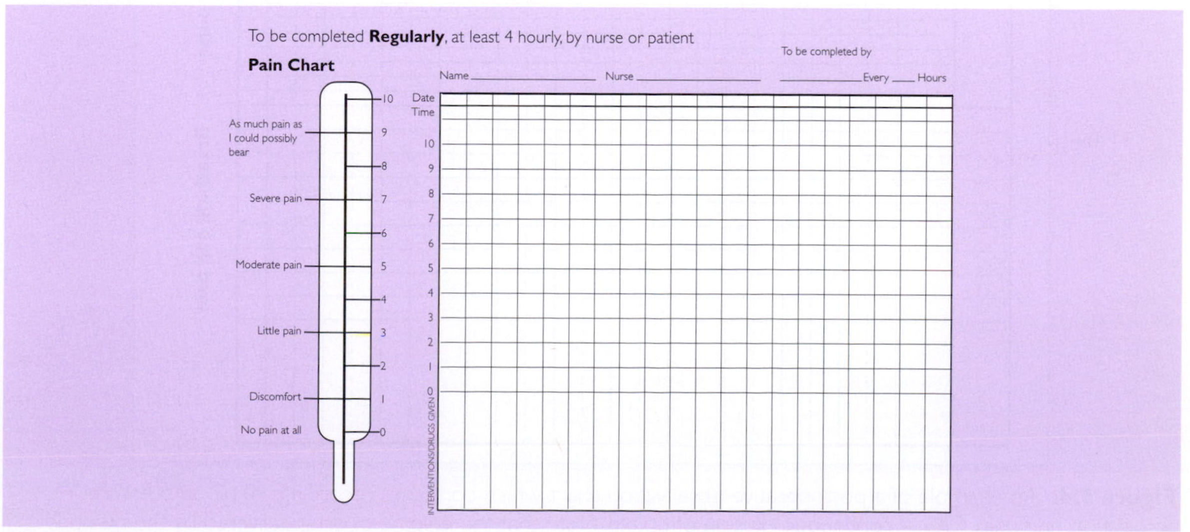


**Figure 5.2.** An example of a postoperative pain chart for adults. (Courtesy of South Cleveland Hospital NHS Trust.)

0 1 2 3 4 5 6 7 8 9 10
No hurt at all
A tiny hurt
A little more hurt
Hurts even more
Hurts a whole lot
Hurts as much as I can imagine

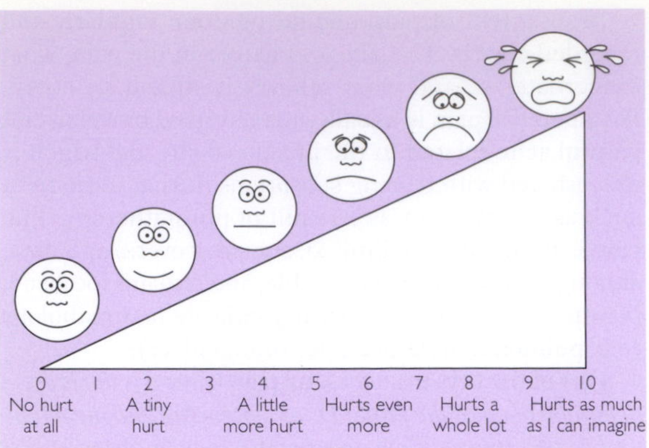

**Figure 5.3.** An example of a postoperative pain chart suitable for use with children. (Courtesy of Birmingham Children's Hospital NHS Trust.)

5.1 and local anaesthetics in Appendix 5.2. Dosing schedules for children are described more fully in Chapter 42. Individual dosing regimens are given where appropriate in other sections of the book. Further details are given under 'Notes on individual drugs' later in the chapter.

One point of great importance is to emphasize that patients should always be looked after in an environment suitable for the pain management prescribed. It is difficult to give rigid advice on this because arrangements differ considerably from hospital to hospital. The golden rule is to ascertain preoperatively what you will do with the patient postoperatively. Sometimes this will be determined by the availability of individual nursing staff, and remember that the night staff are just as relevant as those who receive the patient from the operating room. The advantages, disadvantages and safety

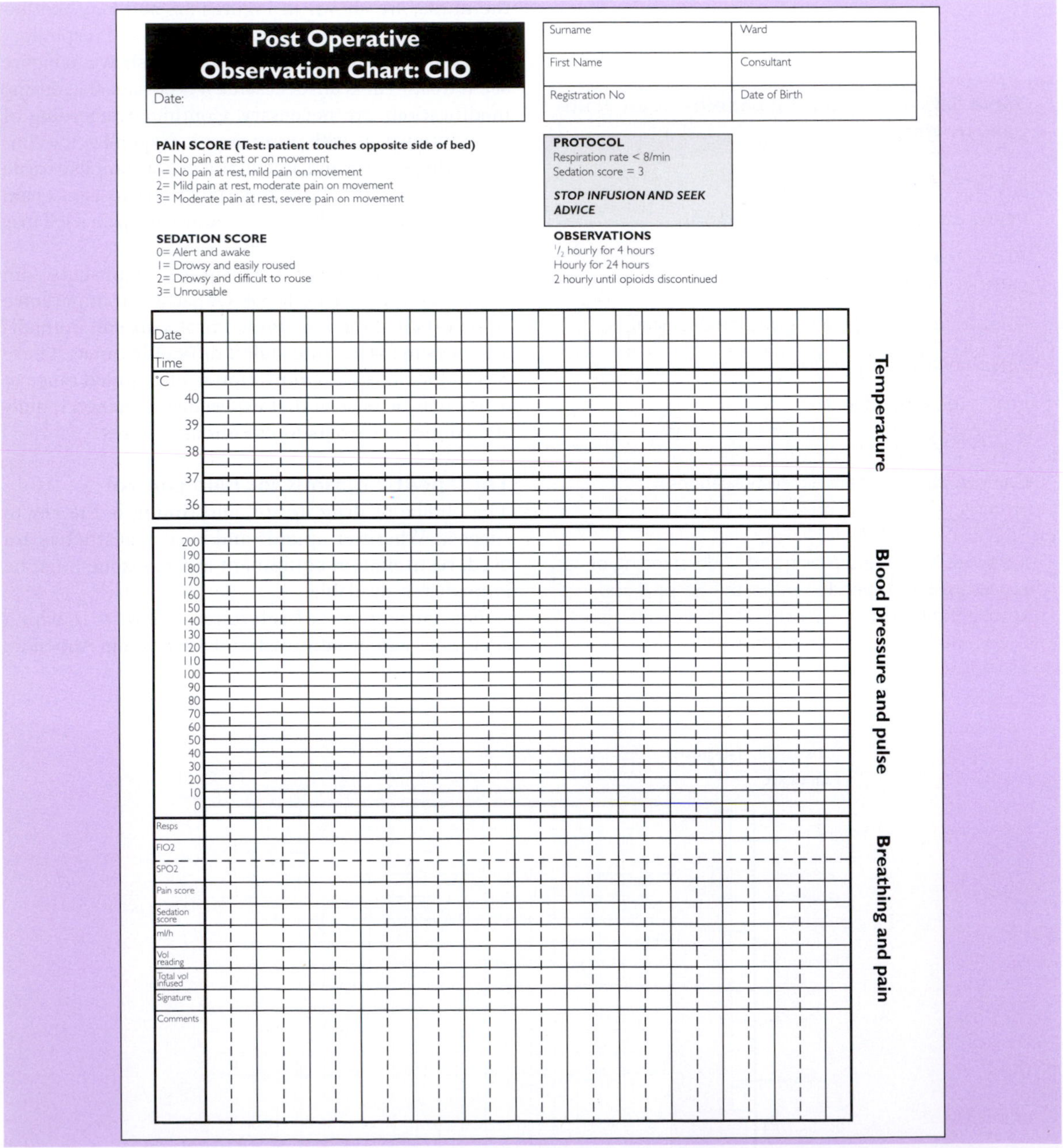

Post Operative Observation Chart: CIO
Date:
Surname
Ward
First Name
Consultant
Registration No
Date of Birth
PAIN SCORE (Test: patient touches opposite side of bed)
0= No pain at rest or on movement
1= No pain at rest, mild pain on movement
2= Mild pain at rest, moderate pain on movement
3= Moderate pain at rest, severe pain on movement
PROTOCOL
Respiration rate < 8/min
Sedation score = 3
STOP INFUSION AND SEEK ADVICE
SEDATION SCORE
0= Alert and awake
1= Drowsy and easily roused
2= Drowsy and difficult to rouse
3= Unrousable
OBSERVATIONS
1/2 hourly for 4 hours
Hourly for 24 hours
2 hourly until opioids discontinued
Date
Time
°C
40
39
38
37
36
Temperature
200
190
180
170
160
150
140
130
120
110
100
90
80
70
60
50
40
30
20
10
0
Blood pressure and pulse
Resps
FIO2
SPO2
Pain score
Sedation score
ml/h
Vol reading
Total vol infused
Signature
Comments
Breathing and pain

**Figure 5.4.** An example of a postoperative observation chart which combines recordings of blood pressure, respiration, and pain. CIO = continuous infusion of opioid. Note that the volume of drug delivered by the pump is recorded. (With permission of University Hospital Birmingham NHS Trust.)

| Table 5.4. The requirements of an acute pain service |
|---|
| Enthusiastic consultant leadership |
| Enthusiastic nursing support: ideal for clinical nurse specialist |
| Effective hospital education programme |
| Establishment of agreed protocols |
| Sufficient equipment and funding to run the service |
| Appropriate on-call cover and lines of responsibility |
| Proper drug dispensing and storage |
| Audit of performance of service |
| Good communication with patients' groups and purchasers |

precautions of the main parenteral methods of pain relief are described below and summarized in Appendices 5.1 and 5.2.

#### *Intermittent intramuscular dosing schedules*

Intermittent, 'as required' intramuscular schedules prescribed at infrequent intervals (e.g. 3–4 hourly pro rata nocte) produce peaks and troughs in pain relief, as shown in Figure 5.5. Despite this, such dosing schedules are still frequently written because of their acceptability to the ward staff and their reputation for the absence of serious respiratory depression. The latter assumption is based on the fact that the patient has to be sufficiently alert to make the request. Such considerations are, however, not necessarily logical because if, for example, the onset of pain prevents effective breathing and promotes hypoxia, this has its own morbidity.

Although frequently criticized, intramuscular opioids can nevertheless be prescribed so as to be quite effective. An example of an effective *hourly* intramuscular schedule is shown in Figure 5.6. The following are the advantages:

- The frequent dosing removes the large peaks and troughs of Figure 5.5.
- The dose can be titrated to patients' needs.
- The pain is measured regularly and doses can be prescribed before moderate or severe pain recurs.
- In visiting the patient to measure pain, other basic signs can be observed (blood pressure, heart rate, colour, respiratory rate, arterial oxygen saturation etc.).
- There is improved communication between patients and ward staff.
- There is enhanced job satisfaction for ward staff.

The negative aspects are:

- Injections are painful.
- Intramuscular injections can lead to haematoma formation in the muscle (especially if the patient is heparinized), cell damage (leading to scarring) and muscle wasting.
- The workload for the ward staff is increased if the method is to be successful.
- Failure of regular assessment can lead to breakthrough pain and cyclical dosing (see Figure 5.5).
- The periods when the patient has inadequate pain relief can be prolonged, especially at night or when the ward is busy.

#### *Intravenous infusion techniques*

Giving drugs by infusion produces steadier conditions, which, if tailored to the patient, are likely to be more satisfactory. However, problems result if the effective serum level is never reached or accumulation occurs. Initiating infusion analgesia is best done in recovery, as described in Chapter 4. Steady infusions should be prescribed only in those patients who can be closely observed and have regular measurements made of their pain management. With these precautions, infusions can be a very safe and effective method of postoperative pain management. The consequences of patients (or relatives) adjusting infusion rates is another hazard not to be forgotten. An example of a protocol in current use is given in Figure 5.7 and the standing orders to ensure safety are given in Figure 5.8.

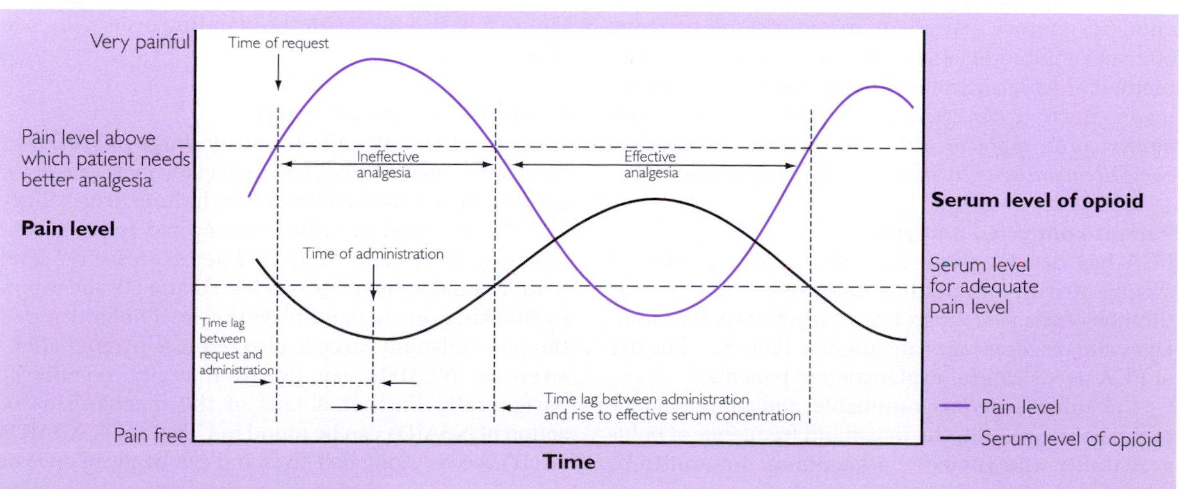


**Figure 5.5.** Diagrammatic representation of the potential for ineffective analgesia when opioids are prescribed on an intramuscular basis as required.

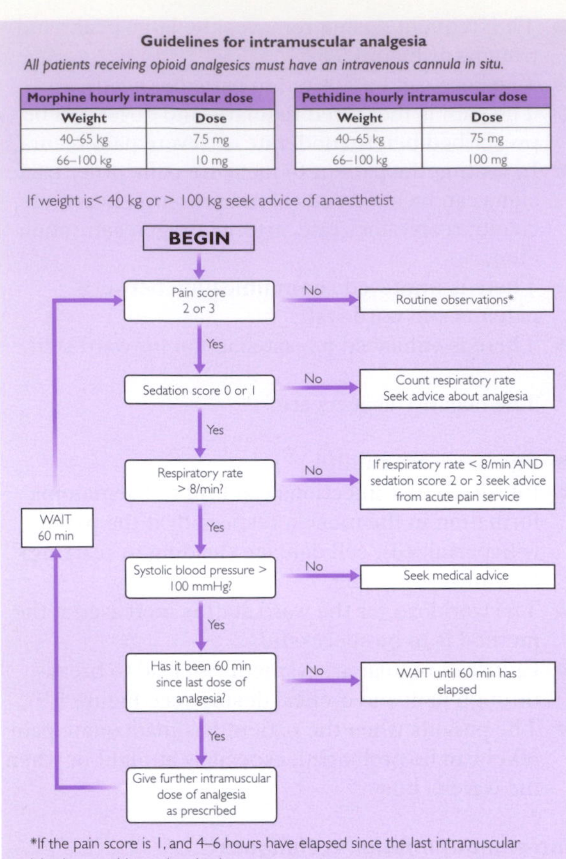


**Figure 5.6.** An example of a protocol for 1-hourly intramuscular opioid analgesia. The sedation and pain scores are as defined in Figure 5.4 and given on the reverse of this protocol form with the recording chart. (With permission from University Hospital Birmingham NHS Trust.)

**Pain relief algorithm for the use of continuous intravenous opioid**

**Pain score = 0 or 1**

***Assess sedation score:*** If sedation score is 0 or 1 adjust treatment if required

Continue to monitor until end of treatment

**Pain score = 2**

***Consider:*** A: Sedation score is 0 or 1, increase infusion rate as per prescription

B: Monitor and reassess in 1 hour

Monitor until pain score is 0 or 1

**Pain score = 3**

***Unacceptable*** Check IV line is patent Check pump

***Rescue analgesia*** Give IV bolus dose of 2 ml via infusion pump (2 ml = 2 mg morphine) (2 ml = 20 mg pethidine) Consider increasing infusion rate as per prescription chart

Review in 10 min If pain score = 3, repeat 2 ml bolus Review in 10 minutes

**If pain score still 3, seek advice**

**If sedation score = 3 or respiration rate < 8/min — STOP INFUSION, SEEK ADVICE**

**Who to contact:**

For inadequate pain control contact:
Acute Pain Team, bleep 1564
On-call anaesthetist

***The re-siting of intravenous cannulae or minor problems should be dealt with at ward level.***

**Figure 5.7.** An example of a protocol for continuous intravenous opioid (CIO) analgesia in current use. The sedation and pain scores are as defined in Figure 5.4 and given on the reverse of this protocol form with the recording chart. (With permission from University Hospital Birmingham NHS Trust.)

### *Epidural and spinal techniques*

These are discussed fully in Chapter 15. There is, however, one important point that deserves emphasis. A fortunately now less common error is to respond to a badly functioning epidural or intrathecal block containing opioids by immediately prescribing additional parenteral opioids. This has caused severe, life-threatening respiratory depression in a number of patients, often at an unpredictable time. Consequently, if a given method of pain control is thought not to be able to be made effective, *change to another only after a careful analysis of the problem and ensure that the patient is very carefully monitored by an adequately trained person.*

### *Patient-controlled analgesia*

PCA has developed as the safety and reliability of syringe driving pumps has improved. It allows self-titration of analgesia apart from during sleep. Its advantages and disadvantages are given in Table 5.5. The use of PCA needs careful explanation to patients.

The pumps are programmable, and allow a choice of the bolus amount, the maximum frequency of bolus availability, and (usually) a maximum amount to be administered in a given time period. These terms are defined in Table 5.6. Background infusions can be used and prevent falls in analgesia during sleep, but they require frequent assessment and possible adjustment to maintain satisfactory baseline analgesia without progressive accumulation of opioid. PCA use should occur only when there is a 24-hour acute pain team, and the ward staff have had training and developed expertise in its use.

An example of guidelines in current use is given in Figure 5.9, together with the standing orders for safe practice.

## Notes on individual drugs

### *Non-steroidal anti-inflammatory drugs (NSAIDs)*

Mild-to-moderate pain, and especially pain related to bone surgery, is well controlled with these drugs. They can also be used to reduce the opioid requirement following more major surgery. They decrease the level of inflammatory mediators released after tissue injury by blocking prostaglandin synthesis. The limiting of the prostaglandin cascade also reduces platelet adhesiveness. NSAIDs can be given orally, rectally or parenterally. Further details of the mechanisms of action of NSAIDs can be found in Chapter 34. NSAIDs often have very long half-lives and can be given once or twice daily. They do not cause respiratory depression or sedation, and have no effect on gastric emptying, small bowel motility, or haemodynamic stability.

**Standing orders**

**When CIO is used please undertake the following:**

| | | |
|---|---|---|
| **1.** | **Oxygen therapy:** | **This is a minimum requirement**<br>2 litres per min via nasal specs for first 24 hours<br>Ideally oxygen therapy should be continued throughout CIO regimen |
| **2.** | **Observations:**<br>For the first 4 hours postoperatively<br><br>Up to 24 hours<br><br>After 24 hours | **Record the following**<br>½ *hourly* pulse, BP, repiratory rate, pain and sedation scoring must be recorded<br><br>*Hourly* BP, pulse, respiratory rate, pain and sedation scores must be recorded<br><br>*Two hourly* BP, pulse, repiratory rate, pain and sedation scores must be recorded until CIO is discontinued |
| **3.** | **Syringe drivers:** | **Record the following**<br>Rate of infusion (ml/h)<br>Volume left in the syringe<br>Volume infused<br><br>Any changes to infusion rate must be signed for by the nurse responsible and recorded on the observation chart<br><br>**This must be recorded hourly for the first 24 hours and thereafter at least 2-hourly** |

- Syringe changes or removal from carriage for dressing/ washing purposes, must only be undertaken by nurses who are deemed intravenous competent
- All infusion lines must be labelled
- Opioids must be administered via a dedicated intravenous line only
- Naloxone must be prescribed as required for all patients receiving opioids
- Syringe drivers must be placed level with patient; lines must be occluded when changing the syringe to prevent backflow

**Figure 5.8.** The standing orders to ensure safety during a continuous infusion of opioids (CIO). (With permission from University Hospital Birmingham NHS Trust.)

NSAIDs are often prescribed for day-care patients to take home because of this beneficial profile of activity. The choice of NSAIDs for routine protocols requires care since some are very expensive for the little clinical advantage, if any, that they offer over others.

NSAIDs also have significant side effects, especially in elderly patients, related to their prostaglandin inhibition. They are associated with an increase in bleeding time, they can cause gastric erosions and bleeding, and they can impair renal blood flow regulation, leading to a deterioration in renal function. This renal damage is made worse by dehydration, which unfortunately can occur commonly even in day-care surgery. Although NSAIDs can reduce opioid requirements by up to 50%, they are usually inadequate for severe or visceral pain and should not be prescribed in isolation for such pain. Finally, NSAIDs can cause bronchospasm in susceptible individuals. This affects 10–20% of asthmatic patients and the bronchospasm, when it occurs, can be very severe.

The perioperative use of NSAIDs has recently been the subject of published clinical guidelines. These are given in Appendix 5.3.

### *Opioids*

Postoperatively, the requirement is for potent, medium- or long-acting drugs. The most commonly used include morphine, papaveretum, pethidine, codeine, and diamorphine. They can be administered by a variety of routes (see Appendices 5.1 and 5.2), but there are differences in bioavailability, duration of action, and

**Table 5.5. The advantages and disadvantages of patient-controlled analgesia**

| Advantages |
|---|
| Psychologically good for patient who feels 'in control' and involved in their own recovery |
| Adjusts automatically to patient's needs |
| Small, frequent boluses reduce fluctuations in plasma level |
| Painless |
| Can reduce nurses' workload |
| **Disadvantages** |
| Requires patient understanding and cooperation. No good for under-5s and confused or demented patients |
| Equipment is expensive |
| Equipment can malfunction |
| Inadvertent administration of full syringe (potentially fatal) |
| Can be misprogrammed |
| Can be wrong concentration of drug |
| Patients with some conditions (e.g. arthritis) may not be able to press button |
| Does not run while asleep |
| Relatives may tamper with it |
| Large doses of drug in syringe or bag may result in self-abuse or theft |
| Solutions may become infected (rare) |

time to peak pain relief. Elderly patients often need lower doses of opioids to achieve effective analgesia because of alteration in their protein binding, plasma volumes, clearance, and receptor function. The oral route is the most comfortable for the patient but most inpatients will require parenteral opioids.

Intramuscular opioids have a very long tradition, and can be effective, but it is very difficult to maintain stable plasma levels without frequent dosing (see Figure 5.5 and above).

Subcutaneous analgesia can, with the right conditions, be as effective as intravenous, but has the same delay as intramuscular, injections. There is usually little pain from subcutaneous injections and low-volume continuous infusions can be used. They are mostly used for terminal care.

Intravenous infusions can, as described above, be very successful, but are not without risk. If there has been effective titration of intravenous opioid in the recovery unit, the delay to reach effective plasma levels on the ward will be avoided and analgesia will be maintained. The initial intravenous titration in such a high-observation area as a recovery unit provides the safety necessary for the period when overdosage with respiratory depression is most likely.

**Table 5.6. The variables in patient-controlled analgesia**

| Variable | Description |
|---|---|
| Analgesic agent | Each hospital needs to standardize on one or two intravenous opioids to optimize experience and familiarity |
| Concentration | Each drug should always be administered in the same concentration. This prevents errors in preparation and programming of the pump. Ideally, drugs should be made up by pharmacy and delivered ready to use |
| Bolus dose | The dose delivered by each patient demand, e.g. 1 mg morphine |
| Lock-out time | The time after one bolus before which the system will allow a second to be delivered, e.g. 5 or 10 min. Should be at least long enough for previous dose to have been effective |
| Dose limit | The maximum dose that can be delivered by the patient in a given time period. Limits the delivery and identifies high-use patients who may require different prescription limits |
| Background infusion | There is little evidence in adults that a background infusion improves the quality of analgesia, but it does increase sedation and respiratory depression; May be of more use in children |

All opioids cause nausea and vomiting (see below), and this is more pronounced if the patient is mobile. Once the patient becomes ambulatory, the balance between complete analgesia and this side effect can become difficult. In the absence of effective antiemetsis, the addition of or change to another form of analgesia often becomes essential.

Epidural administration of opioids can provide excellent stable analgesia with much smaller doses than other routes, and is often combined with local anaesthetic drugs. It provides prolonged analgesia but it has several major disadvantages. For instance, respiratory depression can occur up to 18 hours after the initial injection. This makes close monitoring and assessment essential. Some hospitals only provide epidural analgesia when there is a high dependency bed available, but many others have trained and experienced nursing staff on the surgical wards who can provide a safe environment for this technique. Pruritus can be a major problem with centrally administered opioids, and responds to low-dose intravenous naloxone titrated slowly to abolish the itching without affecting the analgesia.

***Local anaesthetic drugs***

These all act by blocking the central transmission of nociceptive signals from areas of damage. They may be applied to sensory nerves peripherally or more centrally, and can be given by bolus or infusion. Epidural local anaesthetic drugs in combination with opioids can provide satisfactory analgesia for major abdominal, thoracic, and orthopaedic surgery. Bupivacaine, lignocaine (lidocaine), and ropivacaine are the most common drugs used, but the short duration of action of lignocaine limits its use as an effective postoperative analgesic unless given by infusion. Further details of local anaesthetics, their toxicity and regional blocks are described in Chapter 15, to which reference should be made.

The risks of epidural local anaesthetics include blockade of the sympathetic nervous pathways (with the resulting loss of haemodynamic stability) ascending blockade reaching higher centres, local nerve damage, and haematoma formation.

Local anaesthetics, either alone or in combination with opioids, provide optimal analgesia where there are clear segmental distributions of pain such as thoracotomy or abdominal incisions. The analgesia may be given by repeated bolus dosing, a continuous infusion, or be patient controlled. The choice of drug and its concentration depend on the type of surgery and the anatomical extent of the blockade necessary. Concerns about toxicity and cephalad spread of the local anaesthetics have limited the provision of epidural infusions and epidural PCA to areas where close monitoring of the patient is possible. As with opioid PCA, the provision of 24-hour availability of an acute pain team has increased the use of these techniques, and also their management on acute wards.

Subarachnoid administration is more likely to result in ascending blockade, but is also the most effective method for providing a precise level of analgesia. Systems for prolonged intrathecal infusions using fine-bore catheters, are available, but the risks of infection and postdural puncture headache limit the widespread use of the technique.

***$\alpha_2$-adrenoceptor agonists***

$\alpha_2$-Adrenoceptor activation produces a potent analgesic response, involving both supraspinal and spinal sites. The most common available drug is clonidine, which is an imidazoline, and a selective agonist for $\alpha_2$-adrenoceptors with a ratio of 200 : 1 ($\alpha_2 : \alpha_1$). Clonidine is rapidly and almost completely absorbed after oral administration; it can also be given intravenously or spinally. It exerts a potent analgesic effect, but high doses can cause bradycardia, sedation and hypotension. Its potency is enhanced synergistically with concomitant treatment with opioids, and it is in combination with epidural opioids that it most probably has a role in postoperative pain control. Its place in routine practice has yet to be established.

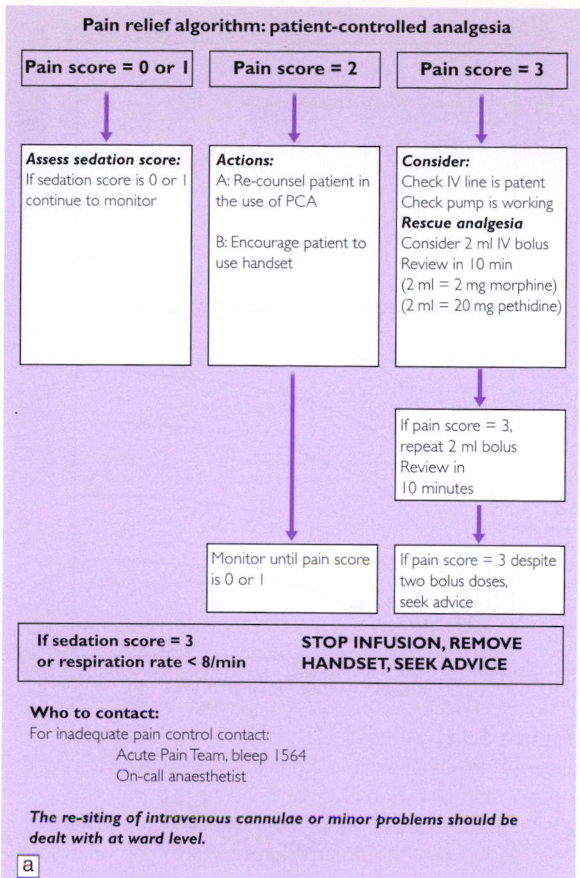


**Standing orders**

When PCA is commenced please undertake the following:

| | | |
|---|---|---|
| 1. | **Oxygen therapy:** | 2 litres per min via nasal specs for first 24 hours |
| 2. | **Observations:** For the first 4 hours postoperatively | **Record the following:** ½ hourly pulse, BP, respiratory rate, pain and sedation scoring, number of good/bad attempts made<br>The amount of morphine/pethidine used |
| | Up to 24 hours | *Hourly* BP, pulse, respiratory rate, pain and sedation scores, number of good/bad attempts made<br>The amount of morphine/pethidine used |
| | After 24 hours | *Two hourly* BP, pulse, respiratory rate, pain and sedation scores, number of good/bad attempts made<br>The amount of morphine/pethidine used<br><br>Record until PCA is discontinued |

**Programming of pumps can be undertaken only by anaesthetist or other designated person**

b

**Figure 5.9.** (a) An example of a patient-controlled analgesia (PCA) protocol in current use, together with (b) the standing orders for patient safety. The protocol requires morphine and pethidine to be prepared at 1 mg/ml and 10 mg/ml, respectively. The pain and sedation scores are as defined in Figure 5.4. (With permission of University Hospital Birmingham NHS Trust.)

### *Other drugs and techniques*

Several anaesthetic drugs have been used to provide analgesia, ranging from ketamine to nitrous oxide, but the difficulties of administering them during the postoperative period makes them unsuitable except for cases such as burns where skilled nursing care is provided and there are predictable, short periods of pain.

Complementary techniques of pain control using physical methods can be effective in mild or moderate pain, and can bolster pain control when the patient is becoming mobile. They include transcutaneous electrical nerve stimulation (TENS), cold, and massage.

## MAINTENANCE OF TISSUE OXYGENATION

Adequate tissue oxygenation requires a supply of oxygenated blood to be pumped through the various vascular beds. When investigating cyanosis or low oxygen saturation readings, first check that oxygen is being administered and the patient is breathing adequately. Then make sure that the patient has an appropriate heart rate and blood pressure and is not hypothermic. Cyanosis accompanied by hypotension and a low cardiac output is usually the result of hypovolaemia from either inadequate replacement (most commonly) or blood loss. As described in Chapters 3, 4 and 14, it is easy to underestimate the ongoing losses of fluid into body cavities and tissue spaces. First-line fluid management in a normal-sized adult is to give up to 500 ml of colloid and observe the response, if necessary repeating it. In the event that reasonable filling pressures are obtained and the blood pressure remains low, it is time for an arterial line, inotropes, and relocation to a high dependency area. Subsequent management should be along the lines described in Chapters 14 and 17. The problems of circulatory management will not be considered further in this chapter.

Immediately after surgery, oxygenation of the blood by the lungs can be adversely affected for any of the reasons given in Chapter 4. The acute management of such disturbances is as described in that chapter. There are, however, two modalities of lung dysfunction that can persist several days into the postoperative period and are regularly seen on the wards. These are alveolar hypoventilation and ventilation–perfusion ($\dot{V}/\dot{Q}$) mismatching. When coupled with sleep disturbances and/or opioids, their effects on postoperative oxygenation can be as shown in Figure 5.10. The problems with ventilation and oxygenation described here should be studied in conjunction with Chapter 21.

### Alveolar hypoventilation

Alveolar hypoventilation is a reduction in the bellows function of the lungs. Mild alveolar hypoventilation is very common in the postoperative period. It can result from some of the factors listed in Chapter 4, Table 4.4. After the immediate recovery period the main causes are sedative and analgesic drugs, pain on ventilation, and airway obstruction during sleep. If severe, the consequent hypoxia and hypercapnia can themselves augment the depression of respiration. Once this situation has been reached, the condition is life threatening.

The relationship between alveolar ventilation, the alveolar oxygen partial pressure ($P\text{AO}_2$), and the inspired oxygen concentration ($F\text{IO}_2$) is shown in Figure 5.11 together with the accompanying changes in alveolar partial pressure of carbon dioxide ($P\text{ACO}_2$). It can be seen that, to correct a low $P\text{AO}_2$, all that is required is to increase the $F\text{IO}_2$. This moves the patient on to a different performance curve, which raises the

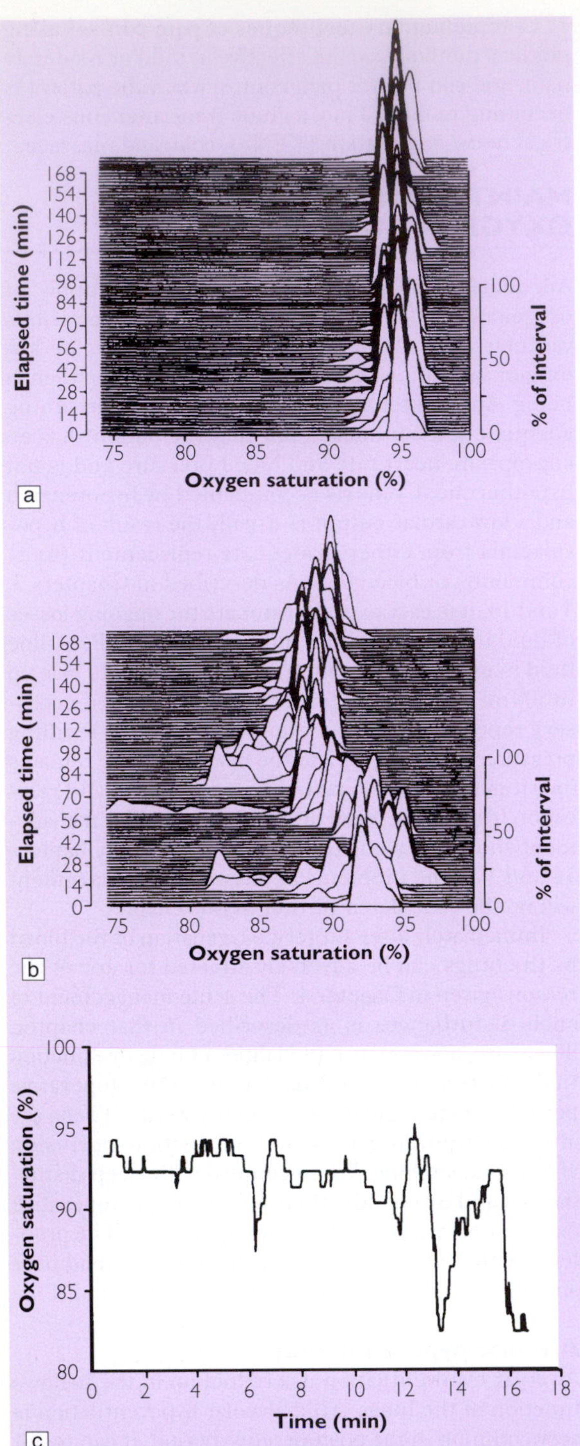


**Figure 5.10.** Oxygen saturations collected over 3 hours in the postoperative period. (a) A patient with satisfactory postoperative saturations; (b) an unstable trace from a patient with ineffective ventilation; (c) a plot of the oxygen saturation against time for the first eight intervals of (b). (Adapted from Roe PG, Jones JG. *Br J Anaesth* 1993;71:48.)

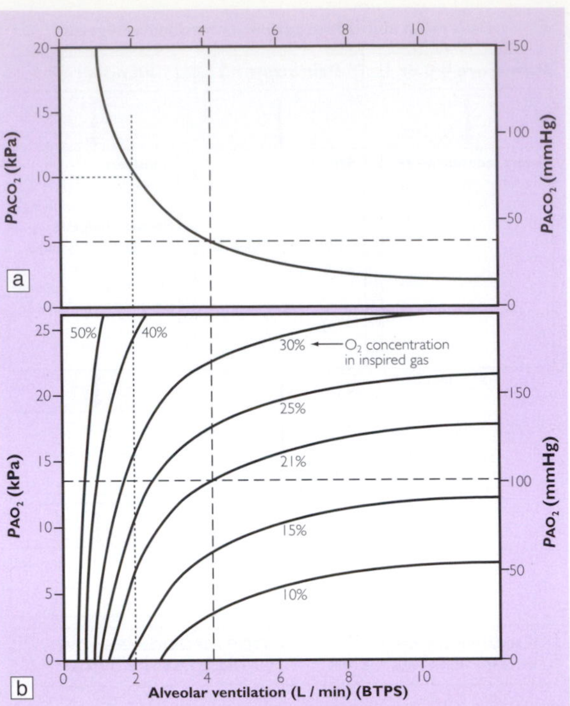


**Figure 5.11.** Alveolar gas tensions produced by different levels of alveolar ventilation. (a) The hyperbolic relationship between alveolar partial pressure of $CO_2$ ($P_{ACO_2}$) and alveolar ventilation. The derivation of this relationship is described in Chapter 9. (b) The relationship between alveolar partial pressure of oxygen ($P_{AO_2}$) and alveolar ventilation for differing oxygen concentrations in the expired gas. The dashed lines represent the normal alveolar ventilation in a healthy adult. It can be seen that if the alveolar ventilation falls by 50% (the dotted line), the $P_{AO_2}$ can be maintained by increasing the oxygen concentration in inspired gas to just below 30%, but this results in a rise in the $P_{ACO_2}$ to approximately 10 kPa. BTPS, body temperature and pressure saturated with water vapour. (Adapted from Nunn JF. *Applied Respiratory Physiology*, 2nd edn, London: Butterworths, 1977: 188.)

alveolar $P_{AO_2}$. It is therefore good practice to give all patients facemask oxygen in the postoperative period. As emphasized elsewhere in this book, it is, however, important to remember *that, in the presence of alveolar hypoventilation, although a high inspired oxygen concentration can correct hypoxia, the poor bellows function of the lungs may allow the* $P_{aCO_2}$ *level to rise to unacceptably high values*. It is consequently essential to measure the respiratory rate and observe the tidal excursion of the chest. *Do not rely on pulse oximeter readings alone*.

### Ventilation–perfusion mismatching

The changes in $\dot{V}/\dot{Q}$ mismatching are likely to persist for several days. These changes are caused by a fall in the functional residual capacity and by alterations in hypoxic pulmonary vasoconstriction. These start with the induction of anaesthesia and take up to 6 days to resolve completely. They are at their most severe during the first postoperative day, and during sleep, and the effects and response to oxygen therapy will vary depending on the relative proportion of shunting and $\dot{V}/\dot{Q}$ abnormalities. If there is predominantly a problem with shunting, such as a bronchial plug of mucus or lobar pneumonia, the response to increasing the inspired oxygen will plateau at lower and lower levels, the effect of raising the $F_{IO_2}$ becoming less and less as the shunt increases.

The reduction in effective lung volume that occurs after anaesthetic induction is largely caused by atelectasis of dependent airways (Chapter 21). Elderly patients are most vulnerable to this process because they are often closing off alveoli at the end of tidal breaths. This encroachment of closing capacity into tidal ventilation predisposes them to $\dot{V}/\dot{Q}$ changes, and these effects are heightened by the supine position. Very large breaths during anaesthesia can reduce the atelectasis that occurs but the clinical benefit in the postoperative period has yet to be demonstrated.

### Oxygen therapy

Oxygen therapy is rarely given effectively. The reasons are legion but, because the uptake of oxygen is continual, any interruption in supply to the patient will be followed by a rapid fall in its alveolar concentration.

The most common method of administering oxygen is via a facemask. Variable performance facemasks vary in design and effectiveness, and deliver oxygen concentrations of up to about 40%. High airflow oxygen entrainment (HAFOE) masks are capable of delivering precise concentrations of oxygen up to 60%, but can be uncomfortable because of the very high gas flows generated by the Venturi system. Nasal cannulae are effective, comfortable and well tolerated by most patients. They are probably the best method of delivering moderate concentrations of oxygen for prolonged periods. Masks and nasal specula and their performance are described in Chapters 6, 7, and 37. It has to be remembered that oxygen is highly supportive of combustion, and patients have died from burns resulting from smoking while on oxygen!

Monitoring of oxygenation by pulse oximetry should be available on all surgical wards for the patients who require it. Patients who will need oxygen therapy and monitoring can be identified before discharge from the recovery unit. Pulse oximetry readings of 93% or less on air is one simple guide, and the observed response to increasing the inspired oxygen concentration identifies both the prescription to be written and the probable underlying cause. Continuous pulse oximetry is necessary in patients who have an unstable pattern of oxygenation, but many patients will require only occasional recordings (as part of the pain assessment observations, for example). *What is essential is that patients should be prescribed oxygen, and have it administered to them, until they have a proven ability to maintain oxygenation on room air.* The following would seem to be reasonable practice guidelines:

- All patients should receive oxygen in the immediate postoperative period.
- After thoracic, abdominal, or major limb surgery, all patients should receive oxygen for 24 hours.
- Even if they are well oxygenated when awake, after thoracic, abdominal, or major limb surgery, patients should receive oxygen on the second and third postoperative nights.
- Oxygen should continue to be prescribed as long as parenteral, epidural or spinal opioids are being given for postoperative pain.

## MAINTENANCE OF FLUID BALANCE

Details of fluid balance management are considered fully in Chapter 14. There are, however, one or two points that will be emphasized so that they are not forgotten.

- The risk of bleeding continues into the postoperative period and a steady but slow loss is often underestimated.
- After major surgery, losses of plasma proteins, water and electrolytes from the vascular to the extravascular space are frequently grossly underestimated.
- Catabolism is common in the postoperative period. Early feeding with glucose (intravenously or enterally) decreases muscle breakdown and nitrogen losses.
- Urine output remains the most useful barometer of adequate volume replacement, and should never be allowed to fall below 0.5 ml/kg/hr.

## POSTOPERATIVE NAUSEA AND VOMITING (PONV)

### Physiology

The physiology of the gastrointestinal tract is described in Chapter 27. PONV is a complex problem, and may be more clearly understood after reviewing the basic mechanisms, which are shown in Figure 5.12. The 'vomiting centre' is an ill-defined area which lies within the medulla, possibly in the region of the nucleus tractus solitarius. It has an afferent supply from the chemoreceptor trigger zone (CTZ), and from many of the cranial nerves and higher centres. Signals from the distribution of the vagus are particularly stimulating. The CTZ lies on the floor of the fourth ventricle in the area postrema.

The 'vomiting reflex' is precipitated by afferent stimulation from the glossopharyngeal, hypoglossal and vagal nerves reaching the vomiting centre. Efferent signals are directed to the glossopharyngeal, hypoglossal, trigeminal, accessory and spinal segmental nerves. There is a coordinated contraction of abdominal muscles against a closed glottis, which raises intra-abdominal and intrathoracic pressures. The pyloric sphincter contracts and the oesophageal sphincter relaxes, and there is active antiperistalsis within the oesophagus, which forcibly expels the gastric contents. This is associated with marked vagal and sympathetic activity leading to sweating, pallor, and bradycardia.

### Clinical effects and incidence of PONV

The results of PONV are listed in Table 5.7 and include embarrassment, retching, wound pain or even dehiscence, dehydration and electrolyte disturbances, aspiration of gastric contents, and failure to take oral medication.

There are identified risk factors for PONV, which are summarized in Table 5.8. These include being young, female, obese, or prone to migraine, as well as the obvious associations of motion sickness or a previous report of PONV. It is most likely in surgery on the gut, ENT, and in gynaecological, orthopaedic, and extraocular eye surgery such as correction of squints. It is especially likely after emergency surgery.

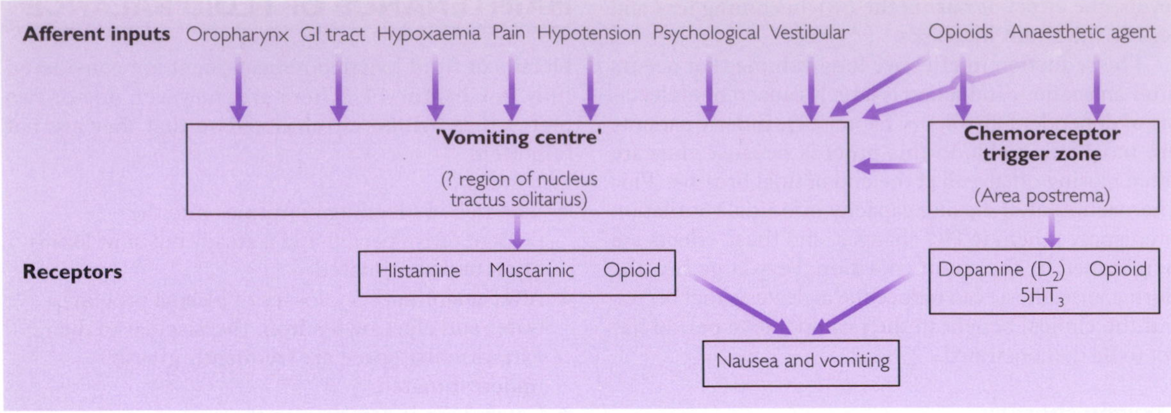


**Figure 5.12.** The inputs and receptors involved in causing postoperative nausea and vomiting. 5HT, 5-hydroxytryptamine/serotonin; GI, gastrointestinal.

**Table 5.7. The harmful effects of postoperative nausea and vomiting**

| Effect on | Consequences |
|---|---|
| The patient | Embarrassment and distress<br>Discomfort; can intensify postoperative pain<br>Can be exhausting and humiliating<br>Adverse psychological effects on any future surgery |
| The surgery and treatment | Can disrupt the wound<br>Can cause aspiration if drowsy<br>Prevents oral medication<br>Can upset fluid and electrolyte balance<br>May prevent early mobilization |
| The hospital | Increased nursing requirement<br>May delay discharge<br>Significant added cost if day-stay patient is hospitalized |

Anaesthetic causes for PONV include the anaesthetic vapours and barbiturates. All opioids cause nausea and vomiting through a direct action on the vomiting centre. Propofol has been suggested as being slightly protective against PONV.

### Drug therapy for PONV

There is no satisfactory drug that will stop or prevent nausea in all patients. The principal neurotransmitters in the vomiting reflex are serotoninergic, dopaminergic, and cholinergic. The rational choices and dosage ranges are very difficult to establish, but use of the drugs related to the predicted stimulus may be more effective than random 'routine' prescriptions. Vagally mediated cholinergic stimuli, such as gut handling, may respond to anticholinergic drugs such as hyoscine. Direct stimulation of the vomiting centre via dopaminergic or serotoninergic pathways is more likely to respond to low-dose droperidol (0.005 mg/kg), phenothiazines, or ondansetron.

Caution with the phenothiazines is necessary in patients with Parkinson's disease because of the risk of greatly increasing their rigidity and tremor.

Drug therapy for PONV is discussed further in Chapter 27.

## OTHER COMPLICATIONS IN THE FIRST 24 HOURS

### Disturbances of glucose homoeostasis

Postoperatively, because of the stress response, catabolism, and (in some cases) disturbed nutrition, patients with existing diabetes usually require more insulin. Those in a prediabetic state may become insulin dependent. Consequently, postoperative bloods should routinely include a glucose estimation. If the level is found to be high, it is best managed by using the hospital protocols that are in place at the time. Details of available regimens are given in Chapter 55.

### Hypothermia

The definition of hypothermia is a core temperature of less than 35°C. This can readily be measured in the recovery unit, and in a mild form affects up to 80% of all surgical patients. The presentation of hypothermia on the surgical wards can imply inadequate observation in recovery. However, patients may be at the borderline of hypothermia before discharge and be precipitated into clinical hypothermia by exposure on transport, the infusion of cold (room temperature) intravenous fluids, or the simple lack of blankets.

**Table 5.8. Factors affecting the incidence of postoperative nausea and vomiting (PONV)**

| Factors | Incidence |
|---|---|
| In the patient | Very strong association with previous PONV<br>Worse if a history of motion sickness<br>Incidence is three times higher in females than in males<br>Worse in obese people<br>Worse if a history of migraine<br>Age: lower at extremes of age<br>More common in pregnant women<br>Nausea worse in prolonged starvation<br>Can be caused by hypotension<br>Can be caused by emotional upsets or sight of other patients in distress<br>Worse with preoperative gastrointestinal tract ileus, obstruction or delayed emptying |
| Drugs | The following drugs are known to be emetogenic in some patients:<br>Opioids and partial opioid agonists<br>Volatile agents<br>Nitrous oxide<br>Neostigmine<br>Some antibiotics |
| Surgery | Higher incidence with:<br>Gynaecological surgery<br>Surgery to middle ear and tonsils<br>Surgery for strabismus<br>Surgery to gastrointestinal tract |
| Other factors | Oropharyngeal suction<br>Nasogastric tube in position<br>Movement (e.g. rapid changes of direction on way to recovery) |

The normal physiological responses to hypothermia are centrally blunted by general anaesthesia and peripherally limited if regional anaesthetia has been used. General anaesthetics also suppress the vasoconstrictive responses, leading to an increased heat loss to peripheral tissues. These reflexes are completely blocked by regional anaesthesia, which removes sympathetic control. General anaesthesia also reduces the shivering reflex, which is the only active method of heat production available to postoperative patients.

Shivering can increase heat production by 500%. On recovery from general anaesthesia, these reflexes begin to return and the vigour of response is partly determined by age. The metabolic cost of shivering is very high, and increases in oxygen consumption have been estimated at five to eight times the normal oxygen uptake. This may be beyond the reserve of the patient's breathing, and will then lead to hypoxaemia and progressive acidaemia. The increased cardiac output necessary to satisfy this oxygen demand may also lead to myocardial ischaemia or even infarction.

Hypothermia increases the stress response and there is a much higher catabolism of proteins than if the patient's temperature had been maintained within normal limits. Complex effects occur with coagulation; platelet function falls with temperature, but plasma viscosity increases as the body temperature falls. The latter may be one of the predisposing factors in the formation of deep vein thromboses (see Chapter 1 and below).

Thermoregulation during anaesthesia is considered in more detail in Chapter 73.

### Routine drug therapy

Many patients for surgery will be on medication (usually oral) for a wide variety of conditions. However, patients undergoing gastrointestinal surgery may be 'nil by mouth' for several days after their surgery. The failure to provide adequate maintenance drug therapy by parenteral routes may then cause problems. Clear instructions for the continuation of routine medication into the postoperative period are essential.

### Patients on steroids

There has been considerable debate about the stopping of steroid therapy and cover for steroids over the operative period. As a result of this, the Medicines Control Agency and the Committee on Safety of Medicines have recently drawn up new guidelines. These are as follows:

- Abrupt withdrawal of corticosteroids can be done if the patient has been taking them for less than 3 weeks and the underlying disease is not likely to relapse.
- In patients who have received systemic corticosteroids for longer than 3 weeks, withdrawal should be gradual and not abrupt.
- Gradual withdrawal should be considered after courses lasting less than 3 weeks in the following groups of patients:

- patients who have had repeated courses of corticosteroids;
- when a short course has been prescribed within 1 year of cessation of long-term therapy;
- patients who have adrenocortical insufficiency for reasons other than corticosteroid therapy;
- patients receiving over 40 mg daily of prednisolone (or equivalent);
- patients repeatedly taking doses in the evenings.

- Patients who encounter stresses such as trauma, surgery, or infection and are at risk of adrenal insufficiency should receive systemic corticosteroid cover during these periods. Those unable to take tablets by mouth should receive parenteral corticosteroid cover. (See Chapter 56 for details of dosage.)

### The central anticholinergic syndrome

This is a severe confusional state that occurs within the early recovery period, and may be seen before discharge to the ward. It is rare and is caused by the action of anticholinergic drugs crossing the blood–brain barrier and affecting the central cholinergic neuronal systems of cortical arousal. The most common precipitating drugs are hyoscine (scopolamine) and atropine. Intravenous physostigmine 1–3 mg is the treatment of choice and there is rapid recovery with little likelihood of recurrence. This syndrome can occur at any age but is more common in the elderly patient. Anticholinergic drugs that do not cross the blood–brain barrier, such as glycopyrrolate, should be used whenever possible.

## LATER COMPLICATIONS

### Postoperative cognitive deficit

Postoperative cognitive deficit (POCD) is a range of associated symptoms and signs, occurring after a surgical episode, which includes the following:

- poor short-term memory;
- reduction in attention;
- disorientation in time and space;
- impairment of the activities of daily living;
- personality changes;
- reduced social skills;
- fatigue.

These changes are most marked in the early postoperative period, but can last for months or even permanently. The exact proportion of patients affected by such features has been the subject of debate for many years.

The causes of POCD have not been clearly identified, but there is no evidence of a specific risk from the choice of anaesthetic technique. Intraoperative hypoxia and hypotension have been blamed but there are no clear data to support this either. Central cholinergic neuronal function appears to be involved, and this is confirmed by the striking similarities between POCD and dementia, which is known to be caused by failure of this central cholinergic system.

### Respiratory complications

One of the most common life-threatening postoperative complications is an acute chest infection. This usually becomes clinically apparent during the second and subsequent days after the operation. Atelectasis during anaesthesia, combined with inadequate pain relief, may lead to secondary infection developing in the collapsed airways. Antibiotic therapy, once microbiological samples have been sent for culture, is essential, as is physiotherapy to encourage coughing and airway expansion. Pulse oximetry should be used to ascertain the need for oxygen therapy. Acute respiratory failure is likely in elderly patients with a history of chronic obstructive airway disease. Serious cases may need relocation to a high dependency unit or even ventilating on an intensive care unit. The decision whether or not to do this is not always easy and must be based on individual patient considerations. It is, however, salutary to remember that hypoxia does not promote wound healing, and multiple organ failure easily supervenes if an anastomosis breaks down.

The patient with poor pulmonary function is considered in greater detail in Chapter 54.

### Deep vein thrombosis

Categories of patients at risk are described in Chapter 1, Table 1.6. Once there is thrombus formation in the deep veins of the leg or pelvis, distant embolization becomes more likely. Pulmonary embolism has a high mortality and is probably underdiagnosed as a cause of death postoperatively.

When it occurs acutely, there is usually severe pleuritic chest pain, dyspnoea, and tachypnoea. Examination may show hypotension, a raised venous pressure, and evidence of right heart strain on the ECG and a low expired $CO_2$. Pulmonary angiography or ventilation perfusion scan is the definitive investigation; if embolism is confirmed, anticoagulation therapy is started with heparin. Frequently, the 'classic' presentation is not seen, and patients with unexplained confusion, breathlessness, or hypoxia should be suspected of having a pulmonary embolism.

The management of postoperative deep vein thrombosis is prophylaxis. It is important to ensure that all patients at risk are anticoagulated as described in Chapter 1, Table 1.7.

### Sleep and disordered breathing

The timing of many of the complications in the postoperative period around the third to the fourth night after surgery led investigators to look for underlying causes. The changes in sleep patterns that follow operations were described in the late 1980s and can be summarized as having two phases.

In the first, there is the physiological response to trauma with loss of most of the deep sleep stages (stages 3 and 4 of non-rapid eye movement [REM] sleep, and nearly all of REM sleep). This lasts for the whole of the first night after surgery, and often for the second night as well. The REM suppression is partly an opioid effect because μ-receptors in the midbrain are involved in the regulation of the REM stage.

The second phase is when these suppressed REM and non-REM sleep stages rebound back on the third and subsequent nights. Then, almost the entire night is spent in very deep sleep. It is during these periods that profound changes in physiology occur. In non-REM sleep hypotension, hypoventilation, and reduced airway tone predominate. In contrast, during REM sleep, although complete loss of airway tone causes obstructive apnoea, there are also marked behavioural drives leading to hypertension, high circulating levels of catecholamines, and hypoxia. Not surprisingly, a number of these changes may lead to myocardial and cerebral ischaemia or even infarction.

Sleep (especially when there is a rebound of the deep stages) can lead to disordered breathing. Usually this is seen as a loss of upper airway patency and obstruction. The duration of the obstruction determines how low the oxygen concentration in the lung falls, and if one episode is rapidly followed by another there is progressive fall in the haemoglobin saturation.

The significance of these episodes of desaturation is unclear. Certainly patients who have compromised circulation within an organ, be it brain, heart, or liver, will have a very high oxygen extraction from the local circulation and any fall in saturation will lead to ischaemia. This mechanism may explain studies showing that episodic desaturations after vascular surgery are associated with ST segment changes on the ECG, and also with mental confusion. The significance in otherwise fit people is less clear. The current recommendations are for the prescription of postoperative oxygen therapy for the first 3 or 4 nights after major surgery, especially in patients who have diagnosed ischaemic vascular disease of the cardiovascular or cerebral systems.

## CONCLUSION

The postoperative anaesthetic care of a patient is often extremely hazardous and may be inadequately unsupervised. The careful assessment and prescription of pain relief, oxygen, antiemetics, and replacement fluids are the responsibility of the anaesthetist. The role of the anaesthetist is increasingly continuing until the patient goes home and is effectively no longer dependent upon specialized hospital care.

**Appendix 5.1. Administration of analgesics (simple analgesics, NSAIDs, and opioids but excluding local anaesthetics)**

| Route | Advantages | Disadvantages | Comments | Agent(s) used |
|---|---|---|---|---|
| Oral | Simple, convenient, painless, can be self-administered | Variable uptake, depends on food, variation in bioavailability, first-pass effect | If satisfactory analgesia can be obtained, probably the preferred route. Requires functioning GIT. No good if vomiting. Gastric stasis can provide reservoir of drug, which is released later with consequent overdosage | Opioids, NSAIDs, simple analgesics |
| Sublingual/buccal | As for oral, no first-pass effect and more rapid onset of action. If swallowed, uptake of active drug limited | Needs specific instructions to patient; dependent upon saliva and positioning of tablet | Apart from very fast-acting preparations (e.g. GTN), problems are dislodgement and swallowing | Buprenorphine |
| Oral transmucosal | As for oral and sublingual | Depends on sucking a lozenge or lollipop, dissolution in saliva, and absorption through mucosa | If patient stops sucking, uptake ceases | Fentanyl |
| Intranasal | As for sublingual | Only at clinical trial stage | | Fentanyl, sufentanil, buprenorphine |
| Transdermal | Painless | As for subcutaneous. Depends on skin thickness and properties. Very slow onset and offset of effect | Not usually suitable alone for postoperative pain | Fentanyl |
| Rectal | Painless, no first-pass metabolism | Disliked by some patients, and can be irritant to rectal mucosa. Requires proper positioning of suppository. Variable uptake | Always obtain patient's permission and record it on the anaesthetic sheet | Paracetamol, NSAIDs |
| Inhalational | Painless, quick onset and offset if insoluble agent | Needs patient to understand and cooperate | Used mainly in obstetrics and in immediate care situations. Often given for safety as Entonox (see Chapter 8) | Nitrous oxide |
| Subcutaneous | Simple, not painful if small volume | Dependent on subcutaneous blood flow which varies with circulatory state, pain, ambient temperature, etc. | Can be administered as bolus or infusion. Frequently used in some centres for terminal care | Diamorphine and other opioids |
| Intramuscular | As for subcutaneous. Well tried, inexpensive, and perceived as safe. No special equipment needed | Normally uptake predictable but varies with muscle movement and poor in shock. Injections painful, especially if large volume | Normally given by intermittent injection; delayed onset of analgesia and 3- to 4-hourly 'as required' dosage lead to 'swings' in pain level. Very dependent on nursing staff. However, vast clinical experience and relative safety from overdosage result in continued use. Can be satisfactory with an hourly dosing schedule (see text) | Mainly opioids |

*(cont.)*

**Appendix 5.1. Administration of analgesics (simple analgesics, NSAIDs, and opioids but excluding local anaesthetics) (cont.)**

| Route | Advantages | Disadvantages | Comments | Agent(s) used |
|---|---|---|---|---|
| Intravenous | Painless with drug delivered directly into bloodstream. Rapid onset of action: titratable. Potentially much 'smoother' action than intramuscular. | Potential for overdosage. Needs careful supervision, assessment, and adjustment. Wide patient variability, special equipment needed, errors can be life threatening | Not practically suitable for intermittent bolus technique unless PCA. Best system is a slow bolus to control pain followed by infusion to maintain serum levels. Patients need regular assessment to ensure both adequate analgesia and that overdosage is not occurring. Dependent upon reliability of syringe driver. Large amount of opioid in syringe at beginning: beware tampering, theft, etc. by third persons | Mainly opioids (PCA described separately in text) |
| Epidural (opioid) | If opioids are used alone there is the potential for analgesia without sensory, motor, or deficits. Able to work on autonomic specific dermatomes. Catheter normally inserted | Potential for delayed respiratory depression. May not control some types of pain. Needs appropriate nursing area | Can be very effective, especially if opioids combined with local anaesthetics. More fat-soluble compounds (diamorphine, fentanyl) produce respiratory depression earlier than less fat-soluble ones (morphine). Other disadvantages are pruritus, urinary retention, nausea, vomiting and reduced peristalsis, and sedation. Can be administered by bolus, infusion, or PCA. Respiratory depression can result from additional opioids given by other (e.g. intramuscular) routes | Many analgesic compounds used but now almost exclusively opioids, which may be combined with local anaesthetics |
| Intrathecal (opioid) | As for epidural but normally 'single shot' | As for epidural | The less lipid-soluble compounds (e.g. morphine) last for up to 24 hours which is an advantage if only bolus dose given. Otherwise as for epidural route. Almost always single-shot but intrathecal catheters are available and used in some centres | Opioids may be combined with local anaesthetics |
| Intra-articular (opioid) | Put in at the end of joint surgery. Low dose with few systemic effects | Effectively one-shot only | Good for procedures such as arthroscopy, etc. | Morphine often combined with local anaesthetic |

GIT, gastrointestinal tract; GTN, glyceryl trinitrate; NSAIDs, non-steroidal anti-inflammatory drugs; PCA, patient-controlled analgesia.

**Appendix 5.2. Administration of local anaesthetics (see Chapter 15 for details of regional techniques and Appendix 5.1 for comment on epidural and intrathecal opioids)**

| Route | Advantages | Disadvantages | Comments | Agents used |
|---|---|---|---|---|
| Topical | Painless | Takes hours to act, limits choice of vein. Depends on skin properties for effect | Most frequently used in paediatric practice for venepuncture sites | EMLA cream[a] Ametop gel[b] |
| Intradermal | Rapid onset of intense analgesia | Can only be used to raise a small 'bleb', e.g. for putting in intravenous cannula | Does not obscure underlying veins | Almost all local anaesthetics can be used like this |
| Subcutaneous | Local infiltration is easy and usually safe. Epinephrine (adrenaline) extends action. Can be effective for up to 12 hours on occasions | May be limited by maximum permitted dose. Really only single-shot technique | For surgical incisions need to infiltrate both superficial and deep layers | Lignocaine (lidocaine), bupivacaine, prilocaine |
| Peripheral nerve/field block | Targeted to specific area | Often need more than one nerve to be blocked. Can be long time to onset of effect | Needs considerable knowledge of anatomy and skilled practice. Potential for nerve damage from injections. Essential not to include epinephrine in ring blocks or ischaemia may develop | Lignocaine, bupivacaine |
| Nerve plexus block | Targeted to specific area | Complications from patchy blocks, different approaches affect different parts of plexus | Can have serious complications both from site of block (e.g. pneumothorax) or from inadvertent intravenous injection of large volume of local anaesthetic. If successful can produce dense analgesia that lasts for many hours | Lignocaine, prilocaine |
| Epidural | Usually dense analgesia over dermatome band. Catheter can be placed for top-ups or infusion | Complications given in Chapter 15. Always produces an accompanying motor and autonomic block. May cause urinary retention | Concentration and volume of solution control effectiveness and side effects. Often possible to achieve satisfactory sensory block with minor motor effects. If the epidural dose goes intrathecally, total spinal; if it goes intravenously, severe toxicity. Often combined with opioids for post-operative pain relief | Lignocaine, bupivacaine, ropivacaine; can all be combined with opioids |
| Intrathecal | Usually dense analgesia below a particular dermatome. Chemically 'transects' the cauda equina and spinal cord | Complications given in Chapter 15 and as for epidural. Usually only single shot. Spread dependent on volume, concentration, baricity, and patient position | Intrathecal catheters available but not widely used | Lignocaine and bupivacaine, normo- and hyper-baric solutions; can be combined with opioids |

*(cont.)*

**Appendix 5.2. Administration of local anaesthetics (cont.)**

| Route | Advantages | Disadvantages | Comments | Agents used |
|---|---|---|---|---|
| Intra-articular | Put in at end of joint surgery. Low dose with few systemic effects | Effectively one shot only | Good for procedures such as arthroscopy, etc. | Local anaesthetic often combined with morphine |
| Intravenous regional | Simple to carry out | See Chapter 15 for complications. Often not completely dense analgesia | Needs careful safety checks of tourniquet and resuscitation equipment. Bupivacaine completely contraindicated because of intravenous toxicity | Prilocaine |

[a]EMLA Cream 5%, eutectic mixture of lignocaine and prilocaine. [b]Ametop gel 4%, topical amethocaine.
Note that all local anaesthetic blocks have the potential to cause inadvertent patient injury because of lack of sensation (e.g. burning hand on stove after brachial plexus block).

## APPENDIX 5.3: SUMMARY OF THE RECOMMENDATIONS OF THE ROYAL COLLEGE OF ANAESTHETISTS' WORKING PARTY ON THE USE OF NSAIDS IN THE PERIOPERATIVE PERIOD (1998)

### Grade A

Based on the strongest evidence available, including at least one randomized trial as part of the body of literature of overall good quality:

1. NSAIDs are not sufficiently effective as the sole agent after major surgery in most patients.
2. They are often effective after minor or moderate surgery.
3. NSAIDs often decrease opioid requirement. Significant reduction in opioid side effects has been noted in only a few studies.
4. The quality of opioid-based analgesia is often enhanced by NSAIDs.
5. NSAIDs increase bleeding time and some studies have shown increased blood loss.
6. In situations where there are no contraindications, NSAIDs are the drug of choice after many day-case procedures.

### Grade B

Based on availability of well-conducted clinical studies but not randomized trials:

7. The clinician should be aware that many important drug interactions have been reported.

### Grade C

Based on the expert consensus of the group in the absence of studies of good quality:

8. The clinical significance of a tendency to increased bleeding time is unclear. It should not inhibit the use of NSAIDs in most cases if there are no specific contraindications. However, NSAIDs should not be given before surgery if there is an increased risk of intraoperative bleeding.
9. NSAIDs should not be used in patients with pre-eclamptic toxaemia, hypovolaemia, or uncontrolled hypertension.
10. Intramuscular diclofenac should be avoided.
11. Gastrointestinal ulceration and bleeding should be a prominent differential diagnosis in any patient receiving NSAIDs.
12. NSAIDs should be avoided in renally compromised patients.
13. Renal function should be monitored regularly in all patients receiving NSAIDs after major surgery. Any upward trend in plasma urea, creatinine, or potassium, or reduced urine output, is an indication for discontinuing NSAIDs.
14. NSAIDs should be used with caution in elderly patients, those with diabetes or vascular disease, and after cardiac, hepatobiliary, renal, or major vascular surgery.
15. NSAIDs are contraindicated in aspirin-sensitive asthma and should be used with caution in other people with asthma.

16. It is impossible to give significantly meaningful recommendations on the safe use of NSAIDs with epidural anaesthesia. More work is required in this area.

## FURTHER READING

Articles in: Breivik H, ed. *Postoperative Pain Management. Baillière's Clin Anaesthesiol* 1995;**9**:403–584.

Breivik H. Benefits, risks and economics of post-operative pain management programmes. *Baillière's Clin Anaesthesiol* 1995;**9**:403–22.

Carpenter RL, Liu S, Neal JM. Epidural anesthesia and analgesia: their role in postoperative outcome. *Anesthesiology* 1995;**82**:1474–506.

Articles in: Frost EAM, Thomson D, eds. *Post-anaesthetic Care. Baillière's Clin Anaesthesiol* 1994;**8**:749–910.

Gould TH, Crosby DL, Harmer M *et al.* Policy for controlling pain after surgery: effect of sequential changes on management. *BMJ* 1992;**305**:517–22.

Hutton P, ed. Mini-symposium – Cardiovascular. *Curr Anaesth Crit Care* 1995;**6**:135–170.

Knill RL, Moote CA, Skinner MI, Rose RA. Anesthesia with abdominal surgery leads to intense REM sleep during the first postoperative week. *Anesthesiology* 1990;**73**:52–61.

McHardy FE, Chung F. Postoperative sore throat: cause, prevention and treatment. *Anaesthesia* 1999;**54**:444–53.

Mayers I, Johnson D. The nonspecific inflammatory response to injury. *Can J Anaesth* 1998;**45**:871–9.

Moller JT, Cluitmans P, Rasussen LS *et al.* (ISPOCD investigators). Long-term post-operative cognitive dsyfunction in the elderly. ISPOCD 1 study. *Lancet* 1998;**351**:857–61.

Murphy WG, Davies MJ, Eduardo A. The haemostatic response to surgery and trauma. *Br J Anaesth* 1993;**70**:205–13.

Owen H, Wheatley RG, eds. Symposium on acute pain. *Curr Anaesth Crit Care* 1995;**6**:67–102.

Roe PG, Jones JG. Causes of oxyhaemoglobin saturation instability in the postoperative period. *Br J Anaesth* 1993;**71**:481–7.

Roe PG, Jones JG. Analysis of factors which affect the relationship between inspired oxygen partial pressure and arterial oxygen saturation. *Br J Anaesth* 1993;**71**:488–94.

Royal College of Anaesthetists. *Guidelines for the use of NSAIDs in the Perioperative Period*. London: Royal College of Anaesthetists, 1998.

Royal College of Surgeons of England and the Royal College of Anesthetists. Report of the Working Party on Pain after Surgery. London: Royal College of Surgeons, 1990.

Welchew E. *Patient Controlled Analgesia. Principles and Practice Series*. London: BMJ Publishing Group. 1995.

# Chapter 6 Airway management I: anatomy and equipment

P. Hutton

## THE ANATOMY OF THE AIRWAYS

The upper airways are innervated by the cranial nerves. Because of their importance, these are described in detail in Chapter 22, Table 22.3. Throughout this section they will be referred to by their number in roman numerals.

### The nose

The nose is one of the two entries to the pharynx (and subsequently larynx), the other being the mouth. The external nares (alae or anterior nares) are oval and their size is a guide to the selection of nasal tubes and airways. The mucosa lining the nose is very vascular and bleeds easily, especially if it is inflamed. Upper respiratory tract infections often cause obstruction of the nasal airways.

#### *Functions*

- Providing the sense of smell and enhancing taste.
- Humidification and heating of inspired gases.
- Filtration by adhesion of particulate material onto mucus-covered surfaces that possess beating cilia.

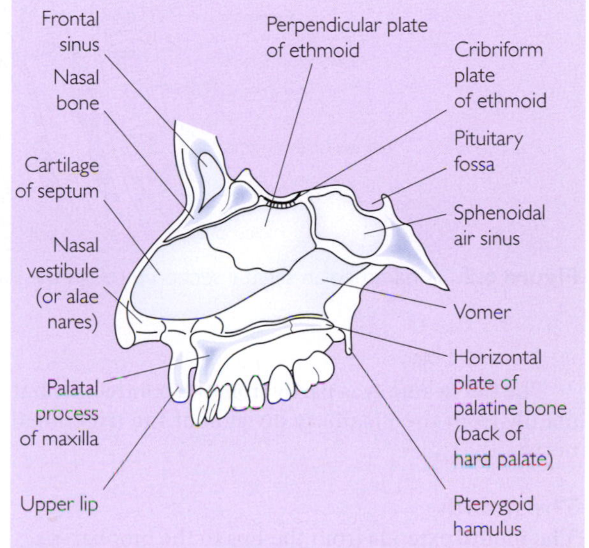


**Figure 6.1.** The structure of the septum of the nose and its immediate surroundings.

#### *Morphological anatomy*

The nose is divided grossly into the external nose and the nasal cavity. The external nose is bony in its upper part, but becomes cartilaginous in the lower part and in the anterior septum.

The nasal cavity is divided into right and left parts by the septum: it opens externally by the alae and posteriorly by the choanae. The septum is cartilaginous anteriorly and bony posteriorly; the major bones are the perpendicular plate of the ethmoid and the vomer (Figure 6.1). The septum is frequently deviated to right or left, making one cavity wider than the other. This is obviously relevant to the passage of nasal tubes, etc.

The floor of the nose is bony anteriorly where it is above the hard palate and soft posteriorly where a tissue flap extends into the nasopharynx and terminates in the uvula. The soft palate closes off the nasal passages during swallowing, speech, blowing, and straining (Figure 6.2).

Anterior to posterior, the roof of the nose initially slopes upwards and backwards, then horizontally (cribriform plate of the ethmoid), and finally downwards towards the pharynx.

The lateral walls of the nose are mainly bony but cartilaginous anteriorly. There are three nasal conchae (superior, middle, and inferior), which increase the surface area available for heating, humidifying, and filtration (Figure 6.2). They are composed of thin curved bones (turbinates) which are easily damaged during airway procedures. The openings into the maxillary, sphenoid, frontal, and ethmoidal sinuses open onto the lateral nasal walls. The presence of infection in the nose, causing sinusitis, can occasionally progress to meningitis or cerebral abscess formation.

The alae nares are constructed from fibrofatty tissue, and immediately behind them the lining is composed of stratified squamous epithelium together with hair and sebaceous and sweat glands. All the rest of the nose is covered with columnar ciliated cells and mucus-secreting goblet cells.

#### *Blood and nerve supply*

There is a generous blood supply to the nasal mucosa, all of which originates from the carotid arteries. The upper sections are supplied by the branches of the ophthalmic artery, the lower by branches of the maxillary artery, and the anteroinferior septum by branches of the facial artery. Venous drainage is by a submucous plexus which drains eventually into the sphenopalatine, facial, and ophthalmic veins. Haemorrhage from the nose can be minor or profuse (in some cases life threatening) and can come from one or many bleeding points. Spontaneous haemorrhage ( nose bleed ) frequently occurs from Little s area on the lower part of the anterior septum.

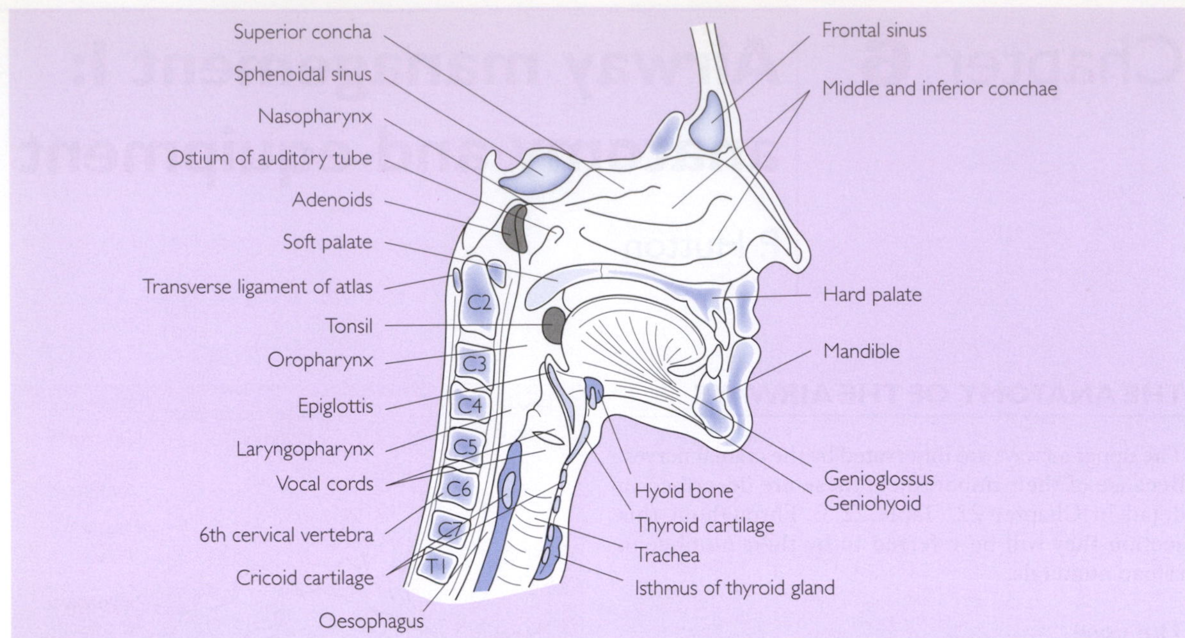


**Figure 6.2.** A paramedian sagittal section through the nasal and oral cavities, pharynx, and larynx.

The nerve supply is partly from the ophthalmic but mainly from the maxillary division of the trigeminal nerve.

## The mouth

The mouth extends from the lips to the oropharynx.

### *The palate*

The morphology of the hard and soft palate is described above and shown in Figures 6.1 and 6.2. The hard palate is made up of bone, periosteum, and a squamous mucosa in which accessory salivary glands are buried. The framework of the soft palate is formed by the aponeurosis of the tensor palati muscle, which adheres to the posterior border of the hard palate and into which are attached the palatine muscles. The whole is covered by epithelium that is squamous on its buccal aspect and ciliated columnar on its nasopharyngeal surface. The sensory supply of the palate is mainly from the maxillary division of nerve V with nerve IX posteriorly. Motor innervation of the palatine muscles is from nerves IX, X and the cranial part of XI; the tensor palati are supplied by the mandibular division of nerve V.

### *The tongue*

#### *Surface structure*

The tongue is essentially a highly sophisticated set of muscles that has the additional functions of taste and dense sensory innervation. It is covered throughout with thick stratified squamous mucosa. The anterior two-thirds of the tongue occupy the mouth and the posterior one-third occupies the oropharynx. Separating these two portions of the tongue approximately is a V-shaped groove (with the point of the V pointing posteriorly), the sulcus terminalis. At the apex of the groove is a shallow depression, the foramen caecum (marking the embryological origin of the thyroid), and immediately in front of the sulcus lies a row of large vallate papillae. As well as the normal sensory innervation, the anterior two-thirds of the tongue have papillae that carry the taste buds, which are sensitive to sweet (anterior), sour (anterolateral), salt (lateral), and bitter (posterior) tastes. The posterior one-third of the tongue has no papillae but carries numerous lymphoid nodules. Under the tongue is the frenulum linguae (frenulum of the tongue), which is covered by a much thinner mucosa through which can be seen the lingual veins.

#### *Muscles and blood supply*

The tongue is divided by a relatively avascular median vertical fibrous septum, often identifiable as a shallow groove on the dorsal surface. The intrinsic and extrinsic muscles are mirrored on each side of this septum with individual vascular and nervous supplies. The muscles of the tongue and the floor of the mouth are shown in Figures 6.3 and 6.4, respectively. Intrinsic muscles have vertical, longitudinal, and transverse bundles, which alter the shape of the tongue.

Extrinsic muscles move the tongue as a whole. Genioglossus arises from the rear of the mandible and passes throughout the length of the tongue. Lower fibres that travel to the hyoid bone are classified as the geniohyoid muscle. Hypoglossus, styloglossus, and palatoglossus pass to the hyoid bone, styloid process, and the soft palate, respectively. Intrinsic tone in the genioglossus muscle is essential to keep the posterior tongue pulled anteriorly away from the posterior pharyngeal wall; without it, unless the tongue is pulled forward or allowed to fall forward (e.g. in the recovery position), the patency of the airway is lost.

The blood supply of the tongue is from the lingual branch of the external carotid artery and does not cross the midline.

#### *Nerve supply*

##### *Sensory*

The anterior two-thirds receives sensory and special sensory nerves from the lingual branch of nerve V, which also transmits the gustatory fibres of the chorda tympani of nerve VII. Common sensation and taste to the posterior third, including the vallate papillae, are from nerve IX, with some further minor innervation provided by nerve X from the superior laryngeal nerve.

*Motor*

All the extrinsic and intrinsic muscles of the tongue except palatoglossus are supplied by nerve XII; the palatoglossus is innervated by nerve XI.

### *The floor of the mouth*

This is principally formed by the mylohyoid muscles which form a sling supporting the tongue and other structures. The arrangement is shown in Figures 6.3 and 6.4. The submandibular gland is described as having superficial and deep parts, which are described in relation to the submental skin. The superficial part lies below the mylohyoid muscle. The gland then curves around the posterior edge of the mylohyoid and this deep part travels forward almost as far as the sublingual gland. The submandibular duct (Wharton s duct) is 5 cm long and emerges in the floor of the mouth on the summit of the sublingual papilla, at the side of the frenulum of the tongue. The sublingual salivary gland lies above the mylohyoid. Its drainage is inconstant, with its excretory ducts ranging from 8 to 20 in number; some open directly on to the floor of the mouth on the summit of the sublingual fold. Sometimes a number form a major sublingual duct and occasionally a few open into the duct of the submandibular gland.

### *The teeth*

The upper teeth are fixed into the maxilla and the lower teeth into the mandible. Human dentition is both diphyodont (temporary and permanent) and heterodont (different types of teeth). Diphyodont dentition allows the jaw to grow without producing wide spacing of the teeth. The temporary or deciduous teeth are 20 in number, the permanent teeth 32. The time of eruption and the type of teeth are shown in Figures 6.5 and 6.6. On dental charts and in a patient s notes, the mouth is represented diagrammatically in quadrants as shown in Figure 6.7. The layout assumes that you are looking at the patient from the front.

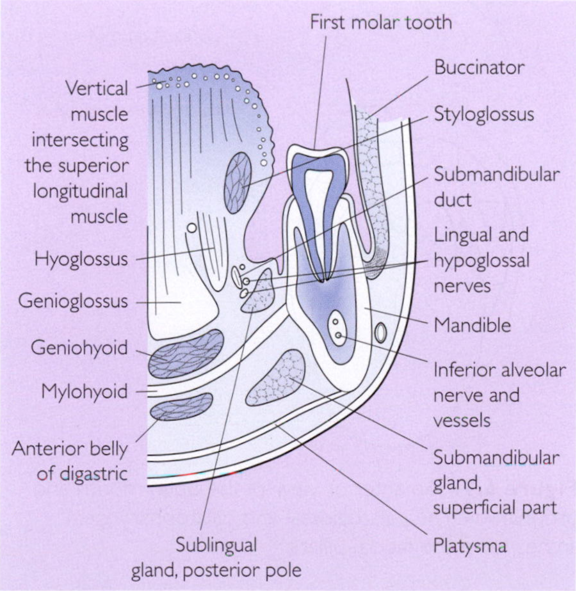

**Figure 6.3.** A coronal section through the floor of the mouth at the first molar tooth. The sublingual gland lies above the mylohyoid. The submandibular gland curves round the posterior edge of the mylohyoid and hence its duct is close to the sublingual gland.

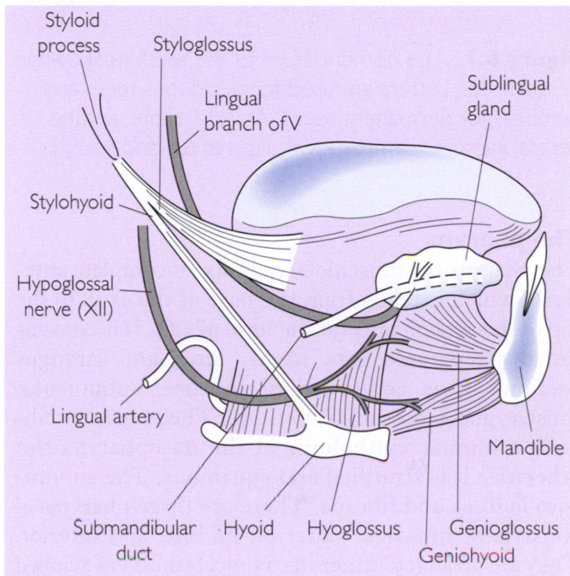


**Figure 6.4.** A paramedian lateral view of the tongue and its associated extrinsic muscles and nerves. The mandible and mylohyoid muscle (see Figure 6.3) have been removed, together with associated structures such as the submandibular gland. The palatoglossus muscle is also omitted.

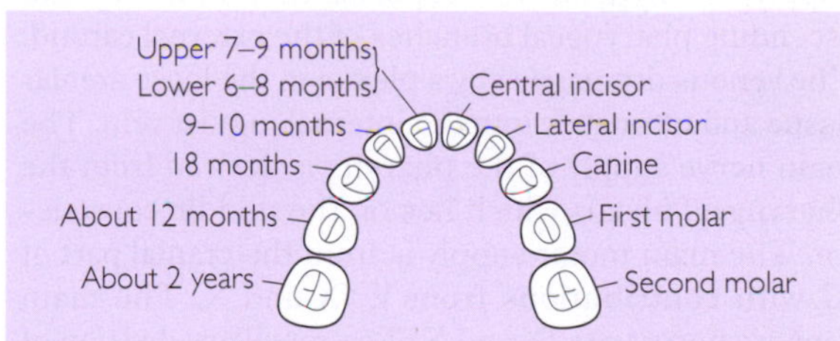


**Figure 6.5.** The average times of eruption of the deciduous teeth.

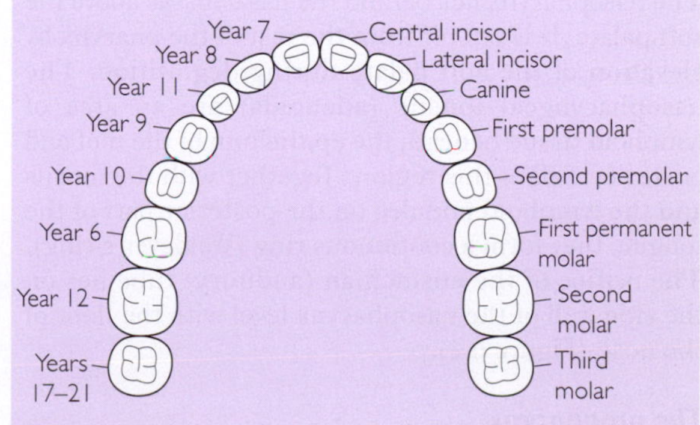


**Figure 6.6.** The average times of eruption of the permanent teeth.

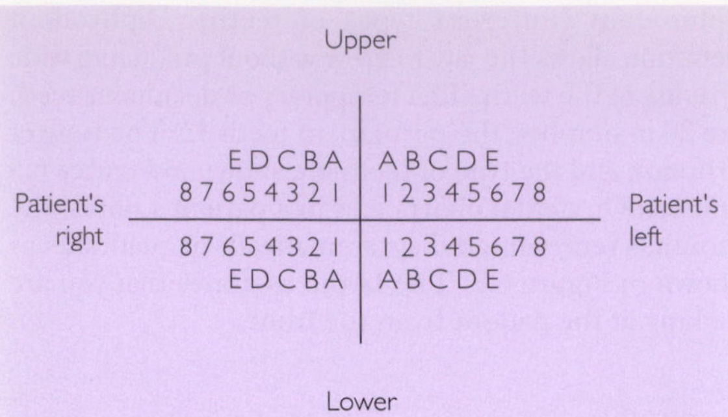


**Figure 6.7.** The nomenclature of the teeth as shown in dental notes. Letters are used for deciduous teeth and numbers for permanent teeth. A and I represent the central incisors. Compare with Figures 6.5 and 6.6.

### The pharynx

The pharynx is a musculofascial tube, incomplete anteriorly, which extends from the base of the skull to the top of the oesophagus (at the level of C6). It is conventionally separated into naso-, oro-, and laryngo-sections. It is composed of mucosa, submucosa, muscle, and a loose areolar sheath. The mucosa is ciliated columnar epithelium in the nasopharynx but otherwise it is stratified and squamous. The submucosa is thick and fibrous. There are three pharyngeal constrictor muscles: superior, middle, and inferior. They are arranged rather like conical tumblers stacked one within the other, but are open at the front at the entries to the nasal, buccal, and laryngeal cavities. Each constrictor muscle is attached anteriorly to rigid structures at the side wall of these cavities, as shown in Figure 6.8, and spreads out posteriorly to insert into a median raphe which extends from the base of the skull to the oesophagus. The pharynx receives its arterial supply mainly from the superior thyroid artery and ascending pharyngeal branches of the external carotid. The venous drainage is by a plexus in the loose areolar tissue and ultimately into the internal jugular vein. The main nerve supply of the pharynx is derived from the pharyngeal plexus which lies on the middle constrictor. The main motor supply is from the cranial part of XI with contributions from V, IX and X. The main sensory nerves are IX and X. The maxillary division of nerve V supplies the sensory innervation of the nasopharynx.

#### *The nasopharynx*

The nasopharynx lies behind the nasal fossae above the soft palate. It is cut off from the rest of the pharynx by elevation of the soft palate during deglutition. The nasopharyngeal tonsils (adenoids) are an area of lymphoid tissue beneath the epithelium of the roof and posterior wall of this region. Together with the tonsils and the lymphoid nodules on the posterior part of the tongue, they form a continuous ring (Waldeyer s ring). The orifice of the eustachian (auditory) tube lies on the side wall of the nasopharynx level with the floor of the nose (Figure 6.2).

#### *The oropharynx*

The oropharynx lies behind the mouth and tongue. It is bounded anteriorly by the anterior pillars of the

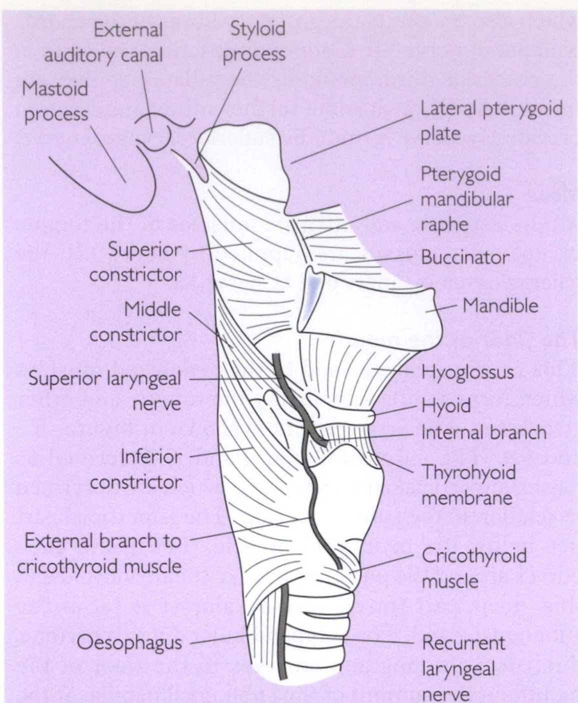


**Figure 6.8.** The constrictor muscles of the pharynx and the nerve supply to the larynx. (The blood vessels have been omitted for clarity.) The internal branch of the superior laryngeal nerve pierces the thyrohyoid membrane with the superior laryngeal artery; the external branch is the motor supply to the cricothyroid muscle. The recurrent laryngeal nerve passes upwards as shown, accompanied by the laryngeal branch of the inferior thyroid artery. It goes deep to the inferior border of the inferior constrictor and enters the larynx behind the cricothyroid joint.

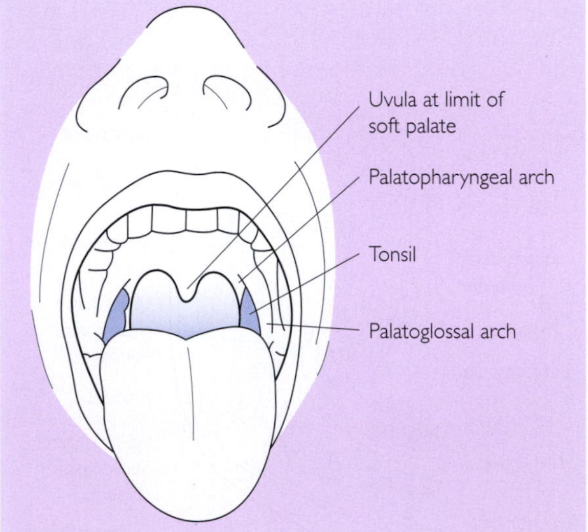


**Figure 6.9.** An anterior view of the open mouth and oropharynx. The palatoglossal and palatopharyngeal arches form the faucial pillars.

fauces, and extends from the palate to the epiglottis. The entrance is shown in Figure 6.9. The anterior pillar, containing the palatoglossus muscle, forms the boundary between the buccal cavity and the oropharynx-

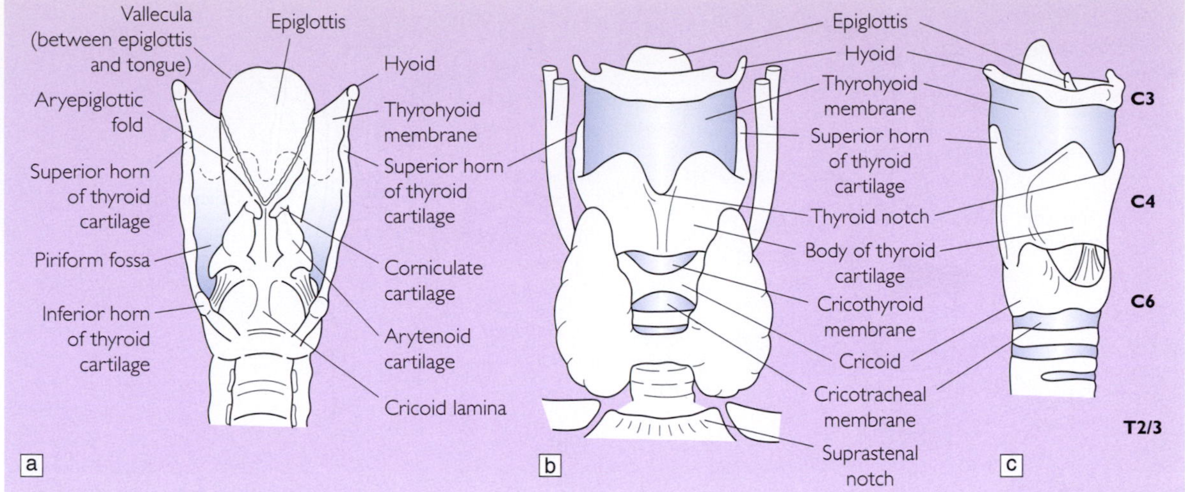


**Figure 6.10.** (a) Posterior, (b) anterior, and (c) lateral views of the larynx. The nerve supply shown in Figure 6.8 is omitted here for clarity.

ynx. The palatine tonsil lies behind the anterior pillar and in front of the posterior pillar, which contains the palatopharyngeus muscle. Posteriorly, the oropharynx is supported by the lower part of the superior, and the middle and upper parts of the inferior constrictor muscles. The tonsil lies at the level of the superior constrictor muscle.

#### *The laryngopharynx*

The laryngopharynx extends from the level of the tip of the epiglottis to the beginning of the oesophagus at the level of C6. It is surrounded laterally and posteriorly by the inferior constrictor muscle. Anteriorly, the larynx itself bulges backwards into the laryngopharynx, leaving deep recesses on either side called the piriform fossae. Below the level of the laryngeal aditus, the anterior and posterior walls of the laryngopharynx are in contact, except during the passage of food, so that the entrance to the oesophageal lumen is via a transverse slit.

### The larynx

The larynx has the following functions:

- when open allows respiration;
- when closed protects the trachea and bronchial tree from soiling;
- allows coughing;
- allows phonation;
- permits straining by allowing a build-up of intrathoracic (and hence intra-abdominal) pressure.

#### *Structure*

The larynx extends from the root of the tongue to the cricoid cartilage and is shown in a variety of views in Figures 6.10–6.12. The structures that form its framework are the hyoid bone, the epiglottis, and the thyroid, cricoid, and arytenoid cartilages.

The hyoid bone is 'U' shaped with the open section posteriorly (Figures 6.4 and 6.8). It is suspended and stabilized by muscular and fibrous attachments to the styloid process, the mandible and tongue, and the pharynx. From it is slung the rest of the larynx by the thyrohyoid membrane and muscle (Figure 6.8).

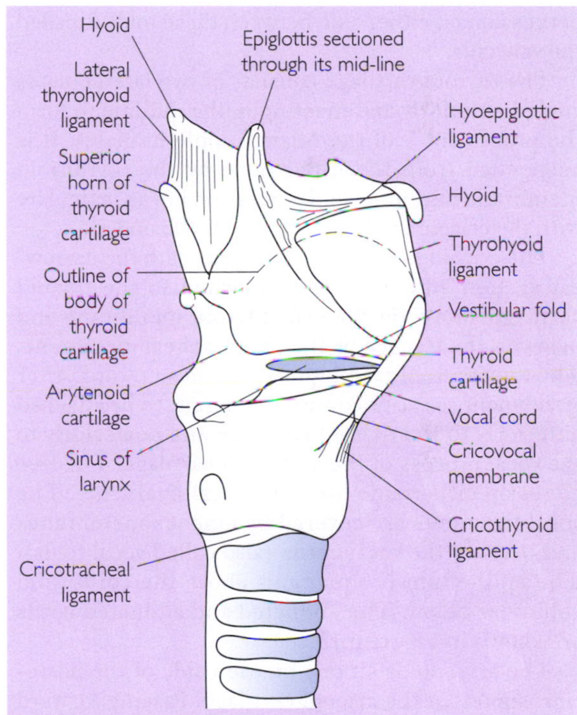


**Figure 6.11.** A paramedian lateral view of the cartilages and ligaments of the larynx.

The epiglottis is a leaf-like plate of cartilage, attached at its base in the midline to the thyroid cartilage via the thyroepiglottic ligament and in its middle section to the rear of the hyoid bone. Its upper section lies free behind the tongue (Figure 6.11). The sides of the epiglottis are connected to the arytenoids by the aryepiglottic folds which run backwards to form the margins of the entrance to the larynx (Figures 6.10a and 6.12b). The anterior surface of the epiglottis is behind the base of the tongue and from this arise mucosal reflections. In the midline is a glossoepiglottic fold and laterally pharyngoepiglottic folds. The

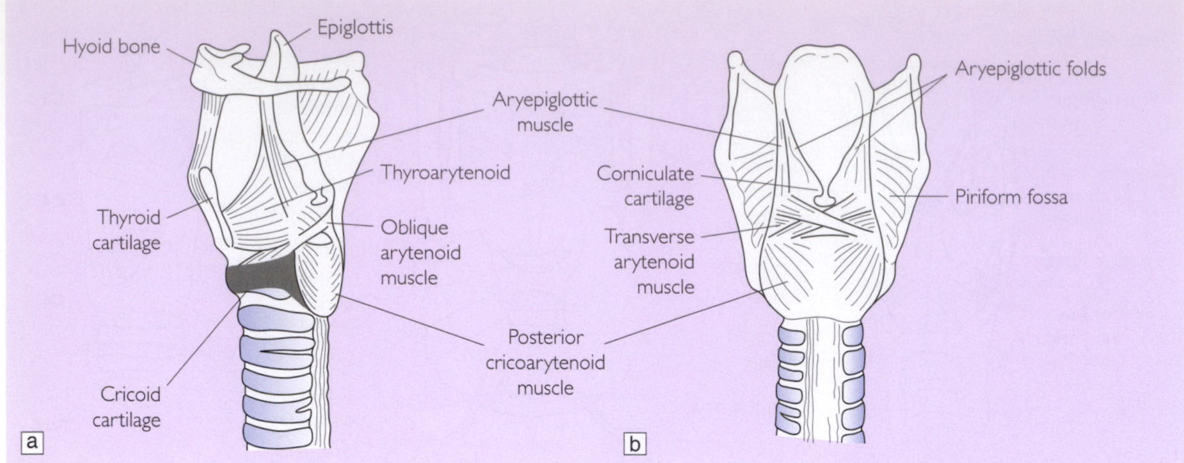


**Figure 6.12.** The intrinsic muscles of the larynx in (a) lateral and (b) posterior views. In (a) the left lamina of the thyroid cartilage has been removed.

depression on either side between these folds is called the vallecula.

The thyroid cartilage consists of two lateral plates angled anteriorly and meeting in the midline to form the prominent V of the Adam s apple in males. It is suspended from the hyoid bone by the thyrohyoid membrane and muscle. Its inferior horns articulate with the cricoid cartilage (Figures 6.10b and c).

The cricoid is signet-ring shaped, with the narrowest section anteriorly. It is attached to the thyroid cartilage above via the cricothyroid membrane and below to the trachea by the cricotracheal membrane. The cricothyroid membrane continues upwards after attachment as the cricovocal membrane to be attached anteriorly to the thyroid cartilage and posteriorly to the vocal process of the arytenoid cartilage. The free edges on either side form the vocal ligaments. The vocal ligaments are covered by mucous membranes and become the vocal cords (also called vocal folds). The epithelium is squamous above the cords, and columnar below. The abducted and adducted cords are shown in Figure 6.13.

The arytenoids sit one on each side of the posterior signet of the cricoid cartilage. Passing forward from the arytenoid to the back of the thyroid cartilage, just below the epiglottic attachment, are two folds of mucosa. The upper is the vestibular fold, containing a small amount of fibrous tissue and forming on each side the false vocal cord. The lower fold (the true vocal fold or cord) contains the vocal ligament. The mucosa is firmly adherent to the vocal ligament without any intervening submucosa. The space between the vocal cords is termed the rima glottidis. The corniculate and cuneiform cartilages lie in the aryepiglottic folds.

### *Muscle action*

The extrinsic muscles pass between the larynx and surrounding structures. They move its position and are important in glutition. The intrinsic muscles of the larynx open the glottis in inspiration, close the vestibule and glottis in swallowing, and alter the tension and position of the vocal cords for speech.

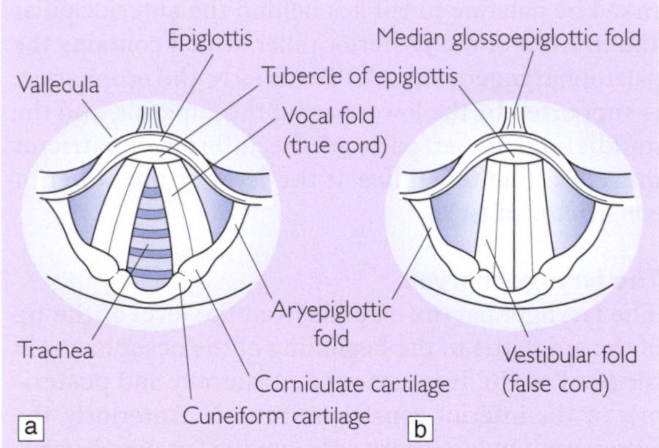


**Figure 6.13.** The (a) abducted and (b) adducted positions of the vocal cords.

The only intrinsic muscle that is on the external aspect of the larynx is the cricothyroid muscle (see Figure 6.8), which tenses the vocal cords by tilting the thyroid on the cricoid cartilage. The posterior cricoarytenoid muscles abduct the vocal cords by rotating the arytenoids outwards. The thyroarytenoid muscles relax the cords. The cords are adducted by the transverse arytenoid muscle and the lateral cricoarytenoids (which rotate the arytenoids inwards).

### *Blood supply*

This is from branches of the superior and inferior thyroid arteries. The vessels enter the larynx with the superior and recurrent laryngeal nerves.

### *Nerve supply*

This comprises the superior and recurrent laryngeal branches of the vagus nerve.

The superior laryngeal nerve divides into internal and external branches. The internal branch pierces the thyrohyoid membrane with the superior laryngeal vessels to supply the mucosa of the larynx down to the vocal cords. The external branch supplies the cricothyroid muscle (Figure 6.8).

The recurrent laryngeal nerve has a different course on each side. The right arises from the vagus as it crosses the subclavian artery, passes round the vessel, and ascends in the tracheo-oesophageal groove with the inferior laryngeal vessels. The nerve enters the larynx behind the cricothyroid articulation below the inferior constrictor muscle of the pharynx (Figure 6.8). The left nerve curves round the arch of the aorta, ascends to the trachea and then follows a similar course to the right. The recurrent nerves supply all the intrinsic muscles of the larynx apart from the cricothyroid, and the mucosa below the cords. For the intrathoracic course of the recurrent laryngeal nerves see later in Figure 6.19.

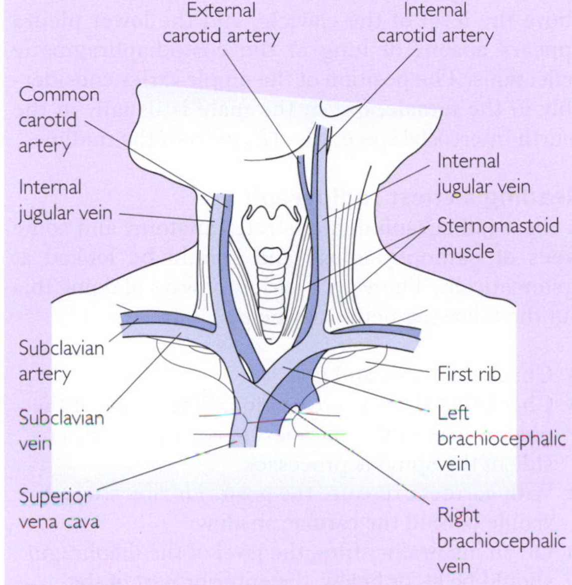


**Figure 6.14.** The surface projection of the great vessels of the neck and their relationship to the sternomastoid muscle and thoracic inlet. (The clavicles have been omitted for clarity.)

## The neck and upper mediastinum

In the midline, from below the chin downwards, can be felt, in order:

1. The hyoid bone, at the level of C3.
2. The notch of the thyroid cartilage, at the level of C4.
3. The cricoid cartilage at C6, immediately below which is the trachea and behind which is the top of the oesophagus.
4. The rings of the trachea. Sometimes, over the third and fourth of these the isthmus of the thyroid can be felt.
5. The suprasternal notch (approximately T2/3).
6. The sternal angle of Louis at the manubriosternal junction at the level of the T4 – 5 junction.

The path, location, and relationships of important structures in the neck and upper mediastinum are shown in Figures 6.14 – 6.17.

The carotid pulsation can be felt at the lateral edges of the laryngeal structures. At the level of the cricoid, the common carotid can be pressed backwards against the long transverse process of C6; between the upper border of the thyroid cartilage and below the hyoid bone, the internal and external carotids are formed and lie just below the deep fascia where they are easy to feel (and may be visible).

The line of the carotid sheath goes from a point midway between the tip of the mastoid process and the angle of the jaw to the ipsilateral sternoclavicular joint. Within this sheath the internal jugular vein lies lateral to the carotid artery.

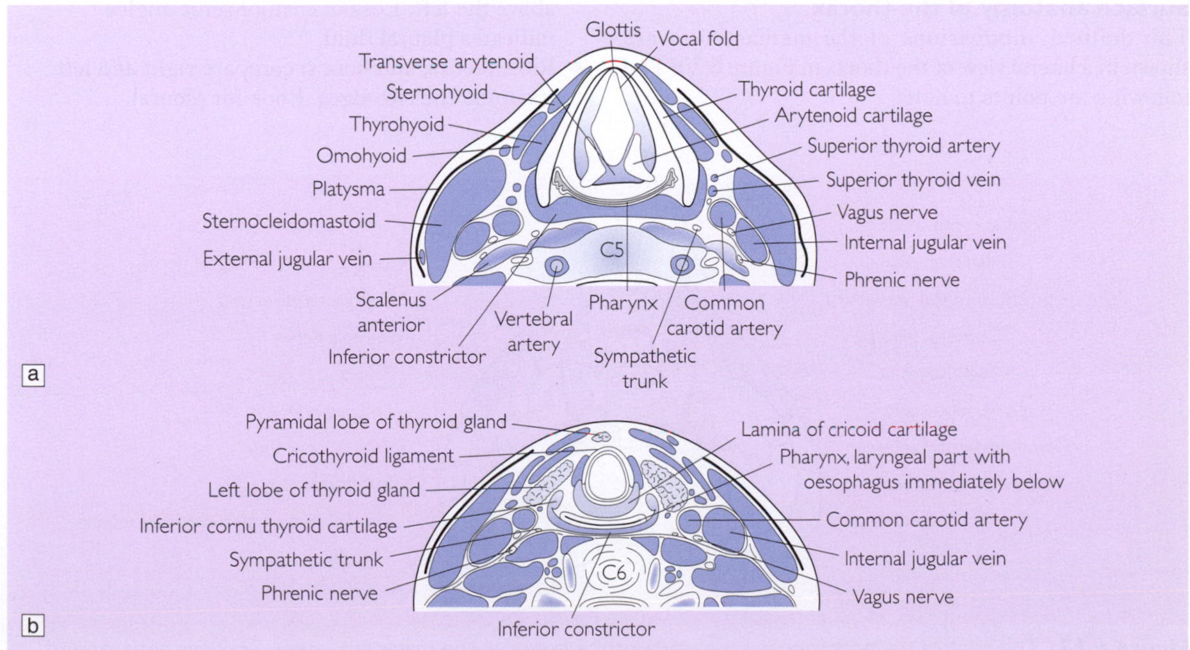


**Figure 6.15.** A transverse section of the ventral region of the neck at the level of (a) the vocal folds and (b) the cricoid cartilage between C5 and C6.

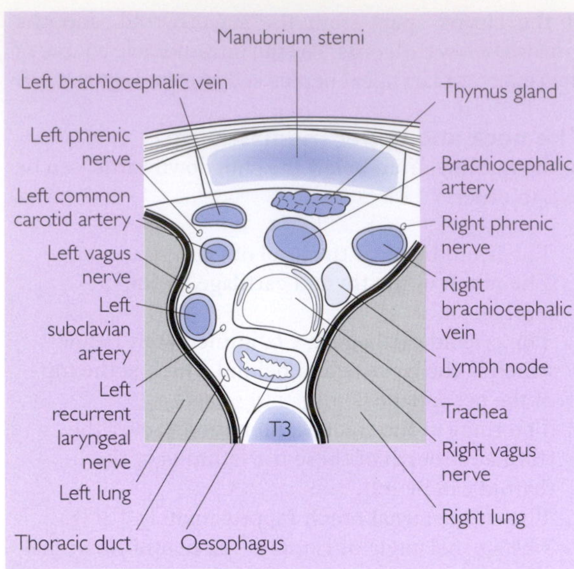


**Figure 6.16.** A transverse section through the manubrium at the level of the third thoracic vertebra.

***The trachea and major airways***
The trachea extends from the lower border of the cricoid cartilage (C6) to its bifurcation into the major bronchi, a distance of 10 – 12 cm. The level of the bifurcation is T4 in expiration and T5 or T6 in inspiration. The external diameter of the trachea in the adult male is approximately 2 cm and 1.5 cm in the adult female. This obviously varies from person to person but can be estimated from the diameter of the root of the index finger. The patency of the trachea is maintained by 15 – 20 U-shaped cartilages which are deficient posteriorly (Figure 6.12) where the trachea is directly anterior to the oesophagus. The trachea and its major branches are shown diagrammatically in Figure 6.18 and their relationship to the heart in Figure 6.19.

**Surface anatomy of the thorax**
The defined subdivisions of the mediastinum are shown in a lateral view of the thorax in Figure 6.20. The following are points to note:

- Vertebrae can be identified by counting downwards from the first spinous process to be felt (C7, vertebra prominens).
- Ribs can be identified by counting downwards from the second costal cartilage which articulates with the sternum at the angle of Louis.
- The suprasternal notch is opposite T2 – 3, and the sternal angle of Louis is opposite T4 – 5.
- The lowest part of the costal margin is formed by the tenth rib and dips to the level of L3.

The surface markings of the pleura and lungs are shown in Figures 6.21 and 6.22. The upper pleura rises above the level of the clavicle, and the lower pleura appears absent of lung at the costodiaphragmatic reflections. The position of the nipple varies considerably in the female, but in the male is usually in the fourth intercostal space, 10 – 12 cm from the midline.

**Reading a chest radiograph**
A chest radiograph demonstrates anatomy and some types of pathophysiology and should be looked at systematically. There are a variety of ways of doing this but the following notes may help:

- Check the name and date.
- Check that there is no rotation. When correct the medial ends of the clavicles lie equally on either side of the spinous processes.
- With correct exposure the posterior ribs are just visible behind the cardiac shadow.
- On an inspiratory film, the level of the diaphragm should be at, or below, the anterior part of the sixth rib and the posterior part of the tenth rib.

Then, on a posteroanterior (PA) film, look at the individual structures:

- Diaphragm: both the right and the left domes should be well defined. The right side is 2 cm above the left. Loss of costophrenic angles indicates pleural fluid.
- Ribs, pleura, and bones: compare right and left. Examine the rib edges. Look for pleural

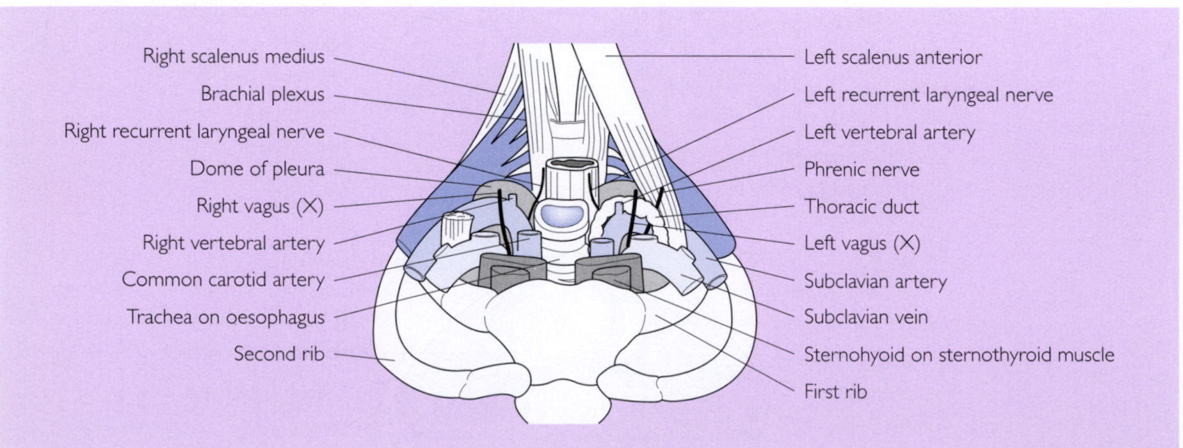


**Figure 6.17.** The root of the neck showing the relationships between the major structures. Scalenus anterior and the phrenic nerve have been removed on the right and scalenus medius on the left of the model. The phrenic nerve lies on the surface of scalenus anterior covered by the prevertebral fascia.

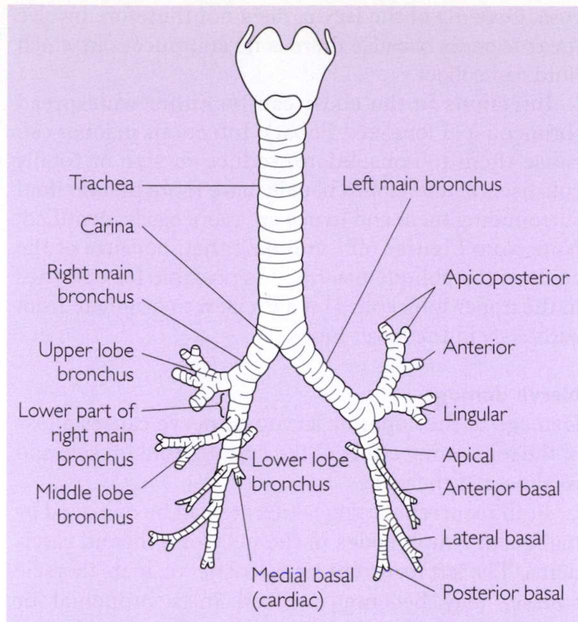


**Figure 6.18.** A diagrammatic picture of the trachea and major bronchi viewed from the front.

thickening. Look at the shoulder joints, clavicles, scapulae, and visible vertebral bodies.

- Mediastinum: this should be centrally situated with a cardiothoracic ratio of less than 50%. The cardiac outline in PA view is illustrated in Figure 6.23.
- Hila: these are made up of pulmonary arteries and upper lobe veins, concave on their lateral aspect with the left 1 – 2 cm higher than the right.
- Trachea: this should be central. The carina is at the lower border of the body of T4.
- Horizontal fissure: this goes from the right hilum to meet the sixth rib in the axilla.
- Lungs: both lung fields should be of equal greyness (as a result of blood in the pulmonary vasculature) with markings extending to the peripheries.
- Other: look at the soft tissues surrounding the chest and below the diaphragm.

On a lateral film:

- One can localize lesions seen on a PA film.
- The oblique fissure runs from T5 to the angle between the diaphragm and the anterior chest wall (see Figure 6.22).
- Look at the dorsal vertebrae.
- Pay particular attention to the area below the lip of the diaphragm which is hidden on PA view.
- Retrosternal and retrocardiac shadows should be approximately equal.

## Relevant applied anatomy

### *Infections*

The tissues lining the nasal cavity become oedematous and very vascular when infected, even if it is just a simple acute viral upper respiratory tract infection. This almost always results in the nasal passages becoming blocked and useless as airways, e.g. for nasal masks in dentistry. In addition, insertion of a nasal airway in an attempt to overcome the blockage can produce profuse haemorrhage.

Tonsillitis is common in children and young adults. The tonsil lies between the pharyngeal pillars (see Figure 6.9) and is shown in cross-section in Figure 6.24. When infected, the tonsils enlarge dramatically and on some occasions meet in the midline. Repeated infections are treated by tonsillectomy, usually during

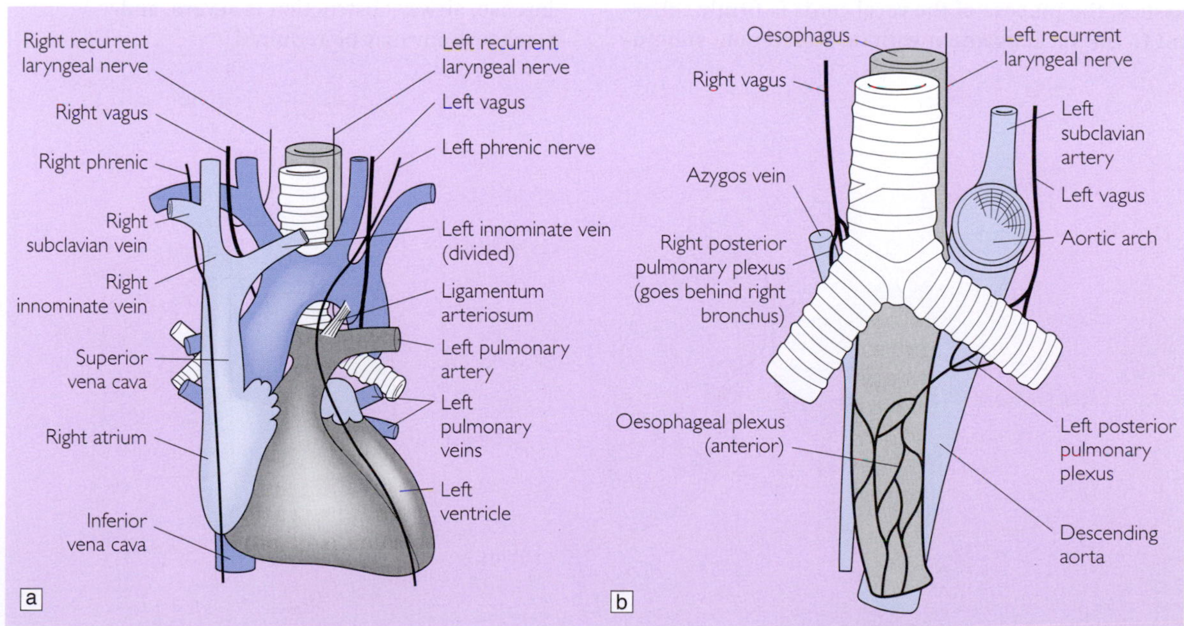


**Figure 6.19.** The interrelationships of the trachea, the major bronchi, the major thoracic arteries, and the heart. Note the difference in path of the right and left recurrent laryngeal nerves in (a).The right and left vagus nerves first form the right and left posterior pulmonary plexuses and then join to form the anterior and posterior oesophageal plexus (b). In (b) the heart and ascending aorta have been removed.

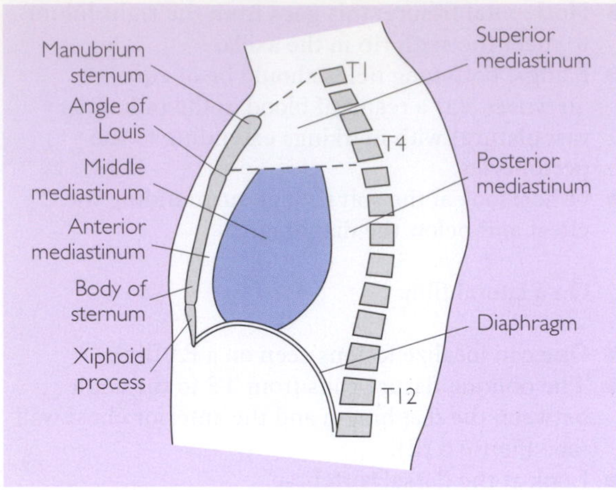


**Figure 6.20.** The major subdivisions of the mediastinum.

a quiescent phase to ensure reduced vascularity. During this operation, the tonsillar branch of the facial artery is cut and can be the cause of subsequent haemorrhage. A quinsy is suppuration in the peritonsillar tissues secondary to tonsillitis. In acute tonsillitis, and particularly with a quinsy, the patient usually has difficulty in opening the mouth properly and there can be reactive spasm in the masseter muscles. Incision and drainage of an acute quinsy under general anaesthesia must be taken very seriously and regarded as involving management of a difficult airway.

Epiglottitis is an acute infection of the epiglottis, usually involving the vestibular folds (false cords) and the aryepiglottic folds surrounding the laryngeal inlet. It can be life threatening and, in severe cases, the entrance to the larynx on laryngoscopy can be identified only by bubbling which shows a narrow slit on expiration. In contrast to the thick submucosa of these tissues, the mucosa of the vocal cords is firmly adherent to the vocal ligament with no intervening submucosa. Oedema of the larynx does not therefore involve the true cords because there is no submucosa in which fluid can collect.

Infections in the chest can be either widespread (broncho-) or localized (lobar). Infections in lobes can cause them to consolidate, reduce in size or totally collapse. Infected lobes usually have more pleural fluid surrounding them and hence are more easily identified. Note from Figures 6.21 and 6.22 that, because of the angle of the oblique fissure, it is possible for opacities in the upper lung zones on a PA view to originate from pathology in the lower lobes.

### *Nerve damage*

Damage to the superior laryngeal nerve causes a loss of the tensioning effect of the cricothyroid muscle and weakness of the voice.

Both recurrent laryngeal nerves can be damaged by malignant lymph nodes in the neck or a thyroid carcinoma. The left recurrent laryngeal nerve, in its thoracic course, may become involved in a bronchial or oesophageal carcinoma, in a mass of enlarged mediastinal glands, or stretched over an aneurysm of the aorta or an enlarged left atrium.

There are three important aspects of damage to the recurrent laryngeal nerves:

1. Complete damage to one nerve produces a cord held midway between the midline and abducted positions. If bilateral, breathing through the partially opened glottis becomes difficult and, on occasions, the flaccid cords may be snapped shut during inspiration.
2. If only one side is affected, the other cord compensates, often remarkably well.
3. If there is only partial damage to the nerve, the abductors are affected more than the adductors and the cord adopts the adducted, midline position. With bilateral partial damage, stridor is intense, airway obstruction is severe, and tracheostomy may be required.

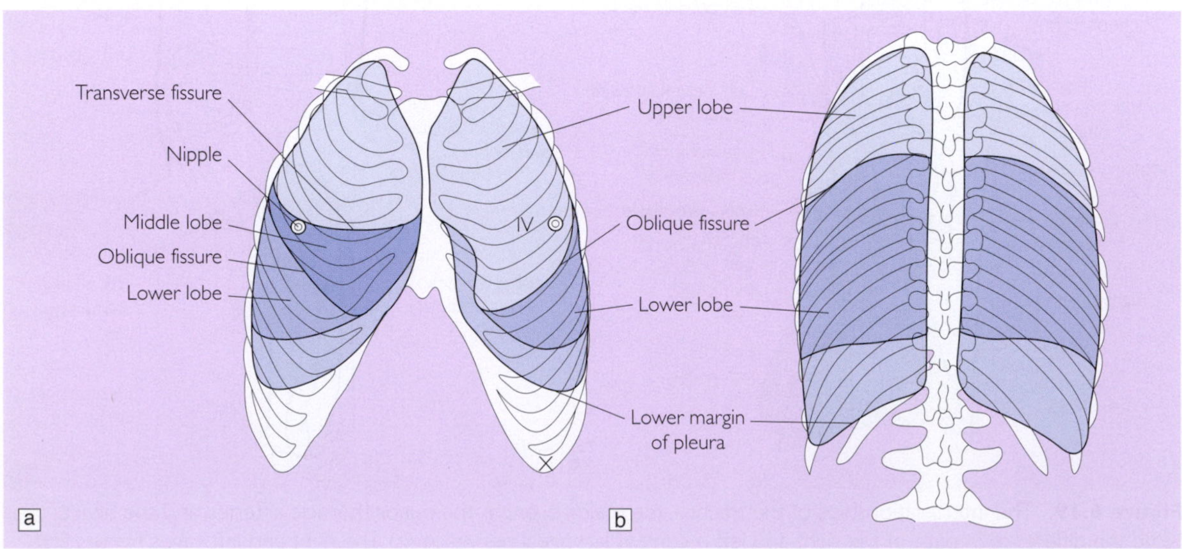


**Figure 6.21.** The surface markings of the lungs and pleurae seen from (a) the front and (b) the back. Note the height of the lower lobe at the back. (IV, fourth rib.)

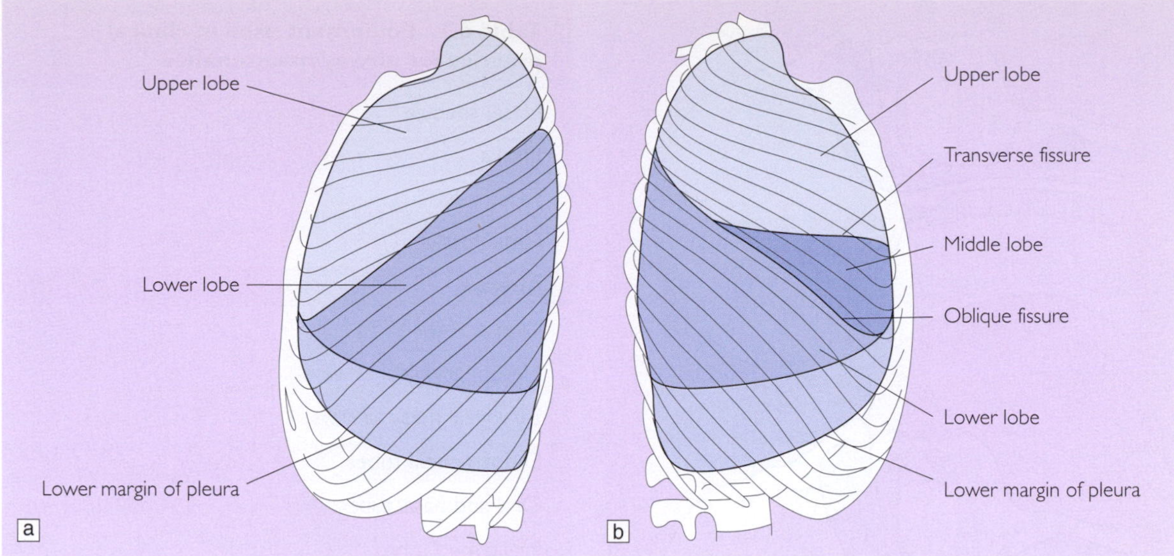


**Figure 6.22.** The surface projection of the lungs and pleurae seen from (a) a left lateral view and (b) the right.

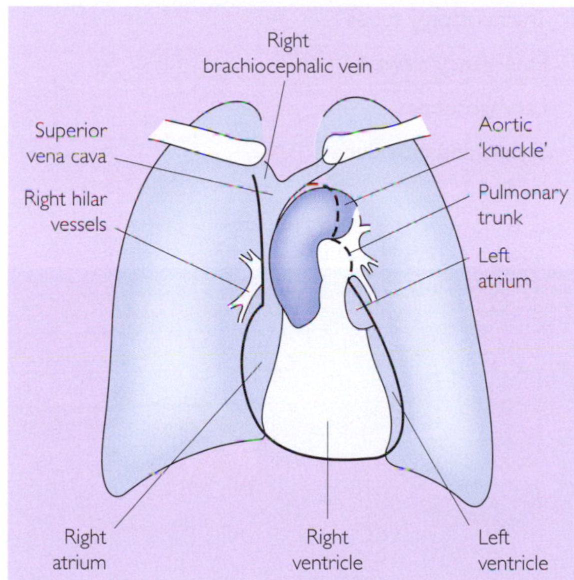


**Figure 6.23.** The radiographic projection of the heart and great vessels in PA view. The aorta and pulmonary trunk show as two curved shadows (dotted line).

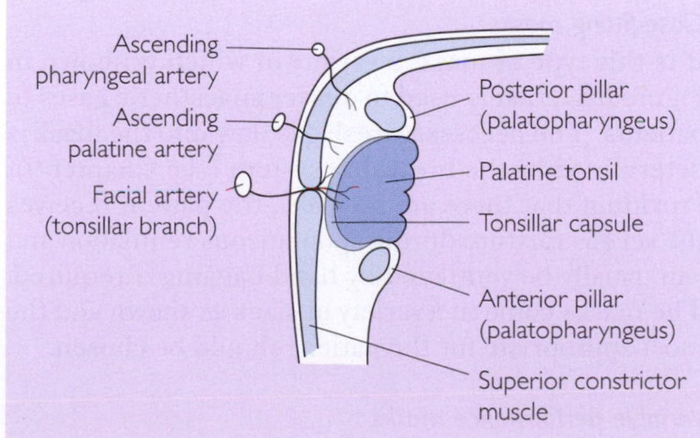


**Figure 6.24.** A diagrammatic representation of the tonsil and its surroundings in horizontal section.

***Airway management***

The nasal and oral airways in a conscious, supine adult are shown in Figure 6.25. After the induction of anaesthesia or when unconscious, the normal tone of the musculature is lost, and the tongue and soft palate fall back against the posterior pharyngeal wall, cutting off the airway. This can usually be alleviated by lifting the lower jaw (and together with it the attached tongue), which also pulls the soft tissues of the pharynx forward as shown.

## EQUIPMENT FOR AIRWAY MAINTENANCE

The appropriate equipment to be used for airway management depends on the individual patient and the exact procedure being undertaken. The items of equipment used in clinical practice are shown in Table 6.1.

More complex airways and equipment such as endobronchial and double-lumen tubes are not considered here.

### Nasal specula

These can be used to raise the level of inspired oxygen after premedication, during sedation, and during recovery (Figure 6.26). They are very well tolerated by most patients provided that the flow is below 5 L/min. The technique is obviously no use unless the nasal passages are patent. In some patients, specula not only dry out the nasal mucosa and thereby cause irritation, but can also cause the patient to mouth breathe.

Nasal specula raise the fractional inspired oxygen concentration ($F\text{IO}_2$) in an unpredictable way and there are no charts or nomograms available as a guide to their effectiveness at a given flow. This is because patients inspire different proportions of their inspiratory tidal volume from the mouth and nose, and their peak inspiratory flow is well above the oxygen delivery rate. This means that specula are unsuitable for reliably delivering anaesthetic agents.

The recommended use of these devices is when modest rises in the $F\text{IO}_2$ would be beneficial in sponta-

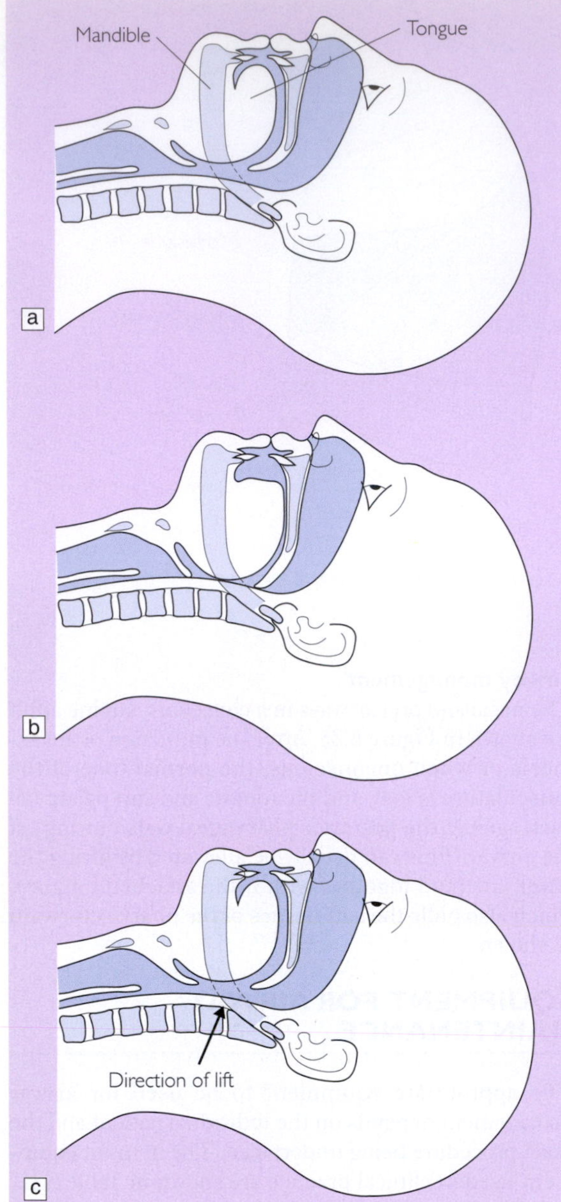


**Figure 6.25.** The relationship of the tongue and soft palate to the posterior wall of the pharynx in the supine patient. When a patient is anaesthetized, the position of the soft structures moves from that shown in (a) the awake state to that shown in (b) the anaesthetized state. This cuts off both the nasal and oral routes to the trachea. (c) The obstruction can be alleviated by lifting the lower jaw forwards. The tongue moves away from the posterior wall because it is attached to the back of the mandible and the lateral soft tissues drag the soft palate forwards.

neously breathing patients in whom precise delivery is not of vital importance. Any patients at risk of becoming hypoxic should be monitored by pulse oximeter.

## Masks

### Facemasks

Facemasks can be broadly divided into those that fit closely with a gas-tight seal and those that do not. Those that do not can be further divided into variable and fixed performance devices.

| Table 6.1. Equipment used in clinical practice for airway maintenance |
|---|
| **Nasal specula** |
| **Masks** |
| Facemasks |
| Nasal masks |
| **Airways** |
| Oral airways |
| Nasopharyngeal airways |
| Laryngeal mask airways |
| **Endotracheal tubes** |
| Oral and nasal tubes |
| Preformed tubes |
| Armoured tubes |
| Special function tubes |
| Tracheostomy tubes |
| **Emergency airways** |
| **Laryngoscopes** |
| **Stylets and introducers** |

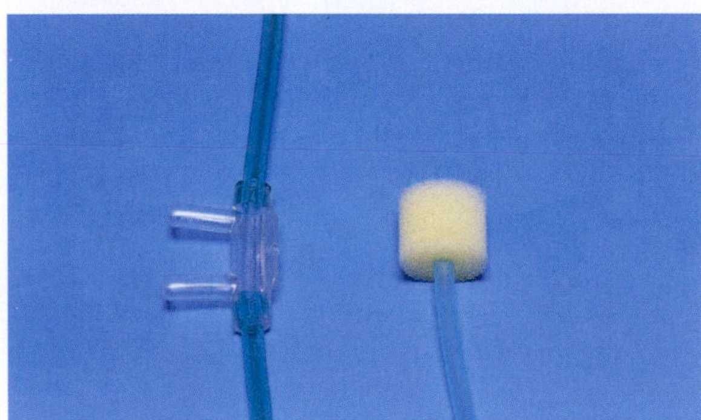

**Figure 6.26.** Nasal specula: on the left is the conventional model in which each prong enters a nostril. The model on the right is for single nostril use. The foam collar maintains the catheter comfortably in position.

*Close-fitting masks*

It is this type of mask, a variety of which is shown in Figure 6.27, that is used to deliver anaesthetic gases to patients. The necessary fresh gas flow into the mask is determined by the breathing system (see Chapter 9). Providing that there are no leaks, the patient receives the set gas mixture during spontaneous ventilation and can usually be ventilated by hand bagging if required. The masks come in a variety of sizes as shown and the most appropriate for the patient should be chosen.

*Variable performance masks*

These masks, which fit loosely over the nose and mouth, are not used for the administration of anaesthesia but for the delivery of oxygen in the conscious

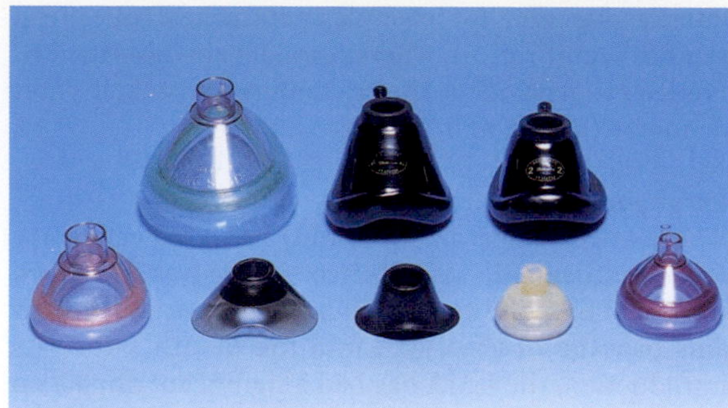

**Figure 6.27.** Close-fitting facemasks for induction and maintenance of anaesthesia. A variety of adult and paediatric models is shown.

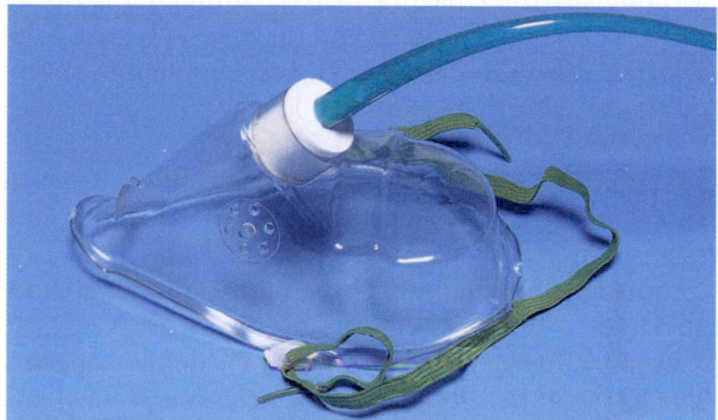

**Figure 6.28.** An example of a variable performance oxygen mask in current use.

or sedated patient. A frequently used model is shown in Figure 6.28. They are variable performance masks because they supply oxygen at a fixed rate which is below the peak inspiratory flow rate, and the effective $F\text{IO}_2$ achieved depends on the patient s individual breathing pattern. The masks have holes to allow air to enter during inspiration and expired gases to leave, although a considerable amount of gas goes around the edges of the mask. There is inevitably a very small (effectively negligible) amount of rebreathing from the dead space of the mask. The dead space effect is greater the lower the flow of oxygen.

In an average-sized adult patient, masks of this type will provide an $F\text{IO}_2$ of approximately 25 – 30% at 2 L/min, rising to 30 – 40% at 6 L/min.

*Fixed performance masks*

As with variable performance masks, these are not used for the delivery of anaesthetic agents. They are termed high airflow oxygen entrainment (HAFOE) devices, or Ventimasks, the latter being the trade name of a particular family of masks. They work on the principle that the net flow of gas over the nose and mouth exceeds the peak inspiratory flow (i.e. > 30 L/min). This high flow rate is produced by the Venturi effect of a jet of oxygen entraining atmospheric air (see Chapter 37). The oxygen flow rate for the mask to produce a given $F\text{IO}_2$ is normally written on it. Typical $F\text{IO}_2$ values available from such masks range from 25% to 40% depending on the model. They are useful when it is necessary to know the administered $F\text{IO}_2$ and there is of course no rebreathing. The Venturi device and a selection of currently available masks are shown in Figure 6.29.

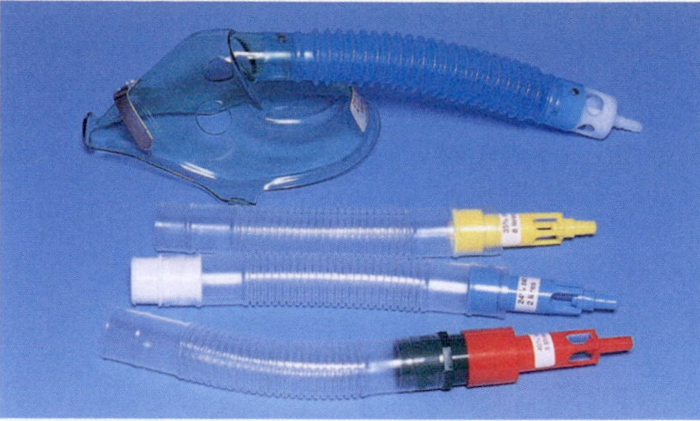

**Figure 6.29.** A high airflow oxygen entrainment (HAFOE) mask shown with a variety of interchangeable Venturi devices to produce different concentrations of inspired oxygen. The white labels on the Venturi devices indicate the delivered inspired oxygen concentration and the minimum oxygen flow required to achieve it.

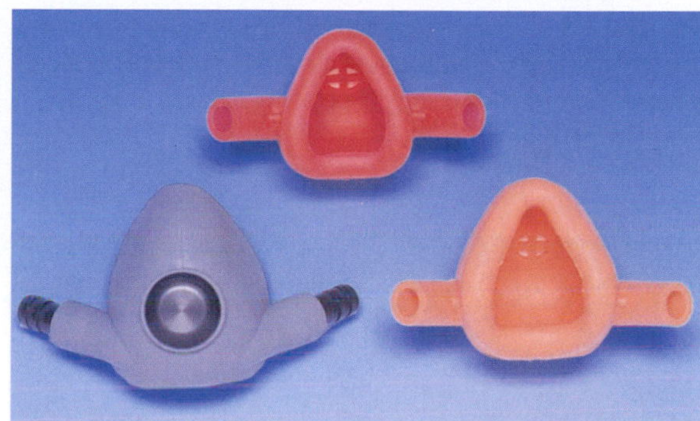

**Figure 6.30.** Examples of small, medium, and large nasal masks in anterior and posterior view. The pink mask has a strawberry aroma and the orange mask has a peach aroma incorporated into their production. The grey mask, for adult use, is odourless.

***Nasal masks***

These are used almost exclusively for dental anaesthesia. They are smaller than the usual facemasks, which cover the nose and mouth and have a different contour for obvious reasons. A variety of nasal masks is shown in Figure 6.30.

## Airways

***Oral airways***

Oral airways are used to hold the tongue away from the posterior pharyngeal wall and prevent the soft tissues of the pharynx collapsing in, as shown in Figure 6.31. For adults, airways come in sizes 3, 4, and 5, corresponding to 80, 90, and 100 mm, respectively. Children s airways number 0, 1, and 2 (50, 60, and 70 mm), with numbers 000 and 00 being used for pre-term babies. Oral airways have a reinforced section immediately behind the flange to prevent clenching of the teeth compressing the lumen. They are usually made of plastic and disposable. A selection is shown in Figure 6.32.

### *Nasopharyngeal airways*

Nasopharyngeal airways (Figure 6.32) are inserted through the anterior nares and the distal tip should lie in the pharynx above the epiglottis as shown in Figure 6.33. Some nasal airways are sized in terms of their internal diameter, for example endotracheal tubes (e.g. sizes 5, 6, and 7 mm), whereas others are described by French gauge which is the circumference of their outer diameter (28, 30, and 32 mm).

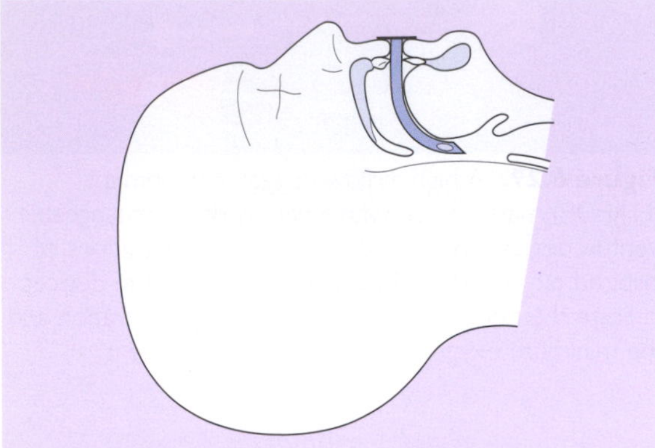

**Figure 6.31.** The use of an oral airway to prevent the collapse of the soft tissues of the mouth and oral pharynx on to the posterior pharyngeal wall. Compare with Figure 6.25.

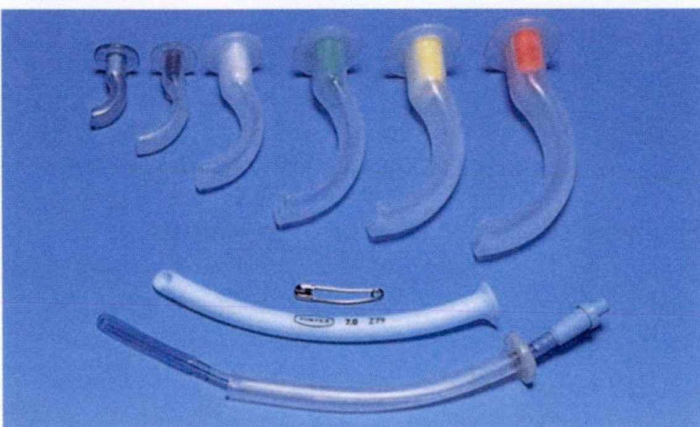

**Figure 6.32.** A variety of adult and paediatric oral airways and two types of adult nasal airway. Note the safety pin, which is often used to transfix a nasal airway and allow fixation to the skin by use of adhesive tape. The lower nasal airway incorporates an inflatable introducer to ease its passage.

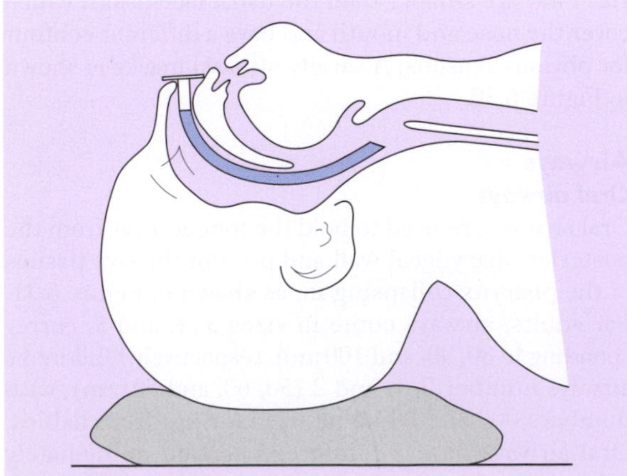

**Figure 6.33.** The ideal position for a nasopharyngeal airway.

### *Laryngeal mask airway*

The laryngeal mask airway (LMA) has now been in use for more than a decade. Its acceptance was helped by the use of propofol as an induction agent, which greatly aids passage of the LMA into the mouth. Since its introduction, the LMA has had a significant impact on anaesthetic practice, and has largely superseded the traditional facemask for spontaneously breathing patients requiring anaesthesia for more than a few minutes.

The principle of the LMA is that it provides an effectively gas-tight seal around the laryngeal inlet without anything having to pass through the vocal cords. It is shown inflated and deflated in Figure 6.34 and in position in Figure 6.35. It is supplied in seven sizes: size 1 for babies up to 5 kg; size $1\frac{1}{2}$ for babies 5 – 10 kg; size 2 for babies and children of 10 – 20 kg; size $2\frac{1}{2}$ for children of 20 - 30 kg; size 3 for young people of 30 – 50 kg; size 4 for small or normal-sized adults, and size 5 for normal- or large-sized adults. The respective volumes for cuff inflation are 4, 7, 10, 14, 20, 30 and 40 ml.

A black line can be seen on the tube on the opposite side to the outlet of the mask, which gives a check on its correct orientation when inserted. The bars across the outlet from the tube are to prevent the epiglottis becoming caught. Reinforced LMAs are available for procedures on the head and neck.

## Endotracheal tubes

### *General principles: oral and nasal tubes*

The original endotracheal (ET) tubes were straight and termed catheters . This small piece of history is preserved in the retention of the term catheter mount for the connector between the ET tube and the breathing system. It is now routine practice to use single-use, disposable tubes for tracheal intubation. This is not always the case with double-lumen endobronchial tubes, but these are not considered in this text. ET tubes now come in a variety of styles but a reasonable classification would be:

- standard curved tube, plain and cuffed;
- preformed tube, plain and cuffed;

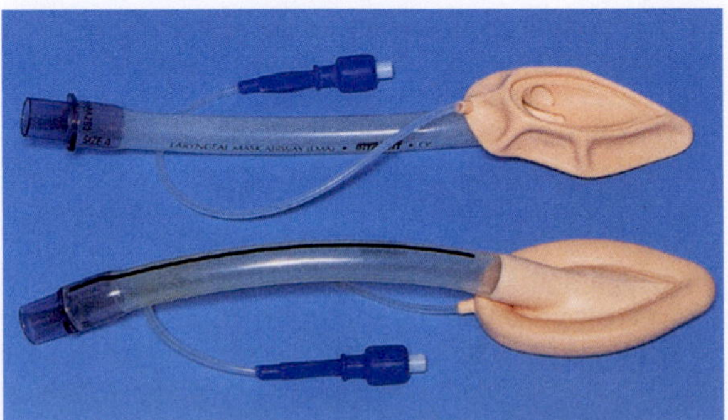

**Figure 6.34.** A laryngeal mask with its cuff inflated and deflated.

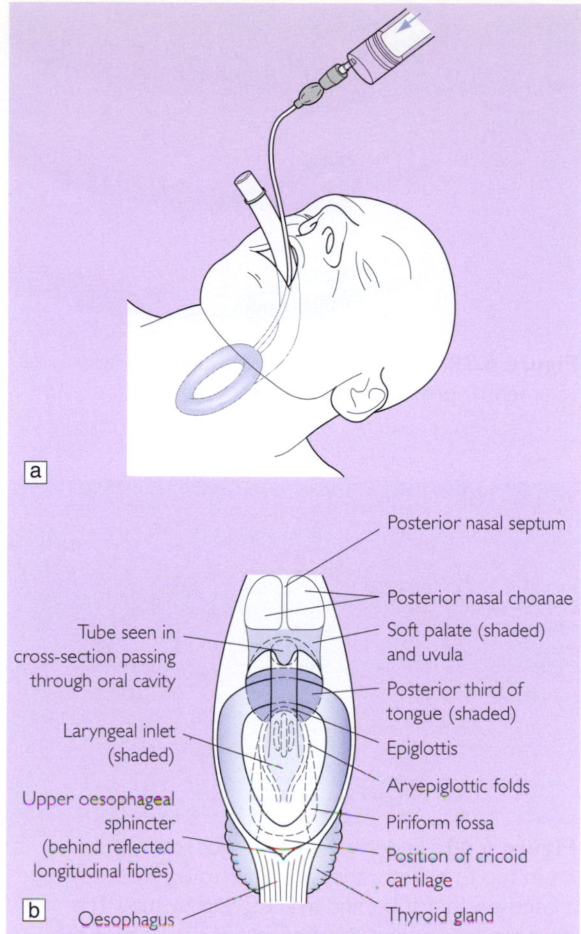


**Figure 6.35.** (a) The laryngeal mask in position and (b) the structures it seals against. Note that the mask lies over the larynx and the bars across its entrance prevent the epiglottis prolapsing into the tube and getting caught.

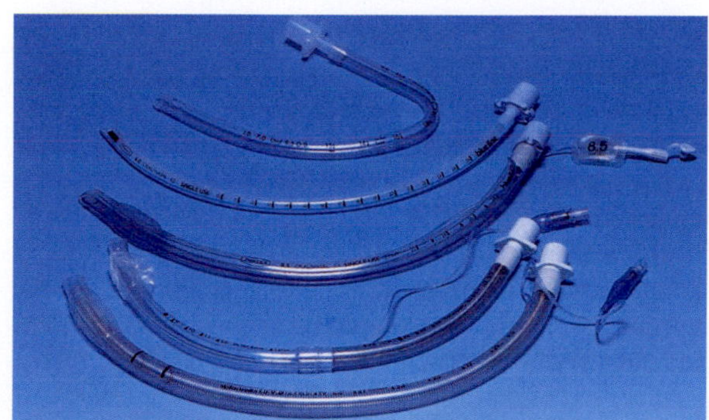

**Figure 6.36.** Examples of endotracheal tubes. From the top downwards they are: a plain preformed 'south pointing' tube; a plain uncut nasotracheal tube; an uncut oral endotracheal tube with a standard cuff; a tube with an armoured upper section intended to prevent kinking at the teeth; and an oral endotracheal tube reinforced against kinking along its whole length.

- reinforced or armoured tube, usually cuffed;
- special function tubes.

Examples of these are shown in Figure 6.36. The 'size' of a tube is a measurement of its internal diameter in millimetres. The size is stamped on the wall of the tube together with the outside diameter or tube thickness, a centimetre scale measuring the distance from the tip, and the implant testing code, which guarantees minimal irritant properties. Some tubes also have two heavy black lines marked, between which the vocal cords should lie; others have a black section at the end to assist with correct positioning (Figure 6.37). The plastic of which ET tubes are made becomes soft at body temperature. Most tubes have a hole cut in the wall opposite the bevel (known as a Murphy's eye), which permits gas flow if the bevel becomes occluded by the wall of the trachea. Tubes can be passed into the trachea by the oral or nasal route: oral intubation is the norm unless there is a specific reason for using the nasal route. The only notable practical difference between a standard oral and nasal ET tube is that the tube from the pilot balloon leading to the cuff comes off more proximally in a nasal tube. This limits the facility for cutting nasal tubes down to act as oral tubes.

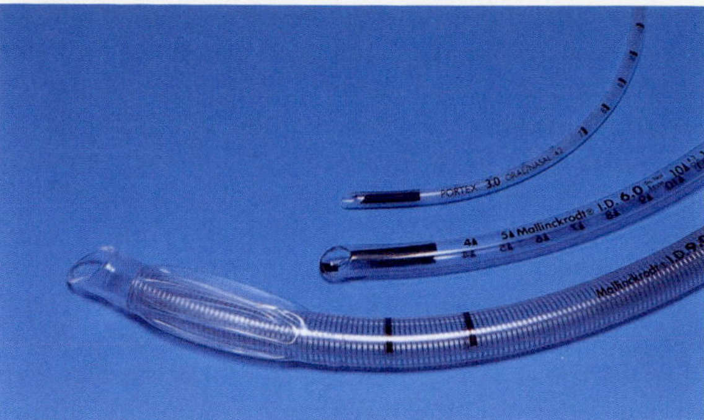

**Figure 6.37.** A close-up of the distal ends of an adult reinforced and two paediatric plain endotracheal tubes. The black sections and lines are designed to make it easier to position the tube below the vocal cords with the tip at the correct distance from the carina. Note that, as shown in this figure, the length of the black section varies with tube size.

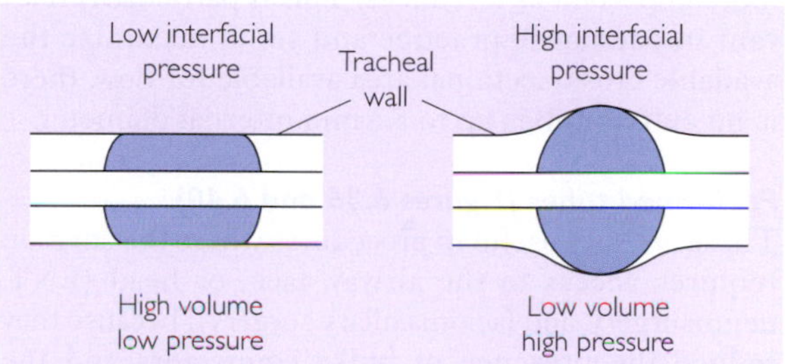


**Figure 6.38.** The difference in contact area between a low-volume and a high-volume endotracheal tube cuff shown diagrammatically.

The tube cuff provides a seal with the tracheal mucosa. Cuffs vary in size and shape, the extremes being represented by the low-volume/high-pressure and high-volume/low-pressure designs (Figure 6.38). High-volume/low-pressure cuffs are designed to accommodate a large change in volume without a marked rise in pressure, thereby allowing the cuff internal pressure to be representative of that applied to the tracheal mucosa. Although cuffs pass stringent quality control procedures, they always need checking for leaks. A guide to the pressure in the cuff can be obtained from the tension of the pilot balloon after inflation. In everyday practice in the operating room, cuffs cause relatively little morbidity and are inflated to the pressure required to prevent an audible leak on ventilation at the selected tidal volume. This allows reasonable protection from aspiration without excessive wall pressure. Cuff pressures are generally in the range of 15–25 mmHg and the perfusion pressure of the tracheal mucosa is 25–35 mmHg. For routine use in the operating room, medium-volume/medium-pressure cuffs are used, high-volume/low-pressure models being reserved for tubes intended to remain in place for over 24 hours (Figure 6.39).

The resistance to flow down an ET tube is dependent upon the length and internal diameter of the tube and the flow characteristics of the gas. The major determinant is, however, the diameter, as described in Chapter 37, and its effect becomes ever more important as it reduces. This is particularly relevant in paediatric practice and so, to maximize the available cross-sectional area available for flow, there is no cuff on tubes up to 5.5 mm internal diameter.

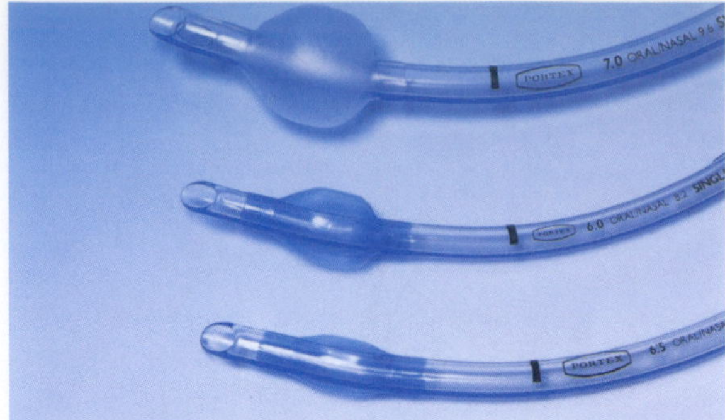

**Figure 6.39.** High- (top), medium- and standard-volume/low-pressure endotracheal tube cuffs.

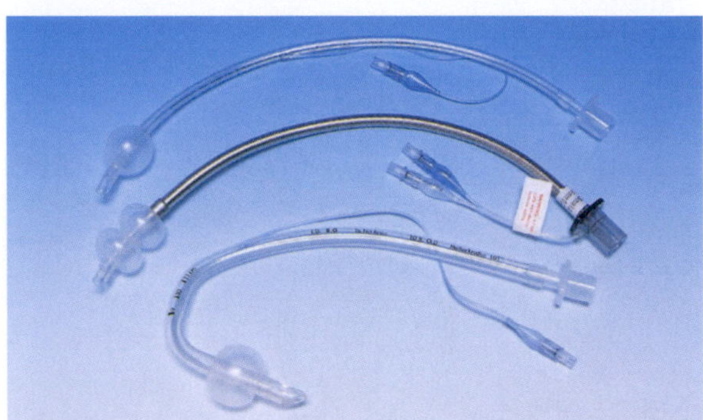

**Figure 6.40.** Endotracheal tubes for specialist use. From top to bottom they are: a microlaryngoscopy tube; a laser-resistant tube; and a laryngectomy tube. The laryngectomy tube is inserted into the trachea in the same way as a tracheostomy tube, with the connector pointing towards the feet. The label on the laser-resistant tube reminds the user to fill the balloons with saline and not air.

### *Preformed tubes (Figures 6.36 and 6.40)*

These are very useful in procedures where the surgeon requires access to the airway, face, or head (ENT, neurosurgery, and faciomaxillary surgery), because they reduce the presence of bulky connectors and the number of connections that can fall apart. They are also less likely to kink. Their great advantage is therefore practical convenience. They have two disadvantages:

1. Passing suction catheters down them is usually impossible because of the tight angled curves.
2. There is a fixed distance from the lips or nares to the tip of the tube which may, because of the variability in patient size, allow the tube to either enter the bronchus or to slip out of the larynx.

### *Armoured tubes (Figure 6.36)*

Armoured (or reinforced) tubes are designed to prevent kinking and are used in circumstances where the anaesthetist has no ready intraoperative access to the airway or where the head or larynx has to be manipulated during surgery. Such circumstances are neurosurgery, face-down positions, thyroid surgery, and faciomaxillary procedures. Armoured tubes cannot be cut shorter because of their construction and hence have to be secured at the appropriate length. As a result of their 'floppy' nature, they have to be placed with the help of an introducer (see below).

### *Special function tubes*

There are a number of highly specialized tubes of which only a few are described briefly below and shown in Figure 6.40.

#### *Microlaryngoscopy tube*

This is a tube designed to allow examination and surgery of the larynx. The tube has a 5- or 6-mm internal diameter with a large low-pressure/high-volume cuff. It is supplied and used uncut for either oral or nasal use. The resistance to flow in these tubes is such that spontaneous ventilation should be used only for very short periods. They are really designed for intermittent positive pressure ventilation (IPPV).

#### *Laryngectomy tube*

This tube is a preformed tube designed to enter a tracheostomy at the same time as removing the bulky connector from the operative site. It has a short, straight section, which resides in the trachea, with a preformed right-angled bend leading to a length of tubing that can be moved around and placed in the most convenient position.

#### *Laser-resistant tubes*

Lasers are used in surgery because they are able to resect unwanted tissue without damaging adjacent structures; this is a particularly useful property when working on the vocal cords. In the airways, lasers are potentially dangerous because they can ignite plastic, puncture cuffs, and damage tissues by reflection. The solution to this has been to produce microlaryngeal tubes that reflect laser light and have modified cuffs. The tube surface is either coated in aluminium foil (some anaesthetists do this themselves on a 'home-made' basis) or constructed of flexible stainless steel.

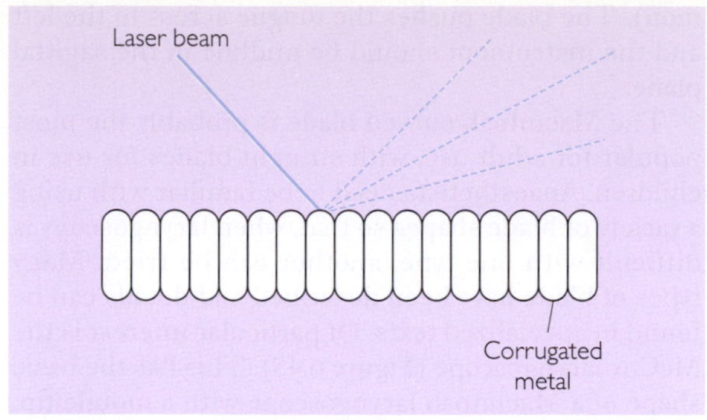


**Figure 6.41.** The reduction of intensity of a laser beam by reflection from an endotracheal tube with a metal surface.

The metal surface essentially 'defocuses' the laser beam by the diffusing effect of its convex surface (Figure 6.41). Some tubes have two cuffs in case one should puncture. For this type of work the cuff, instead of being filled with air, should be filled with saline to prevent combustion. Some anaesthetists put methylene blue in the saline so that leaks can be seen easily and immediately by the surgeon during use. Other tubes have a foam-like substance which prevents complete deflation.

*Injectors and insufflation*

These are not strictly speaking types of tracheal tube but are nevertheless used to oxygenate the anaesthetized patient. They are used mainly for laryngeal examination and bronchoscopy.

Injectors are fine tubes or needles fixed to or built into the wall of a bronchoscope and connected to a high-pressure (usually 100% $O_2$) gas supply (Figure 6.42). The anaesthetist has a valve which he or she opens intermittently to allow flow through the injector. This entrains air via the mouth of the bronchoscope in the same way as a fixed performance mask (see above and Chapter 37), and the pressure generated by the momentum of the gas flow is sufficient to ventilate the lungs of a paralysed patient.

Insufflation is a technique in which a patient is anaesthetized and breathes spontaneously whilst a thin catheter delivers fresh gas into the trachea. The catheter can be adapted from a nasogastric tube, suction catheter, and a variety of other types of thin, sterile tubes. The principle is that the patient breathes in a mixture of the insufflated gases and air, and breathes out normally into the atmosphere. Insufflation methods are not greatly used now because of the developments in tube and injector technology.

***Tracheostomy tubes***

Tracheostomy tubes (Figure 6.43) enter the trachea below the cricoid cartilage just above the suprasternal notch, and reduce the anatomical dead space by 30–50%. The creation of a tracheostomy should be an elective procedure carried out by a surgical or dilational technique. The function of a tracheostomy tube is to bypass the larynx for the following reasons:

- to provide a safe airway in those patients who have upper airway obstruction (e.g. supraglottic tumour) or an incompetent larynx (e.g. neurological disease, prolonged depression of conscious level);
- to provide an airway for patients during and after laryngectomy and other types of major head and neck surgery;

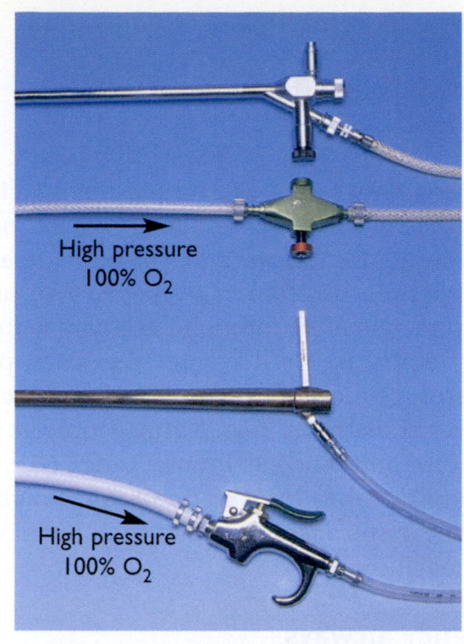


**Figure 6.42.** Two examples of bronchoscopes with injector systems. In each case, the injector is a fine tube inside the bronchoscope immediately beyond the Luer lock connection of the high-pressure hose. The high-pressure hoses that loop in and out of the photograph have on/off valves with which the anaesthetist controls the intermittent airflow and hence the ventilation. Two types of bronchoscope and valve are shown here. The upper post on each bronchoscope is for the attachment of the light source. The larger tube on the upper bronchoscope pointing downwards, which crosses the injector mechanism, is blocked off in this photograph. This tube, when not blocked off, will accept a standard 15-mm connector with the gas flow coming from a conventional circuit. The patient can then either breathe spontaneously or be ventilated using a conventional 2-litre bag.

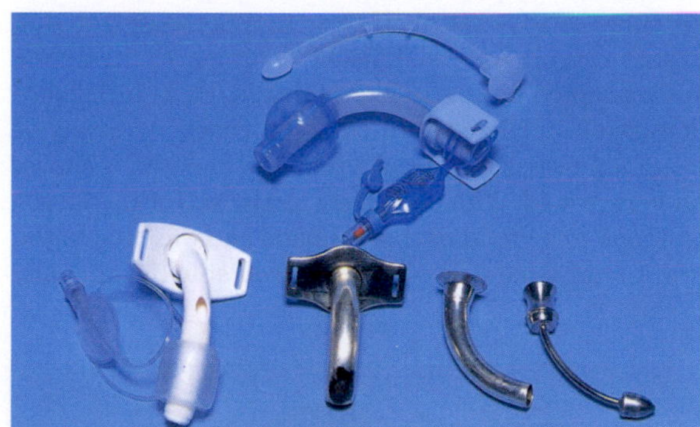

**Figure 6.43.** Examples of plastic and silver tracheostomy tubes. Note the presence of the obturators which are necessary for the smooth passage of the tube into the trachea. The white plastic tube has a fenestration which allows a patient with intact vocal cords to speak. The silver tracheostomy tube has an inner tube which can be removed to clean out secretions, etc.

- to allow long-term IPPV or weaning from ventilation;
- to provide long-term control of bronchial secretions.

Tracheostomy tubes can be plastic, which (apart from paediatric models) are usually cuffed, or metal, which are uncuffed. Both types of tube are available with either a fenestration or a one-way flap valve that allows redirection of air through the larynx so that those patients who are still able to, can phonate. Tracheostomy tubes, like ET tubes, are sized either on their internal diameter (e.g. 8 mm, 9 mm) or on their external circumference as French gauge (e.g. 28, 32). Tracheostomy tubes have an obturator, which acts as an introducer and eases the passage of the device into the tracheal lumen.

### Emergency airways

*It is an undeniable fact that, if the passage of oxygen to the lungs ceases, the human is essentially dying until the flow is restored.* Emergency airways are designed to support life when conventional methods of airway management have failed (e.g. difficult intubation) or cannot be used (e.g. trauma). A large number of devices and methods have been described. Three are outlined in Chapter 7. All involve the insertion of a gas-carrying device through the relatively avascular and easily palpated cricothyroid membrane.

### Laryngoscopes

A laryngoscope is used for displaying the larynx, for either inspection or intubation. Originally they were designed for their tip to be placed under the epiglottis to lift it forwards, but for most instruments in common use today the tip is designed to be placed in the vallecula. Apart from plastic laryngoscopes found in some resuscitation boxes, they have detachable blades that are interchangeable. This allows the device to be adapted to a particular patient's needs and makes it easy to sterilize them between cases. A variety of common blades for use in adults and children is shown in Figure 6.44. The blades are designed for the laryngoscope to be held in the left hand and the tube in the right (right-handed blades are available but uncommon). The blade pushes the tongue across to the left and the instrument should be midline in the sagittal plane.

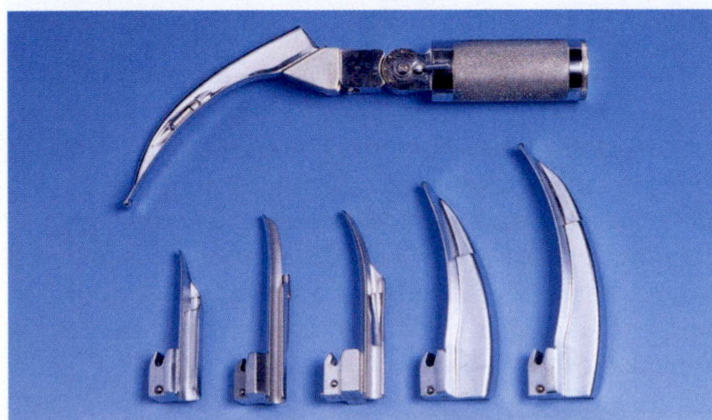

**Figure 6.44.** A variety of detachable adult and paediatric laryngoscope blades. The blade at the top shown attached to the handle is called a polio blade and allows access in those cases where a conventional laryngoscope with the blade at right angles to the handle cannot be introduced into the mouth.

The Macintosh curved blade is probably the most popular for adult use, with straight blades for use in children. Anaesthetists need to be familiar with using a variety of blade shapes so that, when laryngoscopy is difficult with one type, another can be tried. Many types of blade have been described and details can be found in specialized texts. Of particular interest is the McCoy laryngoscope (Figure 6.45). This has the basic shape of a Macintosh laryngoscope with a mobile tip. The tip is placed into the vallecula in the normal way and, when elevated, pulls up the soft tissues and epiglottis, often making difficult intubation much easier.

### Stylets and introducers

Stylets and introducers are frequently used to assist in the passage of ET tubes (Figure 6.46).

A stylet is a malleable but stiff, usually plastic-covered, length of wire. It has an acute bend at the proximal end, which curves over the ET tube connector and prevents the stylet tip emerging from the end of the ET tube. The stylet can be bent to allow the tube

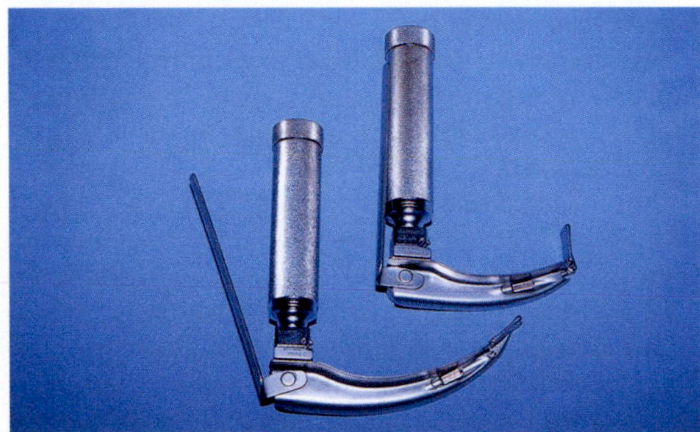

**Figure 6.45.** The McCoy laryngoscope shown with the tip in its normal and elevated positions. The tip is lifted by pressing the lever against the handle as shown.

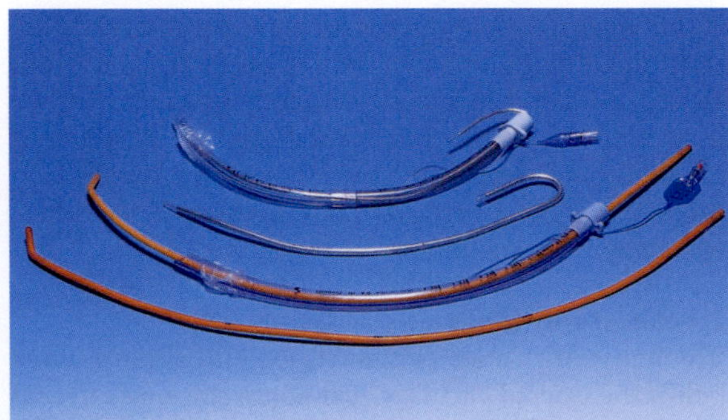

**Figure 6.46.** Stylets (top two) and bougies or introducers (lower two) which assist with the passage of endotracheal tubes. Note that the stylet should be adjusted so that it does not protrude through the tip of the tube and damage the cords at intubation. In contrast, the bougie is intended to be passed into the trachea and the endotracheal tube rail-roaded over it.

to adopt the most advantageous curve when intubation is difficult because of poor visualization of the larynx. It can also be used to give rigidity to a 'snake-like' armoured tube.

An introducer (or bougie) is a long semirigid device with a curved distal end, the most common type in use being the gum-elastic bougie (or Eschman introducer). It is first placed in the trachea and the tube is slid over it. An introducer is probably the most useful intubation aid that there is, and invaluable when only the epiglottis can be visualized (see Chapter 7). The length of the bougie is crucial because the ET tube needs to sit over it outside the mouth, thus allowing an unobstructed view of the epiglottis or larynx.

## FURTHER READING


Brimacombe JR, Brain AIJ, Berry AM. *The Laryngeal Mask Instruction Manual* 4th edn. Reading: Intravent Research, 1999.

Ellis H, Feldman S. *Anatomy for Anaesthetists*, 7th edn. Oxford: Blackwell Scientific Publications, 1997.

Articles in: Jones JG, Hanning CD, eds. *The Upper Airway*. *Baillière's Clin Anaesthesiol* 1995;**9**:213–396.

Pelling MX, Dick R. How to read the chest X-ray – Parts 1 and 2. *Current Anaesth Crit Care* 1994;**5**:102–8, 165–71.

Pennant JH, White PF. The laryngeal mask airway. Its uses in anesthesiology. *Anesthesiology* 1993;**79**:144–63.

# Chapter 7 Airway management II: assessment, control and problems

P. Hutton

## ASSESSING AND CONTROLLING THE AIRWAY

Management of the airway in all groups of patients, whether spontaneously breathing or ventilated, unconscious or awake, is one of the cornerstones of anaesthetic practice. There is no substitute for experience based on sound theoretical knowledge. For the purposes of this chapter and to prevent repetition, standards of good practice described elsewhere in the book (e.g. machine checking, monitoring, intravenous access, etc.) are assumed. As discussed in Chapter 2, preoxygenation before induction of anaesthesia is used routinely by many anaesthetists and is part of many hospital protocols. It is recommended to all trainees in their routine practice, and is assumed in this chapter.

### General principles

Assessment of the airway is paramount in every patient, whether it is the intention to give a general, regional, or local anaesthetic, because complications can occur in the most unexpected way. Not to do the assessment constitutes negligent practice. It must never be omitted. Fortunately, it is usually quick and easy to carry out.

It is important to note the difference between the incidence of difficult intubation (or, more correctly, difficult laryngoscopy) and the incidence of failure to maintain an airway on a mask. Accurate data on the occurrence of both are difficult to establish but it is probably reasonable to say that, for trained anaesthetists, they will find their skills tested in 1–2% of cases requiring intubation, whereas it will be very, very rare that facemask ventilation cannot be maintained. The dreaded combination of unable to ventilate/unable to intubate is mercifully rare for the experienced, but nevertheless must be regarded as a possibility on all occasions that anaesthesia and sedation are administered. Problems with the airway are maximal during the early part of training.

The importance of being prepared cannot be overstated. Published tests, measurement ratios, and other indices can, on occasion, both predict difficult intubation when it turns out to be easy and indicate easy intubation when, subsequently, difficulties arise. No method of assessment has been found to be 100% reliably predictive. It is the responsibility of every anaesthetist to ensure that the intubating environment is properly equipped with laryngoscopes, introducers, emergency airway equipment, etc. before any anaesthetic or sedative agent is given to a patient. Many hospitals now have clear policies as to what should be available and these need to be known beforehand, so that any special requirements for a particular case can be met. It is too late to discover that something is missing the moment it is needed. Some anaesthetists develop, or encourage to be developed, a reputation for being 'lucky' with respect to airway problems. This is a bad attitude. Once, when Joe Davis (15 times world snooker champion) had executed a very difficult shot to pot the black, a member of the audience sitting close to the table shouted out 'you were lucky there Joe!' He walked across to them and said 'You know, the more I practise, the luckier I get.' The lesson here is that proficiency depends upon attitude and practical experience.

There is a voluminous literature on airway assessment and difficult intubation and some of this is referred to later. Much of it can be confusing to trainees so this book takes a more pragmatic approach than is usual. *A crucial point, which is easy to forget in the heat of the moment, is that when difficulties arise, adequate oxygenation of the patient is the most important objective.* The sooner a problem is identified and admitted to exist, the sooner it can be solved. Everyone has difficulties from time to time, no matter how senior. Four points of good practice are:

1. Do not press on repeatedly trying to intubate: the more you try, in general, the worse it gets. After a few attempts, maintain the airway, oxygenate the patient, and rethink the situation before doing any damage.
2. Do not be proud: send for help. Another person may do things in a slightly different way, which on that occasion makes the impossible possible.
3. Do not be reluctant to wake the patient up: safety and absence of brain damage are crucial. In the rare event of being unable to oxygenate the patient, accept that the situation is happening in reality, to you, at that time, and move earlier rather than later to an emergency airway.
4. As a trainee, if intending to intubate the trachea, do not start without the immediate availability of capnography, and use it to confirm the position of the endotracheal (ET) tube.

## Using masks and airways

### Facemasks

A variety of facemasks used to deliver anaesthetic gases is shown in Figure 6.27. It is important to have a gas-tight seal between the mask and the patient's face because, if there is an imperfect fit, either (1) during spontaneous ventilation the reservoir bag will not fill properly during expiration and during inspiration the set gas mixture will be diluted by atmospheric air or (2) facemask ventilation will be ineffective.

If there are problems getting the mask to fit properly, increase the fresh gas flow (FGF) and, if ventilating by hand, use frequent, low-volume bag compressions to maintain oxygenation. Apart from very short procedures (e.g. waiting for a neuromuscular blocking agent to work), a badly fitting facemask should be changed as soon as possible for a better mask or an alternative airway maintenance method.

The principle of establishing an airway by pulling the lower jaw away from the pharyngeal wall is shown in Figure 6.25. In practice, this is done by pressing the mask on to the face with a finger grip while elevating the jaw with the forearms. In many cases, one hand is satisfactory (Figure 7.1). In some patients with full dentition, oral or nasal airways may not be required.

### Oral airways

Oral airways are used to hold the tongue away from the posterior pharyngeal wall and prevent the soft tissues of the pharynx collapsing inwards, as shown in Figure 6.31. As a guide to selecting the size of airway, its length should be approximately equal to the distance from the centre of the mouth to the angle of the mandible. This can, in children, result in the selection of an airway that at first glance looks too large but is usually not. If, however, the selected oral airway fails to provide the easy passage of gas, another should be tried.

Airways cannot usually be tolerated in conscious patients because they cause the patient to gag and spit it out. Immediately after induction of anaesthesia, the patient has to be either at a suitable level of anaesthetic depth or paralysed for airway insertion to be successful. Trying to force an oral airway into an unwilling patient can result in tissue damage, vomiting, and aspiration. When inserting an airway, it is often easiest to introduce it upside down and rotate it once the distal end is well into the oral cavity. Alternatively, the laryngoscope can be used to depress the anterior part of the tongue (so that gagging does not occur) and the airway slipped into position over it. Oral airways have a flange at the front, immediately behind which is a rigid section that must lie between the teeth to prevent biting compressing the airway. The flange can lie in front of, or behind, the lips; care should always be taken to prevent the lips being trapped and damaged between the airway and teeth.

Airways are very useful in the recovery phase while the patient is still unconscious. They do not, however, *guarantee* a good airway. Even with one *in situ,* it is still often necessary to push the jaw forward to get good gas transfer. *It can therefore never be assumed that a patient requiring an airway does not need constant attention.* This is sometimes particularly relevant to the management of head-injured patients.

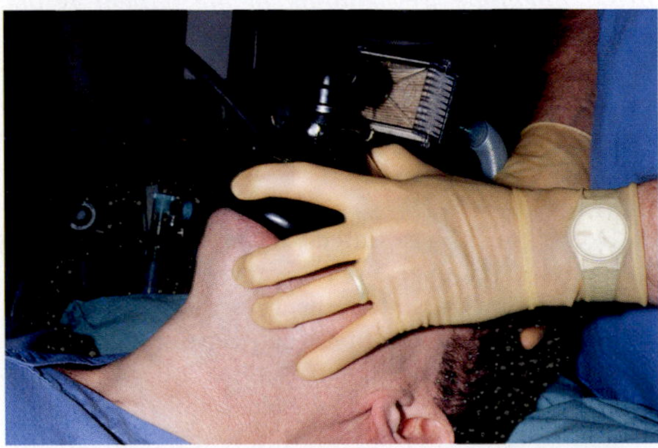

**Figure 7.1.** Holding a facemask with one hand. Note that the little finger is behind the angle of the mandible, and that the ring and middle fingers are applied directly to the ramus of the mandible rather than compressing the soft tissues of the floor of the mouth. The forefinger and thumb press the mask down to form a seal on the face while the jaw is elevated to pull the tongue and soft structures of the oropharynx away from the posterior pharyngeal wall. The anaesthetist's right hand is being applied to the patient's head to steady its position and prevent undue traction on the neck.

### Nasal airways

Nasal airways are inserted through the anterior nares and the distal tip should lie in the pharynx above the epiglottis, as shown in Figure 6.33. The length required is usually equal to the distance from the tip of the nose to the external meatus of the ear. The length of a nasopharyngeal airway is very important because, if too short, it obstructs easily and, if too long, finds its way into the oesophagus, as shown in Figure 7.2. The latter is a particularly important risk if a nasotracheal tube is being used as nasopharyngeal airway.

Before using a nasal airway, it is wise to assess the patency of the nasal passages and to introduce it into the clearest side. Coagulopathies and nasal infections are contraindications to their use. Epistasis is a common complication and it is possible (on occasions), by being too aggressive, not only to break the turbinates but also to breach the mucosa and pass the tip of the airway into the submucosal tissues. If it is known that the nasal route will be used, it is good prac-

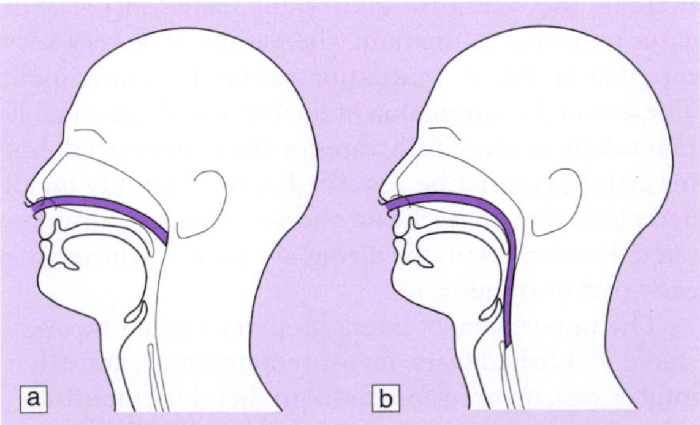


**Figure 7.2.** (a) A short nasal airway which may occlude on the soft tissues of the posterior pharyngeal wall and (b) one that is too long going into the oesophagus. Compare with the ideal length in Figure 6.33.

tice to instil vasoconstricting drops into the nasal passages preoperatively to shrink the mucosa as much as possible.

When inserting the lubricated nasal airway into the supine patient, immediately after introducing it into the entrance of the nares, the direction of travel needs to be changed so that it passes vertically downwards, parallel to the roof of the mouth along the floor of the nasal cavity. Pointing the airway cephalad in the direction of the entrance to the anterior nares directs it towards the turbinates and the cribriform plate in the roof of the nose (causing intense stimulation), behind which is the base of the brain (see Figures 6.1 and 6.2). As a result of the possibility of entering the brain, nasal airways should never be used in head-injured patients until a fracture of this region has been excluded.

Purpose-made nasal airways have a good sized flange at the end (see Figure 6.32). If this does not lie snugly when the airway is in the best position for gas transfer, or if an ET tube is being used as a nasal airway, the airway must be securely positioned at the correct length. This is often best done by transfixing it with a safety pin and taping this to the face. Fixing is particularly important with uncut ET tubes because these are long enough to slip down into the oesophagus.

With a well-functioning nasal airway, it is quite possible to give a satisfactory spontaneously breathing anaesthetic if the other nostril and mouth are closed.

### *Nasal masks*

These are used almost exclusively for paediatric dental anaesthesia and are shown in Figure 6.30. It is obvious that the use of nasal masks is impossible without a patent nasal airway. Consequently, this must be checked on every child before anaesthesia is induced.

The principles of usage are as follows: the patient (usually a child) is induced either by inhalational (common) or intravenous (rare) means while maintaining spontaneous ventilation. The nasal mask is then placed over the nose and the mouth is closed while continuously watching the reservoir bag, as shown in Figure 7.3. With fully patent nasal passages, there should be no change in bag excursion from that during facemask breathing. Anaesthesia is then deepened in the usual way and, when the jaw is slack, the dentist puts in a pack to seal off the oral cavity from the pharynx. Problems of the shared airway are described later (Figure 7.27).

### *Laryngeal mask airways*

*Indications*

The main use of the laryngeal mask airway (LMA) is in spontaneously breathing patients for procedures lasting between 10 and 60 min. It provides good airway control in many patients who would be difficult to handle on a facemask and leaves the anaesthetist's hands free. For the purposes of trainees, it should be regarded as a device for spontaneously breathing patients only.

The LMA (see Figure 6.34 and 6.35) has also been used by experienced anaesthetists together with intermittent positive pressure ventilation (IPPV) to ventilate paralysed patients, provided that there is no hiatus hernia or history of reflux and that they have normal lungs requiring low inflation pressures. *For controlled ventilation, it must only ever be used on elective, starved patients because the LMA does not protect against aspiration and is not a substitute for an ET tube*. Up to 20 mmHg pressure can usually be achieved satisfactorily and adjustment of the head position can resolve a leak at lower inflation pressures.

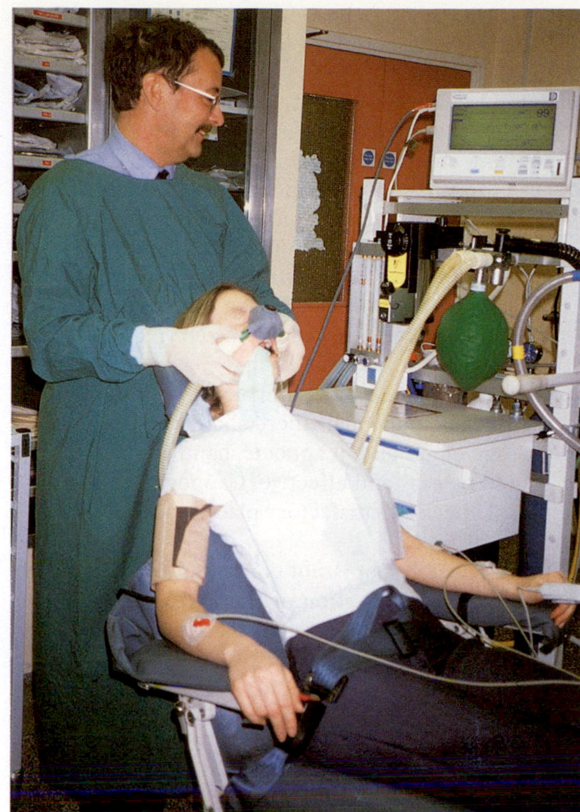

**Figure 7.3.** An example of a nasal mask in use. Note that the anaesthetist is observing the movement of the reservoir bag and adjacent to it are the monitors that can be seen at the same time.

The LMA can also be successful in establishing a reliable airway when facemask ventilation or intubation prove problematic. This is described on page 88 in the section on 'Unexpectedly difficult or failed intubation'.

*Method of use for a spontaneously breathing anaesthetic*

The technique of insertion is as follows:

- Following good practice guidelines, have the patient in a well-equipped environment with appropriate monitoring in use and an intravenous line established. Test the cuff on the LMA, lubricate it lightly, and deflate the cuff as shown in Figure 6.34.
- Induce anaesthesia in a well-oxygenated patient either intravenously (preferably with propofol) or inhalationally (see Chapter 2).
- Wait until the lower jaw relaxes and can be freely moved up and down. A gloved finger slid along the tongue should not elicit a gag reflex; if it does the depth of anaesthesia is insufficient.

- Place the patient's head in the intubating position. Pulling forward on the lower jaw by an assistant can be helpful.
- Stand behind the patient, open the mouth with one hand, and hold the LMA in the other with the air entry side of the mask facing the feet.
- Pass the LMA into the mouth and slide it over the tongue in a continuous smooth movement until it is felt to locate in position. Blow up the cuff. If the mask is in the correct position, blowing up the cuff causes the tube to rise and the neck immediately above the larynx to swell slightly.
- Check the patency of the airway. If continuing to breathe spontaneously there should be free passage of gas and, if apnoeic, hand ventilation should be easy and effective. Capnography is a useful check of satisfactory placement.

If the anaesthetist is not completely satisfied with the position and function of the LMA, it should be taken out immediately and a facemask or ET tube used to continue ventilation.

Removal of the LMA at the end of anaesthesia is discussed in Chapter 4.

*Contraindications to use*

The contraindications are few but important. The most important is that the LMA is not suitable for a patient with a full (or potentially full) stomach or one who has a history of reflux or hiatus hernia.

*Complications*

- The airway can be introduced at too light a level of anaesthesia, resulting in difficulties in passage, trauma to the tissues, coughing, and laryngospasm.
- The epiglottis can become trapped and folded down.
- Malposition results in a compromised airway with the typical signs of obstruction. These are failure of reservoir bag movement, tracheal tug, and intercostal recession in the spontaneously ventilating patient, and high airway pressures and lack of chest expansion on commencement of IPPV. On these occasions the mask must be repositioned or substituted immediately.

As the LMA forms a gas-tight seal with the pharyngeal walls, it should never be connected to a high-pressure gas supply and all the precautions taken when using ET tubes must be adhered to.

## Laryngoscopy and ET intubation

### *Indications for ET intubation*

For oral intubation these are the following:

- when protection of lungs against aspiration of foreign material, especially stomach contents, is necessary;
- when a patient has to be paralysed, e.g. neurosurgery, some types of abdominal surgery;
- when any other form of airway maintenance would be unsatisfactory, e.g. shared airway, prone position;
- when intubation is required to allow certain types of surgery to be possible, e.g. thoracotomies;
- when ventilating unhealthy or damaged lungs intraoperatively.

For nasal intubation the following would be added:

- when an oral tube would be in the way or distort the anatomy, e.g. surgery in or around the mouth;
- when the mouth cannot be opened or its structures are swollen or abnormal;
- also, a nasal tube is more readily tolerated for long-term ventilation in the conscious patient.

*Selecting the right size tube*

Although children obviously differ greatly in size and shape, it is often forgotten that adults are also frequently non-standard. Slavish adherence to rigid rules in selecting tube sizes is therefore bad practice. There are various formulae, nomograms, and charts to help with selection, but they must all be regarded only as a guide.

For adults, men will usually take a size 8 or 9 mm internal diameter (ID) oral tube cut at 22–24 cm, and women an oral 7 or 8 mm ID oral tube cut at 20–22 cm, but there will be obvious exceptions to this rule. Nasal tubes are normally 3–4 cm longer than the correct length oral tube.

Useful formulae as a guide for children are:

- Tube diameter (ID) in mm = 4 + (age in years/4)
- Incisor teeth to carina (cm) = 12 + (age in years ÷ 2)
- Nares to carina (cm) = 15 + (age in years ÷ 2).

In case of difficulty, tubes smaller than the predicted size must be available on all occasions and the correct one selected for the individual patient.

Below 5.5 mm ID, tubes are uncuffed, although uncuffed tubes are also available in larger sizes. The correct size plain tube should pass easily into the trachea, the smallest diameter in its passage in children being the cricoid ring (see Chapter 42). To ensure that there is no compression on the mucosa and cartilage, most books and anaesthetists recommend that there is an audible leak from a plain tube during hand ventilation. This obviously has to be sufficiently small to be compatible with the development of adequate airway pressure and chest expansion.

An apparently increasing trend in current practice is to use uncut tubes and secure them firmly at the appropriate length of insertion. There is nothing against this practice provided that the tube is well secured and not able to slip down into a bronchus or out into the pharynx.

### *Assessing the ease and difficulty of laryngoscopy*

It is impossible to predict absolutely the ease or difficulty of laryngoscopy; all locations where it is undertaken therefore need to be equipped for the worst case scenario. Clinical experience and intuition play a key role in identifying probable difficulties.

Most publications concentrate on predicting difficult intubation, which is obviously important. This account also looks at the prediction of difficulty, but first considers those factors that might indicate that intubation is probably going to be routine. This is not so that a false sense of security is created, but to make it unlikely that trainees will miss a potentially difficult case.

*Prediction of routine intubation*

An adult patient can probably have their larynx visualized and be intubated routinely if:

- he or she can open his or her mouth and protrude the tongue to enable the whole of the uvula and the posterior pharyngeal wall to be seen;
- he or she is not grossly obese;
- he or she has normal dentition or completely absent upper and/or lower dentition;
- he or she has an interdental distance at the incisors of 3.5 cm (approximately two finger breadths in a man);
- he or she looks to have normal external head and neck anatomy;
- he or she can easily adopt the 'sniffing the morning air' position (neck flexion with extension of the head);
- he or she can protrude the lower mandible beyond the maxilla;
- she is not pregnant.

The possession of these features has been found to be very reliable, in the author's clinical practice, for predicting easy laryngoscopy, but it overestimates the number of difficult laryngoscopies encountered. Patients who meet the above criteria can, in the author's opinion, justifiably be given neuromuscular blocking agents immediately after induction of anaesthesia. These guidelines do not of course rule out some rare possibility causing difficulty, for which one should always be prepared.

For the novice anaesthetist, all patients who do not fulfil the above criteria should be assumed to possess a potentially difficult airway, accepting that not all will. It is better to be well prepared for difficulties. The importance of this preparation in terms of both the mind and the equipment cannot be overemphasized. Capnography is essential if a difficult intubation is anticipated. The problems of pregnancy are described separately in Chapter 45.

*The prediction of difficult laryngoscopy*

Like most things in medicine, there is no substitute for taking a history and examining the patient. General features of concern suggesting difficult intubation are given in Table 7.1 and specific medical problems suggesting difficult intubation are given in Table 7.2.

None of the published clinical tests for predicting difficult laryngoscopy has ever been found to have anything close to 100% specificity and 100% sensitivity when applied by subsequent investigators. There are, however, two that provide useful information and have found a place in the clinical practice of many anaesthetists.

*The thyromental distance*

This is the distance between the upper border of the thyroid cartilage and the bony point of the chin measured along the submental surface (Figure 7.4). Short distances indicate an anterior larynx. Given normal mouth opening and neck movements, a distance of over about 7 cm in the adult is usually associated with adequate laryngoscopy. In clinical practice, depending on the size of the hand, this is often approximated as the total width of the anaesthetist's first, middle, and ring fingers (big men) or the first, second, ring, and little fingers (small women).

| **Table 7.1. General features of concern suggesting difficult intubation** |
|---|
| A history of previous difficult intubation |
| Abnormal facial anatomy |
| High palate with crowded teeth |
| Loose teeth |
| Small mouth |
| Reduced jaw opening with small interdental distance |
| Large, protuberant upper teeth, especially if capped |
| Receding chin/short mandible (may be concealed by a beard) |
| Immobile neck and restricted head movement |
| Obesity, especially around the face and if associated with large jowls |
| A short or bull neck |
| A larynx that does not rise and fall normally on swallowing |

| **Table 7.2. Specific medical problems suggesting difficult intubation** |
|---|
| Facial scarring or contractures |
| Acute infections of the mouth: inflamed tissues are swollen and bleed very easily |
| Disease of the upper airways or larynx |
| Ankylosing spondylitis (rigid neck) |
| Rheumatoid arthritis (may be stiff jaw and neck, may be unstable neck) |
| Acromegaly (soft tissue overgrowth with huge tongue) |
| Trauma to the neck (external signs may give little indication of internal soft tissue swelling or haemorrhage) |

*Direct pharyngoscopy*

This useful and easy test is correctly associated with the name of Mallampati who published on it in 1985. He originally described three classes of pharyngeal visibility and this has since been extended to four and contracted to two by other authors. Probably the easiest and most sensible scheme is to sit in front of the

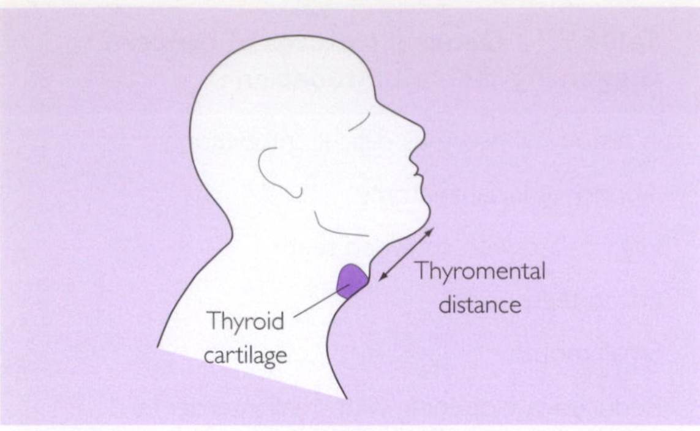


**Figure 7.4.** The thyromental distance. This is measured from the upper border of the anterior part of the thyroid cartilage to the point of the chin.

patient and ask them to open their mouth and stick their tongue out. If the faucial pillars, soft palate, posterior pharyngeal wall and uvula are visible, laryngoscopy will probably not be difficult; if only the hard palate is visible it probably will be difficult (Figure 7.5).

### The technique of laryngoscopy

This section assumes a fit, starved, elective adult patient. Laryngoscopy can begin when the patient is unconscious and paralysed or, if breathing spontaneously, when a suitable depth of anaesthesia has been achieved that obtunds laryngeal reflexes.

#### *Equipment*

The following are required to be present and checked before starting:

1. Masks and airways of appropriate size.
2. Powerful suction.
3. Two laryngoscopes; general principles of using laryngoscopes are:
   - check the intended instrument before use for action and light
   - always have a spare one available
   - have some spare blades available
   - be gentle: do not apply undue force to the tissues and do not lever on the teeth.

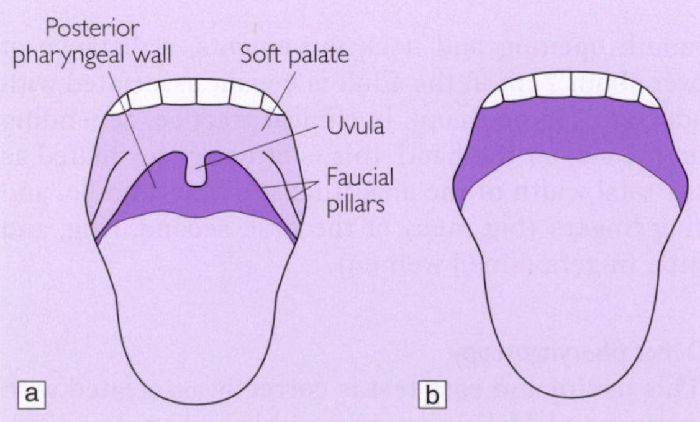


**Figure 7.5.** A view of the mouth and oropharynx with the tongue extended. In (a) the faucial pillars, uvula, and soft palate are visible; in (b) they are not. (Adapted from Mallampati SR. *Can Anaesth Soc J* 1985;32:429.)

4. ET tubes: sized as described earlier, but with smaller sizes always immediately available.
5. Appropriate connections and breathing system.
6. Adjuncts for difficult intubation and emergency airway equipment.

#### *Procedure for oral intubation in an anaesthetized patient*

First be confident that you can maintain an airway easily, with the patient either being ventilated on a facemask or breathing spontaneously. Raise the fractional inspired oxygen to increase the quantity of oxygen in the lungs; if you anticipate difficulty or if you are trying to intubate for a second time, raise it to 100% while ensuring unconsciousness by other means.

Successful laryngoscopy is very dependent on head position. Traditionally, two positions are recognized, as shown in Figure 7.6, originally called the 'classic' and 'amended' positions. The classic position was described by Jackson in 1913 as follows: 'The patient's head must be in full extension, with the vertex firmly pushed down towards the feet of the patient, so as to throw the neck upward and bring the occiput down as close as possible to the cervical vertebrae.' This position is shown in Figure 7.6a. With the possible addition of a sandbag under the shoulders, this is the ideal position for establishing an emergency transtracheal airway or tracheostomy. The drawback to this position is that it involves tension on all the anterior structures of the neck, increases the distance of the larynx from the teeth, and renders the larynx rather immobile.

The amended position (Figure 7.6b) was described some years later. The essential difference is that, although in both the patient lies supine with his or her scapulae flat on the trolley or operating table, in the amended position the head is raised at least 10 cm by a

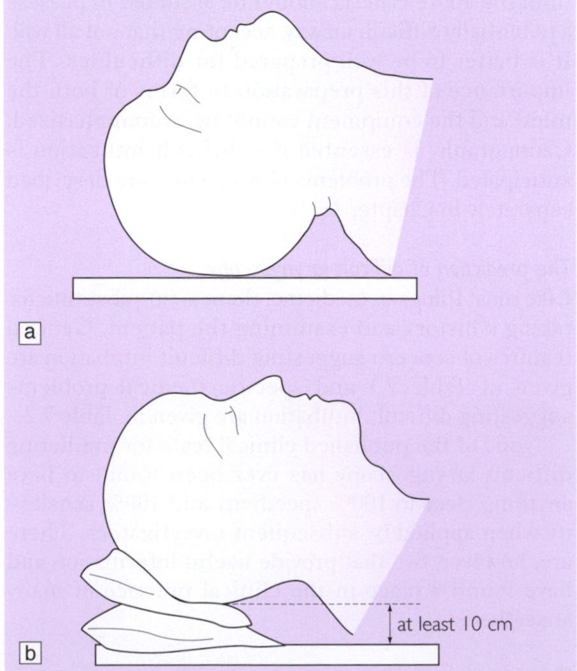


**Figure 7.6.** The position of the head and neck for laryngoscopy and intubation. (a) The 'classic' position and (b) the 'amended' position which is the usual position in current practice.

firm pillow. This allows the lower neck to flex and the intubating position is achieved by extending the atlanto-occipital joint. This technique puts no tension on the muscles of the anterior neck, the distance from the teeth to the glottis is shortened, and, perhaps most importantly of all, the larynx is much more mobile and its position can be adjusted by external manipulation for optimal conditions. It also allows cricoid pressure to be applied more easily. Successful laryngoscopy for insertion of an oral tube occurs when points A, B, and C are in the same line (Figure 7.7). The amended position shown, with the occiput on a pillow, the neck flexed, and the head extended at the atlanto-occipital joint, is the best for routine laryngoscopy and intubation. For rigid bronchoscopy, the trachea has to be in the same axial line as A, B, and C, and for this the classic position with the neck and head extended is required (Figure 7.6a).

Open the patient's mouth by crossing the thumb and first finger of the right hand to push the teeth apart (Figure 7.8) and hold the laryngoscope in the left hand. Avoiding the teeth and not catching the lips, introduce the laryngoscope blade into the right hand side of the mouth, slide it gently down the tongue, and retract the tongue to the left, so that the blade and the handle of the laryngoscope are in the midsagittal plane. Advance the blade until the epiglottis is seen and get the tip into the vallecula (Figure 7.9). Lifting the laryngoscope in the direction of the long axis of the handle (note: not levering on the upper teeth) reveals first the oesophagus as a closed slit and then the laryngeal inlet (Figure 7.10). Backward and upward external pressure on the larynx from an assistant may improve the view. If the larynx cannot be visualized easily, proceed as described later under 'Airway problems'.

Pick up the tube in the right hand, and advance the tip and cuff (if present) through the rima glottidis to the appropriate distance, as determined by the tube markings. Inflate the cuff while ventilating the chest and put in enough air just to prevent a leak.

To test for correct position proceed as follows:

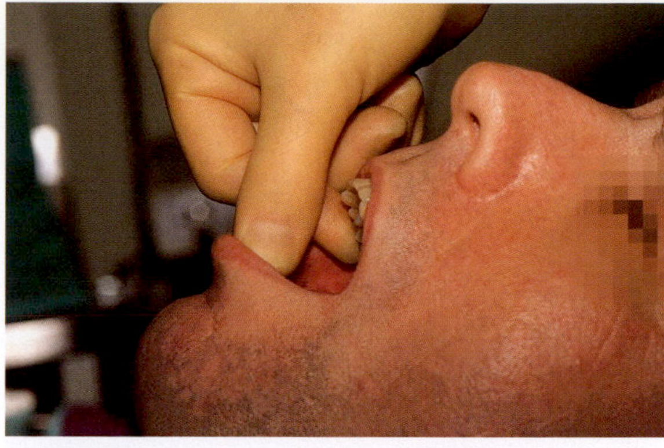

**Figure 7.8.** Opening a patient's mouth before laryngoscopy by use of the thumb and forefinger of the right hand. The thumb is applied to the right lower canine and the forefinger to the right upper premolars. This allows maximum space for introduction of the laryngoscope blade.

- Check that on inflation both sides of the chest rise and that they fall easily when the inflation pressure is removed.
- Auscultate both sides of the chest in the axillae for the presence of breath sounds and the epigastrium for an absence of gurgling.
- Connect the capnograph and observe a normal trace.
- Observe that the oxygen saturation is maintained.

Although the 'gold standard' for confirming ET placement, capnographs still have some drawbacks:

- It is essential to observe an alveolar plateau because the stomach often has a $CO_2$-containing gas bubble which will record on a numerical readout.
- Capnography will not indicate endobronchial intubation.

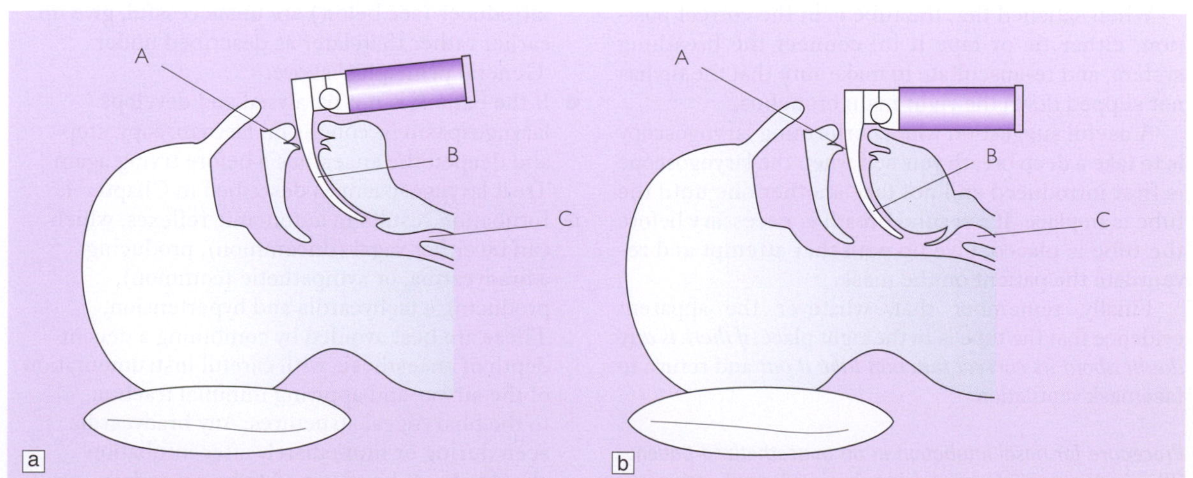


**Figure 7.7.** The line of sight between the interdental space and the larynx (A, incisors; B, horizon of laryngoscope; C, vocal cords). Note that during laryngoscopy in a normal person (a), the mouth opens and the tongue is swept away from the midline by the laryngoscope and hence points A, B, and C can be aligned more easily than appears in the diagram. (b) The obvious effects of a receding chin, which pushes the tongue backwards and provides little space for its retraction by the laryngoscope.

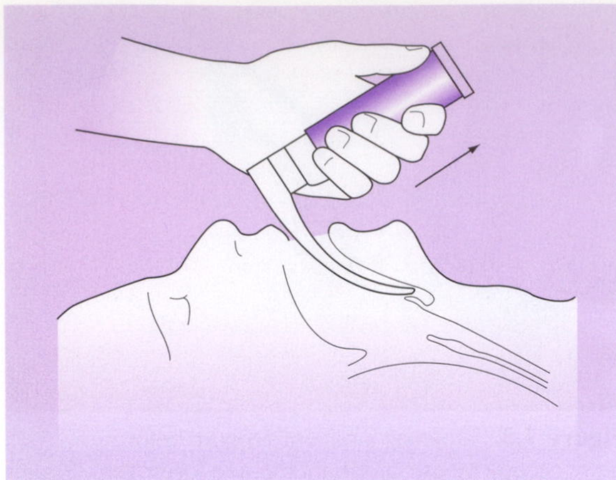

**Figure 7.9.** Diagrammatic representation of the tip of the laryngoscope in the vallecula showing the direction of lift that should be applied along the axis of the laryngoscope handle.

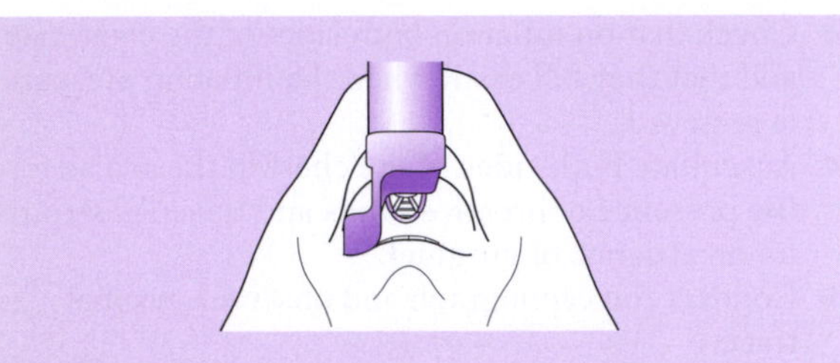

**Figure 7.10.** An ideal view of the larynx at laryngoscopy.

- They sometimes fail to work because of secretions in the sampling line entering the measuring cell.

Another reliable test of ET placement is to aspirate the ET tube with a 50-ml catheter nozzle syringe. If the tube is in the trachea, the syringe will fill with air easily; if it is in the oesophagus, the walls collapse and aspiration is difficult or impossible.

When satisfied that the tube is in the correct position, either tie or tape it in, connect the breathing system, and re-auscultate to make sure that the tip has not slipped down the right main bronchus.

A useful suggestion when performing laryngoscopy is to take a deep breath yourself when the laryngoscope is first introduced and not take another one until the tube is in place. If a second breath is necessary before the tube is placed, give up with that attempt and re-ventilate the patient on the mask.

Finally, remember that, whatever the apparent evidence that the tube is in the right place, *if there is any doubt about its correct function take it out* and return to facemask ventilation.

*Procedure for nasal intubation in an anaesthetized patient*

The indications for nasal intubation have been given earlier. If nasal intubation is planned, the patient should have had some vasoconstricting nose-drops preoperatively to shrink the nasal mucosa. Always lubricate the tube well.

Contraindications to nasal intubation are:

- head injuries, especially to the base of skull;
- obstructed nasal passages, large adenoids, or polyps;
- coagulopathy;
- active sinusitis.

Proceed initially as described above for oral intubation and introduce the nasal tube into the nose and pass it as described earlier for the insertion of a nasopharyngeal airway. In an uncomplicated case, with the laryngoscope in position in the left hand, the tube will be seen to appear in the nasopharynx and can be advanced through the cords by a minor movement of the head or the use of forceps. Once it has negotiated the change of direction into the pharynx at the back of the nose, a nasal tube has a more natural passage to the trachea because the bends required are less acute than for those of an oral tube (Figure 7.11). Locate and test the position of the tube as described above for an oral tube.

***Complications of laryngoscopy and intubation***

- The most dire and serious is unrecognized oesophageal intubation.
- The second is to press on mindlessly if you cannot intubate. Get help early and do not be afraid to wake the patient up. An ongoing battle between the patient's airway and the anaesthetist usually results in damaged tissues and, more seriously, hypoxia.
- The laryngoscope can produce damage to any of the soft tissues that it encounters and can damage the teeth. If a tooth is damaged, rescue it or the fragment before it enters the trachea.
- When introducing the laryngoscope, if the epiglottis cannot be seen either the blade is not far enough in or is too short, or it is in too far and below the epiglottis. If advancing the blade, withdrawing it, or using a longer blade does not result in a satisfactory view, proceed as described later for failed or difficult intubation.
- If laryngoscopy is difficult and simple measures such as repositioning the head or using an introducer (see below) are unsuccessful, give up earlier rather than later as described under 'General principles' above.
- If the patient is not paralysed and develops laryngospasm or coughs on laryngoscopy, stop and deepen the anaesthesia before trying again. Treat laryngospasm as described in Chapter 4.
- Intubation results in autonomic reflexes, which can be either vagal (uncommon), producing a bradycardia, or sympathetic (common), producing a tachycardia and hypertension. These are best avoided by combining a decent depth of anaesthesia with careful instrumentation of the airway and applying minimal traction to the pharyngeal structures. Any bradycardia seen during or immediately after intubation should always be assumed to be secondary to hypoxia until proved otherwise. The usual rule applies to the ET tube: *if in doubt, take it out*.
- People with untreated hypertension are particularly prone to intubation hypertension.

- The passage of the tube can damage the vocal cords and high inflation pressures in the cuff can damage the trachea.
- The tube can always change its position, slipping forwards to irritate the carina or enter a bronchus, or slipping backwards to enter the pharynx.
- The head and neck movements produced during intubation can cause damage to the cervical vertebrae and spinal cord (especially in rheumatoid arthritis and trauma patients).
- There is sometimes difficulty in passing the nasal tube from the direction of the floor of the nose round the bend into the pharynx (Figure 7.11). Force at this point can push the tube under the mucosa of the posterior pharyngeal wall with subsequent haemorrhage, haematoma formation, and swelling. If it will not go easily, remove the tube and re-oxygenate the patient. Then pass a nasogastric tube or flexible introducer through the nasal cavity and, when it appears in the oropharynx, pull it forwards with forceps into the mouth. Slide the nasal tube over the introducer and try to rail-road it into position. If this does not work, seek senior help or abandon the nasal route.

## Elective tracheostomy

Tracheostomy tubes (Figure 6.43) and the indications for tracheostomy are described in Chapter 6. An elective tracheostomy can be undertaken as a surgical operation or carried out percutaneously (either from the skin inwards or the trachea outwards) with a special set of introducers and dilators.

As a surgical procedure, the patient is usually already intubated and anaesthetized and he is positioned supine with his neck extended, often with a sandbag under the shoulders (Figure 7.6a). In principle, the operation proceeds as shown diagrammatically in Figure 7.12. Immediately before incising the trachea, oxygenate the patient on 100% $O_2$ and be sure that the equipment is present to intubate the patient orally again if necessary. Once the trachea is incised (sometimes the ET tube cuff is punctured), or just before it is incised, let down the cuff and pull the ET tube back (but try to keep the tip below the cords) and allow the surgeon to insert the tracheostomy tube. After a successful insertion, inflate the tracheostomy tube cuff and connect the ventilator tubing to the tracheostomy tube. Make sure that the lungs ventilate properly, particularly checking that the tip of the tracheostomy tube is not down the right main bronchus.

Establishing a tracheostomy with a percutaneous kit follows the same principles of safety but is usually carried out on the intensive care unit or at the beginning or end of surgery by the anaesthetist. An example of such a kit is shown in Figure 7.13.

The complications and longer-term management of a tracheostomy are described later, under 'Airway problems' (page 84).

## Emergency airways

It is an undeniable fact that, if the passage of oxygen to the lungs ceases, the person is essentially dying until the flow is restored. Emergency airways are designed to support life in dire situations when conventional methods of airway management have failed or cannot be used. A large number of devices and methods have been described. Three are outlined here. All involve passage of a device to carry 100% $O_2$ through the relatively avascular and easily palpated cricothyroid membrane (see Chapter 6), and all require the patient to be positioned supine with the neck extended. Although only described briefly here, none is without complications. All are much easier to perform in the tall thin person than in the short fat person (Figure 7.14). The golden rule is to stay in the midline. Emergency airways supply inspiratory oxygen below the vocal cords: expiration occurs via the larynx (unless a cuffed tube is inserted).

### *Needle tracheostomy*

The principle of this technique is to pass an intravenous cannula through the cricothyroid membrane and to attach it to a high-pressure oxygen supply for intermittent ventilation. There is obviously a wide range of components that can be combined for this purpose and two suitable systems are shown in Figure 7.15. The procedure is carried out as follows.

Connect two pieces of oxygen tubing to a T or Y connector and the other end of one of the pieces of

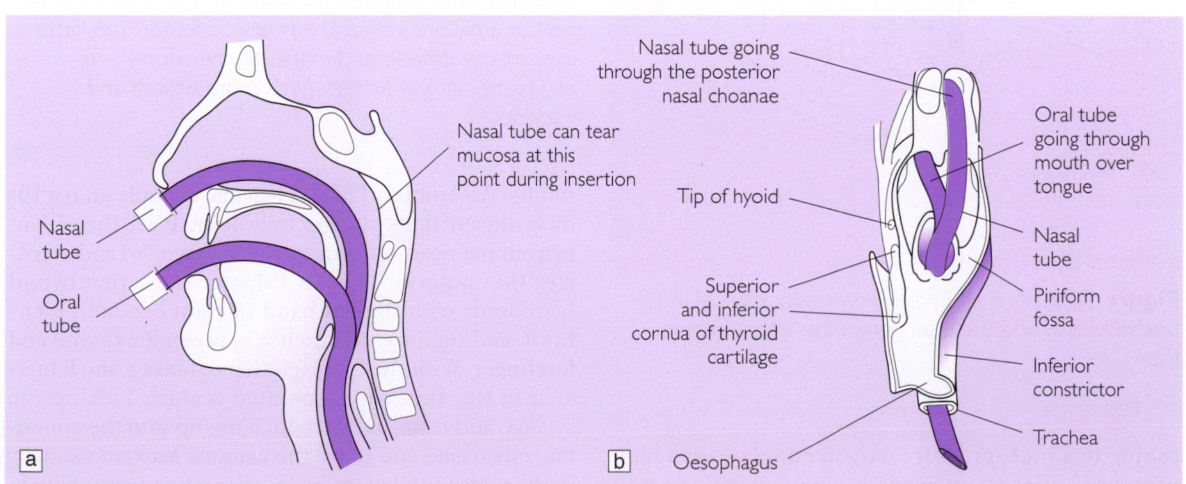


**Figure 7.11.** Nasal and oral tubes seen in (a) lateral and (b) posterior views. Note the more acute angle of the oral tube as it passes from the mouth to the trachea.

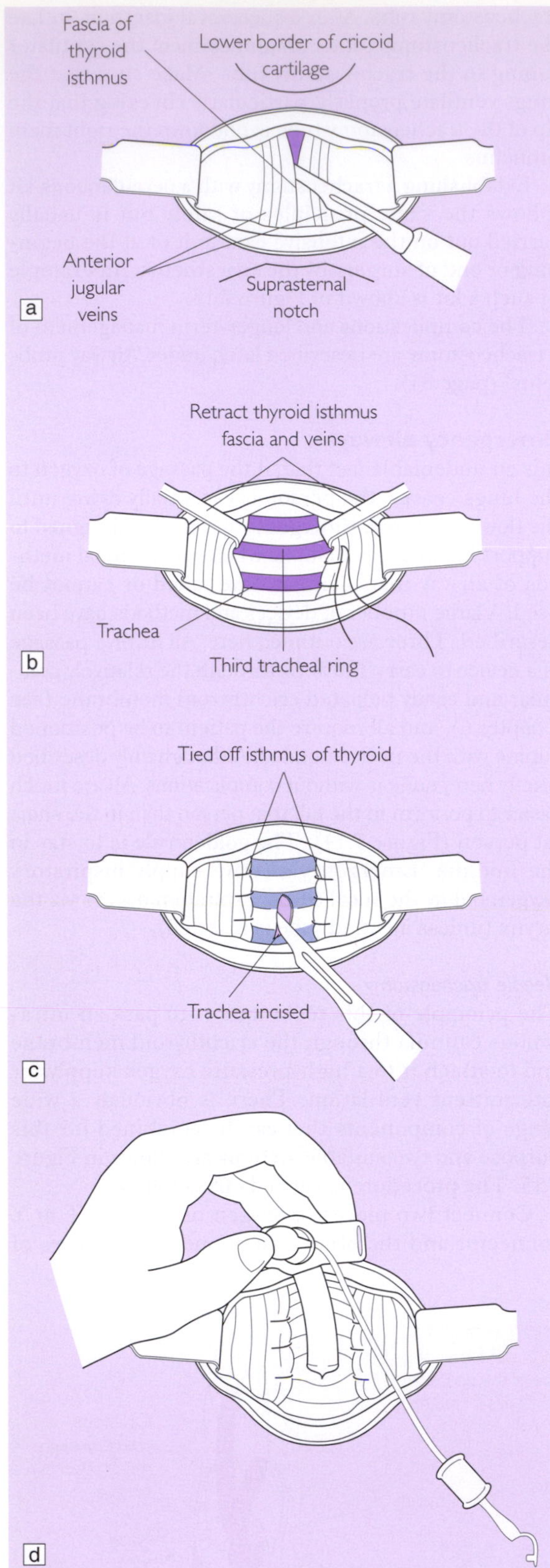


**Figure 7.12.** A diagrammatic representation of a tracheostomy and the insertion of the tracheostomy tube.

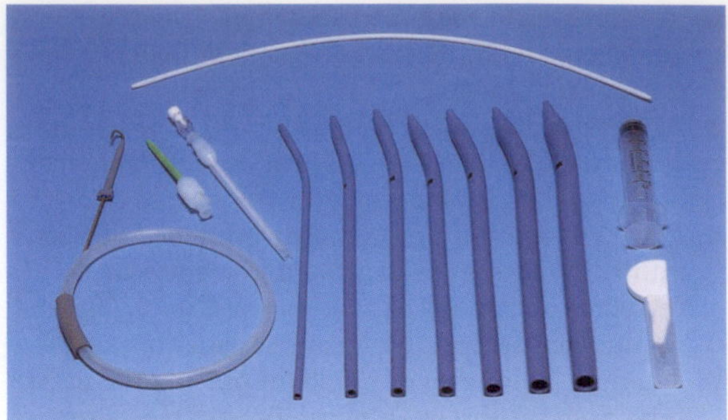

**Figure 7.13.** A percutaneous tracheostomy kit.

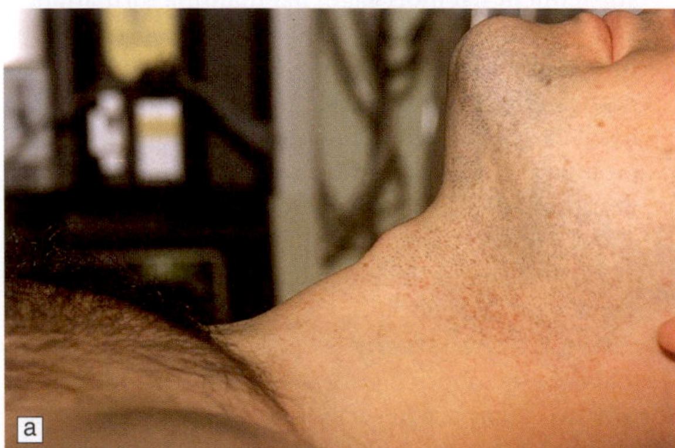


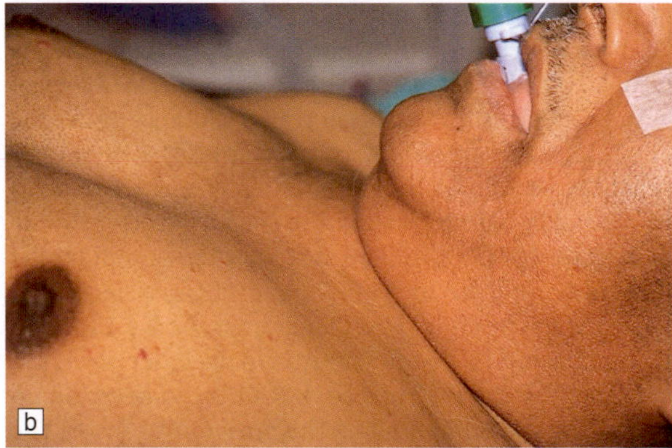


**Figure 7.14.** An example of (a) a long thin neck in extension with well-defined anatomy and (b) a short fat neck in a patient with a fixed cervical flexion. The latter obscures landmarks and makes tracheostomy and emergency airway access much more difficult and hazardous.

tubing to a high-pressure oxygen supply (e.g. a high pressure outlet on an anaesthesia machine or a wall outlet) or the common gas outlet of the anaesthesia machine, and ensure a free flow of oxygen down the tubing. Assemble a 12- or 14-gauge cannula onto a 10-ml syringe with its plunger fully down. Place the patient in a supine position with the neck extended and sterilize the anterior neck. Palpate the cricothyroid membrane with the left hand (if right handed), identify it, and stabilize the trachea between the thumb and forefinger. With the free right hand, make a small incision in the skin with a pointed scalpel. Pick up the syringe and cannula, introduce the tip into the subcutaneous tissue and move the cannula forward caudally in the midsagittal plane at 45°, aspirating continuously. When the trachea is entered, air is aspirated. Release the trachea and, using the left hand, push the plastic

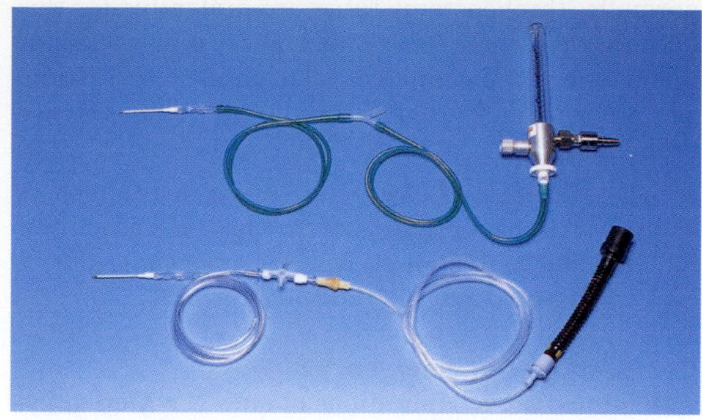

**Figure 7.15.** Examples of two emergency needle tracheostomy kits. The upper one is attached to a high-pressure $O_2$ outlet and the lower one to the common gas outlet on the anaesthetic machine. Note that both arrangements incorporate a T connector. This allows patient ventilation when closed and, when open, prevents the build-up of pressure within the system by allowing the high-pressure $O_2$ to vent to the atmosphere.

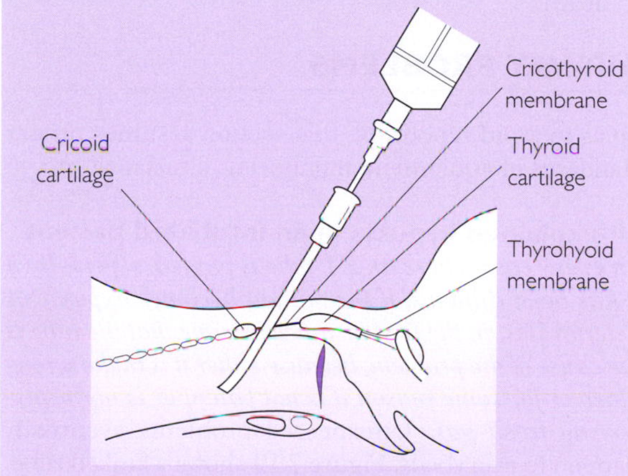


**Figure 7.16.** A diagrammatic representation of the passage of a cannula or Tuohy needle into the trachea through the cricothyroid membrane.

cannula off the metal needle (Figure 7.16). Detach the needle from the syringe and aspirate again from the plastic cannula to confirm tracheal entry. Connect the free end of the oxygen tubing to the cannula. Ventilate the patient by intermittently occluding the free port of the T or Y connector by closing it for 1 second (by thumb) and releasing for 4 seconds. An adequate $Pa\text{O}_2$ can be maintained only for minutes by this method, and it should only ever be used as a temporizing solution.

There are three very important aspects of needle tracheostomy that bear emphasis:

1. The kit must be available for use with components known to fit together before an emergency occurs. Scrabbling around to lash up a system in the heat of the moment is poor practice.
2. After the cannula is introduced into the trachea, an assistant needs to be given the job of holding it in position so that it neither kinks at its entry site nor flies out backwards when the flow is directed through it.
3. There must be a vent in the system that allows the escape of gas in a fail-safe manner to prevent the inadvertent build-up of pressure.

*Mini-tracheostomy*

This is a commercially available set intended primarily for postoperative management of patients after thoracic surgery, which places an uncuffed 4-mm plastic tube into the trachea via the cricothyroid membrane. It has the advantage of all the necessary parts being available as a kit (except the $O_2$ supply connection which can come from the anaesthesia machine common gas outlet). Its insertion follows the principles described above and below. The procedure and insertion of the tube over its introducer are as shown in Figure 7.17.

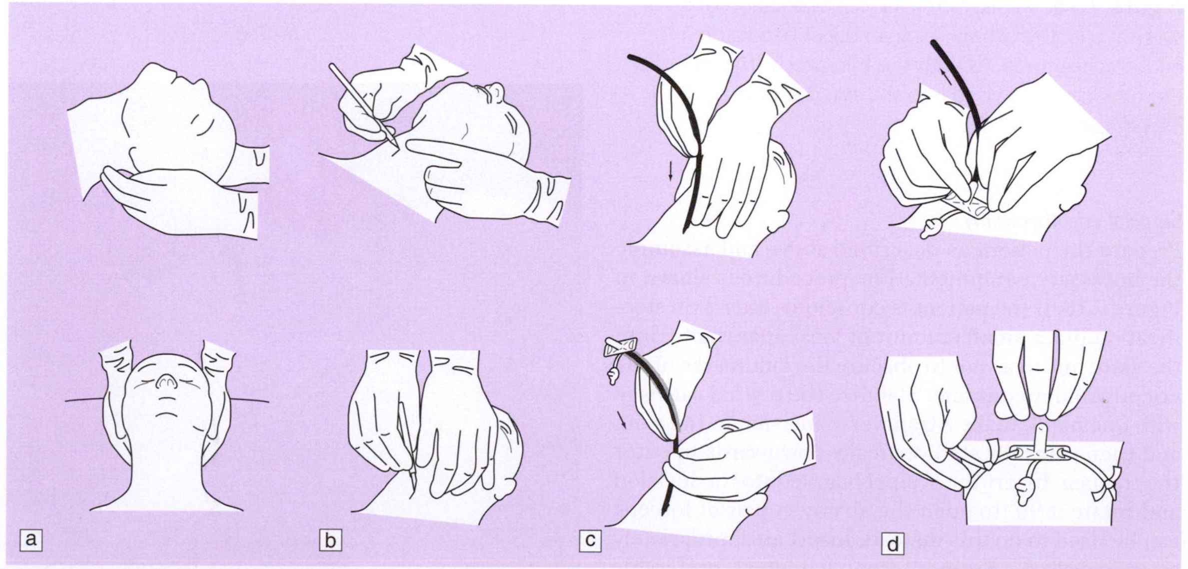


**Figure 7.17.** Establishing a mini-tracheostomy using a Mini-Trach kit: (a) neck extended and straight; (b) marking and incising cricothyroid membrane; (c) inserting the introducer and rail-roading tube; (d) pushing the tube into the trachea and securing. Once inserted, check the position of the tube by passage of a suction catheter or aspirating with a large syringe.

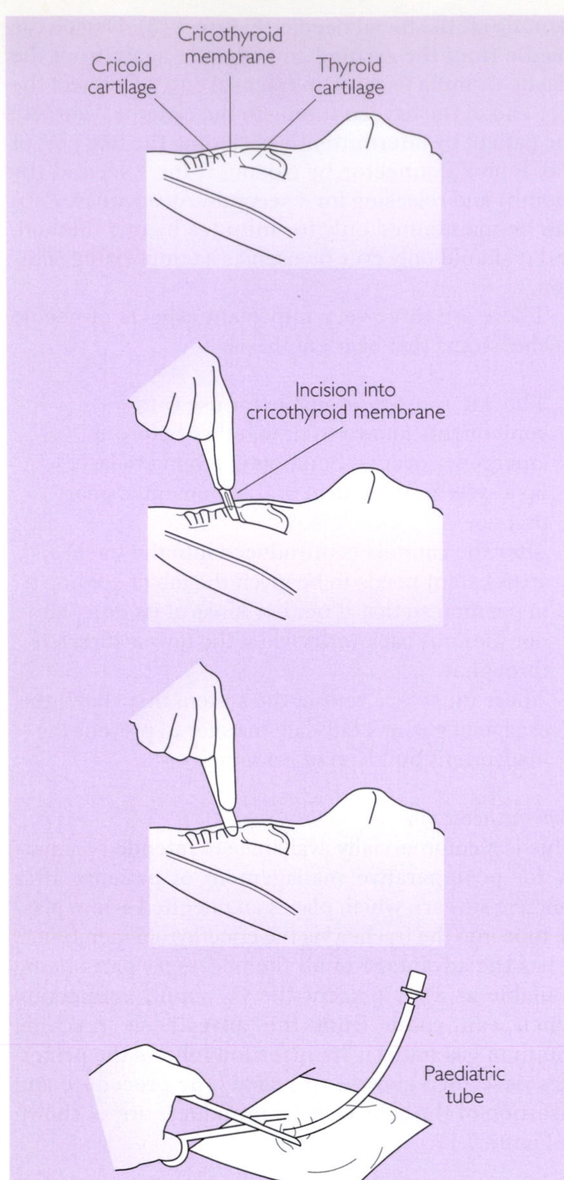


**Figure 7.18.** A diagrammatic representation of a surgical cricothyrotomy using an uncut paediatric endotracheal tube. As with the Mini-trach (Figure 7.17), the tube can be passed into the trachea over an introducer.

*Surgical cricothyrotomy*

Prepare the patient as described above and assemble the necessary equipment. The procedure is shown in Figure 7.18. If the patient is conscious, after skin sterilization put a small amount of local anaesthetic into the skin, but so as not to obscure the landmarks of the cricothyroid membrane. Stabilize the thyroid cartilage with one hand, make a transverse incision in the skin, and then carefully stab vertically downwards to enter the trachea. Insert the scalpel handle into the incision and rotate it 90° to open the airway. A pair of forceps can be used to do this instead. Insert an appropriately sized (usually 4 – 5 mm internal diameter), preferably cuffed, tracheostomy or ET tube vertically through the incision, then direct it downwards into the trachea and advance it the appropriate distance. After checking its patency, attach the oxygen supply and ventilate normally. Tracheostomy tubes are preferable for this because they are better shaped, possess an obturator that reduces the chance of false passage formation, and are less likely to go down too far and intubate a bronchus.

Whatever form of emergency airway is established, always watch the movement of the chest and auscultate for adequate ventilation. Whenever practicable allow a capnograph to sample expired gas.

***Complications of emergency airways***

The immediate complications of emergency cricothyrotomy using the three methods above are as follows:

- incorrect placement and creation of a false passage in the tissues;
- haemorrhage;
- pneumothorax, surgical and mediastinal emphysema, and other forms of barotrauma;
- perforation of the posterior wall of the trachea, oesophagus, and other surrounding structures;
- inadequate ventilation leading to hypoxia and death.

## AIRWAY PROBLEMS

So as to avoid repetition, this section assumes proper standards of equipment, monitoring, assistance, etc.

### Unexplained hypoxia in an intubated patient

*In every case where an ET tube is passed, especially if it has been difficult, if the patient becomes hypoxic or deteriorates, in the first instance assume that the tube is the cause of the problem, because either it is in the wrong place or for some reason it is not patent or is not transferring fresh gas.* Unexpected problems eventually happen to everybody. Figure 7.19 shows a kinked tube. One of the simplest and most reliable tests of tube patency is to pass a lubricated bougie (see Figure 6.46) down the lumen. Remember the maxim: if in doubt, take it out.

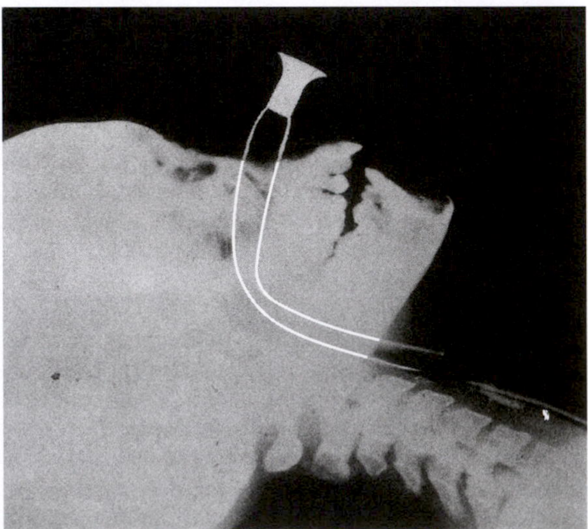

**Figure 7.19.** Example of a kinked endotracheal tube. (Adapted from Gillespie NA. *Endotracheal Anaesthesia*. University of Wisconsin Press, 1941.)

On a number of occasions, hypoxia develops in an intubated patient whose ventilation was previously satisfactory. When this happens, always briefly hand ventilate to ensure the patency of the airway and to check the feel of the lungs. If these are normal, the development of the problem often guides the anaesthetist towards the likely cause. Hypoxia of the tissues can result from respiratory or cardiovascular causes. Table 7.3 is a logical method of classifying the possible difficulties, which is useful as an *aide-memoire* when rehearsing critical incident procedures. Do not forget the option of ventilating the patient on fresh air with a resuscitation bag, if there is any doubt at all concerning the oxygen content of the inspired gas.

### Difficulty with facemasks

There is a wealth of literature on difficult intubation and comparatively little on difficulty with facemasks. Not infrequently, patients who are difficult to handle on a facemask are straightforward to intubate, particularly if edentulous. The following features might suggest that facemask ventilation could be difficult:

- abnormal facial anatomy;
- a beard;
- receding chin;
- large tongue;
- heavy jowls;
- thick-set, stiff, bull neck;
- no teeth, or isolated or loose teeth;
- problems with access to face and ability to hold mask on properly.

Abnormal facial anatomy, isolated teeth, and absence of teeth may make a good fit between the mask and face impossible. In edentulous patients, the absence of teeth allows the mandible to compress soft tissues into the oral cavity and pharynx, and the lips to occlude the anterior nares, rendering airway maintenance virtually impossible without an airway (Figure 7.20).

**Table 7.3. Classification of the causes of hypoxia in an intubated patient**

| |
|---|
| **Failure of oxygen supply** |
| Hypoxic mixture |
| Low fresh gas flow |
| Disconnection |
| Endotracheal tube fallen out |
| **Failure of adequate fresh gas to reach the trachea** |
| Kinked tube |
| Compressed tube |
| Blocked tube or other foreign body |
| Severe respiratory depression or respiratory arrest (spontaneously breathing patient) |
| Ventilator failure (patient on IPPV) |
| **Failure of gas delivered to trachea to reach the blood** |
| Pneumothorax |
| Bronchospasm |
| Asthma attack |
| Pulmonary oedema/collapse/consolidation |
| Surgical retractors |
| Aspiration pneumonitis |
| **Failure of blood to reach the alveoli** |
| Severe hypotension |
| Cardiac arrest |
| Pulmonary embolism (of any cause) |
| Wrongly placed surgical ligature |
| Excessive ventilation pressure |
| Other causes of high intrathoracic pressure |

IPPV, intermittent positive-pressure ventilation

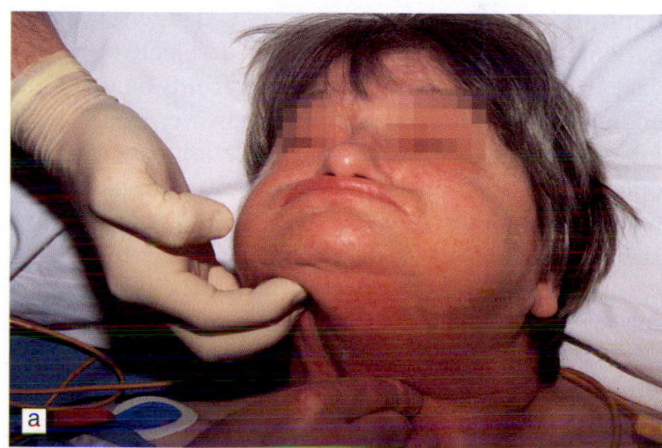


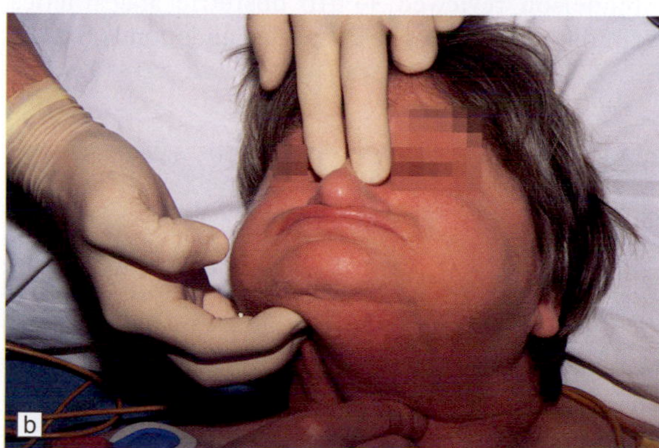


**Figure 7.20.** An edentulous face after induction of anaesthesia. In this patient, cricoid pressure is being applied because of the presence of a hiatus hernia. Note in (a) that traction on the mandible compresses the lower and upper jaws, forcing the lips forwards. This makes the facial anatomy fit badly on to a conventional facemask and the upper lip partially occludes the anterior nares. The fingers compressing the nose in (b) demonstrate the effect of the application of a facemask. It can be seen that there is now complete occlusion of both the oral and the nasal passages. In such a situation, the use of an artificial airway is essential.

Apart from very short procedures (e.g. waiting for a neuromuscular blocking agent to work), a badly fitting facemask needs to be changed for an alternative such as an LMA or ET tube as soon as possible. The situation may be eased temporarily by switching to 100% $O_2$, increasing the FGF, and, if ventilating by hand, using frequent, low-volume bag compressions to maintain oxygenation.

If you are having difficulty maintaining an airway while using a facemask, either with or without an airway, a good first-line manoeuvre (after making sure that an alternative mask does not fit better) is to hold on to the mask with both hands (Figure 7.21) to optimize the head and neck position while, if necessary, an assistant squeezes the bag and adjusts the valve. This is just one example of the importance of always having a *trained* assistant who knows what to do and recognizes the importance of the problem to be overcome.

Any patient who is thought likely to be difficult to manage on a facemask should be preoxygenated thoroughly before induction to allow maximum time to convert to another technique before hypoxia occurs.

## The patient in danger of aspirating

Aspiration of gastric contents is a danger in every patient without a competent larynx. In elective starved cases (who are not in the at-risk group below), the chance of aspiration occurring is, however, sufficiently low that other factors become more important in the optimal management of the patient. An example of this would be the efforts taken to ensure haemodynamic stability in the prolonged induction of a patient with cardiac disease, which renders the larynx incompetent for some time before the ET tube is in place.

### *Incidence of aspiration*

The incidence of aspiration is difficult to estimate, not least because only cases with significant morbidity or mortality are identified. In his original work, Mendelson reviewed 44 016 obstetric anaesthetics administered over a 13-year period and found 66 cases of aspiration. More recent data reported in 1993, including all patient types, suggest an incidence of aspiration of 1 in 8000 anaesthetics for the American Society of Ansthesiologists (ASA) class I and II patients, and 1 in 343 for ASA III and IV, with an overall mortality for all elective and emergency patients of 1 in 71 829. (See Further Reading Warner *et al.* 1993.) Patients at particular risk of aspiration include those who have:

- abdominal pathology, especially obstruction or ileus;
- delayed gastric emptying (pain, trauma, opioids, alcohol, vagotomy, etc.);
- poor oesophageal sphincter function (especially hiatus hernia);
- reduced laryngeal reflexes (already sedated, altered conscious level, elderly);
- neuromuscular or neurological disease (nerve palsies, autonomic neuropathy);
- reduced conscious level (head injury, sedation, etc.);
- pregnancy;
- a difficult airway (from whatever cause, see earlier);
- metabolic disturbances (uraemia, diabetes).

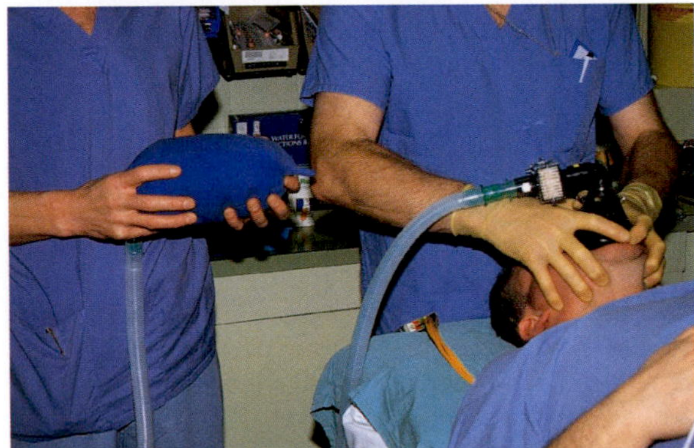

**Figure 7.21.** Two pairs of hands can be better than one. The anaesthetist is using both hands to maintain a difficult airway after an intravenous induction. It is important in this situation to have a properly trained assistant who is able to adjust the gas flows, expiratory valve position, bag compression, etc. and gradually allow the ventilation to be converted from spontaneous breathing to hand ventilation by the reservoir bag.

### *Prophylaxis in routine cases*

Experimental evidence suggests that, if the pH of aspirated material is below 2.5, the lung damage will be much more severe. The pH of the stomach contents can been raised by administration of antacid compounds such as sodium citrate or by histamine $H_2$-receptor antagonists. Both these methods of management do not stop aspiration, but they lessen its consequences. Antacids work directly and immediately. $H_2$-receptor antagonists act within 2 hours of oral administration and within 1 hour of intravenous administration. They do not, however, modify the pH of the existing stomach contents, so they logically should be started 12–18 hours before anaesthesia.

The severity of aspiration pneumonia is greatly dependent on the volume of aspirated material and whether it contains solid food. Low gastric volume with no solid content is therefore preferable. Gastric volume can be reduced by starvation and by the use of gastrointestinal prokinetics (e.g. metoclopramide). There have been innumerable regimens developed and published. The most recent, and most thorough, based on evidence-based medicine, concluded with the recommendations in Table 7.4.

**Table 7.4. Fasting periods to minimize gastric aspiration**

| Ingested material | Minimum fasting period (hours) |
|---|---|
| Clear liquids | 2 |
| Breast milk | 4 |
| Solid food/infant formulae | 8 |

From *Anesthesiology* 1999;90:896

Note that the fasting periods relate to fit patients of all ages with no additional risk factors (see Incidence of aspiration above) and that examples of clear liquids include water, fruit juices without pulp, carbonated beverages, clear tea, and black coffee, but not milk.

Not all hospitals follow these recommendations; trainees should adopt local protocols.

### Prevention of aspiration in at-risk cases

Having taken the prophylactic measures described above (and assuming that there is a nasogastric tube in patients with intestinal obstruction or ileus), there are two approaches:

1. Place a tracheal tube while the patient is still in full consciousness and has a fully competent larynx. Awake intubation is described later.
2. Perform a sitting or rapid sequence induction. A sitting induction, in which gravity is used to prevent passive regurgitation, is not employed frequently in current practice. Rapid sequence induction is considered in detail below.

### Rapid sequence induction

This is a serious undertaking requiring meticulous attention to detail. Proper standards of monitoring and *trained* assistance are assumed. Proceed as follows:

- Check the suction – it must be strong and effective. Have ready:
  - two laryngoscopes, both working;
  - capnograph that is working properly (test on yourself);
  - ET tube, smaller sized ones, and an introducer (Chapter 6, Figure 6.46).
- Make sure that the assistant can perform cricoid pressure correctly. If necessary mark the position of the cricoid on the patient.
- Check that it is the correct patient on a trolley that tips head-down easily.
- Put up a reliable drip.
- Explain the procedure to the patient and let him know what (gentle) cricoid pressure feels like.
- Get the patient to adopt the optimum intubating position.
- Draw up all drugs into labelled syringes. Have spare ampoules.
- Preoxygenate for 3 - 5 min on 100% $O_2$.
- Give the predetermined dose of IV induction agent and, as the patient starts to look drowsy, apply cricoid pressure using the thumb and first finger to push the cricoid vertically downwards to compress the oesophagus (Figure 7.22). Immediately follow with the suxamethonium 1 - 1.5 mg/kg.
- Do not ventilate by mask. As soon as the jaw begins to relax, perform laryngoscopy and intubate.
- Blow up the cuff; ventilate and confirm tube placement clinically and with capnograph.
- When satisfied with the tube position and that the cuff has no leak, release cricoid pressure.
- Fix the tube securely.

The problems that can occur are as follows:

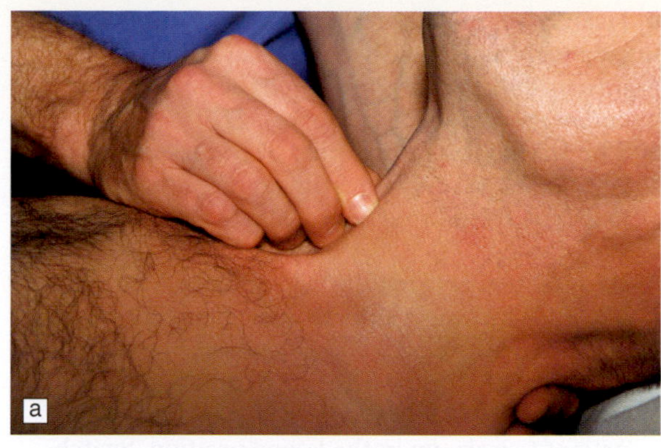


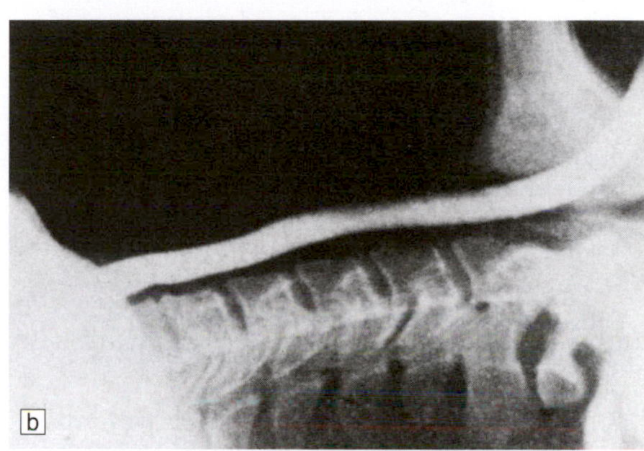


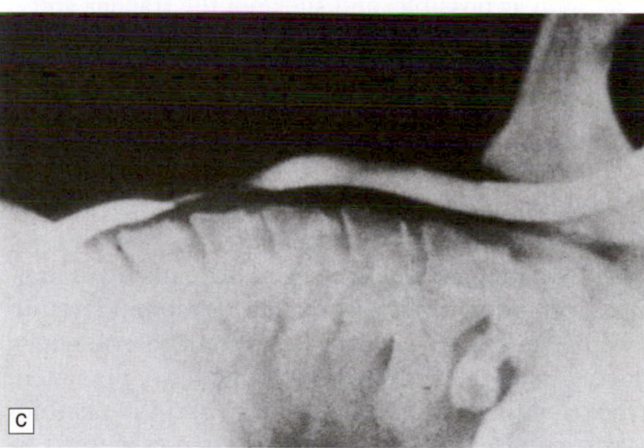


**Figure 7.22.** (a) The application of cricoid pressure. The cricoid is being pressed directly backwards by the thumb and the forefinger of the right hand towards the palm of the left hand, which is supporting the back of the neck. (The fingers of the left hand can just be seen at the bottom of the picture.) Having the second hand behind the neck sometimes makes it easier to move the larynx around at the request of the anaesthetist. Note that the thumb and forefinger are together pushing backwards and are not squeezing the larynx from side to side. If working with an inexperienced assistant, it is often best to mark the position of the cricoid cartilage on the neck before induction of anaesthesia. (b) The oesophagus during a barium swallow and (c) the effect of cricoid pressure. (This technique was originally described by Sellick BA. *Lancet* 1961;ii:404. The radiographs are taken from this article.)

- Haemodynamic instability: treat according to response. The more usual is a fall in blood pressure (especially if shocked), requiring fluids and/or vasopressors/inotropes.
- The larynx may be distorted by badly applied cricoid pressure. If adjusting it, move the assistant s hand yourself to ensure that pressure is maintained.
- If intubation proves difficult and the patient becomes hypoxic, ventilate while maintaining cricoid pressure.
- If two or three good attempts to intubate fail, do not press on. Get immediate help or allow the patient to wake up in the lateral position. Switch on the sucker, ready for immediate use.

#### Management of aspiration

*If aspiration occurs after induction and administration of relaxants and is immediately observed*

- Immediately apply cricoid pressure, suck out the pharynx, and go on to 100% $O_2$. If cricoid pressure is preventing further regurgitation, follow the steps below. If not, turn the patient to the left lateral position, tip the head down and then follow the steps below. The left lateral position makes subsequent laryngoscopy with a left-handed laryngoscope easier than the right-side-down position.
- If the patient is paralysed, immediately perform a laryngoscopy and suck out the trachea and major airways. Then intubate.
- If the patient is not paralysed, maintain oxygenation, wait for relaxation to occur, intubate as soon as possible, and suck out the trachea and major airways. Try not to use vigorous hand ventilation prior to intubation, but ventilation should not be withheld if hypoxia is occurring.
- Consider bronchoscopy if there is any evidence of solid matter or if ventilation is difficult and hypoxia supervenes.

The decision to abandon surgery depends upon individual cases and the reason for the operation. Certainly it would, for example, be unwise to press on with minor, elective surgery if there was immediate, persistent hypoxia with severe bronchospasm and the need for positive end-expiratory pressure. Each case must be assessed on its merits and the balance of priorities.

The subsequent management of aspiration pneumonitis is essentially the same as that for adult respiratory distress syndrome, described in Chapter 17. It should not be forgotten that aspiration may be silent and that the first signs could be unexplained bronchospasm. It can also occur during spontaneous ventilation.

### Unexpectedly difficult or failed intubation

Always remember that the objective of anaesthesia is to enable surgery to occur, and not just to succeed in intubation. Do not press on illogically. If possible, bale out early, and see that the patient comes to no harm. If necessary move quickly to an emergency airway. An awake, unharmed patient is infinitely preferable to an intubated patient with upper airway damage, aspiration, pneumonitis or neurological problems.

There is no universally accepted definition of difficult intubation, but the ASA has defined a difficult intubation as 'insertion of a tracheal tube with conventional laryngoscopy requiring more than 3 attempts and/or insertion requiring over 10 minutes'.

When attempting laryngoscopy, if the full larynx cannot be seen the view can be graded using the classification listed in Table 7.5 and shown in Figure 7.23. If the patient can be neither ventilated on a mask nor intubated, proceed to an emergency airway and wake the patient up. If facemask ventilation is possible, the management can be effectively separated into those patients who are 'elective' and those in whom there is an 'aspiration danger'. *In all cases send for senior help.*

#### Unexpected difficult intubation in elective patients

First get an assistant to move the larynx about; it may come into view. Otherwise, use a McCoy laryngoscope and/or try to place an introducer (see Chapter 6, Figure 6.46) into the trachea by keeping strictly to the midline and the curved tip pointing anteriorly. If you can t see the passage of the tip, *when advancing gently*, if the tip is in the trachea it comes to a stop at less than about 30 cm; if in the oesophagus, it continues beyond 30 cm down into the stomach.

Keep the patient well oxygenated at all times. If intubation remains difficult, try a laryngeal mask. If this is successful, relax and think out the best way forward. There is much to be gained, and nothing to be lost, by allowing the patient to wake up unharmed. Try at all costs not to persist with unsuccessful attempts that are progressively likely to be harmful.

In difficult intubation, the LMA has been used to assist the blind passage of a bougie into the trachea. Also, if a fibreoptic laryngoscope is passed through a properly located laryngeal mask, it may be possible to enter the trachea and slide a previously placed ET tube down the fibreoptic scope, through the LMA and into the trachea. This is not a procedure that should be undertaken lightly and, before proceeding, it must be established that the tube selected will pass over the fibreoptic scope, through the LMA, and be long enough to get the cuff below the cords. One that will do this is the 6-mm Mallinkrodt reinforced ET tube.

**Table 7.5. Classification of laryngoscopic views**

| Grade | View |
|---|---|
| 1 | Most of glottis visible: no difficulty |
| 2 | Only posterior extremity of glottis visible: slight difficulty. Light pressure on the larynx nearly always brings the arytenoids into view, if not the cords |
| 3 | No part of glottis seen, just epiglottis: severe difficulty likely |
| 4 | Not even the epiglottis seen: intubation needs special techniques |

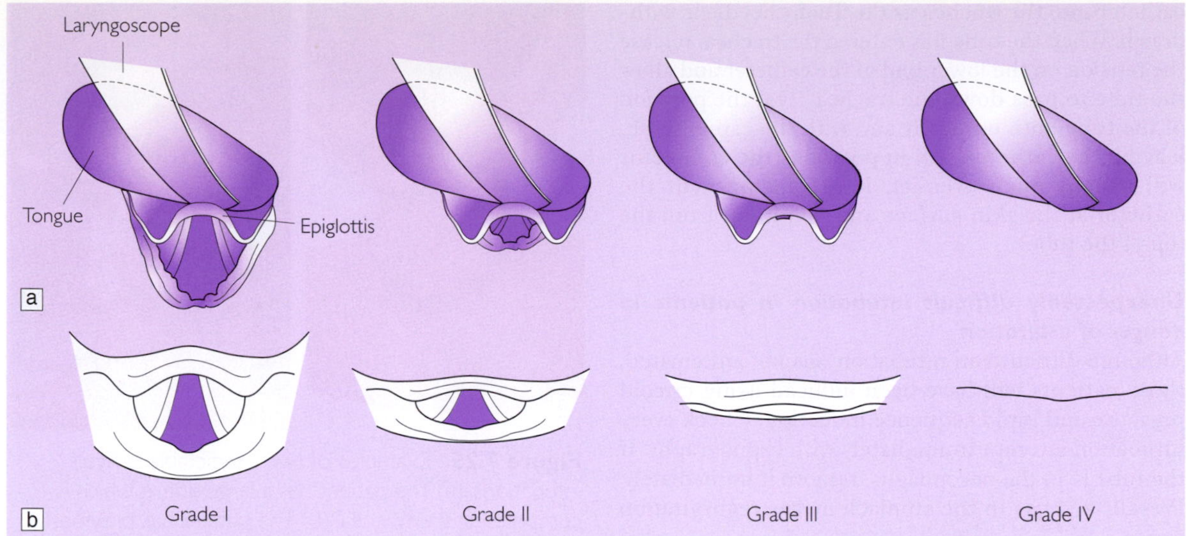


**Figure 7.23.** Various views of the vocal cords at laryngoscopy. (a) A representational view as seen by the anaesthetist which includes the laryngoscope blade (adapted from Cormack and Lehane. *Anaesthesia* 1984;39:1105) (b) Diagrammatic views that are frequently printed on anaesthetic sheets (adapted from Samsoon and Young. *Anaesthesia* 1987;42:487). The incidence of difficult intubation (grades 3 and 4) is probably about 1–3% but, with experienced anaesthetists (not necessarily trainees), the combination of 'can't intubate, can't ventilate', has an incidence measured as a fraction of 0.1%.

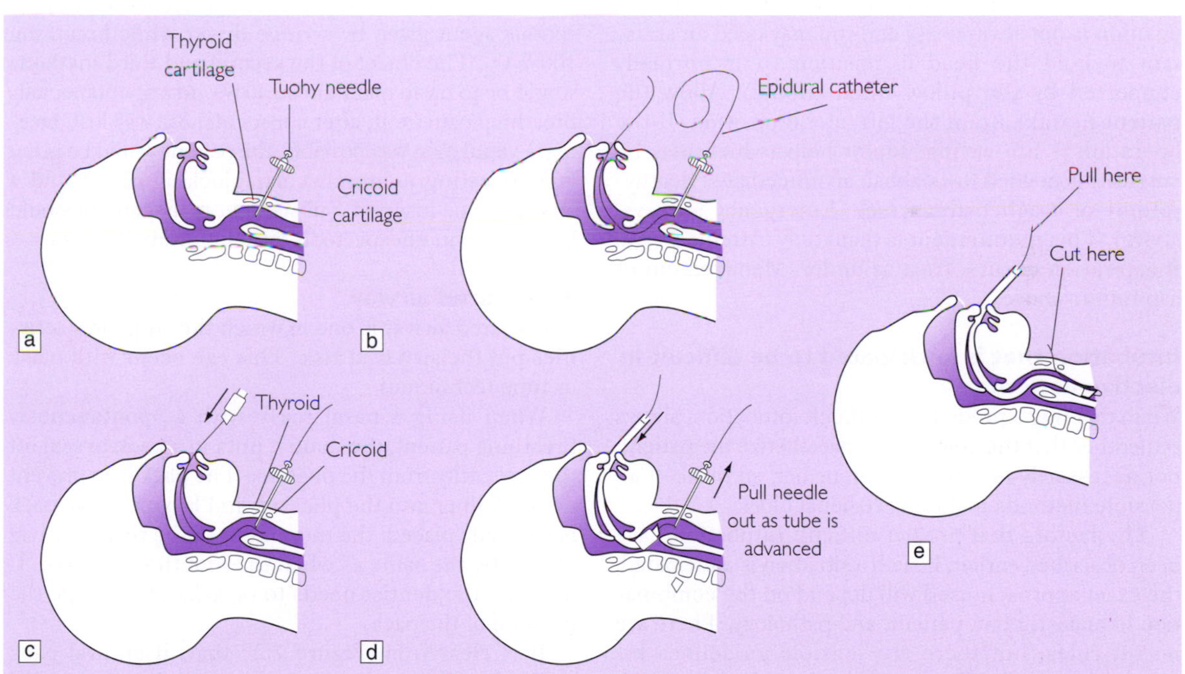


**Figure 7.24.** Endotracheal intubation assisted by retrograde percutaneous guidewire insertion. (See text for details.)

Another method of dealing with difficult intubation, if there is good control of the airway, is to use retrograde percutaneous guidewire insertion. The technique is shown graphically in Figure 7.24. Having got the patient anaesthetized and breathing spontaneously (or being ventilated on a facemask), deepen anaesthesia, extend the neck, and identify the cricothyroid membrane. Put a spot of local anaesthetic on the skin, advance the needle (23 gauge) and inject 2 ml of 2 – 4% lignocaine (lidocaine) during inspiration. This usually stimulates coughing but anaesthetizes the trachea and larynx locally. Introduce a Tuohy epidural needle into the trachea through the cricothyroid membrane (Figure 7.24a) and advance the catheter cephalad as shown in Figure 7.24b. Retrieve the epidural catheter from the mouth with Magill s forceps. Keep the patient well oxygenated by intermittently returning to the facemask. Then feed the tube over the catheter (Figure 7.24c), tension the catheter so that it does not kink, and pull the tube and catheter into the trachea as the Tuohy needle is withdrawn. When the tube has entered the trachea, release the tension on the lower end of the catheter and allow the tube to pass down the trachea. Test the position of the tube both clinically and with the capnograph, leaving the catheter still in position (the connector will usually push over it). If satisfactory, cut the catheter at the skin surface and pull it out from the top of the tube.

### *Unexpectedly difficult intubation in patients in danger of aspiration*

Although difficulty in intubation was not anticipated, these patients will have been induced using cricoid pressure and rapid sequence induction. Check every intubation attempt immediately with capnography. If the tube is in the oesophagus, remove it immediately. Pressurized gas in the stomach makes regurgitation worse.

After attempting intubation in the presence of cricoid pressure, and perhaps trying once or twice with the introducer or bougie and/or the McCoy laryngoscope, the decision to discontinue the attempt must be made. Call for help again if it has not already arrived. Maintain cricoid pressure and ventilate the patient. If the operation is not life-saving, keep cricoid pressure on, turn the patient on to the left-hand side, and tip head down. Ventilating a patient in the lateral position is not always easy and you may need an assistant to hold the head in position (it is normally supported by the pillow when supine). Allow the patient to wake up in the left lateral position. If the operation is life-saving, senior help (which may be surgical) is needed to establish an immediate cricothyrotomy or tracheostomy (see Emergency airways above). This requirement is thankfully extremely rare. If aspiration occurs, treat as under Management of aspiration above.

### Intubation that is anticipated to be difficult in elective patients

When meeting a predictably difficult intubation, always remember that the object is to anaesthetize the patient, not necessarily to intubate him or her, so think of all possible methods including regional blocks.

The factors that predict difficult intubation have been described earlier. If such a situation is anticipated, the exact approach used will depend on the combination of anaesthetist, patient, and pathology. There are no set rules, but there are sensible guidelines for proceeding. In the final analysis, the safest approach may be to do an awake intubation (see below). Examples of two predictably difficult intubations are shown in Figure 7.25.

It is now almost 10 years ago that the ASA designed an algorithm to promote a logical sequence of options in an expectedly difficult intubation. It is shown in Figure 7.26. To the algorithm I would add two important riders:

1. If you are anticipating difficult intubation, get another anaesthetist to be present. This is as true for consultants as it is for trainees.
2. Always send for help early if things go badly; it is never too early.

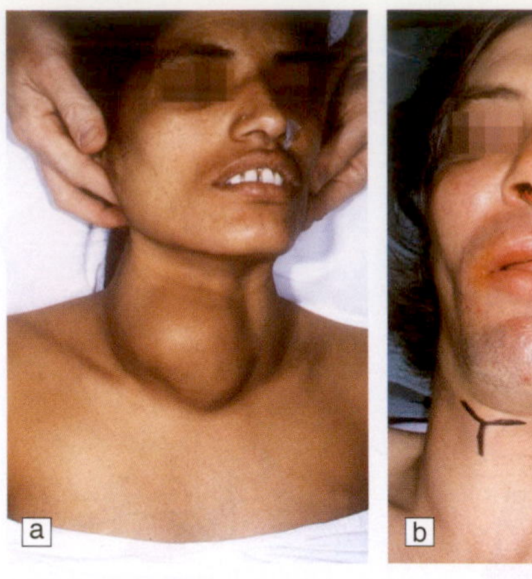


**Figure 7.25.** Examples of two predictable difficult intubations. (a) The patient has a large goitre which is compressing the trachea. (b) The patient has previously had radiotherapy to the throat, which has resulted in fibrosis and tethering of the thyroid cartilage (marked in) some distance from the midline.

The practice of the author in cases of anticipated difficult intubation in an elective patient would be 1) to do an awake intubation, or 2) to do a gaseous induction with sevoflurane in 100% $O_2$ or 3) to induce with an intravenous agent given by syringe driver while breathing 100% $O_2$. The object of the second and third methods would be to try to maintain an airway in a spontaneously breathing patient. If, after consciousness was lost, facemask ventilation was possible, the patient would be given a short-acting neuromuscular blocking agent, and a laryngoscope inserted. Subsequent management would be as above in unexpectedly difficult intubation.

### The shared airway

The shared airway is one in which the surgeon s activities put the airway at risk. This can occur with mask or tube techniques.

When using a nasal mask with a spontaneously breathing patient, the dentist puts in a pack to seal off the oral cavity from the pharynx. The pack is to prevent debris falling into the pharynx and larynx. If the pack is correctly placed, the movement of the reservoir bag should be the same as when the mouth was closed. If it is not, the dentist needs to be asked to change the position of the pack.

It is clear from Figure 7.27 that, if an oral pack pushes the soft palate on to the posterior pharyngeal wall, the patient has no airway. It is also obvious that the use of nasal masks is impossible without a patent nasal airway. Consequently, this must be checked on every patient before anaesthesia is induced if a pack is required. Blocked nasal passages are the usual reason for turning away children with acute coryza.

Although an ET tube will not be obstructed by a pack unless it kinks or compresses it, the tube can nevertheless be disturbed, pulled out, pushed down, kinked, cut, or sewn into position. Meticulous attention to airway patency is vital during procedures requiring a shared airway.

*It is a pity, but morbidity and mortality from oral packs inadvertently left* in situ *continue to occur.* When

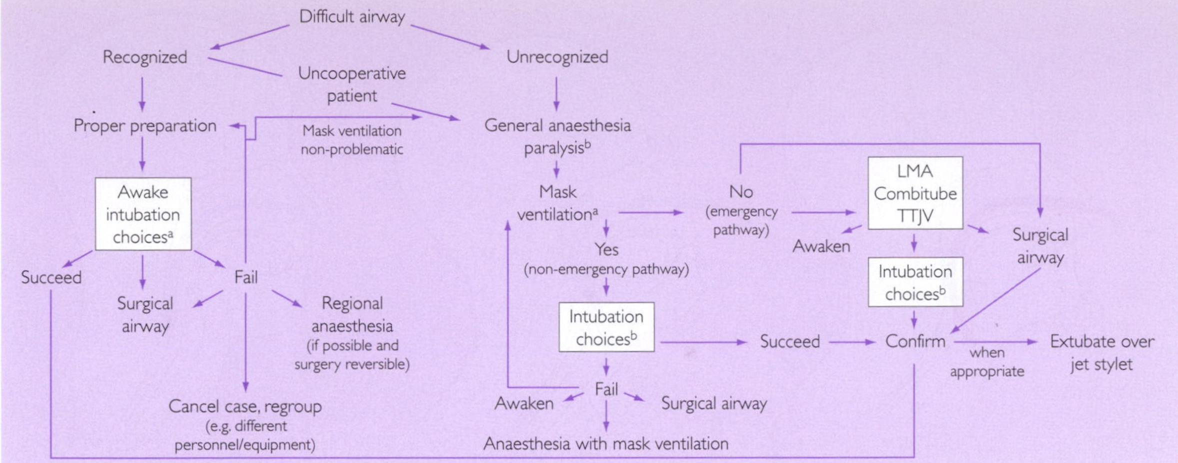


**Figure 7.26.** The American Society of Anesthesiologists' Difficult Airway Algorithm. [a]Always consider calling for help (e.g. technical, medical, surgical, etc.) when difficulty is encountered with mask ventilation and/or tracheal intubation. [b]Consider the need to preserve spontaneous ventilation. LMA, laryngeal mask airway; TTJV, transtracheal jet ventilation. (Adapted from Biebuyck JF. *Anesthesiology* 1991;75:1087.)

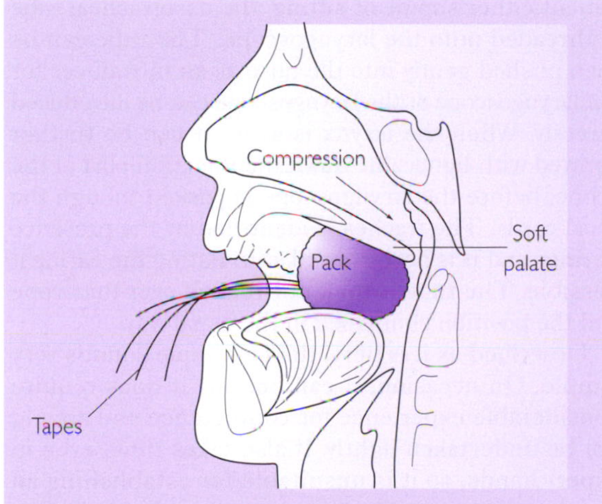


**Figure 7.27.** An oral pack shown in position. It can be seen that if the pack pushes the soft palate on to the posterior pharyngeal wall, both the nasal and oral airways are occluded.

used, they should always have tapes that remain outside the oral cavity and, during their use, clear communication between the anaesthetist and surgeon is very important.

### Blind nasal intubation in anaesthetized patients

This is the passage of a nasotracheal tube into the trachea in the presence of a closed mouth. It can be considered for any condition in which the mouth cannot be opened or laryngoscopy would be difficult or dangerous. *It is unsuitable for patients at risk of aspiration.*

The patient is anaesthetized using an appropriate technique that maintains spontaneous ventilation, and the head placed in the intubating position. The tube is well lubricated and introduced into the nasopharynx as described earlier. The other nostril and mouth are closed and the tube connected to the breathing system; the patient should breathe comfortably. Loud breath sounds from the end of the tube indicate proximity to the larynx.

Anaesthesia is deepened and, with the mandible pulled forward, the tube is advanced swiftly at the start of inspiration. The position and rotation of the head determine its route. At too light a level of anaesthesia, laryngospasm, or breath-holding, may occur. The tube may go into the trachea or the oesophagus or jam into other soft tissues anteriorly, posteriorly, or laterally (Figure 7.28).

When the tube enters the nasopharynx and passes downwards towards the larynx, its natural path is to cross the midline. This means, as shown in Figure 7.29, that the direction of the bevel can optimize the chance of the tube tip passing between the vocal cords. The effect of rotating the nasal end of the tube is to swing the tip laterally in the pharynx, as shown in Figure 7.30. Manoeuvres of this type can be used to reposition the tube tip during a second attempt after an initial failure.

This technique needs practice to be competent. When using it, always confirm the position of the tube by capnography. *The most dire consequence is unrecognized oesophageal intubation.*

### Awake intubation

Many ways have been described of intubating the awake patient. Apart from the retrograde catheter technique referred to above, the only method described here is the use of the fibreoptic laryngoscope using topical anaesthesia, which has revolutionized the approach to difficult intubation. It can of course also be used on anaesthetized patients.

The technique is shown diagrammatically in Figure 7.31. The nasal route is shown and described (which visualizes the larynx more easily), but the oral route can also be used. Contraindications to the nasal route are similar to those for a nasal airway and nasotracheal tube. All patients should first be given a dose of an anticholinergic to reduce secretions, an amethocaine lozenge to suck, and vasoconstricting nasal drops. On arrival, the nose and pharynx are liberally sprayed with either cocaine or a lignocaine/phenylephrine combina-

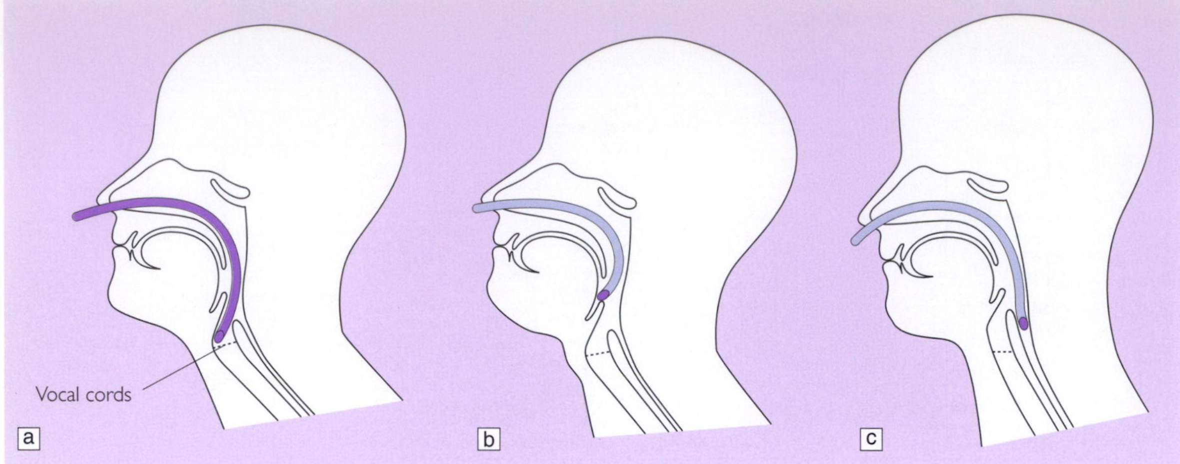


**Figure 7.28.** Unwanted destinations of a nasotracheal tube. At (a) the tip is stuck on the vestibular fold lateral to the rima glottidis, at (b) it is in the vallecula, and at (c) it has entered the oesophagus.

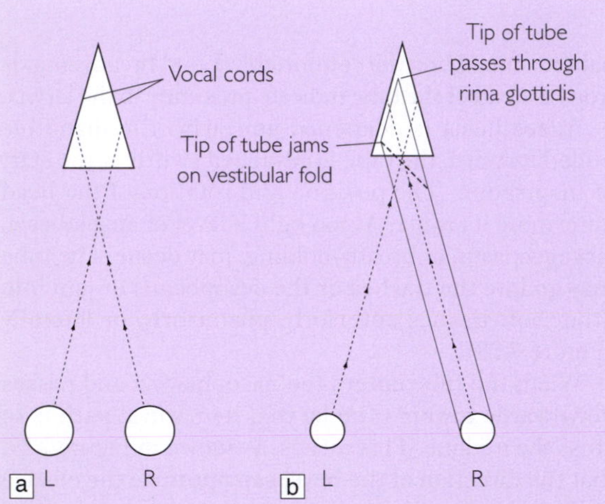


**Figure 7.29.** (a) A diagrammatic representation of the path of a nasotracheal tube in the pharynx. (b) As it approaches the vocal folds, the direction of the bevel can determine whether it passes through the rima glottidis. (Adapted from Gillespie NA. *Endotracheal Anaesthesia*. University of Wisconsin Press, 1941.)

tion and the trachea anaesthetized by the cricothyroid membrane route as described earlier. Then, with the patient either supine or sitting, the nasotracheal tube is threaded onto the laryngoscope. The tube can be then pushed gently into the nose as an introducer for the laryngoscope or the laryngoscope can be introduced directly. When the larynx is seen, it can be further sprayed with lignocaine down the injection port of the scope, before the laryngoscope is passed though the vocal cords. The trachea is identified by the presence of rings and it is best to avoid stimulating the carina if possible. The tube is then rail-roaded over the scope and the position confirmed in the usual way.

Described as it is here, the technique sounds very simple. On occasion, it can be, but it does require considerable experience for competence and should not be undertaken lightly. It also takes time, even in expert hands, so it is unsuitable for establishing an emergency airway. The larynx, in an awake patient, is constantly moving and presents a very different picture to that in the textbooks or in the paralysed patient. Finally, one must not lose contact with the patient during this process. Patients need constant reassurance and the role of assistants is crucial. The patient also needs to be both warned and reminded that they will be unable to speak when the tube is in place.

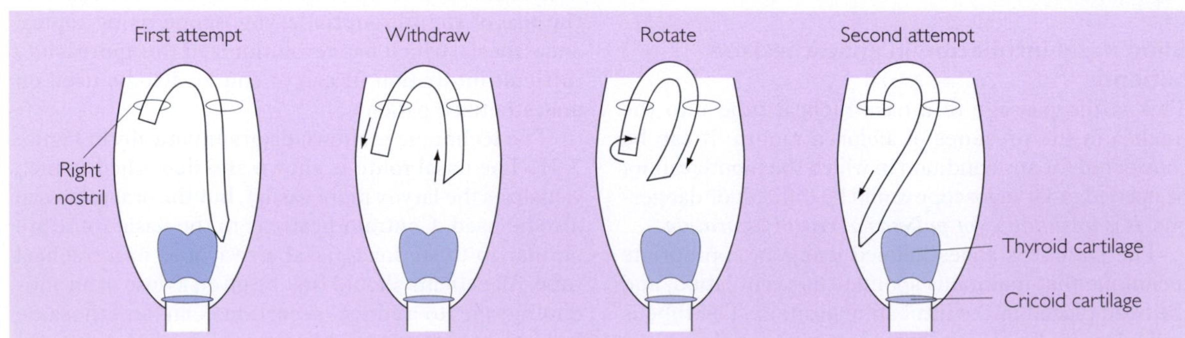


**Figure 7.30.** Effect of rotating the nasotracheal tube on its axis on the position of the tip. (Adapted from Gillespie NA. *Endotracheal Anaesthesia*. University of Wisconsin Press, 1941.)

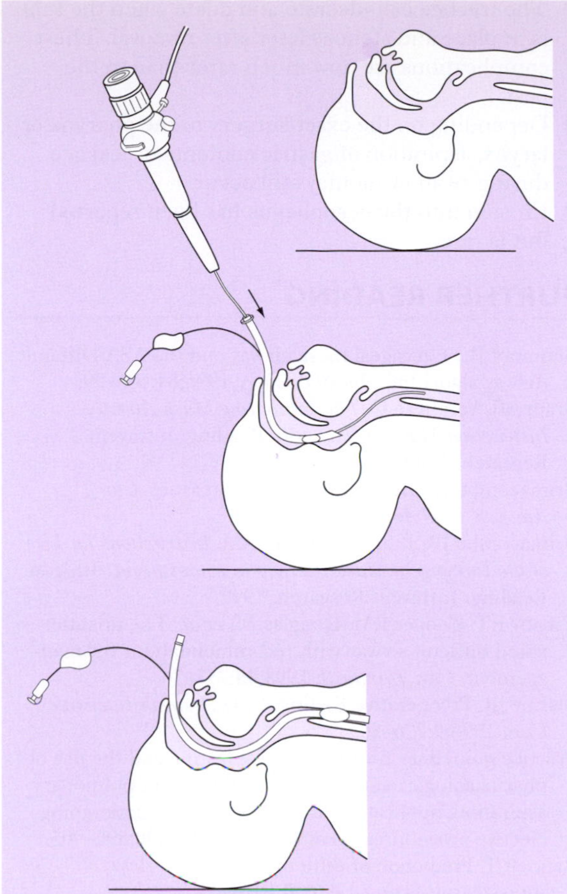

**Figure 7.31.** A diagrammatic representation of fibre-optic intubation via the nasal route. The tube is threaded on to the scope, the scope introduced into the trachea, and the tube 'rail-roaded' over it.

## Complications and management of a tracheostomy

The description of tracheostomy tubes is given in Chapter 6, with examples shown in Figure 6.43. Indications for tracheostomy are given earlier.

### *Early complications (cuffed tracheostomy tube)*

- For the first few hours after tracheostomy, the patient needs to be in an area where immediate re-intubation is possible. If the patient is conscious, he is often reassured by having a bell to hand because he is unable to call for attention.
- It is very important for the tube to be properly secured. Pulling and twisting from hoses erodes the edges of the wound.
- Breathing or ventilation difficulties can arise from the tube becoming blocked (blood or secretions) or twisting, or the tip slipping down the right main bronchus. There have been cases of cuff herniation blocking the tube outlet. If a patient is having a problem with a tracheostomy tube and it is not alleviated immediately by suction, it needs changing.
- Bleeding can occur from the adjoining vessels (jugulars, carotids, and thyroid vessels), thyroid isthmus, or skin. A new bleed after the immediate postoperative period is not usually an ooze and needs surgical exploration. The bleeding may be occult and directly into the trachea.
- Aspiration can still occur.
- Surgical emphysema, mediastinal emphysema, and pneumothorax are all serious signs warranting immediate investigation and resolution.

### *Tracheostomy care*

General principles are:

- Cuff inflation pressure should be below 20 mmHg to minimize mucosal damage.
- In the early phase, and especially if the patient cannot swallow, suck out pharyngeal secretions gently but regularly.
- Humidification of the inspired air is essential to reduce crusting, especially in the first few weeks. Later the tracheal mucosa adapts .
- Patients with tracheostomies cannot cough. They require physiotherapy to propel secretions from the periphery of the lung to the major bronchi, and then suction to aspirate these secretions. This is unpleasant for the patient and should not be done more than is necessary; when it is done it needs to be effective so that the patient has not suffered in vain.
- Changing a tracheostomy tube before a proper track has formed must always be taken seriously. This may need to be done as an emergency so the equipment for doing so must be kept by the patient s bedside. The procedure for the first change (which is potentially the most dangerous) is as follows:
  - have present a member of the medical staff who is skilled in intubation, together with (Figure 7.32): two tracheostomy tubes, one the same size and one smaller than that already *in situ*; a 6-mm ET tube (uncut); a pair of tracheal dilators; long and short bougies over which the tracheostomy or ET tubes can be rail-roaded if necessary; adequate suction (both bronchial and Yankauer attachments); intubation equipment and induction drugs;

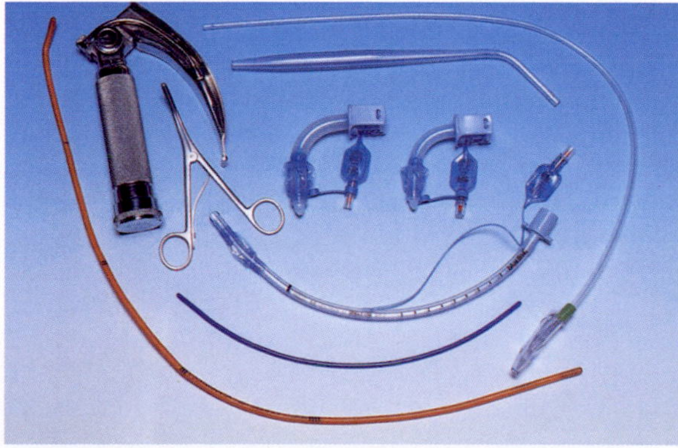

**Figure 7.32.** The equipment required when changing a tracheostomy tube. (See text for details.) Note that intubation drugs not shown here should also be immediately available. (With permission of University Hospital Birmingham NHS Trust.)

- preoxygenate the patient and have him sitting upright, reclining, or lying with the neck extended;
- if it is likely to be a difficult changeover, suck out the tube, and place a catheter or bougie down the lumen to act as an introducer; otherwise, suck out and continue aspiration as the tube is removed; there are often secretions adherent to the tube;
- identify the tracheal lumen; if not rail-roading, use the obturator; you should not need to force the tube into position; doing so often creates a false passage;
- following insertion, check that spontaneous breathing is satisfactory or that the patient can be ventilated easily. Auscultate both lung fields and the epigastrium. *If difficulties occur, or if cyanosis develops, assume that the tube is in the wrong place and take it out.*

- Subsequent changes when a fibrous track has been formed are less hazardous and eventually, if the tracheostomy is permanent, will be able to be done by the patient or a relative.

***Later complications***

- Infection is a perennial problem. The site rapidly becomes colonized by a variety of organisms, often Gram-negative bacteria. When chest infections occur, the inability to cough makes regular suctioning very important.
- Haemorrhage may occur because of infection or erosion into the surrounding vessels. This usually involves the immediately surrounding vessels, as described above, but rarely involves a brachiocephalic vessel with correspondingly catastrophic results.
- The trachea can ulcerate and dilate when the tube is in place and stenose later after removal. These complications are now much rarer than in the past.
- Depending on the exact surgery to the pharynx or larynx, aspiration of gastric contents or leakage during swallowing may still occur.
- Erosion into the oesophagus has been reported but is rare.

## FURTHER READING


Benumof JL. Laryngeal mask airway and the ASA Difficult Airway algorithm. *Anesthesiology* 1996;**84**:686–99.

Brain AIJ, Verghese C. *The Intubating Mask Airway Instruction Manual*, 2nd edn. Reading: Intravent Research, 1999.

Brimacombe JR, Berry AM. Cricoid pressure. *Can J Anaesth* 1997;**44**:414–25.

Brimacombe JR, Brain AIJ, Berry AM. *Instructions for Use of the Laryngeal Mask Airway in Anaesthesia*, 4th edn. Reading: Intravent Research, 1999.

Crosby ET, Cooper RM, Douglas MJ *et al.* The unanticipated difficult airway with recommendations for management. *Can J Anaesth* 1998;**45**:757–76.

Maltby JR. Preoperative Fasting. *Curr Anaesth Intensive Care* 1996;**7**:276–80.

Practice guidelines for preoperative fasting and the use of pharmacologic agents to reduce the risk of pulmonary aspiration: application to healthy patients undergoing elective procedures. *Anesthesiology* 1999;**90**:896–905.

Randell T. Prediction of difficult intubation. *Acta Anaesthesiol Scand* 1996;**40**:1016–23.

Soni N. *Practical Procedures in Anaesthesia and Intensive Care*. Oxford: Butterworth-Heinemann, 1989.

Warner MA, Warner ME, Weber JG. Clinical significance of pulmonary aspiration in the perioperative period. *Anesthesiology* 1993;**78**:56–62.

# Chapter 8 Delivery and disposal of gases and vapours

P. Hutton

## GAS PROPERTIES, STORAGE AND DISTRIBUTION

During anaesthesia patients can be allowed to breathe spontaneously or be ventilated using:

- air (atmospheric or medical) or
- oxygen-enriched air or
- nitrous oxide ($N_2O$) and oxygen (± air).

Although now uncommon, some children are still hyperventilated using $CO_2$-containing gas mixtures and some adults are given $CO_2$ at the end of anaesthesia to stimulate respiration.

This section describes the storage and distribution of the above gases up to their entry into the anaesthesia machine. The basic principles of cylinders and pipelines are considered first and then each gas is examined separately.

### Cylinders

#### *Construction*

At present there are approximately equal numbers of medical gas cylinders in use that are made out of carbon–manganese steel and molybdenum steel. The latter are more modern and weigh less. There are also a very small, but increasing, number of cylinders made from aluminium alloy. Steel cylinders are manufactured in sizes A–J but sizes A and H are not used for medical gases. The sizes and shapes of steel cylinders that contain medical gases are shown compared with the size of a man in Figure 8.1. Aluminium alloy cylinders do not have these proportions and tend to be shorter and wider for a given volume.

Cylinders that are intended to be attached to a machine have a convex base to maximize their strength. Those intended to stand on the floor have a flat bottom rim, the inside of which is curved upwards, similar to that of a champagne bottle and for the same reasons. Most cylinders originate from a solid billet of steel of the appropriate composition, which is then heated, stamped hollow, forged, and spun to the familiar cylindrical form with a teat-like end. Nowadays, some begin life as steel tubing or flat plate, which is heated, moulded, and welded into the necessary size and shape.

#### *Testing*

After a variety of tests that measure the uniformity of wall thickness and check for surface defects, the cylinder is heat treated, hardness and tensile tested, threaded to take a valve, and thoroughly descaled and cleaned. Identification marks denoting the place and date of manufacture, the weight (tare) of the cylinder, its constant safe working (CP) and test (TP) pressures, and the industrial standard to which it has been constructed are stamped on the surface. The volume of each cylinder is measured by filling with water, and this result and the date of the first hydraulic pressure test (to 150% or 167% of its maximum working pressure, depending on the country) are also stamped on the surface. Although these markings differ in detail and position depending on the country and manufacturer, the principles of the information they carry is similar.

After a cylinder enters service, it is subjected to tests at regular intervals. Again the exact method of surveillance varies from manufacturer to manufacturer and country to country, but the principles are constant and can be illustrated by reference to those carried out by BOC. Their system is as follows. For easy reference (instead of having to look at the surface of each cylinder), a plastic ring is put around each valve stem after

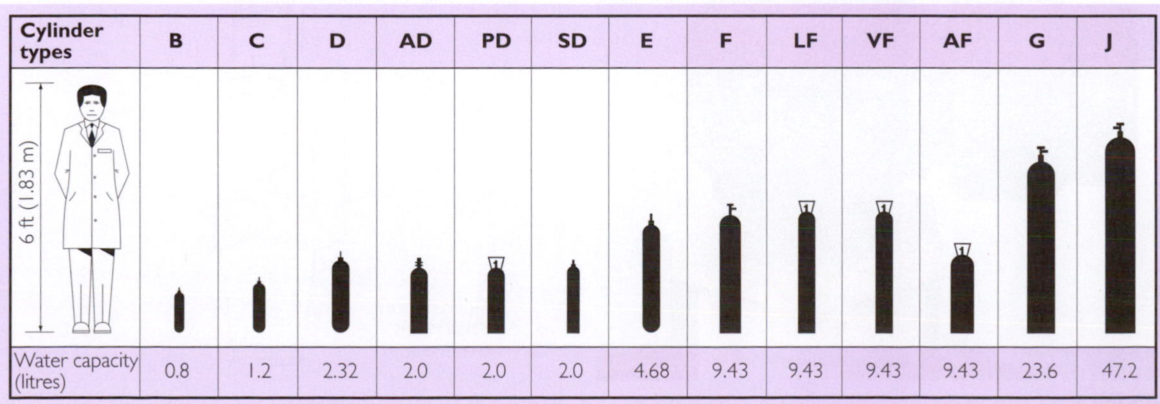

Cylinder types
B
C
D
AD
PD
SD
E
F
LF
VF
AF
G
J
6 ft (1.83 m)
Water capacity (litres)
0.8
1.2
2.32
2.0
2.0
2.0
4.68
9.43
9.43
9.43
9.43
23.6
47.2


**Figure 8.1.** The sizes and shapes of medical gas cylinders compared with a man. (Courtesy of BOC Medical Gases.) Size E cylinders are usually fitted to an anaesthesia machine.

the cylinder is tested. This can be one of six colours or three shapes (i.e. 18 combinations), which identify the year when the cylinder has to be re-tested. The ring is also punched, indicating in which quarter of the year this should be done. This is shown in Figure 8.2.

At 5 years from new or from a previous 10-year hydraulic test, the cylinder is weighed and, if its weight has fallen by over 5%, it is scrapped. If not, it is subject to an external and internal visual check (with a kind of endoscope) and, if this is satisfactory, the date, followed by the letter V, is stamped on the cylinder and it re-enters service for a further 5 years with a new date ring. At the 10-year interval, it receives the same tests followed by a full hydraulic test to 150% of its maximum working pressure and the date, followed by a T, is stamped on. The cycle is then repeated.

### *Colour coding*

Medical gas cylinders must be permanently painted with a colour-coded, non-fading, durable, water-insoluble paint. Each cylinder should also carry a permanently attached label or painted symbol to confirm the composition of the contents. Before colour coding and pin indexing (see below) were introduced, there was more chance for misconnection (indeed a thriller film was made called *Green for Danger* based on such an event in World War II). There is now an international standard for colour coding gases, but a number of countries (e.g. USA and Germany) have their own system. Any anaesthetist working in an unfamiliar country needs to check the local arrangements carefully. A comparison of colour codes is shown in Table 8.1. Examples of cylinders in current use in the UK and the USA are shown in Figure 8.3. At present, a new system of bar coding cylinders and gases (including test dates, etc.) on a collar around the neck of the cylinder (in addition to the ring) is being introduced in the UK and such a cylinder is shown in Figure 8.4.

### *Valves and the pin-index system*

A valve (on a tapered thread) is screwed into the neck of the cylinder for the purposes of both sealing and discharge. The most common type of valve is shown in cross-section in Figure 8.5 and the physical form of it and others in Figure 8.6. The tapered thread is usually wrapped in PTFE (polytetrafluoroethylene) tape to

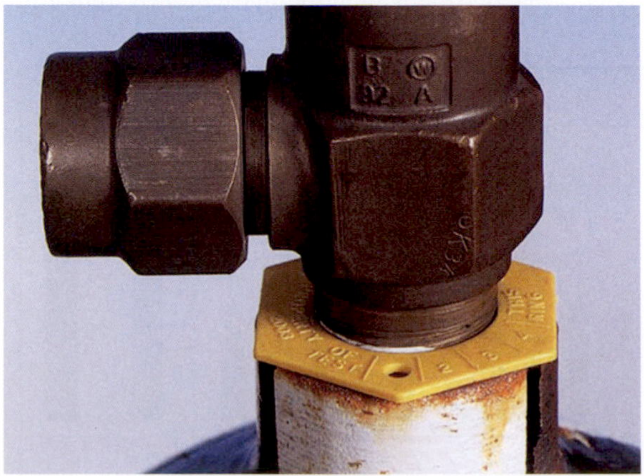

**Figure 8.2.** A cylinder neck ring showing the time at which re-testing should occur. Note the punched hole showing the year and its quarter when re-testing is due.

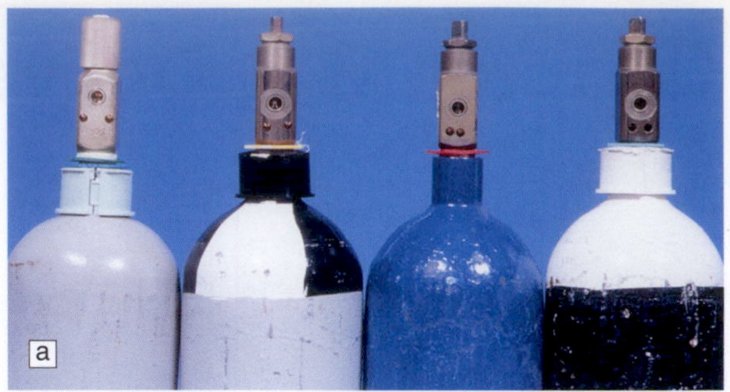


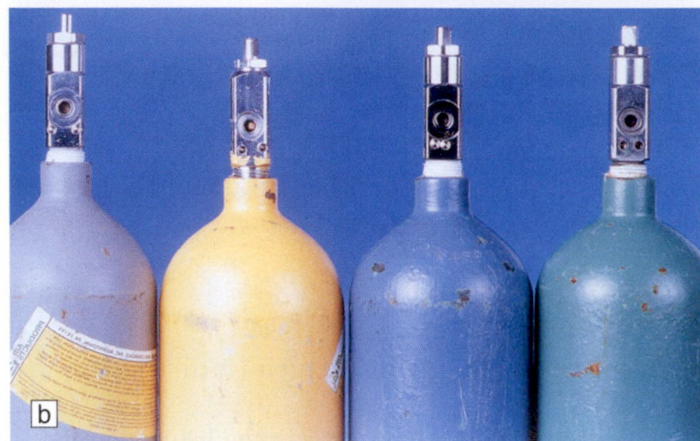


**Figure 8.3.** The colour coding of gas cylinders in the UK (a) and the USA (b). The cylinder contents from left to right are carbon dioxide, medical air, nitrous oxide, and oxygen. The valve on the carbon dioxide cylinder in (a) has a hand grip instead of the conventional spigot.

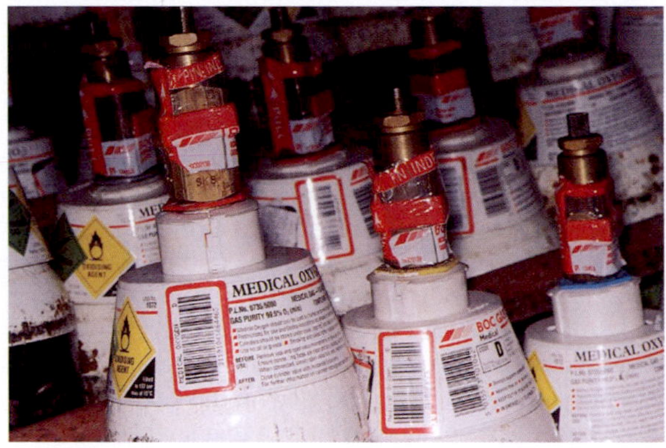


**Figure 8.4.** Bar coding on oxygen cylinder collars.

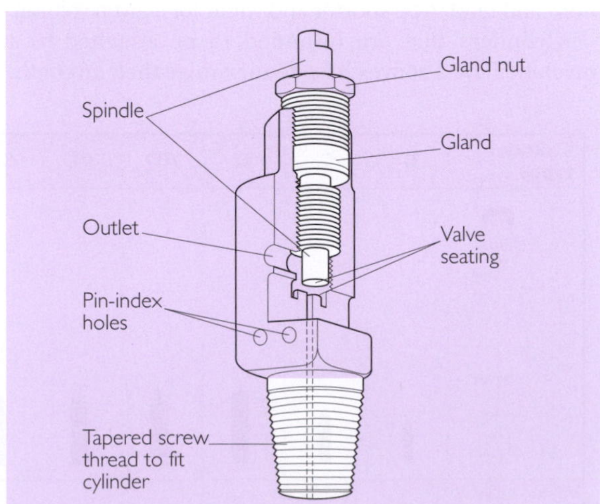


**Figure 8.5.** A diagrammatic cross-sectional view through a pin-index cylinder valve block. The tapered screw is sometimes wrapped in PTFE tape.

**Table 8.1. Colour coding of medical gases (and vacuum) in cylinders and pipelines**

| | UK | | USA | | Germany | | France | | Australia | |
|---|---|---|---|---|---|---|---|---|---|---|
| Content | Cylinder | Pipeline | Cylinder | Pipeline | Cylinder | Pipeline | Cylinder | Pipeline | Cylinder | Pipeline |
| Oxygen | White shoulders on black body | White | Green | Green | Blue | Blue | White | White | As UK | As UK |
| Nitrous oxide | Blue | Blue | Blue | Blue | Grey | Grey | Blue shoulders on white body | Blue | As UK | As UK |
| Entonox* | White and blue shoulder quarters on blue body | Blue/white | Not used | Not used | Not used | Not used | Blue and white shoulders on white body | Not used | As UK | Blue/white |
| Medical air | White and black shoulder quarters on grey body | Black | Yellow | Yellow | Yellow | Yellow | Black and white shoulders on black body | Black and white | As UK | Black with diagonal white lines |
| Carbon dioxide | Grey | Not used | Grey | Not used | Black | Not used | Dark grey | Not used | Green-grey | Not used |
| Vacuum | | Yellow | | White | | White | | Green | | Yellow |

*oxygen and nitrous oxide in a 50/50 mixture.
Note that all European countries are supposed to move to a new standard Euro-Norm EN 1089-3 by 1st July 2006.
Not all countries follow strict nationally accepted colour coding rules.

produce a seal when it is threaded in. It is imperative that no grease is used in any part of the valve or subsequent pressure regulators or pipework. For medical gases, each valve assembly is tested to a pressure that is stamped on to it, together with its chemical symbol (Figure 8.7). To prevent misconnection, the valve block is drilled in two of a possible six locations (Figure 8.8 and Table 8.2), depending on the gas that it controls. These holes mate with projecting pins on the yoke of the anaesthesia machine or free-standing outlet valve (Figure 8.9). The gas port from the valve is on the same side as the pin-index holes and will not seal against the Bodock seal (see The anaesthesia machine , page 111) unless the pins and holes are aligned.

In the USA and some other countries, the valve block has a rupture disc or plug that blows out if the cylinder is overpressurized or subjected to excessive temperature (Figure 8.10). This type of device is not fitted to medical gas cylinders in the UK. If the cylin-

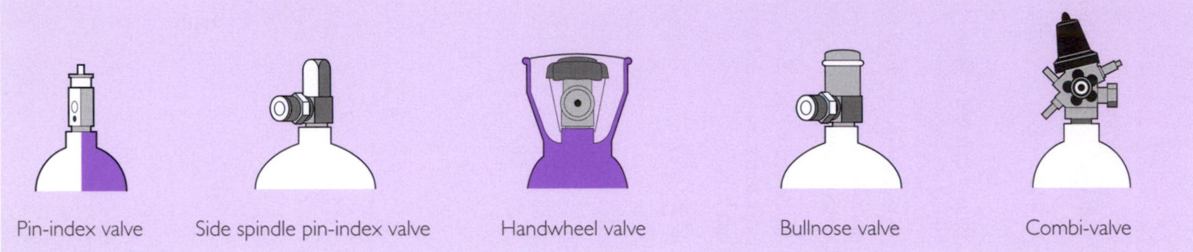


**Figure 8.6.** Different valve types in current use.

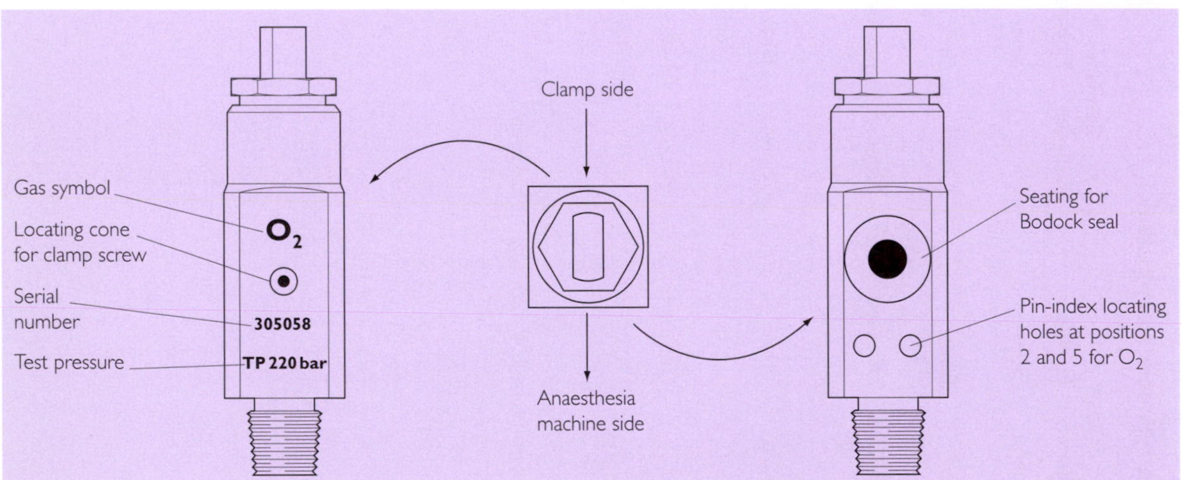


**Figure 8.7.** The clamp and anaesthesia machine sides of a pin-index cylinder valve block. Note the gas symbol, the hydraulic test pressure, and the pin-index holes. On $N_2O$ cylinders, the tare weight (the weight with no contents) is often given. The arrangement of the markings differs from manufacturer to manufacturer.

**Table 8.2. Pressure when full, pin-index positions, and litres of gas (nominal) available from various cylinder sizes when discharged to the atmosphere**

| Cylinder size | | | | C | D | E | F | G | J |
|---|---|---|---|---|---|---|---|---|---|
| | Pressure when full (kPa/bar/psig) | Pin-index positions | Tare wt (kg) | 2.0 | 3.4 | 5.4 | 14.5 | 34.5 | 68.9 |
| Gas | at 15°C | if used | Cylinder volume (L) | 1.2 | 2.32 | 4.68 | 9.43 | 23.6 | 47.2 |
| Oxygen | 13 650/135/1980 | 2, 5 | | 170 | 340 | 680 | 1360 | 3400 | 6800 |
| Nitrous oxide | 4400/43.5/640 | 3, 5 | | 450 | 900 | 1800 | 3600 | 9000 | 18000 |
| Entonox | 13650/135/1980 | Central | | – | 500 | – | 2000 | 5000 | – |
| Medical air | 13650/135/1980 | 1, 5 | | – | – | 640 | 1280 | 3200 | 6400 |
| Carbon dioxide | 5000/49.2/723 | 1, 6 | | 450 | – | 1800 | – | – | – |

Note that numerical data in cylinder tables varies slightly depending on whether it is specified at 15 or 20°C.
psig, pounds per square inch gauge.

der was subjected to unexpectedly very high temperatures, it is true that, as a potential safety feature, the PTFE taper-thread-sealing tape would be degraded

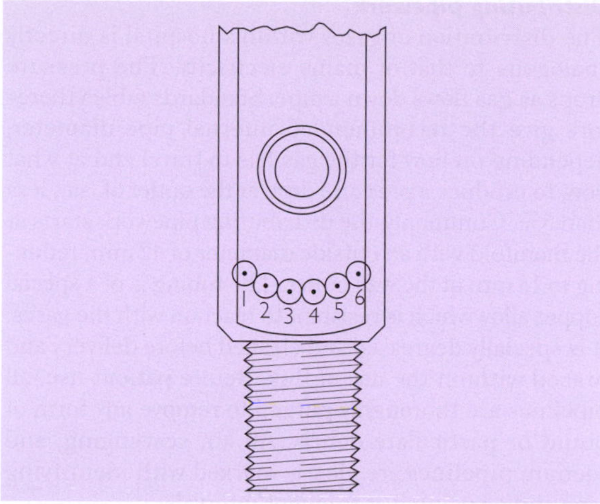

**Figure 8.8.** The various positions in which the pin-index holes are drilled. Entonox has a single central hole between the level of the holes shown and the Bodock seal.

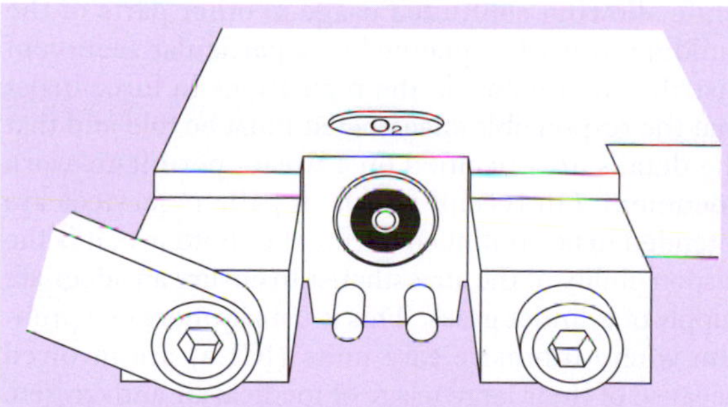

**Figure 8.9.** The yoke of an anaesthesia machine showing the projecting pins that locate with the pin-index holes of the valve block on the cylinder. The example shown is for $O_2$.

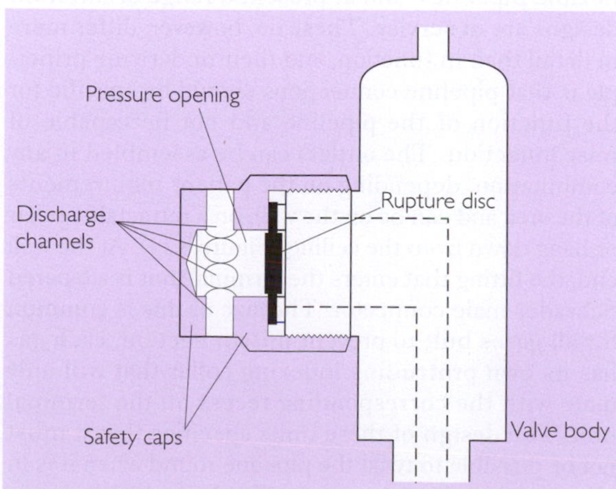

**Figure 8.10.** Diagrammatic representation of a pressure-limiting rupture disc. When the prescribed pressure is exceeded, the disc ruptures and gas discharges to the atmosphere.

and gas would leak round the thread. This is, however, not part of any industrial safety standard, nor should it be relied upon.

Full cylinders come with a plastic wrapping over the valve apparatus, which must be removed before use. Before attachment to the machine the valve should be cracked open briefly to blow out any particles of dust, etc. in the valve outlet. On the anaesthesia machine, it is good practice to open the cylinder to full pressure slowly to prevent pressure surges in the Bourdon gauges and pipelines.

#### *Storage*

Cylinders should be stored in a clean, dry, preferably fire-proof, and well-ventilated room away from flammable materials and other sources of heat. They are not designed to withstand continued dampness or corrosive chemicals or fumes. New cylinders should be stored safely in a rack and used sequentially from their date of arrival, the empty cylinders being stored separately with their valves closed to prevent the ingress of dirt, etc.

#### *Cylinder capacity*

Not all gases are available in all cylinder sizes, and the type of valve assembly also varies. Details need to be obtained from manufacturer's literature. The sizes, tare weights, and volumes of cylinders and their gas capacities are, however, fairly similar. The nominal values are given in Table 8.2.

A practical point of note is to consider the rate at which equally sized cylinders empty during anaesthesia. If two full size-E oxygen and nitrous oxide cylinders are opened at the same time and used to provide a fractional inspired oxygen concentration ($F\text{IO}_2$) of 25%, the cylinders will empty approximately simultaneously. At an $F\text{IO}_2$ greater than this, the oxygen will run out first. In addition, oxygen cylinders exhaust rapidly if, in addition to supplying respiratory gas, they also have to provide pneumatic power for a ventilator.

### Pipelines

#### *General principles*

There is no doubt that, in everyday anaesthetic practice, pipelines have considerable advantages over the use of cylinders. They are more convenient in that cylinders do not have to be changed over, they are more economical if the use of gas is substantial, there is a labour saving from the reduction of movement of cylinders within the hospital, and there is less chance of the introduction of dirt and infection into the operating room complex. A disadvantage is that, if there is a serious misconnection or cross-connection as a result of faulty maintenance, it may be unsuspected and not necessarily be limited to a single operating room. There have been rare instances of this in the past, but regulations for working on pipelines are now very strict. Nevertheless, the responsibility remains fairly and squarely with the anaesthetist at the start of each session to ensure that the gases leaving the anaesthesia machine are those intended and he or she *must always ensure that there is a reserve oxygen supply in the form of an adequately filled cylinder* attached to the machine and available for immediate use in the event of a pipeline supply failure. Although it is generally accepted that the anaesthetist cannot be held responsible for the practical and maintenance aspects of what goes on 'behind the wall', it is his or her responsibility to check the attachments of the hoses within the operating and anaesthetic rooms at the wall and anaesthesia machine ends and that they provide adequate flows within the patient breathing system.

All pipeline systems can be thought of as having three major sections:

1. a central supply of gas or vacuum;
2. a rigid, metal, distributing system of pipes within the hospital;
3. outlets in the anaesthetic or operating room that allow flexible pipes to be attached to the anaesthesia machine or pneumatically powered equipment.

Pipelines for all medical gases are at a pressure of 50 pounds per square inch gauge (psig) (330 kPa, 3.4 atm) in the USA and 60 psig (400 kPa, 4 atm) in the UK. Air is also supplied at 103 psig (700 kPa, 7 atm) for driving pneumatic drills and saws. There are also specific attachments for vacuum and scavenging.

#### *Central supplies of gas or vacuum*

All medical gases can be supplied centrally from banks of large medical gas cylinders, and this process will be considered here. In addition, oxygen can be supplied from liquid oxygen and air from a compressor; these aspects will be considered below under individual gases.

The basic principle underlying the safe design of cylinders supplying a pipeline involves the use of three sets of cylinders at any one time:

1. a set that is actively discharging into the distributing system in response to demand;
2. a set that is attached to the distributing system and that will take over automatically when the active set is exhausted;
3. an emergency set piped in separately from the two sets referred to above for use in the event of a pressure failure from whatever cause. These cylinders can also be used to maintain pipeline supplies when the main manifold is under maintenance or repair.

An example of such a system is shown diagrammatically in Figure 8.11 and in practice in Figure 8.12. The actual number and size of cylinders connected to a manifold bank are determined by the likely usage of gas. In use, all the cylinders are switched on, backflow from one cylinder to another being prevented by check valves and pressure regulators, which are installed on the common outlet manifold. When the duty bank becomes exhausted, the control unit automatically switches to the reserve bank, which now becomes the duty bank. A warning signal or alarm is then transmitted to the maintenance staff who replace the empty cylinders with full ones, which now in turn become the reserve bank. Immediately adjacent to the outlet from the control panel is an overpressure relief valve, which exhausts the pipeline to atmosphere if, for some reason of pressure regulator malfunction, the pipeline pressure exceeds that intended by a specified amount. Central cylinder supplies should be housed in an environment similar to that specified above for individual cylinders.

#### *Distributing pipework*

The distribution of gases within a hospital is directly analogous to that of mains electricity. The pressure drops as gas flows down a pipe. Standards tables therefore give the recommended internal pipe diameter, depending on how far the gas has to travel and at what flow, to produce a pressure drop at the outlet of, say, less than 5%. Commonly, the distributing pipework starts at the manifold with an outside diameter of 42 mm, reducing to 15 mm at the wall outlet. The tubing is of a special copper alloy which is resistant to reaction with the gases. It is specially degreased and cleaned before delivery and brazed without the use of flux. Before patient use, all pipelines are thoroughly purged to remove any form of liquid or particulate debris. All air, scavenging, and vacuum pipelines are clearly marked with identifying tape and/or painted at frequent intervals.

Large installations are usually divided into sections that can be isolated individually by valves, and specific areas (e.g. a ward or operating room) have their own isolating valve in a (usually) locked box (Figure 8.13). These valves allow segmental stoppage of gas flow in the event of pipeline fracture, fire, or maintenance, while allowing continued usage in other parts of the building. If work is planned on a particular section of distributing pipework, the regulations in force insist that the responsible anaesthetist must be told and that the details are specified on a timed, permit-to-work document. On receipt of this, if patient services are intended to be continued during the shutdown, it is the responsibility of the anaesthetist to ensure an adequate supply of cylinder gases. This is usually more of a problem where intensive care units (ICUs) are involved because of their large usage of medical air and oxygen.

#### *Outlets and connections in the anaesthetic room, operating room, ward, and ICU*

The attachment point for a pipeline or flowmeter in a patient area is called a terminal unit. Over the years, improvements have been made to terminal units and flexible pipelines, and at present a range of different designs are in service. These do, however, differ more in detail than in function, and their underlying principle is that pipeline connections should be specific for the function of the pipeline and not be capable of misconnection. The outlets can be assembled in any combination, depending on the patient requirements of the area and can be on the wall, on a retractable pillar or hang down from the ceiling (Figure 8.14). At the wall end, the fitting that enters the terminal unit is a tapered Schrader male connector. The size of this is common for all gases but, to prevent misconnection, each gas has its own protruding indexing collar that will only mate with the corresponding recess on the terminal unit. The design of these units specifies that it must not be possible to twist the pipeline round when it is in place, the unit must seal off when the probe is withdrawn, and it must be possible to insert and remove it with one hand.

At the anaesthesia machine or ventilator end of the hose the inlet should have a check valve (to prevent

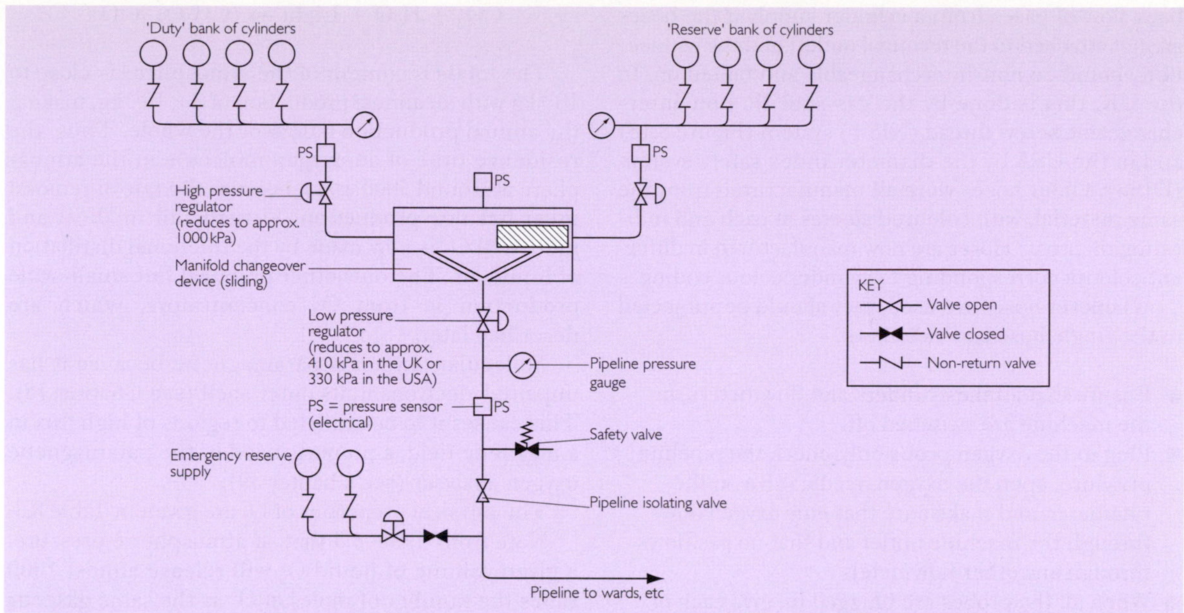


**Figure 8.11.** A diagrammatic and simplified representation of a typical automatic medical gas cylinder manifold. The valve between the emergency reserve supply and the main pipeline opens when the pipeline pressure falls below a set minimum. See text for mechanism of operation. (Adapted from Howell RSC. *Anaesthesia* 1980;35:676.)

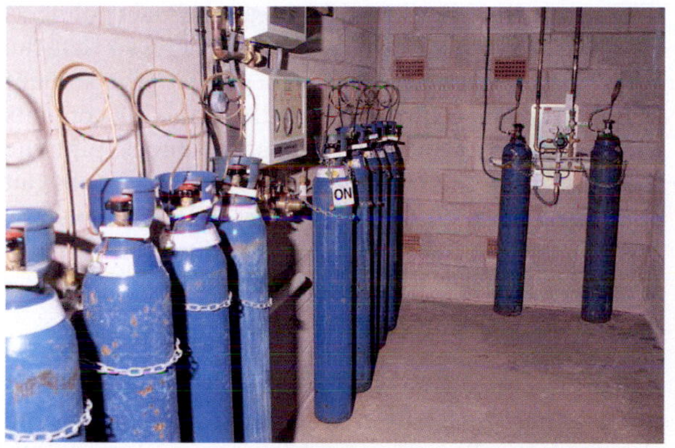


**Figure 8.12.** A bank of $N_2O$ cylinders that supplies part of a large hospital. The bank that is in use is labelled 'on'. When this empties the exchange mechanism on the wall will switch the delivery source to the bank of cylinders in the immediate left-hand foreground. The two cylinders on the far wall are the emergency supply which trip-in should the main supply fail. (Courtesy of the University Hospital Birmingham NHS Trust.)

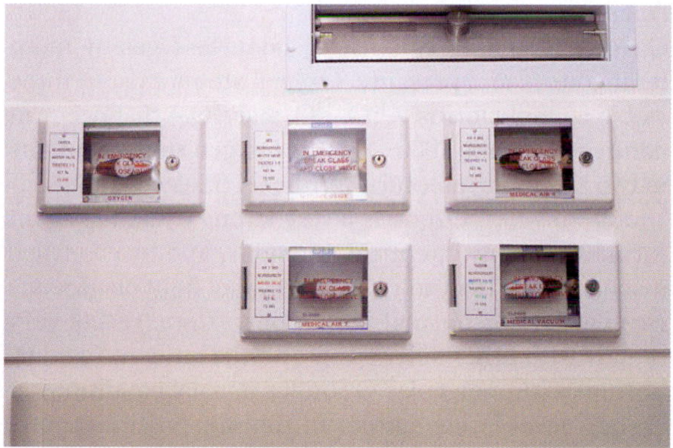

**Figure 8.13.** Isolating valves that permit the switching off of gas flow and suction to a particular area of the hospital. The valves shown are for $O_2$, $N_2O$, medical air at 4 and 7 bar, and mains vacuum. (Courtesy of the University Hospital Birmingham NHS Trust.)

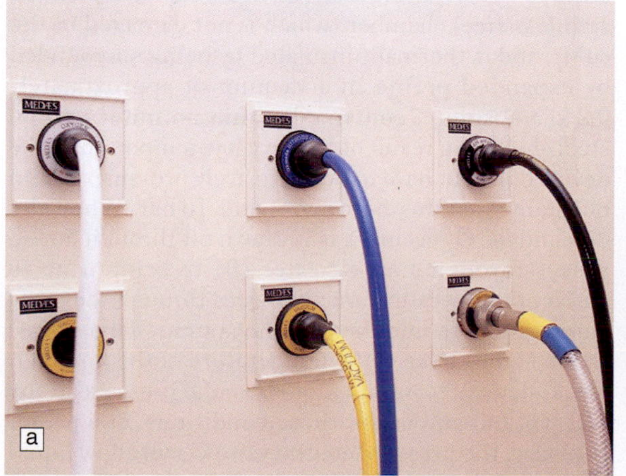


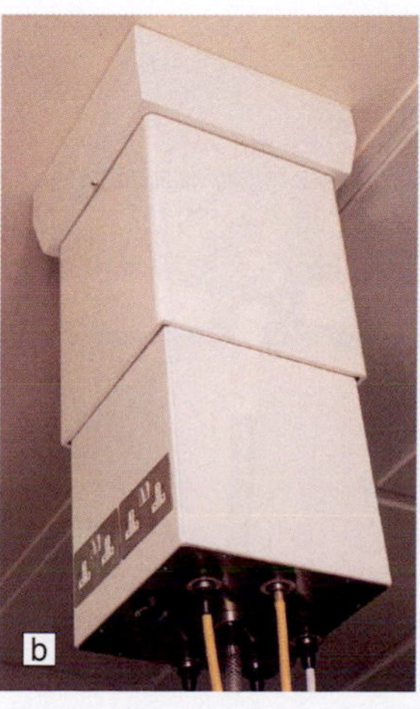


**Figure 8.14.** (a) Wall and (b) ceiling pipeline and vacuum outlets. The ceiling-mounted unit is retractable so that it can be adjusted to the most convenient height. (Courtesy of the University Hospital Birmingham NHS Trust.)

back flow of gases from a cylinder supply if the hoses are not attached to the terminal outlet) and the connection should be non-interchangeable and bolted on. In the UK, this is done by the gas-specific **n**on-**i**nterchangeable **s**crew **t**hread (NIST) system (Figure 8.15) and in the USA by the **d**iameter **i**ndex **s**afety **s**ystem (DISS). Older hoses were all manufactured from the same material, with coloured sleeves at each end indicating their use. Hoses are now manufactured in different colours corresponding to cylinder colour coding.

Whenever hoses are used, they should be subjected to the single hose test as follows:

- Ensure that all the cylinders and flowmeters on the machine are switched off.
- Plug in the oxygen probe only, check the pipeline pressure, open the oxygen needle valve on the rotameter, and make sure that only oxygen flows through the machine outlet and that no gas flows through any other flowmeter.
- When all the probes are plugged in, give each of them a sharp tug to make sure that they are properly engaged.

## Medical gases

### Oxygen

#### *Properties*

Oxygen ($O_2$) is a colourless, odourless gas at room temperature and pressure. Oxygen atoms exist in three stable isotopic forms – $^{16}O$, $^{17}O$, and $^{18}O$ – that occur in nature in the ratio 1000 : 3.7 : 20. Oxygen atoms combine in two allotropic molecular forms: $O_2$ (molecular oxygen) and $O_3$ (ozone). Ozone is a very strong oxidizing agent formed in many chemical reactions, and by electrical discharges and the action of ultraviolet light on gaseous oxygen. Under normal conditions, ozone reacts very rapidly with other substances and the amount in equilibrium with molecular $O_2$ under normal conditions at ground level is negligible. In the upper atmosphere, ozone is formed by the action of high-energy radiation from the sun and its concentration is maximal at an altitude of approximately 25 kilometres.

The free $O_2$ content of our atmosphere effectively arises from the $O_2$ cycle. Photosynthetically produced $O_2$ enters the atmospheric reservoir generated from the dissociation of water molecules and the cycle is closed by the respiration of plants and other organisms:

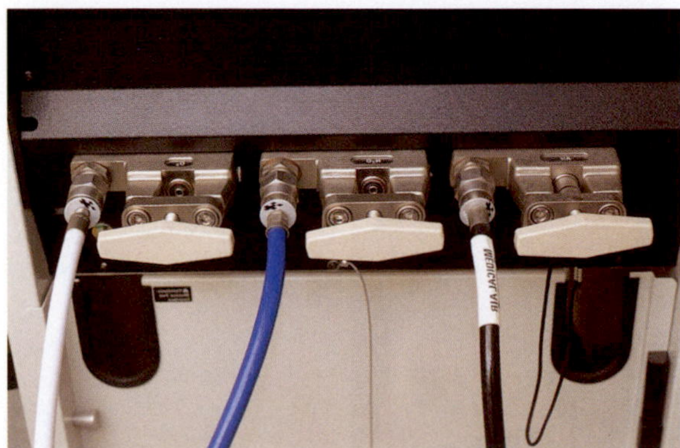

**Figure 8.15.** Gas-specific hoses attached to an anaesthesia machine by non-interchangeable screw thread (NIST) fittings.

$$CO_2 + H_2O + \text{Light} \rightarrow (CH_2O) + O_2.$$

The total $O_2$ content of the atmosphere is close to $10^{18}$ kg with an annual production of $2 \times 10^{14}$ kg, making the annual production 0.02% of the whole. Thus, the residence time of an oxygen molecule in the atmosphere is around 5000 years, because the rate of removal must balance production. Virtually all medical and industrial $O_2$ is now made by the fractional distillation of liquid air. The only other practical but small-scale production is from $O_2$ concentrators, which are described later.

Molecular oxygen is paramagnetic because it has unpaired electrons in its outer shell (see Chapter 18). This causes it to be attracted to regions of high flux in a magnetic field, a property used in the paramagnetic oxygen analyser (see Chapter 39).

The physical properties of $O_2$ are given in Table 8.3.

Note from Table 8.3 that, at atmospheric pressure, a given volume of liquid $O_2$ will release almost 1000 times the number of moles of $O_2$ as the same gaseous volume.

#### *Cylinders*

In cylinders, $O_2$ is stored in its gaseous form and at room temperature it behaves effectively as a perfect gas. The gas in the cylinder undergoes minimal cooling as its pressure drops from continued usage, so that the pressure in the cylinder is a good guide to the amount of gas remaining, when compared with the full contents as specified in Table 8.2. In most instances, pipeline installations are not supplied from cylinder banks but from vacuum-insulated evaporators (VIE) (see below). For pipelines supplied by cylinders, the layout is similar to that for $N_2O$ shown in Figure 8.11.

#### *Liquid oxygen*

This is the most common form of supply for pipelines and a typical installation is shown in Figure 8.16 and diagrammatically in Figure 8.17. It is a much more efficient way of storing $O_2$ (see Table 8.3 above). Not only are these units much greater in actual volume (up to 15 000 kg liquid $O_2$), 1 litre of a full cylinder of $O_2$ will yield approximately 130 L $O_2$ in use, whereas 1 L of liquid $O_2$ will yield approximately 850 L in use. The principle of action is as follows. The liquid $O_2$ is delivered in specially insulated tankers at a temperature of −160°C to −180°C (which is below its critical temperature of −118.4°C). It is stored in a welded, austenitic, stainless steel chamber (which is not damaged by the cold), and is thermally insulated by being surrounded by expanded perlite in a vacuum of approximately 0.2 kPa absolute, contained within an outer carbon steel shell. As a result of the very low temperature, the device does not have to be excessively pressurized and normally operates between 7 and 10 bar. When the demand for $O_2$ occurs, gas is drawn off through line A, passes through a superheater (B) to bring it up to ambient temperature and then goes through the pressure regulators into the pipeline system. This evaporation serves to keep the temperature of the liquid $O_2$ low. If demand continues, or rises, the pressure in the VIE will fall and under these conditions, at a preset pressure, the pressure control valve C will allow liquid $O_2$ to flow through the pressure-raising evaporator D

**Table 8.3. The properties of oxygen**

| Property | Value or description |
|---|---|
| Formula of molecular oxygen | $O_2$ |
| Molecular weight | 32 daltons |
| Density of gas at 1 bar, 15°C | 1.34 kg/m$^3$ |
| Density of liquid oxygen at 1 bar, −183°C | 1140 kg/m$^3$ |
| Boiling point (BP) at 1 bar | −183.1°C |
| Critical temperature | −118.4°C |
| Critical pressure | 50.8 bar |
| Critical density | 430 kg/m$^3$ |

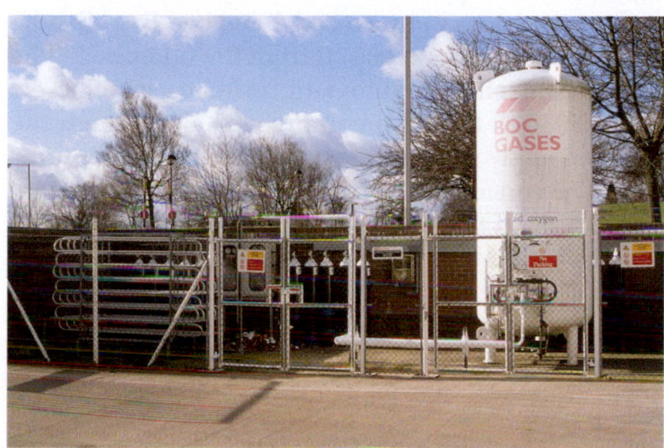


**Figure 8.16.** A liquid $O_2$ installation suitable for supplying a hospital. Note the presence of the emergency cylinder bank at the rear. (Courtesy of the Birmingham Women's Hospital NHS Trust.)

to augment both the flow from and the pressure in the VIE until it reaches its upper preset pressure. In very large VIEs, at times of exceptional demand when there is a pressure drop at the distal side of the flow restrictor E, liquid $O_2$ is added directly to the gaseous withdrawal line (F) before its entry to the superheater. The maintenance of a low temperature depends on continued evaporation because no VIE is a perfect insulator. Most can remain unused for several days before the internal pressure rises sufficiently to lift the pressure-relief valve G. All VIEs are protected against uncontrolled rises in pressure or fracture of the outer skin of the vessel by an additional high-pressure release valve (17 atm) and ultimately by a bursting disc (26 atm).

Older VIEs are mounted on three legs, two of which form a hinge, and the third is a spring balance (Figure 8.18a). The weight of the liquid $O_2$ remaining gives a measure of its level and need for refilling. Modern installations have internal pressure transducers at the

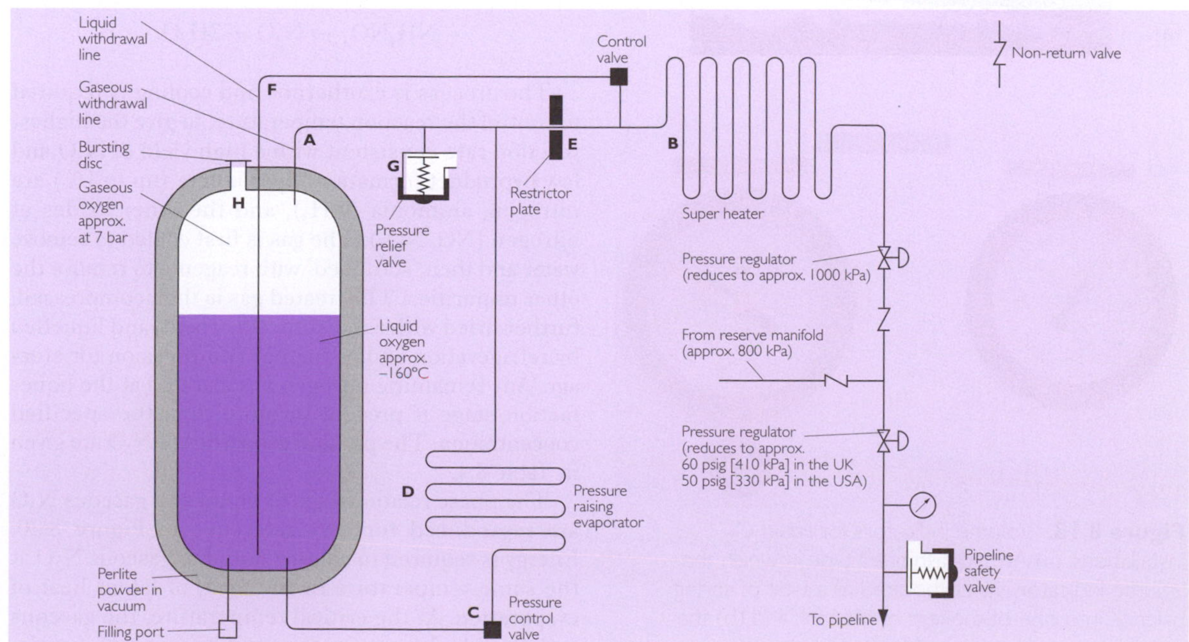


**Figure 8.17.** Diagrammatic representation of the mechanism of action of a liquid $O_2$ supply system (see text for details). (Adapted from Howell RSC. *Anaesthesia* 1980;35:676.)

top and bottom of the tank. The difference between the two gives the depth of the liquid $O_2$ and this, together with the cross-sectional area, allows the volume of liquid $O_2$ to be calculated or read off a calibration chart (Figure 8.18b). All VIE installations have next to them a reserve cylinder bank and enough cylinders on site to supply a typical 24-hour need (Figure 8.16).

### *Oxygen concentrators*

Oxygen concentrators are devices that compress air and pump it through dust-free aluminium silicate, which absorbs nitrogen. The rest of the gaseous components of air pass through unchanged, resulting in a gas mixture containing the residual gases in air (see Table 8.5 later), but consisting principally of up to 95.4% $O_2$ and 4.5% argon. There is a theoretical possibility of argon accumulation in a totally closed circuit.

The absorbent is commonly called artificial zeolite and is sometimes referred to as a molecular sieve. Zeolites are metal–aluminosilicate crystals which occur naturally and can also be synthesized. They have a lattice structure that contains channels running from one surface of the crystal to the other. The maximum diameter of the channels varies from compound to compound (e.g. 0.27–0.9 nm), but it is constant for a particular zeolite. Larger molecules are unable to pass through the channels, which thus act as molecular sieves. An $O_2$ concentrator uses zeolites with a maximum channel diameter of about 0.5 nm. Zeolites are also capable of ion exchange and in this role are used as water softeners.

A typical unit is shown schematically in Figure 8.19. The extraction of nitrogen is extremely rapid but the initial uptake reduces the subsequent efficiency. Fortunately, the recovery of the zeolite is equally rapid. The principle of action is based on the fact that, under pressure, the larger $N_2$ molecules are trapped in the zeolite, but that when the pressure is reduced the zeolite crystals release the $N_2$ and become available again for absorption. As shown in Figure 8.19, the airflow alternates between bed A and bed B, whilst the trapped nitrogen is released from the other bed. The flow is controlled by automatic switches, which cycle every 30–60 s to pump compressed air through the bed and apply suction to extract the unwanted nitrogen. The concentration of $O_2$ in the output gas is very dependent on the flow through the extraction bed, the concentration falling as the flow increases.

Most of the use for $O_2$ concentrators has been to produce domiciliary $O_2$ but there have also been hospital installations. The latter have been used to feed $O_2$ pipelines.

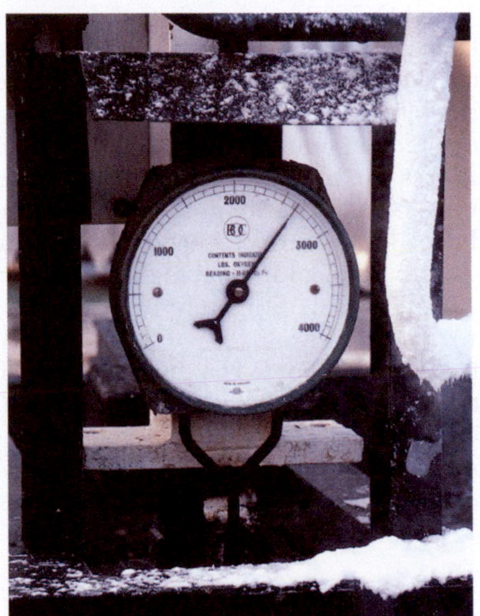


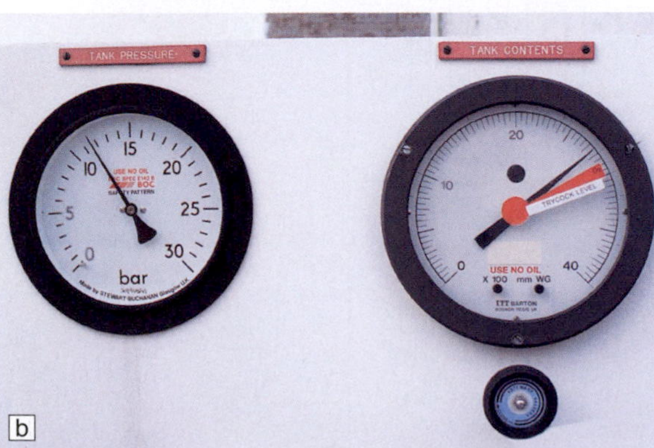


**Figure 8.18.** Volume indicators for liquid $O_2$ installations. (a) An old-fashioned type in which the volume indicator is incorporated as a type of spring balance into one of the legs of the tank and (b) the more modern type where the tank contents are determined from differential pressure transducers in the top and bottom of the liquid $O_2$ container.

### *Nitrous oxide*

$N_2O$ occurs naturally in very low concentrations (approximately 0.4 parts per million [p.p.m.]) in the atmosphere and soils, but this is too low for any form of economic extraction. It is therefore manufactured and this is done almost universally by the thermal decomposition of ammonium nitrate at around 250°C, the process being represented by:

$$NH_4NO_3 \rightarrow N_2O + 2H_2O.$$

The process is exothermic and cooling is required to control the reaction temperature, to give the highest reaction rate consistent with a high yield of $N_2O$ and low byproduct formation. Byproducts (up to 1%) are nitrogen, ammonia ($NH_3$), and the other oxides of nitrogen (NO, $NO_2$). The gas is first cooled to remove water and then 'scrubbed' with reagents to remove the other impurities. The treated gas is then compressed, further dried with a moisture adsorbent, and liquefied by refrigeration and/or further compression for storage. Any remaining nitrogen is separated at the liquefaction stage if present in more than the specified concentration. The physical properties of $N_2O$ are given in Table 8.4.

The phase relationships of liquid and gaseous $N_2O$ are reproduced for easy reference in Figure 8.20. Energy is required to convert liquid to gaseous $N_2O$ at the same temperature in the form of latent heat of evaporation. At the critical temperature, the gaseous and liquid phases are in equilibrium and, as the temperature falls, more energy is required for the conversion (Figure 8.21). When the vapour phase is in

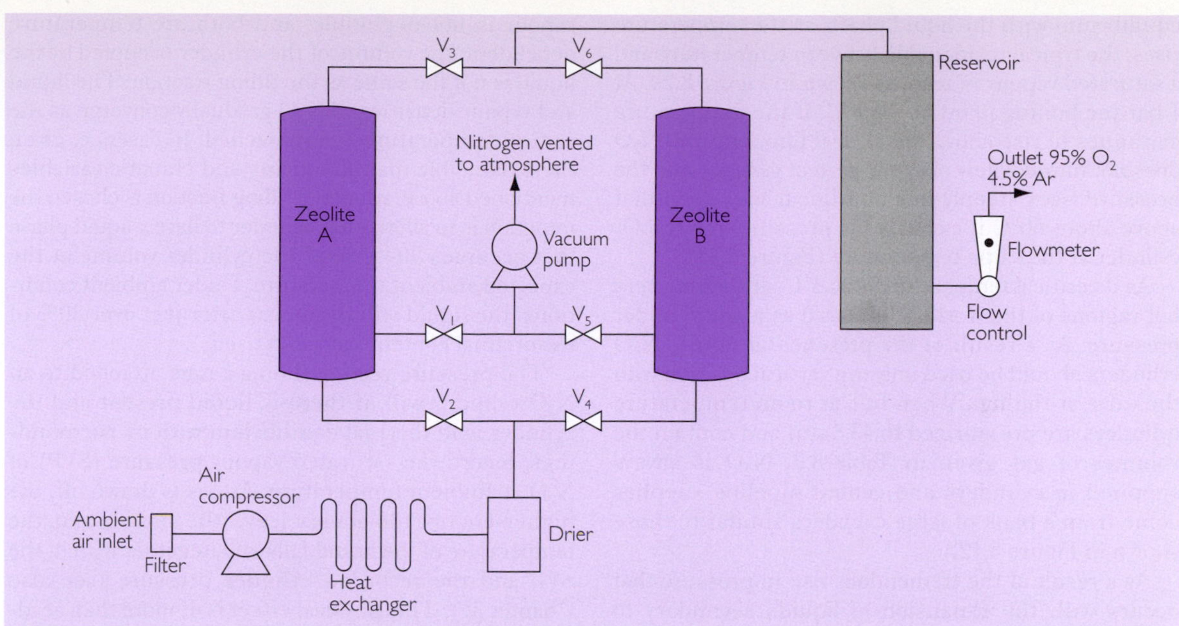


**Figure 8.19.** Diagrammatic representation of an $O_2$ concentrator. Valves $V_1$–$V_6$ are opened sequentially by an automatic control system as described in the text. (Adapted from O'Sullivan J. *Br J Pharm Practice* 1988;9:395.)

**Table 8.4. The physical properties of nitrous oxide**

| Property | Value or description |
|---|---|
| Formula | $N_2O$ |
| Molecular weight | 44.01 daltons |
| Density of gas at 1 bar, 15°C | 1.850 kg/m$^3$ |
| Density of liquid at 1 bar, –88.5°C | 1225 kg/m$^3$ |
| Boiling point, 1 bar | –88.6°C |
| Critical temperature | 36.5°C |
| Critical pressure | 72.5 bar |
| Critical density | 452 kg/m$^3$ |
| Latent heat of vaporization at 1 bar | 375 kJ/kg |

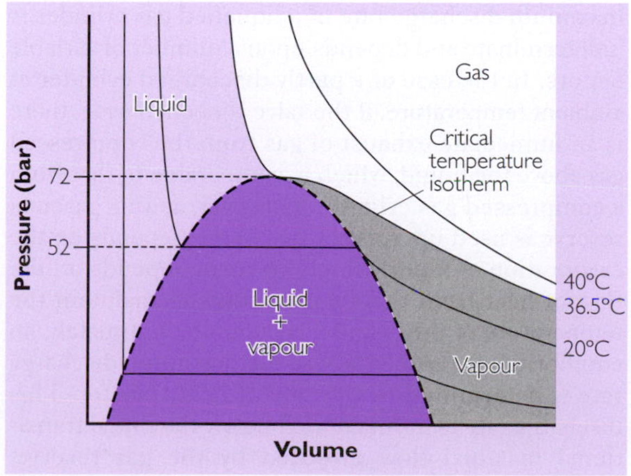


**Figure 8.20.** The phase relationships of liquid and gaseous $N_2O$.

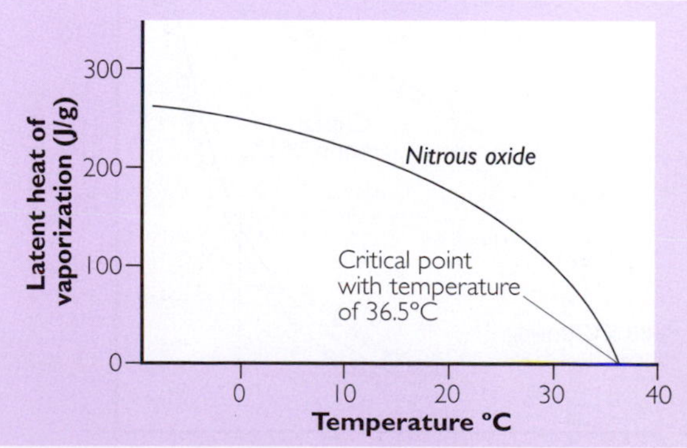


**Figure 8.21.** The relationship between the heat of vaporization and the temperature of $N_2O$. Note that, at the critical temperature, the latent heat of vaporization falls to zero. (Adapted from Mushin WW and Jones PL. *Physics for the Anaesthetist*, 4th edn. Oxford: Blackwell Scientific, 1987: 108.)

equilibrium with the liquid phase, as the temperature rises, the typical relationship between temperature and a saturated vapour is seen, as shown in Figure 8.22. At 1 bar the boiling point is –88.6°C. If the temperature continues to rise above the critical temperature, $N_2O$ does not immediately obey the perfect gas laws and the pressure rises steeply in a non-linear way, such that above about 60°C it exceeds the pressure in a full $O_2$ cylinder at the same temperature (Figure 8.22).

As its critical temperature is 36.5°C, apart from very hot regions of the world, it is stored as a liquid under pressure. As a result of the presence of liquid, $N_2O$ cylinders should be used only in a vertical position with the valve at the top. When full, at room temperature cylinders are pressurized to 43.5 atm and contain the volumes of gas given in Table 8.2. $N_2O$ is always supplied in cylinders and central pipeline supplies come from a bank of large cylinders similar to those shown in Figure 8.12.

As a result of the tremendous rise in pressure that occurs with the expansion of liquids secondary to temperature changes, and the fact that it is gaseous $N_2O$ that is required for anaesthesia, cylinders, when supplied full, always have a gas fraction overlying the liquid phase. The ratio of gas to liquid phase is determined by the filling ratio which is defined as:

$$\text{Filling ratio} = \frac{\text{Weight of liquid and gaseous } N_2O \text{ in the cylinder}}{\text{Weight of water the cylinder could contain}}$$

The filling ratio for liquefied gases is typically specified for temperate climates (maximum expected temperature = 25°C) as 0.75, and for tropical climates (maximum temperature = 35°C) as 0.67. The exact filling ratio used depends on the manufacturer and the particular region of intended use, and includes manufacturing uncertainties such as inaccuracies in gas weight, cylinder volume, etc. As the density of liquid $N_2O$ is less than that of water and the density of its vapour is not negligible, and both are temperature dependent, the volume of the cylinder occupied by the liquid is not the same as the filling fraction. The liquid and vapour densities of $N_2O$ gradually converge as the critical temperature is approached. In essence, given the irreducible manufacturing and climatic variables mentioned above, whatever filling fraction is chosen the intention is to allow a full cylinder to have a liquid phase that occupies 90–95% of the cylinder volume at the expected ambient temperature. Under ambient conditions, the liquid will disappear after just over 80% of the original content has been used.

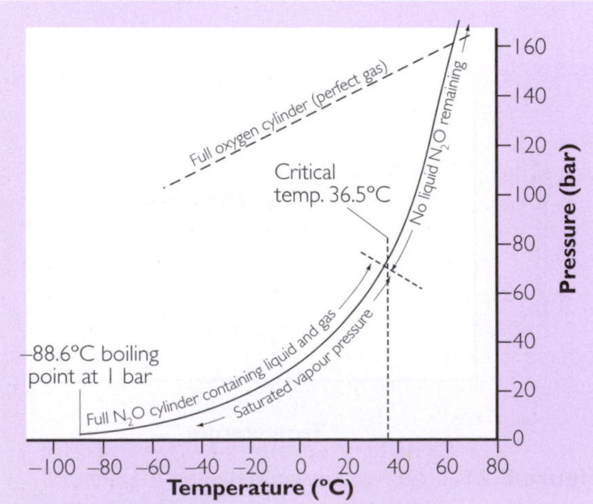


**Figure 8.22.** The variation in pressure with temperature for a full $O_2$ and a full $N_2O$ cylinder. The $N_2O$ cylinder is filled to the normal filling fraction (see text). Plotted from the data in standard gas tables.

The pressure recorded on a gauge attached to an $N_2O$ cylinder will, if there is liquid present and the cylinder is in thermal equilibrium with its surroundings, record the saturated vapour pressure (SVP) of $N_2O$ at ambient temperature. As gas is drawn off, the higher-energy molecules leave the liquid, and the temperature of the liquid falls and, together with it, the SVP and the recorded cylinder pressure (see also Chapter 37). This physical effect is of more than academic value and has two important practical consequences.

Many trainees have the impression that the $N_2O$ cylinder pressure will remain constant until all the liquid has been used up and then fall as if it were an ideal gas. This assumption is untrue because the rate of supply of heat from the surroundings is too slow to maintain isothermal conditions. When using cylinders on the anaesthesia machine, as gas is drawn off, the fall in temperature causes the $N_2O$ pressure gauge to fall, the rate of fall depending on the rate of gas usage. Typical results of this process are given in Figure 8.23; the temperature usually falls sufficiently low for ice to form on the outside of the cylinder (Figure 8.24). From Figure 8.23, it can also be seen that, if there is sufficient content left in the cylinder to maintain the liquid phase, as it warms up back to ambient temperature, the pressure will recover to equal that in the original full cylinder. Consequently, the pressure in an $N_2O$ cylinder bears little relationship to its content and only those cylinders being used to supply low-flow systems at below approximately 2 L/min will empty without undue cooling and approximate to isothermal behaviour.

Unlike a cylinder containing compressed gas, the maximum discharge rate of a liquefied gas cylinder is indeterminate and depends upon a number of variable factors. In the case of a partly discharged cylinder at ambient temperature, if the valve is opened wide, there is an immediate exhaust of gas from the compressed gas above the liquid, which is comparable to that from a compressed gas cylinder. However, as this gaseous reserve is used up, further discharge depends on the evaporation of liquid which, in turn, depends on the flow of heat from the surroundings to maintain the temperature of the cylinder's contents. Ultimately, an equilibrium is reached where the maximum discharge rate is determined by the rate of heat transfer. This discharge rate is normally well below the initial transitional maximal flow provided by the gas reserve. Although this limitation is not a problem when discharging a size-E cylinder on an anaesthesia machine, it represents a major consideration in the provision of pipeline supplies from $N_2O$ cylinders (and

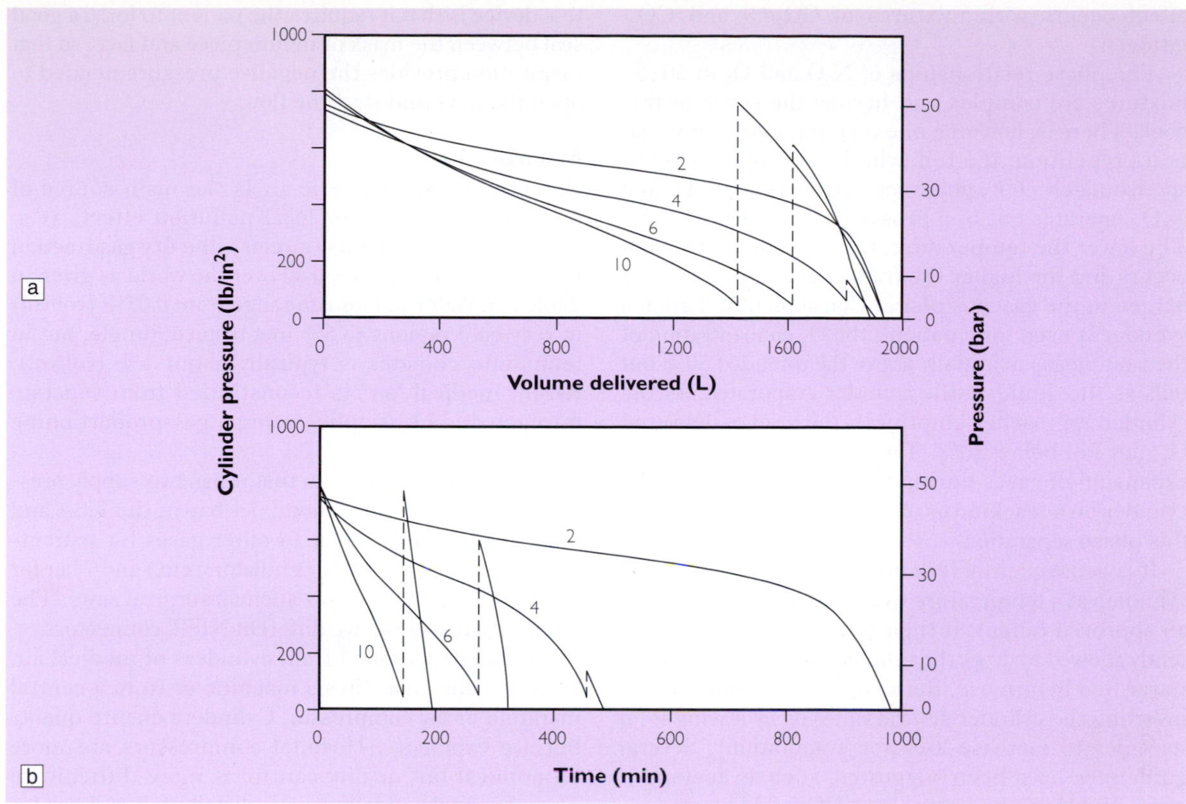


**Figure 8.23.** Pressure changes in an 1800-litre (size E) $N_2O$ cylinder emptying at continuous flow rates between 2 and 10 L/min. The fall in pressure is shown with (a) the number of litres delivered and (b) the time elapsed. Note the speed with which the higher flows decrease the pressure in the cylinder. Each broken line indicates re-warming of the cylinder to room temperature. (Adapted from Jones PL. *Br J Anaesth* 1974;46:534.)

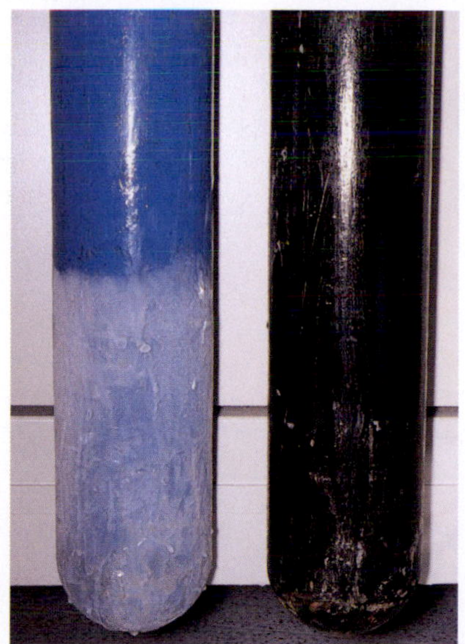

**Figure 8.24.** The formation of ice on the outside of a $N_2O$ cylinder during steady discharge at 6 L/min. At the time that the photograph was taken, the cylinder was about 40% full of liquid $N_2O$ and the pressure gauge on the cylinder was approaching the red 'low contents' zone. This is because the saturated vapour pressure of the $N_2O$ is determined by its temperature, which in this case was sub-zero.

also from liquefied $O_2$ supplies as described above). The difficulty can be overcome in two ways:

1. At times of high demand, liquid can be drawn off directly and vaporized in an external evaporator. This is the method used for $O_2$.
2. Several cylinders can be manifolded together so that flows from individual cylinders are combined, each having an evaporation rate compatible with the thermal flux from its surroundings. Tables are available for the number and volume of cylinders required to match a given maximum flow. This method is used for $N_2O$.

#### *Entonox*

Entonox is a mixture of 50% $N_2O$ and 50% $O_2$. Like $N_2O$, it is supplied only in cylinders. These can be free-standing, attached to an anaesthesia machine, or manifolded for pipeline supplies. The pressures, capacities, and sizes of Entonox cylinders are given in Table 8.2. Etonox is not available in some countries (e.g. USA).

From a consideration of the physics of $N_2O$ it could be apparently assumed that, whenever the gas was at room temperature and at a partial pressure of over approximately 45 atm in a gas mixture, it would be capable of being liquefied. This is not, however, always true. Under pressure, $O_2$ is quite soluble in liquid $N_2O$ and, when in gaseous mixture together, they have a higher SVP than $N_2O$ alone. This non-ideal gas behaviour is described as the Poynting effect, and results in mixtures of $O_2$ and $N_2O$ being capable of being compressed to the normal cylinder pressure of 137 bar at room temperature with no fear of liquefaction. This behaviour is also considered in Chapter 37. A similar effect occurs with mixtures of $CO_2/O_2$ and $CO_2$/nitrogen.

The phase relationships of $N_2O$ and $O_2$ in 50 : 50 mixtures are complex and beyond the scope of this book. There is, however, one very important point that bears repetition. If a full cylinder is cooled to below approximately –6°C, phase separation occurs and liquid $N_2O$ separates out by a process termed 'lamination'. The lower the temperature, the more the separation occurs and the higher the fractional concentration of oxygen in the gaseous phase. Consequently, if such a cylinder is used for a patient, the $O_2$ concentration of the issuing gas is initially above the intended 50% but falls as the liquid in the cylinder evaporates. As the cylinder approaches emptiness, the level of delivered $O_2$ may fall below 20%. Temperature drop from the expansion of gases during the normal emptying of a cylinder on a machine or on a manifold does not cause this phase separation.

It is consequently very important to store Entonox cylinders at a temperature well above –6°C (10–38°C is an approved range). If their temperature is inadvertently allowed to drop, the cylinders must be thoroughly rewarmed before use. Remixing can be enhanced by inverting the cylinder several times or by leaving it on its side (to increase area for evaporation). Several guidelines have been suggested, such as keeping it above 10°C for 2 hours or above 5°C for 24 hours.

For analgesia in conscious patients, Entonox can be delivered by a special two-stage demand pressure regulator. This is shown in Figure 8.25. A practical point of this device is that it requires the patient to form a good seal between the mask or mouth piece and face, so that inspiration provides the negative pressure needed to open the valve and start the flow.

### Medical air

Compressed atmospheric air is the main source of medical air. Except for local pollution effects (e.g. carbon monoxide in busy streets), the dry gas fraction has the same composition all over the world as given in Table 8.5. Water vapour can range from 0.05% (vol/vol) in very cold regions to 5% in a tropical jungle, but in temperate climates is typically about 1% (vol/vol). Rarely, medical 'air' is reconstituted from separate nitrogen and $O_2$ supplies using a gas-proportioning system.

Medical air is unique in that it has two supply pressures in the operating room: 3.4 bar in the USA and 4 bar in the UK (similar to other gases for patient-related use and for driving ventilators, etc.) and 7 bar for powering pneumatic tools such as surgical saws. The different pressures have different NIST connectors.

Air can be supplied from cylinders of medical air, either on the anaesthesia machine or from a central manifold or air compressor. Cylinders ensure quality but are expensive. Hospital compressors are more economical but quality control is more difficult. In many hospitals, pipeline air is distributed at 4 bar for patient use and cylinders are used to drive tools at 7 bar. This methodology represents a good compromise between cost and safety.

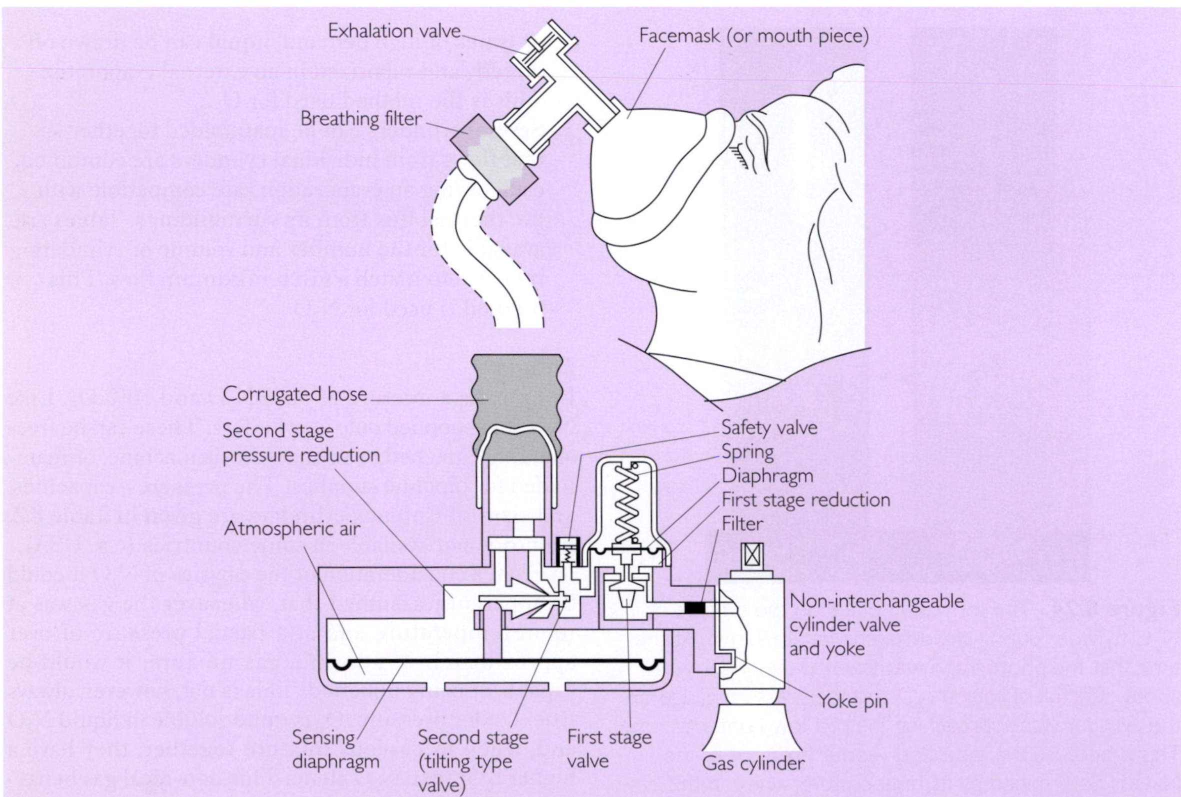


**Figure 8.25.** An Entonox demand valve. The patient has to apply a negative pressure to the outlet of the valve in order to trigger the valve to open. When the patient inhales, the negative pressure deflects the sensing diaphragm and initiates the flow of gas from the cylinder. See later in text for method of operation of pressure-reducing valves. (Adapted from British Oxygen Co. Ltd equipment manual.)

The pressures and volumes of medical air cylinders are given in Table 8.2. A cylinder's contents can be judged directly from its pressure, and cylinder manifolds are constructed from three sets of cylinders as described above for $N_2O$ (Figure 8.11).

Medical compressed air differs from industrial compressed air in that a greater purity is required and that compressor oil must be removed. It should be remembered that medical air, although subject to strict regulations, is not sterile. Its specification is given in Table 8.6.

A medical air compression plant is shown schematically in Figure 8.26. There are two compressors that work alternately (often a week at a time), each of which is capable of producing the maximum required flow on its own, supported by a reserve manifold for emergencies. The air enters through a filter, is compressed and then cooled back to room temperature, before entering a reservoir tank. The tank, which has a working pressure of approximately 10 bar, possesses a water drain and safety valve. It allows the storage of gas during quiet periods and supplies a constant, non-fluctuating head of pressure. On leaving the tank, the compressed air

**Table 8.5. The dry gas composition of atmospheric air**

| Constituent | Percentage by volume (% mole fraction) |
|---|---|
| Nitrogen | 78.08 |
| Oxygen | 20.95 |
| Argon | 0.93 |
| Carbon dioxide | 0.03[a] |
| Neon | 0.0018 |
| Helium | 0.0005 |
| Methane | 0.0002[a] |
| Krypton | 0.0001 |
| Hydrogen | 0.00005 |
| Nitrous oxide | 0.00005[a] |
| Xenon | 0.000008 |

[a]Variable.

**Table 8.6. Specification for medical compressed air**

| A sample of medical compressed air at standard temperature and pressure (STP) shall not contain more than the following concentrations of contaminants: |
|---|
| 0.5 mg/m$^3$ oil mist particulate |
| 5.5 mg/m$^3$ carbon monoxide (5 p.p.m.) |
| 900 mg/m$^3$ carbon dioxide (900 p.p.m.) |
| The humidity should be such that the dew point of the air is below −40°C at 1 bar |

p.p.m., parts per million

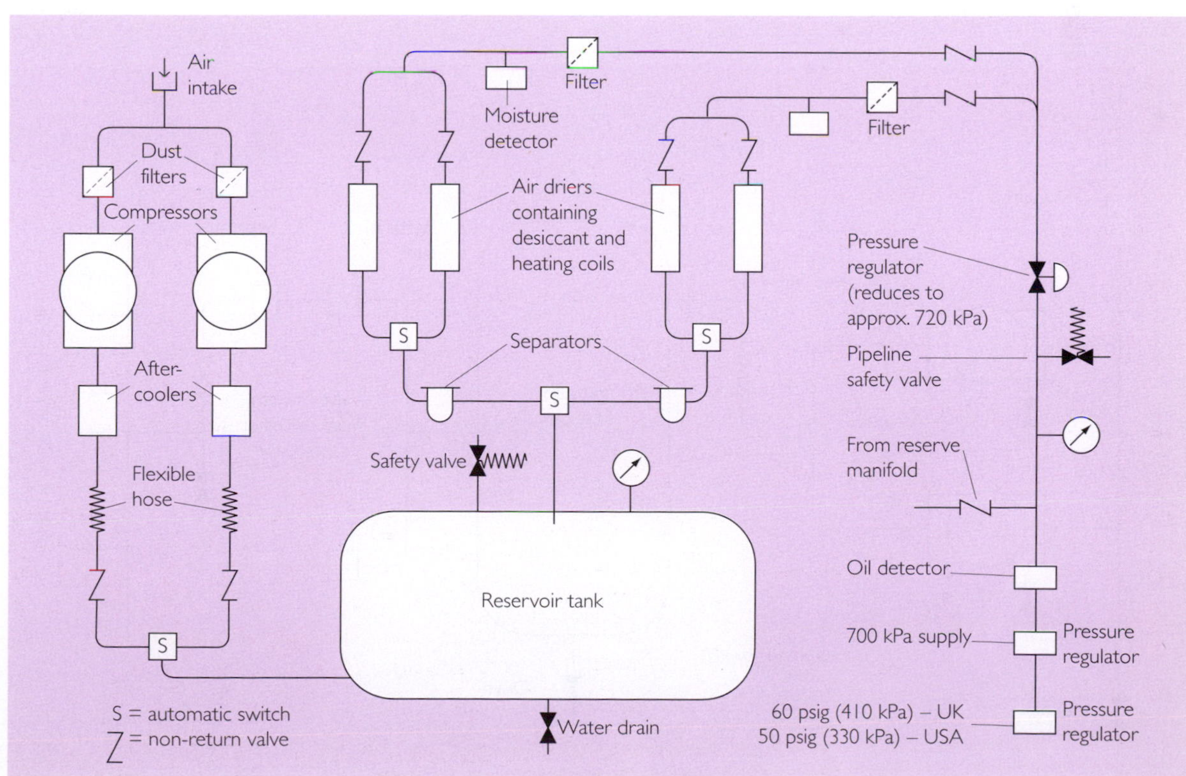


**Figure 8.26.** A diagrammatic representation of a medical compressed air plant. Note the two pressures at which air is supplied. (Adapted from Howell RSC. *Anaesthesia* 1980;35:676.)

passes through a dessicator to remove water vapour, and finally through a further filter to remove any remaining oil or water. The oil and water content of the output gas is checked regularly.

### *Carbon dioxide*

$CO_2$ occurs naturally (see Table 8.5) but in too low a quantity for economic extraction. It is manufactured from three sources: a byproduct in the manufacture of hydrogen, a byproduct from fermentation, and from the combustion of fuels. From whatever source, it is subsequently purified and liquefied for cylinder storage. Its physical properties allow it to be solid at atmospheric pressure and at atmospheric temperature it sublimates directly into the gaseous form. Its properties are given in Table 8.7.

$CO_2$ is stored as a liquefied gas and is available in cylinders as specified in Table 8.2. Its behaviour in cylinders is analogous to $N_2O$ but, because it is used infrequently and at low flows, the temperature effects are not seen in the same way; indeed it is not usual for a $CO_2$ cylinder to have a pressure gauge attached. Some anaesthetists hold very strong and diametrically opposed views about the value of $CO_2$. Many years ago the late Sir Robert Macintosh tried to abolish its use in the operating room. The main problem is when it is on and the anaesthetist does not realize it. This is considered more fully in 'The anaesthesia machine', page 111.

$CO_2$ is also supplied in gaseous mixtures with $O_2$ and nitrogen in certificated cylinders for the calibration of blood gas machines.

**Table 8.7. Properties of carbon dioxide**

| Property | Value or description |
|---|---|
| Formula | $CO_2$ |
| Molecular weight | 44.0 daltons |
| Critical temperature | 31.04°C |
| Sublimation temperature at 1 bar | –78.5°C |

### Vacuum

Efficient suction is a key component of anaesthetic safety. It can be provided locally from isolated vacuum units or centrally from an evacuated reservoir. As a general rule small suction machines do not have the power of pipeline suction. Pipeline suction outlets have their own collars and NIST fittings.

A central vacuum source is basically the same as a compressor system working in reverse, as shown in Figure 8.27. Specifications differ from country to country, but, in the UK, a system should be capable of maintaining a vacuum of at least 53 kPa (400 mmHg) below atmospheric pressure at each outlet, each of which should be able to take a free flow of air at 40 L/min. There should be at least two outlets per operating room, one per anaesthetic room, and one per recovery bed.

The chief practical problem with suction is the fact that the flow of gas is from the patient to the wall. Although there should always be a trap to catch solid and liquid aspirate, this does not stop bacterial and gaseous effluent and water vapour reaching the main pipeline. It is therefore necessary to protect the plant and the people who work on it with filters, separators and inspection windows.

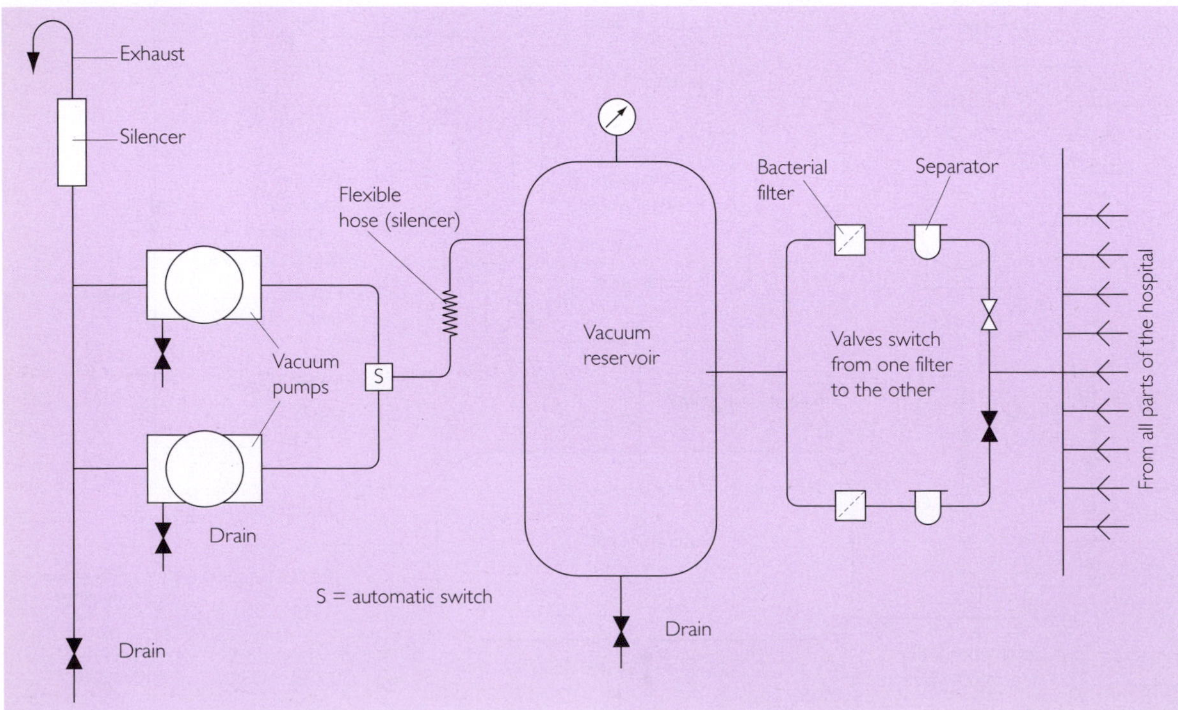


**Figure 8.27.** A diagrammatic representation of a piped medical vacuum plant. (Adapted from Howell RSC. *Anaesthesia* 1980;35:676.)

## THE ANAESTHESIA MACHINE

The anaesthesia machine controls the release of pressurized gases at preset rates, adds vapours to the gases as required, and delivers the mixture to a common gas outlet. It also incorporates a number of safety features that prevent hypoxic mixtures being delivered and dangerous pressures being developed within certain parts of the pipework. Only the principles of the machine itself and those attachments not described in more detail elsewhere are dealt with here. The supply of gases up to the machine is described in the first section of this chapter.

The regulations on performance and safety of anaesthesia machines vary from country to country. The latest USA standard is the F1161-94 standard of the American Society for Testing and Materials (ASTM). This states that a newly manufactured anaesthesia machine must have:

- an oxygen analyser,
- a breathing pressure monitor,
- an exhaled tidal volume monitor, or capnograph, which functions automatically when this machine is in use,
- a prioritized alarm system.

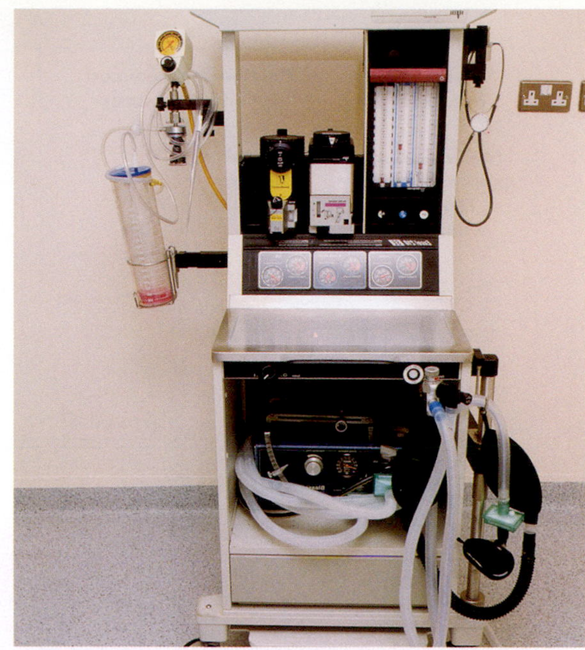

**Figure 8.28.** A basic anaesthesia machine without integrated monitoring. This model is the Ohmeda Excel 200SE. Note the immediate availability of a stethoscope and powerful suction.

It is clear that these recommendations cannot be applied retrospectively, so it is essential to be clear on the performance of the anaesthesia machine to be used, and to check it thoroughly. The method of checking a 'traditional' machine is described in Chapter 12. The more complex modern machines with integrated monitoring cannot always be checked using these guidelines; in these circumstances the manufacturer's handbook should be followed. Whatever checking system is used, before a patient is connected *the anaesthetist must be absolutely certain that when the $O_2$ alone is switched on, 100% pressurized $O_2$ is delivered to the common gas outlet, and that a reserve $O_2$ cylinder is available*. A typical basic machine without integrated monitoring is shown in Figure 8.28 and in schematic block diagram form in Figure 8.29. Specific features of importance are described below.

### Cylinder attachment

The cylinders are specific to the yoke that matches their pin index (see earlier). The gas-tight joint between the cylinder and the yoke is made by a Bodock seal (Figure 8.30). This is an annular piece of neoprene surrounded circumferentially with a ring of aluminium. The neoprene is thicker than the aluminium and compresses down as the cylinder is tightened into position. The difference in thickness between the metal ring and the neoprene ensures an adequate compression of the neoprene to provide a gas-tight joint while the ring prevents over-tightening and destruction of the neoprene.

The path of gas into the machine pipework is shown in Figure 8.31. It can be seen that there is a check valve that permits only forward flow of gas and prevents leakage if there is no cylinder present. A leak of not more than 15 ml/min through an open yoke is acceptable on a new machine. In some unfortunate occurrences on older machines, these check valves have not been working properly, leading to early exhaustion of cylinders and delivery of hypoxic gas mixtures.

### Pressure gauges

The mode of action of pressure gauges is given in Chapters 37 and 39. Bourdon-type gauges are tapped into the yoke and pipeline supplies, and the gauge faces are displayed in a convenient position. The gas entry to the pressure gauge has a constriction to eliminate surges in pressure when hoses are connected and disconnected and cylinders turned on (see flow restrictor, Figure 8.31). Gauges are colour coded for the country of use to match the cylinder and pipeline colour. The markings have to be readable by someone with normal vision at a distance of 1 metre under 20 foot-candles of illumination. The full-scale reading must be 33% greater than the maximum cylinder pressure.

### Pressure regulators

Pressure regulators are important because they provide a constant head of pressure to the rotameter needle valves and hence render the flow, once set on the rotameter, effectively independent of the normal working changes in cylinder pressure until the cylinder is substantially emptied. They possess stringent design criteria: they must not react chemically with the gas being controlled, and they must be capable of withstanding four times the maximum inlet pressure, have a pressure relief valve fitted on the low-pressure side, and have a corrosion-resistant filter fitted upstream of the first valve seat.

There are a number of designs in use, but, whatever the physical arrangement of components, their principle of action is identical. Two designs are shown in cross-section in Figure 8.32. Figure 8.33 represents the valves

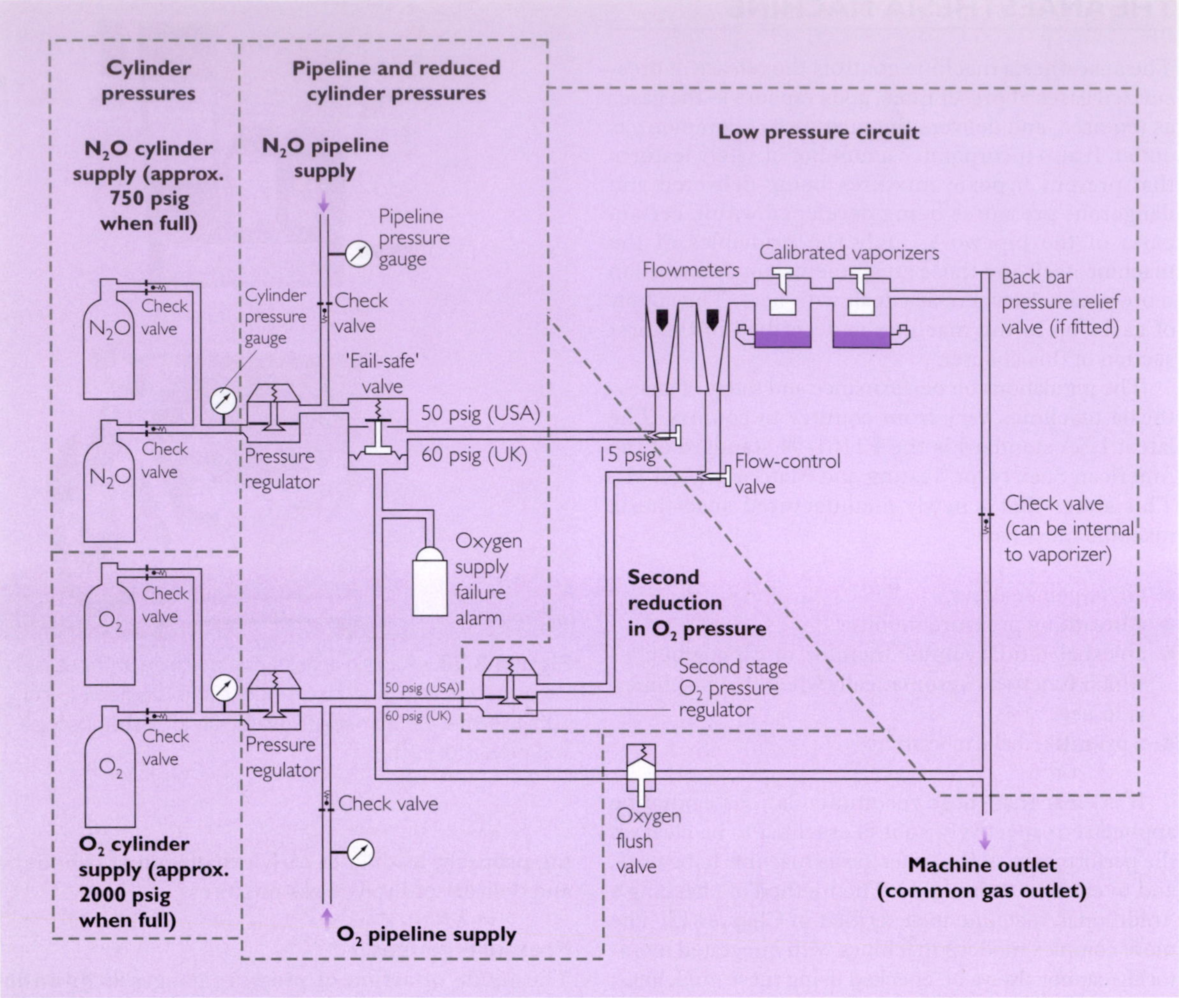

**Figure 8.29.** A schematic block diagram of an anaesthesia machine. Note the variation in pressures in different parts of the machine. Note also that the flowmeters are the wrong way around for UK practice (see text). psig, pounds per square inch gauge. (Adapted from *Check-Out, A Guide for Preoperative Inspection of an Anesthesia Machine*. American Society of Anesthesiologists, 1987.)

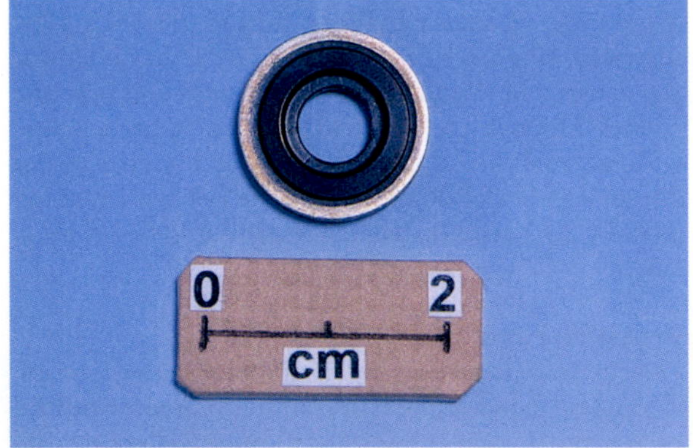


**Figure 8.30.** A Bodock seal which forms a gas-tight joint between the cylinder and anaesthesia machine.

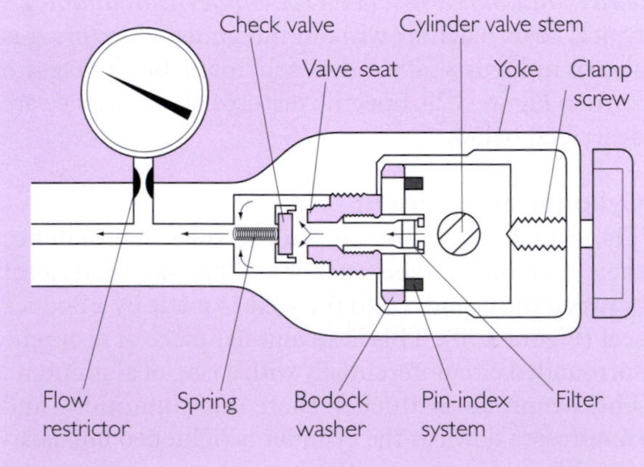


**Figure 8.31** A diagrammatic representation of a plan view of the attachment of a cylinder valve to the anaesthesia machine showing the one-way check valve for preventing the back flow of gas.

in elemental form and gives the mathematical derivation of their performance characteristics. The final equation:

$$\text{Change in outlet pressure} = -\left(\text{Change in inlet pressure} \times \frac{\text{Valve area}}{\text{Diaphragm area}}\right)$$

shows from the minus sign that the outlet pressure rises slightly as the cylinder pressure falls (until the cylinder is substantially empty), and that the relationship between the two is controlled by the valve to diaphragm area ratio. Typical values for this ratio are 1 : 200 or 1 : 300. The performance of a single-stage regulator is shown in Figure 8.34.

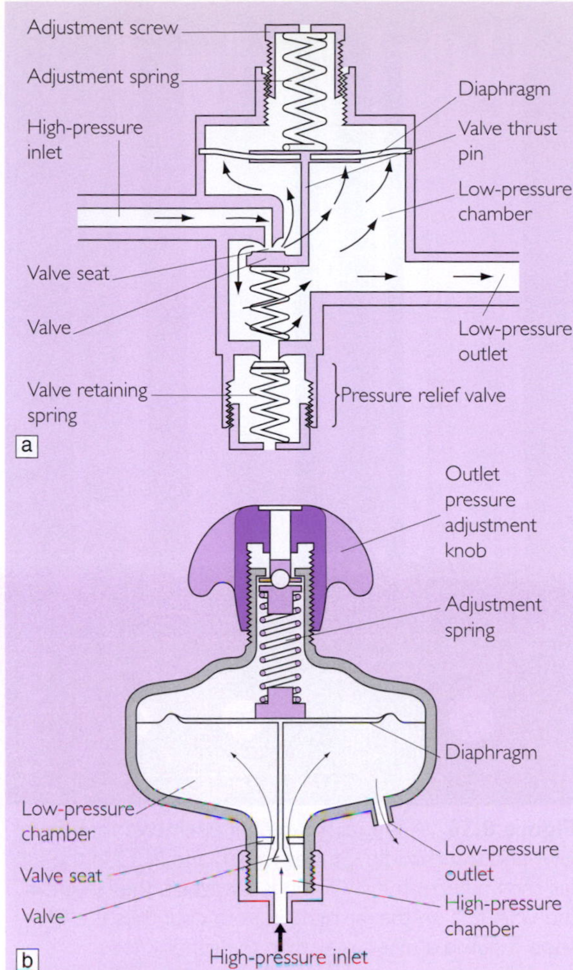


**Figure 8.32.** Diagrammatic cross-sections of typical pressure-regulating valves. Two arrangements are shown but the principle is the same in both.

Many modern machines have a secondary pressure regulator on the $O_2$ supply to the rotameter fitted after the attachment of the pipeline, as shown in Figure 8.29. This is because a number of external factors could otherwise cause the machine working pressure to fluctuate around the nominal $O_2$ supply pressure by up to 20%. Such factors are, for example, changes in pipeline demand in other parts of the hospital and the use of auxiliary outlets on the anaesthesia machine for driving a ventilator. Secondary pressure regulation is also important in machines that incorporate an anti-hypoxia link (see below) because these systems, when designed, assume a steady flow of $O_2$ from a constant pressure head. Typical pressures in anaesthesia machine pipework are shown in Figure 8.29. The exact levels depend on the specific machine and can be found in the manufacturer's service manual.

## High-pressure (auxiliary) outlets

Anaesthesia machines may be fitted with power gas sockets for air and/or $O_2$ that originate from the 50/60 psig piping in the machine. These are used as pneumatic power supplies for ventilators, for suction units, and for Venturi systems and injectors. Typical power outlets are shown in Figure 8.35.

## The rotameter block

The physics of rotameters is described in Chapter 37. A typical flowmeter assembly is shown in Figure 8.36 and in cross-section in Figure 8.37. It is subject to stringent design criteria. For UK practice, these are set down in British Standard BS 4272. The flow is read at the top of the float which should always be spinning freely away from the walls of the tube. Free spinning is seen by rotation of the spot or stripes on the bobbin.

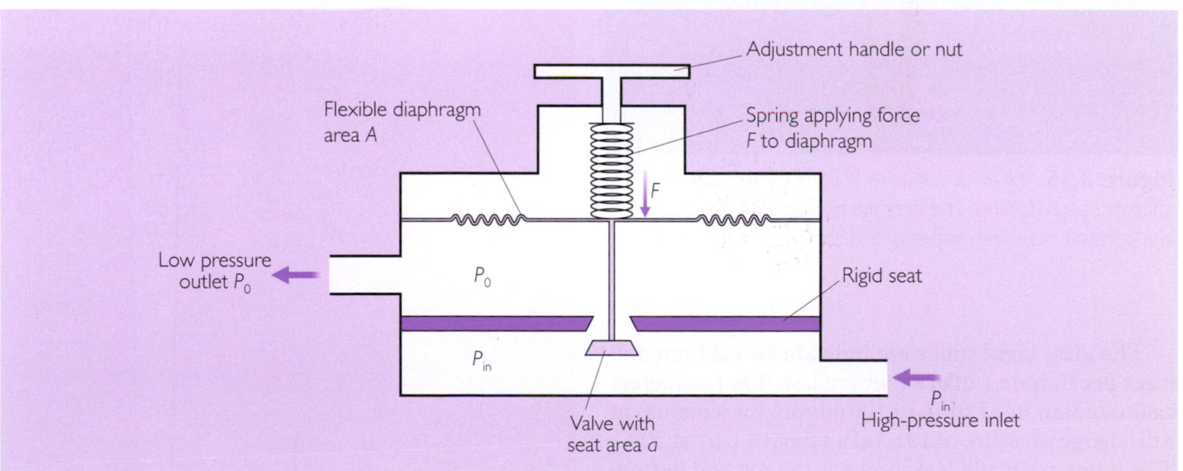


**Figure 8.33.** Diagrammatic representation of a pressure-reducing valve. The physical layout of the components may vary from valve to valve but the principle is identical. The mathematical derivation of its performance characteristics is as follows. Assume that, in the equilibrium position, the valve is just closed or open. Then, at equilibrium:

$$F = P_0 A + P_{in} a$$

and, if the outlet pressure changes by $\Delta P_0$ and the inlet pressure by $\Delta P_{in}$:

$$F = (P_0 + \Delta P_0)A + (P_{in} + \Delta P_{in})a = P_0 A + P_{in} a$$

giving:

$$\Delta P_0 A + \Delta P_{in} a = 0$$

or

$$\Delta P_0 = -\Delta P_{in}(a/A).$$

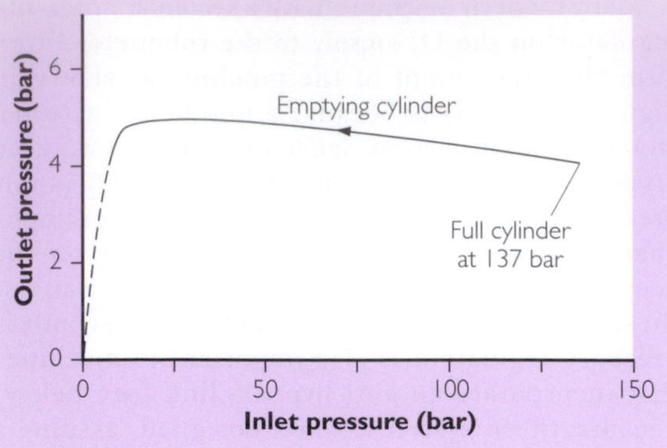


**Figure 8.34.** The relationship between the outlet pressure of a single-stage regulator on an $O_2$ cylinder and its inlet pressure. The inlet pressure is the pressure within the cylinder. It can be seen that, over a wide range of inlet pressures as the cylinder empties, the outlet pressure varies relatively little until the mechanism fails when the cylinder is close to being completely empty. Note the slight rise in outlet pressure during regulation as the cylinder pressure falls.

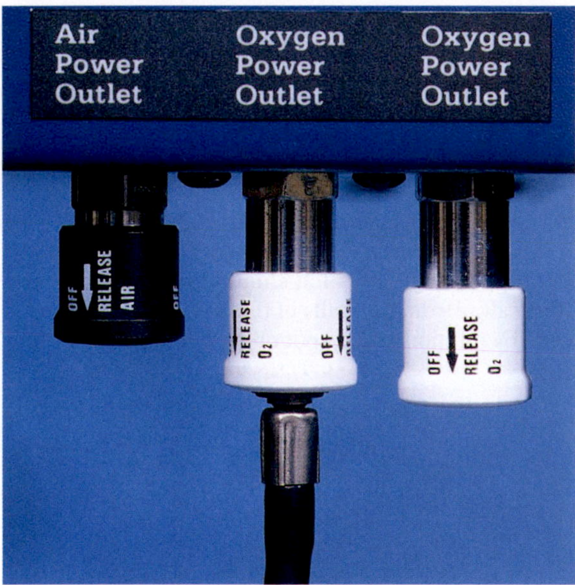


**Figure 8.35.** High-pressure auxiliary outlets on an anaesthesia machine. Their exact position on the anaesthesia machine depends on the particular model.

The glass sight tubes are individually calibrated in litres per minute (unless they are low-flow rotameters calibrated up to 1 L/min in 100 ml/min increments) at a discharge pressure of 101.3 kPa (about 1 bar) at 20°C. The tubes are made leak-proof at the top and bottom by 'O' rings, washers, or some other sealing arrangement, and some manufacturers give different gases different diameters or some other form of indexing system to prevent inadvertent errors of assembly. Details differ slightly from country to country, but the following are a list of factors that feature in BS 4272:

- Flow rates must be accurate to ± 10% of the indicated flow between 10% and 80% of the scale range.

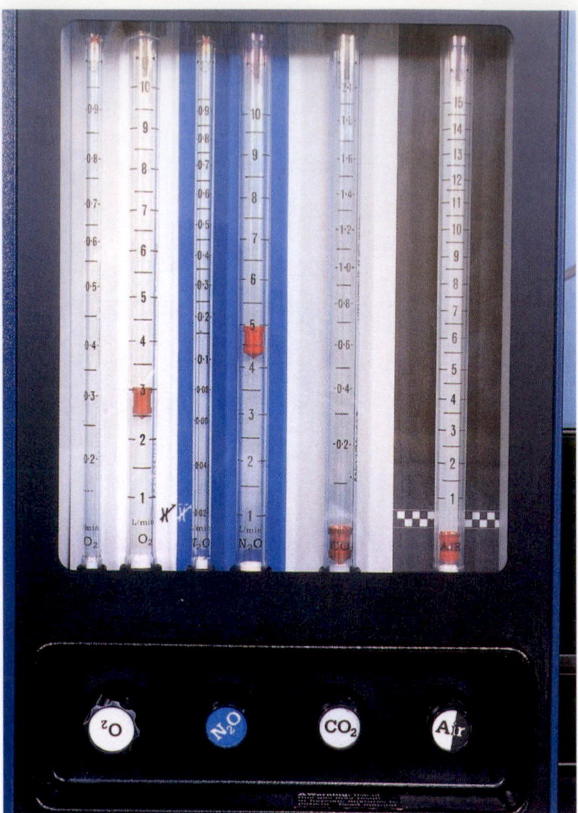


**Figure 8.36.** A typical rotameter assembly. Note the low- and standard-flow tubes for $O_2$ and $N_2O$. In the UK (as shown here) the $O_2$ knob is always on the far left; in the USA it is on the far right. In both countries the $O_2$ knob is fluted and is larger than the other knobs.

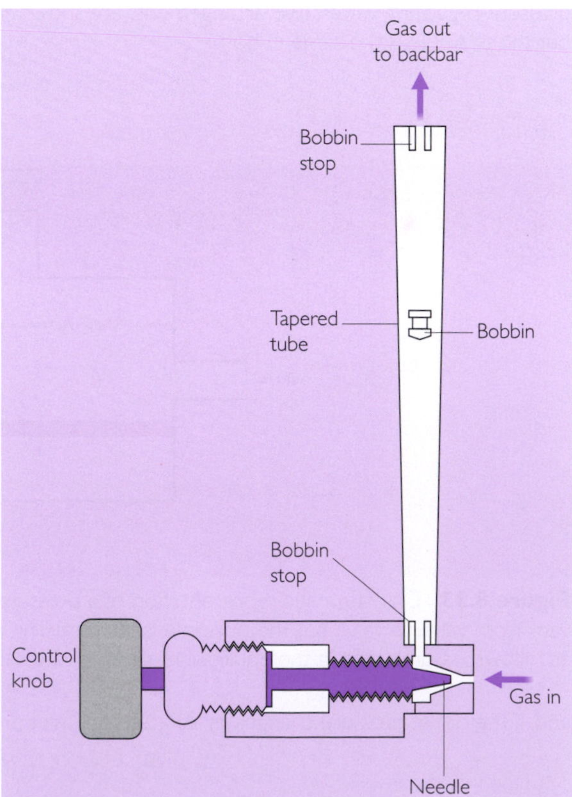


**Figure 8.37.** Diagrammatic representation of a needle valve and rotameter block assembly.

- Each needle valve knob must be clearly marked, indicating the gas it controls, and the $O_2$ knob must have an octagonal profile and be of greater diameter and project beyond the other flow control knobs.
- The twist required to turn the knobs must be sufficient to prevent accidental readjustment from a casual knock.
- When axial push–pull forces are applied to the needle valve spindle, the flow change must not be greater than 10% or 10 ml/min, whichever is the greater.

Many flowmeters exceed this specification and are typically accurate to ±5%.

The order of the flowmeters in the rotameter block is of some importance. If there is a crack in a rotameter tube, especially if it is a gas that is not switched on, there will be backflow of gas through the leak. In order to minimize the generation of hypoxic mixtures, there are several designs which, although having an $O_2$ control knob and rotameter at the extreme left end of the block, deliver $O_2$ downstream of any other gas. One such design and the way it is intended to work is shown in Figure 8.38. It should of course be noted that, if the crack is big enough or if it is in the $O_2$ rotameter itself, the composition and volume of the delivered flow will differ from that set, despite the protective design features shown. As an additional safety feature, modern machines incorporate a chain link system which ensures that an $O_2$ concentration of over 25% is always given, as shown in Figure 8.39. This system will not of course allow for the effect of leaks or other gases in the gas mixture, nor will it compensate for variations in gas supply pressure. It is partly for this latter reason that secondary pressure regulators (see above) are included as part of the design specification because its effectiveness depends on a steady preset upstream pressure for the needle valves.

### Low-flow considerations

As a result of newer expensive volatile agents and the ability to easily monitor gases within a circle easily, there has been an increased interest in low-flow techniques. This has necessitated the introduction of low-flow rotameters because those calibrated up to, say, 10 L/min cannot be used reliably below 1 L/min. The usual design is for the low- and high-flow rotameters to be in series, as shown in Figure 8.40. Consequently, at flows of more than 1 L/min, the bobbin in the low-flow tube is permanently held at the top of its tube.

Another feature of some modern machines is that they have a mechanical stop fitted to the $O_2$ control valve. This ensures a minimum standing flow of 175–250 ml/min of $O_2$, sufficient to provide a basal flow into a totally closed circuit.

### Carbon dioxide flowmeters

The provision of $CO_2$ on machines is somewhat controversial because it has been the cause of considerable morbidity and mortality over the years in the following ways:

- Cylinders have been removed while the flowmeters have been left on, and faulty check valves at the yoke have allowed the escape of other gases such as $O_2$ and $N_2O$.

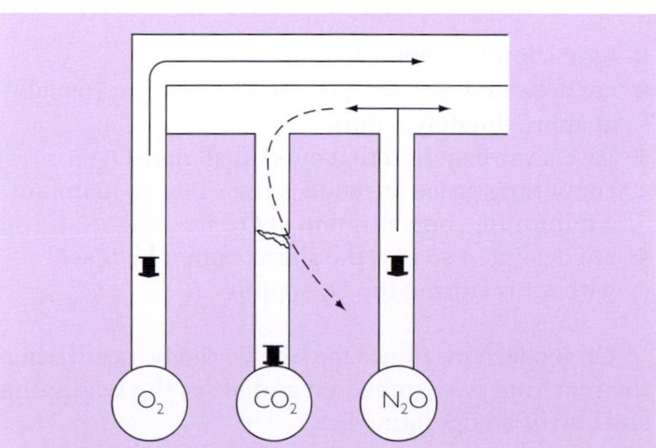


**Figure 8.38.** An example of the design of the outlet to a rotameter block intended to minimize hypoxic events secondary to leakage from the rotameter block. This drawing assumes that the leak is not in the $O_2$ assembly.

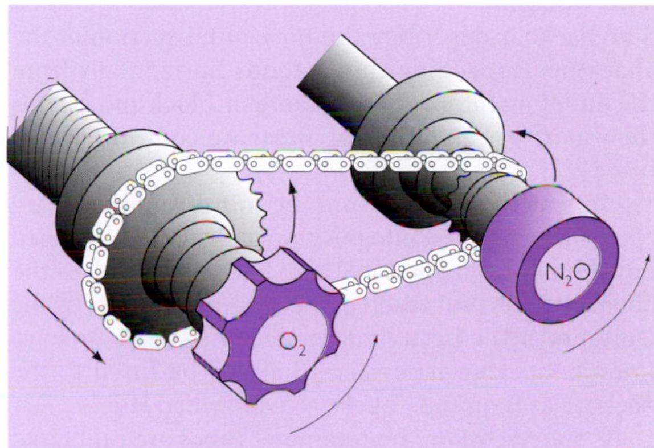


**Figure 8.39.** The Ohmeda $O_2/N_2O$ link system to prevent hypoxic mixtures.

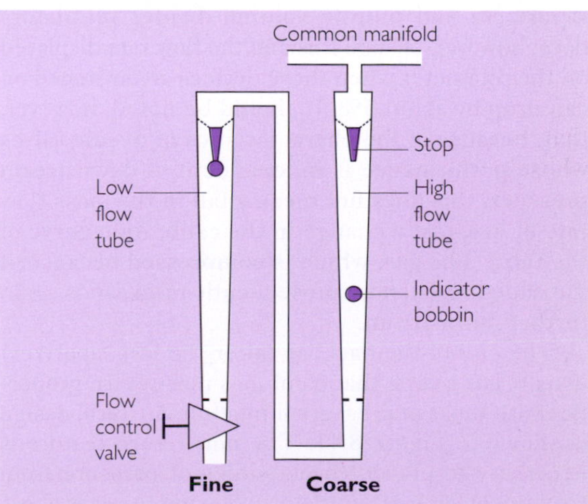


**Figure 8.40.** Diagrammatic representation of flow-meter tubes in series which allow accurate setting of low gas flows. Note that, when a high gas flow is used, the bobbin in the low-flow tube is permanently in the maximum position, often designed to be hidden behind a screen. Such an arrangement is shown in Figure 8.36.

- Cylinders have been put on while the flowmeter was open and $CO_2$ administered inadvertently. In some instances, this has not been noticed because the float immediately went to the top of the tube.
- The gas has been turned off at the cylinder with the needle valve open. When the cylinder was turned on again, inadvertent administration of $CO_2$ occurred unnoticed.

The response to these dangers has been the advice that only the anaesthetist using the $CO_2$ should put it on the machine and should take it off when finished. In addition to this, manufacturers have responded with designs that limit the maximum flow to 600 ml/min, which is displayed in the centre of the tube scale, or have introduced a flow restrictor to limit the flow into a standard flowmeter to about 600 ml/min.

The need for $CO_2$ cylinders on anaesthesia machines, now that hyperventilation is not used routinely and there is wide availability of capnographs, is greatly reduced. Some would say that it was not required at all.

### The backbar

The backbar describes the horizontal section of the anaesthesia machine that extends horizontally from the outlet manifold of the rotameter block and carries the vaporizers and working pressure control valve (if fitted).

On older machines, one or more vaporizers are permanently bolted into position and each can be used individually or in combination. The latter involves the obligatory contamination of the second vaporizer by the contents of the first. The modern method is to have interchangeable vaporizers that can be fitted to the backbar as required. These are described later.

As stated earlier, the rotameter tubes are calibrated at atmospheric downstream pressure. In old-fashioned backbar systems with large 23-mm internal diameter (ID) pipework, the pressure developed at typical flow rates was only marginally above atmospheric. The addition of modern high-resistance vaporizers and minute volume divider ventilators does, however, change this and the flow rate displayed on the rotameter when these devices are switched on can drop by about 5%. It should be noted, however, that, because of the characteristics of needle valves whose performance is independent of downstream pressure, this does not mean a fall in the mass flow rate of gas, just a change in the calibration curve of the tube. The gas, which is compressed because of the added resistance, subsequently re-expands again further downstream.

The end of the backbar (after the last vaporizer) usually has a valve that combines non-return properties with those of pressure limitation. A typical design is shown in Figure 8.41. The non-return feature is necessary to prevent back surges of pressure from equipment such as ventilators allowing re-entry of gas into vaporizers (pumping), and the pressure relief component is necessary to prevent the build-up of pressure, which could damage vaporizers and other equipment.

A typical blow-off pressure is 0.33 atm. It should be noted that this level of pressure relief greatly exceeds that necessary for patient safety and therefore patients' lungs need additional protection.

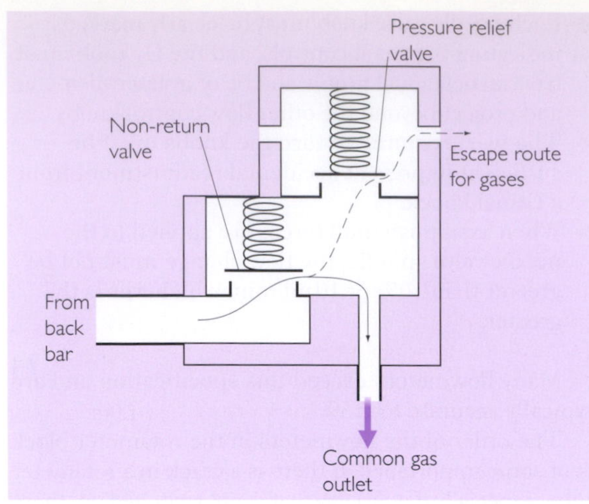


**Figure 8.41.** The valve apparatus on the end of a backbar which combines a non-return feature with a pressure relief system. If the outlet to the anaesthesia machine is obstructed, the gases escape to the atmosphere, preventing damage to vaporizers and other equipment.

### Emergency oxygen

All machines have an emergency $O_2$ flush valve which, when activated, supplies $O_2$ at a minimum rate of 30 L/min. It is connected directly to the common gas outlet from the pipeline and the first-stage cylinder regulator, as shown in Figure 8.29. Older machines have a locking system to allow it to be kept on but, because of inadvertent barotrauma being caused by this, current recommendations are that it should not be capable of being locked on. The knob is also recessed to reduce the chances of accidental activation.

### Oxygen supply warning devices

These were originally introduced to prevent the unobserved emptying of $O_2$ cylinders before piped gases were in common use. There have been a variety of designs over the years, but there are now standards for their performance in most countries. In principle these devices:

- have a loud audible warning;
- are activated by falling $O_2$ supply pressure (usually at approximately 2 atm);
- have a valve system that cuts off all non-$O_2$-containing gases or reduces their flow to maintain a minimum concentration of $O_2$;
- are designed so that the alarm cannot be reset without restoring the $O_2$ supply.

On modern machines the whistle can be heard when the machine is switched on and off at the beginning and end of an operating list.

### The common gas outlet

The common gas outlet is where gases leave the machine (see Figure 8.29). It is a 22-mm male outer diameter /15-mm female internal diameter conical taper that may be fixed or swivelled. It is usually fitted at the front right-hand corner of the machine, but can be at the other side. The preference for the right-hand corner is reputed to result from Boyle (the designer of the original anaesthesia machine) who was left-handed and found this to be the best position for writing a chart while holding on a mask.

## VAPORIZERS

The basic physics of vaporization is covered in Chapter 37. Vaporizers can be broadly classified as follows:

- So-called 'plenum' vaporizers are high resistance and depend upon a pressurized gas supply. They *cannot* be used as draw-over devices and are intended to work with a steady flow of gas.
- Draw-over devices have low resistance, through which the patient can pull the gases when they inspire. Some draw-over vaporizers can be used in plenum mode, but it depends on the individual model.
- More complex injector systems depend on real-time measurement of the vapour concentration in the breathing system and are as yet largely research tools.

### Plenum vaporizers

This section deals mainly with the practical use of commercial vaporizers which have a sufficiently high resistance to gas flow that they require pressurized gas supplies. Patients cannot be allowed to inspire through them, even if it is possible to connect them into a breathing system. Modern devices have the direction of flow marked on them, and have fittings of such a diameter and type that they cannot, without considerable determination, be included into a patient breathing system.

The majority of vaporizers in everyday use are fitted to the backbar of the anaesthesia machine, and the standard on new machines is an interchangeable type of system similar to that shown in Figure 8.42. This allows one or more agent-specific vaporizers to be dropped into place as required by the anaesthetist.

Apart from checking for obvious leaks and routine cleaning, depending on the model, modern vaporizers need calibration checks at 2- to 5-yearly intervals (usually by a refractometer in the manufacturer's premises).

In clinical practice vaporizers are required to provide a set output concentration in the presence of changes in the following factors.

#### *Temperature*

This is the variable with the greatest effect on performance. The effect of not providing any compensation for temperature changes is seen in Figure 8.43. In current designs (Figure 8.44), the effect of a temperature drop caused by evaporation of the volatile agent is compensated for by making the vaporizer a heat sink with a large thermal capacity and/or using a bimetallic strip (Tec series) or gas-filled aneroid bellows (Penlon series) to control a valve that varies the proportion of the set flow rate going through the vaporizing chamber. The typical working temperature range of a modern vaporizer is 15–35°C (Figure 8.45).

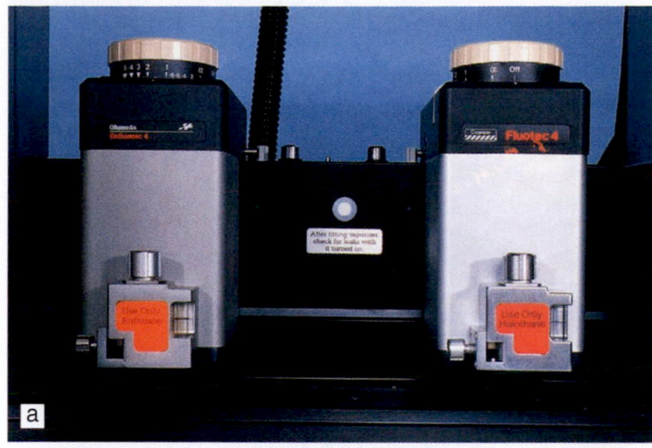


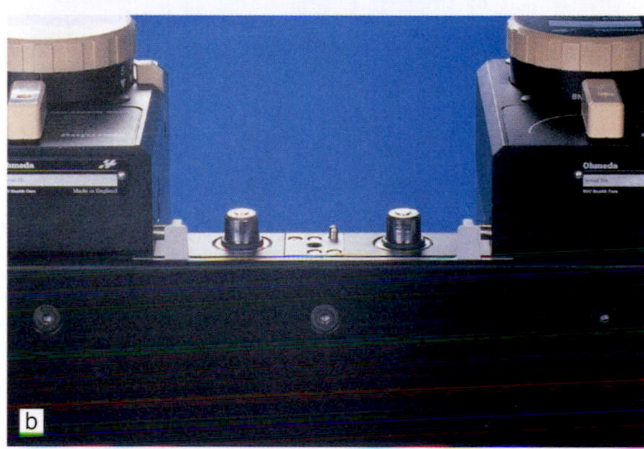


**Figure 8.42.** Interchangeable vaporizer system on the backbar of an anaesthesia machine. (a) Two vaporizers in position with a space for a third between them. (b) A close-up of the alignment pins. When a vaporizer is dropped into place, the axial valve ports in the centre of the pins are opened to the vaporizer and the 'O' rings at the bottom of the pins provide a gas-tight seal. (Reproduced with permission from Ohmeda.)

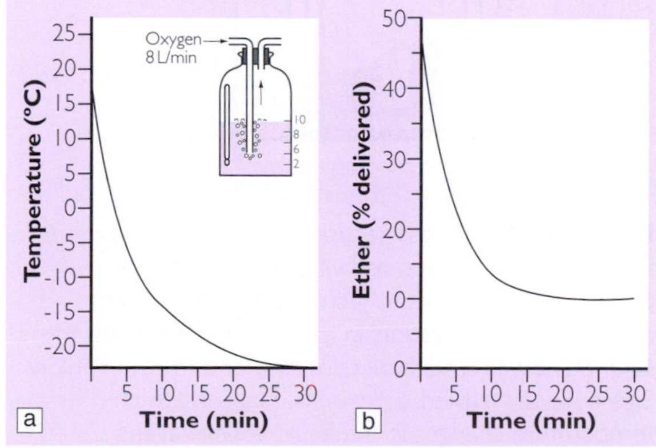


**Figure 8.43.** The fall in (a) temperature and (b) delivered concentration in an uncompensated ether vaporizer during a steady flow of $O_2$ at 8 L/min. (Adapted from Mushin WW and Jones PL. *Physics for the Anaesthetist*, 4th edn. Oxford: Blackwell Scientific, 1987: 143.)

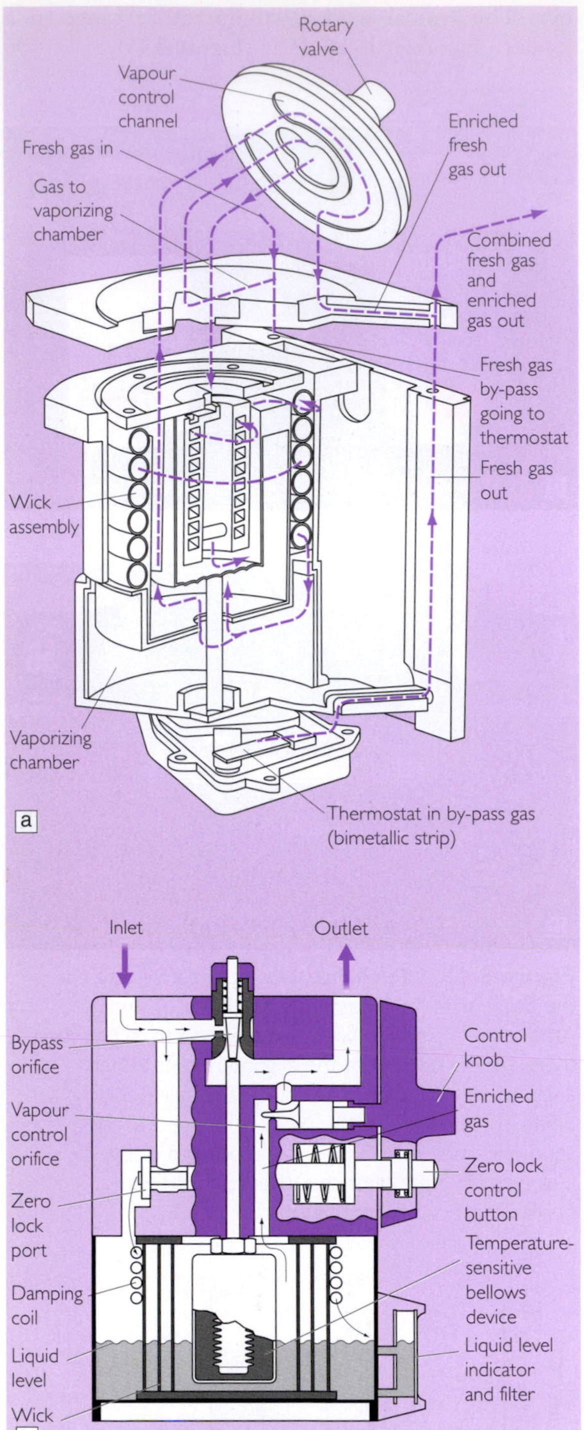


**Figure 8.44.** A cross-sectional diagram of two modern temperature compensated vaporizers. Note the presence of the wicks to increase the surface area available for vaporization. In the models shown, (a) the Ohmeda Tec 5 has a bimetallic strip and (b) the Penlon Sigma has a gas-filled bellows to compensate for temperature changes in the liquid volatile agent. (Adapted from manufacturer's literature.)

### *Gas flow rate*

All vaporizers are affected to some degree by the flow rate, but on current models the vapour concentration supplied by setting the dial is, for clinical purposes, effectively independent of fresh gas flows from 0.5 to 10 L/min. Outside this range, manufacturer's data need to be consulted. When using very low flows, our own practice would be to have a vapour analyser in the breathing circuit and to be guided by that. Typical performance characteristics are shown in Figure 8.46.

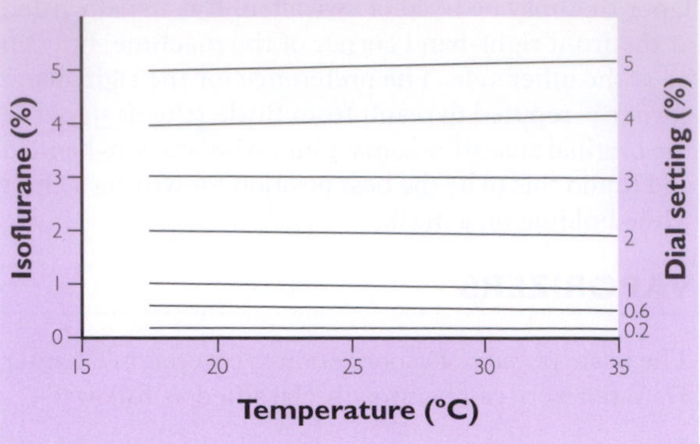


**Figure 8.45.** The typical performance characteristics of a modern vaporizer as the temperature changes. Gas flow rate = 5 L/min of $O_2$. These are taken from the Ohmeda Tec 5. (Data from manufacturer's literature.)

### *The level of liquid anaesthetic agent*

The effect of changes in liquid levels is minimized by the use of wicks, which greatly enlarge the surface for evaporation irrespective of the liquid level (see Figure 8.44).

### *Barometric pressure*

The effect of a change in barometric pressure on vaporizer performance is described in Chapter 37. In summary, it has little effect in clinical practice because the same partial pressure of volatile agent is delivered to the patient.

### *Gas composition*

In practice this is not a problem.

### *Practical problems with vaporizers*

- The wrong agent can still be put in. To prevent this happening, agent-specific keyed fillers have been designed. The bottle of liquid agent has a special cap or collar with lugs, which fits only an agent-specific filling tube. The filling tube itself matches the port on the vaporizer (Figure 8.47). In addition the fillers are colour coded and the recommended method of use ensures that overfilling of the vaporizer does not occur.
- It is sometimes possible (with some models) to position the vaporizers incorrectly on their locating pins so that, when they are switched on, a gas leak occurs at the vaporizer–backbar junction. This should be detected at the time from a hissing sound or during a routine anaesthesia machine check.
- Vaporizers can be accidentally tipped or knocked over before being placed on the backbar. Depending on the model and whether the control knob is in the off or on position, this can result in very high (dangerously so) concentrations of vapour being delivered to the patient. If any vaporizer suffers

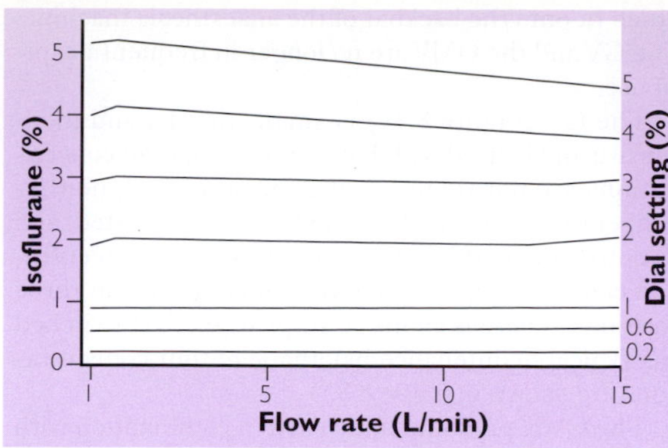


**Figure 8.46.** The typical performance characteristics of a modern vaporizer for a range of flow rates at 22°C with $O_2$ flowing. These are taken from the Ohmeda Tec 5. (Data from manufacturer's literature.)

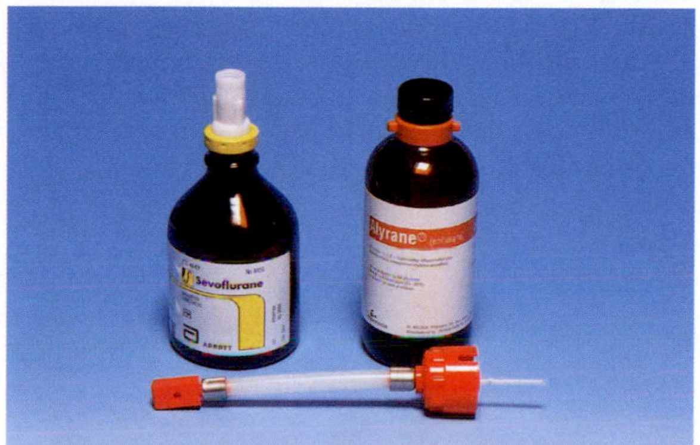

**Figure 8.47.** Examples of keyed filling tubes for volatile agents. The one on the left for sevoflurane is integral with the bottle. The one on the right for enflurane consists of a permanently fixed plastic collar on the bottle neck which has agent-specific lugs. These match the cut-outs on the filler tube shown horizontally in front of the bottle.

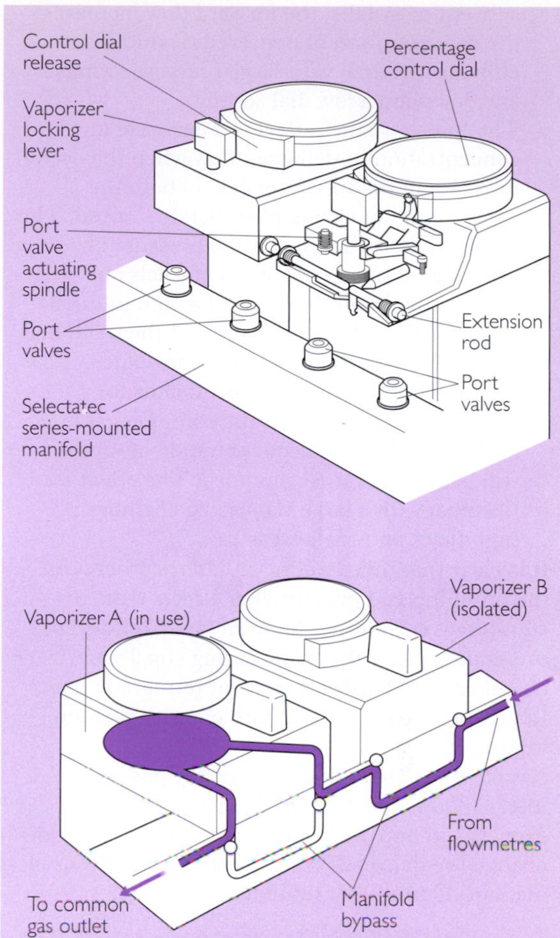


**Figure 8.48.** The Select-a-tec vaporizer interlock mechanism. This ensures that two agents cannot be delivered simultaneously. (Adapted from the manufacturer's literature.)

such an event, unless you are absolutely certain that the manufacturer's literature indicates that there will be no problem, it is best to wait until there is no patient connected to the anaesthesia machine and to flush the vaporizer through, confirming that the output is within the expected range by a gas analyser. For similar safety reasons, vaporizers should be moved or transported only when they are in the off position.

- Overfilling is still possible on several models in current use. This can result in liquid agent entering the bypass chamber and up to 10 times the intended vapour concentration can be delivered. Consequently, the top of the liquid in the level sight tube must be visible before anaesthesia commences.
- The Select-a-tec system with its interlock mechanism is intended to prevent the inadvertent (or deliberate) administration of two agents simultaneously (Figure 8.48). On a backbar with three vaporizer locations, if the middle one is removed, on older models it is possible to simultaneously switch on both of the others because of the missing central interlocking rods. Consequently, if only two vaporizers are in position on a three-vaporizer manifold, they should be placed in adjacent positions.
- Vaporizers are subject to 'pumping' and 'pressurizing' effects. Both were found in relation to the use of devices that alter the pressure in the backbar: they work in opposite directions to change the output concentration from the common gas outlet. In everyday anaesthesia, with modern vaporizers and vapour monitors they are more relevant as examination questions than issues to be considered crucial to everyday practice.
  - The 'pumping' effect is an increase in the delivered concentration when the common gas outlet is connected to a ventilator that produces cyclical and significant changes in backbar pressure. The surge in back pressure forces gas in the backbar (which is not saturated with vapour) back into the vaporizing chamber, and the gas in the vaporizing chamber (which is saturated with vapour) retrogradely into the bypass channel. When the pressure

subsequently falls, the forward flow increases the concentration of delivered vapour. The effect is maximal with large pressure swings, low flows and a low dial setting.

- The 'pressurizing' effect is a decrease in concentration in delivered flow when the overall pressure in the vaporizer (i.e. in both the bypass and vaporizing chambers) is raised. The mechanism is that the partial pressure of vapour generated is dependent solely on temperature, and therefore at a high internal pressure the vapour forms less of the fractional composition of the number of molecules. Consequently, when the gas expands to atmospheric pressure at the common gas outlet, the delivered concentration of vapour will be less than that intended. The effect is maximal with a large vaporizing chamber at high flows and high pressures.

It is clear that there will be an interplay between the pumping and pressurizing effects that counteract each other. Modern vaporizer design overcomes these effects by having small vaporizer chambers and baffles to prevent retrograde flow. In practice they are not a problem with plenum vaporizers.

- A vaporizer (which does not usually possess internal flow-directing valves) is only meant to carry gas in one direction. Reversing the flow can change the delivered concentration by an order of magnitude from that intended.

In summary, modern plenum vaporizers, if used as intended by the manufacturers, are (apart from recommended service schedules) maintenance-free devices that provide accurate concentrations of vapour over the range of conditions encountered in everyday clinical practice.

### Draw-over vaporizers

Although many of these have been described, only the Goldman Vaporizer (GV) and the Oxford Miniature Vaporizer (OMV) will be considered. Both these vaporizers are low-resistance vaporizers which can be placed in the breathing systems of both spontaneously breathing (when they act as draw-over devices) and ventilated patients. Both are less accurate in their settings than the calibrated plenum vaporizers in common use, which fit onto the backbar of the anaesthesia machine. The GV and the OMV are no longer in frequent hospital use.

The GV (Figure 8.49) is small, simple, and inexpensive and is used with halothane when high concentrations are not required. It is uncalibrated, neither temperature nor volatile liquid level compensated, and its output depends on gas flow. The output concentration can be changed by a lever which locates in three positions. There is an initial surge when first switched on. Typical maintenance halothane output concentrations are shown in Table 8.8.

The GV is predominantly used in combination with $N_2O/O_2$ anaesthesia for dentistry or in locations where the supply of pressurized gas is limited.

The OMV is now primarily used with portable anaesthetic equipment and has been very usefully employed in the Triservice apparatus. The direction of the flow of gas is indicated on the model, and can be from left to right across the vaporizer or vice versa. It is shown in Figure 8.50. The concentration is selected by the position of the lever on the top and the scale (which is screwed down) can be changed for use with other agents. The halothane scale goes up to 4.5% and the enflurane scale up to 3.5%.

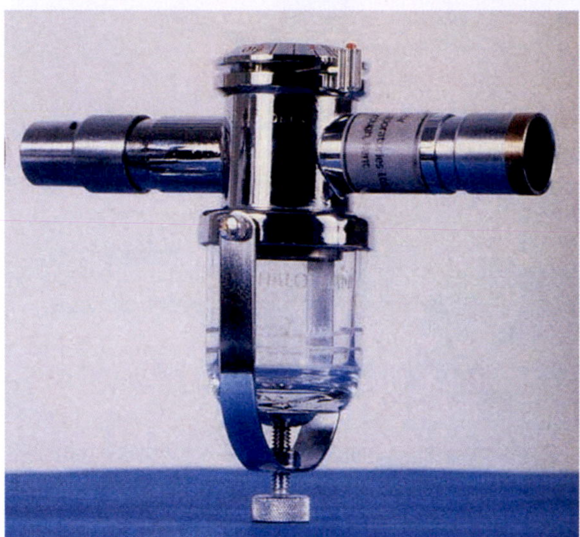

**Figure 8.49.** The Goldman Halothane Vaporizer.

**Table 8.8. Performance characteristics of a Goldman Vaporizer giving halothane output concentrations (%) at different flows and lever settings.**

| Lever setting | Gas flow (L/min) | | |
|---|---|---|---|
| (position number) | 2 | 8 | 30 |
| 1 | 0.1 | 0.1 | 0.1 |
| 2 | 0.5 | 1.0 | 1.0 |
| 3 | 1.5 | 2.5 | 1.5 |
| Full on | 1.5 | 3.0 | 1.5 |

Note that different publications report varying performance characteristics but the ones shown are typical.
From Goldman V. *Anaesthesia* 1962;17:537.

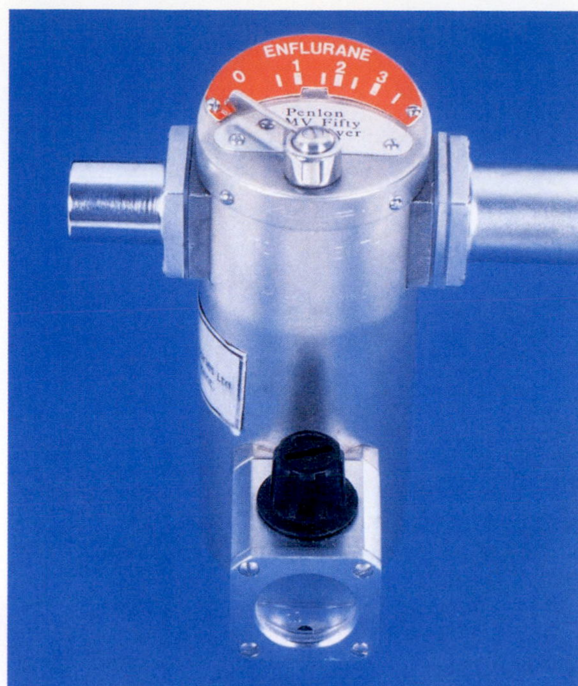


**Figure 8.50.** The Oxford Miniature Vaporizer.

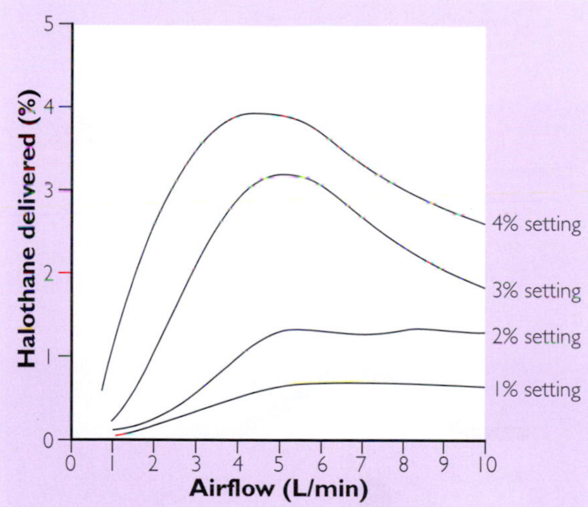


**Figure 8.51.** Typical performance characteristics of the Oxford Miniature Vaporizer filled with halothane under steady flow conditions. (Adapted from Schaefer H-G and Farman JV. *Anaesthesia* 1984;39:171.)

Within the vaporizer are wicks constructed of wire gauze which can easily be cleaned by rinsing with a solvent (e.g. ether), and subsequently dried by blowing air through. It is not temperature compensated, but is buffered by a sealed compartment filled with a solution of water and ethylene glycol, which acts as a heat sink. Although there is some variability in the delivered concentration with temperature, gas flow, and breathing frequency, the delivered concentration always remains below that indicated on the scale. Typical performance characteristics are shown in Figure 8.51. When compared with Figure 8.46, the sophistication of modern plenum vaporizers is clear.

## HUMIDIFICATION

Humidity is relevant to clinical anaesthesia in two ways:

1. The atmosphere of the operating room should be kept at a suitable level of relative humidity (RH; 50–70%) for comfort and suppression of sparks. This is not considered further here.
2. Medical air, $O_2$, $N_2O$, and other gases are supplied dry to protect against corrosion, condensation, bacterial contamination, etc. When these are delivered directly to the lungs by an endotracheal tube or laryngeal mask airway, the normal heat- and moisture-exchanging properties of the upper respiratory tract (which deliver gas at 37°C with 100% RH) are bypassed.

The physics of vaporization and water vapour, and how to measure humidity, are outlined in Chapters 37 and 38.

The pattern of humidification in normal physiology is shown in Figure 8.52. The following are the consequences of removing the normal warming and humidifying processes:

- Compared with normal ventilation there is a net loss of heat from the heating of dry gases and the requirements of the latent heat of vaporization. The effect of this is proportionally greatest in small children.
- Compared with normality, there is a net loss of water from exhaled, saturated gas.
- The dry gases lead to dehydration of the upper airways (including major bronchi), and changes in the alveoli. These include:
  - the production of dry, inspissated secretions;
  - damage to cilia and underlying airway cells, which results in impaired function of the mucociliary elevator with sputum retention, bronchiolar collapse, and atelectasis; the surface of the airways may become dry, inflamed, and ulcerated;
  - surfactant activity is impaired; lung compliance falls.

Humidifiers are devices that compensate for the loss of heat and moisture-exchanging properties of the upper respiratory tract. An ideal humidifier should:

- be safe to the patient with no risk of foreign material being inspired;
- have accurate temperature settings with temperature, electrical, and misconnection and disconnection fail-safe alarms;
- have an adequate moisture output;
- maintain body temperature;
- pose no microbiological hazard;
- be convenient to use, clean, and store;
- have low capital and running costs.

The five most common ways of humidifying inspired air in anaesthesia and intensive care practice are:

1. cold water baths
2. hot water baths

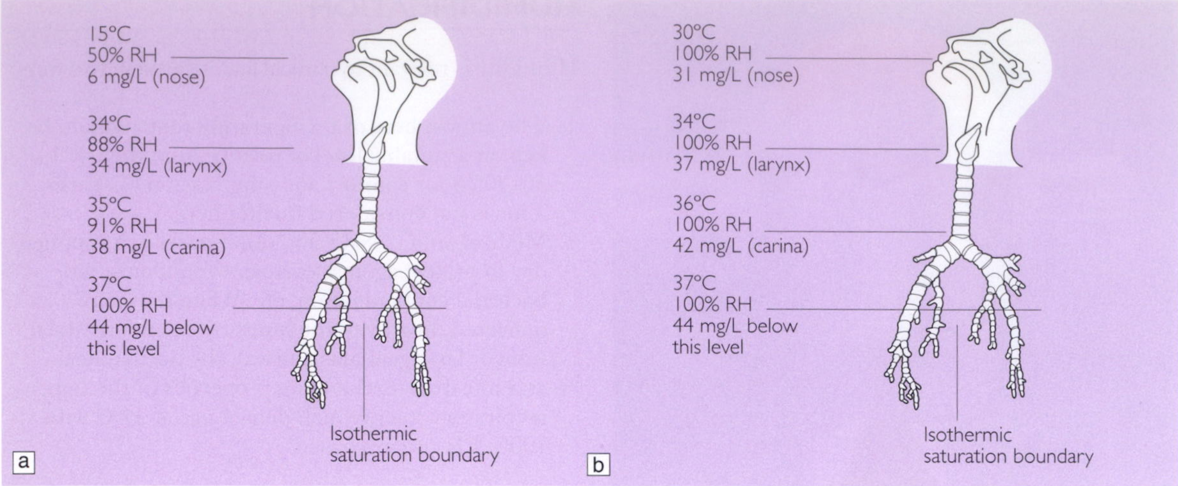


**Figure 8.52.** The pattern of humidification in the human airways during (a) inspiration and (b) expiration. RH, relative humidity. Values represent mg water per litre of air. (Adapted from Shelly MP. *Humidification: Intensive Care Rounds*. Abingdon: The Medicine Group (Educational) Ltd, 1993: 7.)

3. nebulizers
4. heat and moisture exchangers
5. low flows and soda lime.

Each meets some but not all of the desirable criteria above.

### *Cold water baths*

These work by inspired gas being passed over or bubbled through water at ambient temperature. The humidification can be increased by the use of sintered filters or wicks. They are electrically safe, never reach 100% RH, can be contaminated by bacteria, and are only really of use as adjuncts to $O_2$ therapy in the fit postoperative patient.

### *Hot water baths*

These are similar in design to cold water baths, but possess a heating element and usually some form of safety cut-out from a sensor in the patient circuit (Figure 8.53). They are mainly used in ICUs and should be filled with sterile water. They can deliver air at up to 100% RH at 37°C, but some of this moisture condenses in the inspiratory limb of the breathing circuit. Bacterial contamination is a problem. Care must be taken not to tip condensed water that has collected in dependent tubing into the patient's lungs.

### *Nebulizers*

These can be mechanically, gas, or ultrasonically driven. Rather than evaporate water, they break it up into a myriad of tiny droplets within a saturated vapour (Figure 8.54). The size of the droplets is very variable (1–20 μm), their fate in the respiratory tract is poorly understood, and they can produce bacterial contamination. The devices can be at ambient temperature or heated, and can produce so much moisture that the patient becomes water overloaded.

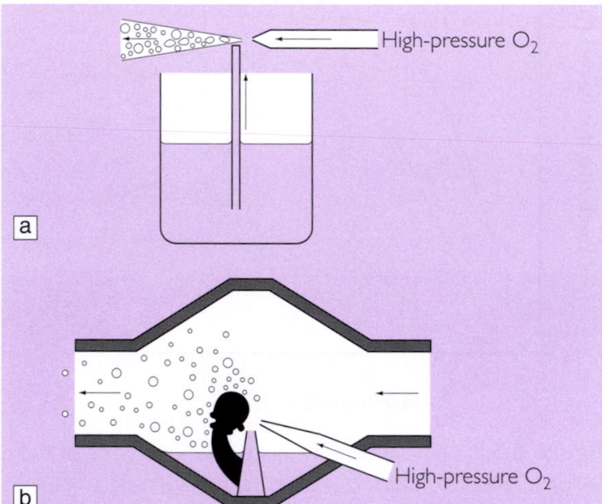


**Figure 8.54.** The principle of a nebulizer. (a) The nebulized spray being produced by the Bernouilli effect; (b) droplets being broken up on an anvil to produce even smaller particles.

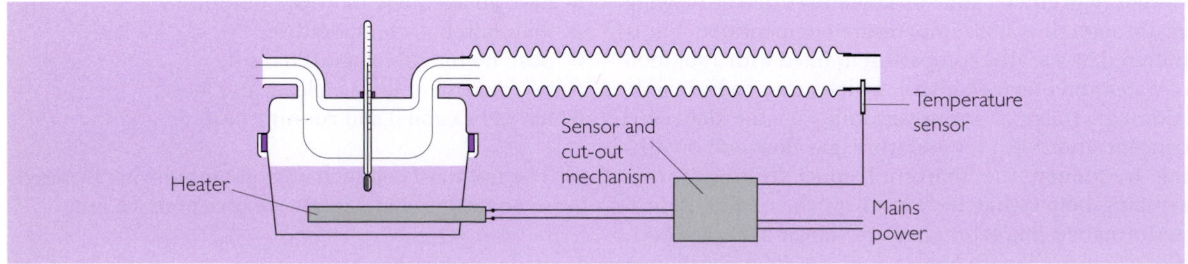


**Figure 8.53.** A basic hot water bath humidifier involving a simple safety cut-out.

### *Heat and moisture exchangers (HMEs)*

These are now widely used both in the operating room and on the ICU. Examples are shown in Figure 8.55 and diagrammatically in Figure 8.56. Their principle of action is that expired gases condense on the material of the element (which can be paper, aluminium, cellulose, foam, or stainless steel fibres). Then, when fresh, dry inspired gas flows over the element, the moisture and some of the heat are returned. They can achieve a RH of 60–70% with gas temperatures of 28°C. The elements can be either hygroscopic or hydrophobic. Hydrophobic filters with a pore size of 0.2 μm can filter out bacteria, virus particles, and dust flowing in either direction. Dead space volumes for HMEs range from approximately 8 ml to 60 ml depending upon their exact design. They provide a small increase in airway resistance of up to 2 $cmH_2O$ depending on the flow rate and model. They should be replaced every 24 hours.

### *Soda lime*

This becomes hot because the process of $CO_2$ absorption is exothermic, and moist because of the passage of expired gas. The process is described in detail in Chapter 10. Its exact contribution to the composition and temperature of inspired gases is very dependent on the fresh gas flow, the length of the procedure, and the age of the lime. The apparatus is also a source of bacterial contamination.

The relevant characteristics of the different humidifying methods are set out in Table 8.9 for easy comparison.

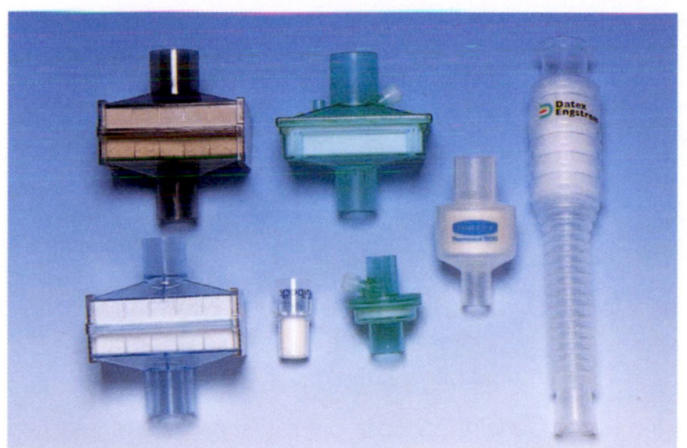

**Figure 8.55.** Examples of heat and moisture exchangers (HME) for use with adults and children.

The clinical applications of the various types of device bear some discussion. Cold water humidifiers are inefficient, and have an insufficient water output to replace normal respiratory function. Hot water humidifiers are relevant to the ICU and long operative procedures where the patient has a high minute volume or abnormal airway function. Nebulizers have now found a regular place in providing large volumes of gas (e.g. $O_2$ tents, continuous positive airway pressure, very high gas flow rates), in enhancing sputum clearance in combination with physiotherapy, and in the administration of bronchodilators. With nebulizers, great care is always needed to prevent over-hydration when the patient's airway is bypassed. HMEs are now the most widely used general-purpose humidification device. They are appropriate for intubated patients without significant chest or airway disease who do not require minute volumes above 10 L/min (which dry them out). A comparison of the uses of the various types of device is given in Table 8.10 and a suggested clinical strategy is shown in Figure 8.57.

It remains true that humidification is a very unresearched subject and relatively little is known about its function in the upper airways in health and disease.

## SCAVENGING AND POLLUTION

Scavenging is the process of removing unwanted gases and vapours from the working environment. It is one of the measures used to control pollution, but is particularly relevant to airway management because scavenging equipment is usually attached to the breathing circuit.

### Effects of long-term exposure

At various times, waste anaesthetic gases have been held responsible for spontaneous abortions in staff and their spouses, infertility, birth defects, impairment of skilled performance, cancer, liver and renal disease, blood dyscrasias, and neurological symptoms. None of these has been confirmed, although there is no doubt that $N_2O$ affects red cell maturation, and some dental surgeons exposed chronically to high levels of $N_2O$ have developed polyneuropathies.

### Pollution levels

Exact knowledge about the chronic effects of trace levels of anaesthetic vapours and gases on humans is virtually non-existent. Those guidelines that have been estab-

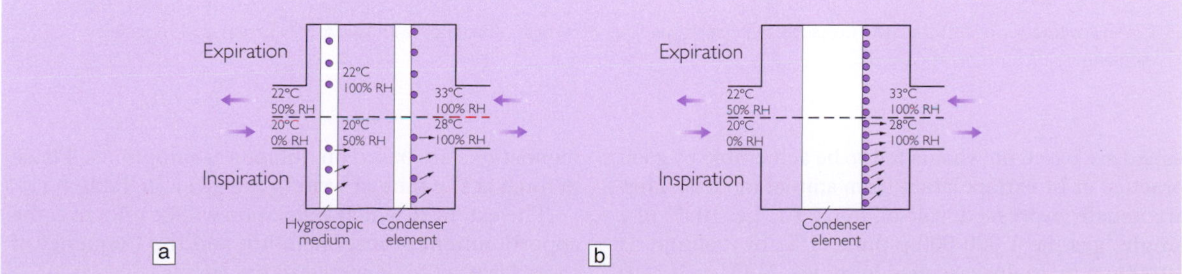


**Figure 8.56.** A diagrammatic representation of (a) hygroscopic and (b) hydrophobic heat- and moisture-exchanging filters. In a hydrophobic model, water condenses onto the condenser element. In a hygroscopic model, in addition to a condenser element, there is a hygroscopic medium that takes up moisture. RH, relative humidity. (Adapted from Shelly MP. *Humidification: Intensive Care Rounds*. Abingdon: The Medicine Group (Educational) Ltd, 1993: 17.)

**Table 8.9. Characteristics of different humidifying methods**

| | Cold water bath | Hot water bath | Nebulizer | HME filter | Soda lime |
|---|---|---|---|---|---|
| Inspired gas temperature (°C) | 18–23 | 34–38 | 23–36 (depends if heated) | 28 | Variable but <37 |
| Relative humidity (%) | <100 | Up to 100 | Can be >100 | 60–80 | 10–65 |
| Absolute humidity (mg/L) | 15–20 | 35–45 | 15–1500 | 25–35 | 5–30 |
| Body temperature maintenance | Poor | Can be good | Depends on temperature of nebulizer | Good | Variable |
| Safety | Good | Can overheat, electrical faults | Can overheat, electrical faults | Blockages, disconnections, cracks | See breathing circuits, Chapter 10 |
| Biological hazards | Reservoir and circuit colonization | Reservoir and circuit colonization | Reservoir and circuit colonization | Protective | Housing and valves can become contaminated |
| Internal compliance | Low/moderate | Low/moderate | Low | Low | See breathing circuits |
| Convenience | Fair/poor | Poor | Poor | Good | Good |
| Cost | Low | High | High | Low | As for soda lime |

HME, heat and moisture exchanger.

**Table 8.10. Comparison of uses of different types of humidifier**

| Humidifier | Restrictions | Clinical applications |
|---|---|---|
| Cold water | Only relevant if breathing normally; no abnormal airway; no high FGF | $O_2$ therapy in spontaneously breathing |
| Hot water | Only for ventilatory support with high FGFs and abnormal lungs | $O_2$ tents, head boxes, ICU, long anaesthetics, CPAP |
| Nebulizers | Only for high-volume humidification or for specific job, e.g. sputum clearance with physiotherapy, administration of drugs | $O_2$ tents, head boxes, CPAP, HFV, physiotherapy. Best in patients without intubation |
| HME | Not suitable for high FGFs and some abnormal lungs | General purpose operating room and ICU use, transport of ventilated patients and infection control |
| Soda lime | Only used in operating room; very variable performance; not to be relied on | Only as part of an anaesthetic technique |

CPAP, continuous positive airway pressure; FGF, fresh gas flow; HFV, high-frequency ventilation; HME, heat and moisture exchanger; ICU, intensive care unit.

lished are based on what is felt to be achievable by good practice or by extrapolation from animal models. They are usually expressed, vol/vol, in p.p.m., i.e. 100% of a single gas is 1 000 000 p.p.m., 1% by volume is 10 000 p.p.m. In unscavenged locations, $N_2O$ levels have been measured on occasions at over 5000 p.p.m.

Several governments have now introduced maximum recommended levels for good practice, some of which are statutory and others advisory. All recommendations are based on dubious assumptions. Those in force at the time of writing are given in Table 8.11.

The extent to which legislation will be effective, the apportionment of responsibility, and the frequency of cases have yet to be tested in the courts.

In line with the setting of safe limits, there are also statutory codes of practice which, although they vary in detail, in principle insist that employers instruct and train employees about:

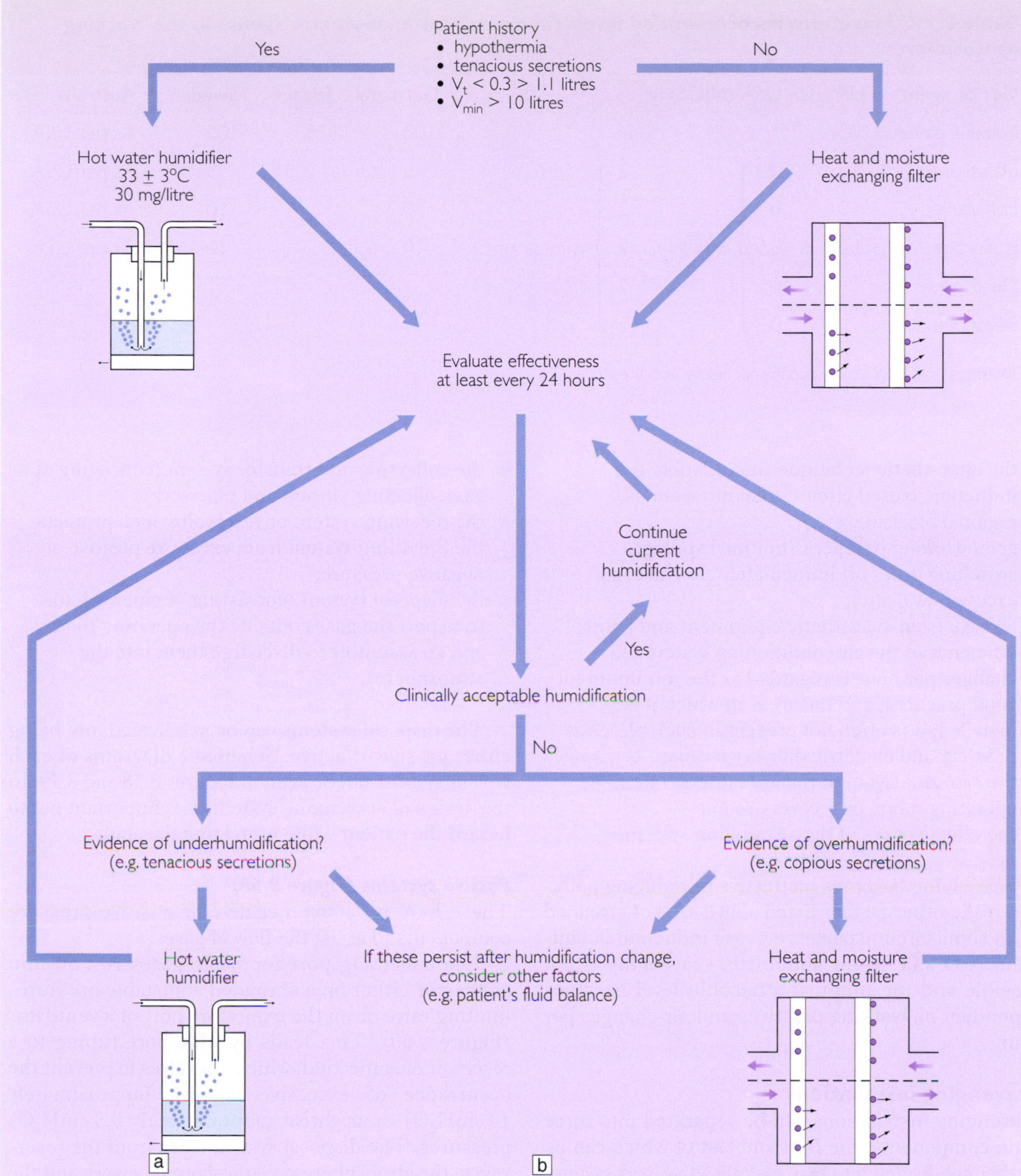


**Figure 8.57.** A suggested clinical strategy for the selection and use of humidifiers. $V_t$, tidal volume; $V_{min}$, minute volume. (Adapted from Shelly MP. *Humidification: Intensive Care Rounds.* Abingdon: The Medicine Group (Educational) Ltd, 1993: 18.)

- the nature of the substances that they work with and the risks created by exposure to those substances;
- the precautions that they should take;
- control measures, their purpose, and how to use them;
- how to use protective equipment and clothing provided;
- emergency procedures.

In most countries, this type of legislation is just in its infancy and its effect has not yet started to 'bite'. The extent to which it will affect the daily life of an anaesthetist, the monitoring systems that will be put into place, and whether or not it will alter the number of volatile and intravenous anaesthetics given is unknown.

### *Causes and control of pollution*

The causes of pollution are multifactorial and there are several ways in which the amount can be reduced. The level of pollution that results at any one time depends upon:

- the frequency with which gases and vapours are used;

**Table 8.11. Maximum recommended levels (in p.p.m.) for anaesthetic agents in the working atmosphere**

| Gas or agent | UK | USA (NIOSH)[a] with $N_2O$ | USA (NIOSH)[a] with air or $O_2$ | Germany | France | Sweden | Australia |
|---|---|---|---|---|---|---|---|
| Nitrous oxide | 100 | | 25 | 100 | 25 | 100 | As per USA |
| Halothane | 10 | 0.5 | 2 | 5 | 2 | 5 | As per USA |
| Enflurane | 50 | 0.5 | 2 | 20 | | 10 | As per USA |
| Isoflurane | 50 | 0.5 | 2 | 10 | | 10 | As per USA |
| Desflurane | | 0.5 | 2 | | | | |
| Sevoflurane | | 0.5 | 2 | | | | |

[a]National Institute for Occupational Safety and Health.

- the anaesthetic technique (insufflation, gas induction, closed circuit, total intravenous, regional blockade, etc.);
- good working practices (minimal spillage, switching gases off immediately after use, no excess flows, etc.);
- leakage from anaesthetic equipment and joints;
- efficiency of the air conditioning system (15 changes per hour is regarded as the minimum for good practice), and the areas in which it is installed; it is often not present in such places as recovery and obstetric delivery rooms;
- the size and layout of the anaesthetic room, operating room, or recovery room;
- the effectiveness of the scavenging system.

Scavenging becomes ineffective in reducing pollution if the other factors listed above are not attended to. In some circumstances, e.g. gas induction in children, $N_2O$ and $O_2$ for childbirth, scavenging is not possible and the minimal attainable level becomes dependent on working practices and air changes per hour.

### Scavenging installations

Scavenging installations can be separated into three main components, the first and last of which can be further subdivided into two, making a five-part system:

- the collecting and transfer system (consisting of a gas-collecting shroud and pipework);
- the receiving system or reservoir which protects the breathing system from excessive positive or negative pressure;
- the disposal system (consisting of pipework to transport the gases outside the operating room and an assembly to discharge them into the atmosphere).

The disposal systems can be subdivided into being either passive or active. Schematic diagrams of each type of system can be seen in Figures 8.58 and 8.59. In the design of scavenging systems it is important not to hazard the patient while protecting the staff.

#### *Passive systems (Figure 8.58)*

These have no active negative or positive pressure components to assist the flow of gases.

The collecting port for waste gases is a 30-mm connector either on a shrouded adjustable pressure-limiting valve or on the expiratory port of a ventilator (Figure 8.60). This leads by wide bore tubing to a reservoir of some kind, which has valves to prevent the occurrence of excessive positive (approximately 10 $cmH_2O$) or negative (approximately 0.5 $cmH_2O$) pressures. The disposal system leads from the reservoir to the atmosphere via large-bore pipework and the

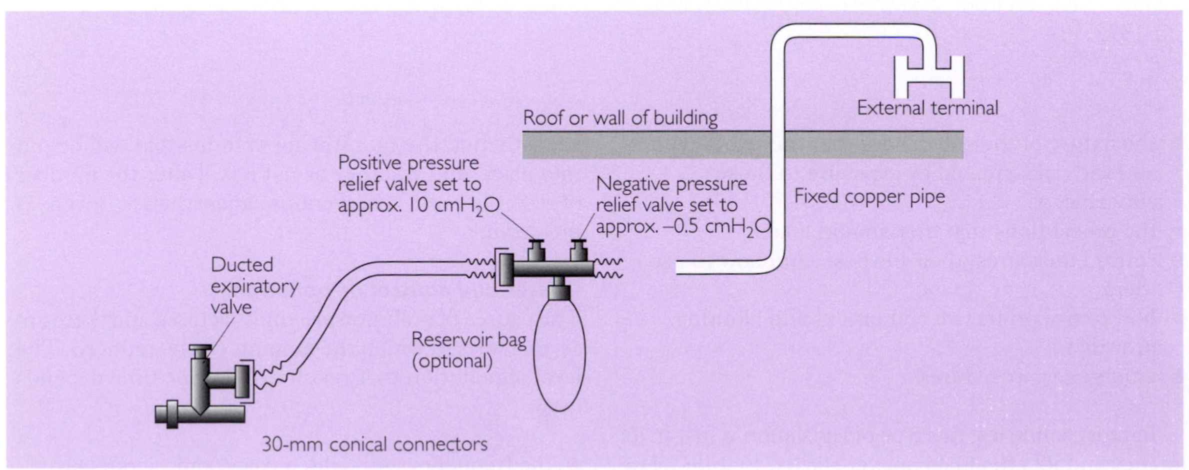


**Figure 8.58.** Diagrammatic representation of a passive scavenging system.

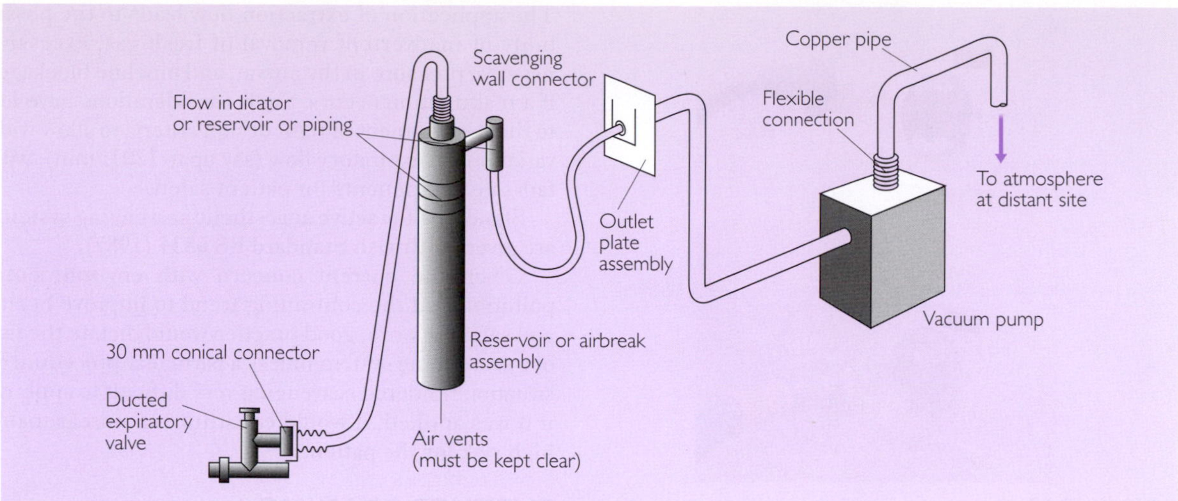


**Figure 8.59.** Diagrammatic representation of an active scavenging system.

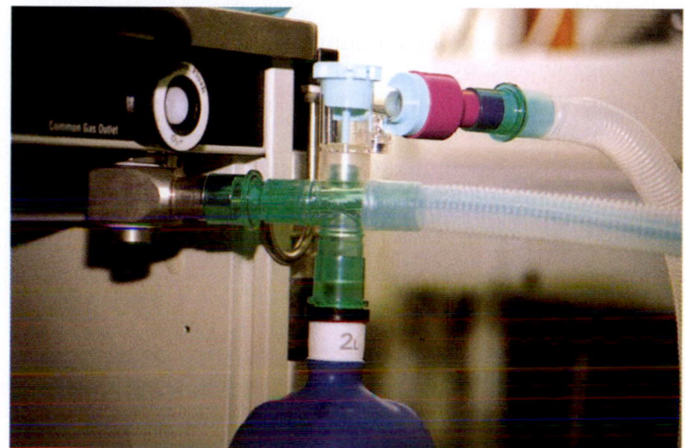

**Figure 8.60.** An example of a shrouded adjustable pressure-limiting (APL) valve, which allows the scavenging of expired gases.

gases are driven along it by the patient's expiratory efforts. The wide-bore tube vents via an exterior wall or on to the roof. The flow down the tubing can be subject to wind changes and may on some occasions even reverse its direction. Some ventilators also direct the driving gas as well as the fresh gas through their exhaust valve, so this needs to be taken into account during design. For the overall system, the resistance to gas flow should not exceed approximately 0.5 $cmH_2O$ at 30 L/min.

The limitations on passive systems are significant because the external terminal, which is usually a T- or H-shaped construction, is subject to a number of adverse factors. Positive or negative pressures can be generated in the pipework by wind conditions, which themselves may be affected by the prevailing direction and adjacent buildings. If outlets from separate operating rooms are close to one another, gases from one operating room may be redirected into another, and birds, ants, or other small animals might try to make a home. It is also necessary to incorporate a water trap to deal with condensation. Passive systems are really only suitable for small installations close to an external wall and are now rarely installed.

Passive systems using activated charcoal, which adsorbs volatile but not gaseous agents, are now very rarely seen in hospital practice.

#### *Active systems (Figure 8.59)*

In active systems, the collecting and reservoir systems are essentially similar to those of passive systems, except that some may employ an air break instead of a reservoir. Such a device is shown diagrammatically in Figure 8.61. The key difference in an active system is that there is pumped removal of the waste gases to a suitable external site via a pipework system and water trap. The disposal system is often plugged into a wall or pendant connector, as shown in Figure 8.62. A commonly used design is that of an open-ended valve-less tube with a float to indicate that it is extracting (Figure 8.63). Depending on the installation, the negative pressure can be provided by a fan, a Venturi system, or an injector flowmeter, or from the mains vacuum.

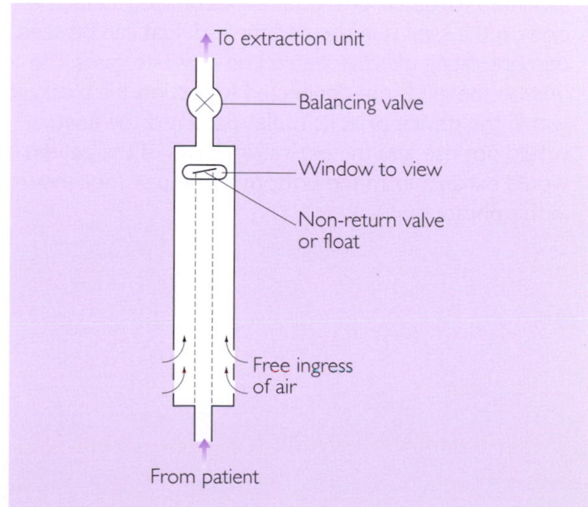


**Figure 8.61.** Diagrammatic representation of a single simple air break, which allows the ingress of air to satisfy excess demand from the extraction system. This is intended to prevent gas from the patient circuit being inappropriately sucked out.

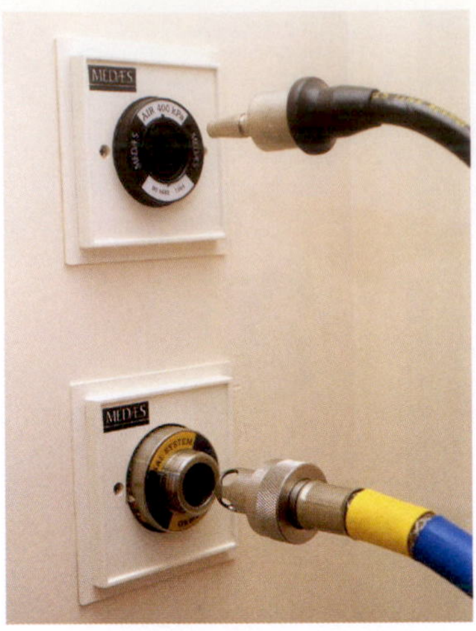


**Figure 8.62.** A wall terminal unit used for a scavenging system (lower) compared with a pipeline air supply. Note the wide-bore, fenestrated, screw-thread attachment of the scavenging system.

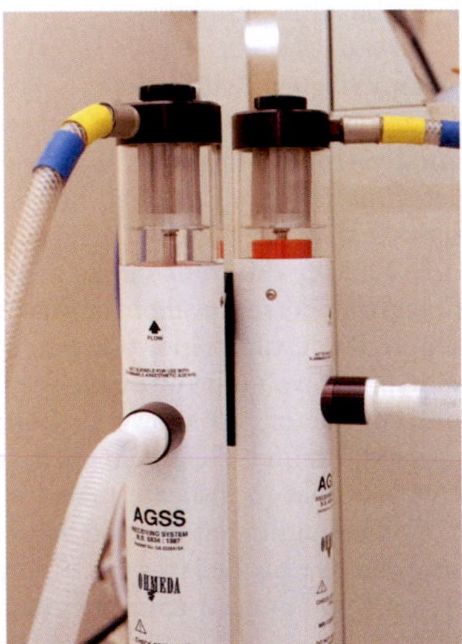


**Figure 8.63.** Two active scavenging units have been mounted together for the purposes of illustration. The one on the right is in use and the red float can be seen demonstrating effective extraction of waste gases. The unit on the left is not connected to suction. If a blockage within the device or at its outlet occurred, the float would not rise and the expiratory gases of the patient would exhaust from the bottom of the unit (not shown in this photograph).

The application of extraction flow leads to the possibility of inadvertent removal of fresh gas, excessive negative pressure in the airway, and pipeline blockages if a malfunction occurs. Such considerations have led to the development of tight design criteria to allow wide variations in expiratory flow (say up to 120 L/min), with fail-safe components for patient safety.

Standards for active anaesthetic scavenging systems are given in British Standard BS 6834 (1987).

Given the current concern with environmental pollution and the continuing trend to improve health and safety at work, good practice would dictate the use of a scavenging system unless a particular procedure or situation rendered scavenging very difficult to apply or, if it was applied, it would constitute an unreasonably high risk for the patient.

## FURTHER READING

Dorsch JA, Dorsch SE. *Understanding Anaesthesia Equipment*, 3rd edn. Baltimore, MA: Williams & Wilkins, 1994.

Gray WM. Scavenging equipment. *Br J Anaesth* 1985;**57**:685–95.

Hedley RM, Allt-Graham J. Heat and moisture exchangers and breathing filters. *Br J Anaesth* 1994;**73**:227–36.

Howell RSC. Piped medical gas and vacuum systems. *Anaesthesia* 1980;**35**:676–98.

Mikatti NE, Healy TEJ. Hepatic injury associated with halogenated anaesthetics. *Eur J Anaesthesiol* 1997;**14**:7–14.

Petty C. *The Anesthesia Machine*. New York: Churchill Livingstone, 1987.

Russell WJ. The anaesthesia machine, circuits and gas supplies: recent developments, complications and hazards. *Curr Opin Anaesthesiol* 1992;**5**:799–805.

Shelly MP. *Humidification: Intensive Care Rounds*. Abingdon: The Medicine Group (Education) Ltd, 1993.

White DC. Vaporization and vaporizers. *Br J Anaesth* 1985;**57**:658–71.

# Chapter 9 Breathing systems I: basic principles and systems without carbon dioxide absorption

P. Hutton

## DEFINITIONS AND FUNCTION

A breathing system connects the oxygen-containing fresh gas supply to the piece of equipment that delivers it to the patient's upper respiratory tract (e.g. endotracheal [ET] tube, facemask, laryngeal mask, injector). Although it does not have to, the oxygenated fresh gas usually comes from the anaesthesia machine and carries anaesthetic gases and vapours.

The basic functions of any breathing system are to:

1. maintain the delivery of oxygen to the patient, and
2. remove $CO_2$ excreted in alveolar gas.

When the patient uses his own muscles of respiration to provide the tidal flow of gas, the system is classified as *spontaneous*; when manual or mechanical means are employed it is classified as *controlled*. Satisfactory spontaneous ventilation requires adequate muscle power and neural control. For reference, the normal spontaneous breathing cycle is shown in Figure 9.1.

Satisfactory controlled ventilation requires the patient not to resist the imposed ventilation; intraoperatively this is usually achieved by the use of neuromuscular blocking agents, but patients will also accept controlled ventilation if their respiratory drive is suppressed by anaesthetic or opioid drugs, brain damage, or illness. Some very cooperative patients will allow controlled ventilation while fully conscious.

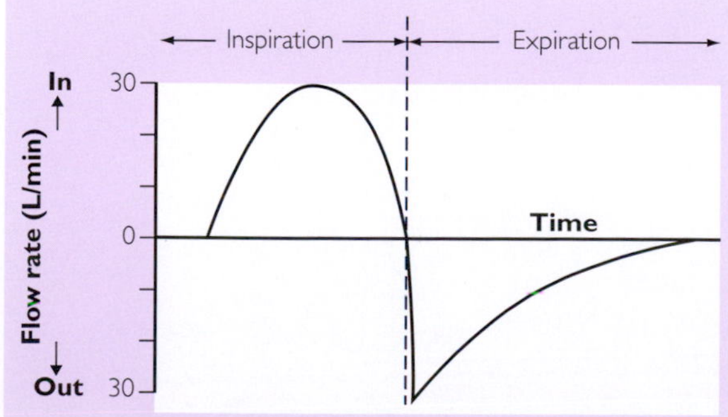


**Figure 9.1.** The normal adult spontaneous breathing cycle at a minute volume of approximately 10 L/min. (Adapted from Sykes MK. *Br J Anaesth* 1968;40:666.)

An ideal breathing system should, in addition to the two basic functions listed above:

- be reliable, easy to use, and fail safe;
- possess safety features to prevent patient morbidity (e.g. pressure limitation, no cross-infection, etc.);
- impose no additional inspiratory or expiratory resistance or compliance that adversely affects breathing;
- provide an adequate peak inspiratory flow during spontaneous ventilation (normally about 30 L/min [Figure 9.1] but on occasions up to 60 L/min, usually from a reserve volume of fresh gas);
- impose no additional anatomical dead space in the form of apparatus dead space; this is the volume within the system that may contain exhaled alveolar gas, which will be rebreathed at the beginning of the subsequent inspiration;
- be adaptable for various sizes and types of patient;
- minimize wastage of gases and permit satisfactory scavenging during spontaneous and controlled ventilation;
- permit easy use of monitoring.

Rebreathing, which is an inexact term, is now accepted in anaesthetic systems to refer to the rebreathing of previously expired gases containing $CO_2$. In other applications (e.g. fire fighting, SCUBA), rebreathing can refer to the recirculation and inhalation of previously exhaled gases that have been purged of $CO_2$ and augmented with fresh $O_2$.

## TYPES OF BREATHING SYSTEM

Breathing systems have been classified in the past in a number of ways, some of which do not obviously aid an understanding of their functional behaviour. This account arranges them in a way that is intended to be most helpful to the trainee anaesthetist and the description is limited to those systems in common use.

Breathing systems can be broadly subdivided into the following:

1. group 1: those that possess no reservoir bag and no valve;
2. group 2: those that have a single reservoir bag and a single adjustable spill valve;
3. group 3: those that in addition have one or more valves that control the direction of gas flow. This group can be further categorized into those with and those without $CO_2$ absorbers.

The breathing systems in groups 1 and 2 will always be linked with the name of Mapleson, and his configurations are shown diagrammatically in Figure 9.2, together with their more modern coaxial equivalents. All these systems provide for cyclical tidal flow from a steady flow of fresh gas. Unless the fresh gas flow (FGF) is equal to or exceeds the peak inspiratory flow, it is necessary for breathing systems to possess a reservoir of gas that can be drawn upon during inspiration and topped up during expiration. This reservoir can take the form of a simple tube possessing a volume greater than that of the maximal breath and communicating with the atmosphere, or a flexible bag of sufficient volume to achieve the same purpose, or a combination of the two.

The connections between the various components of a breathing system are regulated by international standards. Most are push-fit, tapered connections which are pushed and twisted together to form a gas-tight seal. To be leak-proof requires the cross-sections of male and female components to be perfectly circular and to have the same angle of taper.

Current standards specify 22-mm connectors for the intrinsic breathing system components, 15-mm connectors for the attachment of the breathing system to the ET tube and 30-mm connectors for the attachment to a scavenging system. Paediatric systems have a number of separate specifications still in current usage.

Breathing hoses are designed to prevent kinking and the traditional pattern is in black rubber or neoprene with corrugated walls (elephant tubing), which maintain their internal lumen when angled acutely. Various other materials in plastic and silicone, in both corrugated and smooth form, are also used.

The problem of cross-infection from one patient to the next has received considerable attention in the recent past, and disposable circuits for single patient use only have been marketed. Although this may be the ideal, the cost is substantial. Many hospitals, if using

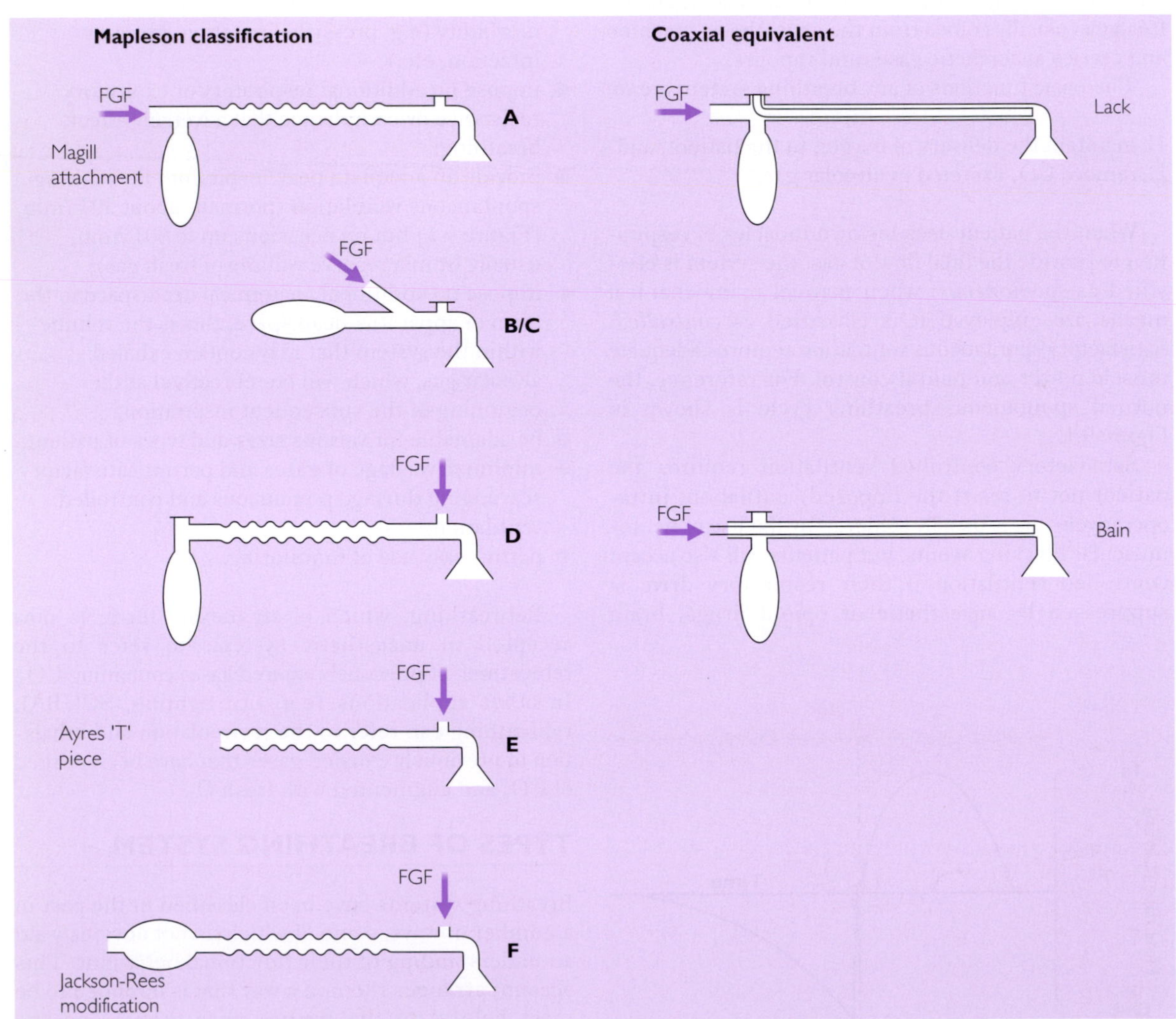


**Figure 9.2.** The Mapleson classification of breathing systems with their coaxial equivalents. FGF, fresh gas flow. Mapleson originally only had classifications A–E; F has been added since and the term is in common usage. The B and C circuits are similar but in B there is a length of corrugated hose between the bag and the FGF connection. (Adapted from Mapleson WW. *Br J Anaesth* 1954;26: 323.)

disposable circuits, compromise by allowing a single circuit to be used for a complete operating list, but insist on fresh breathing filters for each patient. Trainees should follow local guidelines.

Coaxial designs were introduced primarily for convenience. Having a single pipe with the valve at the anaesthesia machine end is particularly helpful when intraoperative access to the airway is difficult. Coaxial systems need careful checking before use to ensure that the inner tube is not kinked and has intact connections. Inner tube disconnections result in the mixing of fresh and alveolar gas with consequent rebreathing of expired $CO_2$. Depending on the system, kinking of the inner tube either cuts off the FGF or severely increases the expiratory resistance. A number of valve attachments are now available (e.g. the Burchett or Humphrey) which are at the machine end of the breathing system and allow the anaesthetist to switch a coaxial system from an A to D mode and vice versa.

The performance of the systems will be described in relation to the 'traditional' Mapleson arrangement; the analysis of their coaxial equivalents (which is essentially identical) has been left for the reader to undertake as an exercise.

## Group 1: systems with no reservoir bag and no valve

This arrangement falls into the Mapleson E category, as shown in Figure 9.2. As there are no valves, very low expiratory resistance is possible which historically makes it a popular system for use in the form of a 'T piece' for anaesthesia of children.

### *Spontaneous ventilation*

At the end of expiration, alveolar gas (mixed with fresh gas flowing into the system during expiration) will occupy the position shown in Figure 9.3a. If inspiration starts immediately at the end of expiration, for there to be no rebreathing of alveolar gas the FGF has to enter the system at a rate that equals or exceeds the maximum inspiratory flow rate. During spontaneous ventilation, this is therefore a wasteful system in which there has to be a steady flow of fresh gas equal to the momentary maximal inspiratory flow rate throughout the whole of the inspiratory and expiratory cycle. If the fresh gas entry is moved further away from the patient to B, as shown by the dotted lines, there is more rebreathing of part of the expired alveolar gas.

In practice, there is sometimes a discontinuity or brief rest between the end of expiration and the beginning of inspiration, known as the expiratory pause. If this is present, the alveolar gas left in the expiratory tubing at the end of expiration is, during this pause, flushed away from the patient, as shown diagrammatically in Figure 9.3b. This creates a small reservoir of fresh gas which, during peak inspiratory flow, can augment the steady FGF, thereby allowing the latter to be decreased from the maximum peak inspiratory flow rate.

The detailed analysis of spontaneously ventilating individual Mapleson E systems is complex and depends on the combination of FGF, minute and tidal volumes, the inspiratory/expiratory ratio (see Chapter 11), the presence and length of pauses, gas mixing, and the length and volume of the expiratory limb. As a guide to routine safe practice, it is reasonable to set the FGF at

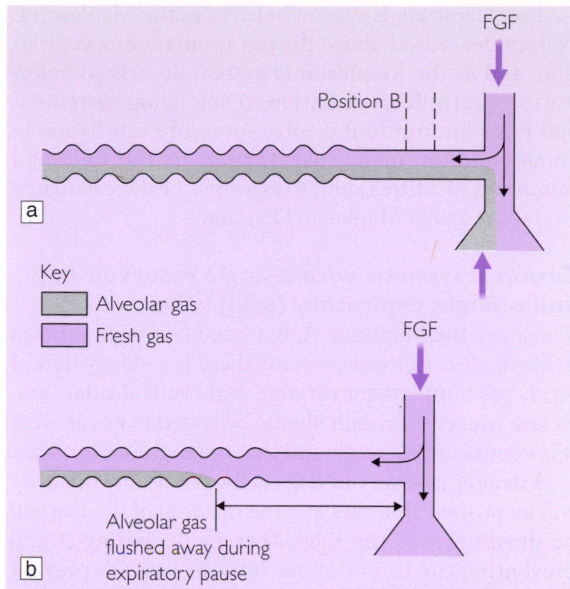


**Figure 9.3.** Performance of the Mapleson E system during spontaneous breathing. FGF, fresh gas flow. (See text for details.) For clarity, fresh and alveolar gas are shown separated; in practice they would be mixed together.

2.5–3 times the predicted minute volume, keeping the volume of the expiratory limb over one-third of the tidal volume. Such a system is very wasteful of gases during spontaneous ventilation, and is almost exclusively used for small children, principally because of its inherent simplicity and very low expiratory resistance.

### *Controlled ventilation*

Controlled ventilation of the lungs can be achieved by intermittent manual or mechanical occlusion of the reservoir tubing. This forces gas down the trachea as the FGF into the system continues. Providing that there is negligible gas mixing, it is efficient in the use of fresh gas. In this system, the tidal volume is dependent on the combination of FGF and occlusion time, and the frequency of occlusion is the respiratory rate. It is, however, not an arrangement that is frequently employed in practice and, if it malfunctions, airway pressure can rapidly build up to dangerous levels because there is a constant flow of fresh gas from a high-pressure source into a small-volume, non-distensible system.

For paediatric use, the Mapleson E is often converted to the Mapleson F system by the addition of a small bag as shown in Figure 9.2. The following are features of this system:

- Occluding the end of the bag temporarily and watching it fill confirms a proper connection to the patient and the presence of FGF into the system.
- During spontaneous breathing it provides visual evidence of inspiration and expiration.
- With practice, ventilation can be controlled by gripping the outlet of the bag between the little finger and the heel of the hand, as the bag is squeezed between the other fingers and the palm.
- It can be used to provide a degree of continuous positive airway pressure or positive end-expiratory pressure.

The Mapleson F system behaves as the Mapleson E system described above during spontaneous ventilation, and as the Mapleson D system described below during controlled ventilation. When using systems E and F for intermittent positive-pressure ventilation in small children, many anaesthetists fix the FGF at a minimum of 3 litres/min, irrespective of the calculated FGF based on a Mapleson D system.

### Group 2: systems with a single reservoir bag and a single expiratory (spill) valve

These are the Mapleson A, B, C, and D systems shown in Figure 9.2. In these systems there is a steady flow of fresh gas supplying a variable and cyclical tidal flow. Before use, every circuit should be tested to ensure that it is connected correctly and that the bag does not leak.

A danger to reservoir bags is the possibility that they will be pushed sideways and the material of the bag will be drawn across the inlet, thereby occluding it and preventing the inflow of gas into the bag. To prevent this, a metal or plastic basket is usually fitted into the connector to ensure that gas flow can enter the bag whatever its orientation to the breathing circuit (Figure 9.4).

Depending on the system, the reservoir bag (usually 2 litres in adult practice) can serve the following functions:

- It allows the breathing system to meet peak inspiratory flows that are greater than the FGF.
- When compressed manually, the patient's lungs can be ventilated.
- During spontaneous ventilation, it provides visual evidence of inspiration and expiration.
- It allows the system to be tested for adequate FGF and evidence of leaks.
- It increases the compliance of the system if there is an obstruction to the outflow of gas.

The older reservoir bags in use some years ago had elastic characteristics such that they were normally unable to exceed an internal pressure of approximately 5 kPa (60 $cmH_2O$). As a result of the relationship between wall tension and internal pressure (Laplace's law, $P = 2T/R$), and the properties of the rubber, after reaching a plateau pressure, the bag merely expanded in volume until it split, as shown in Figure 9.5. This provided some short-term patient safety. Modern bags are, however, made of a wide variety of materials and some are capable of sustaining much greater pressures before they fail. It is therefore wrong to assume that the presence of a reservoir bag automatically limits the system pressure to a safe maximum.

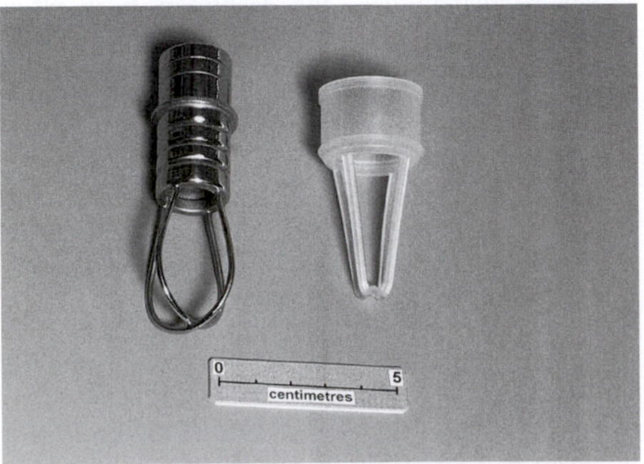

**Figure 9.4.** A basket that is inserted into the outlet of a reservoir bag to prevent occlusion to the flow of gases.

The spill, expiratory, or 'pop-off' valve used in breathing systems, which is more correctly named an adjustable pressure-limiting valve, has the following functions:

- In spontaneous ventilation, it prevents the ingress of atmospheric gases during inspiration and allows the exhaust of breathing system gas at low resistance and pressure during expiration.
- It can be screwed down to increase its opening pressure to allow hand ventilation.
- It will open at a higher preset pressure (usually about 4 kPa or 50 $cmH_2O$) to provide pressure limitation for patient safety.

Several types of valve are available. All provide the first two functions, but some (including the traditional Heidbrink valve) do not provide the third. The normal principle of their design is a spring-loaded, stem-guided, lightweight disc that rests on a knife-edged seating to minimize the area of contact and reduce the risk of adhesion from the surface tension of condensed water vapour (Figure 9.6). Even when fully unscrewed, the valve has to provide some small resistance to opening (about 100 Pa), otherwise the reservoir bag would never fill (it would merely remain flat) and, if scavenging is used, the fully unscrewed valve must prevent the contents of the bag and system being extracted inappropriately. The ideal spill valve would have the characteristics shown in Figure 9.7, the cracking pressure being set by adjustment of the spring, and resistance (measured as pressure drop across the valve) which is independent of the flow rate through the valve. In practice, the resistance of the valve varies with the flow rate, as shown, and the pressure drop across valves is normally specified at a given flow rate, e.g. 30 L/min. It has been suggested that spill valves should not sustain a pressure drop of over 300 Pa at 30 L/min, and many of those in common use operate at half this pressure or below.

#### *Mapleson A*

*Spontaneous ventilation*

The action of the Mapleson A system during spontaneous ventilation is shown in Figure 9.8. It is best understood by beginning at the end of an ideal expiration. This is shown in Figure 9.8a, in which the bag has just completed filling from the FGF, and there is no $CO_2$-containing gas proximal to the spill valve. The shaded section containing alveolar gas represents an obligatory extension to the patient's anatomical dead space. During inspiration (Figure 9.8b), the patient draws gas from both the FGF and the reservoir bag, because the peak inspiratory flow exceeds the FGF and the bag reduces in volume. After inspiration, when expiration commences (Figure 9.8c), expired gas is initially vented into the tubing and the bag begins to fill both from this and from the FGF. As the bag fills, the pressure in the system rises very slightly until the spill

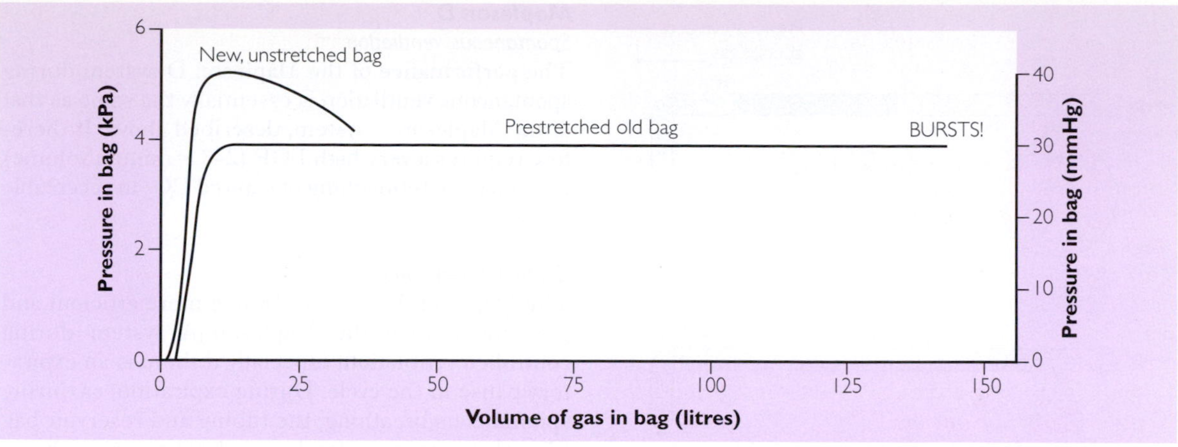


**Figure 9.5.** Behaviour of the internal pressure of a rubber reservoir bag as it is filled from a flow of 8 L/min. (Adapted from White DC, Halsey MJ. Anaesthetic apparatus. In: Gray TC, Nunn JF, Utting GE, eds. *General Anaesthesia*, 4th edn. London: Butterworths, 1980: 983.)

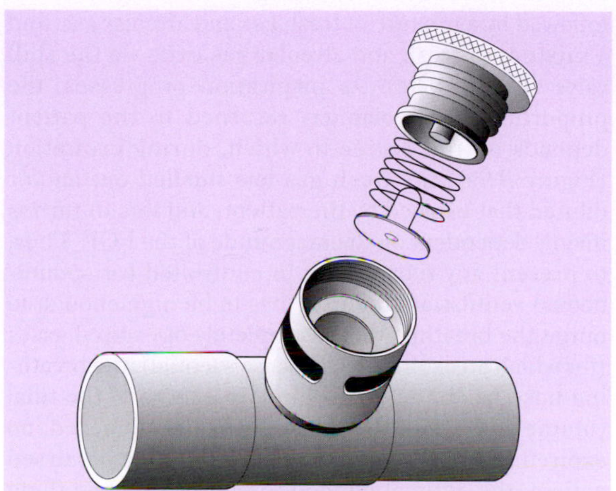

**Figure 9.6.** Diagrammatic representation of an expiratory or 'spill' valve. These are now most commonly made of plastic.

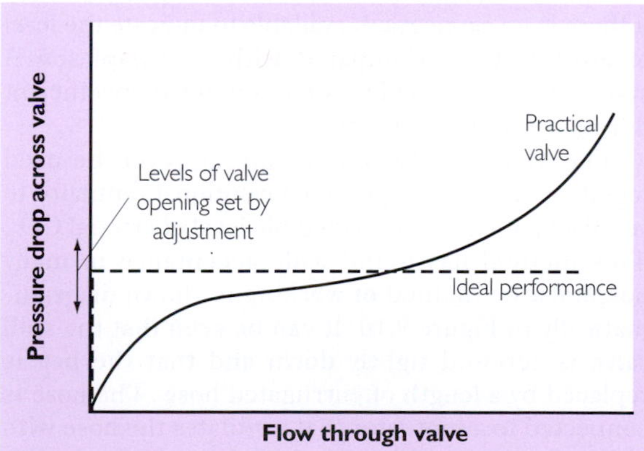


**Figure 9.7.** The ideal and actual characteristics of an expiratory valve in a breathing system.

valve (which is fully unscrewed) opens. The continuing FGF carries on filling the bag and the alveolar gas from the lungs is routed through the valve (Figure 9.8d) with some alveolar gas in the tubing. Under ideal conditions, at the very end of expiration, the FGF would have filled the bag and pushed the anatomical dead space gas back to the valve (Figure 9.8e). With the next inspiration the cycle begins again. In a circuit working at maximum efficiency, with the patient's anatomical dead space gas theoretically lying immediately adjacent to the spill valve as shown in Figure 9.8e, all the alveolar gas would have been exhausted. Consequently, in an ideal system functioning with no leaks and no mixing of dead space and alveolar gas, the FGF needs to equal only the alveolar ventilation, which is usually estimated to be 70% of the minute ventilation. In practice, many systems have small leaks and there is linear mixing of the alveolar, dead space, and fresh gases. Most anaesthetists therefore, for safety, set the FGF just below or at the estimated minute ventilation (100 ml/kg), which produces an FGF of about 6 L/min for a 70-kg patient.

*Controlled ventilation*

During the inspiratory phase of controlled ventilation, the pressure in the upper airways must rise above atmospheric pressure in order to inflate the lungs. This contrasts with spontaneous inspiration, in which the pressure in the mouth is equal to or slightly below that of the atmosphere. To achieve this rise in system pressure, it is necessary to screw down the spill valve, otherwise all the tidal volume would be delivered to the atmosphere. Consequently, the volume displacement resulting from bag compression is divided between the patient and the atmosphere in proportions depending on the resistance of the valve and the compliance and resistance of the patient's airways. Furthermore, during expiration, with a high valve-opening pressure, much of the expired alveolar gas is retained within the breathing system rather than being vented to the atmosphere and consequently forms a significant part of the next tidal volume.

In summary, adequate oxygenation and the removal of alveolar gas during controlled ventilation with a Mapleson A system is inefficient and the performance of the system depends upon the particular combination of patient, FGF, spill valve resistance, and system compliance. It is therefore unpredictable in function and is not 'fail safe'. If such a system is used at the start of an anaesthetic (before adequate spontaneous breathing resumes after induction or while waiting for relax-

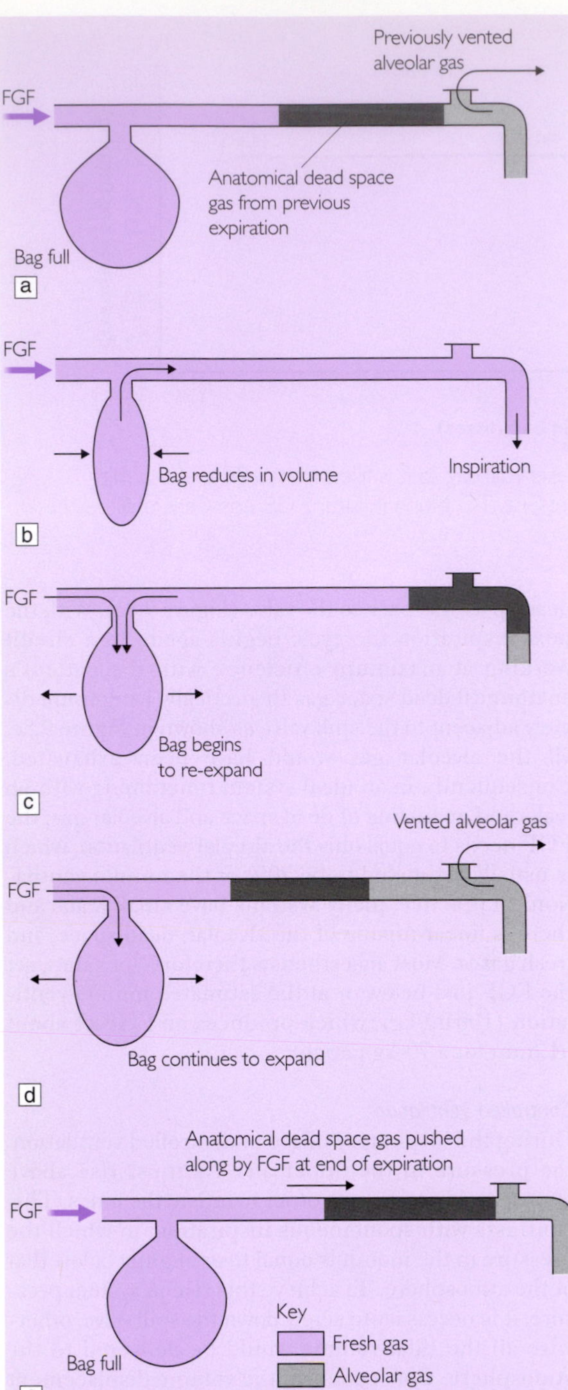


**Figure 9.8.** Performance of the Mapleson A breathing system during spontaneous ventilation. (a) End of expiration; (b) inspiration; (c) early expiration; (d) mid-expiration; (e) end of expiration. FGF, fresh gas flow. (See text for details.) For clarity, clear barriers are shown between the different types of gas; in practice the gases would mix.

ants to be fully effective), it should only be for a short time, with a high FGF (2.5–3 times the minute volume), a high fractional inspired oxygen ($F\text{IO}_2$) and preferably in the presence of a capnograph to warn of inadequate alveolar ventilation and a rising arterial $CO_2$ partial pressure ($P\text{aCO}_2$).

### Mapleson D

*Spontaneous ventilation*

The performance of the Mapleson D system during spontaneous ventilation is essentially the same as that of the Mapleson E system, described above. It therefore requires a very high FGF (2–3 × minute volume) to reduce the rebreathing of expired $CO_2$ to acceptable levels.

*Controlled ventilation*

The Mapleson D system is much more efficient and predictable than the Mapleson A system during controlled ventilation, especially if there is an expiratory pause in the cycle. During expiration, as during spontaneous breathing, the tubing and reservoir bag fill with a mixture of fresh and alveolar gas, as shown in Figure 9.9a. During the expiratory pause, if there is one, fresh gas fills the tubing immediately adjacent to the patient (Figure 9.9b). When the reservoir bag is compressed, initially fresh gas enters the lungs followed by a mixture of fresh gas and alveolar gas, and a mixture of fresh and alveolar gas exits via the spill valve (Figure 9.9c). As inspiration progresses, the proportion of alveolar gas returned to the patient depends on the degree to which, during expiration (Figure 9.9a), the fresh gas has flushed out and/or diluted that exhaled by the patient, and this in turn is mainly dependent on the magnitude of the FGF. Thus, to prevent any rebreathing in controlled (or spontaneous) ventilation, the FGF has to be high enough to purge the breathing hose completely of expired gases (for which an expiratory pause is essential), the breathing hose has to be of a volume in excess of the tidal volume and, when the reservoir bag is squeezed, no expired gas must enter the patient. With a paralysed patient, the optimal method to minimize rebreathing is to use a slow respiratory rate and a long expiratory pause to allow flushing of the alveolar gas along the breathing tube. For safety in practice, when hand ventilating using the Mapleson D system, the FGF should be equal to or above the minute ventilation, especially if there is no capnograph available to indicate the level of alveolar $CO_2$. Compared with the Mapleson A system, the Mapleson D system is much more efficient during controlled ventilation.

The Mapleson D system can, however, be used together with some types of conventional ventilator to ventilate patients to a predictable level of arterial $CO_2$. This method has found wide acceptance in many hospitals. Its method of working is shown diagrammatically in Figure 9.10. It can be seen that the spill valve is screwed tightly down and that the bag is replaced by a length of corrugated hose. The hose is connected to a ventilator that ventilates the hose with either $O_2$ or air, which is termed the 'driving gas'. During inspiration, driving gas moves up the corrugated hose and pushes the gas content of the system tubing back into the patient, together with the FGF, in the same way as would occur if the bag was squeezed. The patient's tidal volume is therefore given by:

$$\text{Patient's tidal volume} = \text{Ventilator tidal volume} + \left(\text{FGF} \times \text{Inspiratory time}\right)$$

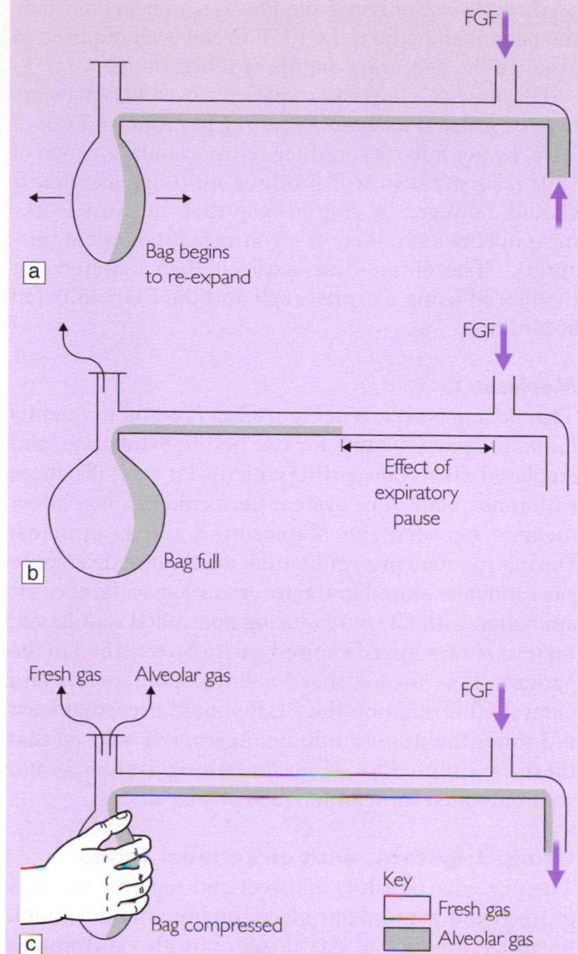


**Figure 9.9.** Performance of the Mapleson D breathing system during controlled ventilation. (a) Expiration; (b) expiratory pause; (c) inspiration. FGF, fresh gas flow. (See text for details.) For clarity, clear barriers are shown between alveolar and fresh gas; in practice the gases would mix.

During expiration, the patient exhales his tidal volume passively down the breathing system and gas is exhausted through the ventilator. The expired volume measured at the exit of the ventilator is given by:

$$\text{'Ventilator' expired volume} = \text{Patient tidal volume} + \left(\text{FGF} \times \text{Expiratory time}\right)$$

For the system to work properly it is essential that the driving gas does not enter the patient's alveolar volume and dilute the anaesthetic-containing fresh gas and rebreathed expired gas. Assuming that the breathing hose is of standard size and length, in practice this is achieved by making the corrugated tubing at least one metre long and at least 0.5 L in volume.

To understand the control of arterial $CO_2$ by the use of this system first requires some understanding of the relationship between alveolar ventilation and $P\text{aCO}_2$. If it is assumed that, for a particular patient, the rate of production of $CO_2$ is constant and equal to $C$, then at a steady state and assuming perfectly mixed inspiratory and expiratory gases:

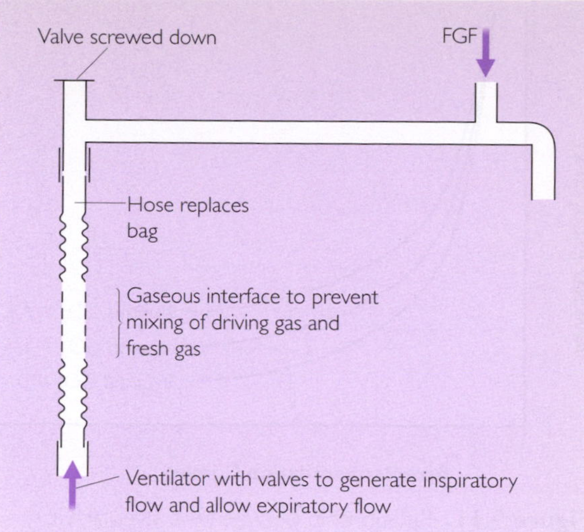


**Figure 9.10.** Diagrammatic representation of a ventilated Mapleson D system. FGF, fresh gas flow.

$$\text{Production of } CO_2 \text{ in body} = C = \text{Removal of } CO_2 \text{ from lungs}$$

In a rebreathing system:

$$C = \text{Wash-out of } CO_2 \text{ from lungs during expiration} - \text{Wash-in of } CO_2 \text{ to lungs during inspiration}$$

Therefore:

$$C = \left(\text{Alveolar ventilation} \times P\text{ACO}_2\right) - \left(\text{Alveolar ventilation} \times P\text{ICO}_2\right)$$

or:

$$C = \text{Alveolar ventilation } (P\text{ACO}_2 - P\text{ICO}_2).$$

Rearrangement gives:

$$P\text{ACO}_2 = \frac{C}{\text{Alveolar ventilation}} + P\text{ICO}_2$$

or:

$$P\text{ACO}_2 - P\text{ICO}_2 = \frac{C}{\text{Alveolar ventilation}}$$

Plotting this relationship gives the hyperbolic curves shown in Figure 9.11. With a zero $P\text{ICO}_2$ (inspiratory $CO_2$ partial pressure), the curve is asymptotic to the horizontal axis. From Figure 9.11, it can be seen that in normality the physiological point (A) is on the bend of the curve where the level of $P\text{ACO}_2$ (alveolar $CO_2$ level) is sensitive to alveolar ventilation, but does not rise or fall to dangerous levels with small changes in alveolar ventilation. This is a good arrangement for a physiological control system. If, however, the patient is hyperventilated, their $CO_2$ falls: initially steeply, then less so. Importantly, as the patient is progressively hyperventilated with non-$CO_2$-containing gas, the curve becomes less steep and his level of $P\text{ACO}_2$ becomes more predictable and less affected by changes in alveolar

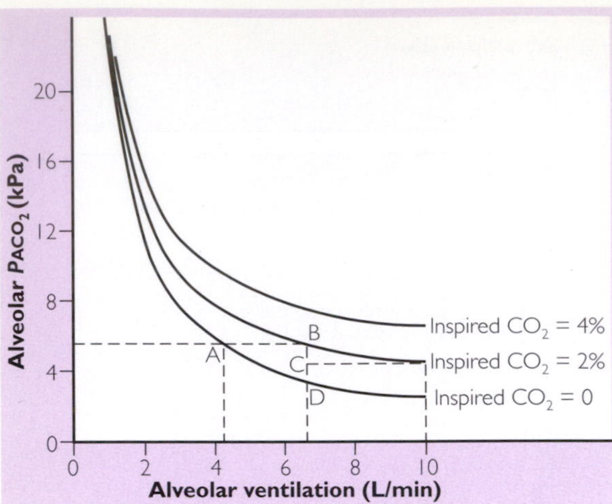


**Figure 9.11.** Relationship between the alveolar $CO_2$ level ($P_{ACO_2}$) and alveolar ventilation. Point A represents the normal physiological point for a 70-kg man with a minute volume of about 100 ml/kg per min, an $O_2$ consumption of 250 ml/min and a respiratory quotient of 1. The alveolar ventilation of B, C, and D approximates to a minute volume of 150 ml/kg per min. The $P_{ACO_2}$ is close to the $P_{aCO_2}$ in healthy lungs: one is then a measure of the other. (See text for details of the principle of ventilating to normocapnia using a Mapleson D circuit.)

ventilation. It also follows that, when underventilated, the $P_{ACO_2}$ rises steeply and becomes very dependent on alveolar ventilation.

If, however, the inspired gas contains a fixed percentage of $CO_2$, the whole curve is moved up by that amount (Figure 9.11). Thus, if a patient is hyperventilated with a known concentration of $CO_2$-containing gas:

- they are on a flatter part of the curve;
- the $P_{ACO_2}$ (and hence $P_{aCO_2}$) is more predictable;
- the $P_{aCO_2}$ is less influenced by changes in alveolar ventilation;
- the $P_{aCO_2}$ is very dependent on the inspired level of $CO_2$.

This contrasts with the situation when the inspired $CO_2$ is zero and normocapnia is more dependent on alveolar ventilation. An example of this is given below.

In the ventilated Mapleson D system, when the minute ventilation is set, the inspired percentage of $CO_2$ depends on the FGF wash-out of the system tubing. With reference to Figure 9.11, if the patient normally at A is hyperventilated by an increase of 50% in his alveolar volume, he will move to position D. If 1% $CO_2$ is added to the FGF, his $P_{aCO_2}$ will rise to C, and if 2% is added it will rise to B. Looking at these changes from the other direction, changing his $P_{aCO_2}$ from B to C at constant alveolar ventilation requires only a 1% change in $CO_2$; on the other hand, without changing the inspired $CO_2$, it requires an increase in alveolar ventilation of over 3 L/min. This leads to the often quoted, but rarely explained, statement that 'in a ventilated Mapleson D system the patient's $P_{aCO_2}$ is controlled almost entirely by the FGF'. In practice this means that, using a ventilated Mapleson D system, the most predictable way of fixing the $P_{aCO_2}$ is to hyperventilate the patient and adjust the FGF to the level required to produce the necessary degree of rebreathing.

For practical purposes in patients over 40 kg who are hyperventilated at about 150 ml/kg per min, an FGF of 70 ml/kg per min will produce normocapnia, and one of 100 ml/kg per min will produce mild hypocapnia. It should, however, be emphasized that these are working guidelines and there is significant interpatient variability. Therefore, the expired $CO_2$ should be monitored using a capnograph and the FGF adjusted accordingly.

#### *Mapleson C*

This system is shown in Figure 9.2. It is still frequently found in recovery units for use before extubation, and employed when transporting patients for short distances within hospitals. The system performs in a way intermediate between the Mapleson A and D systems. During spontaneous ventilation, anatomical deadspace gas cannot be stored in the reservoir bag without contamination with $CO_2$ and, during controlled ventilation, there is always mixed expired gas to be returned to the patient. This means that for both spontaneous and controlled ventilation the FGF should exceed at least 2–3 times the minute volume. Again, it is advised that there is a high $F_{IO_2}$. This breathing system is not recommended for maintenance of anaesthesia.

### Group 3: systems with directional valves

The presence of valves to direct and separate the flow of fresh and expired gas gives the potential for much greater efficiency of gas usage, but also introduces mechanical, pneumatic, and electrical components that can fail, stick, jam, or be misassembled. Whenever a valved system is used, it is vital that the anaesthetist knows how it is constructed and how it should perform. *Malfunction and incorrect assembly can quickly lead to serious morbidity and mortality*.

Valved systems can be subdivided into two major groups: those without and those with $CO_2$ absorption. Those with $CO_2$ absorption are described separately in Chapter 10.

#### *Valved systems without $CO_2$ absorption*

Historically, these were designed to improve the convenience of existing breathing systems (by making the valve accessible) for both spontaneous and controlled ventilation (Figure 9.12). Although now no longer used for this purpose, they are currently employed to control gas flows inside modern ventilators, and they play an important role in the action of manual resuscitators. *It is very important for anaesthetists to know how the ventilator they are using works*; if not, serious mistakes can be made. In particular, considerable attention needs to be paid to the use of the ventilator circuit when switched to manual control. Has it been converted to an A, B, C, D, or E system? Is the patient breathing from the fresh gas supply or from the atmosphere?

One circle without absorption that has been used in a number of ventilators is that shown in Figure 9.13. One of the reasons for this design was that it is possible to give patients large tidal and minute volumes (when it was popularly thought that this reduced atelectasis) while maintaining normocapnia. The tidal

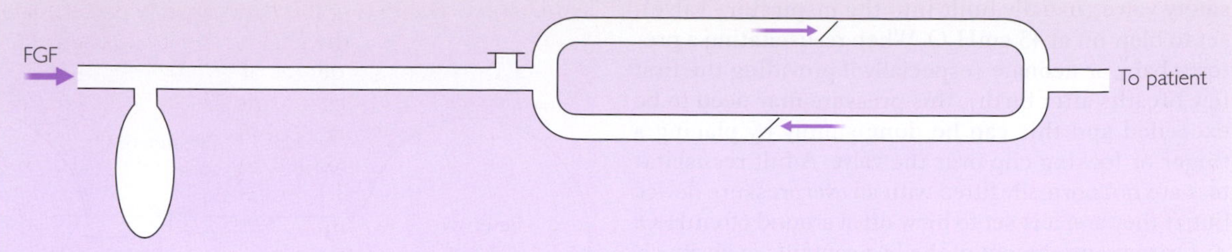


**Figure 9.12.** The use of a valved system to move the expiratory valve of a Mapleson A system away from the patient's airway. The directional valves can be anywhere along the inspiratory and expiratory limbs and were often incorporated into a 'Y' joint at the patient end. FGF, fresh gas flow.

volume and frequency of the bellows are set on the ventilator and the FGF is set on the anaesthesia machine. If the FGF equals or exceeds the minute ventilation, the bellows can (theoretically) fill with fresh gas and the inspiratory flow into the patient contains no $CO_2$. If, however, the FGF is less than the minute ventilation, the bellows draws the balance from the expired gas in the bag, and the patient is ventilated with a mixture of fresh and expired gas. This circle is therefore performing in principle similar to that of a ventilated Mapleson D system. Its ability to control the $P\text{aCO}_2$ can be illustrated by reference to Figure 9.11.

This text will not examine and describe a large number of such possible systems in detail; it is left to the reader to satisfy him- or herself of a system's performance when meeting it in clinical practice. Usually the quickest way to do this, in the case of a ventilator, is to refer to the manufacturer's handbook. Manual resuscitation systems, because of their great importance, are, however, described separately below.

#### *Manual resuscitators*

Manual resuscitators have to be simple to use, robust, and reliable because they are required in emergency situations where device failure could be disastrous. In their simplest form, they consist of a self-inflating bag (so that there is no reliance on pressurized gas), a bag refill valve, and a non-rebreathing valve between the bag and facemask or ET tube. Additional components are an $O_2$ inlet port, a reservoir bag, and a pressure-limiting device. A manual resuscitator is shown schematically in Figure 9.14. They are supplied in three sizes: adult (1500–2000 ml bag volume), child (approximately 500 ml bag volume), and infant (approximately 250 ml bag volume).

The bag refill valve is a one-way (usually simple flap) valve. When the bag is squeezed, the valve closes to prevent the escape of gas back through the inlet. It is opened by negative pressure within the bag as it expands spontaneously after being released at the end of an inspiratory action. The normal arrangement is for the inlet valve to be at the opposite end of the bag from the outlet valve, but this is not invariably the case. There are a few models in which the inlet and outlet valves are physically combined.

The valve connecting the bag to the patient has a 22-mm male connector to fit a facemask coaxial with a 15-mm female connector for attachment to an ET tube. Some are designed to swivel so that the bag can be put at the most convenient angle. During manual ventilation the valve directs flow into the patient and the patient expires to the atmosphere. The major functional difference between individual models of valve is in *how they perform if the patient recovers and starts to breathe spontaneously*. In the simplest type, the spontaneously breathing patient inspires and expires room air through the expiratory port (Figure 9.15a) but in others the patient inspires from the bag and expires to atmosphere just as if he or she was being hand ventilated (Figure 9.15b). It is obviously important to know which type is in use so that separate facemask $O_2$ can be provided if necessary during recovery.

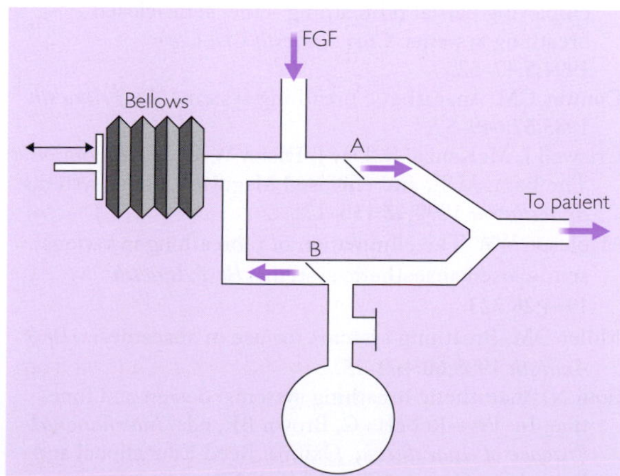


**Figure 9.13.** A ventilated rebreathing circuit without $CO_2$ absorption. FGF, fresh gas flow. A and B are directional valves.

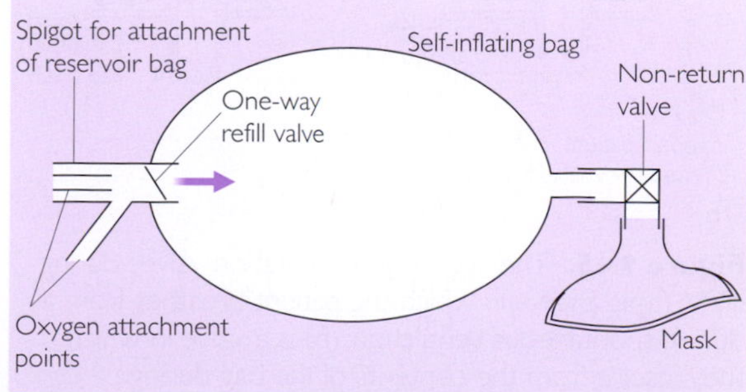


**Figure 9.14.** Diagrammatic representation of a manual resuscitator. The physical design varies from model to model, but the $O_2$ supply should be via the inlet port rather than directly into the bag itself, to prevent excess pressure building up.

safety valve (usually built into the inspiratory valve), set to blow off at 45 $cmH_2O$. When resuscitating a preterm baby or neonate (especially if providing the first few breaths after birth), this pressure may need to be exceeded and this can be done simply by placing a finger or locking clip over the valve. Adult resuscitators are not normally fitted with an overpressure device but, if they are, it is set to blow off at around 60 $cmH_2O$.

Oxygen enrichment of the bag contents is obviously advantageous during resuscitation. A flow of $O_2$ adjacent to the valve (the $O_2$ does not normally enter the bag directly), as shown in Figure 9.14, is a simple way of doing this. The increase in $O_2$ concentration is limited because air will still be drawn into the bag when it expands after being squeezed. American standards require that a manual resuscitator should be capable of delivering an $O_2$ concentration of at least 40% when connected to an $O_2$ supply of not more than 15 L/min. If in doubt, during the resuscitation of an adult, this is the flow that should be set from a bottle or pipeline supply. The flows for a child and infant are correspondingly lower and usually approximate to 10 and 4 L/min, respectively, but this needs to be confirmed for individual devices. Particularly in children and infants, high $O_2$ flows can be the cause of a jammed inspiratory valve. *If ever there is difficulty ventilating the patient and the cause is not obvious, the $O_2$ supply should be disconnected temporarily to see if this relieves the problem.*

Delivery of $O_2$ directly into the bag still allows air entry during bag expansion, unless the flow rate equals the maximum bag expansion rate. If the flow rate is set above this level, there needs to be provision for venting excess $O_2$ and the pressure increase may lock the non-rebreathing valve in the inspiratory position. For these reasons, direct delivery into the bag carries unnecessary risks and, to the author's knowledge, is not used on any commercially available resuscitation bags.

To increase the concentration of inspired $O_2$, a reservoir can be attached at the inlet end to store delivered $O_2$ during bag compression. This store can then subsequently become the inspired gas during bag expansion. The reservoir can either be a long open tube or, which is more usual, a familiar floppy bag as shown in Figure 9.16. Such a system requires both an air intake in case the flow of $O_2$ is insufficient or fails, and a pressure relief valve to prevent high pressure building up if the $O_2$ flow is excessively high. Typical reservoir bag volumes are 2–3 litres for adults and children, and 0.5–1 litre for infants.

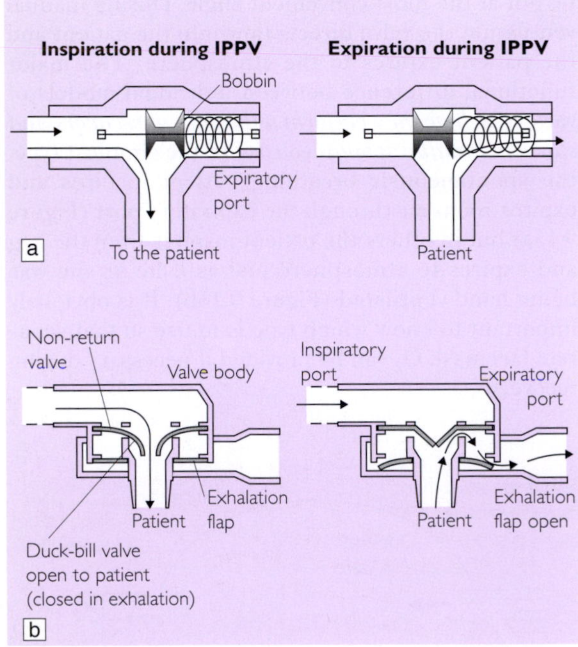


**Figure 9.15.** The action of resuscitation valves during IPPV: (a) is a valve in which the patient breathes from air during spontaneous ventilation; (b) is a valve in which they inspire from the contents of the bag during spontaneous ventilation. In (a) the spring keeps the valve open to air during spontaneous ventilation. In (b) the flap valves ensure inspiration from the bag during spontaneous ventilation.

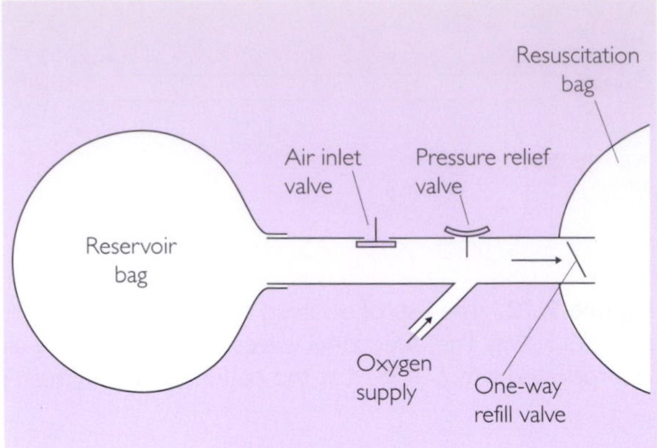


**Figure 9.16.** The addition of a reservoir bag to a resuscitator to allow the delivery of a high concentration of inspired $O_2$. The arrangement shown here is diagrammatic and the physical design varies considerably from manufacturer to manufacturer.

## FURTHER READING

Ayre P. The T piece technique. *Br J Anaesth* 1956;**28**:520.

Barrie JR, Beattie PCW. Anaesthetic breathing systems employing partial rebreathing – the 'semi-closed' breathing systems. *Curr Anaesth Crit Care* 1994;**5**:47–52.

Conway CM. Anaesthetic breathing systems. *Br J Anaesth* 1985;**57**:649–57.

Criswell J, McKenzie S, Day J, Disley W, Bruce E, Soni N. The Bain, ADE, and enclosed Magill breathing systems. *Anaesthesia* 1990;**45**:113–17.

Mapleson WW. The elimination of rebreathing in various semi-closed anaesthetic systems. *Br J Anaesth* 1954;**26**:323.

Miller DM. Breathing systems for use in anaesthesia. *Br J Anaesth* 1988;**60**:469–75.

Soni N. Anaesthetic breathing systems: design and function. In: Prys-Roberts C, Brown BR, eds. *International Practice of Anaesthesia*. Oxford: Reed Educational and Publishing Group, 1996: 2/145/1–13.

Sykes MK. Rebreathing circuits. *Br J Anaesth* 1968;**40**:666.

# Chapter 10 Breathing systems II: low flow and carbon dioxide absorption

P. Hutton

Breathing systems that recycle part of the expired gas and do not employ the use of $CO_2$ absorption have been described in Chapter 9. The need for $CO_2$ removal implies the use of fresh gas flows (FGFs) which are substantially below the minute ventilation. Circle systems with $CO_2$ absorbers can be difficult to analyse both theoretically and in clinical practice. If the principles of action are not understood, there can be unexpected and potentially damaging events, leading to both awareness and hypoxia.

## DEFINITIONS

There are a number of definitions in use in relation to low-flow systems, but the following are probably the most useful.

### *Totally closed systems*

In these the expired gases are purged of $CO_2$ and re-enter the inspired gas. The total volume of the system contracts with $O_2$ uptake and expands with gases that come out of solution in the blood and enter the lungs. The use of such circuits is now confined almost entirely to veterinary practice, where the size of the animal is small compared with the volume of the reservoir bag in the system. The author's advice is that totally closed systems should never be used by trainees.

### *Basal flow systems*

The FGF is reduced to basal levels once equilibrium is reached. The FGF then needs to be 100% $O_2$ only at a flow rate equal to $O_2$ uptake. Their use is infrequent, they require accurate low-flow rotameters, and should be used by trainees only when being supervised by an experienced clinician.

### *Low-flow systems*

These have the FGF set above basal but below the alveolar ventilation of the patient, and thereby necessitate some $CO_2$ extraction in order to maintain the alveolar ventilation with $CO_2$-free gas. Such systems are commonly used in practice. Most clinicians would not frequently use maintenance gas flows below 1 L/min.

In the past, there have been a number of nomograms and rules of thumb published to ensure appropriate levels of $F\text{IO}_2$ (fractional inspired $O_2$), nitrous oxide ($N_2O$), and anaesthetic agent in the circuit. Although these can be used as guides to practice, *it is the opinion of the author that low-flow circle systems should not be used in current practice unless there is the facility to monitor the* $F\text{IO}_2$*, the* $CO_2$*, and the agent concentration in the circle.* The main stimuli for their use are probably economy of expensive volatile agents and ease of pollution control. From the point of view of trainees, they can also provide a valuable learning exercise that helps the understanding of the uptake and elimination of respiratory and anaesthetic gases and volatile agents. This chapter considers first the chemistry of soda lime and then examines the principles of gas transfer in circles with $CO_2$ absorption.

## ABSORPTION OF CARBON DIOXIDE

$CO_2$ is removed chemically using the general principle that a base neutralizes an acid. In this case, the base is the hydroxide of a metal and the acid is carbonic acid formed by the reaction of $CO_2$ with water. The chemical presence of water (not necessarily 'free' water) is therefore necessary, and the end products of the reaction between the hydroxide and $CO_2$ are a carbonate and water. $CO_2$ absorption is not limited to anaesthesia; it is, for example, a vital component of submarine and spacecraft technology and several industrial manufacturing processes. There are therefore many different commercial preparations available that remove $CO_2$. In anaesthesia these fall into two main categories called soda lime and barium lime (Baralime).

### *Soda lime*

The exact composition of soda lime varies, but it is made up of approximately 4% sodium hydroxide (NaOH), 14–20% bound water, with the balance to 100% being calcium hydroxide ($Ca(OH)_2$). The NaOH is included to improve the reactivity the mixture and because of its superior hygroscopic properties. Some manufacturers used to add potassium hydroxide (KOH) to increase the activity of soda lime when cold, but this is now omitted from the majority of preparations.

The reaction is initiated by $CO_2$ reacting with water to form carbonic acid ($H_2CO_3$), a weak acid which is incompletely dissociated into its ionic components.

$$CO_2 + H_2O \rightleftharpoons H_2CO_3$$

$$H_2CO_3 \rightleftharpoons H^+ + HCO_3^- \rightleftharpoons 2H^+ + CO_3^{2-}.$$

In the presence of $H_2O$, NaOH and $Ca(OH)_2$ are similarly dissociated into their ions:

$$NaOH \rightleftharpoons Na^+ + OH^-$$

$$Ca(OH)_2 \rightleftharpoons Ca^{2+} + 2OH^-.$$

The sodium and calcium ions then react with the carbonate ions forming, as end products, sodium carbonate and calcium carbonate. The hydrogen ions produced by dissociation of carbonic acid combine with hydroxide ions to form water molecules. The reactions for potassium hydroxide, if present, are similar.

#### *Barium lime (Baralime)*

Barium lime is made up of 80% $Ca(OH)_2$ and 20% barium hydroxide octahydrate ($Ba(OH)_2 \cdot 8H_2O$). Water is therefore chemically incorporated into the structure of the granules. The chemical reactions occurring are exactly analogous to those with soda lime.

The reactions of both soda lime and barium lime produce more water than is necessary for the reaction to occur, change the pH of the granules and their surface moisture, and produce heat (they are exothermic reactions). Heat is liberated at the rate of 13 700 cal/mol water produced or $CO_2$ absorbed.

#### *Absorptive capacity*

The absorptive capacity of a soda or barium lime canister depends on many factors. Under ideal conditions soda lime absorbs approximately 25 L $CO_2$/100 g and barium lime 27 L $CO_2$/100 g. In continuous use, ineffective removal occurs before these limits have been reached because the outside of the granules becomes exhausted before the whole granule is used up. Another complicating factor is the size of the canister itself. Smaller canisters (which are now often disposable) containing, say, 0.5 kg of lime become disproportionately exhausted in a given time compared with the larger 2-kg canisters. This is probably because the larger canisters provide a greater absorptive area and allow a slower reaction to occur, thereby making better use of the core components of the granules. Three typical canisters are shown in Figure 10.1.

Although the effect is small with modern preparations of soda lime and barium lime, when the system is allowed to stand for a few hours after use, the granules appear to improve their absorptive capacity. This phenomenon is known as regeneration and is thought to result from chemical reactions within the granules in which unused hydroxide ions migrate towards the surface from the granular core. With modern soda lime preparations the absorptive capacity provided by regeneration is minimal and gives no appreciative extension to the life of the absorbent.

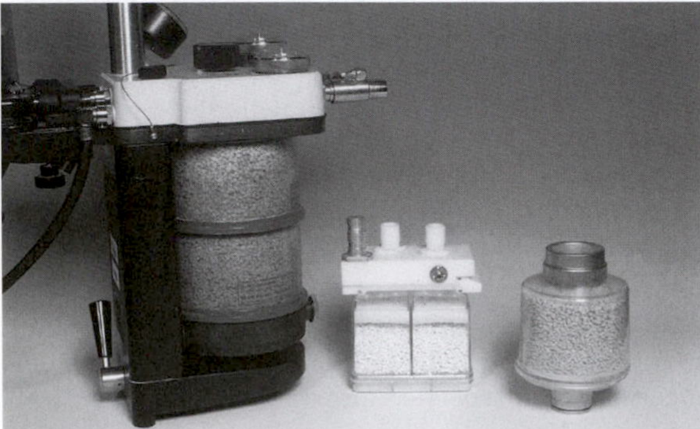

**Figure 10.1.** Examples of soda lime canisters. The large one on the left (sometimes called a 'jumbo') is integral with an operating room ventilator and circle system. The one in the middle is disposable and the one on the right is a small reusable canister.

An important practical point is the need to pack the canister evenly and to shake it to settle the granules. This ensures even absorption of $CO_2$ and prevents the channelling of gas through low-resistance pathways.

#### *Granule size and hardness*

A fully packed absorber consists of approximately 50% granules and 50% intergranular space. The size of the granules is important: larger granules cause less resistance to flow but have a lower total surface area for absorption; smaller granules provide a greater surface area but increase the resistance to gas flow and increase the potential for dust formation. Granule size is therefore a compromise and is measured by mesh number. A 6-mesh strainer has six square openings per linear inch, a 10-mesh strainer ten per inch, and so on. Mesh standards differ slightly between countries because of the gauge of the wire used to construct it. In the USA, granules are supplied between 4 and 8 mesh and, in the UK, between 3 and 10 mesh.

The water of crystallization in barium lime imparts sufficient hardness to the granules to maintain surface integrity, but traditional soda lime granules fragment easily, producing dust. This dust is caustic, and in the little used 'to and fro' system, could enter the patient's airways; this is less likely in proper circle systems because of the length of breathing hose between the canister and patient, and the use of breathing filters. To prevent fragmentation, silica and clay used to be added to soda lime, but modern manufacturing processes no longer require this. The tendency for dust formation (which is now low) is measured by the hardness number (which should be 75 or more).

#### *Indicators*

As the basic hydroxides are gradually used up, there is a shift towards an excess of unreacted $H_2CO_3$. A measure of pH therefore assesses the reserve activity of the soda lime. This is done by incorporating a chemical indicator into the granules which changes colour as the acid accumulates. There are a variety in current use and it is essential to know which is in use because some colour changes are in the opposite direction. Indicators in use are given in Table 10.1.

Although useful as a guide to the state of the soda lime, indicators should not be regarded as foolproof. Capnography is the key to the early detection of $CO_2$ rebreathing because of inadequate absorption by the soda lime. Signs of hypercapnia (increased pulse pressure, increased pulse rate, deepening of spontaneous respiration, increased oozing in the surgical field, and eventual cardiorespiratory collapse) should always be regarded as potentially the result of a problem with the inspired $CO_2$ until proved otherwise. The easiest way of dealing with this, if suspected, is to increase the FGF immediately to more than the minute volume.

| Table 10.1. Indicators in use with soda lime and barium lime | | |
|---|---|---|
| Indicator | Colour when fresh (alkaline) | Colour when exhausted (acid) |
| Ethyl violet | White | Purple |
| Clayton or Titan yellow | Pink | Off-white |
| Mimosa Z | Red | White |
| Phenolphthalein | Red | White |

Ethyl violet and Clayton or Titan yellow are used most frequently.

***Interaction with volatile agents***

The heat and water produced by the reaction of soda lime and water are said to be beneficial in that they warm and partially humidify the inspired gases. It is, however, possible to achieve high temperatures in the centre of a soda lime canister which cannot be felt on the outside. At temperatures above 60°C trichloroethylene is decomposed first to dichloroacetylene and then to phosgene, both of which are highly toxic. This agent, although no longer available for anaesthetic practice, must never be used with soda lime.

Absorbents, especially when dried out, can absorb modern volatile anaesthetics. This theoretically reduces their concentration initially and maintains it later, but is not a clinically important problem. All agents in current use (sevoflurane, isoflurane, desflurane, halothane, and enflurane) have been shown, under extreme laboratory conditions, to be degraded by soda and barium lime at high temperatures as the absorbent becomes exhausted. The magnitude of these reactions is clinically insignificant and there are no reports of human toxicity from degradation products during normal use.

Of much more importance is the production of carbon monoxide (CO) in anaesthetic circle systems, which on rare occasions has been measured at over 1000 parts per million. Fresh barium lime and soda lime do not produce CO but, if the water content is allowed to decrease, the absorbent reacts with agents containing a $CHF_2$ group (enflurane, isoflurane, desflurane) to release CO. Barium lime is the more reactive substance and soda lime does not produce CO until the water content is below 3.2%. The major danger from CO toxicity occurs immediately as the circuit is used for the first time after a period of disuse. It is postulated that, during significant periods of disuse (e.g. over a weekend), especially if there is a basal flow of $O_2$ left on, the absorbent material may become dehydrated, allowing the production of CO during a subsequent anaesthetic.

## PRINCIPLES OF GAS TRANSFER IN CIRCLE SYSTEMS

When a patient is connected to a circle system, the detailed changes in uptake and excretion of the various gaseous and volatile components can be both complex and highly variable, depending on the exact circumstance. Consequently, the description that follows, as an aid to understanding, identifies separately the main concepts and important components that will be present in a variable combination in any given clinical setting. Readers can themselves then consider systems that they have seen in their own clinical practice in the light of these principles. The arguments are developed through a series of scenarios which assume the lung to be a simple, easily stirred, single compartment in communication with a reservoir of inspiratory gas. Although highly artificial, they are intended to provoke thought and to provide a mental picture of the key mechanisms involved.

**Scenario 1** (Figure 10.2)

Imagine that an isolated set of unperfused lungs of volume $V_1$ are connected up to a flexible reservoir of volume $V_2$ containing 100% oxygen (Figure 10.2a). The pumps are switched on and the gas between the lungs and the reservoir begins to be exchanged. Assume that the lungs are composed totally of typical alveolar gas of a composition 5% $CO_2$, 80% $N_2$, and 15% $O_2$ and ignore the presence of water vapour. The changes for each gas, which are gradual, will proceed with time as shown in Figure 10.2b–d. The mixing in such a system approaches equilibrium in an exponential way. The following are the important points to be noted:

- When gas volumes containing different fractional concentrations are connected, the concentration changes are not instantaneous; there is a time delay before they become effective.
- The time delay is described by the time constant of the exponential process.
- The time constant depends on the volume of the two spaces and the mixing flow rate. In principle, rapid changes in lung gas concentration are produced by high minute volumes and large concentration differences.
- The final equilibrium concentrations depend upon the relative magnitude of $V_1$ and $V_2$.
- $N_2$ wash-out from the lung (and to a much lesser extent $CO_2$ wash-out) results in a fall in the partial pressure of $O_2$ in the reservoir.
- As shown with pumps, the mixing between $V_1$ and $V_2$ is steady. With intermittent flow (i.e. spontaneous or controlled ventilation) the curves of Figures 10.2b–d would be sawtooth in shape.

**Scenario 2** (Figure 10.3)

Consider now the system of Figure 10.2a modified to that of Figure 10.3a, in which the patient is connected to a 100% $O_2$ reservoir of volume $V_2$ and in which the lungs exchange $CO_2$ and $O_2$ (but not $N_2$) with the pulmonary blood. The ratio of $CO_2$ output to $O_2$

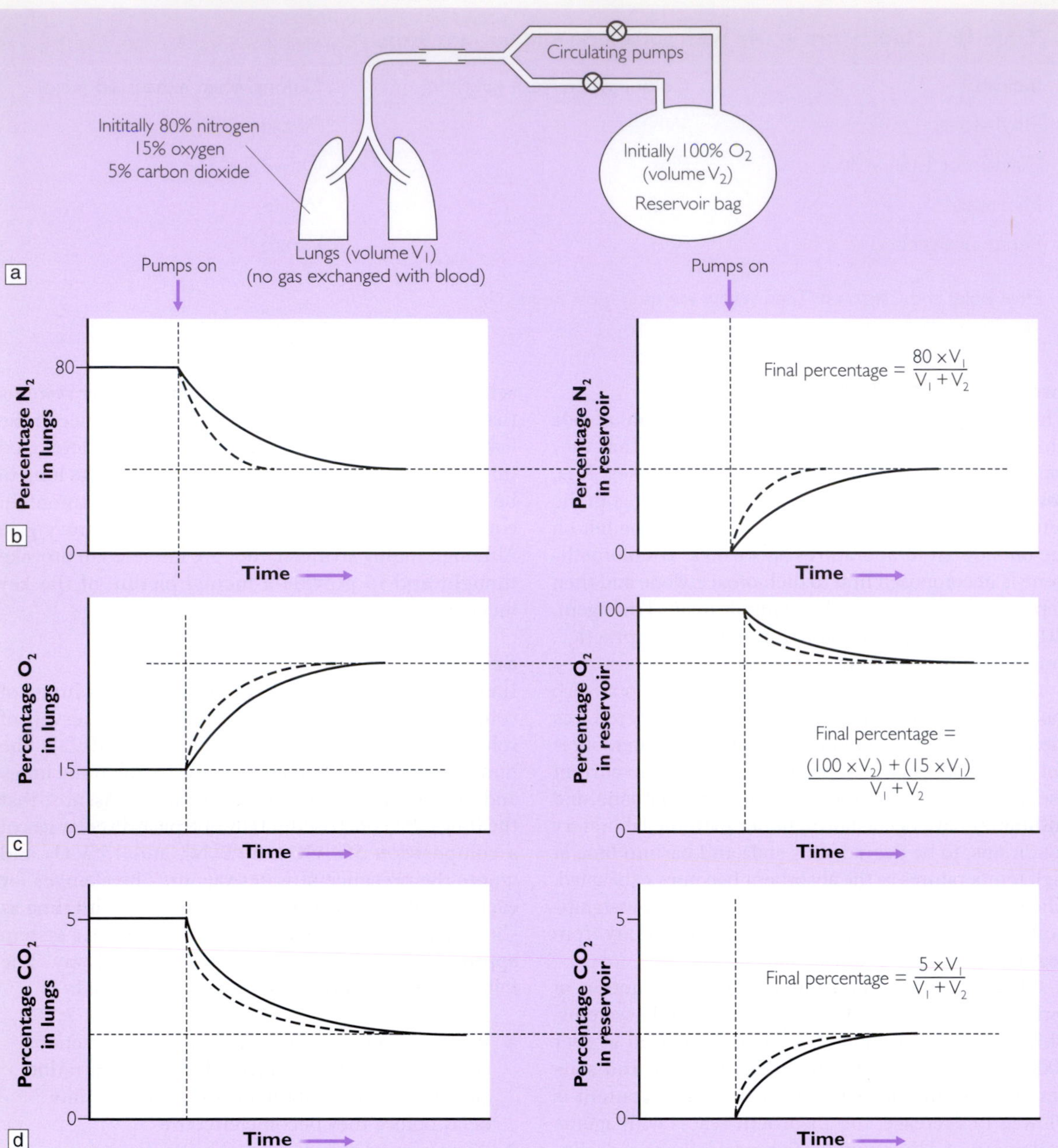


**Figure 10.2.** The behaviour of a completely closed theoretical model in which there is no gas uptake from the lung. The dotted lines show the effect of more rapid mixing. At equilibrium the final percentage composition is the same for both. The figures on the left show the lungs and those on the right the reservoir. The figures indicate trends only. The presence of dead space gas is ignored.

consumption is determined by the respiratory quotient (*RQ*) or respiratory exchange ratio which is defined as:

$$RQ = \frac{CO_2 \text{ produced in unit time}}{O_2 \text{ consumed in unit time}}$$

Normally, the *RQ* is approximately 0.8 because extra $O_2$ is required for the production of water in the metabolism of fat, causing more $O_2$ to be consumed than $CO_2$ produced. If only carbohydrate metabolism is occurring, the *RQ* becomes 1.0 and for simplicity we will assume that this is the case in this example. Typical values of $CO_2$ output and $O_2$ uptake are 180–250 ml/min for a 70-kg adult.

Under the conditions defined after the pumps have been switched on, gas mixing occurs smoothly as before but with the superimposition of a steady input of $CO_2$ and a steady uptake of $O_2$, the total volume of the system remaining constant if the volume of $N_2$ in the system is assumed to remain unchanged.

The gas concentration changes resulting are shown in Figure 10.3b–d. It can be seen that, initially, the direction of concentration changes and the shape of the curves is similar to those in Figure 10.2b–d because gaseous mixing equilibrium of initial concentrations dominates the picture. The initial fall in $CO_2$ and rise in $O_2$ will be as described earlier and depend on the rate of mixing and the size ratio of the two volumes. However, as time continues, $CO_2$ continues to be

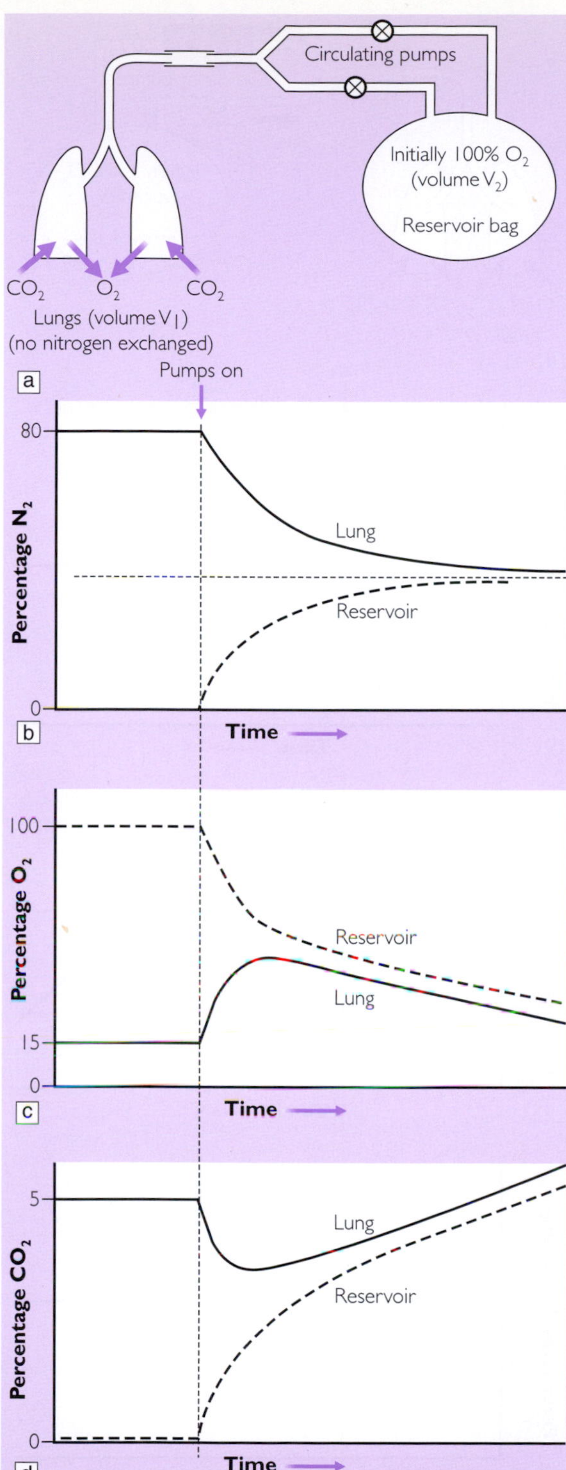


**Figure 10.3.** A theoretical model demonstrating gas exchange when there is $CO_2$ excretion into and $O_2$ uptake from the lungs. The early phase is dominated by mixing, the later phase by gas transfer in the lung. The figures indicates trends only, not accurate numerical changes.

produced, $O_2$ continues to be consumed, and gradually but inexorably the $CO_2$ concentration rises and the $O_2$ concentration falls. This eventually leads to both hypoxia and hypercapnia unless $O_2$ is added and $CO_2$ is removed from the reservoir.

**Scenario 3** (Figure 10.4)
The model of scenario 2 is now further modified to consider the effect of $N_2$. The $N_2$ in the lung is in equilibrium with that in the blood, which is in turn in equilibrium with $N_2$ dissolved in the tissues. In an average man, there is 1500–2000 ml of gaseous $N_2$ in the lung and a further 1000–1200 ml dissolved in the tissues. The diagrammatic representation of this is as shown in Figure 10.4a. Assuming an *RQ* of 1.0 again, in contrast to scenario 2, not only will there be transfer of $N_2$ from the lungs to the reservoir, but there will also be an elution of $N_2$ from the body tissues into the lungs, as the concentration of $N_2$ falls because it is washed out into the reservoir. It follows that, compared with the situation in Figure 10.3, at equivalent times, the concentrations of $O_2$ and $CO_2$ in the lungs will be lower because of the increased concentration of $N_2$ secondary to diffusion from the pulmonary blood into the lung. This is shown in Figure 10.4b–d, where it can be seen that the effect of $N_2$ coming out of solution is to render the gas in the lung hypoxic at an earlier stage. It should be noted that this added 'body' $N_2$ will increase the volume of the closed system. If the bag is not fully inflated, it will gradually expand; if it is fully inflated initially gas will leave the system via the spill valve (Figure 10.4e). The gas that leaves will of course be a mixture of $N_2$, $O_2$, and $CO_2$. Gas loss from the bag does not prevent or affect the onset of hypoxia and hypercapnia. In a totally closed circuit in humans, the washout of the $N_2$ in the lungs is rapid but the gradual loss of $N_2$ from the body tissues takes several hours.

The elution of $N_2$ from the body stores, in addition to potentially causing hypoxia, can also dilute the concentration of anaesthetic gases and volatile agents. Of practical importance are the facts that:

- if air and not pure $O_2$ was used as the reservoir gas, there would be no concentration gradient removing $N_2$ from the body, but the onset of hypoxia would be immediate;
- the $N_2$ elution effect on hypoxia could be overcome by flushing the reservoir continuously with the gas mixture required.

**Scenario 4** (Figure 10.5)
Consider now the effect of introducing a $CO_2$-absorbing canister into the expiratory limb of the connecting tubes between the lungs and reservoir bag, which again is assumed to contain 100% $O_2$ as shown in Figure 10.5a. Under these conditions there would be no build-up of $CO_2$ in the system, the patient eventually becoming hypoxic but not hypercapnic (Figure 10.5b–d) with the reservoir bag reducing in volume as $O_2$ is consumed and not replaced by expired $CO_2$ (Figure 10.5e). Although $N_2$ will elute into the system from the tissues, this will be at a much slower rate than the uptake of $O_2$ and the bag will still deflate.

**Scenario 5** (Figure 10.6)
If the situation in Figure 10.5a is now changed to that in Figure 10.6a, so that the initial gas is air and $O_2$ is added to the reservoir at the rate at which it is consumed and there is an *RQ* of 1, the patient would not become hypoxic, the volume of $V_2$ would remain constant, and the patient would remain normocapnic

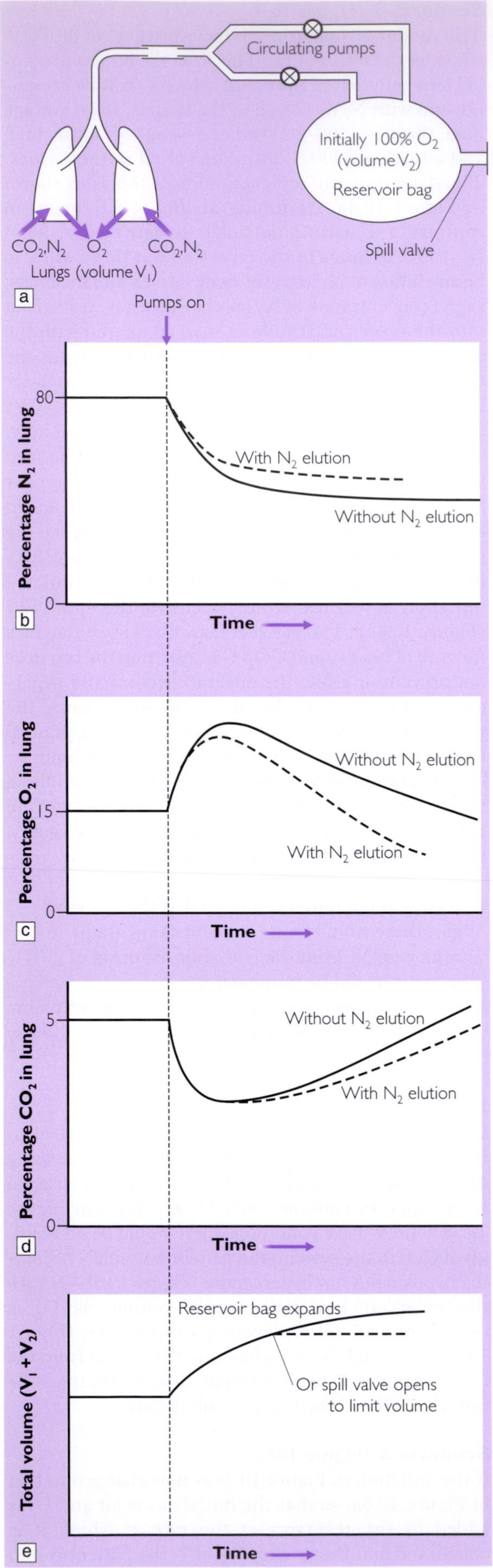

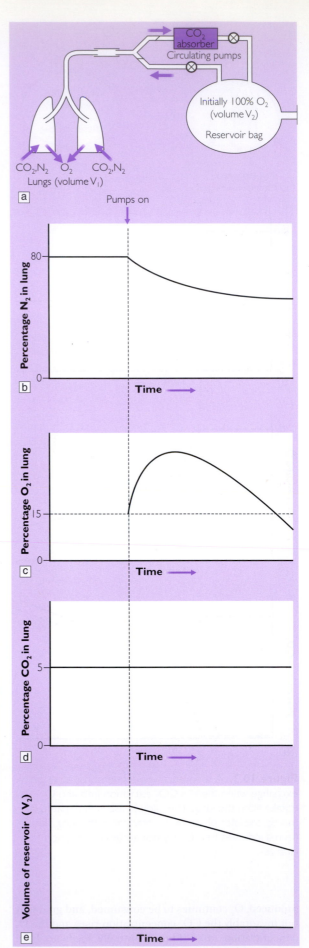

**Figure 10.4.** A theoretical model showing the uptake of gases in the lung in the presence of $N_2$ washout. The figures indicate trends only, not accurate numerical changes.

**Figure 10.5.** A theoretical model showing gas exchange in the lung in the presence of a closed system with a $CO_2$ absorber. The figures indicate trends only, not accurate numerical changes.

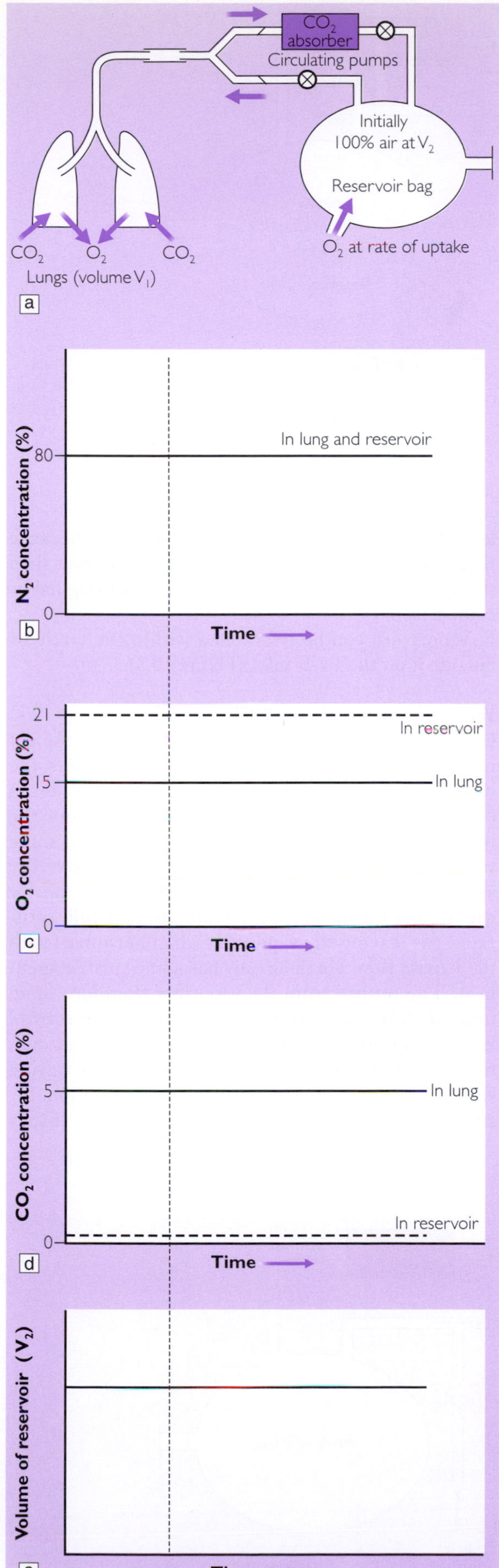


**Figure 10.6.** A theoretical model similar to Figure 10.5, but with $O_2$ added to the reservoir at its rate of uptake in the lungs. The RQ is assumed to be 1.0.

(Figure 10.6b–e). This is because there is no $N_2$ wash-out as a result of its equilibrium with air, and because the gas composition in $V_2$ is effectively unchanging.

If, however, the flow of $O_2$ into the bag exceeded the uptake in the lungs, it would gradually wash out the other gases (including $N_2$) and the concentration of $O_2$ in the bag would eventually rise to 100% and with it the alveolar $P\text{O}_2$. This situation represents a net $N_2$ loss.

It should be noted that $N_2$ loss from body stores when the FGF is composed of, say, 40% $O_2$ in air is much less than when the FGF is 100% $O_2$. At an $F\text{IO}_2$ of 40%, the equilibrium content of $V_2$ at infinite time is a $P\text{O}_2$ of 40.4 kPa (304 mmHg) and a $P\text{N}_2$ of 59.9 kPa (450 mmHg) compared with a $P\text{N}_2$ of 80.9 kPa (608 mmHg) in air. Consequently, with an $F\text{IO}_2$ of 40% rather than 21% (air), the initial partial pressure gradient driving $N_2$ loss into the reservoir will be 80.9 to 59.9 kPa (608 to 450 mmHg). This compares with 80.9 to 0 kPa (608 to 0 mmHg) if the $F\text{IO}_2$ is 100%. Thus, the greater the $F\text{IO}_2$, the greater the $N_2$ loss.

**Scenario 6** (Figure 10.7)

This relates to the effect of $N_2O$ and readers should first read the section on the uptake of anaesthetic gases and vapours (Chapter 33). Temporarily forget about the effect of $N_2$.

Imagine that the patient is suddenly switched from breathing air to a mixture of 75% $N_2O$ and 25% $O_2$ (Figure 10.7) with no FGF into the bag. The alveolar $N_2O$ levels will begin to rise and $N_2O$ will become dissolved in the blood. As it does so its partial pressure (and hence its anaesthetic) effect in the blood will begin to rise. Although classed as an 'insoluble' gas, it nevertheless has to have a net uptake to allow the levels in blood and tissues to rise. These will, in turn, eventually be in an equilibrium potential with the partial pressure in the alveoli. For a typical adult, $N_2O$ uptake declines exponentially as inspiration proceeds, typical uptake figures being about 450 ml/min initially and 100 ml/min after 2 hours. Throughout this time, the uptake of $O_2$ will be constant at approximately 200 ml/min. In the alveoli, the early wash-out effects of $N_2$ are small when compared with the uptake effects of $N_2O$.

The effect of this uptake in the early phase of anaesthesia is to change the composition of the gas in the bag because the proportion (and hence concentration) of $N_2O$ will fall faster than that of $O_2$. Consequently, unless the composition of the bag is maintained by continuous replacement, the maximum partial pressure of $N_2O$ that can be achieved in the blood will be well below that initially present in the bag. Looked at simplistically, the effect of uptake into the blood and tissues is as if some of the $N_2O$ present in the bag initially was removed and the remainder distributed between the bag and the lungs. One danger of $N_2O$ uptake in the early phase of equilibration in a totally closed or very low flow system is therefore failure to achieve anaesthetic partial pressures, with the risk of awareness.

In contrast to this, imagine that the anaesthesia has continued for a number of hours with the bag periodically being recharged with fresh gas and that the patient now is in equilibrium (for $N_2O$) with a concentration of 75% $N_2O$ in the bag. Further imagine that the

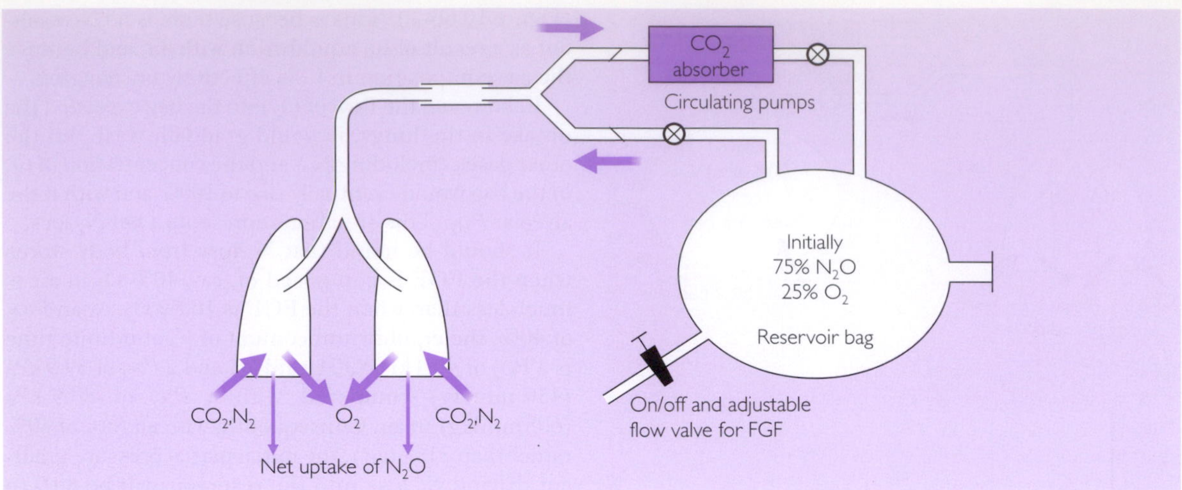


**Figure 10.7.** A theoretical model showing the uptake of gases in the lung in the presence of $N_2O$ and a $CO_2$ absorber. FGF, fresh gas flow.

FGF into the bag is below basal levels or that the bag is actually completely closed. Under these conditions, there will be continued uptake of $O_2$ from the alveoli (and hence from the bag) but no uptake of $N_2O$. The elution of $N_2$ out of the tissues will be small but still present. The volume of the bag will fall and the fractional concentration of $N_2O$ will rise. There is therefore, in theory, a risk of hypoxia developing. In practice, this possibility is offset by other losses of $N_2O$ through the skin and from body surfaces exposed by surgery.

The arguments in this scenario emphasize the unpredictability of the relationship between the administered gas composition and the partial pressures in blood, particularly when $N_2O$ is present and the FGFs are very low or zero.

**Scenario 7** (Figure 10.8)
It is important to consider the addition of volatile agents to circle systems. The reader is directed to Chapter 33 for an account of the kinetics of their uptake. This section will describe the performance of vaporizers essentially under semi-equilibrium conditions. The effects of differing degrees of uptake at different stages of the anaesthetic are, in essence, similar to those set out for $N_2O$ above. However, because their therapeutic concentrations are much lower than those of $N_2O$, their impact on $O_2$ levels is marginal by comparison.

Vaporizers can be positioned within the circle or outside it on the FGF inlet (Figure 10.8).

***Vaporizer in the circle (VIC)***
On the first inspiration, the patient receives the set inspiratory concentration of agent. This enters the lung, where some is taken up and the remainder is expired. On subsequent inspirations, gas from the reservoir enters the vaporizer already possessing some volatile agent. The vaporizer, calibrated under the assumption that there is no volatile agent in the carrier gas, applies the usual splitting ratio, and the fully saturated gas leaving the vaporizing chamber mixes with the bypass flow which already has some volatile agent in it. The output from the vaporizer therefore in an unpredictable way *exceeds* the setting of the control knob. In addition, the lower the FGF into the circuit, the greater the recirculation of gas already carrying vapour, and the higher the inspired concentration. In-circle vaporizers are now used only very rarely. If they

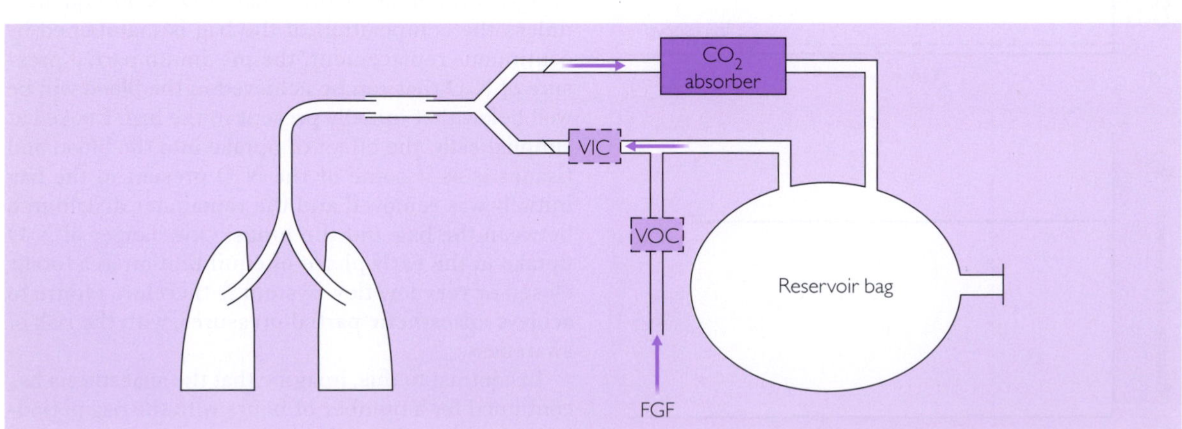


**Figure 10.8.** The positions of vaporizers in and out of circle in a theoretical model. FGF, fresh gas flow; VIC, vaporizer inside the circle; VOC, vaporizer outside the circle.

are used, it should be only when volatile agent monitoring is available.

***Vaporizer out of the circle (VOC)***

VOC is frequently used in routine practice. Consider a situation in which the FGF into the circle (say 1 L/min) was less than the flow round the circle (say 6 L/min). At the end of the first minute, the concentration of volatile agent in the circle (assuming perfect mixing and no uptake or losses) would be one-sixth that set on the vaporizer. As time progressed and uptake reduced, the concentration of volatile agent in the circle would gradually approach that set on the vaporizer. The speed of this approach would depend greatly on the level of the FGF. The basic principle of a VOC is, therefore, that the inspired concentration is unpredictable (unless equilibrium has been reached) and it is always *lower* than that set on the vaporizer unless excessively high flows are used that flush out the reservoir volume rapidly.

## THE PRACTICAL USE OF CIRCLE SYSTEMS

The previous section described the various factors that determine gas transfer and vaporization in circle systems. It emphasized the problems of predicting accurate alveolar concentrations and the dangers of hypoxia and awareness. This section deals with the practical use of circle systems.

### Safety

There are three basic safety factors that the author would advise are present when any circle system is used by a trainee:

1. Make sure that you understand the arrangement of the components, the way the circuit works, and how to test it before using it. There are well over 50 possible ways of connecting two valves, a spill valve, the FGF, and the $CO_2$ absorber.
2. Only use a circle system when it is possible to monitor the $F\text{IO}_2$, the inspired and expired $CO_2$, and the volatile agent concentration (if the technique depends on a volatile agent).
3. Whenever using a circle system, always have available a simple breathing system such as a Mapleson A or D. If, at any time, the patient appears hypoxic or hypercapnic, or the ventilation pressures are abnormal, immediately disconnect the patient from the circle and ventilate by hand on 100% $O_2$.

### Running a circle system

The physical arrangement of components in a circle system is determined as much by practical convenience as by theoretical optimization of economy. Although there is a variety of circle systems available, one of the more common arrangements is that shown in Figure 10.9. Although not the optimal system for either spontaneous or controlled ventilation, it has the following good points:

- Apart from the inspiratory and expiratory hoses, all the other components are away from the patient and can be assembled in a single unit.
- In situations where the FGF is set such that there is a steady loss of excess gas from the circle (the usual situation), it is mixed expired gas that is lost and not fresh gas, hence prolonging $CO_2$ absorber life.
- The FGF is delivered directly to the inspiratory limb. This minimizes the loss of free gas through the relief valve, minimizes the dilution of the vapour, and reduces the total gas flow through the canister. The last increases the efficiency of absorption and prolongs the life of the soda lime.

Such a circle system, when set up on a standard 70-kg patient, typically has a patient with a functional reserve capacity of 2.4 L, breathing hoses and internal piping with a total volume of 1 – 1.5 L and intergranular air space within the absorber of 0.5 – 1 L. This total volume of 4 – 5 L is the volume into which the anaesthetic is diluted at the start of anaesthesia, together with the volume of any reservoir bag or ventilator reservoir.

There have been a variety of guidelines published for the use of circle systems. In essence, they follow two important principles:

1. Give high flow rates into the circle early on in the anaesthetic to replace the volume of the circle with the required gas mixture, to wash out the $N_2$ in the FRC (if there is no or reduced $N_2$ in anaesthetic gas), and compensate for the effects of net uptake of $N_2O$ and volatile agent.
2. For prolonged anaesthesia with very low FGFs, especially in the presence of $N_2O$ and particularly when there is no $N_2$ in the FGF, periodically flush out the system to get rid of the $N_2$ coming out of the tissues, which dilutes the $F\text{IO}_2$.

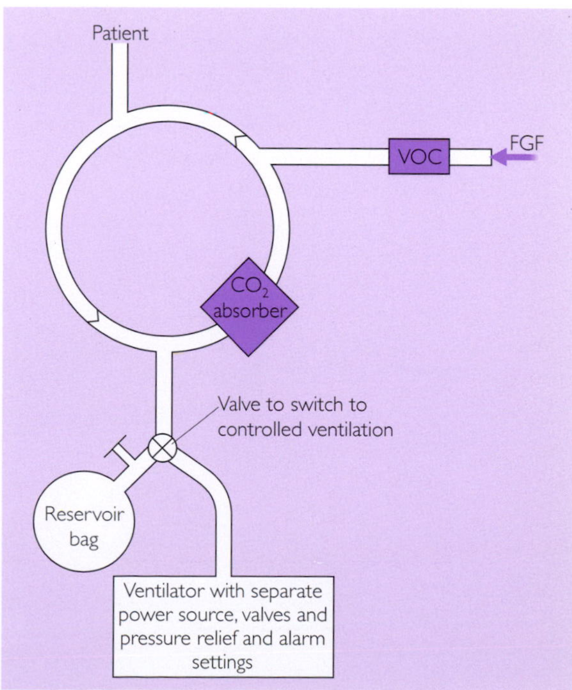


**Figure 10.9.** The position of the various components in a commonly available commercial circle system. FGF, fresh gas flow; VOC, vaporizer outside the circle.

A typical anaesthetic has the FGF reduced in stages as described below.

### *Stage 1*

Wash the system out with an FGF greater than the patient's minute volume for up to 10 min. Under these conditions, most of the expiratory gas will leave via the spill valve before reaching the absorber. If there is no $N_2$ in the FGF, the $N_2$ concentration will fall below 5%.

### *Stage 2*

Put FGF to 70% of minute volume for a further 5 min to ensure purging of the $CO_2$ canister with no major change in gas concentrations.

### *Stage 3*

Select a low flow for maintenance, being aware of the principles described above and the dangers of producing hypoxia or awareness. It is recommended that trainees should avoid the use of basal flows and always keep the $F\text{IO}_2$ in the FGF at 40% or above, whether air or $N_2O$ is being used as the carrier gas. If a change in the concentration of volatile agent is required at any time, the flow needs to be increased for an appropriate period.

### *Stage 4*

At the end of the anaesthetic do not forget that high FGFs (with the vaporizer switched off) are again required to wash out the volatile agent from the lungs and tissues for a rapid return to consciousness.

## FURTHER READING

Conway CM. Gaseous homeostatis and circle systems. Factors affecting anaesthetic gas exchange. *Br J Anaesth* 1986;**58**:1167.

Eger EI II. Anesthetic systems: construction and function. In: Eger EI II ed, Anesthetic uptake and action. Baltimore, Williams & Wilkins, 1974,206.

Liu J, Luster MJ, Eger EI II, Taheri S. Absorption and degradation of sevoflurane and isoflurane in a conventional anaesthesia circuit. *Anesth Analg* 1991;**72**:785.

Morris LE. Closed system anaesthesia: then and now. *Curr Anaesth Crit Care* 1998;**9**:92–8.

Peterson TG, Calkins JM. The circle system: from high-flow to closed-circuit anaesthesia. In: Prys-Roberts C, Brown BR, eds. *International Practice of Anaesthesia*. Oxford: Reed Educational and Publishing Group, 1996: **2**/145/1–10.

Spence AA, Alison RH, Wisheart HY. Low flow and closed systems for administration of inhalational anaesthesia. *Br J Anaesth* 1981;**53**:69s.

# Chapter 11 Ventilators

P. Hutton

A ventilator is a device that provides the bellows function of the lungs.

## THE REQUIREMENTS OF A VENTILATOR

It is customary in introductory texts to itemize the properties of an 'ideal' ventilator and a typical list would approximate to the following:

- reliable and mechanically robust; economical to purchase and use;
- ergonomically designed so that it is difficult to misuse and misconnect;
- ability to monitor airway pressure, expired and inspired minute volumes (MVs), respiratory rate, and inspired oxygen concentration ($F\text{IO}_2$);
- built-in safety features such as alarms;
- if safety features are not integral, easy attachment and interpretation of such things as disconnection, power failure, low fresh gas flow, low $F\text{IO}_2$, high airway pressure, alarms etc;
- easy to clean and sterilize;
- a wide range of tidal volumes (TVs) and breathing frequencies and an adjustable inspiratory to expiratory time (I:E) ratio;
- easy change-over to manual ventilation with a clear indication of the breathing system type to which it converts;
- ability to be used in a number of ventilatory modes (e.g. flow generator, pressure generator, with positive end-expiratory pressure, triggered, etc.).

If ventilation of the lungs is done cyclically via the airways by blowing the lungs up from inside, it is termed 'intermittent positive pressure ventilation' (IPPV). If it is done by applying a negative pressure externally it is termed 'Cuirass ventilation'. Exhalation is normally a passive process with the lungs exhausting to atmospheric pressure. If the pressure to which the patient expires is artificially raised, it is termed PEEP; if it is artificially lowered to below atmospheric pressure it is termed 'negative end-expiratory pressure' (NEEP). *Every method of mechanical ventilation should display the patient's airway pressure clearly and the anaesthetist should ensure that he or she is able to observe the dial or scale throughout the procedure.*

Ventilators can be powered pneumatically or electrically, or require both power sources. There is great variability in design. *It therefore follows that, whenever a ventilator is used, the anaesthetist must be familiar with its mode of action, especially when switching from automatic to manual ventilation via the ventilator. He or she must ensure that a manual breathing circuit is immediately available for substitution in case of difficulty or ventilator failure.*

Although there are ventilators that work at high frequencies with low TVs, only those ventilators delivering physiological TVs at conventional breathing rates will be considered here.

## BASIC DEFINITIONS

### *Tidal volume*

This is the volume of gas entering or leaving the patient during the inspiratory or expiratory phase. The two differ because of water vapour, the respiratory exchange ratio, and temperature effects.

### *Minute volume*

This is the sum of all the inspiratory *or* (not and) expiratory TVs in 1 minute.

### *Respiratory cycle*

This is a complete inspiration followed by a complete expiration.

### *Ventilatory rate or frequency*

This the number of respiratory cycles per minute.

### *Inspiratory (expiratory) flow time*

This is the time period between the beginning and end of inspiratory (expiratory) flow.

### *Inspiratory (expiratory) pause time*

This is the time between the end of inspiratory (expiratory) flow and the start of expiratory (inspiratory) flow. It is sometimes called inspiratory (expiratory) hold.

### *Inspiratory (expiratory) phase time*

This is the period between the start of inspiratory (expiratory) flow and the beginning of expiratory (inspiratory) flow. It is the total of the inspiratory (expiratory) flow and inspiratory (expiratory) pause times.

### *The I:E ratio*

This is the ratio of the inspiratory phase time to the expiratory phase time.

### *The inspiratory flow rate*

This is the volume of gas flowing into the patient in unit time. In spontaneously breathing patients and many ventilators, it is not constant during inspiration but may be so in a constant flow ventilator (see Chapter 9, Figure 9.1).

***The expiratory flow rate***
This is the volume of gas leaving the patient in unit time. It varies throughout the respiratory flow, usually decreasing exponentially (see Chapter 9, Figure 9.1).

***Resistance and compliance***
These are defined later in Chapter 20.

The more complex or specialized the ventilator, the more the parameters listed above can be adjusted. The classification of ventilators is not standardized and varies in detail from publication to publication; their features are described here in a way that is thought will be of the greatest use to the trainee anaesthetist.

## INSPIRATORY CHARACTERISTICS OF VENTILATORS

Ventilators produce a variety of pressure and flow waveforms during inspiration, depending on their mechanism of action and the resistance and compliance of the breathing hoses and lungs. It must not be forgotten that the TV from the ventilator is delivered to both the hoses and the lungs. In health, this is not a problem but, if a patient has high-resistance, non-compliant lungs, connected to the ventilator by compliant, high-volume tubing, the TV set on the ventilator will not be delivered to the patient. There are two main classes of ventilator commonly described: constant-flow and constant-pressure generators. Some ventilators in clinical use do not possess either of these idealized characteristics; others approximate to them.

### Constant-flow generators
These produce a step increase in the inspiratory flow rate. The TV that they deliver is determined by the product of the inspiratory flow and the inspiratory time. The steady rate of rise of airway pressure and the peak pressure attained are determined by the resistance and compliance of the circuit and lungs. A pressure safety blow-off valve is necessary to prevent barotrauma. Such systems have the advantage that variations in lung compliance (e.g. from bronchospasm), respiratory obstruction, or partial or complete disconnections are immediately apparent from the change in airway pressure.

A constant-flow generator produces the constant flow either from a powerful piston displacement or from a very high-pressure gas source, the flow from which is controlled by a variable resistance. The principle of both these methods is that the rise in pressure of the airways is negligible in comparison with the power of the driving source, so that the flow into the lungs will be unaffected by changes in airway pressure, resistance, and compliance. As shown in Figure 11.1, this produces a steady rise in the lung volume. The airway resistance in a constant-flow generator determines the initial step rise in airway pressure and the compliance determines the slope of the airway pressure curve (Figure 11.1). The effect of an inspiratory pause is also shown for completeness. Note that, as drawn, this will change the I:E ratio of the cycle.

### Constant-pressure generators
These produce a step increase in airway pressure to provide inspiratory flow. The resulting inspiratory flow rate depends on the resistance and compliance of the breathing system and lungs, and the TV is determined by all these factors and the inspiratory time. The maximum airway pressure is effectively preset (hence limiting barotrauma), and small leaks are automatically compensated for, although the true TV is often not known. Apart from very specialized situations, pressure generators are mainly used in paediatric anaesthesia. They have the disadvantage that changes in airway properties (e.g. obstruction of a major bronchus or segmental airway by a mucus plug) go unnoticed because the airway pressure remains the same.

A constant-pressure generator imposes a sudden pressure gradient between the mouth and alveoli at the start of inspiration, producing a very high initial flow (see Figure 11.1). The magnitude of the initial flow rate is determined by the airway resistance. As the pressure continues to be applied, flow continues and lung volume increases, but, as it does so, the differential pressure between the mouth and alveoli falls and consequently the flow decreases. Lungs with poor compliance have a greater rise in alveolar pressure for a given volume expansion, so the inspiratory flow is reduced. As the inspiratory cycle progresses, the inspiratory flow and the rate of increase of lung volume both fall, the pattern exhibiting exponential behaviour. The effect of high-resistance, poorly compliant lungs is shown in Figure 11.1.

## CHANGING FROM INSPIRATION TO EXPIRATION

This is often termed cycling from one phase to the other. Cycling which ends inspiration and allows expiration to commence (and vice versa), can be triggered by presetting volume, pressure, or time. Time cycling, which is by far the most common method, in practice applies to any machine in which the duration of the inspiratory and expiratory phases is directly or indirectly set by the anaesthetist.

## EXPIRATORY CHARACTERISTICS OF VENTILATORS

Expiratory flow, as shown in Figure 11.1, is usually independent of the type of ventilator because it occurs under passive forces, as described in Chapter 21. In healthy people, it is essentially an exponential wash-out curve, the flow being driven by the elastic forces in the lung. This is not necessarily so in diseased lungs such as those in chronic obstructive airway disease, where air trapping occurs and the flow is limited by a high airway resistance. In clinical management, when this happens it is sometimes necessary to extend the expiratory time to allow adequate expiration to occur.

The effect of applying NEEP is not considered here.

## FUNCTIONAL STYLES OF VENTILATOR

Arrangements designed to produce IPPV fall into three groupings:

(1) mechanical thumbs ;
(2) MV dividers;
(3) intermittent TV generators.

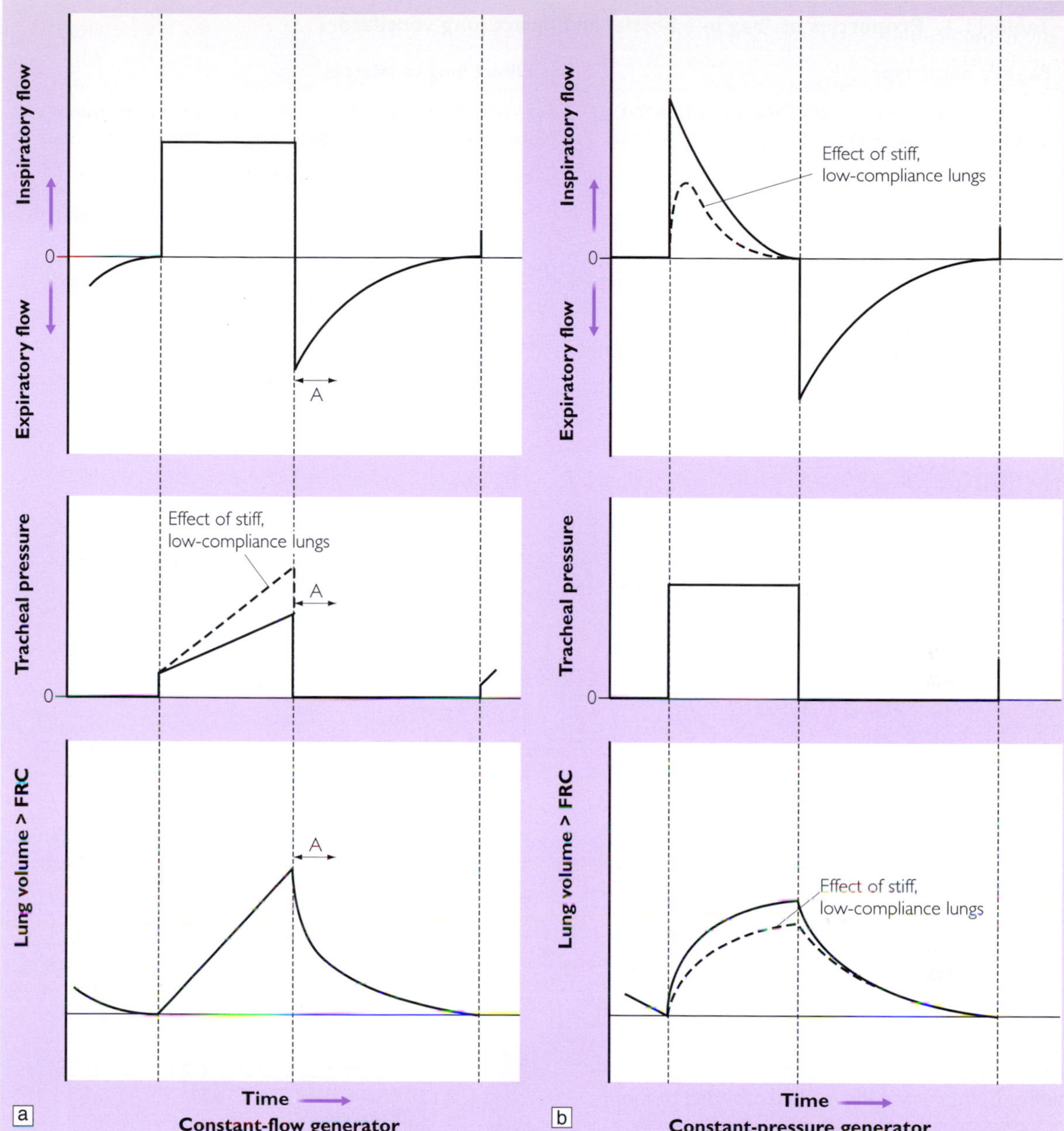


**Figure 11.1.** A diagrammatic representation of (a) constant-flow and (b) constant-pressure generators. The effect of setting an inspiratory hold (A) is shown on the constant-flow generator diagrams. In a constant-flow generator, the initial step increase in tracheal pressure is a measure of resistance, and the following gradient is a measure of compliance. FRC, functional residual capacity. Note the effect of stiff, low-compliance lungs.

The mechanical thumb simply intermittently occludes the expiratory limb of a T-piece breathing system and diverts the fresh gas into the patient (Figure 11.2). Its properties and performance have been described earlier in Chapter 9.

MV dividers and intermittent TV generators can both be subclassified into those that ventilate the patient s lungs directly or those that compress a bag in a bottle . The difference between the two types is shown diagrammatically in Figures 11.3a and b. The main advantages and disadvantages of the two systems are given in Table 11.1.

### Minute volume dividers

These are powered from the pressure of the gas coming from the common gas outlet on the anaesthesia machine. They essentially split the set rotameter flows up into TV-sized chunks and deliver them into the patient or the bottle. The basic principle of action is shown in Figure 11.4. The most common arrangement is that the MV is set on the anaesthesia machine and the TV on the ventilator; the breathing frequency then follows as a derived variable. Superficially, this may be thought to be a volume-cycled system, but usually the valve switch from inspiration to expiration is determined independently. If not enough time is allowed for the set TV to flow into the patient, the bellows will not empty completely, producing a lower than intended TV; if too much time is allowed, the TV will be delivered completely and be followed by an inspiratory pause. The latter of these is the usual working mode of these ventilators and they are therefore time cycled. The

**Table 11.1. Properties of 'bag in a bottle' and direct lung ventilators**

| Bag in a bottle type | Direct lung ventilators |
|---|---|
| Require two sources of gas: fresh gas inside the bellows and driving gas to compress the bellows | Unless pneumatically driven, require only one source of gas, which is the fresh gas going into the patient |
| More connections to come adrift | Have fewer connections to fall apart |
| Easier to autoclave | May be internal ventilator mechanisms which require special treatment to clean and sterilize them |
| Good visual indicator of tidal volume and satisfactory ventilation | Do not always provide visual information concerning adequacy of ventilation |
| If there is an infected case, the ventilator itself is not at risk of contamination | Reduced total volume of gas being compressed, which can be an advantage with very stiff lungs |

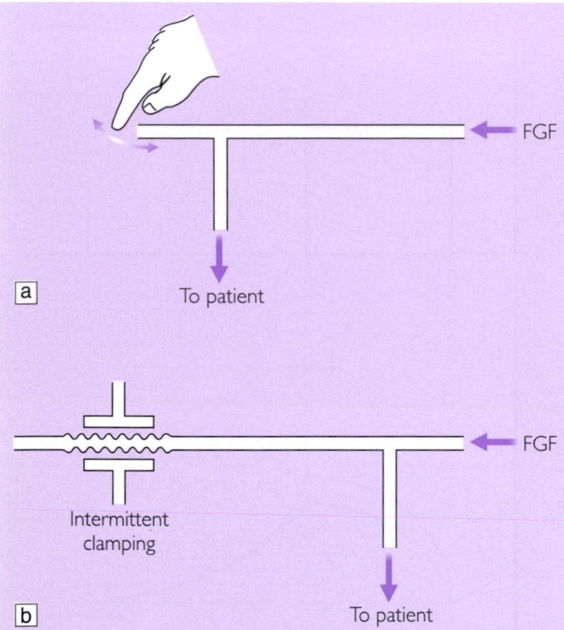


**Figure 11.2.** (a) The basic principle of a mechanical thumb. (b) In practice this is often provided by the compression of flexible tubing. FGF, fresh gas flow.

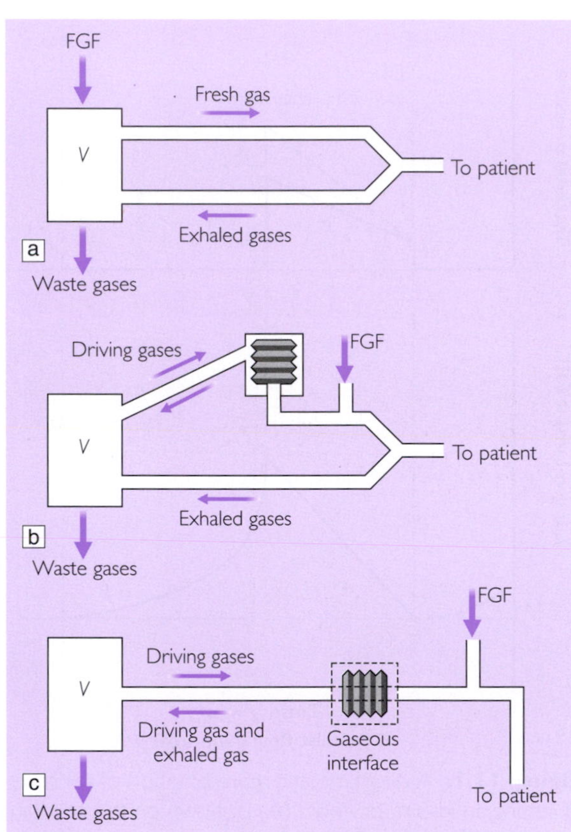


**Figure 11.3.** A diagrammatic representation of (a) a direct lung ventilator and (b) a 'bag in a bottle' ventilator. (c) A 'pseudo bag in a bottle' ventilator, where there is a gaseous interface of driving gas replacing the physical barrier between the driving gas and the inspired gas. V is a ventilator that can be pneumatically or electrically powered. It can be a minute volume divider or an intermittent tidal volume generator. When there is no physical barrier between the driving gas and inspiratory gas, as in (c), the tubing must be long enough and the flow characteristics appropriate to prevent driving gas contaminating the patient gas. FGF, fresh gas flow.

range of adjustments possible with an MV divider depends upon its complexity.

### Intermittent tidal volume generators

These tend to be more complex with a greater variability of settings. Many operating room ventilators and almost all intensive care unit (ICU) ventilators are of this type. The usual way of setting them is to fix the TV and breathing frequency, although several fix the MV and breathing frequency. Two typical operating-room ventilators of this type are shown in Figure 11.5. If the fresh gas supply to the ventilator is not sufficient to meet the delivered MV, entrainment of air occurs. With a suitable breathing system, these ventilators can also usually be set to recycle expired gas, allowing the patient to be hyperventilated while maintaining normocapnia, as described in Chapter 9.

A number of these machines have complex flow and pressure transducers in the inspiratory and expiratory limbs of the breathing system, which give a number of derived variables such as expired MV, peak inspiratory pressure, mean expiratory flow, etc. Photographs of the control panel of two such ventilators designed for ICU use are shown in Figure 11.6.

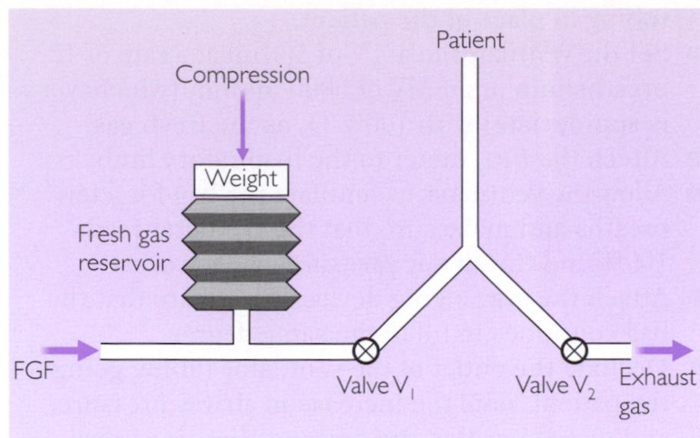


**Figure 11.4.** The principle of the minute volume divider. During expiration, valve $V_2$ is open and the patient expires to the atmosphere, valve $V_1$ is closed, and the fresh gas flow (FGF) enters the reservoir. During inspiration, valve $V_2$ closes, valve $V_1$ opens, and the reservoir bag empties fresh gas into the patient.

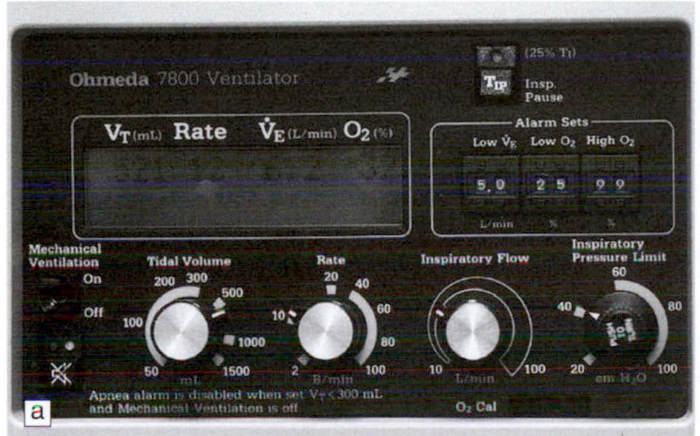


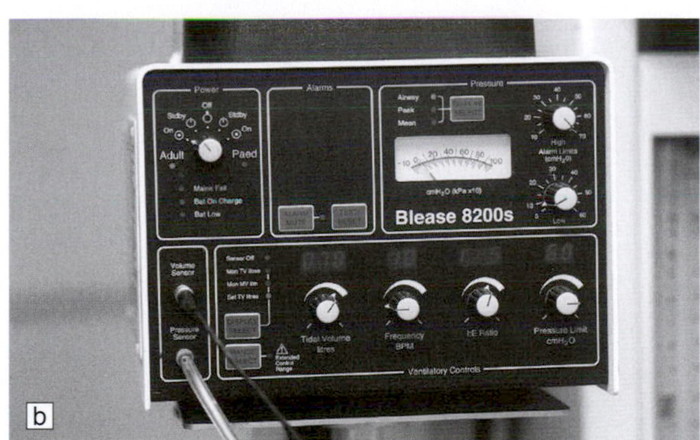


**Figure 11.5.** The control panels of two typical operating room ventilators: (a) the Ohmeda 7800 and (b) the Blease 8200s.

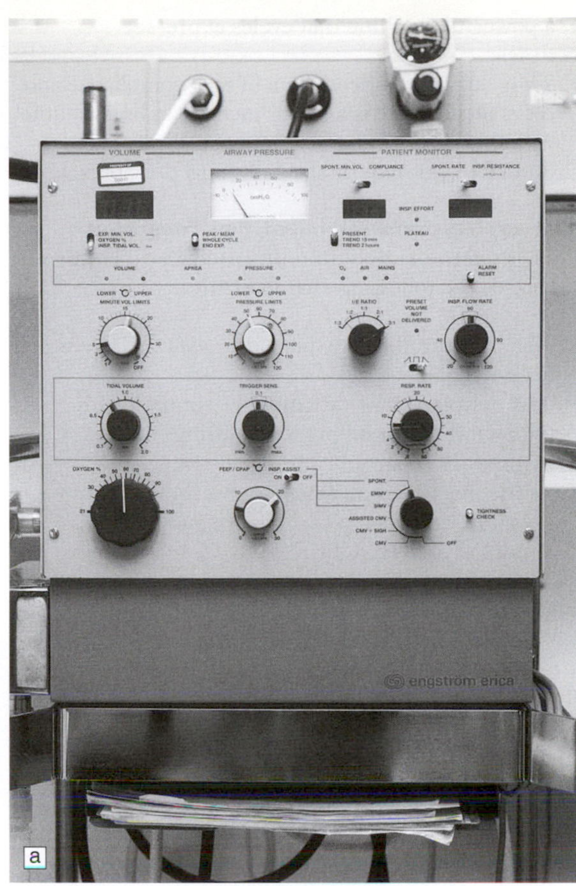


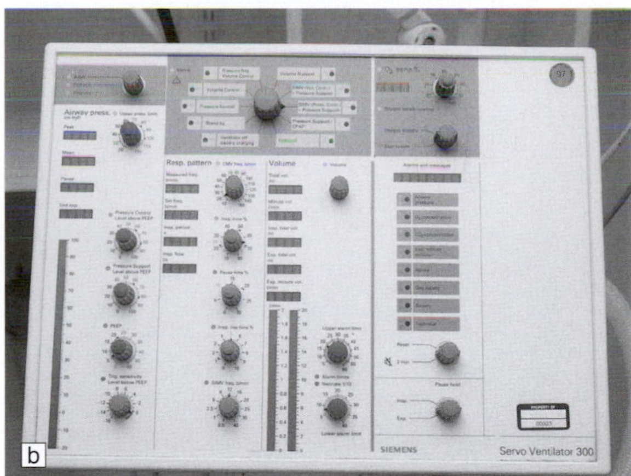


**Figure 11.6.** The control panels of two intensive care ventilators: (a) the Engstrom Erica and (b) the Siemens Servo 300. The latter has a remote screen not shown here which gives a continuous display of measured respiratory parameters.

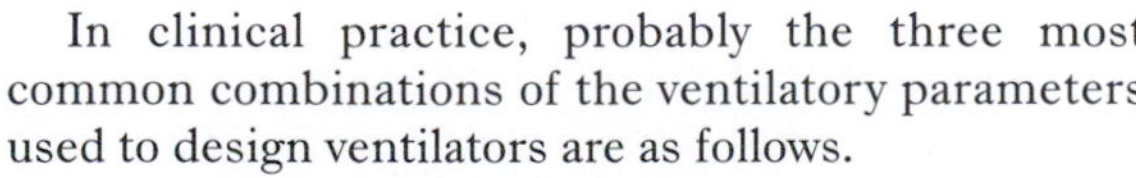

In clinical practice, probably the three most common combinations of the ventilatory parameters used to design ventilators are as follows.

***Time-cycled, pressure generator***

This generator possesses the following characteristics:

- usually powered by a weighted bellows; this produces an initially high inspiratory flow which reduces with time;
- the TV delivered to the patient depends on the ability of the bellows to empty fully (affected by compliance and resistance of lungs) and the volume of the ventilator tubing.

***Time-cycled, volume-set, flow generator***

This generator (commonly used on the ICU) possesses the following characteristics:

- a powerful machine that cycles at pre-set times;
- TV is delivered independent of lung compliance and resistance. There is a steady increase in lung volume with time throughout inspiration. Delivery is only limited by preset permitted maximal pressures.

***Time-cycled, pressure-limited, flow generator***
This generator (commonly used for children) possesses the following characteristics:

- The maximum airway pressure is set and the time for cycling is set.
- The delivered flow rate must be set high enough to reach the desired pressure during the set inspiratory time.
- As the machine ventilates to a preset maximum pressure, changes in compliance and resistance affect the delivered TV.

## SAFETY PROCEDURES

It has been repeatedly demonstrated that ventilator disconnections and problems with the airway constitute the major source of serious critical incidents. As a result of this, checking the ventilator and breathing system is mandatory before use. Checklists vary, but the following is the type of procedure to be followed for a ventilated adult system:

- Make sure that the electrical, high-pressure, and low-pressure gas attachments are secure.
- Put a 2-litre reservoir bag on to the ventilator tubing in place of the patient.
- Set the ventilator to a TV of 500 ml at a rate of 12 breaths/min or an MV of 6000 ml/min (whichever is appropriate) with 100% $O_2$ as the fresh gas.
- Attach the $F\text{IO}_2$ meter to the inspiratory limb.
- Allow the ventilator to ventilate the bag for a few breaths and make sure that the $O_2$ meter reads 100% and the airway pressure gauge works.
- Attach the scavenging device and ensure that the bag continues to fill to the same degree.
- Occlude the outlet of the ventilator tubing going to the patient, note the increase in airway pressure, and make sure that the pressure-limiting valve blows off at the correct setting.
- Switch the ventilator to manual mode and ensure that the bag acting as the patient s lungs can be ventilated easily.

## Further reading

Dorsch JA, Dorsch SE. *Understanding Anesthesia Equipment*, 3rd edn. Baltimore, MA: Williams & Wilkins, 1994: 719—63.

Mushin WW, Rendell-Baker L, Thompson PW, Mapleson WW. *Automatic Ventilation of the Lungs*, 3rd edn. Oxford: Blackwell Scientific Publications, 1980.

Spearman CB, Sanders HG. Physical principles and functional designs of ventilators. In: Kirby RR, Barnney MJ, Downs JB, eds. *Clinical Applications of Ventilatory Support.* New York: Churchill Livingstone, 1990: 63—104.

Sykes K. *Respiratory Support. Principles and Practice Series*. London: BMJ Publishing Group, 1995.

# Chapter 12 Monitoring and safety

P. Hutton

A profusion of electronic monitors is often equated with principles of safe practice but this is erroneous. Monitoring ensures continuous clinical and electronic surveillance of the patient so that adverse conditions can be detected early and corrected before they have done any harm. Safe practice is a wider concept that includes monitoring but which relates to the working environment, training, personnel and resources. Consequently, as well as monitoring, some other important aspects of safe practice are also discussed in this chapter. In addition, critical incidents and other unexpected events are covered in Chapter 13, electrical safety, diathermy and pacemakers in Chapters 38 and 39, and pollution and scavenging in Chapter 8.

## THE OBJECTIVES OF MONITORING

Philosophically, monitoring can be divided into two distinct modalities:

- It can inform that an unexpected or potentially damaging event has occurred irrespective of the procedure being undertaken (e.g. patient disconnected from ventilator, arrhythmias). The accepted professional guidelines for this have now come to be known as minimal monitoring standards .
- It can record anticipated deviations from normality that are secondary to the treatment administered (e.g. blood pressure [BP] fall after sodium nitroprusside), or to surgical trespass (e.g. bradycardia during neurological surgery). The monitors used in these circumstances in addition to those required for minimal monitoring depend on the combination of patient and procedure. The final selection is made on an individual basis by the anaesthetist.

It is clear from the above that current practice dictates a basic minimum standard of monitoring applicable to all patients, which is extended, based on the anaesthetist s professional opinion, by whatever else is in the patient s best interests. This involves an element of judgement and knowledge of the risk – benefit aspects of invasive procedures.

Minimal monitoring standards have been published in most countries, and an International Task Force has broadened their application to under-resourced locations. In many hospitals compliance with the set minimum monitoring standards is a condition of employment and is necessary to obtain professional liability insurance. It should be noted that, in all minimal monitoring guidelines published throughout the world, the most important monitor of all is the trained anaesthetist continuously observing his or her patient.

It is salutary to consider that, for any electronic monitor to be of value, it must detect and relay information faster than the damaging effects of the change that it is recording and present it in a form that is both obvious and interpretable to the anaesthetist. This concept is presented graphically in Figure 12.1. With this concept in mind, it is a useful exercise for the trainee to consider the value and cost-effectiveness of a simple disconnection monitor, an oxygen meter, a capnograph, and a pulse oximeter in detecting a failure of mechanical ventilation or $O_2$ supply in a young fit patient.

The main sources of data on the causes of death, major morbidity, and critical incidents come from voluntary reported surveys and analysis of medical insurance claims. The contribution of electronic monitoring *per se* to patient safety is difficult to assess and there has been only one large randomized study of pulse oximetry involving over 20 000 patients that has tried to assess it. The findings were undramatic and led the accompanying editorial (see Eichorn listed in Further reading) to comment that:

> There were definite positive effects on the process of anaesthesia care . . . but none really on the outcome of the process.

The truth of the matter is probably that the safety of modern anaesthesia is such that the scale of trials necessary to demonstrate significant differences in outcome would have to be so large as to be unmanageable.

One approach to improving patient care is to accept that similar themes continue to repeat themselves in mortality, morbidity, and critical incident studies and to try to minimize the risks that we know occur. As far

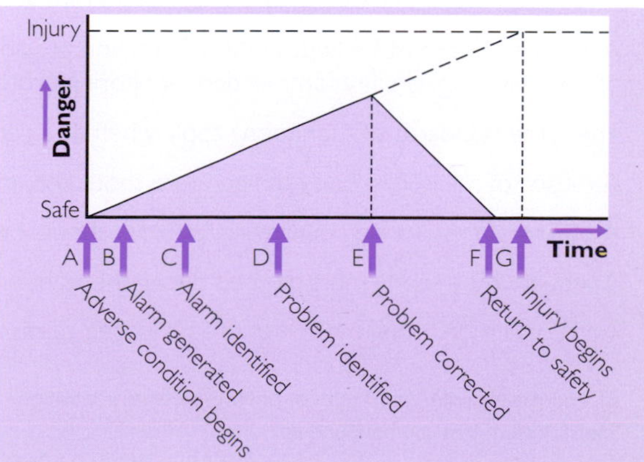


**Figure 12.1.** The anatomy of a critical incident. (Adapted from Schriber P and Schriber J. *Anaesthesia System Risk Analysis and Risk Reduction*. North American Drager, 1987.)

as intraoperative events are concerned, after an exhaustive survey of the available literature, Runciman (see Further reading) concluded the following:

- The hazards that pose most risk to the patient, the anaesthetist, and society at large have been identified. They are problems with hypoxic gas mixtures, gas flows, circuits, endotracheal (ET) tubes, the airway, and ventilation.
- These problems are very common and may constitute up to two-thirds of all potentially disastrous incidents during anaesthesia.
- Most of these problems can be avoided, or their consequences minimized, by following the guidelines and recommendations in minimal monitoring recommendations.

It must not, however, be forgotten that in some series over one-third of events occurred in the recovery period, the most common being respiratory obstruction.

Runciman summarized with a balanced view that:

> . . . safe anaesthesia does not require a mass of complex equipment; the greatest degree of safety for the available resources will be achieved by a careful, conscientious anaesthetist who balances risk, benefit and cost in the context in which he or she works.

Although there are small individual differences between countries and between states within countries, the principles established for minimal monitoring are similar the world over. A summary of the common themes is given in Table 12.1.

## ROUTINE CHECKING

Routine checking of the patient, environment, assisting personnel, and equipment is one of the cornerstones of safe anaesthesia practice. Some of these checks are described in other chapters of the book where they relate closely to the subject matter. Checking the correct functioning of anaesthesia apparatus before use is a mandatory procedure. There is no

| Table 12.1. Important recurring themes in minimal monitoring standards |
|---|
| The most important component of monitoring is the trained clinician, who should be present throughout, using their eyes and ears continuously. |
| Careful preoperative assessment of the patient and a knowledge of the planned procedure are required to determine the optimum method of monitoring the patient. |
| All equipment must be checked before use and alarm limits set appropriately. |
| Both the patient and the anaesthetic equipment must be monitored. |
| Monitoring must begin before induction and continue until the patient has recovered from the effects of anaesthesia. |
| Adequate oxygenation of the patient should be ensured by monitoring:<br>• the concentration of oxygen in the delivered gas mixture<br>• the patient's oxygen saturation clinically and preferably by pulse oximetry. |
| Adequate ventilation of the patient should be ensured by:<br>• clinical observation of the patient, breathing system and/or ventilator<br>• use of a capnograph to confirm placement of an ET tube and to monitor ventilation during IPPV<br>• the use of a disconnection detection device during IPPV. |
| The adequacy of the patient's circulation should be ensured by:<br>• continuous clinical observation augmented by a peripheral pulse meter<br>• continuous display of the electrocardiogram<br>• determination of blood pressure and heart rate at least at 5-minute intervals. |
| A good record must be kept of the information provided by the monitoring devices and a clear statement of the reasons given if recommended monitoring protocols were not complied with. |
| The same standards of monitoring apply whether a general, local or sedative technique is being carried out. |
| A means of measuring body temperature should be immediately available. |
| A means of monitoring neuromuscular block should be readily available. |
| Adequate monitoring must be used during the transfer of patients both within and between hospitals. |
| Additional monitoring may be used as is judged necessary by the anaesthetist. |

ET, endotracheal; IPPV, intermittent positive-pressure ventilation.
Specific references can be found in:
American Society of Anesthesiologists (ASA) Standards for Basic Anesthetic Monitoring. ASA, Park Ridge, Illinois, 60 069–3189
Recommendations for Standards of Monitoring during Anaesthesia and Recovery, 3rd edition (Dec. 2000). Association of Anaesthetists of Great Britain and Ireland, London UK.
International Standards for a Safe Practice of Anaesthesia. *Eur J Anaesthesiol*, 1993, 10 (Suppl 7).

excuse not to do it. Although there are many ways of undertaking these checks, some of which will have been developed because of local factors, the guidelines published by the AAGBI represent sound common sense, and are reproduced in Table 12.2. Some modern anaesthesia machines cannot be checked using generic guidelines as given in Table 12.2. On these occasions, the check will need to be machine specific and the manufacturer's instructions should be followed. Whatever these instructions, before using the machine on a patient, the anaesthetist must ensure that it will deliver a pressurized supply of 100% $O_2$, that there is a reserve $O_2$ cylinder and that a simple manual breathing system is available in case of failure.

## THE ANAESTHETIC CHART

A good record of the preoperative assessment, anaesthetic technique, and postoperative instructions is necessary for a variety of reasons, but most of all because it improves patient care. A well-kept record enables the anaesthetist to observe trends as they occur, and hence to make an early correction if they are adverse. It is also easier to transfer responsibility to another anaesthetist when progress has been well documented, and this is especially so if a second anaesthetist is called to help when difficulties arise with the patient. In a perfect world, the same anaesthetist would see patients preoperatively, anaesthetize them, and look after them postoperatively, but, in practice, this ideal is not always attained. Evidence that a proper preoperative visit has been done, together with its findings, is best recorded specifically on the anaesthetic chart so it can be quickly scanned and interpreted if a different anaesthetist is to administer the anaesthetic. The same is equally true of instructions to recovery and ward staff at the end of surgery. Careful documentation at all stages can be of inestimable value in patient safety to those responsible for providing subsequent anaesthesia at a later date.

The record also allows several types of audit and data collection to be processed more accurately. It allows the departmental production of summary activity information, the ability to ensure that trainees are getting exposure to the right variety of cases and techniques, a database for retrospective research, and the documentation to invoice 'users' of anaesthetic services. Finally, in most countries of the world, it is an essential medicolegal document for internal and judicial enquiries and civil litigation. A full and accurate contemporaneous record can make the difference between the defensible and indefensible when professional negligence is alleged. In the future, the quality of anaesthetic records is likely to play a much more significant role in a hospital's risk-management strategy.

It is worthwhile, for a moment, considering the 'contemporaneous' nature of the intraoperative part of the record. It is the opinion of the author that, in general, although the anaesthetist will be almost continuously scanning key monitors (e.g. ECG, pulse oximeter), it is not usually possible to record data more frequently than approximately every 5 minutes. This limitation is created by the need for the clinical administration of anaesthesia (e.g. observing the effects of induction agents) and other patient-related tasks (e.g. checking blood, drawing up drugs, etc.). The difficulty is partly overcome in some instances by the use of monitoring equipment connected to a printer or a monitoring system with a memory. On these occasions, the data can either be inserted on the chart later or the printout can be attached to the anaesthetic record. It is vital when attaching such a record to make sure that the data it contains are correct and edited appropriately. If it is not, artefactual values will later become the 'true' record of events.

There is therefore an obvious conflict between a 'true' contemporaneous record and the situation when events are changing very rapidly. This is particularly so in a cardiac arrest, when life-saving resuscitation is needed, or when an anaesthetist is called to a crisis that has already occurred. Under these conditions, it is the author's practice to give the whole of his attention to attending to the patient and not to prejudice the outcome by spending time on a perfect record. A solution to this conflict, which works successfully on most occasions, is to identify a person in the group of people that inevitably gathers around a crisis and to get one of them to write down on a separate piece of paper key aspects of management that you tell them to, timed by them on the ward or operating room clock. The data can subsequently be transferred to the proper recording chart and the 'contemporaneous' record stapled to it. If events are changing very rapidly in a patient who is already fully monitored (e.g. unsuccessful attempts to come off cardiac bypass), again it would be my advice to attend primarily to the patient's needs. Someone else can be given the task of temporarily recording data or, if the monitors possess the feature, subsequent display of the stored data as continuously monitored trends can be used to reconstruct the chart. An example of the type of data to be dictated by the anaesthetist and recorded by another person at a cardiac arrest in recovery is given in Figure 12.2. During such a crisis, any ampoules or pre-filled syringes used should not be thrown away immediately into the usual sharps bin, but put safely on one side for later listing and confirmation of usage.

Over the years, ever since Codman and Cushing published on the subject in 1903, there has been a steady contribution to the literature on the design and content of anaesthetic records. It is obvious that what is adequate for the recording of a short manipulation in a fit young person is insufficient for a major neurosurgical procedure. Consequently, there is never likely to be a universal recording sheet devised; indeed it is probably counterproductive to try and produce one. What, however, is possible, and on which there is increasing professional agreement, is to define a minimum data set that should be collected on all patients, for their own and the anaesthetist's benefit. The layout of how this is printed can then be left to individual hospitals to decide. Suggestions about the reasonable content for an anaesthetic record set are given in Figure 12.3. This particular set was developed by the Society for Computing and Technology in Anaesthesia, the AAGBI, and the Royal College of Anaesthetists.

Although most of the record set is self-evident, a few aspects deserve comment. The 'urgency rating' of patients has been described in a number of ways by national audits and anaesthesia societies. The three

**Table 12.2. Checklist for anaesthesia apparatus**

**The following checks should be made before each operating session:**

**1. Check that the anaesthesia machine is connected to the electricity supply (if appropriate) and switched on.**

- Take note of any information or labelling on the anaesthesia machine referring to the current status of the machine. Particular attention should be paid to recent servicing. Servicing labels should be fixed in the service logbook.

**2. Check that an oxygen analyser is present on the anaesthesia machine.**

- Ensure that the analyser is switched on, checked, and calibrated.
- The oxygen sensor should be placed where it can monitor the composition of the gases leaving the common gas outlet.

**3. Identify and take note of the gases that are being supplied by pipeline, confirming with a 'tug-test' that each pipeline is correctly inserted into the appropriate gas supply terminal.**

Note: $CO_2$ cylinders should not be present on the anaesthesia machine unless requested by the anaesthetist. A blanking plug should be fitted to any empty cylinder yoke.

- Check that the anaesthesia machine is connected to a supply of $O_2$ and that an adequate supply of $O_2$ is available from the reserve $O_2$ cylinder.
- Check that adequate supplies of other gases (nitrous oxide, air) are available and connected as appropriate.
- Check that all pipeline pressure gauges in use on the anaesthesia machine indicate 400 kPa.

**4. Check the operation of flowmeters.**

- Ensure that each flow control valve operates smoothly and that the bobbin moves freely throughout its range.
- Check the operation of the emergency $O_2$ bypass control.

**5. Check the vaporizer(s).**

- Ensure that each vaporizer is adequately but not over-filled.
- Ensure that each vaporizer is correctly seated on the back bar and not tilted.

Check the vaporizer for leaks (with vaporizer on and off) by temporarily occluding the common gas outlet.
When checks have been completed, turn the vaporizer(s) off.
A leak test should be performed immediately after changing any vaporizer.

**6. Check the breathing system to be employed.**

- The system should be visually inspected for correct configuration. All connections should be secured by 'push and twist'.
- A pressure leak test should be performed on the breathing system by occluding the patient port and compressing the reservoir bag.
- The correct operation of unidirectional valves should be carefully checked.

**7. Check that the ventilator is configured appropriately for its intended use.**

- Ensure that the ventilator tubing is correctly configured and securely attached.
- Set the controls for use and ensure that an adequate pressure is generated during the inspiratory phase.
- Check that the pressure relief valve functions.
- Check that the disconnect alarm functions correctly.
- Ensure that an alternative means to ventilate the patient's lungs is available.

**8. Check that the anaesthetic gas scavenging system is switched on and is functioning correctly.**

- Ensure that the tubing is attached to the appropriate expiratory port(s) of the breathing system or ventilator.

**9. Check that all ancillary equipment that may be needed is present and working.**

- This includes laryngoscopes, intubation aids, intubation forceps, bougies, etc. and appropriately sized facemasks, airways, tracheal tubes, and connectors.
- Check that the suction apparatus is functioning and that all connections are secure.
- Check that the patient can be tilted head-down on the trolley, operating table, or bed.

**10. Ensure that the appropriate monitoring equipment is present, switched on, and calibrated ready for use.**

- Set all default alarm limits as appropriate.
  (It may be necessary to place the monitors in the stand-by mode to avoid unnecessary alarms before being connected to the patient.)

Published by the Association of Anaesthetists of Great Britain and Ireland (1997), and reproduced with permission.

NAME A. N. OTHER

REGISTRATION NUMBER 123456Y

IN PATIENT History Sheet — RECOVERY

| DATE 14/6/96 | CLINICAL NOTES |
|---|---|
| Time | |
| 16.02 | Called to find patient cyanosed and in VF. Immediate 100% $O_2$ ventilation by facemask. Precordial thump + external massage |
| 16.03 | Defib 200 J. Converted to VT, continue CPR |
| 16.04 | Defib 200 J |
| 16.05 | Sinus bradycardia, spontaneous respiration, palpable femoral pulse. |
| 16.06 | Atropine 0.6 mg |
| 16.08 | Atropine 0.6 mg |
| 16.10 | Patient conscious, BP = 100/50, R = 88 |
| 16.12 | Responds to command, moves all limbs. BP = 110/70, R = 90, Sat$O_2$ = 95% |
| 16.15 | Care transferred to Dr G. M. Cooper (Consultant) |
| | [signature] (SpR 1) |
| | RECORD WRITTEN BY S. BAKER (Student Nurse) |

W20 247

**Figure 12.2.** The record of a cardiac arrest that occurred in recovery. This is an example of the type of data that should be dictated by the anaesthetist resuscitating a patient and recorded by another person at the scene.

categories given in Figure 12.3 represent a simple, user-friendly classification, which carries most of the information necessary for anaesthetic audit, management, and outcome. Some hospitals will use different classifications with more sub-categories. Another key feature of the record is to note the intraoperative position of the patient and any precautions that were taken against injury.

The question of consent for general anaesthesia and regional blocks continues to promote controversy. Everyday practice on this matter differs from country to country, but there are common themes that run through everybody s clinical practice:

- When a patient presents him- or herself for surgical care, it can be assumed that he or she is expecting some sort of anaesthetic and pain relief to be part of the treatment.
- The surgeon is usually allowed to take consent for the patient to submit him- or herself to anaesthesia in principle, at the same time as consent is obtained for the surgical procedure.
- The anaesthetist responsible for the patient must ensure that he or she or another doctor has explained exactly what will happen to the patient when anaesthetized, in a form that is appropriate for the patient s intellectual ability.
- If a local block is to be performed, the anaesthetist must have explained to the patient what this involves and obtained agreement to the procedure.

It is important that the anaesthetic chart is designed to reflect local custom while ensuring that the fact that the patient was adequately informed is recorded.

Finally, any untoward events, complications, etc. need to be specifically recorded, and any that may be repeated in the future, e.g. allergies, difficult intubation, need to be identified by a hazard flag of some sort for future anaesthetists.

## THE CONTRIBUTION OF INDIVIDUAL MONITORS

### The anaesthetist's basic senses

In this technological age, it is easy to forget that every publication there has been on recommendations for minimal monitoring during anaesthesia has emphasized the pivotal role of the trained medical observer, close to and constantly caring for the patient s welfare. It is therefore relevant to review what can be gained from the basic human senses themselves, apart from their role in relaying electronically derived information to the anaesthetist s brain.

#### *Touch*

Touch is a relatively coarse sense which in some instances provides only soft information. Detection of body temperature changes is only possible with large changes and the temperature felt by the hand depends on the hand s existing temperature. Touch will, however, identify the presence of sweating (perhaps indicating light anaesthesia), and the blanching reflex gives a guide to peripheral perfusion. Palpation of the pulse is good for information on rate and rhythm, and when it is weak and thready indicates significant hypotension. Patients who are hypertensive do, however, have a pulse that feels essentially normal.

#### *Hearing*

Hearing allows the almost subconscious monitoring of cyclical events, such as the lift of the expiratory valve, the regularity of the ventilator, and the pattern of breathing. It is probably of greatest discriminatory value when used in the interpretation of sounds from the stethoscope (see below).

#### *Sight*

Sight is a valuable sense that allows both appropriate physiological movements (e.g. the beating of blood vessels, movement of the chest, estimation of tidal volume, etc.) and inappropriate movements (movement of limbs, grimacing, tearing) in the anaesthetized patient to be seen.

Visual estimation of the adequacy of tidal volumes from observations of the reservoir bag, and chest and abdominal movements, is commonly used in clinical practice, particularly at the end of anaesthesia before the patient is extubated. Although easy to do, and quite satisfactory in most patients, its accuracy is highly

**Preoperative information**

*Patient identity*
- Name/identity Number/Gender

*Assessment and risk factors*
- Date of assessment
- Assessor and where assessed
- Weight (kg), [height (m) optional]
- Basic vital signs (BP and heart rate)
- Medication, including contraceptive drugs
- Allergies
- Addiction (tobacco, alcohol, drugs)
- Previous general anaesthetics
- Family history
- Potential airway problems
- Prostheses, teeth, crowns
- Investigations
- Cardiorespiratory fitness
- Other problems
- ASA status ± comment

*Urgency*
- *Scheduled* – listed on a routine list
- *Urgent* – resuscitated, not on routine list
- *Emergency* – not fully resuscitated

**Peroperative information**

*Checks*
- Nil by mouth
- Consent to operation
- Premedication, type, and effect

*Place and time*
- Place
- Date of operation
- Time started and finished

*Personnel*
- All anaesthetists' names
- Qualified assistant present
- Operating surgeon
- Duty consultant informed

*Operation planned/performed*

*Apparatus*
- Checks performed, anaesthetic room, and operating room

*Vital signs recording/charting*
- Monitoring used and vital signs (specify)

*Drugs and fluids*
- Doses, concentrations, and volume
- Cannulation
- Injection site(s), time, and route
- Warmer used
- Blood loss, urine output

*Airway and breathing system*
- Route, system used
- Ventilation: type and mode
- Airway type, size, cuff and shape
- Special procedures, humidifier, filter
- Throat pack
- Difficulty

*Regional anaesthesia*
- Consent
- Block performed
- Entry site
- Needle used, aids to location
- Catheter: yes/no

*Patient position and attachments*
- Thrombosis prophylaxis
- Temperature control
- Limb positions

**Postoperative instructions**
- Drugs, fluids, and doses
- Analgesic techniques
- Special airway instructions
- Oxygen therapy
- Monitoring

**Untoward events**
- Abnormalities
- Critical incidents
- Pre-, per- or postoperative
- Context, cause and effect

**Hazard flags**
- Warnings for future care

**Figure 12.3.** A suggested reasonable content for an anaesthetic record set. (Reproduced, with permission, from the Royal College of Anaesthetists, 1996.)

suspect and depends on many variables such as patient shape and size, the relative contributions of chest and abdomen, and to some extent on observer experience.

Most of all, however, sight allows the detection of cyanosis. This is best looked for in the mucous membranes and within the surgical field. Although there is no question that the detection of cyanosis is fundamental to patient safety and its (even suspected) presence must be taken seriously, it is, however, not without problems of interpretation. For cyanosis to occur, a necessary minimum quantity of reduced haemoglobin has to be present. In patients with anaemia, this occurs only at much more serious levels of desaturation than in those who are polycythaemic. The actual colour of blood as seen is dependent on the spectral intensities of the incident light. If there is a fair amount of red in the incident light (e.g. tungsten filament operating lights), then oxygenated blood looks 'red' and desaturated blood looks significantly more purple; if there is a high concentration of blue wavelengths (e.g. as in some operating lights that mimic the spectral intensity of sunlight), this differentiation is reduced. Perhaps most important of all, however, is the individual variation between observers. Fifty years ago, Comroe studied this problem by making volunteers hypoxic and recording when trained observers thought that they had become cyanosed. These experiments are described in more detail in Chapter 39 (Table 39.3), where it can be seen that there is an enormous individual variation in the detection of cyanosis. The overall conclusion must be that cyanosis, although a very important sign, may not be detected until hypoxaemia is severe. Consequently, if suspected, it must be assumed to be present and everything must be checked until the fault has been recognized and rectified or the anaesthetist is confident (e.g. by use of pulse oximeter, blood gases) that the patient is adequately oxygenated.

### The stethoscope

The stethoscope is the simplest, cheapest, and most valuable addition with which to augment the basic senses in respiratory and circulatory monitoring. Although its use is not universal, and very dependent on local practice, it is difficult to find any single good reason for it not to be used routinely. In either the oesophageal or precordial positions, it gives beat-to-beat information on heart rate, lung sounds, and tidal volumes, and can also give information on arrhythmias, ventilator disconnections or malfunction, wheezing, and quality of heart sounds and murmurs. When monitoring clinically for changes in tidal volume, greater accuracy can be achieved when listening to the breath sounds with a stethoscope than from observation alone. Complications from stethography are rare, but they can affect monitoring during magnetic resonance imaging (precordial), and have been lost into the stomach and known to be ignited by lasers, diathermy, and cautery (oesophageal).

### The ECG

As the heart is a three-dimensional organ, it follows that it is necessary to observe it simultaneously from several locations and directions to be certain of detecting regional abnormalities in cellular function and conduction. This is usually achieved by the standard twelve-lead system, augmented on rare occasions by dorsal and oesophageal electrodes. For intraoperative monitoring, practicability requires that there is a minimum of electrodes and that the surgical field is clear. A compromise is therefore necessary between information obtained and convenience of use.

To be aware of those particularly at risk requires a careful preoperative assessment. A reasonable selection of patients in whom a preoperative ECG should be insisted upon in general anaesthesia practice is given in Table 12.3.

Patients undergoing peripheral arterial surgery are at a high risk of perioperative ischaemic events and infarction because more than half have associated coronary artery disease (which may be asymptomatic). They probably represent the highest-risk cardiac group presenting in non-specialist anaesthetic practice.

Reasons for continuous monitoring of the ECG during anaesthesia and recovery are given in Table 12.4.

The obvious question to ask, as a compromise is necessary, is where should the electrodes be placed for intraoperative monitoring? There are three- and five-electrode systems in common use. Five-electrode systems, although increasingly used in routine practice, still tend to be reserved for cardiac patients and those undergoing major specialist surgery. Such a system allows three of the electrodes to act as limb leads. Traditionally, these are placed on the right arm, left arm, and left leg, and enable leads I, II, and III to be displayed. For convenience, they are often shifted to behind the shoulders and on to the left hip. The fourth electrode can be placed over the V5 or V6 position or as close to this as is practicable. The fifth electrode acts as a ground electrode and can be placed wherever is convenient. Although it is usually possible with these systems to select the leads displayed, the best combination for continuous monitoring is probably a simultaneous display of lead II and V5 (see below for explanation).

Three-electrode systems, which are the most common in everyday practice, are able to display a single lead only, the third electrode being used as the electrical ground to offset overall swings in body electrical potential. The two commonest abnormalities that need to be detected are arrhythmias and left ventricular ischaemia. With the option of displaying only one lead, both cannot be optimized simultaneously. Lead II (left leg to right arm) lies close to the normal cardiac axis, permitting the best discrimination of the P and R waves, and therefore is the most useful lead in the diagnosis of arrhythmias. On the other hand, left ventricular ischaemia is most commonly best seen in V5 on a twelve-lead ECG and lead II gives less than 30% detection of ST segment changes. A good compromise for general purpose use is to use the CM5 lead configuration (chest lead from the manubrium to the V5 position; Figure 12.4). This combines good discrimination of arrhythmias with the ability to detect 80% of left ventricular ischaemic episodes.

Finally there are three important points to be made which should not be forgotten:

| **Table 12.3. Indications for routine preoperative twelve-lead ECG** |
|---|
| Clinical evidence of cardiac disease |
| Hypertension |
| Diabetes mellitus |
| Renal disease or replacement therapy |
| Pacemaker |
| Major and peripheral arterial surgery |
| Age over 60 years |

| **Table 12.4. Reasons for continuous monitoring of the ECG** |
|---|
| Monitoring the heart rate |
| Diagnosis of cardiac arrest |
| Detection of arrhythmia |
| Detection of myocardial ischaemia |
| Detection of hyperkalaemia, hypocalcaemia, and other electrolyte abnormalities |
| Detection of arrhythmias associated with central venous catheters |
| Evaluation of pacemaker function |
| Monitoring myocardial protection during cardioplegic or fibrillatory arrest |

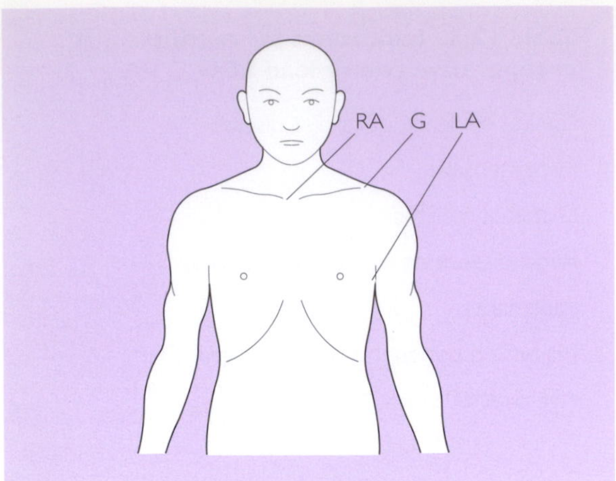


**Figure 12.4.** CM5 lead configuration: the ECG single chest lead system records from the manubrium to the V5 position (CM5 lead). RA, right arm electrode; LA, left arm electrode; G, ground or 'neutral' electrode.

1. The presence of an ECG trace is not evidence of cardiac output or satisfactory contractility.
2. ECG changes intraoperatively can be caused by hypoxia, hypercapnia, or a disconnection, i.e. not cardiac disease itself.
3. Whenever new serious or persisting abnormalities are detected during continuous monitoring, a twelve-lead ECG should be done postoperatively and the patient given the appropriate care.

Further details of ECG abnormalities are given in Chapter 47.

## Non-invasive blood pressure measurement

There are several methods of measuring BP indirectly. They all depend on the compression of an arterial vessel or vascular bed by a pressure cuff, and the subsequent detection distal to or beneath the cuff of blood flow, pressure pulses, or vessel wall movement as the cuff is deflated. The recordings produced are very dependent on the properties of the cuff, which are described separately later. The methods in common use are:

- palpatory;
- auscultatory;
- oscillometric.

### *Palpatory method*

The palpatory method consists of inflating the cuff (usually placed on the upper arm) to above the pressure at which the peripheral pulse (usually the radial) disappears, deflating the cuff, and recording the BP as equal to the cuff pressure at which the peripheral pulse returns. This method records only the systolic BP, and the results are highly operator dependent and usually significantly below the true reading. The accuracy is also strongly affected by the heart rate and the speed of cuff deflation, bradycardia and rapid deflation being the combination with the greatest potential for underestimation of the true figure. However, because of its simplicity, the method is very reliable. It is well suited to measuring gross changes from normality and for judging the response to fluid replacement when other equipment is unavailable or cannot be used (e.g. immediate care of casualties).

### *Auscultatory method*

This is the standard method used in both hospital and general practice for the detection and management of hypertension. There is a substantial literature on its technique and accuracy. The five-phase description of the Korotkoff sounds, introduced by Goodman and Howell in 1911, has now become standard.

*Phase I* – The first appearance of clear tapping sounds which gradually increase in intensity.

*Phase II* – The softening of the sounds which may become swishing .

*Phase III* – The disappearance of swishing and murmurs and the return of sharper thumping sounds.

*Phase IV* – The distinct abrupt muffling of sounds which become soft and blowing.

*Phase V* – The point at which all sounds disappear completely.

These phases are represented graphically in Figure 12.5. The auscultatory gap that can occur during phase II requires a rough estimate of the systolic point to be made by palpation before determining it accurately by auscultation.

Phase I represents the systolic pressure and phases IV and V are related to diastolic pressure. There is considerable debate about the latter. A sensible approach would seem to be the following:

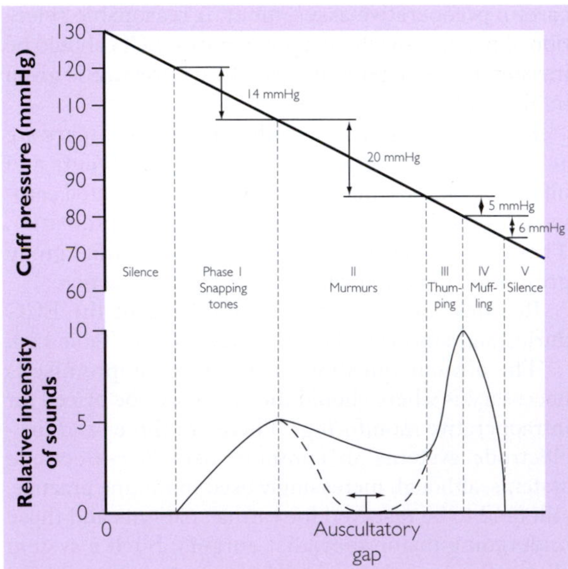


**Figure 12.5.** Characteristics of the auscultatory method of measuring blood pressure. The five phases of the Korotkoff sounds with their approximate times of appearance and disappearance are shown for a typical patient. (Adapted from Geddes LA. *Handbook of Blood Pressure Measurement.* Clifton, New Jersey: Humana Press, 1991; 68.)

- If a patient has a well-defined phase V end-point, record this as diastolic pressure.
- If the patient (with a normal systolic pressure) has a non-existent or absurdly low phase V (this is common in exercise, pregnancy, and other high-output states), record phase IV as the diastolic pressure.

There are several sources of error in the auscultatory method, such as observer variation, individual preference for readings ending in certain digits, and the need to deflate the cuff at 2–3 mmHg per heart beat. Even so, typically, the regression relationships comparing indirect with direct measurements are similar to those for the oscillometric technique (see below).

There have been several automated recorders marketed using the Korotkoff sounds as end-points, but these have been few in number compared with oscillometric machines. One problem with these is that if the microphone is incorporated into the cuff, in order for it to be placed over the brachial artery, the lower edge of the cuff may be in danger of compressing the ulnar nerve (see later).

### *Oscillometric methods*

Oscillometric methods use a single cuff, and the pressure oscillations within this cuff are used to measure the BP as the cuff pressure is reduced. Oscillometric recordings are now almost entirely automated, with an internal algorithm analysing the orderly sequence of changes in transmitted pressure oscillations as the cuff pressure is reduced. Initially, the cuff is pressurized to approximately 160 mmHg (and then subsequently to 30 mmHg above the previous systolic pressure), and the microprocessor lets it down in steps. At each step, the cuff pressure and the oscillations in it resulting from the arterial pulse are sensed and stored electronically. An ideal deflation sequence is shown in Figure 12.6. Systolic and diastolic pressures are estimated where the amplitude of oscillations rapidly increases and decreases, respectively. The mean arterial pressure is usually taken to be the lowest cuff pressure at which the oscillatory pressure component has its greatest amplitude. Typical results comparing oscillometric readings in adults with those from a direct arterial line for systolic pressure are given in Figure 12.7.

It can be concluded from a large number of studies such as this that automated oscillometric devices are very suitable for everyday use during a routine anaesthetic list, and that they produce reliable trend data. The popularity of these machines attests to their convenience, reliability, and robust nature. The limitations of the algorithms and the time it takes for a measurement cycle to be complete do, however, impose some limitations on their use. Unexpected changes in BP need rapid checking, arrhythmias may render the algorithm incapable of interpreting the pressure oscillations, and if the connecting tubes

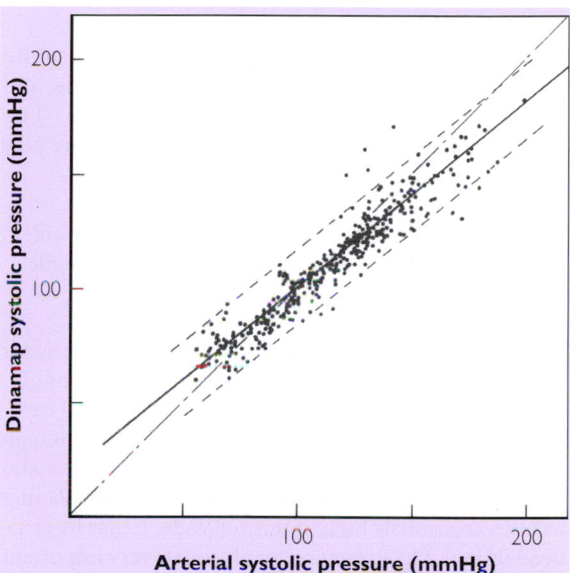


**Figure 12.7.** A comparison of oscillometric recordings from the Dinamap with direct blood pressure recordings for systolic pressure. The dashed lines on either side of the regression line are the 95% confidence limits. (Adapted from Hutton P *et al. Anaesthesia* 1984;39:261–7.)

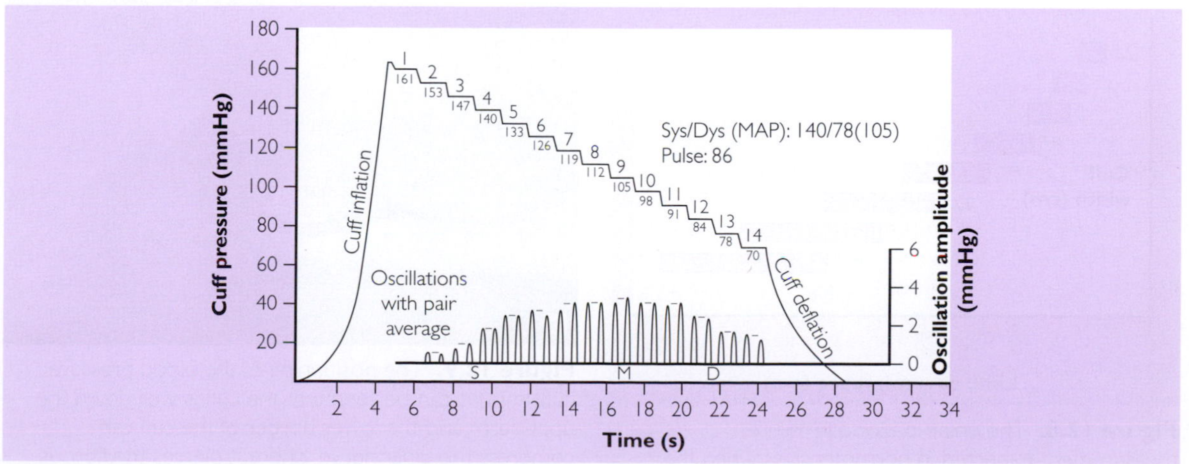


**Figure 12.6.** An ideal deflation sequence of an oscillometric blood pressure determination. (Adapted from Ramsay M. *J Clin Monit* 1991;7:56–67.) The cuff pressure deflation stop numbers are shown above the line, and the cuff pressure (in mmHg) values below the line. S, systolic; D, diastolic; M, mean.

become kinked it will neither inflate the cuff nor allow an inflated cuff to deflate. Oscillometric systems are probably not to be recommended for use in situations where:

- the BP can be expected to change rapidly;
- where the BP has to be maintained at a level with a reduced margin of safety (deliberate hypotension);
- in the presence of very rapidly acting cardiovascular drugs.

Although improvements in cycling capability and artefact rejection are continuously being introduced, it should not be forgotten that algorithms depend on the correct combination of cuff and machine, and that these may not be interchangeable.

### *Cuff-related factors*

The cuff size is a major determinant of the absolute readings obtained with all non-invasive methods, and there is a large literature on its importance. The conclusions of the American Heart Association are now accepted widely and these state:

> The width of the inflatable bladder should be 40% of the mid-circumference of the limb and the length should be twice this width.

This recommendation was determined primarily for use in detecting hypertensive patients in the population. Using a cuff of these dimensions will, with careful use, give accurate results in a normotensive person and detect the presence of clinically relevant hyper- and hypotension. If the cuff is too narrow, the BP reading will be erroneously high; if it is too wide, it may be erroneously low. These factors are obviously very important in children and obese people. The order of magnitude of errors induced by the use of the wrong size cuff is shown in Figure 12.8.

It is unreasonable to expect the indirect cuff readings to maintain equality with direct readings over a wide pressure range, because of the highly non-linear relationship between the pressure in an inflatable cuff and its internal diameter, which is in turn responsible for compressing the enclosed limb. Consequently, almost all the published comparisons of direct and indirect pressures that span a wide pressure range have had regression lines with a gradient that differs from unity. The usual trend is that, at high BP values the indirect readings underestimate the direct arterial pressure, and at low BP they overestimate it (see Figure 12.7).

There is also some morbidity related to the use of cuffs. They have been responsible for skin avulsion, petechiae (including when bleeding disorders are not present), and if left inflated for too long they produce all the complications of an arterial tourniquet. Perhaps the most serious potential common complication is ulnar nerve palsy, caused by the cuff compressing the ulnar nerve as it emerges from the intramuscular septum to go round the lowest part of the humerus. Cases of nerve damage have been reported and the counsel of perfection is to inflate the cuff with the patient fully awake to ensure that paraesthesia does not occur. It must therefore be recommended that, when the cuff is put on the upper arm, it is applied with the lower border well above the elbow joint, as shown in Figure 12.9.



**Figure 12.8.** The error in blood pressure measurement expected in normotensives when the cuff width deviates from a value that is 40% of the arm circumference. (Adapted from Geddes LA, Whistler SJ. *Am Heart J* 1978;96:4–8.)

## Direct blood pressure measurement

Direct BP recording is now a commonplace procedure with a low overall morbidity. For measurements to be

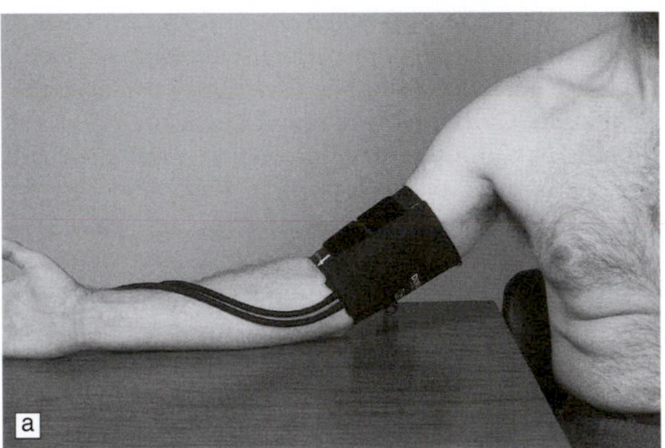


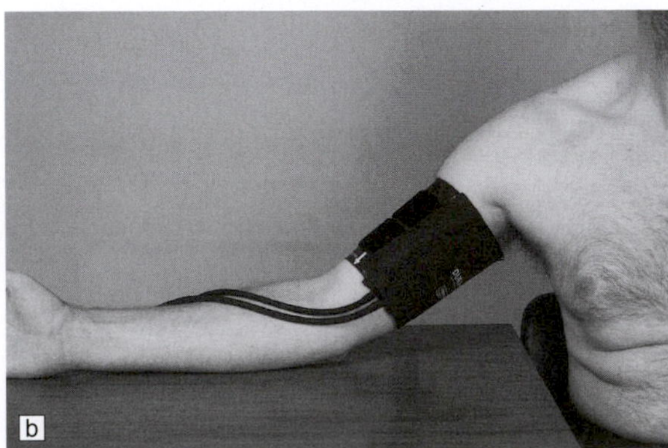


**Figure 12.9.** The positioning of the blood pressure cuff. In (a) it can be seen that the cuff is well down the upper arm and the lower border of the cuff can compress the ulnar nerve where it pierces the fibrous septum just above the elbow. In (b) the cuff is further up the arm and away from where it can damage the ulnar nerve.

made accurately, the overall catheter–transducer–amplifier system must have a proper frequency response and recording system, as described in Chapters 37 and 39. The indications for its use are:

- in those patients for whom accurate pressure information on a beat-by-beat basis is useful;
- patients in whom frequent blood gas analysis is likely to be required.

This allows change to be detected rapidly and the effects of treatment observed. Also, the effect of cardiac arrhythmias (e.g. junctional beats, atrial fibrillation) on haemodynamics can be observed directly and their detrimental effects assessed. In addition to these fundamental aspects, there are also a number of other indices that can be derived from examination of the arterial pressure waveform. These are shown in Figure 12.10 and described below.

- The heart rate can be derived from the arterial pressure wave as well as from the ECG. This may be important if there is a pulse deficit.
- The area under the curve up to the dicrotic notch gives an index of stroke volume.
- The characteristics of the downstroke of the curve (the diastolic decay) give information about the resistance and compliance of the peripheral vascular bed. Decreased arterial pressure associated with peripheral vasodilatation can be identified by an abrupt fall in the pressure wave from its systolic peak and the absence of a sloping diastolic decay. An increased arterial pressure with early limitation of ejection (high dicrotic notch) and a steep diastolic run-off is characteristic of high peripheral resistance occurring either pathologically or secondary to drugs.
- Myocardial contractility (at a known filling pressure) can be assessed from the gradient of the arterial upstroke ($dP/dt$). This still tends to be predominantly used for research work.

As the pressure wave travels through the arterial tree, the mean pressure falls, the pulse pressure increases, the dicrotic notch is lost, and the waveform becomes narrower. It follows from this that, under normal conditions, the closer the cannula is to the aorta, the more accurately the recorded pressure represents that in the central arteries. Typical diagrammatic changes in the waveform shape are shown in Figure 12.11. However, under conditions of significant hypothermia or severe peripheral vasoconstriction, these arguments predicting pulse pressure augmentation no longer apply and the radial artery pressures can be very much lower than those measured in the aorta (Figure 12.12).

It is now normal clinical practice to use the radial artery on the non-dominant hand to measure the BP invasively. Complications of invasive BP monitoring are haemorrhage, local damage, embolism, inadvertent injection, thrombosis, and infection.

## Central venous pressure

Routine clinical examination of the patient includes observation of the central venous pressure (CVP) and estimation of the jugular venous pulsation. Unfortunately, this is only of use in very specialized circumstances (e.g. cannon waves) or when there is

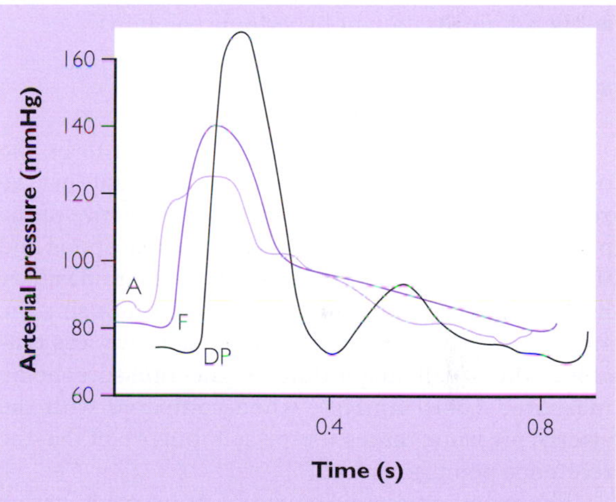


**Figure 12.11.** Typical changes in the waveform of the arterial pressure wave as it moves through the arterial tree. (A) Aortic pressure wave; (F) femoral pressure wave; and (DP) dorsalis pedis pressure wave.

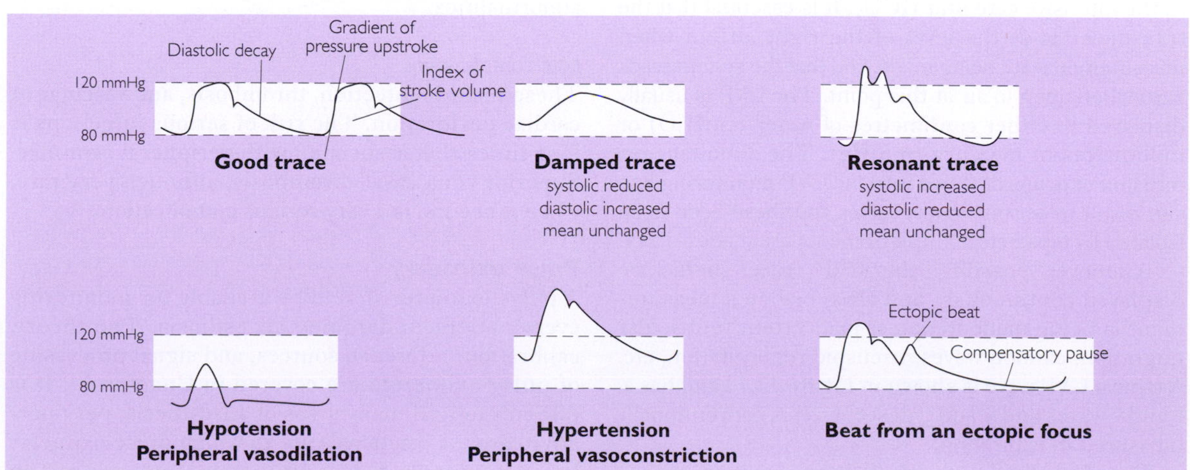


**Figure 12.10.** A variety of directly measured arterial pressure waves. See text for details.

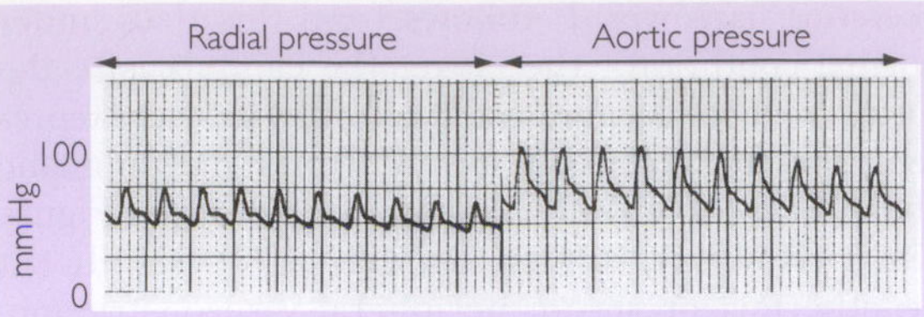


**Figure 12.12.** The effect of severe peripheral vasoconstriction on the relationship between the aortic and radial arterial pressures. (Adapted from Stern DH *et al. Anesthesiology* 1985;62:557.)

gross cardiac failure; in essence, for diagnostic and management purposes, accurate non-invasive measurement is impossible. To measure the CVP, a catheter is inserted via an arm or neck vein and advanced until it reaches the superior vena cava or right atrium. There are four main indications for the insertion of central venous catheters:

- the measurement of CVP;
- the administration of emergency, vasoactive, and/or inotropic drugs;
- the administration of hypertonic solutions (including parenteral nutrition);
- haemodialysis/plasmapheresis.

The measurement of the CVP is taken to be the pressure in the right atrium, so it is important that the zero reference point is at this level, irrespective of the patient's position. In patients with normal spinal and thoracic anatomy, this corresponds to the midaxillary line in the supine position. The practice of using the sternal angle with the patient at 45° is much less reliable. The small magnitude of the pressure being measured (4–10 mmHg), when compared with the arterial pressure, makes it especially important that the reference point is correct.

The pressure measurements can be made with a simple saline-filled manometer, which requires little additional equipment. With this it is, however, difficult to detect inadvertent intraventricular placement of the catheter or to make interpretations of the shape of the CVP wave. It is now commonplace to use electronic transducers for CVP monitoring under anaesthesia and in the intensive care unit (ICU). It is essential that the transducer is at the level of the right atrium when measurements are being made, and that the system reads zero when open to air at this point. The CVP is usually displayed in either centimetres of water (cm$H_2O$) or millimetres of mercury (mmHg). The simultaneous infusion of drugs or fluids into the CVP monitoring line can result in serious inaccuracies and these need to be isolated by taps before measurements are made.

Whenever possible, the CVP trace should be displayed continuously, and always when a measurement is being made to detect inadvertent ventricular migration, cannon waves, tricuspid regurgitation, etc. A typical CVP wave is shown in Figure 12.13 and has a, c and v waves and *x* and *y* descents. It is conventionally measured in expiration.

The clinical importance of these components is as follows:

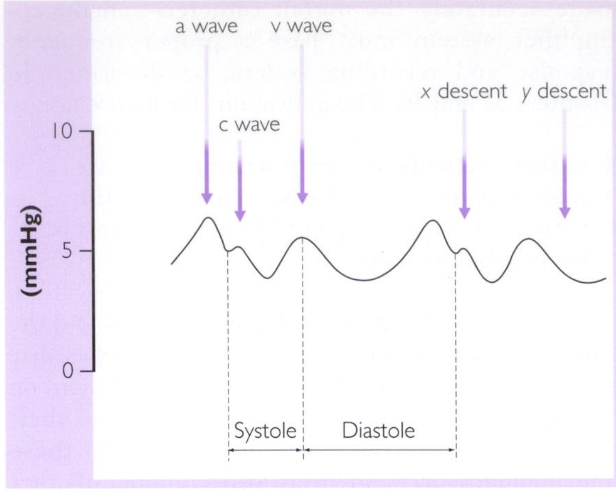


**Figure 12.13.** The central venous pressure wave.

- The a wave is produced by atrial contraction and precedes the first heart sound. It is absent in atrial fibrillation and increased in the presence of tricuspid atresia, pulmonary stenosis, pulmonary hypertension, short PR intervals, and the presence of a non-compliant right ventricle. If the atrium contracts against a closed tricuspid valve, then giant 'cannon' waves result; this is seen in premature atrial depolarization and atrioventricular dissociation, and with junctional rhythms.
- The v wave follows the carotid pulse (c wave) and represents the rise in atrial pressure caused by continued venous filling while the tricuspid valve is closed. If the tricuspid valve is regurgitant, then early, giant v waves may result.

The complications of central venous catheterization are many, but can broadly be divided into early and late.

*Early complications*

At the time of insertion, early complications are inadvertent arterial puncture, arrhythmias (from guidewires and catheters), cardiac perforation (leading to tamponade), air embolization, haematoma, pneumothorax, and haemothorax. Microshock is possible via an electrolyte-filled catheter (Chapter 39), and the risk of all complications is increased in patients with clotting abnormalities.

*Late complications*

These include infection, thrombosis, and vascular or cardiac perforation. The risk of serious infections is four times that associated with peripheral cannulae. Superior vena caval thrombosis, although very rare, when it occurs, is a very serious complication.

## Pulse oximetry

A pulse oximeter should be available for monitoring every patient undergoing anaesthesia. The theory, calibration, reference sources, and signal processing of pulse oximeters are covered in Chapter 39. It is difficult to find many areas of anaesthesia, perioperative care, or intensive care to which pulse oximetry has not contributed and these are summarized in Table 12.5.

**Table 12.5. Uses of pulse oximetry**

| |
|---|
| **Anaesthesia** |
| Routine perioperative monitoring |
| Specific advantages with:<br>• reduced lighting, e.g. endoscopy, angiography<br>• reduced skin and mucous membrane access, e.g. ENT, neurosurgery<br>• altered skin circulation, e.g. head-down position<br>• increased pigmentation, e.g. Negroes, post-lymphangiogram<br>• procedures with known risk of hypoxia, e.g. one-lung anaesthesia, bronchoscopy<br>• patients with known preoperative hypoxia |
| Training of anaesthetists |
| Monitoring routinely in recovery and on the ward for 'at-risk' patients |
| **Intensive care** |
| Monitoring oxygenation during therapeutic procedures, e.g. physiotherapy, respiratory failure, intermittent positive-pressure ventilation, and weaning |
| Staff education |
| **Other uses** |
| Transport of patients |
| Respiratory function tests |
| Preoperative assessment |
| Sleep apnoea studies |
| Angiography, cardiac shunt studies, etc. |

Although invaluable in many ways, pulse oximetry is not without its limitations and there are several clinical situations in which the data it displays can be misleading. All pulse oximeters use an empirical algorithm for the calculation of saturation. As they all have only two wavelengths and are calibrated to the ethical limit for volunteers (above 70% saturation), severe hypoxia and the presence of non-functional haemoglobins (carboxyhaemoglobin, methaemoglobin, fetal haemoglobin [HbF], and sulphaemoglobin), all produce errors.

Methaemoglobin is normally present in a low concentration (< 1%), but this can rise to 8% after the use of prilocaine for a Bier's block. It is absorbed similarly in both the red and infrared bands, and biases the reading to 85%. Low quantities of methaemoglobin reduce a high $O_2$ saturation reading by approximately half the value of the methaemoglobin. HbF behaves very similarly to haemoglobin A and sulphaemoglobin is rarely a problem. Carboxyhaemoglobin is a more variable and common cause of inaccuracy. It comprises 1–3% of the total haemoglobin in city dwellers (and is programmed in at 1.7% in Ohmeda machines), but can reach up to 15% in moderate or heavy smokers, especially those who smoke cigars. After carbon monoxide poisoning or smoke injury, it can of course be much higher. The problem with carboxyhaemoglobin is that it is interpreted by the pulse oximeter as oxygenated haemoglobin. This causes the displayed value for haemoglobin saturation to be approximately equal to the total of the oxygenated haemoglobin and carboxyhaemoglobin, thus displaying normal values in the presence of hypoxia. Although skin pigmentation, and clinical shifts in body temperature, pH, and bilirubin have little effect on the accuracy, very poor peripheral perfusion, nail varnish, and intravenous dyes can have very significant effects. All pulse oximeters are to some extent affected by motion artefact, although the design of lightweight, closely adherent probes has done much to improve this.

Problems can arise when a serious change in the patient's physiology is interpreted as artefact or modified by the algorithm. Examples of this are that a sudden fall in the patient's $O_2$ saturation may take some time to result in a changed reading because the displayed reading is averaged over several seconds; a severe arrhythmia or cardiac arrest can cause the machine to display 'probe off patient'; and the size of the pulse wave on the screen may be normalized to maximize its size and hence mask a gradually reducing pulse volume.

Of all the problems that can occur with these invaluable monitors, two that are based on basic physiological principles deserve special mention:

- Although ideal for confirming that all is well, if desaturation does occur, the pulse oximeter is completely non-diagnostic and measures the final result of the transmission of $O_2$ from the anaesthesia machine or atmosphere via the lungs and cardiac output to the periphery. Furthermore, given the shape of the oxyhaemoglobin dissociation curve (see Chapters 31 and 52) in a previously well-saturated patient, there needs to be a very large fall in the arterial oxygen tension ($P\text{a}O_2$) to produce a measurable fall in the $O_2$ saturation; *the change in $O_2$ saturation therefore occurs late*.
- If the $O_2$ saturation is used as the only measure of the adequacy of breathing (e.g. in recovery), with a high inspired $O_2$ content, it is quite possible to have normal $O_2$ saturations in the presence of a high $CO_2$ and low respiratory rate (see Chapter 5). It is consequently essential that other simple measurements (e.g. counting the respirations) are made to detect the onset of hypercapnia.

## Capnography

A capnograph should be available for use in all patients undergoing anaesthesia. The mode of action of a capnograph and the sources of error are described in Chapter 39. This section deals with the use of the capnograph as a clinical monitor.

### *Capnography during intermittent positive-pressure ventilation (IPPV)*

This is the most common time for the capnograph to be used and, in adults, with the tidal volume set as in normal practice (10–15 ml/kg), there is usually little problem in obtaining a sample of alveolar gas. The capnograph morphology depends considerably on the mode of ventilation. A capnogram from a healthy patient ventilated on a minute volume (MV) divider is shown in Figure 12.14. It is recognizable as being close to an idealized capnogram and a change in paper speed permits monitoring of drift.

Figure 12.15 shows a capnogram derived from a ventilated Mapleson D breathing system (see Chapter 9). This system has no valves to separate inspired and expired gas and allows rebreathing of expired $CO_2$. During normal use, there is a non-zero inspired $CO_2$ pressure ($P\text{ICO}_2$) because the free gas flow (FGF) is below the MV. The inspiratory part of the trace is therefore not flat, but distorted by the mixing of expired and inspired fresh gas during inspiration. The mean level of inspired $CO_2$ cannot be determined from a visual inspection of the capnograph because it gives no indication of gas flow rate; the instantaneous $P\text{ICO}_2$ and inspiratory flow rate have to be combined, integrated, and averaged to do this. The potential mixing of the continuous fresh gas supply with expired gas may also prevent the accurate sampling of alveolar gas, but this artefact is minimal if the sampling site is within or immediately adjacent to the ET tube and there is a catheter mount or elbow joint between the ET tube and the end of the D system circuit.

It is highly likely that the use of capnography will become mandatory during IPPV.

### *Capnography during spontaneous ventilation*

In contrast to capnography during IPPV, the literature on capnography during spontaneous breathing is relatively sparse. There are greater difficulties in obtaining a true sample of alveolar air and, although this is usually satisfactory for clinical purposes in intubated patients or those breathing with a laryngeal mask, within a facemask there can be considerable mixing of inspired and expired gases. If no alveolar plateau is seen, even in young fit patients, the expired levels of $CO_2$ cannot be used reliably to estimate the arterial $CO_2$ pressure ($P\text{aCO}_2$). When a facemask is being used, it is best to push the sampling catheter into the oral or nasopharyngeal airway. Capnograms from spontaneous facemask ventilation using various airways can be found in Chapter 3 (see Figure 3.3).

An example of the error that can occur during facemask ventilation is shown in Figure 12.16. Before A, a capnograph trace has been recorded from within a nasopharyngeal airway supplied by fresh gas from a Bain circuit at 12 L/min. At A, the sampling catheter slipped out of the airway into the deadspace of the facemask, with a resulting artefactual fall in the end-tidal $CO_2$ pressure ($P\text{ETCO}_2$). A quick way of checking to see whether or not the $P\text{ETCO}_2$ is artefactually low is to temporarily disconnect the fresh gas supply as shown at B. If there is an abrupt rise in the $P\text{ETCO}_2$ when the diluting effect of the FGF is removed, then the first breaths that follow will give a measure of the true $P\text{ETCO}_2$. This manoeuvre can obviously be tolerated for only a short time because of rebreathing. At C, the fresh gas supply is reconnected with a prompt fall in the $P\text{ETCO}_2$ to its incorrect level.

### *The relationship between $P\text{ETCO}_2$ and $P\text{aCO}_2$*

A sample of end-tidal gas is assumed to have come from the alveoli where it is in equilibrium with pulmonary capillary blood. In fit young adult patients with healthy lungs, the $P\text{ETCO}_2$ is usually about 0.3–0.6 kPa (2.3–4.5 mmHg) less than the $P\text{aCO}_2$, the difference being least when the patient is ventilated with large tidal volumes. This enables expired gas to be used as an indicator of arterial $CO_2$ (Figure 12.17). When there is a true intrapulmonary shunt, or a right/left shunt in the heart, venous blood bypasses the alveoli and mixes directly with the arterial blood. As shown in Figure 12.18, theoretically with a pure shunt that is not attended by coincident lung damage, the $P\text{ETCO}_2$ still reflects reasonably well the arterial $CO_2$ because the usual difference between venous and arterial $CO_2$ levels is only 0.7 kPa (5.3 mmHg) (see Chapter 21).

The situation is, however, very different in the case of increased deadspace, particularly in the case of constant tidal and minute ventilation. Increased deadspace implies that a greater proportion of the inspired

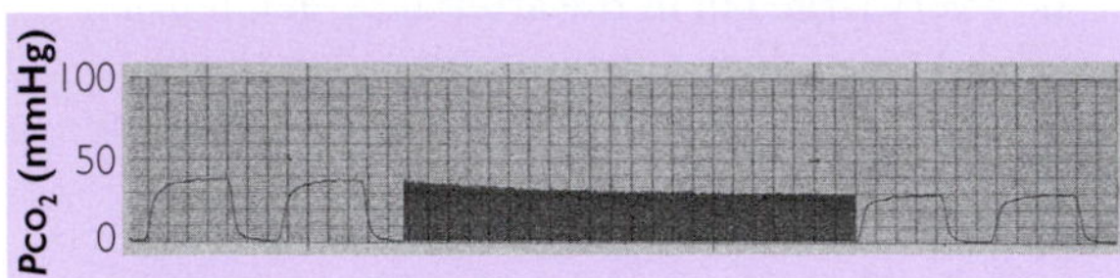


**Figure 12.14.** A capnogram from a healthy adult being ventilated on a minute volume divider. Note the change in paper speed in the central section (from 5 mm/s to 5mm/min and back again). The slower paper speed allows the monitoring of drift. This recording was obtained from a monitor with a paper readout. Many modern monitors continuously display the capnograph trace on the screen, and the drift can be obtained from a display of the variables stored in the memory.

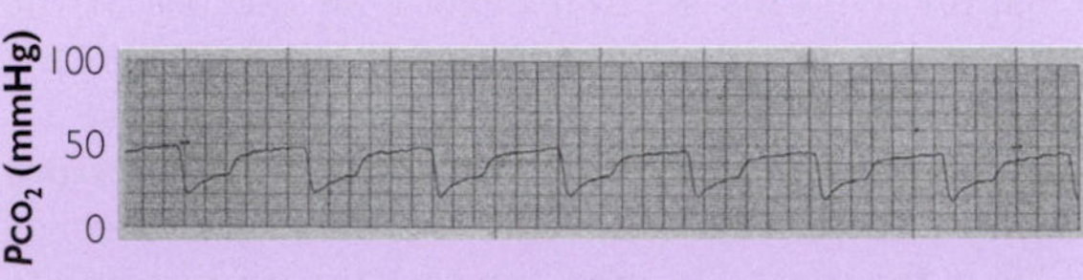


**Figure 12.15.** Capnogram from a patient ventilated on a Mapleson D breathing system. See text for details and explanation of its morphology. (Chart speed = 5 mm/s.)

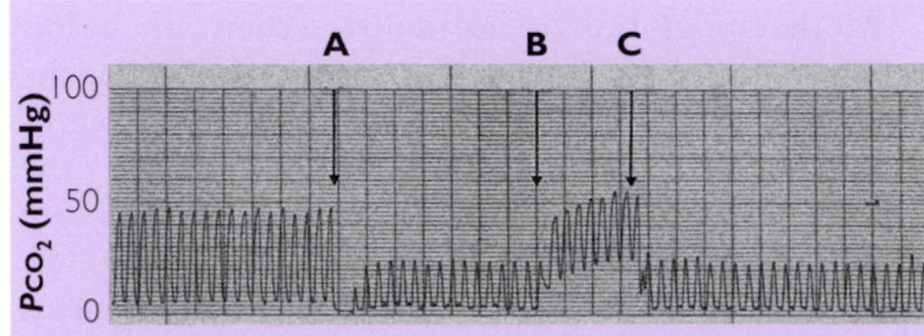


**Figure 12.16.** Capnogram during spontaneous facemask ventilation breathing from a Mapleson D system. Fresh gas flow equals 12 L/min. Note that, even at this fresh gas flow rate, there is still a non-zero inspired $CO_2$ level (chart speed = 1 mm/s). See text for details.

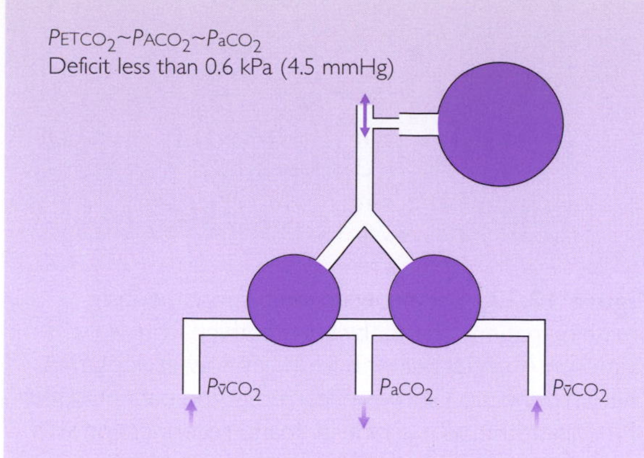


**Figure 12.17.** A diagrammatic representation of normal capnography in a fit patient. Alveolar gas is represented by the shading. As the lungs have a clear division between deadspace and alveolar gas and empty simultaneously, it is as if, at the sampling point, the capnograph is taking gas from a single large lung. $P\bar{v}CO_2$, mixed venous $PCO_2$; $PaCO_2$, arterial $PCO_2$; $PACO_2$, alveolar $CO_2$.

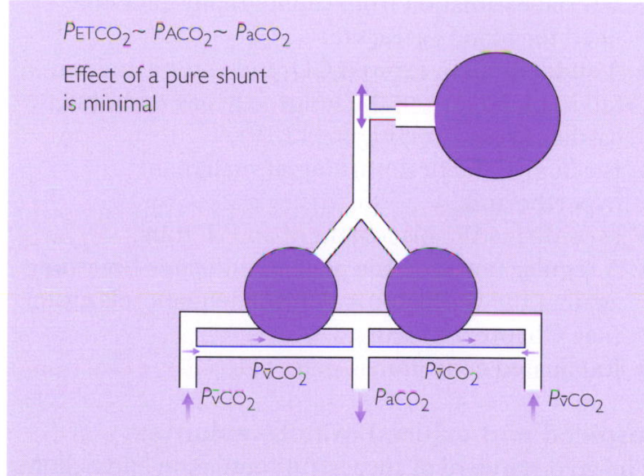


**Figure 12.18.** The effect of a true right-to-left shunt on capnography. See text for details.

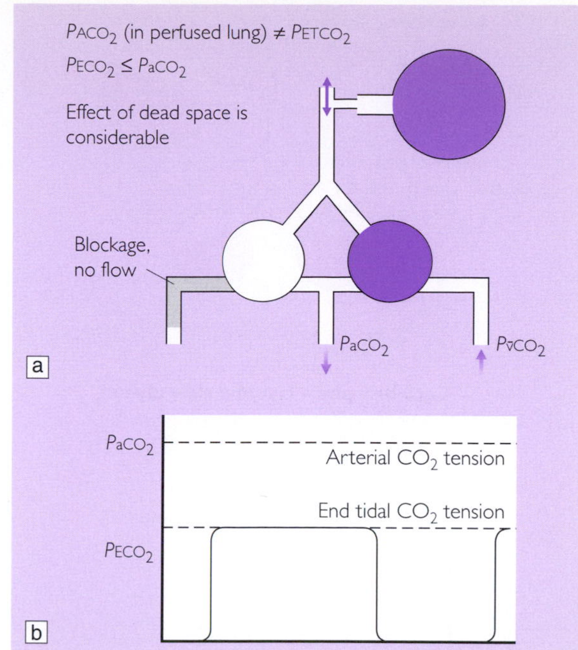


**Figure 12.19.** A diagrammatic representation of a sudden increase in deadspace on the expired $CO_2$ in previously normal lungs. In (a) it can be seen that there is a blockage to the blood flow to one of the lungs, and in this lung there is no exchange of $CO_2$ to the alveolar air. As both lungs exhale together, the alveolar air from this lung and from the other lung mix in the trachea and larger airways, and at the sampling point the capnograph takes in a gas mixture that has a level of $CO_2$ well below that in the pulmonary venous blood. When this occurs rapidly in fit healthy lungs, as shown diagrammatically in (b), the capnograph maintains its shape but the alveolar plateau is well below the arterial $CO_2$.

gas fails to come into contact with capillary blood. When this occurs suddenly, it is usually the result of a sudden failure of lung perfusion, e.g. some type of pulmonary embolus; when it occurs chronically, it is secondary to parenchymal lung damage. Both these produce conditions in which the $P_{ETCO_2}$ is no longer representative of the $P_{aCO_2}$ (Figures 12.19 and 12.20). The management of pulmonary embolus and chronic respiratory disease are described in Chapters 13 and 54, respectively.

### *Applications of capnography*

The capnograph in clinical monitoring practice has the following applications:

- In patients with a normal respiratory and cardiovascular system it can be used as a breath-by-breath estimator of the $P_{aCO_2}$.
- It can give qualitative evidence that rebreathing is occurring, although used alone it cannot quantify the amount.
- It can be used as a disconnection alarm. The change in the capnograph trace during a disconnection depends upon whether the patient is being ventilated or breathing spontaneously. Figure 12.21 shows an accidental disconnection between the catheter mount and the ventilator hoses in a paralysed patient. The capnograph was sampling from the catheter mount distal to the disconnection. It can be seen that there is a sudden loss of cyclical activity (at A) until the patient was reconnected (at B). Most capnographs feature an alarm that indicates when such a disconnection has occurred. Figure 12.22 shows a disconnection in a spontaneously breathing patient when a disconnection occurred at the common gas outlet of the anaesthesia machine. The intubated patient was breathing from a Mapleson A system at 4.5 L/min and the capnograph was sampling at the catheter mount. Note the difference from Figure 12.21. In Figure 12.22 the disconnection occurred at point A and the patient began to rebreathe expired air, with a consequent rise in both the inspired and expired $CO_2$ levels until reconnection was effected at B. Most capnographs will not indicate this series of events as a disconnection. If, in Figure 12.22, the site of the disconnection had been at the junction of the breathing system and the catheter mount

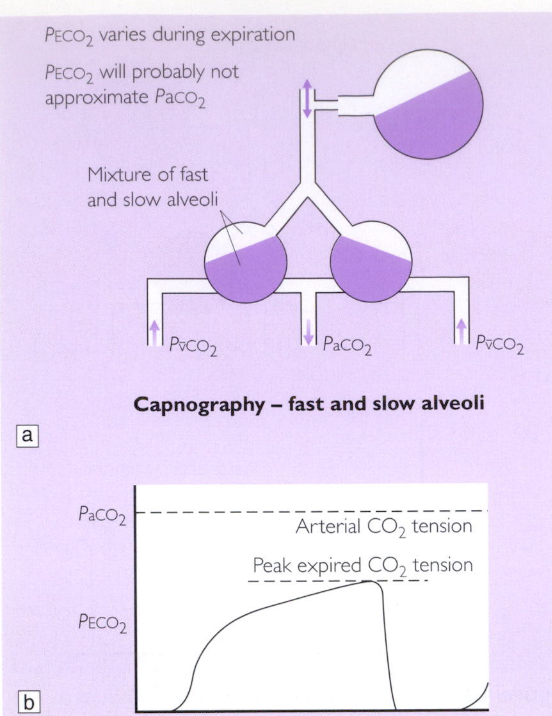


**Figure 12.20.** A diagrammatic representation of the effect of fast and slow alveoli on capnography in the lungs of a patient with chronic lung disease. (a) Diagrammatic illustration that both lungs are equally diseased with a mixture of healthy and poorly functioning alveoli. (b) Diagrammatic representation of the capnogram trace from such a pair of lungs. It can be seen that there is no flat alveolar plateau because the alveoli empty at different times with different concentrations of $CO_2$. Furthermore, the peak expiratory $CO_2$ is still well below the level of the arterial $CO_2$. When a patient without a flat alveolar plateau is encountered, it is necessary to make simultaneous measurements of the peak expiratory $CO_2$ and the arterial $CO_2$ to estimate the difference between them. It is clear from this that ventilating to normocapnia on the $CO_2$ trace in such a patient could lead to significant arterial hypercapnia.

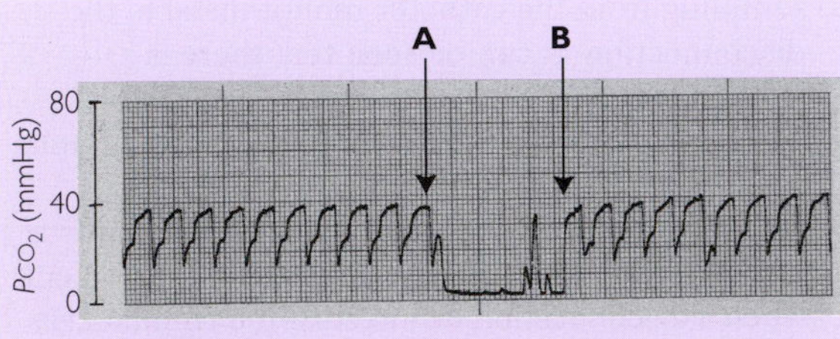


**Figure 12.21.** An accidental disconnection in a paralysed patient being ventilated on a Mapleson D circuit. Disconnection occurred at A and reconnection at B. (Chart speed = 1 mm/s.)

proximal to the capnograph sampling point, there would have been no immediate rise in inspired $CO_2$ because the patient would have breathed from room air. The changes to the capnograph trace would, in this instance, have been much slower to develop

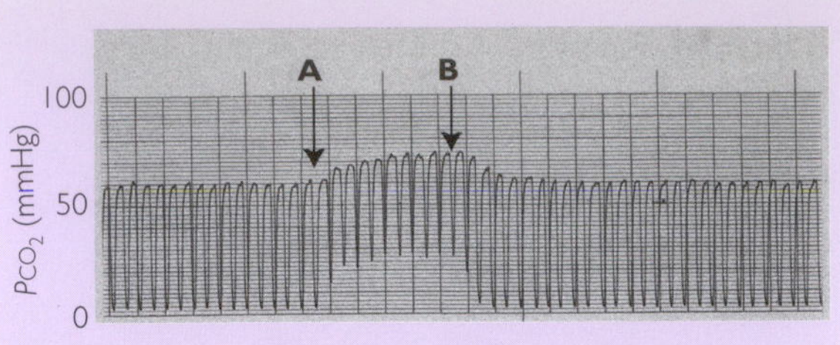


**Figure 12.22.** Disconnection in a spontaneously breathing patient. The patient is breathing from a Mapleson A circuit fed with fresh gas flow at 4.5 L/min. The disconnection shown occurred at the patient outlet of the anaesthetsia machine at A and reconnection was at B. See text for details. (Chart speed = 1 mm/s.)

and simply indicated a lightening of anaesthesia as the volatile agent was blown off.

- It can be used to measure respiratory rate. In spontaneous breathing it gives an indication of the lightening of anaesthesia and/or adequacy of FGF.
- The shape of the curve gives knowledge about ventilation–perfusion ratios and likely accuracy of arterial estimation from capnography, plus the need for blood gases, etc.
- A sudden fall in expired $CO_2$ indicates a sudden fall in blood flow to the lungs, e.g. gas embolus, cardiac arrest (see Figure 12.19).
- It can give the first warning of malignant hyperthermia.
- It confirms the placement of an ET tube.
- A regular notch on the plateau indicates breathing against the ventilator and/or inadequate relaxation (see Chapter 3, Figure 3.4).
- Exhausted soda lime is detected.

### Inspired and expired minute volumes

The gold standard of successful ventilation and bellows function of the lungs is the continuous monitoring of the expired volume. In many instances, the expired MV is assumed to be satisfactory from setting the inspired MV and tidal volume, or is estimated by eye from a bellows or bag. Electronic methods commonly found in current use are described below.

#### *Spirometry/direct volume measurements*

A number of anaesthesia and ICU ventilators incorporate a lightweight calibrated bellows into the breathing system, either as an expiratory volume indicator or as part of a 'bag-in-bottle' ventilator. Some collect the expired tidal volume into a rubber bag-in-bottle system, which is subsequently evacuated by passing gas into the bottle at a fixed rate, the time taken to empty the bag being a measure of the tidal volume, independent of the gas composition.

#### *Turbine flowmeters*

Since its introduction over 40 years ago, the Wright's respirometer has remained the most widely used turbine flowmeter. Gas passes through a slotted stator, is directed through a set of vanes that rotate, and a jewelled watch-like movement converts this into rotations of a dial (see Chapter 37, Figure 37.61). The curve is shifted up and to the left as the density of the gas increases (nitrous oxide is 1.53 as dense as air). At the extremes of performance, these flowmeters under-read at low flow rates as a result of 'slippage' of gas past the rotor and over-read at high flows because of 'over-run' of the rotor. In practice, they do not tend to overestimate expired volumes and are satisfactory for clinical use at normal expired MVs. Paediatric models are also available. Nowadays, a new generation of turbine flowmeters is also used that employ much simpler turbines, mounted axially in a housing that fits into the inspiratory or expiratory limb of the breathing circuit. They usually respond to bidirectional flow, and optical measurement of the rotational velocity has microprocessor-based algorithms to correct for the non-linearity in the response to flow (Figure 12.23). For obvious reasons, if a ventilatory flowmeter is to be used as a disconnection monitor, it is best placed in the expiratory limb of the breathing system during IPPV.

### *Hot wire and hot film anemometry*

A heated wire, film, or coated wire placed in a gas stream will be cooled by the flowing gas. The degree of cooling is determined by the temperature of the gas, the composition of the gas (if its specific heat is changed), and the velocity of the gas over the wire. With temperature and composition constant, the cooling effect becomes a (very non-linear) measure of velocity. This is used in the Spirolog, Drager, and Servo ventilator systems.

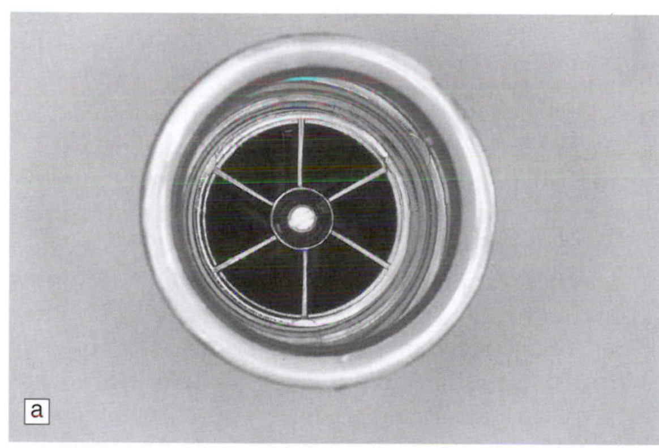


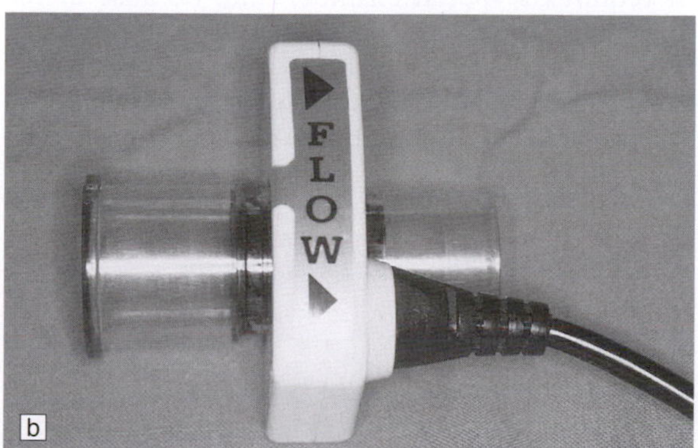


**Figure 12.23.** An example of a turbine flowmeter seen (a) axially and (b) with its external measuring collar. (Courtesy of Ohmeda Limited, Madison USA.)

### *Other methods*

For other methods, such as ultrasonic flowmeters, the pneumotachograph, thermistors, and ionization methods, refer to the basic science section in Chapter 37.

## Ventilatory pressure measurement and pressure alarms

In most operating room ventilators, the pressure gauges are mechanical, using a thin copper bellows or Bourdon-type tube attached via a mechanical linkage to a pointer (see Chapter 37, Figure 37.8). Their frequency response is limited to less than 1 Hz and, with rapid changes in pressure (e.g. when a constant pressure ventilator is used), considerable overshoot arises in the needle movement and exaggerated readings of peak inspiratory pressure can result.

In modern anaesthetic and ICU ventilators, electronic pressure transducers (often solid-state bridge strain gauges) are used (see Chapter 39). These have a high degree of accuracy and a frequency response of up to 100 Hz and the signal can be displayed continuously on a screen or digitized and analysed to give derived variables such as peak pressure, etc. It is common practice for the pressure transducer to be mounted in the ventilator where it is connected to the inspiratory limb of the breathing system. The pressure so measured is the proximal breathing system pressure, which may not always accurately reflect airway pressure. In particular, if there is a large compressible volume in the inspiratory limb, damping of the signal results. In neonatal and infant ventilation, where small-volume high frequencies are used, the pressures measured at the proximal end of the breathing system will significantly overestimate the true pressure applied to the alveoli.

Measurement of the inspired pressure is often used as a disconnection alarm. Depending on the model in use, pressure monitors can be adapted with alarms for pre-set high and low pressures and for failure to fall to atmospheric pressure during expiration. When they are used as disconnection monitors during IPPV, it is important to have their attachment point as close to the patient as possible (Figure 12.24). If it is close to the ventilator outlet on the inspiratory limb, kinked ventilator hoses, external compression on the hoses, or a blocked breathing filter, etc. can all allow the pressure in the ventilator hosing apparently to cycle correctly when no, or substantially reduced, fresh gas is entering the patient. It should also be noted that, even with the attachment point at the catheter mount, if the ET tube is kinked or blocked, a pressure sensor may still cycle satisfactorily without sounding an alarm if the pre-set alarm pressure is not reached.

## Disconnection monitors

Capnographs, flowmeters, and pressure sensors can all be used as disconnection monitors. Each has advantages and disadvantages as described in the relevant sections above.

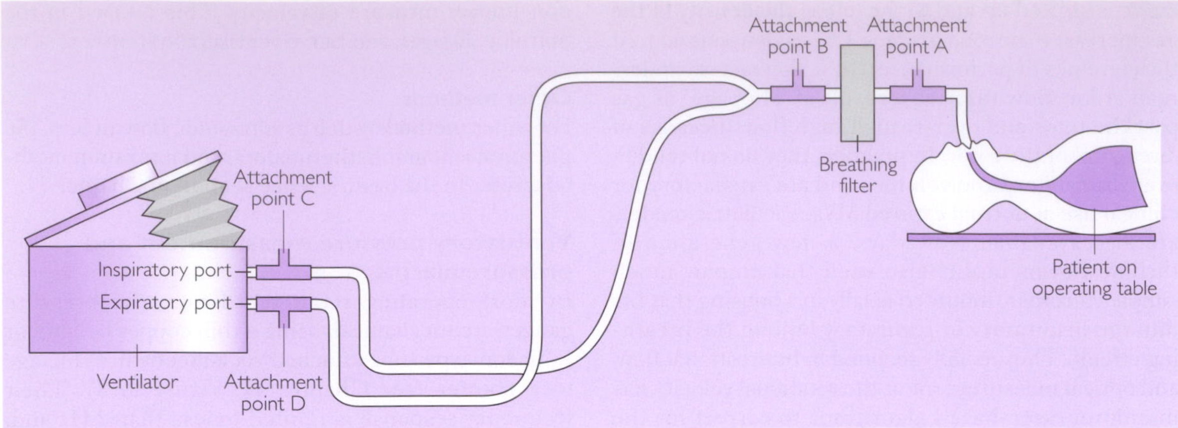


**Figure 12.24.** Possible attachment points for a pressure sensor. Note that the correct attachment point is at A. Attachments at B, C, and D can all show satisfactory pressure cycling with a blocked filter, kinked tube, etc.

## STERILIZATION, DISINFECTION, AND CROSS-INFECTION

### Sterilization and disinfection of equipment

#### *Definitions*

There is uncertainty about the exact terminology in this area, but for the purposes of this book, the following definitions will be used.

*Decontamination*

This is the physical removal of unwanted matter by thorough washing or scrubbing.

*Disinfection*

This is the removal or killing of most or all of the infected matter with the exception of the most resistant such as spores.

*Sterilization*

This implies the killing of all organisms, including the most resistant organisms and spores.

#### *Methods and their application*

*Decontamination*

This can be effected by holding components under running water, manual brushing or wiping, the use of dishwashers, or ultrasonic vibration in a bath of detergent or other chemical solvent. Decontamination must not be regarded as unimportant: the removal of the bulk of the unwanted debris is required to ensure that subsequent disinfection and sterilization are totally effective. Decontamination is now reserved only for those things, such as anaesthesia machine work surfaces, pulse oximeter probes, facemasks, BP cuffs, etc., that come into contact with intact body surfaces.

*Disinfection*

This requires higher temperatures and more reactive chemicals than decontamination. It can be done by pasteurization, which consists of heating the article to 70°C for 20 min or 80°C for 10 min (which can be done in a water bath or low-temperature autoclave) or boiling for 5 min at normal atmospheric pressure. Disinfection in clinical practice is often carried out by use of the many chemicals now available for this purpose. Some of these are 70% ethyl or isopropyl alcohol in water, chlorhexidine in strengths varying from 0.5% to 5%, hydrogen peroxide, phenols, and aldehydes. They can be wiped on, the apparatus can be immersed in them, or equipment is available for them to be formulated as mists or fogs. Some of these compounds, when applied for long enough in sufficient concentration, can act as sterilizing agents.

*Sterilization*

This, particularly of small and metal items, is most usually carried out by autoclaving. The articles are placed in a gas-tight chamber which admits steam for a pre-set period and then usually finishes with a vacuum stage for drying. The time required for sterilization depends on both the temperature and the pressure, as shown in Table 12.6.

Dry heat (approximately 160°C for about 30 min) is also effective and is the method of choice for some types of surgical instrument. If glass items (e.g. syringes) are subject to this, then the temperature has to be raised and lowered gradually to prevent breakages. For equipment that is damaged by heat or temperature changes, ethylene oxide or propylene oxide can be used. It requires a special chamber and, because of the inflammability of the agents, is usually mixed with $CO_2$ or some other gas that will not support combustion. The gas is released into a chamber in which the temperature and humidity are also controlled. With

**Table 12.6. The requirements for sterilization**

| Time (min) | Pressure[a] (psi [kPa]) | Temperature (°C) |
|---|---|---|
| 30 | 15 [101.3] | 122 |
| 10 | 20 [135] | 126 |
| 3 | 30 [202.6] | 134 |

[a]Pressures given are gauge pressure above atmospheric.

rubber or plastics, there can be a period of days required to allow the gas to elute out of the material, although this can be accelerated by the use of an aeration chamber.

Gamma irradiation is widely used for the sterilization of pre-packaged disposable items, but the capital cost of setting the apparatus up renders it an impracticable technique for a hospital's reusable service.

### Routine guidelines for the cleaning and sterilization of anaesthetic equipment

It may seem surprising, but cleaning and sterilization are areas on which there are few nationally agreed guidelines: almost all procedures are derived from locally agreed best practice discussions. Single-use tubes and breathing system components have made some of the problems related to sterility and cross-infection much easier to deal with, but their sensible everyday use is based on what seems to be reasonable opinion rather than experimental fact. Although evidence has been published suggesting that cross-infection can occur from contaminated anaesthesia equipment (see Dorsch and Dorsch, Further reading), well-authenticated cases are extremely rare given the number of anaesthetics administered. One useful way of looking at things is to follow the classification of the American Centers for Disease Control and Prevention. They categorized items into three categories based on the potential risk of infection involved in their use: critical items, semicritical items, and non-critical items.

#### *Critical items*

These are those introduced into the bloodstream or tissues of the body by penetrating skin or mucous membranes, which must be completely sterilized at the time of use. These include all types of needle, indwelling catheters, and their associated tubing and connectors, urinary catheters, and syringes.

#### *Semicritical items*

These are devices that come into contact with intact mucous membranes but do not penetrate the surface. If they do pierce the surface, then they obviously become critical items. This group includes laryngoscope blades, nasopharyngeal and rectal temperature probes, oral and nasal airways, tracheal tubes and suckers, oesophageal stethoscopes, breathing circuits and connectors, resuscitation bags, and facemasks. In most cases, decontamination followed by high-level disinfection for these items is probably adequate but, because of the chance of mucosal damage, several of them are frequently treated as critical items (see guidelines later). Facemasks are an exception in the other direction, in that they are frequently downgraded to non-critical status.

#### *Non-critical items*

These are those that do not normally touch the patient or touch only intact skin. These need only low-level disinfection or thorough decontamination. Examples are precordial stethoscopes, BP cuffs, pulse oximeter probes, ECG electrodes, reusable skin temperature probes, and the surfaces of the anaesthesia machine and monitors.

### Suggested guidelines

With these considerations in mind, the following seem reasonable guidelines to follow:

- As a result of the potential for breaking the mucosal surface, all tracheal tubes, suction catheters, nasal and oral airways, bougies and intubating stylets, probes, etc. placed in the nose or oesophagus should be sterilized. Most of these items are pre-packaged and sterilized anyway; those that are reusable need to be sterilized between cases.
- Laryngoscope blades should be cleaned thoroughly, wiped with disinfectant, and then rinsed and dried.
- Facemasks should be thoroughly washed in soap and water, rinsed, and dried.
- Non-disposable breathing tubing should, whenever possible, be protected by the use of breathing filters that can be changed between cases. It is not uncommon practice to wash non-disposable breathing hoses, valves, reservoir bags, and elbow and catheter mounts in hot soapy water, followed by rinsing and drying, at the end of each day's work. Before using any other detergent or disinfection solution, the compatibility with the hose material needs to be established. At longer intervals they need to be autoclaved.
- Circle valve systems can also be protected by the use of disposable bacterial filters and the manufacturers' instructions followed with respect to cleaning or autoclaving of the component parts.
- Ventilators should be protected by the use of disposable filters on the inspiratory and expiratory ports, and the internal mechanism sterilized by a method approved by the manufacturer at regular intervals. This is very important for ICU ventilators.
- The external surfaces of anaesthesia machines and other equipment (particularly if there are blood or tissue fluid splashes on it) need to be thoroughly cleaned and disinfected.
- Where expired gas sampling is used, it should be taken from the circuit side of the filter.
- In paediatric practice, where the use of a filter would increase the deadspace or resistance unacceptably, filters should not be used but the breathing system changed between patients.
- If immunocompromised patients are being treated, all equipment relating to the airway and its management must be sterile.
- All disposable equipment must be discarded and non-disposable items relating to the airway must be re-sterilized after use on a patient known to be infected.
- The methods and principles described above are adequate to deal with the majority of routine patients. At the time of writing there is, however, considerable uncertainty over the impact and management of prion disease. Prions are extremely resistant to disinfection and sterilization, and have been isolated from tonsillar tissue. Although not firmly established, it is likely to be recommended that all equipment used during tonsillectomies or pharyngeal surgery that

comes into contact with mucosa or blood is either disposable or protected by disposable coverings. It is important that trainees check what the current local recommendations are. To the author's knowledge, no recommendations have yet been made for neurosurgical procedures.

### Preventing cross-infection from patients to staff

Cross-infection from one patient to another via the anaesthetic apparatus has been dealt with above. This section considers cross-infection from the patient to the staff and vice versa. Fortunately, both of these events are rare.

In preventing the transmission of infection from staff to patients, common sense is required. Apart from the rare occasions when a health worker is found to be carrying a nosocomial pathogen contributing to repeated infections (e.g. methicillin-resistant *Staphylococcus aureus*) or has an open infected wound or pustule, simple measures such as repeated hand washing and wearing a mask in the presence of an upper respiratory tract infection are probably satisfactory. Current guidance is that health workers infected with a blood-borne virus can continue to work, provided that they do not carry out exposure-prone procedures. An exposure-prone procedure is defined as 'a procedure where there is a risk that injury to the health worker may result in the exposure of the patient's open tissues to the blood of the worker. These procedures include those where the worker's gloved hand may be in contact with sharp instruments, needle tips or sharp tissues (spicules of bone or teeth) inside a patient's open body cavity, wound or confined anatomical space where the hands or finger tips may not be completely visible at all times'. Perhaps the greatest risk to patients from staff is not cross-infection but when staff continue to work in the face of genuine illness (e.g. flu, migraine, etc.), when they are unable to give the patient their proper attention.

Of more personal importance to anaesthetists is the possibility that they may become infected from the patients with whom they are dealing. Again, good routine practice reduces the risk considerably. All needles and other sharps should be discarded immediately after use into a puncture-resistant container. Appropriate barrier precautions should be taken commensurate with the surgical procedure being undertaken. The wearing of gloves for insertion of lines and management of the airway should be universal. Other measures such as the wearing of masks, plastic aprons, and goggles should be related to the likely risk of splashes and other methods of contamination. Most hospitals have local guidelines which should be followed.

Chapter 60 discusses the management of a patient known to have an infection.

## CONTROLLED DRUGS

Every country in the world possesses legislation to limit the use and control the supply of substances that can produce dependency in the recipient. Although details differ from place to place, the principles of control are very similar. These are based on statute law relating to prescribing and storage, modified for convenience by local agreements to ensure safe and best practice. All anaesthetists should make themselves aware of the exact mechanisms that are current in the place in which they are working. Clinical protocols should ensure that patients receive what is prescribed and make it as difficult as possible for theft and abuse to occur. The following points form the basis of good practice:

- There must be compliance with statutory regulations.
- Medical staff must sign for the controlled drugs received, record the quantity of drug administered, return any unopened ampoules, and ensure safe disposal of any unused drug.
- Controlled drugs must be stored in a secure and locked place.
- Local guidelines should be established to promote good, safe, and legal practice for handling controlled drugs. It must be clear who is allowed to hold the drug cupboard keys, particularly if it is local arrangements rather than professional qualifications that allow them to do so.
- Unused controlled drugs must be disposed of in the approved manner.
- The sharing of the contents of any ampoule between patients, whatever the size of the ampoule, is to be condemned. It greatly increases the opportunities for theft and substitution.
- Whenever possible, syringes for infusion and patient-controlled analgesia should be purchased pre-filled, or should be filled in the hospital pharmacy.

Abuse of controlled drugs continues to be a problem that all anaesthetists should be constantly aware of. Unfortunately, medical, nursing, operating room, and ancillary staff are not immune to addiction. Trainee staff suspicious of any one or more individuals should immediately share their thoughts with a trusted member of the consultant staff. Those addicted need help and patients need protection (both from substitution of ampoule contents and the effects of addiction in staff). Turning a blind eye because of misguided loyalty never produces a solution and may be responsible for allowing a containable problem to escalate.

## PATIENTS IN CLINICAL TRIALS

Experiments on humans raise many ethical questions and stimulate statements such as those given below:

> Among experiments that may be tried on man, those that can only harm are forbidden, those that are innocent are permissible, and those that may do good are obligatory.
>
> Claude Bernard, 1878

> The health of my patient will be my first consideration.
>
> Declaration of Geneva, 1968

> At any time during the course of clinical research the subject or guardian should be free to withdraw permission for research to be continued.
>
> Declaration of Helsinki, 1964

At some point in almost everyone's career they will be asked to assist in a clinical trial: most will become involved in them as part of their training in research methods. Trite statements and moral aphorisms such as those given above help greatly to stimulate discussion; they are less useful when faced with the request from a colleague who pops his head into the operating room half-way through an operation and says 'The patient's in a trial, can you give me 10 ml of arterial blood in an EDTA tube?'. This is especially so when the motivations for some research are not always unrelated to career advancement, and anaesthetized, unconscious patients are far from being able to exercise free will.

The purpose of this section is to offer some practical advice to trainees involved in setting up and taking part in clinical trials. There are few absolute rights and wrongs but the following form reasonable working guidelines:

- All anaesthetists, whether trainees or consultants, should regard it as part of their professional responsibility to assist those who are trying to improve patient care through experimentation.
- When becoming involved in such work, having one's name on a paper or abstract should not be regarded as a right or as a form of currency in agreeing to take part. Inclusion in authorship should follow the guidelines laid down by the International Committee of Medical Journal Editors. Dual publication to increase the back page of the Curriculum Vitae is to be resisted. It only backfires if you are caught out.
- If you are included as an author, insist on seeing the manuscript in time for your comments to be considered before it is sent off for publication.
- When taking part in clinical research, ensure that the proper guidelines with respect to the local ethical committee have been followed and identify the person who has accepted clinical responsibility for the project.
- When recruiting patients, be as honest as possible to them about what is involved, in line with their ability to grasp what is being asked of them. Slick salesmanship is to be resisted.
- Do not, alone, undertake distracting, time-consuming research that will reduce the normal level of care that you would give to a patient (e.g. frequent blood sampling during induction). If this could occur, get a colleague to help to ensure that the patient is not disadvantaged.
- Do not undertake procedures for research that you are not competent to do. For example, it is quite appropriate for a first-year trainee to take a peripheral venous blood sample for a drug assay, whereas it is quite inappropriate for them to insert a pulmonary artery catheter to obtain a true mixed venous sample.

As usual, common sense is the key to protecting the interests and advancing the cause of both the patient and the anaesthetist.

## FURTHER READING


Arnold WP, Hug CC. *Recommendations for infection control for the practice of anesthesiology*. Park Ridge IL: American Society of Anesthesiologists, 1991.

Articles in: Aitkenhead AR, ed. *Quality Assurance and Risk management in Anaesthesia. Baillière's Clin Anaesthesiol* 1996;**10**:237–390.

Association of Anaesthetists of Great Britain and Ireland. *HIV and other Blood Borne Viruses*. London: AAGBI, 1992.

Association of Anaesthetists of Great Britain and Ireland. *Recommendations for Standards of Monitoring during Anaesthesia and Recovery*. London: AAGBI, 1994.

Association of Anaesthetists of Great Britain and Ireland. *Controlled Drugs*. London: AAGBI, 1995.

Association of Anaesthetists of Great Britain and Ireland. *Risk Management*. London: AAGBI, 1998.

Bell MDD, Bodenham AR. Problems and pitfalls of practical procedures: a medico-legal perspective. *Curr Anaesth Crit Care* 1998;**9**:278–89.

Davey A, Moyle JTB, Ward CS. *Ward's Anaesthetic Equipment*, 3rd edn. *Cleaning and Sterilisation*. Philadelphia: WB Saunders, 1992: 306–14.

Davis PD, Parbrook GD, Kenny GNC. *Basic Physics and Measurement in Anaesthesia*, 4th edn. Oxford: Butterworth-Heinemann, 1995.

Articles in: Dinnick OP, Thompson PW, eds. *Some Aspects of Anaesthetic Safety. Baillière's Clin Anaesthesiol* 1988;**2**:243–438.

Dorsch JA, Dorsch SE. *Understanding Anaesthesia Equipment*. Baltimore: Williams & Wilkins, 1994; 74S.

Eichorn JH. Pulse oximetry as a standard practise (editorial). *Anesthesiology* 1993;**78**:423.

Gravenstein JS, Paulus DA, Hayes TJ. *Capnography in Clinical Practice*. Oxford: Butterworth-Heinemann, 1989

Gravenstein JS, Paulus DA, Hayes TJ. *Gas Monitoring in Clinical Practice*, 2nd edn. Oxford: Butterworth-Heinemann, 1995.

Greenbaum R. National and international standards for anaesthetic equipment. *Br J Anaesth* 1985;**57**:709–17.

Hutton P, Prys-Roberts. *Monitoring in Anaesthesia and Intensive Care*. Philadelphia: WB Saunders, 1994.

International Committee of Medical Journal Editors. Criteria for authorship. *Ann Intern Med* 1988;**108**:258–65.

The International Task Force on Anaesthesia Safety. International standards for a safe practice of anaesthesia. *Eur J Anaesthesiol* 1993;**10**(suppl 7):12–15.

Lake CL. *Clinical Monitoring*. Philadelphia: WB Saunders, 1990.

Lindberg LG, Lennmarken C, Vegfors M. Pulse oximetry – clinical implications and recent technical developments. *Acta Anaesthesiol Scand* 1995;**39**:279–87.

Milde LN. Drug dependence among anaesthetists in the United States. *Royal College of Anaesthetists Newsletter* 1998;**39**:12–15.

Moyle JTB. In: Hahn CEW, Adams AP, eds. *Pulse Oximetry. Principles and Practice Series*. London: BMJ Publishing Group, 1994

O'Flaherty, D. In: Hahn CEW, Adams AP, eds. *Capnography. Principles and Practice Series*. London: BMJ Publishing Group, 1994.

Runciman WB. Risk assessment in the formulation of anaesthesia safety standards. *Eur J Anaesthesiol* 1993;**10**(suppl 7):26–32.

Scott WE, Vickers MD, Draper H. *Ethical Issues in Anaesthesia*. Oxford: Butterworth-Heinemann, 1994.

Taylor TH, Major E, eds. *Hazards and Complications of Anaesthesia,* 2nd edn. Edinburgh: Churchill Livingstone. 1993.

White E, Crosse MM. The aetiology and prevention of peri-operative corneal abrasions. *Anaesthesia* 1998;**53**:157–61.

# Chapter 13 The unexpected event

P. Hutton and C. Dodds

This chapter gathers together a number of events, all of which are unwelcome and can occur unexpectedly at any time. They are together simply because they do not fall automatically into other sections of the book. There are obviously many other causes of sudden difficulty (e.g. laryngospasm, impossible intubatation, etc.), but these are dealt with as they arise in the appropriate chapter.

## CRITICAL INCIDENT ANALYSIS

Although every death caused totally or partially by anaesthesia needs careful analysis to try to prevent its recurrence, deaths occur so infrequently that restricting analysis to them alone misses most of the problems. Consequently, it is more profitable to look at morbidity and 'close shaves' to establish patterns of common error. The process of doing this is called critical incident analysis.

The critical incident reporting method was first published in the *Psychological Bulletin* in 1954, but the technique had been used previously by the US military during the Second World War. It has been applied to several medical specialties and the first publications in anaesthesia appeared in the 1970s. There have been several definitions of what constitutes a critical incident. One currently in use and accepted for reporting by the Royal College of Anaesthetists (UK) is:

> 'An event which led to harm, or could have led to harm if it had been allowed to progress. It should be preventable by a change in practice.'

The potential for harm is usually to the patient but could be to the anaesthetist or another member of staff. The adverse event could be caused by the anaesthetist, another member of staff, equipment, or the organizational environment (e.g. the wrong patient arrives in the anaesthetic room). The great majority of critical incidents do not lead to adverse outcomes and much larger quantities of data can be collected than by identification of adverse outcomes alone. All critical incident reporting schemes and reports to date have two major uncertainties:

1. The reporting is voluntary. The anaesthetists who send in reports are probably conscientious doctors who are willing to learn from their experience and to change their practice appropriately.
2. Only the reported cases can be counted. Although common patterns of occurrence can be established, there is no denominator from which to produce incidence figures. It is not possible, for instance, to give a figure for the percentage of cases in which a disconnection occurs.

Despite these drawbacks, the benefits of critical incident reporting have led to its adoption in many departments of anaesthesia around the world. It is now regarded as one of the components of a hospital's risk management strategy, although there is considerable debate about how the information should be used. An obvious problem is that a caring reporter may (wrongly) be regarded as a high-risk doctor if confidentiality is breached. Imposing the threat of this or subsequent disciplinary action will encourage under-reporting. Whether critical incident reporting should be carried out continuously or as a time-limited exercise is another moot point. Continuous reporting is the ideal, but, in a voluntary system, may result in a loss of enthusiasm with time.

Given these limitations, critical incident reports have nevertheless produced very valuable data and they have all identified several common themes. The causes of critical incidents as a percentage of those reported is typically as given in Table 13.1.

The findings of the study shown in Table 13.1, which was published 15 years ago, have been replicated many times since. The uniform findings are that:

- human error is the most frequent cause of critical incidents;
- a problem with the gas supply and/or airway management is the most common site of the difficulty;
- the time of highest risk is during maintenance anaesthesia.

The categories of human error associated with critical incidents are shown in Table 13.2. Note the frequency of problems that involve getting fresh gas into the patient and expired gas safely out. The common occurrence of such problems is one of the strongest arguments for using the combination of a capnograph with a pulse oximeter.

**Table 13.1. Causes of critical incidents as a percentage of the total reported**

| Cause of incident | % |
|---|---|
| Human error | 68.2 |
| Equipment failure | 13.4 |
| Disconnection | 13.0 |
| Others | 5.4 |

Adapted from Cooper JB et al. *Anesthesiology* 1984;60:34.

**Table 13.2. Categories of human error contributing to critical incidents during anaesthesia**

| Category of human error | Percentage of total | |
|---|---|---|
| Problem with airway management | 16 | 49 |
| Problem with breathing system | 11 | |
| Misuse of anaesthesia machine | 22 | |
| Wrong drug administered | 24 | |
| Disconnection of intravenous infusion | 6 | |
| Mismanagement of fluid therapy | 5 | |
| Failure of monitoring | 4 | |
| Others | 12 | |

Adapted from Cooper JB *et al. Anesthesiology* 1984;60:34.

**Table 13.3. Factors minimizing the adverse outcome of critical incidents**

| Factor | % of total |
|---|---|
| Prior experience or awareness of problem | 35 |
| Monitor detection | 35 |
| Recheck of equipment | 15 |
| Skilled assistance | 12 |
| Supervision | 9 |
| Other factor | 8 |
| Staff change | 2 |

Adapted from Williamson JA *et al. Anaesth Intens Care* 1993;21:678.

A large Australian study, published in 1993, identified a list of the factors that minimized the adverse outcome of critical incidents. This is reproduced in Table 13.3. Again note the preponderance of human factors but also the importance of monitors.

Critical incident reporting is now an established tool for looking at clinical practice. The same messages continue to emerge with monotonous regularity. This means that we do not always learn from experience when the incidence of disasters is low. It is therefore important to keep the system going so that each of us is reminded of the things that can go wrong before we injure patients. In reporting the event, it is hoped that we remind our colleagues of the common errors of everyday practice and in so doing improve patient safety.

## ANAPHYLACTIC REACTION

Anaphylactic reactions are rare during anaesthesia. When they do occur, even patients with severe reactions should show a prompt and successful response to the appropriate treatment. Every anaesthetist should therefore know an 'anaphylaxis drill' to optimize the outcome of these uncommon events.

### Definition

Anaphylaxis (or the result of an anaphylactic reaction) is an exaggerated response to a substance to which an individual has become sensitized. Histamine, serotonin, and other vasoactive substances are released from basophils and mast cells in response to an immunoglobulin E (IgE)-mediated reaction. This causes the symptoms and signs in Table 13.4.

An anaphylactoid reaction can be clinically indistinguishable from an anaphylactic reaction, but it is not mediated by a sensitizing IgE antibody.

### Incidence

Estimation of the frequency is difficult but it is probably between 1 in 5000 and 1 in 20 000 anaesthetics and is three to five times more common in women than in men. It can occur with no previous history of drug exposure. The most common triggers are intravenous drugs (Table 13.5). Latex allergy is being recognized more frequently as a cause but no inhalational agent has ever been implicated as a trigger.

### Clinical features at presentation and during anaphylaxis

The presenting clinical features and the predominating clinical consequences are given in Tables 13.6 and 13.7.

### Diagnosis

Diagnosis is made on the presenting clinical picture and treatment should be started immediately.

### Management of a suspected anaphylactic reaction

***General advice***

Send for help; stop administering the offending drug; give 100% oxygen. If there is not one already *in situ*, put in an intravenous cannula and connect a litre of saline or colloid. In life-threatening cases, if this is difficult, do not waste time but press on as described below.

**Table 13.4. Symptoms and signs of an anaphylactic reaction**

| | |
|---|---|
| Pruritus | Erythema |
| Flushing | Urticaria |
| Angio-oedema | Nausea |
| Diarrhoea | Vomiting |
| Laryngeal oedema | Bronchospasm |
| Hypotension | Cardiovascular collapse and death |

**Table 13.5. Incidence of reported anaphylactic or severe anaphylactoid reactions from anaesthesia-related drugs**

| Induction agents | Neuromuscular blocking agents | Local anaesthetic agents |
|---|---|---|
| Thiopentone | Suxamethonium | Bupivacaine |
| Propofol | Alcuronium | Lignocaine (lidocaine) |
| Etomidate | Atracurium | Prilocaine |
| Methohexitone (methohexital) | Vecuronium | |
| | Gallamine | |
| | Tubocurarine | |
| | Pancuronium | |

The agents are listed with the most common reporting incidence at the top of each column. Note that the incidence of reporting depends on the usage of the drug and does not necessarily indicate the tendency to produce serious reactions per administration. Adapted from Watkins J. *Anaesthesia* 1989;44:157.

**Table 13.6. Presenting clinical features of anaphylaxis**

| Presenting feature | Incidence (%) |
|---|---|
| Marked fall in arterial pressure; no pulse detectable | 28 |
| Difficult to inflate lungs | 26 |
| Flushing | 21 |
| Coughing | 6 |
| Rash | 4 |
| Desaturation | 3 |
| Cyanosis | 3 |
| Others (e.g. ECG changes, urticaria, swelling) | 9 |

Adapted from Association of Anaesthetists of Great Britain and Ireland, *Suspected Anaphylactic Reactions Associated with Anaesthesia*, 2nd edn. 1995,8.

**Table 13.7. Clinical features of established anaphylaxis**

| Clinical feature | Incidence (%) |
|---|---|
| Cardiovascular collapse | 88 |
| Cutaneous signs (rashes, urticaria, erythema, etc.) | 66 |
| Bronchospasm | 36 |
| Angio-oedema of the face | 24 |
| Generalized oedema | 7 |

Adapted from Association of Anaesthetists of Great Britain and Ireland, *Suspected Anaphylactic Reactions Associated with Anaesthesia*, 2nd edn. 1995,8.

***Initial therapy***

- Stop administration of drug(s) likely to have caused the anaphylaxis.
- Maintain airway: give 100% $O_2$; intubate if necessary.
- Lay patient flat with feet elevated.
- Give epinephrine (adrenaline); this may be given intramuscularly in a dose of 0.5–1 mg (0.5–1 ml of 1 : 1000) and may be repeated every 10 min according to the arterial pressure and pulse until improvement occurs.
  - Alternatively, epinephrine, 50–100 μg (0.5–1 ml of 1 : 10 000) intravenously over 1 min, has been recommended for hypotension with titration of further doses as required.
  - In a patient with cardiovascular collapse, intravenous epinephrine, 0.5–1 mg (5–10 ml of 1:10 000), may be required and should be given in divided doses by titration. This should be administered at a rate of 0.1 mg/min (1 ml/min of 1 : 10 000), stopping when an adequate response has been obtained.
- Start intravascular volume expansion with crystalloid or colloid.

***Secondary therapy***

- Antihistamines (chlorpheniramine 10–20 mg by slow intravenous infusion).
- Corticosteroids (100–300 mg hydrocortisone i.v.).
- Catecholamine infusions (starting doses: epinephrine 4–8 μg/min [0.05–0.1 μg/kg per min]; norepinephrine 4–8 μg/min [0.05–0.1 μg/kg per min]; isoprenaline (isoproterenol) 4–8 μg/min [0.05–1 μg/kg per min]).
- Consider bicarbonate (0.5–1.0 mmol/kg i.v.) for acidosis.
- Airway evaluation, looking for oedema (*before* extubation).
- Bronchodilators may be required for persistent bronchospasm.

### After resolution

Most reactions will occur in the anaesthetic room or very early into the surgery. As soon as the diagnosis of anaphylaxis becomes a possibility, do not start or, if it has started, halt the progress of surgery. It depends on the patient and the urgency of the operation as to the best course of action. With a severe reaction preceding minor elective surgery (e.g. carpal tunnel release), it would be best to abandon the procedure on that day; with a mild reaction preceding major surgery for a life-threatening condition (e.g. suspected ectopic pregnancy), it is probably in the patient's best interests to press on. Between these two extremes, clinical judgement is required and the decision is probably best taken by more than one person.

### Investigation of a suspected anaphylactic reaction associated with anaesthesia

#### *Immediate*

1. Do not attempt any investigation until the immediate treatment of the emergency has been completed.
2. Diagnosis is made on clinical grounds. It is important to make a detailed written record of events, including timing of administration of all drugs in relation to onset of reaction.
3. Approximately 1 hour after the beginning of the reaction, take 10 ml venous blood into a plain glass tube. Separate serum and store at –20°C until the sample can be sent to a reference laboratory for estimation of serum tryptase concentration. Tryptase is the principal protein in mast cell granules and is released (together with histamine and other amines) during a reaction.

#### *Later*

4. *The anaesthetist is responsible for ensuring adequate investigation and providing advice to the patient*. This responsibility cannot be delegated. The patient should be encouraged to carry an anaesthetic hazard card or to wear a Medic-Alert bracelet.
5. After the patient has recovered, a detailed history including concurrent illness, previous anaesthetic history, and any known allergies should be taken.
6. Skin tests should be performed with all anaesthetic drugs (except inhalational agents) used in the procedure and with other anaesthetic agents that might be used in future procedures.
7. Only a minority of anaesthetists will feel competent to conduct and interpret such tests; the majority will need to obtain specialist advice either from a more expert colleague or from a specialist in allergy and clinical immunology.

#### *Reporting*

The event should be reported to the relevant national drugs regulatory body. In the UK this is the Committee for the Safety of Medicines which supplies specific 'yellow cards'.

#### *Screening*

There is no evidence or support at the present time for the routine screening of patients for specific drug antibodies before anaesthesia.

## CARDIAC ARREST AND RESUSCITATION

All anaesthetists and most other doctors become involved in treating sudden collapse from time to time. Over the past 10 years or so, there has been a gradually increasing uniformity in the way in which these situations are managed. This is very much in the patient's interests because it means that all the personnel at the scene will be targeting their efforts in the same direction and working to a common plan. It is the responsibility of all anaesthetists to be aware of the guidelines on management and to take part, when asked, in the education of others to the same end. Each country has some sort of administrative body that oversees the publication of relevant documentation and ensures that the published advice takes account of the latest developments in knowledge. In some countries this function is under one of the medical colleges: in the UK it is led by the Resuscitation Council (UK), which was a founder member of the European Resuscitation Council. The general thrust of developments in resuscitation has been to keep the algorithms as simple as possible, provided that they are compatible with the optimum outcome. During resuscitation, regular doses of epinephrine are recommended because it is thought to improve cerebral and coronary blood flow and the rate of return of spontaneous circulation. This section briefly outlines the current management pathways, and comments on a few other key aspects of the process. Trainees should always work from the latest version of published guidelines in their country. The management of complex arrhythmias is not considered here.

All resuscitation events can be divided into three phases.

1. Basic life support (BLS):
   (a) airway control;
   (b) breathing support;
   (c) circulatory support.

2. Advanced life support (ALS):
   (a) intubation, ventilation, and $O_2$;
   (b) continued circulatory support;
   (c) defibrillation;
   (d) drugs and fluids;
   (e) management of arrhythmias.

3. Prolonged life support:
   (a) intensive care;
   (b) withdrawal of treatment issues;
   (c) management of neurological deficits;
   (d) quality of life issues.

### Adult resuscitation

For every 10 in-hospital resuscitation events approximately:

- three survive the initial resuscitation procedure;
- two survive for 24 hours;
- one and a half survive to go home;
- one survives for a year;
- two and a half survive for more than a year.

These figures tell a graphic story. In addition, they emphasize that in only a very few patients will the event have been so brief and the recovery so fast that they will not require some time on an intensive care unit (ICU) or other specialized unit. Resuscitation victims are therefore consumers of scarce resources if the immediate resuscitation is successful. The most common cause of brain damage after cardiac arrest is delay in starting resuscitation, so when circulatory arrest has occurred, the time to arrival of the first trained person is crucial. That is the main reason why all staff in a hospital should be capable of instituting BLS.

The signs of cardiac arrest are shown in Figure 13.1. Note that the presence of dilated pupils before, during, or after resuscitation is an unreliable sign of circulatory arrest. Sudden loss of consciousness and absence of breathing and major pulses are sufficient to justify the diagnosis. Intraoperatively, without invasive monitoring it may be difficult to differentiate between profound hypotension and circulatory arrest. If neither anaesthetist nor surgeon can, however, feel a pulse, external massage should be started immediately, whatever the cause of the problem. When in the operating room, do not forget always to make a rapid check of the breathing system in a ventilated patient to make sure that it is not a hypoxic arrest secondary to $O_2$ failure or disconnection, etc. In all situations, whether in or out of hospital, follow the approved local guidelines. The algorithms published in the UK by the Resuscitation Council for BLS and ALS are given in Figures 13.2 and 13.3 (adults) and 13.4 and 13.5 (children). Notes on each are given below. For full information, consult the Resuscitation Council's Handbook referred to at the end of the chapter.

### Basic life support

The algorithm for this is given in Figure 13.2.

- Always first ensure the safety of the rescuer and victim. A dead hero is useless.
- If there might be a cervical injury, stabilize the neck and be careful in tilting the head. Quadriplegia is to be avoided but an airway is a necessity for survival.
- If there are two rescuers, one should start resuscitation while the other goes for help.
- If there is only one rescuer, and the victim is an adult who has not suffered drowning or trauma, and is not breathing, assume that they have a heart problem and summon help immediately. Under these conditions early arrival of equipment to perform advanced resuscitation is crucial. If the victim has suffered drowning or trauma, perform resuscitation for 1 minute before going for help, in the expectation that spontaneous breathing and circulation might be restored.

### Advanced life support

The algorithm for this is given in Figure 13.3.

- Although it is essential to follow the algorithm, when commencing resuscitation, *always think hard about possible reversible causes of cardiac arrest* (especially during anaesthesia or postoperatively). If these causes are not detected and corrected, ALS will fail.
- In adults, ventricular fibrillation (VF) or pulseless ventricular tachyarrhythmia(VT) is the most common primary arrhythmia causing cardiac arrest, and the chances of successful defibrillation decline by 5% per min. The need to minimize delays in defibrillation is obvious.
- During emergency defibrillation, the polarity of the paddles is unimportant but their positioning is crucial.

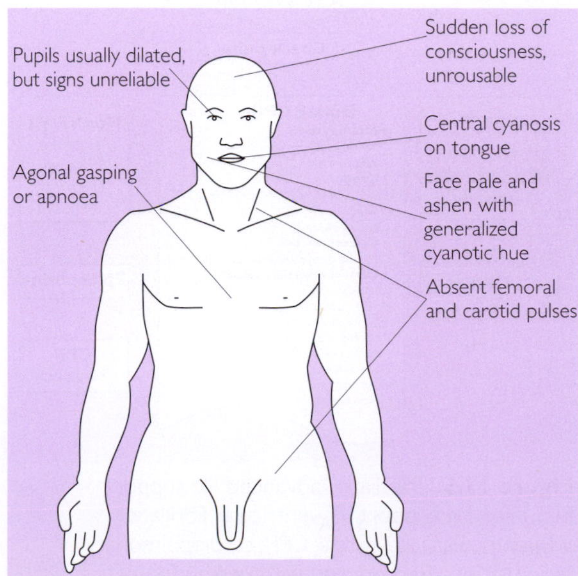


**Figure 13.1.** The signs of cardiac arrest.

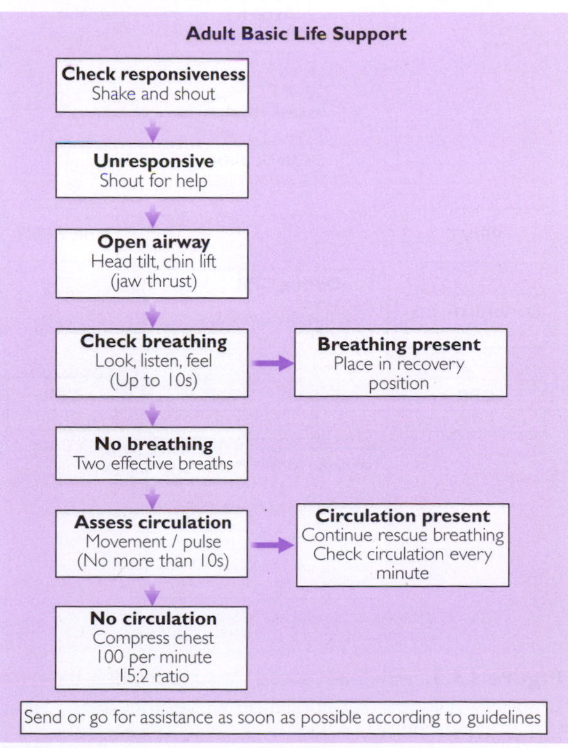


**Figure 13.2.** Adult basic life support. (Reproduced with permission of the Resuscitation Council, UK.)

- Defibrillation should be carried out in the sequence 200 J, 200 J, 360 J, and thereafter 360 J at the times indicated on the algorithm (Figure 13.3).
- Although not stated on the algorithm (Figure 13.3), 1 mg epinephrine should be administered every 3 min, whichever loop you are following, and its effect reviewed before administration of the next dose. Particular care should be taken in the use of epinephrine when resuscitating patients subject to an overdose of sympathomimetic drugs, e.g. solvents, cocaine, Ecstasy.
- All drugs given peripherally should be flushed in with 20 ml of 0.9% saline.
- Treat other rhythms with appropriate drug therapy as they arise.

### Paediatric resuscitation

Resuscitation in paediatric practice differs depending on whether the child is a neonate, an infant (up to 1 year), or a child (up to 8 years). Neonatal resuscitation is not considered here and reference should be made to specialist texts for information on this subject.

Guidelines for the resuscitation of children are as follows:

- As with adults, always ensure the safety of the rescuer and child.
- As with adults, stabilize the neck and avoid head tilt if cervical trauma is suspected.
- If only one rescuer is present, perform BLS for about 1 minute in the expectation of a response before going for assistance. It may be possible to

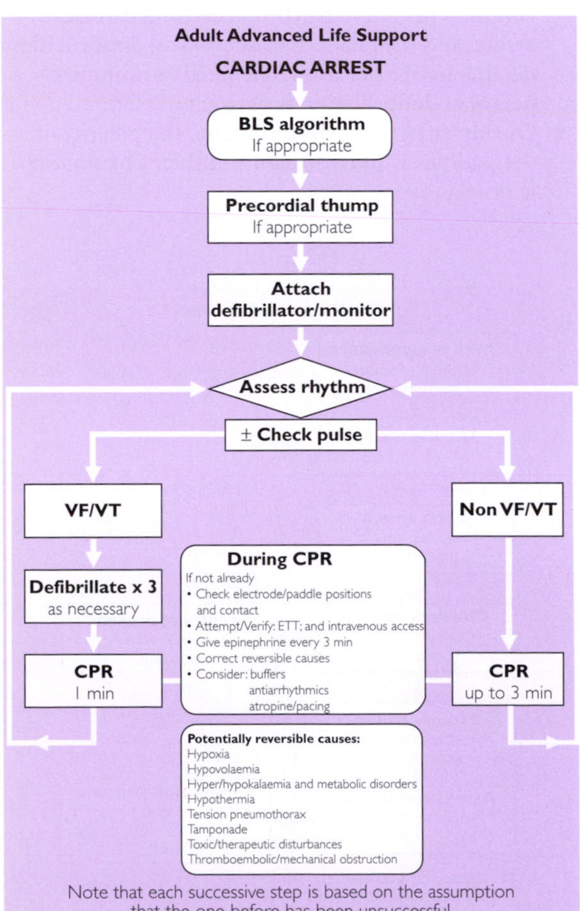


**Figure 13.3.** Adult advanced life support; BLS, basic life support; VF, ventricular fibrillation; VT, ventricular tachycardia; CPR, cardiopulmonary resuscitation; ETT, endotracheal tube. (Reproduced with permission of the Resuscitation Council, UK.)

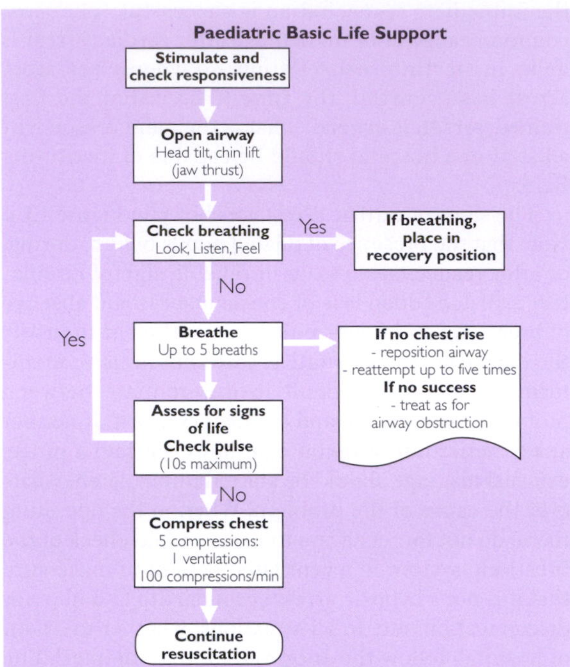


**Figure 13.4.** Paediatric basic life support. (Reproduced with permission of the Resuscitation Council, UK.)

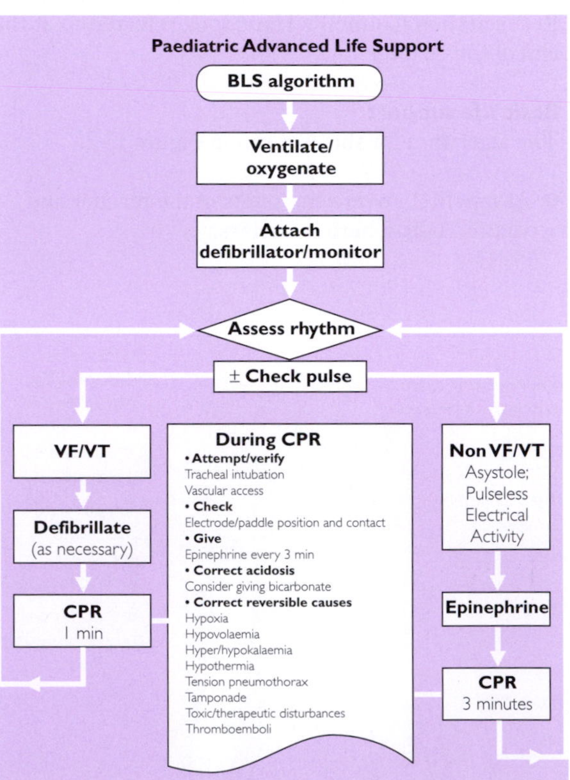


**Figure 13.5.** Paediatric advanced life support. BLS, basic life support; VF, ventricular fibrillation; VT, ventricular tachycardia; CPR, cardiopulmonary resuscitation. (Reproduced with permission of the Resuscitation Council, UK.)

take the infant or child with you while summoning help.

- The same arguments apply to children as to adults with respect to potentially reversible causes of cardiac arrest.
- Asystole and pulseless electrical activity are more common in children and epinephrine is the cornerstone of therapy.
- The first dose of epinephrine should be 10 μg/kg i.v. followed at 3-min intervals by 100 μg/kg i.v.
- If VF/VT do occur, the sequence of shocks is 2 J/kg, 2 J/kg, 4 J/kg, and 4 J/kg thereafter.

Algorithms for basic and advanced paediatric life support are given in Figures 13.4 and 13.5.

## SUXAMETHONIUM APNOEA

The short duration action of the depolarizing neuromuscular blocking agent suxamethonium depends to a large degree on its breakdown by plasma cholinesterase. The normal half-life of suxamethonium is 2–4 min, but this will be increased by falls in the availability or activity of plasma cholinesterase. This reduction in cholinesterase activity may be caused by genetic factors, or by chronic illness such as liver disease, renal failure, hypothyroidism, pregnancy, or a myocardial infarction. Intensive care procedures such as haemodialysis can also reduce the concentrations of cholinesterase. Neuromuscular junction diseases, e.g. myasthenia gravis, will extend the duration of blockade, but the cause is not specific to the relaxant being used. Abnormalities of suxamethonium metabolism are also discussed in Chapter 35 to which reference should be made.

### Plasma cholinesterase

Plasma cholinesterase is synthesized in the liver and is a tetrameric glycoprotein, containing four identical subunits, each having one active catalytic site. The molecular weight of the tetramer is approximately 342 000. Plasma cholinesterase is involved in the metabolism of suxamethonium, mivacurium, procaine, cocaine, and diamorphine. There are several variants of cholinesterase, all arising from alterations in the expression of one gene, which is situated on chromosome 3.

### Clinical features of suxamethonium apnoea

After administration of suxamethonium, the onset of relaxation is normal but there is a very delayed recovery of muscle power. Nerve stimulation, using a train-of-four pattern, shows loss of all four responses, and no post-tetanic facilitation. Recovery is slow and there is no evidence of fade across the four responses. The time to complete recovery will depend on whether the patient is homozygous or heterozygous.

Suxamethonium apnoea only rarely gives rise to anaesthetic problems because the preservation of an adequate airway and depth of anaesthesia do not depend on the duration of action of the depolarizing neuromuscular blocking agent. If it occurs, anaesthesia should be maintained until complete recovery of muscle power occurs. This may take 4 or more hours in severe cases. When a case of suspected suxamethonium apnoea occurs, if not already using one, obtain and attach a neuromuscular block monitor to confirm the diagnosis. In some instances, continuing muscle weakness will not become apparent until the end of surgery when attempts are made to wake the patient. It is extremely distressing for patients to be conscious but paralysed. Therefore, once the problem is recognized, whatever stage the surgical procedure is at, it is important to observe the following principles:

- Keep the patient asleep and well oxygenated until muscle power has returned.
- Do not perform repeated tests of tetanic contraction on awake or semi-conscious patients. They are painful and unpleasant.
- Monitor the expired $CO_2$ to ensure ventilation to normocapnia so that the physiological trigger to breathing is not suppressed.
- Make sure that the ward staff or relatives of the patient who are in the hospital know what has happened so that they can be reassured about the patient's condition.

If suxamethonium apnoea is discovered after induction, surgery can still proceed, and if necessary the patient can be maintained in either the operating room or an ICU depending on the facilities available.

The most common age group presenting with suxamethonium apnoea is children, often for strabismus surgery. In these instances, in particular, reassurance of the family that all is well is vital. They should be told that they and their child appear to have a sensitivity to an anaesthetic drug, and that it is very important for this to be confirmed by a blood test as soon as possible.

### Investigation of possible causes

The genetic causes for deficiencies in cholinesterase can be investigated and diagnosed using the response of the patient's plasma to dibucaine or fluoride inhibition of hydrolysis. More recently, the application of DNA analytical techniques permits precise identification of plasma cholinesterase variants, many of which are difficult or impossible to differentiate using traditional chemical inhibitory techniques. Details of the variants are given in Chapter 35, Table 35.1. It should be emphasized that, following a case of suxamethonium apnoea, it is the responsibility of the anaesthetist to ensure that the appropriate tests are carried out at either the local hospital or regional centre.

#### *Clinical significance*

A family history of anaesthetic problems, specifically suxamethonium apnoea, should always be sought, because unexpected prolongation of relaxation with other drugs such as mivacurium may occur. Provided that these drugs are avoided, there is little clinical significance for the patient, but, where there are imperative clinical reasons for rapidly securing the airway by intubation, a history of suxamethonium apnoea may have to be accepted and the drug still used. Alternative methods of rapid induction and intubation are still less satisfactory and less safe.

## MANAGEMENT OF A SUDDEN PNEUMOTHORAX

Any collection of air within the pleural cavity constitutes a pneumothorax. The severity of the condition depends upon the volume of air present, how fast it develops, and whether there is a direct connection between the pleural cavity and the bronchi. The clinical features may vary from none if the pneumothorax is small, to life-threatening cardiovascular collapse if a tension pneumothorax develops. There may be breathlessness or pleuritic pain, which may be short-lived in mild cases.

The signs of a pneumothorax are of increased percussion resonation with diminished air entry and reduced transmission of breath and vocal sounds on the same side. The trachea may be displaced to the opposite side if the pneumothorax is large or under tension.

A tension pneumothorax occurs when there is a direct leak of air into the pleural cavity on inspiration, but during expiration the leak is sealed. This produces a one-way valve effect which rapidly distends the pleural cavity, causing collapse of the ipsilateral lung, displacement of the trachea and mediastinum, and compression of the major veins, so reducing cardiac filling and engorging the jugular veins. There is a rapid onset of respiratory distress and cardiovascular collapse which if untreated leads to death.

Investigation of a pneumothorax is secondary to the evaluation of its clinical effect. If there is a suspicion of a tension pneumothorax on clinical examination – dyspnoea, tachycardia, hypotension, tracheal deviation, and jugular engorgement – immediate treatment by inserting a large-bore (14-gauge) cannula into the anterior chest wall, usually in the midclavicular line, just over the top of the third rib at the bottom of the second intercostal space, is life-saving. Precise placement is less critical than effective relief of the tension. Summoning more experienced help is essential but must not delay this immediate care. Once the tension has been relieved, a more formal assessment of the pneumothorax may take place. This assessment is the same for all cases, and includes investigations to confirm the side and size of the pneumothorax, whether it is bilateral, whether there are associated injuries such as fractured ribs, and to make a diagnosis of the cause of the pneumothorax. These will then dictate the subsequent treatment of the patient.

A supine portable chest radiograph is not the best upon which to identify a pneumothorax and if a pneumothorax is seen, it is difficult to judge its size. An erect inspiratory chest radiograph will confirm the presence of a pneumothorax by visualizing a cusp of air between the ribs and a clear lung shadow. The size of a pneumothorax may vary considerably and, if there is just a small rim of air seen, no further action may be indicated. Larger volumes need to be aspirated or a drain inserted. If there is doubt about the value of aspiration, go directly to drain insertion.

Aspiration can be done after local anaesthetic infiltration of the anterior chest wall using a 12- or 14-gauge needle, a three-way tap, and a 50-ml syringe. Aspiration of up to 2 litres is safe, but the procedure should be stopped if the patient coughs or if excessive resistance on aspiration is noted. Both of these indicate that the visceral pleura is in contact with the needle, and that further aspiration is likely to make matters worse.

If aspiration is unsuccessful, or if after aspiration there is a further accumulation of air or if there had been a tension pneumothorax, then a chest drain with an underwater seal should be inserted (Figure 13.6). It is essential when doing this not to lacerate the underlying lung, so blunt dissection is important. This has been emphasized in an editorial referred to at the end of this chapter (Hyde *et al*). When the chest drain is satisfactorily in position, there should be a sudden release of air followed by a rapid decrease in the air driven through the water seal. After this the fluid should rise and fall with breathing. If air continues to drain there is either a leak around the drain or there is the possibility of a bronchopleural fistula. An experienced opinion is necessary for further management of the patient if the leakage continues. As long as the patient is still being ventilated, the chest drain bottle must not be attached to a suction pump. If there is a large leak in the lung, the loss of gas can be sufficient to overwhelm the capacity of the pump and it will be prevented from leaving the thorax, causing a build up of intrathoracic pressure.

The drain can be removed after it has ceased to swing for several hours, a chest x-ray confirms lung re-expansion and the patient is well oxygenated.

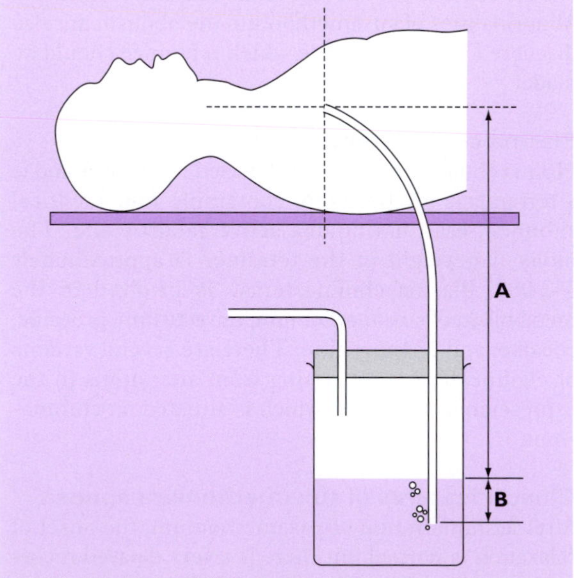


**Figure 13.6.** Diagram of an underwater seal system for a chest drain. The height of the fluid column in the jar determines the resistance (B in $cmH_2O$) that has to be overcome to allow air to escape. The volume of water in the drainage bottle has to be greater than the volume of the chest drainage tubing to the patient. This, together with the difference in height between the bottle and the patient, prevents contamination of the patient's pleural cavity with the fluid in the bottle. For this reason the drainage bottle must always be below the level of the patient (or clamped off). A safe height difference (A) is at least 60 $cmH_2O$ minus the normal maximum inspiratory pressure.

## MALIGNANT HYPERTHERMIA

Malignant hyperthermia (MH) susceptibility is an uncommon inherited disorder of skeletal muscle in which some drugs commonly used in anaesthesia trigger sustained skeletal muscle hypermetabolism. It has an autosomal dominant inheritance, but many cases are sporadic, with less than 25% of patients who experience an MH event having a positive family history. Exposure to a triggering agent is usually necessary but not always sufficient for the susceptible person to experience symptoms. The frequency of MH varies with the patient population, the type of anaesthesia used, and definition of the MH event. The frequency is approximately 1 in 50 000 adults, 1 in 15 000 children, 1 in 250 000 anaesthetics for a fulminant case of MH, and 1 in 6000 for a possible MH event. MH presents with multiple, non-specific, clinical signs of hypermetabolism, and laboratory findings of variable intensity and time course during and after exposure to anaesthetic agents.

The MH syndrome is caused by a deficiency in the re-uptake of calcium ions by the sarcoplasmic reticulum, which results in a failure of muscle relaxation after contraction (see Chapter 24). Consequently, muscle contraction is sustained, the rate of metabolism increases dramatically, and the clinical MH syndrome develops. Although the condition usually presents intraoperatively, if the operation is short and the onset delayed, signs may not be apparent until the patient is in recovery or even back on the ward. The most potent triggers are suxamethonium and halothane, although all volatile agents are potential triggers.

### Presenting features

#### *Those caused by failure of muscle relaxation*

Masseter spasm after giving suxamethonium is associated with MH, but not all patients who get masseter spasm will go on to develop MH. When MH occurs, a generalized increase in muscle tone develops during the anaesthetic even in the presence of adequate neuromuscular blockade. This is because the biochemical abnormality is intracellular and not mediated by the neuromuscular junction.

#### *Those caused by hypermetabolism*

These are often the first indication of the condition and include:

- unexplained tachycardia;
- hypercapnia in the ventilated and hyperpnoea in the spontaneously breathing patient;
- cyanosis and skin mottling;
- arrhythmias, predominantly ventricular;
- a rise in temperature;
- blood tests that show hypoxaemia, hyperkalaemia, hypercapnia, metabolic acidosis, and hypocalcaemia;
- later events are rhabdomyolysis, myoglobinuria, acute renal failure, and cardiac failure.

The most common presentation is increased heart rate (with or without arrythmias) with an accompanying rise in end-tidal $CO_2$ level and a fall in $O_2$ saturation. Temperature changes may be slow or unrecorded. The diagnosis is based on suspicion and clinical awareness.

### Management of the suspected or established case

#### *Stop presenting the stimulus to the patient*

Discontinue all volatile anaesthetics, and change the breathing system and machine. *Send for experienced help immediately and conclude surgery as soon as possible.*

#### *Institute comprehensive monitoring*

This should include direct arterial and central venous pressures, urine output, temperature, clotting, electrolytes, and blood gases.

#### *Treat the consequences of the hypermetabolism*

Hyperventilate on 100% $O_2$, give calcium and insulin/dextrose therapy for hyperkalaemia, sodium bicarbonate as determined by blood gases, and appropriate drugs for persistent and haemodynamically detrimental arrhythmias. Arrhythmias may respond to procainamide (3 mg/kg); remember to avoid calcium channel blockers. The minute volume may have to be three times normal to limit the rise in $CO_2$ tension.

#### *Arrest the progress of the condition*

The only pharmacological therapeutic agent is dantrolene. This is presented as a powder and has a short shelf life (18 months). Because it is needed infrequently and is expensive, dantrolene is kept in only a limited number of locations. The trainee should find out where these are in their hospital.

Give dantrolene (1 mg/kg every 5 min up to 10 mg/kg). Ask an assistant to mix this because it is time-consuming. Institute cooling measures commencing with surface cooling and iced intravenous fluids, progressing to viscus and body cavity irrigation (iced saline bladder and peritoneal lavage), and (in extreme cases) extracorporeal circulation as indicated.

#### *Maintain urine output*

Urine output should be maintained at over 2 ml/kg per min with copious fluids, mannitol, and frusemide (furosemide) to try to minimize the effects of myoglobinuria.

#### *Once the acute episode has subsided*

Monitor the patient carefully on an ICU for the next 12–24 hours, commence oral dantrolene (1 mg/kg 6-hourly for 48 hours), and continue close observation for 48–72 hours.

### Following resolution of the episode

*Do not forget* to refer the patient to a centre for appropriate tests and genetic counselling. Close blood relatives must be screened as well. If they test positive, a Medic-Alert bracelet is advisable.

*In vitro* caffeine and halothane contracture testing is the 'gold standard' on muscle biopsies. However, there is still a lack of clear clinical definition of MH, and the specificity and sensitivity of the tests are under constant refinement.

If a patient turns up with a family history of MH or if they have tested without absolute certainty, the avoidance of triggering agents is mandatory. A vapour-free anaesthesia machine should be used, there should be a second anaesthetist present, and dantrolene should be immediately available.

Safe anaesthetic agents include all opioids and local anaesthetics, non-depolarizing neuromuscular blocking agents, nitrous oxide, propofol, thiopentone (thiopental), and benzodiazepines. Etomidate, ketamine, and droperidol are also thought to be safe.

Prophylaxis with dantrolene is not routinely indicated.

## PULMONARY EMBOLISM

A pulmonary embolus (PE) can originate from many different parts of the vascular system and can have many different causes. Of greatest interest to the anaesthetist are gas embolism, thromboembolism, fat embolism and amniotic fluid embolism. Only the first two will be considered here because of their importance as critical incidents in the operative and post-operative periods, respectively.

The symptoms and signs of a major PE are caused by the reduction in blood flow through the pulmonary arteries, accompanied by a severe fall in left ventricular output. If the patient is conscious they experience a combination of chest pain, dyspnoea, tachypnoea, apprehension and coughing and become hypotensive and cyanosed. The clinical picture depends on the speed and extent of the occlusion and there may be 'air hunger' with cardiovascular collapse. Because areas of lung are ventilated but not perfused, there is a sudden increase in physiological dead space (see Chapter 16) with ventilation/perfusion mismatching. If the patient is anaesthetized and paralysed, expired $CO_2$ monitoring will show a sudden and progressive fall (over a few breaths) in the height of the alveolar plateau. In the face of constant ventilation without cardiac arrest, the fall to a lower but steady value of end-tidal $CO_2$ indicates the proportionate reduction in pulmonary blood flow caused by the embolus.

### Gas embolism

Gas embolism can be caused by air being drawn into open venous channels in the neck, muscles or cerebral sinuses; the ingress of air from a disconnected central venous pressure (CVP) line in the sitting position; air in a pressurized intravenous fluid administration system; or inadvertent intravascular high-flow $CO_2$ from laparoscopic surgery. The clinical consequences depend on the rate and volume of entrained gas, combined with the size and fitness of the patient. Small quantities of gas may go completely unnoticed with routine monitoring. A classic 'mill-wheel' murmur is usually present only with large amounts of gas (1.5 ml/kg per min), the capnograph shows a change at > 0.25 ml/kg per min, and Doppler techniques detect down to 0.1 ml/kg per min. In some operative procedures, for example neurosurgery in the sitting position, air embolus is a recognized complication and specific measures can be taken to monitor for it. This account assumes, however, that this is not the case and that a major embolus (approximately 0.5–1.5 ml/kg per min or > 50 ml bolus) presents unexpectedly in otherwise 'routine' anaesthesia.

On arrival in the right ventricle, a significant gas embolus generates foam and gas bubbles in the heart and pulmonary arteries. In so doing, right ventricular forward flow is reduced because ventricular beats compress gas rather than propelling fluid. The fall in pulmonary blood flow then produces the clinical and physiological changes described above. In addition, a major theoretical problem is paradoxical gas embolization to the arterial circulation through a patent foramen ovale, arteriovenous malformations and the normal pulmonary bed. If this occurs, even small volumes of gas in the coronary or cerebral circulation will produce serious morbidity or mortality.

Unexpected intra-operative gas embolism is rare but should always be considered as a possible cause of a sudden reduction in end-tidal $CO_2$ followed by cardiovascular collapse. ECG changes are non-specific and include both arrhythmias and gross morphological changes. The following is a suggested management plan.

- Look for a potential cause, e.g. insufflation of $CO_2$ during laparoscopic surgery; opening of venous sinuses during laminectomy.
- Take the relevant action to stop the gas embolus continuing, e.g. tell the surgeon to stop insufflating $CO_2$; ask him to flood the bony field with saline.
- Discontinue nitrous oxide; go on to 100% $O_2$.
- Tip the patient head down, preferably with the left side downwards.
- If a CVP or pulmonary artery catheter is present, try to aspirate air.
- Intubate and give intermittent positive-pressure ventilation if not already doing so.
- Resuscitate in the normal way following the adult ALS algorithm (Figure 13.3). Ensure adequate intravascular volume expansion.

The outcome depends on the speedy recovery of cardiac output and effective oxygenation. The prognosis from a $CO_2$ gas embolism is better than that for air because $CO_2$ is highly soluble and is more easily eliminated by continued ventilation. Air is less likely to go into solution and has a much longer period of arterial obstruction. Cerebral effects from gas embolism may occur directly because gas has entered the arterial system, or indirectly from the cardiovascular collapse. Where there is doubt about the extent of neurological dysfunction, cerebral protection strategies need serious consideration.

Although it is unlikely that a Doppler probe will be used during routine surgery, if one is in the locality, whether transthoracic or transoesophageal, it is useful to confirm what is often a presumptive diagnosis.

### Thromboembolism

Pulmonary thromboembolism usually arises from clots that break loose from a deep vein thrombosis (DVT) in the popliteal or ilieofemoral veins. This may occur at any time (including intraoperatively), but most commonly occurs 4–10 days after surgery. Some patients and procedures present specific risks and the only effective management to prevent a PE is to prevent DVT (see Chapter 1). Small emboli may occur frequently, with few symptoms apart from a decreasing arterial oxygen saturation. The clinical signs of tachypnoea, cyanosis, cardiovascular collapse and (later) haemoptysis and pleuritic pain may then be missing.

The classic presentation of a major PE is sudden chest pain and the acute onset of severe breathlessness, accompanied by hypotension and cynanosis, sometimes when straining at stool. Over 10% of patients presenting in this way die in the first hour. Clinical signs are usually non-specific but there can be a fixed splitting of the first heart sound. Simultaneous arterial and end-tidal $CO_2$ estimations show an increased gradient for the reasons given above. The ECG may show the 'classic' signs of right heart strain – deep S waves in lead 1, Q waves in lead 3 and an inverted T wave also in lead 3 (S1, Q3, T3). There may be right axis deviation, right bundle branch block or atrial fibrillation.

If a PE presents intraoperatively, diagnosis is presumptive and treatment essentially supportive. Volume expansion, resuscitation following the adult ALS algorithm and ventilation on 100% $O_2$ with (if necessary) positive end-expiratory pressure are the mainstays of treatment. Diagnosis usually has to wait until the postoperative period. Pulmonary angiography is accurate and has replaced ventilation/perfusion scan as the 'gold standard' for diagnosis. The decision as to whether thrombolysis and/or anticoagulation should begin immediately will depend on the type of surgery.

If a major PE occurs in the postoperative period (the normal time of presentation) and immediate resuscitation is of limited success, surgery and pulmonary embolectomy may be considered if the patient is in a unit capable of open-heart surgery. It is, however, rarely effective if the clot has been broken up and has travelled peripherally during external chest compression.

Provided that the patient survives the initial collapse, urgent anticoagulation is indicated. The site of the DVT should be sought – frequently the calf or pelvic veins. Heparin 10 000 units should be given over 10 minutes, followed by an intravenous infusion of 1000 units/hour. Streptokinase should also be considered if the diagnosis can be confirmed and all risks from surgical bleeding can be excluded. The patient needs high-concentration facemask $O_2$ and intravenous opioids, titrated to effect to provide pain relief.

Once the patient is stable on heparin, s/he should be converted to warfarin, and treatment continued for at least 3 months. Predisposing factors should then be sought, such as malignancy, systemic lupus erythematosus, or polycythaemia, and treated where identified. The patient should then be regarded as very high risk for all subsequent surgery and all prophylactic measures should be taken for even the most minor operation (see Chapter 1).

## AN ANAESTHETIC EVENT WITH AN ADVERSE OUTCOME

Anaesthetic disasters usually occur 'out of the blue', with little warning from the patient's history or examination. They are rapidly progressive, and frightening. Even in experienced hands the patient may die or be left severely disabled. The consequences of such events will be considered here.

During a serious complication, the detailed recording of the physiological events may be neglected. Recall after the event is limited and frequently inaccurate. However, the written record remains the most powerful evidence of what actually occurred. Legible writing of times, problems, actions, and any responses to them have to be detailed. These can be done by, or dictated to, another person at the scene (see Chapter 12, Figure 12.2). Immediate calls for help should be recorded along with the result. Copies of these records should be kept personally in case of future need. The duty or responsible consultant must be informed immediately of the disaster, together with the Clinical Director of Anaesthesia. As soon as possible contact your medical defence organization and take their advice.

Immediately after the event, everyone is shocked and usually supportive, but this is not always the case. If there is aggression or blame is being apportioned, seek senior help and support at once. After the initial shock wears off, self-doubt and blame or denial begins. Your mentor or training supervisor is there to support and advise you, but you may seek the help of any consultant more suited to you. Trying to 'go it alone' is highly unwise and leaves no one the opportunity to give the necessary support. The processes that follow a disaster may take well over a year to resolve, and being able to talk about it, in confidence, helps tremendously.

A realistic view of the adverse event has to be developed to allow recovery of confidence and progression in anaesthesia. There are several questions to answer. Was this a recognized but rare adverse effect? Was it more severe because of inexperienced or inadequate care? Was it solely the result of carelessness? Honesty in answering these questions is the beginning of coming to terms with events.

### Legal issues

Occasionally after a major disaster the doctor involved is suspended by the Medical Director or Chief Executive. This is not, in itself, punitive but is always intensely distressing. As a trainee it will involve a halt to your training until initial reports to the hospital have been received. You may have to give a report of your actions to a number of people. These include the hospital, medicolegal solicitors, the Coroner's Officer and the Police. Your defence organization must be closely involved. They will normally advise you not to admit to any direct fault in the event. You should seek to have your chosen mentor with you on all the occasions on which the issues are considered, and especially if speaking to relatives. If necessary, include solicitors from your defence organization.

If the patient died there will be a Coroner's inquest (in England and Wales). This usually involves an 'Opening' where the patient is formally identified and the Coroner orders further investigations – post-mortem examination, forensic tests, etc. The inquest is then adjourned until a later date, often many months away. The Coroner is legally responsible for deciding how and why the patient died, and once the inquest is reconvened he or she will question all involved about the event. Legal representation may be advisable if there is likely to be direct blame. The verdict that is reached reflects the Coroner's assessment of the event. 'Natural causes' means that the death can be interpreted as being part of the disease process, and that death was unavoidable. A verdict of 'Misadventure' means that, although death was related to the patient's condition, it was by no means likely. The verdict of 'Accidental death' essentially opens the case to the criminal proceedings or the civil action of negligence. The Coroner may also express his wish that the General Medical Council (GMC) investigates the competence of the doctors involved. Legal processes differ from country to country, and trainees need to be aware of the relevant laws.

If the patient is still alive, there may be a civil claim for damages. These will be made to the hospital and the Medical Director will ask for a detailed report from you, and will usually interview you (with your mentor for support). After these preliminary stages, the decision on further action will be taken with advice from the hospital's solicitors. They may not act in your interest at all, because they are not responsible to you. It is obvious that, although you may feel innocent of negligence and resentful of the slight to your professional standing, hard commercial decisions will be taken even if you have done nothing wrong. It may be decided to admit no fault and pay some modest compensation rather than defend the action.

Civil proceedings may take many years to come to Court and can be destructive events because of the adversarial nature of courts. The need to demonstrate facts 'beyond reasonable doubt' does not hold in civil legislation, and it is the 'balance of probabilities' that is used to test the evidence. Retention of your own copy of the event can be seen to be vital in this event. Trainees are not always involved in this process, but may be called as witnesses to support (or otherwise) their supervising, responsible consultants.

Finally, when all settles down, it is vital to review the ordeal with your mentor, to rebuild self-confidence and self-esteem. It also serves to close the book on the event.

## FURTHER READING

Aitkenhead AR. Safety in clinical anaesthesia. In: Aitkenhead AR, Jones RM, eds. *Clinical Anaesthesia*. London: Churchill Livingstone, 1996, 685–728.

Association of Anaesthetists of Great Britain and Ireland. *Suspected Anaphylactic Reactions Associated with Anaesthesia*. London: Association of Anaesthetists of Great Britain and Ireland, 1995.

Baskett PJF, Strunin L, eds. Postgraduate educational issue: Resuscitation. *Br J Anaesth* 1997;**79**:149–59.

Dakin MJ, Yentis SM. Latex allergy: a strategy for management. *Anaesthesia* 1998;**53**:774–81.

Ewan PW. ABC of allergies: Anaphylaxis. *BMJ* 1998;**316**:1442–5.

Articles in: Fisher M McD, ed. *The Anaesthetic Crisis. Baillière's Clin Anaesthesiol* 1993;**7**:199–508.

Medical Devices Agency. Latex sensitisation in the health care setting. *Device Bulletin*, April 1996

Pessah IN. Complex pharmacology of malignant hyperthermia. *Anesthesiology* 1996;**84**:1275–9.

Resuscitation Council (UK). *The 1997 Resuscitation Guidelines for use in the United Kingdom*. London: Resuscitation Council (UK), April 1997.

Roberts G. Is your environment safe? *Curr Anaesth Crit Care* 1995;**6**:255–9.

Runciman WB *et al*. The Australian Incident Monitoring Study. *Anaesth Intensive Care* 1993;**21**:506.

Sigundsson GH, MacAteer E. Morbidity and mortality associated with anaesthesia. *Acta Anaesthesiol Scand* 1996;**40**:1057–63.

Weinberg GL. *Genetics in Anesthesiology: Syndromes and Science*. Newton, MA: Butterworth-Heinemann, 1996.

# Chapter 14 Fluid balance and blood replacement

C. Dodds and P. Hutton

A clear understanding of the distribution of fluids through the intravascular and extracellular volumes is essential to provide safe care of the patient, as is the clinical assessment, measurement, and fluid replacement of these volumes. The cross-capillary and cross-membrane transfer of fluids, oxygen, metabolites, and nutrients to cells is highly dynamic. This chapter briefly examines the physiological basis of these phenomena (which are considered in greater detail in Chapter 19), relates them to patient management, and then considers specific problems of fluid balance and the intravenous solutions available for their correction. The chapter assumes that the patient is a fit adult; differences in very young and elderly people, and in those with specific pathological conditions, can be found in Chapters 41–66.

## FLUID DISTRIBUTION WITHIN BODY COMPARTMENTS

The distribution of water in humans is shown diagrammatically in Figure 14.1. The total body water is 60% of the total body weight in males and 55% in females. This is because females carry a slightly higher proportion of fat that is virtually anhydrous. In elderly people, the total body water falls to approximately 50% of the total body weight. The total body water is kept within tight limits by physiological homoeostatic mechanisms, but there is an obligatory movement of water into and out of the body to allow processes such as transport of nutrients and metabolites, and excretion of waste products, to occur. These are summarized in Figure 14.2. The major component in maintaining tight control of total body water is the urine because all the other methods of loss respond primarily to other requirements, e.g. increased perspiration to keep the body temperature constant or the humidification of inspired gases to prevent inspissation of mucus.

The composition of intracellular fluid (ICF) and extracellular fluid (ECF) is very different, as shown in Figure 14.2. The movement of water and electrolytes between compartments is a mixture of passive and active processes: passive processes do not require an energy source; active processes do. The main passive processes are hydrostatic pressure, diffusion, and osmosis, and the main active processes are membrane pumps and gated channels (see Chapter 19). In certain disease states, e.g. generalized sepsis, the detrimental effect on active processes results in maldistribution of fluids and electrolytes.

The fate of intravenous fluids depends on their ionic composition and their molecular size. An intact vascular endothelium contains within it colloids and molecules larger than about 60 000 daltons (Da). The movement of fluid (which contains electrolytes) between the capillaries and the interstitial fluid is determined primarily by the colloid osmotic forces and the hydrostatic forces across the capillary wall. Cell membranes, on the other hand, are effectively impermeable to sodium ions but highly permeable to water. This means that, in health, solutions with colloid are contained within the intravascular fluid volume; isotonic saline solutions are contained within the total ECF; and water is distributed throughout both the ICF and ECF volumes. These concepts are shown diagrammatically in Figure 14.3 and their fractional distributions are given in Table 14.1.

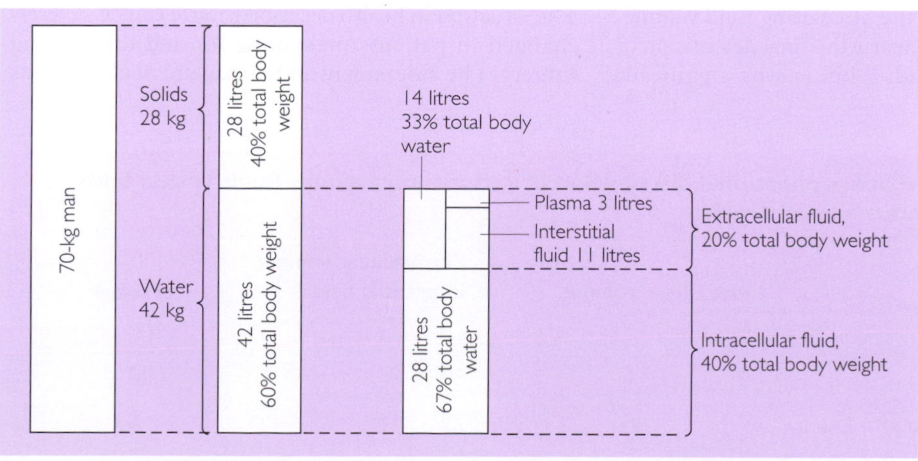


**Figure 14.1.** The distribution of water throughout the body in a human.

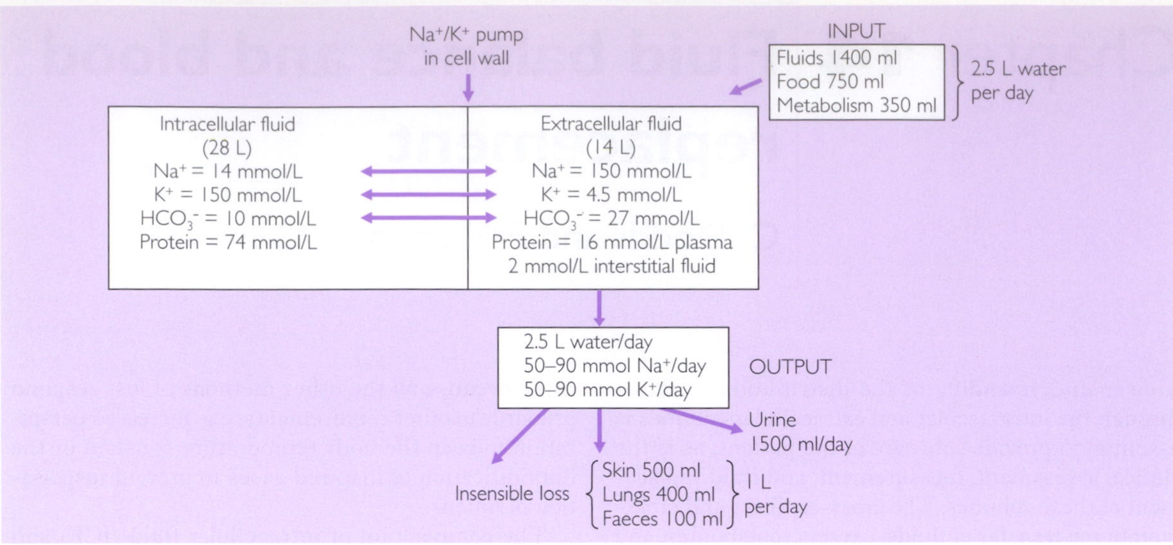


**Figure 14.2.** The electrolyte composition of intracellular and extracellular fluid and approximate daily intake and output. The approximate daily loss of $K^+$ and $Na^+$ is 1 mmol/kg per day in a healthy adult.

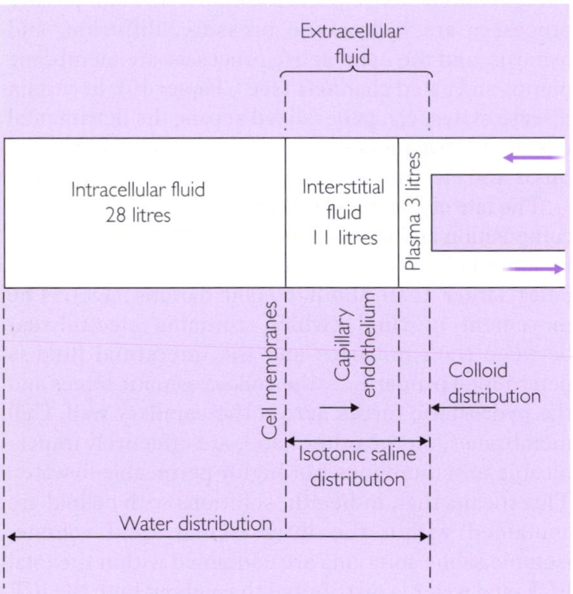


**Figure 14.3.** The distribution of colloid, isotonic saline, and water throughout the body fluid compartment.

Although, in an emergency, any intravenous fluid given rapidly will expand the circulating fluid volume, Table 14.1 demonstrates clearly the final destination of the various types of fluid. This is why significant volumes of crystalloid and even larger volumes of water (dextrose solutions) are required to replace a given blood loss.

If hypotonic saline (e.g. 0.45%) is administered, its distribution will lie between the figures for water and those for isotonic (0.9%) saline given in Table 14.1. The hypotonic solution distributes easily throughout the extracellular volume but reduces its osmolarity. This subsequently causes a shift in water from the ECF to the ICF, with volume expansion of the ICF until they are of equal osmolarity. The effect of hypertonic solutions is the reverse of this process, producing water extraction from the intracellular compartment.

Note that the intravascular fluid volume is identical to the blood volume, but that it excludes the volume of the red blood cells, which are a part of the ICF volume. The blood volume is therefore composed of extracellular and intracellular components, both of which are within the intravascular space. The blood volume varies through life, as shown in Table 14.2.

## EXAMPLES OF PRESENTING ABNORMALITIES OF FLUID BALANCE

The situation in health described above can be severely changed in patients presenting for and undergoing surgery. The assessment and management of fluid loss

**Table 14.1. Approximate proportional distribution of various intravenous fluids within body spaces after intravenous administration**

| Intravenous fluid | Intracellular volume | Extracellular volume<br>Interstitial fluid | Plasma |
|---|---|---|---|
| Colloid (%) | 0 | 0 | 100 |
| Isotonic saline (%) | 0 | 80 | 20 |
| Water (as dextrose solution) (%) | 67 | 25 | 8 |

**Table 14.2. Blood volume and age**

| Type of person | Volume (ml/kg) |
|---|---|
| Neonate (0–4 weeks) | 90–110 (depending on placental transfusion at birth) |
| Infant (4 weeks to 1 year) | 90 |
| Child (1 year to puberty) | 80 |
| Adult male | 70 |
| Adult female | 60 |

are a continuum that begins preoperatively, and concludes when the patient is mobile and drinking normally on the surgical ward. The principles underlying the assessment of loss of circulating volume are identical throughout these periods, and are based on the concept of identifying the percentage of acute volume loss and its physiological and clinical effects. That there are clearly defined classes of shock (see below) should not obscure the fact that these are progressive grades that blur into one another, and clinical judgement is essential. Observation of the patient is mandatory, and will always include the assessment of clinical signs, and measurement of cardiovascular and respiratory variables. Urine output monitoring is essential in most patients. Multisite temperature recording can also be of value in specific instances.

Appropriate volume replacement must always be initiated as soon as early signs of blood or fluid loss are apparent, not when the patient has decompensated and is becoming moribund. There are many sources of fluid loss: the surgical patient will not only have the normal insensible loss (Figure 14.2), but may, for instance, have additional losses from vomiting, bleeding, or leakage into the gut. The content of the fluid lost from the circulation has to be identified and appropriate replacement fluids prescribed and administered. The need for a speedy restoration of normal volumes, in most patients, cannot be overemphasized.

### Water and electrolytes

Pure water loss leads to dehydration and an increase in osmolarity within all fluid compartments that equilibrate rapidly. Electrolytes are also lost with water, and this is the most common type of fluid abnormality in patients presenting for routine or elective major surgery.

The normal physiological insensible loss that occurs through the skin and through the humidification of respiratory gases continues during surgery, and has to be replaced or prevented if surgery is going to be prolonged. Hyperventilation, especially with dry gases, will rapidly increase the rate of loss. Changes in specific electrolytes will depend on the process involved. Sweating leads to the loss of a large volume of water, sodium, and chloride ions. In hot climates, or in pyrexial patients, preoperative deficits of 2–3 litres or more are likely. Vomiting results in the loss of chloride and hydrogen ions with water, and a consequent sodium loss caused by the renal compensatory mechanisms following the resulting alkalosis. Bowel preparation for gut surgery, especially if osmotic laxatives are used, causes large losses of water, potassium, and chloride. These volumes may also be of the order of litres, and lead to a profoundly dehydrated patient.

### Plasma

Plasma is lost in patients who have burns or disrupted basal cell membranes from, for instance, sepsis. The losses may be large and, because of the fall in plasma proteins, there is a corresponding fall in capillary oncotic pressure, with leakage of water and electrolytes from the vascular into the extravascular compartment. The quantitative loss of the plasma binding will increase the free plasma concentrations of highly protein-bound drugs, and increase the concentration at the site(s) of action. Relative overdosage and an increased incidence of side effects can occur. The fall in plasma proteins, especially of immunoglobulins, impairs the immunological responses of the patient. Replacement of the plasma and the proteins will resuscitate the patient and return their vascular volumes to normal. The use of colloids other than plasma increases the intravascular volume, but has variable effects on the oncotic pressure depending on the molecular weight of the protein fragments.

### Blood loss

Blood loss is one of the most serious threats to patients. The assessment of blood loss, and its likely effect on the patient, is a vital part of anaesthetic practice. Blood loss of similar volumes may have very different effects depending on the rate at which it occurs. Chronic blood loss (over weeks, months, or years) leading to anaemia has several compensatory mechanisms to ameliorate the reduction in $O_2$ content in the blood. The cardiac output increases, the dissociation curve for $O_2$ carriage as oxyhaemoglobin will move to the right, and there is an increase in 2,3-diphosphoglycerate (2,3-DGP) in the red cells. This is described more fully in Chapter 52.

The sudden loss of an equivalent blood volume (over minutes or hours) cannot utilize these slow compensatory changes, and several acute compensatory mechanisms become active to protect the vital organs from the blood loss. The development and management of hypovolaemic shock, because of its importance, is discussed more fully in the section 'Blood loss and shock'.

## PERIOPERATIVE FLUID MANAGEMENT IN ROUTINE PATIENTS

### Fit patients for short, minor procedures

A fit patient presenting for elective, minor surgery that does not affect the ability to take oral fluids in the immediate postoperative period can often be managed without the need for any intravenous fluids. *This does not, however, negate the need for intravenous access in every patient during anaesthesia*. In addition, intravenous fluids should not be withheld if they are required to correct significant falls in blood pressure (BP) during the induction or maintenance of anaesthesia or if the patient is slow to recover or has postoperative nausea and vomiting.

### Fit patients for elective procedures requiring intravenous fluids

This section assumes that the adult patient who is fit and apyrexial, is admitted for an elective operation causing negligible blood loss. The procedure is such that the patient may not wish to take oral fluids normally in the first 24 hours. Examples of this could be:

- cholecystectomy;
- hysterectomy;
- major limb surgery;
- laminectomy.

Failure to take oral fluids can be caused by continued sedation, the effect of analgesics, nausea, disinterest in events generally, emotional distress, or any combination of such or similar factors.

#### *Preoperative period*

Depending on the timing of the surgery, the patient will have been fluid depleted for between 4 and 12 hours. By reference to Figure 14.2 the patient's losses will be typically as shown in Table 14.3.

The figures given in Table 14.3 represent the starting deficits for healthy patients. These can easily be made up if the patient were to take oral fluids normally postoperatively, but if he or she is relying on intravenous replacement this needs to be taken into account.

#### *Intraoperative period*

For a patient undergoing body surface surgery with no evaporation from moist cavity surfaces, the losses will continue at the hourly rate specified in Table 14.3 and routine maintenance fluids should reflect this.

It is a reasonable plan in fit patients to replace the estimated pre- and intraoperative water and sodium losses by the end of the operation. This can be conveniently achieved by the use of dextrose–saline solution (4% dextrose, 0.18% saline) which contains 31 mmol/L sodium. Potassium is not required for the first 24 hours in most patients. Any further intraoperative requirements to maintain BP and heart rate within acceptable ranges can be given as isotonic saline, balanced salt solution, or colloid (see later).

In body cavity procedures (e.g. open cholecystectomy), the evaporative losses increase up to about 5 ml/kg/h. Other losses from the skin, lungs, and third space sequestration can take this figure to 10 ml/kg/h. This must be added to the usual maintenance requirements. The exact needs should be tailored for individual patients based on heart rate, BP, tissue perfusion, and an adequate urine output of not less than 0.5 ml/kg/h. Blood or plasma protein replacement, if required, is described later.

#### *Postoperative period*

Postoperatively, the maintenance requirements continue as before but the postoperative patient differs from the 'normal person' in that the stress reaction to surgery modifies homoeostatic mechanisms. In proportion to the severity of the surgical insult, stress-induced release of antidiuretic hormone (vasopressin), aldosterone, and cortisol cause water and sodium retention and increased excretion of potassium (see Chapter 5). Contrary to this, however, tissue damage and catabolism release more potassium into the circulation and ECF is sequestered into tissue spaces.

Opinions vary about the ideal postoperative fluid regimen and some people hold extremely strong views. A reasonable approach is to prescribe fluids as follows:

- no potassium for the first 24–48 hours;
- replace maintenance losses (Table 14.3) with 4% dextrose/0.18% saline solution;
- replace further 'tissue space loss' with isotonic saline or physiological salt solution;
- remove the intravenous line only when the patient is drinking normally and has a satisfactory urine output.

Whatever fluid replacement scheme is chosen, the prescription should be reviewed regularly according to the patient's response, i.e. heart rate, BP, tissue perfusion, plasma electrolytes, and urine output (> 0.5 ml/kg/h). *Poor urine output always necessitates immediate investigation and treatment.*

The most common error is to underestimate fluid requirements. In fit patients, who can handle excess fluids easily, it is a more serious error to underprescribe than to overprescribe replacement fluids.

Fluid requirements in specific conditions with which patients present are described in Chapters 41–46.

## DEHYDRATION

Strictly speaking, dehydration means loss of water, but in the context of patients it also implies the loss of electrolytes because it is impossible to lose these separately.

Dehydration occurs over hours or days, so the symptoms related to it come on gradually and homoeostatic

**Table 14.3. Water, sodium, and potassium losses during preoperative starvation in a 70-kg man**

| Period of starvation (h) | Water loss (ml) | Sodium loss (mmol) | Potassium loss (mmol) |
|---|---|---|---|
| 1 | 105 | 3 | 3 |
| 4 | 420 | 12 | 12 |
| 8 | 840 | 23 | 23 |
| 12 | 1260 | 35 | 35 |

mechanisms have the opportunity to move fluids between different compartments. In essence, the loss of water and electrolytes from the plasma is replaced to maintain plasma volume by taking first from the rest of the extracellular space and then from the intracellular space. The causes of dehydration separate into increased loss and decreased intake (Table 14.4).

Dehydration should always be looked for in sick patients at the preoperative visit and correction started at the first opportunity. On clinical presentation, dehydration is usually classified as mild, moderate, or severe (Table 14.5).

The following additional investigations should be done:

- Full blood count: if the haematocrit is normal in the presence of significant dehydration, consider the possibility of pre-existing anaemia or blood loss.
- Electrolytes: sodium and potassium levels are often abnormal.
- Urea or creatinine: the urea is normally elevated when dehydration is present. If the creatinine is raised, this might indicate incipient or actual renal failure.

When dehydration is present, its correction should be started immediately. The aim should be to effect the correction over a number of hours – 'pushing' fluids too rapidly does not allow time for equilibration between the fluid compartments. The prescription of fluids needs to be tailored to the individual patient in terms of both volume and composition. The electrolyte composition of the fluid can be based to some extent on the plasma electrolyte findings. *Remember that most of the body potassium is intracellular and the plasma levels do not reflect the total deficit.* In addition, potassium cannot be replaced too quickly because of its effect on the heart.

| **Table 14.4. Causes of dehydration** |
|---|
| **Increased loss** |
| Pyrexia (insensible loss increases by 10% for every °C rise in temperature) |
| Vomiting |
| Diarrhoea |
| Acute abdomen (several litres may be sequestered in the abdomen) |
| Excessive diuretic therapy, or normal diuretics continued in absence of fluid intake |
| Excessive exercise in hot conditions (culminating in heat stroke) |
| Metabolic derangements, e.g. diabetes mellitus |
| Some types of chronic renal disease |
| Rarities such as diabetes insipidus |
| **Decreased intake** |
| Reduced oral intake in sick patients because of reduced appetite and thirst |
| Reduced oral intake because of specific lesion (e.g. quinsy, carcinoma of the oesophagus) |
| Patients at extremes of age are less able to maintain fluid balance during illness |
| Prolonged preoperative fasting |

It is difficult to give general guidelines to cover all possibilities because of the variability of patient presentations and the causes of dehydration. Average figures for electrolyte losses from various sites are given in Table 14.6. As an example of the need to tailor therapy to individual needs, compare the following two patients. Volume loss in a young adult with mild dehydration from appendicitis (say loss of 3 litres) could be corrected over 2–4 hours, whereas a moderate-to-severe volume loss in an elderly man vomiting from pyloric stenosis (say loss of 7 litres) may take 12–24 hours.

Because significant fluid loss always implies electrolyte loss, it is usually satisfactory to give the first 3 litres as isotonic saline or balanced salt solution with appropriate potassium additions, *provided that the patient is regularly observed and basic observations recorded, with clear instructions to the nursing staff in case of any problems.* After this, further prescription should be based on plasma electrolyte results and the clinical progress of the patient. *The importance of observing the effects of prescribed fluids cannot be overemphasized.* If treatment is progressing well, the heart rate and BP will return to normal and the urine output will increase. *A steady increase in the rate of urine production towards the normal value of 1 ml/kg/h is the best indicator that the prescribed fluids are achieving their purpose.* In cases of very severe dehydration, treatment may have to be carried out in a high dependency area with the benefit of more invasive monitoring (direct BP and central venous pressure [CVP]), pulse oximetry, and ECG.

## BLOOD LOSS AND SHOCK

The response to chronic blood loss was mentioned earlier. This section deals with the acute loss of blood, either as a steady intraoperative ooze or as an uncontrolled loss, both of which can lead to shock.

Whenever blood loss occurs, there are two major considerations. The first is to correct the loss of circulating blood volume and the second is to maintain the $O_2$ delivery to the tissues. The fall in blood volume activates the volume receptors in the right atrium and large vessels. This causes an increase in catecholamine release, leading to an increased systemic vascular resistance and a reduction in peripheral blood flow (see Chapter 20). The essential organs (the brain and heart) receive proportionately more of the available volume to maintain perfusion. The gut, skin, muscles, liver, and kidneys all become under-perfused. Initially this process results in very little change in commonly measured physiological variables: the BP is maintained, the CVP is normal, and initially there is little change in heart rate. The fall in haemoglobin (Hb) concentration (and hence $O_2$-carrying capacity) causes additional

**Table 14.5. The presentation of dehydration**

| Severity of dehydration | Clinical findings |
|---|---|
| Mild (up to 4% of body weight, 6% of total body water)<br>Up to an approximately 3-litre loss in a 70-kg man | Normal mental state<br>Dry mucous membranes<br>Usually thirsty<br>Blood pressure and heart rate normal<br>Lower than normal urine output<br>Skin turgor almost normal |
| Moderate (up to 7% of body weight, 10% of total body water)<br>Up to an approximately 5-litre loss in a 70-kg man | Disinterest in surroundings, can be drowsy<br>Increased heart rate and respiratory rate<br>Orthostatic hypotension<br>Decreased skin turgor<br>Marked oliguria<br>Decreased intraocular pressure |
| Severe (up to 10% of body weight, 18% of total body water)<br>Up to an approximately 8-litre loss in a 70-kg man | Stuperose<br>Fast pulse and low blood pressure<br>Respiratory distress<br>Sunken eyes<br>Extreme oliguria or anuria |

**Table 14.6. Average figures for the main electrolyte losses in secretions from various sites**

| Site | Sodium (mmol/L) | Potassium (mmol/L) | Chlorine (mmol/L) | Volume/day (ml) |
|---|---|---|---|---|
| Stomach | 60 | 10 | 85 | 1500 |
| Small intestine | 110 | 5 | 100 | 3000 |
| Bile | 150 | 5 | 100 | 1500 |
| Pancreatic juice | 140 | 5 | 80 | 1000 |
| Recent ileostomy | 130 | 10 | 115 | 1000 |
| Established ileostomy | 50 | 3 | 20 | 700 |
| Colostomy | 50 | 8 | 40 | 700 |

Note also that gastric juice has up to 150 mmol/L of hydrogen ions and pancreatic juice has approximately 110 mmol/L of bicarbonate ions in addition to the above. Loss of these fluids has a major impact on acid–base balance.

reflex activity, producing an increase in cardiac output to maintain $O_2$ delivery. The progressive effects of these compensatory changes define the signs associated with the severity of the haemorrhagic shock. When hypovolaemic shock is present, the use of vasopressors should be avoided because they will exacerbate hypovolaemic hypoxic organ damage.

### Steady intraoperative blood loss

In addition to the insensible, interstitial, secretory, and evaporative losses described above, in many operations there is also a loss of blood. In most instances, this occurs gradually throughout the procedure and its volume can be replaced by colloid or crystalloid solutions to prevent hypovolaemia. The question is, when should blood loss be replaced by a transfusion of packed cells?

In fit patients who are able to increase their cardiac output, because of the non-linear relationship of blood viscosity with haematocrit, the maximum $O_2$ delivery to the tissues occurs at a haematocrit of 30%, corresponding to a Hb concentration of 10 g/dl. Some reconstructive and vascular surgeons now request this as a postoperative target level. The combined effect of viscosity and haematocrit is shown graphically in Figure 14.4.

There are no clinical trials of the effects of anaemia in the range 7–10 g Hb/dl. However, the experience of treating Jehovah's Witnesses and patients who have requested no blood transfusion for other reasons (e.g. fear of AIDS) has been that young fit patients will, with adequate fluid replacement, tolerate Hb concentrations considerably lower than 10 g/dl. It is therefore difficult to be definitive in giving didactic advice on routine transfusion. Textbooks have suggested maintaining normovolaemia with crystalloid or colloid until 15% of the blood volume has been lost, after which point blood should be given. Nowadays, this is probably regarded as being far too aggressive an approach.

Reasonable guidelines for intraoperative blood transfusion in current practice are as follows:

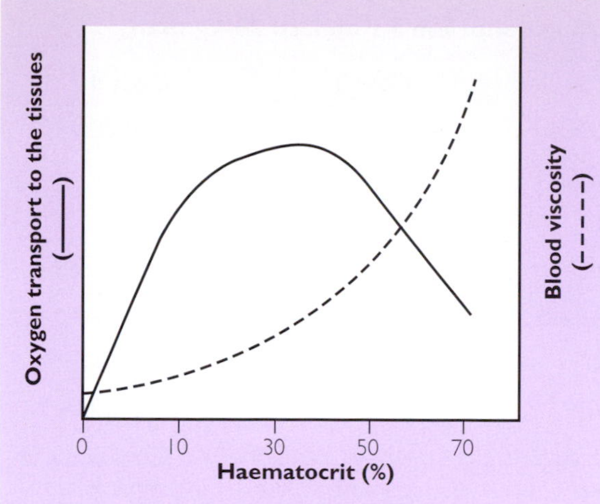


**Figure 14.4.** The relationship between $O_2$ delivery to the tissues, blood viscosity and haematocrit.

- On the basis of the preoperative condition of the patient and the operation, assess the likely need for blood and make sure that the necessary steps (e.g. group and save, cross-match 2 units, etc.) have been taken.
- If the patient is anaemic preoperatively, look for the cause, assess their physiological state at the present Hb concentration, consider the likely operative blood loss, and manage as described in Chapter 52.
- As blood is lost intraoperatively, keep the patient normovolaemic by transfusion of colloid or crystalloid solutions. If a local protocol for fluid replacement exists, use it.
- When deciding whether to give blood, remember that:
  - intraoperative assessments of blood loss often underestimate the true figure;
  - the losses are superimposed on the preoperative Hb concentration;
  - blood loss may continue postoperatively.
- If the response to blood and fluid replacement is not as anticipated, with the heart rate remaining elevated, the BP low, and the urine output poor, assume in the first instance that you have underestimated the blood loss. Blood is often absorbed on to drapes, trickles to the floor and collects in body cavities and, in doing so, goes unnoticed.
- In a fit patient, when the blood loss is estimated to be approaching 10% of the circulating blood volume (about 450 ml in a 70-kg man), if it has not already been done, cross-match grouped and saved serum. When the blood is available or if it has already been cross-matched, ask for it to be brought to the fridge in the operating room.
- In a fit patient, when the blood loss is estimated to be approaching 20% of the circulating blood volume (about 900 ml in a 70-kg man), take a blood sample (arterial or venous) and get an estimate of the Hb concentration. This can often be done most easily by putting the sample through a blood–gas machine.
- On the basis of this reading, the patient's clinical signs, and the need to transfuse fluid to keep the patient's heart rate, BP and urine output normal, estimate the likely postoperative Hb concentration:
  - If this is 10 g/dl or more do not give blood.
  - If it is 7 g/dl or less, give 2 units of packed cells.
  - If it is 7–10 g/dl and the patient is stable, wait for a postoperative blood count and base blood replacement on this and the clinical state of the patient.
- Irrespective of the above:
  - always respect the patient's stated wishes; this will on occasion affect the level at which you begin to transfuse;
  - do not withhold blood if cardiovascular decompensation occurs;
  - remember that what is appropriate for fit patients with good cardiovascular compensation will not apply to others.
- If you ask for a postoperative Hb concentration upon which to base replacement therapy, make sure that either yourself or somebody else follows it up and acts on it appropriately.
- Finally, apply common sense, whatever situation you find yourself in!

## Haemorrhagic shock: presentation and management

Uncontrolled blood loss can occur pre-, intra-, or post-operatively, and its cause can be medical, surgical or traumatic. *Blood loss and the signs of shock should always be treated early and aggressively with fluid replacement.* Get a wide-bore intravenous cannula in early, even it is subsequently not needed. Treatment should follow logical principles and the response to therapy, rather than adhering to rigid rules.

This section should be read in conjunction with 'The injured patient', Chapter 64. If it is recommended that a patient is catheterized to measure urine output, bear in mind that if a patient with pelvic trauma has blood at the urethral meatus, haematoma of the genitalia or a non-palpable prostate, transurethral catheterization is contraindicated until urological advice is available.

### *Presentation*

Haemorrhage is conventionally divided into four classes, the features of which are summarized in Table 14.7.

#### *Class I haemorrhage*

This is defined as a volume loss of up to 15% of the calculated circulating blood volume. It corresponds to the loss of a blood donation. Normally, clinical signs are minimal, and there is little change in heart rate, capillary refill, or pulse pressure. There is little indication for fluid replacement in this patient at this time *if the haemorrhage has been stopped*. An example would be a flesh wound in which the bleeding is well controlled.

If, however, such a haemorrhage is superimposed on an existing deficit (e.g. bleeding duodenal ulcer in a patient who is already severely dehydrated), the effect will be much more dramatic. In addition, those who are

**Table 14.7. Features of the four classes of haemorrhagic shock in a standard 70-kg man**

| | Class 1 | Class 2 | Class 3 | Class 4 |
|---|---|---|---|---|
| Blood loss (ml) | < 750 | 750–1500 | 1500–2000 | > 2000 |
| Blood loss (% blood vol) | < 15% | 15–30% | 30–40% | > 40% |
| Heart rate (beats/min) | < 100 | > 100 | > 120 | > 140 |
| Systolic blood pressure | Normal | Normal | Decreased | Decreased |
| Pulse pressure | Normal | Decreased | Decreased | Decreased |
| Respiratory rate (breaths/min) | 14–20 | 20–30 | 30–40 | > 35 |
| Urine output (ml/h) | > 30 | 20–30 | 5–15 | Negligible |
| Mental state | Slightly anxious/ normal | Moderately anxious | Anxious and/or confused | Confused and lethargic |

Adapted from Alexander RH, Proctor HJ. *Advanced Trauma Life Support Course for Physicians*. American College of Surgeons, 1995;86.

already anaemic or elderly may lack the necessary compensatory mechanisms.

*Class 2 haemorrhage*

This is defined as a 15–30% volume loss, i.e. about 800–1600 ml in a 70-kg adult. Clinical signs result because of decreased $O_2$ delivery and the reflex compensatory changes that try to correct this. There is a tachycardia, and there may also be tachypnoea and a decrease in pulse pressure (related primarily to a rise in the diastolic pressure). These changes, together with anxiety and fear, accompany the high circulating levels of catecholamines. Urine output is a little reduced at approximately 30 ml/h (unless there is renal impairment). Rapid stabilization is by replacement of the predicted lost volume. This can be in the form of colloid or crystalloid; blood itself is not immediately necessary but may become so later.

*Class 3 haemorrhage*

This represents a 30–40% blood volume loss (about 2000 ml in an adult), and is potentially life threatening. There are all the 'classic' signs of shock with inadequate perfusion and $O_2$ delivery. There is pallor, tachycardia, tachypnoea, systolic hypotension, and a prolonged capillary refill time. Mental changes are much more pronounced and may lead to a reduced level of consciousness. Immediate transfusion with 2 litres of crystalloid or colloid is essential, and the majority will require blood later. High-flow facemask oxygen and urinary catheterization are required. There is significant oliguria and the kidneys are at risk.

*Class 4 haemorrhage*

This is immediately life threatening, and occurs where there has been more than 40% of the circulating volume lost. The patient is pale, drowsy, anuric, with a high tachycardia, low systolic and unrecordable diastolic BP, and gasping breathing. Greater losses (over 50%) lead to unconsciousness, an unrecordable pulse and BP, and, unless massive rapid transfusion is given, the patient is likely to die. High-flow facemask oxygen and urinary catheterization are mandatory.

***Management of haemorrhagic shock***

The key to success is early treatment. The aim of fluid resuscitation and blood volume replacement is to regain $O_2$ delivery and organ perfusion with minimal permanent damage to the patient. The evaluation of the patient's responses to fluid replacement is essential, and urinary output gives valuable information on organ perfusion. Work with surgical colleagues to get a diagnosis and management plan as soon as possible.

The choice between using colloids or crystalloid replacement therapy remains debatable. If there is clinical evidence of hypovolaemia, any volume expander is better than none and should be given rapidly. Isotonic saline or balanced salt solutions (see later) are probably the most common fluids used, although many units have protocols that use colloids or a mixture of them both. With crystalloids the three-for-one rule of thumb is often applied, which assumes that patients require, say, 300 ml of fluid for each 100 ml of blood lost. The reasons for this can be seen in Table 14.1 and its associated text.

For patients with symptoms and signs of shock, the volume of crystalloid administered as an initial rapid infusion (over 10 min) should be 20 ml/kg in children or 2000 ml in adults. Once this has been given, the patient is reassessed. There are three possible responses: they may rapidly recover to normal; they may recover but relapse again; or there may be no effect at all. This response will dictate the type and rate of subsequent replacement fluid therapy (Table 14.8). Where there is a restoration of normal organ function (a falling heart rate, normal BP, good urine output), a decision on the need for blood replacement has to be made. Normally, where less than 20% of the blood volume has been lost, blood transfusion is not indicated. This guidance is based on the balance between the drop in blood viscosity as the haematocrit falls, and the need to increase cardiac output to maintain $O_2$ delivery (see Figure 14.4). As discussed above, a common figure for an acceptable acute haemodilution is 10 g/dl.

Where there has been an initial recovery followed by a relapse, inadequate volume replacement is suggested.

| Table 14.8. Responses to initial fluid resuscitation* | | | |
|---|---|---|---|
| | Rapid response | Transient response | No response |
| Vital signs | Return to normal | Transient improvement: BP falls and HR increases again | Remain abnormal |
| Estimated blood loss (%) | Minimal (10–20) | Moderate and ongoing (20–40) | High (> 40) |
| Need for more crystalloid | Low | High | High |
| Need for blood | Low | Moderate–high | Immediate |
| Blood preparation | Type and cross-match | Type specific (ABO and Rhesus compatible) | Emergency group O, Rhesus negative blood |

*2000 ml colloid in a 70-kg man; 20 ml/kg in a child. BP, blood pressure; HR, heart rate. Adapted from Alexander RH, Proctor HJ. *Advanced Trauma Life Support Course for Physicians*. American College of Surgeons, 1995; 88.

Changing to a colloid or to blood is now appropriate, and further rapid infusions of 500 ml of these solutions should be given until stability occurs.

Where there is an ongoing blood loss in a patient who has not responded to 2000 ml of crystalloid, immediate transfusion of blood is essential. Where possible previously ordered cross-matched blood should be used but, if there is none available, 'type-specific' non-cross-matched blood is preferable to the use of group O blood. However, in an emergency it is far better to give O-negative non-cross-matched blood than to wait.

The need for early diagnosis and a management plan cannot be emphasized enough. In serious cases, stopping the bleeding is urgent and cannot always wait for full restoration of blood volume (e.g. ruptured ectopic pregnancy, ruptured aneurysm).

## BURNS

The risk of profound hypovolaemia and hypotension after a thermal injury is related to the extent and severity of the burn. The depth of the damage to the skin determines how the burn is classified. Although there are some variations of classification in use, that used by the Advanced Trauma Life Support (ATLS) manual is well accepted. This is as follows:

1. A first-degree burn is where there is damage only to the epidermis, leading to redness but no blistering (e.g. sunburn). It is intensely painful, is not life threatening, does not require intravenous fluids, and heals within a few days.
2. A second-degree or partial-thickness burn involves damage to the dermis and underlying glands and fat. Blistering occurs, and it weeps, is very painful, and may take 10 or more days to heal.
3. A third-degree or full-thickness burn involves the entire skin down to the subcutaneous fat. There may be charring of the skin, or it may be blanched. It is painless, and only heals by scarring and contracture formation. Where there is circumferential burn, escharotomy is necessary.

Depending on the type of fire, there may be airway burns as well. Clinical indications of this are given in Table 14.9.

| Table 14.9. Clinical indications of airway burns |
|---|
| Facial burns |
| Singeing of the eyebrows and nostrils |
| Carbon deposits and erythema in the oropharynx |
| Carbonaceous sputum |
| Confinement in room with fire |
| Caught in an explosion |

The volume of fluid lost is calculated using standard nomograms often based on the 'rule of nines' (Figure 14.5). These give the percentage of total body surface area damaged and guide replacement therapy. Where there is more than a 15% burn (10% in a child), intravenous fluid therapy should be started. A major burn in an adult is defined as more than 20% of the total body surface area with second- or third-degree burns. This should indicate referral to a specialist centre.

For fluid replacement, the choice of colloid or crystalloid varies across countries, but in the UK colloid is usually given, at least in part. There are several infusion schemes, of which that of Muir and Barclay is one example. This defines the fluid replacement *for specific periods from the time of injury* as given in Table 14.10. Remember that the time of the start of the infusion scheme is the time of the burn, not the time into the accident and emergency department.

These are only guides to fluid resuscitation; careful assessment of the physiological responses is as important as in haemorrhagic shock. Invasive monitoring and urinary catheterization are mandatory to determine the adequacy of therapy. A urine output of 0.5–1.0 ml/kg is essential, and lower rates of production indicate a need for further, rapid intravenous therapy. Blood may be necessary in the later stages of resuscitation but, unless there have been other forms of trauma leading to blood loss, plasma replacement is the major requirement for the first 24 hours.

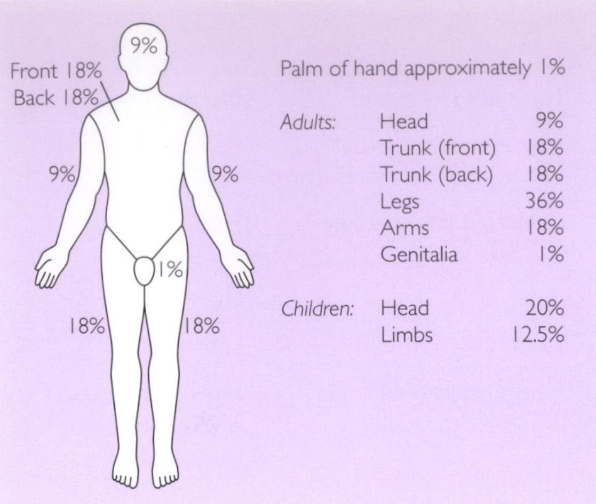


**Figure 14.5.** The 'rule of nines' for assessing the area of burn. Note the difference in the proportion of surface area of the head in children.

| **Table 14.10. Fluid replacement after a burn injury** |
|---|
| Give volume of replacement fluid (at least 50% as colloid) equal to (weight in kg × % burn in ml) in each of the following six periods from the time of burning: |
| 0–4 h<br>4–8 h<br>8–12 h<br>12–18 h<br>18–24 h<br>24–36 h<br>If there are extensive full-thickness burns, some of this will need to be given as blood. |
| Measure haematocrit, haemoglobin, electrolytes, heart rate, and blood pressure, and adjust the above guideline accordingly. |

## PRODUCTS AVAILABLE FOR REPLACEMENT THERAPY

### Crystalloids

Crystalloids are electrolyte-containing solutions that are formulated to match, to a greater or lesser extent, the biochemical and osmotic features of plasma. They contain no high-molecular-weight compounds and rapidly equilibrate (within less than 30 min) throughout the fluid compartments, as described in Table 14.1.

Crystalloids are used to maintain water and electrolyte homoeostasis in the face of measurable and insensible losses, and are also used to replace fluid losses during surgery. Comparative studies on the use of either colloid or crystalloid for rapid fluid resuscitation are equivocal. There is some clinical support for the use of colloids, but some units are reluctant to use them until there has been significant blood loss (10% of the estimated blood volume) because of the risks of anaphylactic reactions (see Chapter 13). The common crystalloid solutions are isotonic saline, balanced salt solutions, and dextrose-containing solutions.

Physiological or 'normal' saline (0.9% NaCl) is both isotonic and iso-osmolar to plasma water and sodium, but has an excess of chloride. It can be used pre- and intraoperatively as described above. If it is used for large volume replacements, hypernatraemia and hyperchloraemia will result. This causes a mild metabolic acidosis. It is especially useful in conditions where plasma concentrations of these ions are low, such as a hypochloraemic metabolic alkalosis resulting from vomiting. It is cheap and has a long shelf-life. Disadvantages include the lack of buffering and other electrolytes.

Balanced salt solutions (Hartmann's or Ringer–lactate solution) are very close to the actual composition of the ECF. They contain a buffering agent, as lactate, citrate, or acetate, which hydrates to carbonic acid and subsequently produces $CO_2$. Although the proportion of electrolytes is balanced, the actual concentration of each is slightly below physiological levels.

Dextrose-containing solutions are used infrequently for resuscitation because the dextrose is metabolized, leaving water as the volume expander. Five percent dextrose is isotonic with plasma. The water rapidly equilibrates throughout the total body water compartments (see Figure 14.3), leading to cellular oedema with only a small amount remaining in the vascular compartment. *Dextrose solutions should never be used for acute high-volume resuscitation.*

A summary of the components of crystalloid solutions is given in Table 14.11.

### Colloids and plasma substitutes

These are solutions that contain high-molecular-weight proteins as well as electrolytes. The large molecules are unable to diffuse through normal capillary membranes and therefore stay in the intravascular volume (see Figure 14.3). For this reason, they are very effective for volume replacement. There are many proteins in use, but most of those manufactured are based on fractionated cellulose or gelatin. They all have an increased risk of anaphylactic reactions compared with crystalloid solutions. Although their benefit is less pronounced when there is damage to the capillary membranes (allowing protein molecules to leak out into the interstitial tissue), for many people colloids remain the cornerstone of fluid resuscitation.

Early colloid solutions led to the binding of citrate and clot formation within the giving set, with the potential for dangerous delays when the need for blood transfusion was urgent. Most current formulations do not have such a disadvantage but it is important for the anaesthetist to know the properties of what s/he is using. Many colloid solutions are slightly hyperosmolar, with values of 310 mosmol/L, compared with the iso-osmotic crystalloid solutions.

#### *Choice of plasma substitute*

The choice of which colloid to use should be made on clinical grounds, but is often influenced by cost as well as clinical factors. The decision is affected by availability of the colloid, the risks of infective transmission, allergenicity, microembolization, and any

**Table 14.11. Composition of some crystalloid solutions**

| Solution | Sodium (mmol/L) | Chloride (mmol/L) | Potassium (mmol/L) | Calcium (mmol/L) | Bicarbonate (mmol/L) | Glucose (g/L)[b] | Tonicity |
|---|---|---|---|---|---|---|---|
| 0.9% sodium chloride | 154 | 154 | | | | | Isotonic |
| Ringer's solution | 147 | 156 | 4 | 2.2 | | | Isotonic |
| Hartmann's solution[a] | 131 | 111 | 5 | 2 | 29 (as lactate) | | Isotonic |
| 4% glucose and 0.18% sodium chloride | 30 | 30 | | | | 40 (164) | Isotonic[c] |
| 5% dextrose | | | | | | 50 (205) | Isotonic[c] |
| 10% dextrose | | | | | | 100 (410) | Hypertonic[c] |

[a]Also called compound sodium lactate solution or Ringer–lactate solution.
[b]Figures in parentheses are kcal/L.
[c]Note that whether isotonic or hypertonic, after metabolism of the glucose, the net effect is hypotonic (see Table 14.1).

other specific adverse effects. Colloid solutions also contain variable amounts of electrolytes, including calcium. Other characteristics such as the duration of plasma expansion are also relevant. Although the average protein fraction size is frequently quoted, there is a wide variation, as shown in Figure 14.6. This, in turn, can lead to a variable duration of volume maintenance because of the differing half-lives of the components, as shown in Figure 14.7. Part of this variability is because the larger proteins are metabolized by amylases to smaller and smaller proteins with molecular weights less than 50 000 Da, which are then readily excreted through the kidney. The details of some colloid solutions are given in Table 14.12.

***Human plasma products***

At present all the plasma removed from the whole blood is pooled and used to provide a variety of plasma products. These include cryoprecipitate, factor VIII, and factor IX concentrates, other plasma proteins, and albumin solutions. Some immunogobulin products are fractionated for use in immunodeficiency states. There is concern about the risk of new-variant Creutzfeldt–Jakob disease contaminating pooled plasma. Some countries, e.g. France, 'quarantine' plasma by re-testing the donor at 3 months.

***Fresh frozen plasma (FFP)***

This is usually pooled from 2–4 individual units of blood (about 150 ml/unit) and defrosted just before use (this takes 20 min). FFP can be stored frozen at −30°C for up to 1 year. It contains all of the clotting factors, albumin, and globulins. It has to be cross-matched, and checked before administration, and can cause transfusion reactions. FFP is indicated for replacement of isolated factor deficiencies, for immediate reversal of warfarin, and in acute disseminated intravascular coagulation. It also has a definite place after massive blood transfusion, where bleeding is continuing during surgery and where there is documented coagulopathy (i.e. the international normalized ratio [INR] is > 1.5). There are no clear reasons for the common practice of

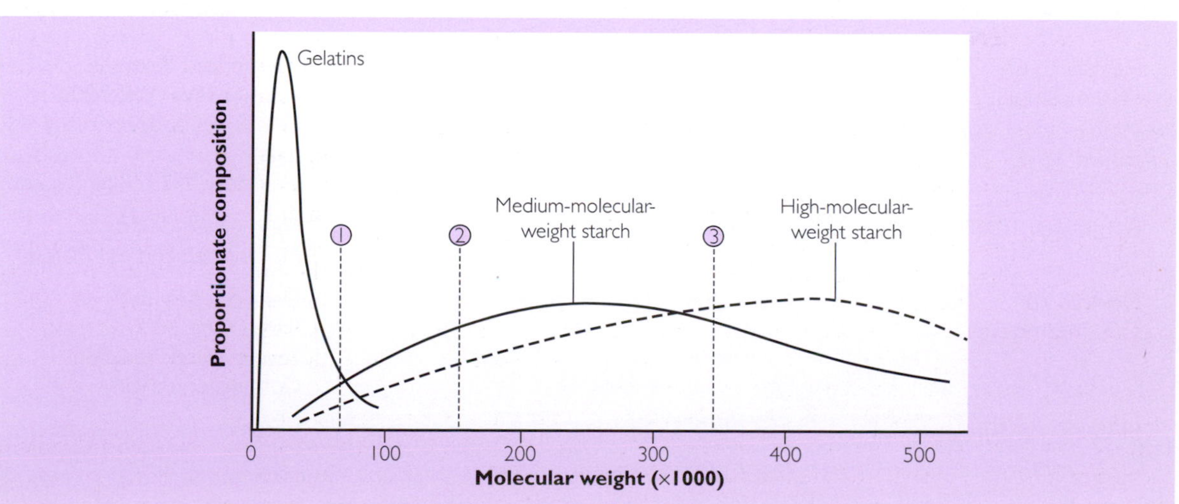


**Figure 14.6.** The approximate molecular weight compositions of various colloid solutions; for comparison the positions of (1) albumin, (2) γ-globulin, and (3) fibrinogen are marked. (Reconstructed from manufacturer's data.)

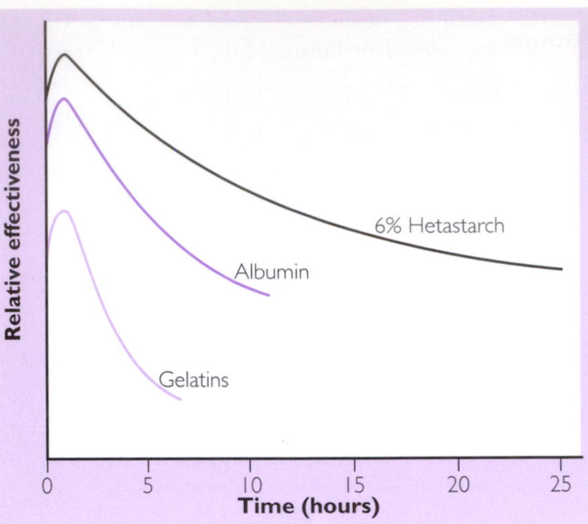


**Figure 14.7.** The relative effectiveness of volume expansion with time of some colloid solutions. (Curves are plotted from manufacturer's data.)

identifying a ratio of FFP to red cells. If there is a likelihood of clotting abnormalities, samples should be sent to the haematology laboratory, and the results discussed with senior colleagues and the haematologist on call.

#### *Platelet concentrates*

These are pooled collections from 5 or 6 units of blood, and contain an equivalent volume of plasma as 1 unit of FFP. They cannot be frozen or pasteurized, and rapidly lose their function. The average shelf-life of these platelets is 5 days. They have the same risks as a unit of red cell concentrates in terms of infections, transfusion reactions, and anaphylaxis. Platelet concentrates are usually provided only after advice from the haematologist, and may have to be transported from a regional transfusion centre. This means that there may be a considerable delay in getting them into the operating room. They have to be given through a non-filtered giving set because the platelets often aggregate during storage and these are too large to pass through a filter. For the patient undergoing surgery, platelet transfusion is indicated when the platelet count decreases to 50 000 or less in the presence of bleeding. For a patient who is otherwise well and *not* undergoing surgery, values as low as 10 000 have been tolerated. Developments in the measurement of platelet function, as yet unavailable routinely, will enable a more rational administration of this scarce resource in the future.

#### *Cryoprecipitate*

This fraction is collected by slowly defrosting FFP from –40°C to +4°C for 16 hours until it precipitates out. It is then separated by 'hard-spin' centrifugation. Cryoprecipitate has very high levels of factor VIII, von Willebrand's factor, and fibrinogen. It is useful in consumptive coagulopathies when there is a reduction in both clotting factors and fibrinogen. It is supplied in bags of 6 or 8 units, and has all the risks of the other plasma-based products. Cryoprecipitate is only indicated if:

- FFP has been ineffective in stopping bleeding;
- the prothrombin time is over 1.8 × control;
- the fibrinogen is below 1.5 g/L.

**Table 14.12. Specific colloid solutions**

| Colloid | Electrolytes contained | Dextrose contained | Comments |
|---|---|---|---|
| Gelofusine 4% (279 mosmol/L) | NaCl 0.9% | N/A | Succinylated gelatin<br>MW = 30 000 da |
| Haemaccel 'isotonic' | Na+ 145 mmol/L<br>$K^+$ 5.1 mmol/L<br>$Ca^{2+}$ 6.25 mmol/L<br>$Cl^-$ 145 mmol/L | N/A | Polygeline: a degraded, modified gelatin 35 g/L<br>MW = 35 000 da |
| Hetastarch 6% (310 mosmol/L) | NaCl 0.9% | N/A | Polymerized dextrose<br>Average MW = 450 000 da<br>Remains in body for many days<br>Max. dose = 20 ml/kg |
| Pentastarch 10% 'isotonic' | NaCl 0.9% | N/A | Polymerized dextrose<br>Metabolized and eliminated |
| Dextran 70[a] (300 mosmol/L) | NaCl 0.9% | 5% | Dextrose polymer<br>Rarely used, 1000 ml max.<br>Severe allergic reactions<br>Coagulation deficits |
| HAS 5% | NaCl 140–150 mmol/L | | Isotonic |
| HAS 20% | NaCl 140–150 mmol/L | | Hypertonic |

[a]Dextran can be in either saline or glucose.
HAS, human albumin solution; MW, molecular weight; N/A, not available.

### *Human albumin solution (HAS)*

This is available as either 5% or 20% solutions of albumin, and is produced from massive pooling and fractionation of plasma, from placental tissue, or from serum. Over 20 000 donations are contained in one bottle of 5% HAS. It is heat treated by pasteurization for 10 hours, and is free from infective risks, even from viruses. Data on prions are unclear at present. HAS is used to raise the plasma oncotic pressure, usually in intensive care units, and has little role in the acute management of blood loss during surgery. HAS was previously supplied as a plasma protein fraction which has a slightly different composition.

### *Specific factor concentrates*

Factors VIII and IX are both produced as concentrates for patients with identified deficiency syndromes. They are sterilized, but in the past have been responsible for transmission of infective agents. Factor VIII is now obtained by recombinant DNA engineering. The factors are used only under the control of a haematology unit, and are given during surgery under this guidance. Activity of these factors is measured as a percentage of normal. As a general guide for surgery, one is aiming at activity of 50% or better.

## Blood and packed cells

The physiology of blood and the clotting process is described in Chapter 31. The storage and distribution of the blood products are managed at a regional level. All donated blood is screened for infectious agents, including hepatitis B and C, syphilis, and HIV-1 and -2. It can also be screened for cytomegalovirus, but this is not routine. The whole blood is stored in either SAG-M (saline, adenine, glucose, and mannitol) or A-CPD (adenine, citrate, phosphate, and dextrose) solutions. SAG-M preserves the red cells for up to 35 days, whereas A-CPD blood lasts for up to 42 days. Fresh whole blood is now very rarely used, and most blood is provided as red cell concentrates.

Whenever blood or packed cells are given, it is important to check that the administration set incorporates a screen filter (170 µm). Some clear-fluid administration sets now have no filter in them.

### *Red cell concentrates*

Whole blood is grouped and concentrated to a haematocrit of about 60%, and is supplied as red cell concentrate in a volume of about 450 ml. It has a reduced concentration of clotting factors and albumin because these have been removed with the plasma. There are no functioning platelets after 48 hours, and the 2,3-DPG level falls after about 14 days. After 3 weeks the serum potassium is 20 mmol/L, the pH is 6.5, and the $P_{50}$ (the $P\text{O}_2$ at which saturation is 50%) is reduced to 2.7 kPa (20 mmHg) (see Chapter 52). It takes 24–48 hours after transfusion for the oxyhaemoglobin curve to be restored to its correct position.

Blood cannot be sterilized chemically or by heat without denaturation, and this leaves the risk of the transmission of infections from the donor. Hb replacement is the prime indication for packed cells, and can be administered simultaneously with equal volumes of colloid or crystalloid replacement to produce a total haematocrit of 30%.

The common blood groups are given in Table 14.13.

The transfusion service issues each unit of blood with a unique identification number for safety and checking procedures. The blood is checked against the cross-match result, the patient's name, date of birth, hospital number and address, from both the patient's arm identification band and from their clinical notes. Two people must sign to show that they have checked these details and confirmed that the blood is within its stated shelf-life. It is only then that the blood can safely be given. *The most common cause of a severe transfusion reaction is human error.*

Cross-matching is a slow process that matches the donor blood to the recipient's serum. The donor blood groups whose blood a patient can receive are given in Table 14.14. Cross-matching can take over an hour if the patient has received blood before and has developed atypical antibodies. Faster, less complete matches can be made if there are overriding clinical needs. The extreme example of this is where there is sudden catastrophic bleeding that needs immediate transfusion. Non-cross-matched blood is then used (and recorded as such). Blood group O rhesus negative is the universal donor because it will not elicit antibody activation with consequent haemolysis. If the cross-matched blood is available before 3 units of universal donor have been given, they should be used, but if more than 3 units of O-negative blood have been given, the risk of isoagglutinins increases to the point where there may be haemolysis of the new blood, and universal donor blood should be continued. The effect of the rhesus factor in pregnancy is described in Chapters 30 and 45.

In controlled situations, or where lost blood is unlikely to have been contaminated, cell salvage and re-transfusion are an alternative method of autotransfusion. The clinical situations where this is most likely to be beneficial include complex orthopaedic surgery,

**Table 14.13. The common blood groups**

| Group | Percentage population | Antigens on red cell | Antibodies in serum | Comments |
|---|---|---|---|---|
| O | 47 | Nil | Anti-A, anti-B | Universal donor |
| A | 42 | A | Anti-B | |
| B | 8 | B | Anti-A | |
| AB | 3 | A and B | Nil | Universal recipient |

In the population the incidence of rhesus D positive is 85% and of rhesus D negative is 15%.

**Table 14.14. The blood groups and fresh frozen plasma (FFP) that a patient can receive**

| Recipient blood group | Donor red cells acceptable | Donor FFP acceptable |
|---|---|---|
| O | O | O, A, B, AB |
| A | O, A | A, AB |
| B | O, B | B, AB |
| AB | O, A, B, AB | AB |
| Rhesus-positive recipients can receive rhesus-positive or rhesus-negative donor blood. | | |
| Rhesus-negative recipients can receive only rhesus-negative donor blood. | | |

cardiac surgery, liver transplantation and some major vascular operations. It may become more widespread as concerns over transfusion with donated blood progressively rise.

### *Transfusion reactions*

Even with safely cross-matched blood there is a risk of a reaction to the transfused blood. The overall morbidity of blood transfusion is 1 in 30 transfusion episodes. Fortunately the majority of these are minor. A transfusion reaction may be an acute response or it may develop over several days. The most severe complication is haemolysis, when an antibody reaction occurs between the transfused red cells and the host immune system. These reactions may lead to anaphylactic shock, renal failure, and disseminated intravascular coagulation or may be less severe with bronchospasm, urticaria, itching, and fever. Treatment is to stop the transfusion, change the giving set, and to give hydrocortisone 100 mg and chlorpheniramine 10 mg intravenously. Specific treatment for the other manifestations, such as hypotension and bronchospasm, should be given immediately as necessary.

Direct transfusion reactions that are less severe and include a fever are usually caused by a host/red cell immune response. Acute lung injury may occur from a similar cause but with the reaction being directed against leukocytes. Microemboli from platelet and cellular aggregates can cause complement activation, thrombocytopenia, and blocking of pulmonary capillaries. The extent of this is directly related to the storage time of the blood, and may be reduced by filtering the blood before transfusion.

Indirect transfusion problems are related either to the other components in the red cell concentrates or to the effects of ageing on stored blood. These include hyperkalaemia and metabolic acidosis from old stored blood although, when transfused, the potassium is taken back into the red blood cells and clinical hyperkalaemia is rare. Excessive citrate may cause acid–base disturbances, as may further leakage of lactate from the old cells. Citrate can also bind with calcium and lead to hypocalcaemia. Finally, unless the blood is warmed before transfusion, the patient is at risk from hypothermia, which further compromises $O_2$ delivery.

Delayed problems with transfusion may be severe and long-standing. Immunization often occurs to antibodies on the cellular components of blood – red cell, leukocytes, and platelets. These may cause minor reactions on subsequent transfusions, and may account for up to 10% of transfusion reactions. Infections from the blood occur rarely but, because they are often diseases of high morbidity and mortality, they are disasters for the patient when they occur. The most common are viral hepatitis B and C, which infect about 1 in 15 000 units of blood. Hepatitis C is the more common at present. HIV infection occurs in less than 1 in 1000 000 units. Immunocompromised patients may be vulnerable to other viruses such as cytomegalovirus and parvoviruses.

The symptoms of an incompatible transfusion (rapid onset of fever, back pain, skin rash, hypotension, and dyspnoea) may not be readily obvious in the anaesthetized patient. Hypotension and oozing from the wound edges might be the only indication of an incompatible transfusion. If haematuria develops mysteriously, suspect a transfusion reaction. The mortality rate from major incompatibility is 50%. At the first suspicion of a blood product incompatibility, recipient and donor blood should be taken and sent for haematological analysis.

Normal cellular immunity is reduced after large transfusions and, because of this, blood transfusion in cancer surgery should, theoretically, be avoided unless it is essential. Transfusion complications are summarized in Table 14.15.

### Massive transfusion

This is a term that describes the administration of such large volumes of blood and plasma (or substitutes) over a short period of time that they cause serious changes in coagulation, temperature regulation, and the biochemistry of the patient. It is defined as the acute replacement of:

- 1.5 times the circulating volume, or
- a single blood volume if this occurs within 24 hours.

There are two occasions when massive transfusion occurs. The first is caused by the surgical procedure, and the second is where the patient presents with massive blood loss and hypovolaemia. The management of the former requires the anaesthetist to maintain normal homoeostasis in coagulation, volume, $O_2$ delivery, temperature, and biochemistry as far as possible. It can be achieved by using a combination of red cell concentrates, crystalloid, colloid and FFP. Regular monitoring and observation of adequate urine output will allow an attempt to maintain normovolaemia. For complex cases, invasive monitoring of the arterial pressure, CVP, cardiac output, temperature gradient, and possibly left-sided pressures is essential.

The second presentation is much less controlled, and requires rapid restoration of the circulating volume, as described earlier and summarized in Table 14.8. The monitoring requirements are identical to the former presentation, but take a secondary place to the transfusion of fluid.

| Table 14.15. A summary of complications of blood transfusion |
|---|
| Transmission of viral and bacterial disease |
| Haemolytic reactions |
| Incompatibility reactions |
| Pyrogenic reactions |
| Allergic reactions |
| Citrate toxicity |
| Hyperkalaemia |
| Metabolic acidosis |
| Hypothermia |
| Air embolism |
| Microaggregate embolism |
| Circulatory overload |

Common complications of massive transfusion are listed below.

### *Hypothermia*

Blood is stored at 4°C to reduce red cell metabolism; large intravenous transfusions of blood at this temperature will profoundly cool the patient. Increasingly sophisticated warming systems prevent the cooling of the patient, and the increased temperature of the blood reduces its viscosity, allowing greater flows for the same pressure gradient.

### *Coagulation deficits*

The usual cause of intraoperative bleeding is surgical, and it is only when this has been excluded that a consumption coagulopathy should be considered. Clotting screens are the essential investigation and may need to be repeated at regular intervals. Coagulation factors should be given only in response to continued bleeding in the presence of an abnormal coagulation screen.

### *Over-transfusion*

There is always the risk that, especially with very efficient pressure infusion systems, excessive volume will be administered to the patient. Pulmonary and peripheral oedema are late complications of massive transfusions and may be the result of low-molecular-weight (< 100 000 da) proteins. Monitoring of the CVP and pulmonary wedge pressures can identify those who are moving over the top of the 'Starling curve' and who would benefit from inotropic therapy rather than simply more volume.

### *Air embolism*

Any system that uses pressure to infuse fluid can cause a massive air embolism. This may be fatal if unrecognized, and there is a Department of Health hazard warning on the replacement of partially used bags of fluids into the transfusion system. These are likely to have entrained air, and this will be pressurized into the patient along with the fluid.

### *Acidaemia*

This occurs after transfusion of old blood because the pH falls from a normal 7.4 to about 6.8 during storage. Large volume transfusion leads to a non-respiratory acidaemia. This is usually short-lived because the citrate is metabolized to bicarbonate.

### *Citrate toxicity*

This occurs if large volumes of A-CPD blood are transfused and may be related to falls in serum calcium. Clinical signs are cardiac output depression, increased bleeding, and, rarely, tetany.

### *Hyperkalaemia*

This is related to the free potassium that leaks out during the storage of the blood, and is most likely if old (> 21 days after donation) blood is used. In clinical practice hyperkalaemia is rarely a problem.

### *Microaggregates*

These form with prolonged storage and are filtered by the pulmonary circulation. They may be vasoactive and lead to histamine and serotonin release. Massive transfusion of these microaggregates can lead to marked increases in pulmonary resistance and ventilation–perfusion mismatching. This can be reduced by the use of in-line filters, but one has to balance their filtering power with the need for a high volume flow.

## Autologous blood transfusion

Risks of transfusion reactions and infection are avoided if the patient donates his own blood. This can be done as follows.

1. Removing and storing up to 6 units of blood over the days or weeks before surgery. Concurrent iron therapy is important to ensure a good bone marrow response. Erythropoietin has also been used.
2. Perioperative haemodilution, which involves simultaneous collection of blood and replacement of removed volume with colloid or crystalloid. Up to 3 units can be collected, the last one containing the lowest Hb concentration. Re-transfusion is in the reverse order.
3. Re-transfusion via a cell saver after washing and filtering of blood collected from the operative site during surgery.

## Artificial haemoglobins

There are several solutions being clinically tested that have the capacity to carry high volumes of $O_2$, with the hope of providing a safe, non-blood plasma substitute. Free Hb solutions can provide $O_2$ delivery in the absence of red cells in animal models, but if these solutions are contaminated by red cell debris they are toxic to humans, so any product intended for human use must be stroma free. However, even pure solutions of human Hb present serious problems. Human Hb is rapidly cleared from the circulation and it has a greater affinity for $O_2$ than red cell Hb, which reduces $O_2$ offloading at the capillary end of the $O_2$ cascade. Free Hb solutions can also cause renal failure. Genetically engineered Hb (rHb1.1 Somatogen) was the first fully synthetic human Hb prepared using recombinant DNA technology. Safety tests are now being performed in anaesthetized surgical patients.

### Perfluorocarbons

Mice have been demonstrated to survive immersion in perfluorocarbon (PFC) through which $O_2$ is bubbled. Although $O_2$ is highly soluble in perfluoro compounds, these compounds have great limitations in clinical practice. They are limited because their $O_2$ carriage is proportional to the partial pressure of $O_2$ and therefore very high inspired (and potentially toxic) $O_2$ concentrations are necessary. PFCs are currently licensed for procedures such as coronary angioplasty where only small volumes are required. Their potential for replacing blood loss is hampered by the potential for adverse reactions and lack of clotting factors. Polyfluoro-octobromide is a new perfluoro compound which is radio-opaque, and has advantages over its predecessors. It can be administered in higher concentrations than other perfluoro compounds because the 100% (w/v) emulsion with phospholipid has a sufficiently low viscosity to be infused without dilution. Also, $O_2$ is more soluble in it than in any other perfluoro compound introduced to date, and is equivalent to a Hb concentration of 7 g/dl for $O_2$ delivery. It has recently entered clinical trials.

## FURTHER READING


American College of Surgeons. *ATLS Handbook*. Chicago: American College of Surgeons, 1995.

Buskard NA. Blood and blood substitutes: Safety of blood transfusion: risks and use of predonation. The Canadian experience. *Can J Anaesth* 1991;**38**:5.

Irving GA. Peri-operative blood and blood component therapy. *Can J Anaesth* 1992;**39**:10

Jones JA. Red blood cell substitutes: Current Status. *Br J Anaesth* 1995;**74**:697–703.

Secher N, Pawelczyk J, Ludbrook J, eds. *Blood Loss and Shock*. London: Edward Arnold, 1994.

Tomson CRV. Basic principles. *Curr Anaesth Crit Care* 1996;7:176–81.

Turner DAB. Blood Conservation. *Br J Anaesth* 1991;**66**:281–4.

# Chapter 15 An outline of regional anaesthesia

J.D. Connolly and P. Hutton

Attempts to induce anaesthesia in specific parts of the body without affecting the level of consciousness have been made for many years. Limbs were subject to nerve compression and cold well before Bier inserted the first spinal anaesthetic in 1899. The potential benefits of regional anaesthesia are significant and have been recognized since its inception. They are summarized in Table 15.1.

Over the last 40 years, advances in needle technology, the appearance of reliable nerve stimulators, and, most importantly, the availability of rapidly acting safe local anaesthetic drugs with an adequate duration of action have all combined to make regional anaesthesia quick, safe, and reliable. The pharmacology of local anaesthetic agents is described in Chapter 36. The advantages of total pain relief both during and after surgery are clear, and regional anaesthesia has gained a permanent position in anaesthetic practice. Although there will always be anaesthetists who are more enthusiastic 'blockers' than others, every trainee anaesthetist should become competent in epidural and spinal anaesthesia and in the more commonly used regional techniques. Failure to gain this expertise deprives patients of the best choices of available treatment.

| Table 15.1. The benefits of regional anaesthesia |
|---|
| Unsurpassed quality of analgesia |
| Within limitations, the duration of analgesia can be tailored to need, especially with the use of catheters |
| Regional blockade can optimize the management of diabetics |
| The unwanted side effects of systemic opioids (nausea, vomiting, respiratory depression, reduced gut motility) can be avoided[a] |
| Sympathetic blockade improves regional blood flow (useful for skin flaps, after amputation or trauma surgery) |
| Reduction in the stress response |
| A minority of patients prefer to remain awake |
| It can be combined with, and reduce the depth of, general anaesthesia |

[a]Spinally or epidurally administered opioids can still produce these effects (see Chapter 5).

## BASIC PRINCIPLES OF REGIONAL ANAESTHESIA

### Selection and assessment of patients for regional anaesthesia

Key points are as follows:

- The same standards of assessment and preoperative investigation apply regardless of the type of anaesthesia contemplated. These are described in Chapter 1.
- Investigations relevant to the patient's condition or the nature of the surgery proposed are required in the usual way.
- Selection of regional rather than general anaesthesia depends on knowledge of the patient, the surgeon, and the proposed operation, as well as one's own knowledge of a particular regional technique.
- The anatomy relevant to the proposed block should be examined preoperatively to ensure that there are no unexpected difficulties, e.g. kyphoscoliosis, lipoma overlying insertion site, etc.
- Not every surgeon relishes the thought of an 'awake patient', and many surgeons fear that regional anaesthesia will prolong the waiting time between operations. Discussion, planning, and practice will dispel or minimize these prejudices.
- Patients too have preconceived ideas about regional anaesthesia, and some may have genuine fears about the techniques.
- A full explanation must be given to the patient, and informed consent obtained. The patient does have an absolute right of refusal and, although refusal of a regional block is rare in the face of reasoned explanations, it will, nevertheless, happen from time to time.
- Although there have been no studies that have shown regional anaesthesia to be less safe than general anaesthesia, it is difficult in most cases to prove that it is safer.
- Certainly the phrase beloved of physicians asked to assess fitness for anaesthesia that the patient 'is not fit for a general anaesthesia but should be suitable for a spinal' indicates ignorance rather than judgement.

Despite the enthusiasm and skill of the anaesthetist there will always remain some absolute contraindications to regional blockade. These are listed in Table 15.2.

| Table 15.2. Contraindications to regional blockade |
|---|
| Patient refusal despite proper information and discussion |
| Surgeon unwilling to undertake the procedure with patient awake (note that a block may still be combined with a general anaesthetic to overcome this problem) |
| A working operating room and ward environment without staff who understand the requirements for, and implications of, regional blockade |
| Uncorrected coexisting condition or other metabolic derangement |
| Full anticoagulation or coagulopathy |
| Infection overlying the site of injection or generalized sepsis |
| Trauma or burns to the site of the block |
| Existing neurological defect in the part to be blocked |
| Mental defect or instability in the patient |

### Premedication

As with premedication before general anaesthesia, many drugs have been used. Oral sedation is preferred to injection by most, and benzodiazepines are currently the most frequently prescribed drugs. Personal choice remains the deciding factor. Regardless of which drug is chosen, many patients benefit from the judicious use of intravenous sedation before insertion of the regional block, which can, on occasions, be an uncomfortable procedure even in experienced hands.

### Preoperative starvation

The preoperative restriction on fluids and solids should be the same as for a patient undergoing a general anaesthetic. If the block does not work properly, general anaesthesia may be required, and some of the complications of local anaesthetics can necessitate full resuscitative procedures, including airway control.

### Sedation and anaesthesia during surgery under regional blockade

Few patients wish to be wide awake during major surgery, and even fewer wish to repeat the experience. The majority will, at least, wish not to remember the procedure. With minor surgery on a limb (e.g. carpal tunnel release), more patients will accept full consciousness. The exception in terms of major surgery is caesarean section, where many women wish and are very motivated to be awake for the delivery of their baby.

The requirement for sedation must be assessed and discussed at the preoperative visit and the patient's wishes taken into account. The level of 'sedation' may therefore vary from none to a light general anaesthetic. The definitions and implications of sedation are discussed in Chapter 3. Increasingly, in some centres, major abdominal and thoracic surgery (e.g. abdominal aneurysm, bowel resection, lung decortication) are being carried out under regional blockade combined with light general anaesthesia. The potential advantages of this are given in Table 15.3.

Although to date there are no firm data to support it, many anaesthetists believe that the reduction in intra- and postoperative opioid requirements results in an improved postoperative recovery. The role of opioids in epidural and intrathecal blockade is considered later and in Chapter 5.

### Monitoring and safety during regional anaesthesia

Exactly the same standards of monitoring apply to regional anaesthesia as to general anaesthesia. These are described in Chapter 12. No matter how minor the procedure, ECG, non-invasive measurement of blood pressure, and pulse oximetry are the minimum requirement. Invasive or more complex monitoring should be used as dictated by the nature of the surgery or the patient's condition. Facilities for resuscitation must always be immediately available and all patients need reliable intravenous access in place throughout.

### Postoperative care and follow-up

Postoperatively, the patients must receive the same standard of care as if they had had a general anaesthetic. Specific points are as follows.

- The extent and duration of the block, and its resolution, together with any residual effects, must be recorded. The regression of analgesia and the return of normal neuromuscular function must be checked and documented. This is usually achieved by questioning, rather than by detailed neurological examination. Other common symptoms, e.g. soreness at insertion site, bruising, headache, etc. should also be sought and the appropriate management, reassurances, and treatment given.

| Table 15.3. The indications and potential advantages for combining general and regional anaesthesia |
|---|
| Patient and surgical preference for unconsciousness |
| Prolonged operation; time lying perfectly still can be distressing, especially if the patient has any form of arthritis or deformity |
| Surgical procedures (e.g. cancer) where intraoperative discussion will be required as to the best course of action |
| Surgical techniques that cause stimulus to an unblocked part of the anatomy (e.g. traction on the viscera) |
| Operations with an unpleasant component (e.g. amputations) |
| Reduction of tourniquet pain |
| Reduction of operating time |

- An anaesthetized limb needs protection from physical injury, e.g. burns or scalds.
- Limbs must be immobilized, eyes covered, etc., until function recovers.
- Ischaemic pain from plaster casts, compartment syndrome, etc. may be masked by a continuing block, so careful observation of the affected part is essential.
- Supplementary analgesia must be introduced before the block wears off completely. This is particularly relevant to day-case patients.
- Patients who have had lower limb or perineal blocks must not be discharged before they have passed urine and can walk properly unaided.
- Day-case patients need careful instructions before being accompanied home to a safe environment.
- Patients who have had regional blockade for more major procedures should be cared for as described in Chapter 5.

## Preparation before undertaking the block

Time and quietness are necessary for the performance of regional anaesthesia, and blocks should therefore be carried out in the anaesthetic room or somewhere relatively undisturbed. The time taken for some blocks to become effective needs to be taken into account to prevent undue delays and unsatisfactory anaesthesia when the procedure starts. The operating room is seldom the ideal environment because it is being prepared for the next case.

As with the induction of any anaesthetic, it is essential that adequate trained help is present, and that full resuscitation facilities are available. *Intravenous access is mandatory in all cases*, and intravenous fluids are necessary for all but the most minor surgery (see Chapter 14). Supplemental $O_2$ is always advisable.

Even when there is a definite reason to combine a block with general anaesthesia (see Table 15.3), most regional blocks are, and should be, performed on patients who are either awake, or only minimally sedated. It is important that the patient understands this when consenting to the block. Care is necessary when positioning the patient, particularly those in pain. Explanation before movement is essential and extra help may be required. Although this degree of care is important for patient comfort, it is also vital in the successful insertion of the block. Incorrect positioning multiplies the difficulties and the likelihood of failure. Practical points not to be forgotten are given in Table 15.4.

**Table 15.4. Practical points during the establishment of regional blockade**

| |
|---|
| 1. Time spent with the patient preoperatively is never wasted. A fully informed, cooperative patient increases the success rate of any regional technique. |
| 2. Time spent on positioning the patient correctly saves time during the performance of the block. |
| 3. If using regional anaesthesia alone, time must be given to allow the local anaesthetic to work. During this time testing should be kept to a minimum, as frequent testing implies doubt, and a lack of confidence is quickly communicated to the patient. Knowledge of the expected time to onset for each block is important. |

## Complications of regional anaesthesia

This section describes complications that can occur during any regional anaesthetic technique. Complications of specific blocks are discussed during descriptions of the technique.

### *Allergy to local anaesthetic*

Genuine allergy to local anaesthetics is rare, and is more commonly associated with amino-ester drugs than with amino-amides. There is no crossover, and amides may be used safely in patients with a known allergy to an amino-ester. The treatment of an anaphylactic reaction is the same as with any other drug (see Chapter 13).

### *Systemic toxicity*

Toxicity occurs as a consequence of a serum concentration that is too high. This can result either from an absolute overdose, or from the inadvertent intravenous administration of the drug. Care must therefore be taken in assessment of the dose to be given, and also by careful repeated aspiration, to ensure its correct placement. All local anaesthetics produce a similar picture of toxicity (Figure 15.1), and treatment is symptomatic and supportive. The degree of disturbance caused by toxicity depends on the potency of the drug (related to lipid solubility), its pharmacokinetic properties (the rate of rise of plasma levels, the peak level, and the fraction of unbound drug in the circulation). Data relevant to the toxicity of common drugs are given in Table 15.5.

During a severe reaction, maintenance of tissue oxygenation will prevent permanent damage, because the drug itself will do no long-term harm. If it is clear that a severe reaction is developing, send for help immediately. It is better to move sooner rather than later to control the airway (if necessary by induction, relaxation, and intubation). Potent drugs should never be used for intravenous regional anaesthesia (see later) and may require very extended periods of cardiac massage after inadvertent intravenous injection.

### *Methaemoglobinaemia*

This is a specific side effect of the absorption of a large dose of prilocaine. The patient appears cyanosed and the lack of true hypoxia must be confirmed by a pulse oximeter. An arterial blood gas sample put into a co-oximeter will confirm both adequate oxygenation and the diagnosis. It is not usually clinically significant and reverts spontaneously. No specific treatment or management is required unless the patient has disordered oxygen-carrying capacity.

### *Neurological damage and neurotoxicity*

Fortunately, the majority of postoperative sequelae are temporary. They are usually manifested as sensory disturbances within the distribution of the blocked nerve and resolve within days or a few weeks.

The most common form of injury is a neuropraxia where the nerve bundles are functionally damaged but

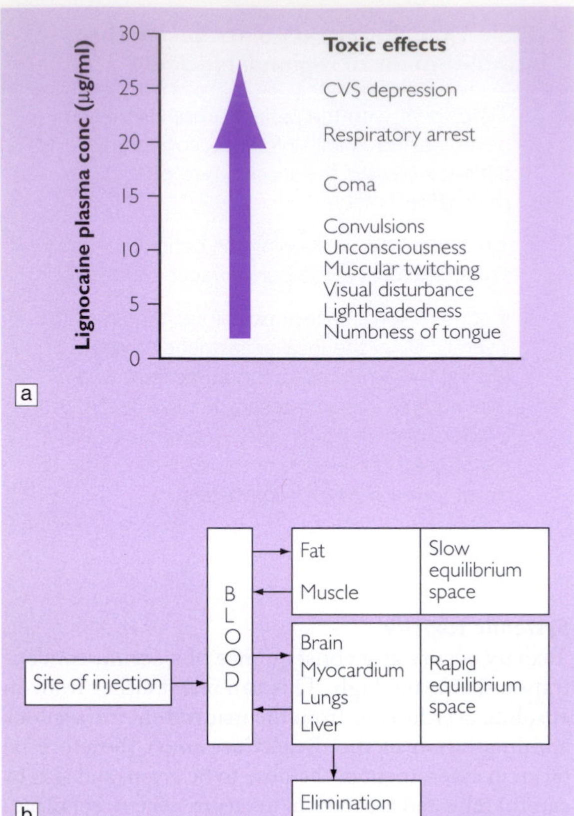


**Figure 15.1.** Pattern of toxicity from rising plasma concentrations of local anaesthetic. (a) The signs and symptoms associated with rising plasma concentrations. These are only approximate figures and there is great individual variation in response. (b) The pattern of uptake of local anaesthetics from the blood. The rapid distribution to the brain and myocardium is responsible for the systemic toxicity. (See also Table 15.12.) (Adapted from Wildsmith JAW, Armitage N. *Principles and Practice of Regional Anaesthesia*. Edingburgh: Churchill Livingstone, 1987, 26.)

anatomically intact. It can be caused by needle damage, pressure from injected solutions, bad intraoperative positioning, or compression from a tourniquet. It has followed blocks at every site, and every local anaesthetic drug has been implicated. Great care must be taken to avoid intraneural injection, for instance by inserting blocks only in awake patients or by careful use of a nerve stimulator. Fortunately, neuropathies are uncommon and rarely permanent.

All local anaesthetics have, however, very rarely been implicated in cases of direct neurotoxicity. It is more likely to occur when high concentrations of drug are used.

### Haematoma formation

Haematomas can be caused by any injection in any site, and usually cause minor effects. However, a haematoma in the epidural space is clearly more dangerous than one of equivalent size in the axilla. Although significant epidural haematomas are rare after epidural injection, the effects may be permanent and disastrous. The anaesthetist must be aware of the possibility, and staff looking after the patient must know the symptoms that a haematoma may cause, and not assume that prolonged or deepening paralysis is the result of the epidural block or epidural infusion.

There is at present considerable debate concerning the establishment of regional anaesthesia in the presence of anticoagulants. Although definite guidelines are not established, Table 15.6 gives what is probably reasonable advice. Trainees should always follow local protocols in the first instance.

### Infection

Considerable debate has taken place around the necessity for scrubbing, gowning, the wearing of masks, etc. during the performance of regional anaesthesia. The authors' practice is to scrub and wear gloves on all occasions, never to touch the needle anywhere but at the hub, and, if a catheter is being sited, to wear a gown. Thorough skin preparation is always necessary. Trainees should follow the guidelines developed in their own hospital.

### Fainting

A vasovagal attack during regional anaesthesia is not uncommon. Its consequences depend on the situation. They are probably worst when they occur halfway through a spinal or epidural block in the sitting position. Whenever it occurs, a vasovagal faint needs to be dealt with quickly, lowering the patient to the horizon-

**Table 15.5. Data related to local anaesthetic toxicity**

| Drug | Relative potency[a] | Approximate protein binding[b] (%) | Onset time | Duration of action | Maximum dose (70-kg man) (mg) |
|---|---|---|---|---|---|
| Prilocaine | 2 | 55 | Fast | Medium | 600 |
| Lignocaine | 2 | 65 | Fast | Medium | 200[c] |
| Ropivacaine | 6 | 95 | Medium | Long | 200[d] |
| Bupivacaine | 8 | 95 | Medium | Long | 150[e] |

[a]Potency is determined by lipid solubility.
[b]Drugs with high protein binding attach strongly to active sites and have prolonged duration of action.
[c]This can be increased to 400 mg with addition of epinephrine for field blocks.
[d]Maximum dose inferred from product data sheet.
[e]This can be increased to 200 mg with addition of epinephrine for field blocks.

**Table 15.6. Guidelines on regional anaesthesia and anticoagulant drugs**

| Anticoagulant regimen | Comment |
|---|---|
| Full anticoagulation with heparin or warfarin | Central neural blockade absolutely contraindicated |
| Subcutaneous heparin, 5000 IU twice daily[a] | Establish regional block before commencing heparin or allow at least 3 hours to elapse from administration of last dose to pass before establishing block or before removing epidural catheter |
| Aspirin 75–100 mg daily | No good agreement; practice differs from centre to centre |

[a]The comments given apply only to this dosing regimen.

tal, giving reassurance, and waiting for any nausea to pass. It needs to be differentiated from a more serious complication such as anaphylaxis (see Chapter 13).

***Positioning***

The intraoperative positioning of patients and the care needed are described in Chapter 3.

## Equipment

***Needles***

Choice of needle for central or peripheral blockade is important, because they can make a difference to the incidence of unwanted effects. Although any 23- or 25-gauge needle may be successfully used for local infiltration, specific nerve blocks are more successful if the correct needle is chosen. A selection of specialized needles is shown in Figure 15.2 and their characteristics are listed below.

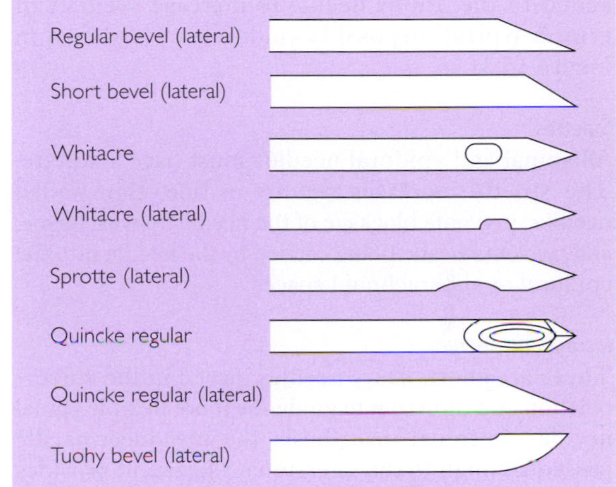


**Figure 15.2.** A variety of needles used for regional anaesthesia.

*Bevel*

Conventional sharp-bevelled needles are associated with a higher incidence of nerve damage than are shorter bevel needles. For regional anaesthesia, a bevel of 18–35° (called short bevel) is recommended rather than the 12° of a hypodermic needle. These needles give more 'feel' as they go through tissues and in so doing improve the accuracy of placement.

*Diameter*

Choice of bore is a compromise between ease of injection, discomfort, and 'feel'. For infiltration, 25-gauge needles or smaller are the least uncomfortable and, for block of nerves close to the skin such as the brachial plexus in the axilla, a 23-gauge needle is optimal. For deeper nerve blocks, where a longer needle is required, the rigidity of a 22-gauge needle improves the control of the tip during passage through the tissues.There are additional factors to take into account for spinal anaesthesia (see below).

*Beaded needles*

Traditionally, needles for regional anaesthesia have a bead, 3–6 mm from the hub of the needle. This security bead is designed to prevent loss of the needle subcutaneously should the needle break at the hub – its most likely point of separation.

*Spinal needles*

A distressing, if not life-threatening, complication of intrathecal anaesthesia is postdural puncture headache (PDPH). Needle design is a major factor in the causation, or prevention, of this side effect. Small needles make small holes in the dura with less leakage of cerebrospinal fluid (CSF). A larger needle, while being technically easier to use, results in an increased incidence of PDPH.

The standard needle for many years has been the Quincke needle with a sharp cutting bevel. These needles are widely available and are still commonly used. To minimize PDPH, it is important to use as fine a needle as possible (25 gauge being a compromise between headache and speed of passage of CSF). It is important that the bevel is inserted parallel to the long axis of the dural fibres.

Pencil-point needles with a side hole for injection of local anaesthetic result in a parting rather than a cutting of the dural fibres, and a lower incidence of PDPH. Their introduction has been one of the factors in repopularizing spinal anaesthesia, especially in obstetrics. They are relatively easy to insert and have an acceptable incidence of PDPH of about 2%. The one drawback is that the side port may straddle the dura and therefore result in an incomplete block. In terms of PDPH, a 25-gauge pencil-point needle is equivalent to a 27-gauge cutting point.

*Epidural needles*

The technique of epidural analgesia requires the use of a larger bore needle, for two reasons:

1. The perception of tissue resistance is much more reliable with a larger, more rigid needle.
2. The needle must be large enough to allow the passage of a catheter into the epidural space.

Consequently most epidural needles are 16, 17, or 18 gauge, all of which will accept a 20-gauge catheter. Smaller gauge needles have been used for single-shot injections, but are not commonly available. The Tuohy needle is almost universally used for epidural anaesthesia. This needle, with an 8-cm shaft, marked in centimetre graduations, has a tip which is contoured so that a catheter comes out directed away from the dura at an angle of about 20°, increasing the likelihood of successful placement. Wings can be added to the Tuohy needle to increase security of grip. A typical disposable epidural set is shown in Figure 15.3.

*Stilettes*

All spinal and epidural needles must have a stilette. The stilette increases rigidity in fine, thin-walled needles, prevents blockage of the needle tip with tissue, and prevents tissue being carried by the needle into the epidural or subarachnoid spaces.

*Introducer needles*

These are short, heavy needles placed in the correct position and direction to guide the more flexible spinal needles. In spinal anaesthesia, the introducer needle passed through to the interspinous ligament provides a straight path for the fine spinal needle over most of its path and minimizes deviation from the midline. In thin patients, care must be taken not to pierce the dura with the introducer needle.

In epidural anaesthesia, introducer needles are available but less commonly used.

### *Peripheral nerve stimulators*

The exact role of peripheral nerve stimulators (PNSs) has not yet been defined and, like other 'new' technology, they have their advocates and critics. The most recent devices do, however, possess characteristics that approach the theoretical ideal, and it is likely that their use will increase.

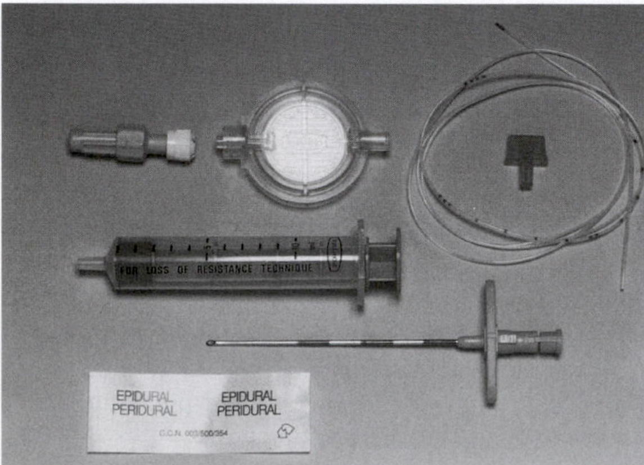


**Figure 15.3.** A disposable epidural kit. Note the printed adhesive label with which the catheter can be clearly marked.

What is agreed is that the PNS is no substitute for proper anatomical knowledge and that it is best used when placed with the needle tip close to but not touching the required nerve. Position is tested by observation of the movement of motor groups. Watching for movement makes them applicable to patients who are sedated or even anaesthetized. The PNS is probably of most use in locating deeply placed nerves. Testing at high power for paraesthesia in sensory nerves can be painful for the patient. The ideal characteristics and approaches that benefit from a PNS have been defined by Pinnock *et al.* and are given in Tables 15.7 and 15.8.

## SPINAL AND EPIDURAL ANAESTHESIA

When performing spinal and epidural blocks, there is no substitute for having a good knowledge of the underlying spinal anatomy. This can really be appreciated only from a three-dimensional study of the skeleton, together with a spinal or epidural needle to observe directly what happens as various approaches are taken and errors made. Time spent doing this is recommended to all trainees. In this chapter the topographical and functional anatomy of the spine is described. Descriptions of blocks outline the important aspects of technique and are intended to be read in conjunction with a study of the skeleton.

### Anatomy

The vertebral column, formed of the vertebral bones, combines strength with mobility. Each vertebra is united to those above and below it by a cartilaginous intravertebral disc and ligaments. Although movement between any two vertebrae is limited, the sum of all the movements makes for considerable mobility. There are seven cervical, twelve thoracic, five lumbar, five sacral, and four coccygeal vertebrae, the sacral and coccygeal ones being fused. They are shown in Figure 15.4.

| Table 15.7. The ideal characteristics of a peripheral nerve stimulator |
|---|
| Portable, battery operated with detachable and sterilizable leads |
| Clearly marked electrodes; cathode (negative) attached to needle |
| Universal alligator clip terminals suitable for many types of needle |
| Digital display of delivered current and/or voltage with linear output |
| Voltage (9 V) and current (5 mA), adjustable and limited to cope with variable resistance of body tissues |
| Short duration of impulse (< 100 μs) at 1–2 Hz so that motor nerves are stimulated in preference to sensory nerves |

Adapted from Pinnock CA, Fischer HBJ, Jones RP. *Peripheral Nerve Blockade*. Edinburgh: Churchill Livingstone, 1996: 12.

**Table 15.8. Nerve blocks that can benefit from the use of a peripheral nerve stimulator**

| |
|---|
| All approaches to brachial plexus |
| Suprascapular nerve |
| Radial nerve at elbow |
| Median nerve at elbow |
| All approaches to sciatic nerve |
| Femoral nerve (including 3 in 1) |
| Obturator nerve |
| Popliteal fossa block |

Adapted from Pinnock CA, Fischer HBJ, Jones RP. *Peripheral Nerve Blockade*. Edinburgh: Churchill Livingstone, 1996: 12.

The vertebral canal is formed by successive vertebral foramina, the ligaments and the discs connecting the vertebrae together, making the canal aligned and continuous. Although there are differences in the anatomy of vertebrae in the various regions, all have the same basic structure, consisting of the following:

- the vertebral body, which supports the weight of the subject;
- the vertebral arch, which surrounds and protects the cord. The arch is made up of a pedicle and a lamina on each side, and a dorsal spine;
- each lamina gives rise to a transverse process, and two articular processes: superior and inferior. The pedicles are notched, creating the intervertebral foramina, through which the spinal nerves pass.

**Figure 15.4.** The adult spine with its characteristic curves seen (a) laterally and (b) posteriorly. On the lateral view, the intervertebral foramina where the nerves leave the spinal canal are shown in black. In the posterior view, the interlaminar spaces are shown in black. Note that the interlaminar spaces in the thoracic region are concealed from view by the spines of the upper vertebrae, which overlap the lamina of the vertebra below.

The morphology of a lumbar vertebra and the way in which vertebrae interlock is shown in Figures 15.5 and 15.6.

***Thoracic vertebrae***

The bodies of the thoracic vertebrae are small, increasing in size from T1 to T12. The intervertebral discs are thicker in front, and the vertebral foramina large and triangular. From T2 to T8 the bodies have upper and lower facets, which retain the rib heads. The pedicles run backwards and have only an inferior notch. The transverse processes are large, passing backwards as well as laterally, and articulate with the corresponding rib. The spinous processes are long; they overlap each other and obscure the interlaminar foramina.

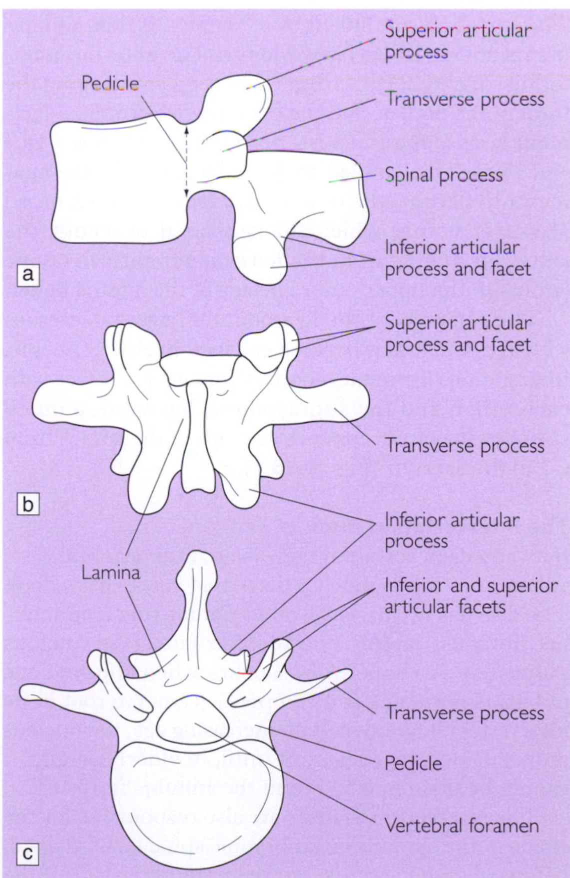


**Figure 15.5.** The morphology of a typical lumbar vertebra. (a) lateral view; (b) posterior view; (c) axial view.

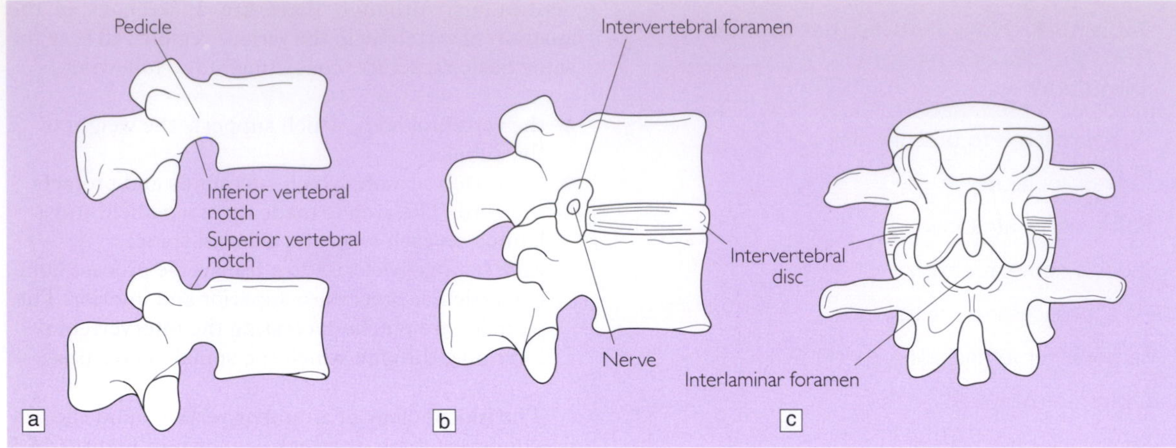


**Figure 15.6.** Two lumbar vertebrae shown (a) to demonstrate the way in which they interlock (b and c).

***Lumbar vertebrae*** (Figures 15.5 and 15.6)
Lumbar vertebrae have large, kidney-shaped bodies, with vertebral foramina that are smaller than those of the thoracic area. The intervertebral discs are thick and wedge shaped, giving mobility to the lumbar region. The transverse processes are slender, the longest being L3, with the length decreasing towards both L1 and L5. The laminae do not overlap and the spinous processes are horizontal, making the interlaminar foramina more accessible from the back.

***Ligaments***
The vertebrae are linked by a complex system of ligaments and articular facetal joints. The anterior longitudinal ligament runs from C2 to the sacrum along the front of the bodies, and the posterior longitudinal ligament runs along the posterior surfaces (Figures 15.7 and 15.8). The laminae are joined together by the ligamentum flavum (the yellow ligament), a strong, broad elastic structure which thickens as it descends the spine, stretching from the lower inner surface of one lamina to the upper outer surface of the lamina below.

The elasticity of the ligamentum flavum decreases with age, and it may become calcified in elderly people. Interspinous ligaments connect spinous processes with each other, and the supraspinous ligament, a much stronger structure, connects the tips of the spines from C7 to the sacrum (Figure 15.8).

***The intervertebral discs***
Between each vertebral body is an intervertebral disc, adherent to the hyaline cartilage that covers each body. The disc has two parts: an outer fibrous ring (the annulus fibrosus) and a central softer core (the nucleus pulposus). A slipped disc occurs when the nucleus pulposus herniates and compresses a nerve root in its intervertebral foramen. With increasing age, the nucleus pulposus becomes less soft until, in elderly people, it cannot be distinguished from the annulus fibrosus.

The intervertebral discs are also responsible for the shape of the spine. The embryonic spine is 'C' shaped, being concave forwards, but the upright posture of the human, with extension of lower limbs and head, introduces secondary curves in the lumbar and cervical regions, both convex forwards. These curves are largely created by moulding of the intervertebral discs, which become wedge shaped.

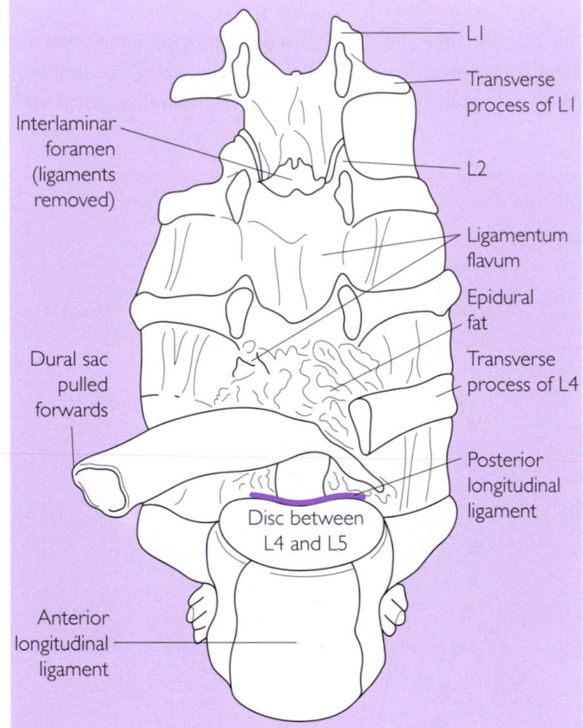


**Figure 15.7.** An anterior dissection of the lumbar spine showing the vertebral canal and ligaments. The dural sac is pulled forwards. The vertebral bodies of L1–L4 have been removed.

***The sacrum***
The sacrum, made up of five fused sacral vertebrae, is a curved wedge between the iliac bones and is concave forwards (Figure 15.9). Posteriorly the laminae are fused to form a rough plate with a median crest created by fused spinous processes, and intermediate crests by fused articular processes.

The lowest articular processes are called the sacral cornua and are two blunt bumps linked to the coccyx by ligaments, often palpable through the skin. In over 90% of people, the arch of the fifth sacral vertebra fails

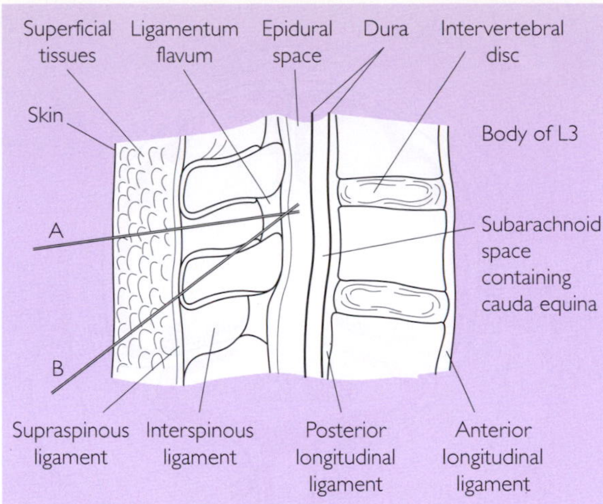


**Figure 15.8.** A diagrammatic midline sagittal cross-section of the lumbar spine. The spinal needle shown in direction A has been passed from the midline or para-midline approach. The spinal needle shown in direction B has been passed from the full lateral position.

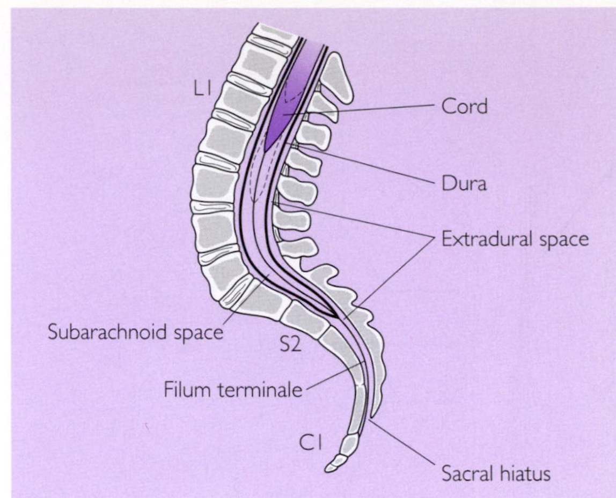


**Figure 15.10.** A midline sagittal cross-sectional view of the lower spine and spinal canal to show the relative positions of the spinal cord and dura.

to fuse in the midline, leaving a triangular gap, the sacral hiatus, about 5 mm above the tip of the coccyx, which allows access to the epidural space.

### *The spinal cord*

The spinal cord is continuous with the medulla oblongata. It is the thickness of a heavy pencil, tapering to its end, the conus medullaris, which in adults is normally at the level of the intervertebral disc between L1 and L2. This level can, however, vary from T12 to L3 (Figure 15.10). A fine thread runs from the conus, the filum terminale, which continues to the coccyx.

In total the spinal cord is about 45 cm long in adults. In newborn babies, the cord is relatively longer than in the adult, and terminates at the lower border of L3. During embryonic development up to the third month, the cord runs the entire length of the canal but, because of the more rapid development of the vertebral bodies thereafter, it terminates higher, until at birth it ends at the lower border of L3.

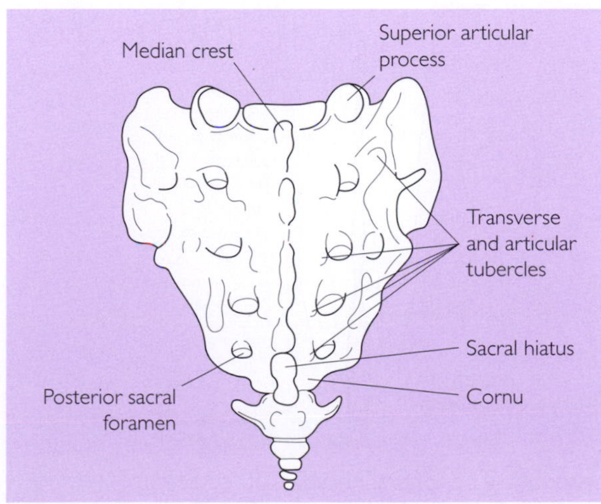


**Figure 15.9.** The posterior view of the sacrum.

As a result of this differential in growth rate, the lumbar and sacral nerves become elongated in order to reach their foramina, and the cauda equina is formed. Subsequently, as the vertebral column is ascended, the spinal nerves become more horizontal. The cross-section of the cord is shown at various levels in Figure 15.11, and the surface representation of the spinal nerves is shown in Figure 15.12.

### *The meninges*

There are three coverings of the spinal cord: the dura mater, arachnoid mater, and pia mater, collectively called the meninges. The spinal dura is a continuation of the inner layer (the cerebral dura) – one of the two dural layers that cover the brain (Figure 15.13). The outer, or endosteal, layer terminates at the foramen magnum, being represented in the spinal canal by its periosteal lining.

The spinal dura is made of dense fibrous tissue and the sac extends to the second sacral vertebra. Individual variations occur, and the sac may terminate as high as L5 or as low as S3. The dura is attached to the edge of the foramen magnum above and to the coccyx below by the filum terminale. It also has loose slender connections to the posterior longitudinal ligament anteriorly. Laterally, the dura extends along the ventral and dorsal nerve roots, being continuous with the epineurium of the spinal nerves. Posteriorly, the dural sac is unattached. The arachnoid mater, a fine membrane, lines the dural sac and extends along each nerve root. The pia mater is a vascular connective tissue that closely covers the brain and spinal cord.

Thus, the spinal meninges divide the spinal canal into the subarachnoid, subdural, and epidural spaces (see Figure 15.14). In the subarachnoid space lie the spinal cord and the CSF. It contains trabeculae, often incomplete and variable in pattern. However, in most people there is a dorsal septum in the midline, extending from the midcervical to the lumbar region. The dorsolateral septa, which atrophy with age, attach the dorsal roots to the arachnoid. Laterally, the spinal cord is supported by the dentate ligaments.

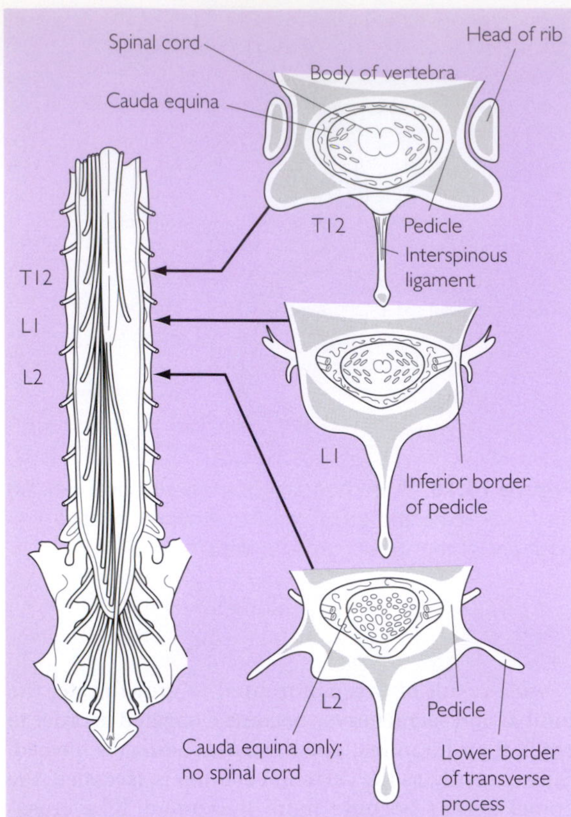


**Figure 15.11.** A diagrammatic representation of the cross-section of the spinal cord at T12, L1, and L2.

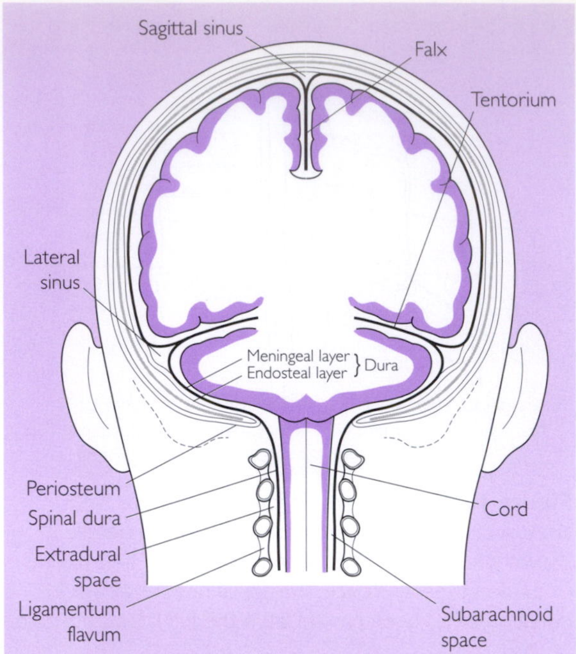


**Figure 15.13.** The cranial meninges.

The subdural 'space' is a potential space only, because the arachnoid is closely applied to the dura. The epidural space lies between the dura mater and the spinal canal, extending from the foramen magnum to

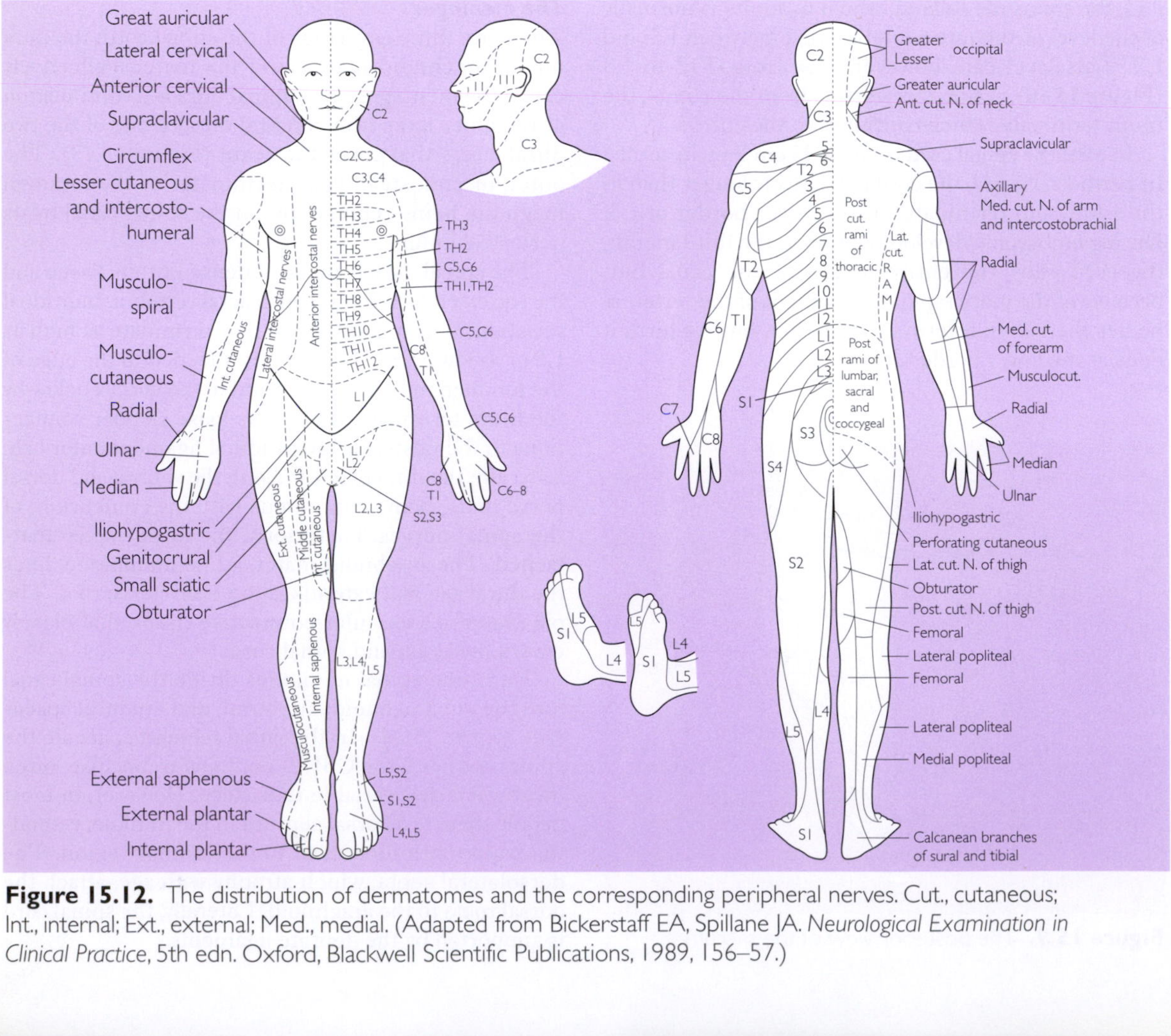

**Figure 15.12.** The distribution of dermatomes and the corresponding peripheral nerves. Cut., cutaneous; Int., internal; Ext., external; Med., medial. (Adapted from Bickerstaff EA, Spillane JA. *Neurological Examination in Clinical Practice*, 5th edn. Oxford, Blackwell Scientific Publications, 1989, 156–57.)

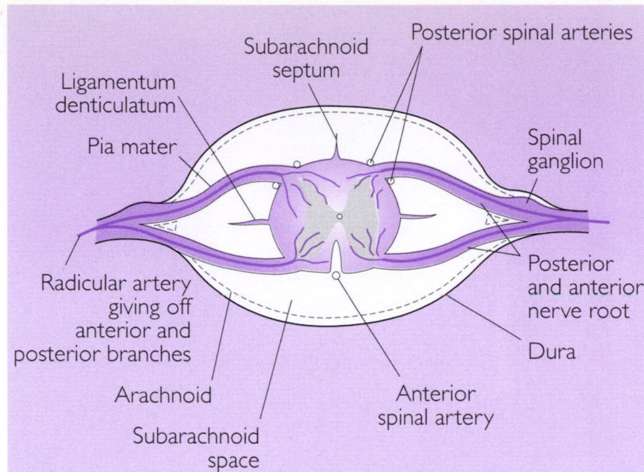


**Figure 15.14.** A cross-section of the spinal cord to show the meninges in transverse section. Note the blood supply from the posterior and anterior spinal arteries and the radicular arteries.

the sacral hiatus. It is filled with fat, blood vessels, and lymph vessels (Figure 15.7). The dural sac usually lies towards the anterior wall of the canal, and therefore the epidural space is smaller anteriorly. The depth of the posterior epidural space varies from approximately 1 mm in the cervical area to 6 mm in the lumbar.

### *Cerebrospinal fluid*

This clear, colourless liquid fills all the cavities and spaces around the central nervous system (CNS). It is secreted by the choroid plexus in the third and fourth ventricles and, although some drains into the connective tissue spaces of the nerves, most is reabsorbed by the arachnoid villi and granulations. There are about 130 ml of CSF, of which 35 ml are in the spinal subarachnoid space. CSF is described in more detail in Chapter 22.

### *Blood supply*

Arterial supply to the spinal cord is from the anterior and posterior spinal arteries (Figure 15.14). The anterior spinal artery is formed at the foramen magnum by branches of each vertebral artery; it is a single vessel that supplies a large part of the anterior cord. There are one or two posterior spinal arteries on each side of the cord, coming from the posteroinferior cerebellar arteries, and their supply is augmented by radicular arteries formed from branches of the vertebral, ascending cervical, posterior intercostal, lumbar, and lateral sacral arteries.

It can be seen therefore that, although occlusion of a posterior spinal artery may be compensated for, occlusion of, or damage to, the anterior spinal artery is likely to be catastrophic. The blood supply of the CNS is considered in more detail in Chapter 22.

## Spinal anaesthesia

In contrast to an epidural injection, which can be performed between any two vertebrae, spinal anaesthesia is always carried out with an injection below the level of the second lumbar vertebra. This tries to ensure that the needle is below the level at which the spinal cord ends, but above the termination of the subarachnoid space contained by the dura to the level of the second sacral vertebra (Figure 15.10).

Approach to the subarachnoid space may be in the midline, or from a lateral direction. In the midline (see Figure 15.8), a spinal needle goes through the skin, supraspinous ligament, interspinous ligament, ligamentum flavum, and the epidural space before piercing the dura to enter the subarachnoid space. Using a lateral approach (Figure 15.8 and 15.15), the needle travels further, piercing skin, subcutaneous tissue, the lumbar aponeurosis, paravertebral muscles, ligamentum flavum, and the epidural space, before entering the subarachnoid space. Compare Figure 15.8 with Figure 15.15.

### *Positioning*

The patient may be either sitting up or in the lateral position, depending on the preference of the anaesthetist and the patient. A trained assistant is always required. If sitting, the patient should be on the edge of the bed or trolley with both feet on a stool. The head is bent so that the chin touches the chest (Figure 15.16). The patient's arms may be folded across his or her thighs, resting on a pillow, or on the shoulders of an assistant, as is most comfortable.

If lying in the lateral position, ask the patient to tuck the chin down on to the chest, and pull the knees up towards the abdomen. The head needs to be on a pillow to keep the vertebral column horizontal. The patient should be helped into position by an assistant, especially if sedated.

After full aseptic preparation and draping, the appropriate interspace is identified. Choice depends on individual anatomical variation, but L2–3 or L3–4 interspaces are those most commonly selected. An imaginary line drawn between the most prominent points of the iliac crests usually crosses the spinous process of L4, or the L4–5 interspace, and is the essential landmark in identifying the level of needle insertion whether in the sitting or the lying position (Figure 15.17).

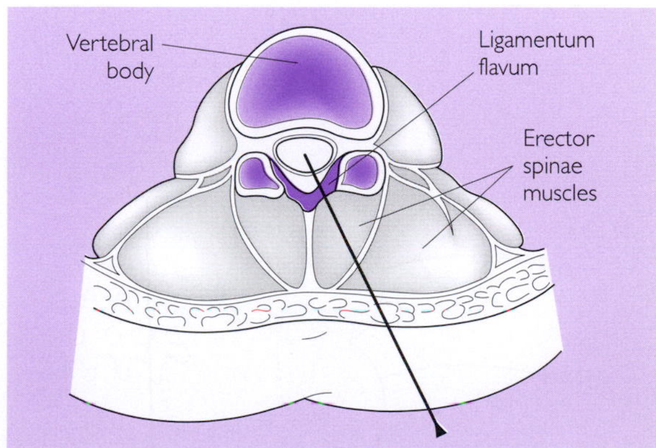


**Figure 15.15.** A cross-section of the lumbar spine showing the adjacent spinal muscles and other soft tissues. The spinal needle is shown piercing the dura and entering the subarachnoid space from the full lateral position. The cross-section is between adjacent spinal processes which are therefore not seen.

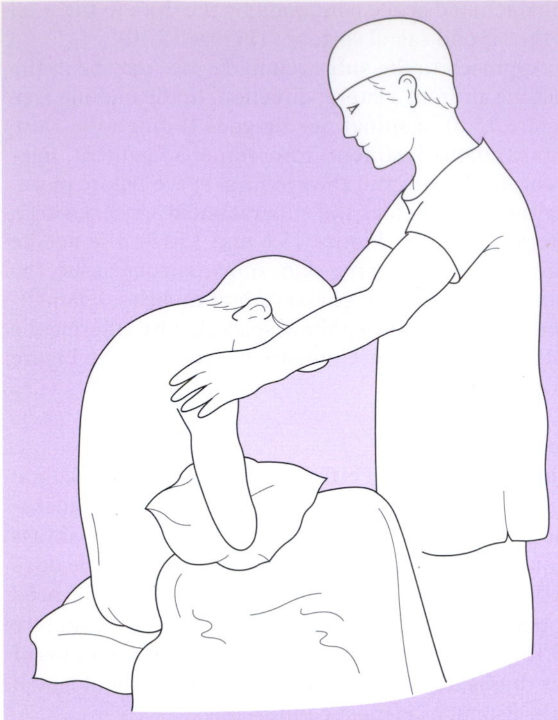

**Figure 15.16.** The sitting position for spinal anaesthesia. Note the position of the assistant.

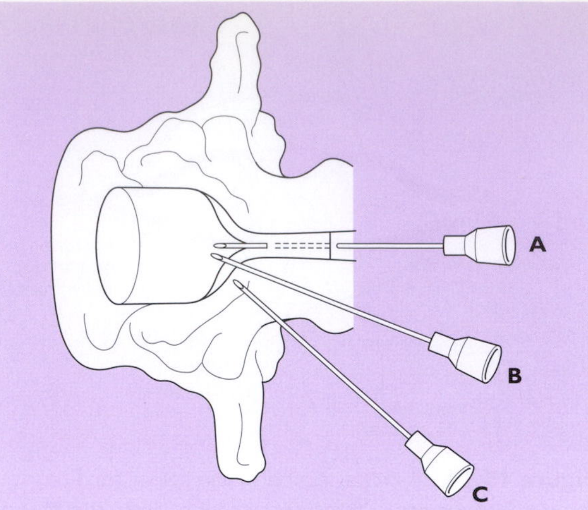


**Figure 15.18.** Diagrammatic representation of the midline (A), para-midline (B), and full lateral (C) approaches to the dura for spinal anaesthesia.

### *Entering the subarachnoid space*

*Midline approach*

This is shown diagrammatically in Figures 15.8 and 15.18. Once the interspace is chosen, 1–3 ml of local anaesthetic is infiltrated into the skin, subcutaneous tissues, and interspinous ligament using a 25-gauge needle.

Stabilize the tissues by using the index and middle fingers of the free hand to 'bracket' the chosen space. As spinal needles are usually 25–27 gauge, they tend to bend as they pass through the tissues, thus deviating from the midline, so an 18-gauge introducer is used to facilitate passage through the supraspinous and interspinous ligaments. The introducer needle is inserted in the midline, midway between the two spinous processes of the chosen space, parallel to the spinous processes, and angling slightly towards the patient's head. Through this the spinal needle is passed, entering the CSF. Before insertion, check that the stilette is fully inserted and, if using a Quincke needle, ensure that the bevel is facing laterally. The correct angulation and adherence to the midline are necessary to avoid (painful) contact with bone.

As the spinal needle is inserted, each tissue has a characteristic 'feel', learned only through experience. The use of an introducer means that only the firm resistance of the interspinous ligament and the ligamentum flavum is noticed before the sudden loss of resistance as the dura is pierced.

*Lateral approach*

This is shown diagrammatically in Figures 15.8, 15.15 and 15.18. The midline approach to the subarachnoid space is the simplest to describe and hence the easiest to teach, but in elderly, stiff, or painful patients it is often not the easiest to perform. There are two lateral

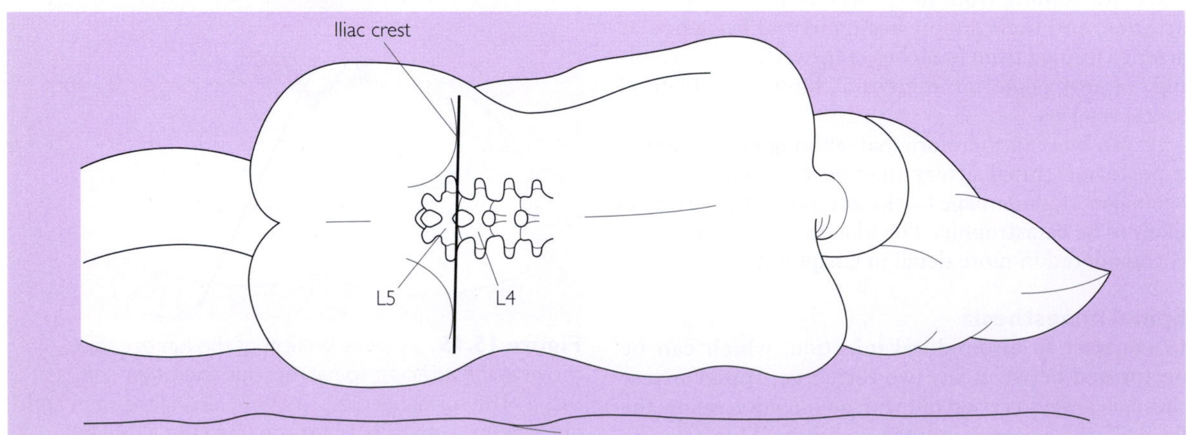


**Figure 15.17.** The lateral position for spinal anaesthesia. The line joining the posterosuperior iliac crests usually crosses the spinous process of L4 or the L4–5 interspace.

approaches that can be used in patients who are difficult to position.

*The para-midline approach*
Simply move the point of insertion 1–1.5 cm laterally, still staying in the same interspace. The path of the needle is then at a slight medial angle, as well as the usual angle towards the patient's head.

If possible, mentally visualize the ligamentum flavum in the midline 4–5 cm away, and aim the needle for that point. This approach bypasses the interspinous ligament, and requires less flexion of the spine to enlarge the space.

*The full lateral approach*
Feel the spinous process below the chosen interspace. From a point 2–2.5 cm lateral to this process, direct the needle at 45° to the midline, and 45° towards the patient's head; the subarachnoid space may then be entered directly via the ligamentum flavum.

Alternatively, from the insertion point, the needle is directed to hit the lamina of the lower vertebra, and then 'walked' over the superior (cephalad) rim of the lamina into the ligamentum flavum.

*Both lateral approaches can cause the patient discomfort, and infiltration of local anaesthetic before insertion of the introducer and spinal needle should be generous.*

Once in the subarachnoid space, the stilette is removed and CSF should appear at the hub of the needle. When CSF is obtained, the needle is held firmly and immobilized by the free hand, while the syringe containing local anaesthetic is attached. Gentle aspiration after attachment, half-way through the injection, and at the end of injection, ensures that the full dose is given and that the needle has not moved. This aspiration must be as gentle as possible to prevent uncontrolled distribution of the local anaesthetic on reinjection (a process known as barbotage).

*Practical points*
*Stop injecting immediately if it produces paraesthesia or pain!*

- Always make sure that the brakes are engaged on the trolley or bed on which the patient is sitting or lying, and adopt a comfortable, controlled posture yourself.
- Obese or pregnant patients may be more comfortable sitting than lying during insertion of the block.
- It is often easier to be sure of the midline if the patient is sitting. In elderly or obese patients in the lateral position, the midline skin crease will drop and may be several centimetres below the true midline (Figure 15.19).
- When positioning the patient in the lateral position ensure that one hip is directly over the other, i.e. that the patient has not rolled forwards, and that the line of transverse processes is parallel to the table.
- Do not forget that the needle has to travel further using a lateral approach, and the subarachnoid space will therefore seem deeper.
- Hold the needle correctly. The hub of the needle is held between the thumb and middle finger, the index finger being used to ensure that the stilette remains in position during insertion. The ring and little fingers rest on the patient's back, giving control.
- If CSF does not appear, it may be because:
    - a nerve root is blocking the needle tip – rotate the needle gently through 90–180°;
    - the CSF pressure may be too low, especially if a lateral approach from the upper side has been used; try gentle aspiration with a 2-ml syringe;
    - the stilette may not have been fully inserted and a tissue plug has blocked the tip; aspirate gently;
    - the bevel or, if using a pencil-point needle, the aperture may still be partially in the epidural space; replace the stilette, advance slowly, and check again for CSF.
- If bone is contacted, the patient may experience considerable pain. Do not force the needle as it may become blunt, bent, barbed, or blocked. Come back to subcutaneous tissue, adjust the angle of the needle, and reinsert. In the midline, the bone contacted may be the spinous process of the vertebra below, or that above or, if using a lateral approach, the lamina of the lower vertebra.
- If paraesthesia is encountered, stop and immobilize the needle instantly. Paraesthesia is usually fleeting, but may be because the needle has strayed from the midline and has hit a nerve root. It is preferable to bring the needle back to subcutaneous tissue, realign, and try again.

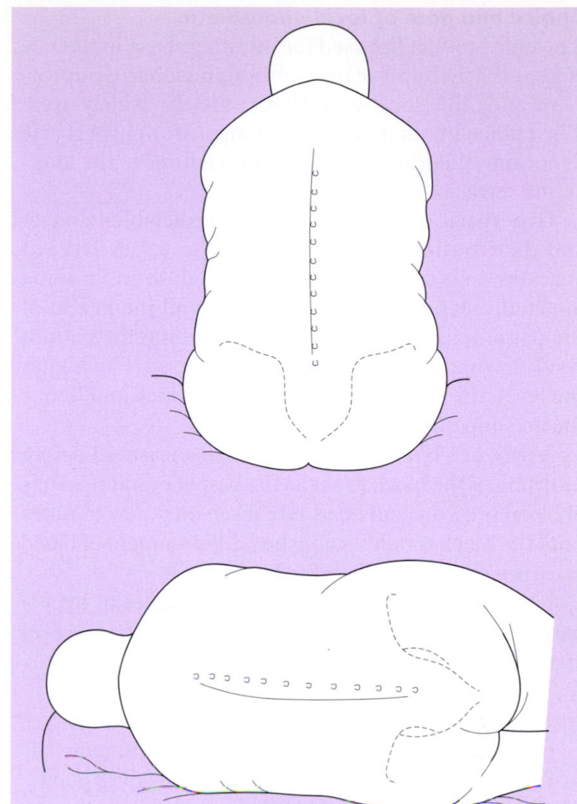

**Figure 15.19.** The midline skin crease in the sitting and lateral positions.

### *Choice and dose of local anaesthetic*

The only product licensed for intrathecal use in the UK is hyperbaric bupivacaine, although isobaric bupivacaine and other local anaesthetics are also widely used. The choice in other countries ranges from hyperbaric lignocaine (lidocaine) for short procedures to the long-acting tetracaine.

Hyperbaric solutions are more predictable in onset and distribution of anaesthesia. The upper level of anaesthesia is dependent on the total dose and volume injected, the position of the patient, and the height of the patient, as well as on baricity. Tipping the patient head-down increases the level of the block. The higher the level, the greater the sympathetic block and hence the accompanying hypotension.

A patient's blood pressure must be measured before insertion of the block to act as the baseline, and readings of blood pressure and heart rate taken every few minutes until the block is fully established. Management of blood pressure changes is described below.

In an average 70-kg man, typical volumes of hyperbaric bupivacaine required to produce specific levels of anaesthesia are as follows:

- 1–1.5 ml produces a 'saddle block' in a sitting patient, useful for perineal or perianal surgery;
- 2–2.5 ml produces a block to T10, providing good anaesthesia for lower limb surgery, transurethral prostatectomy, or hip arthroplasty; it may not, however, prevent discomfort from a thigh tourniquet;
- 3–3.5 ml produces anaesthesia to T4–6 which is necessary for herniorrhaphy, appendicectomy, and abdominal hysterectomy. The patient may, however, be aware of pain or discomfort caused by traction on the peritoneum or gut.

A level of at least T4 is necessary for most women undergoing caesarean section but they require less volume, 2.5–3 ml being a typical dose (see Chapters 45 and 85).

Isobaric and hypobaric solutions are less predictable in their spread of anaesthesia but have the advantage in hip arthroplasty or in patients with a fractured femur, for instance, of greater patient comfort during insertion, and less movement of the patient afterwards, as the procedure can be carried out with the affected limb uppermost.

Although less common than epidural opioids, spinal opioids are used by a number of anaesthetists. Similar precautions should be taken as for epidural opioids (see later and Chapter 5) with respect to monitoring of respiration, etc. A typical dose is morphine 0.03 mg/kg diluted with 0.9% saline. The dose is reduced by 20% per decade for patients over 60 years and the volume increased for very tall patients.

### *Complications of spinal anaesthesia*

#### *Hypotension*

Hypotension is an almost inevitable accompaniment to spinal anaesthesia. It is dependent on the degree of sympathetic blockade and therefore the height of the block. Analgesia to the fourth thoracic dermatome will also involve the sympathetic supply to the gut, and cause dilatation of splanchnic, pelvic, and lower limb blood vessels. Above T4, the supply to the heart becomes involved, causing bradycardia as well as hypotension.

The venous dilatation causes pooling of blood in the peripheral vessels, decreased venous return, and hence a decrease in cardiac output. Decreased peripheral resistance (arteriolar) contributes to hypotension to a lesser extent. As a result of the decreased ventricular afterload, preload, and bradycardia that may occur as the right atrial pressure receptors respond to the decreased venous return, there is a concomitant decrease in myocardial work and $O_2$ requirement. In the healthy patient, this compensates for the decrease in cardiac blood flow that accompanies the drop in mean arterial pressure. In patients with coronary artery disease and critical myocardial perfusion, the fall in blood pressure may, however, produce a severe and disproportionate reduction in coronary blood flow. Such individuals require careful monitoring and prompt management with fluids and vasoconstrictors to ensure adequate coronary perfusion pressure.

Many centres routinely load patients with a litre of crystalloid or colloid to ameliorate the fall in blood pressure as the block takes effect. After this, if the pressure is too low on clinical grounds (the earliest sign of hypotension in the conscious patient is often nausea), vasoconstrictors must be used. Two in common use are ephedrine and methoxamine (see Chapter 23). Ephedrine is a direct- and indirect-acting sympathomimetic which acts on α- and β-adrenoceptors. It produces peripheral vasoconstriction and a rise in heart rate. It is used in obstetrics because it has little vasoconstricting effect on placental blood flow. Methoxamine is a pure α-adrenoceptor agonist which produces peripheral vasoconstriction. Both should be diluted before use. Methoxamine should be given in 1-mg increments and ephedrine in 2- to 5-mg increments.

#### *Headache (PDPH)*

Leakage of CSF after dural puncture may cause PDPH. Reduction in CSF pressure allows the brain to drop, stretching the dura, tentorium, venous sinuses, and nerve endings, and results in the classic post-spinal headache. This is largely occipital but radiates frontally. It is postural, being least or absent when the patient is lying down, and may be associated with nausea, photophobia, dizziness, and sometimes sixth nerve palsy. It may be very severe and distressing, lasting for several days if untreated. Rarely, it may last for weeks and even more rarely be associated with a subdural haematoma. The incidence of headache varies with the size of the needle used to perform the injection, being directly related to the size of the hole produced. Using a 26-gauge needle, the incidence should be less than 1%, and use of pencil-point needles reduces it even further. The incidence is also dependent to a lesser extent on the age of the patient, reducing with increasing age.

#### *Treatment of PDPH*

Patients should be well hydrated, and the headache treated with simple analgesia. If the headache is severe, not settling or not responding to hydration and analgesia, a blood patch should be carried out provided that the patient is apyrexial.

Under full aseptic technique, a sample of the patient's own blood is taken, and 15–20 ml injected into the epidural space. This may cause transient pain in the back, or other neurological effects, but should have no lasting effects.

The patient is asked to lie flat for half an hour, then allowed to mobilize. Treatment is successful in the majority of patients.

It should always be remembered that headaches are common after surgery, and are not always caused by dural puncture. If the headache is relieved by forcible pressing on the abdomen, it is usually because of a CSF leak (Gutsche test).

*Urinary retention*

After spinal anaesthesia, block of the sacral autonomic fibres is long lasting and retention of urine is common. The likelihood is increased by the use of fluids to preload the patient, which may cause over-distension of the bladder.

*Backache*

Backache is equally common after both regional and general anaesthesia, and is more often caused by careless positioning than by spinal anaesthesia.

*Neurological complications*

Fortunately such complications are very rare, but must always be fully investigated. Permanent neurological damage has occurred from hypotension. Other causes identified in the past have been the injection of incorrect drugs or chemicals.

*Significant haematomas and abscesses*

These have been described following both spinal and epidural anaesthesia, and both are very rare. The symptoms and signs are variable. A rapidly spreading haematoma can present as an unexpectedly prolonged block. Abscesses appear 3 or 4 days after the block with pyrexia and a high white cell count. Both are usually attended by back pain and tenderness to palpation. They require urgent referral to a specialist neurosurgical unit. Diagnosis is by scanning and myelography; treatment is surgical.

*Vascular complications*

The classic anterior spinal artery syndrome is very rare but extremely serious. Occlusion of the anterior spinal artery can cause a permanent painless paralysis of the legs and sphincters. It may follow a period of hypotension in elderly patients.

## Epidural anaesthesia

Many of the principles of good practice for epidural anaesthesia are the same as for spinal anaesthesia. All the points made in the list of complications of spinal blocks are equally relevant to epidural blocks. A comparison of some aspects of spinal and epidural block is given in Table 15.9.

Positioning of the patient for epidural anaesthesia is the same as that for spinal anaesthesia and has already been described. As for spinal anaesthesia, both midline and lateral approaches may be used, a lateral approach being more commonly employed for thoracic epidurals because of the long, sloping spinous processes. The methods and approaches have already been described for spinal anaesthesia. Only the midline lumbar approach is outlined here to describe the identification of the epidural space.

### *Entering the epidural space*

*Preparation and initial insertion*

The iliac crests and spinous processes are identified, and marked if desired, to identify and select the interspinous space for injection, usually between L2 and L5.

**Table 15.9. A comparison of some aspects of spinal and epidural anaesthesia**

| Aspect | Spinal block | Epidural block |
|---|---|---|
| Systemic toxicity | Much lower doses, so less dangerous | Large volumes of local anaesthetics, some of which attach strongly to membranes |
| Time to onset | Fast | Slower |
| Reliability of block | Very high if good flow of CSF | Not as high |
| Patchy block | Very rare | Can occur because of incomplete spread |
| Distribution of block | Effectively transects the neural input at the level of the block | Can produce a band of anaesthesia over several dermatomes leaving lower ones free |
| Modality affected | Affects all motor and sensory functions | Dose of some drugs will partially spare motor functions |
| Ability to adjust level of block[a] | After the dose is in, only baricity and positioning are available for adjustment | Easy to achieve if a catheter is in position |
| Test dose | Not required | Recommended by many practitioners |

[a]This assumes that no intrathecal catheter is being used.
CSF, cerebrospinal fluid.

The skin is prepared and the patient draped. The skin at the chosen site is stabilized using the index and middle fingers of the left hand, pressing them firmly against the skin on each side of the space. Local anaesthetic is introduced into the skin and subcutaneous tissues, and the skin pierced with an introducer or pointed scalpel blade. Although not essential, this reduces the pressure necessary to introduce the Tuohy needle, and hence minimizes the risk of misalignment.

Before using the epidural needle (see Figure 15.3), it is essential to check the equipment. In particular, the syringe plunger must move smoothly and seal well, and the catheter must be patent. The Tuohy needle is introduced, as for a spinal injection, in the midline, parallel to the trolley or operating table top (with the patient in the lateral position) and slightly cephalad. The bevel should point towards the head, because this reduces lateral deviation of the needle.

Holding the wings with right and left thumbs and index fingers, and with the hypothenar eminence resting on the patient's back, the needle is advanced until the resistance of the ligamentum flavum is felt. At this point, if the needle is let go, the hub will not drop.

The needle hub is gripped by the fingers of the left hand, the back of this hand resting on the patient's back, the stilette removed by the right hand, and the preferred indicator device attached. Care must be taken not to advance the needle during this procedure.

#### *Identification of the epidural space*

All techniques depend on the loss of resistance that occurs as the needle tip moves out of the ligamentum flavum into the epidural space.

A technique that applies continuous pressure as the needle is advanced is preferable to one in which intermittent pressure is applied, i.e. a saline-filled syringe is preferred to an air-filled syringe. Using an air-filled loss-of-resistance syringe, the pressure must be tested, the needle advanced, and the pressure re-tested. If the syringe is filled with saline, continuous pressure can be applied and the syringe and needle moved as a single unit. When doing this, it is essential to have good control of the needle and syringe and the patient perfectly still. The loss of resistance end-point as the needle tip enters the epidural space is much more clear-cut during continuous motion.

Again, taking care not to move the Tuohy needle, the loss-of-resistance device is removed, the depth of the epidural space noted, and the catheter inserted. The catheter is fed in so that 5–7 cm is in the epidural space. More than this increases the chance of entering an epidural vein or intervertebral foramina. The needle is then pulled back, making sure that it does not drag the catheter out with it. After the needle is fully removed, based on the depth of the epidural space, the catheter is pulled back to leave 3–5 cm in the epidural space. More than this increases the chance of the tip migrating through an intervertebral foramen.

#### *Practical tips*

- If the patient is lying, the midline skin crease may no longer be in the midline (see Figure 15.19).
- The most common fault during needle insertion in the lateral position is to allow the hub to drop towards the floor, lifting the tip above the midline, and therefore missing the ligamentum flavum.
- The catheter must never be pulled back through the needle. This risks amputation of the distal end.
- If blood is seen in the catheter, it can be withdrawn a little, flushed, and aspirated gently, hoping that it no longer resides in a vein. If there is any uncertainty, the epidural must be reinserted. If it is decided to use it, the dose of local anaesthetic (not bupivacaine) must be put in very gradually in small increments, for obvious reasons.
- A bacterial filter should always be incorporated into an epidural system. It also prevents entry of other particles such as glass.
- When securing the catheter, be sure that it is not kinked; curl a loop or two on to the skin and stick down well with an adhesive dressing, ensuring no creases.

### *Choice and dose of local anaesthetic and/or opioid*

#### *The test dose*

Some practitioners use test doses to confirm that the catheter is neither intrathecal nor intravascular. Others do not use them and top up gradually. To be effective a test dose must be large enough to cause detectable effects.

A dose of 2–3 ml of local anaesthetic will produce neurological effects if given intrathecally, but will have little effect if the dose goes intravascularly. For this, epinephrine (adrenaline) has to be added to produce a tachycardia and change in blood pressure. A commercial preparation is available for this purpose. It is 3 ml of 2% lignocaine with 1 : 200 000 epinephrine added.

However, the test dose is not foolproof, and does not remove the need for aspiration before each injection, and giving the first dose and top-ups in small boluses of, say, 5 ml. After *any* injection into the epidural space, measure the blood pressure and heart rate every few minutes until the block is established.

Whether during a test dose, first dose, or top-up, *stop injecting immediately if it produces paraesthesia or pain!*

#### *The anaesthetizing dose*

Several agents can be used and their properties predicted from Table 15.5.

The exact calculation of dosage is difficult because several factors influence spread in the epidural space. The volume and concentration of the local anaesthetic are obviously major variables. In the patient, the age and site of block are the most important factors, but height, weight, and position may also affect the spread. The same volume of agent spreads much further in the thoracic space than in the lumbar space. Pregnant women need considerably less to achieve the same level of anaesthesia.

The advantage of epidural catheter techniques is that more local anaesthetic can be added to adjust the level of the block. Although it is difficult to give firm recommendations on dosage and volume, if undertaking an upper abdominal procedure in a 70-kg man, with the catheter at L2–3, inject 20 ml of solution, and with the catheter at T4–5 inject 5 ml. Then observe the results and adjust accordingly. Give incremental doses until the required height of block is reached.

The block can be maintained with top-ups of one-third to one-half of the initial dose, at intervals determined by the effect of the block. Signs of systemic toxicity may occur if the catheter has migrated intravenously. These are described later under 'intravenous regional anaesthesia' (see Table 15.12). It is also currently popular to keep the block maintained by an infusion of say 10–20 ml/h of 0.100% or 0.125% bupivacaine.

Pregnant women need very much reduced doses and, for a normally sized full-term woman, 10 ml of 0.25% bupivacaine will, in most instances, deal with first-stage pain. Here again, however, the required dose is very variable. In obstetrics there is an increasing trend to move to larger volumes of less concentrated solutions, e.g. 15 ml of 0.125% bupivacaine.

In many centres, local anaesthetics are now mixed with opioids and given by infusion into the epidural space for postoperative pain relief. The drugs can be combined in a number of different formulations, but typically it would be 60 ml of up to 0.125% bupivacaine mixed with 2 μg/ml fentanyl. The principle is to establish the epidural block to make the patient comfortable and then to infuse the mixture at, say, 5–15 ml/h. It is not possible to give tighter guidelines than these, because the optimal dose is very variable and needs to be titrated to the patient. The potential dangers of epidural opioids are described in Chapter 5, and it is essential when this form of analgesia is used that the patient is cared for in a properly equipped area with properly trained staff. An example of a flow chart for the safe management of a postoperative epidural infusion is given in Figure 15.20 and the standing orders that accompany it in Table 15.10. *It is very important that a patient on spinal or epidural opioids is not given parenteral opioids as well.*

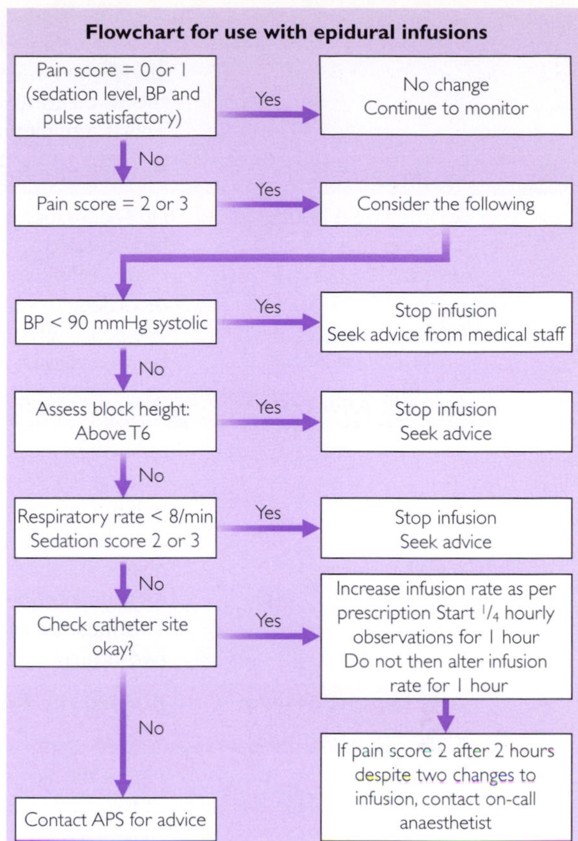


**Figure 15.20.** The flow chart for running a postoperative epidural block. APS, acute pain service; BP, blood pressure. Sedation and pain scores are defined in Figure 5.4. (Reproduced with permission from the University Hospital Birmingham NHS Trust.)

### *Complications of epidural anaesthesia*

These are similar to spinal blockade, to which reference should be made. Specific additional points relevant to epidurals are described below.

#### *Cardiovascular*

The hypotension produced by epidural anaesthesia, being slower in onset than in spinal anaesthesia, can often be compensated for by fluids alone, but in both cases small doses of a vasopressor agent may be needed as described for spinal blockade. Measure the blood pressure and heart rate every 5 min for 20 min after top-ups and every 30–60 min during an infusion.

#### *Dural puncture*

The incidence of dural puncture in experienced hands should be less than 1% for epidural anaesthesia.

Puncture with a Tuohy needle is usually obvious, but that caused by a catheter may not be, particularly if saline has been used in the loss-of-resistance technique to identify the epidural space. If a dural puncture occurs, it is usual to remove the needle or catheter and repeat the injection through another space. In these cases careful administration of the local anaesthetic in fractionated doses is required, as wide spread and rapid anaesthesia may result, presumably because of leakage into the CSF through the punctured dura.

#### *Total spinal anaesthesia*

If dural puncture is not recognized, and a full epidural dose of local anaesthetic is given, a total spinal block may result. *This produces profound hypotension, respiratory depression, convulsions, loss of consciousness, and even cardiac arrest.* Give 100% $O_2$ and send for help early. Once recognized, it is better to move sooner rather than later to control the airway (if necessary by induction, relaxation, and intubation). The surgery will almost certainly have to be abandoned and the patient will need full resuscitative measures, fluids, and vasoconstrictors, probably followed by a period of time on an intensive care unit.

#### *Headache*

The incidence of headache after accidental dural puncture with an epidural needle is high because of the needle size.

Symptoms occurred in 18% of patients after puncture with a 16-gauge Tuohy needle, but in young obstetric patients the incidence may be much higher. It should be treated as described for PDPH after spinal blockade.

#### *Patchy block or unilateral block*

In epidural anaesthesia, missed segments or unilateral block may occur in over 2% of patients. This occurs more often when the catheter is inserted more than

| | | |
|---|---|---|
| **1** | **Oxygen therapy** | |
| | | 2L/min via nasal specula for the first 24 hours. Ideally oxygen therapy should be continued throughout the epidural analgesic regimen. **This is a minimum requirement.** |
| **2** | **Observations** | **Record the following:** |
| | For the first 4 hours postoperatively | *Half-hourly:* pulse, BP, respiratory rate, pain and sedation scoring must be recorded |
| | Up to 24 hours | *Hourly:* BP, pulse, respiratory rate, pain and sedation scores must be recorded |
| | After 24 hours | *Two-hourly:* BP, pulse, respiratory rate, pain and sedation scores must be recorded until epidural is removed. |
| **3** | **Syringe drivers** | **Record the following:** |
| | | Rate of infusion (ml/h)<br>Volume left in syringe<br>Volume infused<br>Any changes to infusion rate must be signed for by the nurse responsible and recorded on the observation chart<br>All lines must be clearly labelled<br>**This must be recorded hourly for the first 24 hrs and thereafter at least two-hourly** |
| **4** | **Assessment of level of block** | **Record the following alongside observations:** |
| | | Assess the skin sensation to cold (use ice or steret) to determine if altered sensation is above or below T6 (xiphisternum), T10 (umbilicus), T12 (groin)<br>Record as T6, T10, T12<br>Enquire if the patient has any tingling or numbness of the chest wall or forearms<br>Refer to flow chart for what to do if above T6 |

- A patent intravenous cannula must be present while the epidural is in use
- Check epidural catheter site for leakage of fluid, catheter misplacement, infection
- Naloxone and ephedrine must be available on each ward where epidurals are used
- Who to contact: acute pain team, Bleep 1564.

**Figure 15.21.** The standing orders in place during the running of a postoperative epidural block to ensure patient safety. (Reproduced with permission from the University Hospital Birmingham NHS Trust.)

5 cm, or when the tip may lie to one side of the space or may have entered an intravertebral foramen. Air bubbles, following use of air in the loss-of-resistance syringe, have also been cited as the cause of missed segments in children.

Usually, missed segments can be anaesthetized by withdrawing the catheter a little and giving more local anaesthetic. Rarely, a midline raphe dividing the epidural space prevents bilateral spread of the block.

*Intravascular injection*

The epidural space is highly vascular, and either the needle or the catheter may enter a vein, although it is more common for the catheter to do so than the Tuohy needle. It is also more common in pregnant women.

Injection of 5–10 ml 0.9% saline through the needle before insertion of the catheter reduces the incidence of intravascular catheter placement. If the catheter enters a vein, it should be withdrawn until no more blood is aspirated, and a test dose of local anaesthetic containing epinephrine (see earlier) given before giving the remainder of the dose incrementally.

*Difficulty in removing catheter*

Very rarely, the catheter will not pull out easily. If this happens, reassure the patient and get them to flex, bend laterally, extend, etc. and try again after each manoeuvre. If this does not work, give up and try again an hour or so later. If there is still no success (which is very rare), the best option is probably to inject some neurocompatible radio-opaque dye and get a radiograph. This can all be done in the radiology department. The next options depend on the findings, and whether or not there is a true knot or if it is just jammed. As it is such a rare event there are no general guidelines. The catheter can be pulled as hard as possible until it breaks, and/or then surgically explored or cut off below the skin. There have been reports of people having a catheter tip *in situ* for several years without problems. The decision about what to do when a catheter will not pull out has to be taken by experienced medical staff at the time. If a catheter tip is left *in situ*, the patient needs to be followed up and instructed to return to the hospital if there are any problems.

## Sacral epidural or caudal block

To approach the epidural space through the sacral hiatus is the easiest but least reliable method of achieving an epidural block. As it is furthest from the nerve roots and is a large potential space, it requires a greater volume of local anaesthetic to obtain a given level of blockade. It also has a higher risk of intravenous injection and, because the anatomy is very variable, has a higher incidence of failure.

### *Anatomy*

Some aspects of the anatomy of the sacrum have already been described (see Figure 15.9). The sacral canal is essentially formed ventrally by the bodies of the vertebrae, and dorsally by the fused posterior laminae. Entry can be achieved only at the fifth sacral vertebra, where the spinous process does not develop and the laminae leave a defect – the sacral hiatus – in the otherwise bony canal roof.

Laterally, the hiatus is bounded by the incompletely developed articular processes – the sacral cornua – and it is covered by the dense sacrococcygeal ligament.

Along the length of the sacral canal, from S1 to S4, there are anterior and posterior foramina through which the sacral nerves emerge. The dural sac ends at S2 level within the canal, but this also is variable and it may extend to within 5 cm of the hiatus.

#### *Entering the sacral epidural space*

The patient may be prone or in the lateral position. The lateral position is generally more acceptable to a patient who is awake, a factor that must always be borne in mind. The hiatus is more easily palpated if the upper leg is flexed at the hip and knee because this helps to spread the gluteal muscles.

The sacral cornua are palpated, lying just above the natal cleft, and the sacrococcygeal membrane is felt as a soft depression between and below the cornua. This point is the lowest point of an equilateral triangle formed by the hiatus and the posterosuperior iliac spines, and is 4–5 cm above the tip of the coccyx (Figure 15.22).

After preparation and draping, infiltrate the skin and subcutaneous tissues with local anaesthetic. The block can be performed with a 21- or 22-gauge 3–5 cm needle in most people, or with an intravenous cannula of similar size. The hiatus is approached at an angle of about 70°, and the needle will 'drop' into the canal. Once in the canal, move the hub of the needle towards the gluteal crease (Figure 15.23), until the needle shaft is almost parallel to the axis of the patient's back. Then rotate the needle so that the bevel faces anteriorly, and advance 2–3 cm, not more than 4 cm. In women, the canal is almost parallel to the skin, whereas in men it is less so. The needle must be advanced in the midline.

If using an intravenous cannula, the needle is removed and only the cannula is advanced, once the combined cannula and needles are in the canal.

It is essential to aspirate carefully before injection, because intravascular and intrathecal placement are both possible. As a result of individual variation in the length of the dural sac, *intrathecal injection is always a possibility. Stop injecting immediately if it produces paraesthesia or pain!*

It is often recommended that, after aspiration, 1–1.5 ml of air is injected to test resistance, which should be minimal, and then 3–5 ml of air while the fingers of the non-injecting hand are rested on the skin over the estimated position of the tip of the needle. If placement is incorrect, crepitus will be felt in the subcutaneous tissues.

In an awake patient, injection of air into the canal may cause discomfort in the back of the thighs as air escapes through the sacral foramina.

If these tests are all negative (no blood or CSF on aspiration, no crepitus on air injection) the anaesthetic dose may be injected.

Although most caudal blocks are single-shot injections, it is possible to use a catheter technique. A longer length of cannula must be inserted (10–12 cm) than by the lumbar route, especially if lower abdominal anaesthesia is required.

#### *Practical points*

- Spirit used during preparation of the skin may cause stinging and discomfort in the perineum.

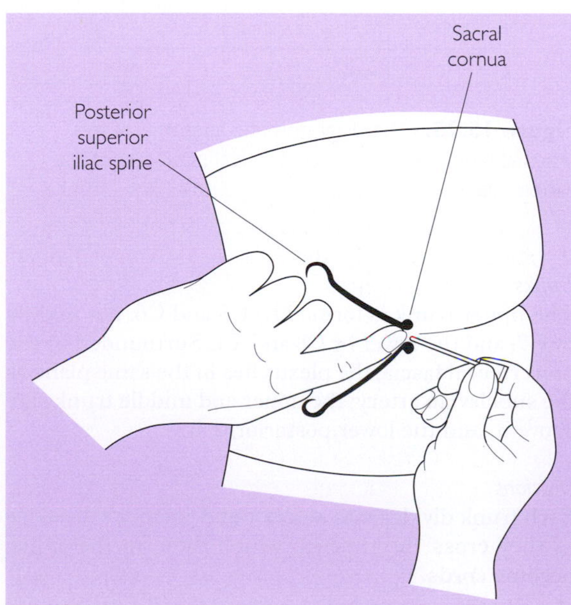


**Figure 15.22.** The method of locating the sacral hiatus.

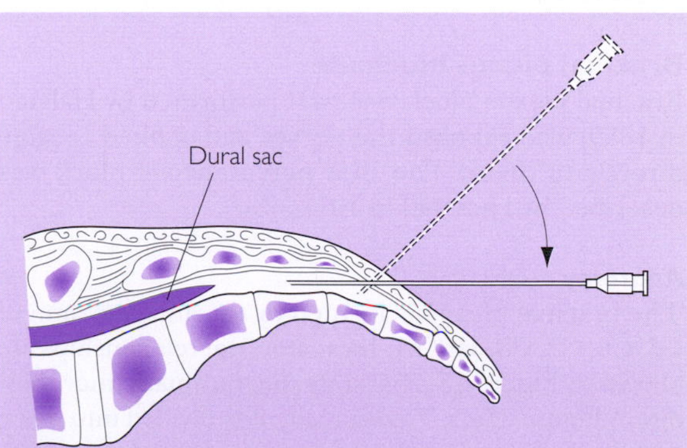


**Figure 15.23.** The initial approach to the sacral hiatus and the rotation of the needle before it is fed along the sacral canal. The end of the dural sac is shown ending at its usual level, but there is considerable variation from person to person in its position. (See earlier text and Figure 15.10.)

Do not use large volumes, but do it properly because of the proximity of the anus.

- The sacral canal is shallow, and it is painful for the patient if the periosteum is hit with the needle.
- Make sure that the patient can pass urine postoperatively. This is particularly important for day-case patients.

#### *Choice and dose of local anaesthetic*

For an adult 70-kg man, a standard dose of 20 ml 0.25% bupivacaine or 1% lignocaine will usually give good anaesthesia of the sacral and perineal nerves.

Sacral anaesthesia can be very successful in children. For this refer to specialized texts, but a general guideline for a lumbosacral block is 0.5 ml/kg of 0.25% bupivacaine.

#### *Complications*

These are as for spinal and epidural blocks, to which reference should be made. Specific additional points relevant to sacral blocks are:

- Intravascular injection is the most common and most serious complication because the canal is highly vascular. Initial careful aspiration and fractionation of the dose with aspiration every 5 ml is essential.
- The sacral hiatus is close to the anus, so sterility is very important.
- Damage to the periosteum can cause pain for several weeks. Analgesia, non-steroidal anti-inflammatory drugs and reassurance are required.
- Intrathecal injection may result in total spinal headache and PDPH.
- Intraosseous injection, which can occur, may cause toxic symptoms within minutes of injection of the anaesthetic, because the drug is rapidly absorbed (see Table 15.12).
- Rectal injection and, in pregnant patients, injection into the baby's scalp have occurred.
- Cardiovascular disturbances have been recorded after too rapid an injection, possibly because of compression of spinal nerves or the cord. This has on occasion caused a hypertensive reaction.

## OTHER SELECTED REGIONAL BLOCKS

### Brachial plexus blockade

Brachial plexus block was first performed by Halsted in 1889, who exposed the nerves and applied cocaine directly to them. The first percutaneous block was described by Hirschel in 1911.

#### *Anatomy*

The brachial plexus is formed by the anterior rami of C5, C6, C7, C8, and T1. Its anatomical relationships are shown in Figure 15.24 and its diagrammatic morphology in Figure 15.25. Traditionally, it is divided into roots, trunks, divisions, cords, and terminal branches.

#### *Roots*

The roots lie in the interscalene groove between scalenus anterior and medius.

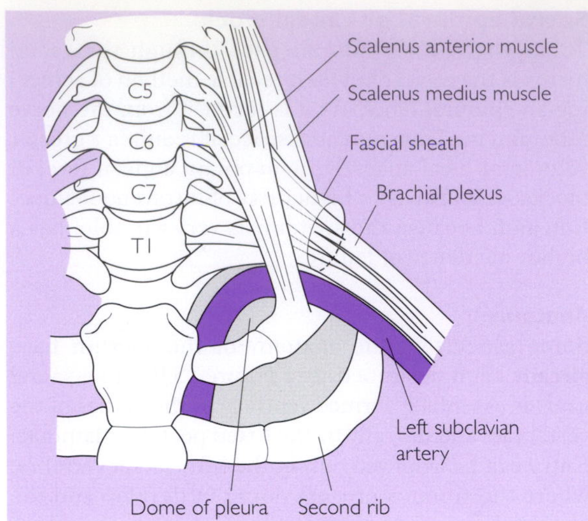


**Figure 15.24.** The immediate relationships of the brachial plexus as it is formed at the root of the neck.

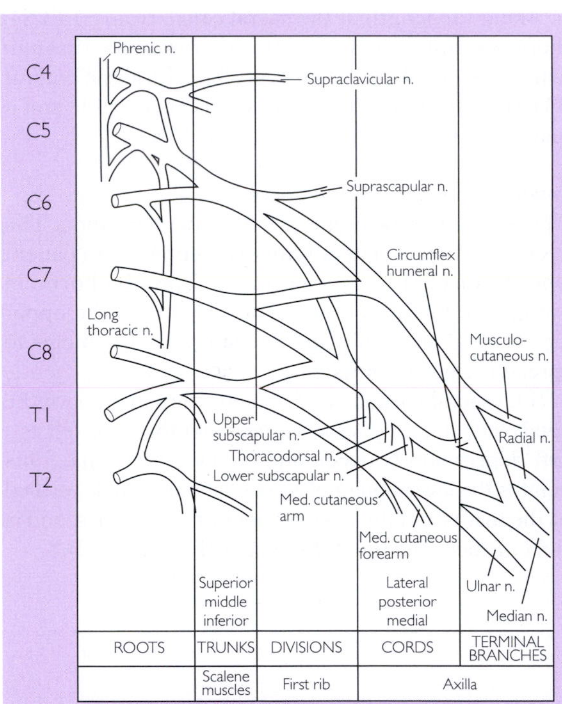


**Figure 15.25.** The diagrammatic anatomy of the brachial plexus. Note the anatomical positions of the various parts.

#### *Trunks*

The upper trunk is formed by C5 and C6, the middle by C7, and the lower by C8 and T1. Surrounded by the prevertebral fascia, the plexus lies in the same plane as the subclavian artery; the upper and middle trunks are above it, and the lower posterior to it.

#### *Divisions*

Each trunk divides into anterior and posterior divisions as they cross the first rib which then, in the axilla, become cords.

*Cords*

The three posterior divisions unite to form the posterior cord, lying under the pectoralis minor muscle, behind the axillary artery. The lateral cord is formed by the anterior division of the upper and middle trunks, and the medial cord by the anterior division of the lower trunk. The cords are named according to their position in relation to the axillary artery.

*Branches*

The median, ulnar, and radial nerves are the three main terminal branches, but many more arise higher in the plexus. From C5 root, branches go to the phrenic nerve, C5 to C7 roots give branches to serratus anterior, and C8 and T1 to rhomboids and levator scapulae. From the upper trunk the suprascapular nerve supplies supraspinatus and infraspinatus.

The lateral cord gives rise to the musculocutaneous nerve, the posterior to the upper subscapular, thoracodorsal, and lower subscapular nerves, and the medial to the medial cutaneous nerves to the arm and forearm. The cutaneous distribution of the main branches and dermatomes is shown in Figure 15.26.

Throughout its length, the brachial plexus lies in a tube of fibrous tissue which is continuous with the prevertebral fascia, and the concept of this sheath, described by Winnie in 1970, is clinically important. Local anaesthetic injected into the sheath spreads both proximally and distally from the point of injection, and the fact that it is continuous with the surroundings of the cervical plexus explains why block of these nerves may occur when a high approach such as the interscalene is used. Cadaveric studies have demonstrated the presence of septa within the sheath, which may explain why, by use of an axillary approach, individual nerves can remain unblocked.

### Dosage, onset, and duration

The brachial plexus can be approached from the side of the neck (interscalene approach), from above the clavicle (subclavian perivascular block), or from the axilla (axillary block). As a result of the volume of the fibrous sheath, the volumes of local anaesthetic solution used are quite large. Although different authors give different figures, there seems a common consensus that the volume injected in a 70-kg man should always be over 20 ml and usually between 30 and 40 ml. This obviously requires some adjustment of the concentration to limit the total dose, and most anaesthetists add epinephrine to limit the rate of systemic absorption (see Table 15.5).

The rate of onset of the block is very variable, but most blocks will be well established within 30 min. Motor blockade often appears before sensory blockade. With any approach, if there is no motor weakness within 10–15 min, the ultimate success of the block is doubtful. Try not to test for sensory loss too soon, because this can undermine the confidence of the patient.

The duration of the block is also inconstant. This results partly from the difference in local anaesthetic agent chosen, but there is also great individual variability. It is particularly important when treating day-case patients that the hazards of an anaesthetized arm are clearly spelt out to both the patient and the accompanying person. For easy reference, the properties of brachial blocks are summarized in Table 15.10.

### Interscalene approach

The interscalene approach described by Winnie in 1970 provides good anaesthesia of the shoulder and upper arm, but may miss individual nerves, most commonly the ulnar to the medial aspect of the forearm and hand.

The patient lies supine, with his head on a pillow and turned away from the side to be blocked. Gentle traction is applied to the arm, pulling it slightly towards the feet.

The cricoid is palpated and a line drawn from it, around the neck, parallel to the clavicle (Figure 15.27). The lateral border of the sternomastoid is palpated, and a finger placed on the line from the cricoid immediately lateral to the muscle. This finger is now on the anterior scalene muscle, and by moving it gently laterally the groove between the anterior and middle scalene muscles is found. This is where the plexus lies (see

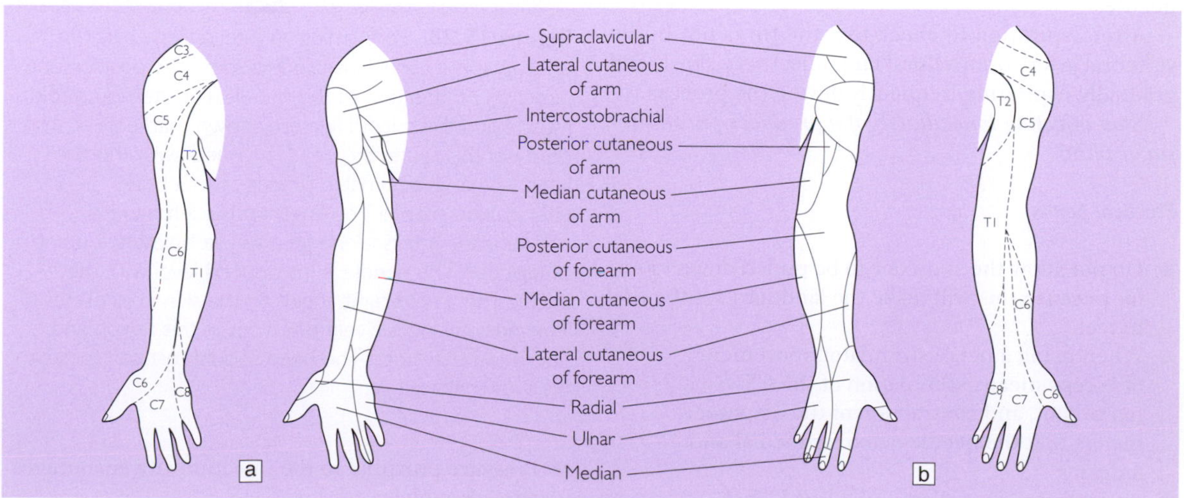


**Figure 15.26.** The cutaneous distribution of dermatomes and superficial nerves in the upper limb. (a) anterior, (b) posterior.

**Table 15.10. Dose, onset, and duration of brachial blocks**

| Approach | Drug | Dose (ml)[a] | Onset (min) | Duration (h) |
|---|---|---|---|---|
| Interscalene, subclavian | Bupivacaine | 30–40 (0.25–0.5%) | 30–45 | 4–18 |
| Perivascular or axillary | Lignocaine | 30–40 (1–2%) | 20–30 | 2–6 |

[a]The higher dose levels need to be used with epinephrine (see Table 15.5); do not exceed the allowed maximum and reduce the concentration for high volumes.

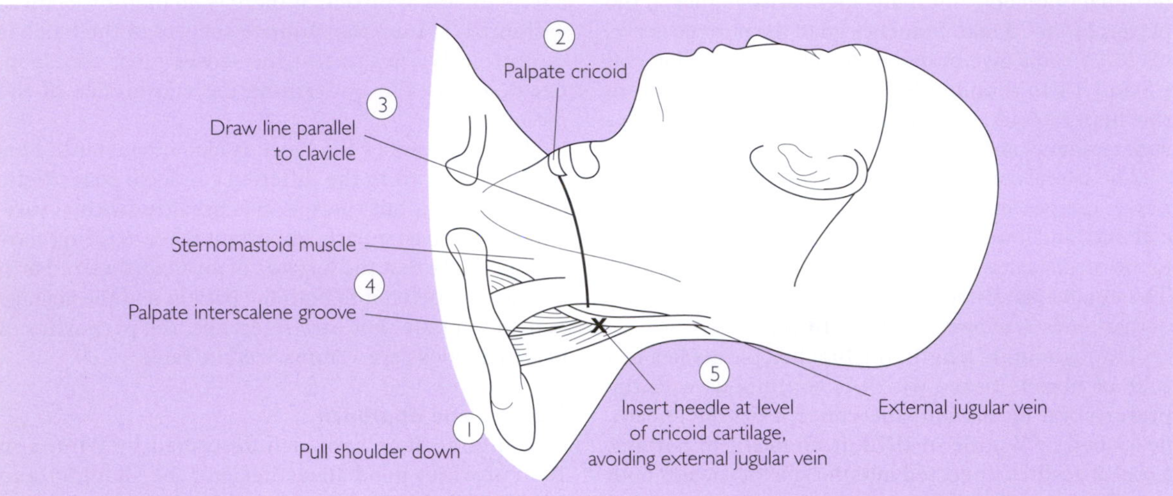


**Figure 15.27.** Landmarks for the interscalene approach to the brachial plexus. Note the position of the external jugular vein, which is at risk.

Figure 15.24). If a nerve stimulator is used, paraesthesia in the elbow or thumb is looked for, or movements of the wrist or fingers occur.

Keeping a finger in this groove, the needle is inserted where the drawn line from the cricoid crosses the interscalene groove. This is often where the external jugular vein crosses the groove, and is at the level of C6. This is shown in Figure 15.27. The needle is introduced at 90° to the skin, and slightly dorsally (Figure 15.28). The sheath is usually entered between 1 and 2.5 cm from the surface and a 'pop' can be felt on occasion with a short bevelled needle.

After aspiration to check that the tip is not in the vertebral artery or in a dural cuff, inject very slowly and gradually, aspirating frequently during the process.

*Stop injecting immediately if it produces paraesthesia or pain!*

*Practical points*

- Do not allow the shoulder to be pulled down too far because this will make the landmarks difficult to feel.
- When using a nerve stimulator, movement of biceps means stimulation of the C5–6 nerve root, and contraction of the diaphragm means that the needle is too far medial and anterior.
- An awake patient allows misplaced local anaesthetic to be appreciated earlier and is therefore safer.

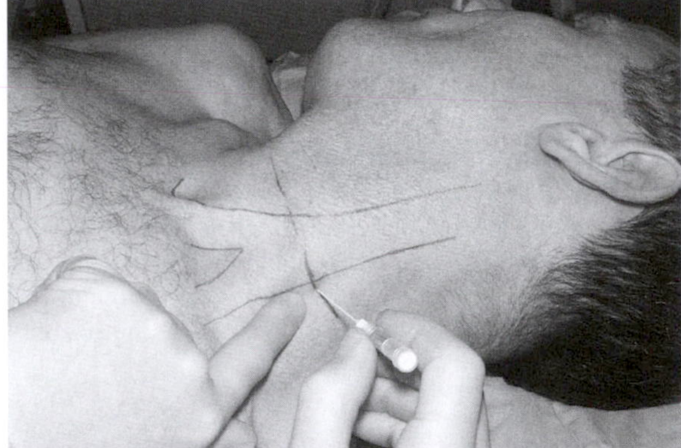

**Figure 15.28.** Performing an interscalene block. In this photograph, a cannula is used to show the position and direction of insertion of the needle. The sternomastoid muscle and the cricoid line are shown marked. For the clarity of this figure, the head is turned away more laterally than is optimal in practice to feel the interscalene groove. The finger of the left hand is palpating the interscalene groove just below the point of injection. The needle is introduced level with the cricoid line and at right angles to the skin in all planes. The external jugular vein often lies in this region and needs to be avoided. The head should rest comfortably on a low pillow.

- Pressure proximal to the injection site encourages spread caudally.
- Injection into the vertebral artery is devastating, producing convulsions and requiring full

resuscitative measures. It is a life-threatening complication.

### *Subclavian perivascular approach*

This technique, although called 'subclavian', describes the position of the point of the needle as the local anaesthetic is delivered; the actual approach is supraclavicular but it differs from the traditional technique normally termed 'supraclavicular'. The risk of pneumothorax is sufficient to contraindicate it as an approach for day-case patients. Of the three approaches described, it is technically the most difficult and should perhaps be avoided in those with poorly defined landmarks, obese patients, and those with significant chest disease.

Locate the interscalene groove as described above and follow it downwards with the index finger, until the subclavian artery is felt. This is usually 1 cm above the midpoint of the clavicle. If the artery is not felt, put the finger in the lower end of the groove. Raise a weal on the skin with local anaesthetic. With the finger palpating the artery or in the groove, insert the needle above the finger and advance it between the scalene muscles in a horizontal plane, caudally and parallel to the axis of the neck (Figure 15.29). A loss of resistance may sometimes be felt as it penetrates the sheath, followed by paraesthesia. If the first rib is contacted with no paraesthesia, withdraw the needle and redirect it more anteriorly or posteriorly. Do not angle it medially because this increases the chance of a pneumothorax.

Aspirate to confirm that the needle is not intravascular and inject slowly but steadily. The sheath may be felt to distend during the injection. This can usually be distinguished from subcutaneous spread because of its shape and direction.

*Stop injecting immediately if it produces paraesthesia or pain!* As with other brachial blocks, a nerve stimulator can be used to identify the correct position.

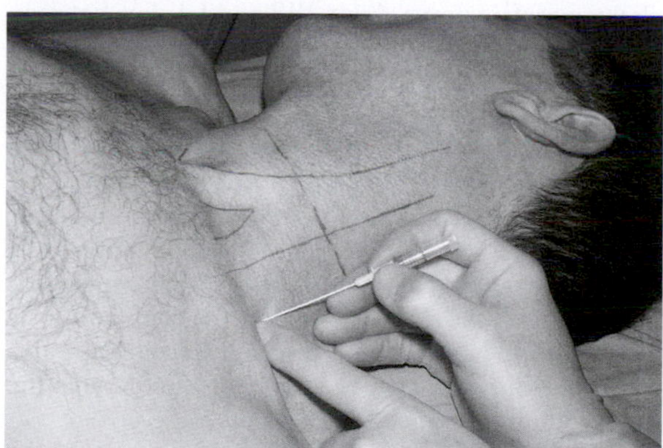

**Figure 15.29.** Performing a brachial plexus block by a subclavian perivascular approach. A cannula is used to show the direction of insertion of the needle. The interscalene groove is located as shown in Figure 15.28 and followed downwards by the forefinger of the left hand. The subclavian artery may be felt pulsating at this point in a thin person. The needle is inserted immediately above the finger and advanced in a caudal direction between the scalene muscles. For the clarity of the figure, the head is turned away more laterally than is optimal in practice to feel the interscalene groove and follow it down to behind the clavicle. The head should rest comfortably on a low pillow.

*Practical points*

- As with the interscalene block, excessive traction on the arm makes the landmarks more difficult to see.
- For the block to be reliable, paraesthesia is necessary.
- The paraesthesia should radiate to the hand or arm. Paraesthesia around the shoulder cannot be relied upon because other nerves may have been encountered outside the sheath.
- If the subclavian artery is inadvertently punctured, withdraw and direct the needle more posteriorly. If arterial puncture occurs, *do not move the tip of the needle from side to side* because it can make a gash on the artery instead of a small pin prick.
- Cough, chest pain, and dyspnoea are all symptoms suggesting a pneumothorax.
- The pneumothorax can develop slowly, sometimes over 24 hours.
- The phrenic, recurrent laryngeal, and stellate ganglion can all be blocked inadvertently.

### *Axillary approach*

This method carries the lowest incidence of serious side effects, but will seldom provide analgesia of the shoulder, and may miss the musculocutaneous nerve. As the intercostobrachial nerve is not part of the brachial plexus, it will also be missed. If a tourniquet is required, these nerves may need to be blocked separately or local infiltration provided to reduce tourniquet pain.

The patient lies supine, with the arm to be blocked abducted to 90° at the shoulder, and flexed to 90° at the elbow (Figure 15.30). At this point the neurovascular bundle within the sheath is well defined (Figure 15.31). The axillary artery is palpated at the level of the lateral edge of pectoralis major. A finger is kept on the artery (Figure 15.32).

A 3–4 cm, 22-gauge, short-bevelled needle is inserted just above the artery at an angle of 30° to the skin, in a plane parallel to that of the artery, until it is felt to enter the fibrous sheath (Figure 15.32). If a nerve stimulator is used, movement of the hand or fingers is

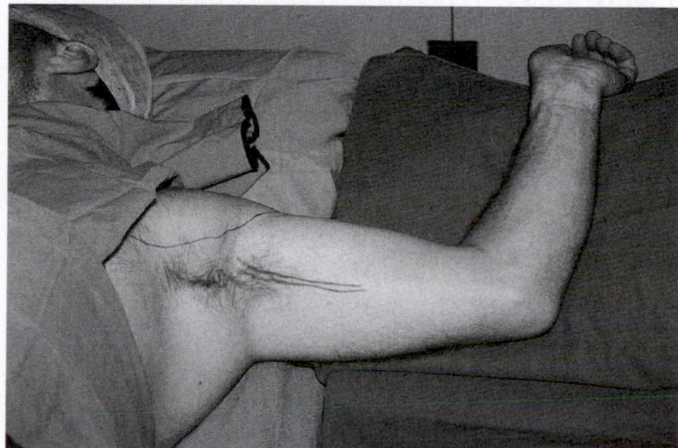

**Figure 15.30.** The position of the arm for an axillary brachial plexus block. Note that the upper arm is approximately at right angles to the body and the forearm is supported comfortably on a pillow, so that the muscles are completely relaxed. The position of the axillary artery is shown.

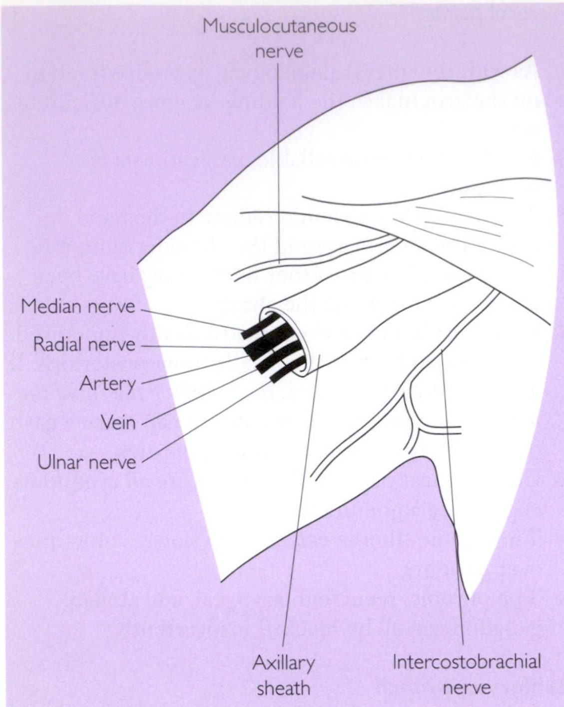


**Figure 15.31.** The brachial plexus in the axilla within its fibrous sheath. Note that the musculocutaneous and intercostal brachial nerves emerge above the point at which the plexus will be blocked.

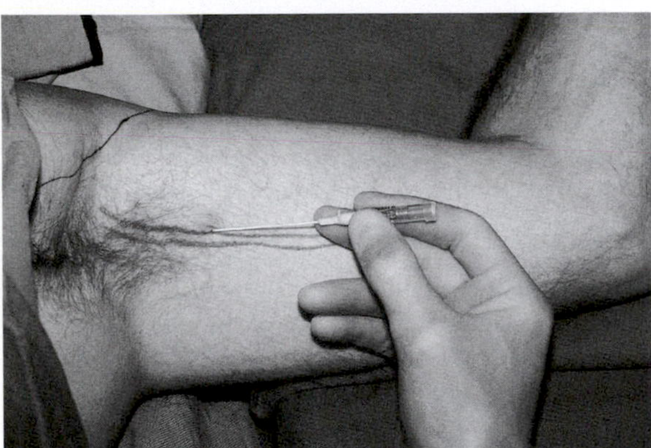

**Figure 15.32.** Performing an axillary brachial plexus block. A cannula is shown to demonstrate the direction of approach. This block can be performed using a needle or the brachial plexus sheath can be cannulated. In practice, the index finger of the other hand is placed over the artery at the position of maximal pulsation. The needle is then inserted immediately above the finger at an angle of about 30° to the skin, directed parallel to and just above the artery. The palpating left hand is not included in this photograph for the sake of clarity.

sought. Otherwise paraesthesia confirms placement. After aspirating to ensure that the needle tip is not in the axillary artery or vein, 30–40 ml of local anaesthetic solution is injected, aspirating after every 5 ml of injection. Maintenance of the needle position is vital for success.

If blood is aspirated, either the needle is removed and repositioned, or deliberately advanced until no more blood can be obtained. The local anaesthetic is then injected deep to the artery.

*Practical points*

*Stop injecting immediately if it produces paraesthesia or pain!*

- Over-abduction of the shoulder will make the artery difficult to palpate.
- The plexus in the axillary approach is shallower than you might think.
- Aspirate repeatedly to ensure that the needle has not drifted into a blood vessel.
- If there is no motor loss at the elbow within 10 min, success is unlikely.
- Pressure distal to the injection site encourages proximal spread of the local anaesthetic solution.
- Generally, lower concentrations of local anaesthetic give adequate anaesthesia, and allow a larger volume to be injected, thereby improving the chances of success.
- Using the axillary approach, a catheter can be inserted into the plexus sheath, allowing prolongation of the block into the postoperative period and providing excellent analgesia.

***Summary***

For easy reference the main features of each of the approaches described is given in Table 15.11 and the nerve distributions blocked are shown in Figure 15.33.

### Ilioinguinal field block

***Anatomy***

The skin of the lower abdominal wall, suprapubic area, and part of the external genitalia is innervated by fibres from nerve roots T12, L1, and L2. This is shown in Figures 15.12 and 15.34. After leaving the pelvis, the iliohypogastric nerve, from T12 and L1, lies between the aponeurosis of the external oblique muscle and the internal oblique. It innervates the skin of the lateral buttock area, and then runs medially, superficial to the inguinal canal, to supply the suprapubic area. The ilioinguinal nerve lies deep to the internal oblique muscle. This relationship is shown diagrammatically in Figure 15.35. The ilioinguinal nerve enters the inguinal canal and runs, in the male, with the spermatic cord to supply the skin at the root of the penis and anterior scrotum. In the female, it supplies the mons pubis and the labia majora. The nerve also innervates the upper and inner aspects of the thigh.

The genitofemoral nerve (L1 and L2) supplies the spermatic cord and skin in a distribution similar to the ilioinguinal via its genital branch, and the skin over the femoral canal via its femoral branch.

***Field block***

Inguinal field block can be used either alone or in combination with a light general anaesthetic for inguinal herniorrhaphy. All three nerves need to be blocked.

The patient is placed supine, and the anteriorsuperior iliac spine is palpated. At a point 2 cm medial and 2 cm caudal to this point, a 22-gauge needle with a short bevel is introduced perpendicularly. The needle is

**Table 15.11. Properties of the interscalene, subclavian perivascular, and axillary approaches to the brachial plexus**

| Approach | Area blocked | Advantages | Complications |
|---|---|---|---|
| Interscalene | Shoulder, humerus, lateral aspect of forearm, and hand | Good landmarks | • Lower dermatomes (C8,T1) may be missed<br>• Possibility of vertebral artery and subarachnoid or epidural injection<br>• High incidence of temporary phrenic nerve palsy and stellate ganglion block<br>• Chance of recurrent laryngeal nerve palsy and pneumothorax |
| Subclavian perivascular | The outer surface of the upper and lower arm, the whole of the forearm, and the whole of the hand | If successful, has the widest distribution of block | • Can be technically difficult<br>• Risk of pneumothorax high<br>• Medium risk of stellate ganglion block and phrenic nerve palsy<br>• Low risk of recurrent laryngeal nerve palsy and subarachnoid or epidural injection<br>• Outside chance of vertebral artery injection |
| Axillary | Medial side of the arm and forearm, and ulnar and median nerves, reliably blocked<br>Lateral aspects of hand and forearm blocked in 75% of cases | Good landmark of the axillary artery<br>Low incidence of complications | • Tracking of solution rarely causes phrenic nerve palsy and stellate ganglion block<br>• Main danger is intravascular injection<br>• Ancillary blockade to radial and lateral cutaneous nerves may be required |

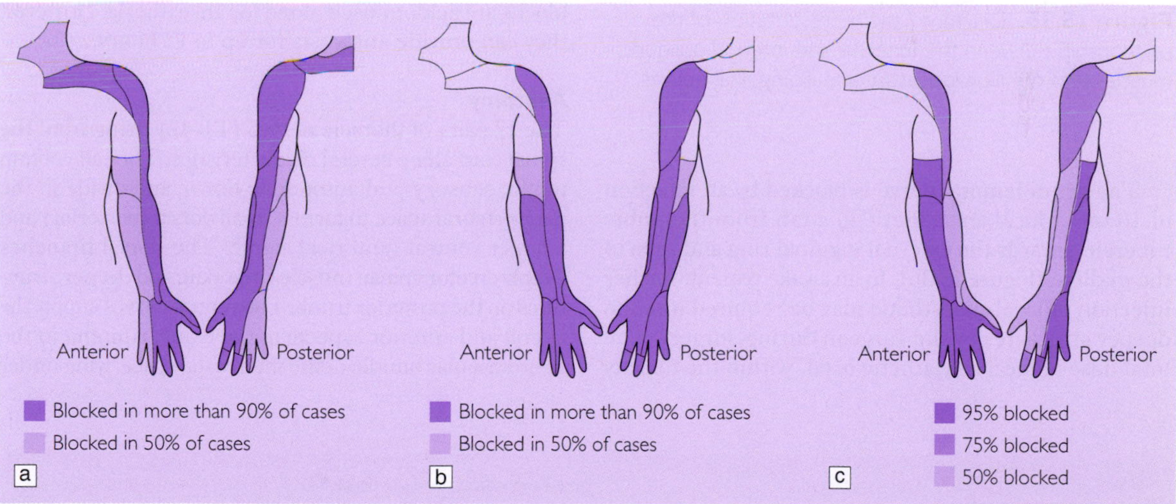


**Figure 15.33.** The probable areas to be blocked by (a) the interscalene, (b) the subclavian perivascular, and (c) the axillary approaches to the brachial plexus. (The quoted success rate of the blocks is taken from Hughes TJ and Desgrand DA. In: Wildsmith JAW, Armitage EN, eds. *Principles and Practice of Regional Anaesthesia*, London: Churchill Livingstone, 1987; 145–8.)

advanced until the aponeurosis of the external oblique is reached, when a slight increase in resistance is noted.

At this point, the needle can be moved freely from side to side and the aponeurosis 'scratched'. This should be done after a small amount of local anaesthetic is injected because it can be painful. The needle is advanced through the aponeurosis, often with a 'pop'. Side-to-side movement of the needle is no longer possible. After aspiration, 5–6 ml of local anaesthetic is injected. The needle is then advanced 1–2 cm through the internal oblique muscle and another 5 ml of anaesthetic injected (see Figure 15.35).

Alternatively, the oblique muscles can be infiltrated in a fan, from the same point, using 10 ml of local anaesthetic. In either case, the needle is then withdrawn to the skin, and a further 10 ml infiltrated in a fan shape subcutaneously, blocking any cutaneous innervation from the subcostal nerve.

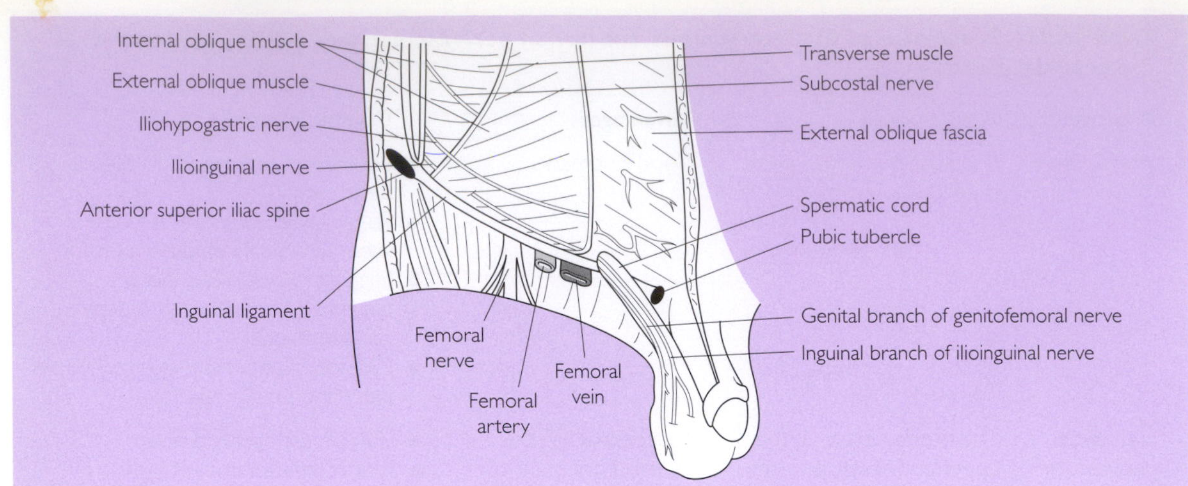


**Figure 15.34.** The nerves supplying the inguinal region.

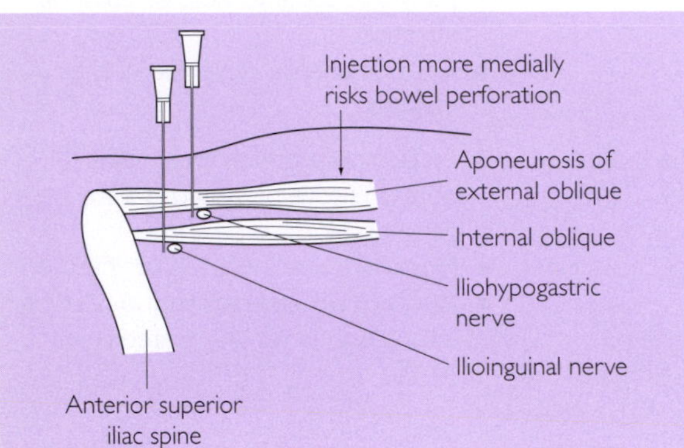


**Figure 15.35.** Diagrammatic representation of the relationship between the external and internal oblique muscles and the iliohypogastric and ilioinguinal nerves.

The genitofemoral nerve is blocked by an injection of 10 ml of local anaesthetic in a fan from the pubic tubercle towards the external inguinal ring and then to the midline (Figure 15.36). In an awake patient, further injection of local anaesthetic may be required into the deeper structures by the surgeon during surgery. The total dose of local anaesthetic used, within the toxicity limits (see Table 15.5) is typically 30–40 ml 0.25–0.50% bupivacaine with epinephrine, or the equivalent in lignocaine. Inguinal field block provides excellent analgesia for 6–12 hours if bupivacaine is used, and is particularly useful for day-case patients.

An inguinal canal block may be used to supplement this block for procedures where analgesia of the scrotal sac is required.

### *Intercostal block*

Intercostal nerve block can be used to provide muscle relaxation or analgesia of the chest wall and abdomen. Visceral anaesthesia is not obtained, hence intercostal blocks are seldom used alone for anaesthesia. However, they can provide analgesia for up to 12 hours.

### *Anatomy*

The 12 pairs of thoracic nerves (T1–12) rising from the spinal cord share several characteristics. They all contain motor, sensory, and autonomic fibres, and divide in the paravertebral space to form a small dorsal (posterior) and a larger ventral (anterior) nerve. The dorsal branches supply erector spinae muscles, the skin, and deeper structures on the posterior trunk. The ventral nerves supply the lateral and anterior aspects of the trunk, running in the neurovascular bundle of the intercostal space, lying under

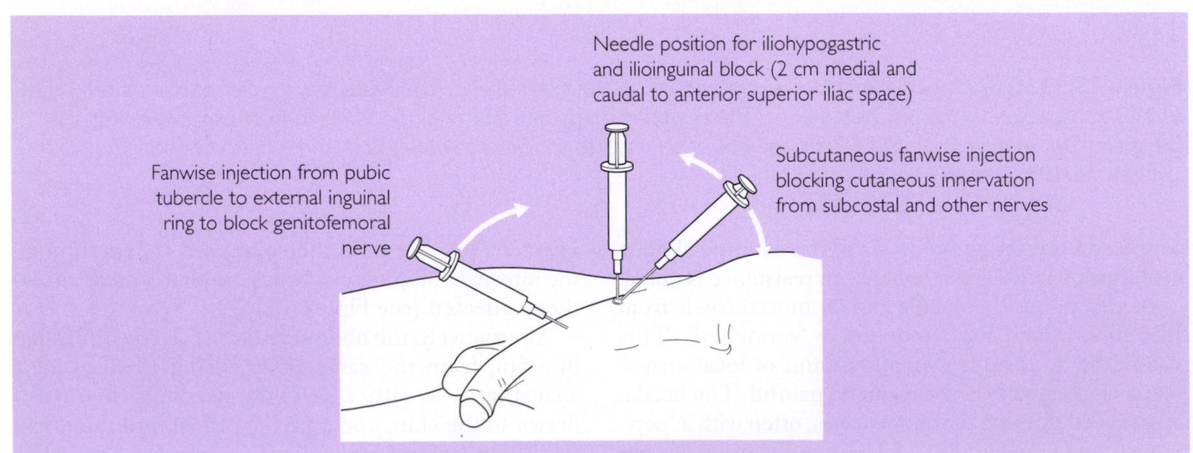


**Figure 15.36.** The infiltration positions used in performing an inguinal field block.

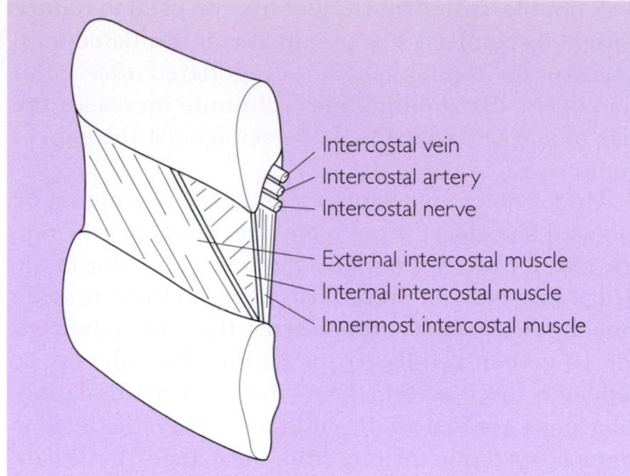


**Figure 15.37.** The anatomy of the neurovascular bundles in an intercostal space.

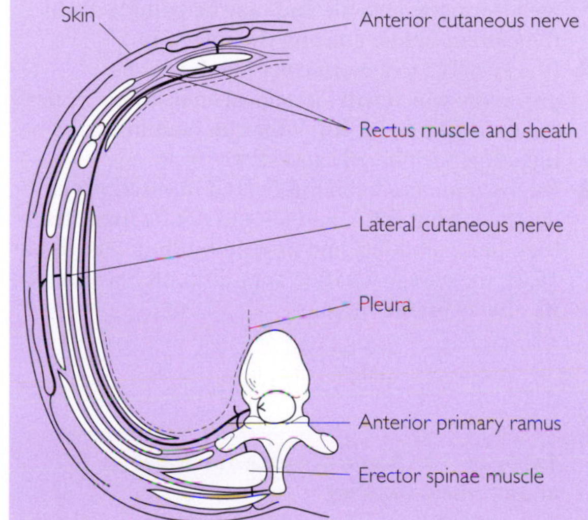


**Figure 15.38.** The anatomy of a typical intercostal nerve.

the inferior aspect of each rib (Figure 15.37). Each ventral nerve gives off a lateral branch and then continues anteriorly to innervate the front of the trunk (Figure 15.38).

There is considerable overlap in the sensory distributions of the nerves, which are depicted as the sensory dermatomes on the skin. The posterior innervation ends at the twelfth thoracic vertebra, but, because the thoracic nerves sweep downwards and forwards, they supply the anterior abdominal wall, with the lateral branch of T12 extending over the iliac crest (Figure 15.12).

### *Technique*

For unilateral blocks the patient can be in the lateral position, for bilateral blocks prone. If not anaesthetized, either unilateral or bilateral blocks may be performed with the patient sitting on the edge of a bed, leaning forwards against support.

Identify the twelfth rib, then count upwards marking each rib. The site of injection is similar in each case – at the angle of the rib, usually 7–8 cm lateral to the spinous process. As the lateral cutaneous branch of each nerve rises at about the midaxillary line, the point of injection must be posterior to this.

Having identified the site of injection, using a 25-gauge needle, a cutaneous bleb of local anaesthetic is raised at the inferior edge of the rib, and infiltrated to the periosteum.

The anaesthetized skin is then pulled cephalad by the left index finger, and a 22-gauge, short bevelled needle is inserted perpendicular to the skin until the rib is contacted. At this point, the needle is firmly held by the thumb and index finger of the left hand, and walked off the inferior edge of the rib, allowing the stretched skin to return to its normal position (Figure 15.39). During the procedure the patient should hold their breath in expiration to stabilize the thoracic wall.

Still under the control of the left (cephalad) hand, which is resting firmly against the patient's back, the needle is advanced 3 mm. A 'give' may be felt as the needle enters the external intercostal muscle. After aspiration, 3–4 ml of local anaesthetic (e.g. 0.5% plain bupivacaine or equivalent in lignocaine) is injected.

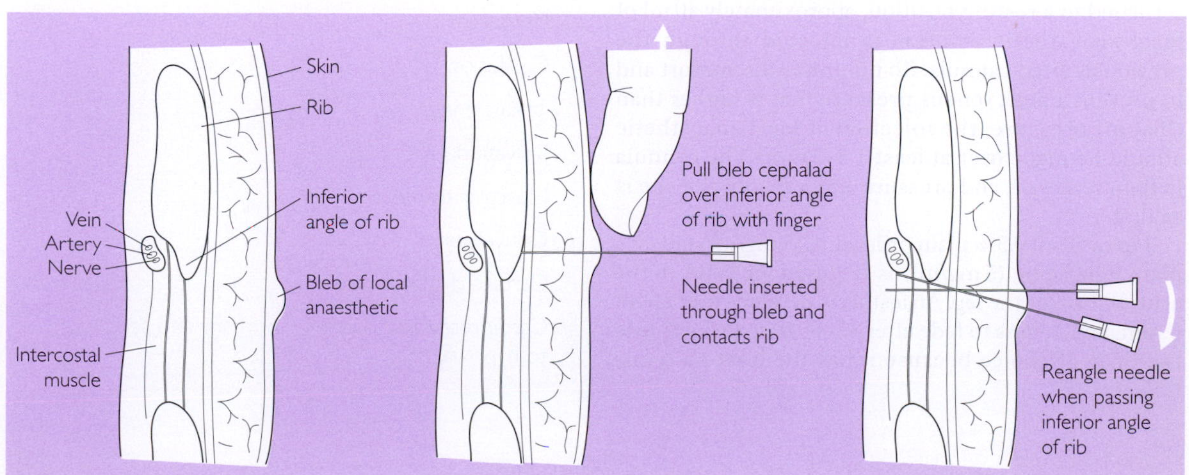


**Figure 15.39.** The method of performing an intercostal nerve block.

*Practical points*

- It is necessary to block one nerve higher and one lower than the estimated analgesic distribution required.
- The most common and most serious complication is pneumothorax.

## INTRAVENOUS REGIONAL ANAESTHESIA

Intravenous regional anaesthesia (IVRA) is one of the simplest and oldest techniques of regional anaesthesia of the limbs, first described by August Bier in 1908 and, after a period of disuse, reintroduced by Holmes in 1963.

Distension of the veins and smaller vessels with local anaesthetic causes diffusion of anaesthetic solution into the nerves, and produces anaesthesia for as long as the venous concentration remains high. This can be achieved by blocking the venous outflow of a limb with a tourniquet, then filling the venous system with a large volume of a dilute local anaesthetic solution. The main advantages are its simplicity and reliability, but it provides no postoperative analgesia and has several dangerous complications.

IVRA is more suitable for arm and hand surgery than for lower-limb procedures, because leakage under the tourniquet is less likely. The size of the thigh and larger volume of local anaesthetic required both cause concern when using IVRA in the leg.

### Technique

The patient is placed supine, with an uninflated proximal tourniquet on the limb to be anaesthetized and an intravenous cannula in the contralateral limb.

A small (20–22 gauge) intravenous cannula is inserted in the hand (or foot) to be operated on, and capped. The limb is then exsanguinated by elevation or, if possible, by 'sausage' exsanguinator or Esmarch bandage up to the tourniquet. The tourniquet is inflated to at least 300 mmHg, or 100 mmHg above systolic blood pressure. It is important that this pressure is maintained throughout, and a constant pressure gas source must be used and the aneroid on the cuff observed throughout.

Once the tourniquet is inflated, and the limb returned to a resting position, approximately 40 ml of local anaesthetic solution is injected through the previously sited cannula. To minimize discomfort and to prevent a peak venous pressure that is higher than the cuff pressure, the injection of local anaesthetic should be made over at least 1.5–2 min. The cannula is then removed, and pressure applied until the site is sealed.

Up to 50 ml 0.5% plain prilocaine (5 mg/ml) or 0.5% plain lignocaine (5 mg/ml) is required for IVRA in the arm, 100 ml for the leg. Anaesthesia develops over about 5 min, and begins to fade after 45–60 min. Prilocaine is the drug of choice because it has the least systemic toxicity.

A double-cuffed tourniquet may be used to reduce patient discomfort. The proximal cuff is inflated until anaesthesia is established, then deflated *after* inflation of the distal cuff. This technique increases the risk of leakage, which must be set against the gain in comfort.

Under no circumstances should the tourniquet be deflated less than 20 min after injection; after 45 min, the risk of toxicity is minimal because of binding of the drug to tissues. For procedures between these times, a staged release is recommended – the cuff is deflated for 10 s, then reinflated for 1 min. This should be repeated three or four times before final deflation, allowing a gradual wash-out of local anaesthetic. The signs of systemic toxicity from local anaesthetics are given in Table 15.12.

*Practical points*

- Systemic toxicity remains the major disadvantage of the technique.
- Injection of local anaesthetic in this technique is usually uncomfortable and may be painful. Warn the patient before starting the injection.
- It is possible to generate very high venous pressures which will force local anaesthetic under the cuff (Figure 15.40). This can be minimized by injecting peripherally and slowly.
- Bupivacaine has been implicated in reactions and deaths during IVRA, and should not be used. Its high lipid solubility and protein binding (see Table 15.5), make resuscitation very difficult because of its effects on the heart.

| Table 15.12. Signs of systemic local anaesthetic toxicity |
|---|
| Apprehension |
| Gastric sensations |
| Visual disturbances – staring episodes |
| Auditory disturbances and tinnitus |
| Olfactory disturbances |
| Sleepiness |
| Confusion |
| Talkativeness |
| Salivation |
| Muscular tremors |
| Convulsions |
| Cardiac dysrhythmias |
| Cardiorespiratory arrest – primary and secondary to hypoxia |

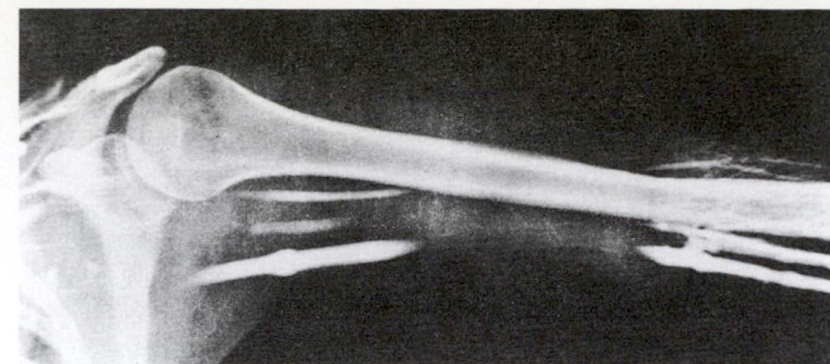

**Figure 15.40.** A radiograph of the upper arm during a Bier's block, showing radio-opaque dye passing beneath the cuff. The passage of dye under the cuff (shown by the arrows) does not appear as clearly in this reproduction as in the original. (From Rosenberg PH *et al. Anesthesiology* 1983;58:95.)

## FURTHER READING


Blomberg RG. Recent insights in the anatomy and physiology of the epidural space and some clinical consequences. In: Van Aken H, ed. *New Developments in Epidural and Spinal Drugs Administration. Baillière's Clin Anaesthesiol* 1993;**7**:535–56.

Bromage PR. Neurological complications of subarachnoid and epidural anaesthesia. *Acta Anaesthesiol Scand* 1997;**41**:439–44.

Breivik H. Neurological complications in association with spinal and epidural analgesia – again. *Acta Anaesthesiol Scand* 1998;**42**:609–13.

Elsenach JC, de Kock M, Klimscha W. $\alpha_2$-Adrenergic agonists for regional anesthesia: a clinical review of clonidine (1984–1995). *Anesthesiology* 1996;**85**:655–74.

Eriksson E ed. *Illustrated Handbook in Local Anaesthesia*. 2nd edn. London: Lloyd-Luke, 1979.

Haljamao H. Thromboprophylaxis, coagulation disorders, and regional anaesthesia. *Acta Anaesthesiol Scand* 1996;**40**:1024–40.

Larson MD, Tait FD, Caglieri GE. The first spinal anaesthetic in America. *Anesthesiology* 1996;**85**:913–19.

McCrae AF, Wildsmith JAW. Prevention and treatment of hypotension during central neural blockade. *Br J Anaesth* 1993;**70**:672–80.

Mulroy M. *Regional Anesthesia: An Illustrated Procedure Guide*, 2nd edn. Chicago: Little Brown, 1995.

Pinnock CA, Fischer HBJ, Jones RB. *Peripheral Nerve Blockade*. Edinburgh: Churchill Livingstone, 1996.

Prithvi Raj. *Clinical Practice of Regional Anaesthesia*. Edinburgh: Churchill Livingstone, 1991.

Wildsmith JAW, Armitage EN. *Principles and Practice of Regional Anaesthesia*, 2nd edn. Edinburgh: Churchill Livingstone, 1993.

# Chapter 16 Surgical requirements of anaesthesia

J.M. Budd

Some types of surgery can be made difficult, if not impossible, if the anaesthesia is inappropriate or substandard. Conversely, if the intentions of the surgeon are unknown, even the most adept anaesthetist can be left glowing with embarrassment. Consequently, knowledge of what the surgeon is likely to do helps in planning the anaesthetic technique and in anticipating events that may require intervention. In this chapter an outline of some of the more commonly encountered operations is given, together with some of the practical implications of these for the anaesthetist.

To avoid repetition, this chapter assumes that the basic standards of pre- and postoperative care, monitoring, and safety described in other chapters will be applied. It is also assumed that the administration of antibiotics and anti-thrombosis regimens will be undertaken routinely (see Chapter 1).

## ELECTIVE GENERAL SURGERY

### Inguinal or femoral hernia repair

The site of the incision depends on the type of hernia. It is above and parallel to the inguinal ligament for an inguinal hernia and below and parallel for a femoral hernia. Dissection follows to expose the sac of peritoneum. The sac is opened and explored and any contents returned to the abdomen. The sac is excised (herniotomy) and the defect repaired either by suture (herniorrhaphy) or with some form of patch (hernioplasty).

*Specific surgical requirements*

These are a supine patient with relaxed musculature in the operative region who does not cough.

*Anaesthetic implications*

- Many methods of anaesthesia are appropriate, including intubation and ventilation, spontaneous ventilation, and regional and field block. The choice of technique depends on patient presentation and personal preference.
- Coughing on extubation may result in stresses on the sutures and the surgeon. Patients who have chronic chest complaints and smokers may warrant a regional technique but coughing can render the surgery very problematic. Clinical judgement is required.
- If the contents of the hernia are suspected to be obstructed or strangulated, the operation may progress to laparotomy. In these circumstances a regional or field block may not be appropriate.
- Surgical traction on the spermatic cord and peritoneum may result in bradycardias and nausea from vagal stimulation.

### Varicose vein surgery

This involves ligation of the saphenofemoral junction, vein stripping, and multiple phlebotomies. An incision is made below and parallel to the inguinal ligament. The long saphenous vein is exposed, then clamped and divided. Any tributaries are ligated and divided. To strip the veins, a metal wire with a head and tip is passed from the knee to the groin, emerging through the upper end of the long saphenous vein. The vein is tied to the stripper at the lower end and the whole lot pulled through. Small incisions are then made over varicosities in the legs, which are then pulled out.

*Specific surgical requirements*

The patient is usually supine but may need to be prone. Head-down positioning may be required to reduce bleeding.

*Anaesthetic implications*

- Although it should be done on the ward or in the preoperative area, marking of veins sometimes occurs in the anaesthetic room and requires the patient to be able to stand and cooperate. Heavy premedication or administration of anaesthetic drugs may interfere with this.
- Patient position: usually supine and head-down. Some surgeons may wish to turn the patient to the prone position during surgery. If this is likely to happen, then the airway must be secured by an endotracheal (ET) tube and provision made for safe repositioning of the patient. Monitoring, e.g. ECG, may have to be repositioned.
- Stripping of veins is very stimulating and may require extra analgesia or deepening of anaesthesia.
- Blood loss can be heavy. It is often concealed on drapes and may be less easy to assess if two surgeons are working simultaneously on the legs.
- Bandaging of the legs at the end may be quite involved and requires the legs to be elevated.
- The inguinal skin incision is often not sutured until the end of the procedure and may be left until after the bandages have been applied.

### Breast surgery

Surgery for benign breast disease may involve local excision of the lesion or, for abscesses, incision and drainage. Small carcinomas may be treated by local excision with breast conservation. For larger tumours, a mastectomy with axillary sampling or clearance is required. In these cases, the arm on the side of the lesion is abducted and an elliptical incision made that includes the skin over the tumour and the nipple. For a simple mastectomy, the breast is dissected off the underlying muscle, the axillary tail is removed, and the lymph nodes sampled. More radical surgery involves removal of pectoralis minor and axillary clearance. Drains are invariably left in after mastectomy and may be left in after local excision of lumps.

*Specific surgical requirements*
A supine anaesthetized patient is needed. The arm on the affected side may be put on a board at right angles to the body. There is potential danger to the brachial plexus (see Chapter 3). Make sure that the arm support is well padded and at the same height as the operating table.

*Anaesthetic implications*
- Women about to undergo mastectomy for carcinoma are frequently very anxious about the severity and implications of the disease and about the impending disfiguring surgery. Anxiety can also be considerable in women undergoing lumpectomy with a frozen section. Consider a sedative premedication on an individual basis.
- Drips are preferably sited in the non-affected arm in order to aid access and because of the possibility of arm swelling postoperatively. The position of the blood pressure cuff and pulse oximeter may need to be considered.
- Blood loss can be considerable, especially in large breasts requiring major dissection.
- Analgesia: breast surgery can be very painful postoperatively. Non-steroidal analgesics (if no contraindications), together with parenteral opioids and local infiltration of the wound with local anaesthetic, may be needed.

## Cholecystectomy
This is done either as an elective procedure for chronic biliary colic secondary to gallstones or as a semi-elective procedure after admission with acute cholecystitis. It is very unusual to operate on an acutely inflamed gallbladder unless to drain pus. Occasionally, the gallbladder can become gangrenous, leading to preoperative sepsis. Laparoscopic surgery is performed in well-selected patients. Obesity and previous abdominal surgery are relative contraindications. If the patient is jaundiced because of stones in the common bile duct, treat as in Chapter 58. This account assumes the patient to be fully recovered from any acute infection or generalized sepsis and is normally hydrated.

### *Open cholecystectomy*
The incision for this is most frequently subcostal but may be midline, especially if the diagnosis is in doubt. The gallbladder is exposed by retraction of the liver upwards and the colon downwards. The peritoneum over the gallbladder neck is incised and dissection occurs to expose the cystic duct and artery. The cystic artery is ligated and the duct explored for stones; it is then ligated close to the gallbladder. An operative cholangiogram may be performed to detect any stones in the cystic duct before it is ligated.

*Specific surgical requirements*
This can be an extremely challenging operation for the surgeon with problems of adequate exposure and complicated anatomy. Keeping the patient still is an absolute necessity in order to create the best conditions.

*Anaesthetic implications*
- Patient positioning: it is important to ensure that the correct part of the patient is over the site of the X-ray plate for the intraoperative cholecystogram. The surgeon may require tilting of the table to improve exposure. The ventilator is turned off briefly for the exposure: *remember to switch it on again!*
- Muscle relaxation is very important. A peripheral nerve stimulator is helpful to guide the accurate use of neuromuscular blocking agents.
- Bleeding can occur intraoperatively from the cystic artery, providing further surgical difficulty.
- Subcostal incisions may be very painful and it is worth considering an epidural for postoperative analgesia.

### *Laparoscopic cholecystectomy*
Laparoscopic surgery minimizes surgical morbidity, with reduced postoperative pain and, hopefully, earlier discharge. Instead of large incisions, the surgical site is accessed by cannulae inserted into the abdominal wall with a port for the endoscope, which has a camera attached to allow viewing. A pneumoperitoneum is required to separate the abdominal wall from the contents and is created by insufflating $CO_2$ through a Verres needle. The intra-abdominal pressure as a result of this should not exceed 15 mmHg. The surgery involves dissecting out the cystic duct and artery by stripping off peritoneum and fat. These are then clipped and divided. The gallbladder is dissected off the liver bed with diathermy being used for haemostasis. It is then extracted through one of the ports. A drain may be left in the gallbladder bed. Operative cholangiograms are done much less frequently than in open cholecystectomies.

*Specific surgical requirements*
As with open cholecystectomy, keeping the patient still is very important.

*Anaesthetic implications*
- Patients are usually supine but may be put in the Lloyd–Davis position, with the surgeon operating from between the legs.
- Avoid inflating the stomach with air when ventilating with a mask before intubation, because this increases the risk of gastric injury with the trocar, decreases surgical access, and leads to the need for a nasogastric tube.
- Insertion of trocars or the Verres needle into the abdomen may lead to damage to intra-abdominal organs and massive haemorrhage if vessels are injured.
- Problems related to the pneumoperitoneum:
  - Intra-abdominal pressure greater than 15 mmHg starts to cause problems. Upward

displacement of the diaphragm leads to reduced functional residual capacity and reduced lung compliance. Compression of the inferior vena cava reduces venous return and therefore cardiac output. Renal blood flow and glomerular filtration rate are reduced.
    - Gas insufflation may cause arrhythmias including bradycardias and asystole, especially if done rapidly. Anticholinergics may be required. Misplacement of the Verres needle may result in surgical emphysema, pneumomediastinum, and pneumothorax. There is a risk of gas embolus if the Verres needle punctures a vessel;
    - $CO_2$ absorption causes a rise in the arterial $CO_2$ pressure; hyperventilation is required to correct this.
- Conversion to open cholecystectomy: difficulties with dissection, uncontrolled haemorrhage, and unexpected findings may lead the surgeon to convert to an open procedure. This has particular implications for postoperative analgesia.
- Good relaxation is important and a nerve stimulator is useful.
- $CO_2$ monitoring is essential, particularly to enable the adjustment of ventilation to prevent hypercapnia.
- Postoperative analgesia: entry wounds are small and not too painful. Local infiltration with local anaesthetics helps. Shoulder tip pain as a result of the pneumoperitoneum may cause some discomfort and some patients experience deep-seated pain from the operative site.

## Gastrectomy

### *Partial gastrectomy*

An upper midline incision is used after which the stomach is mobilized. The duodenum is divided; the stomach is then divided and the remaining portion either anastomosed to the duodenum (Billroth I) or to the jejunum, after which the duodenum is closed (Billroth II or Polya).

### *Total gastrectomy*

This operation is usually done for tumours in the upper third of the stomach. After incision, dissection follows to expose the stomach. The oesophagus is mobilized and the stomach is resected. The oesophagus is joined to the jejunum forming an oesophagojejunostomy. As part of the procedure the spleen may be resected.

*Specific surgical requirements*

The patient should be supine and there should be adequate muscle relaxation to aid surgery.

*Anaesthetic implications*

- Tumours that involve the pylorus may delay gastric emptying, and tumours involving the upper part of the stomach may cause dysphagia. In either case the patient should be treated as having a full stomach and a rapid sequence induction should be used.
- Patient position: supine, but may need to be head-up to allow dissection.
- Fluid losses can be large as a result of evaporative and 'third space' losses.
- A nasogastric tube is required so that the stomach may be aspirated during surgery.
- Be prepared for the possibility of a splenectomy.
- A sternal retractor may be used during a total gastrectomy. This can affect venous return to the heart. The surgeon should be asked to reposition it if there is a drop in blood pressure.

## Large bowel surgery

Indications for this include carcinoma of the colon, colitis, Crohn's disease, and diverticular disease. A vertical incision is usually used although some surgeons may use a transverse incision. Abdomino-perineal (AP) resections also involve incision around the anus. The bowel is mobilized and the mesentery divided and vessels ligated. The relevant portion of bowel is then resected and the remaining bowel anastomosed with staples or sutures, or a colostomy or ileostomy is formed and the bowel oversewn.

*Specific surgical requirements*

The patient should be supine. The Lloyd–Davis (lithotomy–Trendelenburg) position is required for AP resections. Good muscle relaxation and soft undistended bowel aid surgery.

*Anaesthetic implications*

- Patient position: the Lloyd–Davis position involves placing the patient's legs in multi-jointed leg supports with the patient placed head-down. The hips are less flexed than the standard lithotomy position and access is improved by abducting the thighs. The calves should be well supported and the legs held in the supports in such a way as not to cause adverse pressure effects. Extra care should be taken with patients with arthritic hips. For surgery other than AP resections, head-down positioning is often required to reduce the amount of small bowel in the surgical site (see also Chapter 3).
- The instrument trolley (Mayo table) is positioned over the patient's head for AP and anterior resections and left hemicolectomies. This limits access to the patient's head. The ET tube and connections should be well secured. If a nasogastric tube is required, this is much easier to insert before the table is placed. A drip extension is useful because the arms are usually placed at the patient's side. Access to monitoring may also be difficult, and ECG leads and the pulse oximeter should be confirmed to be correct and secure before towelling up.
- Colostomy/ileostomy formation: this may be done to protect a distal anastomosis and is essential if the rectum is removed. It is usually done after the abdominal incision has been sewn up. Anticipation of this is necessary to prevent patients being 'lightened' from anaesthesia or 'reversed' prematurely.
- Prolonged exposure of the bowel results in fluid and heat loss. If possible, the patient's upper body should be covered with a warming device and fluid warmers should be used. A central venous pressure (CVP) line is useful for assessing fluid

balance, particularly for AP resections where losses are higher.
- Blood loss from the perineal wound may not be obvious and inspection of the drapes is necessary.
- The use of nitrous oxide ($N_2O$) may result in unwanted bowel distension and it may be helpful to use $O_2$-enriched air.
- Epidurals provide excellent intra- and postoperative analgesia.

### Thyroidectomy

This is indicated for nodular or diffuse goitres, solitary nodules, and malignancy. A subtotal thyroidectomy takes away enough tissue to cure hyperthyroidism, but plans to leave enough to prevent hypothyroidism. A collar incision is made in the front of the neck. The surgeon may mark the site for this with a piece of suture. Platysma is divided and the sheath of fascia covering the gland incised. The thyroid lobes are then mobilized one side at a time. The superior thyroid vessels in the vascular pedicle of the upper pole are ligated. The lobe is pulled forwards to look for the recurrent laryngeal nerve and inferior thyroid artery. The artery is ligated and the lobe resected. The thyroid remnant is sutured to the pretracheal fascia and the wound closed with a drain left in.

*Specific surgical requirements*

The operation requires a supine patient with an extended neck, often with a head-up tilt on the table. The patient should not cough or gag as surgery proceeds around the trachea.

*Anaesthetic implications*

- Any overactivity of the thyroid should have been treated preoperatively. Recent thyroid function tests must be available.
- Airway: large goitres, especially those with retrosternal enlargement, can compress or displace the trachea and cause stridor. Malignant tumours may erode tracheal cartilage. A thoracic inlet radiograph should show tracheal displacement or deformity and any retrosternal enlargement. Change in voice preoperatively may indicate malignant involvement. Indirect laryngoscopy is often done before surgery to evaluate recurrent laryngeal nerve function. Any airway changes may lead to a difficult intubation and awake fibreoptic intubation may be required. Laryngoscopy and getting a full view of the cords is not usually more or less difficult than usual, but with tracheal compression the airway may become difficult as consciousness is lost. Therefore adequate preoxygenation is necessary and a smaller tube than normal may be required to negotiate the compressed trachea. An armoured tube is recommended to avoid kinking with head movement.
- Eyes should be protected. They are especially vulnerable if there is proptosis.
- The head is covered during surgery, so the ET tube and connections must be well secured.
- Patient position: supine and head-up. A sandbag or equivalent is put under the shoulders to allow neck extension. Head-up tilt may lead to a risk of air embolus.
- $CO_2$ monitoring is essential because it alerts to disconnections and air embolus.
- Recurrent laryngeal nerve damage may occur during surgery. If bilateral, this can lead to marked airway obstruction. The cords should be assessed for movement with laryngoscopy at extubation.
- Tracheal collapse may occur after extubation, especially if there has been any erosion of tracheal cartilage. This may require urgent reintubation and consideration of tracheostomy.
- Haematoma occurring in the wound can lead to pressure on the trachea. Stitch cutters or clip removers should be available to allow rapid reopening of the wound postoperatively.

## URGENT AND EMERGENCY GENERAL SURGERY

### Laparotomy

This is often carried out for obstruction, gastrointestinal bleeding, or peritonitis. A midline incision above and below the umbilicus is done to allow access to most abdominal organs. Opening the peritoneal cavity may give an immediate clue to the diagnosis, especially if it is faecal peritonitis. The abdomen is explored and the specific surgical procedure performed as indicated. A colostomy may be required.

*Specific surgical requirements*

These are as for elective bowel surgery, described above.

*Anaesthetic implications*

- The diagnosis may not be known and this may lead to unanticipated events during surgery.
- The patient is often not in optimal condition. They may be shocked as a result of blood loss or sepsis. A period of preoperative resuscitation may be required. (See also Chapters 60 and 61.)
- A rapid sequence induction is usually indicated because of the high likelihood of food or fluid in the stomach. The preoperative condition of the patient may lead to considerable cardiovascular changes during and after induction.
- A nasogastric tube is needed. This is easier to insert before the patient is fully draped.
- Intraoperative cardiovascular disturbance may occur as a result of large fluid losses or evolving sepsis. A CVP line helps in assessment of fluid balance and an arterial line is indicated if cardiovascular system instability is likely or frequent blood gas analysis is needed.
- Patients are at risk from heat loss. Fluid warmers and warming devices should be used.
- Admission to an intensive care unit (ICU) may be necessary postoperatively. This should be organized as far in advance as possible.

### Appendicectomy

The incision for this is made over the point of maximal tenderness and may only be a few centimetres long. The peritoneum is incised, the caecum found, and the tenia followed to the base of the appendix. Any adhesions are gently divided. The appendix is held up and the mesentery clamped, divided, and ligated, after which the base of the appendix is divided and ligated. A purse-string suture is placed at the base of the appendix and the stump inverted into the caecum while the purse string is tightened.

*Specific surgical requirements*
These are as for elective bowel surgery, described above.

*Anaesthetic implications*
- These patients can be very dehydrated, especially if young and pyrexial. Aggressive rehydration is often required.
- Treat as having a full stomach because an acute abdomen leads to delay in gastric emptying.
- If the diagnosis is wrong, a laparotomy may have to be performed.
- In other ways, the management is as for a laparotomy.

### Repair of obstructed or incarcerated inguinal or femoral hernia

The surgical requirements and the anaesthetic implications are as for the elective inguinal case (see above) with the following additional points:

- If the hernia is obstructed, there may be severe pain (which needs analgesia) and systemic upset with pyrexia, dehydration, tachycardia, etc.
- There may be severe dehydration (particularly in frail and elderly people), which needs urgent correction. Make a particular point of looking at the recent urine output. If there is any doubt, catheterize immediately.
- If an obstructed hernia contains bowel, there may be intestinal obstruction with the need for a nasogastric tube and rapid sequence induction.

### Complications of peptic ulceration

#### *Perforated ulcer*

An upper midline incision is used. Any free fluid in the peritoneal cavity is aspirated. The site of the perforation is located, followed by simple closure with or without omentum covering. A lavage of the abdomen is usually done before closure. Larger perforations may require a definitive operation such as gastric resection.

*Surgical requirements*
These are as for elective bowel surgery, described above.

*Anaesthetic implications*
- Perforation results in a varying degree of shock preoperatively. Patients may need some resuscitation before surgery.
- Perforation is usually very painful and analgesia is needed. This can result in hypotension if the patient is dehydrated and the blood pressure has previously been maintained because of the sympathetic response to pain.
- A nasogastric tube is required if not already in place.
- Treat as having a full stomach.
- There can be a marked fall in blood pressure on induction if not adequately resuscitated with fluids preoperatively. Consequently, induce anaesthesia only with good peripheral intravenous access present and replacement fluids immediately available.
- This should be a short procedure with simple oversew of the perforation, but be prepared for a longer procedure, which may be required for a large perforation or haemorrhage, or in the event of a wrong diagnosis.

#### *Bleeding ulcer*

This will usually have been investigated preoperatively with endoscopy and an attempt made at conservative or endoscopic treatment. Surgery is required if the patient continues to bleed or a rebleed occurs. Surgery involves an upper midline incision, after which the source of the bleeding is located. Appropriate arteries are ligated as necessary and the base of the ulcer is under-run. A definitive operation is then usually performed, i.e. partial gastrectomy for gastric ulcers and vagotomy and pyloroplasty for duodenal ulcers.

*Surgical requirements*
These are as for elective bowel surgery, described above.

*Anaesthetic implications*
- Preoperative resuscitation is invariably required. Adequate venous access is mandatory.
- It may involve a perforation and be very painful.
- Ensure an adequate supply of blood and clotting products preoperatively.
- Endoscopy immediately before surgery may lead to drowsiness from the use of benzodiazepines. This should be accounted for in the preoperative assessment of the patient and in the use of induction agents.
- The patient must be treated as having a full stomach and a nasogastric tube is required to aspirate stomach contents.

### Abscesses

The abscess is incised and pus evacuated. The abscess cavity is explored. Skin and subcutaneous tissue may be excised. The cavity is left open and may be packed with gauze.

*Surgical requirements*
These depend on the site of the abscess. Relaxation is not normally needed for the surgical procedure itself.

*Anaesthetic implications*
- The site of the abscess has implications for the position of the patient. Ascertain the position that the surgeon would like the patient to be in before anaesthetizing, because this may dictate the method of anaesthesia.
- Abscesses can be extremely painful. Often the act of incising the abscess is very stimulating and can provoke laryngeal spasm unless the anaesthesia is sufficiently 'deep'.
- Local anaesthetic infiltration is ineffective because local inflammation renders the tissue pH very low.

## EAR, NOSE AND THROAT SURGERY

### Ear surgery

#### Myringotomy and insertion of grommets

An incision in the tympanic membrane is made in order to remove fluid, usually resulting from secretory otitis media. This is carried out with the aid of the operating microscope and a speculum in the affected ear. The head is inclined away from the operative side. A grommet may be inserted in order to maintain the opening in the drum, allowing drainage.

*Surgical requirements*

These are a supine patient whose head can be turned to gain access to the external auditory meatus.

*Anaesthetic implications*

- This is a short procedure carried out most frequently on children and usually done as a day case. (See Chapters 42 and 46.) Patients often have associated upper respiratory tract infections (URTIs) and active infection may necessitate postponing surgery.
- A facemask may be used but may get in the surgeon's way. The laryngeal mask airway (LMA) is a preferable alternative.

#### Middle ear surgery/reconstruction

This is frequently performed for chronic otitis media where a persistent tympanic perforation may result in conductive deafness and leave the middle ear open to infection. Chronic infection may be associated with cholesteatoma which can invade bone and destroy ossicles. Surgical terminology may be confusing:

- Tympanoplasty refers to repair of the drum with a graft, such as temporalis muscle fascia, and reconstruction of the sound-conducting mechanism.
- Myringoplasty is the simplest form of tympanoplasty with closure of the perforation alone.
- Mastoidectomy is required for more extensive chronic disease, with drilling out of diseased mastoid air cells.
- Tympanomastoidectomy involves drilling out the mastoid cortex with posterior exposure of the tympanic membrane. Diseased tissue is removed and the tympanic membrane grafted. Reconstruction of the ossicular chain may be carried out at the same time or deferred to a second operation, particularly if there is doubt about complete removal of cholesteatoma.
- Stapedectomy is performed for conductive deafness resulting from otosclerosis. The stapes is removed and a prosthesis inserted.

The skin incision for these operations is frequently made behind the ear (postaural), although an anterior incision may be used (end-aural). Prior infiltration with epinephrine and local anaesthetic is usual. The ear is packed at the end of surgery and then covered with crêpe bandaging which encircles the head.

*Specific surgical requirements*

This is classed as microsurgery with intraoperative use of the operating microscope. Small amounts of bleeding are magnified and good operating conditions are those in which bleeding can be minimized.

*Anaesthetic implications*

- A deaf patient can make communication difficult.
- Position of anaesthesia machine: the anaesthesia machine must be placed towards the foot end of the patient to allow the surgeon access. It is therefore important to ensure that there is sufficient length of ventilator and $CO_2$ sampling tubing. Intravenous access should be in the hand nearest the anaesthetist and a drip extension is useful.
- The airway is inaccessible during surgery. The ET tube should be well secured, making sure that the securing system does not get in the operative field. Pre-formed south-facing tubes taped to the chin are useful. Connections must be well secured and $CO_2$ monitoring is essential to aid detection of disconnections.
- The patient's eyes should be well protected.
- Bloodless field: this is aided by employing a 15° head-up position, avoiding coughing, which increases venous pressure in the head and neck, and a neutral head position to prevent engorgement of neck veins. The ET tube should be taped rather than tied because ties can constrict neck veins. Epinephrine is infiltrated by the surgeon to aid local vasoconstriction. Profound hypotension is unnecessary. Lesser degrees of hypotension may be desirable but care should be taken in elderly people and patients with cardiovascular, central nervous system, and renal disease. Maintain the mean pressure above 60 mmHg. Details of hypotensive techniques are outside the scope of this text.
- Surgical preparation: the hair is shaved around the ear. Soap may be applied to the hair to keep it stuck out of the way. The ear is then cleansed with antiseptic solution and drapes are applied. This requires careful lifting of the head by the anaesthetist, avoiding the cleansed areas of skin.
- $N_2O$ can fill the middle ear, causing bulging of the drum and lifting off of the tympanic graft. When it is discontinued, a negative pressure may develop in the middle ear as the gas is reabsorbed. These changes are particularly marked where Eustachian tube function is abnormal, as can occur in patients who have had previous middle-ear surgery or who have chronic otitis media. It is therefore best to avoid $N_2O$ unless having specifically discussed the pros and cons with the surgeon.
- Surgeons may wish to identify the facial nerve while operating on the middle ear. This precludes the intraoperative use of neuromuscular blocking agents. A short-acting neuromuscular blocking agent for intubation with or without spraying the cords with local anaesthetic, increasing depth of anaesthesia with volatile agent, and avoiding manipulation of the head should ensure that intraoperative neuromuscular blocking agent is not required. Neuromuscular monitoring is recommended for such cases.

- Postoperative nausea and vomiting are particularly common after middle-ear surgery.
- These are often lengthy operations. Patients should be kept warm, and thromboembolism prophylaxis may be required (see Chaper 1).

## Nasal surgery

### *Antral wash-out*

This is performed for chronic sinusitis which may result in nasal obstruction, nasal discharge, postnasal drip, and cough. The maxillary sinus is drained by puncturing with a trocar and insertion of a cannula through the antronasal wall. Pus is aspirated and the sinus irrigated. Persistent cases may require more radical drainage procedures as in an intranasal antrostomy, where a permanent opening is created, or a Caldwell–Luc procedure, where an incision into the anterior part of the antrum is made above the canine tooth. A bony window is then made, allowing removal of the contents of the sinus. A drain may then be inserted through an inferior meatal antrostomy and the oral incision sutured.

### *Nasal polypectomy*

Nasal polyps are pedunculated masses of oedematous mucosa usually associated with nasal allergy. They are often multiple and bilateral, and cause nasal obstruction. Polypectomy involves snaring and avulsing the polyp through a nasal speculum.

### *Submucous resection*

This operation is performed to correct nasal obstruction caused by a deviated nasal septum. An incision is made on one side of the septum and the mucoperichondrium dissected off. An incision through the cartilage is then made to allow the mucoperichondrium to be dissected off on the other side of the septum. Deflected cartilage and bone are then removed.

#### *Specific surgical requirements*

These are a supine and slightly head-up positioning of the patient.

#### *Anaesthetic implications*

- Warn the patient that he or she will not be able to breathe through the nose postoperatively.
- As for ear surgery, the anaesthesia machine is placed towards the foot end of the patient.
- Vasoconstrictors such as epinephrine or cocaine are used to provide a bloodless field and to shrink the mucosa. Cocaine has sympathomimetic effects and may result in hypertension, arrhythmias, hypersensitivity reactions, restlessness, and cardiac arrest. The safe maximum dose is 1.5 mg/kg. Moffatt's solution is a mixture of cocaine, epinephrine, and sodium bicarbonate. Avoid in hypertensive patients and those taking monoamine oxidase inhibitors.
- The airway requires protection from blood, mucus, and bony debris. This is usually achieved by using a cuffed ET tube with additional throat packing, although for some surgery a reinforced LMA may be appropriate. A pre-formed south-facing ET tube is useful. Always leave the throat pack tapes out so that they can be seen. It is obviously vital to remember to remove the throat pack before extubation.
- At the end of surgery, the nose is packed and so occluded. An oral airway should be inserted to prevent complete airway obstruction in recovery.

## Throat surgery

### *Adenotonsillectomy*

This is usually performed for recurrent tonsillitis with or without airway obstruction. Chronic airway obstruction may lead to sleep apnoea syndrome and occasionally enlarged tonsils may present with severe airway obstruction and stridor. The tonsils are removed either by dissection and vessel ligation or less commonly with a tonsil guillotine which crushes the tonsillar bed and cuts the tonsil off with a knife blade. For tonsillectomy, the operative site is exposed by extending the head and holding the mouth open with a Boyle–Davis gag, which is then supported by two short poles either side of the head. Adenoids are removed by passing a curette behind the soft palate, pressing it hard against the posterior pharyngeal wall, and pulling it downwards and outwards.

At the time of writing, the likely impact of new-variant Creutzfeldt–Jakob disease on the conduct of anaesthesia for adenotonsillectomy is uncertain. Trainees should follow current local guidelines.

#### *Specific surgical requirements*

The patient is placed supine with head extended, which may be achieved by placing a sandbag or equivalent under the shoulders.

#### *Anaesthetic implications*

- Preoperative assessment: nearly all patients will have a history of recurrent URTIs, and many will have persistent runny noses, which will only improve after surgery is carried out. Surgery should be postponed if there is active infection, particularly if the patient is pyrexial or has evidence of lower respiratory tract infection. Local anaesthetic cream should be applied to children's hands and a benzodiazepine premedication is useful.
- The airway needs protection from blood and debris and access to it during surgery is limited. An oral pre-formed ET tube or reinforced LMA may be used (see Chapter 6). There are pros and cons to spontaneous or positive pressure ventilation techniques. Spontaneous ventilation requires deeper levels of anaesthesia but has advantages where there is a risk of disconnection or accidental extubation during surgery. With either approach the use of end-tidal $CO_2$ monitoring is invaluable.
- Insertion of the Boyle–Davis gag may result in obstruction or disconnection of the ET tube, accidental extubation, or the ET tube being pushed down into a bronchus.
- Good analgesia is essential.
- Intraoperative bleeding may occasionally be marked. Good intravenous access is essential and a cannula must be left in place postoperatively because of the risk of postoperative bleeding.

- Extubation and recovery: the pharynx should be inspected for bleeding at the end of surgery. If there is doubt about the amount of bleeding the surgeon should be informed. Clots may collect in the nasopharynx and gentle elevation of the patient's head should reveal these. Extubation should occur when the patient is either well anaesthetized or awake. Any state in between these two risks precipitating laryngospasm. Again there are pros and cons to either approach. Children should be placed in the 'tonsil position', i.e. on their side, head-down so that blood drains out of their mouth. Patients should be recovered by experienced recovery staff, especially if extubated 'deep', because of the risks of respiratory obstruction and bleeding.

### Oesophagoscopy

Nowadays, rigid oesophagoscopy is usually indicated only to remove food or foreign bodies that are causing oesophageal obstruction.

#### Surgical requirements

For the oesophagoscope to be passed, the oesophagus has to be in direct alignment with the upper airway. This requires the patient's neck to be fully extended in the 'classic position' (see Chapter 6), usually with the head turned to the right.

#### Anaesthetic implications

- It can be a very stimulating procedure.
- Patients should be treated as having a full stomach and so a rapid sequence induction and intubation is required.
- Passing the oesophagoscope usually requires further muscle relaxation using either intermittent boluses of suxamethonium or small doses of non-depolarizing neuromuscular blocking agent.
- The presence of the oesophagoscope can irritate the heart and produce cardiac arrhythmias.

### Laryngoscopy

Direct, rigid-scope laryngoscopy may be indicated in the investigation of altered voice, for evaluation and biopsy of laryngeal malignancy, and in the assessment and treatment of laryngeal papillomas.

#### Surgical requirements

These are as for oesophagoscopy.

#### Anaesthetic implications

- Preoperative assessment: patients are frequently smokers and may have dysphagia leading to malnutrition. An assessment of the severity of any respiratory obstruction is vital, because this will affect the subsequent anaesthetic management. It is helpful to discuss with the surgeon the approximate size of any lesion.
- To prevent obscuring the surgeon's view of the larynx, a small-diameter microlaryngoscopy tube is used (see Chapter 6). This has a high-volume, low-pressure cuff which prevents soiling of the airway and allows positive pressure ventilation with volatile agents to maintain anaesthesia and oxygenation.
- The surgeon may require an unrestricted view of the larynx or may wish to look below the cords, necessitating removal of the ET tube. A rigid laryngoscope with a port for attaching a jet ventilator may be used. $O_2$ is then 'injected' from a high pressure source and air entrained through the laryngoscope. The chest must be observed for adequacy of expansion. Some coordination with the surgeon is required and anaesthesia needs to be maintained using a total intravenous technique (see Chapter 32).
- Good muscle relaxation and adequate depth of anaesthesia are required because passing the laryngoscope can be very stimulating.
- Recovery may be complicated by respiratory obstruction as a result of oedema.

### Laser surgery

Lasers produce a beam of coherent, monochromatic radiation. This can be precisely localized and will ablate tissue in a bloodless manner. The four basic lasers in use are $CO_2$, argon, neodymium : yttrium–aluminium–garnet (Nd : YAG) and potassium titanyl phosphate (KTP). The characteristics of each depend on the wavelength of the laser. The $CO_2$ laser has an invisible infrared wavelength and is coupled to a visible helium–neon beam for guidance. It is absorbed by water and the depth of tissue damage is limited to 0.2 mm with little thermal damage occurring to adjacent tissues. The Nd : YAG laser is absorbed by tissue proteins and requires a helium beam for guidance. It has deep penetrating effects, up to 5 mm, and good haemostatic properties. The KTP laser has a bright-green beam and does not need a separate aiming laser. It penetrates tissue up to 1 mm in depth and the light is absorbed by haemoglobin. The advantages of using lasers include reduced tissue reaction, particularly important in areas such as the larynx, reduced bleeding, greater precision of dissection, and preservation of normal tissue. (See also Chapter 86.)

#### Surgical requirements

These are as for laryngoscopy.

#### Anaesthetic implications

As for laryngoscopy plus the following:

- Airway fires: laser beams easily ignite polyvinylchloride (PVC) ET tubes and, in the presence of gases supporting combustion, such as $O_2$ and $N_2O$, can lead to serious airway fires. A PVC tube can be protected by winding adhesive aluminium tape around it to diffuse the beam (see Chapter 6). Filling the cuff with saline protects it against ignition and gives a warning of cuff penetration. The alternative is to use metallic tubes. All metallic tubes are completely laser proof and can be reused, but do not have a cuff. The Mallinkrodt Laserflex tube has a metal body with a PVC connector and PVC double cuff. Again the cuff may be filled with saline.
- Unwanted tissue damage: areas of the patient adjacent to the surgical field may be damaged directly or indirectly by reflected laser light.

Wet drapes and swabs around the patient's eyes and face will absorb the laser energy. Reflected laser light may also cause corneal damage and staff in the operating room must wear protective glasses or goggles. Staff should be informed when the beam is about to be fired and there should be warning signs outside the operating room.
- Although postoperative oedema is usually minimal, this remains a risk and patients should be observed for signs of airway obstruction.

## UROLOGICAL SURGERY

### Cystoscopy

Cystourethroscopy has been in use for more than 100 years in the investigation and treatment of haematuria, and the management of bladder tumours, with candles as the original light source. More recent development of the flexible fibreoptic cystoscope means that many cystoscopies are now performed without general anaesthesia. Rigid cystoscopes, however, allow better bladder irrigation and direct visualization of the bladder mucosa, and have a large-bore working channel, but the procedure requires general or regional anaesthesia and the patient has to be in the lithotomy position. The well-lubricated endoscope is passed into the bladder down the urethra. The bladder is filled with water or saline and may then be thoroughly inspected. Biopsy forceps can be passed down a cystoscope. A modification of the cystoscope, the resectoscope, is used to resect bladder tumours and a ureteroscope has been developed that enables endoscopic removal of ureteric stones and resection of ureteric tumours.

*Surgical requirements*

These are a supine patient in low or midlithotomy position; head-down tilt may be requested. Relaxation is not usually required.

*Anaesthetic implications*

- Lithotomy position (see Chapter 3): this position is achieved by flexing the patient's hips and knees and placing the feet in stirrups. The legs should be moved together and the sacrum should rest on the operating table, in order to prevent lower back injury and subsequent backache. Particular care should be taken if the patient has diseased hips. The feet should be well supported in the stirrups, with extra padding if necessary, particularly where the leg may be in contact with the pole. Deep vein thrombosis (DVT) and compartment syndrome may occur postoperatively if the lower leg is not protected. Feet and legs must not be in contact with any exposed metal. The lithotomy position is associated with some adverse physiological effects. Increased intra-abdominal pressure and upward movement of the diaphragm results in reduced functional residual capacity and tidal volume, and increases the risk of regurgitation of gastric contents. These effects are exaggerated if head-down (Trendelenburg) positioning is also required. Elevation of the legs increases venous return to the heart. At the end of surgery, when the legs are lowered, venous pooling in the legs may occur. This can result in hypotension, especially if intraoperative volume replacement has been inadequate. Monitoring must therefore be continued throughout this period.
- Patient movement during surgery can be particularly irritating for the surgeon who is trying to look through the cystoscope, is potentially hazardous if resection is taking place, and may significantly damage a ureteroscope.

### Resection of the prostate

#### *Transurethral resection of the prostate*

Transurethral resection of the prostate (TURP) may be performed on prostates that are usually less than 60 g in size. Prostatic size is assessed by bimanual examination and through endoscopic inspection. The operation is done via the resectoscope, through which diathermy cutting loops are passed. The bladder and prostatic area are inspected initially, and then the prostate is resected by advancing and withdrawing the diathermy loop. Cutting occurs as the loop is pulled towards the operator. Continuous irrigation is required during resection to wash away blood and prostatic tissue. At the end of the resection, an Ellik evacuator is used to wash out any remaining prostatic chips and the prostatic bed is inspected for bleeding. A three-way catheter is then inserted and irrigation continued into the postoperative period.

*Specific surgical requirements*

These are as for cystoscopy.

*Anaesthetic implications*

- Lithotomy position: see above and Chapter 3.
- Bleeding: the prostate is a vascular gland and bleeding during surgery may be significant. Blood loss is difficult to estimate because the blood is washed away into a bucket at the feet of the surgeon and mixed with irrigating fluid. Factors associated with increased bleeding are increasing size of gland, increased resection time, and infection associated with long-term indwelling catheters. There are no foolproof methods of quantifying blood loss, so observation and monitoring of vital signs is essential. Deliberate hypotension does not reduce blood loss and is potentially hazardous. Prolonged bleeding postoperatively may be caused by a problem of coagulation as a result of urokinase release from the prostate, leading to fibrinolysis. A haemoglobin estimation is probably the best and easiest test to do in cases of uncertainty.
- Clot retention may occur in recovery, particularly if irrigation is inadequate, and may cause extreme discomfort for the patient. Simple measures such as trying to clear clots with a bladder syringe or milking the catheter may work, but occasionally the patient has to be taken back to the operating room.
- Irrigation fluid and TUR syndrome: as previously mentioned, large quantities of irrigating fluid are used during TURP. The most frequently used fluid is 1.5% glycine because it is iso-osmotic and

non-electrolytic. Saline disperses the diathermy current, glucose caramelizes on the end of the diathermy loop, and distilled water when absorbed into the circulation results in haemolysis and hyponatraemia. Although the severe consequences of the absorption of large amounts of hypotonic solution, including unconsciousness, cardiovascular collapse, and death, are less common with glycine, problems still occur. Any irrigating fluid will be absorbed through the prostatic venous sinuses. The amount depends on the height of the containers above the surgical field, and therefore the hydrostatic pressure, and the length of resection (10–30 ml fluid are absorbed per min of resection). Absorption of large quantities of fluid may result in pulmonary oedema and dilutional hyponatraemia, leading to dyspnoea, hypoxia, ECG changes, and neurological symptoms such as restlessness and confusion. Absorption of glycine, an inhibitory neurotransmitter, and its subsequent metabolism to ammonia may be associated with neurological disturbance. Diagnosis is dependent on thinking about it as a possibility and doing a serum electrolyte estimation. Treatment depends on the severity of symptoms and initially should be supportive, with slow correction of hyponatraemia. Severe cases should be admitted to an ICU.

- Hypothermia may occur during surgery, particularly if cold irrigating fluids are used. The more elderly patients undergoing TURP are less able to cope with heat loss. A warming mattress or blanket should be used and irrigating fluids warmed, ideally using a warmer specifically designed for large quantities of fast-flowing fluids.
- Perforation of the prostatic capsule, urethra, or bladder may occur during surgery. Most are extraperitoneal resulting in periumbilical pain. Intraperitoneal perforations may cause shoulder-tip pain. Small perforations do not usually require treatment, but larger perforations may require surgical exploration.
- Anaesthetic technique: regional and general anaesthesia are both suitable. Advantages of regional anaesthesia include the ability to monitor neurological symptoms that may arise as a result of hyponatraemia. The block should extend to T10 to provide anaesthesia for the discomfort of bladder distension.
- Bacteraemia may occur if urinary tract infection is present. Prophylactic antibiotics may be required.

#### Open prostatectomy

An open prostatectomy, where the prostate is removed via a suprapubic incision, is required for prostates too large to be removed by transurethral resection. This may be done either by approaching the prostate through an incision in the bladder (transvesical prostatectomy) or by approaching it from behind the pubis but without opening the bladder (retropubic prostatectomy). In a retropubic operation, a suprapubic incision is made, the rectus sheath divided, and the anterior capsule of the prostate exposed by gentle dissection. The capsule is opened and the prostate shelled out with a finger. A wedge of tissue is then removed from the bladder neck. A three-way catheter is inserted into the bladder and the capsule closed. A drain is left in the abdominal wound and the bladder irrigated.

*Specific surgical requirements*

These are a supine patient with some head-down positioning, and a relaxed abdominal wall.

*Anaesthetic implications*

- Bleeding may be considerable during open prostatectomy. Ensure good intravenous access and the availability of blood.
- General requirements are similar to elective abdominal surgery.

### Cystectomy

Total cystectomy is most frequently performed for bladder malignancy. It has to be accompanied by a method of urinary diversion either through an ileal conduit to an external opening or by implanting the ureters into the sigmoid colon. After abdominal incision, the bladder, lymph glands, and liver are assessed for the extent of disease. The bladder is then dissected out and mobilized, and the ureters secured and divided. Silastic tubes may be inserted into the ends of the ureters to be brought through the ileal loop later, but before this may be placed in a bag to prevent contamination of the wound with urine. Mobilization of the bladder continues together with removal of surrounding lymph glands. The urethra is then exposed and divided and the bladder removed. The urinary diversion procedure is then performed. For an ileal conduit, the left ureter is tunnelled under the colon and brought through the same peritoneal incision as the right ureter. A loop of ileum is selected that is not too close to the ileocaecal valve and long enough to reach the abdominal wall, with sufficient length for stoma formation. It is then separated with its mesentery from the rest of the small bowel and the continuity of the small bowel restored. The proximal end of the loop is closed and the ureters anastomosed. A stoma site is then created and the conduit fixed to the skin.

*Surgical requirements*

These are similar to major elective abdominal surgery (see above).

*Anaesthetic implications*

- This is a major and lengthy procedure with significant morbidity and mortality, often performed on relatively unfit patients. An assessment of the risks and benefits of surgery must be undertaken preoperatively.
- Large blood and fluid losses can occur and direct arterial and CVP monitoring is justified. Fluids should be warmed and other measures taken to reduce heat loss. The body temperature may fall significantly and should be monitored.
- Epidural anaesthesia supplementing general anaesthesia is desirable because this may be continued into the postoperative period, providing good analgesia.
- Patients should be nursed postoperatively in a high dependency unit or ICU.

### Male genitalia

#### ***Circumcision***

This is indicated for phimosis and recurrent balanitis. The prepuce is first fully retracted, and then returned to its original position after cleaning the glans. The skin is marked at the level of the corona as a guide to the level of dissection. Traction is then applied to the tip of the prepuce and a clamp placed across the prepuce distal to the glans. The excess foreskin is excised, the clamp released, and the skin allowed to retract. The inner layer is then trimmed and bleeding points dealt with. Only bipolar diathermy should be used. The two layers of prepuce are then sutured together with absorbable sutures.

*Surgical requirement*

This is a supine patient.

*Anaesthetic implications*

Circumcision may be associated with considerable postoperative pain and is usually performed as a day-case procedure, particularly in children. A penile or caudal block supplementing general anaesthesia provides good postoperative analgesia. Local anaesthetic solutions for penile blocks should not contain epinephrine. Patients usually need more than simple analgesics for adequate pain relief.

#### ***Torsion of testis***

This can occur when an anatomical anomaly allows the testis to twist, so compromising its blood supply. It occurs most commonly between the ages of 12 and 16 years, and presents with pain and swelling of the scrotum. A scrotal incision is made, the testis rotated, and then fixed to prevent recurrence. The anomaly predisposing to torsion is usually bilateral and the other testis may be fixed at the same time. It is a true emergency that must not be put off. Be prepared to interrupt a planned list if necessary.

*Surgical requirement*

This is a supine patient.

*Anaesthetic implications*

The testis is unable to survive more than about 6 hours of ischaemia and, if the patient presents with a short history, the surgeon may wish to operate as soon as possible. This may mean anaesthetizing a patient with a full stomach with its attendant risks. Preoperative discussion with the surgeon to enable an assessment of the risks and benefits of immediate surgery is very important.

## GYNAECOLOGICAL SURGERY

### Evacuation of retained products of conception

This is performed most commonly after spontaneous abortion where products remain in the uterus, leading to the risk of bleeding or infection. The patient is placed in the lithotomy position, a vaginal examination performed, and the bladder emptied. A speculum is inserted, the cervix grasped with vulsellum forceps, and a uterine sound passed. The cervix is dilated and products are removed.

#### ***Surgical requirements***

These are midlithotomy position, sometimes head-down.

#### ***Anaesthetic implications***

- Although this procedure is usually urgent rather than an emergency, the emotional sequelae to miscarrying are such that the procedure should not be delayed indefinitely, so that the patient can go home at the earliest opportunity. Occasionally, bleeding is so heavy that preoperative resuscitation and emergency surgery are required.
- In a fit, starved patient with a normal body mass index, below 16 weeks into pregnancy and without oesophageal reflux, a facemask or LMA is satisfactory.
- Increasing gestational age at the time of abortion results in increased risk of regurgitation and aspiration. It is advisable to consider rapid sequence induction and intubation where the gestational age is greater than 16 weeks, or at an earlier gestation if the patient is obese.
- Volatile agents cause uterine relaxation, resulting in increased intraoperative bleeding. This is not generally a problem at lower concentrations, but a total intravenous anaesthetic technique with propofol may be more appropriate.
- Dilatation of the cervix is stimulating and may result in bradycardia and laryngospasm, especially if anaesthesia is not of sufficient depth.
- Surgeons generally ask for oxytocin to be given at the end of the procedure to contract the uterus. Transient sinus tachycardias are often encountered with its administration.
- It is not uncommon for the surgeon to perform a vigorous vaginal examination after they have said that they have finished. It is wise to wait for the surgeon to deglove before waking the patient up.

### Hysteroscopy

This procedure is frequently performed in the investigation of abnormal uterine bleeding. It may be done at the same time as laparoscopy if an intrapelvic lesion is suspected, and is often accompanied by dilatation and curettage. The hysteroscope is introduced into the uterus through the cervix after vaginal examination, bladder emptying, and the passage of a speculum. $CO_2$ is usually used as the uterine distending medium and is run as the hysteroscope is introduced. The gas creates a small cavity in the cervical canal into which the scope is slowly advanced until it reaches the internal os. It is then passed through this into the uterine cavity which is then examined.

#### ***Surgical requirements***

These are as for evacuation of retained products of conception.

#### ***Anaesthetic implications***

- $CO_2$ may pass through the Fallopian tubes into the peritoneal cavity, resulting in diaphragmatic irritation and shoulder tip pain.
- Passage through the cervix may result in cervical laceration which should be sutured.

## Laparoscopy/laparosopic sterilization

Laparoscopy is often performed in the investigation of gynaecological symptoms and infertility. Some operative procedures are carried out through the laparoscope such as sterilization, removal of ectopic pregnancy, and hysterectomy. A pneumoperitoneum is induced by insufflation of $CO_2$ through a Verres needle inserted through a small subumbilical incision. The laparoscopic trocar is then inserted through the same incision and directed towards the pelvis. The obturator is removed and the laparoscope inserted. Other instruments may be inserted into the peritoneal cavity through small lower abdominal incisions under laparoscopic guidance. If sterilization is being performed, the Fallopian tubes are identified and clips or rings applied or the tubes are diathermied. At the end of the procedure, the laparoscope is removed and remaining intra-abdominal gas released. Abdominal incisions are often simply covered, although the subumbilical incision may be stitched.

### *Specific surgical requirements*

These are low lithotomy, usually head-down for part of the time.

### *Anaesthetic implications*

- See the section on laparoscopic cholecystectomy for implications of the pneumoperitoneum. Trendelenburg positioning exacerbates the respiratory and cardiovascular effects, as does patient obesity.
- Postoperative pain: shoulder tip pain is frequently encountered after laparoscopy, particularly if intra-abdominal gas has not been adequately released. Diagnostic laparoscopy is not usually as painful as laparoscopic sterilization. The method of sterilization appears to affect the amount of postoperative pain, with rings and clips being associated with more colicky lower abdominal pain than diathermy. Good analgesia is essential, especially as these are often day-case procedures. Local anaesthetics can be applied directly to the Fallopian tubes at operation and non-steroidal anti-inflammatory drugs are helpful.

## Ectopic pregnancy

This condition ranges in severity from presentation with minor lower abdominal pain to life-threatening cardiovascular collapse from acute tubal rupture and arterial haemorrhage. Where there is some doubt in diagnosis, a diagnostic laparoscopy is performed first. An ectopic pregnancy, if present, may then be dealt with laparoscopically or a lower abdominal incision made followed by partial or total salpingectomy. An emergency laparotomy is performed for acutely bleeding ectopic pregnancies. The fundus of the uterus is grasped through the incision and fingers, then clamps applied to the appropriate broad ligament and Fallopian tube at the uterine end to stop bleeding. The pelvis can then be evacuated of blood and salpingectomy or other appropriate surgery performed.

### *Surgical requirements*

This often starts off as laparoscopy in low lithotomy position with the legs later lowered to standard supine.

### *Anaesthetic implications*

- Laparoscopy for ectopic pregnancy is inevitably an emergency procedure. The surgeon should be able to inform the anaesthetist of the likelihood of ectopic pregnancy as the diagnosis, and the cardiovascular status of the patient, so that the urgency of surgery can be assessed. Tubal pregnancies may rupture at any time and it is advisable to insert large-bore intravenous cannulae and have resuscitation fluid available before anaesthetizing.
- Genuine emergency bleeding ectopic pregnancies are less common, but when they occur the only definitive way of controlling bleeding and restoring cardiovascular stability is by clamping the uterine artery. Resuscitation and transfer to the operating room should be done together. A rapid sequence induction in the operating room is the safest approach. Deterioration on induction may occur as a result of loss of the tamponading effect of abdominal muscle tone, so be ready with extra fluids and blood.

## Vaginal surgery for repair and hysterectomy

### *Vaginal repair*

Anterior or posterior vaginal repairs (colporrhaphy) are required for prolapse of the bladder or rectum into the vagina. In an anterior repair a speculum is inserted into the vagina, and the cervix grasped with vulsellum forceps and pulled down to stretch the anterior wall. The anterior wall is opened and separated from the underlying bladder. The bladder is dissected off the cervix and the bladder prolapse repaired by a method of stitching fascia across it. Redundant skin is removed and the vaginal wall closed. In the posterior repair, the posterior wall of the vagina is grasped and elevated and an incision made just inside the vagina. The rectum is separated from the vaginal wall and the rectocele is repaired by closing muscle and fascia across it. Redundant skin is removed and the vagina closed. A Manchester repair consists of anterior and posterior repairs together with amputation of the cervix.

### *Vaginal hysterectomy*

This procedure is performed for vaginal prolapse and other indications for hysterectomy where the uterus is relatively small and mobile. An abdominal wound is avoided so postoperative mobilization is quicker. A dilatation and curettage is usually performed initially. The cervix is then pulled down, an incision made around it, and the vaginal skin separated from it. The bladder is mobilized anteriorly. The uterovesical peritoneum is incised anteriorly and the pouch of Douglas opened posteriorly. Vessels and ligaments have then to be clamped and tied to allow removal of the uterus. The ureters are at risk. The cervix is pulled down, and the cardinal and uterosacral ligaments, then the uterine vessels, are clamped, divided, and tied each side. Further traction on the cervix and uterus exposes the Fallopian tubes, round ligaments, and ovarian ligaments which are clamped and doubly ligated. The peritoneum is closed, leaving the pedicles outside the peritoneal cavity. These are then sutured together to support and close the vaginal vault and the vaginal wall is closed.

*Specific surgical requirements*
These are the midlithotomy position.

*Anaesthetic implications*
- See under cystoscopy for implications of the lithotomy position.
- The surgeon may wish to infiltrate the vaginal wall with epinephrine.
- Bleeding may be considerable and blood loss is not always easy to assess because it is absorbed onto drapes and the area of interest may be obscured by surgical personnel.
- Regional anaesthesia as the sole anaesthetic technique, or in addition to general anaesthesia, may reduce bleeding and is helpful for postoperative analgesia.

### Abdominal hysterectomy
Total abdominal hysterectomy (TAH) is the removal of the uterus together with the cervix. In a subtotal hysterectomy, the cervical stump is left. TAH is most frequently performed for menorrhagia. The ovaries may be removed at the same time depending on the uterine pathology and age of the patient. The more radical Wertheim hysterectomy is performed for carcinoma of the cervix. TAH is usually done through a lower abdominal transverse (Pfannenstiel) incision after initial bladder catheterization and occasional painting of the vagina to aid later identification. Packs and self-retaining retractors are inserted to keep the bowel out of the way. The uterus is elevated and clamps are applied across the fallopian tubes on either side close to the uterus. A second pair of clamps is applied across the broad ligament either medially or laterally to the ovaries, depending on whether they are being removed or not. If they are to be removed, the infundibulopelvic ligament containing the ovarian artery is clamped. The tubes and ligaments between the clamps are cut and tied. The uterovesical fold of peritoneum is incised in front of the vagina. The ureters are identified and the uterine arteries clamped and ligated. The uterosacral ligaments may be clamped and divided and the vagina is then opened. The incision is continued round the vagina and the uterus may then be removed. The vagina is then closed, followed by the peritoneum after securing haemostasis. The abdominal packs are removed and the abdomen closed.

*Specific surgical requirements*
These are standard supine position with head-down tilt on request.

*Anaesthetic implications*
- As this operation is usually performed for menorrhagia, it is wise to check the preoperative haemoglobin and correct anaemia if necessary. This may involve prescribing iron and delaying the procedure for several weeks.
- Intraoperative blood loss may be considerable.
- Patient obesity makes the operation surgically more challenging and blood loss may be heavier.

## ORTHOPAEDIC SURGERY AND FRACTURES

### Anaesthetic implications common to many orthopaedic procedures
- Preoperative condition of patient: patients presenting for orthopaedic surgery are frequently elderly, with many of the disease processes found in this group. Thorough preoperative assessment, optimization of physiological status, and management of medical problems are essential. Joint surgery is often performed on patients with rheumatoid arthritis, presenting particular challenges for the anaesthetist (see Chapter 57).
- Anaesthetic technique: regional anaesthetic techniques are suitable for many procedures in orthopaedics either as a sole method of anaesthesia or complementing general anaesthesia. The condition of the patient may dictate the choice of anaesthetic, but advantages of regional anaesthesia include good postoperative analgesia with reduced use of opioids, reduction of blood loss, and the possible benefit of reduced incidence of DVT. In some patients, regional anaesthesia may be technically difficult as a result, for example, of pain or dementia, and preoperative thromboembolism prophylaxis may preclude its use.
- Infection control: orthopaedic surgeons have particular concerns about bacterial contamination of the wound at the time of surgery, not least because of the serious complication of an infected prosthesis. This often means a zealous approach to the wearing of hats and masks by operating room personnel. Dedicated orthopaedic operating rooms usually contain elaborate airflow systems and, as these are designed to work with the doors closed, leaving the door to the anaesthetic room open may result in surgical irritation. Antibiotic prophylaxis is required and it is usual for this to be given before application of a tourniquet to allow it to reach the affected part.
- Tourniquets: these are used in limb surgery to provide a bloodless field. They should not be used in patients with sickle-cell disease or those with significant peripheral vascular disease (see Chapter 3). The tourniquet should be applied where there is sufficient muscle bulk to protect underlying nerves, i.e. midthigh or midcalf level in the leg and midbiceps level in the arm. The limb is exsanguinated, e.g. by using an inflated rubber sleeve (Rhys–Davis exsanguinator) and the tourniquet inflated. This is usually achieved with an automatic inflator set to the desired cuff pressure. A pressure gauge showing the pressure of the cuff should always be visible and the time of inflation noted. Once inflated the limb becomes ischaemic, anaerobic metabolism occurs, and metabolites accumulate. On deflation of the tourniquet these metabolites are released into the circulation, resulting in a metabolic acidosis, increased end-tidal $CO_2$, and a fall in blood pressure, all of which should be transient. Inflation times of longer than 2 hours should be avoided, and for longer operations the surgeon

may require deflation then reinflation of the tourniquet. Cut vessels are not so obvious in an exsanguinated limb and this may result in large blood loss at the time of deflation.
- Cement: acrylic bone cement (methyl methacrylate) is used to fix prostheses. Its insertion can be associated with cardiovascular instability and even cardiac arrest and death. Several theories exist to explain this, including a systemic response to methyl methacrylate monomer released into the blood, embolism of fat, air and platelet aggregates, and the result of increased intramedullary pressure. Intravascular volume should be optimized before insertion of cement. The use of a cement gun and venting of the femoral shaft reduce the rise in intramedullary pressure. It is, of course, essential that the surgeon warns the anaesthetist before using cement.
- Blood loss: this may be considerable during orthopaedic surgery, especially during reaming of medullary bone and revision surgery. There is some evidence that spinal and epidural anaesthesia reduce intraoperative blood loss.
- Thromboembolism is a significant cause of postoperative morbidity and mortality after orthopaedic surgery, particularly that involving the pelvis, hip, or lower limb. Heparin prophylaxis is frequently used and low-molecular-weight heparins are more effective at preventing DVT after surgery than conventional heparin. Administration of this can be devolved to the anaesthetist at induction, particularly if a regional anaesthetic technique is being used. Spinal and epidural anaesthesia are associated with a reduced incidence of DVT. DVT prophylaxis is considered in more detail in Chapter 1.

## Hip surgery

### Total hip replacement

This operation is performed for pain and disability in the hip joint when conservative measures have failed. The hip joint is usually exposed via a posterior approach with the patient on his or her side and an incision over the greater trochanter. The hip is dislocated and the head removed with an osteotome or reciprocating saw. The acetabulum is prepared by removing soft tissue and remaining cartilage, and is concentrically reamed. Cement is pressed into the bone and the acetabular component inserted with an alignment guide. The femur is then reamed and a trial reduction carried out before cementing in the femoral component. Once the cement has hardened the hip is reduced and the wound closed.

### Fractured neck of femur

This condition occurs commonly and is most frequently seen in a high-risk elderly population with an average age of 75–80 years and pre-existing medical problems. There is significant morbidity and mortality associated with fracture repair, but fracture surgery should not be delayed longer than a few days because of the increased morbidity and mortality associated with long periods of immobilization. Fractures are of two main types: subcapital and intertrochanteric. With subcapital fractures, the blood supply to the femoral head is at risk and avascular necrosis of the head may occur. For this reason, it is usual to replace the femoral head with a prosthesis (hemiarthroplasty). Inter-trochanteric fractures have a good blood supply and heal well. Surgery for these fractures entails open reduction and internal fixation, e.g. with a dynamic hip screw (DHS).

For a hemiarthroplasty procedure, the hip joint is approached either posteriorly or anterolaterally, depending on the type of prosthesis being used and the preference of the surgeon. The joint capsule is opened, the fracture exposed, and the femoral head removed with a corkscrew instrument. The head is measured to size the prosthesis correctly. The neck of the femur is trimmed with a saw and the femoral shaft reamed. The prosthesis is then inserted into the shaft, with or without cement, depending on the type of prosthesis, and is then reduced into the acetabulum. The wound is then closed.

Surgery for an intertrochanteric fracture with a DHS starts with positioning of the patient on an orthopaedic traction table. This has a vertical padded post which prevents movement of the pelvis down the table during traction and two supports for the feet which are held in boots. The image intensifier is then positioned over the fracture site and the fracture reduced by traction to the leg under radiological control. The skin is then cleansed and a drape applied. This takes the form of a large disposable sheet specifically designed for this operation, which is stuck over a horizontal pole held by two vertical ones. A lateral incision is made from the greater trochanter down a line parallel to the femoral shaft. A guide pin is inserted into the femoral neck under radiological control to lie in the centre of the femoral head. When the surgeon is happy with its position, a hole is drilled and the screw inserted. The DHS plate is positioned over the screw and fixed to the femoral shaft with screws. The wound is then closed.

#### *Surgical requirements*

These, apart from the obvious requirement of good anaesthesia, relate principally to positioning. The anaesthetist should be clear preoperatively what position is intended.

#### *Anaesthetic implications*

- Adequate preoperative assessment and treatment of correctable medical problems is essential. Patients with fractured necks of the femur are often hypovolaemic, and perioperative fluid resuscitation and haemodynamic optimization have been shown to improve outcome. Measures for improving the medical condition of the patient preoperatively should not take so long that the period of immobilization itself results in further morbidity.
- Patient position: for a posterior approach to the hip, the patient is placed on his or her side. It is useful to have the drip in the arm on the same side as the fracture. Positioning the patient on the traction table may be difficult. The patient is pulled down the table and care must be taken not to dislodge ET tubes and drips. There should be adequate padding around the vertical pole and no parts of the patient should be touching metal. The

table is elevated to a comfortable working height for the surgeon, which may make access to the patient more difficult for the shorter anaesthetist.
- Revision surgery for total hip replacement is increasingly performed. This is technically more difficult than the initial arthroplasty, takes longer, and is associated with greater blood loss. Good intravenous access and measures to prevent heat loss are obviously important.

## Knee surgery

### Arthroscopy

Arthroscopy is used in the investigation of knee pathology and in the treatment of certain conditions such as meniscal injury and removal of loose bodies. It is frequently performed as a day-case procedure. The limb is exsanguinated and a tourniquet applied to the midthigh. The arthroscope is inserted through a small lateral incision. Other incisions are made to allow irrigation of the knee and the passage of probes or operative instruments. The knee is thoroughly examined and surgery carried out as required. It is now much more common to treat a meniscal tear by arthroscopically guided repair than menisectomy. At the end of the procedure the knee is drained, the incisions closed, bandaging applied, and the tourniquet deflated.

#### *Surgical requirements*

These are a supine position with the ability to flex and extend the knee and otherwise move it around.

#### *Anaesthetic implications*

- Any regional anaesthetic technique, if used, must provide anaesthesia for the area of the tourniquet.
- Good postoperative analgesia may be achieved by the use of intra-articular bupivacaine especially with the addition of morphine, which is injected into the knee joint after it has been drained of irrigating fluid.
- Arthroscopic surgery is highly specialized, requiring a degree of three-dimensional spatial skills. Arthroscopic procedures may therefore take some time, particularly for surgeons gaining experience in the technique.

### Total knee replacement

Knee replacement is indicated for pain and disability in arthritic knees unresponsive to conservative treatment, including loss of excess weight. A tourniquet is applied and the knee joint is approached through an anteromedial incision with the patella moved laterally. Surgical success depends to some extent on correcting any varus or valgus alignment of the knee. Total condylar joints are used, replacing the natural contours of the joint with femoral and tibial components. Femoral and tibial guides are used for correct positioning of these components. The components are usually cemented in place, although some are designed to be used without cement. The under-surface of the patella may also be replaced. A drain is left in the wound, the wound closed, and the tourniquet usually deflated after the application of bandages.

#### *Surgical requirements*

These are as for arthroscopy.

#### *Anaesthetic implications*

- Blood loss during the procedure is minimal because of the tourniquet, but occurs after its release and may then be substantial. It is important to monitor this carefully in recovery, transfuse if necessary, and not to discharge the patient back to the ward until drainage slows.
- Total knee replacement is associated with significantly more postoperative pain than total hip replacement and an epidural for postoperative analgesia is useful.
- Occasionally both knees are replaced at one operation. This takes twice as long and results in greater blood loss. It may not be advisable in the more infirm patients.
- Total knee replacement carries a high risk of thromboembolism.

## Fracture management: general principles

Management of fractures by orthopaedic surgeons will usually entail the need for anaesthesia.

Emergency surgery is required for open fractures and those where there is vascular injury resulting in haemorrhage or ischaemia. If there are signs of compartment syndrome, then prompt fasciotomy is needed. Open fractures provide an entry site for bacteria to an environment suitable for the culture of anaerobes including clostridia. Removal of dead and damaged tissue and any foreign material is essential to prevent infection, which may result in non-union and chronic osteomyelitis. This requires surgical enlargement of the wound with thorough cleaning and débridement of tissues and bones. The fracture is stabilized by external or internal fixation, and the wound is generally left open, to be closed at a later date.

Fractures will often need reducing in order to maintain the function and appearance of a limb and to aid healing. The methods for this are manipulation, traction, and open reduction. Manipulation will require anaesthesia by local infiltration or regional or general anaesthesia. Skeletal traction is applied by a metal pin (e.g. Steinmann or Denham) passing through bone.

Open reduction allows accurate reduction and early mobilization. It is required if fractures cannot be accurately reduced by manipulation or cannot be maintained in reduction. It has the disadvantage of converting a closed fracture to an open fracture with subsequent risk of infection and bleeding. Once reduced, the reduction is held by external or internal fixation. External fixation includes splinting with plaster of Paris, traction, or external fixation devices. This involves inserting pins or screws into bone percutaneously above and below the fracture site. These are then clamped by an external frame forming a rigid splint.

Various techniques are employed in the internal fixation of fractures. Kirschner wires are used to transfix fractures of small bones or small intra-articular fragments. They are inserted using a power drill. They can be used as encircling bands, e.g. in the wiring of olecranon fractures. Screws are used to fix larger fragments, e.g. malleolar fractures. Screws may be self-tapping, with a point designed to cut its own thread, or non-self-tapping. Cortical screws have a shallow thread and cancellous screws a deep thread designed for use where the cortex is thin. When bone is being joined with screws, a hole is first drilled and its depth measured to enable selection of the correct screw length. The hole is tapped if a non-self-tapping screw is being used and the screw inserted with a power or hand-operated screw driver.

Plates and screws, intramedullary nails, and rods are used for long bone fixation and fractures of the femoral neck. Plates are placed along the length of a bone, holding the fracture together and providing some strength. They may be contoured by the surgeon to some extent to fit the curvature of the bone, although some are manufactured with a curve for specific purposes. Intramedullary nailing is used for long bone fractures, e.g. femoral shaft. The Kuntscher nail is clover-leaf-shaped in cross-section and has a tapered end to allow free passage through the medullary canal. The nail may be introduced through the fracture site (open nailing) or more often from one end of the bone (closed nailing) which requires radiological guidance. The nail may be locked to control rotation at the fracture site.

Compression refers to methods that compress the fracture ends together to promote bone healing. Dynamic devices allow for some bone movement to occur so encouraging callus formation.

The initials AO, which prefix the names of many internal fixation devices, stand for *Arbeitsgemeinschaft für Osteosynthesfragen* or the Association for the Study of Problems in Internal Fixation.

#### *Surgical requirements*

These are a well-anaesthetized patient in an appropriate position to reduce and fix the fracture. Check on the necessary position with the surgeon preoperatively if you are not clear on what is intended.

#### *Anaesthetic implications*

- Patients with traumatic injuries may require a period of preoperative resuscitation and stabilization before surgery. Patients with cervical injuries need proper assessment and management before other less important fractures are attended to. Remember the possibility of occult cervical injuries (see Chapter 64).
- Trauma lists are often produced very close to operating room time because of the urgent nature of many procedures. This should not, however, impinge on good anaesthetic care and time must be allowed for adequate preoperative assessment of patients.
- Patients may arrive in the anaesthetic room surrounded by traction devices. It is necessary to ensure that access to the patient is adequate, which may mean the removal of some of the frames. This should be done with the minimum of patient discomfort. Ideally the orthopaedic bed should be tiltable.
- Trauma results in delay in stomach emptying, and it is more helpful to know the time from eating to sustaining trauma than to surgery in guiding the need for a rapid sequence induction and intubation.
- In some hospitals, it is the practice to manipulate fractures under intravenous regional anaesthesia administered by an anaesthetist in the accident and emergency department. In these circumstances, as well as checking the tourniquet, the anaesthetist should ensure that full resuscitation equipment and drugs are available and that there is dedicated anaesthetic assistance.

## FURTHER READING


Badner NH. Anaesthesia for minimally invasive surgery. *Can J Anaesth* 1999;**46**:R101–5.

Hahn RG. The transurethral resection syndrome. *Acta Anaesthesiol Scand* 1991;**35**:557–67.

Morris PJ, Malt RA, eds. *Oxford Textbook of Surgery*. Oxford: Oxford Medical Publications, 1994.

Rintoul RF, ed. *Farquharson's Textbook of Operative Surgery*. Edinburgh: Churchill Livingstone, 1995.

Royal College of Anaesthetists. *Standards and Guidelines for General Anaesthesia for Dentistry*. London: Royal College of Anaesthetists, 1999.

Xue FS, Li BW, Zhang GS, Liao X, Zhang YM, Liu JH, An G, Luo LK. The influence of surgical sites on early postoperative hypoxaemia in adults undergoing elective surgery. *Anesth Analg* 1999;**88**:213–19.

Zorab J, ed. *Surgery for Anaesthetists*. Oxford: Blackwell Scientific Publications, 1988.

# Chapter 17 Principles of high dependency care and intensive care medicine

P. Nightingale and M.P. Shelly

Intensive care units (ICUs) and high dependency units (HDUs) are areas of the hospital designated for the treatment of actual, or prevention of impending, organ failure. The technical facilities available are over and above those in other areas of the hospital, and the staff have specialized knowledge, experience, and skill not automatically acquired by training in other specialties.

In this overview, we show how the basic principles covered in other sections of this book are applied to the care of the critically ill patient. The chapter is not intended to be a mini-textbook of intensive care medicine; it is meant to introduce the trainee to a method of approach and to outline strategies in relation to common problems. Key documents that augment the content of the text are given under 'Further reading'.

## UNITS AND STAFFING

The availability of high dependency and intensive care beds is always limited. As high dependency and intensive care are an expensive resource, it is appropriate to address the suitability and benefit of admission.

### Definitions

High dependency care is an increased level of care and monitoring above that available on the normal ward, which can be achieved with a nurse : patient ratio of 1 : 2.

Intensive care is defined as 'a service for patients with potentially recoverable conditions who can benefit from more detailed observation and invasive treatment than can safely be provided in general wards or high dependency areas'. The nurse : patient ratio is 1 : 1.

The facilities and staffing, patient suitability, and categories of organ support and monitoring are given in Tables 17.1–17.3. The aim should be to place the patient in the appropriate environment at all stages of their care.

Specific recommendations for the care of children, and the future development of paediatric intensive care, have now been made and it is proposed that smaller hospitals will transfer seriously ill children for intensive care to the larger acute hospitals and major specialist centres. Those undertaking such transfers should be appropriately trained or supervised. (See Chapter 62.)

## SCORING SYSTEMS AND PREDICTION OF OUTCOME

Scoring systems enable a complex clinical situation to be expressed numerically. They are usually based on deviations from normal of physiological variables, each of which is weighted.

A number of factors can influence outcome from critical illness (Figure 17.1), and ideally all of them should be included in any prediction of individual outcome, but this is plainly not possible. Consequently, a selection of important variables is combined, the exact combination depending on the scoring system in use. Scoring systems can also be used to predict and assess workload and to cost the treatment given.

A number of scoring systems are in common use. Most are known by their acronyms and include the following.

### Therapeutic Intervention Scoring System (TISS)

This was introduced in 1974 as a method of quantifying nursing, medical, and technological support activity, and for costing. In the present system there are 76 procedures, each assigned a point score of 1–4. It is used as a non-specific system for assessing ICU activity and expenditure.

### Acute Physiology and Chronic Health Evaluation (APACHE)

This system is currently available in two forms: APACHE II and APACHE III.

#### *APACHE II*

This generates a single score from three sources:

1. 12 mandatory physiological variables that give an acute physiology score (APS):
   - creatinine: 0–8 points
   - Glasgow Coma Scale: 0–12 points
   - 10 other variables: 0–4 points
2. age points: 0–6
3. chronic health points: 0–5

The full set of variables is given in summarized form in Table 17.4, and in full as Appendix 17.1. This gives a minimum APACHE score of 0 in health and a maximum of 71 in illness. The score is computed after 24 hours of ICU care, using the worst values recorded for each of the 12 variables. In cohorts of patients, higher scores correlate well with increasing hospital mortality.

Furthermore, it is also possible to calculate the risk of death for each patient, which allows comparisons to

**Table 17.1. Facilities and staffing necessary for an ICU and an HDU**

| Intensive care | High dependency care |
|---|---|
| A designated area where such care is provided | |
| A clear operational policy based on a background of multidisciplinary care and effective communication | |
| A designated consultant as director, supported by consultants with allocated intensive care sessions sufficient to provide continuous (non-resident) availability | A designated consultant as director with continuous consultant cover from either the admitting specialty or intensive care |
| A minimum nurse : patient ratio of 1 : 1 throughout the 24 hours of the day, together with a nurse in charge plus additional nurses, according to patient needs, the total number of beds, and geographical arrangements within the unit. The skill mix of nurses should reflect the physiological instability of the patient | An average nurse : patient ratio of 1 : 2 throughout the 24 hours of the day, together with a nurse in charge plus additional nurses, according to patient needs, the total number of beds, and geographical arrangements within the unit. The skill mix of nurses should reflect the possibility that patients may be physiologically unstable |
| 24-hour dedicated cover by resident trainee medical staff | Continuous availability of trainee medical staff from either the admitting specialty or from intensive care |
| The ability to support common organ system failures, in particular ventilatory, circulatory, and renal failure | Appropriate monitoring and other equipment |
| A sufficient caseload to maintain skills and expertise | |
| Administrative, technical, and secretarial support | |
| Continuing education, training, and audit | |

**Table 17.2. Description of patients suitable for ICU or HDU admission[a]**

| Intensive care is appropriate for | High dependency care is appropriate for |
|---|---|
| Patients requiring or likely to require advanced respiratory support alone | Patients requiring support for a single failing organ system, but excluding those needing advanced respiratory support |
| Patients requiring support of two or more organ systems | Patients who can benefit from more detailed observation or monitoring than can safely be provided on a general ward |
| Patients with chronic impairment of one or more organ systems sufficient to restrict daily activities (co-morbidity) and who require support for an acute reversible failure of another organ system | Patients no longer needing intensive care, but who are not yet well enough to be returned to a general ward |
| | Postoperative patients who need close monitoring for longer than a few hours |

[a]See Table 17.3 for the categories of organ system monitoring and support.

be made between different hospitals. The risk of dying is calculated from the APACHE II score, the primary admission category, and further weighting for emergency surgery.

### *APACHE III*

There were a number of shortcomings with APACHE II and it was further refined and extended to overcome these. APACHE III is considerably more complex than its predecessor, and the expense of purchasing the system has limited its widespread acceptance.

### Simplified Acute Physiology Score (SAPS II)

The original cumbersome APACHE system with 34 variables has been simplified and further modified. SAPS II has 17 variables derived and weighted by statistical modelling.

### The Intensive Care National Audit and Research Centre (ICNARC)

This was established as an independent charity by the Intensive Care Society in 1993, to provide independent, objective audit of, and research into, intensive and high dependency care. The Case Mix

**Table 17.3. Categories of organ system monitoring and support**

| **Advanced respiratory support** |
|---|
| Mechanical ventilatory support (excluding mask CPAP or non-invasive, e.g. mask ventilation) |
| The possibility of a *sudden, precipitous* deterioration in respiratory function requiring immediate endotracheal intubation and mechanical ventilation |
| **Basic respiratory monitoring and support** |
| The need for more than 40% $O_2$ via a fixed performance mask |
| The possibility of *progressive* deterioration to the point of needing advanced respiratory support (see above) |
| The need for physiotherapy to clear secretions at least 2-hourly, whether via a tracheostomy or mini-tracheostomy, or in the absence of an artificial airway |
| Patients recently extubated after a prolonged period of intubation and mechanical ventilation |
| The need for mask CPAP or non-invasive ventilation |
| Patients who are intubated to protect the airway, but needing no ventilatory support and who are otherwise stable |
| **Circulatory support** |
| The need for vasoactive drugs to support arterial pressure or cardiac output |
| Support for circulatory instability resulting from hypovolaemia from any cause and which is unresponsive to modest volume replacement. This will include, but not be limited to, postsurgical or gastrointestinal haemorrhage or haemorrhage related to a coagulopathy |
| Patients resuscitated after cardiac arrest where intensive or high dependency care is considered clinically appropriate |
| **Neurological monitoring and support** |
| Central nervous system depression, from whatever cause, sufficient to prejudice the airway and protective reflexes |
| Invasive neurological monitoring |
| **Renal support** |
| The need for acute renal replacement therapy (haemodialysis, haemofiltration, or haemodiafiltration) |

CPAP, continuous positive airway pressure.

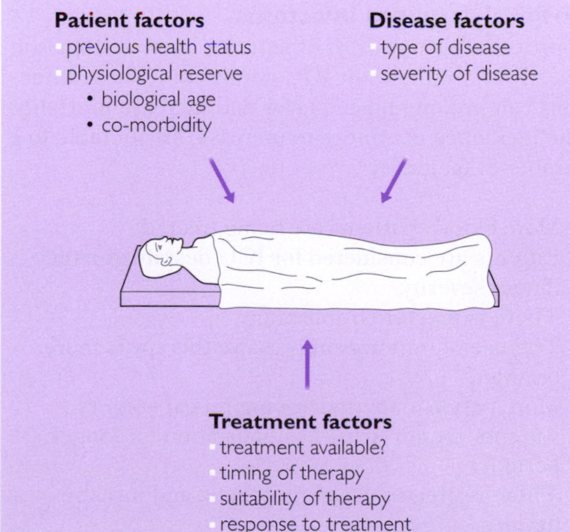


**Figure 17.1.** Factors influencing outcome from a critical illness.

Programme is a national, comparative, patient-outcome audit in which observed mortality differences are adjusted according to severity of illness and other factors.

Although proposed as being a routine part of ICU practice, many questions remain to be answered regarding the use of scoring systems. Despite continued elaboration, these systems should be used only for audit and research, and not for outcome predictions in individual patients.

## SEPSIS AND MULTIPLE ORGAN FAILURE

The most common cause of death in the ICU, and the greatest consumer of unsuccessful resource investment, is multiple organ failure (MOF) associated with sepsis.

Standard definitions are now available for infection, bacteraemia, sepsis, severe sepsis, sepsis-induced hypotension, and septic shock. The terms 'septicaemia' and 'sepsis syndrome' are no longer used, but two new terms have been introduced: systemic inflammatory response syndrome (SIRS) and multiple organ dysfunction syndrome (MODS).

**Table 17.4. The APACHE II scoring system**

| Variable | Maximum points |
|---|---|
| Temperature | 4 |
| Mean arterial pressure | 4 |
| Heart rate | 4 |
| Respiratory rate | 4 |
| Oxygenation | 4 |
| Arterial pH | 4 |
| Sodium | 4 |
| Potassium | 4 |
| Creatinine | 8 |
| Haematocrit | 4 |
| White cell count | 4 |
| Glasgow coma scale | 12 |
| **Acute physiology score** | **60** |
| Age | 6 |
| Chronic health evaluation | 5 |
| **APACHE II score** | **71** |

### Systemic inflammatory response syndrome

This is the systemic inflammatory response to a variety of severe clinical insults. The response is manifest by two or more of the following conditions:

- Temperature > 38°C *or* < 36°C
- Heart rate > 90 beats/min
- Respiratory rate > 20 breaths/min or arterial $CO_2$ pressure ($P\text{aCO}_2$) < 4.3 kPa (32 mmHg)
- WBC > 12 000 *or* < 4000 cells/mm$^3$ *or* > 10% immature forms.

Sepsis is a category of SIRS in which patients have clearly documented infection.

### Multiple organ dysfunction syndrome

This is the presence of altered organ function in an acutely ill patient such that homoeostasis cannot be maintained without intervention. If the underlying problem is not reversed, eventually MOF supervenes, the mortality of which remains high despite major efforts to optimize treatment. MOF also consumes an enormous amount of resources.

The possible aetiologies of MOF include prolonged or severe tissue hypoxia, cytokine release from infected or damaged tissues, and endotoxaemia or secondary bacteraemia resulting from loss of intestinal mucosal integrity.

The MOF syndrome involves one or more of the following:

- respiratory failure: progressively higher levels of inspired $O_2$ and positive end-expiratory pressure (PEEP)
- Hypotension: systemic vasodilatation and inadequate cardiac output unresponsive to fluid therapy alone and requiring vasoactive drugs
- Persisting oliguria: failure of frusemide (furosemide), mannitol, and dopaminergic drugs to maintain a diuresis. Established acute renal failure with the need for renal replacement therapy (renal failure may occasionally be non-oliguric).
- Hepatobiliary failure with intrahepatic cholestasis, jaundice, elevated liver enzymes, acalculous cholecystitis, and coagulopathy
- Hypermetabolic state: muscle wasting, hypoalbuminaemia, and electrolyte and nutritional abnormalities
- Gastrointestinal failure: gastric stasis, ileus, diarrhoea, stress ulceration
- Haematological failure: anaemia and thrombocytopenia
- Neuromuscular complications: encephalopathy, peripheral neuropathy, and myopathy.

The management of MOF involves the following:

- Most importantly, the diagnosis and treatment of the underlying problem;
- Amelioration or prevention of further deterioration by prompt initial resuscitation with rapid reversal of tissue hypoxia;
- Removal of trigger factors by control of infection, prompt recognition and treatment of injuries, with early fixation of fractures and removal of dead tissue, and early recognition and treatment of postoperative complications;
- Supportive therapy: this is the most demanding aspect of management in terms of time and economic implications.

Medical intervention will be designed to maintain the circulation, provide respiratory support, and identify and eliminate sources of infection, especially nosocomial (community-acquired) infections.

### Hospital-acquired infections

Approximately one-fifth of patients have an infection directly related to their ICU admission. These infections can prolong hospital stay and increase mortality. The incidence continues to increase, attributable to a number of factors:

- More elderly patients are being treated.
- Patients are considered for ICU despite greater illness severity.
- There is greater co-morbidity.
- The use of immunosuppressive therapy is more prevalent.
- More patients are undergoing repeat surgery.
- Patients are surviving hospitalization for longer periods.
- There is greater use of prosthetic and invasive devices.

Much of the nosocomial vascular infection related to catheters can be traced to poor hand-washing technique, and poor technique during blood sampling and drug administration.

The use of artificial airways is associated with nosocomial pneumonia, which occurs in up to 60% of high-risk patients. The incidence of respiratory infection can be minimized by regular attention to oropharyngeal toilet and pulmonary secretions, with humidification of inspired gases to reduce the incidence of retained secretions and preserve mucociliary function.

Infection is usually caused by Gram-negative organisms, but the diagnosis of ventilator-associated pneumonia is fraught with difficulty. The presumed route of infection is by microaspiration of organisms from the upper gastrointestinal tract that have colonized the oropharynx.

Oropharyngeal colonization can be reduced by selective decontamination of the digestive tract (SDD). The technique combines the long-term application of an antimicrobial/antifungal paste plus a short course of systemic broad-spectrum antibiotics. This reduces the incidence of ventilator-associated pneumonia, but appears to have little impact on outcome. SDD is not yet recommended for routine use.

Infections such as acalculous cholecystitis and sinusitis may need appropriate treatment with drainage and antibiotics.

### The use of antibiotics

Gram-positive bacteria have become a major problem within the ICU. Methicillin-resistant *Staphylococcus aureus* (MRSA) is now endemic in many hospitals, and the incidence of vancomycin-resistant enterococci is increasing. Vancomycin-resistant staphylococci have also been reported.

Fungal sepsis is becoming more prevalent, and resistant species are becoming more common.

Over the last few years the choice of antibiotics has widened considerably but rational prescribing is needed. It is often difficult to distinguish between colonization and infection of the ICU patient, and it has been suggested that only 30–40% of antibiotics prescribed are for a proper indication.

The selection of an antibiotic regimen depends on a number of factors:

- site of infection;
- known or presumptive organism;
- underlying medical condition and hepatorenal function;
- unit antibiotic policy;
- cost.

The introduction of a hospital antibiotic policy will reduce the emergence of multiply resistant organisms. However, clinicians need to be aware of which organisms are prevalent in the hospital and on their ICU because blind empirical therapy may frequently be needed. Always follow local guidelines when prescribing 'blindly' and seek advice from the microbiologist for specific indications.

## INDIVIDUAL SYSTEMS FAILURE AND SUPPORTIVE THERAPY

### Cardiovascular failure

#### *Pathophysiology*

Shock has classically been recognized as a complex of symptoms and signs. There is agitation, apprehension, dyspnoea, thirst, tachycardia, weak peripheral pulses, low blood pressure, collapsed peripheral veins, and cold peripheries. Arterial blood gas analysis may reveal an acidosis and elevated lactate. Lactate is produced by the incomplete metabolism of glucose and the need to regenerate NAD in the absence of an adequate supply of $O_2$ (Figure 17.2).

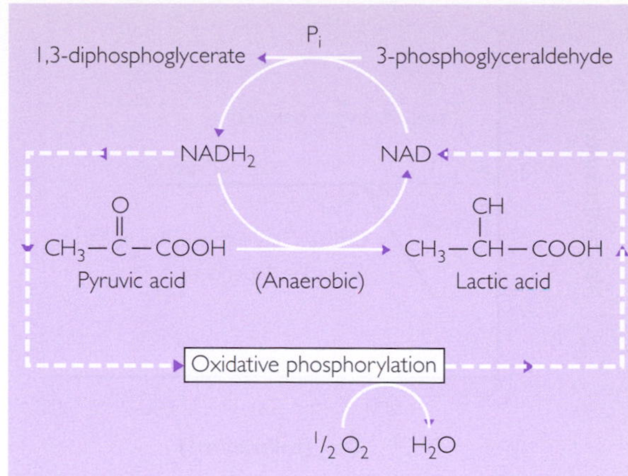


**Figure 17.2.** The formation of lactate when the supply of $O_2$ is insufficient.

Shock is usually classified according to the underlying aetiology into hypovolaemic, cardiogenic, septic, and obstructive, and treatment is directed to the expected physiological disturbances. However, shock is better defined as *failure of the circulation either centrally or peripherally to meet the metabolic demands of the tissues.*

#### *Monitoring oxygen transport*

Oxygen is the single most important substrate carried by the circulation, it is the most flow dependent and has the lowest stores.

The concept of $O_2$ flux ($\dot{D}O_2$) describes the total amount of $O_2$ delivered to the tissues (see also Chapter 21):

$$\dot{D}O_2 = CO \times CaO_2\,\text{ml/min}$$

where CO is the cardiac output (L/min) and $CaO_2$ the arterial $O_2$ concentration (ml/L). Knowing CO, the inverse Fick equation can be used to estimate the oxygen consumption (ml/min), $\dot{V}O_2$:

$$\dot{V}O_2 = CO \times [CaO_2 - C\bar{v}O_2]\ \text{ml/min}$$

where $C\bar{v}O_2$ is the the mixed venous oxygen content (ml/L). The amount of $O_2$ extracted from arterial blood defines the oxygen extraction ratio (OER):

$$OER = \frac{CaO_2 - C\bar{v}O_2}{CaO_2}$$

All the variables needed for these calculations are available at the bedside of critically ill patients with a pulmonary artery flow-directed catheter *in situ*. Clinically, the values for $O_2$ delivery and consumption are indexed to body surface area.

Interest in the calculation and manipulation of these variables stems from a plethora of publications that have examined the relationship between $\dot{D}O_2$ and $\dot{V}O_2$.

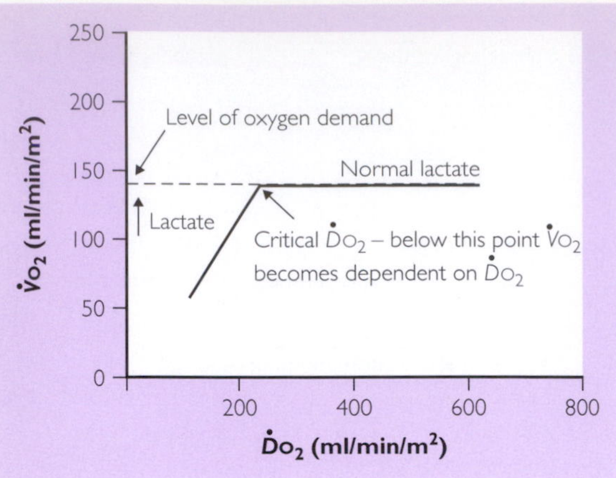


**Figure 17.3.** A diagrammatic representation of the relationship between the consumption of oxygen ($\dot{V}O_2$) and the delivery of oxygen ($\dot{D}O_2$).

Simplistically, there will be a switch from aerobic to anaerobic metabolism at the critical $O_2$ delivery level when supply cannot satisfy demand, and a rise in arterial blood lactate will occur. $O_2$ consumption is independent of supply above this critical level, but below it $\dot{V}O_2$ becomes dependent on $\dot{D}O_2$. This is termed 'physiological flow dependency' (Figure 17.3).

In some patients, the ability to increase OER may be impaired (the exact mechanism being unclear), leading to dependence of consumption on supply at much higher levels of delivery, i.e. the 'knee' of the curve in Figure 17.3 is shifted to the right. This is termed 'pathological flow dependency'.

$O_2$ consumption can also be measured directly using respiratory gas analysis. There is a variety of metabolic computers available for this purpose and the technology is constantly improving, but problems arise mainly from the use of a high inspired $O_2$ concentration ($F_{IO_2} > 0.6$) or air leaks. Measured $\dot{V}O_2$ may, however, fail to increase when $\dot{D}O_2$ is increased, even though calculated $\dot{V}O_2$ does.

The delivery and uptake of $O_2$ in the tissues is a complex, multi-factorial process. The simplified concepts presented here do, however, indicate the basic principles involved and allow a mental picture of the factors involved to be developed. Apart from the obvious need to oxygenate the patient, the value of complex manipulation of $O_2$ tissue delivery in relation to patient outcome is still uncertain.

### *Circulatory shock*

Shock may be caused by:

- an absolute reduction in cardiac output;
- hypotension resulting from excessive peripheral vasodilatation;
- a cardiac output, of whatever level, that is maldistributed.

This last situation can be detected only by direct measurement of regional perfusion, or otherwise inferred from measurements such as mixed venous oxyhaemoglobin saturation and blood lactate.

The arterial lactate concentration represents a balance between its production and clearance. Although lactate rises in shock states, blood levels correlate poorly with mixed venous $O_2$ saturation ($S\bar{v}O_2$), $\dot{D}O_2$, and $\dot{V}O_2$ in critically ill patients. Arterial lactate may be normal in shock, even when an acidosis is present. An elevated lactate in a shocked patient indicates severe or prolonged circulatory failure, and failure of an elevated lactate to fall with treatment is a poor prognostic sign. The mildly elevated arterial lactate levels seen in hypermetabolic states on the ICU does not necessarily indicate tissue hypoxia.

Invasive cardiovascular monitoring can sometimes allow the specific cardiovascular abnormalities in the systemic and pulmonary circulations to be defined precisely. Treatment with volume replacement, vasodilators, inotropes, or vasopressors can then be tailored accordingly, although the use of pulmonary artery catheters to this end continues to generate heated debate.

The various types of shock can be defined in a number of ways. For the purposes of the present chapter, as a result of their occurrence in practice, the following categories will be used:

- hypovolaemic;
- cardiogenic;
- septic;
- obstructive.

*The management of shock always requires the diagnosis and treatment of the specific cause, together with supportive therapy until resolution (or the patient dies).*

### *Hypovolaemic shock*

This is the simplest form of shock to consider. Venous return to the heart and cardiac output are reduced because of loss of circulating blood volume (see Chapter 14), because of:

- inadequate intake;
- haemorrhage: internal; external;
- fluid losses: diarrhoea; vomiting; burns; crush injury.

A clinical diagnosis is often obvious, and the amount and composition of fluid administered can initially be estimated reasonably well by clinical responses such as changes in conscious level, heart rate, non-invasive blood pressure, and urine output.

The debate regarding the use of crystalloid or colloid for resuscitation continues but most clinicians use combinations of both, including blood if haemorrhage is significant. Plasma volume replacement is inevitably accompanied by a degree of haemodilution and the fall in haemoglobin concentration has to be monitored and corrected.

### *Cardiogenic shock*

This is characterized by a low cardiac output state. It can be associated with:

- myocardial infarction;
- acute myocarditis;
- endocarditis;
- valvular lesions: critical aortic stenosis; acute massive mitral regurgitation;
- cardiomyopathy.

The most common cause is myocardial infarction. It is important to identify those cases for which specific medical or surgical treatment is available. Echocardiography will exclude mechanical complications such as ventricular septal defect and limited perforation of the free ventricular wall. Surprisingly, on occasions, the pulmonary artery wedge pressure is not critically elevated when eventually measured.

Hypoventilation and hypoxaemia are common in all acute low cardiac output states, even in the absence of pulmonary oedema, and mechanical ventilation is often necessary. Life-threatening arrhythmias and conduction disturbances are common and may require the use of antiarrhythmic drugs, cardioversion, or temporary transvenous pacing.

Most patients will have received thrombolytic therapy and great care is necessary during central venous cannulation. Angioplasty or acute cardiac surgery may be indicated and in some centres mechanical circulatory assistance may be useful as a 'bridge' to surgery. If inotropic support is used, dobutamine is the initial agent of choice, possibly with the addition of a phosphodiesterase inhibitor such as milrinone. In the final analysis, however, the use of inotropes is ultimately empirical, use being made of those that give the required result.

### *Septic shock*

Sepsis and MOF have been considered earlier. Septic shock is characterized by peripheral vasodilatation with increased capillary permeability. Patients may initially require large volumes of intravenous fluids. With adequate fluid replacement, a hyperdynamic circulation is normally seen, although the increased cardiac output is often not adequate to maintain a normal blood pressure.

In septic shock, the balance between cardiac output and perfusion pressure is crucial. If the calculated systemic vascular resistance is $< 800$ dyne·s/cm$^5$ then excessive vasoconstriction and ischaemia of vital organs will hopefully be avoided, provided that perfusion pressure is adequate. In fact, an increase in blood pressure with controlled vasopressor therapy can improve renal function in sepsis. An adequate blood pressure will also maintain coronary artery perfusion pressure (CPP) and perhaps help to ameliorate myocardial dysfunction. The CPP is normally defined as:

$$\text{CPP} = \begin{matrix}\text{Aortic diastolic}\\\text{pressure}\end{matrix} - \begin{matrix}\text{Ventricular}\\\text{end-diastolic}\\\text{pressure}\end{matrix}$$

This relationship is especially relevant for the right ventricle because patients with sepsis may have a relatively high central venous and right ventricular end-diastolic pressure.

Vasoactive drugs will often be required to restore mean systemic arterial blood pressure and increase and/or maintain cardiac output and tissue $O_2$ delivery. Drugs that act as vasopressors in this situation include dopamine, epinephrine (adrenaline), norepinephrine (noradrenaline), and phenylephrine. Vasopressors are titrated to obtain an adequate mean systemic arterial pressure. An appropriate end-point may be difficult to determine and should be individualized. A value of 80 mmHg is often used, or possibly higher in atherosclerotic patients, although lower values may be acceptable.

Vasopressor agents (except phenylephrine which is a pure α-adrenoceptor agonist) may in fact increase cardiac output by their β-adrenoceptor effects, but the changes are unpredictable and there may even be reflex falls in cardiac output as a result of vasoconstriction. A relatively pure β-adrenoceptor agonist such as dobutamine may be a useful additional agent to maintain cardiac output if deemed necessary. It is important to realize that the use of all inotropes is potentially dangerous because they may cause sinus tachycardia, arrhythmias, and myocardial ischaemia. As a result of its $\beta_2$-adrenoceptor effects, dobutamine may cause peripheral vasodilatation and severe hypotension, if used as the initial agent, especially in hypovolaemic subjects.

Phosphodiesterase inhibitors (such as enoximone or milrinone) may be synergistic with β-adrenoceptor agonists, although they can exhibit profound chronotropic and vasodilating properties, and have a relatively prolonged half-life. The true role of phosphodiesterase inhibitors has still to be established.

Dopexamine may improve splanchnic blood flow, but the issue of a selective increase in renal blood flow in response to dopaminergic agents in critically ill patients remains controversial.

It is not uncommon for patients to depend on sympathomimetic agents for several days or even weeks. Corticosteroids are now no longer used routinely in septic shock, but may be indicated in physiological doses if hypoadrenalism is suspected.

### *Obstructive shock*

This is the result of a mass or pressure effect obstructing venous return to the right or left side of the heart, or impeding outflow from the left or right ventricles. Although none is particularly common, when it occurs, the usual causes of obstructive shock are:

- tension pneumothorax;
- massive pleural effusion/haemothorax;
- massive pulmonary embolism;
- pericardial tamponade;
- constrictive pericarditis;
- inferior vena caval compression;
- acute aortic dissection.

Rapid diagnosis is essential; examination and readily available non-invasive techniques such as ECG, chest radiology, and echocardiography can identify most of the common clinical conditions.

Tension pneumothorax is often difficult to recognize on a supine portable chest radiograph. Valuable clinical signs are diminished air entry and hyperresonance to percussion on the affected side. Once diagnosed, a thoracic drain should be inserted using the fifth intercostal space in the midaxillary line, and connected to an underwater seal drain. In a dire emergency, a wide-bore intravenous cannula is effective in releasing pressurized intrapleural gas while definitive drainage is being organized.

Massive pulmonary embolism should be suspected in high-risk patients. The clinical picture is of circulatory collapse, tachypnoea, cyanosis, grossly elevated jugular venous pressure, and dyspnoea. If invasive monitoring is undertaken, then the usual features are high right atrial, right ventricular, and pulmonary artery pressures, low cardiac output, and high systemic vascular resistance. Management consists of respiratory support to relieve hypoxia and reduce the work of breathing. Circulatory support, guided by haemodynamic measurements, usually involves fluid loading and inotropic support. Definitive therapy is with thrombolytic agents and, in some centres, surgical intervention.

Cardiac tamponade, and severe, rapidly progressing, constrictive pericarditis are treated by drainage and pericardiectomy, respectively. In the interim, patients with tamponade may temporarily respond to careful volume loading. Echocardiography is the investigation of choice. Pulmonary artery catheterization shows equalization of right atrial, right ventricular, mean pulmonary artery, and wedge pressures.

The emergency treatment of aortic dissection includes control of hypertension to limit further progression. Its management is highly specialized and is not considered further here.

## Respiratory failure

### *Pathophysiology*

Two types of acute respiratory failure are described:

- Type 1, where an intrinsic lung problem causes hypoxaemia and, at least initially, compensatory hyperventilation with lowering of $Pa\text{CO}_2$.
- Type 2, where there is impaired alveolar ventilation, and hence an increase in $Pa\text{CO}_2$.

Their causes are outlined in Table 17.5.

This simple classification is useful, especially in patients with chronic lung disease. However, patients referred to the ICU may move from type 1 to type 2 as the underlying disease process evolves, e.g. severe acute asthma.

### *Acute respiratory distress syndrome (ARDS)*

ARDS is a severe form of acute lung injury (ALI). Both terms are used to denote a syndrome of inflammation and increased permeability associated with a constellation of clinical, radiological, and physiological abnormalities that cannot be explained by left atrial or pulmonary capillary hypertension, but may coexist with them. The lung damage can be caused by direct or indirect pulmonary insults, but there will be a degree of overlap in many instances, as indicated in Table 17.6. The principles of management are diagnosis and treatment of the cause, and supportive respiratory therapy until resolution occurs.

Attempts have been made to classify the degree of dysfunction numerically. One of the most common indices calculated is the $Pa\text{O}_2/F\text{IO}_2$ ratio. The $Pa\text{O}_2$ is measured in millimetres of mercury (mmHg) and the $F\text{IO}_2$ as its fractional concentration. Hence, in health, the ratio becomes 100 mmHg/0.2 giving a value of 500. Regardless of the PEEP level, in ALI the $Pa\text{O}_2 : F\text{IO}_2$ ratio is < 300, in ARDS it is < 200.

A semi-quantitative ALI score can also be used to describe the severity of the injury. Each component scores from 0 to a maximum of 4 points, depending on the degree of abnormality as shown below:

- Chest radiograph: 0–4;
- $Pa\text{O}_2/F\text{IO}_2$ ratio: 0–4;
- PEEP level: 0–4;
- Static respiratory compliance: 0–4.

The composition of the score is given in full in Appendix 17.2. Not all components need be scored, and the total score is divided by the number of components utilized. A score of > 2.5 indicates severe lung injury (ARDS). For example, a patient with shadowing in all four quadrants of the chest radiograph, a $Pa\text{O}_2$ of 11.3 kPa (85 mmHg) on an $F\text{IO}_2$ of 0.7 and a PEEP of 2.5 cm$H_2O$ would generate a score of $(4 + 2 + 3)/3 = 3$. In contrast, a patient with one quadrant shadowing on a chest radiograph, a $Pa\text{O}_2$ of 13.3 kPa (100 mmHg) on an $F\text{IO}_2$ of 0.4 and a PEEP of 2.5 cm$H_2O$ would generate a score of $(1 + 0 + 0)/3 = 0.33$. The first patient would obviously have ARDS whereas the second would not.

ARDS follows a precipitating event after a latent interval of up to (usually) 48 hours. Then, respiratory failure ensues, with tachypnoea, intractable hypoxaemia, and ventilatory muscle fatigue. There are bilateral infiltrates on the chest radiograph, but no clinical evidence of left atrial hypertension (cardiac failure or fluid overload). If measured, the pulmonary artery occlusion pressure is less than 18 mmHg. Although of acute onset, these changes persist for days to weeks.

Increased pulmonary capillary permeability leads to non-cardiogenic pulmonary oedema with a variable increase in extravascular lung water. Loss of surfactant activity leads to alveolar collapse. There are functional and anatomical abnormalities in the pulmonary circulation with vasospasm, obstruction, and destruction of vessels. Histological abnormalities include increased cellular infiltration, proliferation of type II alveolar cells, and hyaline membrane formation merging into a recovery phase or progressing to irreversible pulmonary

**Table 17.5. Some causes of type 1 and type 2 respiratory failure**

| Type 1 | Type 2 |
|---|---|
| Pneumonia | Muscle and nerve diseases |
| Cardiogenic pulmonary oedema | Exacerbation of chronic pulmonary diseases |
| Acute lung injury | Morbid obesity |
| Severe acute asthma | Severe acute asthma |

| Table 17.6. Some causes of ARDS (and ALI) | |
|---|---|
| **Direct** | **Indirect** |
| Pulmonary aspiration | Multiple trauma |
| Chest trauma | Severe sepsis |
| Blast injury | Massive blood transfusion |
| Smoke inhalation | Fat embolism |
| Toxic gas inhalation | Amniotic fluid embolism |
| Near drowning | Pancreatitis |
| Pneumonitis | Cardiopulmonary bypass |
| | Disseminated intravascular coagulation |
| | Paraquat poisoning |

fibrosis. There is a wide scatter of ventilation/perfusion ($\dot{V}/\dot{Q}$) ratios with increases in both shunt fraction and alveolar dead space. Functional residual capacity (FRC) and pulmonary compliance are reduced.

### *Management of ventilation in respiratory failure*

Patients should be ventilated only if this is necessary, and the decision to initiate it is based on multiple clinical inputs. The ventilation of patients with poorly functioning lungs can be complex and only the basic principles and consequences are given in this chapter.

#### *Continuous positive airway pressure*

This is a means of providing the beneficial respiratory, and in some cases cardiovascular, effects of PEEP to a patient who is breathing spontaneously.

Continuous positive airway pressure (CPAP) by facemask may be used as a means of avoiding endotracheal intubation and formal mechanical ventilation in patients whose respiratory failure may be expected to recover relatively rapidly, such as is seen in acute cardiogenic pulmonary oedema.

In sick patients, airway protection cannot be guaranteed and gastric distension, which may occur with CPAP, can predispose to aspiration. However, in a patient recovering from a period of mechanical ventilation, CPAP (especially with some degree of pressure support) can be a useful adjunct to weaning.

#### *Indications for initiating intermittent positive-pressure ventilation*

The need to institute intermittent positive-pressure ventilation (IPPV) is sometimes straightforward, as in the sudden onset of apnoea in a patient with head injury. However, more frequently the situation is less clear-cut and a balance has to be struck between the clinical situation, the symptoms and signs, and the arterial blood gases. Clinical conditions requiring ventilation and relevant factors involved in deciding when ventilation is necessary are given in Table 17.7.

#### *Establishing mechanical ventilation for acute respiratory failure*

The most critical period is getting the patient safely on to the ventilator. This takes place in three phases:

1. Securing the airway: this is usually by oral endotracheal intubation using a rapid sequence induction. Hypoxic patients do not tolerate the supine position and may have to be intubated in a semi-erect position. Hypotension caused by induction agents may be minimized by fluid therapy but, not infrequently, judicious small doses of a vasoactive agent are needed at this stage.
2. Setting the ventilator initially: with modern ventilators, patients can usually be allowed to breathe spontaneously, so prolonged deep sedation and paralysis can usually be avoided. However, it is common practice to sedate, and if necessary administer, neuromuscular blocking agents, until the ideal mode of ventilation and the individual ventilator settings have been determined, and circulatory stability achieved.

| Table 17.7. Clinical situations commonly requiring ventilatory support, and indicators of the need for ventilatory support |
|---|
| **Elective or planned ventilation** |
| Postoperative after bypass or major vascular surgery, in pulmonary disease, obesity, gross sepsis, major trauma |
| To ensure oxygenation and control ICP in head injury |
| **Necessitated by the immediate condition** |
| After resuscitation |
| Prolonged shock, of any cause |
| Hypoventilation of whatever cause |
| Hypoxaemia |
| **Clinical signs, and arterial blood gas indices, that may indicate the need for endotracheal intubation and ventilatory support** |
| Obvious fatigue:<br>Paradoxical respiration<br>Variable respiratory rate<br>Impending apnoea |
| Persistent tachypnoea |
| Absent protective reflexes |
| Threat of airway obstruction |
| Hypoxia despite high $F_{IO_2}$ |
| Oxygen saturation < 90% |
| $Pa_{O_2}$ < 8 kPa (60 mmHg) |
| $Pa_{CO_2}$ causing severe respiratory acidosis |
| $Pa_{CO_2}$ > 7 kPa (53 mmHg) and rising from a lower level |
| Metabolic acidosis but $Pa_{CO_2}$ not low |
| $Pa_{CO_2}$ persistently < 3.5 kPa (26 mmHg) |

ICP, intracranial pressure; $Pa_{CO_2}$, arterial $CO_2$ pressure.

Unless dictated by local custom, or clinically inappropriate, ICU ventilators will often be initially set up similarly to Table 17.8.

3. Optimizing the ventilator settings: after arterial blood gas analysis, tidal volume and rate are adjusted according to the desired $Pa\text{CO}_2$, and $F\text{IO}_2$ adjusted according to the desired $Pa\text{O}_2$. An acutely elevated $Pa\text{CO}_2$ should not be normalized rapidly; patients with chronic $CO_2$ retention and an acute respiratory acidosis should be ventilated to a normal pH.

Oxygen toxicity is not an issue during the initial stabilization period. Inspired $O_2$ and PEEP are later adjusted to keep the $Pa\text{O}_2$ at the desired level, usually 10–12 kPa (75–90 mmHg) if possible, although 8 kPa (60 mmHg) or even lower is tolerated, particularly in severe ARDS when high inspired $O_2$ concentrations are required. Once the patient has been stabilized, decisions can be made about the use of other modes of ventilation.

*Positive end-expiratory pressure*

With PEEP, airway pressure in the ventilator circuit is prevented from returning to atmospheric at the end of expiration. When beneficial, PEEP increases FRC by alveolar recruitment and thus improves the distribution of pulmonary blood flow to ventilated lung units. This reduces pulmonary venous admixture and increases $Pa\text{O}_2$ at any given $F\text{IO}_2$. Values of 5–15 $\text{cmH}_2\text{O}$ are usually employed.

PEEP is associated with a number of adverse responses:

- There may be a reduction in cardiac output, especially in hypovolaemic patients. This reduction can be modified by volume loading and inotropic support if required.
- With volume-controlled ventilation, peak inflation pressure will increase.
- In patients with asymmetrical lung disease, there may be over-distension of lung units with short time constants. This may lead to:
  - barotrauma;
  - increased dead space.

**Table 17.8. Initial ventilator settings**

| Mode | SIMV with pressure support |
|---|---|
| Respiratory rate | 10 breaths/min |
| Inspiratory flow rate | 60 L/min |
| PEEP | 5 $\text{cmH}_2\text{O}$ |
| Tidal volume | 10 ml/kg |
| I : E ratio | 1 : 2 |
| Pressure support | 20 $\text{cmH}_2\text{O}$ |
| Inspired oxygen | 100% |

SIMV, synchronized intermittent mandatory ventilation; PEEP, positive end-expiratory pressure; I : E ratio, inspiratory : expiratory ratio.

- Compression of vessels around distended alveoli may:
  - increase pulmonary vascular resistance;
  - divert blood to under-ventilated regions and worsen shunt fraction.
- With pressure-controlled ventilation, there will be a reduction in tidal volume.

The use of inverse ratio ventilation to produce intrinsic PEEP allows a reduction in extrinsic PEEP, and may reduce some of the regional pulmonary effects. The level of intrinsic PEEP must be monitored closely in these circumstances, but few ventilators are able to do this easily.

*Available modes of respiratory support*

Even with the most popular modes of ventilation, currently believed by clinicians to improve outcome in severe ARDS, there are few controlled studies to demonstrate reduction in morbidity and mortality from specific methods in current use. A number of these are described below, and basic definitions of ventilator function are given in Chapter 11.

*Volume preset modes* In these modes the preset tidal volume is always delivered. Flow is often constant but may be decelerating in nature. Minute volume, in the absence of leaks in the respiratory circuit, is therefore guaranteed whatever the level of airway resistance or total thoracic compliance. However, high levels of peak inspiratory pressure may be produced.

Recognition that very high levels of peak and mean inspiratory pressures were associated with barotrauma led to a degree of airway pressure regulation by setting an upper pressure alarm limit above which inspiration was terminated.

There are two types of ventilation in this category:

- Controlled mechanical ventilation: all breaths are mandatory machine breaths, and the estimated minute volume is delivered solely by the ventilator. The term 'assist-control' is used when the patient can trigger a mandatory machine breath.
- Synchronized intermittent mandatory ventilation (SIMV): the patient is allowed to breathe spontaneously between mandatory machine breaths, and mandatory breaths may be initiated by, and synchronized with, patient effort. However, patients with poorly compliant lungs tend to breathe rapidly.

*Inverse ratio ventilation* The usual inspiratory : expiratory (I : E) ratio of 1 : 2 or 1 : 3 is increased to 1 : 1 and then 2 : 1 or greater by prolonging inspiratory time. This theoretically allows for more even distribution of inspired gas to lung units with longer time constants. Inverse ratio ventilation (IRV) can be produced in volume-controlled ventilation by an end-inspiratory pause, or by a slow or decelerating inspiratory flow rate. Because, with IRV, expiration is usually not complete before the next inspiration commences, air trapping occurs with development of intrinsic PEEP. IRV is also commonly employed with pressure-controlled ventilation (see below) by directly prolonging the inspiratory time.

*Pressure preset modes* These modes limit lung inflation to a known pressure level:

- Pressure support ventilation (PSV): this mode is frequently combined with SIMV as the basic ventilator strategy on the ICU. Breaths are patient triggered and an inspiratory pressure is then applied by the ventilator. The level of pressure support is set by the clinician to give an appropriate tidal volume. Usually, airway pressure is maintained at the preset level until the inspiratory flow starts to fall, and at a certain level of flow the expiratory phase commences. As with all triggered modes, it is vital that the response time of the ventilator is rapid or patient work of breathing can be increased.
- Pressure-controlled ventilation (PCV): this mode has become more popular because of its theoretical advantages compared with volume-controlled ventilation. These include:
  - peak airway pressure is lower for the same mean airway pressure;
  - regional over-distension/high regional intrinsic PEEP is avoided;
  - decelerating flow rate may be beneficial;
  - alveolar ventilation may be improved.

  The inspiratory pressure level is preset and expiration is time cycled. Flow rate is initially high to pressurize the respiratory circuit, and then decelerates. It should be noted that this mode is completely different to pressure-cycled ventilation. In clinical practice, for those patients with the most severe forms of respiratory failure, PCV is frequently used to produce IRV by prolonging the inspiratory time.
- Biphasic positive airway pressure (BIPAP): this mode utilizes two levels of CPAP with the ventilator switching between them. The patient can breathe spontaneously at both CPAP levels and this may be synchronized with the patient's inspiratory efforts. The release of CPAP from a supra-ambient level to a lower level augments alveolar ventilation and $CO_2$ clearance. Physiologically, this is equivalent to PCV with set PEEP, but the ability to breathe spontaneously at any time increases comfort and may reduce the amount of sedation necessary.

*Adjuvant therapies to conventional IPPV*

*High-frequency techniques* These include high-frequency positive-pressure ventilation, high-frequency jet ventilation, and high-frequency oscillation. Rates vary up to as high as 3000 ventilatory cycles per minute. Tidal volumes are less than physiological dead space.

As gas distribution may depend on airway resistance rather than compliance, it is possible to ventilate areas with both low and high compliance that are adjacent, e.g. a patient with ARDS and a bronchopleural fistula. Newer machines are capable of providing better humidification and are powerful enough to maintain lung volume in patients with ARDS.

*Prone positioning* Turning patients with severe lung injury into the prone position frequently improves their $Pa\text{O}_2$. There is an improvement in $\dot{V}/\dot{Q}$ matching with a reduction in shunt fraction. This occurs because of changes in the pleural pressure gradient, which becomes more uniform. The manoeuvre should be more widely used because it is not as complex as one would imagine.

*Corticosteroids* These have no role in the prevention or initial treatment of ARDS. In the later fibroproliferative stage of ARDS, steroids can reduce inflammation in the lung, improve oxygenation, and reduce mortality.

*Inhaled nitric oxide* This acts as a selective pulmonary vasodilator. There is frequently a reduction in pulmonary shunt fraction and an increase in $Pa\text{O}_2$ but no substantial long-term benefit has yet been demonstrated in clinical trials. Although an unlicensed drug, guidelines for its use in optimally ventilated patients have been published.

*Ventilator-induced lung injury and lung protective ventilator strategy*

In patients with ARDS, the distribution of alveolar shadowing seen on the chest radiograph is not homogeneous, and a number of thoracic computed tomography studies have confirmed that these areas are gravity dependent. Some lung units remain relatively normal (typically 30%) whereas others are collapsed, consolidated, or fluid filled. The remaining ventilated lung should be viewed as small, not just as non-compliant (the 'baby-lung' concept). Lung injury is thought to occur by:

- relatively large tidal volumes (> 8 ml/kg) which over-distend the small, normal lung areas;
- repeated collapse and opening of distal airways with stress damage to surrounding tissue and surfactant wash-out.

Modern ventilatory management aims to prevent further pulmonary damage based on the concepts of keeping the lung open with PEEP, but avoiding over-distension. Use of the lung's static pressure–volume curve can be helpful here to explain the concept involved. This is shown in Figure 17.4. The upper inflection point represents the point above which over-distension is occurring, and the lower inflection point (seen best in the early stages of ARDS) shows the range of airway pressures below which alveoli are closing. The term 'best PEEP' is sometimes used for the condition when the compliance of the lung is maximal and the patient is being ventilated midway between the upper and lower inflexion points. This is possible by only ventilating on the steep, straight part of the compliance curve. Lung protective strategies are summarized in Table 17.9.

In trying to reduce peak inspiratory pressures, a reduction in tidal volume, even if the respiratory rate is increased, often reduces effective alveolar minute volume and hypercapnia will develop. This is usually well tolerated if there are no contraindications, e.g. raised intracranial pressure (ICP). An acute respiratory acidosis may develop, although arterial pH is normally soon corrected by renal mechanisms and bicarbonate is not generally necessary. This situation is termed 'permissive hypercapnia'.

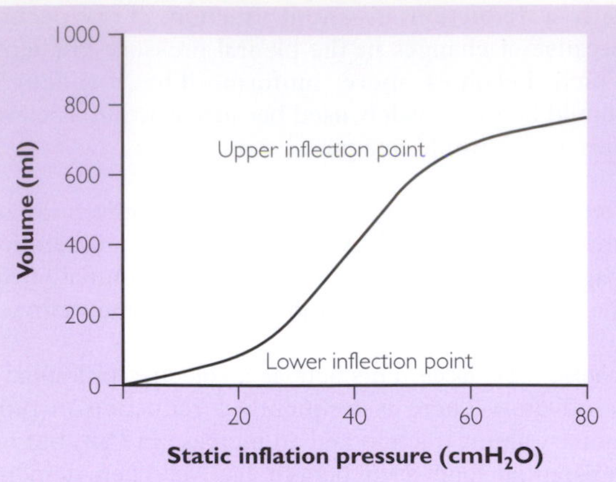


**Figure 17.4.** Static compliance curve from a patient with early ARDS showing the lower and upper inflection points. Tidal volumes should lie between these upper and lower limits.

| Table 17.9. Lung protective ventilator strategy |
|---|
| Alveolar recruitment manoeuvres |
| Avoid alveolar over-distension |
| Positional changes |
| Periodic sustained lung inflation (40 $cmH_2O$ for 20 s) |
| Adequate levels of PEEP to prevent alveolar collapse |
| PEEP levels > 10 $cmH_2O$ commonly required |
| End-inspiratory or plateau pressure < 35 $cmH_2O$ |
| Limit tidal volume (6–8 ml/kg) |
| Pressure-controlled ventilation |
| Avoiding 100% $O_2$ may prevent reabsorption atelectasis |

PEEP, positive end-expiratory pressure.

Such a strategy can be followed using either PCV or volume-controlled ventilation. Although developed with ARDS in mind, a similar approach can be taken when ventilating the asthmatic patient.

*Complications of mechanical ventilation*

The major problems associated with positive pressure ventilation are circulatory depression, pulmonary barotrauma, and nosocomial pneumonia, as described previously.

The complications of prolonged endotracheal intubation include damage to the larynx and vocal cords. Transient hoarseness of the voice is usual when an endotracheal tube is *in situ* for more than 48 hours, and is exacerbated by movement of the tube irritating the vocal cords and laryngeal mucosa. These effects can be minimized by nasotracheal intubation but this can be complicated initially by haemorrhage, and in the long term by purulent maxillary sinusitis.

*Weaning from mechanical ventilation*

Numerous indicators for successful weaning have been proposed although few are useful in clinical practice. In particular, if the patient develops rapid shallow breathing during weaning (the ratio of frequency [in breaths/min]/tidal volume [in litres] is > 100), then weaning is unlikely to be successful in the long term.

The following are important factors to consider during weaning:

- Control underlying illness, pain, infection, and fever.
- Optimize cardiac function.
- Optimize lung function and ensure that $Pa\text{CO}_2$ is normal for the patient.
- Ensure normal serum magnesium, potassium, and phosphate.
- Recognize that patients may have muscle atrophy, myopathy, or a neuropathy.
- Avoid excess $CO_2$ production, particularly from parenteral feeding.
- Avoid exhausting patient and causing sleep deprivation.
- Consider tracheostomy.

Tracheostomy may now be performed on the ICU using percutaneous techniques. There is a distinct learning curve, however, and a cautious approach is recommended. Complications include haemorrhage and malposition of the tube. In the long term, severe tracheal stenosis may occur in about 1% of patients.

Many patients can be weaned rapidly but, remarkably, in those difficult to wean, there is still no consensus as to the best way to do it. When the patient can clear secretions and swallow safely, the endotracheal or tracheostomy tube can be removed.

Patients with poor cardiac reserve may develop acute pulmonary oedema when positive intrathoracic pressure is lost during the weaning process. These patients need aggressive diuretic and vasodilator therapy.

*Mechanical ventilation in severe acute asthma*

The management of severe asthma is a serious business. It is a disease that still causes death in young people and their management needs to be undertaken by experienced clinicians. *Never, ever underestimate the potential for sudden deterioration.*

Bronchospasm and mechanical plugging of the airways by secretions lead to high inspiratory pressures, and expiratory flow obstruction leads to air trapping with high levels of intrinsic PEEP. This is not apparent from the displayed ventilator pressures unless specifically measured. A prolonged expiratory period is needed to allow for passive exhalation to occur. If pressure and flow waveforms can be displayed, these can be used to confirm that expiration is complete before the onset of the next inspiration. Failing this, close clinical observation at the bedside is essential.

To allow a reduction in lung volume, relative hypoventilation has been described. Low tidal volumes of 6 ml/kg can be used with a high inspiratory flow rate (100 L/min) to obtain as long an expiratory time as is necessary for passive exhalation to occur (I : E ratio of at least 1 : 4). The use of pressure-controlled ventilation to limit barotrauma, and the use of extrinsic PEEP to maintain airway patency during exhalation, may also be considered.

Always remember that a pneumothorax is an ever-present danger.

### Acute renal failure

This is simply defined as an abrupt decline in renal function (usually over a few hours to days).

#### *Pathophysiology*

Acute renal failure (ARF) in hospital is now most commonly seen in the ICU, with an incidence of up to 15% of admissions in some series. Although renal function itself is potentially recoverable, in most cases the mortality rate remains high (typically 60–80%), and relates primarily to age and the underlying diagnosis. It is often associated with sepsis and cardiorespiratory failure.

Most cases seen on the ICU are related to surgery and the associated risk factors are shown in Table 17.10.

#### *Diagnosis and investigations*

Patients are usually oliguric, defined as a urine output of less than 20 ml/h for two consecutive hours. Occasionally ARF is non-oliguric and renal hypoperfusion may not produce oliguria if the ability to concentrate is poor, e.g. elderly people and those with prior renal disease or on diuretic therapy. Sudden, total anuria is usually mechanical in origin, e.g. a blocked catheter.

A careful history and examination should establish evidence of precipitating factors and reversible causes. Look specifically for signs of hypovolaemia and poor perfusion, but also for circulatory overload.

It is essential to exclude obstruction, and to check that the bladder is not palpable and the catheter is not obstructed! Catheterize the bladder if not done already.

If the abdomen is tense, then estimation of intravesical pressure may be helpful. Pressures greater than 18–25 mmHg may indicate venous tamponade of the renal vessels and require intervention to relieve the abdominal pressure.

Rarely, one may see evidence of systemic disease associated with nephritis, e.g. fever, haemoptysis, or a vasculitic rash. Urinalysis should be undertaken for blood, protein, and myoglobin (a brownish colour). Serial determination of creatinine clearance is the most sensitive test for detecting the onset of renal dysfunction. This can easily be performed on the ICU and is reliable even over a 2-hour urine collection period. Serum creatinine may not reflect glomerular filtration rate in those with little muscle mass.

Ultrasonography and plain radiographs can be used to check kidney size and for signs of obstruction, renal vein thrombosis, renal parenchymal pattern, and the presence of calculi. Isotope investigations, angiography, and renal biopsy may occasionally be indicated. Urinary indices of function have been used to distinguish pre-renal uraemia from ARF (Table 17.11), but they are relatively imprecise, and become inaccurate after mannitol and loop diuretics. The fractional excretion of sodium is probably the most useful index.

**Table 17.10. Causes of acute renal failure on the ICU**

| Reduced renal blood flow |
|---|
| Sepsis |
| Hypovolaemia |
| Hypotension |
| Low cardiac output states |
| Pre-existing renal damage |
| Renal vascular disease |
| Drugs, e.g. NSAIDs, ACE inhibitors |
| **Intrinsic renal damage** |
| Hypoxia |
| Nephrotoxins: aminoglycosides, amphotericin, radiocontrast media, etc. |
| Tissue breakdown or tumour lysis: myoglobinuria, uric acid |
| Inflammatory nephritides: vasculitis, interstitial nephritis, glomerulonephritis |
| Myeloma |
| **Obstruction to flow** |
| Kidney or ureter |
| Bladder neck or prostate |
| Raised intra-abdominal pressure |

NSAIDs, non-steroidal anti-inflammatory drugs; ACE, angiotensin-converting enzyme.

#### *Prevention and management of ARF*

*Nephrotoxic agents*

Avoid nephrotoxic agents wherever possible, especially combinations of drugs known to be associated with renal impairment, e.g. aminoglycosides and non-steroidal anti-inflammatory drugs (NSAIDs).

*Intravascular blood volume*

Maintain intravascular blood volume. This can be very difficult to assess. Invasive monitoring should be considered early in high-risk groups, especially if there is associated respiratory failure, because clinical estimates of cardiac output and filling pressures in the seriously ill patient are often in error.

Repeated boluses of fluid may be necessary, guided by both cardiovascular monitoring and clinical response, remembering that the central venous pressure (CVP) and even the pulmonary artery occlusion pressure have only a weak relationship to blood volume; trends are more informative.

*Renal perfusion pressure*

Maintain renal perfusion pressure. Knowledge of the premorbid blood pressure is helpful here. In some patients, higher pressures than normal are necessary to ensure adequate filtration, e.g. hypertensive patients with renal artery stenosis.

| Table 17.11. Urinary indices to distinguish prerenal from intrinsic renal dysfunction | | |
|---|---|---|
| | Reduced renal perfusion | Intrinsic renal failure |
| U/P osmolarity | > 1.5 | < 1.1 |
| U/P creatinine | > 40 | < 20 |
| $U_{Na}$ (mmol/L) | < 20 | > 40 |
| $FE_{Na}$ (%) | < 1 | > 3 |

U/P, urine/plasma; $U_{Na}$, urinary sodium concentration, $FE_{Na}$, fractional sodium excretion.

*Diuretics*

Efforts to induce a diuresis are worthwhile because non-oliguric renal failure is easier to manage. Options include mannitol 20 g, frusemide up to 50 mg/h and dopamine 3 μg/kg/h. There is no good evidence that any of these therapies can reverse ARF, and the use of dopamine may be associated with adverse effects.

If myoglobinuria is present, give sodium bicarbonate and acetazolamide to alkalinize the urine. This will increase the solubility of the filtered myoglobin and reduce its toxicity to the tubules. Use mannitol, and frusemide if necessary, to maintain urine output at more than 100 ml/h. If there is a high uric acid level add allopurinol.

*Miscellaneous*

If ARF becomes established then a number of other abnormalities will also require attention:

- fluid overload;
- electrolyte disturbances;
- acidosis;
- anaemia;
- nutrition.

These are described separately in other sections of the book.

### Renal replacement therapy

This may be by conventional intermittent haemodialysis or continuous haemofiltration techniques.

Continuous techniques are said to be associated with less haemodynamic instability but the need for continuous anticoagulation is a hazard. The use of low-molecular-weight heparin or epoprostenol may be safer, although epoprostenol is a potent vasodilator. Bicarbonate haemodialysis, acetate-free biofiltration, and sequential haemodialysis, with the separation of dialysis and ultrafiltration, may help to ameliorate the haemodynamic changes. (See also Chapter 59.)

Some cytokine mediators of sepsis and ARDS are removed by haemofiltration and many clinicians choose to employ this as a method of treatment. There is no good evidence yet that this improves outcome.

It is hard to demonstrate that new techniques of renal support have reduced the mortality from ARF. The most common cause of death in these patients remains infection; however, most survivors recover renal function even after prolonged dialysis.

## Gastrointestinal failure

The gastrointestinal (GI) tract provides nutrients for the body and acts as a barrier to toxins and intraluminal micro-organisms. Failure of the nutrient function results in catabolism and immunosuppression, whereas failure of the GI barrier allows micro-organisms and toxins to enter the portal and systemic circulations. Definitive evidence for translocation in humans is not available but GI tract failure can result in the systemic inflammatory response syndrome and ultimately MODS.

### Pathophysiology

The GI tract has one of the highest rates of cell turnover in the body. This requires considerable energy expenditure and $O_2$ delivery, and makes the GI tract vulnerable to ischaemia. The aetiology of GI failure is multifactorial (Figure 17.5). The most important features are starvation, reduced splanchnic blood flow, and the administration of antibiotics. These lead to an increase in capillary permeability in the GI tract, followed by an increase in mucosal permeability, and finally transmural injury. This reinforces the cycle of poor nutrient absorption, reduced barrier function, and decreased blood flow. Although haemorrhagic shock reduces splanchnic blood flow, flow is preserved in septic shock. Nevertheless, mucosal injury still develops in sepsis because, although mucosal flow is preserved, there is an increase in the effectiveness of the villous countercurrent exchange mechanism, resulting in villous hypoxia.

Drugs and techniques used to treat other organ dysfunctions may influence GI function. For instance, controlled ventilation increases intra-abdominal pressure and reduces splanchnic blood flow, and opioids promote an ileus. The regular use of antibiotics, particularly long-term use and broad-spectrum antibiotics, will alter the GI flora. This, in turn, will change the barrier function of the GI tract and may allow translocation of toxins or micro-organisms. It may also lead to superinfection with *Clostridium difficile* (which causes diarrhoea and results in pseudomembranous colitis) and outbreaks of nosocomial infections.

In the stomach, mucosal ischaemia leads to stress ulceration. This differs from peptic ulceration in that diffuse superficial erosions are produced throughout the stomach, rather than discrete ulcers. Minor bleeding from stress ulceration responds to conservative management, but significant bleeding may be life threatening and responds poorly to surgical treatment.

### Management

GI failure is clinically manifest as an ileus with delayed gastric emptying, vomiting, or diarrhoea, together with reduced nutrition and recurrent sepsis. Diagnosis of an

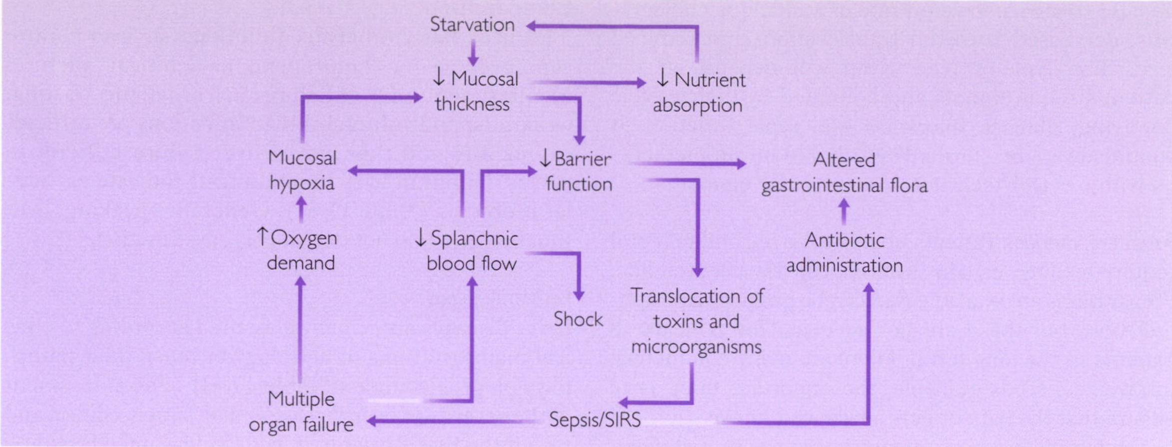


**Figure 17.5.** Pathophysiology of gastrointestinal failure. SIRS, systemic inflammatory response syndrome.

ileus does not depend on the absence of bowel sounds, because air may not be present in the GI tract of ventilated patients. The management of GI failure involves optimization of splanchnic blood flow and adequate nutrition for the GI tract as well as for the rest of the patient.

*Maintenance of splanchnic blood flow*

The maintenance of splanchnic blood flow depends primarily on good quality resuscitation and intensive care. Dopexamine may increase splanchnic blood flow but results have not been conclusive.

Splanchnic blood flow is vulnerable in critical illness and GI hypoxia occurs early in the development of MODS. As a result of this, monitoring of the GI tract is valuable as an indicator of impending deterioration or of the adequacy of resuscitation. Monitoring can be simple, such as the ability to absorb enteral feed or the presence or absence of diarrhoea. More sophisticated monitoring is available in the form of tonometry.

*Tonometry*

A tonometer consists of a PVC tube with a balloon close to its tip. The balloon lumen is filled with saline and left to equilibrate. The $P\text{CO}_2$ of the saline is then determined at the same time as the arterial bicarbonate concentration. These parameters are then applied to the Henderson–Hasselbalch equation:

$$\text{pH}_i = 6.1 + \log \frac{\text{HCO}_3^-}{P\text{gCO}_2 \times 0.003}$$

The $\text{pH}_i$ is interpreted as mucosal pH and $P\text{gCO}_2$ as the gastric $CO_2$ pressure. Mucosal acidosis is thought to indicate poor perfusion and a $\text{pH}_i$ of less than 7.35 in some series has been associated with an increased mortality. The technique assumes that the $P\text{CO}_2$ in the tonometer reflects intramucosal $P\text{CO}_2$, that $CO_2$ diffuses freely, and that the bicarbonate concentration $[\text{HCO}_3^-]$ is similar in arterial blood and intestinal mucosa. These assumptions do not always hold in the changing metabolic states of critical illness. Recently, the technique has been developed to provide semi-continuous readings based on the difference between mucosal $P\text{CO}_2$ and arterial $P\text{CO}_2$.

*Nutrition*

Nutrition can be achieved by several routes in the critically ill patient (Table 17.12). As far as possible the patient's GI tract should be used for feeding to maintain splanchnic blood flow and preserve barrier function. Oral feeding requires the patient to be able to protect his or her own airway. The nasogastric route is simple but gastric stasis may limit its effectiveness. In addition, a nasogastric tube may cause local trauma and lead to sinusitis. It is also contraindicated if the patient has a fractured base of skull. A nasojejunal tube overcomes the problem of gastric stasis but may be difficult to position.

Percutaneous endoscopic gastrostomy is becoming a more popular route for feeding critically ill patients. Complications are operator dependent but include leaks, infection, and obstruction of the tube. If a patient requires a laparotomy, a feeding jejunostomy may be considered. Complications of this include leaks, wound infection, peritonitis, and obstruction of either the bowel or the feeding tube.

Further details of nutritional requirments are given in Chapter 81.

*Enteral nutrition* Nutrients provided enterally improve splanchnic blood flow. Other advantages of enteral feeding over parenteral feeding include: improved nitrogen retention, better weight gain, maintained GI structure and function, normalized GI flora, reduced

| **Table 17.12. Routes available for feeding a critically ill patient** |
|---|
| Oral |
| Nasogastric |
| Nasojejunal |
| Percutaneous gastrostomy |
| Jejunostomy |
| Intravenous |

hepatic steatosis, lowered rate of acalculous cholecystitis, decreased bacterial translocation, and reduced cost. The type of feed given will depend on the patient's requirements and is limited by their gastric emptying, glucose tolerance, and renal function. It should always be sterile. Feed should be supplemented with electrolytes, vitamins, and trace elements.

*Parenteral nutrition* Patients unable to be fed enterally still require feeding, usually intravenously via a central line. Preparations are available that can be given via a peripheral vein, but these are not adequate for critically ill patients in the long term. There are many commercial intravenous feeds available; the important thing is to ensure that the patient gets a balanced intake.

Glutamine has been suggested as an essential nutrient in critical illness. Conventional parenteral nutrition solutions lack glutamine because it does not withstand heat sterilization, so glutamine supplements have been recommended. Glutamine is involved in numerous processes, including nitrogen donation, oxidative fuel, and stimulating protein synthesis in skeletal muscle. Glutamine-containing parenteral nutrition solutions appear to provide better nutrition for critically ill patients and improved outcome at 6 months without increasing cost.

*Drugs* Some drugs stimulate gastric emptying and may promote enteral feeding. It is also important to minimize the use of drugs such as opioids, which reduce gastric emptying and intestinal motility. Cisapride has a structure similar to that of metoclopramide, but it has no dopaminergic activity and therefore no antiemetic effect. It stimulates acetylcholine release in the myenteric plexus, but its effects on GI tract motility are similar to those of metoclopramide. Erythromycin also has a prokinetic action and may be useful in resistant ileus.

### *Stress ulceration*

The management of stress ulceration relies on prophylaxis. Adequate resuscitation and management of the patient will reduce the risk of stress ulceration. Agents used to reduce the incidence of stress ulceration include ranitidine and sucralfate. Sucralfate is generally preferred because the incidence of nosocomial pneumonia is reduced. If GI bleeding occurs secondary to stress ulceration, an ulcer-healing agent, such as omeprazole, may be valuable. Always bear stress ulceration in mind as a cause of unexplained anaemia or cardiovascular instability.

## Liver failure

The liver has numerous functions so liver failure can produce a heterogeneous clinical picture. Manifestations of liver failure such as fatigue, wasting, weakness, and vulnerability to infections are difficult to quantify and this makes liver failure difficult to assess. Different liver function tests indicate particular problems (Table 17.13). Generally speaking, liver function tests do not detect early dysfunction.

*Pathophysiology*

Liver diseases are usually classified according to clinical manifestations or aetiology because their pathophysiology is complex (Table 17.14). The assessment of the severity of liver disease is also largely clinical and two of the five elements in the Child–Pugh classification are clinically derived (Table 17.15).

The aetiology of liver dysfunction in the critically ill patient is multifactorial and its effects are vague (Figure 17.6), with ischaemia often being a significant aetiological factor. Normally the liver has two blood supplies: the hepatic artery supplies 20–35% of the hepatic blood flow, and the remainder is supplied via the portal vein. These supplies have a complementary relationship so hepatic blood flow is preserved. In critical illness, this relationship is altered so that not only is total hepatic blood flow reduced, but also intrahepatic blood flow is disturbed. This is because of changes in cardiac output and regional blood flow caused either by the illness or by treatments such as positive-pressure ventilation or vasopressors. Hepatic ischaemia results in global liver dysfunction and intrahepatic cholestasis. Fortunately, the liver has great powers of regeneration and recovers well after a period of ischaemia.

### *Management of liver failure*

The management of liver failure depends on treatment of the cause, effective resuscitation, physiological support of the patient, and management of the complications. Several aspects of support require consideration. Haemodynamic instability with an increased cardiac output and decreased systemic vascular resistance is a feature of liver failure. Vasopressors may be required, with invasive monitoring of their efficacy, to avoid tissue hypoxia. Assessment of the effects of tissue hypoxia may be difficult clinically. The function of other organs may be impaired and systemic indicators such as acid–base balance and lactate are dependent on liver function. The lungs are also influenced by liver failure, leading to the hepatopulmonary syndrome. The aetiology of this is obscure, but may be a result of infection or oedema and resembles ARDS.

**Table 17.13. Some functions of the liver and indicative tests**

| Function | Example | Test |
|---|---|---|
| Metabolic | Energy production | Alanine transaminase |
| Defence | Kupffer cells | Repeated infections |
| Elimination | Drugs, bile | Bilirubin, alkaline phosphatase |
| Synthesis | Proteins | Albumin, clotting factors |

**Table 17.14. The causes of liver disease**

| | |
|---|---|
| Viral disease | Hepatitis A–E |
| Metabolic disease | Wilson's disease |
| | Haemochromatosis |
| | $\alpha_1$-antitrypsin deficiency |
| | Glycogen storage diseases |
| | Tyrosinaemia |
| | Galactosaemia |
| Cholestasis | Biliary cirrhosis |
| | Sclerosing cholangitis |
| Cardiovascular | Cardiac failure |
| | Budd–Chiari syndrome |
| Drugs and toxins | Paracetamol |
| | Alcohol |
| | Amiodarone |
| | Non-steroidal anti-inflammatory drugs |
| Autoimmune | Chronic active hepatitis |
| Carcinoma | Primary |
| | Secondary |

Renal dysfunction is common with liver failure and produces the hepatorenal syndrome. In this situation, serum urea and creatinine estimations may be poor indicators of renal function, because urea formation depends on liver function and creatinine does not rise in patients with profound muscle wasting. Whatever the aetiology of the liver failure, *N*-acetylcysteine should be considered as a therapeutic option. As a free-radical scavenger, it has been shown to reduce the severity of MODS in patients with liver failure.

Nutrition may be difficult if the patient cannot tolerate a protein load without becoming encephalopathic, but vitamin supplements should always be given. A review of the medication is vital because liver disease profoundly alters the pharmacokinetics of many drugs, particularly those with a high extraction ratio.

Sedation is often necessary for patients with liver disease, but should be stopped regularly to detect encephalopathy. As encephalopathy is associated with an increased ICP, it may be necessary to monitor ICP to reduce the risk of sudden increases with stimuli such as physiotherapy.

Reduction of the barrier and immune functions of the liver lead to recurrent infections. Regular screening should be performed and infections treated early. Laboratory tests of clotting function are almost always abnormal in liver failure as a result of reduced synthesis. A rising prothrombin time is a bad prognostic sign. Routine administration of clotting factors is unnecessary but may be considered for invasive procedures.

Liver transplantation may be the only option for a patient with liver failure. The indications for transplantation in acute liver failure may be discussed with a transplant centre. This should be done earlier rather than later. Contraindications to transplantation include uncontrolled sepsis, refractory hypotension, and advanced disease of another organ.

### Cerebral failure

Cerebral failure is relatively common in the ICU and is an important cause of difficulty to wean from controlled ventilation. This type of cerebral failure is usually manifest as coma or confusion, has an unknown aetiology, and often resolves spontaneously. Patients with cerebral failure caused by epilepsy may also require intensive care if they have an unprotected airway or myocardial depression resulting from either convulsions or their treatment. However, after a head injury or intracranial bleed, aggressive management of cerebral failure is essential and the remainder of this section concentrates on this area (see also Chapter 64).

#### *Pathophysiology*

At the time of injury, the brain suffers a primary injury related to the impact and shear stresses within the brain. The results of this injury include disruption of the blood–brain barrier, microhaemorrhage, and neuronal death (Figure 17.7). A secondary brain injury can then develop related to factors outside the brain,

**Table 17.15. The Child–Pugh classification of the severity of liver disease (Grade A: 5–6 points; Grade B: 7–9 points; Grade C: >10 points)**

| | Points<br>1 | 2 | 3 |
|---|---|---|---|
| Bilirubin (µmol/L) | < 35 | 35–51 | > 51 |
| Albumin (g/L) | > 35 | 28–35 | < 28 |
| Ascites | Absent | Slight | Moderate |
| Encephalopathy (grade) | Absent | I–II | III–IV |
| Prothrombin time (seconds prolonged) | 1–4 | 4–6 | >6 |

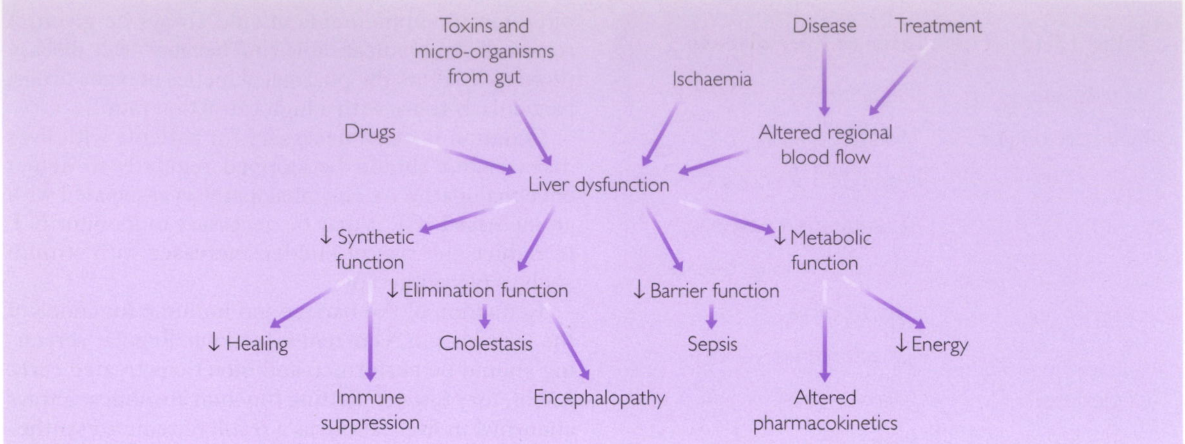


**Figure 17.6.** Some causes and consequences of liver dysfunction in critically ill patients.

such as hypoxaemia, hypotension, hypercapnia, and pyrexia. This second insult compounds the effect of the first. A combination of both causes a rise in the ICP.

### *Management*

The key to the management of brain injuries is to treat any other injuries and normalize intracranial homoeostasis as far as possible. In practice, this involves the usual care of a seriously ill patient plus maintenance of the cerebral perfusion pressure (CPP) and adequate oxygenation of brain tissue. This can be achieved in several ways.

#### *Maintenance of cerebral blood flow*

Cerebral blood flow (CBF) depends on the CPP. As ICP is usually increased by the injury, this effectively means maintenance of mean arterial pressure (MAP) with fluids and vasopressor agents and control of ICP.

$$CPP = MAP - ICP.$$

The effects of CPP on CBF have been investigated using transcranial Doppler ultrasonography. Blood flow is maintained if the CPP is above 70 mmHg but, if it falls to less than 40 mmHg, there are signs of global cerebral ischaemia with reduced jugular venous oxygen saturation ($Sjo_2$) (see Chapter 22).

The ICP can be reduced by reducing the intracranial blood volume, fluid volume, or tissue volume. Intracranial blood volume is reduced by restricting fluid intake and by hyperventilation, which produces cerebral vasospasm. Although this temporarily reduces blood volume and the ICP, it may lead to cerebral ischaemia and requires $Sjo_2$ monitoring to ensure safety. Reduction of the cerebral fluid volume can be achieved by draining cerebrospinal fluid. This is not usually helpful, however, because compression of the ventricles by oedema limits the amount of intracranial fluid available for drainage.

Intracranial tissue volume can be reduced by osmotic diuretics. Mannitol is most commonly used and, given as a bolus, is effective. If used repeatedly, however, it may cross the blood–brain barrier and increase cerebral oedema by increasing the tissue osmotic pressure. Non-osmotic diuretics such as frusemide may also be used; an alternative may be hyperosmolar solutions such as hypertonic saline.

#### *Sedation*

Head-injured patients require sedation, anxiolysis, and analgesia for the same reasons as other patients on an ICU. In addition, sedative agents reduce the increases in ICP with sudden movements. Ideally, sedative agents would be able to reduce the metabolic demands of the brain (cerebral metabolic $O_2$ rate [$CMRo_2$]) without

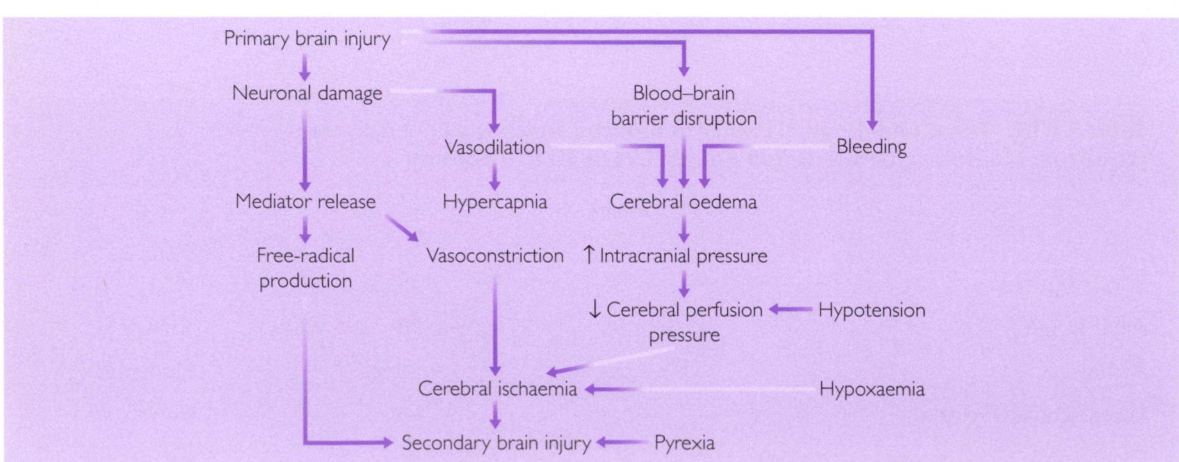


**Figure 17.7.** Pathophysiology of brain injury.

reducing CBF. In practice, this ideal does not exist and, although most sedative agents reduce $CMRO_2$ and have an anticonvulsant action, this is at the expense of an increased ICP, a reduced CPP, or myocardial depression.

The benefits of neuromuscular blocking agents as adjuncts to sedation in the head-injured patient are debatable. Neuromuscular blocking agents reduce the risk of sudden increases in ICP with stimuli such as physiotherapy. However, they may obscure convulsions and have not been demonstrated to improve outcome.

*Other agents*

Steroids are given to reduce ICP and limit the risk of secondary brain injury. Calcium-channel-blocking agents are thought to reduce the reflex cerebral vasospasm that appears after reperfusion. Nimodipine improves CBF after an ischaemic event but this is not accompanied by an improvement in $CMRO_2$.

Free-radical scavengers may have a role in the future. The ischaemia/reperfusion injury to damaged brain tissue results in the formation of free radicals and cellular injury. Various free-radical scavengers are being investigated at present. Other agents currently under investigation include inhibitors of lipid peroxidation and glutamate antagonists.

*Subarachnoid haemorrhage*

The poor outcome after subarachnoid haemorrhage was thought to be caused by rebleeding from the aneurysm. It is now accepted that the haemorrhage is followed by reflex vasospasm, which leads to ischaemia. Current management of subarachnoid haemorrhage is a combination of aggressive neurosurgical management of the aneurysm and anti-ischaemia management using nimodipine and peripheral vasoconstrictors.

## PATIENT COMFORT AND SUPPORT

Attitudes to the sedation of critically ill patients have changed as a result of increased knowledge about the risks of sedative agents and improved nursing care. Sedation is now considered as patient comfort with the individual components of comfort considered separately (Table 17.16). Each patient will have different needs to maintain comfort and these will change with their disease process. The aim of intensive care sedation is to ensure that each patient is comfortable all of the time.

**Table 17.16. The requirements for comfort in a critically ill patient**

| |
|---|
| Relief of pain |
| Relief of anxiety |
| Aiding sleep |
| Anaesthesia for painful interventions |
| Reduction of depression |
| Control of confusion |
| Control of withdrawal reactions |

### Non-drug aspects

The ICU is a frightening place for a critically ill patient, and communication and reassurance will reduce these fears. Discomforts such as prolonged immobility may be helped by regular physiotherapy or massage. Adequate food and fluids will avoid hunger and thirst. Patients should be kept warm and the use of special beds and mattresses may improve patient comfort and ease nursing care. The need for anaesthesia to allow efficient ventilation has been reduced by sophisticated ventilatory modes and early tracheostomy.

### Drug administration

Drugs are frequently necessary to maintain patient comfort but they should be given with care to avoid the consequences of over-sedation. Sedative agents are usually administered by a combination of bolus dosage and continuous intravenous infusion. Bolus dosage provides an intermittent effect to cover occasional stimuli, whereas a continuous infusion is a convenient method of providing a background level of sedation or analgesia.

Sudden withdrawal of opioids or benzodiazepines may produce withdrawal phenomena ranging from mild irritability to frank psychosis. If this occurs, the drug concerned should be reintroduced at a modest dose, then substituted by a longer-acting oral agent such as methadone or diazepam, which can then be progressively reduced. Prophylactic use of this regimen in patients who have received a high cumulative dose of opioids or benzodiazepines will reduce the risk of withdrawal phenomena.

***Sedative agents***

The drugs used to produce sedation or anxiolysis are limited by three main problems.

*Accumulation of active metabolites*

Diazepam and midazolam have active metabolites. Desmethyldiazepam and oxazepam are long acting whereas α-hydroxymidazolam has a short duration of action. Accumulation of these active metabolites may occur in patients with renal failure and cause prolonged sedation. The active metabolite of morphine, morphine-6-glucuronide, also accumulates in patients with renal failure and produces narcosis. Pethidine and phenoperidine are both metabolized to norpethidine, which accumulates to cause anxiety and convulsions.

*Accumulation of parent compound*

The action of midazolam may also be prolonged as a result of decreased metabolism in critically ill patients. Midazolam is extensively metabolized in the liver, but also undergoes extrahepatic metabolism; metabolism is reduced when blood flow to these metabolizing areas is reduced.

The action of anaesthetic induction agents is usually terminated by redistribution rather than clearance. Drugs with a slow clearance, such as thiopentone (thiopental), will accumulate if given by continuous infusion and can have a markedly prolonged action. Fentanyl behaves in a similar way. With prolonged infusions, the large volume of distribution becomes saturated and clearance is slow.

*Side effects of the agent*
Propofol is presented in a lipid emulsion. With high infusion rates, patients receive a significant fat load. Isoflurane is only used as a short-term sedative because of the theoretical risk of renal failure from accumulation of fluoride ions produced by metabolism. The use of NSAIDs is limited by their tendency to produce gastric erosions, clotting abnormalities, and renal and hepatic dysfunction.

## Assessment of sedation

Unfortunately it is frequently impossible to ask critically ill patients about their comfort because their communication is limited. Improved techniques for communicating with intubated patients would significantly improve their comfort.

### *Indirect tests*

Although depth of anaesthesia is usually assessed by haemodynamic measurements, these are unreliable as an index of patient comfort on the ICU. In critically ill patients, haemodynamic changes occur for many reasons. Although discomfort should be excluded, sedative agents should be used only for their sedative effects and not for their haemodynamic effects.

### *Scoring systems*

Several sedation scoring systems have been described that assess the patient's response to a standard stimulus. One of the most widely used systems is a six-point scale (Table 17.17), depending on consciousness and the response to a light glabellar tap or a loud auditory stimulus. Addenbrooke's sedation score defines seven points (Table 17.18). Voice and tracheal suction are the stimuli used, and sedation is not assessed when the patient is asleep, or receiving neuromuscular blocking agents.

Most clinically used sedation scores are a compromise between accuracy and the time taken to assess and record sedation, and most scores do not differentiate sedation, anxiety, depression, and pain, but provide an estimate of overall patient comfort. Sedation scores cannot be used in the presence of neuromuscular blocking agents where the patient cannot respond to a stimulus. Monitoring of the sedation level is vital for the safe use of sedative agents.

Equipment to score or measure the level of sedation of critically ill patients is being developed from technology used to monitor the depth of anaesthesia. The transfer is not simple, and no method described has been used regularly in clinical practice. Most are in the process of development and evaluation, and may prove most useful in the deeply sedated or anaesthetized patient where sedation scores cannot be used.

## Assessment of pain

Awake patients are usually asked about their pain in some detail but critically ill patients are generally unable to give much information. Subjective pain scores rely on communication with the patient, and observer assessment usually reflects the response of the observer. Not infrequently, reliance is placed on the response to painful stimuli, e.g. physiotherapy. Assessment of pain itself is therefore very difficult and depends greatly on the experience and conscientiousness of the observer.

**Table 17.17. The Ramsay sedation scale**

| | |
|---|---|
| **Awake levels** | |
| 1 | Patient anxious and agitated or restless or both |
| 2 | Patient cooperative, orientated, and tranquil |
| 3 | Patient responds to commands only |
| **Asleep levels dependent on response to glabellar tap or loud auditory stimulus** | |
| 4 | Brisk response |
| 5 | Sluggish response |
| 6 | No response |

**Table 17.18. The Addenbrooke's sedation scale**

| | |
|---|---|
| 0 | Agitated |
| 1 | Awake |
| 2 | Roused by voice |
| 3 | Roused by tracheal suction |
| 4 | Unrousable |
| 5 | Paralysed |
| 6 | Asleep |

## Muscle relaxation

The need for neuromuscular blocking agents in critically ill patients has been reduced by the rational use of sedative agents, improved ventilator design, and increased use of early tracheostomy. However, many critically ill patients still require neuromuscular blocking agents at some time during their intensive care stay (Table 17.19). Methods of monitoring the neuromuscular junction are described elsewhere (see Chapter 24) and the monitoring is the same in critical illness.

**Table 17.19. Possible indications for neuromuscular blocking agents in critically ill patients**

| |
|---|
| During intubation and stabilization |
| During anaesthesia for procedures |
| To control ventilation in those with inappropriately high respiratory drive |
| To reduce $O_2$ consumption in critically hypoxic patients |
| To control intracranial pressure in head-injured patients |
| To manage other illnesses, e.g. tetanus |

The main reason to monitor neuromuscular blockade in critically ill patients is to avoid overdosage or drug accumulation. Critically ill patients receiving neuromuscular blocking agents should have their response to a train-of-four stimulus assessed regularly and the dose adjusted to maintain at least one visible twitch. If possible, neuromuscular blocking agents should be stopped each day to allow assessment of the underlying sedation level.

## ETHICS

### Principles

There are four principles of medical ethics: autonomy, beneficence, non-maleficence, and justice.

#### *Autonomy*

This is the right of each person to self-determination. Respect for autonomy reflects the right of others to make their own decisions.

#### *Beneficence*

This principle reflects duty to care for our patients and to achieve good for them.

#### *Non-maleficence*

This enshrines the principle of doing no harm. It is often considered with beneficence so that the duty is to produce a net benefit with minimal risk.

#### *Justice*

Justice reflects the right of all to fair access to resources.

Although these principles are generally agreed, their application may be controversial. For instance, the right to life is considered sacrosanct. But how is this interpreted? Is it the right not to be unjustly killed or does it include a right to be kept alive? Who does this right apply to? Can the right be forfeit if another person has been killed? Does the right apply to the unborn child, patients in a persistent vegetative state, or elderly people who wish to die? It is important to note that these issues do not argue with the basic moral principle of a right to life; instead they reflect the application of that right. The dilemmas that can occur are exemplified by the withdrawal of support in the persistent vegetative state. Similar dilemmas were present some years ago in accepting the concept of brain death. Decisions need to be taken with care, taking due regard to patients' religious and moral beliefs. There are no universal truths, only guidelines and common sense, and what society will sanction and support will vary with time.

### Medicolegal considerations

The law interprets ethics for society. Although there are many grey areas in the interpretation of ethical principles, they are interpreted as black or white in the law. For instance, the issue of withholding or withdrawing intensive care can be considered ethically and legally. Is it ethically justified to withhold or withdraw care if that care has no net benefit to the patient? From a legal perspective, a death is unlawful if it can be shown, beyond reasonable doubt, that another person caused that death and that their intention was to kill or harm that person. The law, however, distinguishes between cases where a doctor decides not to provide or continue treatment that may prolong a patient's life and cases where a doctor administers a lethal drug intending to bring a patient's life to an end. In situations where interpretation is not clear, legal advice should be sought. Decisions should not be taken by a single individual; discussion with others is essential.

### Cultural issues

The different interpretations of ethical principles are enshrined in different laws in different countries where different attitudes prevail. These considerations are very important in multiracial societies where, on occasions, religious beliefs conflict with statute law.

### The doctor/patient relationship

Many medicolegal conflicts have their basis in the doctor/patient relationship. Essentially, the doctor must act as the patient's advocate and the patient must trust the doctor to act in this capacity. Problems ensue if the doctor acts improperly or if the patient or his relatives feel that their trust has been broken or their values are not understood. This is more likely if several doctors are involved in delivering care, because their level of commitment to the patient may differ. There may also be problems if the patient and the doctor have different values, such as with Jehovah's Witnesses. Fundamentally, a clear policy needs to be worked out for each patient and every doctor involved with that patient's care so that all are clear about the therapeutic plan and the procedure to be followed if the patient's condition deteriorates.

## DEATH AND DYING

### Diagnosis

Intensive care, with its sophisticated technology for organ support, has led to a modification of the traditional concept of death. In simple terms, death is the absence of life and a live organism is capable of functioning as a whole and interacting with its environment. At some point in the process of death, the body irreversibly loses these abilities and dies. Death is regarded as an event whereas dying is an irreversible process. This is the basic concept upon which the diagnosis of brain death is made.

The necessary functions that have to be lost for the body to be declared dead are a failure of critical brainstem functions. The diagnosis of death is considered in Chapter 83.

### Withdrawal of treatment

This is a complicated issue and will depend on individual circumstances. The aspects that need to be considered are the expressed wishes of the patient, his or her medical condition, and the ethical and legal framework of the unit in which they are being cared for. The dilemma around whether or not to withdraw treatment usually depends on the balance between the patient's wishes, the feelings of relatives, and medical advice. Rarely are the patient's wishes known directly from the patient. In most circumstances the patient's relatives cannot legally or ethically make decisions for the patient. In the future, living-will legislation may give a nominated person the right to make such decisions, knowing the patient's wishes on the subject and acting as their advocate.

The fear of living in a persistent vegetative state should be approached sympathetically but is not strictly relevant to intensive care. The diagnosis is usually made after 6–12 months with the patient breathing spontaneously. Once the diagnosis of persistent vegetative state has been made, treatment may be withdrawn, but at present a legal opinion should be sought before doing so.

The doctor's duty to act in the patient's best interest means that, if the patient has no realistic chance of recovery, the doctor has a duty not to prolong their death. This decision should include all those involved in the patient's care. The decision needs to be based on care and dignity for the patient, and consideration of the family.

### Bereavement

Working in intensive care, staff deal regularly with death and use their own experiences to comfort bereaved relatives. As the average mortality rate for intensive care in the UK is 18%, facilities are needed for significant numbers of bereaved relatives on every ICU. There is now considerable interest in improving bereavement care in the UK.

The feelings experienced by a bereaved or potentially bereaved family are more than sorrow at their loss and will be dictated by previous experiences and relationships. No two families or family members respond in the same way. The bereavement reaction has been described as stages with initial shock followed by grief, anger, and guilt before resolution. The actual process is more complex and unpredictable, with individual patterns of coping and integration superimposed upon cultural expectations and traditions. Some individuals are likely to suffer a more intense grief response to bereavement than others. This is associated with increased morbidity and mortality and is characterized by the features listed in Table 17.20.

Medical staff frequently regard their job as saving lives, and death may be seen as a failure. The phrase 'there is nothing more we can do' should not apply because much can be done after the inevitability of a patient's death is established. Starting a healthy bereavement process for relatives is vital to their future psychological well-being and the health of society.

| Table 17.20. Risk factors for an abnormal grief response in bereaved individuals |
|---|
| Unexpected loss |
| Sudden loss |
| An unsupportive family |
| A traumatic bereavement |
| An ambivalent relationship between the deceased and the relative |
| Other coincident life crises |

## COMMUNICATION

Communication skills are often taken for granted but, frequently, appropriate skills need to be learned and developed. The importance of effective communication has been repeatedly emphasized as a means of reducing stress and providing support for both patients and relatives. Effective communication on an ICU is also vital so that accurate information is passed on. The communication needs for each group are summarized in Table 17.21.

### Communication with patients

The importance of communicating with patients cannot be overemphasized and is a vital part of the doctor/patient relationship. Critically ill patients are often sedated, intubated, or have other bars to communication. In spite of these, it is important to talk to them about what is happening and to use a tone of voice appropriate to the circumstances. Hearing is an important sense and patients' later reports are often salutary. As patients recover, their need for information can be

| Table 17.21. Communication needs of different groups |
|---|
| **Patient** |
| Information – verbal and written |
| Reassurance |
| To be heard |
| To express anxieties, needs, etc. |
| **Relatives** |
| Information – verbal and written |
| Emotional support |
| Commencing a healthy bereavement reaction |
| **ICU team** |
| Exchange of information – verbal handovers |
| Written notes |
| Guidelines |
| Staff support |
| Meetings with minutes or notes |
| **Other teams** |
| Accurate information – verbal and written |
| Appreciation of skills and needs |
| Mutual exchanges |
| Negotiation |
| **General practitioner** |
| Prompt information |
| Recognition of different role for patient |
| Information to offer support to family |

assessed more easily, although communication may remain difficult and frustrating. Efforts made to understand the patient pay dividends. After discharge, the patient may benefit from written information about their admission and rehabilitation.

### Communication with relatives

Although care is primarily delivered to the patient, their relatives also have communication needs. Although it is inappropriate for the ICU team to deliver medical care to the patient's relatives, support and information can be offered. The patient's own wishes and rights need consideration because breaches of confidentiality may breach the duty of care to the patient. Information booklets on the ICU and on what to do after a death should be available for a variety of religious and ethnic groups.

### Communication with the ICU team

Effective communication is essential for the ICU staff to function as a team. Handovers for staff at all levels should contain information on the patients and should be backed up by written notes. Guidelines help to ensure that everybody knows what to do in given circumstances. Team-building also involves issues such as staff support, staff development, and staff retention.

### Communication with other teams

For a patient to be managed optimally, the ICU team has to communicate effectively with other teams. This ranges from requesting investigations from laboratory services to negotiating transfer to a ward. Keeping teams involved in the patient's care up to date with their progress is essential. Transfer of a patient is a test of communication and information needs to be exchanged at all levels by appropriate members of staff.

### Communication with general practitioners

The patient's general practitioner (GP) is responsible for their long-term care and they need information on the patient that reflects this. Most GPs will treat few survivors of intensive care and they need to know the impact of an ICU stay on the patient and their family. They also need prompt information about the patient's admission, discharge, or death, with a discharge summary following soon after. The GP will often see family members who assume that the GP is aware of the patient's condition. GPs may also welcome the opportunity to be involved in the patient's care or the support of their relatives.

**Appendix 17.1: The APACHE II severity of disease classification system – the APACHE II score is the sum of A + B + C**

| Physiological variables (A) | High abnormal range +4 | +3 | +2 | +1 | 0 | +1 | +2 | +3 | Low abnormal range +4 |
|---|---|---|---|---|---|---|---|---|---|
| Temperature: rectal (°C) | > 41 | 39–40.9 | | 38.5–38.9 | 36–38.4 | 34–35.9 | 32–33.9 | 30–31.9 | < 29.9 |
| Mean arterial pressure (mmHg)[a] | > 160 | 130–159 | 110–129 | | 70–109 | | 50–69 | | < 49 |
| Heart rate (ventricular response) | > 180 | 140–179 | 110–139 | | 70–109 | | 55–69 | 40–54 | < 39 |
| Respiratory rate (non-ventilated or ventilated) | > 50 | 35–49 | | 25–34 | 12–24 | 10–11 | 6–9 | | < 5 |
| Oxygenation: $D_{A}$–$aO_2$[b] or $PaO_2$ (kPa) | | | | | | | | | |
| $FiO_2$ > 0.5 record $D_{A}$–$aO_2$ | > 66.8 | 46.7–66.7 | 26.7–46.6 | | < 26.7 | | | | |
| $FiO_2$ < 0.5 record only $PaO_2$ | | | | | $PaO_2$ > 9.3 | $PaO_2$ 8.1–9.3 | | $PaO_2$ 7.3–8.0 | $PaO_2$ < 7.3 |
| Arterial $H^+$ | < 20 | 21–25 | | 25–32 | 33–47 | | 48–56 | 57–71 | > 71 |
| or pH | ≥ 7.70 | 7.60–7.69 | | 7.50–7.59 | 7.33–7.49 | | 7.25–7.32 | 7.15–7.24 | < 7.15 |
| Serum sodium (mmol/l) | > 180 | 160–179 | 155–159 | 150–154 | 130–149 | | 120–129 | 111–119 | < 110 |
| Serum potassium (mmol/l) | > 7.0 | 6.0–6.9 | | 5.5–5.9 | 3.5–5.4 | 3.0–3.4 | 2.5–2.9 | | < 2.5 |
| Serum creatinine (μmol/l) | | | | | | | | | |
| (double point score for ARF) | > 318 | 180–317 | 136–179 | | 54–135 | | < 54 | | |
| Hb (g/dl) | > 20 | | 16.7–19.9 | 15.4–16.6 | 10.0–15.3 | | 6.7–9.9 | | < 6.7 |
| WBC (total/mm$^3$) (in 1000s) | > 40 | | 20.0–39.9 | 15.0–19.9 | 3.0–14.9 | | 1.0–2.9 | | < 1.0 |
| GCS | | | | | | | | | |
| Score = 15 minus actual GCS | | | | | | | | | |

(cont.)

## Appendix 17.1: The APACHE II severity of disease classification system – the APACHE II score is the sum of A + B + C (cont.)

**Age points (B)**

Assign points to age as follows:

| Age (years) | Points |
|---|---|
| < 44 | 0 |
| 45–54 | 2 |
| 55–64 | 3 |
| 65–74 | 5 |
| > 75 | 6 |

**Chronic health points (C)**

If the patient has a history of severe organ system insufficiency or is immunocompromised assign points as follows:

(a) For non-operative or emergency postoperative patients: 5 points
OR (b) For elective postoperative patients: 2 points.

**Definitions**: organ insufficiency or immunocompromised state must have been evident before this hospital admission and conform to the following criteria:
**Liver**: biopsy-proven cirrhosis and documented portal hypertension; episodes of past upper GI bleeding attributed to portal hypertension, or prior episodes of hepatic failure/encephalopathy/coma
**Respiratory**: chronic restrictive, obstructive, or vascular disease resulting in severe exercise restriction, i.e. unable to climb stairs or perform household duties; or documented chronic hypoxia, hypercapnia, secondary polycythaemia, severe pulmonary hypertension (< 40 mmHg) or respiratory dependency
**Cardiovascular**: NYHA class IV
**Renal**: receiving chronic dialysis
**Immunocompromised**: the patient has received therapy that suppresses resistance to infection, e.g. immunosuppression, chemotherapy, radiation, long-term or recent high-dose steroids, or has a disease that is sufficiently advanced to suppress resistance to infection, e.g. leukaemia, lymphoma, AIDS

[a]Mean arterial pressure = (systolic + [2 × diastolic])/3.
[b]$DA\text{–}aO_2 = (FiO_2 \times 94.8) - PaCO_2 - PaO_2$.
ARF, acute renal failure; GCS, Glasgow Coma Scale; NYHA, New York Heart Association; WBC, white blood cell count.

## Appendix 17.2: Components and individual values of the lung injury score

| **1. Chest Radiograph score** | |
|---|---|
| Alveolar consolidation | Score |
| None | 0 |
| Confined to one quadrant | 1 |
| Confined to two quadrants | 2 |
| Confined to three quadrants | 3 |
| All four quadrants | 4 |
| **2. Hypoxaemia score** | |
| $PaO_2/FIO_2$[a] | Score |
| ≥ 300 0 | |
| 225–299 | 1 |
| 175–224 | 2 |
| 100–174 | 3 |
| < 1004 | |
| **3. PEEP score (when ventilated)[b]** | |
| PEEP ($cmH_2O$) | Score |
| ≤ 5 | 0 |
| 6–8 1 | |
| 9–11 2 | |
| 12–14 | 3 |
| ≥ 15 4 | |
| **4. Respiratory system compliance score (when available)** | |
| Compliance ($cmH_2O$) | Score |
| ≥ 80 0 | |
| 60–79 | 1 |
| 40–59 | 2 |
| 20–39 | 3 |
| ≤ 19 | 4 |
| **The final value is obtained by dividing the aggregate sum by the number of components that were used:** | |
| Final score | Interpretation |
| 0 | No lung injury |
| 0.1–2.5 | Mild-to-moderate lung injury |
| > 2.5 | Severe lung injury (ARDS) |

[a]$PaO_2/FIO_2$, arterial oxygen tension to inspired oxygen concentration ratio.
[b]PEEP, positive end-expiratory pressure.
ARDS, acute respiratory distress syndrome.

## FURTHER READING


Bion J, ed. *Intensive Care Medicine*. London: BMJ Books, 1999.

Articles in: Delooz HH, ed. *Emergency Medicine and the Anaesthetist. Baillière's Clin Anaesthesiol* 1992;**6**:1–208.

Gomez CMH, Palazzo MGA. Pulmonary artery catheterization in anaesthesia and intensive care. *Br J Anaesth* 1999;**81**:945–56.

Granger CE, George C, Shelly MP. The management of bereavement on intensive care units. *Intensive Care Med* 1995;**21**:429–36.

Hinds CJ, Watson D. *Intensive Care – A Concise Textbook*, 2nd edn. London: Saunders, 1996.

Hörmann Ch, Baum M, Putensen Ch, Mutz NJ, Benzer H. Biphasic Positive Airway Pressure (BIPAP) – a new mode of ventilatory support. *Eur J Anaesthesiol* 1994;**11**:37–42.

Intensive Care Society. *Standards for Intensive Care Units*. London: 1997.

Keogh BF. New modes of ventilatory support. *Curr Anaesth Crit Care* 1998;**7**:228–35

Murray JF, Matthay MA, Luce JM, Flick MR. An expanded definition of the adult respiratory distress syndrome. *Am Rev Respir Dis* 1988;**138**:720–3.

NHS. *Guidelines on Admission to and Discharge from Intensive Care and High Dependency Units*. London: NHS Executive, March 1996.

NHS. *Paediatric Intensive Care 'A Framework for the Future'*. London: NHS Executive, July 1997.

Nightingale P. Pressure controlled ventilation – a true advance? *Clin Intensive Care* 1994;**5**:114–22

Prien T. High-dependency units: reducing the cost of intensive care without loss of quality. *Eur J Anaesthesiol* 1998;**15**:753–5.

Oh TE. *Intensive Care Manual*, 4th edn. Oxford: Butterworth-Heinemann, 1997.

Riddington DW, Clutton-Brock TH. Monitoring the severity of illness. In: Hutton P, Prys-Roberts C, eds. *Monitoring in Anaesthesia and Intensive Care*. Philadelphia: WB Saunders, 1994: 415–24.

Ridley S. Severity of illness scoring systems and performance appraisal. *Anaesthesia* 1998;**53**:1185–94.

Royal College of Anaesthetists and Royal College of Surgeons of England. *Report of the Joint Working Party on Graduated Patient Care*. London: Royal College of Anaesthetists and Royal College of Surgeons of England, January 1996.

# Section 2

# Integrated basic sciences

# Chapter 18 Biochemistry, the cell, and genetics

P. Hutton

This chapter, together with Chapter 19, describes the basic building blocks of physiology and pharmacology. Postgraduate trainees vary in their retention and understanding of their undergraduate teaching in these subjects. The content of the chapters therefore reflects our experience of the knowledge base of a 'typical' trainee in anaesthesia and the level to which they need to advance. Consequently, some subjects are dealt with briefly in an almost *aide memoire* way whereas others are developed in considerable detail.

The principle has been to include the material required to underpin the theoretical and clinical aspects of anaesthesia described in other chapters of the book, without losing the link with laboratory science. By doing this, it is hoped that a continuous and logical thread from molecules and cell function via genetics and the properties of specialized tissues to the whole organism will be achieved.

## BASIC CONCEPTS IN BIOCHEMISTRY

### Atomic structure and chemical bonds

#### *Atoms and ions*

An atom is the smallest indivisible unit of an element. The nucleus is composed of protons which are positively charged and neutrons, which have no charge. The nucleus comprises most of the mass of the atom but occupies only $10^{-4}$ of the diameter of its electron cloud. The electron cloud is typically of the order of 0.1–0.2 nm in diameter and the number of electrons in the outer shell has a major impact on the way the atom reacts chemically with other elements.

The stability of the nucleus determines the emission of natural radioactivity. The number of protons in the nucleus is the element's atomic number. The number of neutrons plus the number of protons is its atomic weight. The atomic structure of an atom is conventionally written as:

$$^{\text{Sum of protons and neutrons}}_{\text{Number of protons}}\text{Element}$$

Using potassium as an example, which has 19 protons associated with 20, 21, or 22 neutrons, each atom would be written as:

$$^{39}_{19}\text{K},\ ^{40}_{19}\text{K},\ ^{41}_{19}\text{K, respectively.}$$

Atoms of the same element (i.e. the same atomic number) with different atomic weights (i.e. differing numbers of neutrons) are called isotopes. As the element, when found in its natural state, may include a mixture of isotopes, the atomic weight is not necessarily an integer. Potassium, for instance, has a stated atomic weight of 39.1 which represents the weighted average of its component atoms and indicates an abundance of $^{39}_{19}$K.

Around the positively charged nucleus orbit an equal number of negatively charged electrons of negligible mass. Changes to the number of electrons in the outer shell of the atom lead to the formation of ions.

If an atom combines with oxygen, or loses hydrogen or one or more electrons, the process is called oxidation. Oxidation by electron loss forms positive ions. If an atom loses its combination with oxygen, or gains a hydrogen atom or one or more electrons, the process is called reduction. Reduction by electron gain produces negative ions.

#### *Electron shells*

Atoms possess electrons that orbit around the nucleus at distinct radii. Each orbital has a fixed maximum number of electrons permitted. The first shell has a maximum of 2, the second of 8, the third of 18, the fourth of 32, and so on. As the atomic number increases and the outer shell is being built up, those atoms with eight electrons in the outer shell are particularly stable. These form the inert or noble gases and their electron configuration is given in Table 18.1. The only exception to this is helium which has two electrons in its outer (first and only) shell and is highly stable.

Atoms without this stable outer shell formation have a tendency to donate to or accept electrons from other atoms (either the same or different to themselves) to produce the most stable outer shell formation for the combination. Highly reactive compounds have one or two more or one or two less electrons in the outer shell than the inert gases, and lie on either side of them in the periodic table. Examples are given in Table 18.2.

Those atoms with an atomic number less than an inert gas accept electrons into their outer shell and form negatively charged ions, e.g. $F^-$, $Cl^-$. It is partly the ability of halogens to form stable bonds with carbon that results in the low metabolism of volatile anaesthetic agents (see Chapter 33). Those atoms with an atomic number greater than an inert gas donate electrons and form positive ions, e.g. $Na^+$, $K^+$. In general, metals form positive ions (cations, which move to the cathode) and non-metals form negative ions (anions, which move to the anode).

**Table 18.1 Electron shell configurations of the inert gases**

| Element | Atomic no. | K | L | M | N | O | P |
|---|---|---|---|---|---|---|---|
| Helium | 2 | **2** | | | | | |
| Neon | 10 | 2 | **8** | | | | |
| Argon | 18 | 2 | 8 | **8** | | | |
| Krypton | 36 | 2 | 8 | 18 | **8** | | |
| Xenon | 54 | 2 | 8 | 18 | 18 | **8** | |
| Radon | 86 | 2 | 8 | 18 | 32 | 18 | **8** |

It is conventional to label the electron shells K, L, M, N, etc. Argon comprises just less than 1% of the atmosphere (see Chapter 8) and xenon has anaesthetic properties (see Chapter 33).

**Table 18.2 Outer shell structures for elements adjacent to the inert gases**

| Element | Atomic no. | K | L | M | Bond characteristic |
|---|---|---|---|---|---|
| Hydrogen | 1 | 1 | | | 1-electron acceptor |
| Helium | 2 | **2** | | | Inert gas |
| Lithium | 3 | | 1 | | 1-electron donor |
| Oxygen | 8 | | 6 | | 2-electron acceptor |
| Fluorine | 9 | | 7 | | 1-electron acceptor |
| Neon | 10 | | **8** | | Inert gas |
| Sodium | 11 | | | 1 | 1-electron donor |
| Magnesium | 12 | | | 2 | 2-electron donor |
| Sulphur | 16 | | | 6 | 2-electron acceptor |
| Chlorine | 17 | | | 7 | 1-electron acceptor |
| Argon | 18 | | | **8** | Inert gas |
| Potassium | 19 | | | 9 | 1-electron donor |
| Calcium | 20 | | | 10 | 2-electron donor |

***Chemical bonds between atoms***

Interactions between similar or dissimilar atoms result in a rearrangement of electrons to try to achieve a stable octet in their outer shell. Such an arrangement takes one of two forms:

1. The giving or receiving of an electron until each atom is surrounded by an octet (electrovalency).
2. The sharing of electrons to get similarly stable shells (covalency).

Once bonded, although overall electrically neutral, there may not be a uniform distribution of charge within the molecule. This allows further types of intermolecular attraction to occur which are considered later.

*Electrovalency*

Taking sodium and chlorine as an example, the shell configuration of sodium is 2 : 8 : 1 and that of chlorine 2 : 8 : 7 (see Table 18.2). If the sodium gives its outermost electron to a chlorine atom, the respective shell formations of 2 : 8 and 2 : 8 : 8 result.

Alternatively, writing the outer shell configuration for sodium as $Na^{\bullet}$ and for chlorine as $\overset{\times\times}{\underset{\times\times}{_{\times}Cl_{\times}^{\times}}}$ then the action of sodium on chlorine can be represented as:

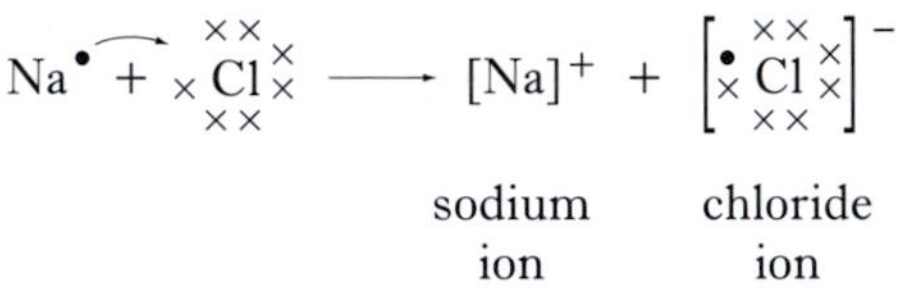

$$Na^{\bullet} + {}_{\times}\overset{\times\times}{\underset{\times\times}{Cl}}{}^{\times}_{\times} \longrightarrow [Na]^{+} + \left[{}^{\bullet}_{\times}\overset{\times\times}{\underset{\times\times}{Cl}}{}^{\times}_{\times}\right]^{-}$$

sodium ion    chloride ion

The electrons of the chlorine atom represented by an '×' are of course identical to the one donated from sodium represented by '•'. The notation is purely to denote the origin of the electrons. A similar representation for the bonding of calcium and chlorine is:

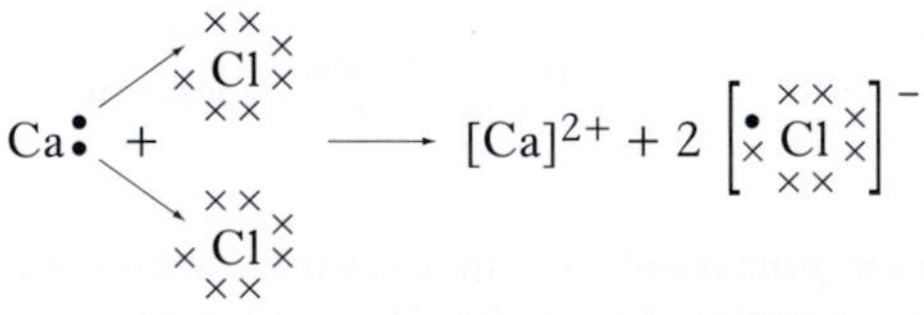

$$Ca\!: + 2\,{}_{\times}\overset{\times\times}{\underset{\times\times}{Cl}}{}^{\times}_{\times} \longrightarrow [Ca]^{2+} + 2\left[{}^{\bullet}_{\times}\overset{\times\times}{\underset{\times\times}{Cl}}{}^{\times}_{\times}\right]^{-}$$

Such chemical combinations resulting from transfer of electrons are known as electrovalent compounds. Electrovalent bonds are also called ionic bonds.

The energy required to remove an electron is known as the ionization energy. It depends on the size of the atom (and hence the distance of the outer shell from the nucleus) and the number of electrons to be given

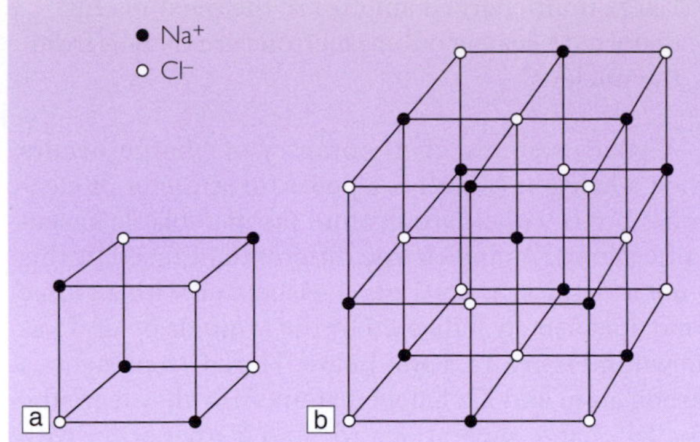


**Figure 18.1** Crystalline sodium chloride. (a) The basic unit and (b) the complete crystalline form.

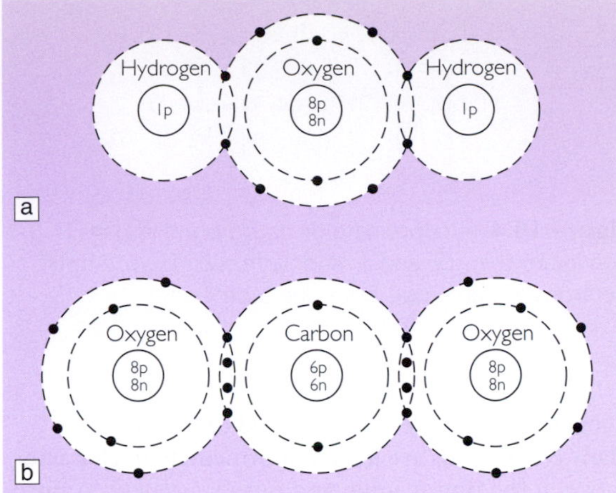


**Figure 18.2** Examples of covalency. The electrons (●) in the outer shells are shared to form stable octets. (a) Water molecule ($H_2O$): the oxygen atom shares two electrons with each hydrogen atom. Both molecules thereby complete the outer shell – the hydrogen atom with two electrons and the oxygen with eight. (b) Carbon dioxide molecule ($CO_2$): the carbon atom shares four electrons with each oxygen atom. All three atoms thereby complete their outer shells with eight electrons. p, proton; n, neutron.

up. Consequently, potassium (atomic number 19) forms ions more easily than sodium (atomic number 11). Also, it is easier to produce the single ionization change from K to $K^+$ rather than the double ionization change from Ca to $Ca^{2+}$ (see Table 18.2).

Ionic compounds often form crystals when not in solution. An example is common salt, sodium chloride, which is shown in Figure 18.1. Figure 18.1a shows the basic unit and Figure 18.1b shows its formation into a crystal. In the cubical crystal unit, sodium and chlorine ions are packed alternately throughout: no one sodium ion is linked to a particular chloride ion. The bonds between the two species are electrostatic.

When the crystal is put into water it breaks up and dissolves. The ions wander about independently, forming an electrolytic solution. The breaking apart of the ions is known as electrolytic dissociation and water is an excellent dissociating solvent. This is very relevant to the movement of ions within the intra- and extracellular spaces and their availability to take part in reactions. Dissociation also occurs when a salt is melted and the liquid again becomes an electrolyte. Ionic solutions do not contain molecules, just electrostatically attracted ions.

*Covalency*

The bonds in covalency consist of pairs of electrons shared between the nuclei of the atoms that they unite. The principle is similar to electrovalency in that each atom attempts to obtain eight electrons in its outer shell, or in the specialist case of hydrogen, two. Examples of this are shown in Figure 18.2.

An atom such as hydrogen or chlorine, which requires a single electron to complete its outer shell, is said to have combining power of one. Oxygen requires two electrons to fill its outer shell and therefore has a combining power of two. Similarly, nitrogen and carbon require three and four electrons respectively to complete their outer orbitals, so they have combining powers of three and four, respectively.

Where a single electron is donated by each atom and the pair is shared by both atoms, the bond is termed a 'single bond'. The donation of two electrons by each atom and the sharing of two pairs of electrons is a double bond, and so on. With its combining power of four (the maximum possible), carbon readily forms covalent bonds with hydrogen, oxygen, nitrogen, and halogens to produce a wide variety of molecules. More importantly, it can combine with another carbon atom to form long chains linked by single, double, or triple bonds. These very long and stable chains are essential to living organisms.

In molecular diagrams, a single bond is represented by a single line and a double bond by a double line, etc. Examples of this are shown in Figure 18.3, which should be compared with Figure 18.2.

As usual, there are exceptions to some of these rules because of the enormous potential for chemical interaction and the space available around a central atom. Also, in some compounds both electrons of a pair are provided by one atom instead of one from each of the pair of combining atoms. An example of this occurs in the stable compound that aluminium chloride forms with ammonia as shown in Figure 18.4. This is called a coordinate or dative bond.

In most covalent compounds, the covalent bonds hold the molecules together strongly. In contrast, the forces between individual molecules (see later) are weaker by orders of magnitude. Thus, many covalently bonded molecules are gases or volatile liquids (e.g. oxygen, carbon tetrachloride). A comparison between electrovalent and covalent bonds is given in Table 18.3.

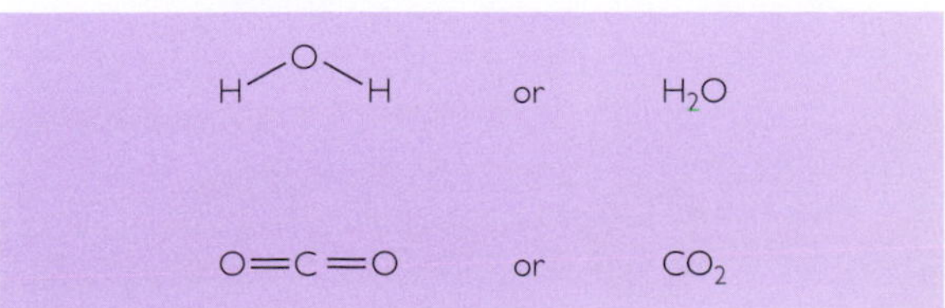


**Figure 18.3** Diagrammatic representations of single and double bonds used in chemical formulae. A single bond contains two electrons, a double bond contains four.

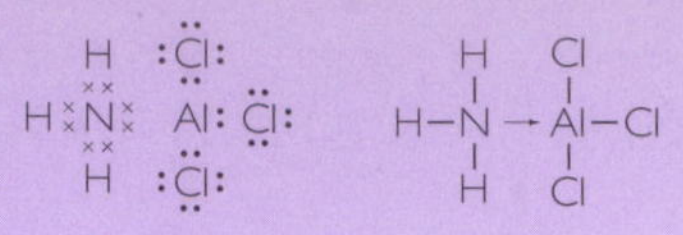

**Figure 18.4** A coordinate or dative bond linking aluminium chloride and ammonia. In such a bond both electrons are provided from one atom.

*Transition between electrovalency and covalency*

Many compounds are in fact intermediate in character between the purely ionic and purely covalent. A pure ionic bond is really found only between metals of low ionization potential and non-metals of high electron affinity. A pure covalent bond is found only in molecules formed by two identical atoms, e.g. $H_2$, $O_2$, $Cl_2$, where the electron cloud is uniform across the two atoms.

Most compounds fit somewhere between these two extremes. If two spherical ions of opposite charge are brought together to form an electrovalent bond, the cation attracts and deforms the electron cloud of the anion. Within a covalent bond, the unequal sharing of electrons can similarly produce an asymmetry of charge in an overall neutral molecule. This continuum of effects is demonstrated diagrammatically in Figure 18.5. As a general rule:

- When two different atoms are joined by a covalent bond the electrons are not shared equally, i.e. their charge cloud is asymmetrical.
- Cations are small and compact, and distortion of the cation by an anion is usually negligible.
- Large multicharged anions are the most readily distorted because outer electrons are distant from the nucleus.

A good example of asymmetry of charge occurs when a halogen (which is a powerful attractor of electrons) binds with a carbon atom (as in a volatile anaesthetic agent). As the charge differential caused by this is not as large as the +1 or −1 associated with an ionic bond, it is usually indicated by the symbols $\delta^+$ or $\delta^-$, as shown in Figure 18.5 and below. Here C represents a carbon atom and X a halogen atom. Also shown are the smaller charge separations ($\delta^+$ and $\delta^-$) that occur with nitrogen, oxygen, and sulphur.

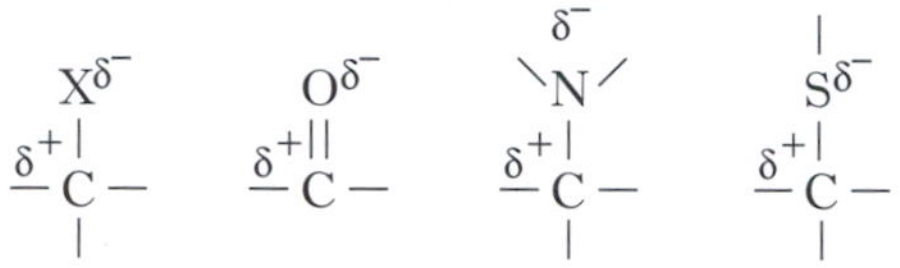

$$\overset{\delta^+}{\text{C}}-\text{X}^{\delta-} \qquad \overset{\delta^+}{\text{C}}=\text{O}^{\delta-} \qquad \overset{\delta^+}{\text{C}}-\overset{\delta^-}{\text{N}} \qquad \overset{\delta^+}{\text{C}}-\text{S}^{\delta-}$$

The partial ionic character of covalent bonds is measured by the dipole moment. The ratio of the measured to the calculated dipole moment of a covalent molecule measures the change in interatomic bond distance caused by ionic effects. This allows the proportion of the bond between the two atoms to be classified as being caused by either ionic or covalent effects. As an example, the HCl molecule has a bond that is 17% ionic and 83% covalent. Bonds with a partial ionic character of over 50% are conventionally classified as ionic.

*Molecules with both electrovalent and covalent bonds*

Many compounds are known in which both electrovalent and covalent bonding occur. These are usually

**Table 18.3 A comparison of electrovalently and covalently bonded compounds**

| Electrovalent compounds | Covalent compounds |
|---|---|
| Component atoms exist as ions | Component atoms exist as part of a molecule |
| Essentially non-directional bond | Bond has well-defined direction |
| Often crystalline solids with a definite geometric crystal structure and high melting point | Often volatile liquids or gases. If solid, usually soft with a low melting point |
| The majority dissolve in water | The majority do not dissolve in water |
| When in aqueous solution or molten, they are electrolytes | Not usually electrolytes |
| Isomerism is not found | Structural and stereoisomerism are common |

Note that some of the generalizations in this table are qualified in the text.

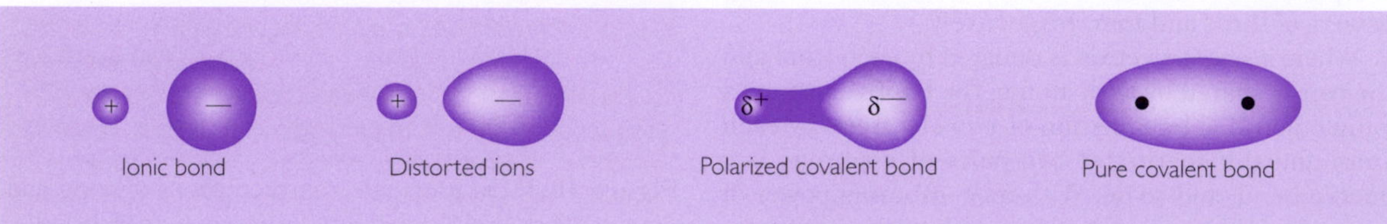


**Figure 18.5** The transition between ionic and covalent bonding: + cation; – anion.

ternary compounds (containing three elements), with oxygen being one of the constituent elements.

Sodium sulphate, $Na_2SO_4$, is such a compound. When solid it consists of sodium ions, $Na^+$, and sulphate ions, $SO_4^{2-}$, arranged in a crystal lattice. When sodium sulphate is dissolved in water, these ions separate and move independently of one another in solution. The sulphate ion is, however, bound together, as a single unit, by covalent bonding. Such polyatomic, covalently bonded ions are common in human biochemistry. Most are polyatomic anions (e.g. $CO_3^{2-}$, $OH^-$, $NO_3^-$, $NO_2^-$, $PO_4^{3-}$, $SO_4^{2-}$) but there are also a smaller number of polyatomic cations (e.g. $NH_4^+$). Some complex ions have a central metal cation surrounded by several anions or other molecular forms (e.g. porphyrins such as haemoglobin).

These molecules, which can exist as effectively unitary entities in aqueous solution, are essential to many of the basic biochemical processes of life (e.g. energy transport processes involving phosphates).

### *Chemical bonds between molecules*

Bonds between molecules, almost by definition, are orders of magnitude less than interatomic electrovalent or covalent bonds. Indeed, if they were not, chemical reactions would occur to optimize bond strength and the original arrangement of molecules would be destroyed. The bonds between molecules contribute to properties such as surface tension and viscosity, and deviations from the perfect gas laws. Quantitatively, the strongest of these intermolecular bonds is the so-called 'hydrogen bond' followed by the much weaker van de Waal's forces. At very low intermolecular distances, the forces between molecules always become repulsive as the negatively charged electron clouds begin to repel. This latter effect is discussed in Chapter 37 and shown in Figure 37.37.

#### *Hydrogen bonds*

As described above, there is a transition from the purely ionically to the purely covalently bonded molecule. This allows adjacent molecules, when orientated appropriately, to have an electrostatic force between them. Such intermolecular attractions of certain hydrogen-containing compounds are particularly strong (5–10% as strong as typical electrovalent or covalent bonds) and, because of this, bonds of this type are generically known as hydrogen bonds.

Significant dipole moments are created when hydrogen is covalently bonded to highly electronegative elements of small atomic size. Examples of this are water and ammonia as shown in Figure 18.6. Here, the hydrogen ions are left almost as exposed protons with a significant positive charge at the opposite end of the molecule to the lone electron cloud(s). Really effective dipole moments and hydrogen bonds are formed only with fluorine, oxygen, and nitrogen compounds. Chlorine forms very weak hydrogen bonds.

The impact of hydrogen bonding can be appreciated by examining the boiling points of various compounds. In general, as hydrogen is sequentially bonded with atoms of greater atomic weight (i.e. with elements of higher groups in the periodic table), the boiling point of the compounds should progressively increase.

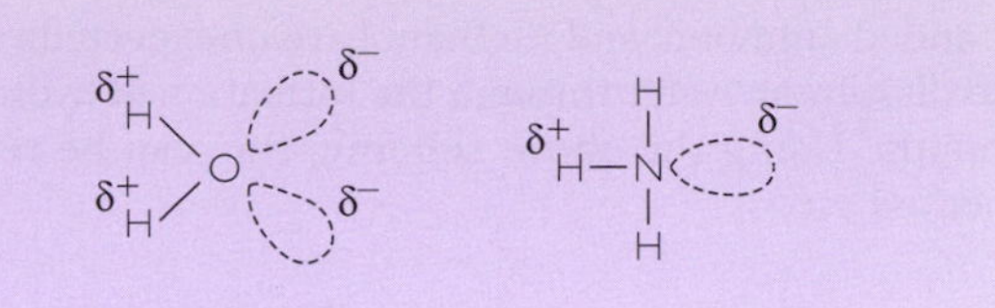


**Figure 18.6** Molecules of water (left) and ammonia (right). The dotted outlines represent the electron cloud of the lone electrons.

Experimental results for such compounds are shown in Figure 18.7.

In Figure 18.7, the progression of the series $CH_4$, $SiH_4$, $GeH_4$, and $SnH_4$, which possess no hydrogen bonds, follows the predicted pattern based on molecular weights. $H_2O$, HF, and $NH_3$, which have strong intermolecular hydrogen bonds, have boiling points well above those predicted on molecular weight alone. The predicted boiling points are shown by the dotted lines in Figure 18.7. As an example, water could be expected to boil at less than −100°C. Consequently, were it not for hydrogen bonding, the properties of water that allow it to be the solvent of life would not exist.

The association of adjacent HF, $H_2O$, and $NH_3$ molecules by hydrogen bonds can be roughly illustrated as follows, the dotted lines representing the hydrogen bonds:

```
                       ⋮          ⋮              H       H
                                                 |       |
H—F···H—F···       H—O···H—O···           H—N···H—N···
                     |      |                  |       |
                     H      H                  H       H
```

Hydrogen bonding also accounts for the unexpectedly high solubilities of some compounds containing oxygen, nitrogen, and fluorine in some hydrogen-

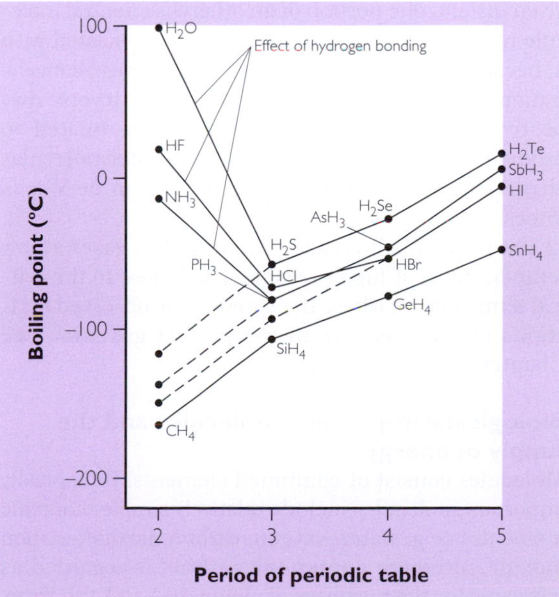


**Figure 18.7** Observed (solid line) and predicted (dotted line) boiling points for hydrogen-containing compounds of increasing atomic weight. (See text for details.)

containing solvents, particularly water. Thus, covalently bonded ammonia and methanol are unexpectedly able to dissolve in water through the formation of hydrogen bonds. Using the above scheme, this can be represented as:

```
    H                  H
    |                  |
H—N····H—O         H—C—O····H—O
    |      |            |   |      |
    H      H            H   H      H
```

In addition to these unexpected solubilities, the hydrogen-bonding properties of water enable rapid dissolution of many other ionic or dipolar compounds. This property is vital for allowing many biochemical molecules essential to life to dissolve in an aqueous medium.

Although individual hydrogen bonds are weak, a vast number of them on large (usually organic) molecules can make them collectively very significant. One of the most important basic functions that compares hydrogen bonding with that of covalent bonding is found in DNA. Here, the relatively weak hydrogen bond between adjacent nucleotides holds together the two strands of DNA, whereas the bonds between adjacent nucleotides forming the back bone of the molecule are covalent diester bonds. The weak hydrogen bonds allow easy cleavage of the molecule for replication, but the strong covalent bonds ensure continued integrity of the structure of the individual strands. This is discussed in more detail later.

*Van de Waal's forces*

Non-polar molecules without dipolar moments also show intermolecular attraction but it is orders of magnitude less even than the hydrogen bond. These extremely weak forces, common to all matter, are thought to be caused by the motion of electrons and are sometimes termed 'fluctuating dipoles'. Hence, at a given instant, one portion of an otherwise neutral molecule may have a small negative charge associated with it, because it has a slightly higher than average concentration of electrons. At the next instant, the reverse may be true. This variation in charge is postulated to produce an ever-changing, very weak intermolecular attraction. Such effects are known as van de Waal's forces.

Van de Waal's forces are important in gases at low temperatures, at high pressures, and close to the critical temperature, where they predict the observed deviations of real gases from the perfect gas laws (see Chapter 37).

### Biologically important molecules and the supply of energy

Molecules consist of combined elements. Biologically important molecules include relatively simple inorganic molecules (e.g. water, oxygen, carbon dioxide; carbon dioxide, although containing carbon, is regarded as inorganic for the purposes of chemistry) and also large, complex organic molecules (e.g. carbohydrates, proteins, fats, and nucleic acids), some of which may carry inorganic ions (e.g. haemoglobin and vitamin B complex).

**Table 18.4 Approximate composition of mammalian cells**

| Element | Percentage of cell mass |
|---|---|
| Oxygen (O) | 60 |
| Carbon (C) | 21 |
| Hydrogen (H) | 11 |
| Nitrogen (N) | 3.5 |
| Calcium (Ca) | 2.5 |
| Phosphorus (P) | 1.2 |
| Chlorine (Cl) | 0.2 |
| Fluorine (F) | 0.15 |
| Sulphur (S) | 0.15 |
| Potassium (K) | 0.1 |
| Sodium (Na) | 0.1 |
| Magnesium (Mg) | 0.07 |
| Iron (Fe) | 0.01 |
| Trace elements | 0.02 |

Elements in all life forms are of low atomic mass and occur readily in the environment. Only about 40% of known elements occur in the molecules of human tissues. The most common are oxygen, carbon, and hydrogen in combination with other elements. The percentages of elements in mammalian cells are as shown in Table 18.4.

Inorganic ions and molecules are relatively small and simple, and with the exception of carbon dioxide do not contain carbon. The three most common inorganic molecules are water, molecular oxygen, and carbon dioxide.

Metals and minerals are also very important as components of inorganic molecules in the body and, although they make up less than 1% of the body weight (Table 18.4), they are essential to its existence. Deficiencies can result in well-defined clinical disorders (e.g. anaemia, goitre). The main inorganic ions and molecules and their functions are listed in Table 18.5.

Organic molecules are based on the unique bonding properties of carbon and are often large and complex. They usually contain a narrow range of elements, mainly oxygen, hydrogen, nitrogen, and sulphur. Organic molecules fall into four main groups: carbohydrates, proteins, lipids, and nucleic acids. The nomenclature of carbon compounds is outlined in Appendix 18.1, which can be referred to as the compounds are described in the text.

***Energy and intermediate metabolism***

Carbohydrates, fats, and proteins are the main sources of energy in the diet. To release energy these food stuffs are broken down to carbon dioxide and water, a process that ultimately requires oxygen. The

**Table 18.5 The functions of inorganic ions and minerals**

| Inorganic ions/minerals | Description | Functions and importance |
|---|---|---|
| Calcium ($Ca^{2+}$) | • Most abundant cation in the body<br>• Appears in combination with phosphorus in ratio of 2 : 1.5<br>• About 99% is stored in bone and teeth<br>• Remainder stored in muscle, other soft tissues, and blood plasma | • Essential for normal muscle and nerve activity, endocytosis and exocytosis, cellular motility, chromosome movement before cell division, glycogen metabolism, and synthesis and release of neurotransmitters<br>• It is a main constituent of bones, teeth, and shells<br>• Needed for the clotting of blood |
| Potassium ($K^{+}$) | • Principal cation in intracellular fluid | • Functions in transmission of nerve impulses and muscle contraction<br>• Helps to maintain the electrical, osmotic, and anion/cation balance across cell membranes<br>• Assists active transport of certain materials across the cell membrane<br>• Necessary for protein synthesis and is a cofactor in respiration |
| Sodium ($Na^{+}$) | • Principal cation in extracellular fluids, some in bones<br>• Principal cation of extracellular fluid | • Helps to maintain the electrical, osmotic and anion/cation balance across cell membranes<br>• Strongly affects distribution of water through osmosis<br>• Cation of bicarbonate buffer system<br>• Functions in nerve impulse conduction<br>• Assists active transport of certain materials across the cell membrane |
| Phosphorus as phosphate ($PO_4^{3-}$) or orthophosphate ($H_2PO_4^{-}$) | • About 80% found in bones and teeth<br>• Remainder in muscle, brain cells, blood<br>• More diverse functions than any other mineral | • Formation of bones and teeth<br>• Constitutes a major intracellular buffer system<br>• Plays important role in muscle contraction and nerve activity<br>• Component of many enzymes<br>• Involved in transfer and storage of energy (ATP)<br>• Component of DNA and RNA<br>• Component of nucleotides, ATP, and some proteins<br>• Used in the phosphorylation of sugars in respiration<br>• A major constituent of bone and teeth<br>• A component of cell membranes in the form of phospholipids |
| Iron ($Fe^{2+}$ or $Fe^{3+}$) | • About 66% found in haemoglobin of blood<br>• Remainder distributed in skeletal muscles, liver, spleen, enzymes | • Component of haemoglobin, myoglobin, and porphyrins<br>• Constituent of electron carriers, e.g. cytochromes, needed in respiration and photosynthesis<br>• Constituent of certain other enzymes, e.g. dehydrogenases, decarboxylases, peroxidases, and catalase |
| Chloride ($Cl^{-}$) | • Found in extracellular and intracellular fluids<br>• Principal anion of extracellular fluid | • Assumes role in acid–base balance of blood, water balance, and formation of HCl in stomach<br>• Helps to maintain the electrical, osmotic and anion/cation balance across cell membranes |

cont.

**Table 18.5 The functions of inorganic ions and minerals (cont.)**

| Inorganic ions/minerals | Description | Functions and importance |
|---|---|---|
| Chloride ($Cl^-$) (cont.) | | • Needed for the formation of HCl in gastric juice<br>• Assists in the transport of $CO_2$ by blood (chloride shift) |
| Sulphate ($SO_4^{2-}$) | • Constituent of many proteins (such as insulin) and some vitamins (thiamine and biotin) | • As a component of hormones and vitamins, regulates various body activities<br>• Sulphur is a component of some proteins and certain coenzymes, e.g. acetyl coenzyme A |
| Nitrogen as nitrate ($NO_3^-$) ammonium ($NH_4^+$) | • Distributed widely through body tissues | • Nitrogen is a component of amino acids, proteins, vitamins, coenzymes, and nucleotides<br>• Some hormones contain nitrogen, e.g. insulin |
| Magnesium ($Mg^{2+}$) | • Component of soft tissues and bone | • Required for normal functioning of muscle and nervous tissue<br>• Participates in bone formation<br>• Constituent of many coenzymes<br>• An activator for some enzymes, e.g. ATPase<br>• A component of bone and teeth |
| Copper | • Some stored in liver and spleen | • Required with iron for synthesis of haemoglobin<br>• Component of enzyme necessary for melanin pigment formation |
| Zinc | • Important component of certain enzymes | • As a component of carbonic anhydrase, important in $CO_2$ metabolism<br>• Necessary for normal growth and wound healing, proper functioning of prostate gland, normal taste sensations and appetite, and normal sperm counts in males<br>• As a component of peptidases, it is involved in protein digestion |
| Iodine | • Essential component of thyroid hormones<br>• Excreted in urine | • Required by thyroid gland to synthesize thyroid hormones, and hormones that regulate metabolic rate |
| Cobalt | • Constituent of vitamin B12 | • A part of vitamin B12 required for maturation of erythrocytes |

energy released from food stuffs is re-stored in a form that is convenient for cellular use – ATP (Figure 18.8). When used as an energy source ATP is broken down into ADP and inorganic phosphate ($P_i$). ATP and ADP molecules coexist in a cycle as shown in Figure 18.9.

Once digestion has broken down carbohydrates, lipids, and proteins into glucose, fatty acids, and peptides, respectively, they all enter the tricarboxylic acid (citric acid or Kreb's) cycle. The tricarboxylic acid cycle produces carbon dioxide and the electron transport chain produces hydrogen ions, $H^+$. This is shown diagrammatically in Figure 18.10. Other acids produced by the body are listed in Table 18.6.

Ultimately, oxygen is required to react with the acidic hydrogen ions to form water. Without this reaction, the pH progressively falls and death of the cell supervenes. All these processes of oxidative metabolism and phosphorylation take place in the mitochondria (see later).

Some methods of releasing energy do not consume oxygen, e.g. the hexose monophosphate shunt. These anaerobic processes are, however, relatively inefficient, short-lived, and ultimately have to be linked with an aerobic pathway to produce the necessary excretion of hydrogen ions as part of water. The energy released by the aerobic metabolism of dietary compounds is given in Table 18.7.

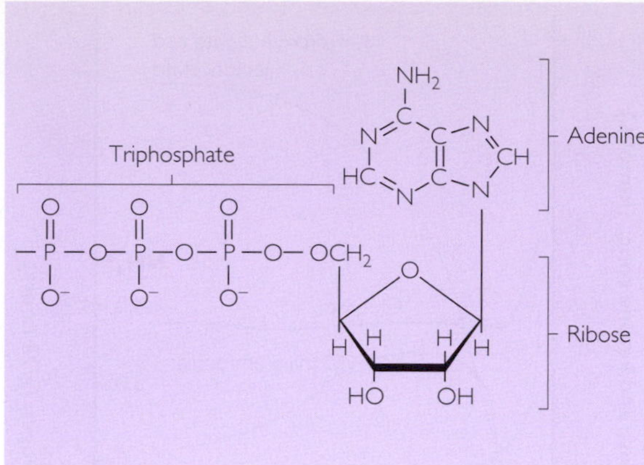


**Figure 18.8** The structure of adenosine triphosphate (ATP). Its three constituents are adenine, ribose, and triphosphate.

| **Table 18.6 Acids produced by the body** |
|---|
| Carbonic acid |
| Lactic acid |
| Citric acid |
| Sulphuric acid |
| Phosphoric acid |
| Ammonium ions |
| Ketone bodies<br>Acetoacetic acid<br>β-Hydroxybutyric acid |

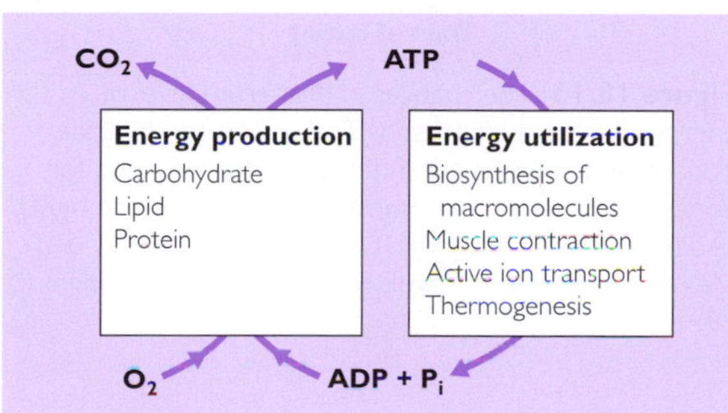


**Figure 18.9** The ATP/ADP cycle ($P_i$, inorganic phosphate).

**Table 18.7 Approximate calorific value of dietary components**

| Dietary components | kcal/g |
|---|---|
| Carbohydrate | 4 |
| Protein | 4 |
| Alcohol | 7 |
| Fat | 9 |

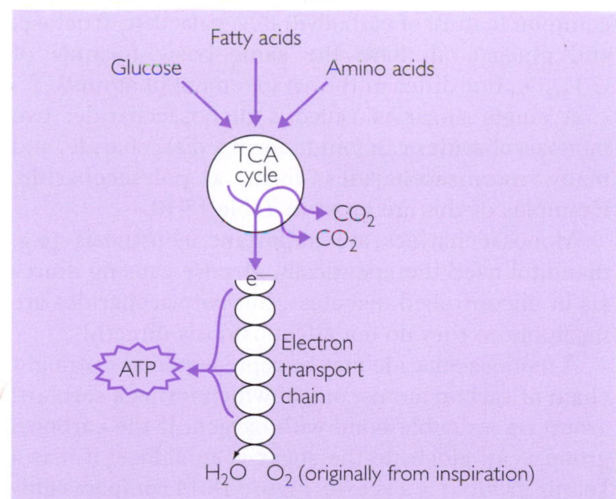


**Figure 18.10** The generation of ATP from glucose, fatty acids, and amino acids (e⁻, electrons; TCA, tricarboxylic acid).

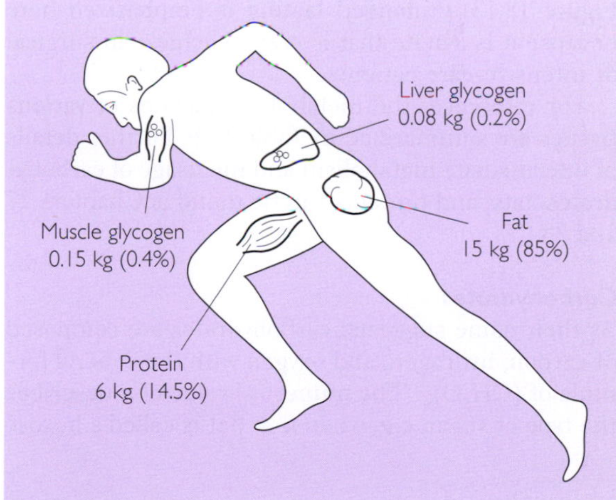


**Figure 18.11** The energy reserves of a 70-kg man after an overnight fast, in kg and as a percentage of total calories.

To enable the intermittent intake of dietary components to be used throughout the day as demand arises, they have to be converted to storage compounds when energy intake exceeds demand. Fats are stored as adipose triacylglycerol (triglyceride), carbohydrates as glycogen, and amino acids as protein. The typical fuel reserves of an average 70-kg man after an overnight fast are shown in Figure 18.11.

The body uses its energy stores as appropriate. The major processes occurring during the absorptive and post-absorptive (fasting) states are summarized in Chapter 27, Figure 27.9. During exercise, muscle glycogen is metabolized first, followed by blood-borne fatty acids and glucose (Figure 18.12).

During prolonged starvation (after a few days), the pattern of fuel utilization changes. If it did not, the body's protein reserves would be quickly reduced to

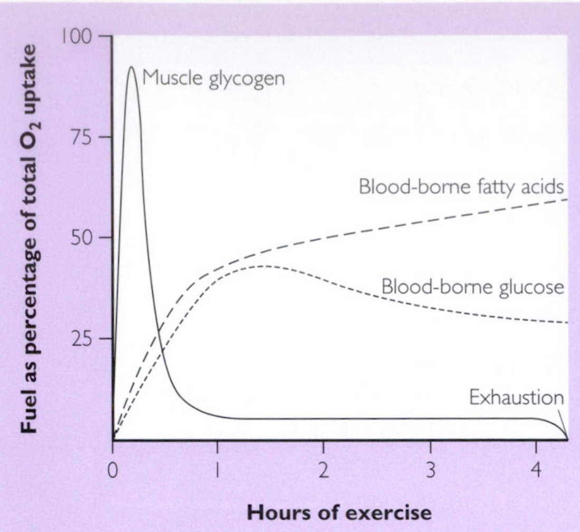


**Figure 18.12** The order of substrate utilization during exercise. (Adapted from Felig P. *Endocrinology and Metabolism*. New York: McGraw Hill, 1981: 796.)

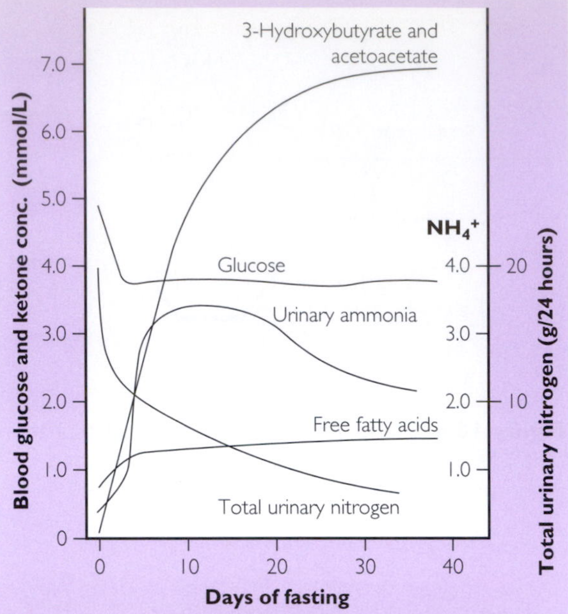


**Figure 18.13** The changes in the serum level of energy sources during fasting. The units for fatty acids, glucose, and ketones are mmol/L (on the left), and for urinary nitrogen and ammonia g/24 hours (on the right). (Adapted from Linder MC. *Nutritional Biochemistry and Metabolism*, 2nd edn. Stamford CT: Appleton & Lange, 1991: 103.)

dangerous levels. As starvation progresses, there is a steady generation of ketone bodies from fat and the brain begins to oxidize them. As a result of the increased utilization of ketone bodies, glucose is 'spared' and the liver needs to produce less. Consequently, the demand for amino acids (produced by the breakdown of protein) for gluconeogenesis is reduced and accordingly less muscle protein is degraded. The metabolic changes occurring during prolonged fasting are summarized in Table 18.8 and Figure 18.13. Prolonged fasting is emphasized here because it is a state that is easy to achieve in surgical or intensive-care patients.

For reference, the metabolic capacities of various tissues are summarized in Table 18.9. Further details of intermediate metabolism and the usage of carbohydrates, fats, and proteins can be found is Chapters 27 and 28.

### *Carbohydrates*

As their name suggests, carbohydrates are composed of carbon, hydrogen, and oxygen with the general formula of $(CH_2O)_n$. The numerical value of $n$ describes the type of sugar, e.g. when $n = 6$ it is called a hexose sugar. Glucose is a hexose sugar with the chemical formula $C_6H_{12}O_6$. Isomerism (see Chapter 19) is a common feature of carbohydrates: galactose, fructose, and glucose all have the same basic formula of $C_6H_{12}O_6$, but differ in the arrangement of atoms.

A single sugar is called a monosaccharide; two monosaccharides can join to form a disaccharide, and many monosaccharides form a polysaccharide. Examples of this are given in Table 18.10.

Monosaccharides are important in osmosis (e.g. mannitol used therapeutically, glucose causing diuresis in uncontrolled diabetes), but polysaccharides are insoluble so they do not affect osmosis directly.

A monosaccharide may be represented as a straight chain of carbon atoms, one of which forms a carbonyl group via a double bond with oxygen. If the carbonyl group is an aldehyde the sugar is an aldose; if it is a ketone group it is a ketose. Figure 18.14 compares glucose (an aldose) with fructose (a ketose).

Although monosaccharides are often represented by a straight chain, they exist in solution mainly as ring structures in which the carbonyl group has reacted with a hydroxyl group in the same molecule, forming a ring. Hexoses form either six-membered rings (pyranoses) or five-membered rings (furanoses) (Figure 18.15). The ring structures can be represented more accurately as chair or boat forms (Figure 18.16), the chair form predominating in solution.

All disaccharides are sweet, soluble in water, and readily converted into monosacharides by the addition of a water molecule. The process is called hydrolysis (Figure 18.17).

**Table 18.8 Metabolic changes during prolonged fasting**

| | | |
|---|---|---|
| Brain | ↑ | Increased utilization of ketone bodies |
| Muscle | ↓ | Reduced utilization of ketone bodies and reduced protein breakdown; depends mainly on fatty acids |
| Liver | ↓ | Reduced gluconeogenesis and reduced production of urea |

**Table 18.9 Metabolic capacities of various tissues**

| Process | Liver | Adipose tissue | Renal cortex | Muscle | Brain | Red blood cells |
|---|---|---|---|---|---|---|
| Tricarboxylic acid cycle (acetyl-CoA $\rightarrow$ $CO_2$ + $H_2O$) | +++ | +++ | +++ | +++ | +++ | – |
| β-Oxidation of fatty acids | +++ | – | +++ | +++ | – | – |
| Ketone body formation | +++ | – | + | – | – | – |
| Ketone body utilization | – | + | ++ | +++ | – (fed)<br>+++<br>(prolonged starvation) | – |
| Lipogenesis (glucose $\rightarrow$ fatty acids) | +++ | + | – | – | – | – |
| Gluconeogenesis (lactate $\rightarrow$ glucose) | +++ | – | + | – | – | – |
| Glycogen metabolism (synthesis and degradation) | +++ | + | + | +++ | (+) | – |
| Lactate production (glucose $\rightarrow$ lactate) | + | + | + | +++<br>(in exercise) | (+) | +++ |

From Marks DB *et al. Basic Medical Biochemistry*. Baltimore, MA: Williams & Wilkins, 1996: 33.

**Table 18.10 Carbohydrates and their properties**

| Carbohydrate group | Chemical structure | Formula | Examples | Function |
|---|---|---|---|---|
| Monosaccharides (simple sugars) | Consist of a single chemical group | $C_6H_{12}O_6$ | Glucose<br>Fructose<br>Galactose | Soluble; basic units for making larger carbohydrates such as glycogen |
| Disaccharides (more complex sugars) | Two monosaccharides joined by a glycosidic bond with the loss of a water molecule | $C_{12}H_{22}O_{11}$ | Maltose = glucose + glucose (malt sugar)<br>Sucrose = glucose + fructose (cane sugar)<br>Lactose = glucose + galactose (milk sugar) | Soluble; easily converted to monosaccharides |
| Polysaccharides (large, complex sugars) | Consist of many joined monosaccharides (i.e. they are polymers) | $(C_{12}H_{22}O_{11})_n$ | Starch<br>Glycogen<br>Cellulose | Insoluble; used as food store in plants (starch) or animals (glycogen); used as structural material in plants (cellulose) |

Carbohydrates are broken down during digestion and rebuilt for energy storage and structural needs. The interrelationships of glucose metabolism are shown in Figure 18.18. There are four important processes:

1. Glycolysis: strictly speaking the chemists' definition refers to the anaerobic breakdown of glucose to lactate, but the term is, in medical use, extended to cover aerobic metabolism as well. Anaerobic glycolysis occurs in erythrocytes, the renal medulla, and for short periods of high demand in skeletal muscles. Aerobic breakdown occurs in the central nervous system, skeletal muscle, and most other organs.
2. Gluconeogenesis: this occurs in the liver and the renal cortex, and is the synthesis of glucose from non-sugars (i.e. amino acids, lactate, and glycerol).
3. Glycogenolysis: this is the process by which glycogen is broken down to glucose.
4. Glycogenesis: this is the process of glycogen formation in liver and muscle. Unlike the liver, the glycogen stored in muscle is for the exclusive use of the muscle itself. Glycogen is a long, branching molecule that consists of glucose residues linked together (Figure 18.19)

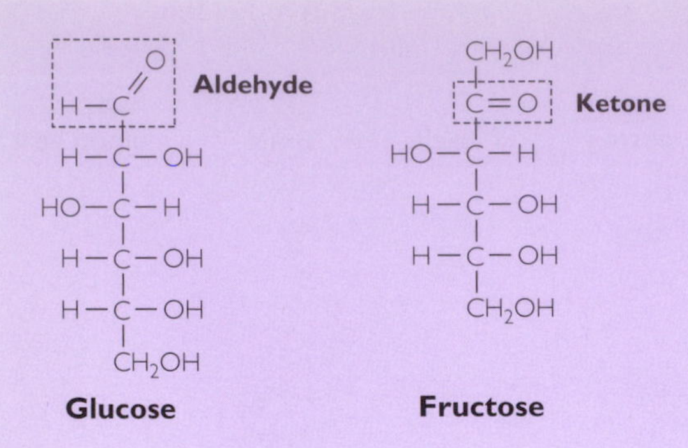


**Figure 18.14** The comparison of glucose (an aldose sugar) with fructose (a ketose sugar).

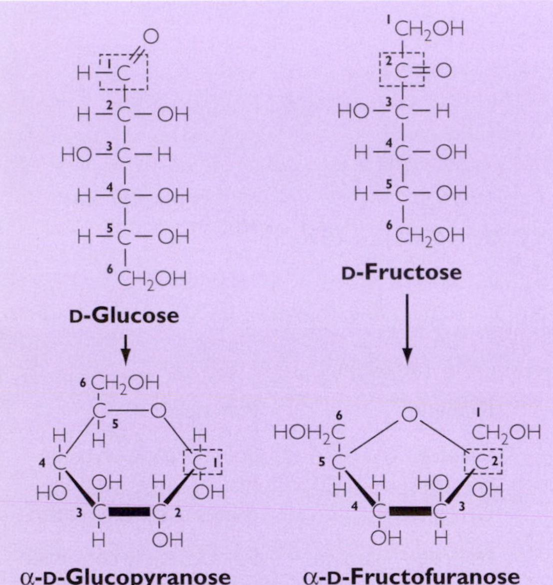


**Figure 18.15** Six-membered (pyranose) and five-membered (furanose) forms of a hexose sugar. The dotted lines around the carbon atom indicate the method of ring formation. The carbon atom that forms the ring is called the anomeric carbon.

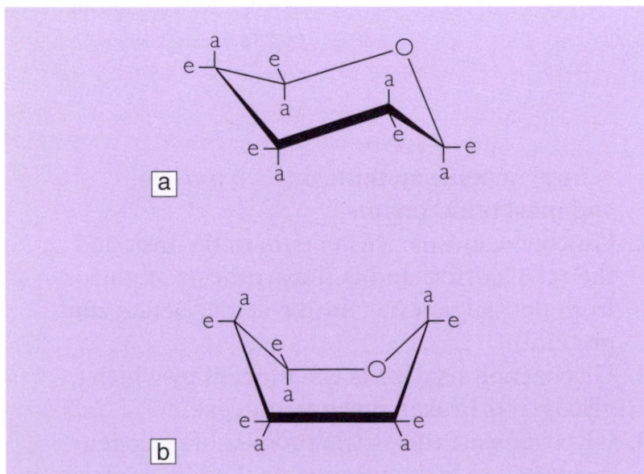


**Figure 18.16** (a) Chair and (b) boat forms of the pyranose ring. Substituents (a) are essentially perpendicular to the plane of the ring whereas equatorial substituents (e) are parallel.

### *Lipids*

Lipids, like carbohydrates, contain carbon, hydrogen, and oxygen but the relative amount of oxygen is low. The words lipids, fats, and oils are rather inexact terms, which describe a set of compounds that are characterized by being insoluble in water but soluble in many organic solvents. Fats are solid at room temperature; oils are liquids. Lipids can be classified as in Table 18.11.

When complexed with more polar compounds, the resulting molecule may have both hydrophilic and hydrophobic regions. Such compounds are often found at the interface between lipids and water, e.g. cell membranes, or at the surface of chylomicrons, e.g. bile salts.

The principal roles of lipids are:

- forming part of cell membranes;
- provision of energy by aerobic metabolism;
- storing energy in the form of fat where it also protects and insulates.

As a result of their hydrophobicity, lipids have to be carried in the blood by attachment to more polar compounds (usually proteins), or enclosed within a hydrophilic envelope (chylomicrons). These lipid-carrying components within the blood are classified by centrifugal separation. This is shown diagrammatically in Figure 18.20 and the properties of each layer are described in Table 18.12.

#### *Fatty acids*

These are straight aliphatic chains with a methyl group at one end and a carbonyl group at the other (Figure 18.21). In humans, most fatty acids have an even number of carbon atoms, usually 16, 18, or 20. Saturated fatty acids have no double bonds, monounsaturates have one double bond, and polyunsaturates have two or more double bonds (Figure 18.22). Fatty acids in the plasma are also called free fatty acids and non-esterified fatty acids.

#### *Triglycerides*

Triglycerides (triacylglycerols) are the major source of fat in the diet and the major storage lipid in adipose cells. They are formed from a condensation of three fatty acids (usually not all the same) (Figure 18.23) and broken down by hydrolysis.

After ingestion, the action of lipases in the gut is to cleave the fatty acids from positions 1 and 3 of the glycerol molecule, leaving a monoglyceride (2-monoacylglycerol). The monoglyceride and the fatty acids are absorbed by the intestinal cells and reassembled into triglycerides for transport as chylomicrons. A summary of the utilization of triglycerides and fatty acids after a meal is shown in Figure 18.24.

#### *Phospholipids*

Phospholipids (phosphoacylglycerols) have a substituted phosphate group at position 3. The most common is lecithin (phosphatidylcholine), shown in Figure 18.25, which is a major component of cell membranes (see later). The presence of a phosphoryl group creates a molecule with a hydrophilic 'head' and two lipid 'tails'.

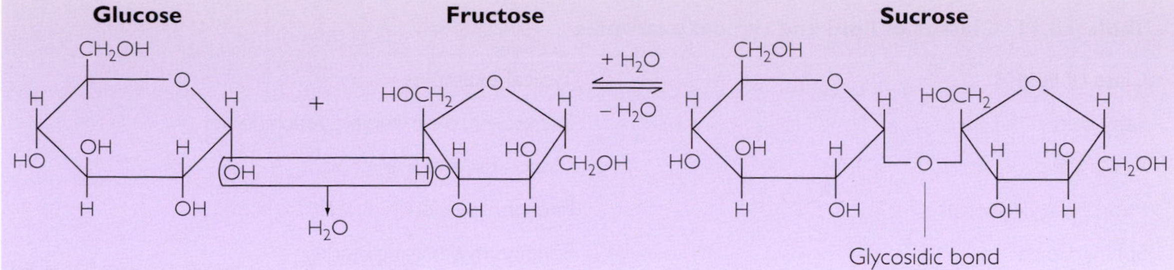


**Figure 18.17** The breakdown and formation of a disaccharide by hydrolysis.

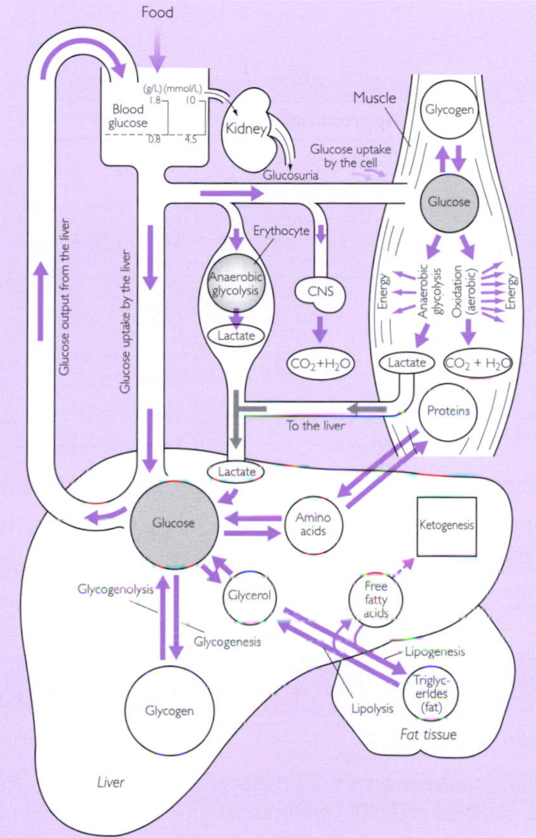


**Figure 18.18** The interrelationships of glucose metabolism in various organs. (Adapted from Despopoulos A and Silbernagi S. *Colour Atlas of Physiology*, 4th edn. New York: Thieme, 1991, 247.)

*Cholesterol*

This is a steroid. Steroids are a group of substances that contain a structure with four rings, which together are called the steroid nucleus. In naturally occurring steroids, virtually all the rings are in the 'chair' form (see Figure 18.16) which is the more stable configuration.

Cholesterol, which is manufactured from acetyl-Coenzyme A, is shown in Figure 18.26. The 3-hydroxyl group allows it to react with acids, forming cholesterol esters. Cholesterol adds stability to the phospholipid bilayer of membranes (see later), and serves as the precursor for bile salts (see Chapter 28) and steroid hormones (see Chapter 29).

***Proteins***

Proteins consist of long chains of amino acids; the basic formula of the latter is shown in Figure 18.27. The nature of the R group determines the amino acid. Amino acids contain carbon, hydrogen, oxygen, nitrogen, and in some cases sulphur or phosphorus.

There are 20 amino acids used to form proteins: ten are termed 'essential' because the carbon skeleton cannot be synthesized by the body and they have to be ingested. Amino acids relevant to human metabolism are listed in Table 18.13.

Nine of the non-essential amino acids can be synthesized from glucose. Tyrosine is synthesized from phenylalanine.

Two amino acids may be linked together by a condensation reaction to form a covalent peptide bond. This is shown in Figure 18.28. Peptide bonds are very stable and chemical hydrolysis requires extreme condi-

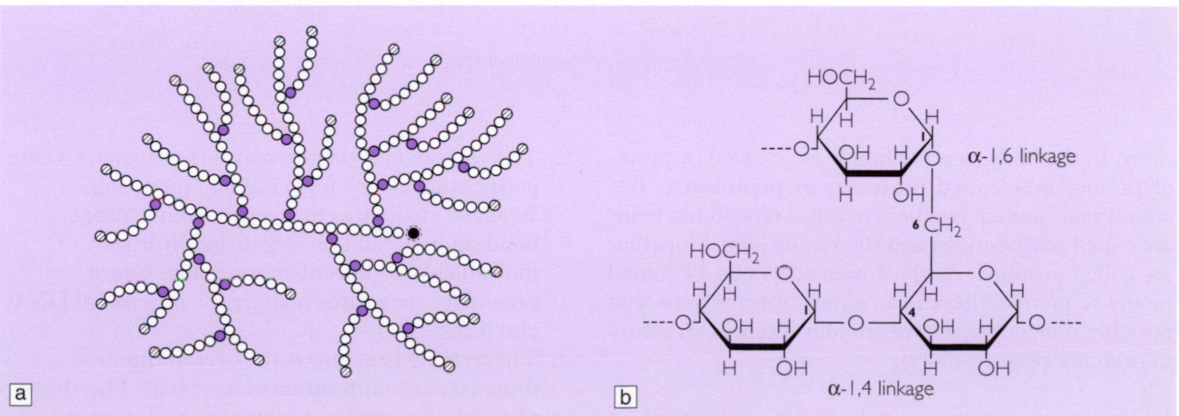


**Figure 18.19** The structure of (a) glycogen and (b) the α-1,4 and α-1,6 linkages between glucose residues. Glucose residue linked (○) α-1,4 and (●) α-1,6; (●) reducing end; (⊘) non-reducing ends.

**Table 18.11 Classes of lipid and typical examples**

| Class of lipid | Typical examples |
|---|---|
| Fatty acid | Palmitoleic, oleic, linoleic, arachidonic[a] |
| Acylglycerols | Mono-, di-, and triglycerides |
| Phosphoacylglycerols | Phospholipids such as lecithin |
| Sphingolipids | Sphingomyelin, gangliosides |
| Eicosanoids[a] | Prostaglandins, thromboxane, leukotrienes |
| Steroids | Cholesterol |

[a]See Chapter 29.

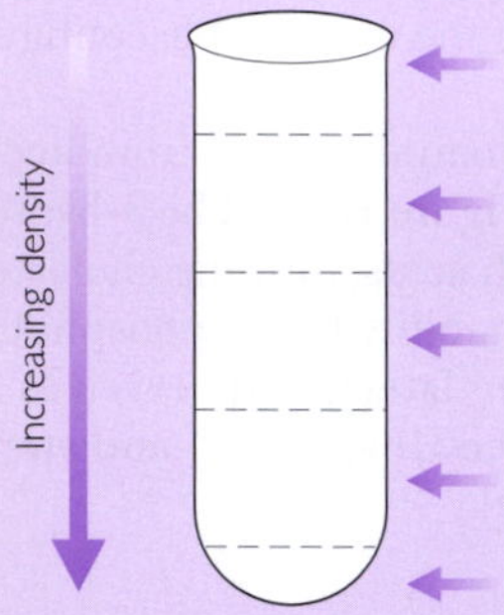

Increasing density

| Description | Approximate size | Life span |
|---|---|---|
| Chylomicrons | 100—1000 nm | Minutes |
| Very-low-density lipoproteins (VLDLs) | 50 nm | Up to 1 hour |
| Low-density lipoproteins (LDLs) | 20 nm | Days |
| High-density lipoproteins (HDLs) | 10 nm | Days |
| FFAs released from adipose tissue and carried as albumin—FFA complex | Molecular | Seconds—minutes |

**Figure 18.20** The lipid-carrying components in the blood and their classification following centrifugal separation. The free fatty acid (FFA) pool, which accounts for only 1–5% of the plasma lipids, is the most metabolically active. The properties of each layer are given in Table 18.12.

**Table 18.12 Blood lipoproteins**

| Lipoprotein | Source and function |
|---|---|
| Chylomicrons | Produced in intestinal epithelial cells from dietary fat<br>Carry triglycerides in blood (80–90% of content) |
| Very-low-density lipoprotein (VLDL) | Produced in liver mainly from dietary carbohydrate<br>Carries triglycerides in blood (50–60% of content) |
| Low-density lipoprotein (LDL) | Contains high concentration of cholesterol and cholesterol esters<br>Endocytosed by liver and peripheral tissues |
| High-density lipoprotein (HDL) | Produced in liver and intestines<br>Functions in the return of cholesterol from peripheral tissues to the liver.<br>Exchanges proteins and lipids with other lipoproteins |

tions. In the body, peptide bonds are cleaved by proteolytic enzymes called proteases or peptidases. Two amino acids joined together are called dipeptides, many are called polypeptides and thousands joined together are called proteins. As the amino acids may be joined in any sequence, there is an almost infinite variety of possible molecules. There are four levels of structure in proteins (Figure 18.29):

1. The *primary structure* is the linear sequence of amino acids linked together by peptide bonds. Branching of chains does not occur.
2. The *secondary structure* consists of regions where polypeptide chains form regular, recurring, localized structures that result from hydrogen bonding between the oxygen and hydrogen molecules on different amino acids. These secondary structures include the α helix (of DNA) and β sheets.
3. The *tertiary structure* is the overall three-dimensional composition of a protein. The shape of a globular protein involves interactions with amino acids widely separated on the primary structure. These interactions include

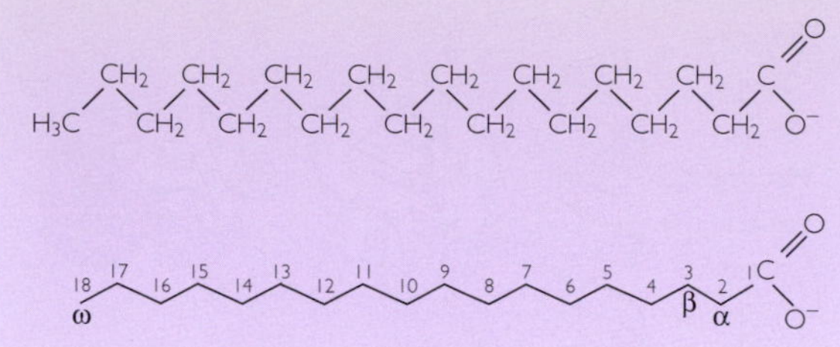


**Figure 18.21** Stearic acid, a typical fatty acid. The molecular nomenclature of fatty acids is described in Appendix 18.1.

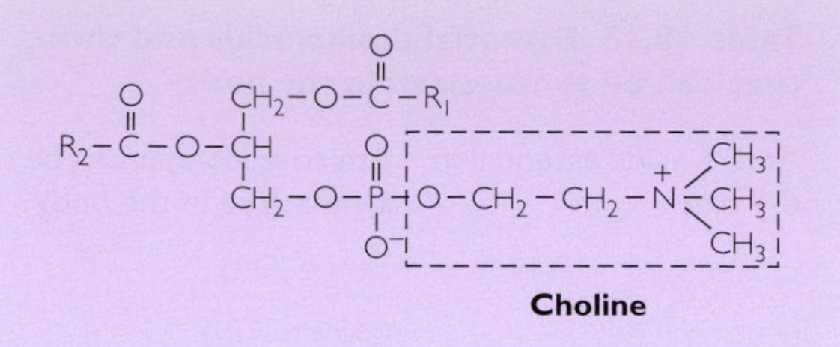


**Figure 18.25** Phosphatidylcholine, a typical phospholipid. The addition of the choline molecule produces a polar component to the otherwise non-polar molecule.

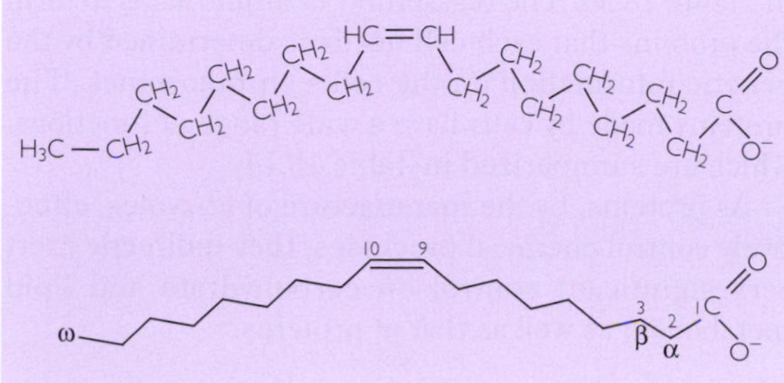


**Figure 18.22** Oleic acid, a monounsaturated fatty acid with a double bond.

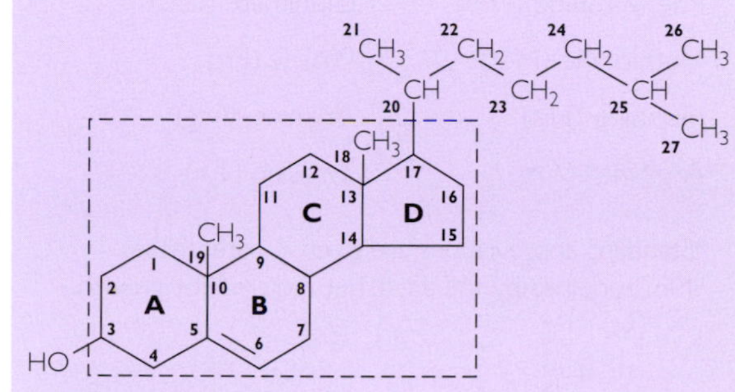


**Figure 18.26** Cholesterol: the steroid nucleus is shown outlined. The conventional numbering system for the carbon atoms is also given.

$CH_2OH$ — $CHOH$ — $CH_2OH$ + 3 Fatty acids → (Condensation) / ← (Hydrolysis) $CH_2O$ — Fatty acid, $CHO$ — Fatty acid, $CH_2O$ — Fatty acid + $3H_2O$

**(Glycerol)** **(Triglyceride)**

**Figure 18.23** The formation of a triglyceride molecule from glycerol and fatty acids.

Amino group | Carboxyl group | Side chain

**Figure 18.27** The basic formula of an amino acid.

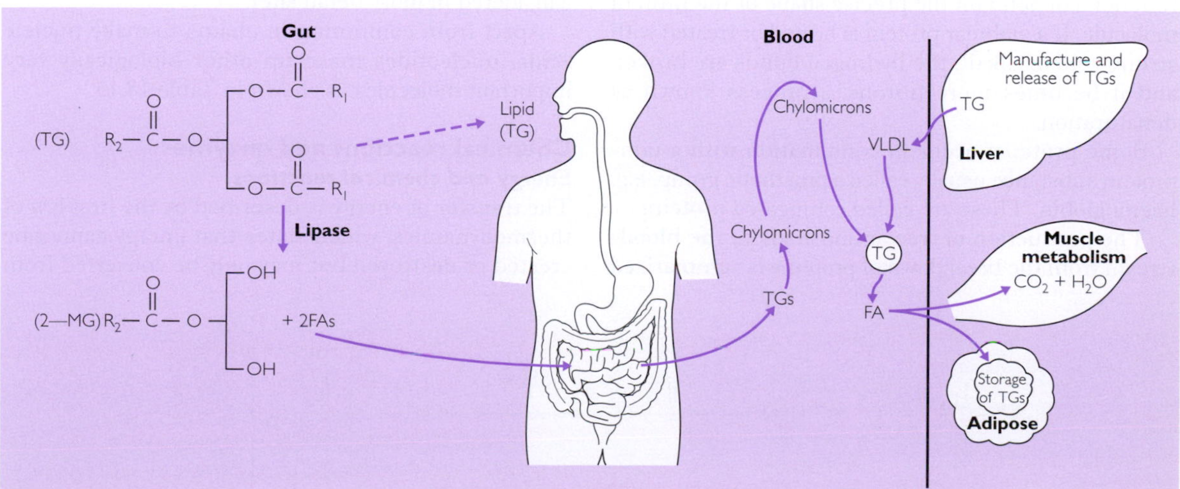


**Figure 18.24** The utilization of triglycerides and fatty acids after a meal. TG, triglyceride; 2-MG, monoglyceride; FA, fatty acid; (TG), triglycerides in VLDL and chylomicrons.

**Table 18.13 Essential amino acids and those that can be synthesized in the body**[a]

| Amino acids essential in the diet | Amino acids that can be synthesized in the body |
|---|---|
| Lysine (Lys) | Serine (Ser) |
| Leucine (Leu) | Glycine (Gly) |
| Isoleucine (Ile) | Cysteine (Cys) |
| Threonine (Thr) | Alanine (Ala) |
| Valine (Val) | Aspartate (Asp) |
| Tryptophan (Trp) | Asparagine (Asn) |
| Phenylalanine (Phe) | Glutamate (Glu) |
| Methionine (Met) | Proline (Pro) |
| Histidine (His) | Arginine (Arg) |
| Arginine[b] (Arg) | Tyrosine (Tyr) |

[a]Standard abbreviations are given in parentheses.
[b]Not required by the adult, but required for growth.

hydrophobic, electrostatic, and hydrogen bonds, together with covalent disulphide linkages between the cysteine residues. Proteins tend to fold so that their peptides are packed close together. Hydrophobic amino acids tend to collect in the interior of globular proteins with hydrophilic amino acids on the surface, thereby allowing aqueous solubility.

4. The *quaternary structure* is the three-dimensional structure of a protein composed of multiple tertiary subunits. These subunits are held together by similar forces that form the tertiary structure.

Some proteins have long parallel chains with multiple cross-links. These are the fibrous proteins, e.g. collagen in cartilage, keratin in hair, actin and myosin in muscle. Most proteins are, however, globular and these form all enzymes and some hormones. Their functions depend on the precise shape of the protein molecule. If a globular protein is heated or treated with strong acid or alkali, the hydrogen bonds are broken and it becomes more fibrous, a process known as denaturation.

Some proteins occur in combination with a non-protein substance usually called a prosthetic group, e.g. haemoglobin. These are called conjugated proteins.

The production of free amino acids in the bloodstream from the breakdown of proteins is summarized in Figure 18.30. The reassembly of amino acids to form the proteins that each cell needs is determined by the genetic information on the cell's chromosomes. The proteins made by cells have a wide range of functions, which are summarized in Table 18.14.

As proteins, by the manufacture of enzymes, effectively control chemical processes, they indirectly exert very significant control on carbohydrate and lipid metabolism as well as that of proteins.

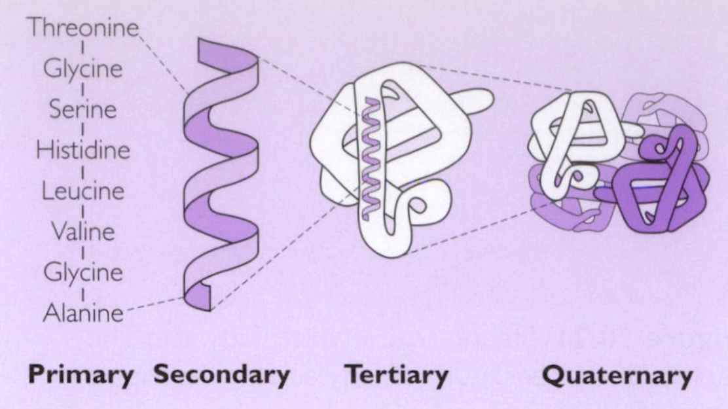


**Figure 18.29** The levels of structure in a protein.

### *Nucleic acids*

There are two main nucleic acids: ribonucleic acid (RNA) and deoxyribonucleic acid (DNA). They are of large molecular mass and composed of units called nucleotides. Each nucleotide comprises three parts:

- phosphoric acid (phosphate) – $H_3PO_4$;
- a pentose sugar – either ribose ($C_5H_{10}O_5$) or deoxyribose ($C_5H_{10}O_4$);
- an organic base – a pyrimidine (single-ring structure), e.g. cytosine, thymine, or uracil, or a purine (double-ring structure), e.g. adenine or guanine.

The basic structure of a nucleotide is shown in Figure 18.31. The bases are not involved in the sugar phosphate back bone and are therefore free to interact with other bases or proteins. A portion of an RNA molecule is shown in block diagram form in Figure 18.32. Because of their importance, DNA and RNA are considered in more detail later.

Apart from combining in chains to make nucleic acids, nucleotides make up other biologically very important molecules as shown in Table 18.15.

## Chemical reactions and enzymes

### *Energy and chemical reactions*

The transfer of energy is described by the first law of thermodynamics, which states that energy cannot be created or destroyed but may only be converted from

$$H_3N^+-\underset{R_1}{\overset{H}{C}}-\overset{O}{\overset{\|}{C}}-O^- + H_3N^+-\underset{H}{\overset{R_2}{C}}-\overset{O}{\overset{\|}{C}}-O^- \xrightleftharpoons{H_2O} H_3N^+-\underset{R_1}{\overset{H}{C}}-\overset{O}{\overset{\|}{C}}-\underset{H}{N}-\underset{H}{\overset{R_2}{C}}-\overset{O}{\overset{\|}{C}}-O^-$$

Peptide bond

**Figure 18.28** The formation of a peptide bond between two amino acids.

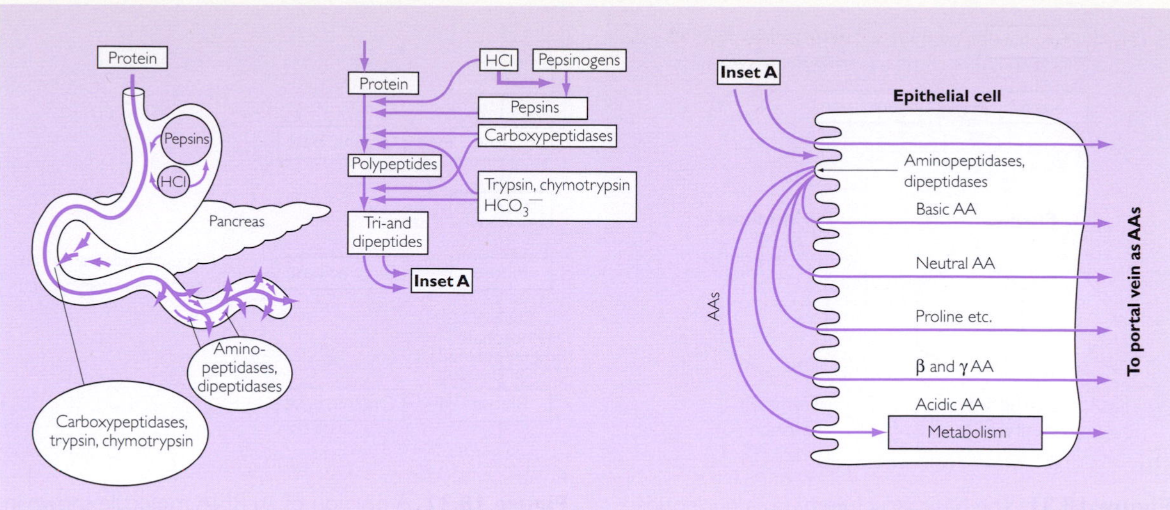


**Figure 18.30** The production of free amino acids and oligopeptides from the digestion of proteins. AA, amino acid. (Adapted from Despopoulos A and Silbernagi S. *Colour Atlas of Physiology*, 4th edn. New York: Thieme, 1991, 225.)

**Table 18.14 The functions of proteins**

| Physiological activity | Protein example | Function |
|---|---|---|
| Nutrition | Digestive enzymes, e.g. | |
| | Trypsin | Catalyses the hydrolysis of proteins to polypeptides |
| | Amylase | Catalyses the hydrolysis of starch to maltose |
| | Lipase | Catalyses the hydrolysis of fats to fatty acids and glycerol |
| | Storage compounds e.g. | |
| | Ovalbumin | Storage of protein in egg white |
| | Casein | Storage of protein in milk |
| Respiration and transport | Haemoglobin | Transport of oxygen |
| | Myoglobin | Interacts with oxygen in muscle |
| | Prothrombin/fibrinogen | Required for the clotting of blood |
| | Mucin | Keeps respiratory surface moist |
| Defence | Antibodies | Essential to the defence of the body, e.g. against bacterial invasion |
| Growth and metabolism | Thyroxine | Controls growth and metabolism |
| | Muscle protein | Energy source under severe starvation |
| Excretion | Enzymes | Catalyse reactions in protein, fat, and carbohydrate breakdown, urea cycle, drug handling, renal tubules |
| Support and movement | Actin/myosin | Needed for muscle contraction |
| | Ossein | Structural support in bone |
| | Collagen | Gives strength with flexibility in tendons and cartilage |
| | Elastin | Gives strength and elasticity to ligaments |
| | Keratin | Tough for protection, e.g. hair, nails, skin |
| Internal environment | Hormones, e.g. | |
| | Insulin/glucagon | Control blood sugar level |
| | Vasopressin | Controls blood pressure |
| | Rhodopsin/opsin | Visual pigments in the retina, sensitive to light |
| Reproduction | Hormones, e.g. | |
| | Prolactin | Induces milk production in mammals |
| | Chromatin | Gives structural support to chromosomes |

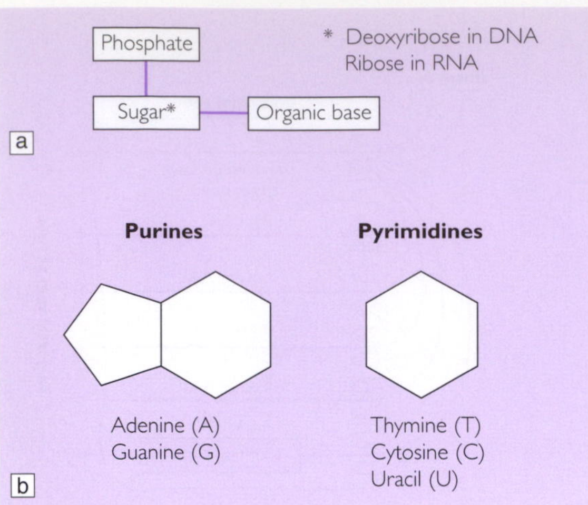


**Figure 18.31** The basic structure of (a) a nucleotide and (b) the organic bases that can be part of the nucleotide molecule.

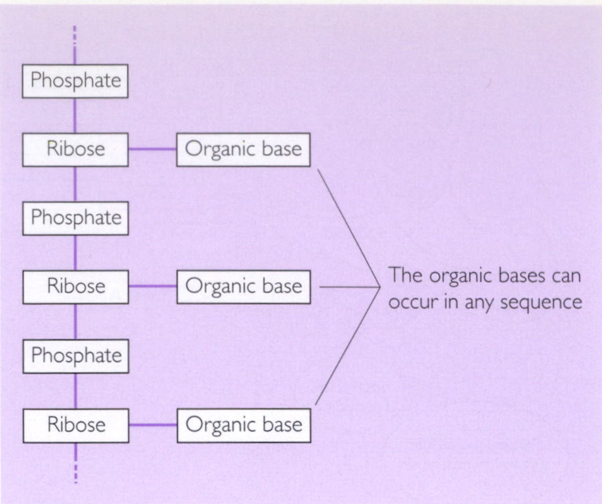


**Figure 18.32** A portion of an RNA molecule shown in diagrammatic form. The organic bases can occur in any sequence.

**Table 18.15 Biologically active molecules which are nucleotides**

| Nucleotide | Abbreviation | Function |
|---|---|---|
| Adenosine monophosphate<br>Adenosine diphosphate<br>Adenosine triphosphate | AMP<br>ADP<br>ATP | Molecules important in making energy available to cells for metabolic activities, osmotic work, muscular contractions, etc. |
| Nicotinamide adenine dinucleotide<br>Flavine adenine dinucleotide | NAD<br>FAD | Electron (hydrogen) carriers important in respiration in transferring hydrogen atoms from the tricarboxylate cycle along the respiratory chain |
| Nicotinamide adenine dinucleotide phosphate | NADP | Necessary for fatty acid synthesis, pentose phosphate pathway, and glucose 6-phosphate control |
| Coenzyme A | CoA | Coenzyme important in respiration in combining with pyruvate to form acetyl-CoA and transferring the acetyl group into the tricarboxylate cycle |

one form to another. Some molecules, e.g. ATP (see Figure 18.8), are designed to contain energy in the form of chemical bonds that can be easily accessed by a large number of substrates. To create a molecule of ATP requires the provision of excess energy over the basal energy levels of its components ADP and $P_i$. This must come from an external source.

There is a tendency in reactions that occur spontaneously for energy to be released, so that the total internal energy of the products is less than that of the reactants. The energy released is, however, now in a form that is less usable and may be difficult to recover (e.g. light emission or heat). These spontaneous reactions decrease the 'orderliness' of the chemical system and increase its randomness or disorder. The degree of disorder is measured by the quantity known as entropy, which is described and defined in the second law of thermodynamics (see Chapter 38).

The question may then be asked: if entropy tends to increase, why do all substances not breakdown continuously? Some do, of course, but most do not. This is because, although the products of a reaction may have less internal chemical energy and greater entropy than the constituents, a small amount of energy, called the activation energy, is required to produce the conditions to allow them to react. This is shown graphically in Figure 18.33.

To reverse the reaction and re-form the original reactants from the products requires more specialized conditions, with the provision of higher levels of available free energy to overcome the activation energy. This is apparent from Figure 18.33, where the direction the reaction takes depends on the free (usable) energy available and the concentration of reactants and products.

Chemical reactions that occur within a living organism are called metabolism. They are divided into two types:

1. Anabolism is the build-up of complex molecules from simple ones: it usually consumes energy, i.e. Figure 18.33 goes to the left.

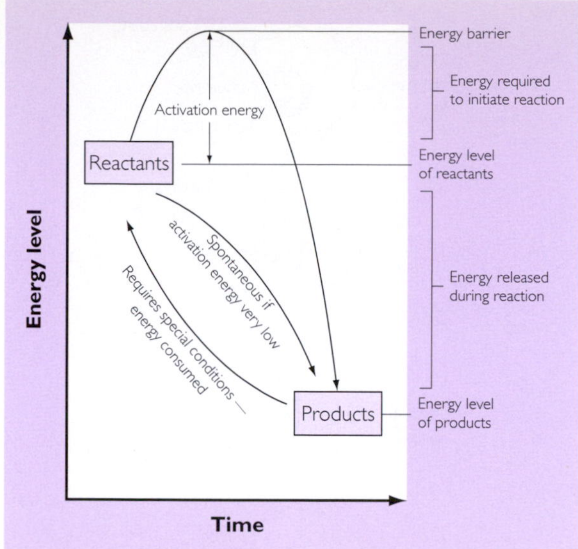


**Figure 18.33** The activation energy of a chemical reaction.

2. Catabolism is the breakdown of complex chemicals into simple ones: it usually releases energy, i.e. Figure 18.33 goes to the right.

***Enzymes and their function***

Enzymes are biological catalysts that alter the rate of a reaction, after which they themselves are unchanged. The vast majority are large globular proteins, although a few (known as ribosomes) are composed of RNA. Enzymes are made by protein synthesis within cells. Extracellular enzymes are secreted outside the cell where they have their effect (e.g. digestion in gut cavity by amylase, lipase, etc.). Intracellular enzymes are retained within the cell (e.g. respiratory enzymes on mitochondria). Different cellular organelles carry different sets of enzymes. These are summarized in Table 18.16. The organelles themselves are described later.

The effect of enzymes on chemical reactions is dramatic and they can increase the rate of reaction by up to $10^{10}$ times or more. This can be put into perspective by considering a bottle of wine. After it has finished fermenting and is put in cellar to mature, under non-enzymatic conditions, a good claret can take 20 years to reach its peak. Were it possible to do this with an enzyme, the time would fall to less than 75 ms. This would perhaps reduce its charm, but be a great investment for venture capitalists. An alternative approach is to consider volume. If the products of a reaction lasting 1 min were equal to the volume of a standard wine bottle (0.75 L), in the same minute the presence of an enzyme would increase the volume to that of a small lake 7.5 metres deep with a surface area of 1 square kilometre! That these changes are of such magnitude makes the biochemistry of life possible and emphasizes the dramatic results of enzyme malfunction or absence.

Enzymes achieve this enormous increase in the rate of reaction by lowering the activation energy, as shown in Figure 18.34. One way of looking at this is to say that they allow reactions to take place at much lower temperatures than would be the case without them. The way in which enzymes reduce the activation energy required for a spontaneous reaction is demonstrated pictorially in Figure 18.35. It can be seen from this that the active site provides a match for the substrate to attach to and, although the enzyme may undergo an intermediate transitional change, at the end it is returned to its original structure. Figure 18.35 shows an enzyme breaking a substrate down into two smaller components. Had the situation been different, with a large excess of smaller components, the reaction would have progressed in the reverse direction.

***The naming of enzymes***

Enzymes are classified and named in two ways: systematically and with a common or trivial name. The systematic classification, approved internationally, recognizes six major groups according to the type of reaction catalysed. These are shown in Table 18.17.

Common names are shorter than systematic ones and are more convenient. Glucokinase, the enzyme in which kinase refers to the transfer of a phosphate group from ATP to glucose, is formally known as ATP : D-glucose-6-phosphotransferase. All formal names end in -ase and so do most common names. There are, however, some exceptions, e.g. chymotrypsin, which is the common name for peptidyl hydrolase or protease.

***Characteristics of enzymes***

The following are the characteristics of enzymes.

**Table 18.16 The location of metabolic activity within the cell**

| Metabolic process | Organelles involved in process |
|---|---|
| Tricarboxylic acid cycle (acetyl-CoA → $CO_2$ + $H_2O$) | Mitochondria |
| β-Oxidation of fatty acids | Mitochondria |
| Ketone body formation | Mitochondria (liver) |
| Ketone body utilization | Mitochondria (muscle, kidney; not liver) |
| Lipogenesis (glucose → fatty acids) | Cytosol and mitochondria (mainly liver) |
| Gluconeogenesis (lactate → glucose) | Cytosol and mitochondria (liver) |
| Glycogen metabolism (synthesis and degradation) | Cytosol |
| Lactate production (glucose → lactate) | Cytosol |

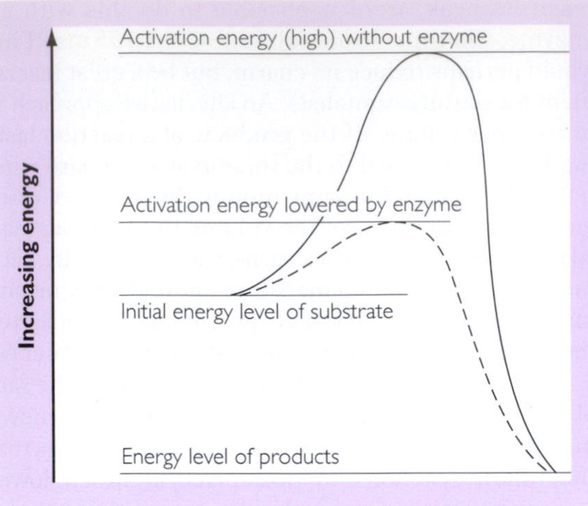


**Figure 18.34** The reduction of activation energy by the presence of an enzyme.

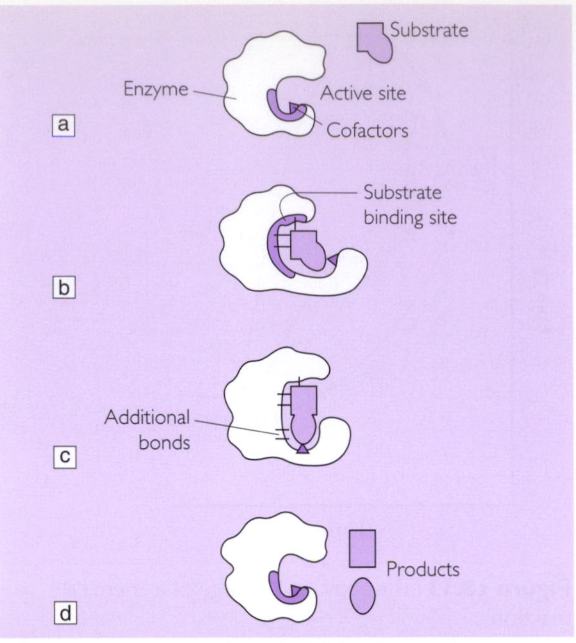


**Figure 18.35** The role of the active site in an enzyme-catalysed reaction. (a) Free enzyme; (b) enzyme–substrate complex; (c) transition state complex; (d) original enzyme with substrate split into products.

*Specificity*

Each enzyme is specific to only one reaction and is frequently limited to specific molecules rather than molecules of a class of compounds. An example of this is that separate enzymes are used by glucose and galactose.

*Reversibility*

Enzymes do not alter the equilibrium of a reaction, only the speed at which it is reached. They catalyse forward and reverse reactions equally. The direction of reaction is determined by the proportional supplies of substrate, the pH, and the available energy. A good example of this is carbonic anhydrase working in the tissues and the lungs:

$$CO_2 + H_2O \xrightarrow[\text{(Tissues)}]{\text{Lower pH}} H_2CO_3$$

$$CO_2 + H_2O \xleftarrow[\text{(Lungs)}]{\text{Higher pH}} H_2CO_3$$

**Table 18.17 Enzyme classification**

| Enzyme group | Reaction catalysed | Examples |
|---|---|---|
| 1. Oxidoreductases | All reactions of the oxidation–reduction type<br>Transfer of electrons (as an $e^-$, hydrogen atoms, or hydride ion) from one compound to an acceptor | Dehydrogenases, oxidases |
| 2. Transferases | The transfer of a group from one substrate to another, e.g. a functional group, such as an acetyl, amino, methyl, or phosphate group | Transaminases, phosphorylases |
| 3. Hydrolases | Hydrolytic reactions<br>Cleavage of a C–O, C–N, or C–S bond by the addition of water across it | Phosphates, peptidases, amidases, lipases |
| 4. Lyases | Additions to a double bond or removal of a group from a substrate without hydrolysis, often leaving a compound containing a double bond | Decarboxylases |
| 5. Isomerases | Reactions where the net result is an intramolecular rearrangement, i.e. transfer of groups within molecule to yield isomeric forms | All-*trans*-retinal converted to all-*cis*-retinal |
| 6. Ligases | The formation of bonds between two substrate molecules using energy derived from the cleavage of a pyrophosphate bond such as ATP, e.g. formation of C–C, C–S, C–O, and C–N bonds | Acetyl CoA carboxylase<br>Glutamine synthetase |

*pH dependence*

The effective functioning of an enzyme depends on its shape and hence on the characteristics of binding between proteins, which is determined in part by ionic and hydrogen bonding. Such bonds are very dependent on the concentration of $H^+$ ions and hence the pH. Enzymes are designed to work optimally at their own environmental pH. An example of this, comparing pepsin and amylase, is shown in Figure 18.36.

*Temperature dependence*

As the temperature increases, the molecules move faster, their internal energy is high, and collisions leading to reactions are more likely. Consequently, as the temperature increases, the substrates are more likely to meet the enzyme and the rate of reaction increases. However, together with the likelihood of a reaction occurring as temperature increases, the more likely it is that the hydrogen and ionic bonds, which hold the enzyme in its particular shape, will be broken. The molecular structure is then disrupted and the enzyme ceases to function because the active site no longer accommodates the substrates. The enzyme is then said to be denatured. The conflicting effects of these influences is shown in Figure 18.37.

### *The rate of reaction*

If an enzyme is working in its optimal environment, the rate of reaction depends on both the enzyme and the substrate concentrations.

*Enzyme concentration*

Enzymes, even at very low concentration, function efficiently because they can be used again and again. Provided that there is an excess of substrate, an increase in enzyme concentration will lead to a corresponding increase in the rate of reaction, until the supply of substrate becomes limiting. This is shown graphically in Figure 18.38. Conversly, when the substrate is in short supply and there is unused enzyme, it is clear that an increase in enzyme concentration will have no effect.

*Substrate concentration*

Variation in substrate availability is the most common situation in clinical practice. The graphic representation of increasing the substrate concentration in the presence of a fixed enzyme concentration is shown in Figure 18.39. The Michaelis constant ($K_m$, a rate constant specific for the enzyme–substrate–product combination) is defined as the substrate concentration that produces half the maximum possible rate of reaction ($V_{max}$).

With a fixed enzyme concentration, an initial increase in substrate concentration will immediately find enzyme with which to interact. When this substrate concentration is doubled, there will be twice the number of enzyme molecules occupied. Consequently, the rate of reaction is initially proportional to the concentration of substrate. This is the situation known as first-order kinetics, defined because the rate of reaction is proportional to the substrate concentration. This relationship is an underlying assumption of the majority of pharmacokinetic theory as described in Chapter 19. Most anaesthetic and anaesthetically related drugs are assumed to undergo

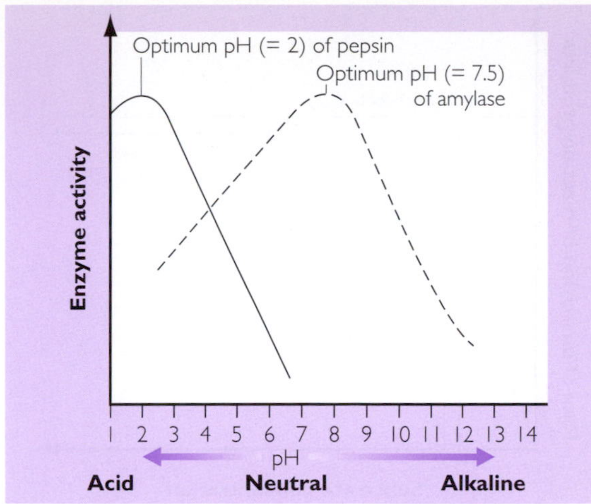


**Figure 18.36** The effect of pH on the activity of pepsin and amylase.

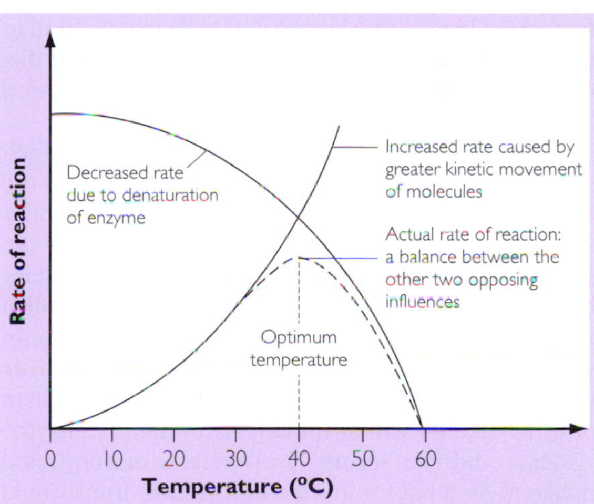


**Figure 18.37** The effect of temperature on an enzyme-catalysed reaction.

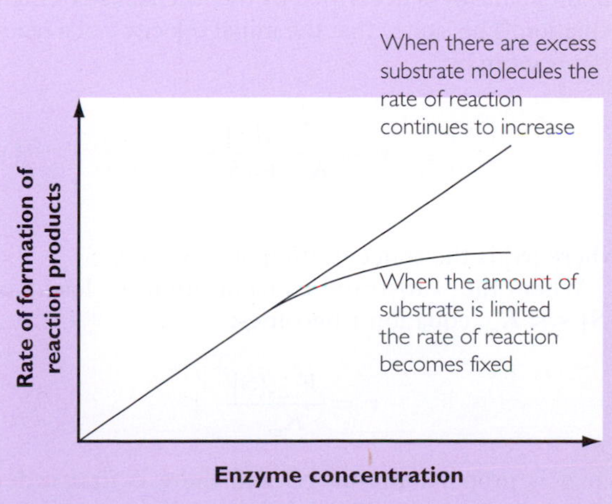


**Figure 18.38** The effect of enzyme concentration on the rate of production of reaction products in the presence of limited and excess substrate molecules.

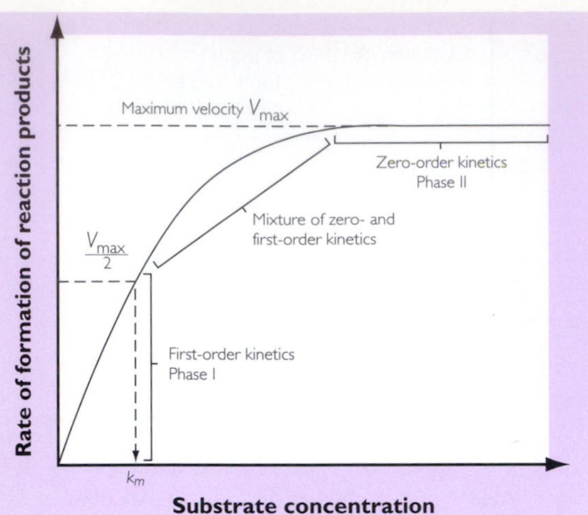


**Figure 18.39** The effect of substrate concentration on the rate of production of reaction products, assuming that the enzyme concentration is constant. $K_m$, the Michaelis constant.

first-order kinetic breakdown and to be metabolized in the presence of excess enzymes. Deviations from this model in terms of drug metabolism are considered later in Chapter 19.

The other form of limiting condition is that which occurs when the substrate concentration exceeds the capacity of the enzymes present (Figure 18.39). Under these conditions, whatever the concentration of the substrate the rate of formation of product is constant because all the enzyme is in use. This situation is called zero-order kinetics because there is no dependency on substrate concentration, i.e. the rate of reaction is constant. The best example of this is the metabolism of ethyl alcohol which quickly saturates its enzyme systems and the serum levels rise with continued intake. Were it not for this feature, getting drunk would be very difficult! Zero-order kinetics can be achieved by any drug that saturates its metabolic pathway enzymes: a situation that is often termed 'accumulation'. Infusions of thiopentone (thiopental) are a good example of this.

The curve shown in Figure 18.39 when analysed mathematically is described by the Michaelis–Menten equation. This states that the initial velocity $v$ of a reaction is given by:

$$v = \frac{V_{max}[S]}{K_m + [S]} \qquad (1)$$

where $[S]$ is the concentration of substrate.

When the substrate concentration is low, i.e. $[S] << K_m$, equation 1 becomes:

$$v = \frac{V_{max}[S]}{K_m}$$

i.e. $v$ is proportional to $[S]$ and there is first-order kinetic behaviour. When $[S] >> K_m$, equation 1 becomes:

$$v = V_{max}$$

i.e. $v$ is independent of $[S]$, and there is zero-order kinetic behaviour.

Isoenzymes are different enzymes capable of catalysing the same reaction. They do not all have the same $K_m$ and so consequently produce different rates of product. A good example of this is the family of hexokinase isoenzymes. Hexokinase I, found in the erythrocyte, and hexokinase IV (better known as glucokinase), found in the liver, are compared in Figure 18.40. It can be seen from this that, at 6.5 mmol/L, glucokinase is working at 50% of its maximum velocity whereas hexokinase is already fully saturated.

A common mathematical transformation to make $K_m$ easier to measure graphically is to perform the Lineweaver–Burke transformation. This produces a reciprocal of equation (1) such that:

$$\frac{1}{v} = \frac{K_m + [S]}{V_{max}[S]} \qquad (2)$$

which, on simplification, results in:

$$\frac{1}{v} = \frac{K_m}{V_{max}[S]} + \frac{1}{V_{max}} \qquad (3)$$

This describes a straight line relationship of the type $y = ax + b$, with $y = 1/v$, $x = 1/[S]$, $a = K_m/V_{max}$ and $b = 1/V_{max}$. (See Chapter 37 for the properties of equations of the type: $y = ax + b$.)

When equation (3) is plotted it results in Figure 18.41. From it $K_m$ and $V_{max}$ can be determined from intercepts on the abscissa and ordinate respectively.

### *Cofactors and coenzymes*

A large number of enzymes require an additional component to carry out their function. The general term 'cofactor' encompasses these compounds. Cofactors are sometimes termed 'activators', e.g. $Cl^-$ ions are required for the activation of salivary amylase. Cofactors are metal or non-protein organic compounds that participate in the reaction, but are not a compo-

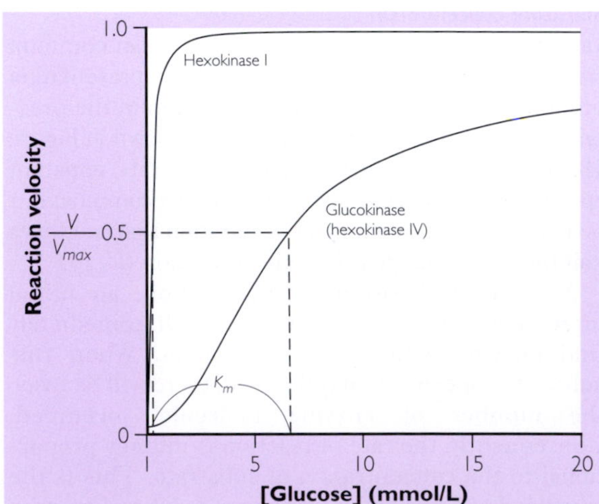


**Figure 18.40** A comparison of the two hexokinase isoenzymes, hexokinase I (found in the erythrocyte) and hexokinase IV (also called glucokinase, found in the liver). This demonstrates the importance of the value of the Michaelis constant ($K_m$) on reaction kinetics.

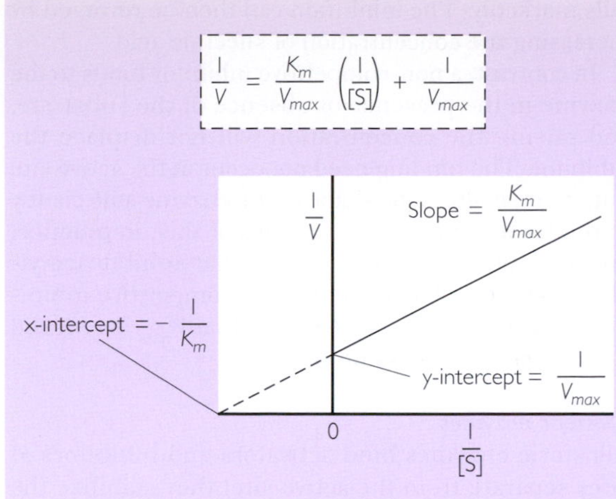


**Figure 18.41** Michaelis–Menten enzyme kinetics plotted after a Lineweaver–Burke transformation. $K_m$, the Michaelis constant; [S], substrate concentration; $v$, velocity; $V_{max}$, maximum rate of reaction.

nent of the substrate or products. They can be divided loosely into three groups:

1. Prosthetic groups, e.g. porphyrin moiety in haemoperoxidase. They are usually covalently bonded to the enzyme.
2. Metal activators, e.g. $K^+$, $Mn^{2+}$, $Mg^{2+}$, $Ca^{2+}$, or $Zn^{2+}$.
3. Coenzymes, which are small, heat-stable organic molecules.

Coenzymes are organic compounds that can be classified as either activation–transfer coenzymes or oxidation–reduction coenzymes (which transfer hydrogen ions). Most activation–transfer coenzymes are synthesized from vitamins, especially the B group, and oxidation–reduction coenzymes work with metals to transfer electrons to oxygen. Vitamins E and C are oxidation–reduction coenzymes that can also act as antioxidants.

It is often helpful to regard coenzymes almost as cosubstrates, because the changes in the coenzyme exactly counterbalance those taking place in the substrate, and hence their own changes may be of greater physiological significance. Examples of coenzyme are given in Table 18.18 and their mode of action is shown diagrammatically in Figure 18.42. Coenzyme A is often bound to acetate (acetyl-CoA) or succinate (succinyl-CoA) to enter metabolic pathways. Acetyl-Co-A is also a precursor of cholesterol.

**Table 18.18 Examples of coenzymes**

| Reduction–oxidation coenzymes | Transfer coenzymes |
|---|---|
| NAD | ATP, ADP, AMP |
| FAD | Coenzyme A |
| NADP | Vitamins of the B group |
| Vitamins C and E | Folate coenzymes |

#### ***Factors affecting enzyme performance and enzyme regulation***

The rate at which a particular enzyme forms its product is dependent on a number of factors, in addition to the quantity and intrinsic optimal function of the enzyme itself (pH, temperature, etc.) and the substrate concentration. These are now considered and for easy reference are listed in Table 18.19. The quantity of enzyme and the substrate concentration have been discussed above.

##### *Multi-substrate reactions*

Some enzymes, such as hexokinase, have more than one substrate and the binding of one facilitates the binding of the other. Often there is a preferred ordered sequence of substrate binding, and the first substrate changes the conformation of the enzyme in a way that permits the second substrate to bind

As a consequence of multi-substrate binding, the apparent value of $K_m$ and $V_{max}$ for one substrate will depend on the concentration of the cosubstrate. However, at a constant concentration of cosubstrate, the behaviour of the substrate under examination frequently generates a simple Michaelis–Menten curve for those given conditions.

##### *Competitive and non-competitive inhibition*

An inhibitor is a compound that decreases the velocity of a reaction by binding to the enzyme. All reaction products are reversible inhibitors of the enzymes that produce them if present in sufficient concentrations.

A competitive inhibitor which is not a reaction product competes with a substrate for binding at its substrate binding site, and binds to exactly the same form of the enzyme as does the substrate. It is usually a close structural analogue of the substrate with which it competes. Increases of substrate concentration can overcome competitive inhibition. When the substrate

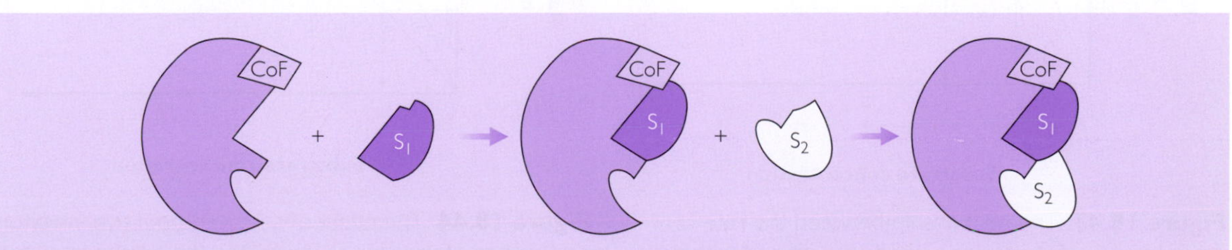


**Figure 18.42** A representation of the adsorption of a coenzyme (CoF) and two substrates ($S_1$ and $S_2$) to an enzyme to allow a reaction to occur. The coenzyme is assumed to carry a group essential for the binding of the first substrate which, in turn, facilitates the binding of the second.

**Table 18.19 Mechanisms of control of enzymatic reactions**

| |
|---|
| Quantity of enzyme |
| Concentration of substrate |
| Multisubstrate reactions |
| Competitive and non-competitive inhibition |
| Allosteric activation and inhibition |
| Phosphorylation |
| Modulator proteins |
| Product inhibition |

concentration is increased to a high enough level, the substrate-binding sites are occupied only by substrate and no inhibitor molecules can bind. Competitive inhibition increases the $K_m$ of the enzyme but not the $V_{max}$. These effects are shown on a Michaelis–Menten plot in Figure 18.43. An example of competitive inhibition is succinic dehydrogenase and its relationship with succinic and malonic acids.

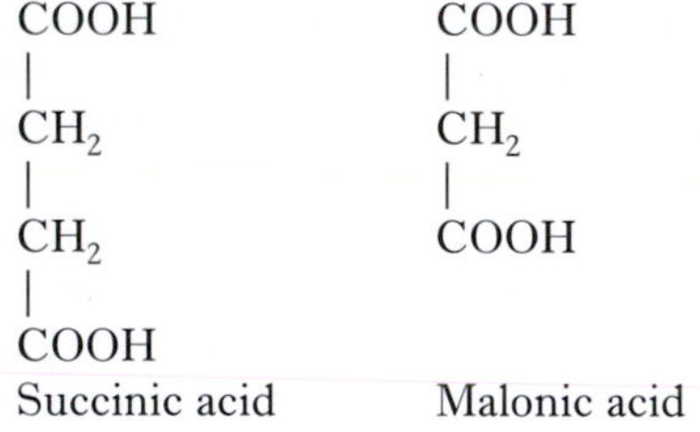


Succinic dehydrogenase readily oxides succinic acid to form fumaric acid. If increasing concentrations of malonic acid, which resembles succinic acid in structure, are added, the activity of succinic dehydrogenase falls markedly. The inhibition can then be reversed by increasing the concentration of succinic acid.

In contrast, a non-competitive inhibitor binds to the enzyme in the presence or absence of the substrate, and raising the concentration will not displace the inhibitor. The binding need not occur at the active site but, if not, it alters the shape of the enzyme sufficiently to render it ineffective. Examples of this, in practice, are penicillin, and nerve gases that inhibit acetylcholinesterase. The effect of non-competitive inhibition is seen in Figure 18.44. Note that $V_{max}$ is reduced but $K_m$ remains the same.

*Allosteric enzymes*

Allosteric enzymes bind activators and inhibitors at sites separate from the active site; they stabilize the conformational change and either increase or decrease the rate of reaction. Allosteric sites can have a powerful effect on the performance of an enzyme. An example of allosteric control is isocitrate dehydrogenase, a regulatory enzyme in the tricarboxylate cycle. As the ATP concentration in the cells starts to rise, the concentration of ADP falls. ADP is an allosteric activator of isocitrate dehydrogenase and, as its levels fall, it decreases the activity of the enzyme, thus regulating the formation of ATP.

*Phosphorylation*

Many hormones affect enzymes by regulating a protein kinase that transfers the phosphate group from ATP. The phosphate released can interact with the enzyme and produce a conformational change at the active site to increase or decrease enzyme activity. Enzyme phosphorylation is the major mechanism by which hormones control the rate of metabolic pathways.

*Modulator proteins*

Modulation proteins regulate the activity of another protein by binding to it. An example is calmodulin which, when activated by the $Ca^{2+}$ released from the sarcoplasmic reticulum during muscle contraction,

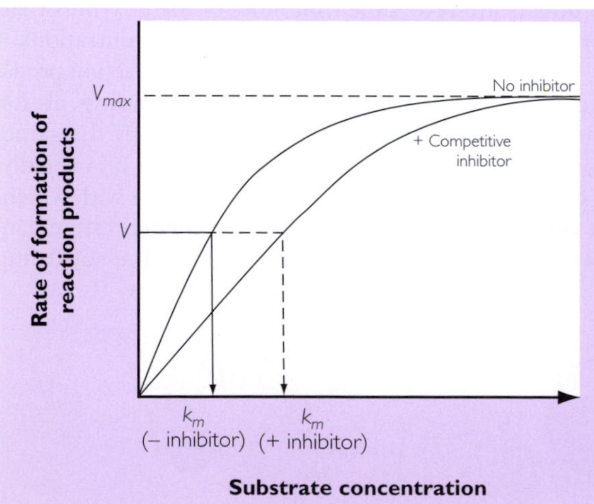


**Figure 18.43** The relationship between the rate of reaction and substrate concentration with and without a competitive inhibitor. Note that, in the presence of the inhibitor, there is a change in the value of the Michaelis constant ($K_m$) but no shift in $V_{max}$.

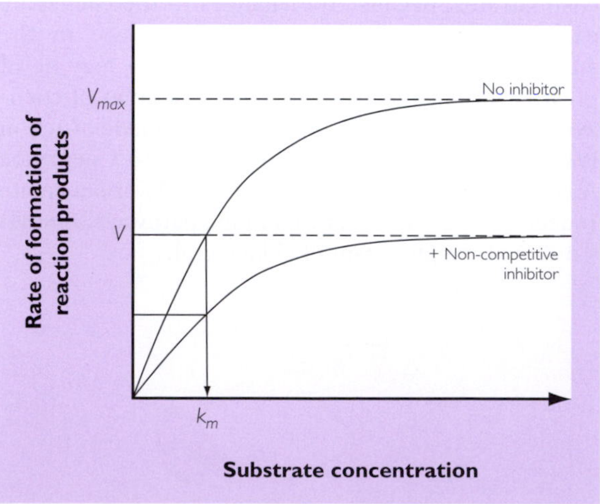


**Figure 18.44** The effect of a non-competitive inhibitor on the rate of reaction. Note that in the presence of the non-competitive inhibitor there is a large change in $V_{max}$ but no change in $K_m$.

forms $Ca^{2+}$ calmodulin. The $Ca^{2+}$ calmodulin binds to glycogen phosphorylase kinase and activates it, thereby degrading more glycogen to provide further energy for muscle contraction.

*Product inhibition*

This occurs in two ways:

1. The product directly inhibits enzyme activity. An example of this is the phosphate group of glucose-6-phosphatase competing with ATP for the active site, thereby inhibiting the continued formation of glucose 6-phosphate by hexokinase. This system works in erythrocytes.
2. The end-product of a pathway may induce or repress the gene for the transcription of the enzyme. This is a much slower system to respond.

## THE CELL

### Cell types and generalized structure

Cells are divided into two major groups: prokaryotes and eukaryotes. All animal cells are eukaryotes; bacterial cells are prokaryotes. Prokaryotes are very much simpler and contain no membrane-bound subcellular structures. Prokaryotes and eukaryotes are compared in Table 18.20. The organelles of eukaryotes have membranes which, like the cell membrane, determine which substances may enter or exit from the region that they enclose.

The ultrastructure of a generalized animal cell is shown in Figure 18.45. Cells are basically spherical in shape but modified to suit specialized needs. In size, they mostly range from 10 to 30 μm in diameter. Their size is restricted by:

- The surface area-to-volume ratio which must be large enough to allow exchange of metabolic substances.
- The capacity of the nucleus to exercise control over the rest of the cell. The function of each part of the cell is described below.

### The structure and function of cellular components

***Cell membrane***

The cell membrane (also known as the plasma membrane or unit membrane) acts as a boundary between the cell and its environment. It is composed of a lipid bilayer with embedded proteins (Figure 18.46). The bilayer is arranged with the hydrophilic

**Table 18.20 A comparison between prokaryotes and eukaryotes**

| Prokaryotes | Eukaryotes |
|---|---|
| No distinct nucleus | Distinct membrane-bound nucleus |
| DNA is a single circular strand | Chromosomes on which DNA is located |
| No spindle forms at cell division (binary or multiple fusion) | Mitosis or meiosis |
| No membrane-bound organelles | Several subcellular organelles |
| Cell wall of protein and polysaccharide | No cell wall |
| Spores sometimes formed | Do not form spores |
| Small ribosomes | Large ribosomes |
| Flagella, if present, lack internal fibril arrangement | Flagella have internal fibril arrangement |
| Cilia absent | May have cilia |

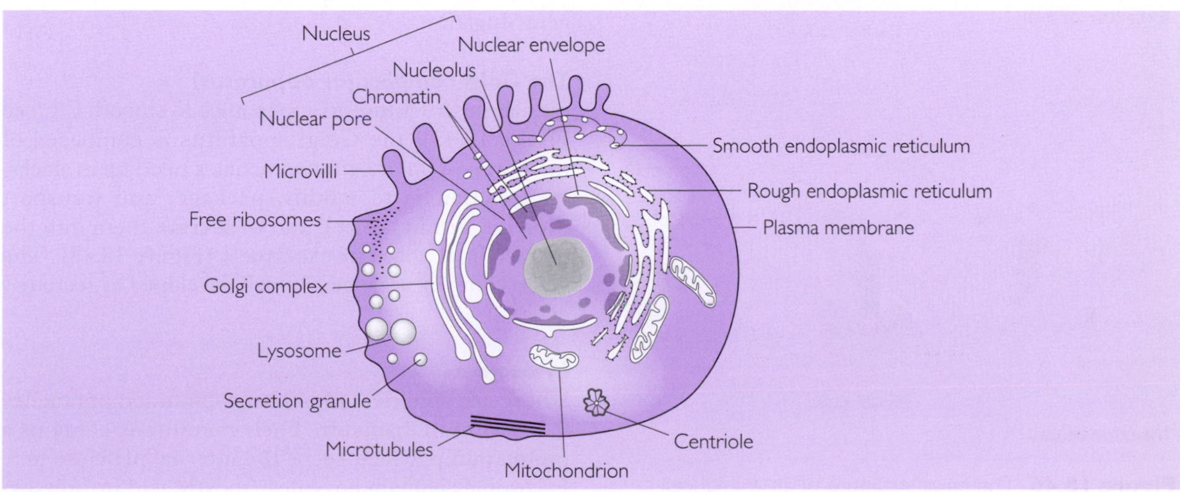


**Figure 18.45** The ultrastructure of a generalized animal cell.

phospholipid heads on the outside and the lipid tails on the inside. In addition to phospholipids, and especially in neural tissue, the membrane may contain sphingolipids. The proteins that span the membrane are called integral membrane proteins; those embedded on one side only are called peripheral proteins. Membrane proteins can act as enzymes, transport proteins, structural components, and receptors. Some of the proteins and lipids also carry carbohydrate chains. Transport across the cell membrane is considered in more detail in Chapter 19.

### *The nucleus*

The nucleus (see Figure 18.45) is a prominent organelle bounded by a double plasma-type membrane which has pores 40–100 nm in diameter. The outer membrane is granular and continuous with the rough endoplasmic reticulum (ER), and contains ribosomes. Within the inner membrane is a mesh of nuclear plasm interspersed with nuclear ribosomes and chromatin (DNA bound to protein). The pores in the membrane allow the passage of large molecules such as mRNA (see later) on its route from transcription on the DNA into the cytoplasm of the cell. Within the nucleus may be one or more small round bodies, the nucleoli which store RNA. The functions of the nucleus are to:

- act as a control centre for the cell;
- contain genetic material of the cell;
- produce ribosomes and RNA;
- play a role in cell division.

### *Mitochondria*

Mitochondria (Figure 18.47) are organelles 1 μm in diameter and 2–5 μm in length, which are the main site of energy production for the cell. Each has an inner and outer membrane, the inner having invaginations known as cristae. The cristae provide a large surface area for enzyme attachment. The space enclosed by the inner membrane is known as the matrix. Mitochondria contain DNA, and they reproduce by replicating their DNA and dividing. This division is not related to cell division and the life cycle of the cell. The proteins within mitochondria are synthesized partly from mitochondrial DNA and also from importation from the cytoplasm. The enzymes of the tricarboxylate cycle are located in mitochondria and components of the electron transport chain are on the inner mitochondrial membrane. Cells that expend a lot of energy, e.g. muscle cells, have numerous mitochondria.

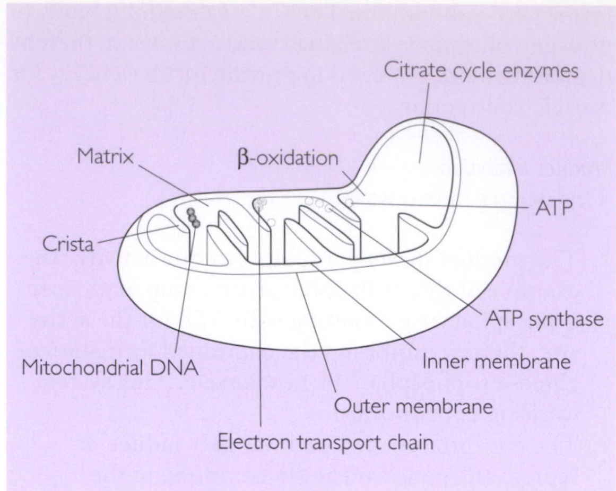


**Figure 18.47** The structure of a mitochondrion.

### *Endoplasmic reticulum*

The ER is a net of tubules in the cytoplasm. Some parts are studded with ribosomes and called 'rough' ER, and others lack ribosomes and are called 'smooth' ER (see Figure 18.45). The membrane of the ER is an extension of the outer nuclear membrane. The functions of the ER are to:

- form a transport network throughout the cell;
- provide a large surface for chemical reactions;
- play a role in protein synthesis (rough ER);
- collect and store manufactured material;
- form a structured skeleton to help maintain the shape of the cell;
- produce lipids and steroids (smooth ER).

The adjective 'microsomal' is sometimes used for processes that occur on or within the ER. Microsomes do not exist as cell organelles; they are a product of centrifugation.

### *The Golgi complex (or apparatus)*

Similar in structure and appearance to smooth ER (see Figure 18.45), the Golgi apparatus is composed of membrane-bound flattened vesicles piled up in stacks. Its function is to modify, package, and transport proteins within the cell and to secrete them into the extracellular space by exocytosis (Figure 18.48). The Golgi complex is especially well developed in secretory cells.

### *Lysosomes*

These are spherical membrane-bounded organelles 0.2–0.5 μm in diameter. Their membrane contains a proton pump, which keeps the internal pH close to 5. Lysosomes contain enzymes (mostly acid hydrolyses) which digest biological molecules, including lipids,

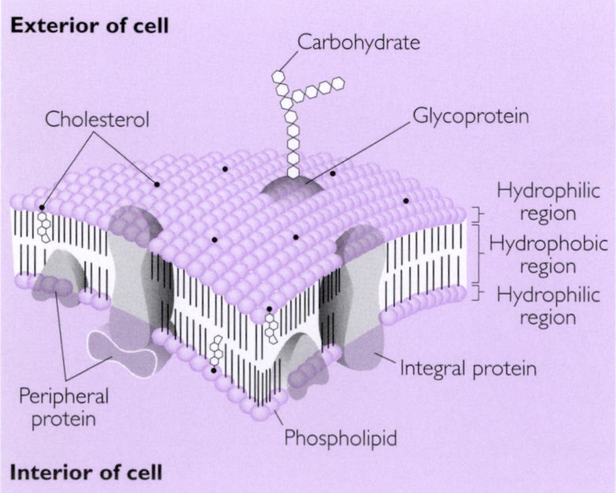


**Figure 18.46** The basic structure of an animal cell membrane shown in diagrammatic form.

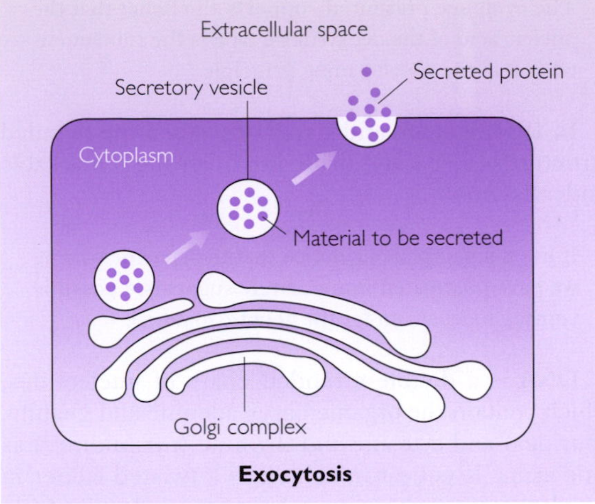


**Figure 18.48** The Golgi complex and the process of exocytosis of proteins.

proteins, polysaccharides, and nucleic acids, and convert them into basic biochemical units (Figure 18.49). Their functions include:

- destruction and recycling of unwanted or worn out cellular organelles;
- digestion of material engulfed by the cell, e.g. bacteria in leukocytes;
- release of enzymes outside the cell (exocytosis) to digest external material;
- normal turnover of cells and digestion of cell after its death (autolysis);
- involvement in tissue remodelling, e.g. the return of the lactating breast to normal.

The lysosomal membrane is impermeable to both lysosomal enzymes and molecules in the cytoplasm, and therefore prevents autolysis occurring. The transfer of material and active actions of lysosomes are shown in Figure 18.50.

### *Ribosomes*

These are small cytoplasmic granules 20 nm in diameter, made up of small RNA molecules and proteins. They are important in protein synthesis. Polysomes are groups of ribosomes attached to messenger RNA (see later), each of which is producing a protein (Figure 18.51).

### *Peroxisomes*

These are small spherical membrane-bound organelles 0.5–1.5 μm in diameter which are similar to lysosomes. They contain enzymes that oxidize many long-chain fatty acids (> 20 carbon units long) to shorter-chain fatty acids, which are then transferred to mitochondria for complete oxidation. Their reactions produce hydrogen peroxide, which is catalysed into water and oxygen preventing cell damage from peroxide.

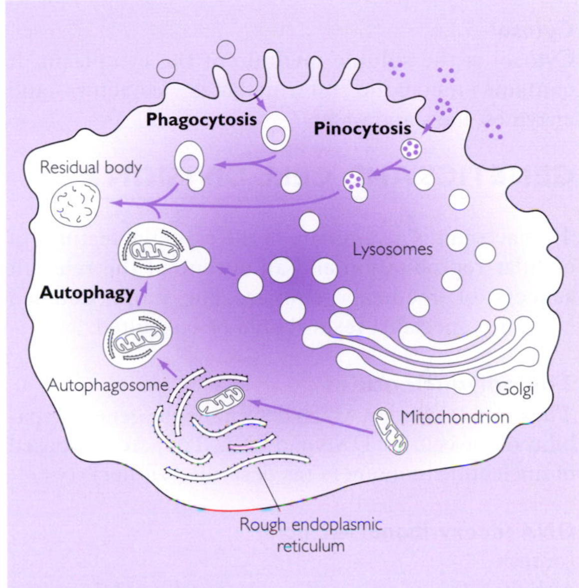


**Figure 18.50** Phagocytosis, pinocytosis, and autophagy taking place in a lysosome.

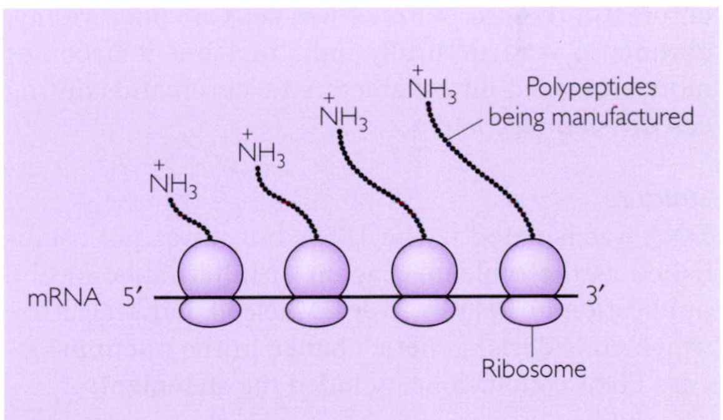


**Figure 18.51** A schematic diagram of a polysome.

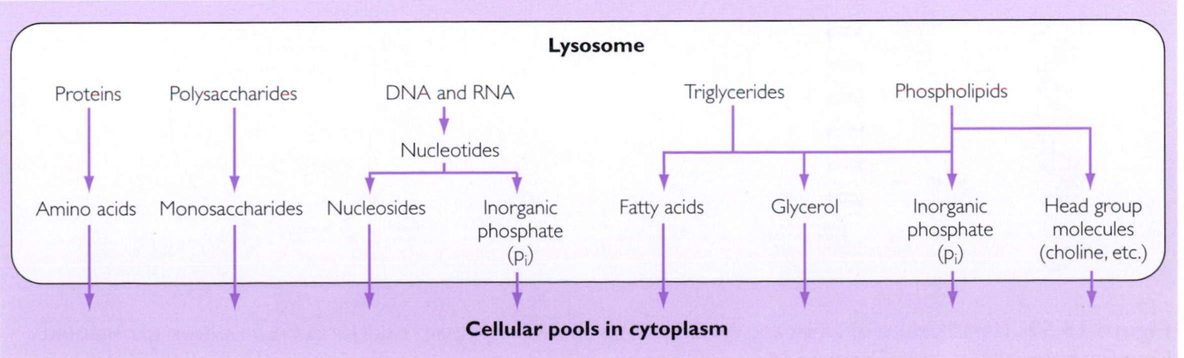


**Figure 18.49** The digestive process of lysosomes.

#### Cytoskeleton

'Cytoskeleton' is a general term for a complex arrangement of actin filaments and microtubules which:

- maintain the cell shape;
- produce cellular movements, e.g. flagella;
- produce movement of organelles within the cell;
- form the spherical apparatus of cell division.

Microtubules are polymerized spirals of a protein called tubulin.

#### Cytosol

Cytosol is the soluble medium of the cytoplasm. It contains metabolic intermediates, cofactors and enzymes, ions, and water.

## GENETICS AND CELL DIVISION

This account is a summary of the essential features of cellular reproduction and an outline of the relevant aspects of medical genetics. For more detailed accounts, specialist texts should be consulted.

### The polynucleotides

The polynucleotides, which determine the genetic capability of the cell, are DNA and RNA. They are composed of nucleotide monomers (as described earlier).

#### DNA (deoxyribonucleic acid)

*Location*

Although there is a small amount of free DNA in the mitochondria (see earlier), it makes up less than 0.1% of the total DNA in a cell. The rest of the DNA (> 99.9%) is located within the nucleus and bound to proteins (e.g. histones), forming a complex known as chromatin (Figure 18.52). When cells are not dividing, chromatin is structurally indistinct but it becomes more organized into characteristic chromatids during cell division (see later).

*Structure*

DNA was isolated in the 1850s but it was not established as the molecular agent of inheritance until a publication in 1944 by Avery, Macleod and McCarthy, which considered genetic change in the pneumococcus. Their conclusions included the statement:

> The evidence presented supports the belief that the nucleic acid of the deoxyribose type is the fundamental unit of the transforming principle.

In 1953, Watson and Crick described the detailed structure of DNA and made the following remarkable understatement:

> It has not escaped our notice that the specific pairing we have postulated immediately suggests a possible copying mechanism for the genetic material.

DNA is a double-stranded chain of nucleotides, which contain the organic bases adenine and guanine (purines) and cytosine and thymine (pyrimidines) as side arms. It is best imagined as a twisted ladder in which the deoxyribose and phosphate molecules form the uprights and the organic bases form the rungs (Figure 18.53). Each rung of the ladder must be of the same length. As the purines and pyrimidines are of different sizes (see Figure 18.31), cytosine (C) bonds with guanine (G) and adenosine (A) with thymine (T). The bonds between the bases are weak hydrogen bonds, but between the phosphate and deoxyribose molecules they are strong covalent diester bonds. Note that, in the way the bases pair, the two corresponding strands of DNA are anti-parallel, i.e. the order of bases is reversed (Figure 18.53).

*Replication of DNA*

The replication of DNA depends on a number of enzymes. The process is the same in principle in both prokaryotic and eukaryotic cells, but is more complex in eukaryotic cells. The differences between them has led to the development of a number of antibiotic drugs that affect bacterial but not human cell replication. DNA replication is shown in schematic form in Figure 18.54. It can be seen that the hydrogen bonding of the base-pairs is broken by DNA polymerase and individual nucleotides present in the local environment link with their base pairs, forming a complementary anti-parallel strand. The bend in the 'Y' during replication is known as the replication fork. During this process, the strong covalent phosphodiester bonds of the back bone retain its integrity and hence the order of the bases. The replication process and the replication fork are shown in more life-like form in Figure 18.55. As

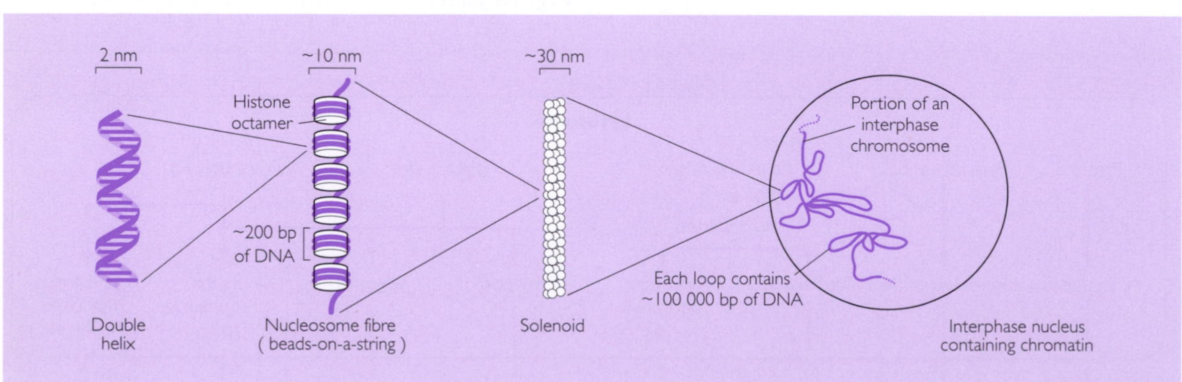


**Figure 18.52** The structure of DNA and chromosomes shown in diagrammatic form. bp, base-pair(s). (Adapted from Thomson MW *et al.* In: Thomson MW and Thomson ME, *Genetics in Medicine*, 5th edn, Philadelphia: Saunders, 1991.)

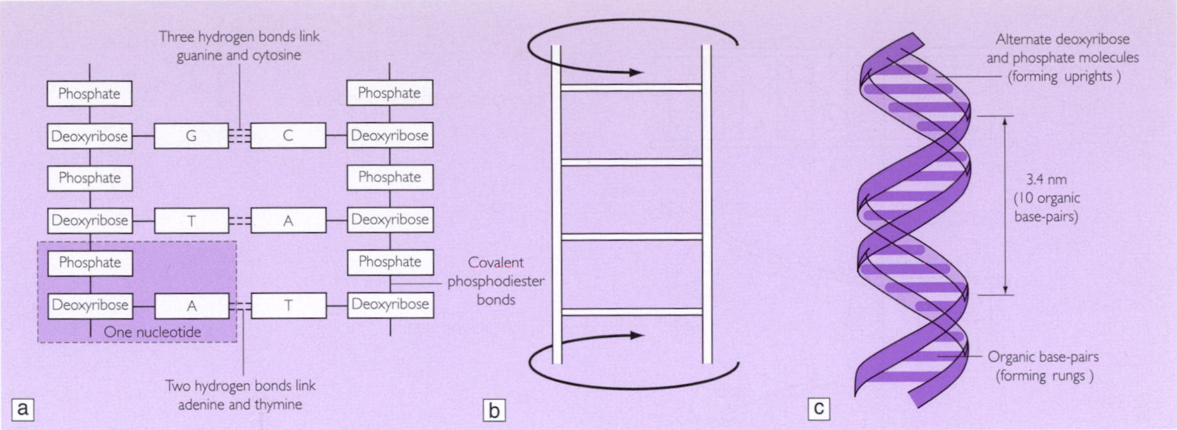


**Figure 18.53** The construction of the double-helix structure of DNA from the basic DNA strands. (a) The links between bases in diagrammatic form; (b) the way in which they are twisted, and (c) a diagrammatic form of the helix of DNA.

the new DNA strands retain half of the original DNA, this form of replication is described as semi-conservative.

### *RNA (ribonucleic acid)*

*Structure*

RNA is a single-stranded chain of nucleotides, which contains the organic purine bases adenine and guanine and the pyrimidines, cytosine and uracil (see Figures 18.31 and 18.32). Complementary binding occasionally produces double-stranded regions. In RNA, adenine pairs with uracil rather than thymine.

*Types of RNA*

There are three types of RNA: messenger (mRNA), transfer (tRNA), and ribosomal (rRNA):

- Messenger RNA is composed of up to several thousand nucleotides in the form a single-stranded helix. It is manufactured in the nucleus as an anti-parallel DNA strand. Once made, mRNA traverses the pores of the nuclear membrane and goes to the ribosomes where it is used as a template for protein synthesis.
- Transfer RNA is much smaller than mRNA, being made up of about 80 nucleotides formed into a clover-leaf shape. Each molecule of tRNA carries a specific amino acid for the construction of a protein molecule.
- Ribosomal RNA is a large molecule manufactured in the nucleus by DNA, which moves to the ribosomes to undertake its function. It actually comprises a large portion of the ribosome itself. Ribosomes are the subcellular structures on which protein synthesis occurs, and they are found in the cytoplasm and mitochondria of eukaryotes (see earlier). The rRNAs, of which there are several types, contain many loops and show base pairing.

In addition to the three main forms of RNA, there are other RNAs present in cells, including oligonucleotides that serve as primers for DNA replication and small ribonuclear proteins in nuclei involved in maturation of RNA precursors. RNA also serves as the genome for certain types of viruses known as retroviruses (including HIV). A summary of the differences between DNA and RNA is given in Table 18.21.

## The genetic code and protein synthesis

Each cell has its own, often unique, combination of proteins that determines its structure and function. A major factor in this is the production of proteins that are enzymes which, by accelerating specific reactions, indirectly determine the products of a cell's chemical activity. As a consequence, protein synthesis can profoundly affect fat and carbohydrate metabolism. Estimations are that a typical cell synthesizes approximately $10^5$ different proteins during its life cycle.

### *The genetic code*

DNA is essentially a set of instructions for protein synthesis comprising four variables: adenine, guanine, cytosine, and thymine. Given that there are four variables the number of possible combinations of any three bases is $4 \times 4 \times 4 = 64$. Apart from three of these combinations, each combination of this triplet code determines an amino acid. The three combinations that do not code for an amino acid on mRNA are known as stop, termination, or nonsense codons that terminate protein synthesis. As there are only 20 amino acids commonly present in proteins, it is clear that more than one combination might code for a single amino acid. Table 18.22 lists the triplet codes found on DNA. Each triplet on DNA is called a codagen and its complementary expression on mRNA is a codon.

It can be seen from Table 18.22 that many amino acids are specified by more than one triplet. This is described by the terms 'degenerate' and 'redundant'. Although a single amino acid may be specified by more than one triplet, each codon specifies only one amino acid. The genetic code is therefore totally unambiguous.

One of the more surprising features is that, in all organisms studied to date, almost all of them use the same genetic code (prokaryotes and eukaryotes). Less than 10 exceptions to this have been found in the whole of genetic science. Three of these are in human mitochondria.

The way in which proteins are constructed from this triplet code is described in the next section.

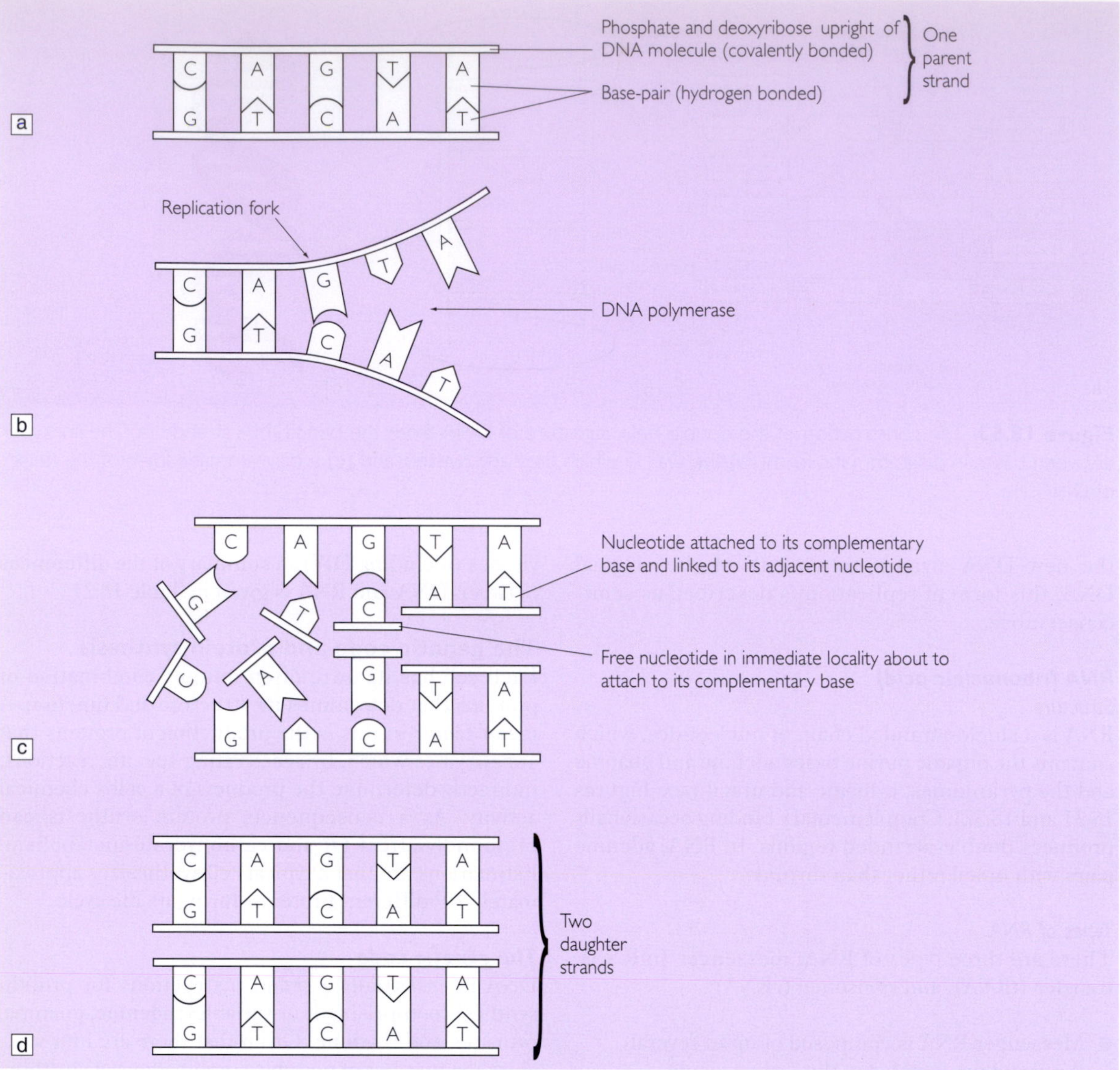

**Figure 18.54** The replication of DNA shown in schematic form. (a) Portion of a DNA molecule; (b) the enzyme DNA polymerase breaks down the bonds between the base-pairs causing the two strands of the DNA molecule to separate; (c) free nucleotides bond with their complementary bases on each strand of the DNA molecule; (d) when the nucleotides are lined up, they join together to form a polynucleotide chain. Two identical strands of DNA are thus formed. Each new DNA molecule retains half of the original DNA material; this form of replication is therefore described as semiconservative.

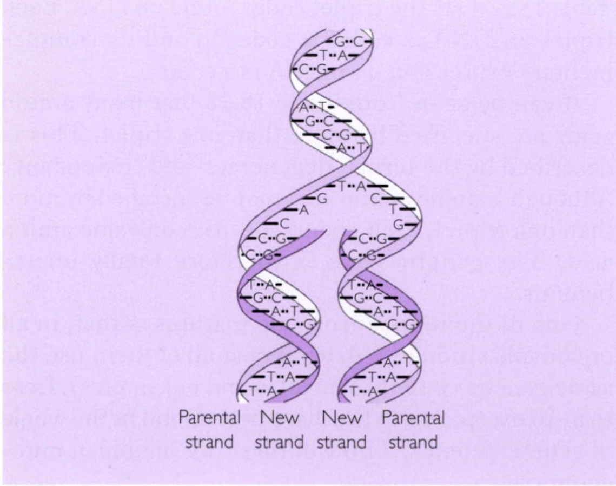


**Figure 18.55** DNA replication showing the replication fork.

### *The synthesis of proteins*

There are four main stages in the synthesis of a protein:

- formation of amino acids;
- transcription of triplet codes to the mRNA;
- attachment of amino acids to tRNA;
- translation of the code into a protein molecule on the ribosome.

#### *Formation of amino acids*

Humans have to obtain ten of their amino acids from their diet, but can synthesize the remainder (see Table 18.13). The individual amino acids are obtained from ingested protein by the process of digestion (see Figure 18.30).

**Table 18.21 The main differences between RNA and DNA**

| DNA | RNA |
|---|---|
| Organic bases are adenine, thymine, guanine, cytosine | Organic bases are adenine, uracil, guanine, cytosine |
| Double helix | Single strand |
| Deoxyribose | Ribose |
| Mostly nuclear | Throughout the cell |
| More stable | Less stable |
| Permanent | Temporary |
| Insoluble | Soluble |
| One basic type | Three types: messenger, transfer, ribosomal |
| Concentration constant | Concentration varies according to cell type |
| Adenine + thymine : cytosine + guanine ratio about equal | Adenine + uracil : cytosine + guanine ratio more variable |
| Very large molecular mass (100 000–120 000 000) | Smaller molecular mass (20 000–2 000 000) |

**Table 18.22 The genetic code**

| First base | Second base | | | | Third base |
|---|---|---|---|---|---|
| (5') | U | C | A | G | (3') |
| U | Phe | Ser | Tyr | Cys | U |
| | Phe | Ser | Tyr | Cys | C |
| | Leu | Ser | Stop | Stop | A |
| | Leu | Ser | Stop | Trp | G |
| C | Leu | Pro | His | Arg | U |
| | Leu | Pro | His | Arg | C |
| | Leu | Pro | Gln | Arg | A |
| | Leu | Pro | Gln | Arg | G |
| A | Ile | Thr | Asn | Ser | U |
| | Ile | Thr | Asn | Ser | C |
| | Ile | Thr | Lys | Arg | A |
| | Met | Thr | Lys | Arg | G |
| G | Val | Ala | Asp | Gly | U |
| | Val | Ala | Asp | Gly | C |
| | Val | Ala | Glu | Gly | A |
| | Val | Ala | Glu | Gly | G |

Abbreviations for the individual amino acids are given in Table 18.13. U, uracil; C, cytosine; A, adenine; G, guanine.

*Transcription*

Transcription is the synthesis of mRNA from a DNA template. The process is initiated by the binding of RNA polymerase to the promoter region of DNA. This causes DNA to unwind and separate within a region that is 10–20 nucleotides in length. As the polymerase transcribes the DNA, the untranscribed region continues to separate while the transcribed DNA region rejoins its partner. The process continues until a termination sequence occurs on the DNA. This process, which occurs in the nucleolus, is demonstrated schematically in Figure 18.56. Two of the functions of RNA polymerase are to zip together the nucleotides, and then to peel them off the DNA. Each codagen on the DNA is matched by a codon on mRNA. The primary mRNA transcripts are then modified and trimmed to produce mature mRNA. This is called post-transcriptional modification. The mature mRNA so formed then passes out of the nucleolus via its pores into the cytoplasm (Figure 18.56), where it binds and becomes incorporated into ribosomes. The region of a DNA molecule that codes for a whole single protein is called a cistron.

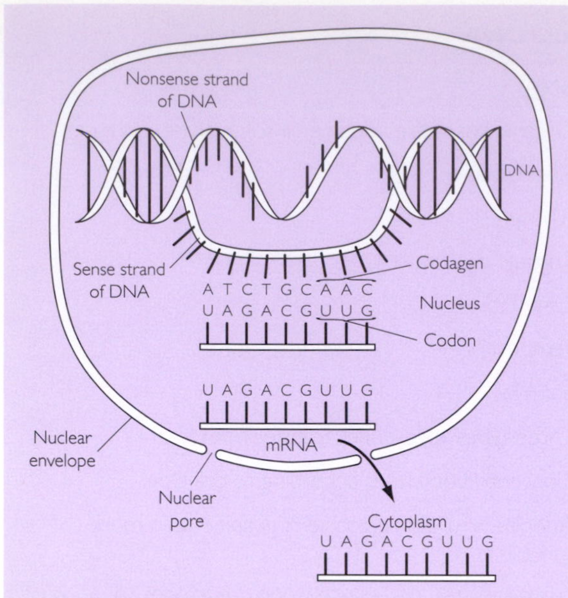


**Figure 18.56** Transcription: the synthesis of mRNA from a DNA template.

*Amino acid assembly using tRNA*

Transfer RNA is a clover-leaf molecule, which at one end carries an amino acid and at the other carries three complementary base-pairs known as an anti-codon. The anti-codon matches the codon on the mRNA (Figure 18.57). Each amino acid is carried by a specific type of tRNA, and the tRNA is free in the cytoplasm to react with mRNA.

*Translation*

Translation is the process of production of a protein from mRNA and tRNA. Each molecule of mRNA is usually bound to a string of ribosomes collectively known as a polysome (see Figure 18.51). A ribosome acts as a framework on which to assemble tRNA on to mRNA. This is shown diagrammatically in Figure

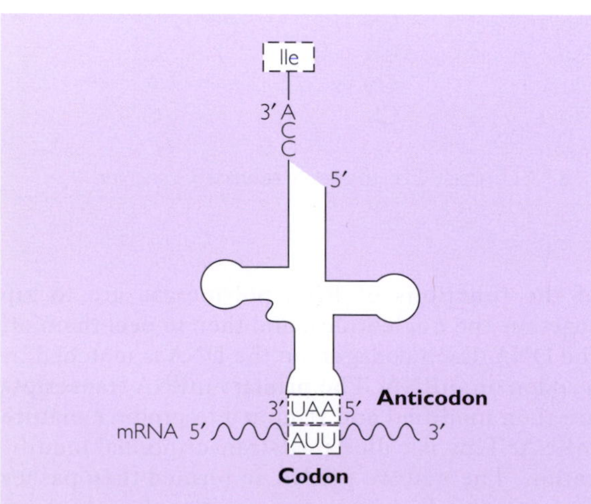


**Figure 18.57** The clover-leaf-shaped molecule of tRNA binding to a codon on mRNA. Note that the codon–anticodon pairing is complementary and anti-parallel. AUU on mRNA codes for isoleucine on tRNA.

18.58. As the protein begins to be assembled, the first two amino acids are brought together and a peptide bond forms (Figure 18.58a); the ribosome then moves along to join the third amino acid, and so on. The rate of polymerization is thought to be four to eight amino acids per second. As the amino acids become incorporated, the tRNA is released back into the cytoplasm to attach to another amino acid molecule (Figure 18.58b). The ribosome continues to pass along mRNA until the stop code is reached when the complete polypeptide is cast off. Several ribosomes pass along the mRNA at the same time (Figure 18.58c).

In this way, the protein chains are made which subsequently form into secondary, tertiary, and quaternary structures – called post-translational modification.

Once synthesized, proteins leave the ribosomes to be transported to wherever they perform their function.

## The cell cycle and cell division

### *The cell cycle*

Definitions of the nomenclature of the cell cycle differ slightly from book to book. What is presented here is that which seems most logical.

The cell cycle of a eukaryotic cell (Figure 18.59) consists of five main phases:

$G_0$: period during which the cell undertakes routine metabolic activity;
$G_1$: cell growth and normal metabolic activity;
S: DNA replication;
$G_2$: preparation for cell division;
M: mitosis or meiosis.

The first four phases together constitute interphase, i.e. the period between cell division. $G_0$ and $G_1$ are sometimes combined together as an extended $G_1$ phase that constitutes normal metabolic activity and preparation for cell division.

The first phase $G_0$ (gap nought) is the most variable in length. During this the cell carries out its routine metabolic function. $G_1$ (gap one or the first gap phase) prepares the cells for chromosome duplication by, for instance, the production of nucleotide precursors. In S phase, DNA replicates and the manufacture of histones and other proteins associated with cell division is increased. During $G_2$ (the second gap phase), the cells prepare to divide, synthesizing tubulin for construction of the microtubules of the spindle apparatus. Division itself occurs in M (the brief mitotic phase).

In humans, many cells (e.g. hair follicles, skin cells, duodenal cells) cycle almost daily. Others such as precursors of red blood cells divide a number of times, then lose their nuclei when they become mature blood cells. Other cells, such as liver cells, may spend days, weeks or months in $G_0$ before being stimulated to enter $G_1$ by hormones, growth factors, or adjacent cell death. Some cells cease to divide at all.

The average mammalian cell cycle spans 18 hours, and a typical schedule is 9 hours for $G_1$, 5 hours for S, 3 hours for $G_2$, and 1 hour for M. After mitosis, cells may re-enter $G_1$ directly or enter $G_0$ for ever and never divide again.

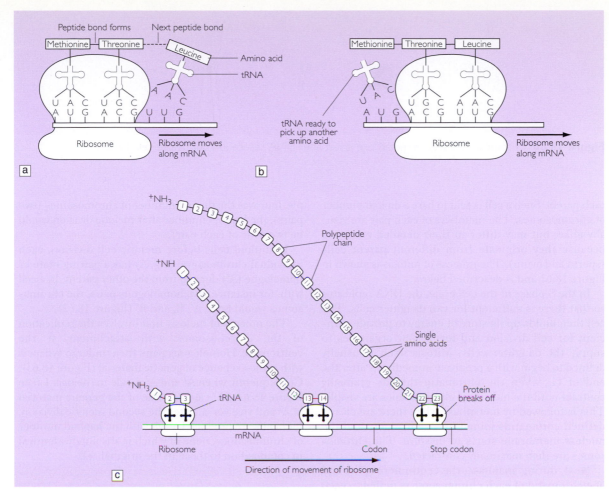

**Figure 18.58** The process of translation; tRNA, transfer RNA.

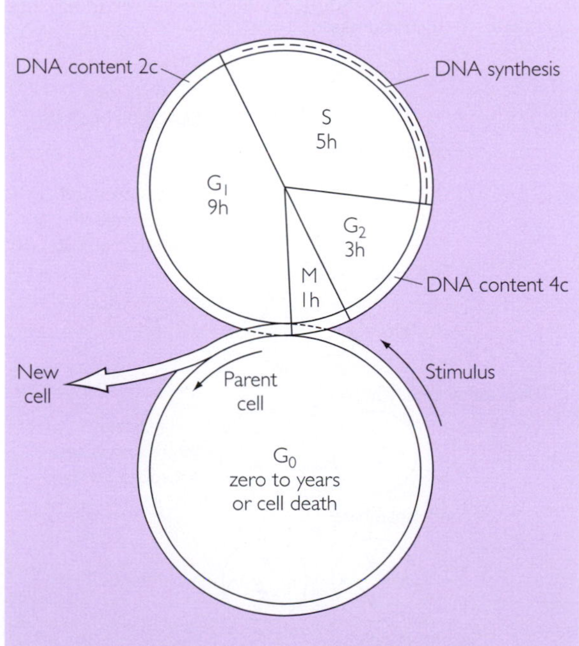


**Figure 18.59** The cell cycle of a eukaryotic cell. Mitosis commences with prophase, continues through metaphase, anaphase, and telophase, and ends with cell division. The times shown for each component of the cell's cycle are averages for a mammalian cell, but can vary enormously depending on the cell's function.

### *Chromosomes*

In all cells, DNA is organized into chromosomes. Chromatin is a non-specific name for the material from which chromosomes are made and consists of DNA, histones, and a variety of other proteins. Chromosomes can be seen by the light microscope only when a cell is dividing. An interphase chromosome is shown in Figure 18.52. During the process of cell division, chromosomes contract and become much more organized. After DNA replication but before cell division, they are seen as paired chromatids joined by a centromere (Figure 18.60). Each chromatid contains a complete strand of DNA. It is in this paired state (metaphase arrest) that they are normally photographed and displayed. The number and length of chromosomes are specific to a given species, but give no indication of the cell's level of organization or the position of the organism in the hierarchy of a phylum. For instance a pigeon (bird brain!) has 80 chromosomes, compared with 46 in humans.

There are two major forms of cell division: mitosis and meiosis.

#### *Mitosis*

Mitosis is the normal process of cell division in which one cell reproduces itself to form two identical cells. In the human cell (see later), the chromosomes (apart from the sex chromosomes) are present in identical pairs, one member from each pair being derived from

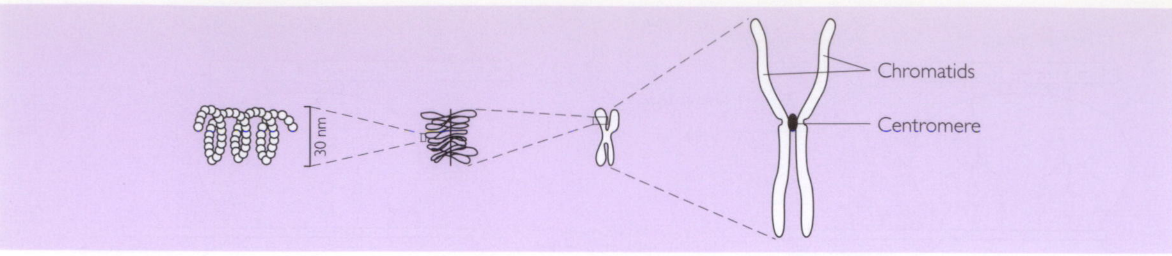


**Figure 18.60** Chromosomes seen in metaphase arrest after DNA replication but before cell division.

each parent. Such a cell is said to have a diploid number of chromosomes. The members of each pair are visually alike, but may differ in their detailed structure because they originate from different parent cells (sperm and ovum). The process of mitosis is shown in Figure 18.61 and is described below.

In the S phase of the cell cycle, the DNA replicates so that there is sufficient for two daughter cells. The cell then builds up its store of energy to provide sufficient for cell division and forms new organelles to supply the daughter cells. Mitosis itself is usually defined to begin with a prophase immediately after the end of $G_0$, when the chromatin threads gradually contract until the individual chromosomes are visible. This is followed by metaphase when there are clearly defined chromatids joined by a centromere and the nuclear membrane starts to dissolve. The chromosomes are then maximally contracted.

Next, during anaphase, the centromere splits and one chromatid of each chromosome is pulled to each pole of the cell by spindle fibres. Telophase represents the situation when chromatids reach their poles, the nuclear membranes re-form, and the cell starts to divide. The daughter cell is diploid, i.e. has the same number of chromosome pairs as the parent.

### *Meiosis*

Meiosis is a type of cell division occurring in sperm and ova, which results in the formation of haploid cells carrying only one of each type of chromosome instead of a pair.

As discussed above, the cells produced by mitosis are diploid, i.e. have a pair of each chromosome. In meiosis, the cells produced are haploid. If, for example, four was the diploid number of chromosomes (two pairs), the haploid number after meiotic division would be two (one of each pair).

In diploid cells before meiotic cell division, each individual chromosome (e.g. A) has a pairing mate or homologue (A′) derived from the other parent. In a cell with, for instance, two homologous pairs, the chromosomes would be A, A′, B, and B′ (Figure 18.62).

The process of meiosis first involves the replication of the chromosomes with attachment at the centromere. Homologous pairs then undergo synapsis with some exchange of genetic material (Figure 18.63). Consequently when $A^1$ and $A^2$ divide in meiosis 1 (see Figure 18.62), $A^1$ carries some of the genetic material of $A^2$ and vice versa. After the second meiotic division, four cells are produced, each with the haploid number of chromosomes, none of which is absolutely identical in composition to those in the original cell.

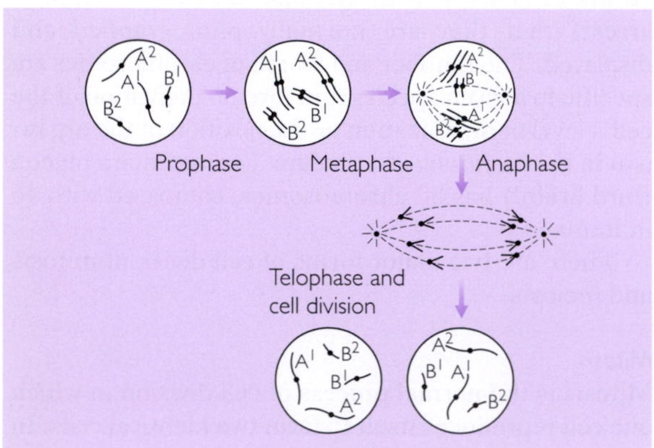


**Figure 18.61** The process of mitosis. (See the text for details.)

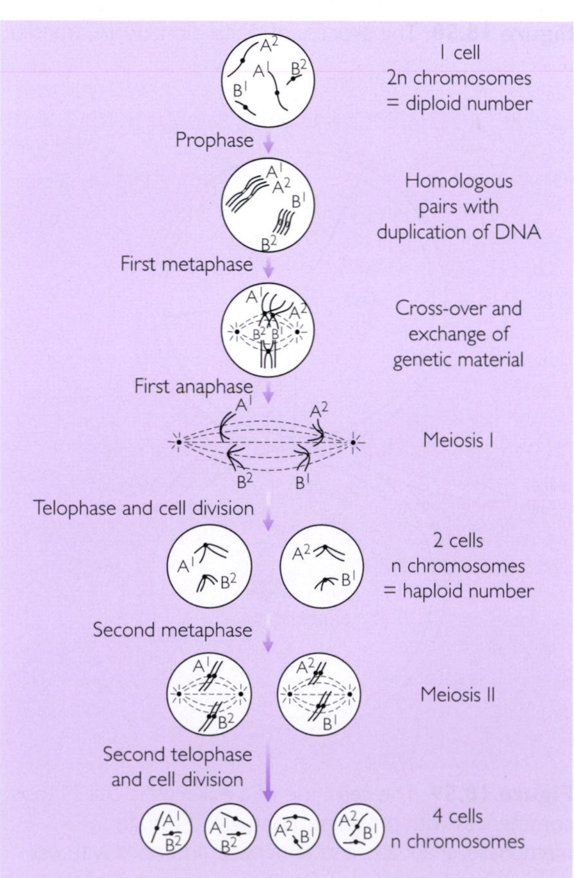


**Figure 18.62** The process of meiosis. (See the text for details.)

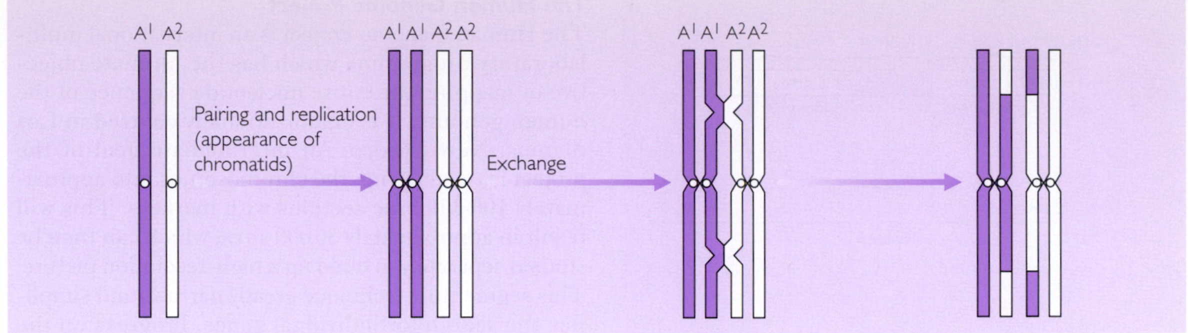


**Figure 18.63** Homologous pairs of chromosomes undergoing synapsis or cross-over with some exchange of genetic material.

Fertilization is the event in which two haploid cells (one from each parent) join to re-form a diploid cell.

## The human karyotype, gene structure, and gene expression

### *The normal human karyotype*

Other than gametes, the typical human cell (e.g. brain, stomach, kidney) contains 46 chromosomes. Two of these are sex chromosomes grouped as XX or XY. The other 44 chromosomes form 22 visually identical pairs. One of each pair will have been derived from each parent. The normal male is described as 46 XY and the normal female as 46 XX. It should be noted that the XY and XX are included within the 46 chromosomes. The 44 non-sex chromosomes are called autosomes; 22 autosomes and one sex chromosome are obtained from each parent. It should be noted that some cells, e.g. muscle cells, have more than one nucleus and so, although each nucleus is identical, in total the cell possesses more than 46 chromosomes. Other cells that lose their nucleus as they mature, such as platelets and red blood cells, of course have no chromosomes.

Under normal working conditions the chromosomes in the human cell cannot be identified by their familiar shapes. To display them, the cells are cultured in an artificial medium and arrested in the metaphase stage of mitosis by colchicine. At this time, the DNA has replicated so two chromatids joined at their centromere are seen. The normal male karyotype is shown in Figure 18.64.

The total length of DNA in a human diploid cell is over 2 m and contains $6\times10^9$ base pairs per haploid cell. The longest single chromosome has DNA over 7 cm in length. The attachment to chromatin and contraction into chromatids can thus be seen to be essential for the practical and reliable transfer of the DNA component into daughter cells during division.

It is clear from this account that all human cells must have the same synthetic and metabolic potential because they all have the same DNA. This is true of all the cells that form by mitosis immediately after fertilization of the ovum by sperm. Early in the first days and weeks of fetal life, cells differentiate into their specialized types (e.g. nerve, muscle, liver, etc.). The exact mechanism of this is still not known, but it is clear that every cell is working in a selective way well below its total synthetic capacity when performing its specific function.

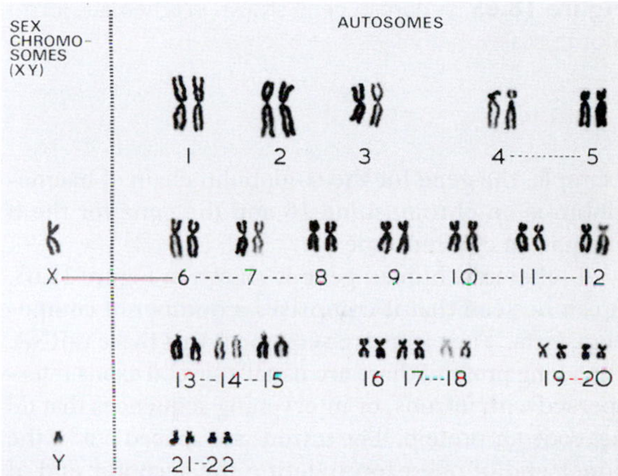


**Figure 18.64** The normal male karyotype.

### *Gene structure*

The genome is the total genetic material. The definition of a single gene is by no means universally accepted. It is, however, essentially a strip of DNA that is required to synthesize a single protein or functional molecule of RNA together with its regulating proteins. No more than 3–5% of the DNA in the human genome codes for protein. Most of the DNA appears to have no function and is called redundant.

As each diploid cell contains duplicated haploid chromosomes, it is the number of protein-coding genes in the haploid human genome that estimates the cellular potential. The number of genes in the human haploid genome has been estimated to be between 14 000 and 300 000 with a consensus figure of about 70 000. The number of base-pairs of DNA in a gene measures its size. They range from 1 kilobase to several megabases. In human DNA, there is roughly one gene for every 40 000–50 000 base-pairs.

The structure of genes, and in particular their organization and regulation, differs considerably between prokaryotic and eukaryotic cells. In bacteria, genes for protein involved in performing a specific function are often grouped together in the genome in units known as operons. They are switched on and off by small molecules called inducers and co-repressors. Such operons are not present in eukaryotes. In eukaryotic cells, genes encoding proteins that function together are usually located on different chromosomes. For

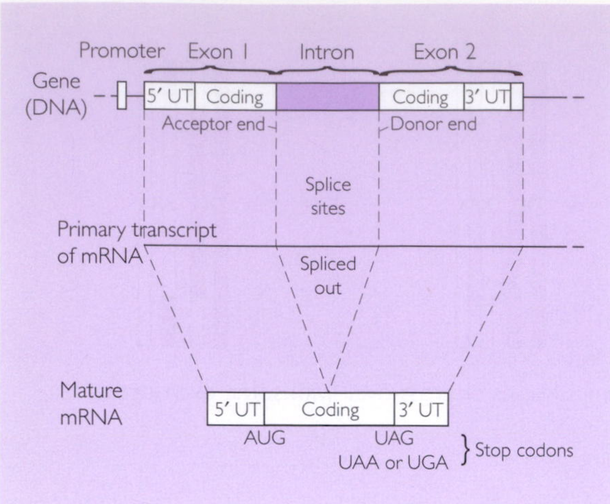


**Figure 18.65** A human gene shown in schematic form (not to scale).

example, the gene for the α-globulin chain of haemoglobin is on chromosome 16 and the gene for the β chain is on chromosome 11.

A schematic human gene is shown in Figure 18.65. It can be seen that it comprises a number of component parts. The exons are sequences that make mRNA. For a long protein, there are usually several exons interspersed with introns, or intervening sequences that do not code for protein. The introns are spliced out by the donor end of one exon meeting the acceptor end of another before mature mRNA is released. Both sides of the gene have regulatory regions. Control sequences can lie several kilobases outside the coding region.

Promoters are present at the 5′-end of all genes. They control the start position of the mRNA and govern the level of transcription activity. They bind other regulatory proteins to switch on the gene. Exons are limited by stop triplets (Table 18.22 and Figure 18.58). The gene, when activated, may be read in multiple frames and use both DNA strands, and there may be alternative combinations of splicing sites to code for a variety of proteins or a single precursor of many proteins. As a typical example, albumin is coded by an average size gene of 25 kilobases. It has 14 introns and produces a mature mRNA message of 2.1 kilobases. The sizes of human genes for various compounds and conditions are given in Table 18.23 as examples.

**Table 18.23 Sizes of some human genes**

| Gene | Size (kilobases) | No. of exons |
|---|---|---|
| Preproinsulin | 1.2 | 2 |
| HLA class I antigen | 3.5 | 8 |
| Factor VIII | 186 | 26 |
| Duchenne muscular dystrophy | 2000 | ~70 |

### *The Human Genome Project*

The Human Genome Project is an international multilaboratory programme which has the ultimate objective of mapping the entire nucleotide sequence of the human genome. It is organizationally centred in Los Alamos, New Mexico. An intermediate goal of the project is to 'chop-up' the chromosomes into approximately 100-kilobase sections with markers. This will result in approximately 30 000 sites, which can then be studied separately to build up a high-resolution picture. This segmenting technique greatly narrows and simplifies the search for individual genes. Progress on the Human Genome Project will advance knowledge about the understanding of embryonic development, control of gene expression, normal chromosomal structure, triggers, promoters, and mutations.

### *Gene expression*

The regulation of gene expression is under the control of a number of mechanisms.

#### *Alteration in genes*

If genes are deleted or lost, functional proteins cannot be formed. An example of this is the mature red blood cell that can produce no mRNA (it has no nucleus) and hence is limited to its initial supply of haemoglobin. Hypochromic anaemia can be treated only by producing more new cells, not by modification of those that exist.

The effect of a single gene can be enhanced by many copies of the gene being produced and incorporated elsewhere – a process known as gene amplification. It is mainly relevant to certain stages of normal cellular development. Genes, or segments of DNA, may also move to another location in the genome, a process known as gene rearrangement. This allows different proteins to be produced and is relevant to antibody production and maturation of B cells.

#### *Regulation of transcription*

Condensed chromatin is less able to produce mRNA than diffuse chromatin. Long-term changes in the activity of genes can be produced by chromatin going from a diffuse to a condensed state and vice versa. It is by the condensation of chromatin that erythroblasts cease to continue dividing.

Perhaps the most important regulation of gene expression is the ability of specific genes to be activated (or inactivated) in minutes or hours by specific compounds, such as steroid hormones, that enter the cells and bind to receptor proteins. Thyroid hormone, cholecalciferol, and retinoic acid act similarly. Polypeptide hormones and growth factors regulate gene expression by reacting with receptors (see Chapter 19) on the cell surface. These generate second messengers which then activate genes.

The same inducer may activate several different genes and, furthermore, one of these products may activate another set of genes. The net result is that one inducer can set off a whole series of events.

It should also be noted that a single gene may be activated by a number of regulatory proteins. Indeed, a small number of regulatory proteins can generate a wide variety of responses for different genes. It is also possible that a combination of promoting molecules have to act together on a single gene to stimulate transcription maximally.

*Post-transcriptional effects*

As has been seen earlier, processing mRNA involves the removal of introns, and joining of the initial and final sections of the gene (Figure 18.65). In certain circumstances, different splicing and modification of the end sections causes different proteins to be produced by the same gene. The mRNA can also be 'edited' after transcription. When the mRNA is travelling through the nuclear pores to the cytoplasm, it is bound to proteins that help to protect it. It is, however, subject to the action of nucleases which, if they act, prevent the mRNA coding properly. The mRNA of eukaryocytes has a half-life measured in hours to days, so controlling its lifespan can consequently affect the amount of protein produced. This can be done by the binding of protective proteins that are specifically induced. An example of this is the binding of a protective molecule to transferrin mRNA when iron levels are low, thereby promoting its function.

*Regulation of translation*

Certain mRNAs can bind proteins that inhibit translation. The subunits that initiate translation (particularly eukaryotic initiation factor 2) can be inhibited by phosphorylation. Haem acts by preventing phosphorylation of this factor. When haem levels are high, globin is synthesized. As haem levels fall, globin is not produced.

*Post-transcriptional regulation*

After proteins are synthesized, their lifespan is regulated by proteolytic degradation. Protein lifespans go from hours to years. The level of protein breakdown is itself indirectly under the control of those genes that produce proteases and lysosomal enzymes. Some proteins appear, at some stage of their lifespan, to be attached to a very stable, highly conserved protein known as ubiquitin which marks them for degradation.

## Genetics and inheritance

### *Heredity and variation of the genotype*

The genotype is the exact make-up of the genome. The phenotype is the actual expression of the genome in the individual. The difference between them is caused by the interaction of the genotype and the environment.

Diploid human cells contain 22 pairs of autosomes and each chromosome of the pair carries the same set of genes. Under normal conditions, both chromosomes produce proteins. However, the genes on the two chromosomes are not necessarily a matching set. This is because individual genes can exist in different forms or alleles. An allele is an alternative form of a gene occupying the correct position but expressing a different characteristic. For example, the gene for eye colour may be for brown on one chromosome and blue on the other. Similarly there are single genes for curly hair and for blood groups. This is shown diagrammatically in Figure 18.66.

During mitosis, both alleles will be transmitted to the daughter cells. This is, however, not the case with meiosis where they will be separated. The resultant final genotype of the offspring is also dependent on the additions from the other parent as a result of 'cross-

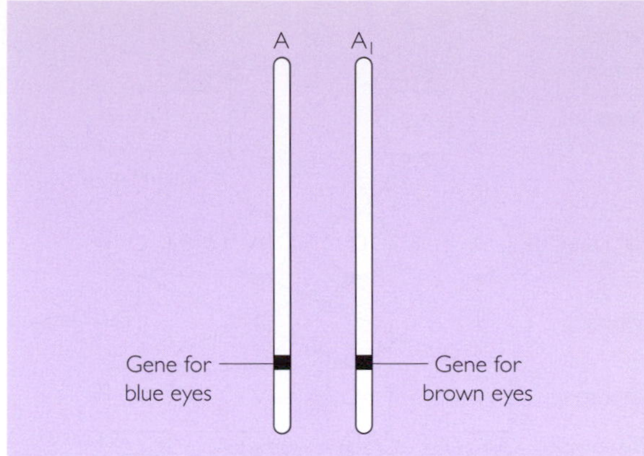


**Figure 18.66** Two alleles of the same autosome providing alternative genes for eye colour.

over' (see Figure 18.63). The way in which alleles are actually expressed in the offspring depends upon whether one allele is dominant over the others. The consequences of this are important in genetic disease.

The principles can be illustrated by considering the inheritance of blood groups. As an example, a parent could have in his or her appropriate chromosomal pair either the gene for blood group A or that for blood group O. The combinations possible would be AA, AO, or OO. Combinations of the same type of allele (AA or OO) are homozygotes; the combination of different alleles (AO) produces a heterozygote. If the gene for group A is present in either chromosome, the blood group expresses the A antigen and is therefore group A. This gene is called dominant, and appropriately the gene for group O is called recessive.

Using the example of blood groups, the meiosis and fertilization of two heterozygote gametes is shown in Figure 18.67. It can be seen that, with this combination of two heterozygote (AO) parents, the chance of having group O blood is 25%. Cystic fibrosis is expressed in the same way as blood groups. It requires two heterozygote parents to have affected offspring, and on average one in four of their offspring will be homozygous for the condition.

A similar genetic tree demonstrating the reproduction ratio of males and females is shown in Figure 18.68. Note that the single Y chromosome of the two parents is expressed in half the children, keeping the sex ratio overall at 1:1.

### *Mutations*

Mutations are permanent changes in the genotype of an organism. Mutations can occur spontaneously within the dividing cell because of internal factors but much more frequently are the result of external influences such as chemicals and radiation. Mutations include single base substitutions, deletions, or insertions. A single base insertion or deletion can change the transcription starting point and cause synthesis of a non-functional protein. Mutations can also cause a single codon change, producing an amino acid alteration or an inappropriate stop codon. Under certain circumstances, because of faulty cell division, there is extra chromosomal material inserted into a cell, forming a genotype compatible with life, e.g. trisomy 21.

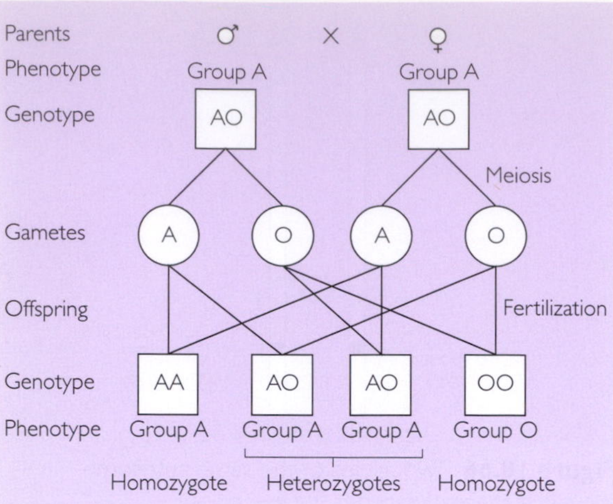


**Figure 18.67** The inheritance of blood groups from two heterozygote parents by the processes of meiosis and fertilization.

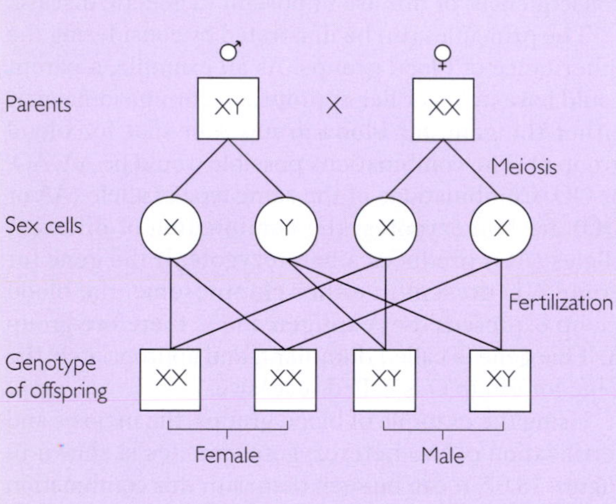


**Figure 18.68** The inheritance of sex chromosomes and the reproduction ratio of males to females.

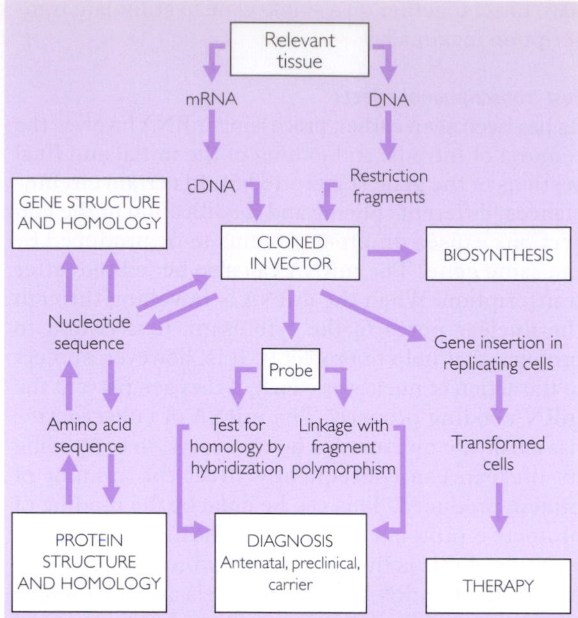


**Figure 18.69** The principles of gene technology. (Adapted from Emery A and Mueller R. *Elements of Medical Genetics*, 8th edn. New York: Churchill Livingstone, 1992.)

The correlation between mutations of various types and disease processes has been recognized for many years, with new findings being announced on an almost weekly basis.

## Gene therapy, recombinant DNA technology, and oncogenes

### *Gene therapy and recombinant DNA technology*

The possibilities of successful gene therapy are truly breathtaking. It is possible, in some people's view, that its effect on therapies will be so widespread that it will markedly affect the need for conventional drugs, surgery, and of course anaesthesia.

The principle of recombinant technology is illustrated in Figure 18.69. It depends on a number of crucial steps:

- identification of the disease clinically;
- identification of abnormal gene or genes;
- the introduction of the desired gene into a modified retro- or adenoviral genome or other plasmid;
- infection by the virus of affected cells with replication gene expression to counter the effect of the imperfect untreated gene.

To date, perhaps the greatest impact of recombinant gene therapy has been the production of drugs, in particular human insulin and hepatitis B vaccine. The methods of their production are summarized in Figure 18.70.

The first successful gene therapy for a genetic deficiency was that of a young girl with adenosine deaminase deficiency, which causes a severe immunodeficiency syndrome. Her T cells were plasmapheresed, infected with a virus containing the adenosine deaminase gene, and reinjected. Other methods considered have been targeting a specific cell system (e.g. inhalation in cystic fibrosis), hepatic arterial injection (e.g. for familial hypercholesteraemia), or engineering the virus surface to recognize particular surface markers on given organs. A large number of clinical trials across a wide range of conditions are currently under way.

In animals, gene therapy has also been used to improve the myocardial response to inotropes by introducing a vector that expresses β-receptors on the cell surface. This may well be of great relevance in the future to patients with heart failure.

### *Oncogenes and anti-oncogenes*

Oncogenes are genes the abnormal expression of which can transform a cell into a tumour cell. They are conserved across species and their normal function is to control cell growth. Over 30 are known in humans. Anti-oncogenes are genes the loss of which leads to the neoplasia because they fail to suppress abnormal cellular activity, e.g. the retinoblastoma gene. In practice, oncogenes and anti-oncogenes are much the same in effect because both

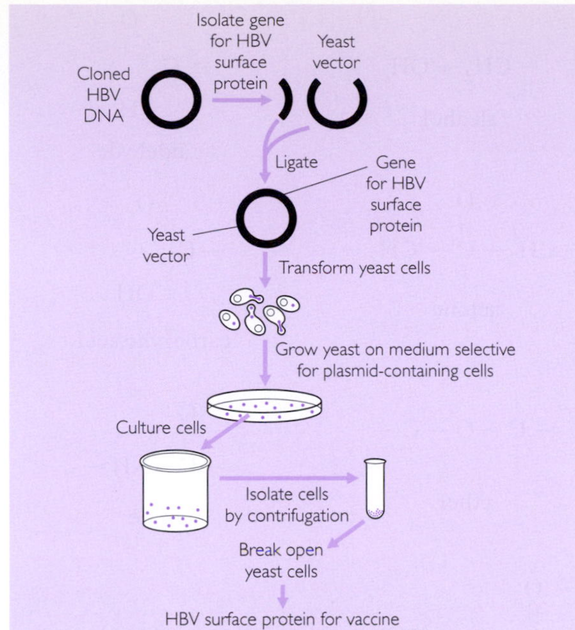


**Figure 18.70** A diagrammatic representation of the production of hepatitis B virus (HBV) vaccine by recombinant DNA. (Adapted from Marks DB *et al. Basic Medical Biochemistry*. Baltimore: Williams & Wilkins, 1996, 253.)

are the sites of mutations leading to cancer. It has been estimated that up to 50% of human cancers may be caused by a change in the suppressor gene known as p53.

It is now accepted that all cancer is genetic although not all cancer is hereditary. Every malignant change does, however, result from a change in genetic machinery. The acquired forms are different from those with a predictable pattern of genetic penetrance by whether or not the genetic mutation occurs in the germline (hereditary) or only in a somatic (sporadic) cell.

### Anaesthesia and genetic disease

These are relevant to each other in the following ways:

- If the promise of gene therapy is fulfilled, the need for conventional anaesthesia may, in the long term, significantly reduce. This depends on the impact that gene therapy has on the prevention of environmental, genetic, and acquired disease.
- Some diseases may be expressed only because of the effects of anaesthesia (e.g. malignant hyperpyrexia and plasma cholinesterase deficiency) or because of preoperative screening or postoperative complications (e.g. sickle-cell trait, porphyria). On these occasions, it is the anaesthetist's responsibility to ensure proper follow-up of the genetic condition.
- There is good evidence to suggest that anaesthetic agents and opioids can have significant effects on gene transcription. The clinical relevance of this is as yet unknown, but it may prove a fertile area for the study of mechanisms of anaesthetic action.
- There are a number of genetic conditions that cause problems in anaesthesia and perioperative management. A number of these are listed in

| **Table 18.24 Some genetic diseases relevant to anaesthesia** |
|---|
| Achondroplasia |
| Acute intermittent prophyria |
| Cystic fibrosis |
| Duchenne muscular dystrophy |
| Haemophilia A |
| Idiopathic hypertrophic subaortic stenosis |
| Malignant hyperthermia |
| Marfan's syndrome |
| Myotonic dystrophy |
| Osteogenesis imperfecta |
| Plasma cholinesterase deficiency |
| Sickle-cell disease |
| Trisomy 21 |

Table 18.24. The implications of some of these diseases are considered in Section 3 of the book. For others more specialized texts should be consulted.

## APPENDIX 18.1: NAMING HYDROCARBON MOLECULES AND FUNCTIONAL GROUPS

### Nomenclature

Many hydrocarbons, which frequently take part in biological reactions, had their own common (or trivial) names that made no reference to their structure, e.g. pyruvate, lethicin, glutamate, etc. Eventually, as more compounds were identified, common names were abandoned in favour of more systematic methods of describing molecules. There are a number of such systems in use.

The most fundamental and precise method is that known as the IUPAC (International Union of Pure and Applied Chemistry) system. It is unambiguous but cumbersome. It is applied as follows:

- Name the longest unbranched chain (this goes at the end of the name).
- Name the substituent groups (these go in the middle of the name).
- Give the positions of the substituent names (these go at the front of the name).
- Count from the end which will give the lower (locant) number for the position of the substituent groups.

Hence:

$$CH_3-CH_2-CH_2-\underset{\displaystyle CH_3}{\underset{|}{CH}}-CH_3 = \text{2-methylpentane}$$

It is important always to select the longest unbranched chain for the basic name. Hence:

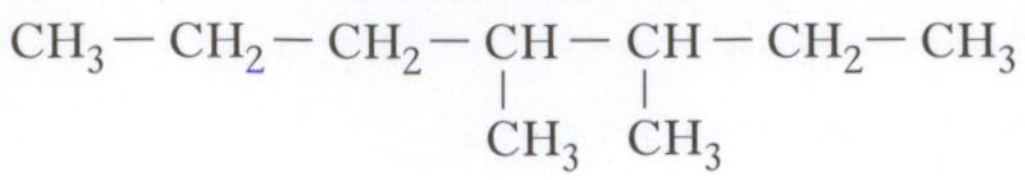

$$CH_3-CH_2-CH_2-\underset{CH_3}{\underset{|}{CH}}-\underset{CH_3}{\underset{|}{CH}}-CH_2-CH_3$$

= 3,4,dimethylheptane

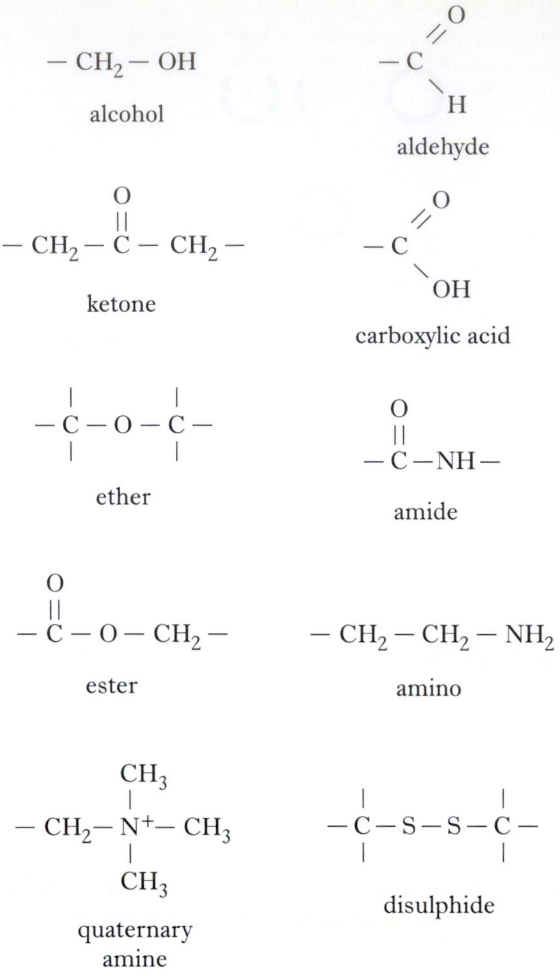

***Single, double, and triple bonds***

Hydrocarbons with single bonds are called alkanes. Hydrocarbons with double bonds are called alkenes. Hydrocarbons with triple bonds are called alkynes. These families of molecules are called aliphatic hydrocarbons. They are tabulated in Table 18.25.

In naming alkenes and alkynes the positions of double and triple bonds are stated. Counting is always done in the direction of minimizing the number of the double or triple bonds. The double bond is numbered before the triple if both are present. Examples of this are:

$CH_2=CH-CH_2-CH_2-CH_3$ = pent-1-ene

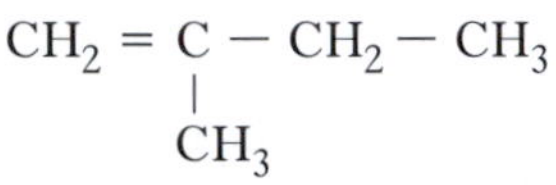

$CH_2=\underset{CH_3}{\underset{|}{C}}-CH_2-CH_3$ = 2-methylbut-1-ene

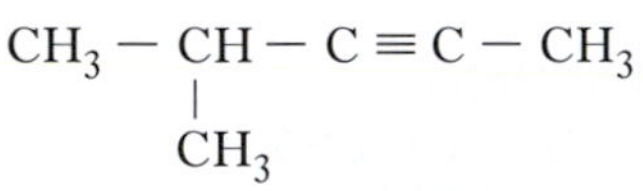

$CH_3-\underset{CH_3}{\underset{|}{CH}}-C\equiv C-CH_3$ = 4-methylpent-2-yne

$-CH_2-OH$ alcohol

$-C(=O)H$ aldehyde

$-CH_2-\overset{O}{\overset{||}{C}}-CH_2-$ ketone

$-C(=O)OH$ carboxylic acid

$-\underset{|}{\overset{|}{C}}-O-\underset{|}{\overset{|}{C}}-$ ether

$-\overset{O}{\overset{||}{C}}-NH-$ amide

$-\overset{O}{\overset{||}{C}}-O-CH_2-$ ester

$-CH_2-CH_2-NH_2$ amino

$-CH_2-\underset{CH_3}{\underset{|}{\overset{CH_3}{\overset{|}{N^+}}}}-CH_3$ quaternary amine

$-\underset{|}{\overset{|}{C}}-S-S-\underset{|}{\overset{|}{C}}-$ disulphide

***Functional groups and named compounds***

The stability of the double and triple bonds produces functional groups with the basic structure:

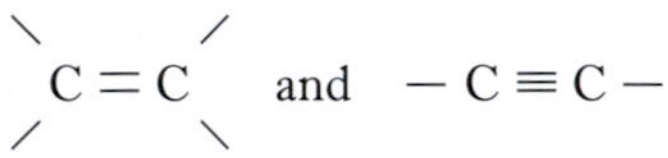

$>C=C<$ and $-C\equiv C-$

$^+NH_3-\underset{R_1}{\underset{|}{H}}-C-\overset{O}{\overset{||}{C}}-NH-\underset{R_2}{\underset{|}{HC}}-C(=O)O-$

peptide bond

- When substitutions are made to these functional groups, or on to a single bonded carbon atom, other named compounds occur. Examples of these are given below.
- When such groupings are present in a molecule, they are often included in the common name of the compound, e.g. methanol, acetaldehyde, phentolamine, etc.

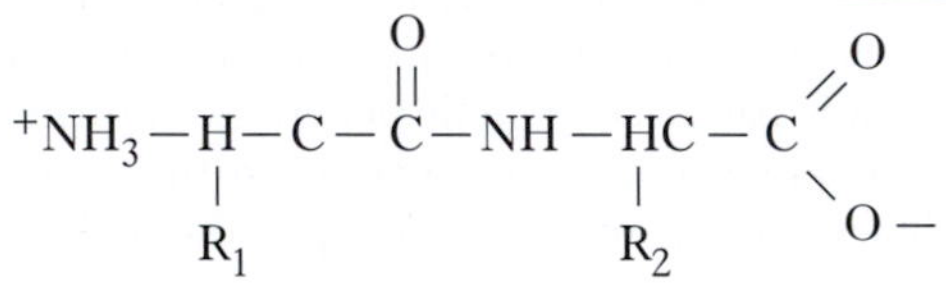

**Table 18.25 Names of aliphatic hydrocarbons**

| No. of C atoms | Alkane | Alkene | Alkyne | Alkyl group |
|---|---|---|---|---|
| 1 | $CH_4$ methane | | | $CH_3$- methyl |
| 2 | $C_2H_6$ ethane | $C_2H_4$ ethene | $C_2H_2$ ethyne | $C_2H_5$- ethyl |
| 3 | $C_3H_8$ propane | $C_3H_6$ propene | $C_3H_4$ propyne | $C_3H_7$- propyl |
| 4 | $C_4H_{10}$ butane | $C_4H_8$ butene | $C_4H_6$ butyne | $C_4H_9$- butyl |
| 5 | $C_5H_{12}$ pentane | $C_5H_{10}$ pentene | $C_5H_8$ pentyne | $C_5H_{11}$- pentyl |
| $n$ | $C_nH_{2n+2}$ | $C_nH_{2n}$ | $C_nH_{2n-2}$ | $C_nH_{2n+1}$ |

### *Other systems of nomenclature*

One system applied to chain hydrocarbons gives the carbon atom in the most oxidized group a number 1 but the second a greek symbol and so on. An example is:

$$\begin{array}{ccccccc} & & OH & & & & O \\ & & | & & & & || \\ CH_3 & - & CH & - & CH_2 & - & C \\ 4 & & 3 & & 2 & & 1 \diagdown O^- \\ \gamma & & \beta & & \alpha & & \end{array}$$

which can be called 3-hydroxybutyrate or β-hydroxybutyrate.

Fatty acids have yet another system in common use in which the numbering begins at the carboxyl group but, whatever the length of the acid, the last carbon is ω. This is shown below in oleic acid which has an 18-carbon chain with one double bond at C9 and is classed as an ω9 fatty acid.

ω 9 10 4 3 γ β 2 α 1 C O O−

## FURTHER READING

Bello EA, Schwinn DA. Molecular biology and medicine: a primer for the clinician. *Anesthesiology* 1996;**85**:1462–78.

Hayflick L. Biologic and theoretical perspectives of human aging. In: *Geriatric Surgery: Comprehensive Care of the Elderly Patient*. Baltimore, MA: Urban & Schwarzenberg, 1990: 3–21.

Weinberg GL. *Genetics in Anesthesiology: Syndromes and Science*. Oxford: Butterworth-Heinemann 1996.

Yost CS. Potassium channels. *Anesthesiology* 1999;**90**:1186–203.

# Chapter 19 General physiological and pharmacological principles

P. Hutton

## BODY FLUID COMPARTMENTS AND TRANSPORT BETWEEN THEM

### The composition and volume of body compartments

Approximately two-thirds of the fluid in the body is located in the cells and is termed 'intracellular fluid'. The other third is called extracellular fluid (Figure 19.1). Note that in the blood the fluid of the red cells is intracellular so that the extracellular compartment of the blood is the total blood volume minus the volume of red and white cells. The volumes of the major body compartments and clinical fluid balance are described in Chapter 14 to which reference should be made for details.

Body fluids contain a variety of dissolved chemicals that are broadly divided into those with covalent bonds (e.g. mainly organic compounds, carbohydrates, proteins, lipids, urea, and creatinine) and those with at least one ionic bond (e.g. mainly inorganic compounds, NaCl, $CaCl_2$, $NaH_2PO_4$, etc.) (see Chapter 18). When dissolved in water, the former group maintain their molecular integrity and form non-electrolytes; the latter dissociate and form electrolytes. Some proteins, when put into a solution, may lose one or two ions, thereby having both covalent and ionic properties.

Dissociating molecules or electrolytes have three main functions:

1. Many are essential minerals (see Chapter 18, Table 18.5).
2. They have a major effect on osmosis (see later).
3. They help to maintain acid–base balance (see later and Chapter 26).

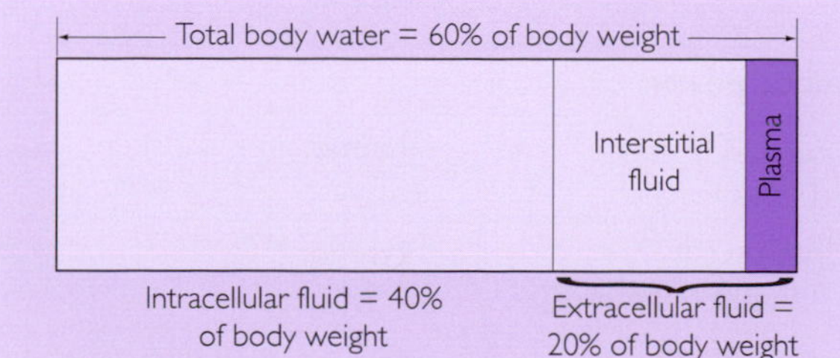


**Figure 19.1** Summary of the relative sizes of body fluid compartments.

Very significant differences exist between the chemical constituents of plasma, interstitial fluid, and intracellular fluids. These are shown in Figure 19.2. It can be seen from this that the main difference between interstitial fluid and the plasma is the concentration of protein (balanced by small changes in $Na^+$ and $Cl^-$ ions). There are, however, very significant differences between the electrolyte compositions of intracellular and those of extracellular fluids in terms of both protein and ion content. In particular, almost all of the potassium and phosphate are intracellular and almost all of the sodium and chlorine are extracellular. This segmentation of ionic species leads to the creation of osmotic and transmembrane potentials (see below).

The main source of body fluid is water derived orally from liquids (1600 ml/day) and foods (1700 ml/day). This is sometimes called pre-formed water. A second, much smaller source is called metabolic water (200 ml/day), which is produced through metabolism and the reaction between $H^+$ and $O^{2-}$ ions in the respiratory chain. The loss of water is from the kidneys, lungs, gastrointestinal tract, and skin. Regulation of intake and output is under complex physiological and hormonal control, as described in detail in Chapters 14, 25 and 29.

### Filtration

Filtration is the bulk flow of liquid through the walls of a container, and is caused by hydrostatic pressure. A semipermeable membrane, depending on pore size, allows the movement of a solvent (such as water) and dissolved substances (such as ions, glucose, urea, etc.) by hydrostatic pressure. The pressure can be generated by the circulation or from gravity. Such movement is always from a high- to a low-pressure region and continues as long as the pressure difference exists. Examples are dependent oedema, the movement of blood through the liver sinusoids, and the filtration of plasma in the glomerulus. In the last, cells and large proteins are retained, but water and small molecules (urea, glucose) pass through the cell membranes into the kidney tubules.

### Osmosis

Water constitutes the bulk of all body fluids and osmosis is the primary way in which water *alone* moves from one body compartment to another. Details of the physics of osmosis can be found in Chapter 38. The concentrations of dissolved solutes on either side of a

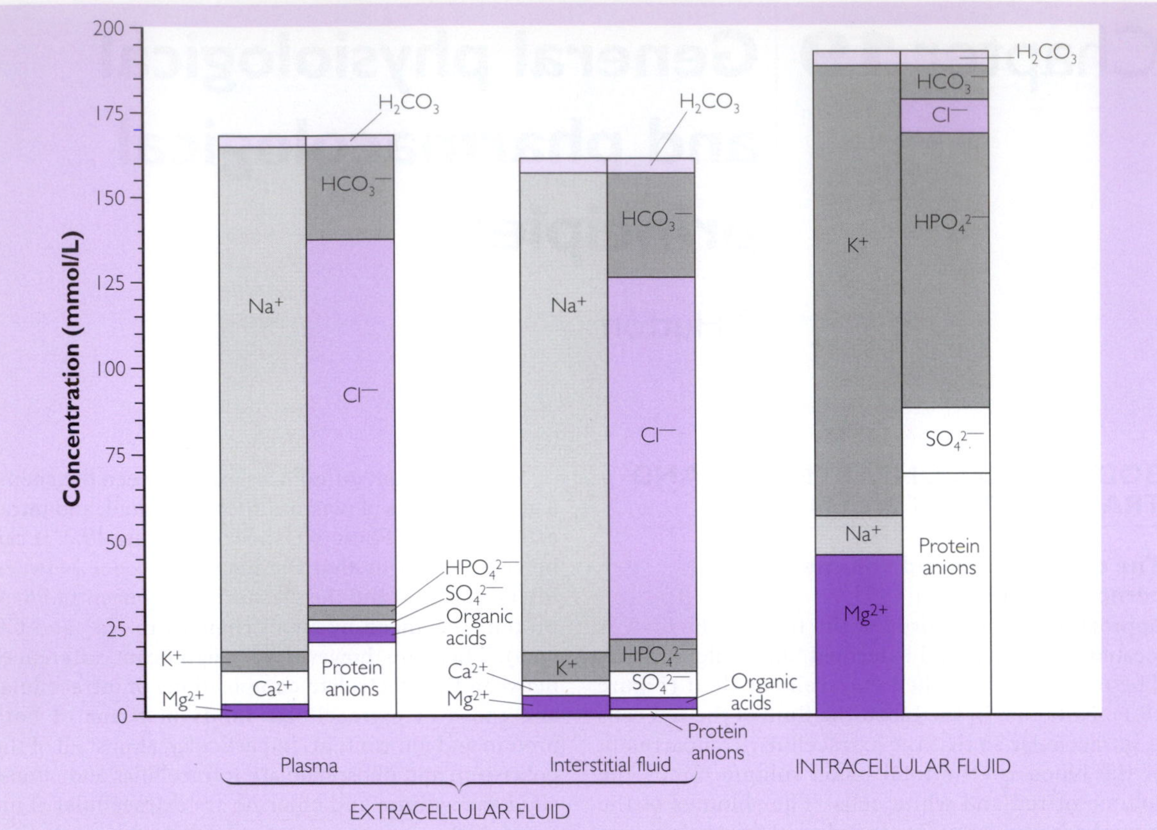


**Figure 19.2** A comparison of the electrolyte compositions of plasma, interstitial fluid and intracellular fluid. $Na^+$, sodium; $K^+$, potassium; $Ca^{2+}$, calcium; $Mg^{2+}$, magnesium; $HCO_3^-$, bicarbonate; $Cl^-$, chloride; $HPO_4^{2-}$, monohydrogen phosphate; $SO_4^{2-}$, sulphate; $H_2CO_3$, carbonic acid. (See text for details.)

membrane are therefore a major determinant of the water balance across it. Most solutes in the body are dissociated into ions and there are additional processes (see later) to maintain differential concentrations of these across membranes.

The osmotic power of a solute depends on the number of molecules or ions in solution rather than on their structure or size. This is called a colligative property. Size is relevant only in that, for the particle to be osmotically active, the effective pore size of the membrane should be less than that of the particle, and the membrane should be permeable to water. Electrolytes, as a result of dissociation, are far more effective than non-electrolytes in producing an osmotic gradient. This can be seen by comparing glucose, sodium chloride, and calcium chloride. They dissociate in water, as shown in Table 19.1.

Although the osmotic power of a molecular species depends on its dissociation properties, it also depends on its concentration. Clinical examples of massive osmotic effects being caused by non-dissociating molecules in high concentration are hyperosmolar diabetic coma, glycosuria, and the action of mannitol.

### Buffering systems and pH effects

Maintenance of the correct pH value is vital for body function. Not only does it allow chemical processes to progress normally, it also regulates the function of enzymes (see Chapter 18) and controls the shape of proteins (see Chapter 18). The pH can be controlled

**Table 19.1 A comparison of the dissociation properties of glucose, sodium chloride and calcium chloride**

| Pure compound | Solvent | Dissolved | Osmotic power |
|---|---|---|---|
| $C_6H_{12}O_6$ (1 mmol) | $H_2O$ | $C_6H_{12}O_6$ 1 mmol | 1 mmol |
| NaCl 1 mmol | $H_2O$ | $Na^+ + Cl^-$ 1 mmol + 1 mmol | 2 mmol |
| $CaCl_2$ 1 mmol | $H_2O$ | $Ca^{2+} + 2Cl^-$ 1 mmol + 2 mmol | 3 mmol |

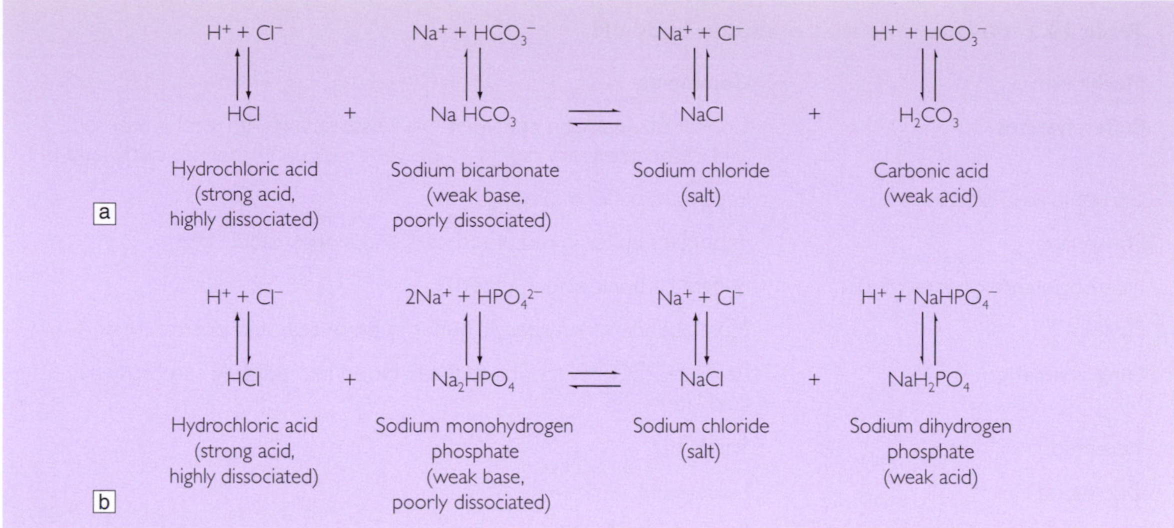


**Figure 19.3** The bicarbonate (a) and phosphate (b) buffer systems. When the pH is normal, bicarbonate molecules outnumber carbonic acid by 20 : 1.

by the excretion of acid ($H^+$) and the retention of bicarbonate ($HCO_3^-$) or by 'soaking up' those ions that are formed during metabolism to prevent them from exerting their effect. The gain and loss of $H^+$ and $HCO_3^-$ ions is controlled by urine formation and breathing: the 'soaking up' for transfer to the lungs or kidney with minimization of their effects is the purpose of a buffer system.

The physiological importance of buffers is that they work within fractions of a second. Most buffer systems in the body consist of weak acids or bases that tend to associate with strong bases or acids, respectively, to remove $H^+$ or $HCO_3^-$ ions out of solution. The most important *inorganic buffers* are the bicarbonate and phosphate systems. There are various ways of representing their action chemically but perhaps the most satisfactory is shown in Figure 19.3.

The two most important *organic buffer systems* are related to proteins. The first is the haemoglobin system. Here the $H^+$ ions from cellular metabolism associate with reduced haemoglobin such that:

$$2H^+ + 2HbO \rightarrow \underset{\substack{\uparrow \\ \text{(released)}}}{O_2} + 2Hb^- + 2H^+ \rightarrow \underset{\text{(weak acid)}}{2HbH}$$

This reaction also helps to explain why haemoglobin gives up its oxygen more easily in acidic conditions.

The second is produced collectively by non-specific proteins that form the most abundant buffer in body cells and plasma. This is because the carbonyl and amine groups in the amino acid bases weakly dissociate to form:

$$NH_2\text{—}\overset{\displaystyle R}{\underset{\displaystyle H}{\overset{|}{\underset{|}{C}}}}\text{—}COO^- + H^+$$

and

$$OH^- + NH_3^+\text{—}\overset{\displaystyle R}{\underset{\displaystyle H}{\overset{|}{\underset{|}{C}}}}\text{—}COOH$$

respectively. The $H^+$ of the COOH group can react with excess $OH^-$, and the $OH^-$ group of the $NH_3^+ + OH^-$ can dissociate and react with excess $H^+$ ions.

The range of pH in the body ranges from 2.5 (in the stomach) to 8.0 (alkaline urine). In contrast, intracellular pH is very tightly controlled for obvious reasons. Differences in intra- and extracellular pH can have a major impact on the transport of substances between the two compartments, especially drugs (see later).

The full significance of buffer base reactions is described in detail in Chapters 21, 25, and 26. For ease of reference, Table 19.2 summarizes buffer systems and routes of excretion of excess $H^+$ and $OH^-$ ions.

### Ionic distribution and transmembrane potentials

Cells are negative internally with respect to their outside by 60–90 mV. This section aims to explain why.

If an equal number of $K^+$ and $Cl^-$ ions were introduced into one half of a tube of water (Figure 19.4a), initially the whole of the tube would be electrically neutral. Then, ions would start to diffuse down the tube through the water. If there was a difference in the speed of diffusion (as there is because $Cl^-$ diffuses faster than $K^+$), an electrical potential will develop between the ends of the tube (Figure 19.4b). Finally, as time passes, the $K^+$ ions will catch up with the $Cl^-$ ions and electrical neutrality will be restored (Figure 19.4c). This property of differential rates of diffusion to separate charges is called a diffusion potential; almost all potentials in living cells are generated by this mechanism.

Now consider the situation in which the KCl is introduced into a container that has a membrane that is permeable to $Cl^-$ but not to $K^+$ ions (Figure 19.5).

**Table 19.2 Mechanisms that maintain body pH**

| Mechanism | Comments |
|---|---|
| **Buffer systems** | Consist of weak acid and weak base associating with strong base or acid, respectively; act rapidly to prevent sudden changes in body fluid pH |
| Carbonic acid–bicarbonate | Important buffer in blood |
| Phosphate | Important buffer in red blood cells and kidney tubule cell |
| Haemoglobin/oxyhaemoglobin | Buffers carbonic acid in blood |
| Protein | Most abundant non-specific buffer in body cells and plasma |
| **Lung ventilation** | Regulates $CO_2$ level of body fluids: blood immediately, cerebrospinal fluid later |
| Increased | Raises pH |
| Decreased | Lowers pH |
| **Urine formation** | Excretes $H^+$ and $NH_4^+$ and conserves bicarbonate as required |

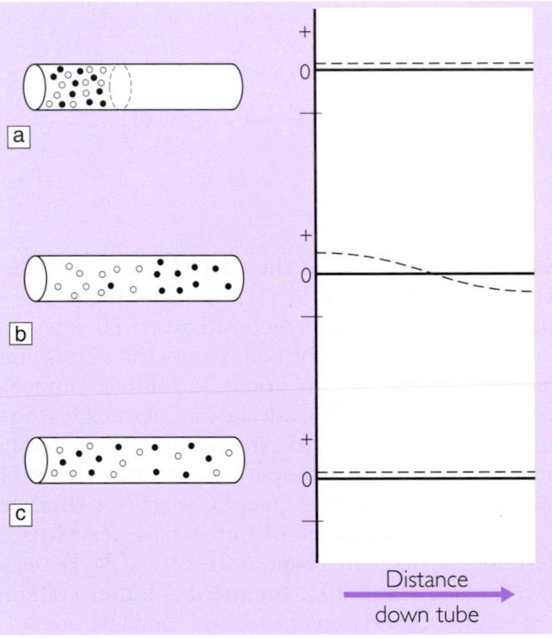


**Figure 19.4** Separation of charge by differential rates of diffusion. •, $Cl^-$; ○, $K^+$. (See text.)

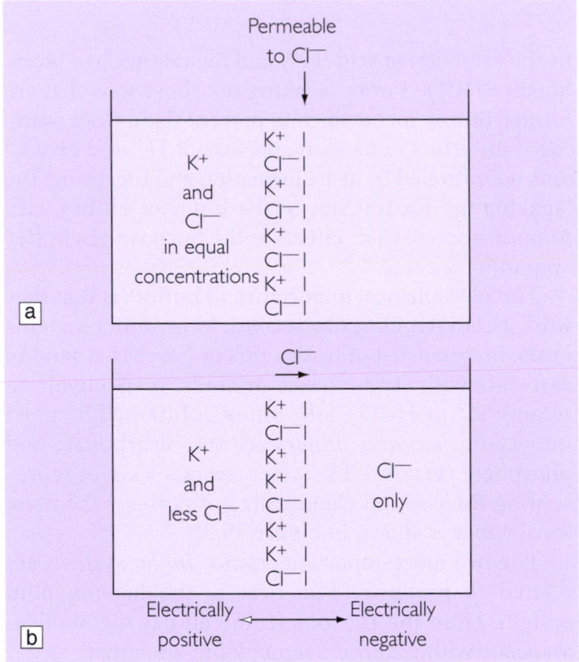


**Figure 19.5** The effect of a membrane permeable to chloride ions but not to potassium ions on the separation of charge. (See text.)

This process of transport across a selectively permeable membrane is called dialysis. Initially, both parts of the cell would be electrically negative (Figure 19.5a), then gradually, because of the concentration gradient, $Cl^-$ ions will move through the membrane and the cell will develop an electrical gradient (Figure 19.5b). At some stage, as the gradient builds up it will exert sufficient back-potential to prevent further diffusion under the concentration gradient of $Cl^-$ ions. At this point, when concentration effects are balanced by electrical effects, the cell is said to be in electrochemical equilibrium and the membrane potential reached is the equilibrium potential.

The phenomenon resulting from the differential separation of charged ions has the name Gibbs–Donnan equilibrium. The potential developed is described by the Nernst equation:

$$\text{Transmembrane potential (mV)} = \frac{60}{Z} \times \log_{10} \frac{[C_o]}{[C_i]}$$

where $Z$ is the ionic charge per ion and $C_o$ and $C_i$ are the concentration of ions on either side of the membrane (o = out and i = in). If there is more than one species of an ion involved, or if an osmotic force comes into play, this equation remains similar in principle but with a series of terms in the numerator and denominator related to each species, their ionic concentration, and the osmotic potential.

The internal and external cellular concentrations of the three major ions, $K^+$, $Na^+$, and $Cl^-$, are shown in Figure 19.2 and numerical values are given in Table 19.3.

**Table 19.3 The relative intra- and extracellular concentrations and equilibrium potentials for chlorine, potassium, and sodium**

| Ions | Approx. extracellular concentration (mmol/L) | Approx. intracellular concentration (mmol/L) | Equilibrium potential (mV) | Permeability of cell membrane |
|---|---|---|---|---|
| $Cl^-$ | 125 | 10 | –70 | Very permeable |
| $K^+$ | 5 | 150 | –90 | Moderately permeable |
| $Na^+$ | 150 | 15 | +60 | Relatively impermeable |

The equilibrium potential for $K^+$ is calculated by substituting into the Nernst equation above:

$$\text{Transmembrane potential (mV)} = \frac{60}{Z} \times \log_{10} \frac{[C_o]}{[C_i]}$$

$$= \frac{60}{+1} \times \log \frac{5}{150} \simeq -90 \text{ mV.}$$

The equilibrium potentials of the other ions are calculated similarly and given in Table 19.3. Also given in Table 19.3 are the relative membrane permeabilities of each of the ions. This means that $Cl^-$ will achieve its equilibrium potential faster than the other two and $Na^+$ will be the slowest. It will be seen later (see Chapters 22–24) that one of the features of neural tissue and muscle is the ability of action potentials to alter these permeability conditions dramatically by opening ion-specific channels, leading to sudden changes in the transmembrane potential.

The total combination of all the ionic species on either side of a nerve cell membrane produces a transmembrane potential of about –70 mV inside with respect to the outside. Comparing this with the equilibrium potentials of Table 19.3 this means:

- little effect on $Cl^-$ ions;
- a steady balance in favour of a net efflux of $K^+$ ions out of the cell (–70 compared with –90 mV);
- a steady balance in favour of a net influx of $Na^+$ ions into the cell (–70 compared with +60 mV).

Why, then, is the cell able to retain a resting –70 mV transmembrane potential? Why do $K^+$ and $Na^+$ ions not move down their ionic and concentration gradients gradually, in time, to reduce their concentration gradients? The answer is that there is a $Na^+/K^+$ pump in the cell membrane which steadily pumps out $Na^+$ and in exchange pumps in $K^+$, thereby countering the physical forces described above. This is represented diagrammatically in Figure 19.6.

The $Na^+/K^+$ pump contains adenosine triphosphatase (ATPase) which catalyses the hydrolysis of ATP to ADP, and is itself activated by intracellular levels of $K^+$ and $Na^+$. Consequently, it is known as the $Na^+/K^+$-activated ATPase pump. The pump extrudes three $Na^+$ from the cell in return for the two $K^+$ that it takes in. Active transport of $Na^+$ and $K^+$ is one of the major energy-using processes of the body and probably

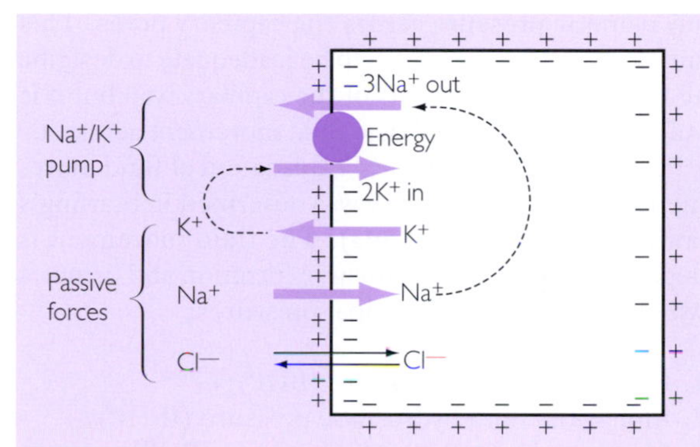


**Figure 19.6** A diagrammatic representation of the sodium/potassium ATPase pump and the fluxes of sodium, potassium, and chloride ions across the cell membrane.

accounts for a large part of basal metabolism. The pump is composed of α and β subunits (Figure 19.7) with binding sites for $Na^+$ on the intracellular surface and for $K^+$ on the extracellular surface. It also has binding sites for ATP and cardiac glycosides.

### Transport across capillaries

The circulatory system uses bulk flow to transport blood around the body. Bulk flow is also relevant in

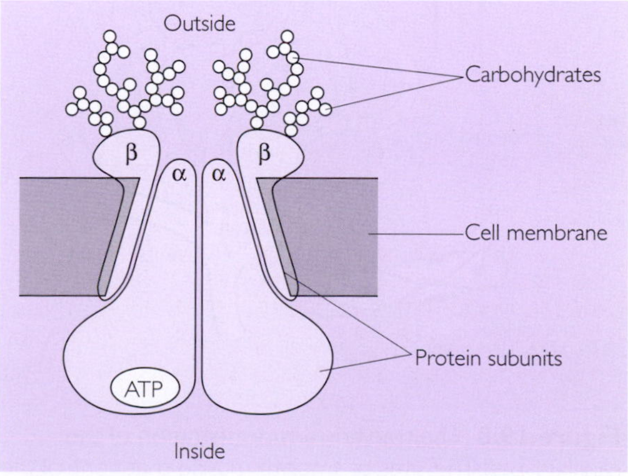


**Figure 19.7** The proposed structure of the sodium/potassium ATPase pump. (See text for details.) (Adapted from Sweadner KJ and Goldin SM. *N Engl J Med* 1980;302:777.)

special areas such as the sinusoids in the liver, spleen, and bone marrow, which have no basement membrane, and large intracellular gaps that allow the free flow of fluid, solutes, and cells. Similarly, arachnoid villi have valves that open and allow the passage of unmodified cerebrospinal fluid into the cerebral veins. In most organs, however, transmission out of the circulating fluid volume is via the capillaries

Transport across and between capillary cells and their basement membranes controls the movement of fluid between the blood plasma and the interstitial compartment of the extracellular fluid. The capillary bed is shown diagrammatically in Figure 19.8. Traditionally, the capillary wall is regarded as having pores of 3.0–5.0 nm in diameter through which water and ions, but not protein, can pass. As a result of this, ions do not exert any osmotic pressure across the capillary pores. This simple model is now known to be inadequate to describe all the observed functions of the capillary wall but it is still a useful model for basic fluid movement across it.

The classic physiological explanation of fluid movement across this boundary was described in Starling's law of the capillaries (1895). The fluid movement is dependent on two mechanisms: filtration and osmosis which generate four principal pressures:

1. blood hydrostatic pressure (BHP);
2. interstitial fluid hydrostatic pressure (IFHP);
3. blood (or plasma) oncotic pressure (BOP);
4. interstitial fluid oncotic pressure (IFOP).

The normal pattern of blood pressure changes through the vascular bed is shown in Chapter 20, Figure 20.25. The oncotic pressure (the osmotic pressure of plasma proteins) is given in Table 19.4.

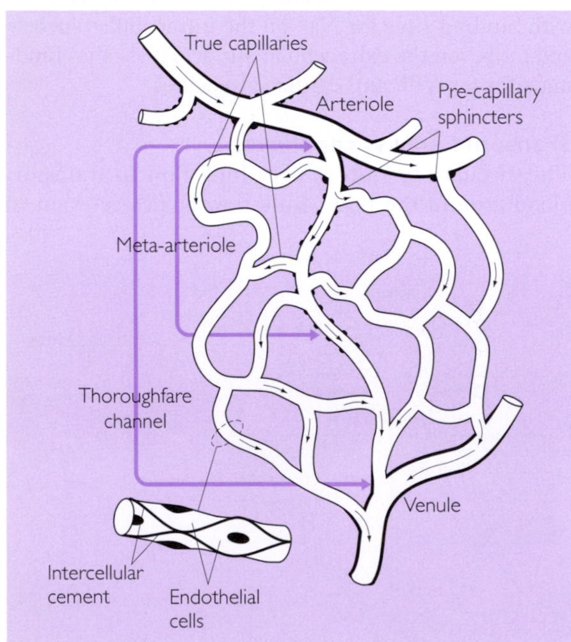


**Figure 19.8** The traditional representation of the capillary bed. The sites of smooth muscle that control the calibre of the channels are indicated for the arteriole, meta-arteriole and pre-capillary sphincters. (Adapted from Rushmer RF. In: Ruch TC and Patton HD, eds. *Physiology and Biophysics*, 19th edn, 1966: 605.)

The net filtration force out of the capillary into the interstitial fluid is BHP + IFOP and the net absorption force into the capillary is IFHP + BOP. Normal transcapillary exchange is shown in Figure 19.9. In this figure it can be seen that at the arterial end the pressures combine to produce a net outward filtration force from the capillary of approximately +10 mmHg, followed by a net inward absorption force of −10 mmHg at the venous end. This balance of forces can be upset by changes in plasma oncotic pressure, arteriolar constriction, venular constriction, arterial blood pressure, venous blood pressure, and the integrity of the capillary wall. These effects are summarized graphically in Figure 19.10.

It should be remembered that the entry pressure to the capillary is under much tighter control by arterioles than the venous pressure, which is dependent on venous filling, posture, and cardiac function. When there is a net flow of fluid from the capillaries into the interstitial space, oedema develops.

## Transport across cell membranes

The movement of fluid across the capillary bed to the interstitial space has already been described. This section considers the much more complex movement across the cell membrane, a schematic cross-section of which is shown in Chapter 18, Figure 18.46. It can be seen that the membrane is a phospholipid bilayer studded with proteins and gated channels possessing cholesterol and carbohydrate attachments. Classifications of transport processes across the membranes differ a little from text to text, but they all divide them into passive systems (which occur under concentration and physicochemical gradients) and active systems that require the expenditure of ATP or some other energy source. For the purposes of this account, the classification summarized in Table 19.5 has been used. Each method is considered in turn.

### *Passive processes*

#### *Filtration*

Filtration has been described above. In transmembrane transport, it is relevant only to those cells with pores (capillaries) and the few specialized areas mentioned (e.g. glomerulus, liver sinusoids).

#### *Osmosis*

This process of movement of water from a lower to a higher concentration of solutes is described in Chapter 38 and above. It is the most important factor in the transmembrane movement of water itself. Osmosis is relevant because if the extracellular osmotic pressure falls, the cell will swell and, if it rises, the cell will shrink. Osmotic changes across cell membranes are the cause of cerebral oedema, which occurs if the serum osmolarity is reduced more quickly than can be compensated for by the blood–brain barrier system. This situation can be produced by the rapid infusion of hypotonic intravenous solutions or rapid reduction of serum glucose by insulin in the presence of longstanding hyperglycaemia.

#### *Dialysis and the Gibbs–Donnan equilibrium*

Dialysis is the diffusion of solute particles across a selectively permeable membrane that separates mole-

**Table 19.4 Osmotic pressure of plasma proteins**

| Protein | Molecular weight | Concentration (g/100 ml) | Oncotic pressure[a] (mmHg) |
|---|---|---|---|
| Albumin | 68 000 | 5.0 | 20 |
| Globulins | 200 000 | 1.5 | 5 |
| Fibrinogen | 500 000 | 0.5 | 1 |

[a]The oncotic pressure is the sum of the osmotic pressures of all the plasma proteins.

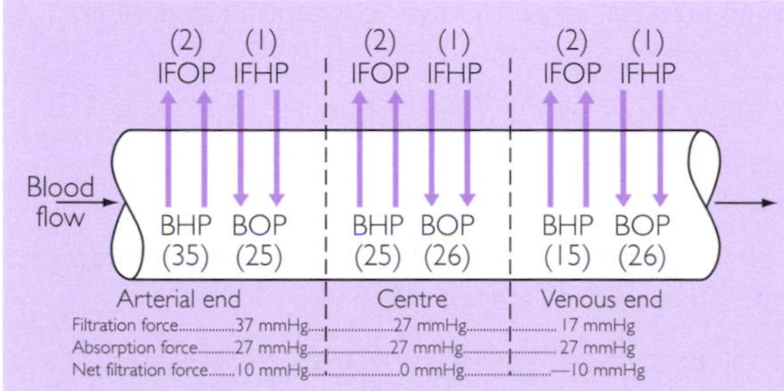


**Figure 19.9** The forces involved in transcapillary exchange. (Values in parentheses are in mmHg.) IFHP, interstitial fluid hydrostatic pressure; IFOP, interstitial fluid oncotic pressure; BOP, blood (plasma) oncotic pressure; BHP, blood hydrostatic pressure.

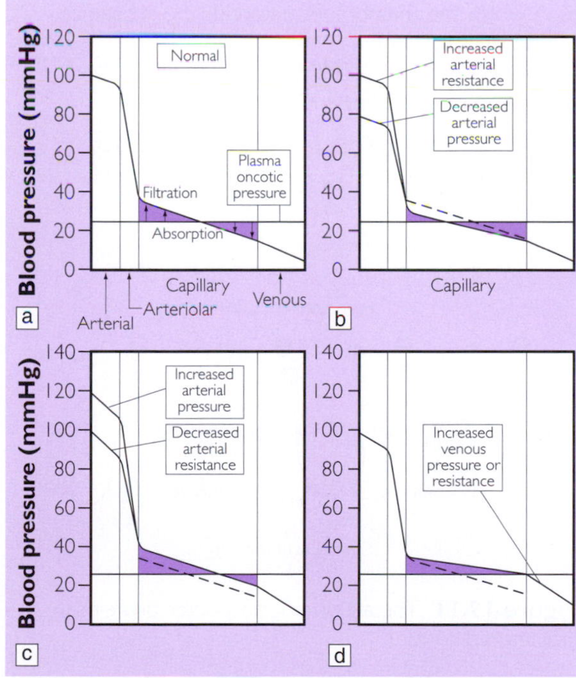


**Figure 19.10** The balance of forces across the capillary wall. (a) Normal conditions; (b) increased arterial resistance or decreased arterial pressure; (c) increased arterial pressure or decreased arterial resistance; and (d) increased venous pressure or resistance. In each of these diagrams the plasma oncotic pressure is the same at the normal value of 25 mmHg. The dashed line in each of the diagrams represents the normal pressure gradient through the capillary. The effect of changes in oncotic pressure can be obtained by changing its level on the graphs. This exercise is left to the reader.

cules on the basis of size. The Gibbs–Donnan equilibrium describes the resulting distribution of charge. This combination of processes, described above, has great importance in the transmembrane transport of ions.

### *Diffusion*

Small (molecular weight [MW] < 60 daltons) uncharged molecules (e.g. $O_2$, $CO_2$, $H_2O$, $N_2O$, NO) can cross membranes easily under a concentration gradient. It is probably one of the most important safety features in cellular respiration that the vital substrate ($O_2$) and the most common waste product ($CO_2$) do not require energy for their transport in and out of cells. Small molecules such as ions which are not lipid soluble ($Na^+$, $K^+$, $Cl^-$) are able to diffuse though channels provided by the integral proteins in the membrane (see Figure 19.6). They are also, under certain circumstances, transferred by active processes (e.g. by the $Na^+/K^+$ ATPase pump, or during the action potential).

A lipid-soluble substance can diffuse through a phospholipid membrane providing that its MW is less than 1000 Daltons and preferably less than 600 Daltons. The greater the lipid solubility (i.e. the bigger the oil/water partition coefficient), the faster the diffusion progresses for a given concentration gradient. Diffusion is how steroid hormones and most drugs used in anaesthesia enter cells. Above a MW of 1000, lipid transfer virtually ceases and other active methods, e.g. pinocytosis (see below), are necessary. Diffusion is the most important route for drugs to cross membranes.

A pH change across a membrane can make a great difference to drug diffusion because, depending on the drug's $pK_a$, it can alter the lipid solubility of the molecule. This effect is used in the forced alkaline diuresis to remove aspirin via the renal tubules. At a urine pH of 4, aspirin is almost 100% un-ionized and, after filtration, is largely reabsorbed back into the circulation in the renal tubule (see Chapter 25). At a pH of 8, it is 99.999% ionized and remains in the tubule after filtration to pass out in the urine. This process is called ion trapping and is covered in more detail below under 'Drug uptake'.

### *Facilitated diffusion*

Although some substances are large molecules (MW > 100 Daltons) and not lipid soluble, they are still able to pass through the cell membrane under a concentration gradient. This is done by a process called facilitated or carrier-mediated diffusion (shown diagrammatically in Figure 19.11) which depends on specific carrier systems. Facilitated and normal diffusion are compared in Figure 19.12. It can be seen that

**Table 19.5 A summary of processes by which substances move across membranes**

| Process | | Description |
|---|---|---|
| *Passive processes:* substances move on their own down a concentration gradient from an area of higher to lower concentration or pressure; cell does not expend energy | Filtration | Net movement of water and solutes through a porous membrane under hydrostatic pressure<br>What passes depends on pore size |
| | Osmosis | Net movement of water molecules as a result of kinetic energy across a selectively permeable membrane from an area of lower to higher solute concentration until an equilibrium is reached |
| | Diffusion | Net movement of molecules or ions as a result of their kinetic energy from an area of higher to lower concentration until an equilibrium is reached |
| | Facilitated diffusion | Diffusion of larger molecules across a selectively permeable membrane with the assistance of integral proteins in the membrane that serve as carriers |
| | Gibbs–Donnan | Separation of charge across a selectively permeable membrane secondary to differences in rates of diffusion |
| | Dialysis | Diffusion of solute particles across a selectively permeable membrane in which small molecules are separated from large ones |
| *Active processes:* substances move against a concentration gradient from an area of lower to higher concentration; cell must expend energy | Active transport | Movement of substances, usually ions, across a selectively permeable membrane from a region of lower to higher concentration by an interaction with integral proteins in the membrane; the process requires energy expenditure in the form of ATP |
| | Endocytosis | Movement of large molecules and particles through plasma membranes in which the membrane surrounds the substance, encloses it, and brings it into the cell<br>Examples include phagocytosis ('cell eating'), pinocytosis ('cell drinking'), and receptor-mediated endocytosis |
| | Exocytosis | Export of substances from the cell by reverse endocytosis |

at low and moderate concentration gradients the rate of transport is higher for the facilitated method, but that, as the concentration gradient continues to increase, a 'ceiling' effect occurs whereby no further increase in the rate of transport is possible and the 'normal' diffusion process again overtakes it.

The best known example of facilitated diffusion is glucose which complexes with a protein carrier (Figure 19.11) and travels down the transmembrane gradient into the cell. The rate of facilitated diffusion depends on:

- the concentration gradient;
- the amount of carrier protein available – this determines the 'ceiling' level of transport;
- the rate of combination of the carrier and substance.

One of the functions of insulin is to accelerate the rate of uptake of blood glucose into the cells, thereby lowering the blood glucose level. Facilitated diffusion systems are selective to optical isomerism (see later), will only function with an appropriate concentration gradient, and are very specific to a particular molecule or groups of molecules.

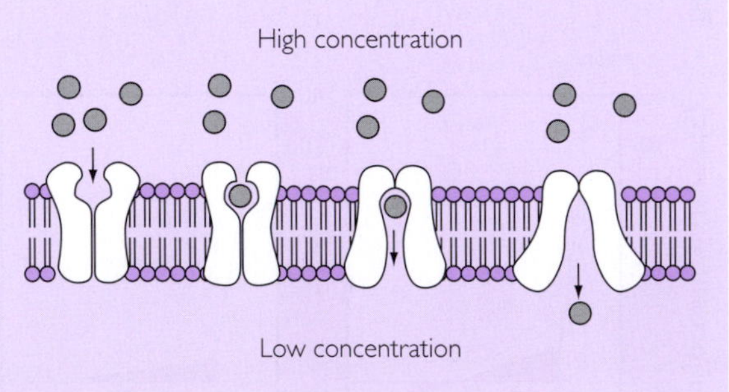


**Figure 19.11** The action of transporter proteins in facilitated diffusion.

### *Active processes*

#### *Active transport*

Active transport is the passage of substances into or out of a cell and has the following properties:

- Membrane proteins that bind or receive the molecule are involved, i.e. it is specific for a molecular type.
- Energy is required for the process to occur.
- It can work against a concentration gradient.

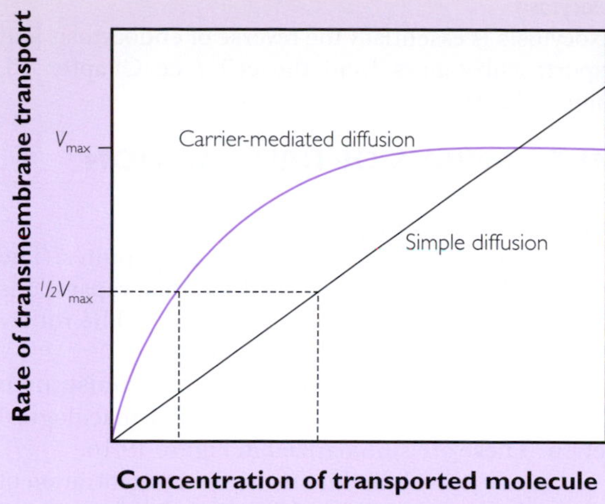


**Figure 19.12** A comparison between simple diffusion and facilitated diffusion. $V_{max}$, maximum rate of reaction. (Carrier mediated and facilitated are equivalent terms.) Note the difference in concentrations required to produce $^1/_2\,V_{max}$.

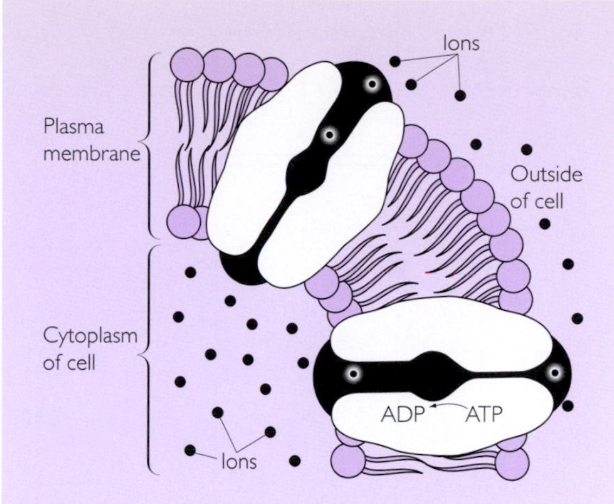


**Figure 19.13** The proposed mechanism of active transport. The upper form of the transporter protein represents an earlier stage of the transport process than the lower one.

The system is shown diagrammatically in Figure 19.13. The fundamental difference between active transport and facilitated diffusion is the ability to work against a concentration gradient. They are compared in Figure 19.14. The following are examples of active transport systems:

- the $Na^+/K^+$ ATPase pump which transports $Na^+$ against a concentration gradient of 10 : 1 and $K^+$ against a concentration gradient of 30 : 1;
- amino acids are transported into cells against gradients of 2–20 : 1;
- sugars, transported into most cells by facilitated diffusion, are actively transported into intestinal and kidney cells;
- iodine uptake in the thyroid;
- catecholamine re-uptake (see Chapter 23);
- secretion of $H^+$ and urate in the renal tubule.

Some drugs similar in molecular structure to endogenous ligands can attach to and compete for active transport. The following are examples:

- Acidic drugs (e.g. salicylates, thiazides, penicillins) compete with urate and may precipitate hyperuricaemia and gout.
- Adrenergic blockers can use norepinephrine (noradrenaline) uptake processes.

A subdivision of active transport systems is sometimes described as secondary active transport. This occurs when a cell joins or shares two extracellular compartments and is shown diagrammatically in Figure 19.15. On one side of the cell there is active pumping of the solute into the cell against a concentration gradient and then, when the concentration in the cell has been achieved, the substance moves passively down the established concentration gradient to the second extracellular compartment. The concentration in the second extracellular compartment is, however, higher than that of the first, a situation that could not have been achieved by passive forces alone. Two examples of this

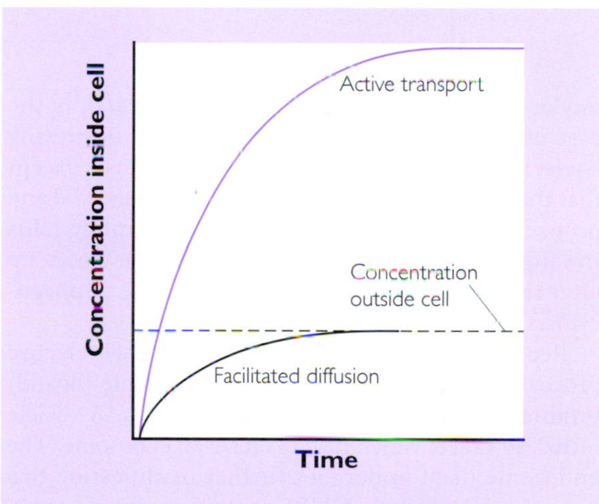


**Figure 19.14** A comparison of active transport and facilitated diffusion into a cell in relation to concentrations inside and outside the cell.

type of system are the movement of nutrients from the gut into the bloodstream, and the reabsorption of glucose into the bloodstream from the renal tubules.

#### *Endocytosis*

Large molecules and particles unsuitable for passive or active transport mechanisms can enter cells by a process called endocytosis, in which a segment of the plasma membrane surrounds the substance, encloses it, and absorbs it into the cell (Table 19.5). The reverse mechanism is called exocytosis. There are three basic types of endocytosis: phagocytosis, pinocytosis, and receptor-mediated endocytosis (see Chapter 18, Figures 18.48 and 18.50).

In phagocytosis, literally cell-eating projections of the cell, called pseudopodia, move around the particle (or other cell), surround it, and form an internal membranous sack called a phagocytic vesicle. The solid material within the vesicle is then broken down and digested. It is an important process for all substances

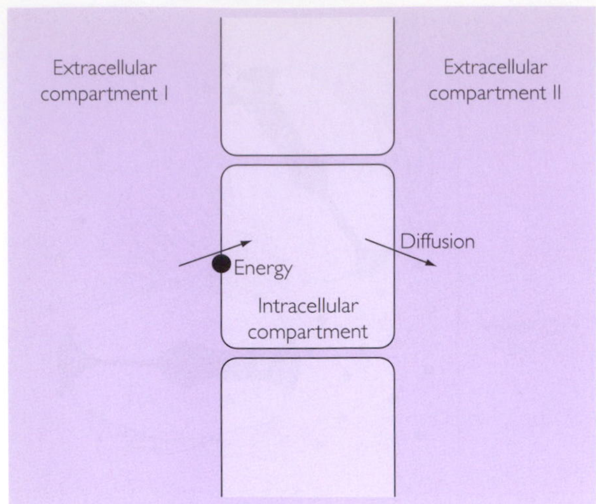


**Figure 19.15** Secondary active transport. There is active transport from extracellular compartment I into the cell and then diffusion from the cell into extracellular compartment II, thereby allowing the concentration in compartment II to be greater than that in compartment I.

too large for other transport mechanisms and, in the case of white blood cells, is one method of destroying bacteria. Pinocytosis is similar to phagocytosis except that the ingested material is fluid rather than solid and no pseudopodia form. The membrane simply folds inwards or there is an existing channel that closes up after the fluid enters. Few cells are capable of phagocytosis but many carry on pinocytosis.

Receptor-mediated endocytosis is a highly selective process which is initiated by a large molecule (ligand) binding to a specific cell surface receptor. A vesicle forms, several of which fuse to create an endosome. The endosome itself undergoes further modification to a large structure called a CURL (compartment of uncoupling of receptor and ligand). In a CURL, the receptors and ligands are separated and compartmentalized into two membrane-bound compartments. The compartment containing receptor proteins is recycled and that containing the ligands is digested by the lysosomes.

*Exocytosis*

Exocytosis is essentially the reverse of endocytosis and exports substances from the cell (see Chapter 18, Figure 18.48).

## MECHANISMS OF DRUG ACTION

### Routes of drug administration

Drugs can be administered by a variety of routes. The route of choice depends on the drug, the preparations in which it is available, and convenience. The routes available are summarized in Table 19.6.

There are many steps between the administration of a drug and the expression of its pharmacological action. These are summarized in Figure 19.16.

In intact animals and humans, the concentration of drug at its site of action is dependent on the route of administration, absorption, distribution, metabolism, and excretion. Under some conditions, it is difficult to obtain meaningful dose–response data. In most of the literature describing results in humans, the serum concentration is taken as the 'dose' level. As will be seen later under 'Pharmacokinetics', only under carefully controlled, specified, steady-state conditions does the serum concentration represent the concentration at the site of action. The relationship between dose and pharmacological action is least well defined for preparations of group I (Table 19.6). The amount of the administered drug that enters the circulation is measured by its bioavailability, a concept that is discussed in greater detail later.

In summary, the message is, when interpreting dose–response data, to look carefully at the mode of administration and all the other factors shown in Figure 19.16.

The pharmacological effects of a drug are usually measured by the use of dose–response curves. Dose–response curves are of two fundamentally different types: graded and quantal. These are described below.

#### *Graded dose–response curves*

A graded dose–response curve results from administering a number of doses over a given range and observing the response. The relationship is typically

**Table 19.6 Routes of drug administration**

| Group | Route | Features |
|---|---|---|
| I | Oral<br>Intramuscular<br>Subcutaneous<br>Inhalational<br>Transdermal/topical<br>Intranasal/transmucosal<br>Rectal | Require absorption to reach blood first and then travel to target tissues |
| II | Intravenous<br>Intra-arterial | Injected directly into blood but need to travel to target tissues |
| III | Local infiltration<br>Epidural<br>Intrathecal | Delivered directly to target tissues |

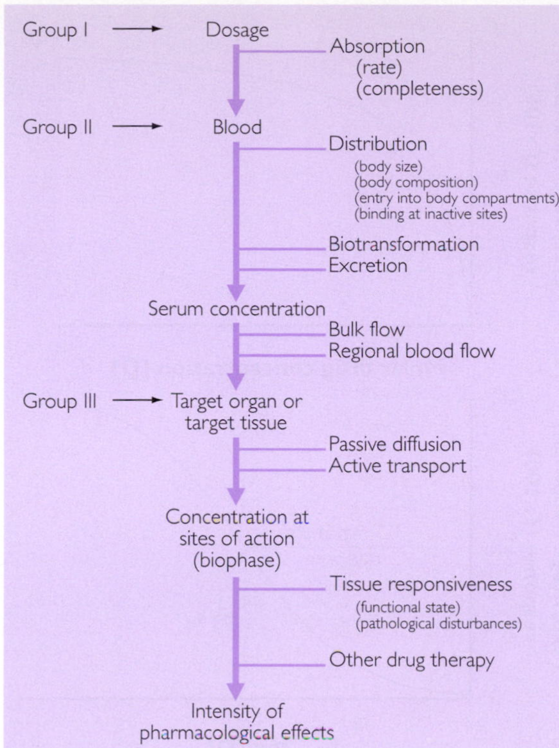


**Figure 19.16** The steps between the administration of a drug and the expression of its pharmacological action. Drug groups I, II, and III are explained in Table 19.6. Note that, often, distribution, biotransformation, excretion, and bulk flow all essentially occur simultaneously but at rates dependent on the individual patient, the cardiac output, and regional blood flows.

subject to a maximal response, assumed to be the condition when the receptors are fully occupied. The drug can be administered *in vitro* in an isolated preparation in a tissue bath, or given *in vivo* to the intact animal or human. The initial assessment of the drug during its development tends to be on *in vitro* preparations with *in vivo* studies being required before its release for human use.

The morphology of the response is as shown in Figure 19.17a. Drug A is more potent than drug B because the same response is produced by a lower dose. When the dose scale is replotted logarithmically, the curves are changed to those shown in Figure 19.17b. Logarithms of dose–response curves are used almost universally for plotting the results of pharmacological measurements for three main reasons:

1. Similar substances and the effects of antagonists (see later) give parallel curves, so potency is easier to measure.
2. If the middle response range (25–75%) is used, a straight line provides a reasonable fit. This is useful when only a limited number of data points are available.
3. A logarithmic scale gives weighting to all dose levels and allows a wide range of doses to be plotted on a single graph without undue compression of data.

Following the recognition of receptors by Langley (1905) and Erlich (1913), the two main classic theories of drug action, the occupancy theory (Clarke) and the rate theory (Paton), were proposed to explain the charateristics of drug action. Both have advantages and disadvantages. The occupancy theory is outlined here because it gives a good mental picture of drug–receptor action and is the most frequently used model. Despite its limitations, which are discussed later, this concept is useful in that it applies to many drugs and provides helpful insights into, and understanding of, agonists, antagonists, and partial agonists.

The occupancy theory assumes that the drug (D) binds through a receptor (R) and that the D–R combination produces a response determined by α, a measure of efficacy. If D, R, and DR are expressed as molar concentrations, and $K_1$ and $K_2$ are velocity constants, such that:

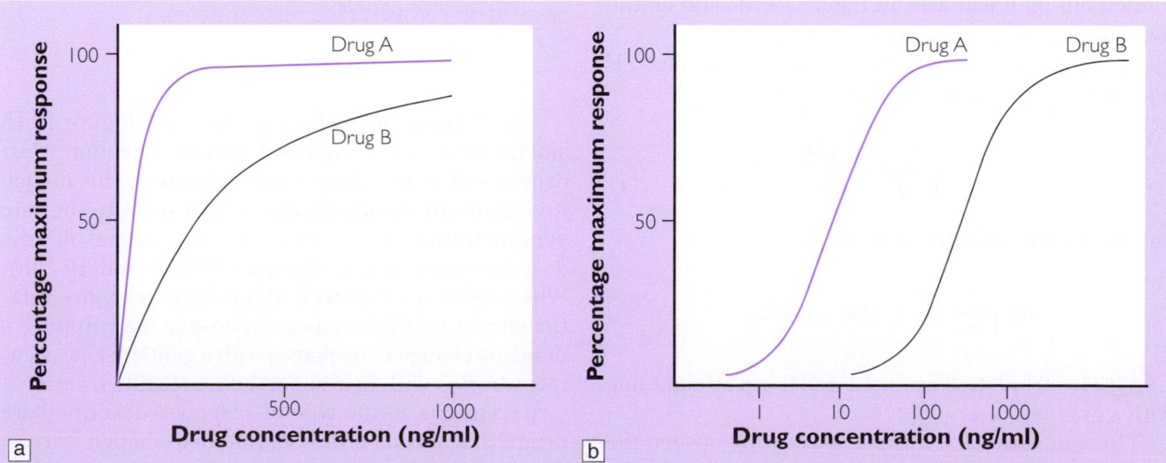


**Figure 19.17** Graded dose–response curves plotted on (a) linear and (b) logarithmic scales. In this example, drug A is acetylcholine and drug B propionylcholine. The pharmacological response is the contraction of guinea-pig ileum in an *in vitro* preparation. (Adapted from Burgen ASV and Mitchell JF. *Gaddum's Pharmacology*, 6th edn. Oxford: Oxford Medical Publications, 1968: 3.)

$$[D] + [R] \underset{K_2}{\overset{K_1}{\rightleftharpoons}} [DR] \xrightarrow{\alpha} \text{effect} \qquad (1)$$

then at equilibrium:

$$K_2\,[DR] = K_1\,[D]\,[R];$$

applying the law of mass action:

$$\frac{[D]\,[R]}{[DR]} = \frac{K_2}{K_1} = K_D \qquad (2)$$

where $K_D$ is the equilibrium dissociation constant. This classic view assumes three properties of receptors:

1. They are specific for the drug or ligand.
2. There is a measurable affinity for the drug to bind to the receptor expressed by the value of $K_1/K_2$, i.e. the reciprocal of $K_D$.
3. The drug–receptor complex has the ability to produce a pharmacological response. This response is called intrinsic activity or efficacy. The degree of pharmacological response would be predicted by the value of α in equation (1). Drugs with different efficacies have different values of α.

Classic occupancy theory continues with the assumption that there is a fixed number of receptors and that the number occupied determines the response. It can be shown by a rearrangement of equation (2) that the fraction of receptors occupied ($f$) is given by:

$$f = \frac{[D]}{(K_D + [D])} \qquad (3)$$

It follows that, because the response is proportional to the number of receptors occupied, $f$ in equation (3) is also the fraction of the maximum response possible produced by drug concentration [D].

Equation (3) is a rectangular hyperbola with identical properties to the Michaelis–Menten equation for enzymes kinetics (see Chapter 18, Figure 18.39). It is plotted out on linear axes in Figure 19.18a and on the familiar log–linear axes in Figure 19.18b.

Classic theory also produces so-called Hill plots. If equation (3) is rearranged, it results in:

$$\frac{f}{1-f} = \frac{[D]}{K_D} \qquad (4)$$

and taking logs of both sides gives:

$$\log \frac{f}{1-f} = \log\,[D] - \log K_D.$$

Log $[f/(1-f)]$ plotted against log [D] is a straight line with a gradient of 1.

Thus, in summary, if the relationship between the response and drug concentration is as described by the assumptions of equation (1), the response curve is hyperbolic (Figure 19.18a) and the Hill plot is linear with a gradient of +1 (Figure 19.18c). Hill plots are undertaken to simplify the analysis of results.

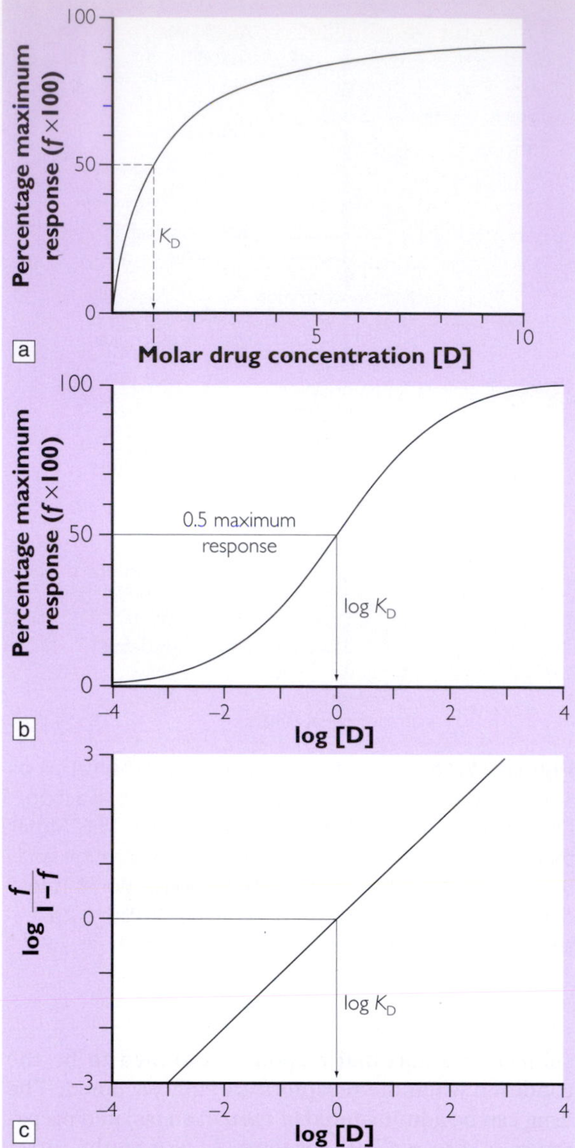


**Figure 19.18** The occupancy model of drug–receptor response. Response plotted on (a) a linear scale; (b) a logarithmic scale; and (c) the corresponding Hill plot. $f$, the fractional value of the maximum response; $K_D$, the dissociation constant. (See text for details.)

Very many drugs behave as shown in Figure 19.18 and the model has served well since its inception. Most drugs used in anaesthesia approximate to this model. An important clinical aspect with respect to the safe administration of a drug is the slope of the dose–response curve (Figures 19.17b and 19.18b). When there is a relatively steep dose–response relationship, a small increment in dosage may produce a dramatic change in response; with a gentler slope accurate titration with incremental doses is much easier.

Exceptions to the type of response described are drugs that produce bimodal or bell-shaped curves. These are not often seen in clinical use because of their obvious practical implications. Other response curves plotted on linear axes for nicotinic, glutamic, and GABAergic receptors (GABA is γ-aminobutyric acid) are sometimes sigmoidal rather than hyperbolic. This can, on occasion, imply an allosteric effect of one receptor on another in a similar way to that for enzymes. The attachment of the four molecules of oxygen to haemoglobin is an example of allosteric binding, in that the presence of the first molecule makes it easier for the second to bind and so on.

Another way in which classic occupancy theory fails is that it is now known that 100% receptor occupancy may not be required for maximum effect. For instance, at the neuromuscular junction, only 25% of the receptors may be required to produce a maximal twitch response and only 50% for a sustained tetanic response. As most receptors have an endogenous ligand targeted by an endogenous transmitter, this phenomenon can be interpreted teleologically by saying that maximal response from occupation of a fraction of receptors provides an important margin of safety under normal conditions.

### *Quantal dose–response curves*

The previous section considered the response of a patient or *in vitro* preparation to a variation in the dose of drug. An alternative approach is to specify a required effect, e.g. loss of consciousness, change in absolute blood pressure by 10 mmHg, etc. and to see what dose is required to achieve it. This is a quantal rather than a graded response, because the specified effect is either present or absent.

When experiments of this type are done and the log of the dose is plotted on the *x* axis, the result is usually a bell-shaped, normal distribution curve as shown in Figure 19.19. Each bar of the curve represents the percentage of individuals for whom a specified dose would be effective but not too much. If this is then integrated, as shown in Figure 19.19, the cumulative frequency curve results.

The cumulative frequency or quantal dose–response curve gives information on the proportion of a population who will respond if a particular dose is given. In the example of a hypnotic shown in Figure 19.20, if 100 mg is given, 50% of the population will respond by going to sleep and, if 150 mg is given, 90% will respond. These are termed the $ED_{50}$ and $ED_{90}$ respectively, meaning the effective dose for 50% and 90% of the population. Examples of $ED_{50}$ values in anaesthetic use are minimum infusion rate $(MIR)_{50}$ (see Chapter 32) and minimum alveloar concentration (MAC; see Chapter 33). The $ED_{50}$ is often termed the 'median effective dose'. It should also be noted that any particular chosen dosage given, e.g. the $ED_{95}$, although effective in 95% of the population, is unnecessarily large for 94% of the population and ineffective in 5% of the population.

Another useful interpretation from such plots is the predictability of drug action. This is illustrated in Figure 19.21. If drug A, with a very narrow bell-shaped distribution, is given at dose $D_1$, 50% of the population will respond. The same is true of drug B. If, however, dose $D_2$ is given, almost 100% of the population will respond to drug A, whereas there will be only a small increase in the number of responders to drug B. Consequently, drug A has an effective dose that is easily predictable whereas drug B requires careful titration. The cumulative frequency distribution is also drawn in for the two drugs in Figure 19.21.

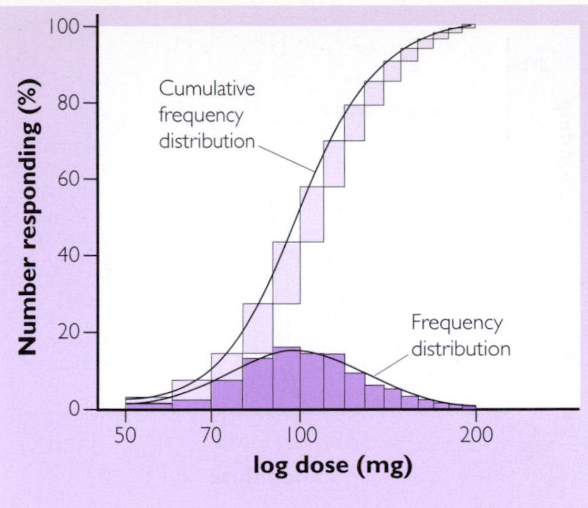


**Figure 19.19** A quantal dose–response curve and the associated cumulative frequency distribution. (Adapted from Fingl E and Woodbury DM. General principles. In: Goodman LS and Gilman A, eds. *The Pharmacological Basis of Therapeutics*, 5th edn. New York: Macmillan 1975: 27.)

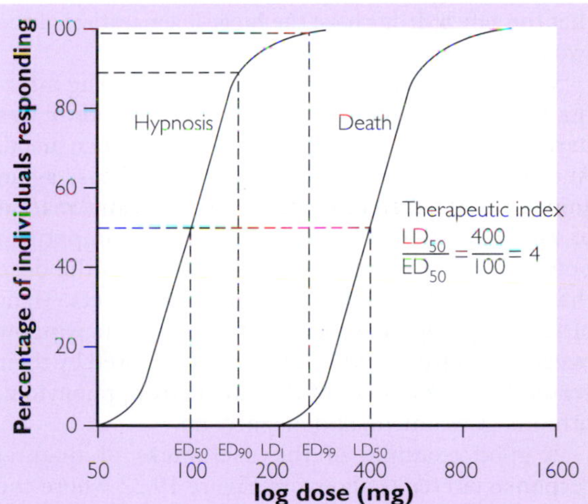


**Figure 19.20** Cumulative dose–response curves of a hypnotic drug for hypnosis and death. Also shown is the calculation of the therapeutic index. (Adapted from Fingl E and Woodbury DM. General principles. In: Goodman LS and Gilman A, eds. *The Pharmacological Basis of Therapeutics*, 5th edn. New York: Macmillan 1975: 27.)

The safety of drugs is sometimes expressed as a therapeutic ratio or therapeutic index. This relates the effective dose for a given percentage of a population to a toxic or lethal dose (LD) for the same percentage. Using a hypnotic, sedative, or induction agent as an example, cumulative frequency distributions can be plotted for both the effective dose for hypnosis and the lethal dose, as shown schematically in Figure 19.20. In the past, these have been determined by animal experiments in which the dose was increased until death occurred. The therapeutic ratio, defined here as $LD_{50}/ED_{50}$, is derived on the graph. It can be seen from the way Figure 19.20 is drawn that the $ED_{99}$ for hypnosis is higher than the $LD_1$ for death, i.e. there is a crossover between hypnosis for the most resistant subjects

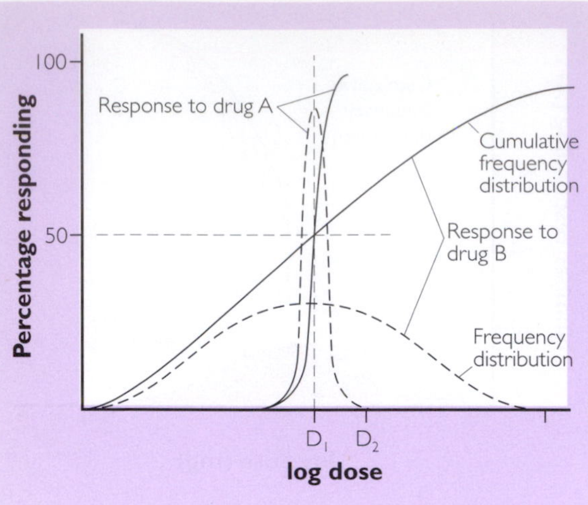


**Figure 19.21** The effect of quantal dose–response curves on the predictability of drug action. -----, frequency distribution; —, cumulative frequency distribution. (See text for details.)

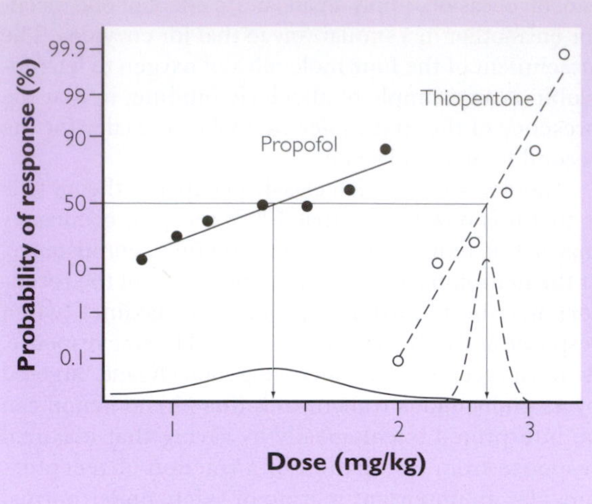


**Figure 19.22** The dose–response curves of propofol and thiopentone. (See text for details.) (Adapted from Leslie K and Crankshaw DP. *Br J Anaesth* 1990;64:734.)

and death for the most sensitive. It is therefore clear that the safest drugs have the biggest separation of the two curves on the *x* axis.

When the therapeutic ratio is quoted in drug information, it is very important to know exactly how it was derived because several methods have been used. Another application of this type of analysis, again sometimes referred to as the therapeutic ratio, margin of safety, or therapeutic window, is the comparison between the effective therapeutic dose and the dose that causes not death but unwanted side effects. Many of the drugs that have a narrow therapeutic window because of adverse side effects are monitored by their serum level. Examples of this are digoxin, phenytoin, lithium, gentamicin, and magnesium.

A good example of the usefulness of quantal response curves is shown in Figure 19.22 where the two induction agents propofol and thiopentone (thiopental) are compared. It can be seen that, for loss of consciousness, thiopentone has a much steeper dose–response curve than propofol. The less-steep dose–response curve for propofol demonstrates that greater multiples of the $ED_{50}$ are required to induce anaesthesia in the more resistant members of the population. These data make thiopentone a more suitable agent to give in situations such as rapid sequence induction, when a fixed milligram per kilogram drug dose aimed at 95% of the population has to be administered blindly rather than being titrated to effect.

Figure 19.22, has, on the *y* axis, not the number responding but the probability of response. This plot is a variation of the quantal dose–response curve constructed using 'probit' analysis. Probit can be thought of as 'the probability of it happening'. An example of how such data are produced is shown in Table 19.7. Dose-ranging studies on a new induction agent require a range of doses to be given to a group of subjects and the response observed. This process is represented by the first three columns of Table 19.7. The fourth column is the probability of sleep occurring at the given dose level. This can be expressed as a fraction of one (as shown) or as a percentage.

The probability of sleep is then plotted against the logarithm of the dose as shown in Figure 19.22 for propofol and thiopentone. The type of graph paper used is called logarithmic probit paper. It has the effect of linearizing the ends of the sigmoid-shaped quantal dose–response curves of Figures 19.19 and 19.20, thereby allowing interpolation for identification of the $ED_{50}$, $ED_{95}$, etc. In practice, the doses of induction agent recommended in product literature approximate, at their upper limit, to the $ED_{95}$ for the population.

A different way of establishing the $ED_{50}$ for induction agents given by infusion was that developed by Kenny's group in Glasgow. They used computer-driven infusion pumps to produce target blood propofol concentrations in the presence or absence of nitrous oxide. After a standard incision, if the patient responded, the next patient received a higher target concentration. This procedure was continued until there was no response. Then, the next patient had a reduced target concentration. Depending on their response, the next patient received a higher or lower target concentration, and so on. In this iterative way, when a given level produced as many responders as non-responders, the $ED_{50}$ was established. The method is shown in Figure 19.23, which also indicates the effect of nitrous oxide on the required dose of propofol.

### Factors that alter the dose–response curve

The factors that alter the position, slope, or maximum height of the dose–response curve in a given subject can be classified as:

- antagonists;
- partial agonists;
- inverse agonists;
- tolerance or tachyphylaxis.

This account will consider these effects on the graded dose–effect relationship as shown in Figure

**Table 19.7 An example of a dose-ranging study for a new induction agent**

| No. of subjects (*n*) | Dose of new agent (mg) | Patients going to sleep (*x*) | Probability of sleep (*x*/*n*) |
|---|---|---|---|
| 50 | 50 | 16 | 0.32 |
| 50 | 75 | 20 | 0.40 |
| 50 | 100 | 24 | 0.48 |
| 50 | 125 | 34 | 0.68 |
| 50 | 150 | 39 | 0.78 |
| 50 | 175 | 42 | 0.84 |
| 50 | 200 | 49 | 0.98 |

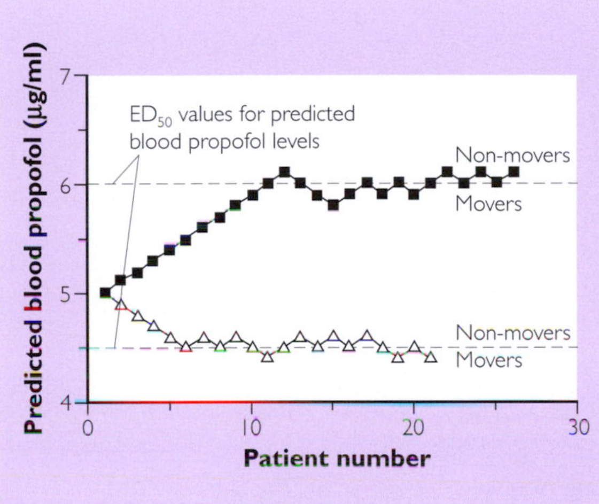


**Figure 19.23** Establishing the $ED_{50}$ for propofol and $O_2$ with (△) and without (■) nitrous oxide using an iterative technique. (See text for details.) (Adapted from Davidson JAH *et al. Acta Anaesthesiol Scand* 1993;37:458.)

19.17. The consequences on the quantal dose–response curve (see Figure 19.19) can be inferred by the reader.

***Antagonists***

When a drug binds to a receptor, its attraction to the receptor is called its affinity. In the analysis above in equation (1), for a high-affinity drug, the combination [DR] will form easily and, once formed, will be stable. The ability of the drug when bound to exert a pharmacological effect is its intrinsic activity or efficacy.

Antagonists are drugs that bind to a receptor but that, once bound, do not produce the appropriate pharmacological response, i.e. they possess affinity but no intrinsic activity. Antagonists can be classified in a variety of ways. Here we have chosen the following:

- competitive reversible antagonists;
- competitive irreversible antagonists;
- non-competitive antagonists.

*Competitive reversible antagonists*

A competitive reversible antagonist combines reversibly with the same receptor as the agonist but induces no pharmacological response. It can be displaced from receptors if the dose of agonist is high enough. An antagonist typically displaces the log dose–response curve to the right in a parallel manner, but the maximum possible response is unaffected. Examples of this are shown in Figure 19.24 where epinephrine (adrenaline) and norepinephrine are compared in the presence of different concentrations of propranolol. A number of competitive reversible antagonists are used in anaesthetic practice. They are listed in Table 19.8.

*Competitive irreversible antagonists*

This group is similar to reversible antagonists, but the drug and receptor dissociate very slowly and there may be some covalent bonding. Alternatively, the antagonist may distort the receptor site, preventing subsequent successful competition by the agonist. Such agents not only displace the dose–response curve to the right, but also reduce the maximum efficacy possible. If only a small dose of irreversible agonist is given and there are spare receptors, the initial effect may

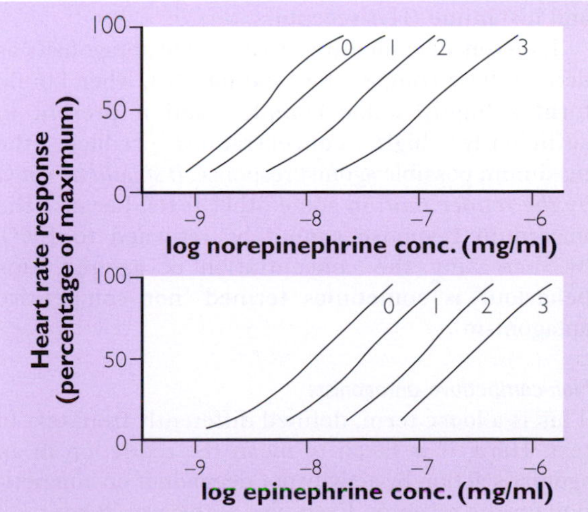


**Figure 19.24** The heart rate of an isolated cat heart preparation to norepinephrine and epinephrine in the presence of increasing concentrations of propranolol (0 = zero; 1 = 0.001 mg/ml; 2 = 0.005 mg/ml; 3 = 0.025 mg/ml). (Adapted from Carlsson E and Hedberg A. In: Popper PJ *et al.*, eds. *Beta Blockade and Anaesthesia*. Molndal: Lingren, 1980: 17.)

**Table 19.8 Competitive reversible antagonists used in anaesthesia practice**

| Drug | Endogenous compound antagonized |
|---|---|
| Atropine<br>Glycopyrrolate<br>Hyoscine | Acetylcholine (at muscarinic sites) |
| Atracurium<br>Pancuronium<br>Rocuronium<br>Vecuronium | Acetylcholine (at the motor end-plate) |
| Trimetaphan | Acetylcholine (at autonomic ganglia) |
| Atenolol<br>Esmolol<br>Propranolol | Epinephrine and norepinephrine (β effects) |
| Phentolamine | Epinephrine and norepinephrine (α effects) |
| Chlorpromazine<br>Domperidone<br>Metoclopramide | Dopamine |
| Cimetidine<br>Ranitidine | Histamine |
| Ondansetron | 5-Hydroxytryptamine (serotonin) |
| Naloxone | Endorphins |
| Flumazenil | ? Endogenous benzodiazepines |

appear to be reversible antagonism but, as the concentration of antagonist increases, the maximum response gradually deteriorates, eventually approaching zero. These features are demonstrated in Figure 19.25. Examples of competitive irreversible antagonists are agents such as α-bungarotoxin, benzynylcholine mustard, phenoxybenzamine, and cimetidine, which respectively block skeletal muscle nicotinic receptors, muscarinic receptors, α-adrenoceptors, and histamine ($H_2$)-receptors.

In essence, competitive irreversible antagonists as defined here compete for binding sites, when bound form a highly stable complex, and if present in sufficiently high concentrations reduce the maximum possible agonist response. *It should be noted by the reader that*, in some other texts, because the maximum response cannot be returned to 100% by increasing the concentration of agonist, this behaviour is sometimes termed 'non-competitive antagonism'.

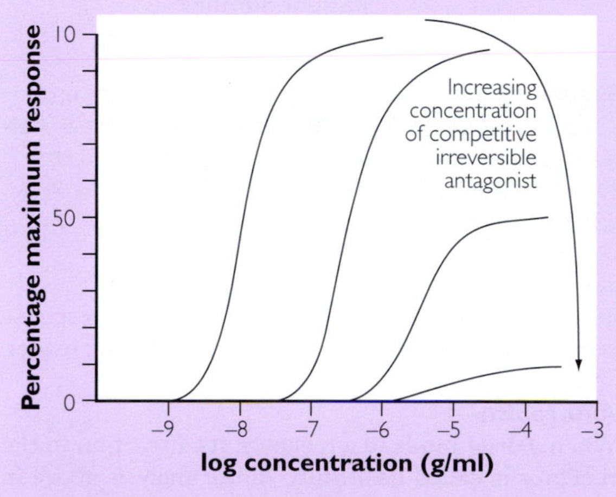


**Figure 19.25** A diagrammatic representation of competitive irreversible antagonism.

*Non-competitive antagonists*

This is a loose term, defined differently from text to text. Here, it is taken to mean the reduction in an agonist's action by activity not dependent on competition for the receptor. Examples of this would be:

- the actions of histamine and epinephrine acting via separate receptors on bronchial musculature;
- reduction of metal poisoning effects by chelating agents;
- action of protamine on heparin to form a stable salt;
- action of calcium ions in milk complexing with oral drugs to prevent uptake (e.g. tetracycline).

***Partial agonists***

Partial agonists are drugs that possess both agonist and antagonist properties, depending on the experimental conditions at the time. Partial agonists possess receptor affinity and compete with a full agonist for receptors but, when bound, have reduced intrinsic activity. Their possible combinations of action are given in Table 19.9 and illustrated graphically in Figure 19.26.

**Table 19.9 Possible interactions between partial agonists and agonists[a]**

| Agonist receptor occupancy | Partial agonist concentration | Effect |
|---|---|---|
| Zero | Zero–high | Agonist effect of partial agonist |
| Small–moderate | Moderate | Additive effects |
| High | High | Reduced effect of full agonist |

[a]Compare this table with Figure 19.26.

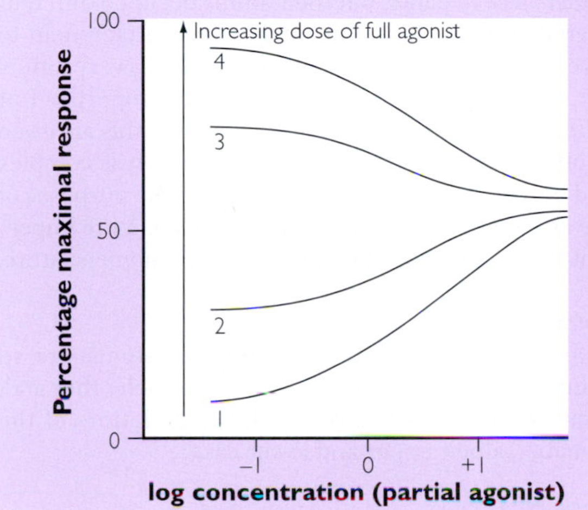


**Figure 19.26** The response resulting from combinations of agonist and partial agonist drugs. 1, 2, 3, and 4 are increasing, fixed levels of agonist in the presence of which the partial agonist is working.

Although some β-adrenoceptor blockers possess intrinsic sympathomimetic activity, it is not clinically of great relevance. Partial agonist activity at opioid receptors has, however, resulted in a therapeutic class of drugs. Examples are nalorphine, pentazocine, and buprenorphine.

#### *Inverse agonists*

Inverse agonists are drugs with high receptor affinity but which, when bound, produce the opposite pharmacological effect to full agonists. The best examples of this are the β-carbolines. These are competitive antagonists of benzodiazepines and reduce their pharmacological effects but, when given alone, they have excitatory proconvulsant or even convulsant effects.

#### *Tolerance or tachyphylaxis*

This is also sometimes called receptor desensitization. It refers to the situation when the response of a tissue declines spontaneously both in the continued presence of an agonist and/or on repeated agonist application. It can occur acutely or chronically; the former may be reversible, the latter usually is not.

Acute desensitization was first described for repeated agonist application to nicotinic acetylcholine receptors in skeletal muscle. It is thought to result either from the formation of an inactive drug–receptor combination, e.g. repeated doses of suxamethonium, or from exhaustion of transmitter with an indirectly acting sympathomimetic or blocking agent, e.g. ephedrine, amphetamine, trimetaphan.

Chronic desensitization may be the result of:

- the failure of intracellular regulatory mechanism (e.g. cAMP, G proteins);
- sequestration of receptors and internalization by endocytosis;
- a diminution of the number of receptors (down-regulation), possibly from failures in mRNA synthesis.

The most closely studied group of drugs have been β-adrenoceptor blockers in which all these three mechanisms have been found to be present.

### Isomerism

Isomers are different compounds with the same molecular formula, molecular weight and elemental composition. Their properties may be almost identical or very different. Isomerism is usually described in two main categories: structural isomerism and stereoisomerism.

#### *Structural isomerism*

Structural isomers have the same molecular formula but their atoms are arranged differently. A standard example in anaesthetic practice is the comparison of enflurane and isoflurane (Figure 19.27). Structural isomers are recognized as different drugs with different names. The pharmacological properties of structural isomers may be very similar or very different. Examples of some structural isomers that might be encountered in clinical anaesthesia are given in Table 19.10.

A subdivision of structural isomerism called dynamic isomerism or tautomerism is of relevance to anaesthesia. In this, two isomeric forms are in reversible equilibrium and local conditions determine which form predominates. The best examples are thiopentone and methohexitone (methohexital).

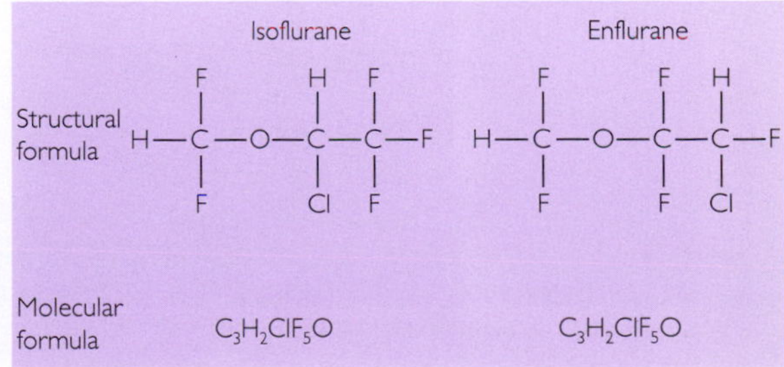


**Figure 19.27** The structural and molecular formulae of isoflurane and enflurane, which are structural isomers.

**Table 19.10 Structural isomers of drugs that may be used in anaesthetic practice**

| Molecular formula | Structural isomers |
|---|---|
| $C_3H_2ClF_5O$ | Isoflurane, enflurane |
| $C_8H_{11}NO_2$ | Dopamine, octopamine |
| $C_{10}H_{16}ClNO$ | Edrophonium, ephedrine |
| $C_{11}H_{17}NO_3$ | Isoprenaline (isoproterenol), methoxamine |
| $C_{11}H_{18}N_2O_3$ | Amylobarbitone, pentobarbitone |
| $C_{13}H_{20}N_2O_2$ | Procaine, monocaine |
| $C_{14}H_{22}N_2O_3$ | Atenolol, practolol |
| $C_{17}H_{19}NO_3$ | Morphine, hydromorphine, norcodeine |
| $C_{17}H_{20}N_2S$ | Promethazine, promazine |
| $C_{17}H_{21}NO_4$ | Hyoscine, cocaine |
| $C_{18}H_{22}N_2$ | Cyclizine, desipramine |
| $C_{18}H_{23}NO_3$ | Dihydrocodeine, dobutamine |
| $C_{21}H_{28}O_5$ | Cortisone, prednisolone, aldosterone |

Thiopentone is ionized and water soluble at a pH of 10.5. On injection into plasma (pH 7.4), the $Na^+$ is replaced by $H^+$ at the sulphur anion. The resulting molecule (Figure 19.28; see also Chapter 32, Figure 32.6) is then in equilibrium with an alternative structure where the $H^+$ is transferred to the N of the barbiturate ring. This secondary isomer is much more lipid soluble and is able to cross membranes easily. Analogous reactions occur with methohexitone.

In a similar manner, the structure of midazolam is transformed from a water-soluble molecule at pH 4 into a liquid-soluble one at pH 7.4 (Figure 19.29). Some enthusiasts may argue that this is not strict isomerism because $OH^-$ ions are required and $H_2O$ is removed. The molecular species are, however, in dynamic equilibrium. Drug classification is full of anomalies.

### *Stereoisomerism*

Stereoisomers have considerable significance in anaesthetic practice. They are isomers of the same chemical and structural formula when drawn on a two-dimensional piece of paper, but their atoms occupy a different spatial arrangement. This makes their attachment to receptors and carrier molecules potentially very different. Stereoisomers often have similar properties but different potencies. Individual examples of this are given in other chapters. Their detailed chemistry is complex and only an overview is given here. For the purposes of the anaesthetic trainee, the principles are more important than the details. A major problem is nomenclature.

#### *Nomenclature*

This is confusing. At least three systems are in common usage. They are unrelated to each other and, even worse, occasionally use the same letters of the alphabet, albeit upper and lower case:

- Optical rotation is one method of classification where the molecules are described as *dextro* or *laevo*, (*d*) or (*l*), or (+) or (–), depending on the direction of rotation of polarized light after transmission.
- The relative spatial configuration of simple sugars and amino acids is described as D or L isomers by comparison to the configuration of D-glyceraldehyde. There is absolutely no correlation between big D and little *d* and big L and little *l*: optical rotation bears no resemblance to stereochemical configurations.

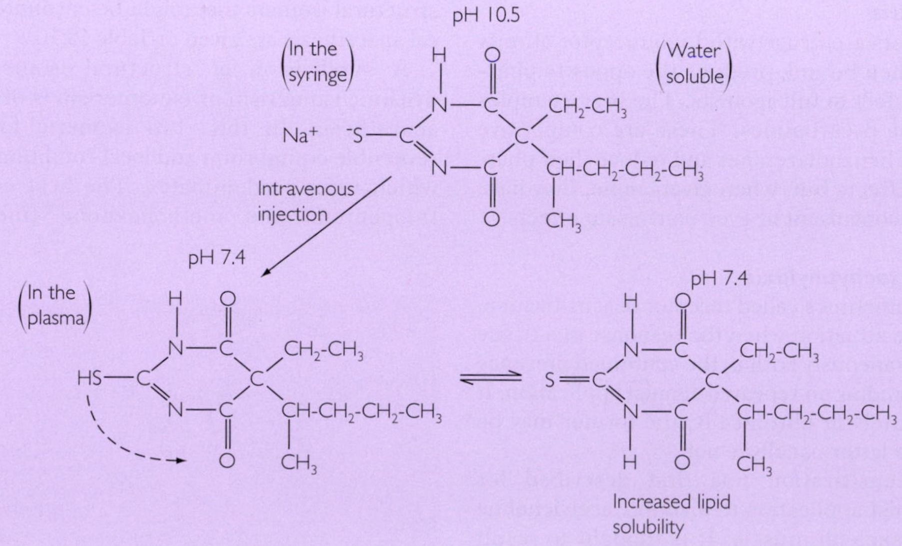

**Figure 19.28** Dynamic isomerism (tautomerism) of the thiopentone molecule. (See text for details).

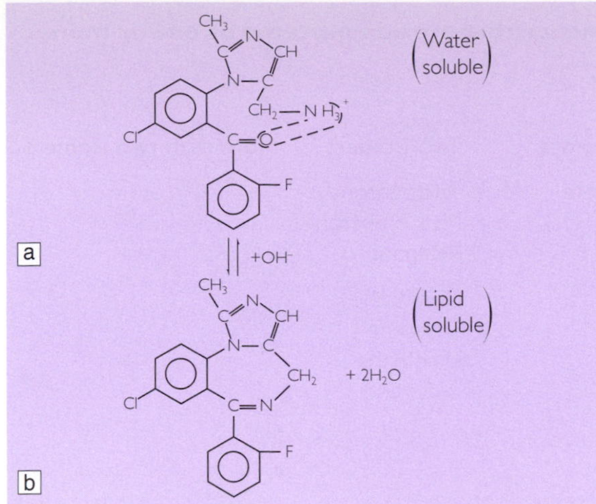


**Figure 19.29** The structure of midazolam at pH 4 in the ampoule (a) and pH 7.4 in the plasma (b) showing a form of dynamic isomerism.

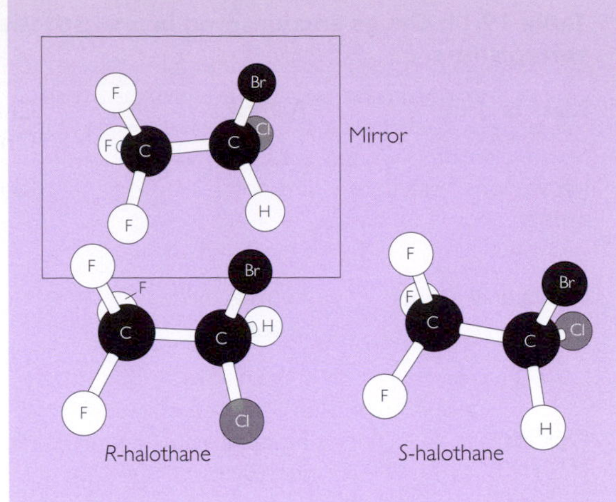


**Figure 19.30** The *R* and *S* enantiomers of halothane. The mirror in the background shows the mirror image of the *R*-halothane molecule. This image is identical to the molecule of *S*-halothane. It is impossible to rotate the *R*-halothane molecule in any orientation to make it *identical* in three-dimensional space to the *S*-halothane molecule.

- Finally, the third and unambiguous classification is that of absolute configuration working to a set of internationally agreed rules that describe drugs and/or atoms as right-handed (*R*) or left-handed (*S*).

In addition to this, as molecules get longer with more carbon atoms, an entirely different nomenclature begins to be used where, when two identical groups are on the same side of a given bond, they are called *cis* and, when on different sides, they are called *trans*. The *cis* is sometimes replaced with *Z* (the German *zusamenon* = together) and *trans* with *E* (the German *entogenon* = across). The *cis* and *trans* concepts are important in the neuromuscular blockers atracurium and mivacurium.

Stereoisomerism is usually separated into two main groupings: enantiomers and diastereoisomers.

*Enantiomers*

Enantiomers are isomers that are mirror images of each other. A good example is halothane which is a mixture of *R* and *S* isomers (Figure 19.30). The property that permits the existence of *R* and *S* isomers is chirality. A chiral centre in a molecule is an atom that has asymmetry in its bonds (usually in three bonds around the axis of the fourth). The principle is demonstrated in Figure 19.31. If the positions of $R_2$, $R_3$ or $R_4$ are interchanged, no rotation around the $R_1$–C bond can restore the original three-dimensional structure.

*Diastereoisomers*

Diastereoisomers are isomers that are not simple mirror images. They arise when drugs have more than one chiral centre (so more rotational combinations are possible) and when *cis* and *trans* arrangements occur. Good examples are methohexitone, tramadol, atracurium, and mivacurium, and compounds containing a carbon–carbon double bond or a heterocyclic ring.

Drugs that are administered in anaesthesia practice as one or more stereoisomers (enantiomers or diastereoisomers) are listed in Table 19.11. For reference, and to save confusion, a summary of the classification of isomers is given in Figure 19.32.

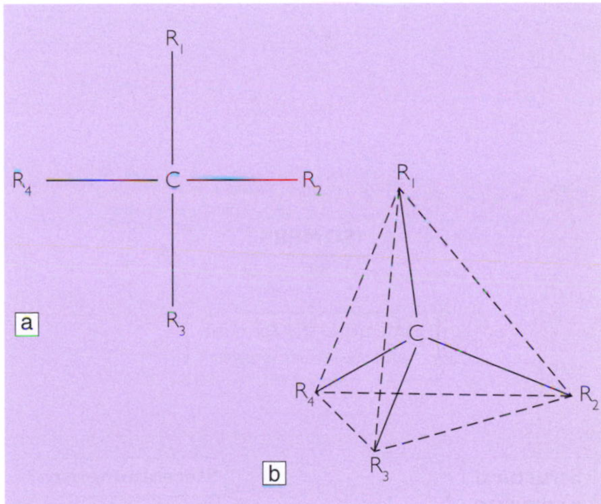


**Figure 19.31** A chiral centre shown in (a) two dimensions and (b) three dimensions. $R_1$, $R_2$, $R_3$, and $R_4$ are *different* chemical groups. (See text for details.)

## The ways in which drugs act

Literature on drug action is complex and often confusing. Classification systems vary from book to book. This account is simplified so that the trainee can obtain an overview without (hopefully) getting lost in too much detail. The content is not encyclopaedic and for greater detail on specific topics more specialized texts should be consulted.

Drug action can be divided into three broad groups, plus that of nitric oxide (NO):

1. direct physical or chemical reactions;
2. reactions involving enzymes;
3. actions on receptors;
4. nitric oxide mediated reactions.

**Table 19.11 Drugs encountered in anaesthesia practice that are administered as one or more stereoisomers**

| Class of drug | Achiral | Chiral | | |
|---|---|---|---|---|
| | | One isomer | Two isomers | More than two isomers |
| Intravenous induction agents | Propofol | Etomidate | Thiopentone<br>Methohexitone<br>Ketamine | |
| Inhalational agents | Nitrous oxide<br>Sevoflurane | | Desflurane<br>Enflurane<br>Halothane<br>Isoflurane | |
| Opioids | Fentanyl<br>Pethidine | Morphine | | |
| Neuromuscular blockers, etc. | Neostigmine | Cisatracurium<br>Pancuronium<br>Rocuronium | | Atracurium<br>Mivacurium |
| Local anaesthetics | Lignocaine (lidocaine) | Ropivacaine | Bupivacaine<br>Etidocaine<br>Prilocaine | |
| Vasoactive drugs | Dopamine | | Epinephrine<br>Norepinephrine<br>Dobutamine<br>Glycopyrrolate<br>Atropine | |

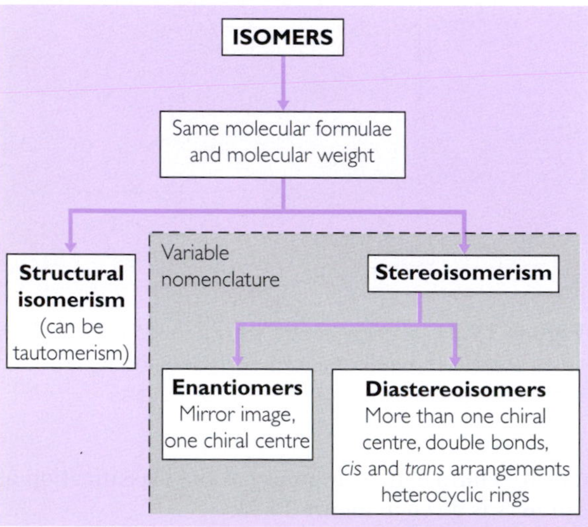


**Figure 19.32** A classification of isomers. (See text for details.)

Although acting via receptors, NO is classed separately because of its individual features. These classes are set out in Figure 19.33 together with their subdivisions. Reference can be made to Figure 19.33 from time to time while reading this section to clarify where a particular process is in the overall order of things.

#### *Direct physical or chemical reactions*

These involve a drug being directly dependent on its own physical or chemical properties to react with or influence another molecule. Chemical reactions essentially result in the target molecule being converted to an inactive form or chemically bound to prevent its action. Examples of this type are given in Table 19.12. Direct chemical reactions are straightforward in both mechanism and understanding and are not discussed further.

Osmotic diuretics, although not reacting chemically, use their physical properties to extract water from cells and then to hold it in the renal tubules. Similarly to direct chemical reactions, they depend on their own innate properties for their effect.

#### *Reactions involving enzymes*

These can be classified in three ways:

1. enzyme induction;
2. enzymes as drugs;
3. enzyme inhibition.

##### *Enzyme induction*

This is the increase in activity of a particular enzyme system as a result of continued stimulation. It is considered in more detail in Chapter 18, Figure 18.38 and Chapter 29. What it does is to provide more enzyme and hence increase the rate of reaction. In many instances, enzymes are not specific so that the induction secondary to one drug (e.g. barbiturates) affects the actions of another (e.g. warfarin).

##### *Enzymes as drugs*

Enzymes, being proteins, are easily broken down when outside their normal environment. Consequently, their use as drugs is limited. When they are used as drugs,

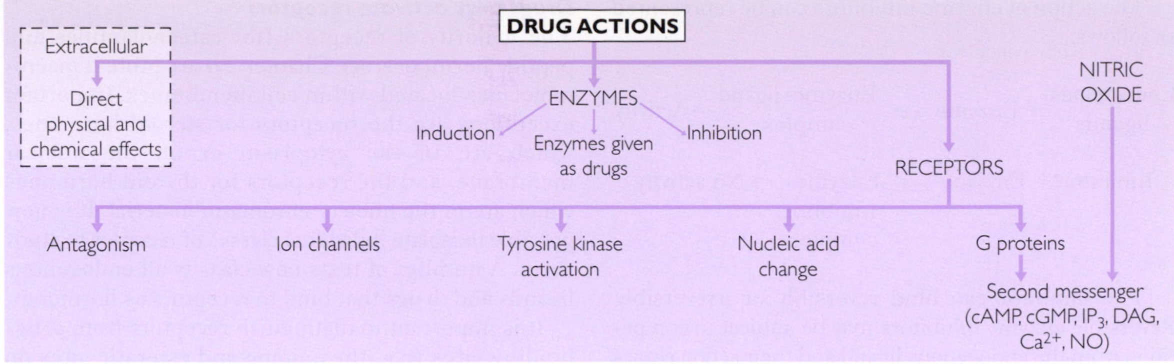


**Figure 19.33** A schematic representation of the ways in which drugs act. $IP_3$, inositol triphosphate; DAG, diacylglycerol; cAMP, cyclic adenosine monophosphate; cGMP, cyclic guanosine monophosphate; NO, nitric oxide; $Ca^{2+}$, calcium ions.

**Table 19.12 Drug actions that are directly dependent on chemical properties**

| Drug | Mode of action |
|---|---|
| Antacids | Neutralize gastric acid directly |
| Desferrioxamine[a] | Binds iron in ferritin and haemosiderin: used in haemochromatosis |
| Sodium EDTA[a] | Binds calcium, anticoagulates stored blood |
| Penicillamine[a] | Binds metals and carries them with it into urine |
| Hydrogen peroxide | Strong oxidizing agent: sterilizes wounds by its direct chemical activity |
| Protamine | Complexes directly with heparin to form stable inactive salt |

[a]These are chelating agents.

it is principally to break down tissue rather than to improve or modify synthetic reactions. The following are examples:

- Chymotrypsin produces dissolution of the zonule of Zinn in intracapsular cataract extraction.
- Streptokinase and streptodornase are used for desloughing skin ulcers and dissolving clots in the urinary bladder.
- Streptokinase, urokinase, alteplase, and related preparations are used intravenously and intra-arterially to activate plasminogen to plasmin, which subsequently degrades fibrin to break up thrombi. Applications are in acute myocardial infarction, clotted arteriovenous shunts, pulmonary embolism, and thrombosis of the eye.
- Pancreatin provides protease, lipase, and amylase activity for patients with inadequate pancreatic function.
- Hyaluronidase catalyses the hydrolysis of hyaluronic acid, the 'cement substance' of the tissues. It is used to promote absorption and diffusion of the subcutaneous route.

Fresh frozen plasma (FFP) contains a number of enzymes and it has been used to administer plasma cholinesterase to reverse suxamethonium apnoea. Its effects are, however, limited and the preservation of cholinesterase in FFP is poor.

*Enzyme inhibition*

A number of drugs produce their effect by inhibiting enzymes which perform part of a cell's normal metabolic activities. Often the drug's structure is very similar to the endogenous ligand (see 'Regulation of enzymes' in Chapter 18). Examples of structural similarity are given in Table 19.13.

**Table 19.13 Examples of drugs with structural similarity to an endogenous ligand**

| Endogenous ligand | Structurally similar drug that blocks enzyme |
|---|---|
| Purine base | Allopurinol |
| Para-aminobenzoic acid | Sulphonamides |
| Uracil | Flurouracil |
| Dopa | Methyldopa |

Dopa, dihydroxyphenylalanine.

The action of enzyme inhibitors can be represented as follows:

$$\text{Endogenous ligands} + \text{Enzyme} \rightleftharpoons \text{Enzyme–ligand complex} \rightarrow \text{Activity}$$

$$\text{Inhibitor} + \text{Enzyme} \rightleftharpoons \text{Enzyme–inhibitor complex} \rightarrow \text{No activity}$$

The inhibitor can bind reversibly or irreversibly. Reversible enzyme inhibitors may be subject to competition from the endogenous ligand and their action ceases when they are metabolized or excreted. Their action is not dependent on permanent bonds, they have to be administered regularly or by infusion (e.g. aminophylline), and their actions stop with cessation of treatment. Conversely, irreversible inhibitors usually form stable (sometimes covalent) bonds with the enzyme. In such a case, deactivation may depend on cellular turnover and synthesis of new enzymes. Examples of such drugs are organophosphorus compounds and monoamine oxidase inhibitors. It may be weeks before the action of these drugs is overcome by normal cellular mechanisms. Drugs encountered in anaesthetic practice which inhibit enzymes are given in Table 19.14.

### *Drugs that activate receptors*

The majority of receptors (for catecholamines and peptide hormones, see Chapter 29) are protein macromolecules located within cell membranes. Important exceptions are the receptors for steroid hormones, which are in the cytoplasm or on the nuclear membrane, and the receptors for thyroid hormones which are in the nuclear chromatin material. It is now possible to isolate individual classes of receptor to study them. A number of texts now classify all endogenous ligands and drugs that bind to receptors as hormones.

It is important to distinguish receptors from drug-binding sites (e.g. the anionic and esteratic sites on acetylcholinesterase) on enzymes and other molecules. These are sometimes loosely referred to as receptor sites because of their binding characteristics, but they are not. They bind drugs but do not possess the properties of a receptor.

The role of receptors is twofold:

1. to recognize the endogenous ligand (or drug) so that only intended actions occur; these are agonist actions;
2. to convert the binding of the ligand into a cellular activity.

**Table 19.14 Commonly used drugs whose effects are partly or totally caused by enzyme inhibition**

| Drug | Enzyme system inhibited |
|---|---|
| Allopurinol | Xanthine oxidase |
| Aminophylline<br>Enoximone<br>Milrinone | Phosphodiesterases |
| Acetylsalicylic acid (and other NSAIDs) | Prostaglandin synthetase (cyclo-oxygenase) |
| Captopril<br>Enalapril<br>Lisinopril | Angiotensin-converting enzyme |
| Methyldopa | Amino acid decarboxylase |
| Edrophonium<br>Neostigmine<br>Pyridostigmine<br>Organophosphates | Acetylcholinesterase<br>Plasma cholinesterase |
| Benzylpenicillin | Bacterial wall transpeptidase |
| Phenelzine<br>Tranylcypromine | Monoamine oxidase |
| Sulphonamides | Folate synthase |
| Glycosides | $Na^+/K^+$ ATPase |
| Warfarin | Vitamin K epoxide reductase |
| Anticancer agents | DNA polymerase |
| Aprotinin | Proteolytic enzymes |

NSAIDs, non-steroidal anti-inflammatory drugs.

Substances that mimic the ligand and bind but produce no effect are called antagonists. They have been considered earlier and reference should be made to this section for their use as drugs (see Table 19.8 and Figures 19.24 and 19.25). The theory of drug–receptor action is described in 'Graded dose response curves' (see Figure 19.18). Most drug–receptor combinations are rapidly reversible. An example of an exception is phenoxybenzamine.

The following are the properties of a receptor.

*Selectivity*

Most receptor systems show great selectivity. The majority of the effective drugs are structurally similar to naturally occurring hormones or neurotransmitters. There are well defined structure–activity relationships and often stereospecificity.

*Sensitivity*

Only small numbers of receptors are present and usually not all are needed for a full response from tiny quantities of drugs (mg/kg body weight or less, nanomolar at the active site). Receptor binding is therefore the beginning of a process that is subject to subsequent intracellular amplification.

*Saturatability*

The number of receptors on a cell is normally constant and there is a maximum cellular response when all receptors are occupied (saturated). This can be reduced by down-regulation (see above) or increased by up-regulation from shortage of endogenous ligands (e.g. denervation hypersensitivity).

*Specificity*

The same agonist binds to receptors in the same types of cell to produce the same effect.

There are four main classes of receptor activation:

- ligand-gated ion channels;
- those dependent on G proteins (or second or intermediate messenger systems);
- those that activate tyrosine kinase;
- those that modify nucleic acid synthesis.

*Ligand-gated ion channels*

Once triggered, this type of receptor is characterized by its speed of action which is in *the order of micro- or milliseconds*. The ion channels and receptors form part of the same macromolecular complex. They are important in neural and neuromuscular transmission. Examples of ligand-gated ion channels are:

- the nicotinic cholinergic (acetylcholine) receptor (see Chapter 24);
- the GABA receptor (see Chapter 23);
- the *N*-methyl-D-aspartate (NMDA) receptor; the endogenous ligand for this receptor has not yet been properly identified but could be glutamate or glycine.

Ion channels all produce changes in the intracellular potential but, in addition, in some cells they may also modify the synthesis of intermediate messengers.

*Receptors acting through G proteins*

These receptors produce a response *within 100 ms to a few seconds*. Their importance cannot be over-emphasized. G proteins are proteins of approximately 450 amino acids in length, which have α, β, and γ subunits. They are called G proteins because the α subunit binds and hydrolyses guanosine triphosphate (GTP) to guanosine diphosphate (GDP). Several different types of G proteins (e.g. $G_s$ = stimulatory, $G_i$ = inhibitory) have been described.

Arrival of a ligand at the receptor causes GDP in the α subunit to be replaced with GTP. The G protein then separates and the α subunit carrying the GTP binds to adenylyl cyclase, guanylyl cyclase, or phospholipase (C or $A_2$) either to stimulate or to inhibit their action. After the enzymes are activated, GTPase converts the GTP to GDP and the α, β, and γ subunits re-form. The sequence is shown schematically in Figure 19.34. This type of cascade, which results in the accumulation of intracellular metabolites, is called an intermediate or second messenger system. The most important intermediate messengers are cyclic adenosine 3′ : 5′-monophosphate (cAMP), cyclic guanosine 3′ : 5′-monophosphate (cGMP), phosphoinositides, calcium ions, and NO.

After cAMP is synthesized it activates protein kinases. The system with cGMP is similar. The action of G proteins on phospholipase results in the mobilization of both protein kinases and calcium. A dependence on G proteins and intermediate mssengers is found with ACTH, adrenergic, angiotensin, glucagon, GABA, histamine, 5-HT, muscarinic and opioid receptors.

*Tyrosine kinase activation*

This produces a pharmacological effect in *minutes to hours*. It is typified by the receptors for insulin and

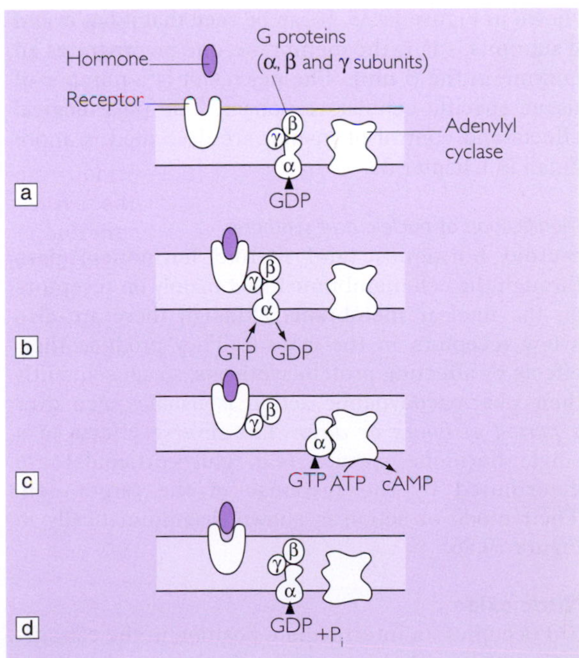


**Figure 19.34** A diagrammatic representation of the action of G proteins. (a) Before hormone binds; (b) after hormone binds; (c) G proteins dissociate; (d) GTPase cleaves GTP to GDP and inorganic phosphate (Pi).

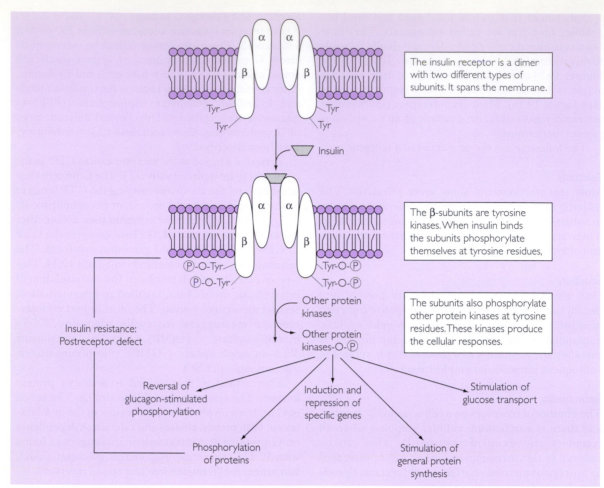

**Figure 19.35** The insulin receptor. (Adapted from Marks DB *et al. Basic Medical Biochemistry*. Baltimore, MA: Williams & Wilkins, 1996: 386.)

epidermal growth factor. The insulin receptor is shown in Figure 19.35. It can be seen that it has α and β subunits, spans the membrane, and incorporates an enzyme in the β unit. The net result is a number of tissue-specific cellular responses. The physiological effects and control of insulin are described in more detail in Chapter 29.

*Modification of nucleic acid synthesis*

Steroid hormones (and thyroid hormones) pass through the cell membrane to act mainly on receptors on the nuclear membrane, although there are also a few receptors in the cytosol. They produce their effects by affecting protein synthesis, so consequently their pharmacodynamic action is usually seen over *a period of hours or days*. The diverse effects of a single hormone species (e.g. glucocorticoids) are determined by the response of the target cell. Their mode of action is shown diagrammatically in Figure 19.36.

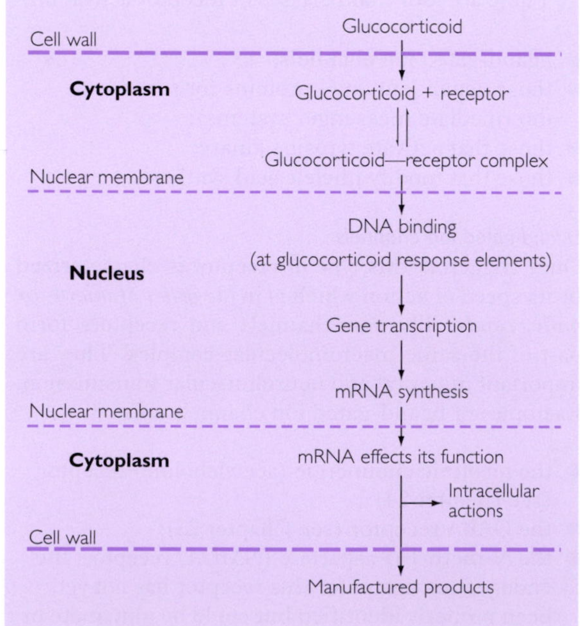


**Figure 19.36** The mode of action of steroid hormones (e.g. a glucocorticoid).

***Nitric oxide***

NO occupies an intermediate position in the classification of ligands because it is both an endogenous ligand produced in the endothelium by intrinsic NO synthase and a drug metabolite of vasodilating agents such as glyceryl trinitrate and sodium nitroprusside. It can also be administered directly into the pulmonary tree. Once formed it diffuses rapidly into vascular smooth muscle and then activates soluble guanylyl

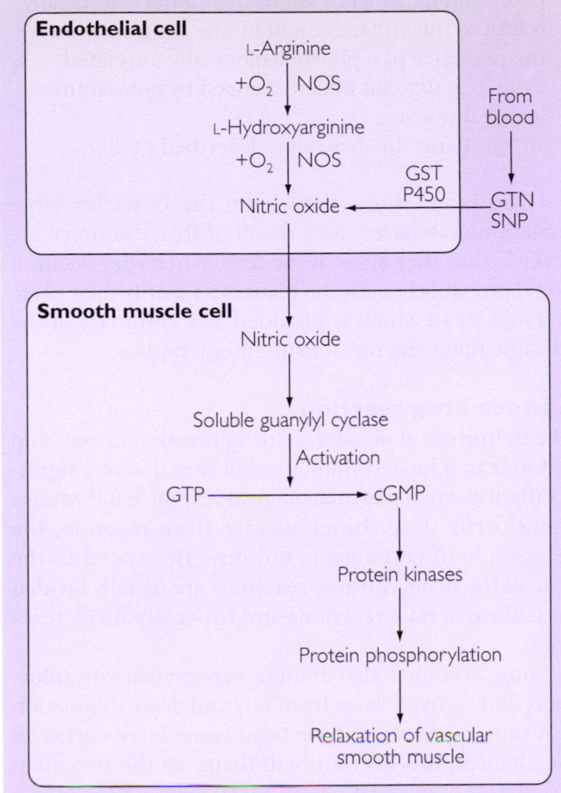


**Figure 19.37** The synthesis of nitric oxide in an endothelial cell and its action in smooth muscle. NOS, nitric oxide synthase; GTN, glyceryl trinitrate; SNP, sodium nitroprusside; GST, glutathione-S-transferase; P450, cytochrome P450.

cyclase, which subsequently produces relaxation of the smooth muscle. Its action is shown in Figure 19.37.

### Variability in drug response

There is a wide variability in the response of different patients to the same dose of drug. The various steps between administration and pharmacodynamic action are shown in Figure 19.16. In addition, in real patients, there are other factors that depend on social, physiological, pharmacological, and pathological influences. They are listed in Table 19.15. How to manage these in any individual patient is described in the appropriate chapters of Section 3 of the book.

The net effect of all these confounding variables on the log dose–response curve is shown schematically in Figure 19.38. Examples of the variability in quantal dose–response data for common inhalational and intravenous anaesthetic agents are given in Table 33.7. In summary, it is reasonable to say that for almost all drugs there is a wide variation in their dose–response relationships in the population and the golden rule is to titrate the dose to the required response.

### Drug interactions

Drug interactions are the modification of one drug's action by another. There are thousands of them and they may be harmless, dangerous and unwanted, or used therapeutically. They broadly separate into pharmaceutical, pharmacokinetic, and pharmacodynamic interactions.

#### *Pharmaceutical interactions*

These occur before the drug enters the body, e.g. while it is still in the syringe or the stomach. They can be subdivided into drug instability (e.g. deterioration of sodium nitroprusside by ultraviolet light), direct chem-

**Table 19.15 Causes of variability in drug response**

| Grouping | Expression of effect |
|---|---|
| Social | Patient compliance<br>Alcohol<br>Tobacco<br>Drug use (recreational and therapeutic)<br>Prescribing errors |
| Physiological | Age<br>Sex<br>Pregnancy |
| Pharmacological | Concurrent drug therapy<br>Modified receptor function<br>Tolerance or tachyphylaxis<br>Idiosyncratic sensitivity<br>Enzyme induction<br>Adverse drug reaction<br>Rate of elimination |
| Pathological | Cardiac disease<br>Liver disease<br>Renal disease<br>Respiratory disease<br>Neurological disease |

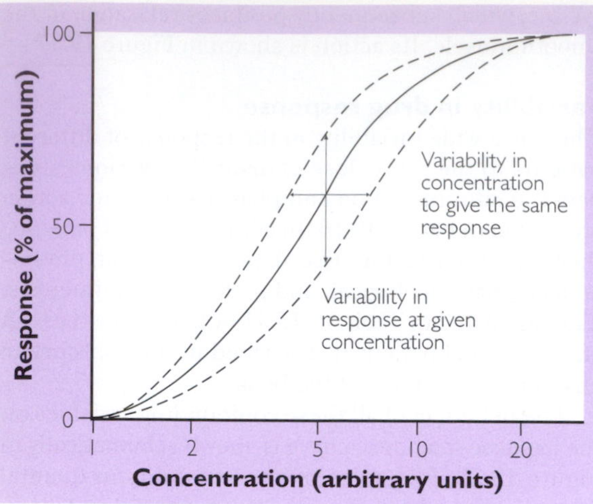


**Figure 19.38** A diagrammatic representation of the variables that shift the position of the concentration–response curve. The solid line represents the average concentration–response curve; the broken lines represent the variability within the population.

ical combination (e.g. mixing induction agents and neuromuscular blockers), or a change to an inappropriate pH (e.g. if the pH of atracurium is changed to 7, it breaks down spontaneously).

***Pharmacokinetic interactions***

These are an alteration in the distribution or bioavailability of one drug by another that modifies its concentration at the site of action. The interactions may be classified as affecting the process of getting the drug into the bloodstream (absorption), distributing it (including protein binding), and metabolizing and eliminating it. Further details of pharmacokinetic effects are given later in the Chapter.

***Pharmacodynamic interactions***

These are caused by a second drug interfering with the expected effect of a given serum level of the first at the site of action. The effects can be any of the following:

- additive: not a true drug interaction but combined similar effects from two different drugs, e.g. nitrous oxide reduces the MIR of propofol (see Figure 19.23);
- synergistic: a response of two drugs that is greater than the sum of their individual actions; this is very rare;
- potentiation: this is a slight misnomer – it usually refers to the enhancement of one drug's action by the presence of a pharmacologically unrelated drug, e.g. digoxin toxicity caused by potassium-losing diuretics;
- antagonism: this has been described earlier.

Drug interactions have been the basis for large books and databases. As a result of this, examples are described as they arise in the text. When they occur, it would probably benefit the reader to identify their place in Table 19.16 which is provided as a summary of the possible mechanisms of drug interactions.

### Adverse drug reactions

The definition of an adverse drug reaction varies from text to text. The definition used here is that of a significantly abnormal pharmacological response following a typical drug dose. In an adverse drug reaction, the magnitude of response is not directly related to the dose of the drug. Adverse reactions are usually divided into: idiosyncratic reactions and hypersensitivity reactions.

Some accounts also include supersensitivity, tolerance, and tachyphylaxis from up- and down-regulation of receptors. As these have been considered earlier in the chapter, this account will focus on the two main divisions.

***Idiosyncratic reactions***

These can be defined as genetically determined abnormal reactions to a drug. They do not require a previous 'sensitizing' dose. Important examples in anaesthetic practice are:

- the genetic variants of cholinesterase (see Chapters 13 and 35);
- malignant hyperpyrexia (see Chapters 13 and 24);
- acute hepatic porphyria;
- abnormal *N*-acetyltransferase causing slow acetylation in the liver;
- autosomal dominant resistance to oral anticoagulants;
- neutropenia after a variety of drugs.

***Hypersensitivity***

Hypersensitivity responses are abnormal reactions to drugs that involve immune mechanisms, usually with the formation of antibodies, and they may or may not involve cell lysis. They usually occur on second and subsequent exposures to the drug. They are classified

**Table 19.16 Mechanisms of drug interactions**

| Pharmaceutical (direct interaction) | Pharmacokinetic (effect of second drug on) | Pharmacodynamic (combined actions as) |
|---|---|---|
| Chemical instability | Absorption | Additive effects |
| Chemical combination | Distribution | Synergy |
| Wrong pH | Metabolism | Potentiation |
| | Elimination | Antagonism |

**Table 19.17 Types of hypersensitivity reaction**

| Reaction type | Features |
|---|---|
| I | Mediated by IgE<br>Antigenic drug–protein complex<br>Involves most cells of skin, bronchial and intestinal mucosa, vascular capillaries<br>Degranulation of mast cells releases histamine, heparin, 5HT, leukotrienes, platelet-activating factor<br>Responsible for anaphylactic drug reactions |
| II | Cytolytic reactions resulting from reaction of circulating antibodies (IgE + IgM) with antigens, usually on blood cell membranes<br>Antigen–antibody reactions in presence of complement cause cell lysis<br>Can produce haemolytic anaemia, thrombocytopenia, agranulocytosis |
| III | Immune complexes (circulating antibody + circulating antigen) called precipitins deposit in small blood vessels, glomerular tissue, and connective tissue of joints<br>Complement is involved<br>Responsible for Arthus reaction, acute glomerulonephritis, acute rheumatoid arthritis, and serum sickness |
| IV | Delayed cell-mediated hypersensitivity in which antibody is not involved<br>Reaction results from combination of antigen with T-cell (killer) lymphocytes and macrophages attacking the foreign material<br>Responsible for Mantoux reaction, contact dermatitis, and graft rejection |

5HT, 5-hydroxytryptamine (serotonin)

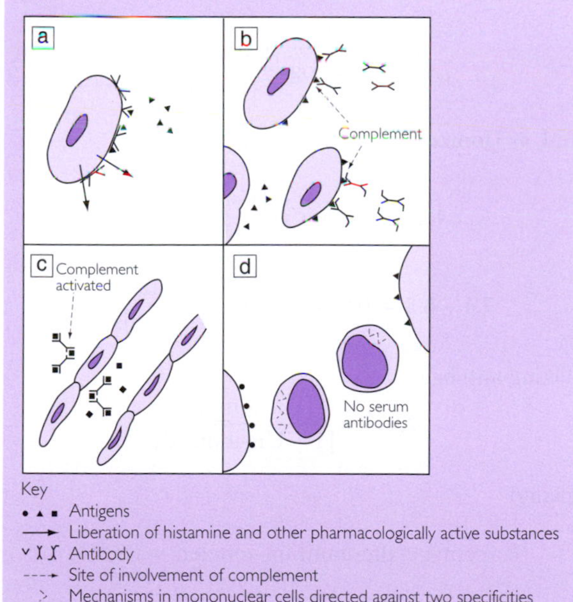


**Figure 19.39** The four types of hypersensitivity reaction: (a) type I, (b) type II, (c) type III, and (d) type IV. (Adapted from Gell PGH. In: Curran RC and Harnden DG, eds. *The Pathological Basis of Medicine*. Oxford: Heinemann Medical Books Ltd, 1972: 172.)

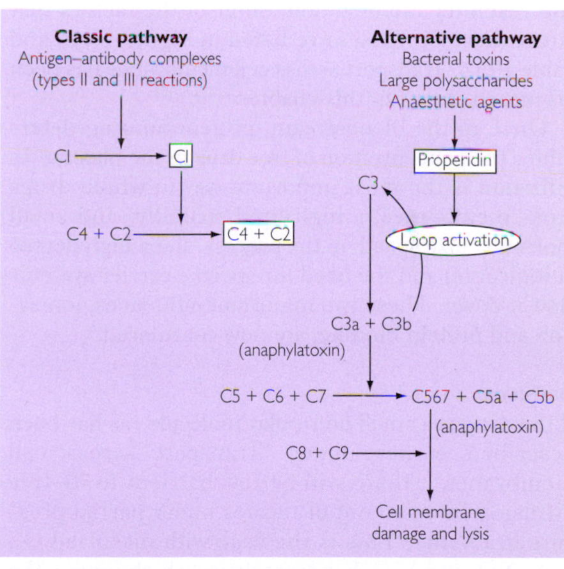


**Figure 19.40** The classic and alternative complement pathways. C1, C2 , C9 etc. indicate components of the complement system. Boxes indicate activation.

into four types (Table 19.17), illustrated in Figure 19.39.

The pathways of types II and III reactions involve activation of complement. Complement is a system of enzymes, present in normal mammalian serum, that can be activated in series (and then subsequently destroyed) by the reaction of antigen with antibody, i.e. it 'complements' the reaction. When the antigen is on the surface of a cell, the cell may be lysed. Complement can also be activated directly without previous exposure to the drug. This is called the alternative pathway. The classic and alternative pathways of complement activation are shown in Figure 19.40.

Type I hypersensitivity and alternative pathway activation can result in an anaphylactic reaction. Anaphylactoid reactions, although being clinically indistinguishable, result from the direct release of vasoactive substances (histamine, serotonin/5-HT, etc.) from circulating basophils or mast cells without the intermediate formation of a drug–protein complex which induces the formation of IgE. The incidence, causes, and management of serious hypersensitivity reactions are described under 'Anaphylaxis' in Chapter 13.

## PHARMACOKINETICS

Pharmacokinetics is the study of what happens to the dose of an administered drug and the determination of its concentration at the site of action. Defining the site of action is not always easy. Warfarin exerts its effect in the blood, neuromuscular blockers at the end-plate, and opioids deep inside the nervous system across the blood–brain barrier. The actual zone at which a drug (or endogenous ligand) comes into intimate contact with its molecular site of action is termed the 'biophase'. Apart from the few drugs that have their site of action in the blood, the true concentration at the site of action cannot be determined. Instead, the concentration in blood or plasma is taken as the best surrogate for the biophase concentration. The problems inherent in doing this are described later.

### Drug uptake, bioavailability, and hysteresis

#### *Drug uptake*

To reach its site of action, a drug has first to be absorbed or injected and then to leave the circulation and reach its site of action. Some of the factors that affect these processes are listed in Figure 19.16 and Table 19.15. Transport across cell membranes has been discussed earlier in this chapter.

Once in the bloodstream, protein binding determines the concentration of free drug in the plasma. As diffusion is the most important way in which drugs cross membranes, a high lipid solubility and small molecular size speed up the process, and a high degree of ionization and the need for specific carrier systems slow it down. These two important influences, ionization and protein binding, are now considered.

##### *Ionization*

If the drug is a small non-polar molecule (as has been described earlier under 'Transport across cell membranes'), there will be few barriers to its free diffusion into and out of tissues under partial pressure gradients. This is the case with dissolved $O_2$, $CO_2$, NO, and $N_2O$. For most drugs which ionize, the molecular polarity is, however, determined by chemical structure and the pH of plasma.

Many drugs are weak acids or bases. A weak acid dissociates in the form:

$$\text{R-COOH} \rightleftharpoons \text{R-COO}^- + \text{H}^+$$

which, applying the law of mass action defines the dissociation constant as:

$$K_a = \frac{[\text{H}^+]\,[\text{R-COO}^-]}{[\text{R-COOH}]}.$$

Rearranging and taking logarithms results in:

$$\text{pH} = \text{p}K_a + \log \frac{[\text{R-COO}^-]}{[\text{R-COOH}]}$$

where pH = – log [$H^+$] and p$K_a$ = – log [$K_a$] or, re-writing:

$$\text{pH} = \text{p}K_a + \log \frac{[\text{Ionized}]}{[\text{Un-ionized}]}$$

which is in the familiar form of the Henderson–Hasslebalch equation (see Chapter 26). An analogous expression can be derived for a weak base:

$$\text{pH} = \text{p}K_a + \log \frac{[\text{Un-ionized}]}{[\text{Ionized}]}$$

Consequently, when pH = p$K_a$, whether acidic or basic, 50% of the drug is in the ionized form. The actual value of p$K_a$ does not determine whether the dissociation is to an acid or a base: both acids and bases can have p$K_a$ values greater or smaller than 7. The degree of dissociation determines the proportion of the plasma concentration of free un-ionized drug that is available for diffusion across cell membranes. The dissociation constant is highly temperature dependent and, in the pharmaceutical literature, most are quoted at 37°C. In physical chemistry tables it is usually quoted at 25°C. Examples of how to determine the degree of ionization mathematically are given below for alfentanil and thiopentone.

Alfentanil is a weak base with a p$K_a$ of 6.5. At a pH of 7.4:

$$7.4 = 6.5 + \log \frac{[\text{Un-ionized}]}{[\text{Ionized}]}$$

and, as [Ionized] + [Un-ionized] = 1:

$$7.4 = 6.5 + \log \frac{[\text{Un-ionized}]}{[1 - \text{Un-ionized}]}$$

$$7.4 - 6.5 = 0.9 = \log \frac{[\text{Un-ionized}]}{[1 - \text{Un-ionized}]}$$

Taking antilogs:

$$7.943 = \frac{[\text{Un-ionized}]}{[1 - \text{Un-ionized}]}$$

giving:

Percentage alfentanil un-ionized = 88.8%.

Thiopentone is a weak acid with a p$K_a$ of 7.6. At a pH of 7.4:

$$7.4 = 7.6 + \log \frac{[\text{Ionized}]}{[\text{Un-ionized}]}$$

$$= 7.6 + \log \frac{[1 - \text{Un-ionized}]}{[\text{Un-ionized}]}$$

$$7.4 - 7.6 = -0.2 = \log \frac{[1 - \text{Un-ionized}]}{[\text{Un-ionized}]}$$

Taking antilogs:

$$0.631 = \frac{[1 - \text{Un-ionized}]}{[\text{Un-ionized}]}$$

giving:

Percentage thiopentone un-ionized = 61.3%.

The ionization characteristics of some drugs in common use in anaesthesia at a pH of 7.4 and a temperature of 37°C are given in Table 19.18.

*Protein binding*

Apart from very small non-polar molecules, most drugs bind to proteins in the blood, but the degree of binding is very variable. The percentage protein binding of some common drugs is given in Table 19.19.

Under normal conditions, the dissociation constants of most drug–protein interactions are greatly in excess of the therapeutic range. This means that an approximately constant fraction of drug in plasma is bound to protein at all times. Albumin plays an important role in the binding of drugs. It has a number of potential sites of variable affinity for drugs and mainly binds neutral or acidic compounds (see Table 19.18). Basic compounds are carried by γ-globulin, glycoproteins, and lipoproteins. The main exception is diazepam, which is bound to albumin.

The component of the drug available to enter the tissue *is only the un-ionized unbound fraction*. The greater this diffusible fraction, the steeper the concentration gradient and the faster the drug will diffuse. The diffusible fraction can vary considerably within the same class of drugs. The diffusible fractions of, for instance, morphine, alfentanil, and fentanyl are 16%, 8%, and 2%, respectively. The rate of diffusion also clearly depends on the solubility of the drug in the tissue. The diffusible fraction, although it determines the rate of diffusion, does not determine the total amount of drug distributed to any specific tissue. As tissue entry occurs, a constant equilibrium is maintained between the bound and unbound fractions and the quantity of bound drug decreases. This equilibrium is shown diagrammatically in Figure 19.41.

Figures are often quoted for the fat or tissue solubility of drugs dissolved in plasma. In the case of drugs that are essentially 100% un-ionized (e.g. volatile agents, diazepam, propofol), the situation is unambiguous and the blood–tissue or plasma–tissue partition coefficients can be determined in a way exactly analogous to that described for blood–gas partition coefficients in Chapter 33. When, however, the drug is

**Table 19.18 Values of p$K_a$ and percentage of drug un-ionized at pH 7.4 (37°C) for some commonly used drugs**

| Drug | p$K_a$ | Percentage un-ionized |
|---|---|---|
| **Intravenous anaesthetics (acids and bases)** | | |
| Etomidate (base) | 4.2 | 99.9 |
| Ketamine (base) | 7.5 | 44 |
| Methohexitone (acid) | 7.9 | 80 |
| Propofol (acid) | 11 | 99.9 |
| Thiopentone (acid) | 7.6 | 61 |
| **Inhalational anaesthetics** | | |
| Desflurane, Enflurane, Halothane, Isoflurane, Sevoflurane, Nitrous oxide | Not recorded: essentially not dissociated | Essentially 100% un-ionized |
| **Local anaesthetics (all bases)** | | |
| Bupivacaine | 8.1 | 17 |
| Etidocaine | 7.7 | 33 |
| Lignocaine | 7.9 | 25 |
| Prilocaine | 7.9 | 25 |
| Ropivacaine | 8.1 | 17 |
| **Benzodiazepines (all bases)** | | |
| Diazepam | 3.3 | 99.9 |
| Midazolam | 6.2 | 94 |
| Temazepam | 1.6 | 99.9 |
| Flumazenil | 1.7 | 99.9 |

| Drug | p$K_a$ | Percentage un-ionized |
|---|---|---|
| **Neuromuscular blocking agents** | | |
| Atracurium, Cisatracurium, Mivacurium, Pancuronium, Rocuronium, Suxamethonium | Not recorded: very highly dissociated | Very little un-ionized drug |
| **Opioids and antagonists (all bases)** | | |
| Alfentanil | 6.5 | 89 |
| Diamorphine | 7.6 | 40 |
| Fentanyl | 8.4 | 9 |
| Morphine | 7.9 | 24 |
| Pethidine (meperidine) | 8.5 | 7 |
| Remifentanil | 7.3 | 58 |
| Sufentanil | 8.0 | 20 |
| Naloxone | 7.9 | 24 |
| **Other drugs** | | |
| Ethyl alcohol | Not recorded | Virtually 100 |
| Mannitol | Not recorded but non-electrolyte | Virtually 100 |
| Heparin (acid) | Not recorded | Virtually zero |
| Warfarin (acid) | 5.0 | 0.4 |

The data in this table are taken from Hull CJ. *Pharmacokinetics for Anaesthesia*. Oxford: Butterworth-Heinemann, 1991: 70; White PF. *Ballière's Clinical Anaesthesiology*, vol. 5. London: Ballière-Tindall, 1991; Stoelting RK. *Pharmacology and Physiology in Anesthetic Practice*, 3rd edn. New York: Lippincott-Raven, 1999; Dundee JW and Wyant GM. *Intravenous Anaesthesia*, 2nd edn. Edinburgh: Churchill Livingstone, 1988; Manufacturers' Data Sheets; and from the Pharmaceutical Information Service, University Hospital Birmingham.

**Table 19.19 Percentage protein binding in plasma of some common drugs**

| Drug | Percentage protein binding | Drug | Percentage protein binding |
|---|---|---|---|
| **Intravenous anaesthetics** | | **Neuromuscular blocking drugs** | |
| Etomidate | 76 | Atracurium | 50 |
| Ketamine | 12 | Cisatracurium | Not recorded |
| Methohexitone | 80 | Mivacurium | Not recorded |
| Propofol | 98 | Pancuronium | 20 |
| Thiopentone | 80 | Rocuronium | Not recorded |
| | | Vecuronium | 30 |
| | | Suxamethonium | 30 |
| **Inhalational anaesthetics** | | **Opioids and antagonists** | |
| Desflurane | Negligible | Alfentanil | 90 |
| Enflurane | Negligible | Diamorphine | 40 |
| Halothane | Negligible | Fentanyl | 85 |
| Isoflurane | Negligible | Morphine | 40 |
| Sevoflurane | Negligible | Pethidine (meperidine) | 70 |
| Nitrous oxide | Negligible | Remifentanil | 80 |
| **Local anaesthetics** | | Sufentanil | 92 |
| Bupivacaine | 95 | Naloxone | 50 |
| Etidocaine | 95 | **Other drugs** | |
| Lignocaine | 65 | Ethyl alcohol | Negligible |
| Prilocaine | 55 | Mannitol | Not recorded |
| Ropivacaine | 95 | Warfarin | 99 |
| **Benzodiazepines** | | | |
| Diazepam | 98 | | |
| Midazolam | 96 | | |
| Temazepam | 96 | | |
| Flumazenil | 50 | | |

The data in this table are taken from Hull CJ. *Pharmacokinetics for Anaesthesia*. Oxford: Butterworth-Heinemann, 1991: 70; White PF. *Ballière's Clinical Anaesthesiology*, vol. 5. London: Ballière-Tindall, 1991; Stoelting RK. *Pharmacology and Physiology in Anesthetic Practice*, 3rd edn. New York: Lippincott-Raven, 1999; Dundee JW and Wyant GM. *Intravenous Anaesthesia*, 2nd edn. Edinburgh: Churchill Livingstone, 1988; Manufacturers' Data Sheets; and from the Pharmaceutical Information Service, University Hospital Birmingham.

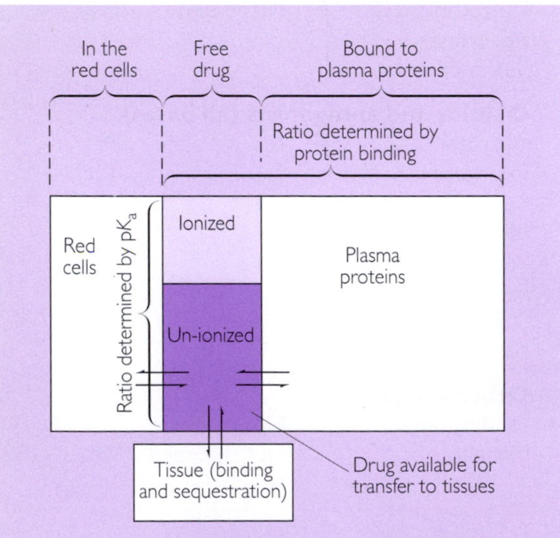


**Figure 19.41** A diagrammatic representation of the distribution of a drug in the blood. Note the importance of the un-ionized : ionized ratio and the effect of plasma proteins and red cells.

ionized, the diffusible fraction depends on the pH. Furthermore, the assay technique can measure the total drug in plasma or blood, the unbound drug in plasma, or the ionized or un-ionized part of the unbound drug. There is, therefore, a range of values that are possible for the partition coefficient depending on the pH, the temperature, the assay, and the lipid medium used for equilibration (e.g. octanol, *n*-heptane, erythrocyte, fat, etc.). Unfortunately, in both papers and textbooks, this level of definition is often omitted. Most assay techniques, if unqualified, usually measure the total blood or plasma concentration. All the tissue solubilities given in Table 19.19 are directly comparable within the drug grouping.

It is sometimes possible to saturate the protein-binding sites if sufficient drug is given or if two drugs that share the same sites are given concurrently. In this way, unexpectedly high concentrations of unbound drug result and toxicity is possible. This is more likely to happen the more protein bound the drug(s) involved. A good example is aspirin producing warfarin toxicity. In practice, it is only a practical problem with drugs that are more than 80% protein bound.

Protein binding does not occur only in the plasma. It can also occur in the red blood cell. Fentanyl is a good example of this, with almost as much fentanyl inside the red cells as in the plasma. Binding in the red cells does not, however, affect the proportional partitioning of free and bound drugs in the plasma. If a drug has been delivered to a particular tissue when the plasma concentrations are high and does not diffuse back when the plasma levels fall, it is said to be sequestered. This can be caused by a strong chemical bonding of the drug in the tissue (e.g. iodine in the thyroid, tetracycline in bone) or because the tissue has made the drug non-diffusible, usually by a change in the pH. Again, fentanyl can be used as an example in that it is 90% ionized in the plasma (pH = 7.4) and 99.999% ionized in the stomach (pH = 2.5).

### *Bioavailability*

Bioavailability is an important concept relating to the uptake of drugs. It can be defined as the ratio of the effective dose (i.e. the amount that reaches the blood) to the administered dose. Put simply, it represents the proportion of the prescribed dose that reaches the systemic circulation. When estimating bioavailability, it is conventional to regard the bioavailability of an intravenous dose as 100%.

Bioavailability can be determined by giving the same dose orally and intravenously (with time for complete clearance between doses) and following the serum concentration with time. This will produce two elimination curves as shown in Figure 19.42. The ratio of the area under the oral elimination curve ($AUC_o$) to the area under the intravenous elimination curve ($AUC_{iv}$), up to when the curves return to the *x* axis, gives the bioavailability. If a drug is not available in an intravenous preparation, then another route may have to be used as the reference standard. In the past, bioavailability has been estimated by measuring the total excretion of unchanged drug in the urine after oral and intravenous administration. This has obvious disadvantages compared with the method shown in Figure 19.42.

The two main causes of low bioavailability are poor absorption from the method of administration (particularly oral and transdermal) and high first-pass metabolism in the liver (see Chapters 27 and 28). The reason for poor bioavailability can often be determined by the isolation and identification of drug metabolites in plasma or urine. When high concentrations of metabolites are present, poor systemic bioavailability is usually caused by high first-pass and flow-limited hepatic clearance; if few metabolites are identified, poor absorption or breakdown in the gastrointestinal tract is probably responsible.

### *Hysteresis*

Some of the factors (e.g. fat solubility, concentration gradient) which cause drugs to reach their target receptors at different speeds were described above. This variability in transmission time between plasma concentration and biophase contributes to a phenomenon known as hysteresis. Hysteresis is the time lag between the time of administration of a drug and the observation of its effect. It has three components:

1. time for the administered dose to reach the blood;
2. time for the drug to go from blood to the biophase;
3. time for the pharmacological effect to occur.

For orally administered drugs, (1) is likely to be the greatest component but it is reduced to zero in intravenous administration. The transfer of drug from the plasma to the biophase and vice versa is shown diagrammatically in Figure 19.43. It can be seen that, as the plasma concentration is rising, the biophase concentration lags behind in time and is lower. After the plasma concentration has peaked and is falling, the biophase concentration is higher. This means that a single plasma concentration P could represent a biophase concentration of $B_1$ or $B_2$ (Figure 19.43), depending on when it was taken. Consequently, it should always be borne in mind that interpretation of concentration–effect data when the plasma concentration is rising or falling is fraught with difficulty.

An example of fentanyl hysteresis in clinical practice is shown in Figure 19.44. A derivative of the EEG, the spectral edge frequency, was measured during a 6-minute fentanyl infusion and for a time after the infusion was stopped. It can be seen that the serum concentration increases to approximately 20 ng/ml before there is any substantial change in the spectral edge frequency. When the infusion ends, the serum

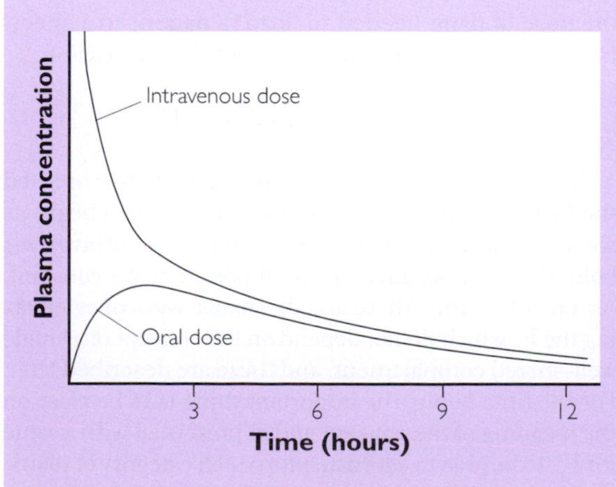


**Figure 19.42** The concept of bioavailability. The graph shows the plasma concentrations with time for both intravenous and oral dosing. Bioavailability = (Area under oral curve)/(Area under intravenous curve).

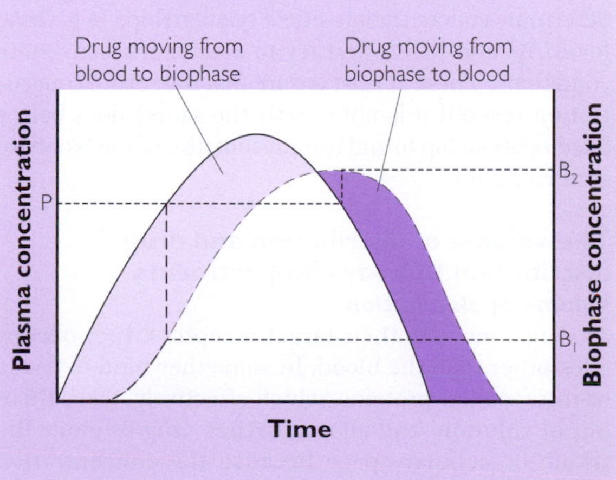


**Figure 19.43** The relationship between the plasma concentration (——) and the concentration at the site of action of a drug (- - - - -) (the biophase concentration). (See text for details.)

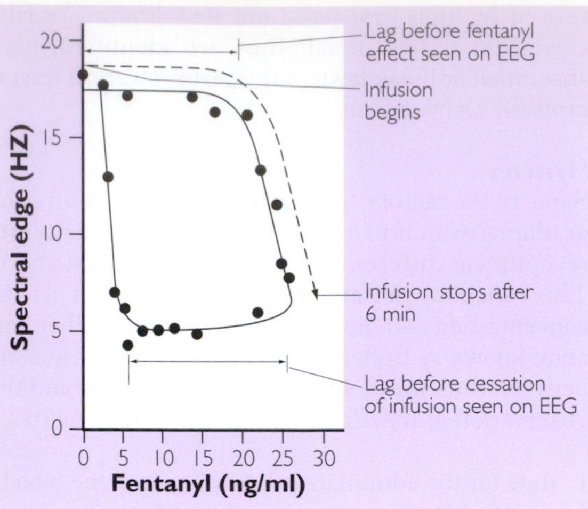


**Figure 19.44** A demonstration of hysteresis. The spectral edge frequency is taken to be a measure of the pharmacodynamic effect of fentanyl. It can be seen that, after the infusion begins, there is a lag before any effect is seen on the spectral edge. The same phenomenon is true in reverse when the infusion stops. (See text for details.) (Adapted from Scott JC *et al. Anesthesiology* 1985;62:234.)

concentration similarly decreases from approximately 25 to 7 ng/ml without significant measurable change. If a line is drawn across the graph at 10 Hz, it can be seen that this spectral edge frequency can be present at plasma fentanyl concentrations of either 5 or 25 ng/ml, depending on whether the concentration was increasing or decreasing at the time. Experiments such as those shown in Figure 19.44 have demonstrated that the half-time for plasma–brain equilibration is about 1 min for alfentanil and 6 min for fentanyl. This would be expected from their diffusible (un-ionized) fractions (see Table 19.19), which are a major determinant of the rate of diffusion. Similar time lag phenomena are seen in the dependence of induction dose on speed of infusion with intravenous induction agents (see Chapter 32).

It is because of hysteresis that many studies trying to determine concentration–effect relationships (e.g. those for MAC and MIR) first try to establish steady-state conditions. These at least ensure that the serum concentration (even if it is not exactly the same) does bear a fixed relationship to and is representative of the biophase concentration.

## The volume of distribution and drug distribution to body compartments

### *Volume of distribution*

As drugs move to their target receptors, they occupy sites other than the blood. In some they bind to tissue or intracellular proteins, which effectively 'takes them out of solution' and allows further drug to enter the tissue or cellular space because the concentration gradient is maintained. In others, because of pH changes (see above), they change their ionization characteristics and become 'trapped'. To calculate the serum concentration resulting from a given dose of drug would therefore require a knowledge of all the various binding characteristics, tissue types, blood flows, dissociation constants, and solubilities.

An alternative approach (assuming for the moment that no drug is metabolized or leaves the body) is to assume that the space that the drug occupies is equivalent to a single well-stirred compartment. For example, if we give 50 mg of drug and record a plasma concentration of 1.0 mg/L, the volume of the hypothetical well-stirred compartment is 50 mg/1.0 mg per L = 50 litres. This virtual volume is called the apparent volume of distribution ($V_d$).

The $V_d$, although a rather imprecise concept, does provide a useful insight into how drugs are distributed within the body. Although there is obviously a continuum of values, there are some general principles that can be established:

- If the drug is very tightly bound to the plasma proteins and/or highly charged, it is likely to have a $V_d$ approximating to the plasma volume, 0.05 L/kg or 3.5 litres in a 70-kg man (e.g. heparin).
- If the drug passes through capillary pores, but does not enter the intracellular space, the $V_d$ will be approximately 0.2 L/kg or 14 litres in a 70-kg man, corresponding to the extracellular volume (e.g. mannitol, inulin).
- If the drug enters the cells, but is not concentrated in any tissue component, the $V_d$ will approximate to the total body water – 0.6 L/kg or 42 litres in a 70-kg man (e.g. ethanol).
- If there is specific cellular uptake, tissue binding, or ion trapping, the $V_d$ will be more than 0.6 L/kg, i.e. larger than the volume of fluid that it can possibly dissolve in. Such values for $V_d$ imply extensive sequestration in the intracellular compartment.

Typical values for a variety of common drugs are given in Table 19.20. The values in the table can be compared with the broad classification described above to gauge the spaces into which the drugs are distributed.

In its simplest form as described above, within its limitations, $V_d$ provides the data necessary to estimate the dose of drug needed to 'load' a patient to a specified concentration by application of the expression:

$$\text{Dose} = \text{Concentration} \times V_d.$$

This account of $V_d$ has of course completely omitted the fact that elimination and metabolism also begin as soon as a drug is injected. After an oral or intravenous bolus dose, the serum concentrations are never constant. As a result of this, there are alternative ways of calculating the $V_d$ which do not depend on the concept of a single well-stirred compartment, and these are described later. For the time being, the important thing is to be clear on the meaning of the concept and, if presented with a value for $V_d$, to be able to estimate into which category of distribution pattern a drug is likely to fit.

### *Drug distribution to body compartments*

This examines the clinical application of the concept of $V_d$. Reference can be made to Table 19.20 to exam-

**Table 19.20 Typical values for the apparent volume of distribution ($V_d$ in litres) and lipid/fat/tissue solubility based on a 70-kg man for drugs encountered in anaesthetic practice**

| Drug | $V_d$ | Lipid solubility | |
|---|---|---|---|
| **Intravenous anaesthetics** | | | |
| Etomidate | 250 | High | |
| Ketamine | 200 | Very high | |
| Methohexitone | 200 | High | |
| Propofol | 750 | Very high | |
| Thiopentone | 200 | High | |
| **Inhalational anaesthetics**[a] | | | |
| | | Blood–gas | Fat–blood |
| Desflurane | > 1200 | 0.42 | 30 |
| Enflurane | > 1700 | 1.9 | 36 |
| Halothane | > 2500 | 2.3 | 62 |
| Isoflurane | > 2000 | 1.4 | 52 |
| Sevoflurane | > 2000 | 0.68 | 55 |
| Nitrous oxide | > 150 | 0.47 | 2.3 |
| **Local anaesthetics**[b] | | | |
| Bupivacaine | 75 | 10 | |
| Etidocaine | 130 | 50 | |
| Lignocaine | 100 | 1 | |
| Prilocaine | 250 | 0.33 | |
| Ropivacaine | 50 | 3 | |
| **Benzodiazepines** | | | |
| Diazepam | 95 | All highly fat soluble | |
| Midazolam | 100 | | |
| Temazepam | 90 | | |
| Flumazenil | 70 | | |
| **Neuromuscular blocking agents** | | | |
| Atracurium | 10 | No published figures but lipid solubility low because highly ionized | |
| Cisatracurium | 12 | | |
| Mivacurium | 12 | | |
| Pancuronium | 12 | | |
| Rocuronium | 18 | | |
| Vecuronium | 12 | | |
| Suxamethonium | NA but approx. 10 | | |
| **Opioids and antagonists**[c] | | | |
| Alfentanil | 30 | 130 | |
| Diamorphine | 350 | 250 | |
| Fentanyl | 330 | 1000 | |
| Morphine | 250 | 1 | |
| Pethidine (meperidine) | 350 | 30 | |
| Remifentanil | 30 | 15 | |
| Sufentanil | 120 | 1700 | |
| Naloxone | 140 | NA | |
| **Other drugs** | | | |
| Blood transfusion: very large-molecular-weight colloids | 5 | NA | |
| Heparin | 5 | NA but highly ionized so very poor fat solubility | |
| Warfarin | 8 | NA | |
| Insulin | 11 | NA | |
| Mannitol | 15 | NA | |
| Ethyl alcohol | 40 | NA but un-ionized so highly fat soluble | |

The data in this table are taken from Hull CJ. *Pharmacokinetics for Anaesthesia*. Oxford: Butterworth–Heinemann, 1991: 70; White PF. *Ballière's Clinical Anaesthesiology*, vol. 5. London: Ballière-Tindall, 1991; Stoelting RK. *Pharmacology and Physiology in Anesthetic Practice*, 3rd edn. New York: Lippincott-Raven, 1999; Dundee JW and Wyant GM. *Intravenous Anaesthesia*, 2nd edn. Edinburgh: Churchill Livingstone, 1988; Manufacturers' Data Sheets; and from the Pharmaceutical Information Service, University Hospital Birmingham.
[Lipid solubility values depend enormously on the method of determination and the lipid phase chosen: the data here are presented in the most useful way to aid an understanding of drug action. For actual numerical values of, say, octanol–water or *n*-heptane–water coefficients, specialized texts should be consulted. Values for the volume of distribution can easily vary by over ± 50%, depending on the method of calculation: the values here should be regarded as comparative guides.] NA, no numerical data available.

[a] $V_d$ estimated from uptake data by author: solubility coefficients given for comparative data.
[b] Lipid solubility presented in comparison with lignocaine.
[c] Lipid solubility presented in comparison with morphine.

ine the properties of a particular drug not specifically mentioned below.

*Drugs that stay in the circulating volume*
As seen above under 'Transfer across membranes', there have to be special conditions that prevent a substance leaving the blood and passing to the tissues. These are the following:

- The drug must be so large that it cannot be filtered through capillary fenestrations (see 'Transport across capillaries'). Examples of this are volume expanders such as albumin, dextrans, starches, and gelatins (see Chapter 14).
- The drug must be so tightly bound to plasma proteins that the unbound fraction is very, very small with poor diffusion characteristics. Examples of this are warfarin and heparin.

*Drugs with a limited distribution*
These are drugs that are able to leave the circulation by filtration but which then find their onward passage into distant cells difficult. The following are the factors that affect this:

- molecular size (the bigger the worse);
- ionization state (the more ionized the worse);
- protein binding (the higher the binding the less free drug);
- tissue perfusion (the lower the blood flow the lower the drug supply).

These factors describe bulky, highly ionized molecules with poor lipid solubility. Examples of such drugs are xanthine salts, penicillins, amino glycosides, non-depolarizing neuromuscular blocking agents, and salicylates. The delivery of these drugs becomes very dependent on the blood flow per gram of tissue and the degree of 'leakiness' of the capillaries. Neuromuscular blocking agents succeed in reaching relatively poorly perfused motor end-plates through leaky capillaries. They can also be isolated from well-perfused visceral tissue (liver, kidney, and thyroid) but are virtually prohibited from entering fat or crossing the blood–brain barrier.

*Drugs with an extensive distribution*
These drugs characteristically are either small, non-polar molecules or have a high lipid solubility. Their concentration in tissues is again a combination of the blood supply to the tissue and the organ's capacity to take it up. Even with high lipid solubility, some tissues (e.g. storage fat) are so poorly perfused that they can take days to reach equilibrium.

Most of the drugs used in anaesthesia fall into this category of extensive distribution. They include inhalational and intravenous anaesthetic agents, opioids, local anaesthetics, and benzodiazepines. Perhaps the most extreme example of a fat-soluble drug is amiodarone which, after cessation of treatment, has a half-life measured in months because of its storage in fat. It is self-evident that, when given by infusion, any drug with the potential for significant peripheral storage must have an initial loading dose to achieve satisfactory plasma concentrations during the early period.

## Extraction ratio, clearance, and elimination

This section describes the theoretical pharmacokinetic aspects of these three closely related topics. Apart from volatile anaesthetic agents that are eliminated via the expired air, the majority of drugs used in anaesthesia are metabolized and excreted by either the liver or kidney, or a combination of the two. Details of the ways in which this is done can be found in Chapters 25 and 28, to which reference should be made.

### *Extraction ratio*

Extraction is the removal of a drug from the circulation by an organ. It is conventionally measured by the extraction ratio (ER) and the relevant variables are shown diagrammatically in Figure 19.45. The ER for an organ is defined as the fraction of drug extracted from each unit volume of perfusing blood and is represented mathematically as:

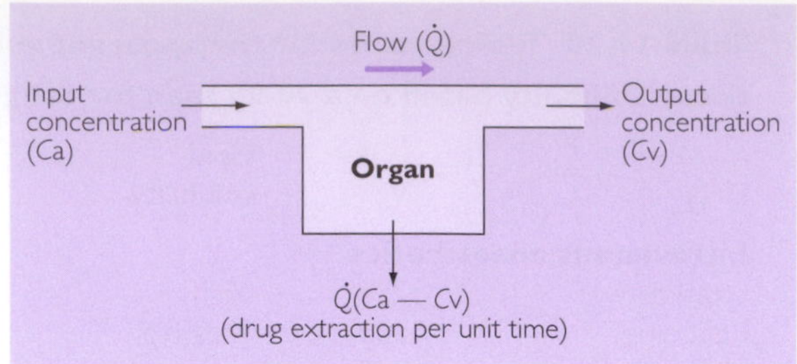


**Figure 19.45** A diagrammatic representation of the extraction of a drug from blood perfusing a given organ. $\dot{Q}$ flow; Ca, arterial concentration; Cv, venous concentration. (See text for details.)

$$\mathrm{ER} = \frac{\text{Quantity of drug removed in unit time}}{\text{Quantity of drug perfusing organ in unit time}}$$

$$= \frac{\text{Flow} \times (\text{Input concentration - Output concentration})}{\text{Flow} \times \text{Input concentration}}$$

As flow cancels out, and if the input concentration is represented as the arterial concentration (*C*a) and the output concentration as the venous concentration (*C*v), the expression becomes:

$$\mathrm{ER} = \frac{[C\mathrm{a} - C\mathrm{v}]}{C\mathrm{a}}$$

This equation will require obvious modification in the case of portal supplies (e.g. liver and pituitary) with *C*a being changed to the input venous concentration. Although the ER is valuable in knowing what proportion of drug will be removed, it does not, however, define the absolute quantity of drug removed per unit time. Although the ER is a useful concept when looking at individual organs, *it is necessary to link it with flow to estimate the rate or efficiency of drug removal per unit time*. This is done in the concept of clearance. The influence of ER on the rate of drug removal is described in Chapter 28 and reference should be made to Figures 28.14 and 28.16.

### *Clearance*

The ER is the fraction of drug removed from each unit volume of blood as it passes through the organ. In its simplest definition the *clearance (Cl) is the product of the ER and the flow rate* ($\dot{Q}$):

$$\mathrm{Cl} = \dot{Q} \times \mathrm{ER}.$$

As ER is a ratio, clearance has the units of flow.

This concept can be applied to single organs (liver, kidney, lung, etc.) or the whole body can be interpreted as a single unit from which the drug is removed in its passage through the vascular bed. When listed without qualification, clearance data usually apply to whole-body clearance.

Now, assume that after passing through the extracting organ and leaving with a concentration *C*v, the output blood (total flow $\dot{Q}$) is now separated into two parts so that it is either completely free of blood (i.e. zero concentration) or returned to its original arterial concentration *C*a. This is shown in Figure 19.46.

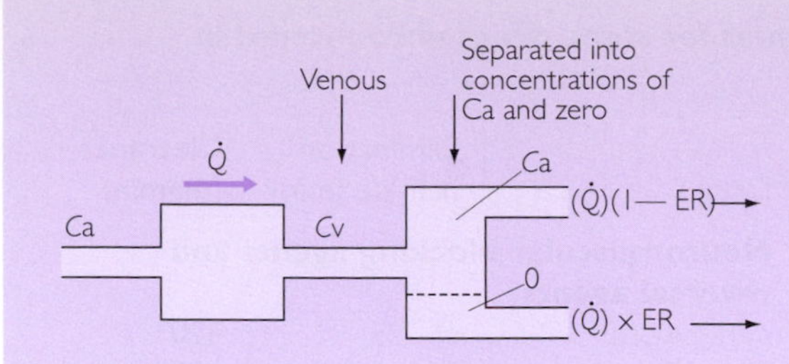


**Figure 19.46** A schematic representation of the concept of clearance. (See text for details and Figure 19.46.)

From the original definition of the ER given above, the volume with zero concentration will be ($\dot{Q} \times$ ER) and the volume with concentration *C*a will be $\dot{Q}$ (1 – ER). Comparing this figure with the definition of clearance given above (Cl = $\dot{Q} \times$ ER) gives a second definition of clearance as *the volume of perfusing blood completely cleared of the drug in unit time*.

Substituting for ER and again referring to Figure 19.46:

$$\mathrm{Cl} = \frac{\dot{Q}\,(Ca - Cv)}{Ca}$$

As the rate of drug extraction is $\dot{Q}$ (*C*a – *C*v), clearance can also be defined as *the rate of drug elimination per unit (input) concentration*. This can be restated *as the extraction of drug per unit time per unit concentration*. These four definitions of clearance are simply different descriptions of an identical process.

A general expression for clearance can also be derived graphically from observations of the serum level after administration following a single intravenous bolus dose ($x_d$). Such an idealized concentration–time curve, extending to zero serum concentration (i.e. all the drug has left the circulation), is drawn in Figure 19.47.

The average rate of removal over the period of observation (*T*) is given by:

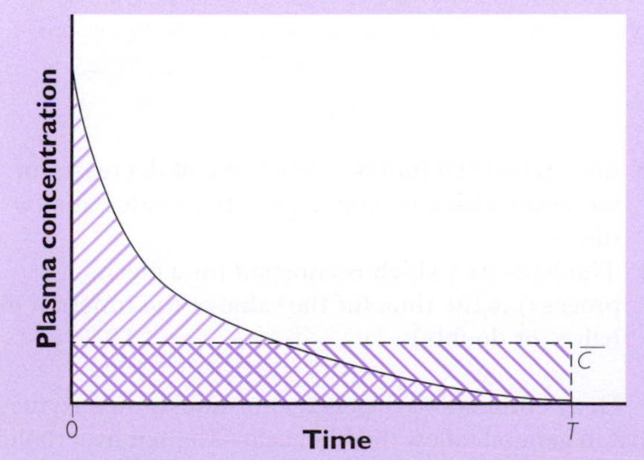


**Figure 19.47** The plasma concentration–time curve following a single dose of drug continued to time *T* when the concentration of drug (*C*) has reached zero (or is at the limit of the assay). When the two shaded areas are equal, $\bar{C}$ is the average concentration.

$$\text{Average rate of removal} = x_d/T.$$

The average concentration during this period can be obtained from the graphic integration of Figure 19.47 (see Chapter 37 for methodology) to give:

$$\text{Average concentration} = \frac{\text{AUC}}{\text{T}}$$

where AUC = area under curve.

From the definition of clearance:

$$\text{Clearance} = \frac{\text{Rate of removal}}{\text{per unit concentration}}$$

$$= \frac{\text{Average rate of removal}}{\text{Average concentration}}$$

$$= \frac{x_d}{T} \times \frac{T}{\text{AUC}}$$

$$= \frac{x_d}{\text{AUC}}$$

This gives us a fifth definition of clearance as *the dose divided by the area under the concentration–time curve*. This derivation, with its assumptions of 'average' values representing complex processes, has obvious limitations. It does, however, represent a simple 'model independent' method of clearance estimation. When the concentration–time curve can be fitted with mathematical equations that can be integrated properly, the expression for clearance has AUC replaced by a precise exponential derivative. This will be seen later under 'Pharmacokinetic modelling'.

In summary, clearance is a very important derived parameter of pharmacokinetics which can be represented by five equivalent definitions:

- Clearance is the flow rate (Q) multiplied by the extraction ration (ER).
- Clearance is the rate of drug elimination per unit (input) concentration.
- Clearance is the extraction of drug per unit time per unit (input) concentration.
- Clearance is the volume of perfusing blood which could be regarded as being entirely cleared of drug per unit time.
- Clearance is the dose of drug divided by the area under the concentration–time curve.

Examples of values of clearance for drugs used in anaesthesia are given in Table 19.21.

Clearance, as discussed above, has not taken into account body size. It is obvious that the numerical value of clearance of a small child will be different from that of an adult and that the value for a small, lean adult will be different from that of a large, fat adult. How are these to be compared? This is often done by dividing the whole-body clearance by the weight, thereby giving clearance in units of litres per minute per kilogram. Although superficially convenient, this is fundamentally flawed because the clearance is dependent on many variables such as regional blood flow, enzyme activity, cardiac output, and coincidental drug therapy, none of

**Table 19.21 Elimination half-lives and clearance values for some drugs encountered in anaesthesia practice**

| Drug | Elimination half-life (min) | Clearance (ml/min) |
|---|---|---|
| **Intravenous anaesthetics** | | |
| Etomidate | 30–300 | 1000 |
| Ketamine | 20–180 | 1200 |
| Methohexitone | 20–200 | 1000 |
| Propofol | 30–350 | 2500 |
| Thiopentone | 50–500 | 220 |
| **Inhalational anaesthetics** | | |
| Desflurane | Dependent on minute volume, cardiac output, and blood-gas solubility | |
| Enflurane | | |
| Halothane | | |
| Isoflurane | | |
| Sevoflurane | | |
| Nitrous oxide | | |
| **Local anaesthetics** | | |
| Bupivacaine | 150–200 | 500 |
| Etidocaine | 150–180 | 1000 |
| Lignocaine | 90–120 | 900 |
| Prilocaine | 80–120 | 2500 |
| Ropivacaine | 100–150 | 500 |
| **Benzodiazepines** | | |
| Diazepam | 1200–5500 | 40 |
| Midazolam | 90–300 | 550 |
| Temazepam | 300–400 | 100 |
| Flumazenil | 60 | 1000 |
| **Neuromuscular blocking agents and reversal agents** | | |
| Atracurium | 15–25 | 420 |
| Cisatracurium | 20–30 | 450 |
| Mivacurium | 10–20 | 4000 |
| Pancuronium | 80–110 | 130 |
| Rocuronium | 70–150 | 250 |
| Vecuronium | 30–70 | 350 |
| Suxamethonium | 5–10 (estimated) | NA |
| Atropine | 60–180 | 330 |
| Glycopyrrolate | 35–65 | 900 |
| Neostigmine | 20–80 | 700 |
| **Opioids and antagonists** | | |
| Alfentanil | 70–110 | 300 |
| Diamorphine | 15–30 | 220 |
| Fentanyl | 100–350 | 1200 |
| Morphine | 100–200 | 1000 |
| Pethidine (meperidine) | 150–350 | 1000 |
| Remifentanil | 8–20 | 2800 |
| Sufentanil | 100–240 | 1000 |
| Naloxone | 30–80 | 1750 |
| **Other drugs** | | |
| Warfarin | 1500–2500 | 5–100 |
| Heparin | 30–150 | 90 |
| Insulin | 2–8 | 250 |
| Mannitol | 50–100 | 500 |
| Ethyl alcohol | Zero-order elimination | |
| Amiodarone | 10–100 days | Extremely low |

The data in this table are taken from Hull CJ. *Pharmacokinetics for Anaesthesia*. Oxford: Butterworth-Heinemann, 1991: 70; White PF. *Ballière's Clinical Anaesthesiology*, vol. 5. London: Ballière-Tindall, 1991; Stoelting RK. *Pharmacology and Physiology in Anesthetic Practice*, 3rd edn. New York: Lippincott-Raven, 1999; Dundee JW and Wyant GM. *Intravenous Anaesthesia*, 2nd edn. Edinburgh: Churchill Livingstone, 1988; Manufacturers' Data Sheets; and from the Pharmaceutical Information Service, University Hospital Birmingham.
The data are taken from many sources and represent the range of published figures. Pharmacokinetic data are very variable, differing by orders of magnitude on occasions. Depending on the technique of estimation, some published half-lives include $\alpha$ and $\beta$ effects. The majority measure $\beta$ effects alone. It is almost as important to note the published variability and the importance of treating patients individually rather than bothering to remember a mean value. The figures are affected by the method of drug administration, age, sex, timing of samples, and assay technique. NA, not available.

which is directly proportional to body weight. Despite these obvious drawbacks, clearance per kilogram of body weight continues to be listed in tables. When taking data from such tables, before multiplying up to get total body clearance, it is first necessary to know the population from which the figures were derived.

#### *Elimination*

This chapter has tried to explore the processes of drug handling, combining basic physiology and pharmacology with the minimum recourse to mathematics. Although this principle continues, readers unfamiliar with logarithms and exponential processes are advised to read Chapter 37 first. The two most important things to remember for the purposes of this chapter are as follows:

- An exponential function has a rate of decrease (or increase) which is proportional to its value at all times.
- The half-life (which is constant for a given process) is the time for the value of the function to halve (or double).

Drug elimination depends enormously on enzymes that in general follow the Michaelis–Menten hyperbolic relationship. This has been described earlier in Chapter 18 and is shown in Figure 18.39, to which reference should be made.

As described in Chapter 37, many biological processes are characterized by the equation:

$$dx/dt = -k(x)^n$$

where $dx/dt$ is the rate of decay, $k$ is the rate constant, and the integer value of $n$ determines the 'order' of the equation. Such an equation produces an exponential curve if $n = 1$.

The most important division of elimination processes is into zero- and first-order reactions. These terms result from mathematical definitions.

*Zero-order elimination*

This is defined to occur when $n = 0$, and, as $x^0 = 1$:

$$dx/dt = -k.$$

This equation describes a process in which *there is a steady decrease in* x *with time that is constant (at the rate of* k*) and independent of the drug concentration.* This is the pharmacological consequence of zero-order elimination.

Zero-order elimination describes the situation in drug metabolism when there is a gross excess of substrate and all the binding sites on the enzyme are fully occupied. In Figure 18.39, it represents the flat asymptotic section of the Michaelis–Menten curve. The best common example of this is the metabolism of alcohol. Ingested alcohol absorbed from the stomach quickly saturates the enzyme alcohol dehydrogenase. Continued intake results in a steady rise in the serum level of a small, completely uncharged molecule that rapidly equilibrates throughout the body's tissues (see Table 19.20). Without these special properties, getting drunk would be much more difficult. Were it not absorbed rapidly, forward planning would be necessary for a social function!

Zero-order drug kinetics are shown graphically in Figure 19.48a. Note again that the rate of fall of serum concentration is steady and independent of the actual serum level.

Zero-order kinetics can be achieved by almost any drug given to excess. Two examples in clinical practice are thiopentone and salicylates which are considered later.

*First-order elimination*

In first-order elimination, in $dx/dt = -k(x)^n$, the exponent $n = 1$ makes the equation:

$$dx/dt = -kx.$$

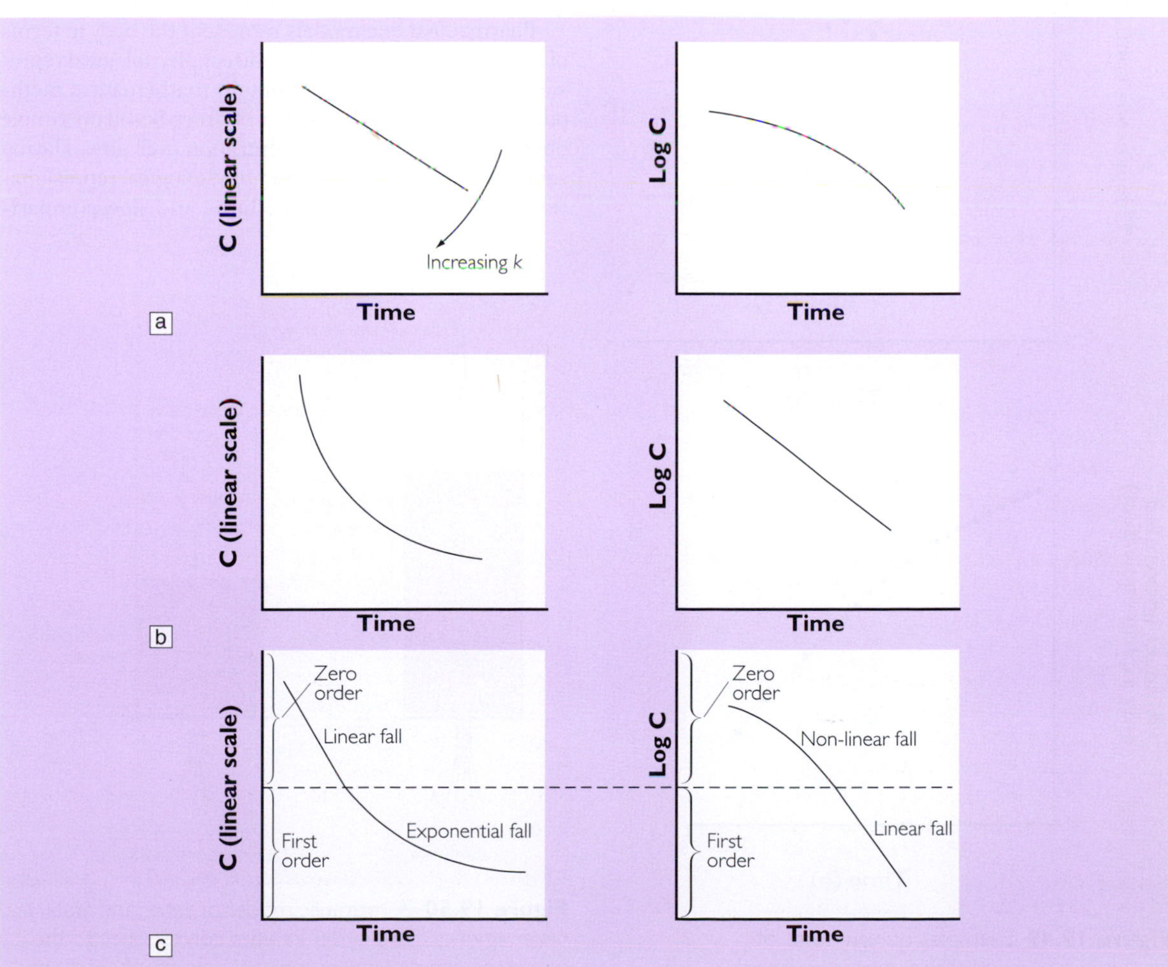


**Figure 19.48** Various pharmacokinetic curves shown plotted on linear and logarithmic axes. (a) Zero-order kinetics with a linear fall on a linear plasma concentration scale; (b) first-order kinetics with linear fall on logarithmic concentration scale; (c) combination of zero- and first-order kinetics from the metabolism of a drug that initially had a saturated enzyme system. C, plasma concentration.

This means that the rate of change of $x$ is proportional to $x$ itself (i.e. it is an exponential process). In terms of drug concentrations and enzyme action, with reference to Figure 18.39, it implies that the enzymes are working on the initial, approximately linear section of the hyperbolic Michaelis–Menten equation, i.e. the concentration of the drug is much smaller than $K_m$ (the Michaelis constant). In practical terms, it implies that there is plenty of free capacity in the enzyme system. Consequently, as the drug concentration rises, so more enzyme sites are proportionally occupied, thereby making the rate of breakdown proportional to the concentration. Most drugs administered in therapeutic doses behave in this way.

Integrating up the basic differential equation above gives:

$$x = x_0 e^{-kt}$$

where $x_0$ is the initial concentration and $k$ is the rate constant.

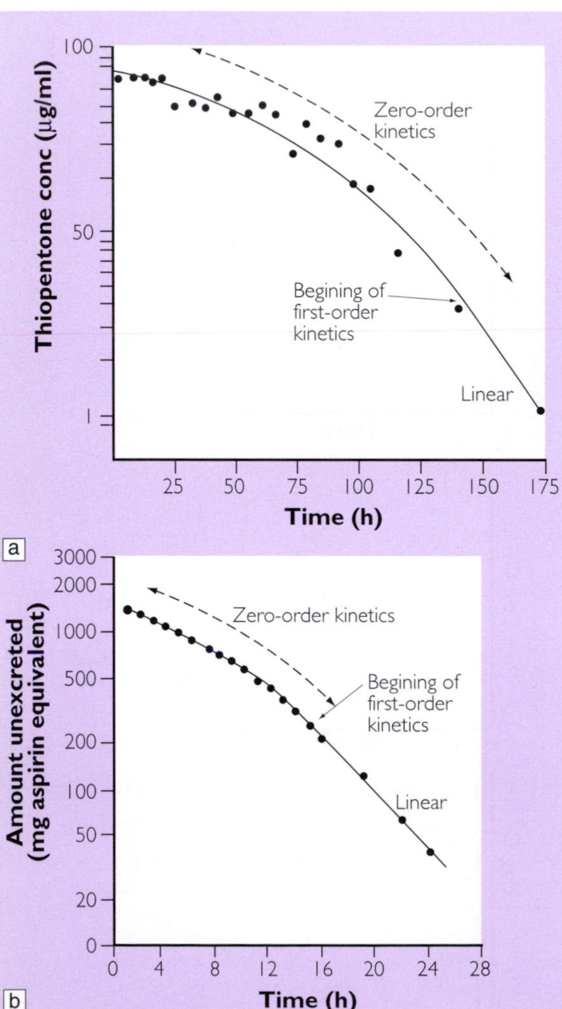


**Figure 19.49** Examples of high doses of (a) thiopentone and (b) salicylate showing the transition from zero- to first-order kinetics. Compare the shapes of the curves with those in Figure 19.48. (Adapted from (a) Stanski DR *et al. Anesthesiology* 1980;53:169; (b) Levy G. *J Pharm Sci* 1965;54:959.)

This relationship is plotted in Figure 19.48b. Its exponential properties are discussed in Chapter 37.

It is clear that, if a drug is present in overdose and the concentration falls steadily under zero-order elimination to a level at which not all the enzyme sites are occupied, there will thereafter be a gradual change to first-order elimination. This situation is represented for enzyme function in Chapter 18, Figure 18.39 and for plasma concentrations in Figure 19.48c. Clinical examples of the transition from zero- to first-order kinetics are high doses of thiopentone and salicylate. The pharmacokinetic behaviour of these is shown in Figure 19.49.

Students often find hydraulic models a useful analogy for explaining pharmacokinetic changes of drug concentration. These are shown for a zero-order converting to a first-order process in Figure 19.50.

### Pharmacokinetic modelling

This section has so far tried, whenever possible, to relate pharmacokinetic behaviour to physiological events. The physiological factors that determine the drug concentration at the site of action are summarized for convenience in Figure 19.51. If the mathematical links between the tails and the heads of all the arrows were known, a true physiological model could be derived mathematically. This detail does not, however, exist and because of this, pharmacokinetic models have been developed.

Pharmacokinetic models represent the body in terms of compartments that have no direct physiological representation. They are fundamentally mathematical methods of predicting the behaviour of drugs based on sample observations of plasma concentration over time. Having said this, there is some limited physiological representation of the body into fast, medium, and slow compart-

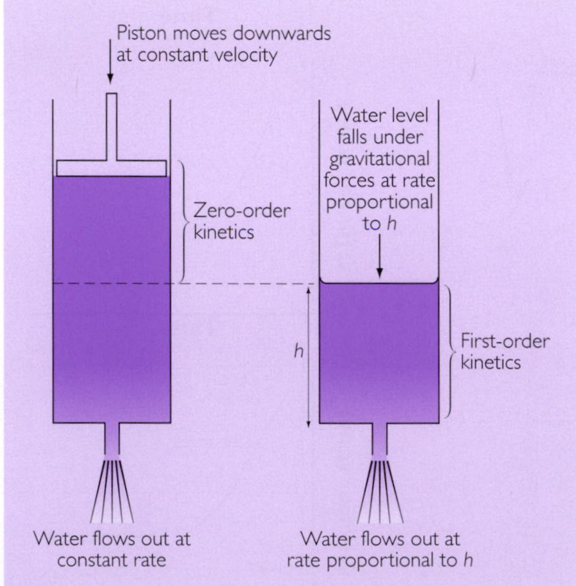


**Figure 19.50** A hydraulic model of zero- and first-order kinetics. Zero-order kinetics corresponds to the piston moving down at a constant velocity and water flowing out at a constant rate. First-order kinetics corresponds to the water flowing out under gravity at a rate that is proportional to $h$. ($h$ = height of water column above outlet.)

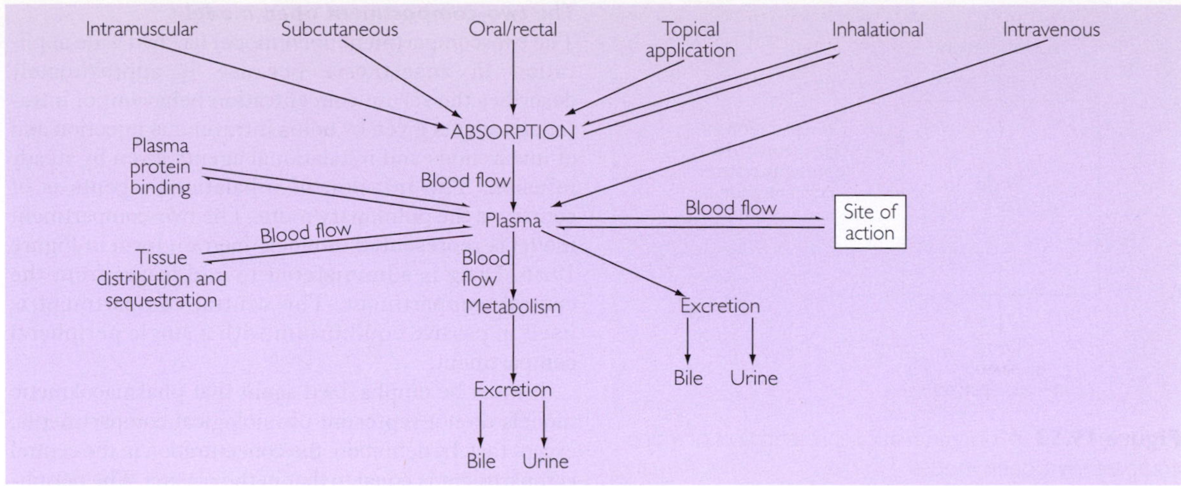


**Figure 19.51** A diagrammatic summary of the physiological factors that determine a drug's concentration at the site of action.

ments that can be made under certain conditions, which aids understanding. This is described in Chapters 32 and 33 for intravenous and inhalational anaesthetic agents. It must, however, be emphasized that these are only useful mental images rather than precise physiological entities.

Only one- and two-compartment open models will be considered here. An open model is one in which the drug can leave the system in a predictable manner with time. All the exponential models used in pharmacokinetics are said to be 'linear'. As a result of the confusion that it causes for many people, the term 'linearity' will be described first.

*Linearity*

How, one may ask, can an exponential drug process show linearity? The answer is that linearity is a mathematical expression which defines the effect of changing the magnitude of the initial value of a wash-out exponential function (see Chapter 37 and later). In a linear model, if the distribution volume and rate constant do not change, at every given time period from zero to infinity the serum concentration of a drug will be in proportion to the initial dose. Put another way, following a single bolus dose, if the initial bolus dose is halved, the serum concentration extrapolated back to zero will be halved, and so will the serum concentration at every other subsequent time period. This is demonstrated in Figure 19.52.

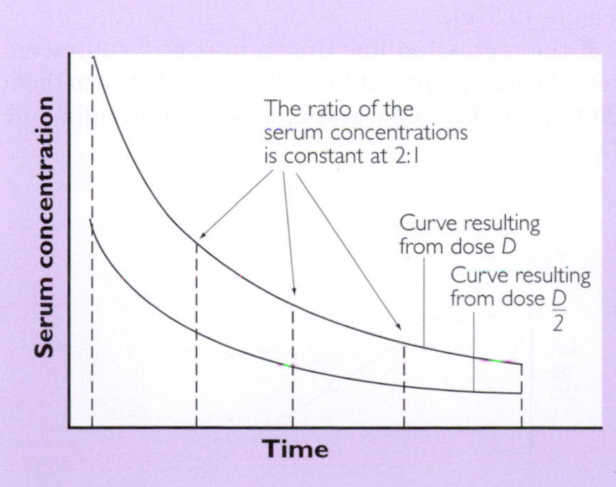


**Figure 19.52** A representation of the concept of linearity. At each point in time the serum concentration resulting from dose *D* is twice that resulting from dose *D*/2.

***The one-compartment open model***

The one-compartment open model assumes a single volume of distribution and a first-order relationship of drug concentration with time. This is represented in Figure 19.53. The one-compartment open model approximately describes the decrease in plasma concentrations in two clinical situations:

- those drugs with a small $V_d$ which are almost confined to the circulating fluid volume (e.g. heparin and warfarin, see Table 19.20);
- many drugs administered by intramuscular injection. This is because the rapid uptake compartment (see 'The two-compartment model' below) is essentially absent.

The linear and logarithmic plots for a one-compartment model are shown in Figure 19.54. Figure 19.54b shows the regression plot extrapolated backwards to obtain the theoretical maximum serum concentration ($C_0$) which would have occurred if the drug was distributed immediately to all parts of its distribution volume. Provided the model represents the changes in serum concentration with time, this allows calculation of $V_d$ such that:

$$V_d = \frac{\text{Dose}}{C_0}$$

Estimation of the gradient in Figure 19.54b gives a value for $-k$, the rate constant.

The one-compartment open model also allows an estimation of clearance (in two ways). The first is the graphical model-independent method described earlier, where the area under the curve (AUC) is measured directly and clearance (Cl) is calculated from:

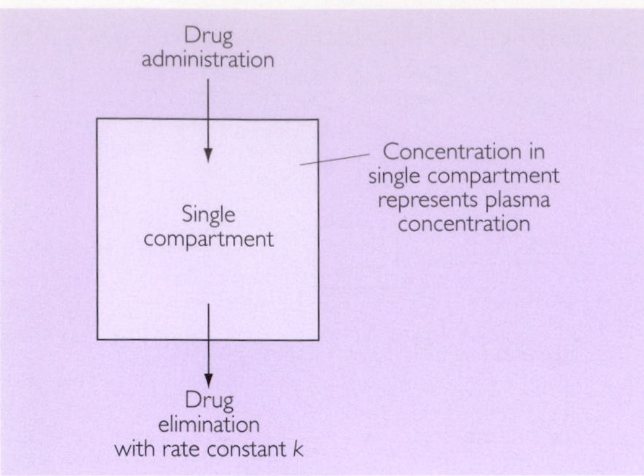


**Figure 19.53** A diagrammatic representation of a one-compartment open model.

$$\mathrm{Cl} = \frac{\mathrm{Dose}}{\mathrm{AUC}}$$

The second method depends on the properties of exponentials (see Chapter 37). Integrating up a single wash-out exponential ($C = C_0\,\mathrm{e}^{-kt}$) mathematically from zero to infinity gives:

$$\mathrm{AUC} = \frac{C_0}{k}$$

and given that Cl = Dose/AUC, substituting gives:

$$\mathrm{Cl} = \frac{k\ \mathrm{Dose}}{C_0}$$

$C_0$ and $k$ can be derived from an analysis of the semi-logarithmic concentration–time plot of the same type as Figure 19.54b. Using this type of analysis does not require the measurements to be continued to zero concentration or the tail of the linear plot (Figure 19.55) to be followed to 'infinity' to integrate the area.

Rearranging the equations for Cl again, by putting $V_\mathrm{d} = \mathrm{Dose}/C_0$ gives:

$$\mathrm{Cl} = V_\mathrm{d} \times k.$$

This expression allows a further way to calculate Cl, $V_\mathrm{d}$, or $k$ if the other two are known. The effect of variations in absorption rate, dose level, and elimination are shown graphically in Figure 19.55.

### *The two-compartment open model*

The two-compartment open model has had wide application in anaesthesia because it approximately describes the serum concentration behaviour of intravenous agents given by bolus intravenous injection and of intravenous and inhalational agents given by steady infusion. The infusion of inhalational agents is of course via the pulmonary route. The two-compartment model is represented in block diagram form in Figure 19.56. Drug is administered to and leaves from the central compartment. The central compartment is itself in passive equilibrium with a single peripheral compartment.

It must be emphasized again that pharmacokinetic models do not represent physiological compartments, except that, by definition, the concentration in the central compartment is equal to that in the plasma. The peripheral compartment as such has no exact anatomical analogue. In explaining the behaviour of the plasma concentration with time, the movement of drug into and out of vessel-rich and vessel-poor tissues (e.g. as done in Chapter 32, Table 32.2 and Chapter 33, Table 33.9) is often considered. Although this is useful for understanding from a physiological viewpoint, these physiological compartments are not specifically represented in the two-compartment model. The drug concentration in the peripheral compartment of Figure 19.56 is not a measurable entity; it is a mathematical derivation. Some other, more complex, multi-compartment models have tried to imitate individual body spaces more accurately but these are not considered here.

The two-compartment model will be studied in its response to intravenous bolus doses and constant rate infusions.

#### *Intravenous bolus doses*

The serum concentration following administration of a single intravenous bolus dose is shown in Figure 19.57a. When this is transposed to a semi-logarithmic plot (Figure 19.57b) and the best line of fit drawn in, it can be seen that, unlike the one-compartment model (see Figure 19.54), it does not translate into a single straight line. If the later points are considered alone, they approximate to a straight line with intercept $B$ and rate constant β, but the early data are well off the line (Figure 19.57c).

If the regression line drawn in is now subtracted from the data points and the difference between them plotted on the same graph, a second straight line

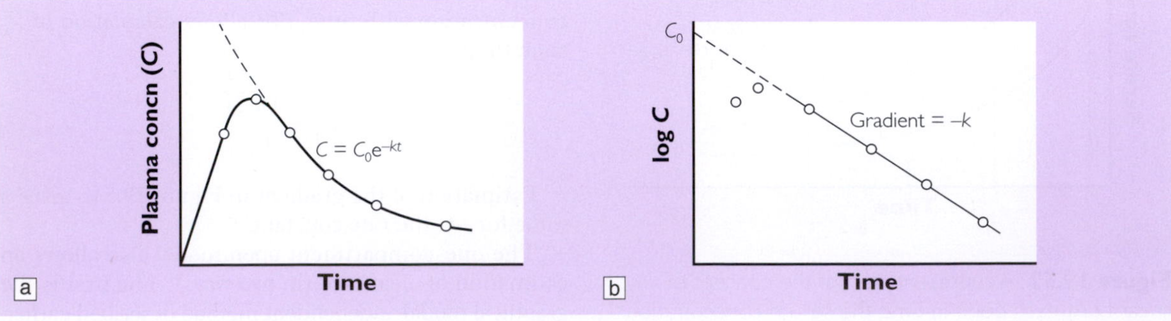


**Figure 19.54** Linear (a) and logarithmic (b) plots of the plasma concentration–time relationship for a one-compartment open model.

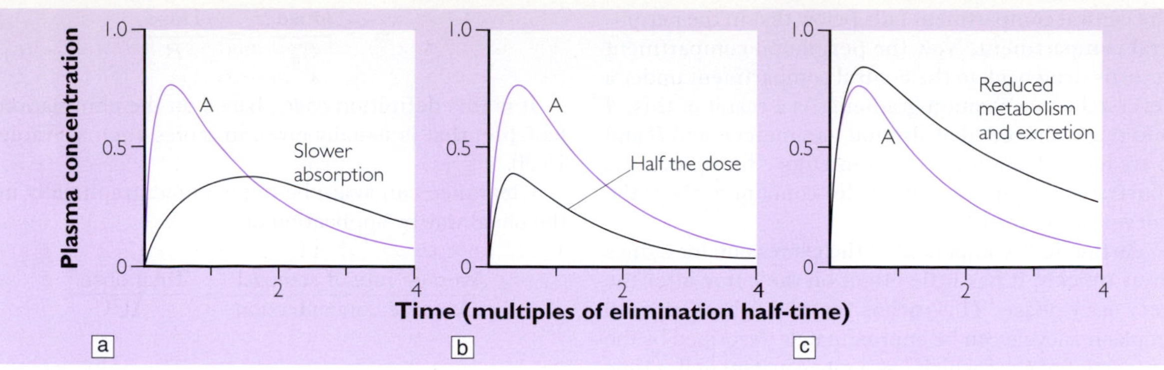


**Figure 19.55** A representation of the effects of changes in (a) absorption, (b) the dose, and (c) metabolism and excretion on the plasma concentration–time curves for a one-compartment open model. In these examples, the plasma concentration is on a linear scale. (A = original curve.)

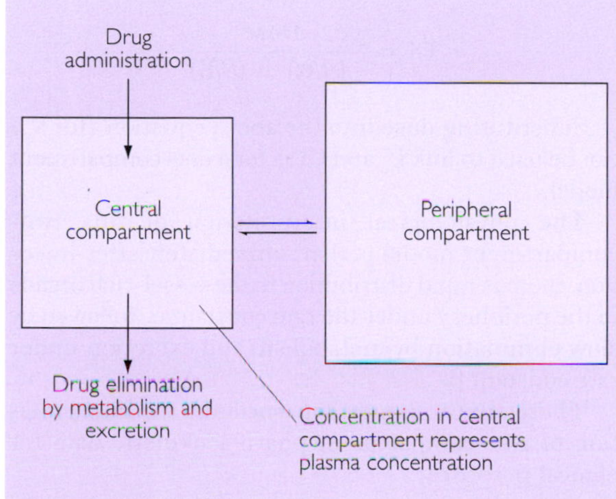


**Figure 19.56** A two-compartment open model. Drug administration and elimination are from the central compartment only.

results with intercept $A$ and rate constant α (Figure 19.57d). When these two lines are added together, they combine to produce a good fit to the original semi-logarithmic plot of Figure 19.57b. The two-compartment model therefore has a central compartment (plasma) concentration (C) that is the sum of two semi-logarithmic exponential functions.

This can be represented mathematically as:

$$C_t = Ae^{-\alpha t} + Be^{-\beta t}$$

where $C_t$ is concentration at time $t$ in the central compartment.

If the concentrations of the drug in the central and peripheral compartments, as determined by the model, are plotted out they are as shown in Figure 19.58. It can be seen that initially the central compartment (where the drug is injected) has the higher concentration and drug distributes to the peripheral compartment. At some point they become equal. Then, as elimination continues from the central compartment, the level in

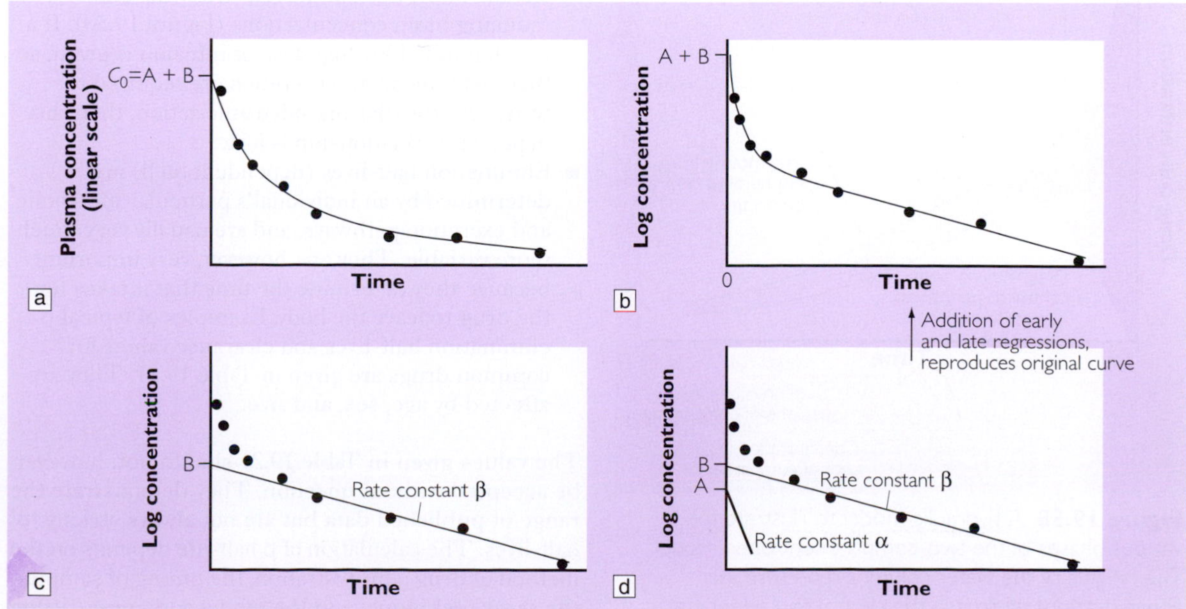


**Figure 19.57** Plasma concentration–time curves for a two-compartment open model. (See text for details.)

the central compartment falls below that in the peripheral compartment. Now the peripheral compartment returns drug back to the central compartment under a reversed concentration gradient. As a result of this, $A$ and $\alpha$ are termed 'distribution parameters' and $B$ and $\beta$ are termed 'elimination parameters'. This process is illustrated graphically with water containers above the curves of Figure 19.58.

As the $Ae^{-\alpha t}$ component of the expression for $C_t$ dies away quickly, it has little effect on the curve after the very early phase. This means that the subsequent fall in plasma levels can be approximately described by the properties of $Be^{-\beta t}$ which has a rate constant of $\beta$, a time constant of $1/\beta$ and a half-life of $0.69/\beta$. These terms are explained in Chapter 37.

Calculating the apparent $V_d$ for a two-compartment model can be done in a number of ways, which emphasize the importance, when looking at values of $V_d$, to be clear about how it was determined.

The initial apparent $V_d$ can be obtained by extrapolating the curve of Figure 19.57b back to zero to obtain the initial theoretical concentration which would be equal to $(A + B)$. Then, as defined earlier:

$$V_d = \frac{\text{Dose}}{C_0} = \frac{\text{Dose}}{(A + B)}$$

Alternatively, the initial sudden fall in serum concentration could be regarded as a transient feature that can be disregarded. Instead the body could be regarded as a single well-stirred compartment, which eliminates drugs with the rate constant, $\beta$. If this was the case, then the initial concentration would be $B$ (Figure 19.57c). Applying the same methodology as above:

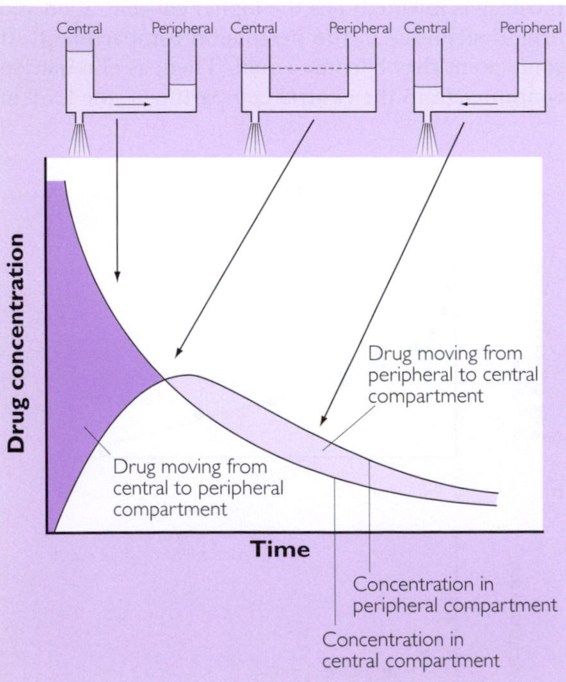


**Figure 19.58** A hydraulic model to illustrate the various phases of the two-compartment open model. The heights of the water columns represent the concentrations of drug in the central and peripheral compartments.

$$V_d = \frac{\text{Dose}}{C_0} = \frac{\text{Dose}}{B} \quad (6)$$

It is this definition of $V_d$, based on the elimination half-life, that is usually given in tables such as Table 19.20.

Clearance can again be determined graphically in the usual way by application of:

$$\frac{\text{Average rate of removal}}{\text{Average concentration}} = \frac{\text{Total dose}}{\text{AUC}}$$

Alternatively, the mathematical properties of the bi-exponential process can be applied. The area under the linear concentration time curve is given by:

$$\text{AUC} = (A/\alpha) + (B/\beta)$$

giving:

$$\text{Cl} = \frac{\text{Dose}}{(A/\alpha) + (B/\beta)}$$

Substituting dose into the above equation (for $V_d$) can be used to link $V_d$ and Cl as for a one-compartment model.

The physiological interpretation of this two-compartment model is that, immediately after injection, there is rapid distribution to the vessel-rich organs in the periphery under the rate constant $\alpha$, followed by slow elimination by metabolism and excretion under rate constant $\beta$.

There are two important aspects to the interpretation of two-compartment pharmacokinetic data for clinical purposes:

- Distribution half-lives (dependent on $\alpha$) usually result from passive concentration gradients and are very predictable. As such the distribution half-life determines the wake-up time from a single bolus dose of intravenous induction agent and, when consciousness returns, very little drug has left the body; it is simply redistributing and reducing brain concentrations (Figure 19.58). If a very big initial loading dose or infusion is given, so that metabolism and excretion are required to terminate the pharmacodynamic action, then this dependable relationship is lost.
- Elimination half-lives (dependent on $\beta$) are determined by an individual's particular metabolic and excretion pathways, and are usually very much more variable. They are, however, very important because they determine the time that it takes for the drug to leave the body. Examples of typical elimination half-lives and clearance values for common drugs are given in Table 19.21. They are affected by age, sex, and size.

The values given in Table 19.21 should not, however, be accepted without question. They demonstrate the range of published data but are not always strictly '$\beta$' half-lives. The calculation of $\beta$ half-life depends on the method of drug administration, the timing of samples, the assay technique, and the model and curve-fitting analysis used. The upper limit of the half-life of propofol may, for instance, be the result of uptake into red blood cells and consequent transfer back into the plasma. How does this affect the pharmacodynamics of a single induction dose? Furthermore, the upper half-life ranges of the drugs quoted may be measurable pharmacokinetically but whether they have any pharmacodynamic relevance is less certain. Does it matter that the serum level can be measured and modelled at a value of 100 times less than the minimum therapeutic concentration for a given patient? By the same token, the lower limit of the quoted half-lives may well represent elements of continued distribution (α effects) rather than true elimination (β effects).

*Constant rate infusions*

The result of an infusion is often best understood by reference to repeated bolus dosing. If a drug is given by repeated doses as shown in Figure 19.59, each dose produces an increase in serum concentration until there is eventually an oscillation about a steady value. Part of the first dose is distributed to the periphery after injection. When the second is administered, less of this goes to the periphery because the periphery is already partly occupied by the first dose. The serum concentration is therefore higher when the third dose is given and so on. Eventually the serum concentration will oscillate around the steady-state concentration when the periphery is filled and the average rate of drug administered is equal to its elimination. This process for intermittent dosing and a steady intravenous infusion is shown in Figure 19.59.

One of the unique properties of the plateau phase is that there is a constant relationship between the plasma concentration and the biophase concentration. All effects of hysteresis (see above) are therefore removed and this is why the steady state is often sought in experiments to measure pharmacokinetic parameters.

Figure 19.59 also illustrates the concept of accumulation. Unless the whole of a single bolus dose is allowed to be eliminated, subsequent doses will produce an increase in the serum concentration until an equilibrium is reached between dosing and elimination. As it needs approximately five elimination half-lives for the drug level to become effectively zero (see Chapter 37), any dosing regimens prescribing more frequently than this will theoretically produce accumulation.

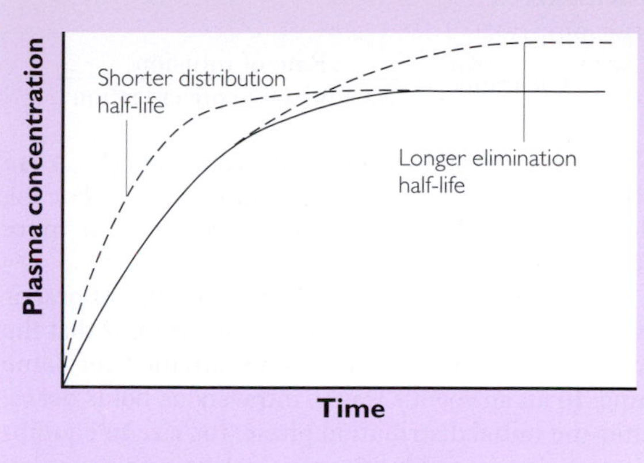


**Figure 19.60** The effect on the plasma concentration of a steady infusion of drug caused by differences in the distribution half-life and the elimination half-life.

If a given drug is infused into the same model at the same constant rate, Figure 19.60 shows the effect of changes in α and β alone. If the distribution half-life is shorter, the periphery fills up quicker but the final plateau level is unchanged. If the elimination half-life is increased, the rate of loss of drug is less and equilibrium is found at a higher plateau level.

The plateau phase of a steady intravenous infusion allows a unique method of calculating the clearance. Given that (see earlier):

$$\text{Clearance} = \text{Rate of drug elimination per unit (input) concentration}$$

this becomes:

$$\text{Clearance} = \frac{\text{Rate of elimination}}{\text{Steady-state concentration}}$$

and in the plateau phase

$$\text{Rate of elimination} = \text{Rate of infusion}$$

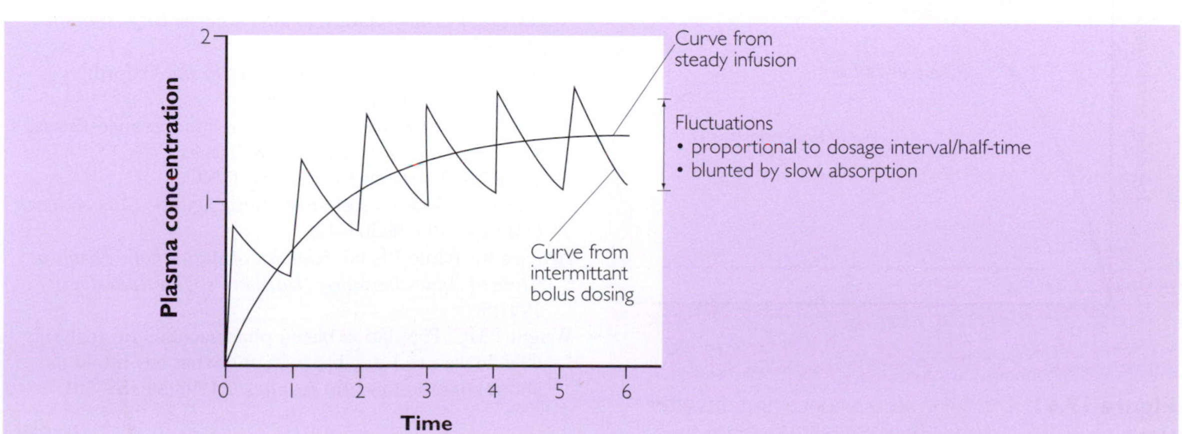


**Figure 19.59** The rise in plasma concentration after repeated bolus doses and a steady infusion.

Therefore:

$$\text{Clearance} = \frac{\text{Rate of infusion}}{\text{Steady-state concentration}}$$

The volume of distribution at steady state ($V_{dss}$) can also be calculated from steady-state kinetics. For the derivation of this the reader is referred to more advanced texts.

The kinetics of infusions have a number of practical implications. One of the most important is that the final plasma concentration is not attained for some time. In an analogous way to intravenous bolus doses, after the initial distribution phase, the rise to equilibrium is dominated by the elimination rate constant. The properties of 'wash-in' exponential curves are described in Chapter 37. As there is a gradual rise to the plateau concentration, in order to achieve a rapid rise in serum concentration it is necessary to increase the infusion rate in the initial stages of the infusion regimen. This is done for volatile agents by applying 'overpressure' (see Figure 33.17), and for intravenous agents by starting the infusion rate high and stepping it down (see Chapter 32, Figure 32.11). There is always the possibility, when giving a single bolus followed by a steady infusion, that there may be a window in which the plasma levels fall below the therapeutic threshold (see Chapter 32, Figure 32.10).

When an infusion is stopped, the decrease in serum concentration depends on how long the infusion has been running and at what rate. If the peripheral compartments have been relatively little filled, there will be an initial steep fall under a rate constant of α caused by continued redistribution, followed by a less steep fall as elimination proceeds under a constant of β. On the other hand, if the peripheral compartments are essentially saturated, the rate of fall of serum level will be determined totally by β, the elimination rate constant (Figure 19.61). It is clear from consideration of Figure 19.61 that, in clinical practice, the time of fall to a given plasma concentration after cessation of an infusion is very dependent on the combination of infusion rate, time of infusion, and patient.

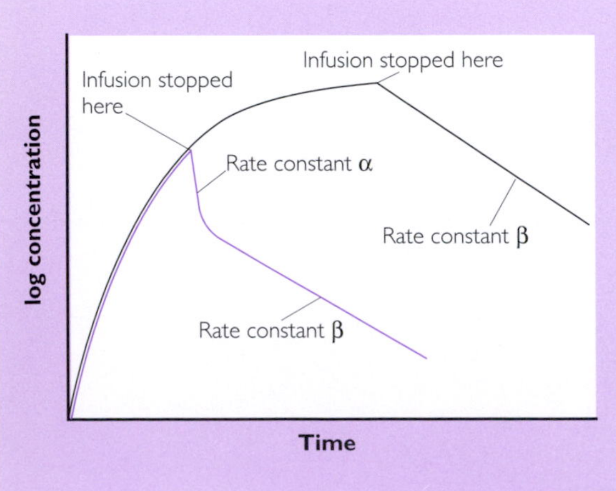


**Figure 19.61** The fall in serum concentrations after stopping an infusion at different times. (See text for details.)

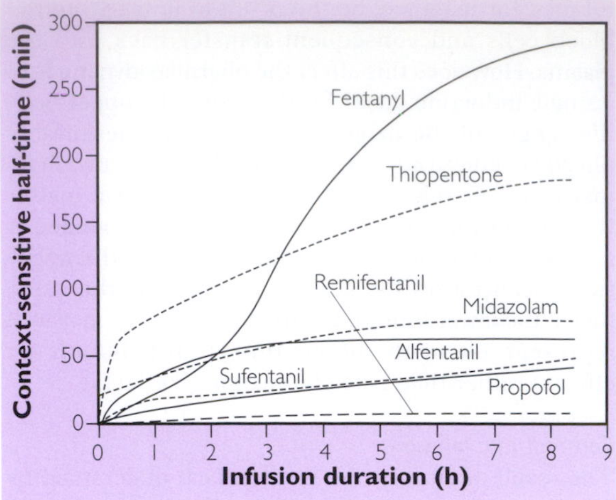


**Figure 19.62** Context-sensitive half-times as a function of infusion duration for a variety of drugs used in anaesthesia. Remifentanil, which was not present on the original figure, has been drawn in for comparison. (Adapted from Hughes MA *et al. Anesthesiology* 1992;76:334.)

As a result of this difficulty, the concept of 'context-sensitive half-time' was introduced. Here 'context' refers to the manner and time in which the infusion had been given before it was terminated. The method therefore takes into account the uncertainties demonstrated in Figure 19.62. The context-sensitive half-time is the time taken for the serum concentration to halve, after cessation of an infusion designed to maintain a constant plasma concentration. Using computer modelling, Glass's group at Duke University compared a number of common drugs; their results are shown in Figure 19.62. It can be seen that there is a wide variation in results, making some drugs much more suitable for use by infusion than others. In particular, the context-sensitive half-lives bear little relation to the elimination half-lives. This has obvious implications for clinical practice.

## FURTHER READING

Calvey TN, Williams NE. *Principles and Practice of Pharmacology for Anaesthetists*, 3rd edn. Oxford: Blackwell Scientific, 1997.

Ciccone GK, Holdcroft A. Drugs and sex differences: a review of drugs relating to anaesthesia. *Br J Anaesth* 1999;**82**:255–65.

Hull CJ. *Pharmacokinetics for Anaesthesia*. Oxford: Butterworth-Heinemann, 1991.

Schwilden H. Pharmacokinetics as related to anaesthesia. *Curr Anaesth Crit Care* 1997;**8**:202–6.

Sutcliffe NP, Murdoch JAC, Kenny GNC. Pharmacodynamics of anaesthetic agents. *Curr Anaesth Crit Care* 1997;**8**:207–13.

Articles in: White PF, ed. *Kinetics of Anaesthetic Drugs in Clinical Anaesthesiology. Baillière's Clin Anaesthesiol* 1991;**5**.

Wright PMC. Population based pharmacokinetic analysis: why do we need it; what is it; and what has it told us about anaesthetics? *Br J Anaesth* 1998;**80**:488–501.

# Chapter 20 Cardiovascular physiology and pharmacology

R.O. Feneck

The cardiovascular system consists of the heart and pulmonary and systemic vasculature. The physiology of these is considered first, followed by the relevant pharmacology.

## ELECTROPHYSIOLOGY OF THE HEART

### Cell types

Cardiac fibres can be divided into two types: pacemaker (automatic) and non-pacemaker (quiescent) fibres. Pacemaker tissue is found in the sinoatrial (SA) and atrioventricular (AV) nodes. Non-pacemaker tissue (the bulk of the myocardium) refers to the muscle cells of the atria and ventricles, and the cells of the His–Purkinje conducting system. Depolarization in cardiac fibres occurs as a result of the net inward movement of positively charged ions, and repolarization involves the net outward movement of positively charged ions. The details of the ion fluxes involved in depolarization and repolarization are different in pacemaker and non-pacemaker tissue, but the direction of ionic movements remains the same for both types of cell.

The cell membrane, or sarcolemma, is important because it is involved in transmembrane ionic movements during an action potential (AP). The sarcolemma is a phospholipid bilayer with a hydrophobic core, and acts as a high-resistance insulated wrapping around the cardiac cell. It is selectively permeable to ions, including sodium, potassium, chloride, and calcium, and is therefore able to create electrical gradients across the cell membrane (see Chapter 19). Ions cross the sarcolemma through specific, voltage-gated membrane–protein channels that span the phospholipid bilayer. In addition, other membrane–protein complexes serve as receptors for neurotransmitters or hormones, or as supplementary ion transport systems. Myocardial muscle fibres differ from skeletal muscle fibres in that they form a syncytium with intercalated discs separating adjacent cells (Figure 20.1). The process of contractility by the cross-linking of actin and myosin is described in detail in Chapter 24. Also included there is a comparison of the APs and subsequent contraction of cardiac and skeletal muscle.

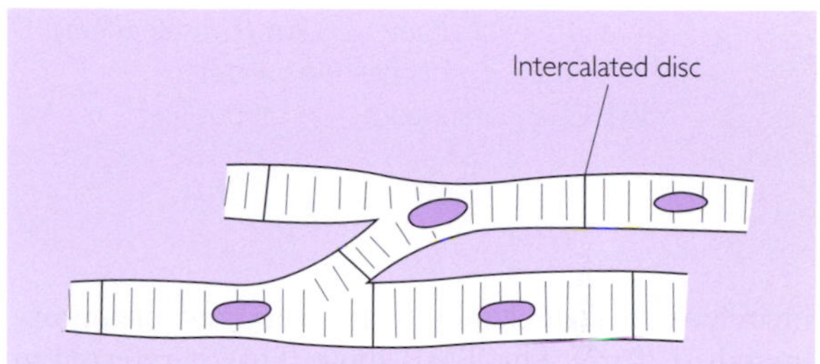


**Figure 20.1** Cardiac muscle showing the intercalated discs that divide the apparent syncytium. Each cell has only one large nucleus.

### Action potential phases

#### *Non-pacemaker tissue (muscle cells)*

The phases of the AP and the ionic changes involved in pacemaker and non-pacemaker tissues are shown in Figure 20.2 and summarized in Table 20.1.

*Phase 0*

Phase 0 depolarization occurs when the depolarizing stimulus is able to raise the level of the resting membrane potential from −90 mV to approximately −65 mV. At this point, the threshold potential has been achieved and an 'all or none' AP response occurs. This AP will propagate to excite other cardiac tissue; smaller stimuli that fail to attain the threshold will not result in APs.

Phase 0 depolarization occurs as a result of a rapid inflow of $Na^+$ ions through ion-specific channels, raising the transmembrane potential (TMP) from approx-

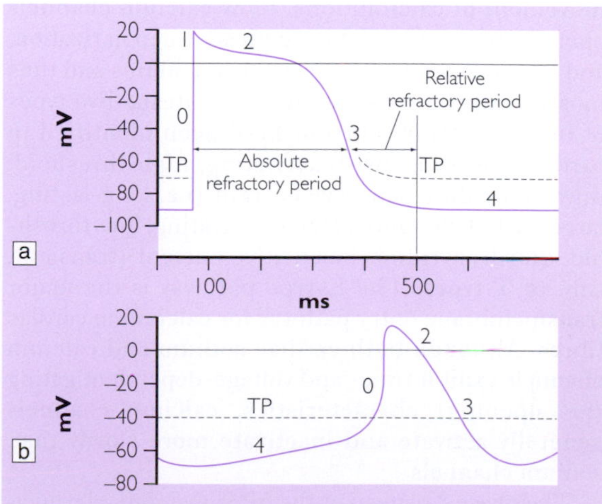


**Figure 20.2** The action potential recorded from (a) a ventricular contractile cell and (b) an atrial pacemaker cell. The five phases of depolarization (0, 1, 2, 3, 4) are shown. TP, threshold potential.

**Table 20.1 Ion movement during phases of the cardiac action potential**

| Phase | Ion | Movement across cell membrane |
|---|---|---|
| 0 | Sodium | In |
| 1 | Potassium<br>Chloride | Out (transient)<br>In |
| 2 | Calcium<br>Sodium<br>Potassium | In (main effect)<br>In (minor)<br>In (minor, anomalous) |
| 3 | Potassium<br>$Na^+/K^+$ exchanger | Out (main)<br>Out (overall effect) |
| 4 | $Na^+/K^+$ exchanger<br>$Na^+/Ca^{2+}$ exchanger<br>ATP $Ca^{2+}$ transport | Out (overall effect)<br>In or out<br>In or out |

imately –65 mV(threshold) to an 'overshoot' of approximately +20 mV. The TMP above 0 mV is referred to as the overshoot. Both the phase 0 upstroke velocity (referred to as $V_{max}$) and the conduction velocity in non-pacemaker tissue are much faster than in pacemaker cells. The value of $V_{max}$ is sometimes taken as a reflection of myocardiac contractility. A sodium 'window' current has also been described during the early phase 2 plateau (see later), possibly representing the activity of two different sodium channel populations or two different modes of operation within the same sodium channel.

*Phase 1*

The early steep part of repolarization, phase 1, occurs as a result of the rapid termination of the inward sodium current and a transient outward potassium current, in addition to an inward chloride current.

*Phase 2*

The phase 2 plateau is produced primarily by inward movement of calcium ions. Slow calcium channels open at about –40 mV during phase 1 depolarization, and remain open for between 30 and 300 ms and thus mostly contribute to the phase 2 plateau. Two types of inward calcium current have been identified in cardiac fibres: a slow-inactivating, high-threshold, dihydropyridine-sensitive current (i.e. long-lasting, large, or L-type) and a fast-inactivating, low-threshold, dihydropyridine-insensitive current (transient, tiny, or T-type). The L-type pathway is the major transmembrane entry pathway for calcium in cardiac fibres. Although both cardiac sodium and calcium channels exhibit time- and voltage-dependent gating (i.e. opening) characteristics, calcium channels generally activate and inactivate more slowly than sodium channels.

The phase 2 plateau of the AP is maintained principally by calcium, assisted to a much lesser extent by sodium, and also by the inward (anomalous) potassium-rectifying current. During phase 2, the TMP is maintained at or near 0 mV, and no stimulus is able to re-excite cardiac fibres – i.e. they are absolutely refractory (see Figure 20.2). For fast sodium channels to reopen and a further AP to be generated, repolarization must first occur. It is the plateau characteristic of phase 2 that allows the sustained contraction of cardiac muscle, prevents tetanic contraction and differentiates it from skeletal muscle.

*Phase 3*

This is characterized by the slowing of the inward calcium flux and the cell starts to repolarize. Outward (delayed) and inward (anomalous) rectifying potassium currents and the outward current generated by the $Na^+/K^+$ exchanger (see Chapter 19) are responsible for the rapid period of repolarization.

In addition, other potassium currents operating in special circumstances may be relevant including:

- a calcium-activated potassium current during calcium overload;
- a sodium-activated current during sodium overload;
- an ATP-sensitive current which opens during energy depletion;
- an acetylcholine-activated current which responds to vagal stimulation and results in hyperpolarization of resting cells;
- a current activated by arachidonic acid and other fatty acids at low pH.

All these currents further the process of repolarization during phase 3. In addition, potassium conductance increases as the TMP becomes more negative, thereby speeding repolarization.

Between the end of the absolute refractory period and the recovery of full excitation, the fibres are relatively refractory (Figures 20.2 and 20.3). During this period, a stimulus may generate a local non-propagated response, or it may generate a propagated AP that is more slowly conducted than normal. Stimuli occurring after the relative refractory period (RRP) will generate normal propagated APs. The absolute refractory period of atrial muscle is shorter than that of ventricular muscle, such that the rhythmic rate of contraction of the atria can be much faster than that of the ventricles.

*Phases 3 and 4*

During phase 3 and phase 4, the membrane-bound ATP-dependent $Na^+/K^+$ exchange pump re-establishes the baseline or resting membrane potential (RMP), with two potassium ions moving inwards for every three sodium ions moving outwards. Thus a net outward movement of positive charges is generated, and the intracellular concentrations of sodium and potassium at rest are low and high respectively. In addition, a non-ATP-dependent $Na^+/Ca^{2+}$ exchanger can be run in either forward or reverse modes, thus enabling either ion to be moved into or out of the cell, and an ATP-dependent calcium transport system also exists. These systems are responsible for maintaining a stable electrical baseline during phase 4 in non-pacemaker tissue until a further stimulus raises the RMP to threshold and a further AP is generated.

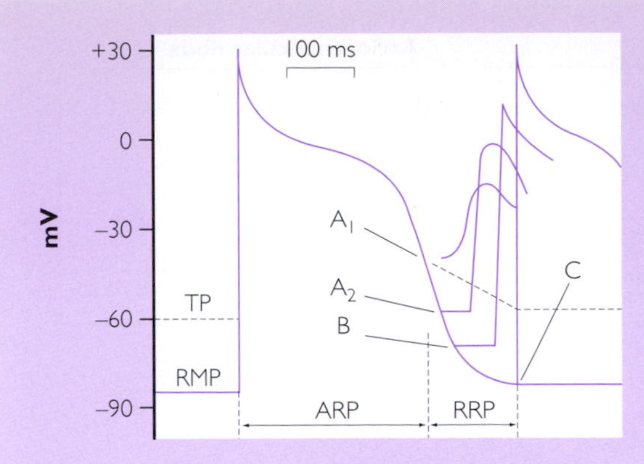


**Figure 20.3** Refractory period during an action potential (AP). ARP, absolute refractory period; RRP, relative refractory period; TP, threshold potential; RMP, resting membrane potential. Stimuli at $A_1$ and $A_2$ produce local, non-propagated APs. The stimulus at B is sufficient to generate an AP that has a slower rising phase 0 and different subsequent morphology. A stimulus at C produces a normal action potential.

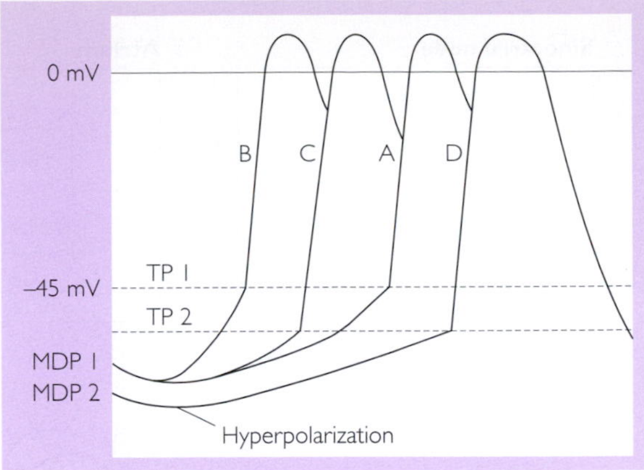


**Figure 20.4** Automaticity in a pacemaker cell. TP 1 and TP 2 represent different threshold potentials; MDP 1 and MDP 2 represent different maximum diastolic potentials. The heart rate may be increased by increasing the slope of phase 4 depolarization (B) or lowering the threshold potential (C). Heart rate may be slowed by raising the threshold potential (A) or by hyperpolarization, i.e. lowering MDP (D).

#### *Pacemaker tissue*

The RMP in non-pacemaker tissue is relatively stable but, in pacemaker tissue, phase 4 is a constant but slow process of depolarization (see Figure 20.2). This process of diastolic depolarization may be influenced by a number of factors, including:

- hyperpolarization (i.e. more negative baseline);
- alteration in the rate of phase 4 depolarization;
- alteration in the threshold potential.

These may all influence the rate of AP generation in pacemaker tissue (Figure 20.4). As the electrical baseline is unstable and the RMP is changing, the most negative value of the TMP is usually measured as the maximum diastolic potential (MDP). There can be different combinations of MDP and drift rate during phase 4 which determine the time to threshold potential. Vagal action, acetylcholine, and β-adrenoceptor blockers stabilize the membrane, reducing the rate of drift and slowing down the heart rate; epinephrine (adrenaline), norepinephrine (noradrenaline), and sympathetic action increase the rate of drift and speed up the heart. These drugs also have more complex actions on contractility and arrhythmogenesis.

The threshold potential in pacemaker tissue is less negative than in muscle fibres and, at a level of approximately −50 mV, sodium channels are refractory and so L-type calcium channels are responsible for initiating phase 0 depolarization resulting in a slow rising AP. At −40 mV, a secondary phase of rapid depolarization occurs associated with inward sodium currents, and potassium currents are also thought to be involved. There may be differences in the relative importance of the potassium and sodium currents in SA nodal tissue and other conducting tissue, and repolarization is associated with the termination of inward cation movement and the efflux of potassium ions.

Once initiated, propagation of an AP will depend on its strength and on the resistance to propagation through the surrounding tissue. Excitation of nearby fast-response fibres is more likely to result in successful impulse propagation than excitation of slow-response fibres, and the excess of activation current over the minimum that is required to ensure successful impulse propagation may be considered as the safety factor of conduction. Fast-response fibres have a higher conduction safety factor than slow-response fibres.

### Normal atrial and ventricular conduction

Normal intracardiac conduction follows a well-described sequence of events. For reference, the way that this occurs in various parts of the heart is shown in Figure 20.5, together with the accompanying APs.

The heart beat begins when phase 4 depolarization of pacemaker tissue in the SA node reaches the threshold potential and calcium-dependent phase 0 depolarization occurs. This depolarization potential is propagated outside the SA node and spreads through atrial tissue. A number of transatrial conduction pathways have been described, including Backman's bundle, which is responsible for the transmission of conduction from the SA node in the right atrium to the left atrium. However, a wave of atrial depolarization may spread through normal atrial muscle cells as well as via specialized conducting pathways. The conducting velocity through atrial tissue is relatively brisk and the wave of depolarization rapidly reaches the AV node. The chief function of the AV node is to slow down electrical conduction and thereby allow atrial emptying to be complete before the onset of ventricular contraction. The speed of electrical conduction through the His–Purkinje system is rapid, and the speed of ventricular contraction in the normal heart is rapid and relatively independent of heart rate, in contrast to diastole which is markedly shortened by tachycardia.

Waves of depolarization can be measured as they spread through myocardial tissue using surface electrodes, and electrocardiography has become the mainstay of the measurement of cardiac conduction and

**Sinoatrial node**

| RMP/MDP (mV) –50 to –60 |
|---|
| AP duration (ms) 100–300 |
| $V_{max}$ phase 0 (V/s) 1–10 |
| Conduction (m/s) <0.05 |

**Atrium**

| RMP/MDP (mV) –80 to –90 |
|---|
| AP duration (ms) 100–300 |
| $V_{max}$ phase 0 (V/s) 100–200 |
| Conduction (m/s) 0.3–0.4 |

**Atrioventricular node**

| RMP/MDP (mV) –60 to –70 |
|---|
| AP duration (ms) 100–300 |
| $V_{max}$ phase 0 (V/s) 5–15 |
| Conduction (m/s) 0.1 |

**Purkinje fibre**

| RMP/MDP (mV) –90 to –95 |
|---|
| AP duration (ms) 300–500 |
| $V_{max}$ phase 0 (V/s) 500–700 |
| Conduction (m/s) 2–3 |

**Ventricle**

| RMP/MDP (mV) –80 to –90 |
|---|
| AP duration (ms) 200–300 |
| $V_{max}$ phase 0 (V/s) 100–200 |
| Conduction (m/s) 0.3–0.4 |

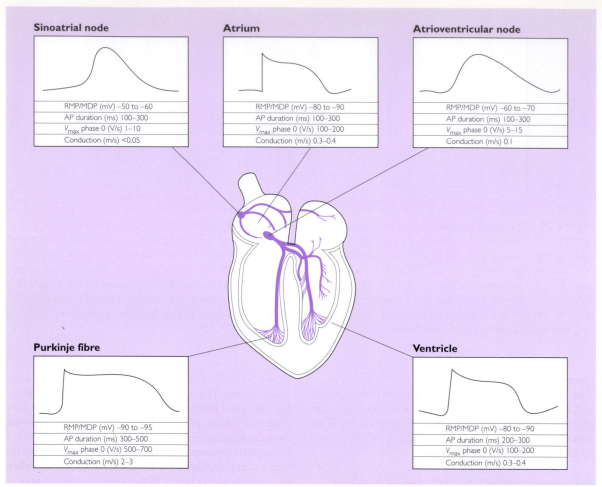

**Figure 20.5** The action potential in various regions of the heart. RMP, resting membrane potential; MDP, maximum diastolic potential; AP, action potential; $V_{max}$ phase 0, action potential upstroke velocity.

diagnosis of myocardial events that have an electrical impact.

## Electrocardiography

A wave of depolarization moving through the myocardium may be recorded as an electrical signal moving between two recording electrodes. As the signal moves towards the exploring electrode (Figure 20.6), the signal records as a positive deflection. As it moves away from a recording electrode, it records a negative deflection. If the signal moves at right angles to the electrode, it may show a biphasic response, first positive as it moves towards the electrode, and then negative as it moves away.

Thus, surface electrodes can record myocardial electrical events that have magnitude and direction, and a series of different 'electrical views' of the heart may be obtained by placing a number of surface electrodes with different zero reference points.

This is the basis of electrocardiography. The father of modern electrocardiography is Willem Eindthoven who was awarded the Nobel Prize in 1924 for his research. In fact, August Waller recorded the first human electrocardiogram (ECG) in 1887, using a glass capillary electrometer previously described by Lipmann in 1875. Eindthoven completed his most successful work using the string galvanometer. The signal (P–QRST) was named based on the standard geometric convention of the time for describing points on curved lines and has no other significance.

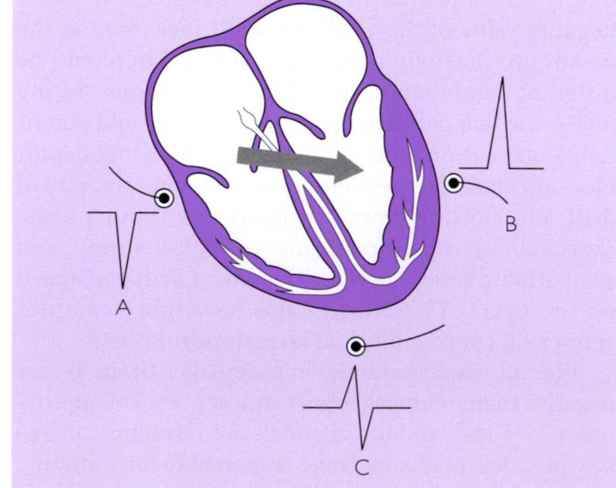


**Figure 20.6** The principle of ECG recording. The large arrow shows the wave of depolarization. Electrode A receives a negative deflection, electrode B a positive deflection, and electrode C a biphasic wave.

Despite its apparent simplicity, the modern ECG machine may be considered as a multitasking microcomputer, able to be programmed to interpret the ECG signal and provide diagnostic information. The ECG has a 'power spectrum', based on a mathematical analysis of the harmonic components, demonstrating sine waves of varying amplitude and frequency (see Chapters 37 and 39).

There are conventionally four limb leads, of which one is a reference electrode. The limb leads are used to derive leads I, II, and III (Figure 20.7a). The positions of the six chest leads are shown in Figure 20.7b. The standard ECG, as monitored in lead II in a normal patient, is shown in Figure 20.8. The derivation of the ECG, its normal morphology, the time relationship of its components, and a consideration of its abnormalities can be found in Chapters 47 and 48, to which reference should be made.

The temporal relationship between the T wave and the arterial pressure waveform is interesting. The peak radial arterial pressure occurs at the same time as the T wave, even though the ventricle is then undergoing repolarization. This apparent discrepancy in timing, with a temporal delay between electrical and mechanical events, is caused by the finite velocity with which the arterial pulse wave travels through the arterial tree.

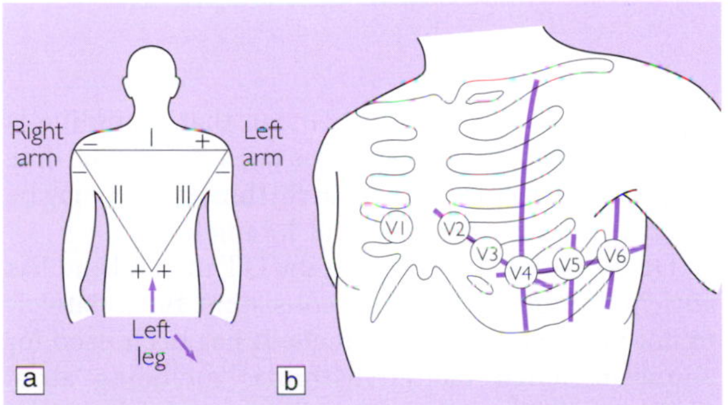


**Figure 20.7** Electrode positions for a standard 12-lead ECG: (a) the limb leads and (b) the chest leads. It is usual for a fourth lead to be attached to the right leg (or elsewhere) to act as a reference electrode and eliminate overall swings in the body's potential (see Chapter 47).

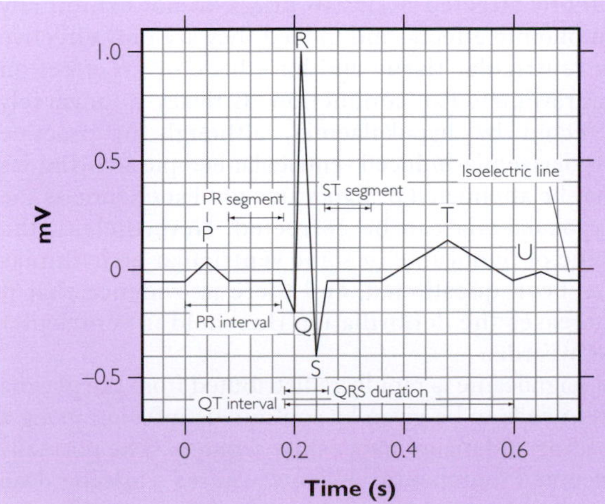


**Figure 20.8** The diagrammatic morphology and nomenclature of a normal recording in lead II. A detailed description of the various components can be found in Chapter 47.

### *Abnormalities of rhythm, conduction, and morphology of the ECG*

A valuable use of electrocardiography is the diagnosis of abnormal electrical heart action. The term 'arrhythmia' is sometimes used synonymously with arrhythmia, and it is not clear what, if anything, differentiates the two. In fact, as arrhythmia means 'absence of normal sinus rhythm', the term arrhythmia is redundant, although it is frequently used even in current literature.

Arrhythmias occur as a result of abnormal cardiac electrophysiology. The main cellular mechanisms responsible for arrhythmia development include:

- loss of membrane potential;
- depressed fast response;
- altered normal automaticity;
- abnormal automaticity;
- after-repolarizations and triggered activity;
- re-entry.

Other problems arise from abnormalities of conduction, ectopic pacemakers, and ischaemia. These are all considered in detail in Chapters 47 and 48.

Many arrhythmogenic processes are relevant to surgery and anaesthesia, simply because provoking factors are common even during uncomplicated surgery (see Table 47.2). In general, we should consider anaesthesia and surgery to be arrhythmogenic, and previous studies have shown a high incidence of arrhythmia during surgery. However, most of these arrhythmias are benign, and will respond to simple manipulations of anaesthesia, fluid and electrolyte balance, and vagal activity. In healthy patients, the need for antiarrhythmic drugs in the perioperative period is rare. However, when necessary such drug therapy may be life-saving, and a clear understanding of the pharmacology of antiarrhythmic drugs is essential.

## Antiarrhythmic drug action

Arrhythmias may be simply classified as follows:

- arrhythmias of sinus origin;
- ectopic rhythms;
- conduction blocks;
- pre-excitation syndromes.

Although attempts have been made to classify antiarrhythmic drugs according to their efficacy in different clinical situations, the variety of drugs that are effective against each arrhythmia has made such a classification almost valueless. The most conventional current classification of antiarrhythmic drug therapy is that of Vaughan-Williams, shown in Table 20.2.

However, even this system has its problems. Most notably, it fails to accommodate drugs with more than one mechanism of action (e.g. amiodarone, sotalol), and assumes that all antiarrhythmic effects are caused by blocking and not activating either receptors or ion channels. Also, it has been unable to classify either digoxin or adenosine, and may also fail to classify accu-

| Table 20.2 The Vaughan-Williams classification of antiarrhythmic drugs | |
|---|---|
| Class | Type of drug and examples |
| I | Membrane-stabilizing drugs |
| Ia | Quinidine, disopyramide, procainamide |
| Ib | Lignocaine (lidocaine), mexilitene |
| Ic | Flecainide, encainide |
| II | β-Adrenoceptor antagonists: propranolol, metoprolol, esmolol |
| III | Drugs that increase the action potential refractory period (antifibrillatory drugs): amiodarone, bretylium |
| IV | Calcium channel blockers: verapamil, diltiazem |
| Others | Cardiac glycosides (sometimes called class V)<br>Adenosine |

| Drug | Vaughan-Williams class | Channels | | | | | | Receptors | | | | Pump |
|---|---|---|---|---|---|---|---|---|---|---|---|---|
| | | Na+ | | | $Ca^{2+}$ | $K^+$ | $I_f$ | α | β | $M_2$ | $A_1$ | $Na^+/K^+$ ATPase |
| | | Fast | Medium | Slow | | | | | | | | |
| Lignocaine | IB | Low | | | | | | | | | | |
| Mexiletine | IB | Low | | | | | | | | | | |
| Tocainide | IB | Low | | | | | | | | | | |
| Moricizine | | | I (high) | | | | | | | | | |
| Procainamide | IA | | A | | | Medium | | | | | | |
| Disopyramide | IA | | A | | | Medium | | | | Low | | |
| Quinidine | IA | | A | | | Medium | | Low | | Low | | |
| Propafenone | IC | | A | | | | | | Medium | | | |
| Flecainide | IC | | | A | | Low | | | | | | |
| Encainide | IC | | | A | | | | | | | | |
| Bepridil | IV | Low | | | High | Medium | | | | | | |
| Verapamil | IV | Low | | | High | | | Medium | | | | |
| Diltiazem | IV | | | | Low | | | | | | | |
| Bretylium | III | | | | | High | | P | P | | | |
| Sotalol | III | | | | | High | | | High | | | |
| Amiodarone | III | I (low) | | | Low | High | | Medium | Medium | | | |
| Alinidine | | | | | | Medium | High | | | | | |
| Nadolol | II | | | | | | | | High | | | |
| Propranolol | II | Low | | | | | | | High | | | |
| Atropine | | | | | | | | | | High | | |
| Adenosine | | | | | | | | | | | Agonist | |
| Digoxin | V | | | | | | | | | Agonist | | High |

Relative potency

Low  Medium  High  A Activated state blocker

Agonist  P Partial agonist  I I Inactivated state blockers

**Figure 20.9** Antiarrhythmic drugs classified according to their effects on channels, receptors, and ion pumps: the so-called Sicilian Gambit.

rately other antiarrhythmic drugs that are developed in the future.

One alternative classification has been provided by the Task Force of the European Society of Cardiology. It is known as the 'Sicilian Gambit' – Sicilian after the location of the international meeting at which it was first published, and 'Gambit' after the Queen's Gambit in chess representing an opening or potential way forward rather than a finished entity. Essentially, it seeks to classify antiarrhythmic drugs according to the molecular targets on which a drug acts (i.e. cell membrane ion channels and/or receptors), the mechanisms responsible for arrhythmogenesis that may respond to therapy, and relevant clinical considerations (Figure 20.9). The combination of mechanisms relevant to various drugs is clearly complex and it is not intended that trainees memorize them all. Figure 20.9 is included for reference and to give a more representative picture of reality than some of the simpler classifications described. In addition, the schematic structure of the Task Force classification is fluid and may change, but the receptors and ion channels that are involved as potential arrhythmogenic mechanisms are important. For convenience, however, the descriptive pharmacology of the antiarrhythmics is dealt with below with drugs grouped according to the classic Vaughan–Williams classification.

#### *Class I: membrane-stabilizing drugs*

*Class Ia: quinidine, procainamide, disopyramide*

These drugs all depress phase 0 and 4 depolarization, and prolong the AP duration and hence the effective refractory period. Quinidine may reduce or enhance AV nodal conduction and may also prolong the QT interval. Both quinidine and disopyramide have anticholinergic effects, and this may provoke unwanted side effects, particularly with quinidine.

These and other features mean that quinidine is now rarely used. Procainamide is used as a second-line drug for ventricular ectopic arrhythmias, and may be given in an intravenous dose of 1.5 mg/kg.

Disopyramide may prolong the QT interval and has anticholinergic effects and consistent but relatively minor negative inotropic effects. It has been used for supraventricular tachyarrhythmias including atrial fibrillation. All of the above drugs undergo partial hepatic and renal metabolism.

*Class Ib: lignocaine (lidocaine), mexiletine*

The main effects on class Ib drugs are on the AP duration and the effective refractory period/AP duration ratio.

In addition, phase 0 and phase 4 conduction are slightly affected. Class Ib drugs do not exhibit any autonomic effects, and indeed they are only effective in ventricular tissue and have little or no effect on supraventricular conduction. Efficacy is adversely affected by hypokalaemia, although in practice hypokalaemia-induced ventricular ectopic arrhythmias may be attenuated by lignocaine until such time as the hypokalaemia can be corrected. Nevertheless, the value of lignocaine in some ventricular arrhythmias has been questioned, and there is evidence that it increases the defibrillation threshold in ventricular tachycardia.

Lignocaine is rapidly redistributed from the plasma and needs to be given by continuous infusion using a loading and maintenance dose regimen. The normally accepted therapeutic scheme requires a loading dose of 1.0–1.5 mg/kg followed by an infusion of 150 μg/kg per min for 20 min and a final infusion rate of 3 μg/kg per min. This dosing schedule should be reduced by 50% for patients in congestive heart failure. Therapeutic plasma concentrations of lignocaine lie within the range 1.5–5.0 μg/ml and concentrations above 9 μg/ml are likely to produce toxic effects. Lignocaine has important side effects particularly on the central nervous system (CNS), including tinnitus, and eventually convulsions. These occur more frequently when lignocaine is used for its local anaesthetic rather than its antiarrhythmic properties, and there is a particular risk during intravenous regional anaesthetic techniques. If signs of overdosage occur, lignocaine should be immediately discontinued and appropriate supportive measures, and if necessary an intravenous anticonvulsant, given. Cardiac toxicity may also occur with depression of contractility and conduction. Other local anaesthetics may be more toxic in this regard, and bupivacaine should *never* be used for intravenous regional anaesthesia because of its toxic effects on cardiac conduction.

Mexiletine generally has the same pharmacological profile as lignocaine but it is active when given orally.

*Class Ic: flecainide, encainide, propafenone*

This is a controversial class of antiarrhythmic agents. The drugs concerned have effects on fast-response sodium channels and cause a significant reduction in phase 0 activity and a reduction in phase 0 $V_{max}$. However, clinical studies of arrhythmia suppression in the setting of postmyocardial infarction discovered an excess mortality with flecainide and encainide. The cause was not fully clear. Possible aetiologies include proarrhythmia, the development of a re-entry mechanism, and myocardial depression. However, class Ic drugs are effective antiarrhythmics, and after review flecainide is still available for AV nodal reciprocating tachycardia and paroxysmal atrial fibrillation.

***Class II: β-adrenoceptor antagonists (propranolol, esmolol, metoprolol)***

β-adrenoceptor antagonists exhibit a number of electrophysiological effects, of which the most important are a decrease in automaticity, an increase in the AP duration especially in ventricular conduction tissue, and an increase in the effective refractory period at the AV node. The resting rate of the SA node may be slowed and transatrial, and AV nodal and intraventricular conduction are also slowed.

β-adrenoceptor antagonists also exert other effects which may have some limited clinical application. Although useful as antiarrhythmic agents, β-adrenoceptor antagonists are used as antianginal and antihypertensive agents. These are common conditions, and thus a large number of these drugs have been developed. The main differences between β-adrenoceptor antagonists are as follows:

- their ability to penetrate the CNS (propranolol);
- cardioselectivity (metoprolol, atenolol, esmolol);
- membrane-stabilizing effects (propranolol);
- intrinsic sympathomimetic activity (oxprenolol);
- pharmacokinetics and clinical duration of action (esmolol – ultrashort; metoprolol – short; propranolol – medium; atenolol – long);
- combined α effects (labetolol).

β-Adrenoceptor antagonists are also discussed later.

***Class III: bretylium, sotalol, amiodarone***

Bretylium has effects on the postganglionic adrenergic nerve terminal, first displacing and then blocking the release of norepinephrine.

Amiodarone is the most commonly used drug in this class, and is now widely used in the perioperative setting. Amiodarone is a di-iodinated benzofuran derivative originally developed as an antianginal. However, it is a useful antiarrhythmic, used to treat supraventricular and ventricular tachyarrhythmias and pre-excitation syndromes. The electrophysiological effects of amiodarone are complex. It decreases phase 0 conduction, reduces SA nodal rate, and prolongs the refractory period in all cardiac tissues. With intravenous administration, this occurs chiefly within ventricular tissue and there is no prolongation of the QT interval, in contrast to oral dosing. Amiodarone has other effects on calcium and potassium channels and adrenergic receptors. This may be related to inhibition of thyroxine 5'-deiodinase, which produces an antithyroid effect. Amiodarone may also produce hepatic damage and alveolitis mimicking adult respiratory distress syndrome. Rashes, corneal deposits, and photosensitivity have also been reported. It is because of its side effects that amiodarone is not used for first-line maintenance.

The pharmacokinetics of amiodarone are complex. Although the oral dosing schedule is such that effective concentrations may take days to achieve, intravenous dosing is simpler and rapidly effective. Intravenously, 5 mg/kg over 30 min should be followed by a maintenance infusion giving a total dose of up to 1200 mg over 24 h. Much less than this may be required in some surgical patients.

Amiodarone is clearly not without haemodynamic effects, causing a reduction in heart rate and vascular tone and, in some cases, in contractility also. Rapid intravenous administration usually causes hypotension and bradycardia; ideally amiodarone needs to be given by infusion.

***Class IV: calcium channel blockers (verapamil)***

The classification of calcium channel blockers and the effect of such drugs on calcium channels generally, and calcium channels involved in vascular smooth muscle in particular, are dealt with elsewhere. Of the calcium channel blockers available in the UK, only verapamil has any significant antiarrhythmic activity, although diltiazem has been recommended for antiarrhythmia prophylaxis after cardiac surgery.

Verapamil causes a potent blockade of calcium channels, and also possesses adrenergic and fast sodium channel-blocking activity. These effects are seen primarily in pacemaker tissue, and verapamil slows AV conduction and prolongs the effective refractory period in AV tissue. This may produce AV dissociation and, on occasion, heart block. Verapamil is highly effective for treating supraventricular arrhythmias including atrial fibrillation, and may be useful when used in combination with digoxin. Despite early reports, the combination of verapamil and β-adrenoceptor antagonist is not as dangerous as once supposed, although the two drugs will summate to slow AV nodal conduction further.

Calcium antagonists are also discussed on page 398.

### Others

*Digoxin*

Digoxin is still used as an antiarrhythmic, but much less than previously. It acts by inhibiting the $Na^+/K^+$ pump and has agonist (cholinergic) effects at muscarinic ($M_2$) receptors, particularly in the AV node. It decreases the conduction velocity in all conducting tissues, but less in the His–Purkinje system than elsewhere. It also changes the slope and duration of phases 2 and 3 of the AP, slows phase 4 repolarization and thus the heart rate, and raises the resting potential. The effects of digoxin are sensitive to changes in serum potassium concentration.

Digoxin is now primarily used to control ventricular rate in atrial fibrillation and vagal activity is enhanced, making it effective at inducing partial AV block. However, toxicity may develop, particularly if rapid dosing schedules are adopted, in elderly patients or those with renal failure. Resting ventricular rate is more easily controlled than the effects of exercise.

*Adenosine*

Adenosine is a naturally occurring compound with interesting haemodynamic effects.

It is formed by two mechanisms: dephosphorylation of cAMP (adenosine cyclic 3′ : 5′-monophosphate) and breakdown of *S*-adenosyl homocysteine. Adenosine acts on adenosine (purinergic) receptors and activates both $A_1$ (high-affinity) or $A_2$ (low-affinity) receptors. Activation of $A_1$-receptors in the human myocardium stimulates $G_i$ protein, causing inhibition of adenylyl cyclase and reduction in cAMP formation. Activation of $A_2$-receptors mediates vasodilatation.

Adenosine acts as an agonist at $A_1$-receptors, causing an increase in potassium conductance, which leads to hyperpolarization of the cell membrane and reduction or absence of spontaneous activity, particularly in the AV node. Ventricular standstill may occur.

Adenosine has an ultra-short duration of action and is mostly used as a diagnostic test for supraventricular tachyarrhythmias; however, it may be effective at converting to sinus rhythm, particularly in patients with pre-excitation syndromes.

Adenosine also has potent vasodilator effects on the coronary vasculature, and local adenosine regulation may be important in the ischaemic myocardium.

## CARDIAC MUSCLE AND ITS CONTRACTION

### Structure and specific features

Cardiac cells resemble branched filaments in their structure. They are approximately 10–20 μm in diameter and 50–100 μm long. They are attached to one another by intercalated discs. T tubules penetrate the cells and allow for rapid activation. These tubules occur every 2 μm. The ultrastructure of a cardiac muscle cell is similar to that of a striated muscle cell (see Chapter 24, Figures 24.5 and 24.9), with the cells arranged in a syncytium (see Figure 20.1). Some cardiac cells, notably those of the nodal regions and the Purkinje cells of the conducting system, contain relatively few myofibrils.

The molecular structure of cardiac actin and myosin is similar to that of skeletal muscle. However, there are some important differences, as well as similarities between cardiac and skeletal muscle. The functional syncytium in cardiac muscle allows for the easy propagation of an impulse, and the larger T-tubule system is important in that it provides a means of rapidly distributing a depolarizing current inwards. In contrast to skeletal muscle, cardiac muscle cannot recruit more fibres to improve performance, but performance is improved by enhancing contractility in response to autonomic activation, drugs, and the movement of calcium ions. Such contractile force in both is dependent on resting sarcomere length. Also, cardiac muscle is relatively non-compliant at resting lengths, in contrast to skeletal muscle. The APs of cardiac muscle are longer than those of skeletal muscle. This prevents tetanic summation and ensures rhythmic activity. The excitation/relaxation cycle of cardiac muscle is similar to skeletal muscle. The properties of skeletal and cardiac muscle are compared in Chapter 24, Figure 24.14.

### The contractile process

In many ways, the process of contraction is similar to that in skeletal muscle, as described in Chapter 24 to which reference should be made. The salient features and points requiring emphasis in cardiac muscle are given here for convenience and completeness.

To initiate the contractile process, the myosin head is associated with ATP, and hydrolysis of ATP leads to the formation of ADP and phosphate ($P_i$), which are transiently stored in the myosin head. The myosin head, having been previously angulated, now becomes realigned but completion of the cross-bridging process with the actin helix is prevented by troponin I. However, calcium ions are released from intracellular stores following membrane depolarization and become bound to troponin C. This induces a protein interaction which results in the liberation of the troponin I-induced inhibition of the actin–myosin interaction, probably through a process of reconfiguration of the troponin–tropomyosin complex, which exposes the actin-binding sites. The myosin head, still containing the stores of ADP and $P_i$, becomes aligned to the actin-binding site as a result of flexion of the tail of the myosin, and thus activated myosin and actin are attached and the cross-bridge is formed. The next step is the force-generating step, in which the myosin head, still attached to the actin in the form of the cross-bridge, flexes and thus moves the actin relative to the myosin molecule, initiating the sliding process that results in contraction of the myofibril without change in the actual length of the actinomysin filaments. With this step energy is consumed, leaving the cross-bridge flexed and the actinomysin complex deactivated. Further ATP combines with the myosin head and the cross-bridge is broken, leaving the myosin–ATP complex ready for the next cycle. Figures representing the process can be found in Chapter 24, Figures 24.7 and 24.8.

Normal contractile processes are therefore heavily dependent on calcium and high-energy phosphates for their function. The invaginations of the sarcolemma in the myocardial cell are broader than in skeletal muscle cells, and thus allow extracellular or sarcolemmal calcium to be more rapidly transported into the cell. The thin filaments containing the troponin–tropomyosin complexes are calcium dependent in respect of cross-bridge formation, which can occur only in the presence of calcium ions. These ions effectively alter the tropomyosin–troponin complex.

Troponin complexes, particularly the T and I varieties, are found in blood after myocardial damage; they are valuable markers because they are highly specific for damage to cardiac muscle, in contrast to other non-specific biochemical markers, e.g. creatine phosphokinase (CPK). Even the myocardial isoenzyme CPK-MB is thought to be less specific for myocardial damage than either of the troponin complexes.

### Contractility and calcium

Calcium is uniquely important in the process of cardiac contraction, and many inotropic mechanisms are involved in directly or indirectly increasing the availability of calcium to the myofibrils. The process can be described as follows (reference should also be made to the 'Action potential phases' earlier in the chapter).

The large T tubules (see Chapter 24, Figure 24.5) abut on the Z bands of the sarcomeres and carry electrical depolarization inwards. They are in close proximity with, but not directly connected to, a complex system of microtubules that surround the sarcomeres and are called the sarcoplasmic reticulum. This microtubular system contains a high concentration of calcium as a result of the activity of an ATP-utilizing calcium pump.

Despite the obvious importance of calcium, the initiating process is the rapid opening of sodium channels during the phase 0 depolarization in non-pacemaker cardiac tissue. However, calcium channels open at –60 mV, and remain open for some time, allowing calcium ions to enter the cell.

The sarcolemma contains L-type voltage-gated channels, and the nature and duration of their open state can be altered by drugs and other factors.

Calcium starts to enter the myocardial cell during the later stage of phase 0 depolarization, but the slow L-type channels in the sarcolemma remain open for 30–300 ms, generating a calcium inflow that is maintained and is responsible for the phase 2 plateau. This relatively modest calcium inflow across the sarcolemma generates a larger release of calcium, both from sarcoplasmic reticular stores and from other intracellular subsarcolemmal sites. Calcium released in this fashion is able to interact with the troponin–tropomyosin complex as described earlier, generating myofibril excitation and contraction. A small portion of the calcium contained within the sarcoplasmic reticulum or at subsarcolemmal sites is released during activation under normal circumstances. The remainder of the calcium stores constitutes a reserve, which may be utilized to enhance contractility when necessary.

Calcium is removed predominantly by reuptake into both the sarcoplasmic reticulum and subsarcolemmal binding sites. Reuptake into the sarcoplasmic reticulum is responsible for the termination of contraction by removing calcium from its troponin-binding complex, troponin C. This reuptake process is an active ATP-dependent process and in the myocardium is facilitated by phospholamban, a protein that spans the membrane of the sarcoplasmic reticulum.

Further removal of calcium from the myoplasma occurs as a result of activation of an energy-dependent sarcolemmal exchange mechanism. During diastole, reuptake of calcium into the sarcoplasmic reticulum and elsewhere means that the concentration of calcium is relatively high outside the cell. This produces a concentration gradient for the inward movement of calcium ions during diastole (a 'leak current'). If the activation process of contraction is to be maintained, calcium ions must be removed.

Calcium ions are exchanged for sodium ions (three sodium ions for each calcium ion), and the energy for this exchange is provided mainly by the sodium gradient from inside to outside the cell. This is generated by sarcolemmal $Na^+/K^+$ ATPase which maintains a high intracellular sodium concentration. Thus, the calcium-exchange mechanism is necessary to remove calcium that enters the cell during both the AP and diastole (the leak current).

The sodium gradient is also important. If this is increased, the removal of calcium will be facilitated; reduction in the sodium gradient will result in intracellular calcium accumulation. The sodium gradient can be influenced by increasing intracellular sodium, thereby resulting in a reduction in calcium exchange, enhanced levels of intracellular calcium, and thus an enhanced level of contractility.

In addition to the sodium exchange pump there is a calcium-stimulated ATP-dependent pump which is also involved in calcium efflux.

### Contractility and inotropic state

Cardiac muscle exists in a state of incomplete activation at rest. All muscle units respond when stimulated, but the initiation of the response (the AP), and particularly the magnitude of the response, are dependent on calcium flux. The interrelationship of calcium, initial resting length, and developed tension in cardiac muscle is shown in Figure 20.10. Although the developed tension is affected by resting sarcomere length, it is particularly affected by calcium concentration. The timing of the force generated by a contracting myofibril is intimately related to the timing of open-state calcium channels and the calcium concentration in the myoplasma.

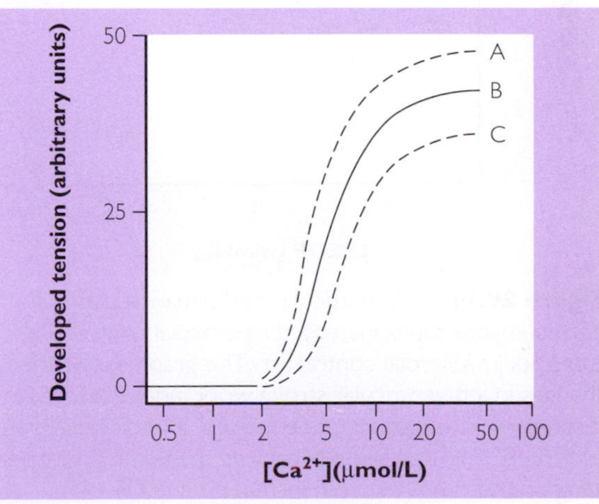


**Figure 20.10** The relationship between increasing the availability of calcium ions and developed muscle tension. Curves A, B, and C represent different preloads (A > B > C).

The relationship between increased myofibril length and force of contraction has been the subject of numerous studies, and was initially described by E.H. Starling in 1915 who wrote 'The energy of cardiac contraction is dependent on the resting length of the cardiac muscle fibre'. This is often described as Starling's law of the heart, although similar observations were made by Otto Frank (1895), and hence the relationship is more accurately described as the Frank–Starling mechanism. As the resting fibre length before contraction is dependent on the ventricular end-diastolic filling pressure (left or right VEDP), the Frank–Starling relationship for the intact heart is generally drawn as shown in Figure 20.11, in which curves are given for normal, increased, and decreased contractility.

Experiments exploring the relationship between resting fibre length and contractility have usually made use of the concept of isometric contraction, i.e. the muscle length is held fixed throughout the contraction and the force developed is measured using a tension transducer. Thus, with no change in length, tension rises, peaks, and falls away as the muscle is activated and relaxed (Figure 20.12). Furthermore, when the initial resting myofibril length, or preload, is varied, the increased force of contraction manifests itself as an increased rate of rise of tension and the actual time to achieve maximum tension varies very little (Figure 20.13). However, the shape of the tension–time curve is altered if we make an intervention that increases (positive inotropy) or depresses (negative inotropy) contractility.

Another factor that affects the contractile performance of a myofibril is the afterload. This is shown in Figure 20.14. In this experiment, the stop and lever are arranged in such a way that, having reached a given tension, the muscle starts to shorten and therefore lifts the load in the pan. The afterload is the load after the muscle starts to shorten. It will include the preload, but it also includes the force necessary to lift the load upwards. The ensuing contraction is termed 'isotonic' because, once the weight is lifted and moved, the muscle will shorten and then lengthen while maintaining the same tension.

The terms 'preload' and 'afterload' are derived from experimental physiology, but they are widely used in cardiovascular medicine. When we use the terms preload and central venous pressure (CVP) interchangeably, we are making a number of assumptions about the effect of increasing CVP on left ventricular (LV) end-diastolic fibre length which may not be true in disease.

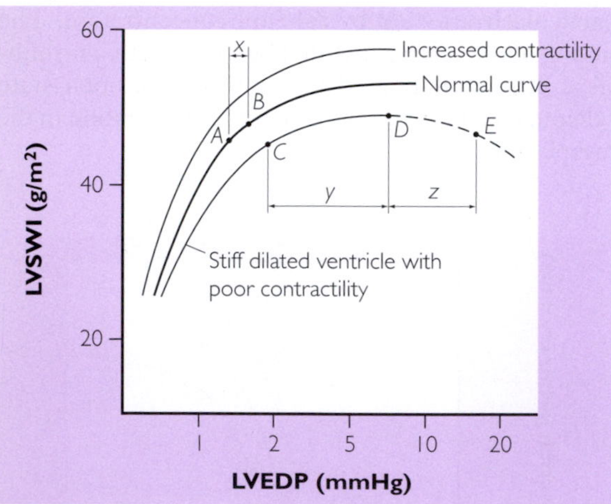


**Figure 20.11** Left ventricular performance curves for normal myocardium, increased myocardial contractility, and poor myocardial contractility. The graph shows the changes in left ventricular stroke work index (LVSWI) in response to changes in left ventricular end-diastolic pressure (LVEDP). The effects of moving the ventricular operating point from *A* to *B* (an increase in LVEDP of *x* mmHg) and from *C* to *D* and *D* to *E* (increases in LVEDP of *y* and *z* mmHg respectively) are shown in Figures 20.18 and 20.19 respectively. (See page 378 for details.)

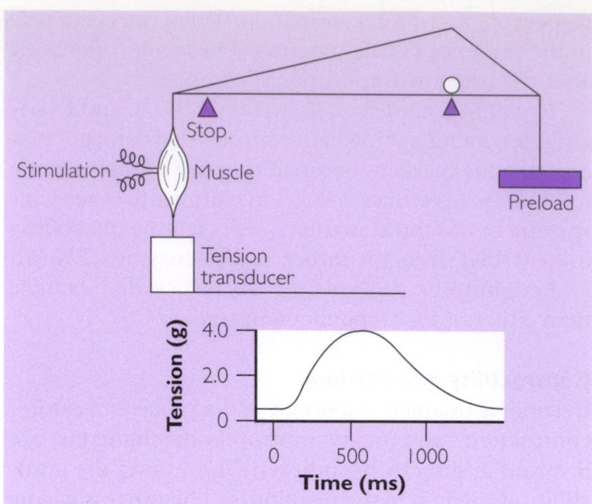


**Figure 20.12** A study of isolated cardiac muscle using a lever arm arranged so that the muscle will contract isometrically. The muscle is stretched by a given weight (preload) and a stop positioned so that, when stimulated, it cannot shorten. The tension–time graph produced by such an arrangement is shown.

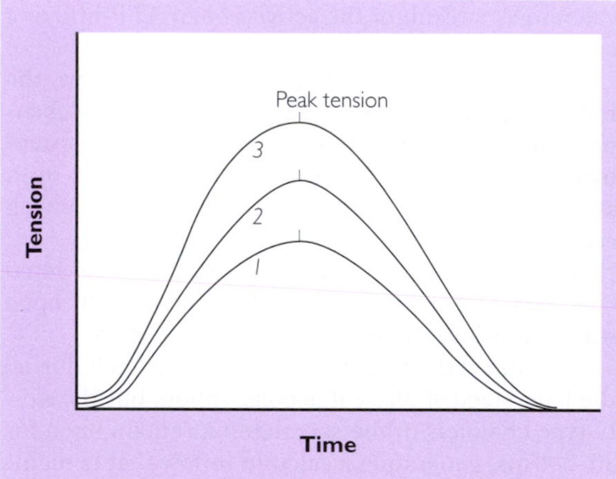


**Figure 20.13** The peak tension obtained by isometric contraction at different preloads (3 > 2 > 1). Note that the time to peak tension remains constant irrespective of the preload.

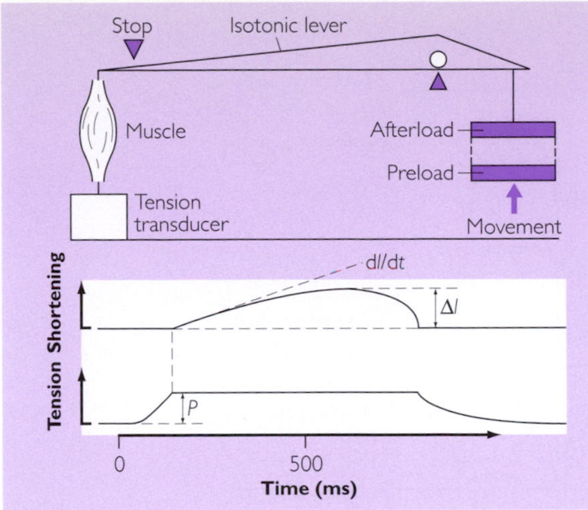


**Figure 20.14** Isotonic contractions with preload and afterload. The stop on the left determines the initial muscle length, but does not prevent the muscle from contracting when it develops tension. The shortening and tension resulting from such an isotonic contraction are shown below the experimental set-up. *P*, afterload, d*l*/d*t*, initial shortening velocity. (See text for details.)

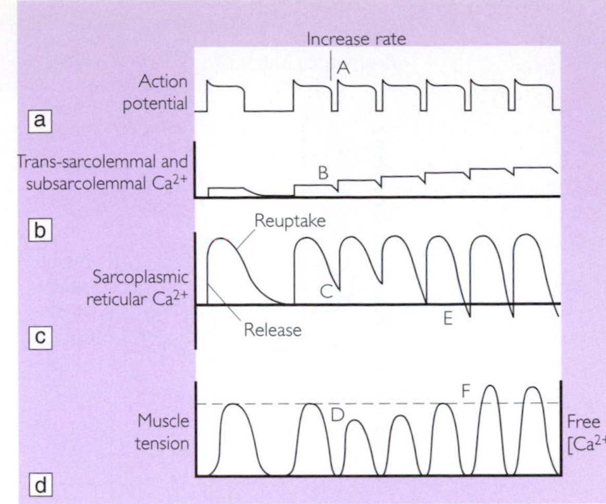


**Figure 20.15** The Bowditch staircase (or force–frequency relationship). As the rate of firing increases (A in graph a) the calcium movement across the sarcolemma begins to increase (B in graph b). Initially, less calcium is released as a result of incomplete re-uptake (C in graph c), resulting in initial reduction in developed tension (D in graph d). As calcium re-uptake and release improves (E in graph c) so tension improves (F in graph d).

The rate of stimulation may also affect the contractile state of a myofibril. This effect is related to calcium flux and storage, and is demonstrable in both isolated myofibrils and the intact heart. If the myofibril is stimulated electrically at an increased rate, contractility during the initial beats is reduced as a result of a reduction in calcium availability from rapid release sites, in part because of a lack of full recovery of calcium stores from the sarcoplasmic reticulum. Shortly thereafter, an increase in calcium available from the sarcoplasmic reticulum leads to an enhancement of contractility – termed the 'Bowditch effect' (Figure 20.15).

Thus there are four major factors that can affect the force, speed, and extent of shortening of cardiac muscle:

- resting muscle length (preload);
- level of afterload;
- inotropic state;
- frequency of contraction.

Although preload and afterload may alter cardiac performance, alterations in these parameters do not affect contractility and may be considered only as mechanical determinants of muscle performance. A change in inotropic state produces a change in the performance of heart muscle, which is independent of loading conditions and will result in a shift of the function curve of cardiac muscle. Measurements used to determine the effects of drugs on contractility are made under different loading conditions. It is important to recognize that many of the changes seen after drug therapy may produce a beneficial effect in the patient (i.e. increased cardiac output), but that the mechanism that produces the effect may be mechanical (i.e loading-related) rather than an improvement in contractility.

In conclusion, a number of parameters may be measured as a means of assessing myocardial contractility, but many of these may be altered by changes in loading, particularly preload.

The ejection fraction (EF) given by:

$$EF = \frac{ESV - EDV}{ESV} \times 100$$

where ESV is the end-systolic volume and EDV the end-diastolic volume, is a useful measurement, commonly used in clinical practice, but it is afterload sensitive. Both the EF and fractional shortening (echo-derived data) are indices of fibre shortening.

### Timing of cardiac contraction: the link between electrical and mechanical events

Let us first consider events on the left side of the heart, starting at the beginning of diastole. The interrelationship between electrical and mechanical events is shown in Figure 20.16 to which reference should be made.

After the end of diastole, there is an initial rapid phase of ventricular filling. Flow from the left atrium to the left ventricle is rapid and ventricular volume increases quickly. During mid-diastole, transmitral flow rate is reduced and ventricular volume increases more slowly. However, in late diastole, atrial contraction occurs, shown on the ECG as the p wave, and results in an increased transmitral flow and a rapid increase in ventricular volume. This 'atrial kick' may account for 20% of the ventricular filling volume; the proportion is increased if the ventricular muscle is poorly compliant and fills less effectively during passive mid-diastolic filling.

The wave of depolarization through the myocardium is slowed at the AV node (see Figure 20.5), and septal,

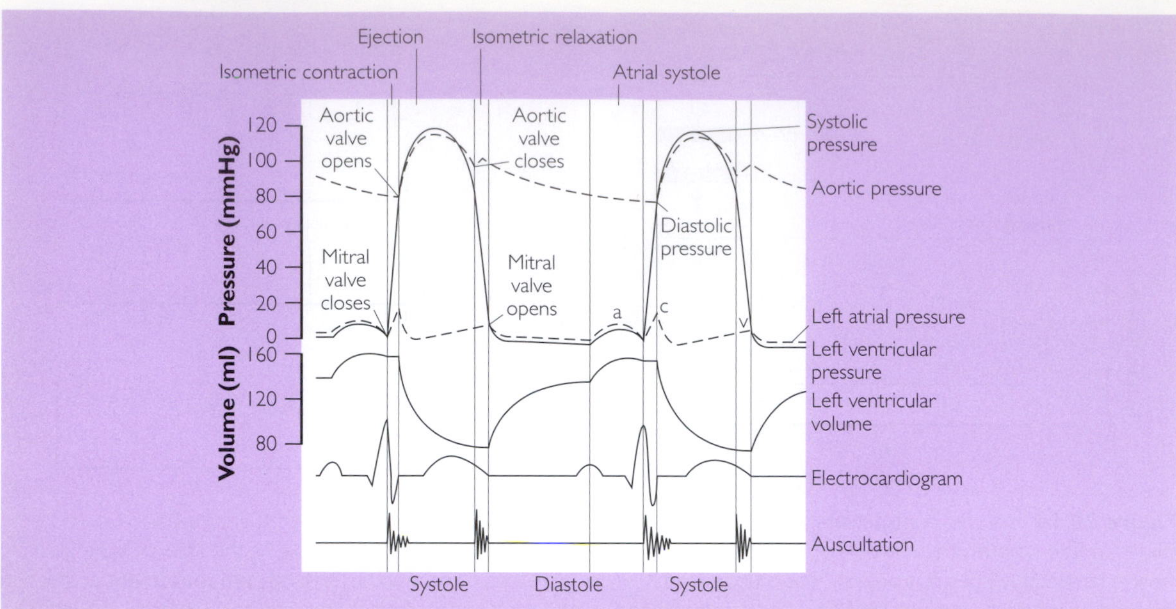


**Figure 20.16** The events of the cardiac cycle. Note the phases of the cycle and compare them in this diagram with their representation in Figure 20.18. The a, c, and v waves of the left atrial pressure wave are shown more clearly in Figure 20.30.

left, and right ventricular depolarization follow. On the normal surface ECG monitoring, on standard lead II, the AV nodal delay is represented by the PR segment, septal depolarization by the initial Q deflection, and left and right ventricular depolarization by the R and S waves, respectively. After a delay of approximately 50 ms, ventricular muscle starts to contract, thereby compressing the blood contained within the LV cavity, and this causes rapid deceleration of blood across the mitral valve, leading to mitral valve closure as the intraventricular pressure rises. Left atrial pressure stays relatively constant and much lower. Although left ventricular muscle starts to contract just before mitral valve closure, it is the point of mitral valve closure that is usually taken as the onset of systole.

After closure of the mitral valve, there is a period where the intraventricular pressure increases before the opening of the aortic valve without any change in ventricular volume. This is the period of isovolumic contraction, and it continues until the pressure in the left ventricle reaches the pressure in the aorta, at which point the aortic valve opens and aortic flow rapidly commences and ventricular volume falls. When the aortic valve is open, aortic and LV pressure changes are identical, continuing to rise to a peak that corresponds to the peak rate of flow across the aortic valve. After this peak the LV muscle is not shortening any further and has started to relax, but transaortic valve blood flow continues albeit at a rapidly reducing rate. Aortic and LV pressure fall, and the rate and magnitude of fall in pressure in the aorta is determined by peripheral circulatory factors. As soon as the pressure in the aorta exceeds the pressure in the LV cavity, the aortic valve closes and, as pressure changes at this point are large and rapid, the aortic valve snaps shut. The point of aortic valve closure is usually taken to be the start of diastole, but the pressure in the left ventricle is still considerably greater than that in the left atrium. LV pressure falls rapidly until such time as the pressure in the left atrium exceeds the pressure in the left ventricle, at which point the mitral valve opens and transmitral flow commences. The period between aortic valve closure and mitral valve opening is called the isovolumic relaxation phase.

Similar pressure and flow relationships exist in the right side of the heart. However, the pressures reached in the right ventricle and pulmonary vasculature are approximately 20% of those in the left ventricle and aorta. The duration of systole, and the duration of the isovolumic contraction and relaxation phases, are also shorter in the right ventricle. As the pressure in the right atrium exceeds the pressure in the right ventricle, flow commences across the tricuspid valve. The filling dynamics of the right ventricle are similar to those of the left, with one or two important differences. Atrial contraction begins marginally earlier in the right atrium than in the left, the SA node is located in the right atrium, and left atrial (LA) enlargement may cause a bifid appearance of the p wave, as contraction of first the right and then the left atrium can be separately identified. The wave of depolarization from the right atrium is again slowed by the AV node giving right ventricular (RV) filling time for completion, and RV contraction commences with an initial isovolumetric phase, which continues until such time as RV pressure exceeds pulmonary artery diastolic pressure. At this point, the pulmonary valve opens and flow continues across the pulmonary valve, accelerating until peak flow rate is reached and then decelerating until RV pressure is identical to pulmonary artery pressure.

RV and pulmonary artery haemodynamics are particularly susceptible to changes in the pulmonary vasculature. The pulmonary arterioles are relatively poorly endowed with smooth muscle, in contrast to the systemic circulation, and the pulmonary circulation represents a considerably more compliant vascular bed for ventricular ejection. Thus, the same flow rate is achieved across the pulmonary valve as across the aortic valve, despite the fact that peak systolic RV pressure is 20–25% of peak systolic LV pressure. Measurements of pulmonary artery pressure and the use of pulmonary artery flotation catheters is described in Chapters 48, 50 and 76.

Factors that increase pulmonary vascular resistance may have a profoundly adverse effect on RV output. Pulmonary vasoconstriction may be produced by hypoxia, acidosis, hypercapnia, and sympathetic activation via a variety of mechanisms. Furthermore, the relatively less muscular RV may be unable to cope with a markedly increased pulmonary vascular resistance, leading to RV failure. This may result in a bulging of the tricuspid ring into the right atrium during RV contraction, or frank tricuspid regurgitation and 'cannon' waves – peaked CVP waves both increased in amplitude and timed to coincide with ventricular systole. Another cause of such waves is the asynchronous contraction of the atria and ventricles, such that the atria are contracting against a closed AV valve. In this situation, atrial filling of the ventricles is lost and the pressure changes in the atrium during atrial contraction are markedly enhanced in both the left and right atria. This may occur with any arrhythmia associated with AV disassociation, e.g. AV nodal rhythm, complete heart block.

The dynamics of RV contraction differ from those of the left ventricle. The right ventricle consists of two functionally linked areas: an inflow and an outflow tract. The right ventricle is crescent shaped, and the septum and attached LV wall are important contractile components for RV function. Septal contraction during LV contraction contributes extensively to RV emptying. During the early phase of systole, the inflow tract contracts and the outflow tract dilates, thereby acting as a compliant volume storage area, perhaps protecting the relatively non-muscular pulmonary circulation from acute rises in pressure. The function of the inflow and outflow tracts may be affected by numerous interventions including positive end-expiratory pressure (PEEP).

The effects of raised intrathoracic pressure may be best demonstrated by the Valsalva manoeuvre (Figure 20.17). This involves making a forced expiratory effort against a closed glottis or obstruction. Normally, this will involve contraction of the abdominal and thoracic muscles, and the pressure gradients within the thoracoabdominal circulation are maintained more than might be anticipated, albeit at higher absolute values. Venous return from other areas (head and neck, limbs) is, however, markedly decreased. The circulatory consequences of the Valsalva manoeuvre are shown in Figure 20.17. It is usually described in four phases:

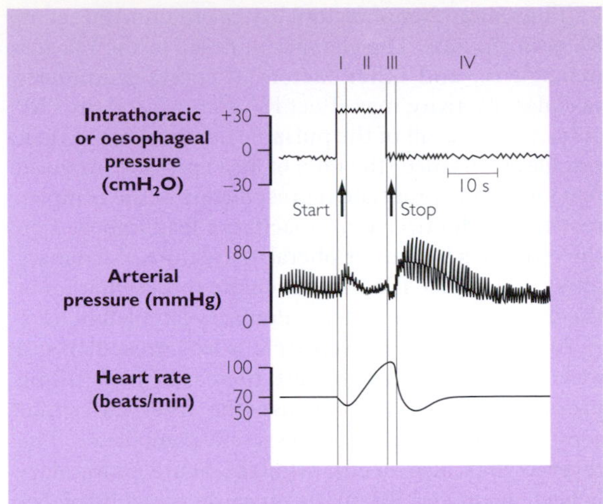


**Figure 20.17** The effects of a Valsalva manoeuvre in humans. (See text for description of phases I–IV.)

1. The initial compression of the thoracoabdominal veins leads to an increase in venous return to the left atrium and a transient increase in blood pressure.
2. As the increased intrathoracic pressure is maintained, blood flow from the right ventricle through the pulmonary circulation to the left ventricle is markedly reduced and cardiac output and blood pressure fall. The CVP remains elevated. This acute fall in blood pressure activates baroreceptor mechanisms (see later), which cause vasoconstriction and a gradual restoration of blood pressure. There is also a reflex tachycardia, which serves partially to restore the cardiac output.
3. As the high intrathoracic pressure is released, there is a transient reduction in blood pressure as a result of the reduction in external compression of the pulmonary vessels that fill with blood.
4. There is then an overshoot in blood pressure as compensatory mechanisms continue to operate with venous return restored. This may be accompanied by a reflex bradycardia.

In patients with autonomic neuropathy (e.g. those with diabetes), activation of the various vascular reflexes is not seen. Thus the initial fall in blood pressure is maintained without any ensuing reflex vasoconstriction and gradual increase in blood pressure, nor is there a reflex tachycardia. The overshoot in pressure after release of the Valsalva manoeuvre may also be absent.

The circulatory effects of the Valsalva manoeuvre are also dependent on the pulmonary circulation being acutely compressible by increasing intrathoracic airway pressure. Where the pulmonary vasculature is less compressible, the effects of the Valsalva manoeuvre may be negligible. This may occur in heart failure or pulmonary arterial hypertension from whatever cause.

Intermittent positive pressure ventilation may be said to mimic the Valsalva manoeuvre partially, in that intrathoracic airway pressure is increased and therefore the resistance to transpulmonary blood flow is also increased, leading to a reduction in left atrial filling and cardiac output. Simply altering the loading conditions of the heart (i.e. increasing RV filling by giving fluids) should restore the situation to normal, but in clinical practice other factors, such as the myocardial depressant effects of anaesthetics and other drugs, may serve to limit the response. The effect may be more marked if intrathoracic pressure is more markedly increased by other mechanisms including PEEP and gas trapping (e.g. asthma, pneumothorax).

Thus a number of factors have a profound effect on RV performance. The changes imposed by the Valsalva manoeuvre, and other factors affecting pulmonary vascular reactivity, may affect RV afterload and thus RV output. As a result of the pulsatile nature of blood flow, vascular resistance (the ratio of mean pressure to mean flow) is an inappropriate representation of the complex resistive, inductive, and capacitative load imposed on the ventricles by the peripheral vasculature. Pulmonary input impedance is a more accurate representation of the dynamic effects of the pulmonary circulation.

Although the right ventricle is less muscular and more compliant than the left, increases in LV filling pressure may serve to cause the interventricular septum to be displaced and lessen RV compliance. The reverse may also occur, whereby acute pulmonary hypertension and RV dilatation cause septal displacement into the left ventricle with reduced LV output.

### Measurements of ventricular function and pressure/volume (dimension) loops

One of the most sensitive methods (in theory) of measurement of ventricular contractility can be obtained by constructing pressure/volume loops which allow measurements that are both preload and afterload independent. Pressure/volume (or dimension) loops exhibit four segments: isovolumetric contraction, ejection, isovolumetric relaxation, and filling (Figure 20.18). This figure should be compared with Figures 20.11 and 20.16 to obtain an overall view of ventricular function.

Although isovolumetric contraction and relaxation are usually represented as straight lines, in practice early shortening and/or lengthening may occur in normal individuals. Severe displacement of the pressure/dimension loop is pathological; poor ventricular function is shown in Figure 20.19. Note the displacement along the horizontal axis when compared with Figure 20.18. In ventricular dilatation (usually associated with LV failure) the EDV is greatly increased, producing a fall in the EF. In summary, a shift of the curve upwards and to the left indicates an enhancement of cardiac function, whereas a shift downwards and to the right indicates a depression. However, the function curve is afterload sensitive and similar changes may be caused by changes in outflow resistance.

The area of the pressure/volume loop represents the external work of the ventricle. By expressing this area as a function of EDV, ventricular function curves may be obtained. This relationship, termed 'preload-recruitable stroke work', is considered to be a superior index of contractility because of its load independence.

The pressure/volume relationship at the end of systole in health has been shown to be approximately linear. Ventricular tissue may be considered to behave in a similar fashion to an elastic bag, generating pressure when filled beyond its unstressed volume and returning to its unstressed volume at the end of systole. This is the concept of time-varying elastance, i.e. the elastance of the ventricle varies during the contraction/relaxation phase of each beat. At successive instants in the cardiac cycle, there is a defined relationship between ventricular pressure and volume,

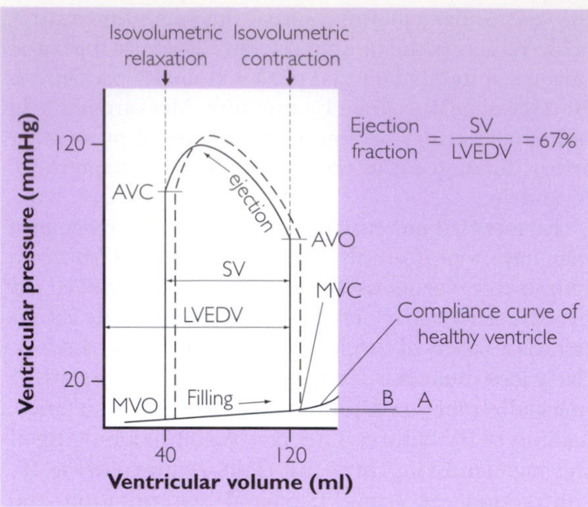


**Figure 20.18** Left ventricular pressure/volume loops representing normal ventricular function. MV, mitral valve; AV, aortic valve; O, opens; C, closes. The stroke volume (SV) and left ventricular end-diastolic volume (LVEDV) used to determine the ejection fraction are marked. The effect of fluid loading, which increases the LVEDP from A to B (see Figure 20.11), is shown by the broken line.

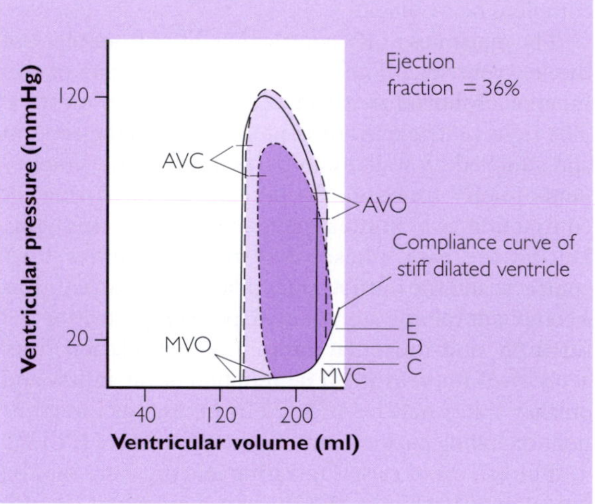


**Figure 20.19** Poor left ventricular function demonstrated on a pressure/volume loop. This figure shows the pressure/volume loop for a stiff dilated ventricle. Note the change in scale on the *x*-axis compared with Figure 20.18. MV, mitral valve; AV, aortic valve; O, opens; C, closes. The change in left ventricular end-diastolic pressure (LVEDP) required to increase the left ventricular stroke work index (LVSWI) by the same amount as moving from A to B in the normal ventricle (see Figures 20.11 and 20.18) is represented by the movement from C to D. The fall in LVSWI in moving from D to E (see Figure 20.11) is shown by the reduced area enclosed on the pressure/volume loop. A reduction in LVSWI with an increase in LVEDP (often termed 'decompensation') is now thought to result mainly from mitral incompetence from a stretched valve ring, rather than over-extension of the myofibrils. As a result of mitral incompetence, in contracting from an LVEDP of E (above), there is no isovolumetric contraction. Decompensation is more common in right ventricular failure where the tricuspid valve stretches easily because of the thinner ventricular wall.

which represents the time-varying elastance. At end-systole, the relationship is such that it is insensitive to changes in preload and afterload. Thus this index, the end-systolic pressure volume ratio (ESPVR), has been recommended as a useful and accurate measure of contractility that is both preload and afterload independent. However, there may be circumstances where measurements of ESPVR are not a good estimate of global contractility, for example, when contractility is impaired as a result of regional ischaemia.

The main drawback in the clinical use of cardiac pressure/volume loops is that they are difficult to measure in routine practice. Although pressure can be measured accurately, the left ventricle is difficult to access, and pressure measurements have to be made through catheters advanced from a peripheral site across the aortic valve, or via the pulmonary vein across the mitral valve. Transducer-tipped intraventricular catheters have been developed with a good dynamic response and enhanced accuracy over saline-filled catheters.

The biggest difficulty is in measuring ventricular volumes. Ventricular stroke volume (SV) can be calculated from a measurement of cardiac output (CO) and heart rate (HR):

$$SV \times HR = CO$$

This does not, however, reveal ventricular dimensions and is therefore of little value. A modern development of thermodilution is a technique based on the use of ultra-fast-response thermistors, which calculate ESV and EDV. However, this technique measures RV flow and volume and, although the outputs of the right and left ventricles are similar, the ventricular volumes are not. The LV conductance catheter has also been used experimentally to provide accurate LV volume data, but this is again largely restricted to cardiac surgical patients.

The estimates of ventricular volume and EF made in practice most commonly involve imaging the ventricle, by either radionuclide techniques or echocardiography. Although transthoracic echocardiography may be useful, transoesophageal echocardiography is the most reliable echocardiographic technique for measuring ventricular volumes, particularly with software to define the endocardial border. Contrast ventriculography is also highly accurate in measuring LV volume, but the cost and invasive nature of the technique restrict its use. Pressure/volume loops remain instructive tools for understanding ventricular function, but outside the animal laboratory their practical contribution to patient care has yet to be realized.

### Effect of the autonomic nervous system

The autonomic nervous system (ANS; see Chapter 23) plays a vital role in regulating the circulation. Adrenergic innervation is important in regulating cardiac activity and peripheral vascular tone, and the parasympathetic nervous system is important in regulating heart rate. These effects and those of sympathomimetic and parasympathomimetic drugs are considered in more detail above in the text relating to Figures 20.2, 20.3, and 20.4, later in this chapter and in Chapter 23.

## CORONARY BLOOD FLOW AND MYOCARDIAL METABOLISM

### Anatomy

The topography of the main coronary arteries (which arborize on the surface of the heart) and the transmural flow are shown in Chapter 48, Figures 48.1 and 48.2, respectively.

Functionally, the coronary vasculature has traditionally been divided into three groups:

- large-conductance, low-resistance epicardial vessels;
- small, high-resistance vessels 10–250 μm in diameter;
- veins.

Previously it was thought that coronary vascular resistance was determined by the tone in the small coronary arteries. More recently, it has become apparent that up to half the resting coronary vascular resistance may be determined by the larger diameter vessels, and this may vary because of physiological conditions and pharmacological interventions.

The structure of coronary arteries is well defined. The outer layer, or adventitia, consists of elastin, collagen, fibroblasts, mast cells, macrophages, and Schwann cells with nerve axons. Nerves within small arteries are contained within the adventitia and do not penetrate the media.

The tunica media is made up of circumferentially arranged smooth muscle cells. The number of layers is determined by the diameter of the vessel, e.g. from six in 300-μm vessels to one in 30- to 50-μm arterioles. The smooth muscle cells are spindle-shaped, have centrally located nuclei, lack striations, and are joined together mechanically at desmosome-like junctions. Electrically they behave like a syncytium, and are specialized for long slow contractions.

The lumina of blood vessels are lined by a continuous sheet of endothelial cells which, in arterioles, are 2 μm thick, 10–20 μm wide, and 30–50 μm long. These endothelial cells project into the media and are in contact with vascular smooth muscle; they are thus able to regulate many of the functions of vascular smooth muscle, including muscle tone.

### Vascular muscle tone

Smooth muscle cells contain a greater ratio of actin to myosin than skeletal muscle, but contractile forces are not significantly diminished. Contraction may be from electrical activity or by the action of neurotransmitters. In both cases, contraction is triggered by an increase in intracellular concentration of calcium ions, which is released from the sarcoplasmic reticulum in response to increased calcium entry through voltage-gated or receptor-operated calcium channels in the cell membrane. In contrast to skeletal and cardiac muscle, vascular smooth muscle does not contain the calcium-binding protein troponin C. A troponin-like protein, leiotonin, may play a similar role but this is not clear. Myoplasmic calcium combines with calmodulin, and the calcium–calmodulin complex activates myosin light chain kinase, which catalyses the phosphorylation of myosin P light chain, allowing actin to activate myosin

ATPase. Cross-bridge formation then continues as in skeletal muscle, with the exception that smooth muscle is able to arrest a cross-bridge cycle in the attached state, termed 'latch'. This results in the capability of sustaining tonic contractions with a very low rate of energy expenditure.

### Determinants of coronary blood flow

Coronary blood flow is proportional to the pressure gradient across the coronary circulation. This gradient is calculated by subtracting downstream coronary pressure from the pressure in the root of the aorta. However, the determination of downstream pressure is complicated because the intramural vessels are compressed with each heartbeat (see Chapter 48, Figure 48.2). Intramural vessels are most effectively compressed during systole, and it is therefore not surprising that coronary blood flow is significantly affected by the phases of the cardiac cycle. During systole, flow into the left coronary artery is markedly reduced, and the major part of blood flow occurs during diastole. Blood flow into the right coronary artery is better maintained throughout the cardiac cycle, but in pulmonary hypertension right coronary blood flow assumes a phasic pattern similar to that of the left coronary artery (Figure 20.20).

During systole, flow is impeded in small vessels by both direct compression and twisting of vessels as the heart contracts. Blood is expelled forwards into the coronary sinus, and backwards into the epicardial coronary arteries, which therefore act as capacitors. In this way the coronary arteries act as systolic storage reservoirs and receive systolic backflow.

Although zero inflow at the coronary ostia may occur, intramural forward flow has been shown to continue until pressures little greater than those in the coronary sinus have been reached. However, the compressive force acting on the subendocardium from the LV cavity (the LV end-diastolic pressure or LVEDP) will resist blood flow into the subendocardium. Consequently, when the LVEDP is raised, subendocardial compression and ischaemia may ensue. In clinical practice, LVEDP may be estimated by measuring the pulmonary capillary wedge pressure (PCWP) or left atrial pressure (LAP).

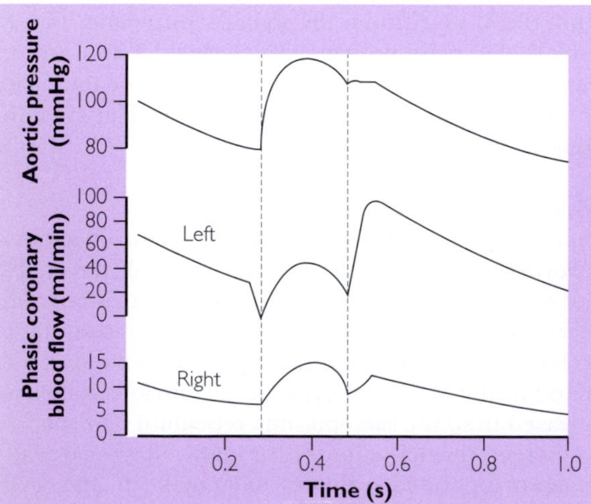


**Figure 20.20** Phasic blood flow in the right and left coronary arteries and the aortic pressure that fills them. Note that the majority of left coronary flow occurs during diastole, whereas right coronary flow is spread throughout the cardiac cycle. (Adapted from Berne RM and Levy MD. *Review of Medical Physiology*, 18th edn. Norwalk, CT: Appleton & Lange, 1997.)

As the coronary arteries fill during diastole, an averaged aortic diastolic pressure may be considered as the input pressure. This may be different from the diastolic pressure measured at the radial artery, owing to distortion of the pressure waveform as it is propagated through the vascular tree, and inaccuracies associated with the hydraulic and electronic components of the monitoring system. In these circumstances, the mean radial arterial pressure may be a more accurate estimate of coronary driving pressure. Finally, as the coronary arteries fill during diastole, factors that shorten the duration of diastole (i.e. tachycardia) may reduce coronary blood flow.

Myocardial blood flow is primarily under metabolic control. Even when cut off from external neural and hormonal control, the heart maintains its ability to match blood flow to metabolic need. The main determinants of the heart's oxygen requirement are:

- the intraventricular systolic wall tension and compression (reflected by the systemic blood pressure in the absence of aortic stenosis);
- the heart rate;
- preload;
- myocardial contractility (influenced by the patient's own sympathetic activity and by drugs).

Good control of coronary blood flow is essential. The heart takes approximately 5% of the cardiac output through the coronary circulation and consumes just over 10% of the body's oxygen uptake. In contrast to average venous blood, which is 25% less saturated with oxygen than arterial blood, the heart, even at rest, removes over twice as much. Extraction rates of up to 70% have been measured in some studies. As resting myocardial oxygen extraction is normally very efficient, only a small amount of extra oxygen extraction is available during exercise. Any extra oxygen requirements must therefore be met by increased blood flow.

Hypotheses of metabolic control suggest that vascular tone is linked either to depletion of a substrate (e.g. oxygen, ATP) or to the accumulation of a metabolite such as carbon dioxide or hydrogen ions. Potential mediators that have been investigated therefore include oxygen, carbon dioxide, hydrogen ions, potassium, hyperosmolarity, calcium, and adenosine. It is likely that a combination of local factors (oxygen, carbon dioxide, adenosine) act together, probably with differing importance depending on the situation. It is unlikely that any one factor will dominate.

The specific influence of neural control is difficult to establish because sympathetic or parasympathetic activation can cause profound changes in heart rate, blood pressure, and contractility, and these alterations will provoke changes in myocardial metabolic requirements and hence in blood flow.

The heart is supplied with branches of the sympathetic and parasympathetic nervous systems. Thicker vagal fibres end in the adventitia of coronary vessels, and fine, non-medullated fibres end on vascular smooth muscle cells. Vagal stimulation causes bradycardia and reductions in contractility and blood pressure. The resultant fall in myocardial oxygen consumption causes a metabolic-induced coronary vasoconstriction. However, if myocardial metabolism is held constant, cholinergic activation causes coronary vasodilatation. The effects of acetylcholine on coronary vascular tone also differs in health and disease: in normal individuals, acetylcholine produces vasodilatation, whereas in the presence of coronary atheroma constriction is observed.

β-Adrenoceptor activation causes coronary vasodilatation independent of blood flow changes; $\beta_1$- and $\beta_2$-adrenoceptors are involved, $\beta_1$ predominating in the conductance (large) vessels and $\beta_2$ in the resistance vessels. Activation of the sympathetic nerves to the heart results in increases in heart rate, contractility, and blood pressure which will result in metabolism-induced coronary vasodilatation and an increase in blood flow. However, activation of α-adrenoceptors causes coronary vasoconstriction; this may oppose the metabolic-induced effects. Both $\alpha_1$- and $\alpha_2$-adrenoceptors have been identified in the myocardium.

Regarding the humoral control of coronary blood flow, vasopressin (AVP), atrial natriuretic peptide (ANP), vasoactive intestinal peptide (VIP), neuropeptide Y (NPY), and calcitonin gene-related peptide (CGRP) have all been studied. AVP can cause vasoconstriction in experimental animals, but may also provoke opposing release of endothelium-derived releasing factor (EDRF), particularly in large vessels. ANP may also cause endothelium-dependent vasodilatation in the experimental setting. Angiotensin-converting enzyme (ACE) is present on vascular endothelium and converts angiotensin I to angiotensin II, resulting in coronary vasoconstriction. Angiotensin II also facilitates the release of norepinephrine from presynaptic adrenergic nerve terminals. Bradykinin, which can attenuate vasoconstriction via EDRF stimulation, is inactivated by ACE. Despite these observations, ACE inhibition has not been shown to be beneficial through mechanisms other than afterload control.

## Coronary pressure/flow relationships

### *Autoregulation*

Flow autoregulation is the tendency for blood flow to remain constant over a wide range of perfusion pressures (Figure 20.21). Many vascular beds demonstrate autoregulation, and the pressure/flow relationship in the coronary circulation is shown in Figure 20.21. There are three separate areas:

1. A high-pressure region, where flow increases with coronary perfusion pressure (CPP) (Figure 20.21, points C and D);
2. An intermediate-pressure range where flow alters little with changes in CPP (Figure 20.21, points B and C);
3. A low-pressure region where flow decreases with decreasing CPP (Figure 20.21, points A and B).

In the autoregulatory range, sudden changes in perfusion pressure will autoregulate within 30 s, and

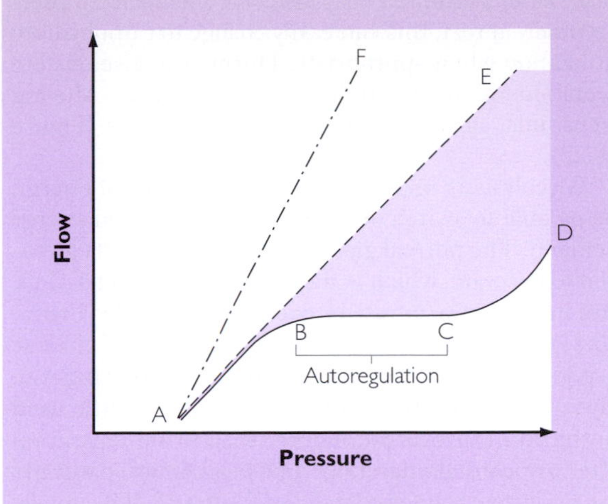


**Figure 20.21** The concept of autoregulation. A tissue that autoregulates has a flow–pressure curve that has a horizontal section, as shown above from B to C. If autoregulation fails, flow becomes directly proportional to pressure as shown by the line A–E. In the presence of drugs and severe hypoxia, the tissue may dilate further making the flow–pressure relationship even steeper (A–F).

autoregulatory capacity is greater in the subepicardium than in the endocardium, with little variation between right and left ventricles.

In the presence of a controlled level of myocardial oxygen demand, coronary blood flow remains relatively stable at mean arterial pressures (MAP) of between 60 and 140 mmHg.

### *Reserve*

As resting myocardial oxygen extraction is high, any increase in oxygen demand (e.g. as in exercise) needs to be met by an increased myocardial blood flow. The increase possible can be seen in concept in Figure 20.21 (see Figure 20.26 for numerical changes). The resting autoregulatory state may also be changed and elevated, thus encroaching on the reserve, by diseases including left ventricular hypertrophy and chronic anaemia.

Transient coronary occlusion produces a reactive myocardial hyperaemia, which is a useful method of estimating coronary flow reserve experimentally; if there is no hyperaemia then there is no physiological flow reserve under the prevailing conditions. However, further coronary vasodilatation may be induced pharmacogically using a coronary vasodilator such as adenosine, or dypyridamole.

Some anaesthetics have also been shown to be effective coronary vasodilators. This mechanism has, on occasion, been shown to cause coronary steal and luxury perfusion of non-ischaemic areas of the myocardium in experimental and clinical studies. Its relevance to the incidence of perioperative ischaemia during routine surgery is less clear.

### *Myocardial metabolism*

The heart needs a continuous and effective source of oxygen and high-energy fuel for its metabolism. The major substrates for cardiac metabolism are carbohydrates and lipids, although in truth the heart is not a fussy eater. Although fatty acids are metabolized preferentially at rest, this can easily change to carbohydrate utilization when appropriate. During exercise, lactate metabolism may predominate. However, during ischaemia, carbohydrate usage predominates (Figure 20.22).

Glycolysis is important as a rapid source of energy, being able to switch on within 5 s of increased energy demand. The normal glycolytic pathway converts glycogen to pyruvate, which is then converted to acetyl-CoA, and hence to the citrate or tricarboxylate cycle (Figure 20.23). The pentose shunt – the conversion of glucose 6-phosphate to riboses and then re-entering the glycolytic pathway or used to form RNA – is little used in the adult myocardium other than to aid reparation after myocardial infarction. The biochemical pathways are described in more detail in Chapter 18. The uptake and use of lactate are clearly important and may identify the state of aerobic or anaerobic metabolism.

Free fatty acid (FFA) metabolism is an important source of fuel. FFAs in the circulation are bound to albumin, and the FFA–albumin complex needs to bind to the sarcolemmal receptor before FFAs can translocate into the plasma. Oxidation converts the FFA to acyl-CoA; this is then carried into the mitochondria under the influence of carnitine, which acts as a carrier. Acyl-CoA is eventually oxidized in the citrate cycle with the release of ATP.

During hypoxia, activated long-chain fatty acids may accumulate in the myoplasm and in the mitochondria. This may lead to the build-up of acylcarnitine, which has been implicated in the development of arrhythmias and inhibition of the $Na^+/K^+$ pump.

After formation, acetyl-CoA enters the citrate cycle and $NADH_2$ is formed. This yields the hydrogen atoms for the cytochrome chain, where ADP is converted to ATP by the process of oxidative phosphorylation. Produced in the mitochondria, ATP is then transported to the cytosol and is thus available as a source of energy for cellular processes.

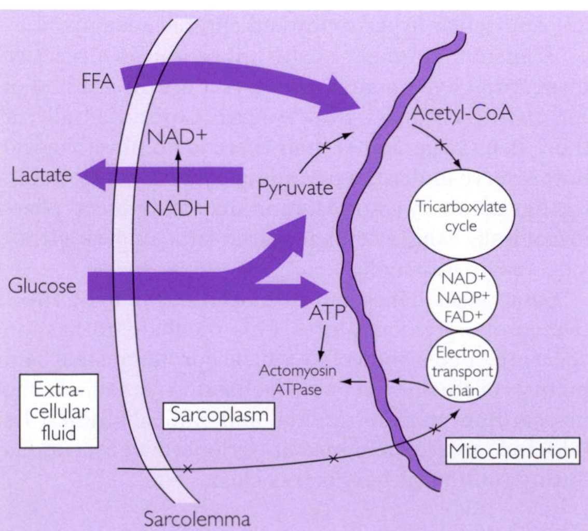


**Figure 20.22** A schematic representation of metabolic uptake and excretion by a myocardial cell. During aerobic metabolism the heart extracts lactate; during anaerobic metabolism it produces lactate. FFA, free fatty acid.

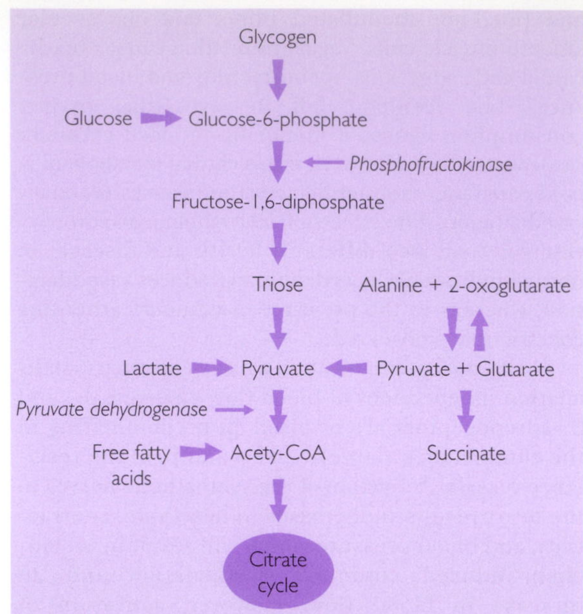


**Figure 20.23** Myocardial metabolism. During normal aerobic cardiac metabolism pyruvate is transformed by pyruvate dehydrogenase into acetyl-CoA, which is then used for ATP production. Under hypoxic conditions, oxidative phosphorylation is reduced and acetyl-CoA levels are increased, leading to inhibition of pyruvate dehydrogenase and increased pyruvate levels in the sarcoplasm. Increased hydrogen ion production leads to the conversion of pyruvate to lactate.

### *Measurement of coronary blood flow and myocardial energetics*

Measurement of coronary blood flow and myocardial metabolism is useful in assessing the safety of anaesthetic drugs and techniques, particularly in patients with ischaemic heart disease. However, measurement of coronary blood flow in patients is very difficult, although it can be done in experimental animals. It demands a number of assumptions and approximations that make the techniques vary greatly in accuracy both within and between patients.

#### *Radioactive microspheres*

This method involves injecting radioactive microspheres into the blood stream, and relies on the assumption that, although larger than red blood cells, they are distributed to the tissues in the same manner. Microspheres then become trapped in the myocardium and tissue biopsies can reveal the level of uptake. This technique is confined to experimental animals.

#### *Inert gas clearance*

This method is theoretically simple, relying on the arteriovenous difference in gas content. Coronary blood flow can then be calculated from the Kety–Schmidt equations. The gas indicator must be physiologically inert, and coronary blood flow must be stable during the period of saturation and desaturation. This may take up to 20 min. Also, venous blood from the entire region in question must be sampled (for the global myocardium, coronary sinus samples are used) and the partition coefficients for the gas in fat, red blood cells, plasma, and the myocardium must be known. Radioactive xenon has been used successfully, and this technique, although cumbersome, is used in human studies.

*Electromagnetic flowmeters, and Doppler flowmeters*
The physical principles dealing with these are described elsewhere (see Chapter 37, Figures 37.67 and 37.69). Electromagnetic flowmeters have been used to measure flow in humans, and devices that circumscribe coronary grafts have been used. The Doppler flow probe is more exciting, and probes have been developed that are small enough to enter epicardial coronary arteries.

*Thermodilution*
Despite initial enthusiasm and hence wide usage, the technique of coronary sinus reverse thermodilution produces results of widely varying accuracy and reproducibility. The technique relies on cannulation of the coronary sinus, and the injection of indicator at known temperature and flow rate. From the change in temperature in the blood/injectate mixture measured downstream, the coronary sinus blood flow rate can be calculated. In practice, this technique is critically dependent on accurate and fixed placement of the catheter within the coronary venous system, and this may vary even with small changes in heart size.

*Other techniques*
Newer imaging techniques, including positron emission tomography (PET), digital subtraction angiography (DSA), and ultra-fast-computed tomography (CT), may be effective in measuring global coronary blood flow in humans, but have yet to be proved.

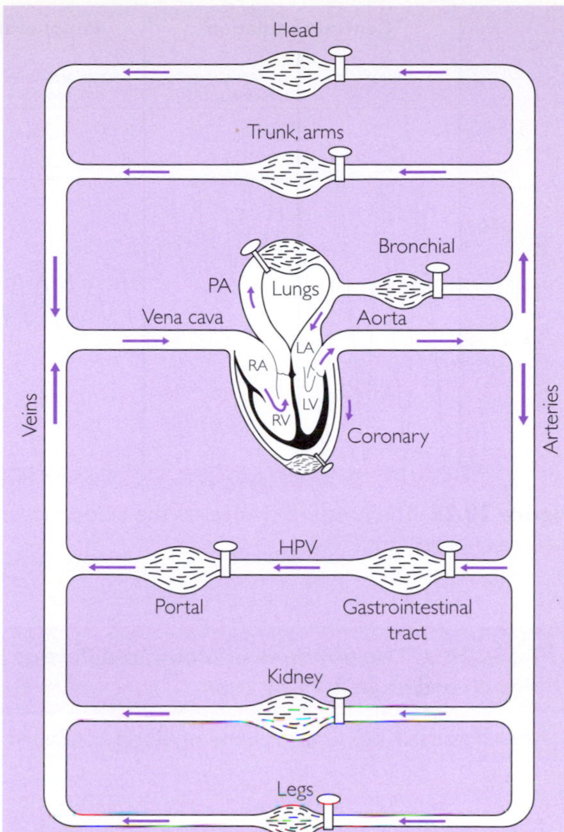


**Figure 20.24** The arrangement of the blood flow to the major organs. LA, left atrium; LV, left ventricle; PA, pulmonary artery; HPV, hepatic portal vein; RA, right atrium; RV, right ventricle.

## THE PERIPHERAL VASCULATURE AND PERIPHERAL BLOOD FLOW

### Blood flow distribution

The heart, major vessels, and arterioles effect the transport of blood to all the organs. The capillary network allows nutrients, dissolved gases, and excretory products to be exchanged and other systems (e.g. the immune response) to function properly. Waste products are transported to specialized organs of excretion for exchange and elimination. The blood flow to each organ is controlled by numerous factors, including each organ's metabolic needs. Blood flow to the major organs is arranged in parallel from the aorta and major vessels as shown in Figure 20.24. Individual organ blood flows can be measured by the Fick principle (see Chapter 37, Figure 37.68) or by other specialized techniques as described in their respective chapters.

### Components of the circulation

The pressure changes as blood moves through the circulation are shown in Figure 20.25. After ejection of the SV, the elastic nature of large arteries allows them to act as blood and energy storage sites. Consequently, when blood enters the aorta during systole, the aorta dilates slightly under pressure and then elastic recoil during diastole dissipates the stored energy and maintains the pressure, forcing the blood onwards and ensuring effective transport. This accessory pump has been termed the 'Windkessel effect'.

The small arteries and arterioles determine the systemic vascular resistance. The terminal arterioles and small arcade arterioles open and close to regulate capillary blood flow. These vessels may therefore act as physiological sphincters and determine the area of capillary bed perfused. They are under neural, hormonal, and local control (see later). The small venules also help to regulate capillary hydrostatic pressure and thereby affect fluid exchange in the capillaries. The larger venules and veins contain most of the blood volume and act as capacitance vessels, with the ability to dilate and accommodate even more blood volume, thereby controlling venous return to the heart. The proportionate volumes of various parts of the circulation and their cross-sections are given in Table 20.3.

Average blood flow ($\dot{V}$ in cm/s) in each part of the vascular bed can be easily calculated by dividing the volume flow by the cross-sectional area. Thus the aorta, with a small cross-sectional area (3.5–4.5 $cm^2$) will have a high average flow velocity (approximately 30 cm/s). The cross-sectional area of the capillary network is huge and thus the flow velocity is very small. This allows gases and metabolites to be exchanged easily across a relatively short length of capillaries. The flow velocity increases as the blood drains into the venous network, and blood returning to the right atrium via the

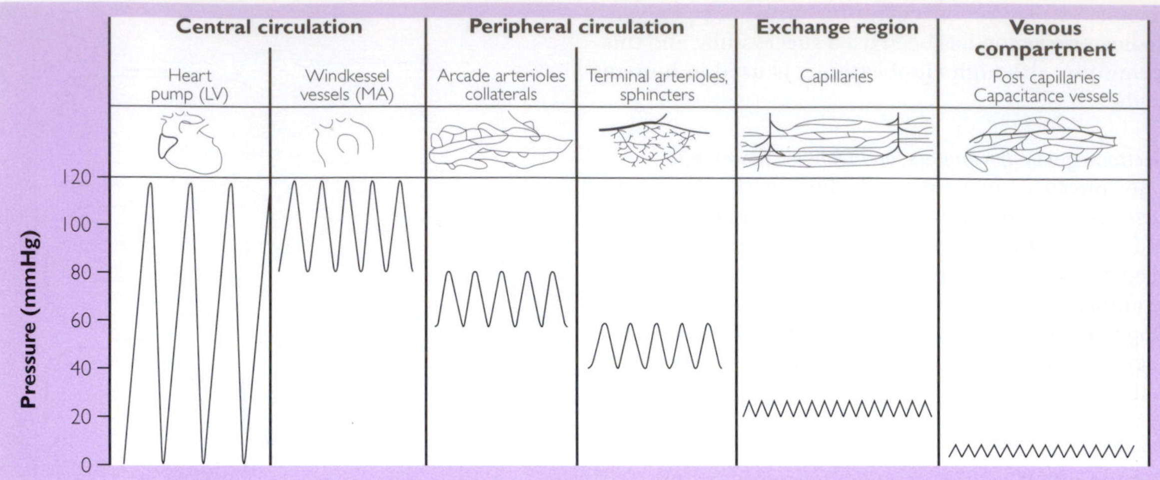


**Figure 20.25** The pressure changes as the blood moves from the left ventricle (LV) through the systemic circulation. MA, major arteries.

**Table 20.3 The volumes of blood in different parts of the circulation as a percentage of the total blood volume in a 70-kg man**

| Vessel/vascular bed | Volume of blood contained (%) | Approximate cross-sectional area ($cm^2$) |
|---|---|---|
| Aorta | 2 | 4 |
| Major arteries | 8 | 20 |
| Arterioles | 1–2 | 400 |
| Capillaries | 5 | 4200 |
| Venules | } | 4000 |
| Major veins | } 50–60 | 40 |
| Vena cava | } | 18 |
| Cardiac vessels | 8–10 | |
| Pulmonary vessels | 12–15 | |

The two most important messages are that most of the blood volume is in the venous system and to note the large cross-section of the microvasculature. These data should be regarded as guidelines rather than precise figures.

superior and inferior vena cavae has a velocity approximately half of that in the aorta, albeit at a much reduced pressure.

The blood flow into the pulmonary artery is also equal to the blood flow into the ascending aorta, but at approximately 20% of the pressure. The concept of high blood flow at reduced pressure is central to our understanding of the haemodynamics of the venous circulation and the right side of the heart.

The organ blood flow at rest and under conditions of exercise or high metabolic activity may vary greatly, and the flow reserve available under such conditions also varies greatly between different organs. The extremes are seen between the kidney, whose high resting blood flow simply represents a reflection of its necessary filtration and excretory functions, and the salivary glands, whose resting blood flow may be increased dramatically during a meal. Variability in blood flow in different organs is summarized in Figure 20.26. Note the variations possible in the myocardium and skeletal muscle: without this facility physical exercise would be impossible.

The capillary network from target organs usually drains into venules, then into veins, and finally into the superior and inferior vena cavae, before returning to the right atrium. There are three exceptions:

1. The bronchial circulation arises from the aorta and the capillaries drain into the left atrium, thereby ensuring that the left side of the heart pumps marginally more blood than the right side.
2. The hepatic portal circulation receives its blood supply (70% of total hepatic blood supply in health) from postcapillary network draining the gastrointestinal tract, before draining into venules contributing to the inferior vena cava (see Chapter 28).
3. The pituitary portal system (see Chapter 29) is numerically a very small flow but functionally very important.

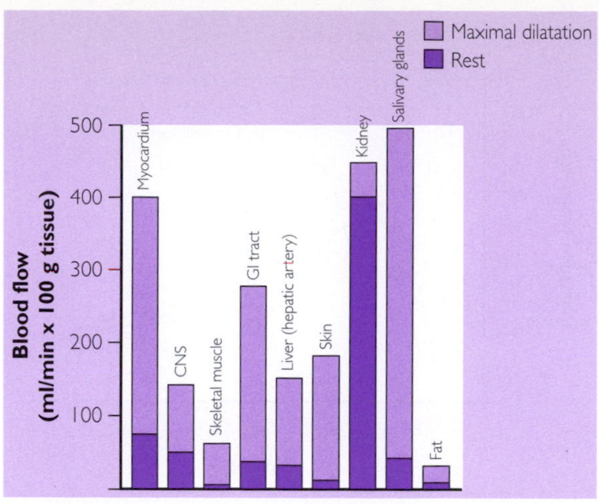


**Figure 20.26** Regional blood flows at rest and at maximum dilatation per 100 g tissue for each organ shown. Note the lack of reserve in the kidney.

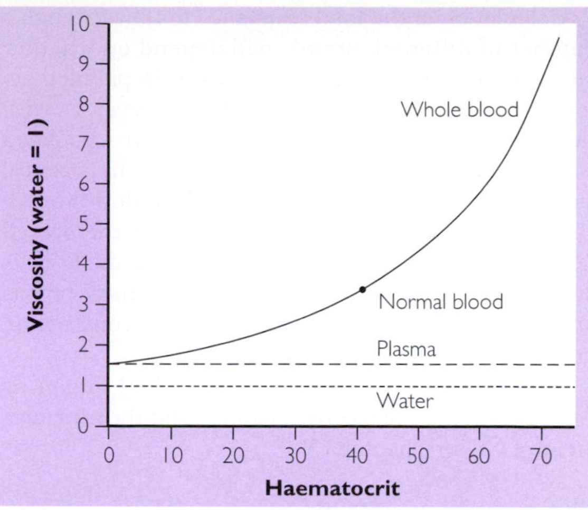


**Figure 20.27** A comparison of the viscosities of water, plasma, and whole blood. Note the dependence of whole blood viscosity on haematocrit. (See also Chapter 37, Figures 37.44 and 37.45).

### The dynamics of peripheral blood flow

A number of well-defined physical properties govern the flow of liquids through tubes. However, blood vessels are not simple rigid tubes and blood is not a clear fluid. The solid content of blood, namely the blood cells, has an important influence on blood flow through small vessels and capillaries. The cell and protein content of blood render it relatively viscous in comparison with water. The flow of fluids through pipes and the viscous behaviour of blood are described in Chapter 37.

The SI unit of viscosity is Pa·s, and the cgs unit is the poise. The practical unit is the centipoise (cP); water at room temperature has a value of 1 cP (10 Pa·s). Relative viscosity refers to the viscosity of a liquid compared with the viscosity of water at the same temperature. At normal haematocrit, blood has a relative viscosity of 40–200 Pa·s (4–20 cP), depending on its flow properties (see Figures 37.44 and 37.45). The comparison of blood viscosity with that of water and plasma at a typical shear rate is shown in Figure 20.27.

Although whole blood does not behave like a newtonian fluid, the deformability of red cells under normal conditions tends to limit the increase in viscosity. Under certain conditions (e.g. sickle-cell disease) the red cell becomes much less deformable as a result of polymerization and gel formation of the haemoglobin, and viscosity may increase. Similarly, white cells are much less deformable and large increases in white cell count, as well as red cells and proteins, may increase viscosity.

Although described fully in Chapter 37, it is relevant to remind readers of two important principles of laminar flow:

1. Flow is inversely related to viscosity, i.e. if viscosity is doubled and other factors held constant, flow is halved.
2. If the radius of the tube doubles and other factors are held constant, flow will increase 16-fold. Perhaps more importantly, if the radius is halved, for example as a result of vasoconstriction, flow is reduced 16-fold.

A non-dimensional number, the Reynold's number (see Chapter 37) determines the transition from laminar to turbulent flow. When the Reynold's number exceeds 2000, blood flow usually changes from laminar to turbulent. Turbulence will tend to occur with increasing flow velocity (in larger blood vessels) and with decreasing viscosity. If the size of a large blood vessel is artificially reduced by compression, then turbulent conditions may be created and an audible signal detected. This is one theory of the basis of blood pressure measurement by sphygmomanometry, which detects tapping Korotkoff's sounds beyond the cuff. Arterial bruits may be heard in areas of arterial disease for similar reasons. Also, if blood flow is high (e.g. high CO) or viscosity very low (e.g. anaemia), or there is a combination of the two, then turbulent conditions may be created and cardiac flow murmurs become apparent in the absence of vascular pathology.

The resistance to liquid flow through a tube is related to the driving pressure and flow rate through the tube. This relationship is analogous to the flow of current through an electrical circuit as defined by Ohm's law:

$$E = I \times R$$

where $E$ is the electromotive force (pressure), $I$ the current (flow), and $R$ the resistance.

In the context of the resistance of blood flow through a vascular bed, the equation may be written:

$$\text{Flow } (\dot{Q}) = \frac{\text{Input pressure} - \text{Output pressure}}{R}$$

This equation holds good for cardiac output or regional blood flow where it can be summarized as:

$$\text{Flow} = \frac{\text{Pressure drop across vascular bed}}{\text{Resistance of vascular bed}}$$

Calculation of the total resistance to flow through a number of different circuits will depend on whether these circuits are arranged in series or in parallel. In-series resistances simply summate. However, as with electrical circuits, resistances in parallel are calculated by calculating the sum of their reciprocal. In practical terms, this means that resistance to blood flow through one organ may change markedly without the overall vascular resistance being greatly affected. This is important because vasodilatation to one or more organs may not be accompanied by balancing vasoconstriction to others.

Measurement of flows to individual organ is described in their respective chapters and the measurement of CO in Chapter 77.

### The arterial waveform

With the use of intra-arterial blood pressure monitoring in clinical anaesthesia, understanding of the arterial waveform, its variants, and the factors responsible for change are important if blood pressure is to be measured correctly. The methodology of intra-arterial measurement is described in Chapter 39, Figure 39.53. The arterial pressure wave is shown in Figure 20.28, together with some of its variations.

One factor that is often not appreciated is that the peak systolic pressure is higher and the pulse pressure larger in the distal circulation (e.g. femoral, radial artery) when compared with the aorta (Figure 20.29). This occurs because pulse pressure waves are reflected back towards the central aorta and these returning wavefronts interact with oncoming waves. Factors that tend to cause summation of these waveforms are the stiffness and elasticity of the blood vessels, the diameter of the vessel, and phase synchronicity. As the waveform progresses down the vascular tree, there is a progressive increase in the amplitude of the systolic pressure and the pulse pressure, the time to the peak pressure diminishes, the systolic component of the waveform narrows, and a secondary positive wave appears. Harmonic analysis shows an increasing amplitude as the distance from the arch of the aorta increases. These combine to produce a wider pulse pressure, and an apparently elevated peak systolic pressure, but with a gradually decreasing mean pressure. Under some conditions however, for example severe peripheral vasoconstriction or damping, the peripheral pulse pressures may be much lower than that of a pulse waveform measured at the aorta (see Chapter 12, Figure 12.22). As a practical point, if the arterial pressure wave shows no signs of resonance and displays the dicrotic notch, it is usually recording accurately.

The outcome of altering systemic pressure, vascular compliance, pulse pressure, heart rate, and SV depends enormously on the circumstances. For example, in health, an increased SV is likely to be associated with a modest increase in pulse pressure whereas, if vascular compliance is reduced, as in an elderly ather-

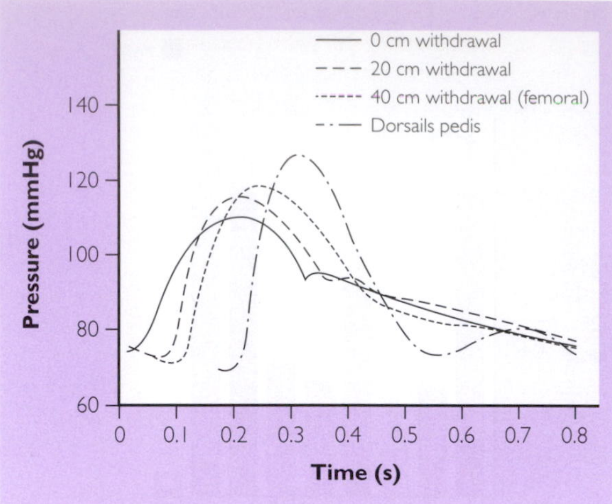


**Figure 20.29** The blood pressure recorded as a cardiac catheter is withdrawn from the left ventricle through its entry point in the femoral artery. The dorsalis pedis trace is taken from a second line. (Adapted from Guyton AC. *Textbook of Medical Physiology*, 4th edn. Philadelphia: WB Saunders, 1971,222.)

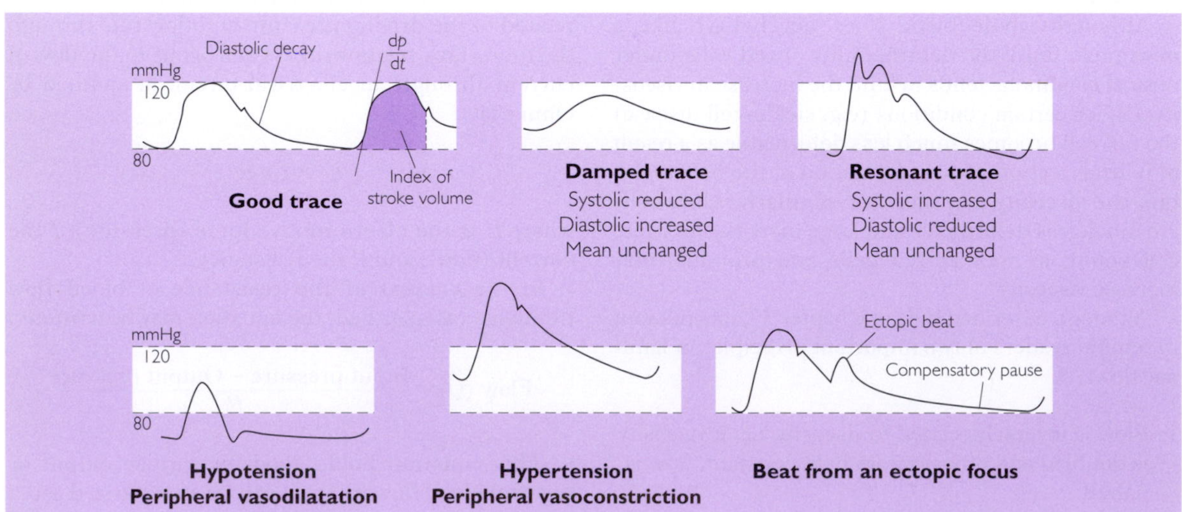


**Figure 20.28** A selection of recorded arterial pressure waves. A good trace from a normotensive patient is shown at the top left.

osclerotic person, the same SV is associated with a much larger increase in pulse pressure. There are innumerable combinations of such effects which need to be analysed on an individual basis.

MAP usually remains relatively constant, is unaffected by resonance or damping (Figure 20.28), and falls with distance from the heart. For this reason, on some occasions, MAP is a more useful measurement than systolic blood pressure (SBP), even though peak systolic pressure is more closely related to other important haemodynamic indices, e.g. myocardial oxygen demand. In modern equipment the MAP is usually calculated electronically by integration of the pressure wave (see Chapter 37, Figure 37.22b), but it can be approximated by the equation:

$$\text{MAP} = \text{DAP} + \frac{1}{3}(\text{SAP} - \text{DAP})$$

where DAP is diastolic arterial presssure.

The interrelationship of pressure, flow, and resistance, outlined by the modified Ohm's law and applied to circulatory physiology, assumes that pressure and flow are constant. When pressure and flow are pulsatile, the term 'resistance' should be replaced by impedance, which may be thought of simply as the resistance to flow in a pulsatile circuit. When flow is pulsatile, the impedance includes not only the opposition to flow afforded by friction but also that caused by vascular compliance and the mass of blood. Calculations of aortic impedance are complicated and require Fourier analysis of high-fidelity aortic pressure and flow data.

### The right atrial (central venous) pressure

The right atrial pressure (approximately 5 mmHg mean) is used as a surrogate for the filling pressure of the right ventricle and, in health, can also be used to estimate the left atrial pressure which is usually 4–5 mmHg higher. It must be measured relative to a fixed point because of its dependence on gravity. The usual convention is to take it at the midaxillary line with the patient lying supine.

Poor correlation between right and left atrial pressures has been noted in:

- patients with a history of LV failure or low EF (< 40%);
- patients with LV dys-synergy (especially after myocardial infarction);
- bundle-branch blocks;
- patients with tamponade or constrictive pericarditis;
- patients with pulmonary hypertension.

The normally accepted morphology of the CVP wave is shown in Figure 20.30. The source of the named waves is given in the caption. Although this is the classic description, it has to be said that, in clinical practice, the separate components are not always easily identified. Its temporal relationship to other parts of the cardiac cycle can be seen in Figure 20.16.

Abnormalities of the CVP wave occur in clinical practice for a variety of reasons. They are summarized in Table 20.4.

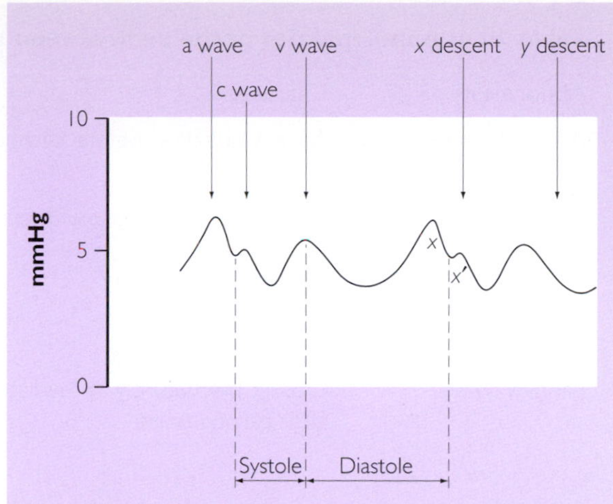


**Figure 20.30** The central venous pressure wave. Two peaks (a and v) and two troughs (*x* and *y*) are classically described during every cardiac cycle. The a wave is the result of atrial contraction and precedes the carotid pulse. The v wave follows the carotid pulse and represents the rise in atrial pressure caused by continued venous filling while the tricuspid valve is closed. The c wave is an inconstant and variable feature, which is associated with transmitted atrial pulsation and/or deformation of the atrium from bulging of the tricuspid valve during early systole.

## BLOOD PRESSURE REGULATION AND NEUROHUMORAL CONTROL OF THE CIRCULATION

The circulation is regulated by local, neural, and hormonal control systems. Local controls are described in the chapters for individual organs. Neural and hormonal influences form a complex series of systems, which respond both regionally and globally to maintain a level of CO that meets the body's demands. Neural control is able to react as changes occur whereas hormonal control is essentially more long term.

### Neural control

This may be divided into afferent (input) and efferent (output) limbs. The afferent limbs are shown in Figure 20.31. The efferent supply travels by the sympathetic and parasympathetic nervous systems which are described in detail in Chapter 23. For convenience of reference they are reproduced diagrammatically in Figure 20.32.

#### *The afferent system*

This comprises five inputs:

1. The carotid sinus baroreceptors consist of a dilatation at the base of each internal carotid artery close to the junction of the external carotid artery. Fibres run in a branch of the glossopharyngeal (cranial IX) nerve.
2. The carotid body chemoreceptors are small organs consisting of rounded clumps of polyhedral cells near the carotid sinuses. They are highly vascular and respond to chemical stimuli. Afferent signals run in fibres passing to the cranial nerve IX.

**Table 20.4 Abnormalities of the central venous pressure wave**

| Abnormality | Character | Significance |
|---|---|---|
| Absent 'a' wave | Absent pulsation before carotid pulse | No coordinated atrial contraction, atrial fibrillation |
| Large 'a' wave | Occurs before systole with every cardiac cycle<br>Requires sinus rhythm | Powerful atrial contraction to force blood through narrow orifice (tricuspid valve stenosis or atresia) or into stiff, hypertrophied ventricle (pulmonary valve stenosis or pulmonary hypertension) |
| Large 'v' wave | Occurs prematurely, immediately after carotid pulse | Represents reflux of blood into the right atrium during right ventricular systole because of tricuspid incompetence; usually secondary to cardiac failure |
| 'Cannon' waves | Large, abrupt waves synchronous with the carotid pulse (i.e. at the timing of the 'c' wave) | Implies atrial contraction against a closed tricuspid valve<br>If regular is the result of nodal rhythm and retrograde atrial conduction; if intermittent, complete heart block |

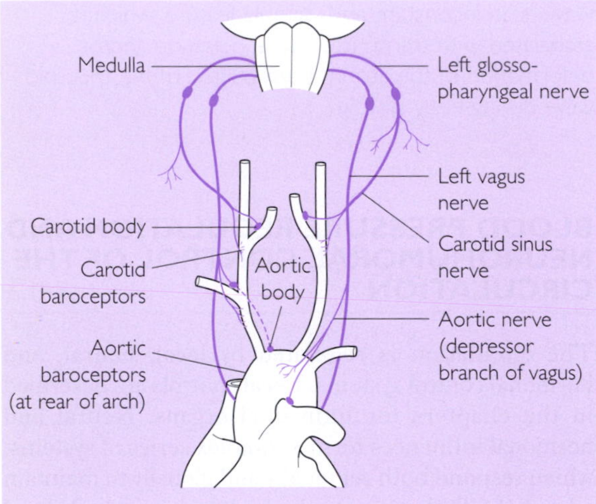


**Figure 20.31** The afferent neural connections of the aortic and carotid sinus baroreceptors and chemoreceptors. The baroreceptors and chemoreceptors are close to but distinct from each other.

3. The aortic baroreceptors are a network of branching nerves, which innervate the aortic wall in the region of the aortic arch, and the carotid and subclavian arteries. They are similar to the carotid sinus receptors, but their afferent fibres run via the vagus (cranial nerve X).
4. The aortic body chemoreceptors lie mainly near the aortic arch and the pulmonary artery, but are also found on the coronary arteries. Structurally, they resemble the carotid bodies. Afferent fibres run via the vagus nerve
5. Finally, baroreceptors and chemoreceptors can be found in the lungs, atria, and ventricles, and at the junctions of the vena cavae and pulmonary veins. Afferent fibres run via the sympathetic and parasympathetic trunks.

#### *The efferent system*

As indicated above, this consists of sympathetic and parasympathetic fibres and is described in detail in

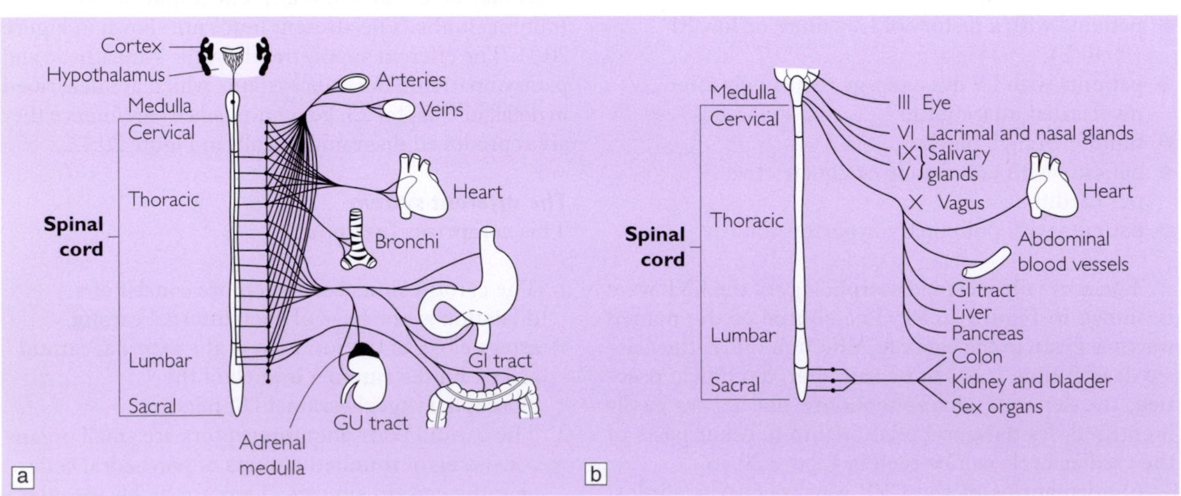


**Figure 20.32** A diagrammatic representation of (a) the sympathetic nervous system and its connections, and (b) the parasympathetic nervous system and its connections.

Chapter 23. A summary is presented here and reference should be made to Figure 20.32.

*Cardiac actions*

Sympathetic fibres from the CNS traverse the spinal cord and synapse in the sympathetic chain, and in cervical and paravertebral ganglia. Efferent fibres from these ganglia provide a rich network of postganglionic nerve endings innervating the atria, ventricles, sinus, and atrioventricular nodes. The parasympathetic (vagal) fibres synapse in ganglia in the heart and innervate the atria, sinus, and atrioventricular nodes, with a few fibres also supplying the ventricles.

Heart rate control is closely regulated by autonomic innervation. At rest, parasympathetic tone predominates on the sinus node, the rate of the denervated heart being approximately 100 beats/min. Thus, parasympathetic blockade may produce a significant increase in heart rate. The AV node is also richly innervated by sympathetic and parasympathetic fibres, but the balance between the two appears to be more evenly spread.

*Peripheral actions*

The efferent connections to the peripheral circulation consist of vasoconstrictor fibres, discovered by Claude Bernard in 1852. Constrictor fibres, arise from groups of nerve cells situated in the intermediolateral columns of the spinal grey matter, extending from the first thoracic to the second or third lumbar segments. Axons from these cells synapse with neurons lying in the sympathetic ganglia outside the cerebrospinal axis. Vasoconstrictor fibres to the head and neck are conveyed from the sympathetic chain through the plexus and via peripheral nerve trunks, including cervical and certain cranial nerves. The vessels of the abdomen and pelvis are supplied with fibres that pass along the vascular walls from the plexus surrounding the aorta and its branches.

*Postganglionic adrenergic nerve endings*

These contain norepinephrine as the neurotransmitter, and they have been identified in all blood vessels except true capillaries. Vasoconstrictor fibres are of major importance in the short-term homoeostasis of blood pressure, and are the mechanism whereby baroreceptors have their effect. The normal resting state involves a degree of vasoconstriction, and vasodilatation is predominantly the result of inhibition of constriction. Some vasodilator fibres have, however, been identified, either as parasympathetic fibres innervating cranial (cerebral vessels, sweat glands) and sacral (external genitalia, bladder, rectum) structures or in some species as a separate sympathetic cholinergic system.

The anatomy of the central connections important in circulatory control is complex. Five areas of the CNS are of major importance: the spinal cord, medulla oblongata, hypothalamus, cerebellum, and cerebral cortex. The role of these areas is to integrate different inputs and adjust the tonic autonomic outflow appropriately.

### Humoral control

Endocrine systems and the controls that they exert are described in detail in Chapter 29; a summary is given below of the main points relevant to circulatory regulation.

A reduction in blood pressure leads to the sympathetically mediated release of renin from the granular cells of the juxtaglomerular apparatus. Renin acts on angiotensinogen to produce a decapeptide, angiotensin I. Angiotensin I is an inactive prohormone, but is converted into angiotensin II by removing two amino acids. This is brought about by ACE. Angiotensin II has two important actions: first, it stimulates the adrenal cortex to secrete aldosterone, to cause salt and water retention and, second, angiotensin II is a powerful vasoconstrictor that may serve to increase peripheral vascular resistance and hence elevate blood pressure.

Other hormonal regulatory mechanisms include antidiuretic hormone (ADH; vasopressin) and atrial natriuretic factor (ANF). ADH is secreted by the posterior pituitary in response to an increase in plasma osmolality brought about by dehydration. It acts as a powerful vasoconstrictor. ANF, on the other hand, is secreted by the atria in response to atrial distension, as may occur as a result of fluid overload in congestive heart failure. ANF produces a diuresis and loss of circulating fluid.

Finally, other endocrine organs are essential for the maintenance of blood pressure. Although these do not constitute direct blood pressure control mechanisms, normal function of the anterior pituitary, adrenal cortex, adrenal medulla, and thyroid is essential for blood pressure homoeostasis. Uncorrected complete adrenal failure is incompatible with life.

### Regulation of blood pressure

Neural control mechanisms are responsible for the short-term control of blood pressure whereas long-term control of blood pressure and blood volume is brought about by humoral mechanisms.

Regulation via baroreceptors is the most important method of short-term blood pressure control and an example of negative feedback. Increased blood pressure causes stretching of the blood vessel wall, which leads to an increased rate of discharge and increase in nerve traffic from the baroreceptors to the brain stem, particularly the medulla. This is shown in Figure 20.33. The integrating centres in the medulla and on the floor of the fourth ventricle then inhibit sympathetic action on the heart and peripheral vasculature (Figure 20.34). Cardiac contractility and heart rate decrease, and the degree of vasoconstrictor tone on both the resistance and capacitance vessels is decreased, and hence the traditional tetralogy of reduced cardiac vigour, bradycardia, vasodilatation, and venodilatation. It is important to remember that vasodilatation occurs predominantly as a result of the inhibition of vasoconstriction. Falls in blood pressure produce the reverse of these changes.

Baroreceptors show adaptation to sustained changes in blood pressure over 2–3 days. Sensitivity is greatest within the physiological blood pressure range (50–170 mmHg) and responds to both absolute pressure and rate of change of pressure. Baroreceptor sensitivity may be affected by a number of factors, including drugs, disease (hypertension, heart failure), and anaesthetics.

Chemoreceptors are not as important as baroreceptors in the control of blood pressure because they predominantly respond to hypoxia, carbon dioxide, and

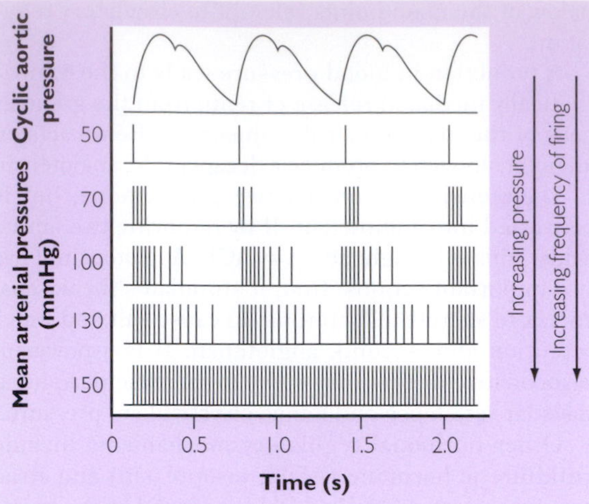


**Figure 20.33** The firing rate of a single afferent nerve fibre from the carotid sinus at various arterial pressures. Normal aortic pressure cycles are shown to demonstrate the changes in firing rate throughout the cycle.

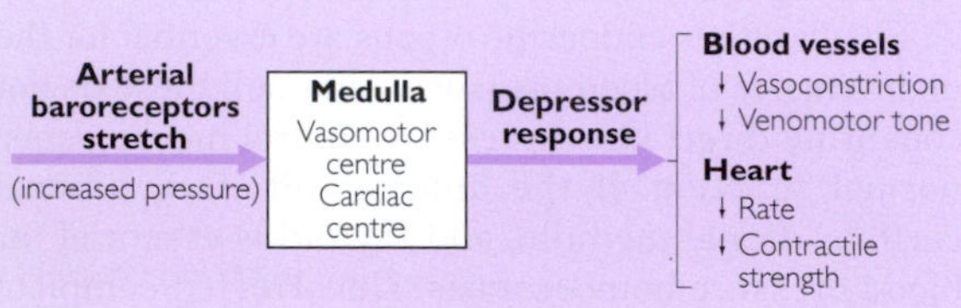


**Figure 20.34** A diagrammatic representation of the response and integrating functions of the medulla to a change in signal from the arterial baroreceptors.

pH changes. They begin to contribute to control when the blood pressure is below 80 mmHg, possibly secondary to changes in blood chemistry associated with hypotension. The chemoreceptor regulation of respiration is dealt with elsewhere (see Chapters 21 and 26). There is also some cross-reactivity in the CNS between baroreceptor and chemoreceptor input.

The body's response to haemorrhage is described in Chapter 14. The effect of secreted catecholamines is covered in Chapter 23 and later in this chapter. When hypotension is very severe, what is often termed the 'CNS ischaemic reflex' can be triggered. This reflex is not responsible for regulation of normal blood pressure, does not become active until the blood pressure has fallen to 50 mmHg, and is maximal at 20 mmHg. It consists of massive sympathetic nervous system activity with maximal vasoconstriction and is thought to be initiated by the failure to remove carbon dioxide from the vasomotor centre.

The blood pressure can be affected over minutes and hours by three hormonal mechanisms, as described in Chapters 23 and 29:

1. catecholamine release;
2. renin–angiotensin-induced vasoconstriction;
3. antidiuretic-induced vasoconstriction.

Long-term mechanisms for the regulation of systemic blood pressure occur slowly but do not adapt. Resetting of the 'set point' is one theory of the cause of essential hypertension. The predominant role in long-term control is carried out by the renal system via its control of total body fluid and sodium. This is described in Chapter 25.

### Myocardial receptors

Endogenous neurohumoral ligands and drugs may affect the contractile state of the myocardium and tonic state of vascular smooth muscle.

Up to five components can be involved in transmembrane signalling, including:

- receptor interaction;
- G protein coupling;
- effector producing a second messenger;
- phosphorylation of regulator protein;
- physiological effects.

These are described in detail in Chapters 18, 19, and 69. Particular aspects relevant to myocardial cells are described here.

A large number of cell membrane receptors have been shown to be present in the human myocardium, as shown in Figure 20.35. Work on receptors is, however, constantly revealing new aspects of their function and this account should essentially be regarded as a summary of the more important facets of the subject.

Myocardial receptors may be linked to $G_s$, $G_i$, or $G_q$ proteins. Interaction with $G_s$ proteins causes the hydrolysis of GTP to GMP and the activation of adenylyl cyclase (described in Chapters 19 and 69), leading to the conversion of ATP to cAMP. Interaction with $G_i$ protein leads to an inhibition of hydrolysis of GTP and inhibition of activation of adenylyl cyclase. This is important, because it establishes that myocardial contractility can be enhanced and inhibited by activation of the appropriate G proteins, and not simply inhibited by receptor-blocking drugs that prevent interaction with $G_s$ proteins. Interaction with $G_q$ protein leads to activation of phospholipase C and the subsequent hydrolysis of phosphoinositol diphosphate as described. So far no G protein inhibiting phospholipase C activation has been identified.

Of the different cell-membrane receptors that have been identified in the human myocardium, β-adrenoceptors, histamine $H_2$-receptors, VIP, prostaglandin $E_1$, and 5-hydroxytryptamine (serotonin) $5HT_4$ receptors have all been shown to interact with $G_s$ protein, leading to the activation of adenylyl cyclase and the production of cAMP. However, the distribution of these receptors within the myocardium, and the results of activation, are not uniform. Although the effects of activation of other receptors may be significant in disease when β-receptors have been down-regulated and reduced in number, the effects of β-receptor activation far outstrips that of others in the normal adult.

Myocardial β-receptors may become desensitized by continuous receptor occupancy. This may initially involve uncoupling of the receptor from the G protein, a process that occurs in seconds to minutes and is aided by second messenger kinases and β-adrenergic

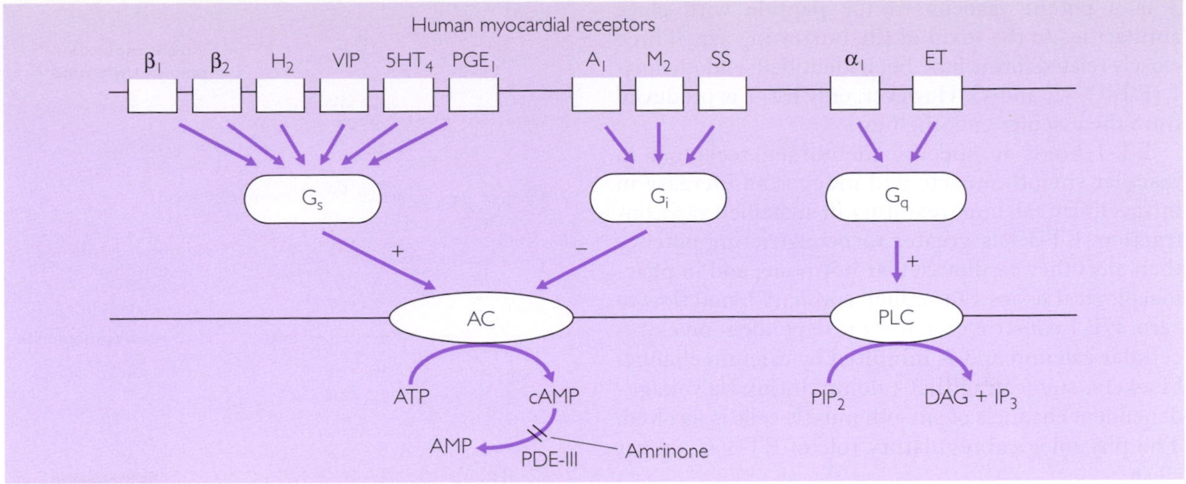


**Figure 20.35** G-protein-coupled receptors and signal transmission pathways in the human myocardium. α and β are adrenoceptors; $H_2$, histamine receptor; VIP, vasoactive intestinal peptide receptor; $5HT_4$, serotonin receptor; $PGE_1$, prostaglandin receptor; $A_1$, adenosine receptor; $M_2$, muscarinic receptor; SS, somatostatin receptor; ET, endothelin receptor; AC, adenylyl cyclase; PLC, phospholipase C; $PIP_2$, phosphatidylinositol diphosphate; DAG, diacylglycerol; $IP_3$, inositol triphosphate; PDE, phosphodiesterase. (See text for details.)

receptor kinase. The receptor is then internalized (or sequestrated) and, if this process continues for days, actual receptor numbers fall (down-regulation). Both increased sequestration and decreased receptor synthesis may cause down-regulation, which is commonly seen in patients with chronic heart failure and high circulating catecholamine levels. However, desensitization is a more acute phenomenon and explains the relative insensitivity to the heart after cardiopulmonary bypass.

$M_2$ (muscarinic), $A_1$ (adenosine), and SS (somatostatin) receptors are also present and activation of these receptors activates $G_i$ protein, which inhibits the hydrolysis of GTP and hence reduces the activation of adenylyl cyclase. Agonist binding at $\alpha_1$-adrenergic and endothelin receptors leads to activation of $G_q$ protein and activation of phospholipase C.

Activation of adenylyl cyclase and the subsequent hydrolysis of ATP to cAMP lead to a variety of intracellular effects, including activation of protein kinases and phosphorylation at a number of sites. These processes have a significant influence on myocardial energy mobilization and utilization. In addition, cAMP production leads to phosphorylation of the cell membrane voltage-gated L-type calcium channel, leading to an increase in open state probability and calcium entry into the cell. Diacylglycerol (DAG) has similar effects via activation of protein kinase C. Entry of calcium ions into the cell facilitates calcium release from the sarcoplasmic reticulum, which may also be directly influenced by inositol triphosphate, and more calcium becomes available for attaining the activated form of tropomyosin– troponin, thus leading to an increase in contractility. Mechanisms that interfere with the reuptake or extrusion of calcium may also enhance the effects of calcium intracellularly. However, interference with mechanisms of calcium homoeostasis may also lead to high intracellular calcium and calcium overload, and to adverse effects including arrhythmias.

### Endothelium

The endothelium is very far from an inert blood vessel lining and further details of it can be found in Chapter 67. It has synthetic and metabolic capabilities, and may respond to a variety of substances that may induce vasodilatation.

The first vasoactive substance identified from endothelium was prostacyclin ($PGI_2$), a product of arachidonic acid metabolism. $PGI_2$ production is activated by a variety of factors, including shear stress, pulsatility of flow, and hypoxia, and produces cAMP-mediated vasorelaxation. More recently, the endothelium has been shown to be essential for acetylcholine-induced vasodilatation. A labile diffusible non-prostanoid molecule has been implicated in many vasodilatory mechanisms. This molecule, called EDRF, has since been identified as nitric oxide (NO), although it is possible that there may be more than one EDRF. EDRF is continuously released from the vascular endothelium, producing a constant background of vasodilatation.

An intact endothelium may also be essential in determining the vasoactive response to a transmitter. Agents such as acetylcholine cause vasoconstriction when directly applied to the vascular smooth muscle membrane, whereas when applied to the intact endothelium the result is vasodilatation. In some circumstances, the net effect may be the result of differing and opposing actions, and EDRF activity is not confined to large or small vessels.

The endothelium can also facilitate vascular smooth muscle contraction. Endothelium-dependent vasoconstriction can be stimulated by endogenous agents including arachidonic acid and norepinephrine, pharmacological agents including calcium agonists and nicotine, physical forces (stretch, pressure), high serum potassium, and hypoxia. Three different endothelium-derived contracting factors (EDCFs) have been identified: EDCF-1 is an arachidonic acid metabolite; EDCF-2 is released by hypoxia; and EDCF-

3 is a potent vasoconstrictor peptide with close similarities to the toxin of the burrowing asp. Three closely related forms have been identified: endothelins-1 (ET-1), -2, and -3. However, only ET-1 is produced from the vascular endothelium.

ET-1 binds to specific membrane receptors in vascular smooth muscle and induces an increase in intracellular calcium, resulting in sustained vasoconstraction. ET-1 has greater vasoconstricting potency than any other cardiovascular hormone, and in pharmacological doses can reduce coronary blood flow to zero. ET-1 constrictor activity is dependent on extracellular calcium and is inhibited by calcium channel blockers, suggesting that calcium influx via voltage-dependent channels of smooth muscle cells is involved. The physiological regulatory role of ET-1 is not yet clear.

## INOTROPIC MECHANISMS AND INOTROPIC DRUGS

From 'Myocardial receptors' above, it is clear that G-protein-mediated effects play a vital part in the modulation of cardiac contractility. Drugs that have effects on cardiac contractility work through the same receptor systems, or act intracellularly on processes that are the consequence of receptor activation. For that reason it is simplest to classify inotropic mechanisms and drugs as cAMP dependent and cAMP independent

### cAMP-dependent mechanisms

#### *β-Adrenoceptor-mediated stimulation of adenylyl cyclase*

This occurs by activation of intermediate processes and second messengers after the administration of drugs such as catecholamines. β-Adrenoceptors are G-protein-coupled cell membrane receptors that activate adenylyl cyclase to produce cAMP (see Figure 20.35 and Chapters 19, 67 and 69). β-Adrenoceptor antagonists reduce contractility by competitive antagonism at the β-adrenoceptor. In this case, inhibition of $G_s$ activity, not stimulation of $G_i$ activity, reduces adenylyl cyclase activity and hence reduces contractility. Although possibly implicated in modulation of inotropic activity, inositol triphosphate ($IP_3$) and DAG are more closely involved with factors affecting vascular smooth muscle tone via the release of calcium ions and activity of calmodulin.

It should be noted that receptor activity is not constant. After activation, myocardial β-receptors may become rapidly desensitized to further stimulation. This can occur in minutes. Further adaptive changes including receptor down-regulation and alteration in density occur over a period of days.

#### *β-Adrenoceptor agonists*

β-adrenoceptor agonists that act on human myocardial receptors are principally the catecholamines, e.g. norepinephrine, epinephrine, dopamine, dobutamine, isoprenaline (isoproterenol), and dopexamine. These drugs share a number of features: they have some structural similarities (Figure 20.36), containing a benzene ring with an ethylamine side chain of varying length and complexity. A catecholamine is a sympathomimetic drug whose benzene ring portion has hydroxyl group substitutions at positions 3 and 4. They all activate different adrenoceptors to a varying degree, dependent on both the nature of the drug and the dosage used. A comparison of the effects of sympathomimetic drugs is given in Chapter 23, Table 23.11. For reference, the effects of the three oldest drugs, epinephrine, norepinephrine, and isoprenaline, given in a low therapeutic dose, are shown in Figure 20.37. At higher dose levels the α effects of epinephrine cause the blood pressure to rise considerably.

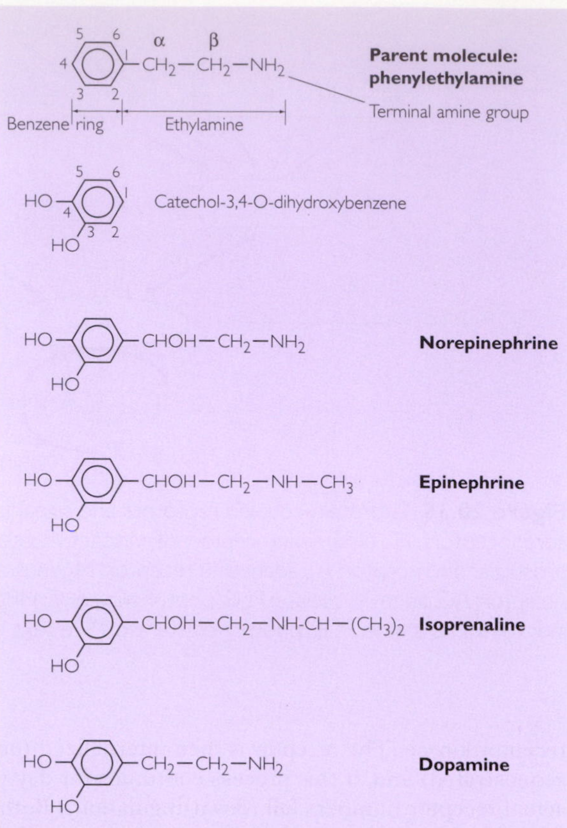


**Figure 20.36** The chemical structures of catecholamines.

#### *Norepinephrine*

Norepinephrine is a naturally occurring neurotransmitter at postganglionic neurons and in the brain, and is secreted by the adrenal medulla. Norepinephrine primarily exhibits $\alpha_1$ and $\alpha_2$ agonist activity (causing peripheral vasoconstriction in the systemic and pulmonary circulations), with significant $\beta_1$ effects also. The $\beta_1$ effects can be best observed either by infusion at very low dosage (< 0.05 μg/kg per min) or, if the dose exceeds 0.1 μg/kg per min, by simultaneous administration of an α-adrenoceptor blocker (e.g. phentolamine) to antagonize the α-agonist effects.

Norepinephrine causes an increase in indices of contractility (LV $dP/dt_{max}$) as well as increases in mean, systolic, and diastolic blood pressure, right atrial pressure, and pulmonary artery pressure. Left atrial pressure (or pulmonary capillary wedge pressure) is also usually increased. Heart rate is usually reduced as a reflex result of the increase in blood pressure. Vascular resistances (systemic, pulmonary, and coronary) are usually increased, although the effects on coronary

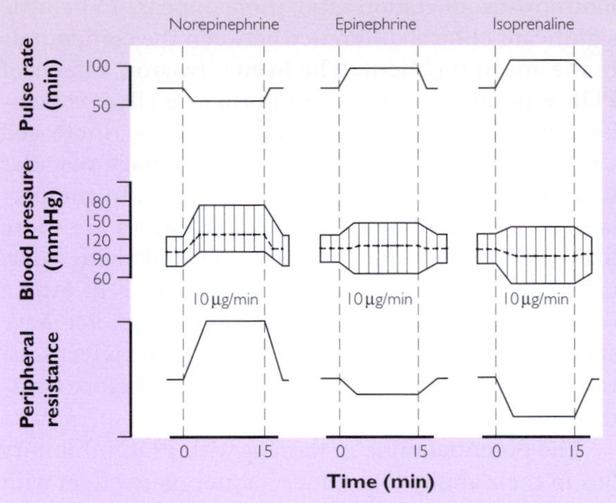


**Figure 20.37** The effects of comparable low-dose intravenous infusions of norepinephrine, epinephrine, and isoprenaline. (Adapted from Allwood MJ, Cobbold AF, Ginsburg J. *Br Med Bull* 1963;19:132.)

blood flow may vary. Myocardial oxygen demand and consumption are usually increased. Norepinephrine also causes splanchnic vasoconstriction and a reduction in renal and mesenteric blood flow. The effect on CO is usually a small increase, the increase in contractility being offset by a large increase in afterload.

The physiological responses described above may, however, be different in clinical practice, particularly in septic patients when norepinephrine infusions have been used effectively to improve vital organ perfusion. The effects on blood pressure and CO are, however, qualitatively similar.

*Epinephrine*

This is synthesized in the adrenal medulla, where it represents 80% of the catecholamines present (see Chapters 23 and 29). It is derived from the amino acid phenylalanine, and the synthetic pathway also leads to the synthesis of dopamine and norepinephrine. Epinephrine is metabolized by either oxidation by monoamine oxidase or conjugation by catechol-*O*-methyl transferase. Epinephrine is mostly secreted in the urine as vanillylmandelic acid.

Epinephrine has dose-dependent effects on α- and β-adrenoceptors. Initially $\beta_1$ effects predominate (1–2 µg/min), then mixed α and β effects are seen (2–10 µg/min), and finally α effects predominate (10–16 µg/min). Thus, the haemodynamic effects seen are dose dependent. CO is increased, but at low dosage systemic and pulmonary blood pressure may be little affected. Heart rate may not increase markedly. As the dose is increased and the α effects become more apparent, there are increases in systemic and pulmonary vascular resistance and blood pressure. Myocardial oxygen consumption is increased and splanchnic vasoconstriction occurs at high dosage. Increases in heart rate and in conduction abnormalities, including ventricular irritability, may also be seen. Epinephrine is a first-line resuscitation drug and may be given intravenously, intramuscularly, intradermally, or transtracheally as appropriate.

*Dopamine*

This has cardiovascular effects on peripheral dopaminergic ($DA_1$ and $DA_2$) and adrenoceptors. Dopaminergic (predominantly $DA_1$) effects are seen at low doses (3–4 µg/kg per min), with α-adrenergic effects becoming predominant at 10 µg/kg per min. In the intermediate dose range, $\beta_1$-adrenergic effects predominate, thus giving the drug the appearance of a stepped response from vasodilatation, inotropy, and finally vasoconstriction. However, there is considerable between-patient variability, and vasoconstrictive effects may predominate at a lower dose in some patients. Increases in CO and blood pressure can also occur with low and intermediate doses. Cardiac filling pressures show an initial fall, an effect that is more marked in clinical practice, but which at higher doses may increase.

Controversy still surrounds the role of low-dose dopamine as a diuretic or nephroprotective agent. There is no doubt that repeated studies have shown that low-dose dopamine is associated with an increase in urine output in surgical patients. However, whether this is the result of $DA_1$-mediated increase in renal blood flow, inhibition of aldosterone secretion, or inhibition of tubular $Na^+/K^+$ ATPase activity, or simply as a consequence of an increase in CO is not clear.

*Dobutamine*

This is a synthetic catecholamine, modified from isoprenaline. The intention was to create a catecholamine molecule, and by suitable side-chain substitution, render it highly $\beta_1$ specific and with little arrhythmogenic effect. Although it is primarily $\beta_1$ specific, α and $\beta_2$ effects are still seen but at substantially increased doses. Dobutamine causes an enhancement of indices of contractility, and an increase in CO. Heart rate is increased particularly in hypovolaemia. Cardiac filling pressures and pulmonary artery pressure may fall, particularly in acute or chronic heart failure. Although measurement of vascular resistance shows a decrease, dobutamine has very little direct effect on the vasculature and reductions in vascular tone are brought about reflexly via an increase in cardiac output. Although dobutamine has no effect on $DA_1$-receptors, dobutamine is associated with improvements in urine production quantitatively similar to dopamine (in some studies).

*Isoprenaline*

This is a synthetic catecholamine with strong $\beta_1$ and $\beta_2$ effects and is devoid of clinically relevant α-adrenergic activity. The combined β effects cause an increase in indices of contractility and reductions in cardiac filling pressures, pulmonary artery pressure, and systemic and pulmonary vascular resistance. Blood pressure may fall unless filling pressure is restored. The heart rate increases, often markedly, as a result of the combination of a direct chronotropic effect and a reflex response to the hypotension. Coronary blood flow may be reduced and hence myocardial oxygen balance impaired.

*Dopexamine*

This is a synthetic catecholamine with marked dopaminergic and $\beta_2$-adrenergic affects. Cardiac output is increased as a result of a reduction in afterload and some mild degree of inotropy. Cardiac filling pressures and pulmonary artery pressures are reduced, and blood pressure may also fall. Heart rate increases significantly. The effects on $DA_1$-receptors have led to speculation that dopexamine may be an effective nephroprotective agent and diuretic.

#### *Inhibition of phosphodiesterase isoenzyme*

Phosphodiesterase (PDE) is present as several isoenzymes in mammalian tissues, including myocardium, vascular and bronchiolar smooth muscle, the gastrointestinal tract, the CNS, and platelets. In the myocardium, PDE is responsible for the breakdown of cAMP, and inhibition of PDE leads to an increased intracellular cAMP concentration. This, in turn, increases the activity of protein kinases, leading to enhanced phosphorylation of membrane L-type calcium channels, enhanced calcium entry into the cell, and enhanced myocardial contractility (Figure 20.38).

The combination of a drug to activate adenylyl cyclase with another to inhibit PDE will markedly enhance contractile mechanisms. Thus, catecholamines and PDE inhibitors have summative effects.

Previously, PDE inhibitors were used for their effects as bronchodilators (e.g. aminophylline), and the cardiac effects were largely side effects (i.e. arrhythmias).

In contrast, modern myocardial PDE inhibitors are inhibitors of that fraction referred to as PDE-III, previously termed peak IIIc, type IV, F3, and PIII. These drugs not only enhance contractility but also cause vasodilatation by a direct effect. Activation of protein kinases causes the phosphorylation of phospholamban, which in turn promotes the reuptake of calcium into the sarcoplasmic reticulum, and vascular smooth muscle relaxation. This combined inotropic and vasodilator effect has led to the use of the term 'inodilators' (which could in fact also be applied to a number of catecholamines).

There are two clinically useful classes of PDE inhibitor: the bipyridine derivatives (amrinone, milrinone), and the imidazole derivatives (enoximone). Despite theoretical considerations, including the inotropy/vasodilatation ratio, there appears to be little significant clinical difference between the compounds in the surgical patient. The haemodynamic effects of PDE inhibitors tend to be uniform as a class: venodilatation (reduced cardiac filling pressures), increased CO, and reduced systemic and pulmonary vascular tone, with little direct effect on heart rate. In comparison with catecholamines, PDE inhibitors are more likely to drop the blood pressure, less likely to cause tachycardia, and produce similar changes in stroke volume. Studies on myocardial oxygen balance have suggested little change overall, although the effect seen will depend on the state of the circulation before treatment.

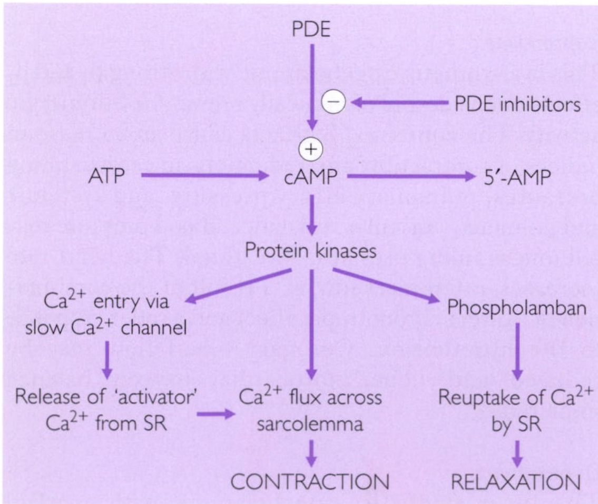


**Figure 20.38** The action of phosphodiesterase (PDE) and PDE inhibitors. SR, sarcoplasmic reticulum.

The potential value in therapy with PDE inhibitors lies in their ability to produce a synergistic effect with catecholamines as described earlier, or by being able to produce an inotropic effect by a mechanism that bypasses the β-adrenoceptor altogether. This may be particularly important in chronic heart failure, when chronically elevated levels of circulating catecholamines have led to the down-regulation and desensitization of β-receptors, rendering β agonists less effective. This may explain the reports of marked haemodynamic improvement in patients awaiting cardiac transplantation when given PDE-III inhibitors. However, the desensitization phenomenon may also occur acutely, and this is particularly relevant in situations when catecholamine levels are elevated, e.g. during and after cardiopulmonary bypass.

#### *Direct activation of adenylyl cyclase*

Forskolin acts directly on the catalytic subunit of adenylyl cyclase without first interacting with membrane-bound adrenoceptors. It is of interest as a mechanism but not currently available or relevant to clinical pharmacology.

### cAMP-independent mechanisms

A number of drugs and mechanisms are involved in cAMP-independent inotropic activity. Some of these are well established (e.g. digoxin) but a number are of theoretical interest only at the moment. Nevertheless, an understanding of their potential as inotropes is important because it underscores an understanding of ionic mechanisms that may lead to inotropic effect.

#### *Inhibition of the ATPase-dependent $Na^+/K^+$ pump*

This causes an increase in intracellular sodium and concomitant increase in calcium. Two examples of drugs in this class are digoxin and DPI 201-106. The chemical structure of cardiac glycosides uses the steroid skeleton to combine an aglycone with between one and four sugar molecules (Figure 20.39a). The pharmacological activity is determined by the aglycone moiety whereas the sugar molecules determine lipid and water solubility, attach to the membrane, and affect potency. The pharmacology of cardiac gylcosides is complex. They have direct effects on force of contraction and on electrophysiology, in addition to a number of secondary effects.

Sodium is actively extruded and potassium imported into cardiac cells. The energy for this process comes from hydrolysis of ATP by membrane-bound $Na^+/K^+$ ATPase. Cardiac glycosides bind to $Na^+/K^+$ ATPase

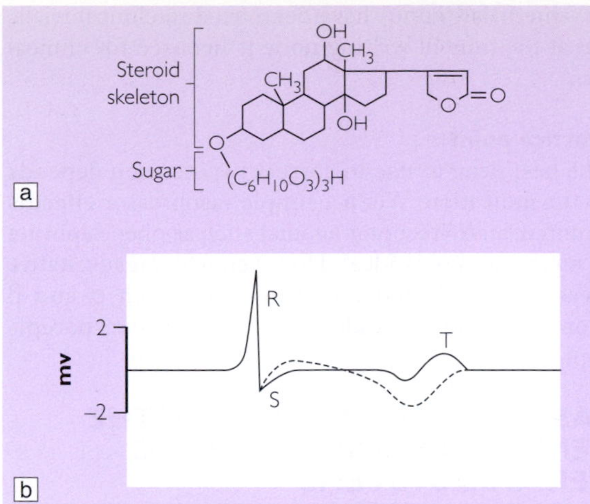


**Figure 20.39** (a) The digoxin molecule and (b) its effect on the ECG as seen in lead II. — Normal ECG; - - - - digoxin effect.

and inhibit its activity, thereby leading to a gradual increase in intracellular sodium. This in turn leads to a reduction in the exchange of intracellular calcium for extracellular sodium, and therefore the intracellular calcium concentration increases. This has the consequence of increasing calcium stores in the sarcoplasmic reticulum, thereby ensuring that more calcium is available for interaction with tropomyosin–troponin complexes, thereby enhancing contractility.

In addition, the increase in intracellular calcium leads to an increase in the slow inward current during the AP, thereby reinforcing the calcium-dependent phase 2 plateau of the AP in myocardial cells. Other modes of action have been proposed to explain digoxin's inotropic effect, including stimulation of the $Na^+/K^+$ pump and alterations in calcium binding by sarcolemmal phospholipids. However, it does appear that an effective inotropic effect is dependent on inhibition of active transport of sodium and potassium. The changes in ionic flux can be seen in phases 2, 3, and 4 of the AP and affect the ECG, as shown in Figure 20.39b.

The concept of enhancing intracellular calcium concentrations as a consequence of loading the cell with sodium is an elegant concept, and other inotropes have been developed that exploit this effect. One agent, DPI 201-106, is a piperazinyl–indole derivative that maintains the open state of the sodium channels during the AP, thus transiently loading the cell with sodium, and leading to an eventual increase in intracellular calcium. Both the cardiac glycosides and sodium-channel openers are more effective as oral therapy in chronic heart failure than as intravenous therapy in the acute setting, an observation that is probably related to the kinetics of sodium–calcium exchange in the myocardial cells. The real value of digoxin in the surgical patient probably lies in the fact that, in contrast to other antiarrhythmic agents, it has no significant negative inotropic effect.

#### *Direct activation of $Ca^{2+}$ channels*

A number of drugs have been developed that have partial agonist activity at the dihydropyridine receptor on the L-type calcium channel, thus potentially enhancing the likelihood of the channel being maintained in the open state, and potentiating calcium entry into the cell. However, because of their partial agonist activity, such drugs are not yet used in clinical practice.

#### *Calcium sensitizers*

These increase the sensitivity of contractile processes. Examples are pimobendan and levosimendan. Myofilament calcium sensitizers augment calcium binding to the calcium-specific regulatory site of cardiac troponin C, and stabilize calcium-induced conformational changes in this protein, thus causing positive inotropic effects without altering the intracellular calcium concentration, but by promoting prolonged interaction of actin and myosin filaments during systole. Levosimendan acts in this manner, but the calcium-sensitizing effect is concentration dependent, i.e. it is greater during systole than during diastole, in contrast to earlier agents. Levosimendan also has cardiac and vascular PDE inhibition activity, and these effects become more apparent at higher doses. This is a novel class of drugs and further development is awaited with interest.

#### *$\alpha_1$-Adrenoceptor stimulation*

$\alpha_1$-Adrenoceptor agonists, e.g. phenylephrine and methoxamine, will interact with myocardial $\alpha_1$-adrenoceptors, thus activating $G_q$ protein and phospholipase C, causing hydrolysis of phosphatidylinositol diphosphate ($PIP_2$) and leading to the activation of DAG and $IP_3$. $IP_3$ causes an increase in calcium release from the sarcoplasmic reticulum and thus enhances contractility, in part by sensitizing the contractile proteins also. The major therapeutic use of $\alpha_1$ agonists is, however, their ability to produce peripheral vasoconstriction.

## VASOPRESSOR DRUGS

Vasopressor or vasoconstrictor agents used or encountered in clinical practice fall into five groups:

1. $\alpha_1$-receptor agonists;
2. ergot alkaloids;
3. ADH (vasopressin);
4. angiotensin;
5. NO synthase antagonists.

### $\alpha_1$-Adrenoceptor agonists

The effects mediated by $\alpha_1$-adrenoceptor agonists are arteriolar constriction, venular constriction, sphincter contraction, contraction of the pregnant uterus, and proximal tubular reabsorption of sodium. $\alpha_1$-adrenoceptor agonists can be selective for $\alpha_1$-adrenoceptors or may also produce some $\alpha_2$ or $\beta$ effects. The majority of the inotropes based on the catecholamine skeleton (see Figure 20.36 and Chapter 23, Table 23.11) express both $\alpha$ and $\beta$ agonist activity, but the proportions differ from drug to drug.

Norepinephrine is the catecholamine with the greatest $\alpha_1$ action although it also possesses $\alpha_2$ and $\beta_1$ effects. It is a potent vasoconstrictor and, if the cardiac output is maintained, it causes a rise in both the systolic and diastolic pressures. Its effect is shown in Figure 20.37 where, at equipotent doses, it is compared with epinephrine and isoprenaline.

Metaraminole, phenylephrine, and methoxamine are all highly selective for $\alpha_1$-adrenoceptors. Metaraminole also has some indirect effect. The action of these drugs on the peripheral vasculature is similar to that of norepinephrine. They are widely used in anaesthesia to increase the blood pressure in the presence of other drugs that have vasodilator side effects (e.g. propofol, intrathecal and epidural local anaesthetics).

Ephedrine has both $\alpha$ and $\beta$ ($\beta_1$ and $\beta_2$) effects. It actions are partly dependent on the displacement of norepinephrine from sympathetic nerve endings and partly result from direct stimulation of adrenoceptors. Ephedrine is usually preferred for obstetric anaesthesia because the combined $\alpha$ and $\beta$ effects are less likely to compromise placental perfusion.

### Ergot alkaloids

Ergotamine has 300 times the affinity of norepinephrine for $\alpha$-receptors; prolonged administration can lead to vascular insufficiency of the extremities. The principal use of ergotamine is in anti-migraine preparations. Ergometrine, a related compound, is used in obstetrics to control postpartum bleeding. Both drugs are potentially dangerous in hypertensive patients or those with pre-existing cardiac disease.

### ADH (vasopressin)

ADH has well-recognized effects on the kidney (see Chapter 25) and is also a potent vasoconstrictor. Vasopressin $V_1$-receptors are located on vascular smooth muscle cells and are linked to phospholipase C. When given exogenously, ADH has marked arteriolar and venoconstrictor actions but it is unlikely to have a major role in physiological blood pressure homoeostasis.

Large intravenous doses of ADH cause hypertension and skin pallor from cutaneous vasoconstriction. There is, however, a disproportionately marked effect on the portal circulation which enables a dose range to be found that is effective in controlling haemorrhage from oesophageal varices while producing only a moderate rise in blood pressure.

Octapressin (or felypressin), a related vasoconstrictor compound, is added to some preparations of local anaesthetic to prolong their action.

### Angiotensin

The renin–angiotensin system is described in Chapters 25 and 29. Angiotensin II is the most potent pressor substance known. It has direct and indirect actions. Indirectly it augments sympathetic tone; directly it acts on angiotensin (AT) receptors. $AT_1$-receptors show greater affinity for angiotensin II and mediate their effects by G-protein coupling. $AT_2$-receptors (at which angiotensin I and II have equal potency) are linked to protein tyrosine phosphate activity.

Angiotensin was previously available as a prescribable preparation but to the author's knowledge has now been withdrawn.

### Nitric oxide synthase antagonists

It may be anticipated that in those conditions in which NO is being produced to excess (e.g. septic shock), blockade of NO synthase might improve haemodynamics. NO synthase antagonist compounds (e.g. L-*N*-methylarginine) have been used in clinical trials, but at the time of writing none is licensed for clinical use.

***Practice point***

The best drug to use to correct hypotension depends on the indication. When a simple vasopressor effect is required, an $\alpha_1$-receptor agonist such as phenylephrine or methoxamine is ideal. However, when resuscitative measures are called for, drugs with both $\alpha$ and $\beta$ agonist effects are indicated (epinephrine, norepinephrine).

## VASODILATORS ACTING ON THE CENTRAL AND SYMPATHETIC NERVOUS SYSTEMS

Drugs that have a vasodilator effect may act at a number of different sites. These include the CNS, the sympathetic outflow, the autonomic ganglia, postganglionic adrenergic neurons, and adrenergic nerve terminals. Other drugs may be more specific in their effects, particularly at the effector site. These include drugs acting at adrenergic, dopaminergic, and serotoninergic receptors, calcium channel blockers, and ACE inhibitors. This section considers those active in the CNS and sympathetic nervous system.

### Vasodilators acting via the CNS

Many drugs that are used in anaesthesia and have CNS effects will lower blood pressure. This frequently occurs as a result of reduction in higher centre activity causing a reduction in medullary vasomotor centre activity, and resulting in a reduction in resting sympathetic tone. Opioid analgesics, sedatives, hypnotics, and intravenous and volatile anaesthetics all reduce higher centre input to the vasomotor centre. However, many of these drugs also have peripheral effects, including effects on myocardial contractility, and on specific peripheral tissues, including vascular smooth muscle.

Methyldopa, clonidine, dexmedetomidine, medetomidine and other related compounds act as partial agonists at the preganglionic $\alpha_2$-adrenoceptor in the CNS. Many $\alpha_2$ agonists have cross-activity with imidazoline receptors. Two types of receptors have been identified: $I_1$ and $I_2$. Drugs that have an effect on $I_1$ receptors tend to cause less sedation, but have a centrally mediated hypotensive effect. The exact site of action for the central haemodynamic effect is not fully clear. $\alpha_2$-Receptors have been found in the nucleus tractus solitarius and the lateral reticular nucleus. The locus coerulus in the upper brain stem has been identified as a major site for the hypnotic and sedative effects.

Clonidine, and in particular dexmedetomidine, have effects on central $\alpha$-receptors, resulting in both sedation and haemodynamic stability, manifested by less vasoreactivity to noxious stimuli. Dexmedetomidine is the *dextro*-stereoisomer of medetomidine and is effective in reducing the anaesthetic and analgesic requirements in surgical patients. However, $\alpha_2$-receptors are located peripherally as well as centrally, and agonist effects at peripheral postjunctional $\alpha_2$-receptors result in a long-lasting, slow-onset vasoconstriction. In addition, there may be cross-activity with $\alpha_1$-receptors. $\alpha_2$ Agonists may produce a degree of acute vasoconstriction when given intravenously, followed by sedation and vasodilatation.

### Vasodilators acting via the sympathetic outflow

The sympathetic outflow from the spinal cord runs from T1 to L2–3. Spinal anaesthetic techniques (epidural, subdural) using local anaesthetic drugs lignocaine, bupivacaine) may serve to block conduction in preganglionic sympathetic fibres and thus reduce the activity of sympathetic nerves, resulting in vasodilatation. This is of great clinical relevance, and vasodilatation resulting in hypotension is an important component of this type of anaesthesia. The pharmacology of the local anaesthetic drugs concerned is covered in Chapter 36.

### Vasodilators acting at autonomic ganglia

The neurotransmitter at the autonomic ganglion is acetylcholine. However, the subset of receptors on which acetylcholine acts are nicotinic receptors, i.e. they are blocked by a nicotinic antagonist (hexamethonium, pentamethonium) and are unaffected by muscarinic antagonists such as atropine (see Chapter 24). The effects of ganglion blockade are both important and complex, and a full understanding of them is valuable because it demonstrates a clear understanding of both the qualitative and the quantitative interactions of the ANS, and the effects of parasympathetic/sympathetic activity and blockade (see Chapter 23, Table 23.5).

Autonomic blockade is, however, now very rarely used as a therapeutic mechanism for producing vasodilatation or controlling blood pressure. A number of drugs that were previously available have been withdrawn, and even those drugs with ganglion-blocking side effects such as *d*-tubocurare are now virtually unobtainable. Trimetaphan remains available: it is relatively short acting and is usually given by a continuous infusion.

### Vasodilators acting on postsynaptic adrenergic neurons

Drugs acting at postsynaptic adrenergic neurons include guanethidine, bethanidine, debrisoquine, and reserpine. These are actively transported into nerve endings and combine with storage vesicles to stabilize the granules. The result is inhibition of norepinephrine release, and a reduction in vasoconstrictor tone. After more prolonged exposure, vesicle destruction takes place with metabolic degradation of the norepinephrine contained within the vesicles by monoamine oxidase and catechol-*O*-methyl transferase.

The effects of these drugs, which are now only very rarely used, may be very long lasting. The anaesthetic management of patients taking such drugs may be difficult for a number of reasons. After prolonged depletion of norepinephrine stores, there is an up-regulation of synthesis and expression of new adrenergic receptors. This synthesis of new receptors is a compensatory mechanism consequent on the chronic reduction in transmitter release that may result in apparent sensitivity to either exogenous or endogenous norepinephrine; this leads to severe hypertensive episodes during the perioperative period.

Also, as we have seen, norepinephrine is a transmitter within the CNS, and chronic depletion of central norepinephrine stores may produce sedation and sometimes severe depression.

### Vasodilators that act at peripheral receptors

#### *$\alpha_1$-Adrenoceptor antagonists (e.g. phentolamine and phenoxybenzamine)*

$\alpha_1$-Adrenoceptors are present in all vascular smooth muscle except true capillaries. Stimulation of these receptors will produce vasoconstriction, and thus vasodilatation is produced by antagonism. The mechanism of action is well understood. Interaction with an $\alpha_1$-cell membrane receptor activates $G_q$ protein (and possibly also $G_o$ protein), phospholipase C hydrolyses $PIP_2$ leading to the secondary activation of two second messengers. DAG activates protein kinase C, and $IP_3$ enhances the release of calcium from the sarcoplasmic reticulum, thereby increasing cytosol calcium concentration and activating contractile proteins, resulting in muscular contraction.

Phentolamine is a non-specific ($\alpha_1$ and $\alpha_2$) receptor antagonist. It is ultra-short-acting, and is widely used for acute short-term vasodilatation in clinical anaesthesia. Phenoxybenzamine is slightly more specific for $\alpha_1$-receptors but with a profoundly long-lasting effect. It combines irreversibly with the receptor and its effect is terminated only after the affected receptor has been sequestered and new receptor synthesized and expressed.

Of the newer drugs, doxazosin has a long half-life and effective blood pressure control may be achieved with a single daily dose. Thus, it may be an effective replacement for phenoxybenzamine, for example, in the preoperative management of phaeochromocytoma. Urapidil is a weak adrenoceptor antagonist, with some activity (probably weak partial agonist) at the serotonin $5HT_{1a}$ receptor. It is also an effective hypotensive agent.

#### *$\beta_2$-Adrenoceptor agonists*

Skeletal muscle arterioles have a predominance of $\beta_2$-receptors and therefore $\beta_2$ agonist activity will result in vasodilatation (e.g. isoprenaline, salbutamol, dopexamine). This vasodilator effect may be pronounced, but such drugs are rarely used for reducing blood pressure because of their inotropic effects. Interaction with $\beta_2$-receptors results in the formation of cAMP and activation of physiological effector mechanisms as described earlier. In vascular smooth muscle, the most important mechanism is the phosphorylation of myosin light chain kinase. This results in reduction of its affinity for the calcium–calmodulin complex and dephosphorylation of myosin light chains, and leads to vasodilatation.

#### *Dopaminergic receptor agonists*

Peripheral dopaminergic receptors have been identified. $DA_1$-receptors activate adenylyl cyclase and $DA_2$-receptors inhibit it. $DA_1$-receptors are found distributed throughout the splanchnic, mesenteric, and renal circulations, and have also been identified in the renal tubule, and coronary and cerebral circulations. $DA_1$ agonists include the parent compound dopamine, as well as dopexamine and fenoldopam. Both dopamine and dopexamine are able to interact with adrenoceptors, producing a variety of effects.

The haemodynamic effects of dopamine are well described. At low dose, only vasodilatation is seen; at intermediate doses, an inotropic effect is apparent; at high doses, interaction with $\alpha_1$-receptors produces peripheral vasoconstriction.

Dopexamine interacts with $\beta_2$-adrenoceptors only. Although the only effect seen is vasodilatory, activation of $\beta_2$-receptors may lead to blood diversion away from the splanchnic bed to skeletal muscle. Also, the $\beta_2$ effects may produce a mild degree of inotropy.

Fenoldopam is a synthetic $DA_1$ agonist with no cross-activity with adrenoceptors. The effects seen are only vasodilatory, and it has been shown to be effective in the management of essential, accelerated, and post-operative hypertension. It has effects on the renal tubule and causes a diuresis, supposedly by natriuretic mechanisms, as well as by improving renal blood flow.

## ANGIOTENSIN-CONVERTING ENZYME INHIBITORS

Angiotensin I is formed via the actions of renin on angiotensinogen. Angiotensin I is an inactive prohormone, but it is converted into angiotensin II by the action of ACE. Angiotensin II stimulates the adrenal cortex to secrete aldosterone, causing salt and water retention, and acts as a powerful vasoconstrictor that may increase peripheral vascular resistance and hence elevate blood pressure (see above). ACE inhibitors will therefore lead to a reduction in angiotensin II formation. This is an effective vasodilator mechanism even in patients with normal or low renin hypertension.

ACE inhibitors have been shown to be a group of drugs with enormous clinical potential, particularly in patients with severe congestive heart failure. They have also been shown to be of benefit after myocardial infarction and may have favourable myocardial protective properties after periods of ischaemia. The reduction in afterload favours myocardial oxygen balance and LV emptying, thus reducing LVEDP and pulmonary venous pressure. ACE inhibitors appear to be very well tolerated, particularly in hypertension and heart failure once patients are established on stable therapy. ACE inhibitors should, however, not be used in patients where renal perfusion is pressure dependent, i.e. renal artery stenosis.

ACE inhibitors also have effects on bradykinin metabolism, which may give rise to bradykinin accumulation in the lungs and a persistent dry cough. Discontinuation of medication effectively treats the cough, which may not return when treatment is restarted. Earlier compounds such as captopril contained a sulphydryl moiety which was thought to be responsible for side effects that were probably the result of relative overdosage. Unwanted side effects have been reduced with second-generation drugs. ACE inhibitors are named with the ubiquitous suffix -pril.

Longer-acting agents have been formulated (e.g. lisinopril) which are particularly useful in heart failure. There is debate as to whether ACE inhibitors should be stopped before general anaesthesia.

ACE is not the only enzymatic pathway available for the conversion of angiotensin I to angiotensin II, and production of angiotensin II may become re-established after some weeks with resulting poor control of hypertension – 'ACE escape'. For this reason, newer drugs have been developed that produce a fall in blood pressure by direct antagonism of angiotensin II at its receptor site. These drugs (irbesartan, losartan) have no effect on bradykinin metabolism.

## CALCIUM ANTAGONISTS

Calcium antagonists are used as antiarrhythmic agents and as antihypertensive drugs. Their use and place in the classification of antiarrhythmic agents was described earlier in the chapter.

Calcium enters the cell through at least four types of calcium channel: L, T, N, and P. Different types of calcium channel may coexist in the same cell. The features that characterize the cell type are the activating voltage and sensitivity to depolarization, the unitary conductance, the inactivation kinetics, and the susceptibility to various blockers, including drugs.

The two main types of myocardial calcium channels are the T type and L type. T-type channels are activated by a low voltage and are rapidly inactivated leading to tiny conductance and transient current. L-type channels are slow, activated by a high voltage and not inactivated rapidly, leading to large conductance and a long-lasting current. L-type channels are virtually ubiquitous, and make up the major route for voltage-gated calcium entry into most cardiovascular and muscle cells. T-type channels are mainly found in the myocardium. N- and P-type channels are found primarily in the CNS.

The opening and closing of calcium channels is sudden and stochastic (i.e. all or nothing) and can be predicted only in terms of probability. The overall calcium flux is dependent on the density of calcium channels, the size of the single-channel current, and the probability of the open state. Calcium channels are activated (opened) in response to depolarization within a few milliseconds. Deactivation occurs in response to repolarization and intracellular calcium levels. Channels can exist in three modes:

0: closed or unavailable;
1: resting (brief bursts of opening, mostly closed);
2: open (prolonged bursts of opening with brief closures).

Four specific groups of calcium channel blockers are defined:

- the phenylalkylamines (e.g. verapamil);
- the benzothiazepines (e.g. diltiazem);
- the dihydropyridines (e.g. nifedipine);
- the piperazines (e.g. flunarizine).

Of these, the dihydropyridines (e.g. nifedipine) are particularly useful as arteriolar vasodilators in the management of high blood pressure. They have mostly vascular effects with very little effect on intracardiac conduction or inotropy, although detailed studies *in vivo* have revealed a negative inotropic effect. Reflex sympathetic activation usually compensates. Different drugs demonstrate selectivity for different vascular beds; nimodipine is almost cerebral selective, whereas isradipine and nicardipine have effects on the vasculature in skeletal muscle, brain, kidney, and coronary circulations. Dihydropyridines are much less effective as venodilators and have less potency on the pulmonary circulation, although there are reports of efficacy in idiopathic pulmonary hypertension.

Two classes of calcium channel blockers are widely used in chronic angina. The dihydropyridines interact with the dihyropyridine receptor on the L-type calcium channel, causing coronary vasodilatation and reducing afterload, LV work and myocardial oxygen demand. Diltiazem, a benzothiazepine, has more specific myocardial effects and less specificity for vascular smooth muscle, and is highly effective in the treatment of angina. Neither diltiazem nor the dihydropyridines produce significant conduction disturbances in therapeutic dosage, but mild myocardial depression may occur, particularly with diltiazem. However, this may also serve to limit myocardial work and oxygen requirements and thus aid control of angina. Myocardial depression with diltiazem or the dihydropyridines is not as great as with β-adrenoceptor.

Recently, a new class of T-type calcium channel blockers has been introduced for the treatment of hypertension and angina. Mibefradil is available as an oral preparation, needing once-daily administration. The effects of therapy, including side effects, appear to be qualitatively similar to diltiazem, with a potential risk of heart failure and conduction abnormalities if the dosage is excessive.

The antiarrhythmia activity of agents such as verapamil is described earlier.

## NITRIC OXIDE RELEASING DRUGS

NO is the final common effector molecule of nitrovasodilators, including sodium nitroprusside (SNP) and glyceryl trinitrate (GTN). The activation sequence for the release of NO and subsequent vasodilatation is summarized in Figure 20.40. It is also discussed in Chapter 19, Figure 19.38.

As is shown in Figure 20.40, interaction between an agonist and a membrane-bound receptor coupled to phospholipase C is the initial step. Physiological stimuli for activation include not only the products of platelet aggregation (adenosine, serotonin, thrombin) but also histamine and kinins, and haemodynamic change in wall stress. Ligands first interact with $G_q$ protein; the consequence of activation of phospholipase C is the hydrolysis of $PIP_2$ to produce DAG and $IP_3$. $IP_3$ causes the release of calcium from the endoplasmic reticulum. Calcium becomes bound to the protein calmodulin, and the calcium–calmodulin complex activates NO synthase which catalyses the production of NO from L-arginine. NO is a small lipophilic molecule that diffuses easily across biological membranes and into the cytosol of adjacent cells, where it combines with thiol groups to form a nitrosothiol compound. This in turn activates guanylyl cyclase, which catalyses the conversion of guanosine triphosphate (GTP) to cyclic guanosine monophosphate (cGMP). Cyclic GMP then activates protein kinase G, resulting in the dephosphorylation of phosphorylated myosin light chains and smooth muscle relaxation.

The half-life of NO is 5 s, therefore only the local environment is affected and levels are very difficult to assay directly. Different isoenzymes of NO synthase have been identified. However, the calmodulin-linked form is the most important in vascular smooth muscle, and may be inhibited by methylated L-arginine derivatives. Calmodulin may be inhibited by calmidazolium.

NO binds to the iron moiety on guanylyl cyclase, and this binding is essential for enzyme activation. Inhaled NO is rapidly bound to the iron residues in haemoglobin and deactivated and therefore, although NO is active when inhaled, its duration of action is so short as to limit it to an effect on the pulmonary but not the systemic vasculature. It is increasingly used in the management of severe pulmonary hypertension and adult respiratory distress syndrome, although there are difficulties in administering and monitoring inhaled NO. An example of its action in the lungs is shown in Figure 20.41.

Vascular smooth muscle is in a constant state of NO-induced vasodilatation, and abnormalities in the ability of the endothelium to produce NO may play a role

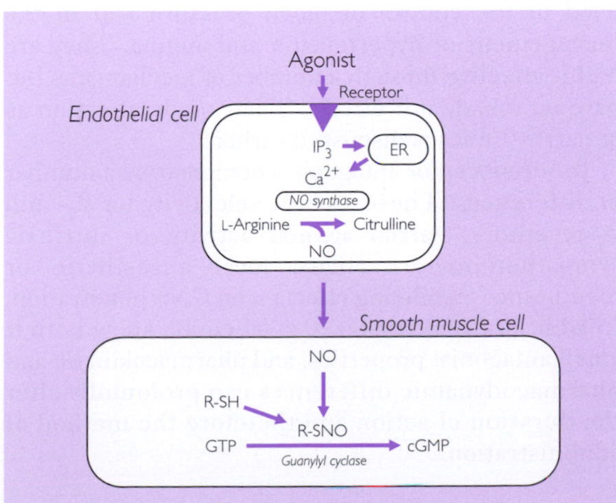


**Figure 20.40** The activation sequence and effects of nitric oxide (NO). ER, endoplasmic reticulum; $IP_3$, inositol triphosphate; R-SH, thiol group; cGMP, cyclic GMP.

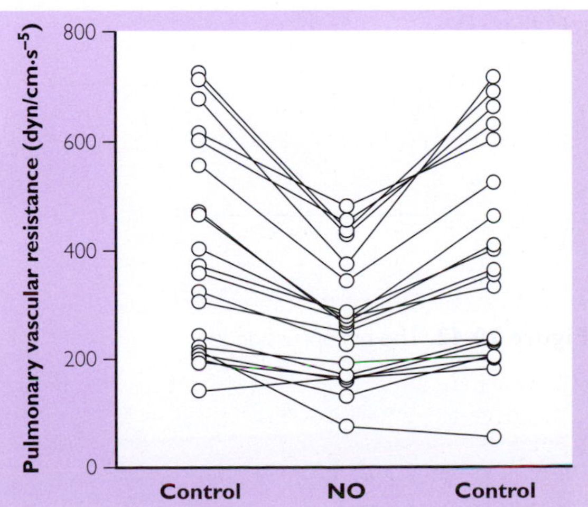


**Figure 20.41** The effect of inhaled nitric oxide (NO) on pulmonary vascular resistance. (Adapted from Rich GF, Murphy GD, Roos CM *et al. Anesthesiology* 1993;78:1028.)

in diseases such as diabetes, hypertension, and atherosclerosis. The venous circulation has a lower basal release of NO than the arterial circulation, and nitrovasodilators are more effective venodilators than vasodilators. This increased venous sensitivity reflects a higher concentration of guanylyl cyclase, a form of up-regulation.

### Sodium nitroprusside

SNP is a potent vasodilator, and is probably the gold standard against which other intravenous vasodilators are compared. It consists of a ferrous iron atom bound with five cyanide molecules and one nitric group (Figure 20.42). Contact with red blood cells decomposes the molecule, releasing NO, and thus mediating vasodilatation as described above. SNP is a highly potent drug and, although tachyphylaxis does develop, it is usually possible to reduce arterial blood pressure to profoundly low levels. Veno- and vasodilatation occur, almost invariably with a significant reflex tachycardia unless steps are taken to minimize this (i.e. β blockade). SNP administration is associated with the activation of physiological reflexes to compensate for the hypotension (tachycardia, increased plasma renin, and catecholamine levels) and the hypotensive effect will be potentiated if these reflexes are in any way obtunded.

The ferrous iron reacts with sulphydryl groups in the blood to release cyanide, which is reduced to cyanate in the liver and excreted in the urine. Prolonged administration with SNP, particularly at high doses, carries the risk of thiocyanate toxicity, which may manifest itself as severe hypotension, vomiting, tremors, convulsions, and psychotic behaviour. This should be treated with sodium thiosulphate, 12.5 mg in 50 ml 5% glucose over 5–10 min, repeated if necessary, or dicobalt edentate, 300 mg in 20 ml over 1 min, and by supportive measures as appropriate.

### The nitrates

The nitrates (GTN – Figure 20.43 – and isosorbide mono- and dinitrate) are widely used, although they are more effective as antianginal drugs than in the treatment of hypertension. Nitrates reduce venous and arterial tone, but the reduction in venous tone is more pronounced when the drug is given by any route other than as an intravenous bolus. Reflex tachycardia is seen. The effects on cardiac output will vary, but in normal individuals cardiac output is little altered. With both nitrates and SNP, CO is increased in patients in whom afterload is elevated before treatment (facilitated LV ejection) and reduced in patients with normal filling pressures (reduced LV filling leading to reduced SV).

In contrast to SNP, nitroglycerine will form NO only in the presence of other factors. Thiol-containing compounds such as cysteine must be present to act as a cofactor, which may then act as a rate-limiting step. If sulphydryl groups are absent, conversion of organic nitrates to NO is impaired and this may be an explanation for the development of nitrate tolerance. *N*-Acetylcysteine has been shown to reverse nitrate tolerance partially.

Nitrates are widely used in the treatment and prophylaxis of angina. GTN is short acting and effective as an antianginal agent. Extensive hepatic first-pass clearance makes it unsuitable for oral use; it may be used sublingually (tablet or spray), transdermally (patch), or intravenously. Isosorbide does not undergo hepatic first-pass clearance and is available orally. Tolerance to nitrates is well described and most authorities recommend a nitrate-free period during every 24-hour cycle when isosorbide is used for antiangina prophylaxis.

As described above, nitrates are effective blood pressure-lowering agents and may substantially reduce venous tone. This reduction in preload (LVEDP) is thought to be partly responsible for the antianginal effect. Nitrates also dilate large epicardial coronary arteries, but not small coronary resistance vessels; thus they do not cause coronary steal. Reduction of LVEDP and epicardial coronary dilatation causes flow redistribution with beneficial effect in patients with ischaemic heart disease.

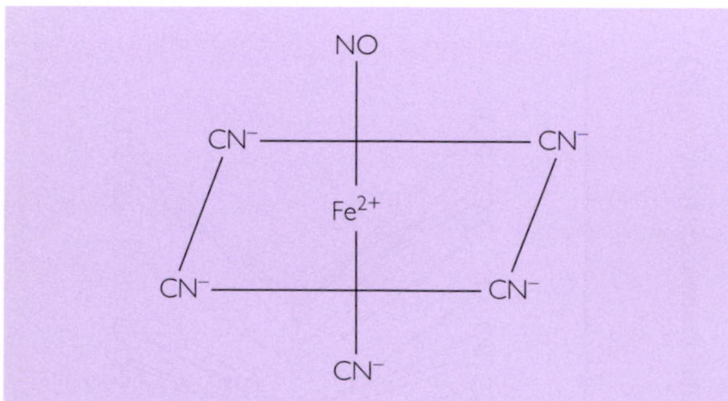


**Figure 20.42** The nitroprusside ion.

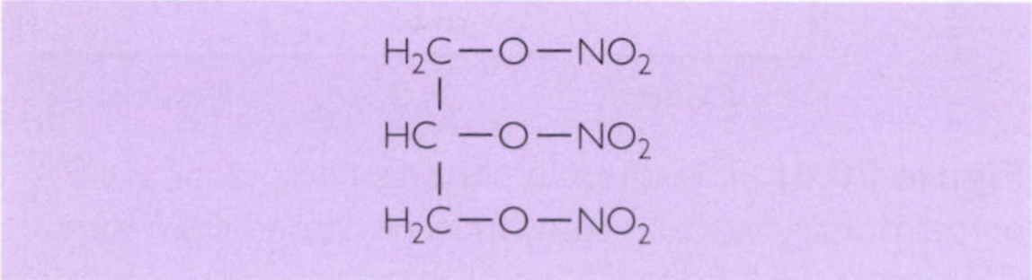

$$\begin{array}{l} H_2C-O-NO_2 \\ \quad | \\ HC-O-NO_2 \\ \quad | \\ H_2C-O-NO_2 \end{array}$$

**Figure 20.43** The nitroglycerin molecule.

## β-ADRENOCEPTOR ANTAGONISTS

These are an important group of drugs that are widely used in the control of blood pressure and in the management of hypertension and angina. They are highly effective through a number of mechanisms but have no vasodilator effects. Their mode of action as antiarrhythmics is discussed earlier.

β-Adrenoceptor antagonists demonstrate a number of differences. These include selectivity for $\beta_1$- and $\beta_2$-receptors, partial agonist activity, or intrinsic sympathomimetic activity, local anaesthetic or membrane- stabilizing effects, and CNS penetration. In addition, some drugs, e.g. labetolol, show both α and β antagonist properties, and pharmacokinetic and pharmacodynamic differences can profoundly alter the duration of action and therefore the method of administration.

### Chemical structure

The chemical structures of the β-adrenoceptor antagonists are closely related to the structure of the agonists (Figure 20.44). The steric configuration of the

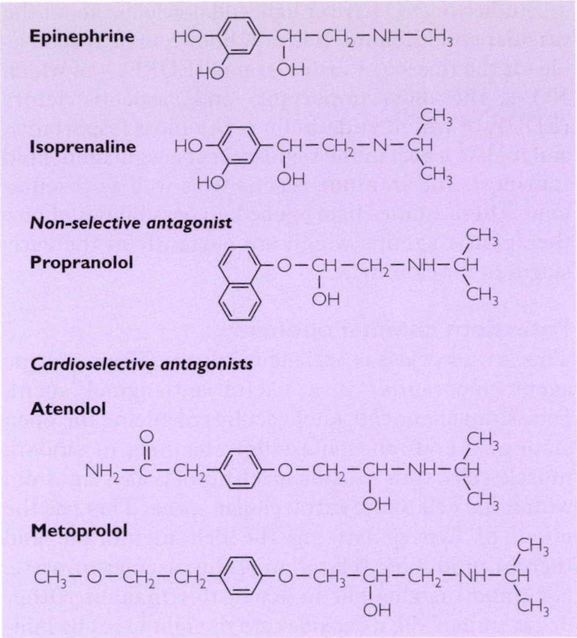

Epinephrine

Isoprenaline

*Non-selective antagonist*

Propranolol

*Cardioselective antagonists*

Atenolol

Metoprolol

**Figure 20.44** A comparison between epinephrine, isoprenaline, and some β-adrenoceptor antagonists.

OH-bearing β carbon atom in the side chain confers specific β-receptor affinity; alkyl or aralkyl substitution on the terminal amine radical is associated with an increased β-receptor affinity, and methyl substitution on the α carbon atom increases the duration of action.

### Receptor selectivity

Although different receptor types will predominate in different tissues, it is clearly over-simplistic to assume that only one receptor subtype exists in each tissue. Similarly drugs described as 'cardioselective' will in fact have some $\beta_2$-antagonist activity, but it will be significantly less than the $\beta_1$-antagonist activity and also profoundly less than those drugs not classified as cardioselective. For example, although propranolol is more effective at $\beta_1$ blockade than atenolol, atenolol has very much less $\beta_2$ blockade, making it the preferred cardioselective drug. Another drug with mixed actions is labetolol, which is approximately seven times more potent at β-receptors than at α-receptors. It should be remembered that β-adrenoceptor antagonists have no vasodilator effects and, indeed, drugs that combine $\beta_2$ with $\beta_1$ antagonism would tend to have a constrictive effect in skeletal muscle vessels.

### Intrinsic sympathomimetic activity

One of the original compounds, dichloroisoprenaline, was shown to have partial non-specific β-agonist activity. Other drugs have also been identified, including oxprenolol and pindolol. Much attention has been directed towards exploiting this effect, by trying to instigate a therapeutic regimen that would be antihypertensive but have less adverse effect on cardiac contractility and even, perhaps, be of therapeutic benefit in heart failure. In fact large-scale studies have shown β-adrenoceptor to be of value in chronic congestive heart failure using drugs without intrinsic sympathomimetic activity (i.e. metoprolol). Although there is a risk of acute heart failure, the sympatholytic effects of β-adrenoceptor in patients with severe heart failure often predominate and are beneficial.

### Local anaesthetic activity

Although this can be demonstrated in a number of compounds, the membrane-stabilizing effect does not appear to have predictable therapeutic benefit.

### Action as anti-hypertensive agents

The main haemodynamic effects of β-adrenoceptor blockade are reduction in heart rate and blood pressure. The mechanism for the reduction in blood pressure is still debated. One explanation is as follows. β-Adrenoceptor blockade is likely to cause a reduction in CO. The physiological response to this to maintain blood pressure is a baroreceptor-induced increase in peripheral vascular tone. This increase in vascular tone is also attenuated by β-adrenoceptor antagonists (how is not exactly clear), thus maintaining the fall in blood pressure. Possible mechanisms include baroreceptor resetting, central inhibition of sympathetic drive, reduction in renin release, alteration in the autoregulatory response to a reduced CO, and blockade of presynaptic β-adrenoceptors. $\beta_1$-Receptor blockade is essential for a blood pressure-lowering effect; experimentally, $\beta_2$-receptor blockade does not reduce blood pressure.

Clinically, β-adrenoceptor blockade has been used in a wide variety of settings. The consequences are reduced exercise tolerance, breathlessness, bradycardia, hypotension, cold extremities, fatigue, and vivid dreams. In certain circumstances, interference with carbohydrate and fat metabolism may cause persistent hypoglycaemia as a result of inhibition of $\beta_2$-receptor-mediated glycogenolysis. Furthermore, the sympathetically mediated signs and symptoms of hypoglycaemia may be masked. This is particular relevant during anaesthesia.

### Action as antianginal drugs

The value of β-adrenoceptor antagonists in the management of chronic angina pectoris is well established, but recent trends have swung away from their use. β-adrenoceptor antagonists have receptor-mediated effects on coronary arteries that tend to oppose $\beta_1$- and $\beta_2$-agonist-induced vasodilatation. The effect of sympathetic activity on resting coronary vascular tone is, however, more than just these opposing actions. This is discussed earlier.

The main value of β-adrenoceptor antagonists is that they tend to reduce many of the factors that increase myocardial oxygen demand, including LV systolic tension, systemic blood pressure, heart rate, and the resting level of myocardial contractility. They will also tend to reduce the exercise-induced changes in these haemodynamic indices, thus preventing exercise-induced myocardial oxygen imbalance and ischaemia. As exercise-induced tachycardia is better controlled, the duration of diastolic coronary blood flow is maintained and myocardial oxygen supply is preserved. Centrally acting β-adrenoceptor have been particularly useful in the control of angina (e.g. propranolol) and their use is particularly beneficial when angina occurs in conjunction with systemic hypertension.

β-adrenoceptor antagonists have no coronary vasodilating effect, and their use may be associated with unwanted effects, including poor peripheral circulation, erectile dysfunction, fatigue, and depression. As a result, their use as oral prophylaxis is less widespread than previously.

However, in surgical patients at risk from ischaemic heart disease, there is some evidence that β-adrenoceptor blockade for the duration of hospital stay improves survival up to 2 years after discharge. Whatever the merits of antianginal prophylaxis with β-adrenoceptor antagonists in other settings, their value in the surgical patient appears to be becoming more established.

## DIURETICS

Diuretics are discussed in more detail in Chapter 25. They can be classified as follows:

- thiazides;
- loop diuretics;
- osmotic diuretics;
- potassium-sparing diuretics;
- aldosterone antagonists;
- carbonic anhydrase inhibitors.

Their relevance to cardiovascular medicine (other than simply enhancing fluid loss) is limited to their use as antihypertensive agents. This role is almost confined to the thiazide group, sometimes with the addition of a potassium-sparing agent.

The antihypertensive effect of thiazide diuretics is thought to be an initial decrease in the interstitial fluid volume followed by a sustained peripheral vasodilatation, which can take weeks to develop. The mechanism of this vasodilatation may be a reduction in total body sodium, which attenuates the receptor response to normal sympathetic activity.

Thiazide diuretics induce a hypokalaemic, hypochloraemic, metabolic alkalosis. Cardiac arrhythmias may develop in response to hypokalaemia and hypomagnesaemia, especially in patients on digoxin. Orthostatic hypotension may indicate over-treatment and effective hypovolaemia. They also cause hyperglycaemia and precipitate gout.

In clinical maintenance therapy, thiazide diuretics are often combined with a potassium-sparing diuretic or aldosterone antagonist to prevent hypokalaemia.

## OTHER DRUGS

### Other receptor-based vasodilator agents

Many endogenous compounds, including histamine, kinins, serotonin, and thrombin act through receptors linked to phospholipase C and $G_q$ protein to produce $IP_3$ and DAG as intermediates in the production of NO. Although these are important mechanisms, especially in pathological processes, the compounds described are not utilized therapeutically.

Studies on NO have enhanced knowledge about the vascular endothelium. It is now known to be responsible for the release of vasorelaxants (EDRFs – of which NO is the most important) and vasoconstrictors (EDCF, of which endothelin is the most important), and it plays a part in the regulation of coagulation, lipid transport, and immune reactivity as well as vascular tone. These studies have opened up possibilities of new therapeutic agents, which are currently in the early stages of development.

### Potassium channel openers

This is a new class of antianginal drugs. The prototype agent, nicorandil, is a useful antianginal agent. Potassium channel openers act by enhancing the open state of membrane potassium channels in smooth muscle cells, thus causing an efflux of potassium from within the cell to the extracellular space. This has the effect of hyperpolarizing the cell membrane and thereby producing relaxation of the vascular myocyte. Nicorandil is thought to act in this manner. Other drugs (minoxidil, diazoxide) are thought to act by inhibition of ATP-dependent potassium channels.

Nicorandil has a nitrate group that also confers nitrate-like activity, and is effective as a coronary vasodilator in large coronary vessels, thus increasing coronary blood flow. Veno- and vasodilatation are also seen, but, as a result of the relative lack of a potent effect on small coronary arteries, nicorandil has not been associated with the development of a coronary steal syndrome, in contrast to other coronary vasodilators (excluding the nitrates). However, development of an associated tachycardia is not uncommon.

#### *Dipyridamole*

Dipyridamole is a drug with two actions:

1. It affects platelet function by potentiating the effects of prostacyclin or by inhibiting PDE activity.
2. It acts to dilate the small resistance vessels of the coronary circulation, but has little effect on those vessels already maximally dilated. This may be the result of its ability to prevent the cellular uptake of adenosine.

Both these actions are used therapeutically: the first orally for prophylaxis against thromboembolism, the second intravenously to promote dilatation of healthy coronary vessels during radionuclide scanning.

#### *Prostaglandin $E_1$ ($PGE_1$)*

$PGE_1$ is a smooth muscle neuromuscular blocking agent which can be administered in neonates with congenital heart disease to maintain patency of the ductus arteriosus while the patient is awaiting corrective surgery.

#### *Adenosine*

Adenosine has been described under antiarrhythmic drug action earlier.

## FURTHER READING


Bennett DH. *Cardiac Arrhythmias*, 3rd edn. Bristol: Wright, 1989.

Feneck RO. Anti-arrhythmics. *Curr Opin Anaesthesiol* 1990;**3**:110–16.

Ganong WF. *Review of Medical Physiology*, 18th edn. Stamford, CA: Appleton & Lange, 1997.

Hull CJ. *Pharmacokinetics for Anaesthesia*. Oxford: Butterworth-Heinemann, 1991.

Kanmura Y. Pharmacological and clinical use of vasodilators. *Curr Anaesth Crit Care* 1998;**9**:242–8.

Articles in: Skarvan K, ed. *Vasoactive Drugs. Baillière's Clin Anaesthesiol* 1994;**8**:1–292.

# Chapter 21 Ventilation, gas exchange and gas transport

M. Manji

The principal function of the lungs is to maintain appropriate levels of oxygen and carbon dioxide within the body. This need arises as a direct result of cellular aerobic metabolism which consumes oxygen and which, in turn, creates a constant demand to eliminate carbon dioxide. This constant gas exchange between venous blood and inspired air is one of the key factors in maintaining an optimum intracellular pH. Table 21.1 highlights some of the other functions of the lungs.

The physiology and functional anatomy of the lung are intrinsically linked. The latter will be considered before detailed examination of respiratory physiology.

## THE BELLOWS FUNCTION OF THE LUNGS

### Functional anatomy

The anatomy of the upper airways and lungs is also considered in Chapter 6. The lungs are bordered by the rib cage, mediastinum, and diaphragm, which form the thoracic cavity. Contraction of the diaphragm (C3–5 innervation, the principal respiratory muscle) and movements of the ribs upwards and outwards by the external intercostal muscles increase the volume of the thoracic cavity, causing its contents (the lungs) to expand. This can be augmented by the use of accessory respiratory muscles (sternomastoid, scalene, and pectorals) during increased respiratory effort. Expiration, which is normally passive, can also be facilitated by muscles aiding the downward movement of the ribs. The accessory expiratory muscles include the inner intercostals, rectus abdominis, and the external and internal oblique.

The lungs are surrounded by the visceral pleura. This is in close contact with the parietal pleura, which lines the inner surface of the chest cavity. The space in between the two pleura is thus only potential. The volume of the lungs is maintained by dynamic equilibrium between the tendency of the thoracic cage to expand and the lungs' elastic recoil, which pulls the diaphragm and ribs upwards and inwards respectively, thus opposing thoracic cage expansion. These forces create a subatmospheric pleural pressure which maintains uninterrupted contact between the pleural surfaces. A leak into the pleural cavity allows the ingress of air and lung collapse, generating a pneumothorax.

The lower airway begins at the trachea and ends with the alveolar sacs. In the process, approximately 23 generations of dichotomous division take place. The first 16 generations, which are made up of bronchi, bronchioles, and terminal bronchioles, form the conducting zone. The remaining seven generations form the transitional and respiratory zones, where gas exchange takes place; they are made up of respiratory bronchioles, alveolar ducts, and alveolar sacs. The total cross-sectional area therefore increases dramatically from the beginning of the lower airway (Figure 21.1) to the alveoli. By comparison, if the

**Table 21.1 Functions of the lungs**

| | |
|---|---|
| Metabolic | Gas exchange<br>Tight control of pH |
| Endocrine | Production of angiotensin-converting enzyme<br>Secretion of vasoactive peptides (APUD system) |
| Immunology | Production of secretory IgA and alveolar macrophages |
| Other | Sequestration of microaggregates<br>Removal of prostaglandins, bradykinin, serotonin |

APUD, amine precursor uptake decarboxylase.

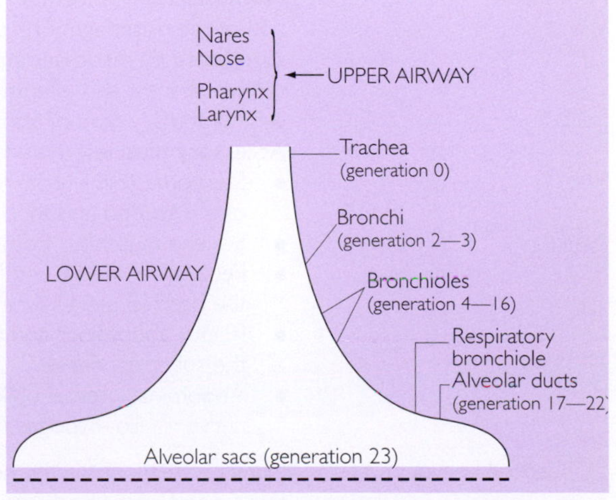


**Figure 21.1** 'Trumpet' model: cross-sectional area of airways.

cross-sectional area of the trachea is approximately equal to that of a 2.5 cm disc then that of the alveolar sacs is equal to the area of a tennis court.The resistance to airflow is greatest in the trachea and major airways, where airflow is turbulent and rapid, and much less in the smaller airways where flow is slow and laminar.

The mucosal lining gradually changes from ciliated columnar epithelium in the trachea to cuboidal and finally to flat alveolar epithelium. Gas exchange can take place only across the latter, which begins to appear on respiratory bronchioles. In parallel to the change in the mucosal lining of the supporting wall, there are also changes with a gradual loss of cartilaginous support at the bronchioles, followed later by smooth muscle. The patency of the smaller airways thus becomes dependent on the radial traction of the elastic recoil of the surrounding tissue. At this level, airway diameter depends on the total lung volume, being greater in inspiration and least in expiration.

Lung action is under autonomic, central and voluntary control. These neural mechanisms are summarized in Table 21.2.

### Alveoli

The size of an alveolus averages about 0.2 mm in diameter and is subject to the influence of gravity and lung volumes. In the upright position, the largest alveoli are at the apex of the lung and slowly decrease in size towards the base. The alveoli are surrounded by pulmonary capillaries. In most areas, the distance between the alveolar epithelium and capillary endothelium is extremely small – approximately 0.4 µm – which provides good gas exchange. Alveoli first begin to appear at the respiratory bronchiole (zones 17–19) and increase in numbers as the dichotomous division continues through the alveolar duct (zones 20–22), and finally ending in blind alveolar sacs (zone 23). Each of the last contains an aver-

**Table 21.2 Nerve supply of the respiratory system**

| Structure | Nerve supply |
|---|---|
| Pharynx | **Efferent and afferent** supplies from pharyngeal plexus, formed from pharyngeal branch of vagus, glosso–pharyngeal and branches from the cervical sympathetic chain. (See 'The pharynx', Chapter 6, and Figure 6.8.) |
| Larynx | **Efferent and afferent** supplies from the vagi on either side give rise to the superior and recurrent (inferior) laryngeal nerves. (See 'The larynx', Chapter 6, and Figures 6.8 and 6.19.) |
| Lungs | **Efferent:** parasympathetic fibres are supplied by the right and left vagi; sympathetic fibres are supplied from the second to fifth thoracic ganglia.The parasympathetic and sympathetic fibres form anterior and posterior pulmonary plexuses at the root of the lungs (see Chapter 6, Figure 6.19).The fibres from these are distributed via pulmonary blood vessels and the bronchial tree. Sympathetic stimulation constricts blood vessels but dilates bronchioles. (Note the use of sympathomimetic drugs in asthma.) Parasympathetic stimulation causes bronchoconstriction and stimulates secretion from mucous glands but has little effect on blood vessels.<br>**Afferent:** nerves run from the epithelium of the bronchial tree with the vagus to its origin and with sympathetic nerves to cell bodies in the posterior thoracic root ganglia. |
| Pleura | **Efferent:** there is none.<br>**Afferent:** there is none from the visceral pleura.There is a rich supply from the parietal pleura, which travels with the phrenic nerves and the intercostal nerves. |
| Muscles | **Main muscles:** The right and left phrenic (C3–C5) are the sole motor nerves to each side of the diaphragm.The phrenic nerves are also sensory to the diaphragm, augmented by the lower intercostal nerves at the periphery.The intercostal muscles receive afferent and efferent supplies from the intercostal nerves formed from the ventral primary rami of spinal nerves T1–T12. (See Chapter 15, Figures 15.37 and 15.38.)<br>**Accessory muscles:** the efferent and afferent supplies are:<br>• Sternomastoid – from the spinal accessory nerve and the anterior primary rami of the second and third cervical nerves<br>• Scalene muscles – from the anterior primary rami of the cervical plexus<br>• Pectorals – medial and lateral pectoral nerves from medial and lateral cords of the brachial plexus (see Chapter 15, Figure 15.25)<br>• Rectus abdominus and abdominal external oblique – lower five intercostals and the subcostal nerve<br>• Abdominal internal oblique and transversus – as external oblique plus first lumbar nerve via ilio–hypogastric and ilio–inguinal nerves (see Chapter 15, Figure 15.34) |
| Central nervous system | Many connections via the nerves listed above and from chemoreceptors in the carotid and aortic bodies, and the medulla. |

age of 17 alveoli, providing an estimated $300 \times 10^6$ alveoli with an enormous surface area (50–100 $m^2$) for gas exchange in the average adult.

The alveoli are lined by two types of epithelial cells: type 1 pneumocytes are flat and are the primary lining cells responsible for gas exchange; type 2 pneumocytes are granular and thicker, and their main function is to secrete surfactant. Other types of cells present include pulmonary alveolar macrophages, lymphocytes, plasma cells, APUD (amine precursor uptake and decarboxylation), and mast cells.

### Lung volumes

Lung volumes during spontaneous respiratory activity can be shown by simple spirometry (Figure 21.2). These vary according to body height, age, and sex. Further detail on the measurement of lung volumes is given in Chapter 39, Figures 39.1–39.5. The average adult tidal volume at rest is approximately 500 ml. The additional air inspired by a maximal inspiratory effort is the inspiratory reserve volume and, similarly, the additional volume expelled by active expiratory effort is the expiratory reserve volume. The two combined, together with the tidal volume, define the vital capacity, which is normally 70–80 ml/kg. The anatomical dead space (approximately 30% of the tidal volume at rest) is the air distributed in the upper airways (trachea and bronchi) that cannot participate in gas exchange. Alveolar dead space is the result of ventilation/perfusion mismatch, when gas exchange fails at the alveolar level. Then, effectively, ventilated alveoli are not perfused. The sum of the two is called the physiological dead space ($V_D$):

$$V_D = \text{Anatomical dead space} + \text{Alveolar dead space}$$

The alveolar dead space is very small in a healthy conscious person. The relationship between VD and tidal volume ($V_T$) is expressed as a ratio and calculated using the Bohr equation:

$$\frac{V_D}{V_T} = \frac{(Pa_{CO_2} - P_{ECO_2})}{(Pa_{CO_2} - P_{ICO_2})}$$

where $Pa_{CO_2}$ is the arterial $CO_2$ tension, $P_{ECO_2}$ is the mixed-expired $CO_2$ tension and $P_{ICO_2}$ the inspired $CO_2$ tension.

The volume at end of passive expiration reflects an equilibrium between the lung recoil and the thoracic cavity expansion. At this point the average pleural pressure is least negative. This volume remaining at end expiration is the functional residual capacity (FRC: about 2800 ml), which remains relatively constant in healthy people throughout adult life. As small airways and alveoli depend on the elastic recoil forces of the lung for their patency, if lung volume is reduced below normal FRC, radial traction may become insufficient, resulting in small air spaces collapsing. The volume at which the airway begins to collapse is called the closing capacity. This volume is normally below the FRC but increases with age.

The closing capacity equals FRC at an average age of 44 years in the supine position and 66 years in the erect position (Figure 21.3). This causes some lower airway closure during tidal respiration and probably contributes to the normal age-related decline in oxygen tension. Pathological conditions can decrease FRC (or increase closing capacity) and promote airway closure, as can change in position, increases in intra-abdominal pressure, and administration of general anaesthetic agents (Figure 21.3). The last produces a further 15–20% reduction of FRC above that which occurs in the supine position alone. The FRC is the single most important factor in relation to pathological conditions such as acute lung injury. Figure 21.4 shows the relationship of lung volumes and FRC to lung compliance, pulmonary vascular resistance, and airway resistance.

The concept of preoxygenation before induction of anaesthesia is based on FRC and 'oxygen stores'. When the continual replacement of oxygen ceases, as in apnoea, existing oxygen stores are depleted at the rate equivalent to the body oxygen requirement. The aver-

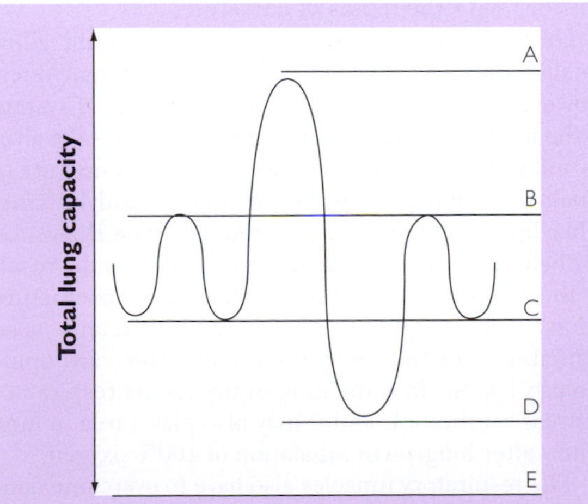


**Figure 21.2** Spirometry tracing showing normal lung volumes. A–B, inspiratory reserve volume; B–C, tidal volume; C–D, expiratory reserve volume; A–D, vital capacity; A–E, total lung capacity; D–E, residual volume; C–E, functional residual capacity.

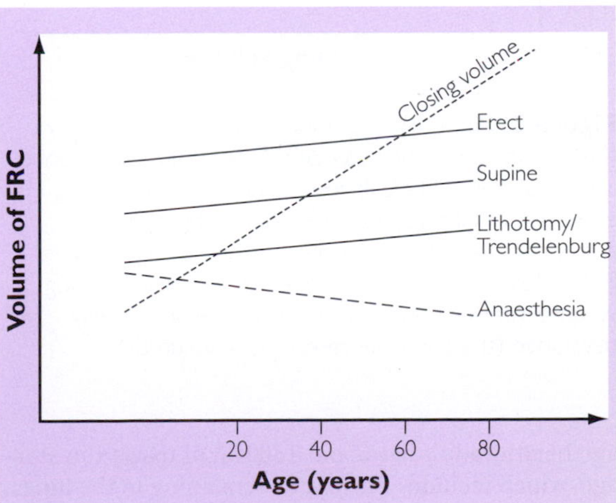


**Figure 21.3** Relationship of functional residual capacity (FRC), age, and closing volume. Note how the closing volume increases with age whereas the FRC is relatively constant.

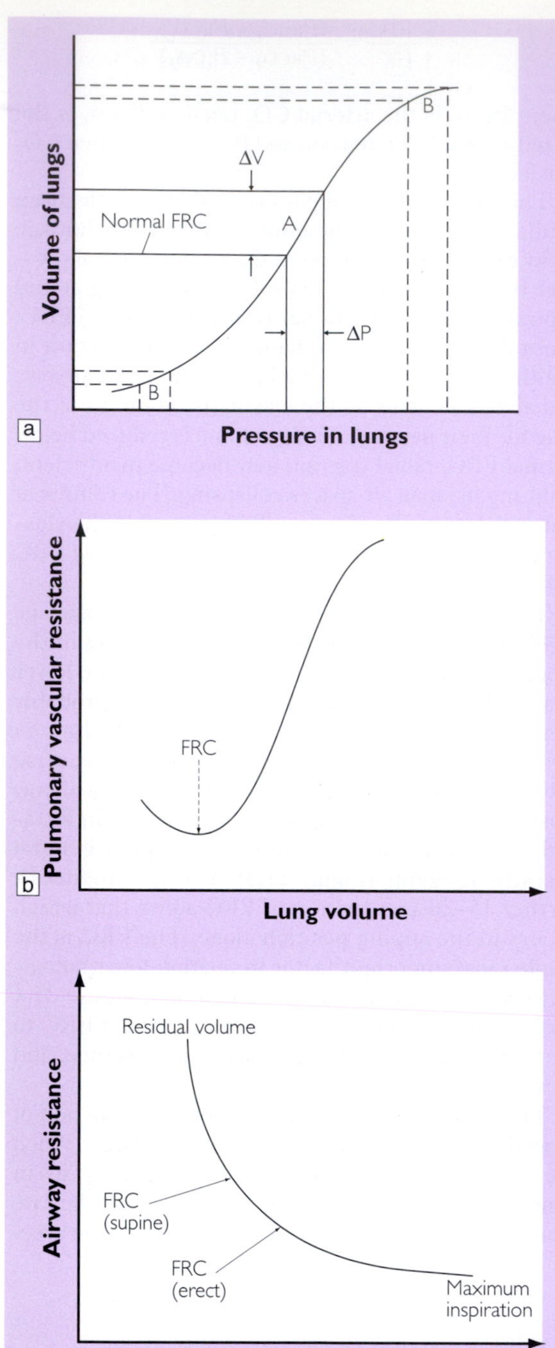


**Figure 21.4** (a) Normal functional residual capacity (FRC) and compliance ($\Delta V/\Delta P$). A, optimum compliance is seen at normal FRC; B, low compliance seen at extremes of lung volume. (b) Relationship between pulmonary vascular resistance (PVR) and lung volume. PVR is least at FRC and increases at extremes of lung volume. (c) Relationship of lung volume and airway resistance (the curve represents lung volumes).

age healthy adult has about 1500 ml of oxygen in storage, which includes the oxygen remaining in the lungs, that bound to haemoglobin and myoglobin, and that dissolved in body fluids. That remaining within the lungs at FRC is the most important source of fresh oxygen. Following apnoea after breathing room air, there is approximately enough oxygen to support metabolic activity of tissues for about 90 seconds before hypoxaemia ensures. After a full nitrogen purge by breathing 100% oxygen for several minutes (preoxygenation), the FRC oxygen store is greatly improved and, under these conditions, the onset of hypoxaemia is delayed for 3–4 minutes.

## Work of breathing, lung compliance, and airway resistance

The work of breathing is determined by elastic and non-elastic components. The elasticity of the respiratory system is measured in terms of compliance ($C$), expressed by the ratio of the volume of gas moved per unit change in distending pressure ($\Delta V/\Delta P$):

$$\underset{(\text{ml/cmH}_2\text{O})}{\text{Compliance}} = \frac{\text{Change in volume (ml)}}{\text{Change in pressure (cmH}_2\text{O)}}$$

Total compliance is the sum of the reciprocal of lung and chest wall compliance. Normal total compliance is 100 ml/cm$H_2O$.

$$C_{\text{Lung}} = \frac{\Delta\text{Lung vol}}{\Delta\text{Transpulmonary pressure}} = 200\ \text{ml/cmH}_2\text{O}$$

$$C_{\text{Chest wall}} = \frac{\Delta\text{Chest volume}}{\Delta\text{Transthoracic pressure}} = 200\ \text{ml/cmH}_2\text{O}$$

$$\frac{1}{C_{\text{Total}}} = \frac{1}{C_{\text{Lung}}} + \frac{1}{C_{\text{Chest wall}}} = 100\ \text{ml/cmH}_2\text{O}.$$

Two main forces act to determine lung compliance: the elastic fibres of the lung parenchyma and the surface tension of the liquid/air interface in the alveoli.

According to Laplace's law, as the radius of curvature of the alveolus falls, the pressure inside the alveolus rises. Laplace's equation states:

$$P = 2T/r$$

where $P$ is the pressure within a bubble, $T$ the surface tension, and $r$ the radius of curvature.

Under normal circumstances, this would allow smaller bubbles (alveoli) to empty into larger ones. However, this does not occur in the biological system of the lungs because of surfactant, which lines the alveoli and reduces these forces. Surfactant is a mixture of dipalmitoyl phosphatidycholine, phosphatidylglycine, other lipids, and proteins, secreted by type II alveolar epithelial cells. Hyaline membrane disease is the result of the inability to produce surfactant in premature lungs. Deficient or abnormal surfactant also contributes to the atelectasis seen after cardiopulmonary bypass, in acute lung injury (acute respiratory distress syndrome), and it may also play a role in lung injury after long-term inhalation of 100% oxygen.

The respiratory muscles also have to overcome non-elastic components: moving inelastic tissues (viscous resistance) and airway resistance. Both influence the pressure required to generate flow into the alveoli.

The flow pattern in the respiratory tree and the pressure–flow relationship depend on whether the flow is turbulent, laminar, or by molecular diffusion. The flow is turbulent in the upper airways and trachea, becomes laminar in the smaller airways and bronchioles, and is by diffusion down concentration gradients at the alveolar cell surface level. Details of the characteristics of turbulent and laminar flow can be found in Chapter 37, Figures 37.46–50. Very importantly, in laminar flow resistance is inversely proportional to the fourth power of the radius and in turbulent flow the density of the gas becomes a major factor. It is because of the latter that a gas mixture of low density (such as the use of helium in upper airway obstruction and in underwater breathing apparatus) reduces the intensity of turbulent flow, thus reducing the work of breathing.

An increase in airway resistance has dramatic effects on normal lung mechanics. Examples include obstruction to the upper airway by the tongue or foreign bodies, external compression of the airway, increased bronchial smooth muscle tone, and mucosal oedema. In acute asthma, in order to maintain tidal flow the normal passive expiration becomes active as a result of airway narrowing. There is also an increase in inspiratory muscle activity and a tendency to increase lung volume such that tidal breathing occurs at an abnormally high FRC with markedly reduced compliance (see Figure 21.4a). This has profound effects on the work of breathing and leads to respiratory muscle fatigue and exhaustion if unresolved.

## PULMONARY BLOOD FLOW

### Pulmonary circulation

The total pulmonary blood flow is equal to the cardiac output, averaging 5 L/min at rest. The pulmonary vascular system is a distendable low-pressure system accommodating blood flow that is equal to the sum of all the other organs in the body. The normal pulmonary artery pressure (PAP) is about 20/10 mmHg with a mean of 13 mmHg. These pressures are about five to six times lower than systemic pressures, because of the high wall compliance and low vascular resistance of the pulmonary vasculature. It is imperative that these low pressures are maintained to enable the right ventricle to function optimally. Both perfusion pressure and vascular resistance are important determinants of blood flow distribution within the pulmonary circulation. In disorders that result in disruption of this homoeostasis, the right ventricle becomes dysfunctional and may contribute to inadequate oxygenation and low cardiac output. Chronic disorders of perfusion can result in 'cor pulmonale' – right ventricular failure secondary to pulmonary pathology.

The volume of blood in the pulmonary vessels at any one time varies between 500 ml and 1000 ml. Large increases in cardiac output or intravascular volume can be accommodated with minimal changes in pulmonary vascular pressures as a result of high compliance and recruitment of collapsed pulmonary vessels.

In addition to the normal pulmonary blood flow, approximately 1% of cardiac output is directed into the bronchial circulation. The bronchial arteries provide the vaso-vasorum of the pulmonary arteries and may be responsible, in part, for determining pulmonary arterial tone. The origins of the bronchial arteries are inconstant and include the aorta and the intercostal, subclavian and innominate arteries. Two-thirds of the bronchial blood supply empties into the pulmonary veins, and the remainder into the azygos system. The former creates a shunt by depositing deoxygenated blood into the left side of the heart.

### Distribution of pulmonary blood flow

Pulmonary blood flow is not uniform; it is influenced by the effect of gravity and hydrostatic pressure differences within the lungs. In the normal lung, the dependent or lower portions of the lung receive greater blood flow than the non-dependent areas. To understand the influence of hydrostatic gradient on pulmonary blood flow, the upright lung may be divided into three zones depending on alveolar ($P_A$), arterial ($P_a$), and venous ($P_v$) pressures (West's lung zones: Figure 21.5). Zone 1 is the upper zone where PAP is normally just sufficient to maintain perfusion, but, if it is reduced (e.g. hypovolaemic shock) or if alveolar pressure is increased (e.g. positive pressure ventilation), the pulmonary artery capillaries become occluded. Under these circumstances this area represents alveolar dead space.

In the middle portion of the lungs (zone 2), PAP exceeds alveolar pressure which, in turn, exceeds pulmonary venous pressure. However, because respiration and pulmonary blood flow are cyclic, blood flow in zone 2 is intermittent and varies with the artery–alveolar pressure gradient. As arterial pressure increases down the zone, blood flow also increases.

In zone 3, pulmonary venous pressure exceeds alveolar pressure. As both vascular pressures are greater than alveolar pressure, the potentially collapsible vessels are now held permanently open and blood flow becomes continuous, determined by the arterial–venous pressure difference. In descending zone 3, the vascular pressure splinting the blood vessels open increases more than the opposing outside pressure, so that the transmural distending pressure increases. This results in increased calibre of vessels, reduction in vascular resistance, and further increase in blood flow.

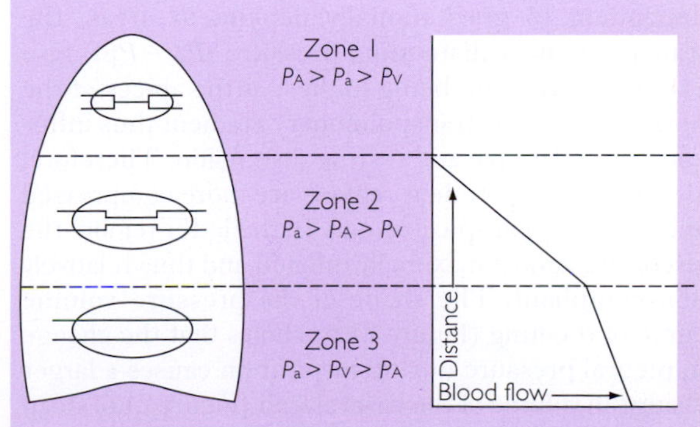


**Figure 21.5** Distribution of pulmonary blood flow in the three-zone model of the vertical lung. The upper zone is drawn as having no perfusion; in practice a basal perfusion is maintained. Pa, alveolar pressure; Pc, arterial pressure; Pv, venous pressure.

## THE INTERFACE BETWEEN GAS AND BLOOD

### Ventilation

Ventilation is usually measured as minute ventilation (MV) given by:

$$MV = V_T \times f$$

where $V_T$ is the tidal volume and $f$ the respiratory rate (frequency in breaths/min).

As mentioned above, the $V_D$ represents the gas unable to participate in gas exchange. The relationship between $V_D$ and $V_T$ is expressed as a ratio ($V_D/V_T$) and calculated using the Bohr equation (see above). In normal healthy lungs this ratio is usually less than 30% ($V_D$ amounting to 150 ml in a 70-kg adult – approximately 2 ml/kg). A variety of factors affects the dead space, including posture, age, artificial airway, intermittent positive pressure ventilation, drugs, pulmonary perfusion, and intrinsic lung disease. In severe obstructive airway disease, $V_D/V_T$ may increase to 60%. Under these conditions ventilation is grossly wasted or inefficient.

Alveolar ventilation ($\dot{V}_A$) is the part of MV that takes part in gas exchange, defined as

$$\dot{V}_A = f \times (V_T - V_D).$$

As a result, the average adult's MV of 6 L/min (500 ml tidal volume, 12 breaths/min) results in actual alveolar ventilation of 4.2 L/min. Rapid but shallow breathing produces much less alveolar ventilation than does slow, deep breathing at the same total MV volume because of the disproportionate effect of anatomical dead space at low tidal volume.

During spontaneous ventilation, the dependent regions are better ventilated than the non-dependent ones. This inequality is the result of the gravitational induced intrapleural ($P$pl) and transpulmonary pressure gradient. The pressure in the intrapleural space is normally subatmospheric (negative). The pull of the gravitational force creates a relatively more negative intrapleural pressure at the top of the thoracic cavity, where the lung tries to pull away from the chest wall. Because internal alveolar pressure is constant, as the intrapleural pressure becomes less negative from non-dependent to gravitationally dependent areas, the transpulmonary distending pressure ($P_A - P$pl) also exhibits a gradient, being highest at the apices of the upright lung. The transpulmonary gradient thus influences alveolar size and resting distension. Therefore, alveoli in the dependent regions are more compressed and smaller than apical alveoli. In the latter region, the alveoli are almost maximally inflated and thus relatively non-compliant. The shape of the pressure–volume curve of the lung (Figure 21.6) shows that the change in pleural pressure during inspiration causes a larger change in volume of the basal alveoli (Figure 21.6, steep slope) than the apical alveoli (Figure 21.6, flat slope).

### Ventilation–perfusion ratio

The alveolar ventilation ($\dot{V}_A$) is approximately 4.5 L/min and pulmonary blood flow ($\dot{Q}_A$) is 5 L/min. This gives an overall $\dot{V}_A/\dot{Q}_A$ (commonly abbreviated to $\dot{V}/\dot{Q}$) of 0.9. However, this relationship is not constant and can theoretically vary from one extreme to the other: from infinity (no perfusion – as in zone 1) to 0 (no ventilation). The former is referred to (theoretically) as alveolar dead space and the latter as intrapulmonary shunt.

The difference between the rate of increase in blood flow and ventilation from top to the bottom of the upright lung results in regional differences in gas exchange. The $\dot{V}/\dot{Q}$ ratio decreases from zone 1 to zone 3 (Figure 21.7), resulting in alveoli at the top of the lung over-ventilated in relationship to their perfusion. Lung units with a low $\dot{V}/\dot{Q}$ ratio have low alveolar oxygen partial pressure ($P_{AO_2}$) and a high alveolar $CO_2$ partial pressure ($P_{ACO_2}$). Conversely, those units where ventilation is in excess to perfusion (high $\dot{V}/\dot{Q}$ ratio), the $P_{AO_2}$ is high with low $P_{ACO_2}$. It follows that pulmonary venous blood from units with low $\dot{V}/\dot{Q}$ ratios has a low arterial oxygen tension ($P_{aO_2}$) and high arterial $CO_2$ tension ($P_{aCO_2}$) and vice versa. A compensatory increase in oxygen uptake cannot take place in remaining areas with high $\dot{V}/\dot{Q}$ ratios because of the shape of the oxyhaemoglobin dissociation curve – in this region the effluent blood is normally already maximally saturated with oxygen (Figure 21.7). However, because the $CO_2$ dissociation curve is linear, over-ventilated but perfused alveoli give off an excessive amount of $CO_2$ with a compensatory decrease in $P_{aCO_2}$. In the normal

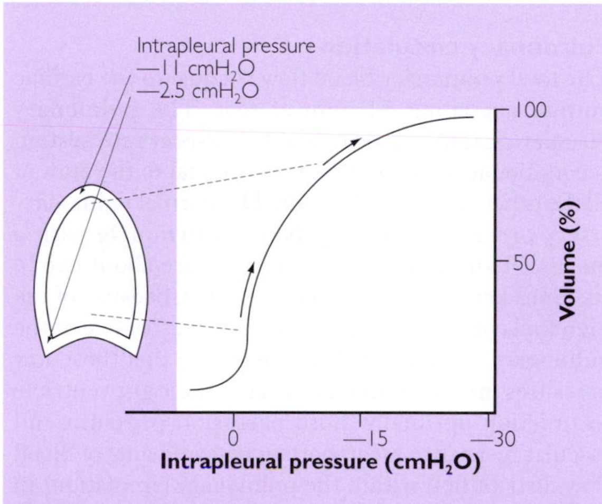


**Figure 21.6** Intrapleural pressure and ventilation in the upright lung.

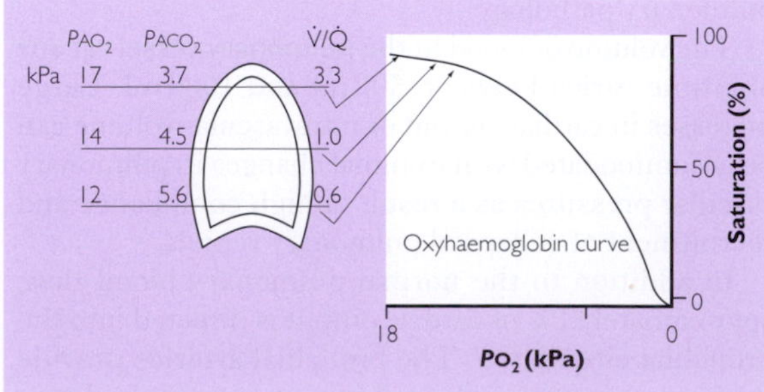


**Figure 21.7** Regional differences in ventilation–perfusion ($\dot{V}/\dot{Q}$) ratio and its effect on normal haemoglobin saturation

lung this produces mixed pulmonary venous blood with $Pa\text{O}_2$ and $Pa\text{CO}_2$ of 13.3 and 5.3 kPa respectively. Deviation from this is accompanied by adjustment of overall ventilation (thus, overall $\dot{V}/\dot{Q}$ ratio) from the respiratory centre via the $Pa\text{CO}_2$. There is, however, some control over local $\dot{V}/\dot{Q}$ ratios from a process called hypoxic pulmonary vasoconstriction. By this mechanism, decreased regional alveolar $P\text{O}_2$ causes regional pulmonary vasoconstriction, which diverts blood away from hypoxic sections of the lung to better ventilated normoxic sections, thereby minimizing venous admixture.

In the diseased lung, the $\dot{V}/\dot{Q}$ ratio inequality may be so severe that no amount of increase in ventilation can return the $Pa\text{O}_2$ to its normal level, although the $P\text{CO}_2$ is brought down. This is the blood gas definition of type I respiratory failure. Sometimes with advanced disease or when the respiratory muscles are unable to keep up with the increasing demand in ventilation, hypercapnia develops (type II respiratory failure – Table 21.3).

### Shunt

The overall effect of shunting is to reduce arterial oxygen content. Some of the blood in the thoracic branches of the aorta, and bronchial and coronary arteries, is returned directly to the left side of the heart, bypassing the pulmonary capillaries. This constitutes the true anatomical shunt and, together with 'shunt-like' effect from areas of low $\dot{V}/\dot{Q}$ ratio, adds to the overall venous admixture.

| Anatomical shunt | + | 'Shunt' from low but finite $\dot{V}/\dot{Q}$ ratio | = | Venous admixture |
|---|---|---|---|---|

The anatomical shunt (normally 1–2% of cardiac output) is made up of arteriovenous connections, as described above, and, when present, right-to-left intracardiac shunts.

The normal $\dot{V}/\dot{Q}$ variation is exacerbated in pulmonary disease and results in an increase in pulmonary venous admixture. Quantitatively, this can be calculated using the shunt equation that expresses the amount of shunted blood ($\dot{Q}\text{S}$ in L/min) as a percentage of the total cardiac output ($\dot{Q}\text{T}$):

$$\frac{\dot{Q}\text{S}}{\dot{Q}\text{T}} = \frac{Cc'\text{O}_2 - Ca\text{O}_2}{Cc'\text{O}_2 - C\bar{v}\text{O}_2}$$

where $Cc'\text{O}_2$ is the end-capillary oxygen content (ml/dl), $Ca\text{O}_2$ the arterial oxygen content and $C\bar{v}\text{O}_2$ the mixed venous oxygen content

The ideal $Cc'\text{O}_2$ is calculated from the ideal alveolar gas equation. It is assumed that the alveolar oxygen tension is in equilibrium with end-capillary oxygen tension and therefore of the same value. The alveolar air equation calculates the $P\text{AO}_2$ by subtracting from the dry gas fraction of inspired air, the water vapour and the uptake of oxygen which exchanges for $CO_2$ in the alveolus depending on the respiratory quotient.

$$P\text{AO}_2 = P\text{IO}_2 - \frac{P\text{ACO}_2}{R}$$

where $P\text{IO}_2 = F\text{IO}_2 \times (P_B - P\text{H}_2\text{O})$. $F\text{IO}_2$ is the fractional inspired oxygen concentration, $P_\text{B}$ is the barometric pressure, and $P\text{H}_2\text{O}$ is the saturated vapour pressure of water at body temperature (5 kPa). R is normally 0.8.

If hypoxaemia results from a reduction in $\dot{V}/\dot{Q}$ ratios, i.e. relative underventilation, then an increase in $Pa\text{O}_2$ can be brought about by an increase in $F\text{IO}_2$ as shown in Figure 21.8. This is the situation that occurs commonly in the immediate postoperative period when hypoxaemia can be corrected by facemask oxygen. Conversely, as the shunt fraction increases, the resultant hypoxaemia is less likely to be corrected by an increase in $F\text{IO}_2$. This is because the blood leaving the well-oxygenated units, although it has a high $Pa\text{O}_2$,

**Table 21.3 Causes of respiratory failure**

| Type I[a] | Type II[b] |
|---|---|
| Pneumonia | Sleep apnoea |
| Asthma (early) | Asthma (late stage – exhaustion) |
| Emphysema ('pink puffers') | COPD and acute exacerbation ('blue bloaters') |
| Pulmonary embolism | Respiratory muscle fatigue/polio/myasthenia |
| Pulmonary oedema | Neuropathy (late) (Guillain–Barré) |
| Pneumothorax | Opioid overdose |
| Pulmonary fibrosis | Head injury |

[a]Hypoxaemia without hypercapnia.
[b]Hypoxaemia with hypercapnia.
COAD, chronic obstructive airway disease.

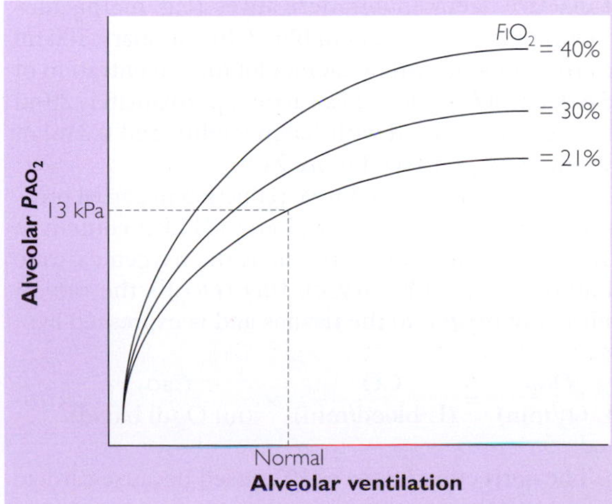


**Figure 21.8** Relationship between hypoventilation and $Pa\text{O}_2$. Normal alveolar ventilation is 60 ml/kg/min. $F\text{IO}_2$, fractional inspired oxygen concentration.

carries little extra content of oxygen because the haemoglobin is already maximally saturated. Consequently, when this mixes with poorly oxygenated blood from poorly ventilated units the resulting $PaO_2$ remains low. For practical purposes, with a shunt of greater than 50% an increase in $FIO_2$ results in almost no increase in $PaO_2$.

The alveolar–arterial oxygen partial pressure difference (A–a$PO_2$) reflects the amount of $\dot{V}/\dot{Q}$ ratio inequality. Normally, this is less than 2 kPa (15 mmHg) but it increases progressively with age. Clinically, this is often used as an approximation for venous admixture. However, the A–a$PO_2$ is dependent not only on the amount of right-to-left shunting, but also on the mixed venous tension, cardiac output, and oxygen consumption. Although $PaCO_2$ remains essentially constant throughout life (except in the case of pregnancy), the $PaO_2$ falls steadily because of the increasing alveolar–arterial difference associated with age. There is a variety of expressions available to calculate this trend. A typical equation to approximate arterial tension in otherwise normal lungs is:

$$PaO_2 = 102 - (0.33 \times \text{age})\ \text{mmHg}$$

or

$$PaO_2 = 13.6 - (0.44 \times \text{age})\ \text{kPa}.$$

## TRANSPORT OF RESPIRATORY GASES

### Oxygen

Oxygen is carried in the blood mainly in reversible association with haemoglobin. A small proportion is also carried dissolved in solution. The solubility coefficient of oxygen at normal body temperature and barometric pressure is 0.0225 ml/dl per kPa. Thus, the maximum amount of oxygen dissolved in blood at normal arterial tension is very small (0.3 ml/dl) compared with that in association with haemoglobin.

By comparison, the theoretical maximum oxygen-carrying capacity of haemoglobin is given by the Hufner's constant and is 1.39 ml/g (or 139 ml/dl). However, for practical purposes this constant is reduced to 1.36 ml/g to take account of small amounts of inactive haemoglobin derivatives (e.g. methaemoglobin) normally present in blood. In summary, 100 ml of arterial blood with a haemoglobin concentration of 15 g/dl and a $PaO_2$ of 13 kPa carries approximately 20 ml of oxygen combined with haemoglobin and 0.3 ml of dissolved oxygen (see Figure 21.9).

There is a normal stepwise reduction in partial pressures of oxygen from atmospheric (21 kPa) content to the tissues. This is referred to as the oxygen cascade (Figure 21.10). The oxygen flux ($DO_2$)is the rate of delivery of oxygen to the tissues and is expressed by:

$$\underset{(\text{L O}_2/\text{min})}{DO_2} = \underset{(\text{L blood/min})}{\text{CO}} \times \underset{(\text{ml O}_2/\text{dl blood})}{CaO_2} \times 10$$

The correction factor of 10 is used because cardiac output (CO) is expressed as litres/minute, whereas oxygen content ($CaO_2$) is normally calculated as millilitres/decilitre:

$$CaO_2 = (0.0225 \times PO_2) + (SaO_2 \times \text{Hb} \times 1.36\ \text{ml/g})$$

where Hb is the haemoglobin concentration in g/dl, $SaO_2$ is the normal arterial oxygen saturation (99%) and 1.36 is the corrected Hufner's constant oxygen-carrying capacity. Oxygen flux is therefore dependent on $PaO_2$, haemoglobin concentration, and cardiac output , and approximates in health to 1 L/min at rest.

At rest, total oxygen consumption ($\dot{V}O_2$) is approximately 250 ml/min, resulting in a mixed venous oxygen saturation of 75% ($PO_2$ = 5.3 kPa). The normal oxygen extraction ratio (OER) is therefore 25%, which at times of increased demand or reduced delivery can increase with resultant drop in mixed venous saturation. The OER is given by:

$$\text{OER} = \frac{CaO_2 - C\bar{v}O_2}{CaO_2} \times 100\%$$

where $C\bar{v}O_2$ is the mixed venous oxygen content.

It can be seen that there is a relationship between oxygen consumption, oxygen content, and cardiac output. This is expressed by the Fick equation (Chapter 37, Figure 37.68):

$$\dot{V}O_2 = \text{CO} \times (CaO_2 - C\bar{v}O_2).$$

By rearranging, it can be seen that arteriovenous oxygen content difference is a good indicator of the global adequacy of oxygen delivery:

$$CaO_2 - C\bar{v}O_2 = (\dot{V}O_2/\text{CO}).$$

With normal oxygen consumption, the arteriovenous oxygen difference is approximately 5 ml/dl. This is equivalent to the normal extraction fraction for oxygen (see above) of 25%.

Although the cardiac output, content of oxygen per 100 ml of blood and the concentration of haemoglobin are very important, the $PaO_2$ (which above about 13 kPa has little effect on content – Figure 21.10) does have another important effect. It can be seen from the oxygen cascade (Figure 21.10) that the $PO_2$ in the mitochondria is very low (0.13–1 kPa). It is, however, the partial pressure gradient of dissolved oxygen that provides the 'driving' force for the displacement by diffusion of oxygen from the blood to the mitochondria.

### Haemoglobin and the oxygen dissociation curve

Haemoglobin is a large complex molecule (molecular weight of 64 500 Da) containing four protein subunits, each of which contains a haem moiety. The protein subunits consists of two α and two β chains, held together by weak bonds. The ferrous ($Fe^{2+}$) iron–porphyrin (haem) units form a loose reversible compound with oxygen. Thus, one molecule of haemoglobin binds up to four oxygen molecules. The reaction is oxygenation and not oxidation as the iron remains in the ferrous state.

The characteristic sigmoid oxyhaemoglobin dissociation curve (ODC – see Figure 21.9) results from a complex interaction between subunits reflecting a non-linear affinity for oxygen binding. Four separate chemical reactions are involved in binding the four

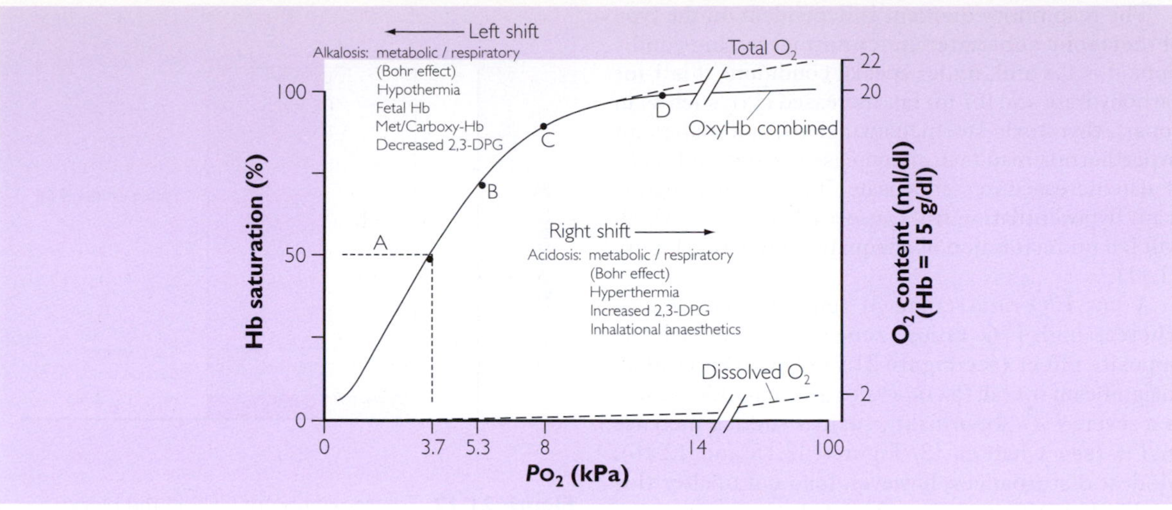


**Figure 21.9** Oxygen ($O_2$)–haemoglobin (Hb) dissociation curve. A, $P_{50}$; B, $P\bar{v}O_2$; C, 90% saturation; D, arterial point (98% saturation) (see text). 2, 3-DPG, 2, 3-diphosphoglycerate.

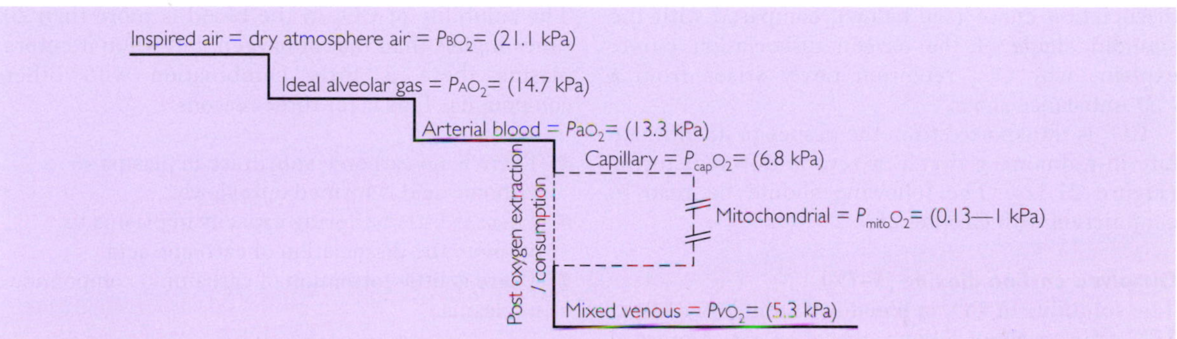


**Figure 21.10** The oxygen cascade.

oxygen molecules. The oxygen affinity of haemoglobin increases as it combines with increasing numbers of molecules, so that the affinity of haemoglobin for the fourth oxygen molecule is many times that for the first.

The position of the steep slope of the ODC on the horizontal axis is defined by the oxygen tension when the haemoglobin is 50% saturated (Figure 21.10 – point A, $P_{50}$). In normal subjects, this is 3.7 kPa. The affinity of haemoglobin varies according to the position of the ODC. Factors causing an increase in $P_{50}$ value, as occurs in metabolizing tissues, shift the ODC to the right. For any given $PaO_2$ the corresponding haemoglobin saturation is lower than that when the $P_{50}$ is 3.7 kPa. This therefore encourages oxygen release. Conversely, a decrease in $P_{50}$ causes a left shift and encourages oxygen binding as occurs in the lungs.

It can be seen from Figure 21.9 that, at a normal $PaO_2$, haemoglobin is 98% saturated. If the $PaO_2$ falls to less than 8 kPa (point C, approximately 90% saturated), the saturation begins to fall steeply, so that for a further given reduction in $PaO_2$ there is a disproportionately greater decline in haemoglobin saturation. Mixed venous blood has a $P\bar{v}O_2$ of about 5.3 kPa resulting in a saturation of 75% (point B). As can be seen, when giving 100% oxygen to normal individuals, dissolved oxygen increases to 2 ml/dl, but with very little increase in oxygen carriage by haemoglobin and in overall oxygen content.

The oxygen delivery to the peripheral tissues is 1000 ml/min. Of this total there is a limit to which oxygen can be extracted because it would lower the tissue $PO_2$ below the level at which vital organs can survive. In an extreme case, if the oxygen saturation of haemoglobin falls to 40% with normal cardiac output and normal haemoglobin level, then the oxygen availability is just sufficient to meet demands at rest. Increased demand can then be met only with an increase in cardiac output or haemoglobin (polycythaemia).

### Carbon dioxide

The normal mixed venous ($P\bar{v}CO_2$) and arterial ($PaCO_2$) carbon dioxide tensions are about 6.1 kPa and 5.4 kPa respectively. This is a function of both $CO_2$ production according to the respiratory quotient ($R$):

$$R = \frac{\text{Rate of } CO_2 \text{ production}}{\text{Rate of } O_2 \text{ consumption}}$$

and elimination which is inversely related to alveolar ventilation:

$$P\text{ACO}_2 = \frac{\dot{V}CO_2}{\dot{V}A}$$

This results in a hyperbolic curve (Figure 21.11).

The respiratory quotient is dependent on the type of metabolic substrate; under normal resting conditions it is 0.8 and, under special conditions it is 1 for carbohydrate and 0.7 for fat. Increased $\dot{V}CO_2$ such as in sepsis, thyrotoxic storm, convulsions, and malignant hyperthermia results in an increase in $PaCO_2$ unless $\dot{V}A$ is also increased to compensate. It follows that significant hypoventilation will cause a rise in $PaCO_2$ which will fall on restoration of adequate ventilation (Figure 21.11).

A low $\dot{V}/\dot{Q}$ ratio (zone 3) tends to raise $PaCO_2$ whereas high $\dot{V}/\dot{Q}$ ratios (zone 1) tend to have the opposite effect (see Figure 21.7). This results in an insignificant overall $PaCO_2$–$PACO_2$ gradient unless there is a severe $\dot{V}/\dot{Q}$ abnormality, such as sudden increase in $VD$ (see Chapter 12, Figures 12.15 and 12.16). Modest disturbances, however, tend not to alter this gradient significantly because of the reflex increase in $\dot{V}A$ (to a rise in $PaCO_2$) and the fact that diffusion capacity for $CO_2$ across the alveolar membrane is significantly greater (approximately 20 times) than that of oxygen. The relative linearity of the carbon dioxide dissociation curve (see below), compared with the sigmoid shape of the oxygen dissociation curve, explains why $CO_2$ retention rarely arises from a $\dot{V}/\dot{Q}$ imbalance alone.

$CO_2$ is transported from the tissues to its ultimate fate in pulmonary alveoli in several different forms (Figure 21.12). The following should be read in conjunction with Chapter 26.

***Dissolved carbon dioxide (5–7%)***

The solubility of $CO_2$ in blood is 0.5 ml/dl per kPa at 37°C which is about 20 times that of oxygen. At normal arterial $CO_2$ tension (5.3 kPa), this amounts to 2.65 ml/dl with a corresponding increase of 0.4 ml/dl in mixed venous blood. Therefore, there is considerably more $CO_2$ than oxygen in simple solution at equal partial pressures. Forty percent of dissolved $CO_2$ is in the erythrocytes.

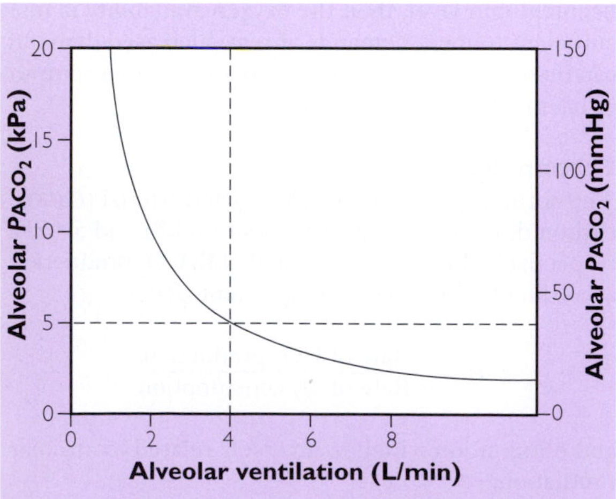


**Figure 21.11** The hyperbolic relationship between alveolar $CO_2$ tension and alveolar ventilation (at body temperature and ambient pressure, and saturated with water vapour). Normal alveolar ventilation is 4.0–4.5 L/min.

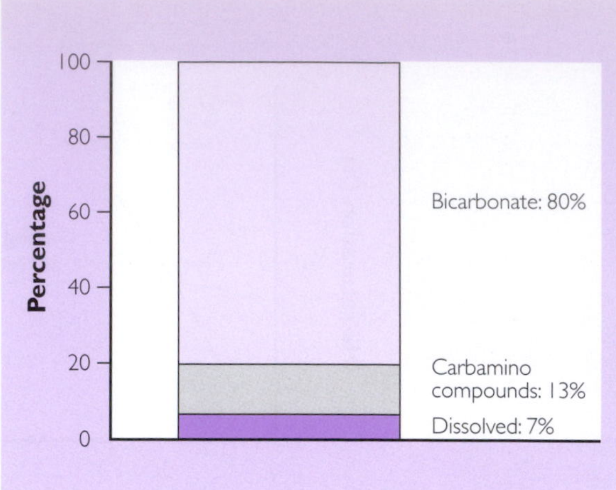


**Figure 21.12** Transportation of $CO_2$ in the blood.

***Bicarbonate (80–85%)***

The solubility of $CO_2$ in the blood is more than 20 times higher than that of oxygen, but when it enters plasma there is little combination with other compounds. This is for three reasons:

- There is no carbonic anhydrase in plasma so carbonic acid is formed only slowly.
- There is little buffering capacity in plasma to promote the dissociation of carbonic acid.
- There is little formation of carbamino compounds in plasma.

$CO_2$ does however diffuse freely into the erythrocytes, where there are carbamino compounds (see below) and carbonic anhydrase, which is associated with haemoglobin (and is not found in the plasma). Carbonic anhydrase specifically catalyses the formation and breakdown of carbonic acid as shown below:

$$CO_2 + H_2O \overset{\text{carbonic anhydrase}}{\rightleftharpoons} H_2CO_3 \rightleftharpoons H^+ + HCO_3^-$$

Once formed, carbonic acid spontaneously breaks down into bicarbonate ions; at a pH of 7.4 the ratio of bicarbonate ions to carbonic acid molecules is 20:1. The bicarbonate thus produced then passes into the plasma. In this way the bicarbonate system carries the majority of $CO_2$ produced in the tissues to the lungs. Subsequently, to maintain electrical neutrality, chloride ions move into the erythrocytes in equimolar quantities. This is referred to as the chloride shift or the Hamburger effect. The reverse reactions occur in the pulmonary capillaries, where bicarbonate re-enters the erythrocytes, with liberation of $CO_2$. At any one time approximately three-quarters of the bicarbonate ions are in plasma and one-quarter in the erythrocytes.

***Carbamino compounds (10–13%)***

A small amount of $CO_2$ also combines directly with amino residues on proteins:

$$R\text{-}NH_2 + CO_2 \rightarrow RNH\text{-}CO_2^- + H^+.$$

During normal conditions, only a small amount of $CO_2$ is carried in this form, of which the majority is in combination with haemoglobin. The hydrogen ions produced are buffered by the histidine residues of haemoglobin itself. The greater carbaminohaemoglobin formation in venous blood increases deoxyhaemoglobin affinity for $CO_2$. Thus venous blood carries more $CO_2$ than does arterial blood. Almost all the carbaminohaemoglobin is in the erythrocytes.

#### *Christian–Douglas–Haldane effect*

Deoxyhaemoglobin, a weak acid and buffer, promotes bicarbonate formation by its ability to buffer hydrogen ions. As a result, the total amount of $CO_2$ that is carried in venous blood (as bicarbonate) is increased. The reverse happens when reduced haemoglobin is oxygenated and converted to the stronger acid, oxyhaemoglobin. This shift in relationship of $P\text{CO}_2$ to total $CO_2$ as a result of a left shift of $CO_2$ dissociation curve in venous blood is referred to as the Haldane effect. The carbon dioxide dissociation curve for whole blood, demonstrating the Haldane effect, is shown in Figure 12.13.

## CHANGES IN POSITION AND THE EFFECTS OF ANAESTHESIA

When a person is awake and in the supine position, the diaphragm is high in the chest (presumed to be secondary to pressure from the abdominal contents), with a consequent reduction in the FRC of 0.5–0.75 L (see Figure 21.4). By analogy with the upright position, the tidal flow of gases now gradually increases down the lungs from anterior to posterior (assuming no atelectasis). As with the upright lung, the increase in blood flow is in the same direction, with the dependent parts receiving the most. These changes produce a similar spread of $\dot{V}/\dot{Q}$ values.

When a supine patient is anaesthetized, there is a further reduction of the FRC by 0.4–0.5 L, putting the FRC close to the residual volume. This change is likely to be caused by a reduction in muscle tone because it is accompanied by a further cephalad movement of the diaphragm, a decrease in the ventilation of the most dependent parts of the lung, and an increase in airways resistance. In addition, it has been known for some time that, during anaesthesia, there is an increase in venous admixture of 10–15%. Computerized tomography scanning has now shown that this is the result of atelectasis occurring at the most posterior dependent sections of the lung, as shown in Figure 21.14. This atelectasis occurs during both spontaneous breathing and IPPV. After anaesthesia, the FRC does not return to normal until some hours after recovery to consciousness. This requires specific management in the post-operative period (see Chapter 5, Figures 5.10 and 5.11 and accompanying text).

During spontaneous ventilation in the lateral position, the lower dome of the diaphragm is pushed higher into to chest, whilst the upper dome is flattened. In this position the lower dome can contract more effectively than the upper dome, and ventilation of the lower lung is approximately twice that of the upper. Gravity causes a similar disparity between the blood flow to the two lungs, thereby making ventilation–perfusion ratios

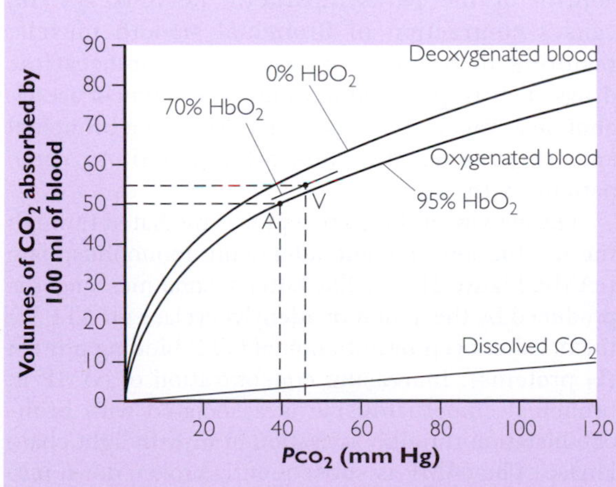


**Figure 21.13** The carbon dioxide ($CO_2$) dissociation curve, demonstrating the Haldane effect. The arterial point (A) and the venous point (V) indicate the total $CO_2$ found in arterial and venous blood, respectively, in a resting human. (Adapted from Kinney, *Anesthesiology* 1960;10:4.)

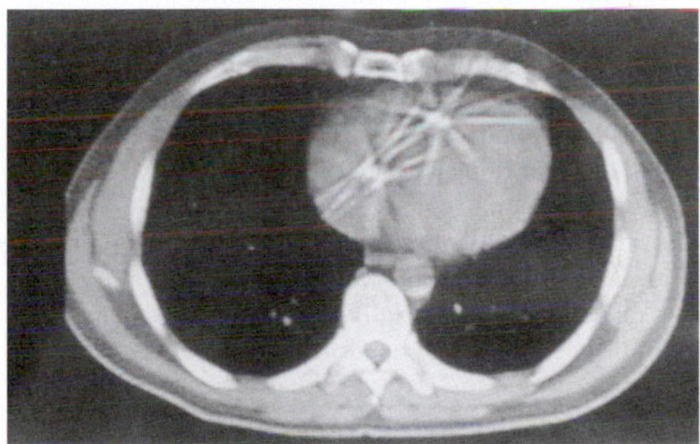

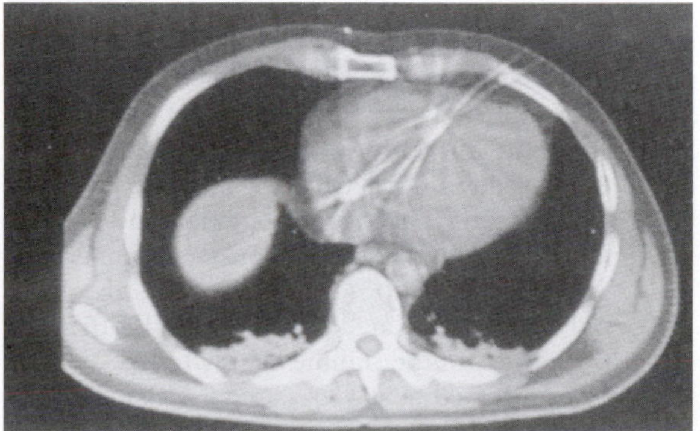

**Figure 21.14** Computerized tomography scans of awake (top) and anaesthetized (bottom) patient. During anaesthesia, dense regions in the dependent parts of each lung can be seen, corresponding to atelectasis. In addition, in the anaesthetized state, a grey–white, egg-shaped region can be seen in the middle of the right lung field. This is caused by cranial shift of the diaphragm during anaesthesia. (From Hedenstrierna G. *Clin Anaesthesiol* 1996,10:4.)

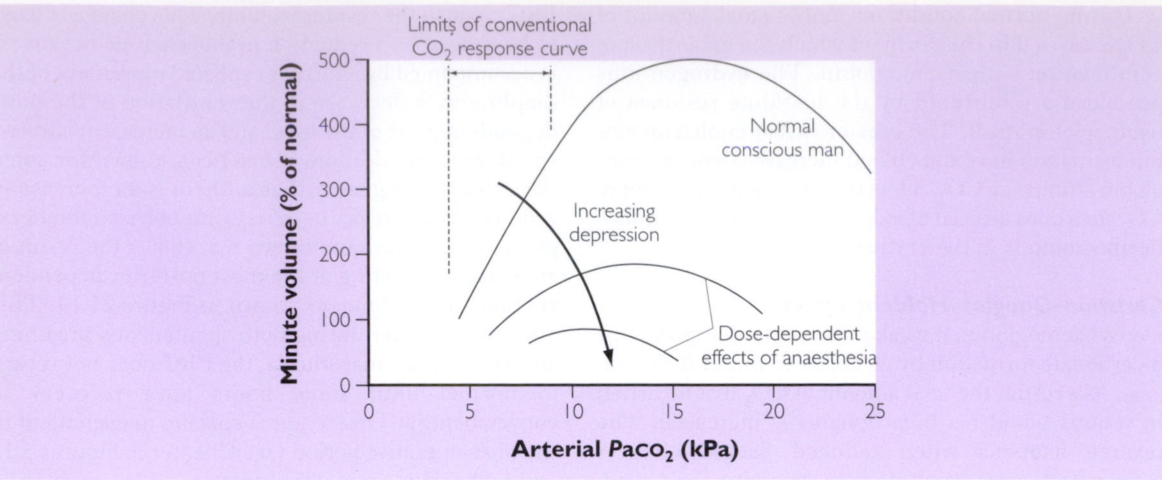


**Figure 21.15** The effect of anaesthesia on the normal $CO_2$ response curve. These curves are usually obtained by the subject inhaling gas mixtures that contain $CO_2$.

more constant throughout. When a patient is anaesthetized, breathing spontaneously in this position, the FRC falls, the tone of the diaphragm is lost, and the position of the lungs changes. This results in preferential ventilation of the upper lung, with increased pulmonary blood flow to the lower lung.

IPPV changes the distribution of ventilation. In the supine position it increases the air flow to the anterior part of the lung and in the lateral position increases air flow to the upper lung. IPPV can also reduce pulmonary blood flow, particularly if cardiac output is low. Detailed discussion of the regional gas and blood flows during thoracotomy, one-lung ventilation and other complex situations is beyond the scope of this book.

Anaesthesia can also affect breathing because of the techniques and drugs used. Inadvertent hyperventilation can reduce the $Pa_{CO_2}$ to below the threshold that triggers spontaneous breathing, and the drugs used can significantly reduce the minute volumes achieved in spontaneous breathing. This can be either a direct effect of residual neuromuscular blockade or the result of central depression of the medullary neurones and respiratory centre.

The normal response of a healthy conscious non-medicated human to a rise in arterial $CO_2$ tension is a prompt linear increase in minute volume. This produces the conventional $CO_2$ response curve (Figure 21.15). It is assumed from animal models and isolated observations in man that this response continues until very high levels of $Pa_{CO_2}$ (15–20 kPa), the toxicity of $CO_2$ and subsequent acidosis depress the drive to breath, and the minute volume begins to fall – a state sometimes referred to as $CO_2$ narcosis. The effect of volatile anaesthetic agents, opioids, and all sedative drugs is to shift the curve to the right and lower the gradient (see Figure 21.15). This means that a higher threshold is needed to trigger breathing and there is a reduced response to a rising $CO_2$. Slopes and intercepts of $CO_2$ response curves show wider intersubject variability, both in the medicated and non-medicated state. Further details of the effects of drugs and diseases on the control of ventilation and acid–base balance are given in Chapters 4, 5, 22, 23, 25, 26, 34 and 54.

## BRONCHIAL PHARMACOLOGY

### Bronchomotor tone

The ratio of smooth muscle to cartilage increases in the walls of the conducting airway from the trachea to bronchioles. Beyond the terminal bronchiole, the airway is devoid of cartilage. The walls of the bronchi and bronchioles are innervated by cholinergic and adrenergic fibres of the autonomic nervous system. Cholinergic discharge from the vagus causes bronchoconstriction and an increase in respiratory tract secretion, both mediated via muscarinic receptors. In addition there are $\beta_2$-adrenoceptors in the bronchial smooth muscle which, on stimulation, cause bronchodilatation. The majority of these $\beta_2$-receptors appear not to be innervated.

A series of second messengers trigger intracellular events leading to the change in the bronchial smooth muscle tone. Cyclic guanosine monophosphate (cGMP), a second messenger under the control of the parasympathetic nervous system, causes contraction of bronchial smooth muscle, resulting in bronchoconstriction. Antimuscarinic drugs such as ipratropium inhibit the action of acetylcholine at vagal nerve endings to constrict bronchial smooth muscle, and thus offer benefit to some patients with asthma.

The activity of the $\beta_2$-receptor is mediated through the production of cyclic adenosine monophosphate (cAMP; Figure 21.16). The latter second messenger is produced by the action of adenylyl cyclase on ATP via the $\beta_2$-adrenoceptor initiation of GTP-binding protein (G proteins). Increasing concentration of cAMP in bronchial smooth muscle is associated with bronchodilatation through activation of myosin light chain kinase. The cAMP is subsequently broken down into 5′-adenosine monophosphate (5′-AMP) by phosphodiesterase. Thus bronchodilatation can be pharmacologically mediated by:

- stimulation of $\beta_2$-adrenergic receptors, and thus increased production of cAMP, e.g. salbutamol, terbutaline, epinephrine (adrenaline);

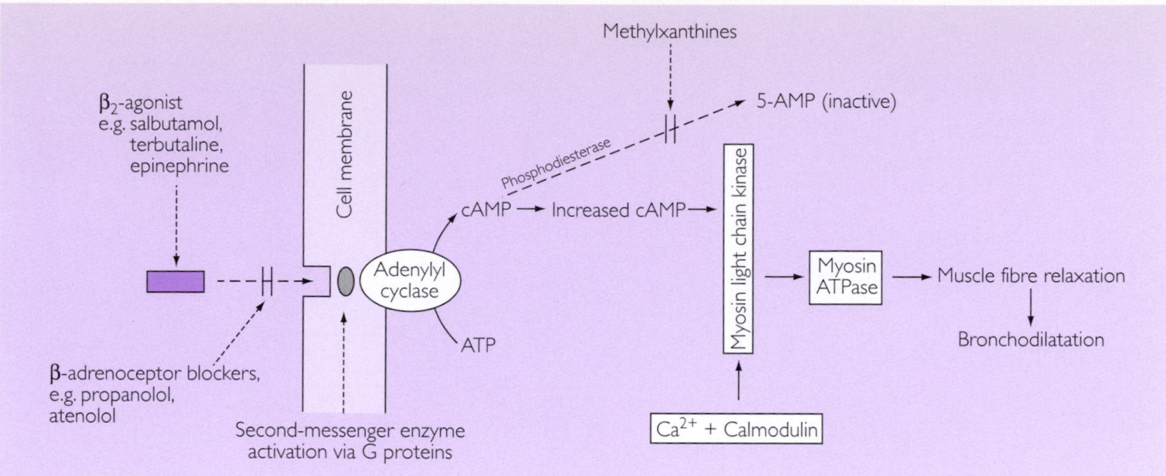


**Figure 21.16** Role of the β-adrenergic system and phosphodiesterase in relaxation of airway smooth muscle.

- inhibition of cAMP breakdown, e.g. methylxanthines;
- inhibition of cGMP production by antimuscarinic agents, e.g. ipratropium.

The bronchodilatation action of theophylline purely by inhibition of the intracellular phosphodiesterase is unlikely to be the major factor because this action would require a serum level ten times greater than that producing maximal bronchodilatation in humans. Selective inhibition of an isoenzyme relatively specific for cAMP breakdown (phosphodiesterase F-III) may be one of the possible modes of action. Other mechanisms, such as theophylline-mediated endogenous release of catecholamine, alterations in intracellular calcium, and synergistic pharmacological interaction with $\beta_2$-agonists may all contribute to the improvement in airflow.

### *Glucocorticoids*

Although popular and the most powerful group of systemic drugs for the treatment of reversible airflow obstruction, their exact mode of action is still not fully understood. They appear to have a small effect on the acute reaction and more effectively inhibit the delayed, late phase of the inflammatory response, and therefore are also commonly used prophylactically in moderate-to-severe asthma. The clinical effects are the result of a combination of several effects: reduction of inflammatory mucosal swelling, bronchial smooth muscle relaxation, and reduction of bronchial capillary permeability. At the molecular level, glucocorticoids bind to a cortisol–receptor complex in the cell cytosol, leading to synthesis of new protein. Phospholipase $A_2$ inhibition is seen which may, in turn, impair production of leukotrienes and prostaglandins. Inhibition of the antigen-presenting cell, T-cell function, and impaired production of inflammatory cytokines (interleukin IL-1) also contribute to the anti-inflammatory effects. Furthermore, glucocorticoids increase both the number and affinity of $\beta_2$-agonist receptors on the cell surface. The side effects of long-term systematic delivery are considerable and frequently encountered.

### *Sodium cromoglycate*

Like low-dose inhaled corticosteroid, cromoglycate has prophylactic action and has no place in the acute treatment of acute severe asthma. It stabilizes mast cell membranes and thus prevents release of chemical mediators of bronchospasm from these sensitized cells. Inhaled cromoglycate is very useful in childhood asthma and is of particular value in preventing exercise-induced bronchospasm.

## FURTHER READING


Benumof JL. *Anaesthesia for Thoracic Surgery*, 2nd edn, Chapters 3 and 4. Philadelphia: WB Saunders, 1995.

Black AMS. Old hat and old hands in controlled breathing (part 1): the drives to breathing and (part 2): translating ventilatory drive into breathing. *Curr Anaesth Crit Care* 1997;**8**:214–20, 221–30.

Flenley D, ed. *Respiratory Medicine*, 2nd edn. London: Baillière Tindall, 1990.

Ganong WF. *Review of Medical Physiology*, 18th edn. Stamford, CA: Appleton & Lange, 1997.

Nunn JF. *Applied Respiratory Physiology,* 3rd edn. London: Butterworths, 1987.

Pearl RG, ed. The lung in Anaesthesia. *Clin Anaesthesiol* 1996;**10**:4.

Pereira P, Loxley M, Orrett FA, Balbirsingh M. Physiological responses of therapy in bronchial hyperreactivity. *Can J Anaesth* 1996;**43**:700.

Wahba R. Airway closure and intraoperative hypoxaemia: twenty five years later. *Can J Anaesth* 1996;**43**:1144.

# Chapter 22 Physiology and pharmacology of the central nervous system

A.A. Tomlinson and L. Bromley

The organization of the central (CNS) and peripheral nervous system (PNS) is shown schematically in Figure 22.1. The CNS comprises the brain and spinal cord. Its principal function is to obtain appropriate information about the external environment and, after analysis, produce an appropriate integrated response.

The cells in the nervous system are broadly classified into:

- neurons, the true 'nerve cells', which are specialized for the reception, integration, transformation, and onward transmission of coded information;
- neuroglia, the supporting cells, which are essential for the correct functioning of neurons.

## NEURONS AND NEUROGLIA

### Neurons

A primitive nerve cell differentiates into the specialized neurons found in the CNS and PNS. There are three main avenues of differentiation, as shown in Figure 22.2. Each neuron possesses a nucleated cell body (the cyton), and one or more branching processes. In the adult these branches can vary in length from a few micrometres to a metre or more. The longest connect the brain and lower spinal cord or extend from the cord to the hands and feet. There are approximately $10^{12}$ neurons in the CNS.

A receptive field of dendrites conducts impulses to the cyton and an axon conducts them away from the cyton to a specialized ending. These endings interface with another nerve cell or effector organ via a synaptic cleft. The transmission of impulses across a synaptic cleft is effected by the release of specialized chemical transmitters. Details of synaptic transmission are

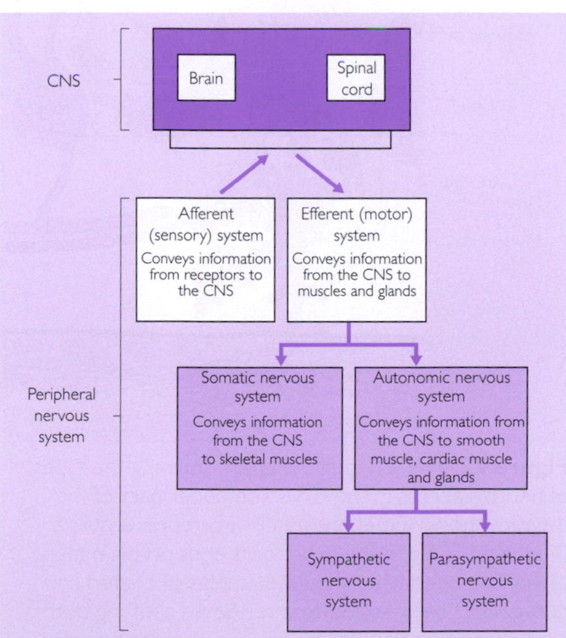


**Figure 22.1** A block diagram representing the organization of the human nervous system, which shows its major component divisions. CNS, central nervous system.

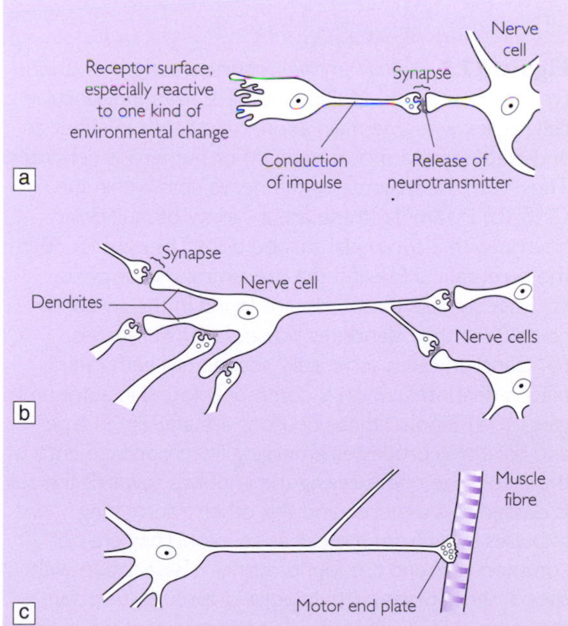


**Figure 22.2** The three main avenues of differentiation that can be followed by a primitive nerve cell: (a) a receptor neuron shown synapsing with another nerve cell; (b) an interneuron showing its role in connecting together a large number of other nerve cells; (c) a motor or effector neuron with an end-plate on a target organ shown here as a muscle fibre. (Adapted from Warwick R and Williams PL. *Gray's Anatomy*, 35th edn. London: Longman, 1973.)

given in Chapters 23 and 24. Considerable variations exist in cell size and shape in both the CNS and the PNS. The main types of neuron are shown in Figure 22.3. The functions of motor and sensory neurons (types a and f in Figure 22.3) are described in detail in Chapter 23.

A nerve fibre is the name given (when it is present) to the long axonal projection of a nerve. A collection of axons is termed a 'tract' within the CNS and a 'peripheral nerve' in the PNS. The axons are protected and insulated by myelin. Ganglia are collections of nerve cell bodies grouped together within the brain and spinal cord. Ganglia are also found in the PNS in association with both afferent and efferent peripheral nerves. Macroscopically, sections of the CNS appear to consist of grey and white matter. Grey matter is composed largely of cell bodies (cytons) whereas white matter contains the axonal processes.

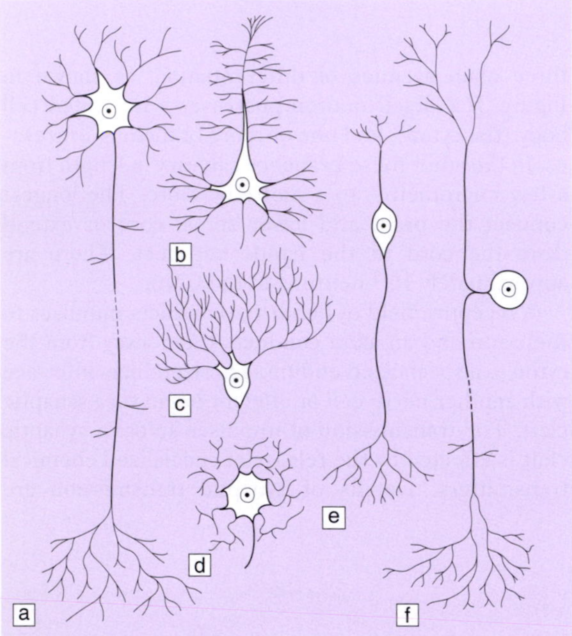

**Figure 22.3** A diagrammatic representation of various types of neuron. (a) Multipolar: these have multiangular cell bodies with one main axon, which ends in either an end-plate (as in a motor neuron) or numerous dendrites. They form the majority of the nerve cells within the CNS. (b) Pyramidal: these are a variety of multipolar neuron with a pyramidal shaped body. They are found in the cerebral cortex and the precentral motor gyrus. (c) Flask shaped: these cells are found in the cerebellar cortex and their dendrites possess many branches. (d) Ganglion cell: a spherically shaped cell with radially placed dendrites, which is commonly found in autonomic ganglia. (e) Bipolar: these neurons are afferent in type and have two processes emerging from opposite ends of the cyton. The one carrying the impulses towards the cell is classed as a dendrite and the other transmitting impulses away from the cell as an axon. They are not common cells and are found mainly in association with special sense organs. (f) Unipolar or pseudo-unipolar: these are cells in which the two processes of the bipolar cell have become fused over a short distance. This single process soon bifurcates in a T-shaped fashion. These cells are afferent in function and are found mainly in the ganglia on the dorsal roots of the spinal nerves. The longer process can extend peripherally to a receptor ending in skin, muscle, ligament, blood vessel, or viscera, which transmits impulses to their cyton. The shorter process conveys these impulses from the cyton to the spinal cord or brain, functioning as an axon.

### Neuroglia

Neuroglia is a collective name for the cells that support the functions of the neurons. Neuroglia are generally smaller than neurons and outnumber them by a factor of 5–10 times. As with neurons, a number of different classifications have been proposed and the functions of all cell types are, as yet, not completely established. A summary describing the main cell types is given in Table 22.1 and they are shown diagrammatically in Figure 22.4. Neuroglia are the cause of approximately 50% of tumours found in the CNS.

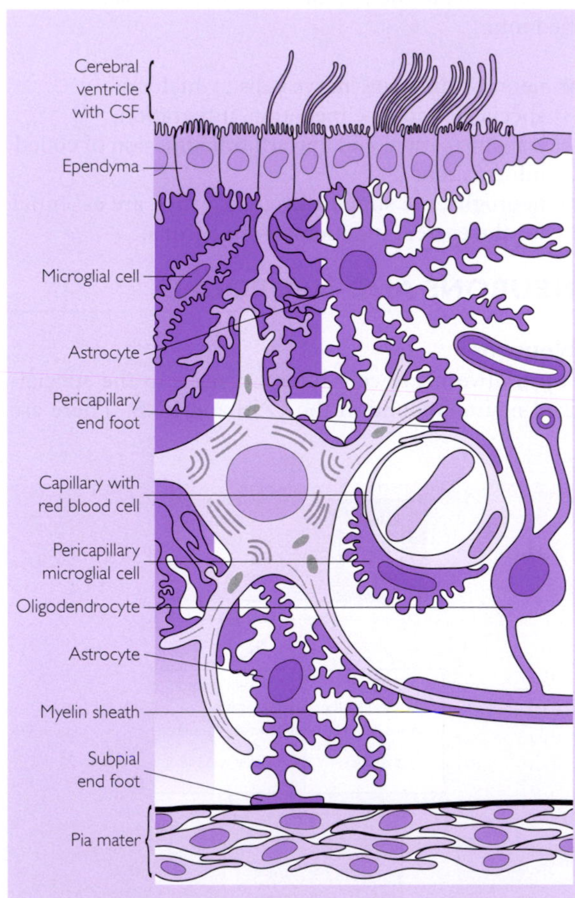


**Figure 22.4** A schematic diagram showing the types of neuroglial cells in the CNS. The upper part of the diagram shows the ependyma in a cerebral ventricle filled with CSF and the lower part ends on pia mater tissue. The ependyma shows examples of ciliated and non-ciliated cells. Astrocytes are shown abutting both capillaries and nerve cell bodies. An oligodendrocyte provides the myelin sheaths for two axons, the upper axon being sectioned across a curve in its length. (Adapted from Warwick R, Williams PL. *Gray's Anatomy*, 35th edn. London: Longman 1973.)

**Table 22.1 Main types and functions of neuroglial cells in the CNS**

| Cell type | Description | Function(s) |
|---|---|---|
| Astrocyte (*astro* = star, *cyte* = cell) | Star-shaped cell with numerous processes<br>Protoplasmic astrocytes (with many dendrites) are found in the grey matter of the CNS and fibrous astrocytes (with fewer dendrites) in the white matter of the CNS | Attach neurons to blood vessels and as such are part of the blood–brain barrier<br>Curl around nerve cells to provide supporting network in brain and spinal cord<br>Metabolic and regulating functions for biochemical environment |
| Oligodendrocytes (*oligo* = few, *dendro* = tree) | Resemble astrocytes but, as their name suggests, they have fewer and less arborizing dendrites<br>A single oligodendrocyte may be applied to several neurons | Support the CNS neurons physically by forming a semi-rigid connective tissue structure<br>They produce the phospholipid myelin sheaths around axons in the CNS<br>Represented in the peripheral nervous system as Schwann cells |
| Microglia (*micro* = small, *glia* = glue) | Small cells with few processes, which are derived from monocytes<br>Also called brain macrophages<br>May migrate to the site of injury | Phagocytose and destroy cell debris and infective organisms<br>Essentially function as macrophages<br>Regarded as part of the reticuloendothelial system |
| Ependyma or ependymocytes (ependyma = blouse or upper garment) | Epithelial cells in a single layer which range from squamous to columnar; many are ciliated | Form the lining of the ventricles and the central canal of the spinal cord<br>Secrete substances into and absorb them from the CSF<br>In some areas form specialized cells of the choroid plexus |

Note that astrocytes and oligodendrocytes are often classified together as types of macroglial cells.

## ANATOMY OF THE BRAIN

The brain is divided into two basic parts by the tentorium cerebelli (commonly just called the tentorium). This is a crescent-shaped lamina of dura mater, the concave anterior border of which is free. Above the tentorium lies the forebrain and below it the hindbrain, with the midbrain lying at their junction in the tentorial notch – the opening left by the free anterior border of the tentorium – which allows the fore- and hindbrains to connect. These divisions, together with the major intracerebral structures, are shown in Figures 22.5 and 22.6.

The forebrain comprises the cerebral cortex, thalamus, and hypothalamus; the hindbrain consists of the cerebellum, pons, and medulla; the midbrain joins the two together. A clinically important grouping of structures, called the brain stem, comprises the midbrain, pons, and medulla. Its importance lies in the fact that, in the absence of brain-stem function, despite artificial maintenance of circulation and gas exchange, cardiac arrest inevitably results together with death of the whole organism. The subdivisions, components, and functions of the brain are summarized in Table 22.2.

The reticular formation (or the reticular activating system) is very important. It is not a discrete anatomical entity, but occupies the central core of medulla, pons, and midbrain with complex links to ascending pathways, cerebellum, limbic system, and cerebral cortex. Its function is to transmit sensory impulses that stimulate and activate the cortex, thereby helping to maintain consciousness and the waking state.

The nuclei of cranial nerves III–XII lie in the brain stem; Figure 22.7 depicts the functions of all the cranial nerves. The cranial nerves are detailed in Table 22.3.

The clinical subdivisions of the cerebrum into lobes is shown in Figure 22.8. The approximate locations of the motor and sensory areas are demonstrated in Figure 22.9. Language-related functions (e.g. speech) are largely localized to the dominant cerebral hemisphere. This is the left hemisphere in 96% of right-handed people but also 70% of left-handed people.

An important but loosely defined area of the cortex is the limbic system. It includes a rim of inner cortex (the cingulate gyrus) surrounding the corpus callosum and associated deeper structures, including the hippocampus, uncus, and hypothalamus (Figure 22.9b). The limbic system is concerned with the integration of emotional responses. Benzodiazepines depress the excitability of this system by facilitating the effects mediated by γ-aminobutyric acid (GABA), thus producing sedation and hypnosis (see later).

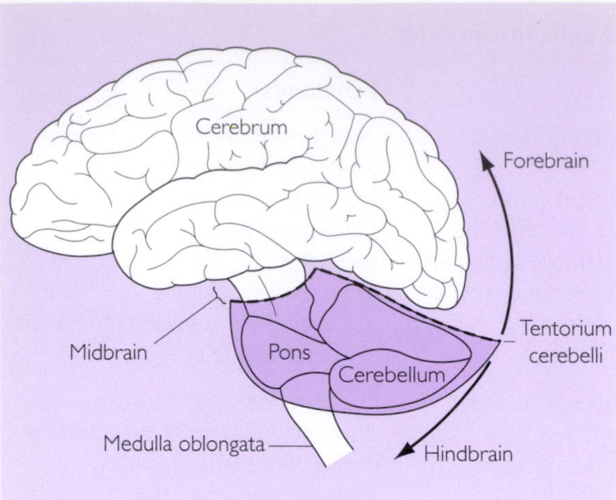


**Figure 22.5** A lateral view of the brain showing its division into the forebrain, midbrain, and hindbrain by the tentorium cerebelli.

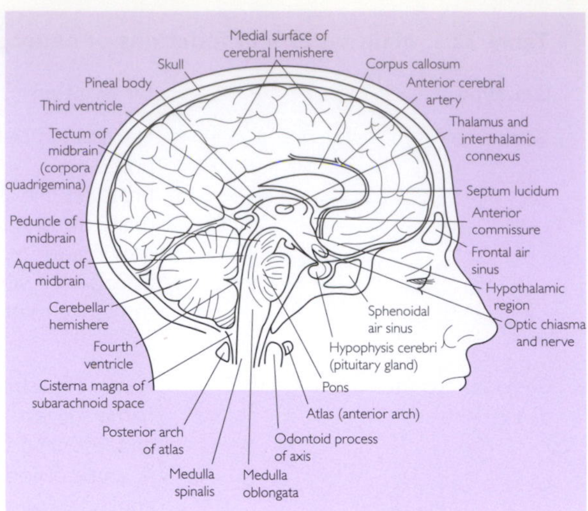


**Figure 22.6** A median sagittal section through the head. The falx cerebri has been removed to show the medial surface of the left cerebral hemisphere.

Details of the nerve tracts in the spinal cord and their route to the cortex are described in Chapter 23.

## THE BLOOD SUPPLY TO THE BRAIN AND SPINAL CORD

### Brain

In health, the adult brain weighs 1400 g (2–3% of body mass) and receives 15% of the resting cardiac output (700 ml/min), giving rise to a global cerebral blood flow (CBF) of about 50 ml/100 g brain tissue per min. There are wide variations in resting regional blood flow. Flow in grey matter (80 ml/100 g per min) is considerably higher than that in white matter (20 ml/100 g per min).

The blood supply to the brain (Figure 22.10) is delivered by the two internal carotid arteries (67%) and two vertebral arteries (33%). The vertebral arteries combine to form the basilar artery, which anastomoses with the internal carotids to form the circle of Willis. From the circle of Willis arise the anterior, middle, and posterior cerebral arteries, the distribution of which is shown in Figure 22.10. These major branches progressively divide into multiple smaller branches over the surface of the cerebral hemispheres. The posterior communicating arteries join the posterior cerebral arteries to the middle cerebral arteries, and the anterior communicating artery joins the two anterior cerebral arteries. The arterial supply to the mid- and hindbrain is from branches of the basilar and vertebral arteries.

The principal venous drainage is by a system of superficial and deep veins, which drain into intra- and extradural venous sinuses (endothelialized channels in folds of dura mater) and from these to the internal jugular veins. This is shown in Figure 22.11. There can, however, be considerable variations in venous drainage.

The total cerebral blood volume (CBV) in adults is approximately 150 ml. Of this 60–70% is in the veins and venous sinuses, and 30–40% in the arterial system, although these values may vary considerably because cerebral vessel capacities are influenced by a number of factors (see later). Venous and arterial vessels with diameters smaller than 300 μm are probably the main contributors to CBV, because their large total cross-sectional area makes them the major cerebrovascular compartment.

### Spinal cord

The spinal cord is supplied by a single anterior and two pairs of posterior spinal arteries which descend through the foramen magnum. The single anterior spinal artery arises from the fusion of a branch from each vertebral artery (see Figure 22.10) and supplies the anterior two-thirds of the cord. It lies along the line of the anterior median fissure.

The two pairs of posterior spinal arteries arise from the corresponding vertebral or posteroinferior cerebellar arteries (themselves branches of the vertebral arteries) (see Figure 22.10). Each pair lies on either side of the posterior nerve roots. They supply the posterior third of the cord.

Both the anterior and posterior spinal arteries can be traced down to the lower end of the cord, but in their course they receive regular reinforcements from small radicular arteries which travel with the anterior and posterior nerve roots. This arrangement of arterial vessels is shown in Figure 22.12. Except in the upper cervical segments, the supply from the origins of the anterior and posterior arteries is not adequate for the cord's blood supply. Superiorly therefore, the blood supply to the cord is dependent on the vertebral arteries, but the lower two-thirds are relatively dependent on the 'booster' supplies from the radicular arteries – this is particularly so anteriorly because of the single vessel supply. There is a 'watershed' around T4–5 where these two supplies meet and where the supply from each may be tenuous. One of the major radicular feeder arteries usually enters (sometimes just on the left) between T9 and L2, and this is known as the artery of Adamkiewicz.

Disruption of the anterior supply produces the anterior cord syndrome, which is a predominantly motor lesion with loss of corticospinal and spinothalamic tracts. The posterior columns are spared so

**Table 22.2 Subdivisions, components, and functions of the brain**

| Subdivision | Components | Functions |
|---|---|---|
| **Forebrain**<br>The forebrain consists of the telencephalon and the diencephalon<br>The cerebral hemispheres, including the corpus striatum, comprise the telencephalon | Cortex | Generates *content of consciousness*<br>Memory, language, conscious thought<br>Some function localization present, e.g.<br>• sensory (postcentral gyrus)<br>• motor (precentral gyrus)<br>• vision (towards occipital pole)<br>• auditory (superior aspect of temporal lobe) |
| The diencephalon comprises the thalamus, the hypothalamus, the medial and lateral geniculate bodies, | Thalamus | Relay centres for all types of information going to cortex<br>Correlation and integration of signals occurs but conscious interpretation of peripheral sensory stimuli, except for pain, does not occur at this level<br>The optic nerves (II) travel to the right and left lateral geniculate bodies |
| and the immediately surrounding structures | Hypothalamus | Closely linked to the endocrine system<br>Linked with control of thirst, appetite, temperature, autonomic nervous system, and pituitary<br>Integrates stress response |
| **Midbrain**<br>(mesencephalon) | Midbrain[a] | Short segment between pons and diencephalon<br>Traversed by cerebral aqueduct (which joins third and fourth ventricles – Figure 22.6), all the major ascending and descending tracts, and the reticular formation<br>It contains many important nuclei and gives off the oculomotor (III) and trochlear (IV) nerves |
| **Hindbrain**<br>The pons and cerebellum comprise the metencephalon | Pons[a] | Lies between midbrain and medulla oblongata in front of the cerebellum (pons = bridge)<br>Consists of nuclei, ganglia, and longitudinal and transverse tracts, and receives and sends fibres to the cerebellum<br>Boundaries of pons and cerebellum form the fourth ventricle<br>Gives off trigeminal (V) nerve<br>The abducent (VI) and facial (VII) nerves leave at the junction of the pons and medulla in the cerebellopontine angle |
| | Cerebellum | Occupies most of the posterior cranial fossa<br>Attached to pons, medulla, and midbrain by peduncles at the sides of the fourth ventricle<br>Superior surface against tentorium cerebelli<br>Responsible for muscle synergy and coordination so that movements are performed smoothly<br>Malfunction of the cerebellum leads to ataxia, tremor, nystagmus, and hypotonia |
| The medulla comprises the myelencephalon | Medulla[a] (medulla oblongata) | Pivotal role in integration of neural function<br>Includes centres for autonomic reflex control of respiratory and cardiovascular function (the so-called 'vital centres')<br>Swallowing and gag reflexes are other examples of medullary integrated reflex responses<br>Chemoreceptor trigger zone located in the area postrema (lateral walls of fourth ventricle)<br>The cranial nerves VIII to XII originate here |

[a]The midbrain, pons, and medulla make up the brain stem.

vibration, proprioception, and fine touch are left intact. The anterior spinal artery syndrome may occur after profound hypotension, or after surgery that disrupts the supply from the artery of Adamkiewicz (e.g. aortic aneurysm surgery or surgery to the lower thoracic spine). The description of spinal tracts is given in Chapter 23.

## THE BLOOD–BRAIN BARRIER

Under normal circumstances only water, carbon dioxide ($CO_2$), and oxygen ($O_2$) enter the brain easily. The exchange of all other substances between blood and brain is much slower. The anatomical sites of this barrier are the cerebral capillary endothelium and

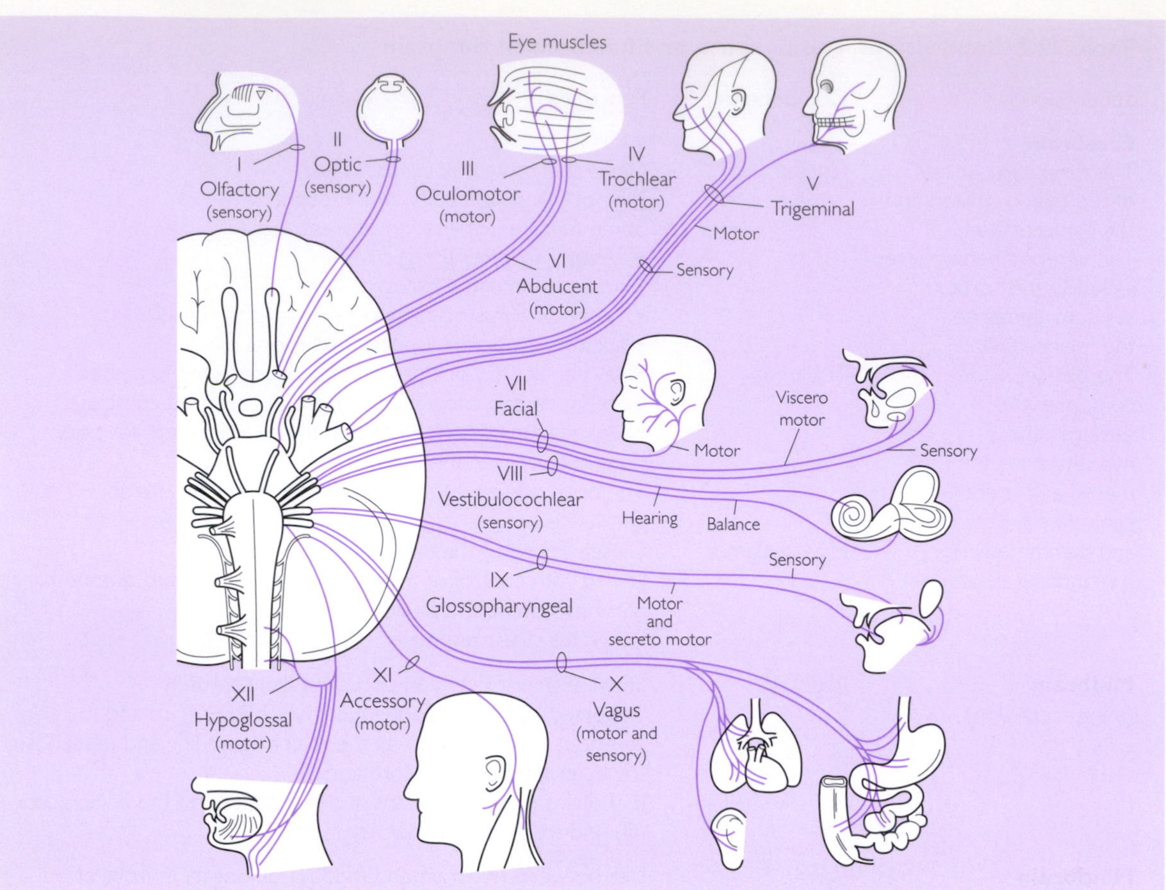


**Figure 22.7** The cranial nerves arising from the ventral surface of the brain and their distribution to various anatomical regions. The visceromotor and sensory nerves going through the submandibular, sublingual, and lacrimal glands originate from the nervus intermedius branch of the facial nerve as it emerges from the lower border of the pons at the cerebellopontine angle. (Adapted from MacKenna BR and Callander R. *Illustrated Physiology*, 5th edn. London: Churchill Livingstone, 1990,226).

choroid plexus epithelium, which collectively are known as the blood–brain barrier (BBB). These cells are structurally and functionally unique (compared with systemic capillary endothelia) in that they lack fenestrations and endothelial clefts, while developing tight junctions (occlusive zones) between adjacent cells (Figure 22.13). There are also large astrocyte foot processes surrounding the basement membrane (see Figure 22.4). This 'barrier' is selectively permeable to some substances and impermeable to others.

The rate of transfer of substances across an intact BBB depends on molecular size, lipid solubility, and active bidirectional transport mechanisms (e.g. for glucose, sodium [$Na^+$], chloride [$Cl^-$], and bicarbonate [$HCO_3^-$]). Transport mechanisms require significant amounts of metabolic energy. The pores of cerebral capillaries are approximately one-tenth the size of those in peripheral capillaries, so that even small molecules contribute to the osmotic movement of water. This is shown diagrammatically in Figure 22.14. In neuroanaesthetic practice, it is important to maintain the plasma osmolality by using intravenous fluids containing a high number of osmotically active particles. This minimizes the flow of water into the brain extracellular compartment *provided* that the BBB is intact.

The BBB has multiple functions. It maintains a constant environment for neuronal function, which is dependent on the concentration of specific ions (e.g. potassium [$K^+$], calcium [$Ca^{2+}$], hydrogen [$H^+$], magnesium [$Mg^{2+}$]) – even minor variations may have significant effects. It protects the brain from many exogenous toxins and it retains internally produced neurotransmitters (e.g. dopamine), so reducing the load on central synaptic pathways. One disadvantage of the BBB is that many therapeutic agents are excluded and the only way that they can gain access to brain extracellular fluid is by injection into the ventricles, the cisterna magna, or the lumbar cerebrospinal fluid (CSF) – all routes that cannot be used long term.

There are seven small areas (known as the circumventricular organs) that lie outside the BBB. These include the posterior pituitary (neurohypophysis), the median eminence (the area postrema), the subfornical organ, and the organum vasculosum of the lamina terminalis or supraoptic crest). These lie in the midline and have dense, permeable, capillary beds in proximity to the CSF. They transduce chemical signals in blood and CSF to new neural information (or vice versa) and so have a role in general homoeostasis. Some function as neurohumoral organs, i.e. substances are secreted by neurons into the circulation such as oxytocin and antidiuretic hormone from the posterior pituitary. Other circumventricular organs contain receptors for many different peptides and other substances, and function as chemoreceptor zones, i.e. areas where substances circulating in blood

Table 22.3 The cranial nerves and their functions

| Number | Name | Type | Main distribution | Chief functions |
|---|---|---|---|---|
| I | Olfactory | Special sensory | To olfactory epithelium of nose | Nerve of smell |
| II | Optic | Special sensory | To retina of eye | Nerve of vision |
| III | Oculomotor | Motor | To muscles of eye (except superior oblique and lateral rectus), including sphincter pupillae and ciliary muscles<br>Also to levator palpebrae superioris | Turning eye upwards, downwards and medially<br>Constriction of pupil and accommodation<br>Lifting eyelid |
| IV | Trochlear | Motor | To superior oblique muscle of eye | Assists in turning eye downwards and laterally |
| V | Trigeminal | Sensory and motor | (a) Ophthalmic division: to eye, nose and scalp<br>(b) Maxillary division: to upper jaw and teeth, face, nose, and palate<br>(c) Mandibular division: to lower jaw and teeth, face, and mucosa of mouth cavity and tongue; muscles of mandible and tensor palati and tensor tympani<br>Meningeal branches from each division | Main sensory nerve of head<br>Moving mandible (e.g. for mastication and speech), assisting swallowing and tensing soft palate and tympanic membrane |
| VI | Abducens | Motor | To lateral rectus muscle of eye | Turning eye laterally |
| VII | Facial (with nervus intermedius which branches off later and forms majority of chorda tympani) | Motor, secretomotor, and special sensory | To muscle of face, ear, scalp and m.m. platysma, digastricus (posterior belly), stylohyoid and stapedius<br>Nervus intermedius distributed with fifth nerve to lacrimal and salivary glands and taste buds | Facial expression and lip movements of speech<br>Nervus intermedius promotes lacrimation and salivation and is a pathway for taste sensation from tongue (oral part) |
| VIII | Vestibulocochlear | Special sensory | To vestibule, semicircular canals and cochlea of internal ear | Pathways for sense of position and movement of head (vestibular part) and for hearing (cochlear part) |
| IX | Glossopharyngeal | Sensory and special sensory; motor and secretomotor | To mucosa of pharynx and posterior third of tongue; to carotid sinus, parotid salivary gland and stylopharyngeus | Sensory nerve of pharynx and pharyngeal part of tongue; pathway for taste sensation from the latter; carries impulses from carotid sinus influencing blood pressure; assists swallowing and promotes salivation |

cont.

**Table 22.3 The cranial nerves and their functions (cont.)**

| Number | Name | Type | Main distribution | Chief functions |
|---|---|---|---|---|
| X | Vagus | Sensory, special sensory and motor | To: (a) meninges in posterior cranial fossa;<br>(b) heart and great vessels within thorax;<br>(b) respiratory system – larynx, trachea, bronchi, and lungs;<br>(4) much of the alimentary canal (pharynx to midcolon) and associated glands (liver, pancreas, etc.) | Supplies the structures mentioned with afferent and efferent fibres, including some special sensory (taste) fibres from the epiglottis and back of tongue<br>It has much the most extensive distribution of all the cranial nerves |
| XI | Accessory | Sensory and motor | On leaving cranium it divides into an internal ramus and external ramus<br>Internal ramus joins vagus and is distributed with it<br>External ramus supplies trapezius and sternomastoid muscles | Assists vagus and innervates the muscles mentioned |
| XII | Hypoglossal | Motor | To muscles of tongue | Motor nerve of tongue |

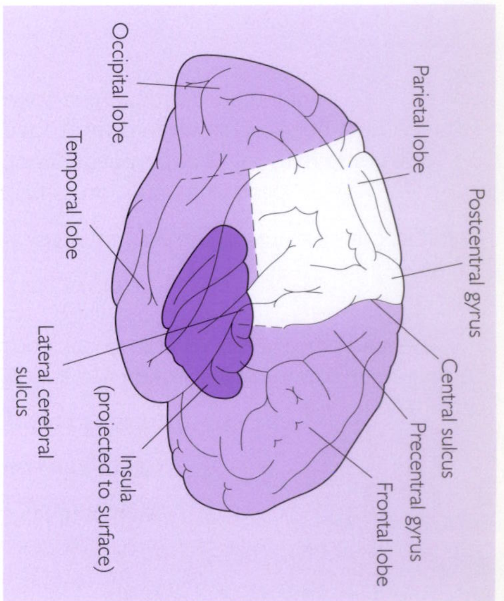


**Figure 22.8** The lobes and fissures of the cerebrum shown in a right lateral view. As the insula cannot be seen externally, it has been projected on to the surface.

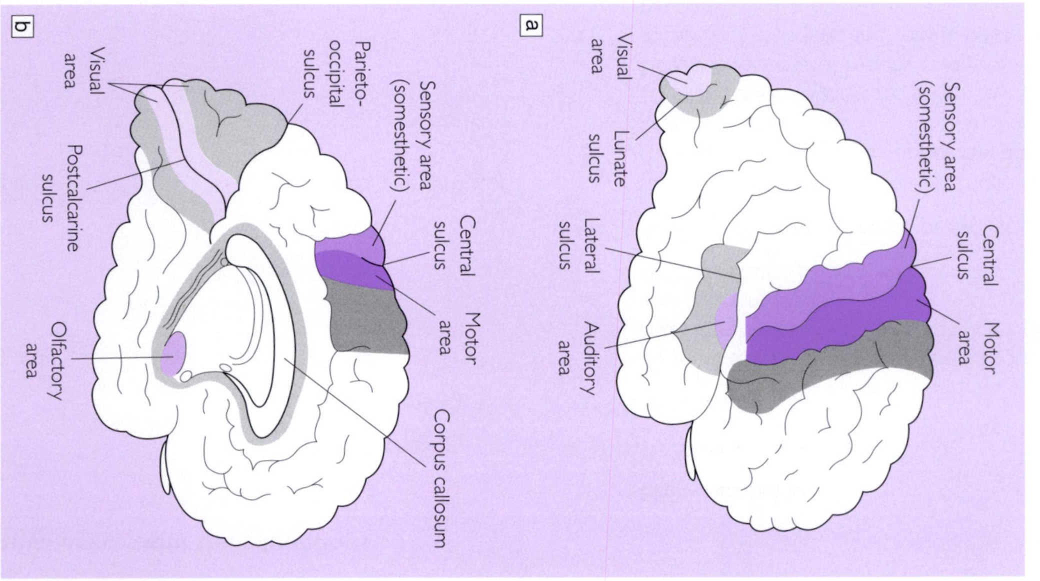


**Figure 22.9** The approximate cortical localization of motor, somatic sensory, auditory, and visual functions on (a) the lateral and (b) the medial surfaces of the cerebral hemispheres. The areas shown in grey, which comprise part of the singular gyrus above the corpus callosum, and the areas shown in grey going down around the third ventricle to the hypothalamus are parts of the limbic system.

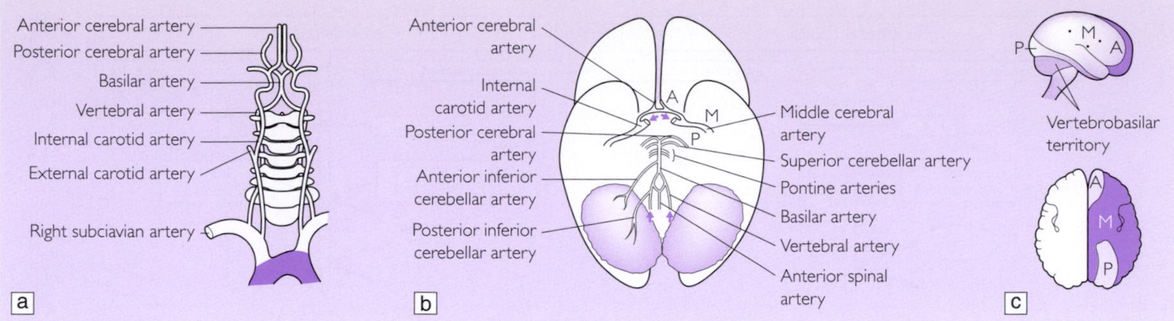


**Figure 22.10** The blood supply of the brain. (a) The origins of the carotid and vertebral vessels. The internal carotid arteries are a branch of the common carotid arteries and the vertebral arteries arise from the right and left subclavian arteries before following their path through fenestrations in the transverse processes of the cervical vertebra. (b) The arrival of these arteries at the base of the brain. The vertebral arteries fuse to form the single basilar artery and the basilar artery, together with the two internal carotid arteries, form the feeder vessels for the circle of Willis. The main named branches of arteries on the base of the brain are given. (c) The areas of distribution of the anterior (A), posterior (P), and middle (M) cerebral arteries. Note the formation of the anterior spinal artery from the two vertebral arteries before they fuse to form the basilar artery. (Adapted from Scadding JW and Gibbs J. Neurological disease. In: Souhami RL and Moxham J, eds. *Textbook of Medicine,* 2nd edn. London: Churchill-Livingstone 1994, 896.)

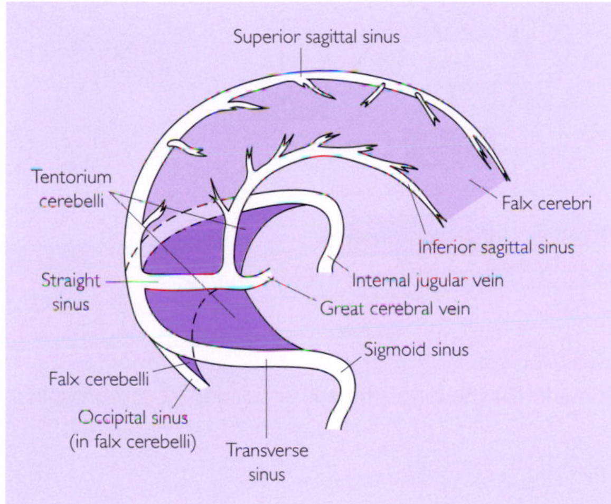


**Figure 22.11** Diagrammatic representation of cerebral venous drainage.

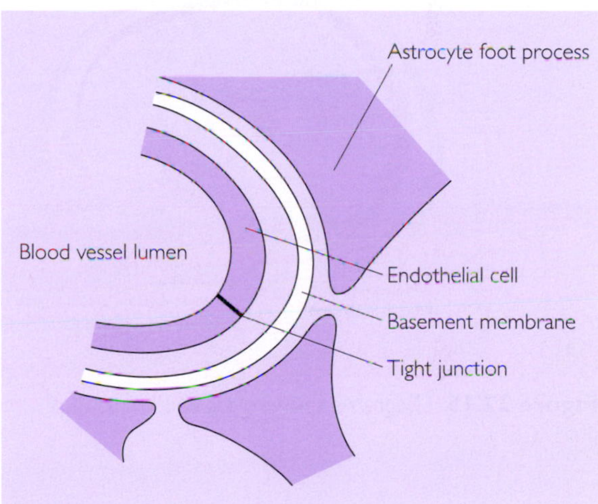


**Figure 22.13** Diagrammatic representation of the cellular structures that form part of the blood–brain barrier. (From Inglis A, Fitch W. Physiology and metabolism of the central nervous system. In: van Aken H, ed. *Neuro-anaesthetic practice*. London: BMJ Publishing Group, 1995, 13.)

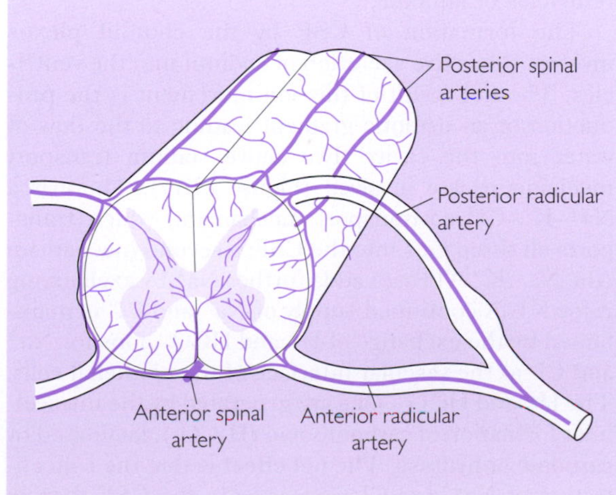


**Figure 22.12** The blood supply of the spinal cord.

can trigger changes in brain function without penetrating the BBB. In or near the area postrema is a chemoreceptor trigger zone that initiates vomiting in response to chemical changes in the plasma. Another example is that of angiotensin II acting on receptors in the subfornical organ to increase water intake.

## CEREBROSPINAL FLUID AND INTRACRANIAL PRESSURE

### Cerebrospinal fluid

CSF fills the ventricles and subarachnoid space and, together with the meninges, provides some protection for the brain. Although a very small quantity is formed by ultrafiltration, the majority of the CSF is formed by secretion from choroid plexus in the two lateral and third

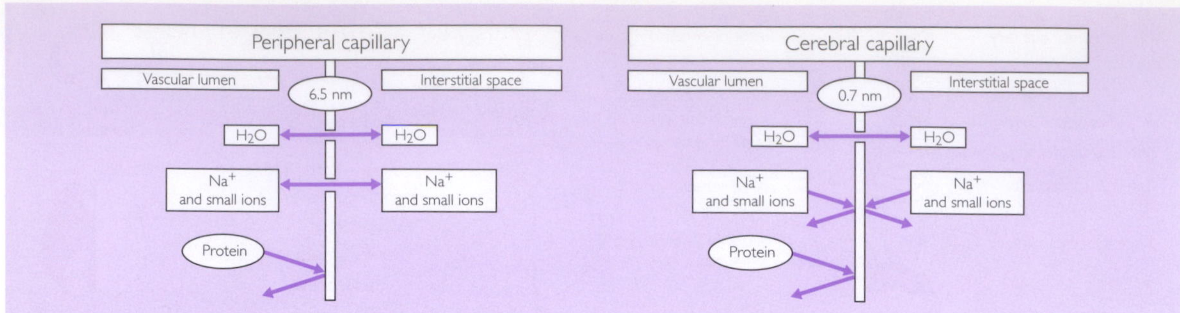


**Figure 22.14** A schematic diagram showing the differences between peripheral capillaries in the systemic circulation and cerebral capillaries. Note that in the periphery the approximate pore size is 6.5 nm, which makes the vessel wall permeable to both water and small ions but not to protein. The pores in the cerebral capillary are 0.7 nm, approximately one-tenth of the size of those in peripheral capillaries. This renders the blood–brain barrier impermeable to both small ions and protein but not to water. (Adapted from Tommasino C and Todd MM. Fluid management in neurological patients. In: *Neuro-anaesthetic practice*. van Aken H, ed. London: BMJ Publishing Group, 1995, 135.)

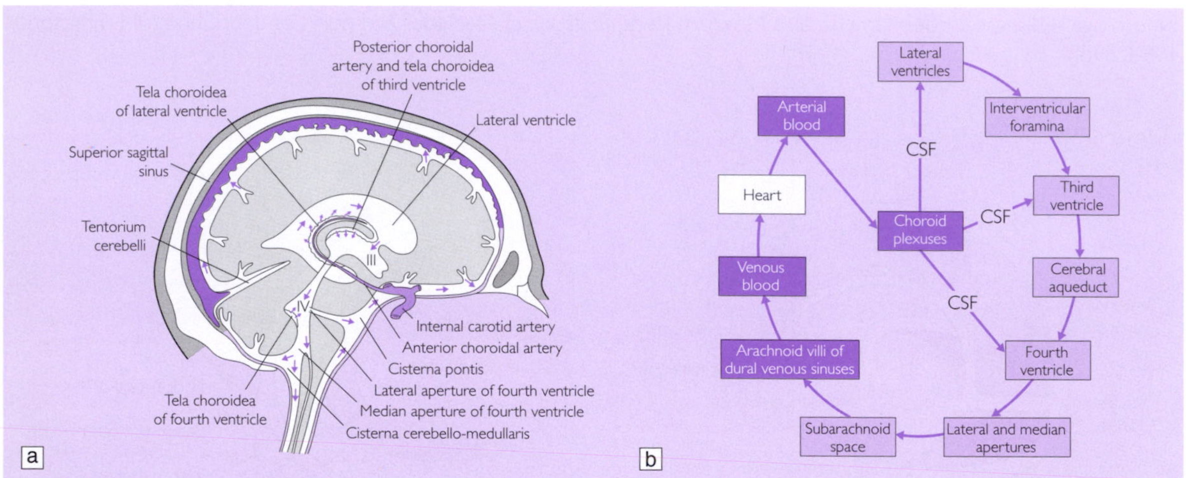


**Figure 22.15** Diagrams showing (a) the anatomical circulation and (b) the diagrammatic circulation of cerebrospinal fluid (CSF).

ventricles. These choroid plexus are formed from invaginations of ependymal cells, which are pushed inwards by vascular pial tissue on the surface of the brain.

The circulation of the CSF is shown in Figure 22.15. CSF traverses the lateral and third ventricles passing through the aqueduct to the fourth ventricle. From the fourth ventricle, the ventricular system communicates with the subarachnoid space through the laterally placed foramina of Luschka (two) and the midline foramen of Magendie. The subarachnoid space is continuous over the cerebral hemispheres and spinal compartment.

The CSF is reabsorbed into the central venous system principally via the arachnoid villi (areas where the arachnoid space has invaginated into the large venous sinuses) as shown in Figure 22.16. The reabsorption is driven by the pressure gradient that exists between the CSF in the subarachnoid space and the venous blood. If the CSF pressure falls below the venous pressure, the villi collapse so reducing reabsorption. In addition, small amounts are reabsorbed by the cerebral and spinal veins.

The average volume of CSF is around 140 ml (range 80–200 ml). It is produced at approximately 0.5 ml/min and 550 ml is excreted per day. Total exchange occurs between 8 and 24 hours. The resting pressure depends on the balance between production and reabsorption and it fluctuates with respiration and blood pressure. Hydrocephalus results from either reduced reabsorption or blockage within the ventricles or aqueduct.

The formation of CSF by the choroid plexus involves the active secretion of sodium into the ventricles. The net result of this ion movement is the production of an osmotic gradient leading to the flow of water into the cavity. Two active sodium transport mechanisms are involved (Figure 22.17). There is a $Na^+$–$K^+$–$Cl^-$ co-transport mechanism, which transports all three ions into the CSF; a second mechanism (the $Na^+/K^+$ ATPase) adds further $Na^+$ by exchanging it for $K^+$. A continued supply of $Na^+$ and $Cl^-$ is maintained by the exchange of $H^+$ and $HCO^-_3$ ions for $Na^+$ and $Cl^-$ at the vascular interface of the epithelial cells. The $H^+$ and $HCO^-_3$ ions are generated by the intracellular formation of carbonic acid ($H_2CO_3$), facilitated by carbonic anhydrase. The net effect is that the concentration of $Na^+$ and $Cl^-$ is greater in the CSF than in plasma, whereas the $K^+$ concentration is reduced.

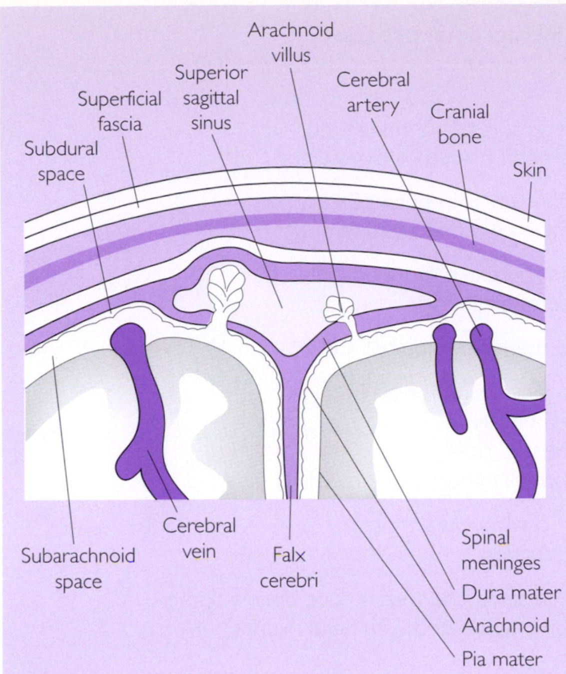


**Figure 22.16** A section through the top of the cranium showing the arachnoid villi and their relationship to the superior sagittal sinus.

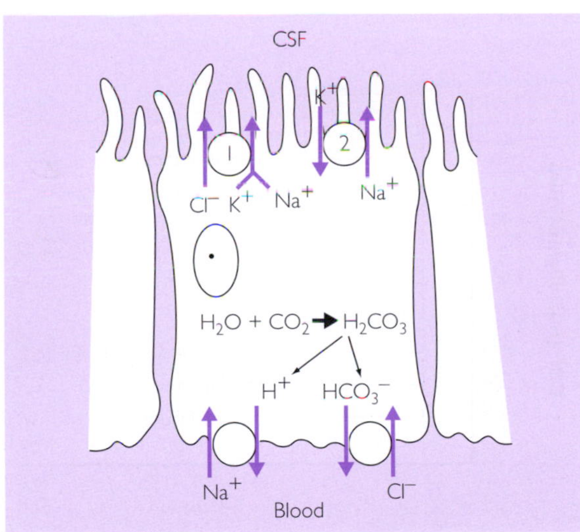


**Figure 22.17** Sodium transport mechanisms involved in the production of CSF by the choroid plexus: (1) the $Na^+$–$K^+$–$Cl^-$ co-transport mechanism: (2) $Na^+/K^+$ ATPase. Reciprocal processes occur at the cell's interface with blood.

**Table 22.4 Constituents of plasma and cerebrospinal fluid**

| Constituent | Blood plasma (mmol/L) | Cerebrospinal fluid (mmol/L) |
|---|---|---|
| Urea | 2.5–6.5 | 2.0–7.0 |
| Glucose (fasting) | 3.0–5.0 | 2.5–4.5 |
| Sodium | 136–148 | 144–152 |
| Potassium | 3.8–5.0 | 2.0–3.0 |
| Calcium | 2.2–2.6 | 1.1–1.3 |
| Chloride | 95–105 | 123–128 |
| Bicarbonate | 24–32 | 24–32 |
| Protein | 60–80 g/L | 200–400 mg/L |

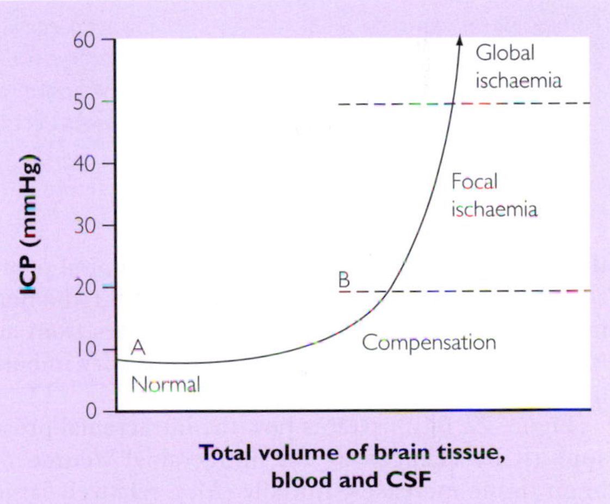


**Figure 22.18** The relationship between intracerebral pressure and the volume of the contents of the skull. (From Inglis A and Fitch W. Physiology and metabolism of the central nervous system. In: van Aken H, ed. *Neuro-anaesthetic Practice*. London: BMJ Publishing Group, 1999, 18.)

The constituents of CSF are summarized in Table 22.4. CSF has a pH of 7.33 and a specific gravity of approximately 1.005. The protein content of CSF is a fraction of that found in plasma and indicates the barrier to protein movement across the BBB. Protein levels are significantly raised in bacterial infections (as is the number of white cells), and high levels are seen with carcinomatous involvement of the meninges.

The production of CSF can be altered by drugs. The carbonic anhydrase inhibitor acetazolamide reduces CSF production by reducing intracellular $H^+$ and $HCO^-_3$ formation and therefore the turnover rate of $Na^+$ and $Cl^-$. This has not proved to be an effective treatment, however, for hydrocephalus. High doses of frusemide (furosemide) and bumetanide may reduce CSF production by inhibiting the $Na^+/K^+/Cl^-$ co-transport mechanism.

### Intracranial pressure

The brain, blood, and CSF are all contained within a closed cranial cavity. The whole of the intracranial contents adhere to the Monro–Kellie doctrine – i.e. the total volume of the skull must remain constant at any one time. As brain tissue is virtually incompressible, the only volumes that can change readily are those of the CSF and blood (CBV). CSF can be diverted from the intracranial to the intraspinal compartment. The CBV can be reduced by cerebral vasoconstriction of the arterioles. The veins and capillaries do not take part in active vasoconstriction, although their

**Table 22.5 Treatment modalities used to reduce intracranial pressure**

| Treatment modality | Comments |
|---|---|
| Head-up position | Approximately 20° – ensures CVP minimized<br>Minimal effect on cerebral MAP, thus maintaining CPP |
| Hyperventilation | Vasoconstriction secondary to reduced $Paco_2$<br>Should not reduce $Paco_2$ < 4.0 kPa (30 mmHg) |
| Moderate hypothermia | Reduces $CMRO_2$ and therefore required CBF<br>(Also reduces release of excitatory amino acids) |
| Barbiturates and propofol | Reduce $CMRO_2$ and therefore required CBF |
| Mannitol | Osmotic diuretic 0.5 g/kg as 20% over 20 min<br>Extracts water from the brain<br>Beware frequent repeated doses<br>If BBB damaged, will cross into brain extracellular fluid |
| Frusemide (furosemide) | Mechanism of action controversial<br>May reduce CSF production |
| Steroids | Reduce peritumoral oedema and thus reduce brain volume<br>Do not reduce oedema associated with head injuries |
| Tapping of ventricle | Direct surgical intervention |

BBB, blood–brain barrier; $CMRO_2$, cerebral metabolic rate for oxygen; CPP, cerebral perfusion pressure; CSF, cerebrospinal fluid; CVP, central venous pressure; MAP, mean arterial pressure; CBF, cerebral blood flow, $Paco_2$, $CO_2$ partial pressure.

thin walls may collapse under high transmural pressure and this may contribute to the overall reduction in CBV. This ability to buffer pressure rises from an increase in the volume of brain tissue is very important in disease.

Figure 22.18 illustrates how the intracranial pressure (ICP) changes as the intracranial volume of brain tissue increases. Initially (A), a relatively large increase in volume (in the order of 25 ml) can be accommodated with little increase in ICP (also called the compensation phase), but as the volume increases a critical point is reached (B) where the pressure-buffering system is exhausted. Small increases in volume (approximately 5 ml) then produce large increases in pressure. Once on the steep part of the curve, increases in ICP can affect the CBF profoundly by reducing cerebral perfusion pressure (CPP) to critical levels (see later). In this situation, the mean arterial pressure (MAP) should be increased in an attempt to maintain the CPP, although this may itself increase the ICP further. Alternatively, strategies aimed at reducing the ICP can be introduced as detailed in Table 22.5. Conversely, if in the presence of a raised ICP the MAP should decrease (e.g. on induction of anaesthesia), active measures must be taken to restore it to appropriate levels.

## FACTORS AND DRUGS AFFECTING CEREBRAL HAEMODYNAMICS

### Cerebral blood flow

CBF is produced by the CPP. This is determined by the MAP, the ICP, and central venous pressure (CVP) as follows:

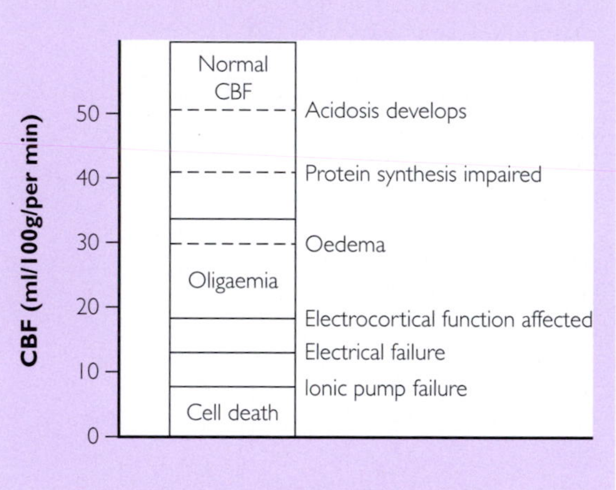


**Figure 22.19** Thresholds for cerebral ischaemia. CBF, cerebral blood flow. (From Menon DK. Monitoring the central nervous system. *Curr Anaesth Crit Care* 1997;8:255.)

$$CPP = MAP - (ICP + CVP)$$

The venous pressure is usually assumed to be zero, but it may be raised if partial obstruction to drainage of cerebral venous blood occurs (e.g. jugular venous compression, raised intrathoracic pressure, coughing, and straining). The normal ICP is 10 mmHg and therefore the CPP is normally 70–80 mmHg; the critical level for cerebral ischaemia is 30–40 mmHg.

As described earlier, the normal CBF is 50 ml/100 g of brain tissue per min. As it falls from this level, various adverse sequelae occur, which are summarized in Figure 22.19.

A number of physiological factors have the ability to alter global and regional CBF.

## Measurement of cerebral blood flow and oxygenation

### *Cerebral blood flow*

Most methods described are based on applications of the Fick principle (see Chapter 39). Kety and Schmidt used this principle in 1945, and are credited with the first quantitative measurements of CBF in humans. At steady state they used a form of the equation:

$$CBF = \frac{\text{Quantity of substance removed by the brain from the circulation per unit time}}{\text{Arteriovenous difference}}$$

In the Kety–Schmidt method, nitrous oxide ($N_2O$) is used as the diffusible tracer (15% in air is breathed for 10–15 min), and its *wash-in* is followed by taking frequent paired peripheral arterial and jugular venous bulb samples to measure the $N_2O$. These are then plotted and the speed at which the two curves equilibrate measures the rate at which $N_2O$ is being delivered to the brain. At equilibrium it is assumed that the brain and venous concentrations are equal. The disadvantages of this method are that it:

- is invasive;
- is slow (i.e. it takes at least 10–15 min);
- provides an averaged value only;
- measures only global flows (and only flows to the *perfused* brain).

The measurement of regional CBF (rCBF) with xenon-133 clearance uses the same principles described by Kety and Schmidt, except that it is based on monitoring of the *wash-out* of xenon-133, which is given by inhalation or intravenous injection. Scintillation counters are used to plot the wash-out and, depending on the number of counters used, global or regional flows may be obtained.

Tomographic information regarding rCBF may be obtained using modern imaging techniques that quantify the wash-in of radiodense contrast agents. Single photon emission computed tomography and positron emission tomography (PET) are two such techniques. PET utilizes flow–metabolism coupling and tracks the local uptake of 2-deoxyglucose labelled with a short half-life positron emitter, whose regional cerebral concentration is monitored by tomography.

None of the above methods is suitable for measuring CBF in clinical practice, although they are used in research. Transcranial Doppler ultrasonography, which measures the *velocity* of red blood cells flowing through large vessels in the brain, is used, however, in clinical practice. The middle cerebral artery is most commonly insonated, because it is easy to detect, receives a substantial proportion of the blood flow from the internal carotid artery, and allows easy probe fixation.

The diameter of the middle cerebral artery and other basal arteries is not affected by common physiological variables, such as MAP and $CO_2$ partial pressure ($Pa\text{CO}_2$), and so the flow velocity in these vessels provides an index of flow. Provided the angle of insonation, the velocity profile, and the diameter of the vessel remain unchanged, changes in CBF velocity correlate closely with changes in CBF. The principal reason for interest in CBF is that clear ischaemic thresholds have been identified for various physiological processes in the neuron (Figure 22.19).

### *Cerebral oxygenation*

Normal CBF may provide inadequate metabolic substrates in the presence of hypermetabolism associated with excitotoxicity or fits, and subnormal CBF may be adequate when the cerebral metabolic rate of $O_2$ ($CMRO_2$) is reduced by anaesthetic agents or hypothermia. The measurement of cerebral oxygenation by jugular bulb oximetry is one method of assessing the adequacy of CBF. A sample of jugular venous blood will normally contain blood representative of the venous drainage of two-thirds of the ipsilateral and one-third of the contralateral hemispheres, although there may be marked asymmetry in the venous drainage. In addition, extracerebral contamination of jugular bulb blood is usually present, but is less than 5%.

A catheter is inserted into the internal jugular vein so that it lies above the point of entry of the common facial vein (at the level of the C1–2 vertebral bodies). The superior sagittal sinus typically drains via the right sigmoid sinus into the right internal jugular vein; cannulation of this vessel therefore allows assessment of global flow to the cerebral hemispheres. Normally the brain removes about 30% of oxygen delivered and therefore the normal jugular bulb oxygen saturation ($Sjv\text{O}_2$) is 65–70%. Increases in $CMRO_2$ will result in decreases in $Sjv\text{O}_2$ when, for whatever reason, oxygen uptake is greater than its supply. $Sjv\text{O}_2$ can be measured continuously using a fibreoptic catheter or, intermittently by drawing blood samples through the catheter. Major disadvantages of this technique include its invasiveness and poor signal reliability (frequent false-positive readings occur when $Sjv\text{O}_2$ falls below 50%).

## Physiological factors affecting cerebral blood flow

### *Global cerebral blood flow*

#### *Autoregulation*

Autoregulation is the ability of a tissue to regulate its own blood flow despite changes in perfusion pressure. It is a fundamental property of the cerebral and other (e.g. myocardial and renal) circulations. Reference to Figure 22.20 shows that, within ranges of MAP between 50 and 150 mmHg, autoregulation maintains CBF at a constant value. However, once the lower limit of autoregulation is reached, further reductions in MAP result in a progressive decline in CBF, leading to ischaemia. Conversely, increases in MAP above the upper limit result in hyperaemia and increased CBV (and, importantly, potentially increased ICP).

In patients with chronic hypertension, the whole curve shifts to the right and such patients require a higher MAP to maintain CBF (Figure 22.20) . In reality, such clear-cut autoregulatory thresholds are not observed – the acute changes at either end tend to be more gradual, and there may be regional variations. These responses may be affected by the rate of change in perfusion pressure – i.e. a sudden fall in pressure may result in a transient reduction in flow as

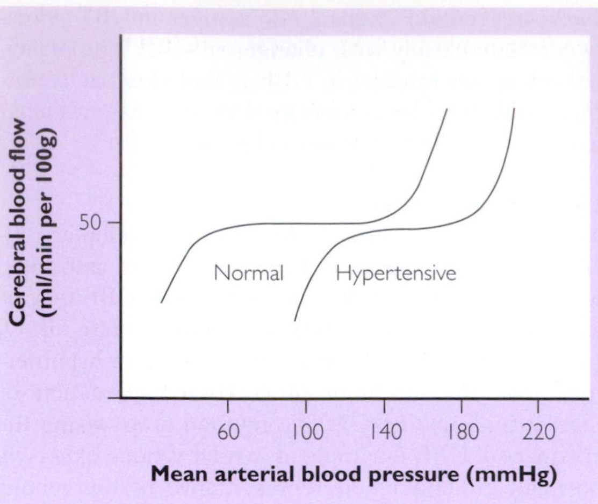


**Figure 22.20** Thresholds for autoregulation in normal and hypertensive patients.

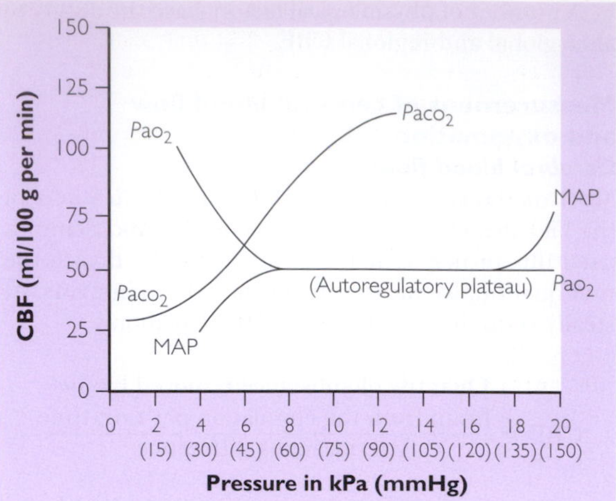


**Figure 22.21** The effect of changes in oxygen partial pressure ($PaO_2$) and $CO_2$ partial pressure ($PaCO_2$) and the mean blood pressure on cerebral blood flow.

the compensatory reflexes take longer to respond. Normal individuals autoregulate at a rate of 20%/s and the process is complete in 5–8 s. This time is, however, prolonged in patients with pathological changes. In addition, autoregulation at the lower limit appears to be better preserved when falls in CPP result from increases in ICP rather than because of decreases in MAP caused by hypovolaemia.

Myogenic reflexes are thought to be the major mechanism of autoregulation. This is an example of Starling's law as applied to vascular smooth muscle – the force of contraction of a muscle is proportional to its initial fibre length. Inevitably this mechanism is not acting in isolation and is modulated by other factors, such as local vasodilating substances.

Autoregulation is lost in damaged areas of the brain such as that surrounding tumours, abscesses, and haematomas. There is global loss of autoregulation following generalized cell disruption, as after severe head injury and widespread brain ischaemia. Wherever autoregulation is lost, CBF becomes largely pressure dependent.

#### *$CO_2$ partial pressure*

CBF is directly proportional to the $PaCO_2$ between 3.5 and 10 kPa (26 and 75 mmHg) (Figure 22.21). In the physiological range, a 1-kPa change in $PaCO_2$ produces a change in CBF of approximately 15 ml/100 g tissue per min. Below 3.5 kPa (26 mmHg), vasoconstriction results in increasing tissue hypoxia and leads to reflex vasodilatation (resulting from accumulation of local metabolites), whereas above 10 kPa maximal vasodilatation occurs, giving flows of about 120 ml/100 g tissue per min. It is possible that nitric oxide (NO) may be the principal mediator of this effect. Mild hyperventilation ($PaCO_2$ 4–4.5 kPa; 30–34 mmHg) will help reduce CBV in patients with raised ICP, but lower values than this should be avoided because of the risk of inducing tissue hypoxia secondary to reduced CBF.

#### *Oxygen partial pressure*

CBF is unchanged until the oxygen partial pressure ($PaO_2$) falls below 7–8 kPa (53–60 mmHg), but increases sharply with further decreases in $PaO_2$ (Figure 22.21). The exact mechanism has not been elucidated but, because tissue oxygen delivery is a major function of CBF, metabolites resulting from hypoxia must be a significant factor.

#### *Autonomic activity*

Vasomotor plexuses exist around the cerebral arteries with adrenergic (constrictor) and cholinergic (dilator) receptors on cerebrovascular smooth muscle. The adrenergic neurons arise from the superior cervical ganglia and the cholinergic fibres may originate in the reticular formation in the medulla. Their action is mainly on the proximal parts of the anterior, middle, and posterior cerebral arteries, with maximal sympathetic stimulation reducing flow by only 5–10%.

#### *Temperature*

Temperature affects cerebral metabolic rate. Overall, the $CMRO_2$ changes by about 7% for every 1°C change in temperature and, with this, appropriate changes in CBF occur. Thus, hyperthermia is detrimental to patients with raised ICP because it increases CBF and demand for $O_2$. Hypothermia reduces CBF and $O_2$ needs, although this is not the only mechanism by which it provides cerebral protection; mild hypothermia also reduces the release of glutamate, which may confer neuronal protection.

#### *Haematocrit*

A decreased plasma viscosity and haematocrit improve cerebral capillary blood flow (see Chapter 31). This must be offset against the reduced $O_2$-carrying capacity as the haemoglobin concentration falls. The optimum haematocrit value for cerebral perfusion/$O_2$ delivery is 30–40%. Haematocrits above 50% decrease CBF.

### *Local and regional cerebral blood flow*

Increases in local neuronal activity are accompanied by increases in the rCMR. This linked increase in rCBF is referred to as flow–metabolism coupling. The increases in rCBF that occur during functional activation tend to track glucose use, which may be far greater than the increase in $O_2$ consumption – i.e. regional *anaerobic* glucose utilization occurs.

Perivascular $H^+$, $K^+$, and adenosine concentrations are major metabolic mediators. NO may also play an important role in local neurogenic control of flow–metabolism coupling. One hypothesis is that NO (released from neurons containing NO synthase) diffuses rapidly into vascular smooth muscle cells and causes a reduction in free intracellular calcium (via a cGMP-mediated action), leading to dephosphorylation of myosin and consequent relaxation.

### The effects of drugs on cerebral haemodynamics

The intravenous induction agents thiopentone (thiopental), etomidate, and propofol all reduce $CMRO_2$ and CBF together, but without affecting autoregulation. Ketamine, however, increases CBF principally because of its effect on MAP.

All inhalational agents increase CBF while reducing $CMRO_2$. With the exception of sevoflurane, they all have a dose-dependent direct vasodilatory effect, which predominates but can be reduced by hyperventilation. Autoregulation is abolished by 1.5 MAC of isoflurane, enflurane, halothane, and desflurane, because of these direct vasodilatory effects (MAC is the minimum anaesthetic concentration). Sevoflurane appears to have less of a vasodilatory effect and therefore up to 1.5 MAC does not increase CBF or affect autoregulation.

Neuropharmacological effects of drugs used in anaesthetic practice are summarized in Table 22.6.

$N_2O$ increases CBF secondary to an increase in $CMRO_2$, although the exact reason for this remains unclear to date. The opioids fentanyl, alfentanil, and remifentanil have no direct effect on cerebral haemodynamics, although they will have a significant secondary effect if the $Pa\text{CO}_2$ increases as a consequence of respiratory depression. Case reports have suggested that bolus doses of alfentanil and remifentanil have been associated with increases in ICP. The mechanism may be cerebral autoregulatory vasodilatation in response to a fall in MAP caused by the rapid administration of these potent opioids. Alfentanil and remifentanil should be administered by infusion to avoid these secondary effects.

It is important to remember that in areas of damaged brain, where CBF is dependent on MAP because of loss of autoregulation, cerebral vasodilatation produced by inhalational agents may produce 'steal' – perfusion to the undamaged brain is enhanced at the expense of that to the damaged brain. Conversely, hypocapnia induced by hyperventilation will result in vasoconstriction and reduced flow to 'normal' cerebral vasculature – as a consequence 'luxury perfusion' will occur in areas of damaged brain provided that the MAP is maintained. This effect is known as 'inverse steal'.

## NEUROTRANSMITTERS IN THE CNS

Our understanding of neurotransmitters and chemical messengers is currently expanding as a result of cloning and related molecular biological techniques. Some idea of the complexity of the subject is gained from the summary of information of neurotransmitters and their receptors given in Table 22.7.

Three common themes have emerged:

- For each transmitter, there are many subtypes of receptor (some of which are currently being identified and investigated). Examples include the $\alpha_1$-, $\alpha_2$-, $\beta_1$-, $\beta_2$-, and $\beta_3$-receptors for norepinephrine (noradrenaline). However, it is now clear that there are many different kinds of $\alpha_1$- and $\alpha_2$-receptors, which increases the variety and selectivity of possible responses.

**Table 22.6 Effects of drugs on cerebral haemodynamics**

| | $CMRO_2$ | CBF | ICP | $CO_2$ reactivity | Cerebral autoregulation |
|---|---|---|---|---|---|
| Isoflurane (MAC) | ↓ | ↑ | ↑ | ↑ | Impairs |
| Sevoflurane (1.5 MAC) | ↓ | ↑[a] | ↑[a] | →<br>← | →<br>← |
| Nitrous oxide | ↑ | ↑ | ↑ | →<br>← | Impairs |
| Thiopentone, propofol | ↓ | ↓ | ↓ | →<br>← | →<br>← |
| Fentanyl | →<br>← | →<br>← | →<br>← | →<br>← | →<br>← |
| Alfentanil, remifentanil | →<br>← | →<br>← | →<br>← | →<br>← | →<br>← |
| Mannitol | →<br>← | →<br>← | ↓ | →<br>← | →<br>← |

[a]Early studies suggest direct vasodilator effect at 1.5 MAC sevoflurane is 30% of the effect seen with isoflurane.
MAC, minimum anaesthetic concentration; $CMRO_2$, cerebral metabolic rate for oxygen; CBF, cerebral blood flow; ICP, intracranial pressure.

**Table 22.7 Neurotransmitters in the central nervous system**

| Substance | Locations |
|---|---|
| Acetylcholine | Ubiquitous |
| *Amines* | |
| Dopamine | Hypothalamus, limbic system, neocortex, retina |
| Norepinephrine (noradrenaline) | Cerebral cortex, hypothalamus, brain stem, cerebellum, spinal cord |
| Epinephrine (adrenaline) | Hypothalamus, thalamus, periaqueductal grey |
| Serotonin (5-hydroxytryptamine) | Hypothalamus, limbic system, cerebellum, retina |
| Histamine | Hypothalamus |
| *Excitatory amino acids* | |
| Glutamate | Cerebral cortex, brain stem |
| Aspartate | Spinal cord, ?elsewhere |
| *Inhibitory amino acids* | |
| Glycine | Direct inhibiting neurons, retina |
| GABA | Cerebellum, cerebral cortex, presynaptic inhibitors, retina |
| *Purines* | |
| Adenosine | Neocortex, olfactory cortex, hippocampus, cerebellum |
| ATP | Not established |
| *Polypeptides* | |
| Substance P | Ubiquitous, retina |
| Vasopressin | Posterior pituitary, medulla, spinal cord |
| Oxytocin | Posterior pituitary, medulla, spinal cord |
| CRH | Median eminence of hypothalamus, other parts of brain |
| TRH | Median eminence of hypothalamus, other parts of brain, retina |
| GRH | Median eminence of hypothalamus |
| Somatostatin | Median eminence of hypothalamus, other parts of brain, retina |
| GnRH | Median eminence of hypothalamus, circumventricular organs, retina |
| Endothelins | Posterior pituitary, brain stem |
| Enkephalins | Ubiquitous, retina |
| β-Endorphin | Hypothalamus, thalamus, brain stem, retina |
| CCK | Cerebral cortex, hypothalamus, retina |
| VIP | Postganglionic cholinergic neurons, hypothalamus, cerebral cortex, retina |
| Neurotensin | Hypothalamus, retina |
| GRP | Hypothalamus |
| Gastrin | Hypothalamus, medulla oblongata |
| Glucagon | Hypothalamus, retina |
| Motilin | Neurohypophysis, cerebral cortex, cerebellum |
| Secretin | Hypothalamus, thalamus, olfactory bulb, brain stem, cerebral cortex, hippocampus |
| CGRPα | Taste pathways, medial forebrain bundle |
| Neuropeptide Y | Medulla, periaqueductal grey, hypothalamus |
| Activins | Brain stem |
| Inhibins | Brain stem |
| Angiotensin II | Hypothalamus, brain stem, spinal cord |
| Galanin | Hypothalamus |
| ANP | Hypothalamus, brain stem |
| BNP | Hypothalamus, brain stem |

GABA, δ-aminobutyric acid; CRH, cortisol-releasing hormone; TRH, thyroid-releasing hormone; GRH, growth-hormone-releasing hormone; GnRH, gonadotrophin-releasing hormone; CCK, cholecystokinin; VIP, vasoactive intestinal polypeptide; GRP, gastrin-releasing peptide; CGRPα, calcitonin-gene-related peptide α; ANP, atrial natriuretic peptide; BNP, brain natriuretic peptide. (Adapted from Ganong WF. *Review of Medical Physiology*, 1st edn. Stamford: Appleton and Lange 1997, 89.)

- There are receptors on the pre- as well as the post-synaptic elements at many synaptic junctions. The presynaptic receptors (also called autoreceptors) often inhibit further secretion of the transmitter, providing feedback control. This is, for example, true of $\alpha_2$ presynaptic receptors which inhibit norepinephrine secretion. However, autoreceptors can also facilitate the release of neurotransmitters.
- The types of transmitter and receptors tend to group in large families as far as structure and

**Table 22.8 Mechanism of action of selected neurotransmitters**

| Neurotransmitter | Receptor (gene on chromosome) | Second messenger | Net channel effects |
|---|---|---|---|
| Acetylcholine | Nicotinic | – | ↑ $Na^+$ |
| | $M_1$ | ↑ $IP_3$, DAG | ↑ $Ca^{2+}$ |
| | $M_2$ (cardiac) | ↓ cAMP | ↓ $Ca^{2+}$ |
| | $M_3$ | ↓ cAMP | |
| | $M_4$ (glandular) | ↑ $IP_3$, DAG | |
| | $M_5$ | ↑ $IP_3$, DAG | |
| Dopamine | $D_1$ | ↑ cAMP | |
| | $D_2$ | ↓ cAMP | ↑ $K^+$, ↓ $Ca^{2+}$ |
| Norepinephrine | $\alpha_{1A}$ | ↑ $IP_3$, DAG | ↓ $K^+$ |
| | $\alpha_{1B}$ (C5) | ↑ $IP_3$, DAG | |
| | $\alpha_{1C}$ (C8) | ↑ $IP_3$, DAG | |
| | $\alpha_{1D}$ (C20) | ↑ $IP_3$, DAG | |
| | $\alpha_{2A}$ (C10) | ↓ cAMP | ↑ $K^+$, ↓ $Ca^{2+}$ |
| | $\alpha_{2B}$ (C2) | ↓ cAMP | |
| | $\alpha_{2C}$ (C4) | – | |
| | $\beta_1$ | ↑ cAMP | |
| | $\beta_2$ | ↑ cAMP | |
| 5HT (serotonin) | $5HT_{1A}$ | ↓ cAMP | ↑ $K^+$ |
| | $5HT_{1B}$ | ↓ cAMP | |
| | $5HT_{1C}$ | ↑ $IP_3$, DAG | ↓ $K^+$ |
| | $5HT_{1D}$ | ↓ cAMP | ↓ $K^+$ |
| | $5HT_2$ | ↑ IP3, DAG | |
| | $5HT_3$ | – | ↑ $Na^+$ |
| | $5HT_4$ | ↑ cAMP | |
| Adenosine | $A_1$ | ↓ cAMP | |
| | $A_2$ | ↑ cAMP | |
| Glutamate, aspartate | NMDA | – | ↑ $Na^+$, ↓ $Ca^{2+}$ |
| | AMPA | – | ↑ $Na^+$ |
| | Quisqualate | ↑ $IP_3$, DAG | – |
| | Kainate | – | ↑ $Na^+$ |
| GABA | $GABA_A$ | – | ↑ $Cl^-$ |
| | $GABA_B$ | ↑ $IP_3$, DAG | ↑ $K^+$, ↓ $Ca^{2+}$ |

AMPA, alpha-amino-3-hydroxy-5-methyl-4-isoxazolepropionate; cAMP, cyclic adenosine monophosphate; DAG, diacylglycerol; GABA, γ-aminobutyrate; 5HT, 5-hydroxytryptamine; $IP_3$, inositol triphosphate; M, muscarinic; NMDA, N-methyl-D-aspartate. (Adapted from Ganong WF. *Review of Medical Physiology*, 1st edn. Stamford: Appleton and Lange 1997, 91.)

function are concerned. Many are serpentine receptors, which act via G proteins and protein kinases to produce their effects. Others are ion channels. The receptors, their principal second messengers, and, where known, the net effect on channels for a group of selected established neurotransmitters are given in Table 22.8.

## DRUGS ACTING IN THE CNS

The large number of transmitters in the CNS that have been identified (see Table 22.7), and more that are suspected, give huge potential for significant pharmacological modification of neurotransmitter function. To be effective, the drug needs to be able to cross the BBB. Examples are the action of anaesthetic agents, opioids, serotonin (5-hydroxytryptamine) 5-$HT_3$ antagonists and L-dopa. The only drugs that will be considered here are antidepressants, lithium, anticonvulsants, major tranquillizers, and calcium channel blockers. For details of other drug actions, apart from those covered in other sections of this book (e.g. opioids, benzodiazepines, anaesthetic agents, antiemetics, etc.), the reader should consult more specialist texts.

### Antidepressant drugs

Depression affects 5–6% of the population at any given time, and 10% of the population will suffer from depression during their lives. Therefore, it is likely that anaesthetists will encounter patients undergoing treatment for this condition. The hypothesis that depression is a result of impaired turnover of brain amines is undoubtedly simplistic, but it has been the basis for the pharmacological approach to the disease.

***Amine neurotransmission***
The mode of action of antidepressants can be understood only by first considering the physiology of neuroamine transmission (described in detail in Chapter 23). The action of amine neurotransmitters is partly terminated by the reuptake of the amines into the nerve terminal. There is also a degradation pathway involving the action of the enzyme monoamine oxidase (MAO) on the amine. The uptake of amines is under the control of serotonin, and serotonin itself is taken up into the terminals of interneurons. Increased serotonin availability results in more norepinephrine being available and this elevates mood. Norepinephrine is the presynaptic final common pathway. Preventing its breakdown can also increase norepinephine levels; this is the purpose of the MAO inhibitors. MAO-A is selective for norepinephrine and serotonin whereas MAO-B is more selective for dopamine.

The postsynaptic effects of this increase in neurotransmitters has again attracted interest recently. The amines released act on β-adrenoceptors in the CNS, and the consequence of prolonged exposure to increased levels of the amine is a down-regulation of these β-receptors and a decrease in cAMP concentration in the cell. This down-regulation seen in animals follows a similar time course to the delay in clinical onset of the action of these drugs. It is difficult to demonstrate a similar effect on central β-receptors in patients, so only inferences can be made. However, attention has become focused on the postsynaptic changes that these drugs produce as a result of their presynaptic action.

The drugs used to treat depression fall into four categories based on their mode of action:

1. tricyclic antidepressants;
2. heterocyclics;
3. selective serotonin-reuptake inhibitors (SSRIs);
4. MAO inhibitors (MAOIs).

*The tricyclic antidepressants*
These drugs (Table 22.9), all chemically related to a three-nucleus ring structure, have been in use for 30 years. An example of their basic structure is shown in Figure 22.22a. They resemble the phenothiazine drugs and have some antihistaminic, antimuscarinic,

| Table 22.9 Tricyclic antidepressants |
|---|
| Amitriptyline |
| Imipramine |
| Desimipramine |
| Clomipramine |
| Nortriptyline |
| Doxepin |

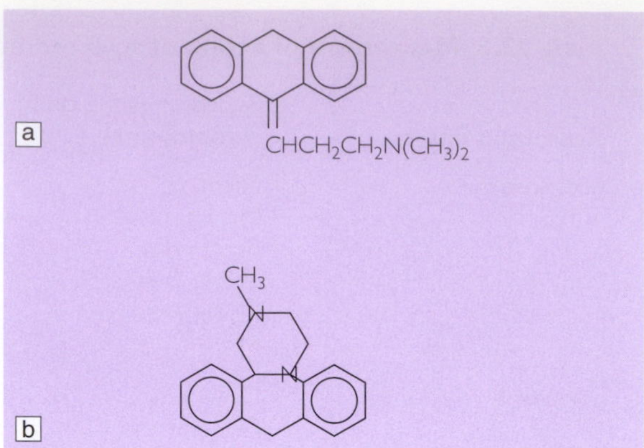


**Figure 22.22** Examples of (a) a tricyclic (amitriptyline) and (b) a tetracyclic (mianserin) antidepressant .

and α-receptor-blocking actions. Imipramine and amitriptyline are the original drugs in this class. The later drugs were developed to reduce the incidence of side effects.

Tricyclics have a varying degree of selectivity for the amine reuptake pumps. Their clinical action is not manifest until 15–17 days after the commencement of treatment. They have a large number of unwanted effects. They can be sedative and this action can be additive to other sedative drugs. Their sympathomimetic actions include tremor and insomnia, and as antimuscarinics they produce blurred vision, constipation, urinary hesitancy, and confusion. Orthostatic hypotension, conduction defects, and arrhythmias can occur, as can aggravation of psychosis and withdrawal syndrome.

Overdose of tricyclics, deliberate or accidental, is a medical emergency. Coma, metabolic acidosis, respiratory depression, neuromuscular irritability and seizures, hyperpyrexia, and a large variety of cardiac problems, including conduction defects and arrhythmias, are seen. Intensive care treatment with supportive measures is required, but there remains a significant mortality.

The tricyclics have been used in the management of depression and panic disorders, in the treatment of enuresis, and for chronic pain states.

*The heterocyclic drugs*
These second-generation drugs (Table 22.10) are similar to the tricyclics in their onset of action, and their potency, but differ significantly in their unwanted and toxic effects. Amoxapine, maprotiline, and mianserin are the commonly used drugs in this group. Mianserin is a tetracyclic and is shown compared with a tricyclic in Figure 22.22b.

| Table 22.10 Heterocyclics |
|---|
| Amoxapine |
| Maprotiline |
| Mianserin |

The cardiac toxicity of these drugs is much lower than that of the older tricyclics, but neurological symptoms are more common. The seizure threshold is lowered, and these drugs cannot be used in people with epilepsy. They should not be given within 14 days of stopping MAOIs. It is recommended that these drugs should be continued up to the morning of surgery, as a safer option than stopping the drug before surgery. Amoxapine is more prone to produce convulsions in overdose than maprotiline, but rarely causes more than a sinus tachycardia in its effect on the heart.

*The selective serotonin reuptake inhibitors*

Serotonin release is part of the feedback mechanism for norepinephrine release, and these drugs, with a very specific action, are free of many of the unwanted effects of the tricyclics. Fluoxetine, paroxetine, fluvoxamine, and sertraline are available in the UK.

Fluoxetine (Prozac) (Figure 22.23) was the first of these drugs to be introduced, and the newer drugs differ only in having shorter half-lives. The combination of the SSRIs and MAOIs can result in a marked increase in serotonin in the synapse, producing the so-called serotonin syndrome. This syndrome is characterized by hyperthermia, muscle rigidity, myoclonus, and rapid changes in mental status. Fourteen days should be allowed after stopping MAOIs, and before starting SSRIs. These drugs are metabolized by hepatic cytochrome P450 enzymes and can interact with drugs also metabolized by this system. The effect persists for 5 weeks after stopping the drug.

Seizures have been reported with these drugs, but they have a very wide safety margin, and reports of death from overdosage of SSRIs alone are rare.

*The monoamine oxidase inhibitors*

These drugs are of two groups: the hydrazines such as phenelzine and the non-hydrazines such as tranylcypromine. They are mainly non-selective and bind with both forms of the enzyme, MAO-A and MAO-B. MAOIs prevent the breakdown of norepinephrine, serotonin, and dopamine, resulting in the accumulation of norepinephrine in nerve terminals. The older MAOI drugs have fallen out of use with the introduction of the new generation of heterocyclics and SSRIs. They had a wide spectrum of interactions with other drugs, which made their use difficult, and the patient also had to avoid tyramine-containing foods.

MAOIs enjoy an infamous reputation in their interaction with drugs during anaesthesia. As a result of the increased norepinephrine stores, the greatest danger of unpredictable changes in blood pressure is with sympathomimetic agents (e.g. ephedrine; Chapter 23, Table 23.11). Perhaps most important is the interaction with pethidine. Agitation, restlessness, hypertension, rigidity, convulsions, and hyperpyrexia may result. The primary opioid effects of pethidine may also be potentiated, causing coma, depressed ventilation, and hypotension. Morphine appears to be safe. Adequate analgesia is important to prevent excess sympathetic drive as a result of pain. The advice in the past was to stop MAOIs 2–3 weeks before surgery, but some anaesthetists continue them and avoid triggering agents perioperatively.

Moclobemide is a second-generation drug, which reversibly blocks MAO-A. It causes less potentiation of tyramine than traditional MAOIs and does not require special dietary restrictions, although patients are still advised not to eat large quantities of tyramine-rich food. The use of pethidine in patients taking moclobemide is still contraindicated because of consequent CNS excitation or depression with hypertension or hypotension. The drug is extensively metabolized, and some patients have a genetic variation of liver function that results in slow metabolism and therefore high levels of the drug.

The relative potencies of various antidepressant drugs as inhibitors of the uptake of norepinephrine or serotonin is shown in Figure 22.24.

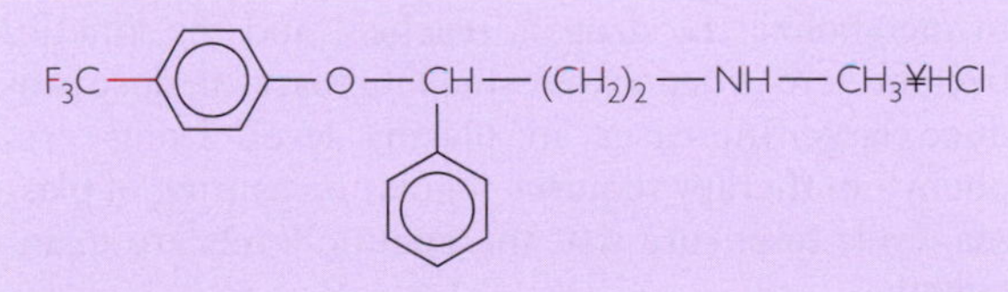

$F_3C$—C₆H₄—O—CH—$(CH_2)_2$—NH—$CH_3$¥HCl (with phenyl ring on CH)

**Figure 22.23** The structure of fluoxetine.

### Lithium

Lithium (administered orally as the carbonate or citrate) is effective in bipolar illness, preventing both mania and depression. Its exact mode of action is not clear. It has a narrow therapeutic range

**Table 22.11 Benzodiazepines in common use in anaesthesia**

| Drug | Typical dose (mg) | Potency ratio | Half-life of parent drug | Active metabolites | Half-life of metabolites |
|---|---|---|---|---|---|
| Nitrazepam | 10 | 3 | 18–36 | No | |
| Temazepam | 20 | 1.5 | 5–10 | No[a] | |
| Midazolam | 10 | 3 | 1–3 | No | |
| Lorazepam | 1 | 30 | 10–20 | No | |
| Diazepam | 10 | 3 | 24–48 | Yes | Up to 5 days |
| Oxazepam | 30 | 1 | 5–15 | No | |

[a]Minor amounts of temazepam may be metabolized to oxazepam.

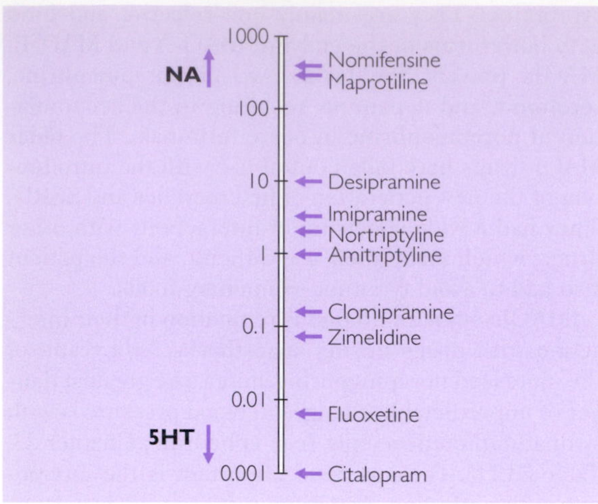


**Figure 22.24** The relative potencies of various antidepressant drugs as inhibitors of the uptake of norepinephrine (noradrenaline, NA) or 5-hydroxytryptamine (5HT).

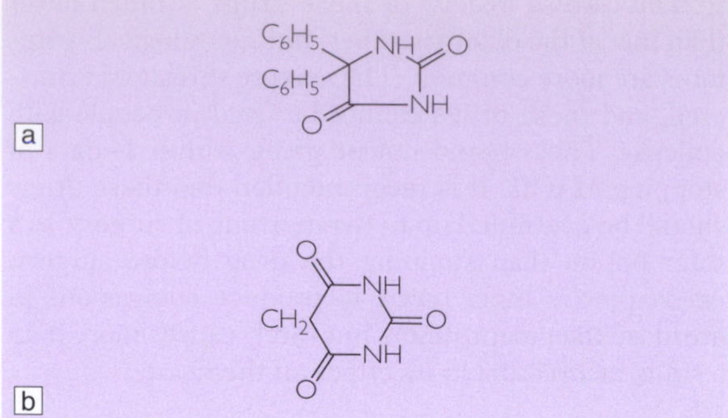


**Figure 22.25** The anticonvulsant drug phenytoin (a) compared with barbituric acid (b).

(0.8–1.2 mmol/L) and should be monitored by plasma estimations. Even in the therapeutic range T wave changes can occur in the ECG (intracellular $K^+$ is replaced by lithium), and myocardial infarction and failure are contraindications to its use. It is a dangerous drug in overdose. If plasma concentrations rise to 1.5–3.0 mmol/L, diarrhoea, weakness, drowsiness, thirst, and ataxia can occur. Further rises to 3.0–5.0 mmol/L can cause confusional states, convulsions, coma, and death.

Longer-term dose-dependent toxicity occurs with thyroid deficiency and nephrogenic diabetes insipidus. Thiazide diuretics can precipitate toxicity by reducing lithium clearance. Although lithium interferes with acetylcholine release, there is no strong evidence that it has a major clinical effect on neuromuscular blocking agents.

## Anticonvulsant drugs

These drugs are used in the management of epilepsy, and in seizures of other causes. Seizures result from abnormal discharge of cerebral neurons and consist of finite episodes.

The first pharmacological treatment of seizures was with barbiturates. Phenobarbitone (phenobarbital) was first used in 1912, and chemical analogues were investigated for antiseizure activity. Phenytoin was discovered in 1938. Drug development slowed in the subsequent 20 years, but several new drugs have been introduced in the last decade.

A better understanding of the complex conditions that make up epilepsy has led to a rationalization of drug therapy. The major seizures, partial and generalized, are treated with different drugs. Generalized seizures can be tonic–clonic (grand mal), absence (petit mal), tonic, atonic, and clonic–myoclonic. Seizure control is aimed at modifying ionic conductance particularly of $Na^+$ and $Ca^{2+}$. This enhances GABAergic transmission, which is inhibitory, or diminishes excitatory (usually glutaminergic) transmission.

### *Phenytoin*

This drug is a hydantoin derivative. It is a chemical relative of the barbiturates (Figure 22.25). It alters $Na^+$, $K^+$, and $Ca^{2+}$ conductances, and changes membrane potentials and the concentrations of a number of neurotransmitters. It blocks sustained high-frequency firing of neurons in a dose-dependent manner. The drug binds to inactivated sodium channels in the axon, a property that it shares with carbamazepine and sodium valproate. Phenytoin reduces $Ca^{2+}$ permeability in neurons, which accounts for its effects in reducing the release of a number of neurotransmitters.

Phenytoin is well absorbed orally, but less reliably from the intramuscular route. When given intravenously, it should be given slowly to minimize cardiovascular depression. It is highly protein bound, and its free plasma level can be altered in states where binding is altered. It is metabolized in the liver in a two-stage process to inactive metabolites. Its elimination is dose dependent. It undergoes first-order kinetics at low doses, but, as the plasma level rises within the therapeutic range, the maximum capacity of the liver to metabolize the drug is reached, and the kinetics become zero order so that small increases in dose produce large increases in plasma level. Long-term phenytoin therapy requires regular measuring of plasma levels to ensure that therapeutic levels are maintained.

Overdose produces nystagmus, diplopia, and ataxia and, at higher levels, sedation. Gingival hypertrophy, hirsuitism, and coarsening of the facial features are the distressing long-term effects of using the drug.

### *Carbamazepine*

This drug is chemically related to the tricyclic antidepressant drugs, but produces its anticonvulsant action via a mechanism similar to that of phenytoin. It is commonly used for partial seizures, but it may be used in combination with phenytoin for grand mal epilepsy. It is used in the treatment of trigeminal neuralgia, often in doses that cause sedation. Diplopia and ataxia are common side effects. Rarely, fatal blood dyscrasias have occurred.

Carbamazepine is an enzyme-inducing drug, and may increase the metabolism of other anticonvulsant drugs, notably phenytoin, clonazepam, ethosuximide, and sodium valproate.

#### *Ethosuximide*

This drug is used primarily in the control of absence-type seizures, although now such seizures are often managed by a combination of drugs. Its mode of action probably involves the $Ca^{2+}$ channel, the inhibition of $Na^+/K^+$ ATPase, and some depression of GABA aminotransferase. Most important is its effect on $Ca^{2+}$ channels. This depresses thalamic neurons which produce rhythmical cortical discharges during absence attacks.

Ethosuximide can cause abdominal pain, nausea, and vomiting, which are dose-related symptoms. It has a wide margin of safety.

#### *Sodium valproate*

This drug is fully ionized at body pH and it is the valproate ion that is the active moiety. It blocks sustained high-frequency firing, probably by an effect on $Na^+$ channels. It also increases brain GABA levels, although the mechanism of the therapeutic implication of this is unclear, because this occurs only at high concentrations, well above those required for its anticonvulsant effect. It is commonly used where absence and tonic–clonic seizures occur together.

Sodium valproate is highly protein bound and highly ionized, so its distribution is confined to the body water; 20% is conjugated and excreted and the remainder is metabolized to inactive metabolites. The tablets are hygroscopic and are packed in sealed foil. It can produce nausea and vomiting, abdominal pain, and heartburn, all of which are dose dependent. Idiosyncratic hepatotoxicity has been reported, and can be severe. At greatest risk are small children and those on combinations of drugs. The hepatotoxicity occurs early in the treatment, and careful monitoring of liver function is required for the first few months.

#### *Lamotrigine*

This new anticonvulsant drug has its action on $Na^+$ channels. It blocks use-dependent channel opening, and inhibits the release of glutamate. It is used alone, and as an add-on therapy to sodium valproate.

It is 55% plasma protein bound and the displacement from binding sites does not increase toxicity. It induces enzymes, and its own metabolism, but does not affect the kinetics of the other anticonvulsants. Its own half-life is reduced by enzyme-inducing drugs.

#### *Gabapentin*

This is a drug marketed to supplement standard anticonvulsants in the management of partial seizures. It is not effective in absence seizures. It is structurally related to GABA, but the binding site of gabapentin has not been defined. It appears to be non-toxic and well tolerated. It is available in an oral preparation only. It does not interfere with the kinetics of the standard anticonvulsant drugs. It is not metabolized and is excreted through the kidney following zero-order kinetics. Care must be taken with the drug in patients with renal impairment.

### Benzodiazepines

Benzodiazepines are the most commonly prescribed drugs in the Western World. They are generally considered to produce sedation and hypnosis by depressing the excitability of the limbic system (see above). Consequently they generally produce:

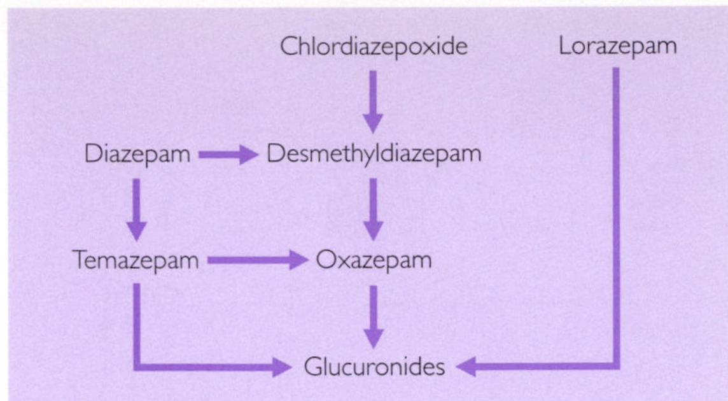


**Figure 22.26** Metabolic pathways of benzodiazepines.

- a reduction in emotional responsiveness and behaviour;
- a decrease in alertness and arousal;
- anterograde amnesia under some conditions;
- anticonvulsant activity;
- suppression of polysynaptic reflexes in the spinal cord and reduction of spasms.

Benzodiazepines in common use in anaesthesia are listed in Table 22.11. They are metabolized in the liver through common pathways via intermediate metabolites (which may be pharmacologically active or inactive), and excreted in urine as inactive glucuronide conjugates. The metabolic pathways are shown in Figure 22.26.

Specific binding sites for benzodiazepines have been found in the cortex, cerebellum, hippocampus, and spinal cord. They have been subclassified into $BZ_1$- and $BZ_2$-receptors and are found in close relationship to $GABA_A$-receptors. Benzodiazepines probably work by facilitating the $Cl^-$ channel in GABA-receptors as shown in Figure 22.27. Neurons that release GABA are essentially small interneurons that induce hyperpolarization at pre- and postsynaptic sites, possibly making up 20–40% of all synapses within the CNS. Five different $GABA_A$-receptor subunits have now been described, which may account for the different clinical responses to the various benzodiazepines currently marketed. There is also marked interpatient variability in response to the same drug.

A benzodiazepine antagonist, flumazenil, is now available for intravenous use and is shown compared with diazepam in Figure 22.28. It is an almost pure antagonist devoid of agonist activity, which acts rapidly but has a relatively short duration of action (up to 1 hour). Consequently, it may need to be repeated or given by infusion to antagonize the sedation and respiratory depression of the longer-acting benzodiazepines. Reported side effects are nausea, vomiting, flushing, anxiety, and convulsions in epileptic patients.

In chronic users, a benzodiazepine withdrawal syndrome is now recognized and may occur within a few hours or up to 3 weeks after stopping the drug. Characteristically, it includes sleep disturbances, anxiety, tremors, perspiration, tinnitus, and loss of appetite.

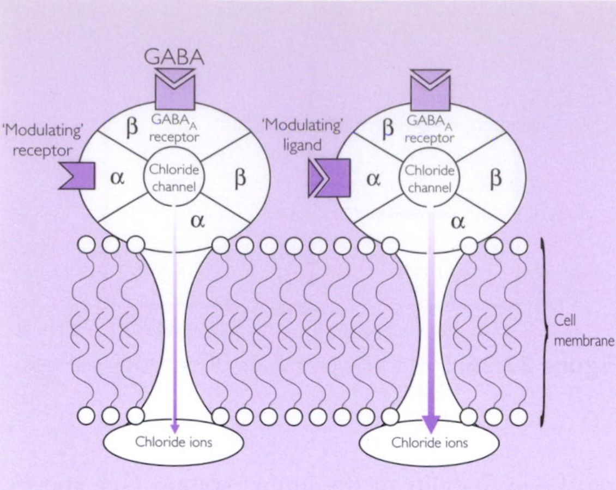


**Figure 22.27** A diagrammatic representation of the GABA receptor, which controls chloride channels across the cell membrane. The endogenous ligand GABA binds at the GABA receptor on the β subunit. Modulating ligands such as benzodiazepines, barbiturates, and intravenous induction agents bind to a separate modulating receptor which is on the complex (on the α subunit), but separate to the endogenous GABA receptor. When the modulating receptor is activated, it enhances GABA-mediated chloride conductance through the membrane, which results in a hyperpolarization of the cell, thereby making it less excitable. (From Salonen MA and Maze M. Molecular mechanism of action for hypnotic and sedative drugs. In: Feldman SA, Paton W, Scurr C. *Mechanisms of Drugs in Anaesthesia,* 2nd edn. London: Edward Arnold, 1993, 205.)

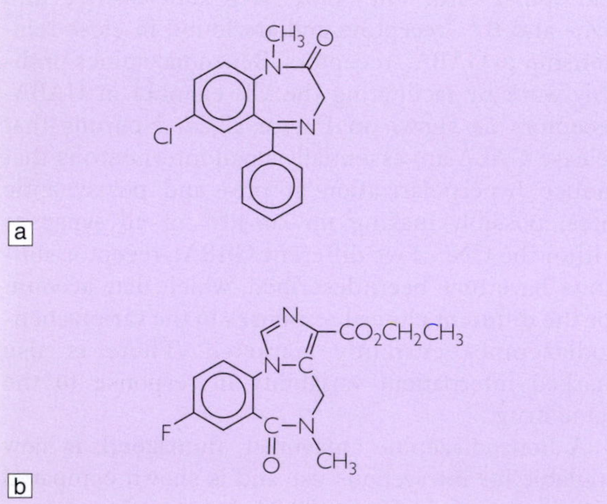


**Figure 22.28** The structures of (a) diazepam and (b) flumazenil.

### Antipsychotic drugs

Antipsychotic drugs are also known as neuroleptics and major tranquillizers. They ideally exert their effects without impairing consciousness or causing paradoxical excitement or other side effects. In the short term, they are used to quieten disturbed patients of all types, irrespective of the underlying pathophysiology, and are prescribed selectively for maintenance.

Antipsychotic drugs are considered to act by interfering with dopaminergic transmission in the brain by blocking dopamine receptors. This may give rise to extrapyramidal symptoms and blockade of cholinergic, adrenergic, histaminergic, and serotinergic receptors. Consequently, they have a wide spectrum of side effects. Extrapyramidal symptoms consist of:

- parkinsonian symptoms, including tremor;
- dystonia (abnormal face and body movements);
- akathisia (unremitting restlessness);
- tardive dyskinesia.

They can be broadly classified into phenothiazine derivatives, the butyrophenones, and 'atypical antipsychotics'.

Phenothiazine derivatives, in addition to their neuroleptic properties, also have anticholinergic and antihistaminic effects. These produce hypotension and antiemesis, respectively, the intensity of the effect varying from drug to drug. They can be divided into three main groups:

1. Chlorpromazine and promazine: pronounced sedative but moderate antimuscarinic and extrapyramidal side effects.
2. Thioridazine, pericyazine, and pipothiazine: moderate sedative effects, marked antimuscarinic but low extrapyramidal side effects
3. Prochlorperazine, perphenazine: low sedative effects, fewer antimuscarinic but pronounced extrapyramidal side effects

Note that, in appropriate doses, a number of these drugs are used in anaesthesia practice as antiemetics, antihistamines, and antihypertensives.

Hypotension and interference with temperature regulation are especially dangerous in elderly patients. A severe adverse reaction called the neuroleptic malignant syndrome includes hyperthermia, altered level of consciousness, muscular rigidity, autonomic instability, labile blood pressure, and incontinence. It is fortunately very rare but can be fatal.

The butyrophenones (droperidol and haloperidol) resemble phenothiazines of group 3. They are also very effective in low dosage as antiemetics.

The newer 'atypical antipsychotics' include risperidone, amisulpride, and clozapine. They may be effective in patients refractory to other treatments and extrapyramidal symptoms may be reduced.

## CALCIUM CHANNEL BLOCKERS

The only drug considered here is nimodipine. The source of $Ca^{2+}$ necessary for the contraction of large cerebral arteries is extracellular. This differs from systemic arteries which use an intracellular pool of $Ca^{2+}$. Consequently, cerebral arteries are theoretically susceptible to therapeutic attack by calcium channel-blocking drugs.

Nimodipine has been used in animal and human trials to try to reduce ischaemia secondary to vasospasm. It has been most extensively studied for the management of subarachnoid haemorrhage.

Evidence to date indicates that it can ameliorate the extent of neurological damage but its use is not universal. One of its problematic side effects is hypotension (from actions on the heart and systemic vasculature) which may need to be countered with vasoconstrictor drugs in an effort to maintain CPP.

Nimodipine is also being used in clinical trials as an antihypertensive for pre-eclampsia.

## FURTHER READING


Bradley PB. *Introduction to Neuropharmacology*. Bristol: Wright, 1989.

Durieux ME. Muscarinic signalling in the central nervous system. *Anesthesiology* 1996;**84**:173–89.

Ganong WF, ed. *Review of Medical Physiology*. Stamford: Appleton & Lange, 2001.

Gunawardana RH. Cigarette smoking and anaesthesia. *Ceylon Med J* 1999;**44**:180–3.

Gupte S, Heath K, Matta BF. Effect of incremental doses of sevoflurane on cerebral pressure autoregulation in humans. *Br J Anaesth* 1997;**79**:469–72.

Hsia CC. Respiratory function of haemoglobin. *New Engl J Med* 1998;**338**:239–47.

Inglis A, Fitch W. Physiology and metabolism of the central nervous system: anaesthetic implications. In: Van Aken H, ed. *Neuroanaesthetic Practice. Fundamentals of Anaesthesia and Acute Medicine Series.* London: BMJ Publishing Group, 1995.

Janssens JP, Pache JC, Nicod LP. Physiological changes in respiratory function associated with ageing. *Eur Resp J* 1999;**13**:197–205.

Kam PCA, Chang GWM. Selective serotonin reuptake inhibitors. Pharmacology and clinical implications in anaesthesia and critical care medicine. *Anaesthesia* 1997;**52**:982–8.

Koeppen BM, Stanton BA, eds. *Physiology*. St Louis: Mosby, 1998.

Lees G. Receptors for neurotransmitters and neuromodulators and their roles in drug action. *Curr Anaesth Crit Care* 1997;**8**:192–7.

Lumb AB, ed. *Nunn's Respiratory Pharmacology*. Oxford: Butterworth–Heinemann, 2000.

Matera MG. Nitric oxide and airways. *Pulmon Pharm Ther* 1998;**11**:341–8.

Mawer GE. New antiepileptic drugs. *Curr Anaesth Crit Care* 1997;**7**:126–32.

Menon DK. Cerebral circulation. In: Priebe H-J, Skarvan K, eds. *Cardiovascular Physiology. Fundamentals of Anaesthesia and Acute Medicine Series.* London: BMJ Publishing Group, 1995.

Menon DK. Monitoring the central nervous system. *Curr Anaesth Crit Care.* 1997;**8**:254–63.

Scurr C, Feldman F, Soni N, eds. *Scientific Foundation of Anaesthesia. The Basis of Intensive Care*. Oxford: Heinemann, 1990.

Stanford SC, Stanford BJ. Drugs acting in the brain. In: Kaufman L, ed. *Anaesthesia Review 9*. Edinburgh: Churchill Livingstone, 1992: 127–44.

Tindall GT, Cooper PR, Barrow DL. *The Practice of Neurosurgery*, Vol 1: Part 1 *CNS Physiology*. Baltimore, MA: Williams & Wilkins, 1996.

West JB, ed. *Pulmonary Pathophysiology – the Essentials*, 5th edn. Baltimore: Williams & Wilkins 1997.

West JB, ed. *Respiratory Physiology– the Essentials*, 6th edn. Baltimore: Williams & Wilkins 1999.

Zacny JP, Galinkin JL. Psychotropic drugs used in anesthesia practice. *Anesthesiology* 1999;**90**:269–88.

Zaugg M, Lucchinetti E. Expiratory function in the elderly. *Anaesth Clin North Am* 2000;**18**:47–58.

# Chapter 23 Physiology and pharmacology of the peripheral somatic and autonomic nervous systems

L. Bromley, P. Hutton, and G.M. Cooper

The peripheral nervous system (PNS) has three functions: sensory, somatic motor, and autonomic (see Chapter 22, Figure 22.1). By the action of reflex arcs, an appropriate motor reaction can occur in the periphery without necessarily involving higher centres in the central nervous system (CNS). Sensory information arriving in the spinal cord can be amplified or diminished at the level of the dorsal horn and/or relayed to higher centres. The traditional concept of the nervous system as a series of wiring diagrams for sensory information is now seen as somewhat simplistic. The integration of information in the dorsal horn of the spinal cord has led to a picture of a more plastic and responsive sensory nervous system and the introduction of the term neuroplasticity.

In this chapter, the general structure and function of the PNS are discussed first, together with relevant aspects of motor and sensory function. This is followed by basic and applied physiology and pharmacology related to the autonomic nervous system (ANS). The blood supply to the spinal cord and the circulation of cerebrospinal fluid are described in Chapter 22.

## STRUCTURE AND FUNCTION OF MOTOR AND SENSORY NEURONS

### Basic neuronal structure

A typical motor efferent neuron is shown in Figure 23.1 (see also Chapter 22, Figure 22.3). It has three main components:

1. A cell body in the CNS (the cyton), which has all the normal cellular components and integrates the effect of impulses received from synapses on its dendrites and cell body; Figure 23.1b shows the application of end-bulbs (bouton termineaux) to a cell body;
2. Dendrites, which are involved as postsynaptic components of synapses from other cells and transmit information to the cell;
3. An axon, which arborizes at its periphery. It conducts information away from the cell body and ends in presynaptic end-bulbs or specialized end-plates. An axon can synapse primarily with one cell, or, more commonly, with several.

A typical sensory afferent neuron is shown diagrammatically in Figure 23.2 (see also Chapter 22, Figure 22.3). Specialized endings on the dendrites of this cell are able to respond to different sensory modalities. Impulses generated by these sensory modalities are carried to the cell body, which lies in the dorsal root ganglion of the spinal cord, outside the

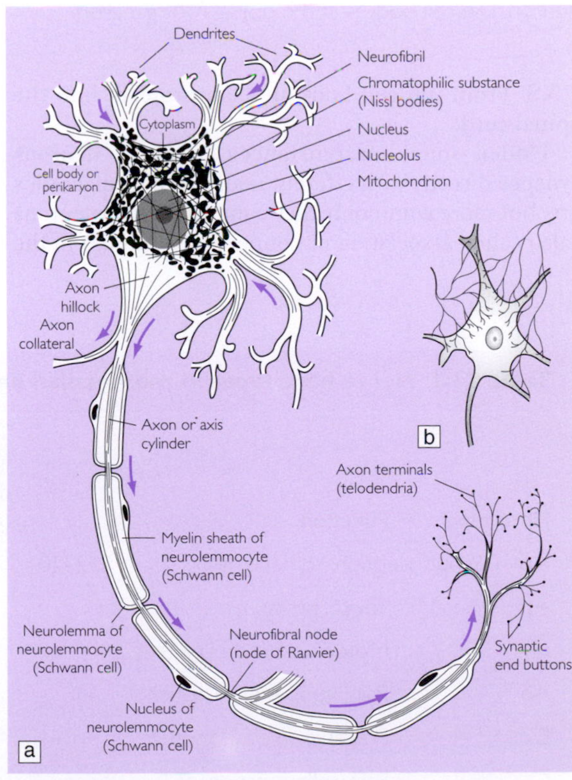


**Figure 23.1** The structure of a typical motor (efferent) neuron. (a) An entire neuron the cell body of which would be in the CNS. (b) The way in which terminal buttons impinge on the cyton and dendrites.

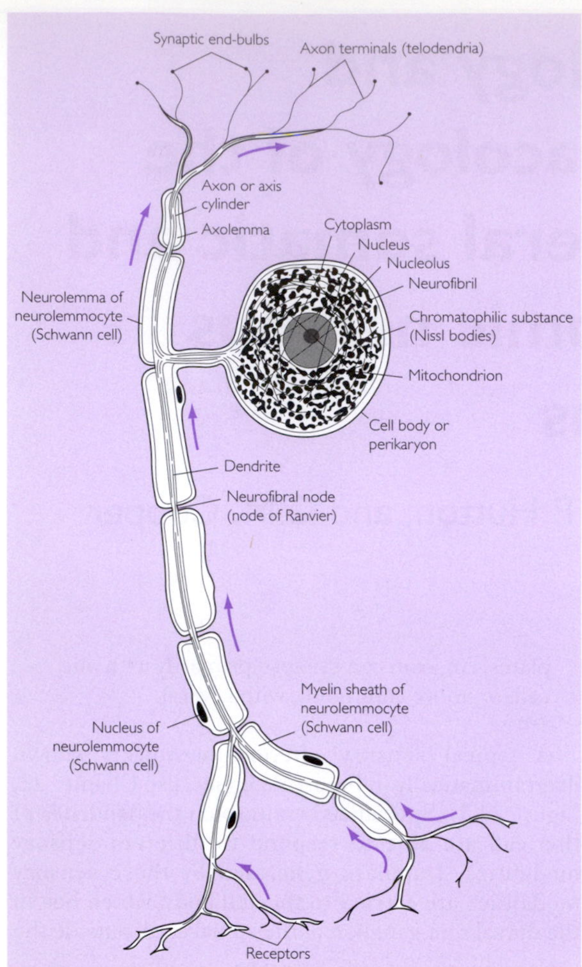


**Figure 23.2** The structure of a typical sensory (afferent) neuron. The cell body is in the dorsal root ganglion.

CNS. From the cell body an axon projects into the spinal cord.

Under some circumstances, afferent neurons synapse directly with efferent neurons to form a reflex arc, but more commonly they connect by interneurons (also called association or connecting neurons) in the spinal cord and brain. Up to 90% of neurons in the nervous system are interneurons.

Neurons are classified in relation to their structure and function, and whether or not they are myelinated (Table 23.1). Larger neurons have their axons enveloped in a sheath of myelin, formed from the cell membranes of the Schwann cells which wrap around the circumference of the axon (Figure 23.3). Schwann cells (or neurolemmocytes) are of neural-crest origin and are the chief non-excitable cells of the PNS, enfolding and wrapping axons around most of their surfaces. In addition to their importance in conduction, they may perform local nutritive and energy-supplying roles for neurons. Axons less than 0.5–1.0 μm in diameter share a single Schwann cell and are said to be unmyelinated (Figure 23.3).

At the junction between adjacent Schwann cells there is a gap where the axolemma is exposed, called the node of Ranvier. It will be seen later that nodes of Ranvier facilitate transmission of the action potential. The distance between nodes (150–1500 μm) varies directly with the diameter of the nerve fibre. Where fibres branch, they do so at nodes.

### Generation of the action potential

In its resting state, the interior of the nerve is maintained at a potential of –70 millivolts (mV) with respect to the exterior. The membrane potential is created by the difference in ionic concentrations across the membrane. The sodium concentration is far greater outside the cell, whereas potassium is present in a high concentration within the cell. There are therefore concentration gradients which will cause the passage of these ions across the membrane when it is permeable to the particular ions. These concentration gradients are maintained via the $Na^+/K^+$ ATPase pump. This, as its name implies, consumes energy to pump sodium ions out of, and potassium ions into, the cell against their concentration gradient. As the pump exchanges three sodium ions for two potassium ions, the inside of the cell becomes relatively negative. In its resting state, the membrane is said to be polarized. Nerve tissue is classified as excitable because the

**Table 23.1 Nerve fibre types in mammalian nerve**

| Fibre type | Function | Total fibre diameter (μm)[a] | Conduction velocity (m/s) | Spike duration (ms) | Absolute refractory period (ms) |
|---|---|---|---|---|---|
| Aα | Proprioception; somatic motor | 12–20 | 70–120 | | |
| Aβ | Touch, pressure | 5–12 | 30–70 | 0.4–0.5 | 0.4–1.0 |
| Aγ | Motor to muscle spindles | 3–6 | 15–30 | | |
| Aδ | Pain, temperature, touch | 2–5 | 12–30 | | |
| B | Preganglionic autonomic | <3 | 3–15 | 1.2 | 1.2 |
| C | Pain, reflex responses | 0.4–1.2 | 0.5–2 | 2 | 2 |
| Sympathetic | Postganglionic sympathetics | 0.3–1.3 | 0.7–2.3 | 2 | 2 |

[a]Total fibre diameter includes the axon and its myelin sheath. Types A and B are myelinated; C fibres are unmyelinated.

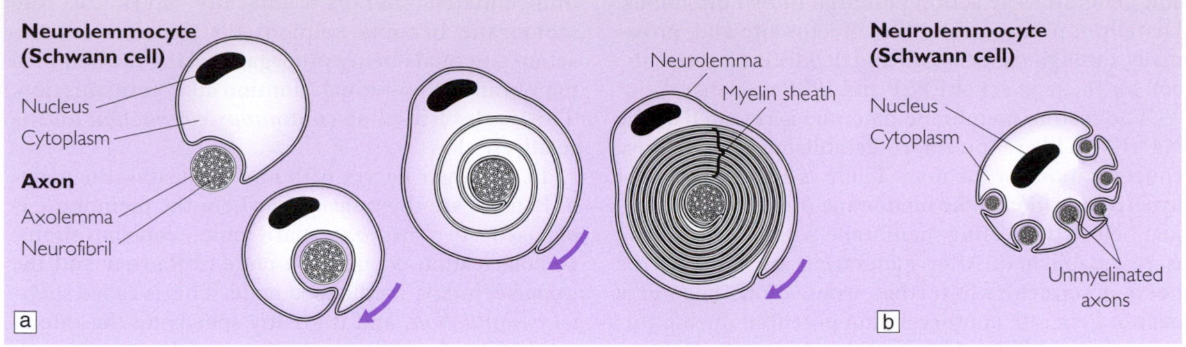


**Figure 23.3** Myelin sheaths. (a) Development of a myelin sheath by a Schwann cell continually wrapping itself around an axon. (b) Axons embedded in a single Schwann cell: these are known as unmyelinated axons.

membrane can have its permeability to sodium and potassium altered in response to chemical stimulation.

Transmission from nerve to nerve or nerve to effector cell involves the passage of a chemical substance across the synaptic cleft between the two. (Details of transmission across the neuromuscular junction can be found in Chapter 24 and are not considered further here.)

Transmitter substances diffuse across the narrow synaptic gap between nerves and combine with receptors on the dendrites or cyton of the postsynaptic nerve. A single stimulus from a single synapse does not usually lead to the propagation of an action potential in the postsynaptic cell. Instead it produces either a transient depolarization or hyperpolarization. This depolarizing response reaches a peak after 1–2 ms and then decays with a time constant of 4 ms. Responses that depolarize are called excitatory postsynaptic potentials (EPSPs); those that hyperpolarize are called inhibitory postsynaptic potentials (IPSPs) (Figure 23.4).

The EPSP is caused by depolarization of the membrane immediately below the synaptic knob on a cell body or dendrite that is receiving multiple signals from many other synaptic knobs. The EPSP lasts only a few milliseconds. The effect of multiple EPSPs from hundreds of synaptic end-bulbs can be combined to initiate a nerve impulse, an effect known as *summation*. When the summation is the result of accumulation of neurotransmitter from several different presynaptic end-bulbs, it is known as *spatial summation*. When it is the result of repetitive firing of a single presynaptic end-bud it is known as *temporal summation*. Both these processes can act simultaneously. Activity at one site is said to *facilitate* activity from others to enable the postsynaptic threshold potential to be reached.

On the other hand, IPSPs work against the effect of EPSPs to decrease the sensitivity of the neuron to other excitatory stimuli. These also summate in time and position. Whether or not a cell body reaches its threshold potential of −50 to −60 mV is therefore the result of the effect of many EPSP and IPSP responses.

Once the threshold has been reached, an action potential is generated and the neuron 'fires', the sodium channels open, and the membrane potential very rapidly rises to +30 mV. At this voltage, potassium channels open and potassium flows out of the cell along its concentration gradient. This is shown in Figure 23.5.

In a motor neuron the portion of the cell with the lowest threshold for the generation of an action potential is the initial segment just beyond the axon hillock (see Figure 23.1). The initial segment is unmyelinated

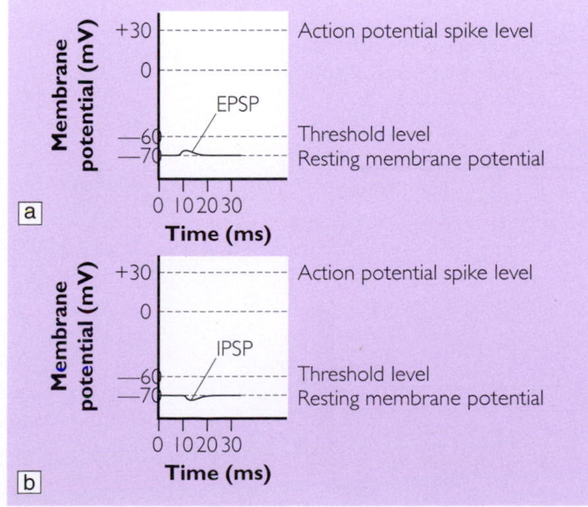


**Figure 23.4** A diagrammatic representation of (a) an excitatory postsynaptic potential (EPSP) and (b) an inhibitory postsynaptic potential (IPSP).

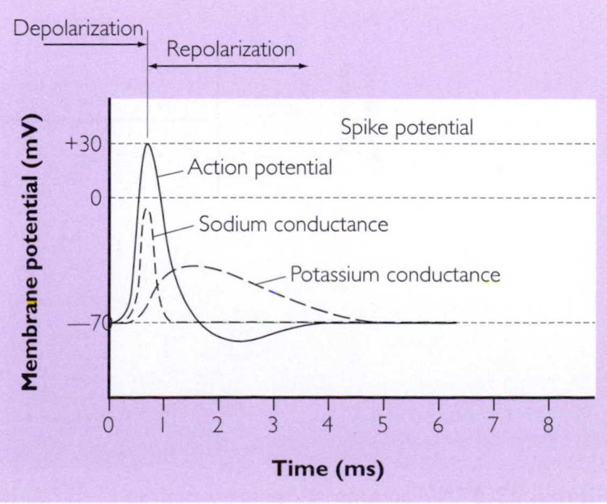


**Figure 23.5** The electrical changes during an action potential and the accompanying ionic movements.

and generates the action potential in two directions. Distally, it propagates to the effector site and, proximally, through the cell body and dendrites, it resets the cell for the next set of EPSP and IPSP responses.

The resting membrane potential is restored as the $Na^+/K^+$ ATPase pump re-establishes the relative concentrations of the ions. There is a short period of hyperpolarization of the membrane (duration 0.4–4 ms) just before the resting membrane potential of −70 mV is re-established. After generating an impulse, the nerve is refractory to further stimulation. The nerve cannot generate another action potential during this refractory period, which is divided into two distinct phases:

1. The absolute refractory period roughly corresponds to the period of sodium permeability changes. During this period, a second potential cannot be generated whatever the stimulus size (see Spike duration, Table 23.1). Larger fibres repolarize faster than smaller fibres.
2. During the relative refractory period a second action potential can be initiated but only by a stronger than normal stimulus. This corresponds to the period of increased potassium permeability.

Under normal circumstances, the frequency of impulses conducted over nerve fibres may range from 10 to 500 impulses per second.

The sodium and potassium ions which leak across the membrane as the action potential is transmitted have to be returned to their original position by the $Na^+/K^+$ ATPase pump. It is, however, not necessary to do so after each nerve impulse because the number of ions actually exchanged with each impulse is very small. The $Na^+/K^+$ pump essentially balances ionic transmission over thousands of nerve impulses. The creation and generation of an action potential are summarized diagrammatically in Figure 23.6.

### Conduction and transmission velocity

Conduction along nerves differs according to the diameter and with the degree of myelination. In small unmyelinated nerves, adjacent areas of the membrane become sequentially depolarized, the action potentials being propagated along the neuronal membrane in a gradual 'domino-like' transmission. This is described as *continuous conduction* and is relatively slow.

In the larger nerves with myelin sheaths, the nodes of Ranvier are the only areas where the membrane is exposed to the external ionic concentrations. Depolarization occurs at a node of Ranvier and the impulse 'jumps' to the next node. This is called *saltatory conduction*, and it greatly speeds up the rate of conduction. In addition, saltatory conduction prevents the depolarization of large areas of the membrane, thus preventing large movements of sodium and potassium ions.

### Transmitters and synaptic transmission

Impulses are conducted across a synapse from one neuron to another by a chemical transmitter (Figure 23.7). At a synapse, there is one-way conduction from a presynaptic axon to a postsynaptic dendrite, cell body,

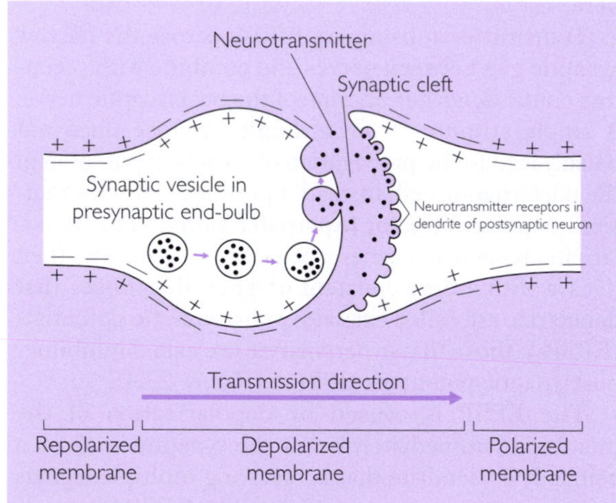


**Figure 23.7** Diagrammatic representation of conduction at a synapse.

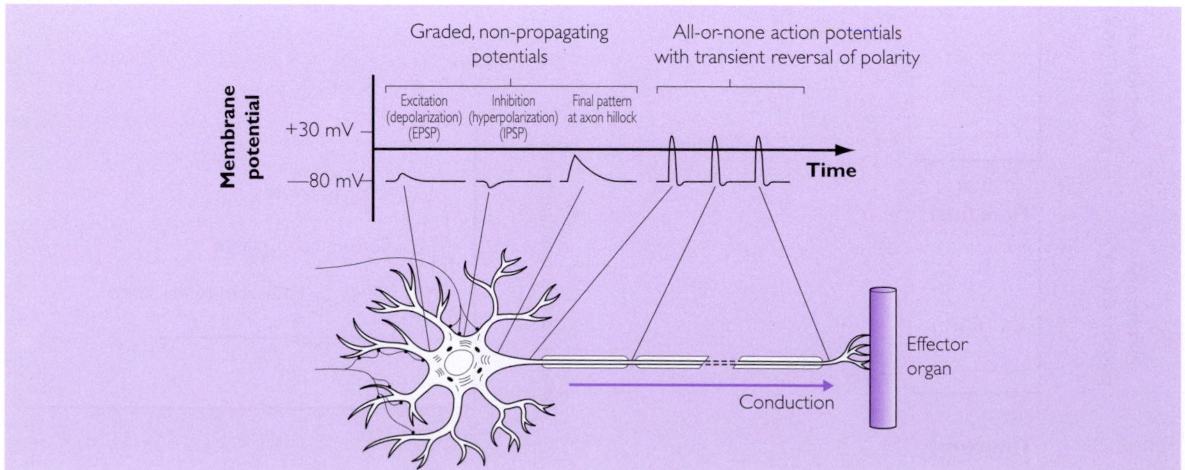


**Figure 23.6** A diagrammatic representation of the various electrical potentials occurring within a motor neuron. EPSP, excitatory postsynaptic potential; IPSP, inhibitory postsynaptic potential. (From Warwick R and Williams PL. *Gray's Anatomy*, 35th edn. London: Longman 1973, 770.)

or axon hillock. The presynaptic end-bulb has thousands of synaptic vesicles, which contain transmitter substance. Whether or not an impulse is transmitted is dependent on neurotransmitter substances being present in the terminal bulb in sufficient amounts. Each of the thousands of synaptic vesicles may contain $10^4$–$10^5$ neurotransmitter molecules and many vesicles are discharged from the presynaptic membrane when a neuron 'fires'.

There are many transmitters identified and postulated in the human nervous system, and these are listed in Chapter 22, Table 22.7. The noradrenergic and cholinergic nerves provide examples of neurotransmitter action. For a substance to be a neurotransmitter it must fulfil the following conditions:

- be synthesized within the neuron;
- be stored in granules which are discharged into the synaptic cleft on arrival of the action potential;
- interact with the postsynaptic membrane usually at specific receptors;
- be rapidly destroyed or removed from the synaptic cleft after its release.

### *Acetylcholine (cholinergic neurons)*

Acetylcholine is synthesized from acetyl-CoA and choline in the nerve in the presence of the enzyme choline acetyltransferase:

$$\text{Choline} + \text{Acetyl-CoA} \xrightarrow[\text{Choline acetyltransferase}]{\uparrow} \text{Acetylcholine} + \text{Reduced coenzyme A}$$

Approximately 50% of the acetylcholine synthesized is transferred to small synaptic vesicles (about 50 nm in diameter), for storage. Of these vesicles, 1% are located at release sites close to the presynaptic membrane and constitute the 'easily available' store of the neurotransmitter. The remainder are distributed throughout the cytoplasm as a reserve store. When released from storage granules, acetylcholine enters the synaptic cleft and binds with acetylcholine receptors on the postsynaptic membrane.

The arrival of the nerve action potential releases 100–200 synaptic vesicles into the synaptic cleft. After binding with the α subunit of the postsynaptic acetylcholine receptor, ion channel opening occurs and lasts for 5–10 ms, resulting in transient permeability to small ions. The acetylcholine receptor is described fully in Chapter 24. Normally, each molecule of acetylcholine activates only one receptor before it diffuses away and/or is broken down.

Only a very small amount of acetylcholine is taken up again by the presynaptic terminal, the majority being broken down by the action of acetylcholinesterase which is present in all cholinergic junctions. It has two binding sites for acetylcholine: one anionic, the other esteratic. The rapid destruction of neurotransmitter is essential in order to prevent repetitive firing of the postsynaptic cell. The reaction is as follows:

$$\text{Acetylcholine} \xrightarrow[\text{Acetylcholinesterase}]{\uparrow} \text{Choline} + \text{Acetate}$$

The choline released is actively taken up into the presynaptic terminal and recycled.

Acetylcholinesterase (true or specific cholinesterase) is probably synthesized locally in the synapse. Miniature end-plate potentials (< 1 mV) are produced by random release of acetylcholine from single vesicles (10 000–12 000 molecules) and are too small to initiate an active impulse.

A less specific cholinesterase (found in plasma, skin, intestine, placenta, and other tissues), butyrylcholinesterase (also known as pseudocholinesterase, plasma cholinesterase), can also metabolize acetylcholine. It has little importance in normal cholinergic transmission, but is relevant in anaesthesia because it breaks down suxamethonium and mivacurium.

The synthesis and breakdown of acetylcholine are shown in Figure 23.8 and the nerve terminal is shown diagrammatically in Figure 23.9a.

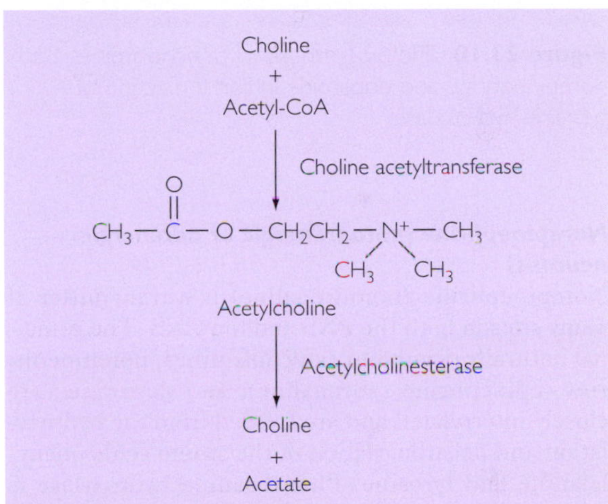


**Figure 23.8** The biosynthesis and catabolism of acetylcholine.

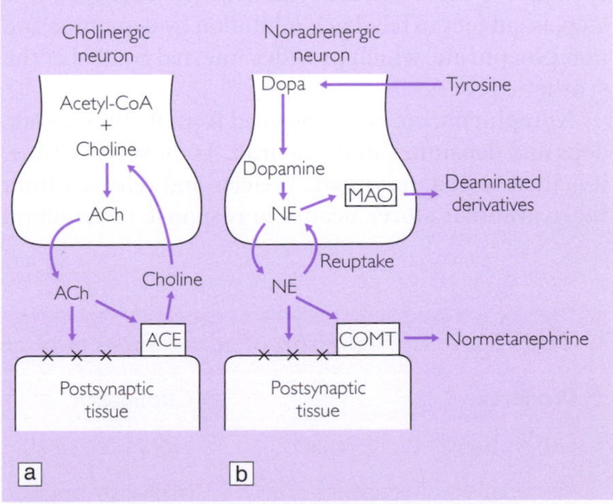


**Figure 23.9** A comparison of the biochemical events occurring at (a) cholinergic endings and (b) noradrenergic endings. ACh, acetylcholine; NE, norepinephrine (noradrenaline); X, postsynaptic receptor. Note that monoamine oxidase (MAO) is intracellular but catechol-*O*-methyltransferase (COMT) and acetylcholinesterase (ACE) are in the synapse.

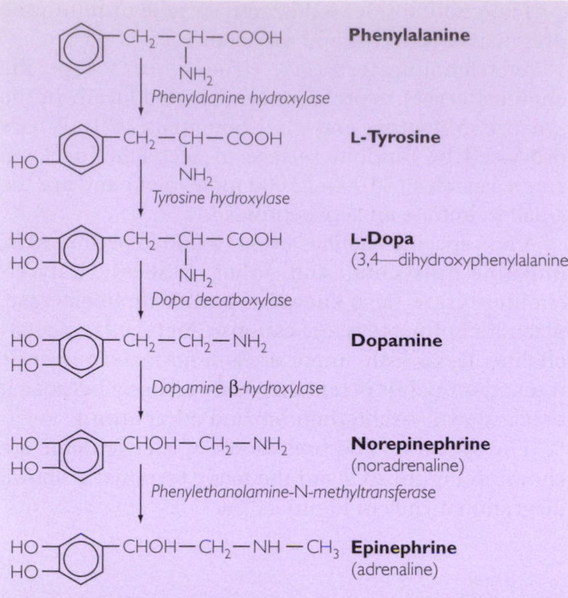


**Figure 23.10** The biosynthesis of catecholamines. Both norepinephrine and dopamine inhibit the action of tyrosine hydroxylase.

### *Norepinephrine (noradrenergic or adrenergic neurons)*

Norepinephrine (noradrenaline) is a transmitter at many sites in both the PNS and the CNS. The principal naturally occurring catecholamines, norepinephrine, epinephrine (adrenaline), and dopamine, are closely interrelated and are formed from the hydroxylation and decarboxylation of the amino acids phenylalanine and tyrosine. Phenylalanine hydroxylase is found predominantly in the liver. Tyrosine is transported into catecholamine-secreting neurons by an active concentrating mechanism. The metabolic pathway for their synthesis is shown in Figure 23.10. The rate-limiting step is the formation of dopamine from tyrosine. Tyrosine hydroxylase, which catalyses this step, is subject to feedback inhibition by dopamine and norepinephrine, which provides internal control of the synthetic process.

Norepinephrine is synthesized from its precursors, dopa and dopamine, in the neuron. As for acetylcholine, it is then stored in synaptic vesicles and released from these granular stores occurs in response to an action potential. It combines on the postsynaptic membrane with adrenoceptors which are classified into different subtypes: α and β (see later). These postsynaptic receptors can also be activated by circulating catecholamines secreted by the adrenal medulla or administered therapeutically. Evidence suggests that autoregulation of norepinephrine release occurs and that it inhibits its own release by adrenoceptors located at presynaptic sites.

The action of norepinephrine is largely terminated by active reuptake into the presynaptic membrane. Any left in the synaptic cleft is destroyed by an enzyme – catechol-*O*-methyl transferase, which metabolizes it to normetanephrine. Any taken up into the presynaptic terminal is either directly recycled or deactivated by monoamine oxidase, which destroys it.

The cycle of synthesis, release, and uptake is summarized diagrammatically in Figure 23.9b. Some aspects of cholinergic and noradrenergic transmission are compared in Table 23.2.

As stated above, there are many other transmitters described acting in both the CNS and the PNS, such as dopamine, serotonin, γ-aminobutyrate, histamine, and several amino acids. These can, in the CNS and dorsal horns, combine in a complex way to modulate synaptic transmission. An example of this from the CNS is shown in Figure 23.11, where serotonin receptors affect noradrenergic transmission. This mechanism is used in the administration of serotonin reuptake inhibitors for the treatment of depression (see Chapter 22).

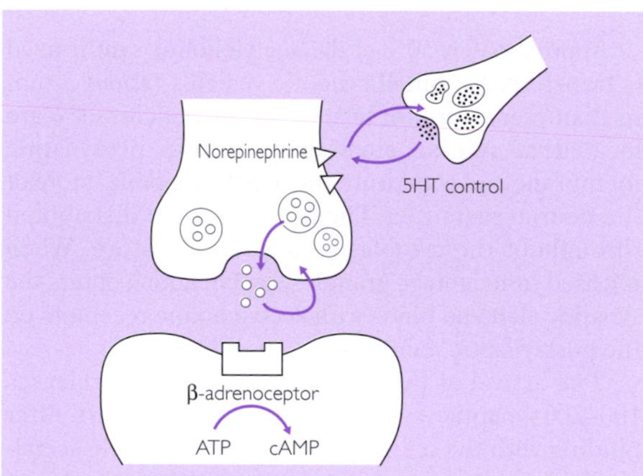


**Figure 23.11** An example of presynaptic control of noradrenergic function by serotonin (5HT).

**Table 23.2 Comparison of some aspects of cholinergic and noradrenergic transmission**

| Property | Cholinergic | Noradrenergic |
|---|---|---|
| Site of transmitter formation | Nerve terminal | Nerve terminal |
| Termination of action | Mainly by breakdown of transmitter | Mainly by uptake of transmitter |
| Postsynaptic receptor activated therapeutically by drugs | Muscarinic or nicotinic agonists<br>Action of acetylcholine increased by anticholinesterases | α and β agonists, direct or indirectly acting |
| Postsynaptic receptor blocked therapeutically by drugs | Yes | Yes |

### Postsynaptic receptors

Postsynaptic receptors for a given transmitter can often be subdivided further by finding some that are, or are not, activated by substances other than the endogenous ligand. Receptor classification using this methodology is summarized in Figure 23.12. Further details are given later, but the general principles are briefly set out here.

#### *Cholinergic receptors*

These are classically regarded as being activated by either nicotine or muscarine. In clinical practice, the anticholinergic agents such as atropine block muscarinic receptors by competitive antagonism.

#### *Adrenergic receptors*

On the basis of investigations by Ahlquist in 1948, these were divided into two main types:

1. α-adrenoceptors which produced vasoconstriction;
2. β-adrenoceptors which vasodilated, relaxed bronchial and intestinal smooth muscle, and increased the force, rate, and conduction velocity of the heart.

These have now been subdivided further as described later.

### Integrated neuronal function

The final output from any neuron is the result of a complex interplay of excitatory and inhibitory neurons. Inhibition can be pre- or postsynaptic. Postsynaptic inhibition is produced as described above by IPSPs. Presynaptic inhibition reduces the amount of synaptic mediator liberated by action potentials arriving at excitatory synaptic knobs. Thus, there is less excitation of the postsynaptic cell. These two arrangements are shown diagrammatically in Figure 23.13.

Presynaptic and postsynaptic inhibition is usually produced by stimulation of neuronal systems converging on to a given postsynaptic neuron. Neurons may also inhibit themselves in a negative feedback fashion. An example of this is the Renshaw cell. This is an inhibitory interneuron activated by a recurrent collateral from a motor neuron which terminates on its original cell and other spinal motor neurons. Impulses generated in the motor neuron activate the inhibitory interneuron to liberate inhibitory mediator, and this slows or stops the discharge of the original and accompanying motor neurons. The arrangement is shown in Figure 23.14.

Groups of neurons are organized into neuronal pools (Figure 23.15). These are broadly classified into *discharge zones*, which result in action potentials being

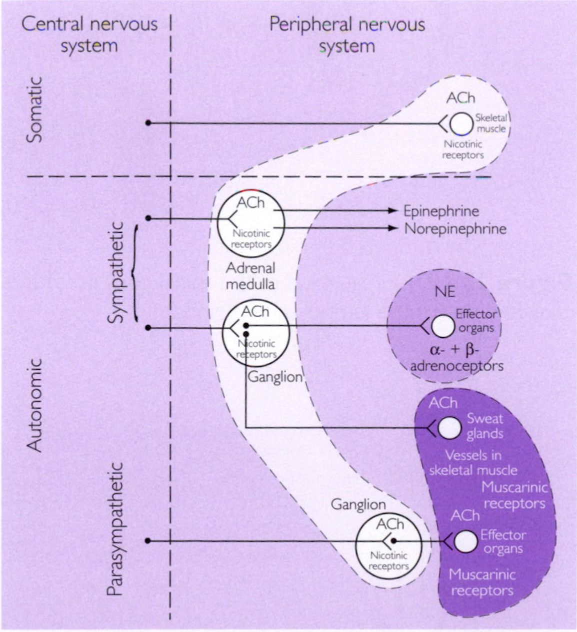

**Figure 23.12** A diagrammatic representation of transmitters in the parasympathetic nervous system. ACh, acetylcholine; NE, norepinephrine. Note the long preganglionic neurons in the parasympathetic system and the short preganglionic neurons in the sympathetic system. Note the distribution of nicotinic and muscarinic receptors and α- and β-adrenoceptors.

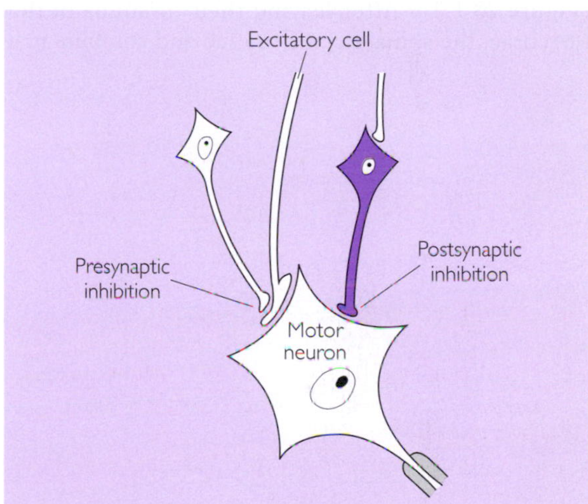


**Figure 23.13** Pre- and postsynaptic inhibition. The neuron producing presynaptic inhibition is shown ending on an excitatory synaptic knob. Many of these neurons actually end further up along the axis of the excitatory cell.

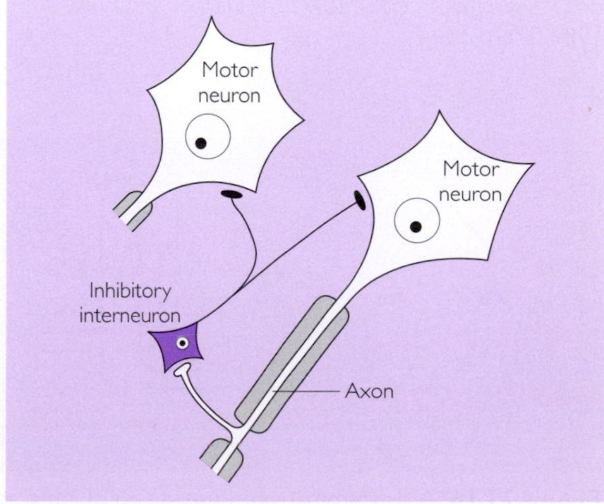


**Figure 23.14** Self-inhibition of a spinal motor neuron via an inhibitory interneuron (Renshaw cell).

propagated, and *facilitation zones* where the postsynaptic neuron will fire if supporting stimuli are received from other neurons.

Neurons are also defined as having diverging and converging behaviour. Divergence is the property of a neuron to influence several other postsynaptic pathways. Convergence is the ability of a number of terminal buttons from one neuron or from several neurons to work synergistically to trigger the postsynaptic cell membrane (Figure 23.16).

## SOMATIC SENSORY AND MOTOR SYSTEMS

Sensory (dorsal) and motor (ventral) nerve roots arise in the cervical and thoracic regions as shown in Figure 23.17a. The dorsal and ventral roots fuse to form a spinal nerve. In the lumbar and sacral regions, the roots leave the cord at a more acute angle and pass downwards beyond the end of the cord, before they leave the spinal canal. In doing so they form the cauda equina (Figure 23.17b). After leaving their foramina in the vertebrae, the spinal nerves branch and combine in a number of ways to reach all parts of the body. Their distribution follows predictable patterns (e.g. formation of intercostal nerves, cervical, brachial, and sacral plexus, etc. – see Chapter 15), in named peripheral nerves, most of which carry both sensory and motor fibres.

### Sensory systems

Sensory neurons have their cell bodies in the dorsal root ganglia (Figure 23.17 and see Figure 23.2). From the cell body, a dendrite projects along a spinal nerve to the area of the body where sensations are to be detected. Irrespective of the path through plexus and peripheral nerve formation, the sensory fibres from each spinal nerve are in a dermatomal distribution as shown in Figure 23.18. There is some overlap between dermatomes such that it may, for instance, be necessary to block three intercostal nerves to produce a band of anaesthesia the width of a single dermatome.

At its periphery, the nerve endings of the dendrite are often surrounded by non-neuronal cells to form a sense organ. These sense organs transduce mechanical, thermal, light, and chemical energy into electrical

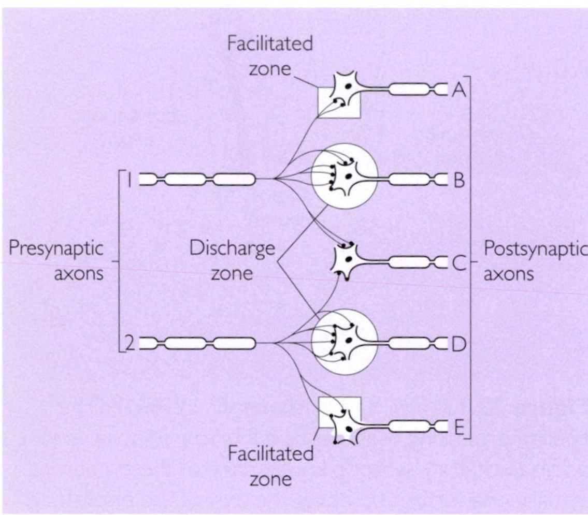


**Figure 23.15** Neurons grouped into pools with discharge zones and facilitation zones. (Adapted from Tortora GJ and Anagnostrakos NP. *Principles of Anatomy and Physiology*, 5th edn. New York: Harper and Row, 1987, 276.)

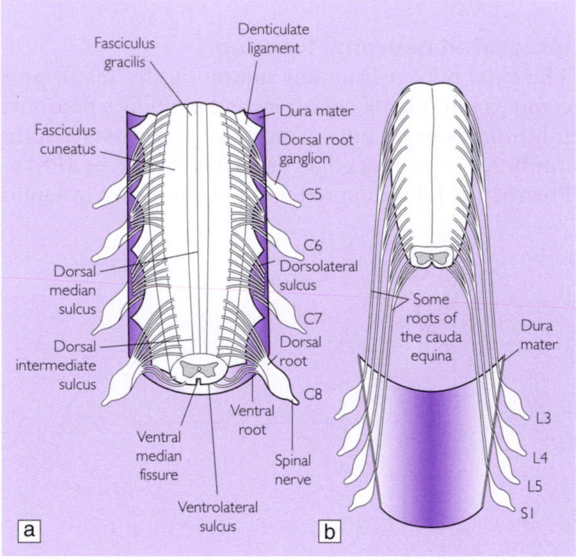


**Figure 23.17** Dorsal views of the spinal cord in (a) the cervical and (b) the lumbosacral regions.

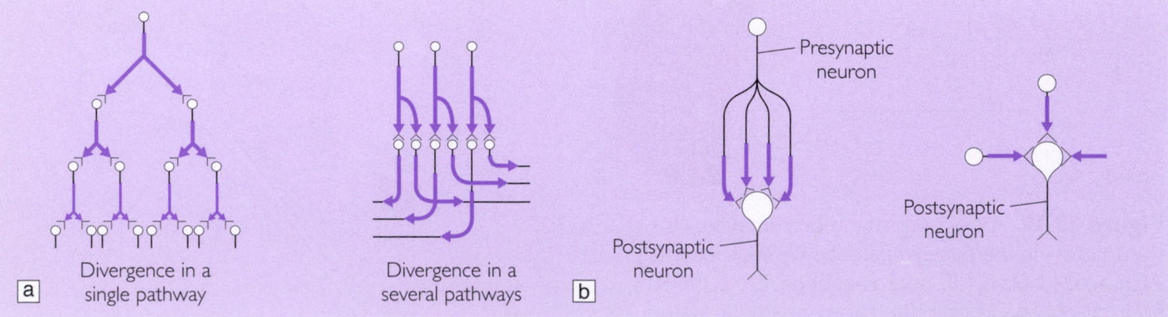


**Figure 23.16** A diagrammatic representation of integrated neuronal function showing (a) divergence and (b) convergence. (Adapted from Tortora GJ and Anagnostrakos NP. *Principles of Anatomy and Physiology*, 5th edn. New York: Harper and Row, 1987, 277.)

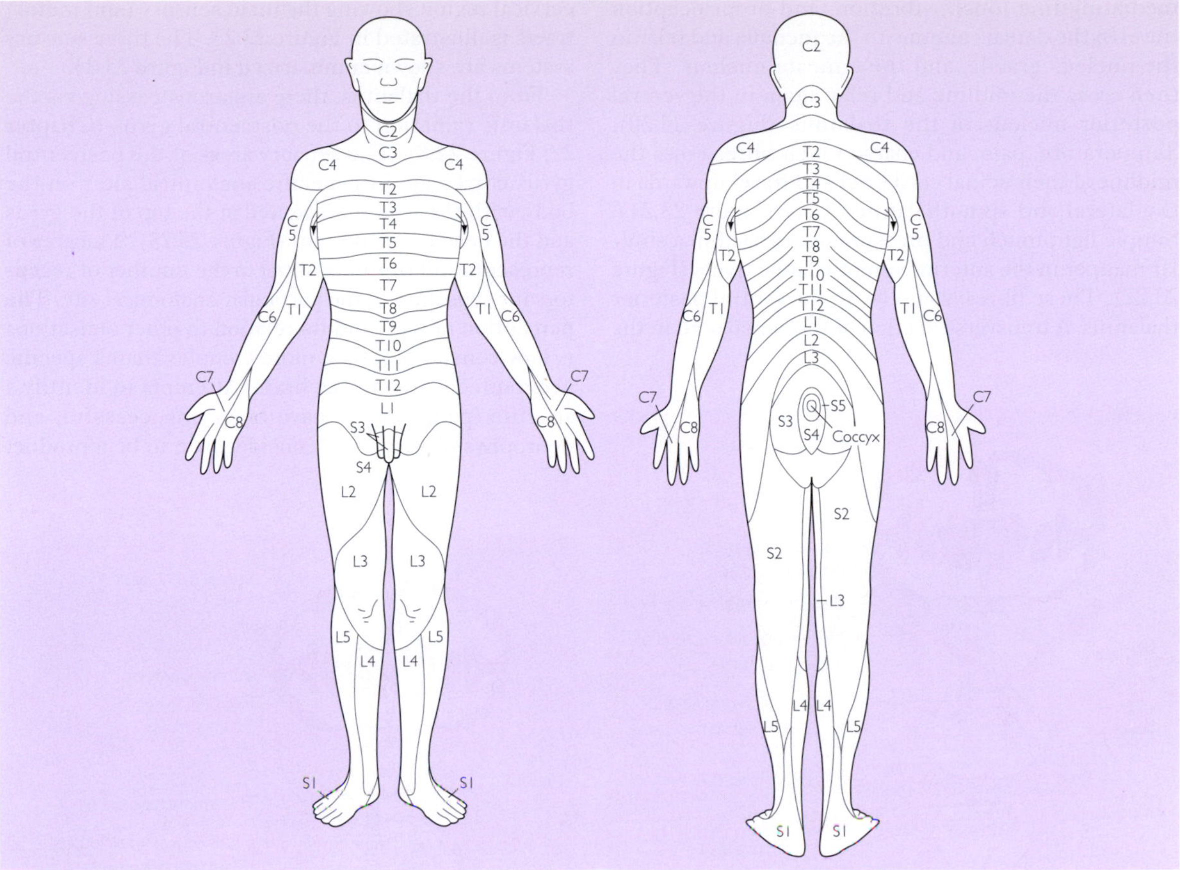

**Figure 23.18** The cutaneous projection (dermatomes) of the sensory spinal nerves.

energy in the form of the action potential in the nerve. In general, the receptors at sensory nerve endings are adapted to have a lower threshold for one form of stimulus, although they will respond to other forms of stimulus at a very much higher threshold. This principle applies to all sense organs, including the eye, the ear, the taste buds, and the sense of smell.

Cutaneous and deep visceral sensation is largely made up of touch (pressure), temperature, and pain. There is clearly an overlap in the perception of information from these receptors, because pressure and thermal stimuli can both be painful. The generation of an action potential in a peripheral nerve is dependent on the summation of smaller generator currents produced at the receptor/nerve complex in the sense organ. Small generator currents of relatively long duration are generated in response to the stimuli; it is the number of these currents that will fire the action potential and which sets the threshold of the nerve.

The cell body also gives out an axon, which passes centrally and ends in a synapse with other cells in the dorsal horn of the spinal cord (see Figure 23.2). The sensory impulse is transmitted from the periphery, along the dendrite, across the cell body, and down the axon into the dorsal horn of the spinal cord. The dorsal horn is an extremely complex neuronal network with many interneurons and axonal connections, both at the dermatomal level of the sensory nerve and at layers above and below. The dorsal horn has been divided, by anatomists, into a number of laminae – the laminae of Rexed (Figure 23.19). Afferent neurons which subserve different sensory

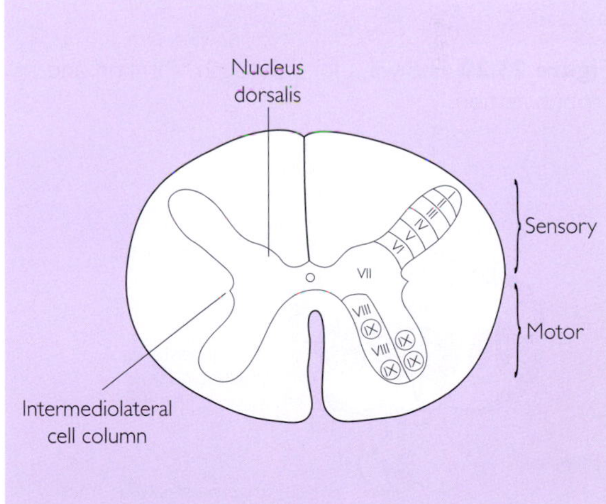


**Figure 23.19** Rexed's laminae of the spinal cord grey matter.

modalities end in different laminae of the dorsal horn. Mechanoreceptors, which transduce touch and pressure, have axons of relatively large size (Aβ fibres) and relay in laminae III, IV, V, and VI. Pain sensation is carried in fast Aδ fibres which relay in laminae I and V, and slower C fibres which relay in laminae I and II.

Cell bodies in the dorsal horn project axons to the higher centres, with further synapses in the thalamus and specialized nuclei in the brain stem. The fibres mediating fine touch, vibration, and proprioception travel in the dorsal columns to the medulla and relay in the nucleus gracilis and the cuneate nucleus. They then cross the midline and relay again in the ventral posterior nucleus of the thalamus (Figure 23.20). Temperature, pain, and coarse touch fibres cross the midline at their spinal cord level and travel upwards in the lateral and spinothalamic tracts (Figure 23.21). Simple light touch and pressure are carried in a similar manner in the anterior spinothalamic tracts (Figure 23.22). These fibres also relay in the ventral posterior thalamus. A transverse section of the spinal cord in the cervical region showing the main sensory (and motor) tracts is illustrated in Figure 23.23. The three sensory systems are shown summarized in Figure 23.24.

From the thalamus, there are axons passing via the thalamic radiation to the postcentral gyrus (Chapter 22, Figure 22.8). The sensory areas of the postcentral gyrus correspond to specific anatomical sites on the body, with the legs represented at the top of the gyrus and the head at the bottom (Figure 23.25). The area of representation is proportional to the number of receptors for sensation in the particular anatomical site. The perception of pain and its relation to other sensations is now considered to be more complex than a specific geographical area in the brain. Attempts to identify a specific 'pain centre' have been unsuccessful, and neurophysiologists now consider pain to be a product

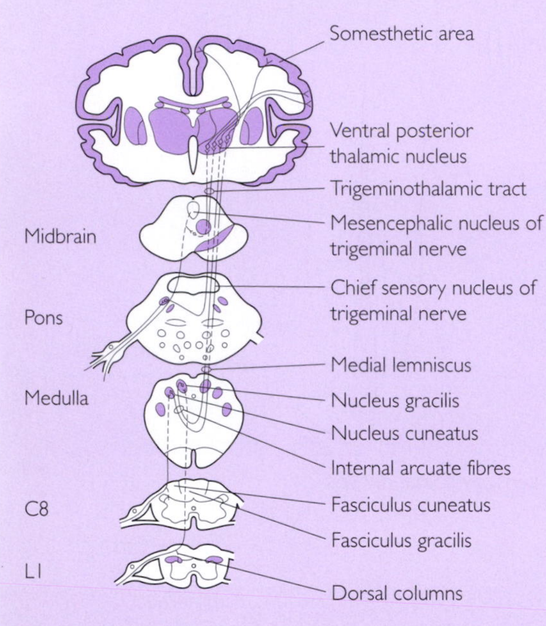


**Figure 23.20** Pathways for fine touch, vibration, and proprioception.

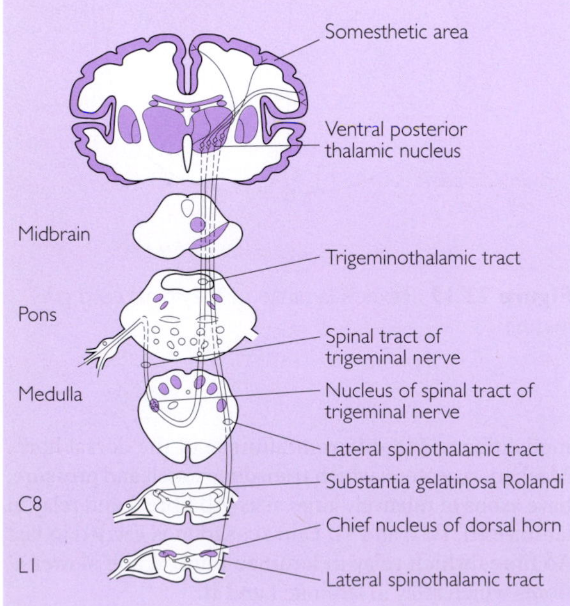


**Figure 23.21** Pathways for pain, temperature, and coarse touch.

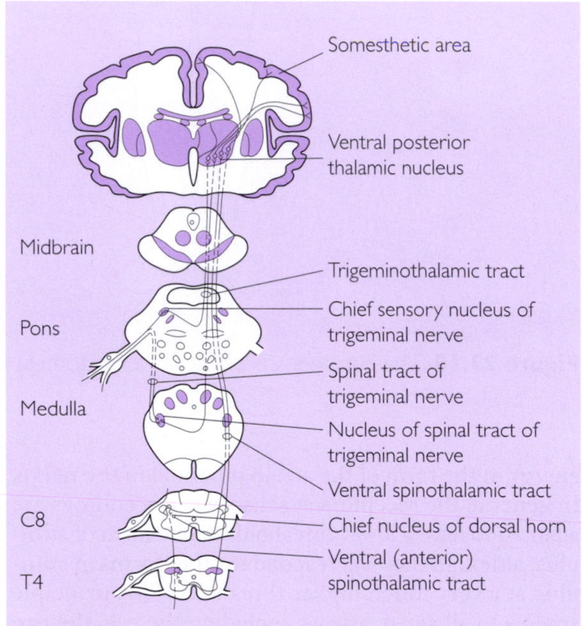


**Figure 23.22** Pathways for simple light touch and pressure.

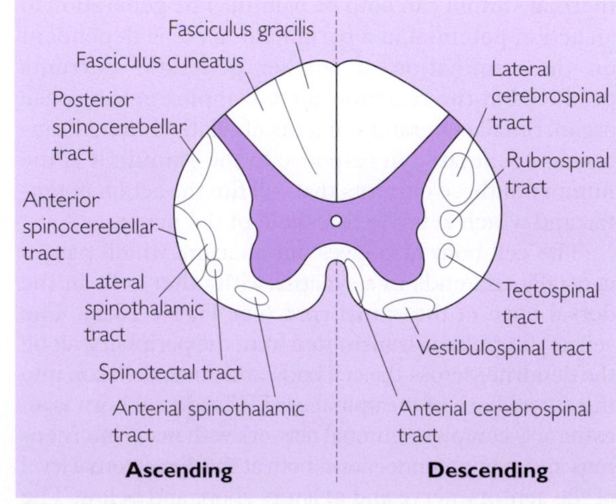


**Figure 23.23** The main ascending (sensory) and descending (motor) tracts on a cross-section of the spinal column.

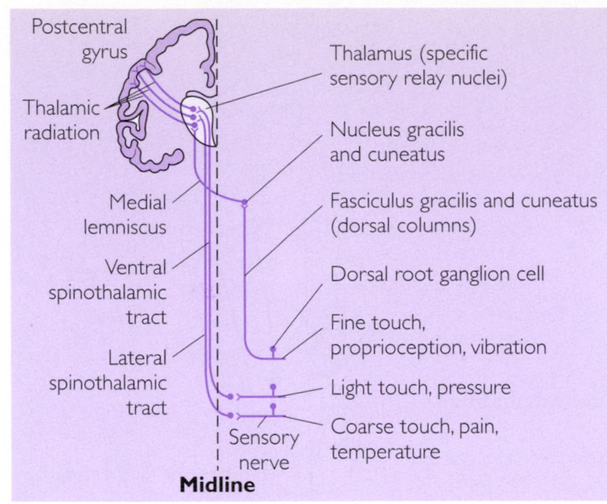


**Figure 23.24** A diagrammatic summary of the three main sensory systems.

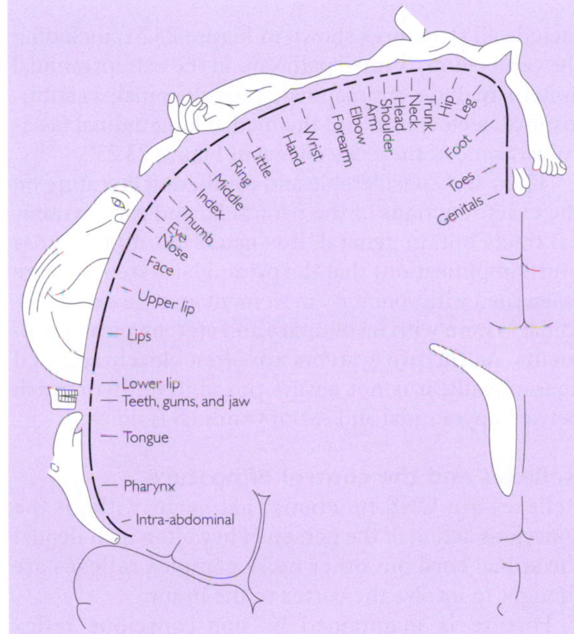


**Figure 23.25** Sensory homunculus, drawn overlying a coronal section through the postcentral gyrus. The area of cortex represents the sensitivity of that part of the body.

of multiple neuronal associations, which are dynamic in time and space.

## Motor systems

The motor cortex is on the precentral gyrus (Chapter 22, Figure 22.8) and has an analogous representation of the body to the sensory system as shown in Figure 23.26. Motor commands from the brain travel downwards from the motor cortex, and are integrated and refined in the basal ganglia and by inputs from the lateral cerebellar hemispheres. The basal ganglia comprise the caudate nucleus, the putamen, and the globus pallidus. They are related to the thalamus, as shown in Figure 23.27. There are also direct connections from the cortex to the brain stem, shown diagrammatically in Figure 23.28. In general, in the descending pathways, fibres situated ventrally in the tracts control proximal muscles, whereas fibres descending laterally control distal limb muscles.

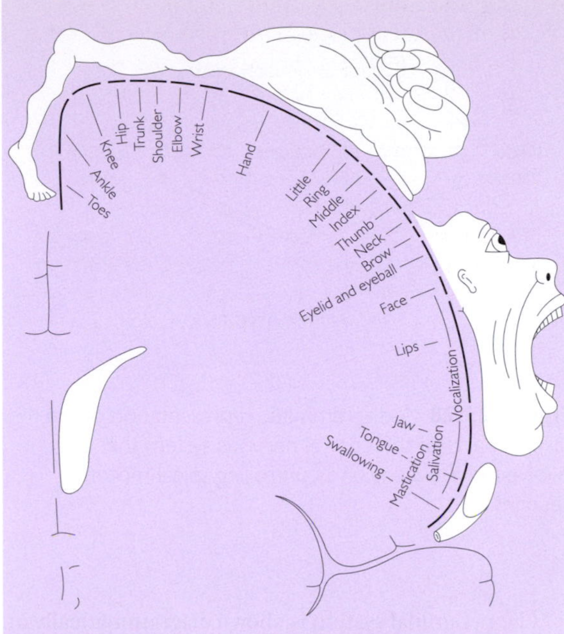


**Figure 23.26** Motor homunculus. The figure represents, on a coronal section of the precentral gyrus, the localization of the cortical representation of the various parts of the body. The area of representation is proportional to the skill and control required in the various muscles.

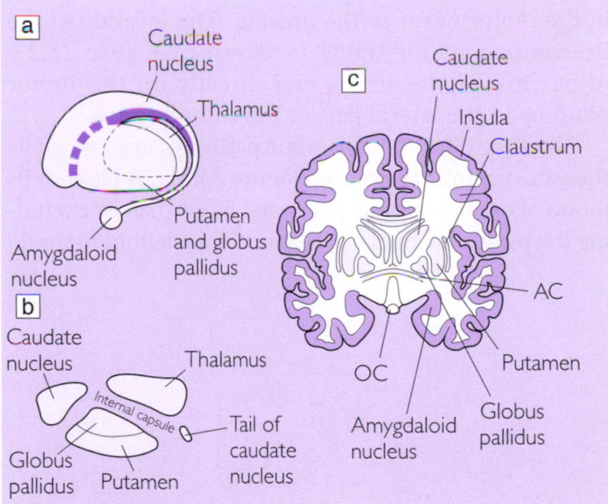


**Figure 23.27** A diagrammatic representation of the basal ganglia: (a) lateral view; (b) horizontal section; (c) frontal section. AC, anterior commissure; OC, optic chiasm. (Not to scale.)

The descending motor pathways are grossly divided into *pyramidal* and *extrapyramidal* systems. The pyramidal system consists of the following:

- the corticospinal tracts which form the pyramids of the medulla;
- the corticobulbar tracts which travel together with the fibres of the corticospinal tract, but which synapse in the brain stem and pons.

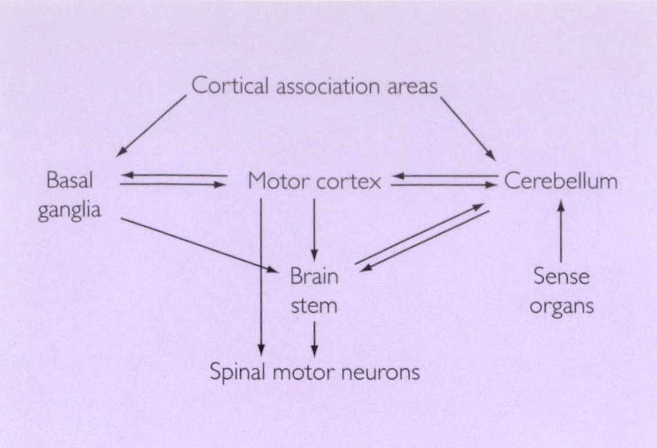


**Figure 23.28** A diagrammatic representation of the various parts of the central nervous system that are involved in activating and controlling spinal motor neurons.

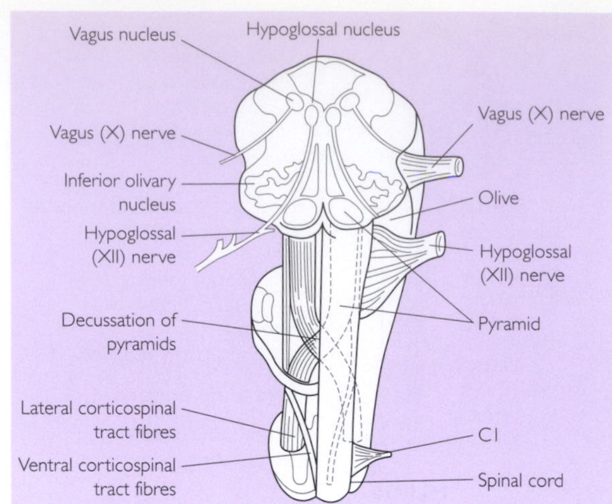


**Figure 23.30** Details of the medulla oblongata showing the decussation of the pyramids.

The pyramidal system is shown diagrammatically in Figure 23.29, and the decussation of the pyramids in more detail in Figure 23.30. About 80% of the motor fibres cross the midline in the medulla to form the lateral corticospinal tract; the other 20% do not, forming the anterior (ventral) corticospinal tract. Fibres travelling downwards in the ventral tracts end on interneurons, which synapse on anterior horn cells in the medial part of the anterior horn of the spinal cord. The anterior horn cell gives off an axon, which travels in the motor nerve to the muscle. The location of the descending motor tracts is shown in Figure 23.23. About 5% of the fibres end directly on the motor neurons in the lateral part of the anterior horn.

All other descending motor pathways are known as the extrapyramidal system (Figure 23.31). A clear definition of extrapyramidal pathways, other than by excluding the pyramidal tracts, is lacking. This definition would include all structures shown in Figure 23.31, including the cerebellum. Named pathways in the extrapyramidal system include rubrospinal, reticulospinal, vestibulospinal, tectospinal, and the medial longitudinal fasciculus. Some of these are shown in Figure 23.23.

There is a considerable and conflicting literature on the exact functions of the pyramidal and extrapyramidal tracts but, in general, it is usually said (as a gross over-simplification) that the pyramidal system is more concerned with voluntary movement and the extrapyramidal system with involuntary and stereotypical movements. As the two systems are often closely apposed anatomically, it is not always possible to distinguish between pyramidal and extrapyramidal lesions.

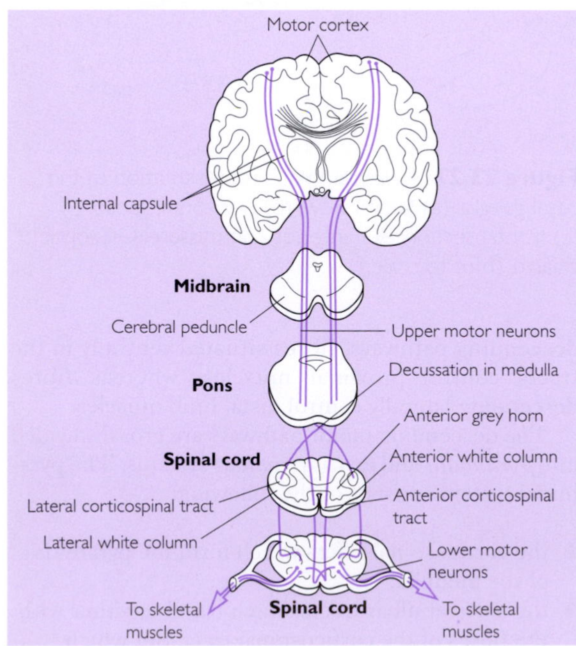


**Figure 23.29** The pyramidal system.

### Reflexes and the control of posture

Reflexes are CNS functions that occur without the conscious action of the person. They often include just the spinal cord but other more complex reflexes are thought to involve the cortex of the brain.

Posture is maintained by non-conscious reflex actions which keep the individual upright and provide constant adjustment for balance. Overriding this system, voluntary actions can adjust posture.

A *reflex arc* consists of a sense organ, an afferent neuron, a central integration point, an efferent neuron, and an effector organ, as shown diagrammatically in Figure 23.32. As we have already seen, the afferent, sensory limb enters through the dorsal horn of the cord and the efferent motor limb leaves via the anterior horn. The integration point, within the CNS, can be in the spinal cord or the brain. Reflex arcs can be monosynaptic or polysynaptic. Clearly a polysynaptic reflex arc has multiple opportunities for modification.

The *stretch reflex* constitutes a monosynaptic reflex and clearly influences the control of posture. This is the only known monosynaptic reflex in the human and is the basis of the knee-jerk reflex, shown in Figure 23.33. The following is the sequence of events in this reflex:

- Stretching of the muscle is sensed in the muscle spindle.

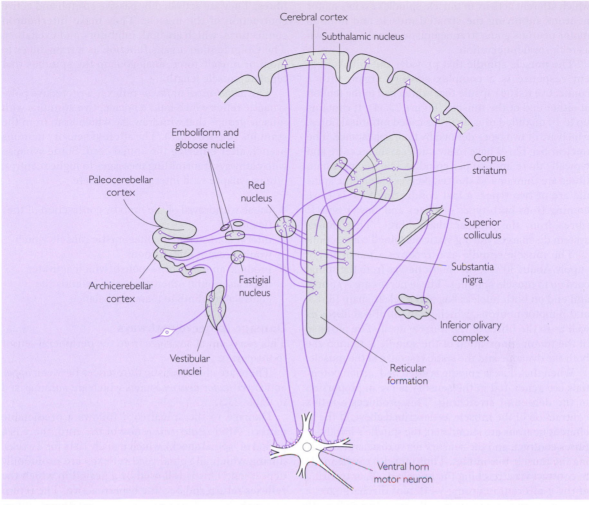

**Figure 23.31** Components of the extrapyramidal system shown projecting to lower motor neurons. (From Barr ML. *The Human Nervous System*. New York: Harper and Row, 1972, 324.)

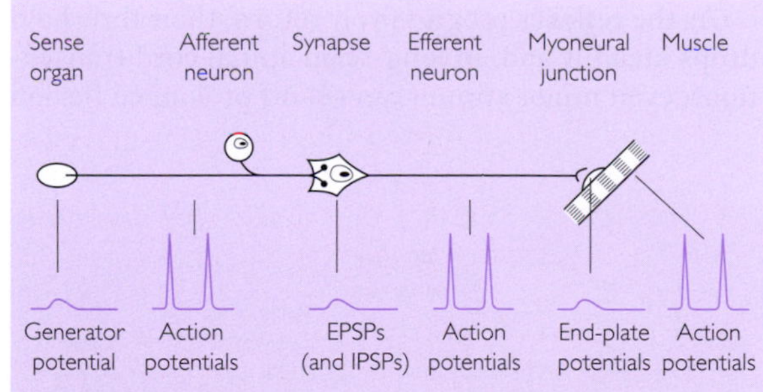


**Figure 23.32** A diagrammatic representation of the simplest form of reflex arc. (From Ganong WF. *Review of Medical Physiology*, 10th edn. Los Altos: Lange Medical, 1981, 88.)

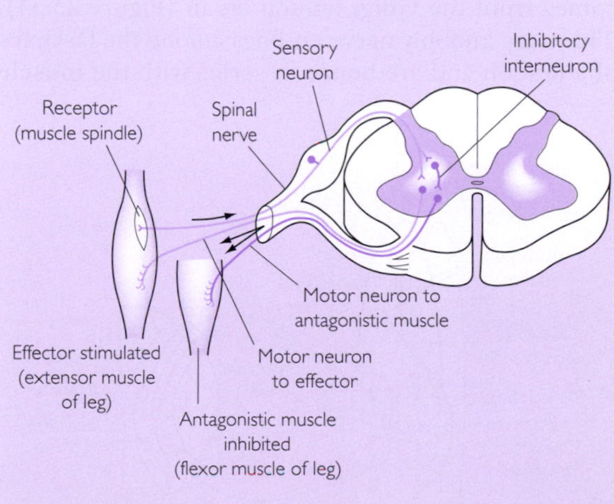


**Figure 23.33** The stretch reflex. Note that the stretch reflex is monosynaptic because there is only one synapse joining the sensory neuron to the motor neuron in the effector muscle. There is an interneuron connecting to the motor neuron to the antagonistic muscle, which is inhibitory.

- The afferent neuron from the spindle passes into the spinal cord through the dorsal root.
- The afferent neuron synapses in the anterior horn with the motor neuron to that muscle fibre. The transmitter at the synapse is glutamate.
- The motor neuron stimulates the muscle to contract.

At the same time as activating the motor neuron to the stretched muscle, the afferents, via inhibitory interneurons, inhibit the antagonistic muscles by the secretion of inhibitory transmitters. This process, by which afferent activity in muscle spindles excites motor neurons supplying the striated muscle and inhibits motor neurons going to antagonistic muscles, is known as reciprocal innervation.

The muscle spindle that provides the initial afferent response is a complex sensory organ, with a connective tissue capsule that is attached to the tendon at either end of the muscle (Figure 23.34). It contains up to 10 modified muscle fibres called intrafusal fibres, which are of two types defined by their appearance. The nuclear bag fibres have many nuclei at their centre and typically there are two per spindle. The nuclear chain fibres are thinner and shorter. Nerves leaving the spindle are of two types: a fast conducting type Ia fibre coming from both types of fibres and slower type II fibres from the nuclear chain fibres. This slower system discharges during static sustained contraction.

The muscle spindle also receives a motor nerve supply. About 30% of the motor nerves from the spinal cord go to muscle spindles. These nerves are Aγ fibres and end on both nuclear bag and nuclear chain fibres, and β motor neurons, which go to intrafusal fibres as well as to the fibres of the muscle itself. The purpose of the motor innervation of the spindle is to increase both the dynamic and the static response of the muscle.

When the muscle spindle is stretched, action potentials are generated in the sensory nerve in proportion to the degree of stretching. This produces a reflex contraction of the muscle as described above. If the γ-efferent neurons are stimulated, the spindle's intrafusal fibres contract, and the sensory nerve discharges causing the muscle to contract. Thus muscles can be made to contract via stretching the muscle itself, or by firing of the γ-efferent neurons; γ-efferent discharge has a role in setting the sensitivity of the muscle spindles. All these reflexes are integrated at a spinal level under the control of descending motor pathways.

In addition to the muscle spindles, an important component of the postural reflex monitoring system comes from the Golgi tendon organ (Figure 23.34). These are knobbly nerve endings among the fascicles of a tendon and are hence in series with the muscle fibres. They are activated by passive stretch and active contraction of the muscle. They make interneuron connections, which are both inhibitory and excitatory. The Golgi tendon organs function as a transducer to monitor muscle force, analogous to the spindles that regulate muscle length.

The *withdrawal* or *flexor* reflex is a protective polysynaptic reflex which links a nociceptive stimulus with muscle groups that withdraw the whole limb from the stimulus (Figure 23.35). The afferent sensory neurons branch after entering the spinal cord. Some synapse with pathways transmitting messages to higher centres, others synapse with interneurons which:

- cause withdrawal of the limb by contraction of the flexors;
- inhibit contraction of antagonistic muscle which would prevent limb flexion;
- produce an extensor response, which activates muscles around other joints and extends the contralateral limb to maintain balance.

### Damage to nerve pathways

This can occur at any stage from the peripheral sensor to the cortex.

There are characteristic differences between *upper* and *lower motor neuron lesions* which are summarized in Table 23.3.

Damage to the spinal cord follows a predictable pattern. After *acute transection* of the cord, there is a period of 'spinal shock', which usually lasts for 2 weeks, during which all spinal cord reflexes are profoundly depressed. This is followed by a period in which the reflexes return and become hyperreactive. The return of the hyperreactive reflexes may be the result of changes in the now denervated muscles, combined with sprouting of collateral neurons in the reflex pathway. The first reflexes to be seen are usually leg withdrawal reflexes.

As the reflexes progressively return, their threshold drops steadily and, in long-term spinal cord transections, even minor stimuli can set off prolonged flexion

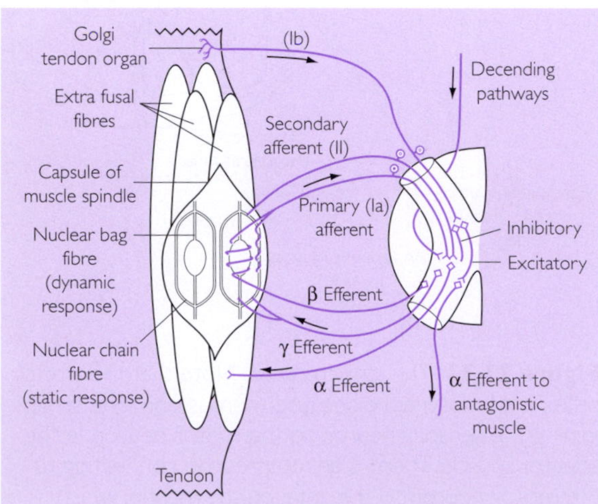


**Figure 23.34** A muscle spindle illustrating the two types of intrafusal fibres (nuclear bag fibres and nuclear chain fibres) and the associated reflex arcs. (See text for details.)

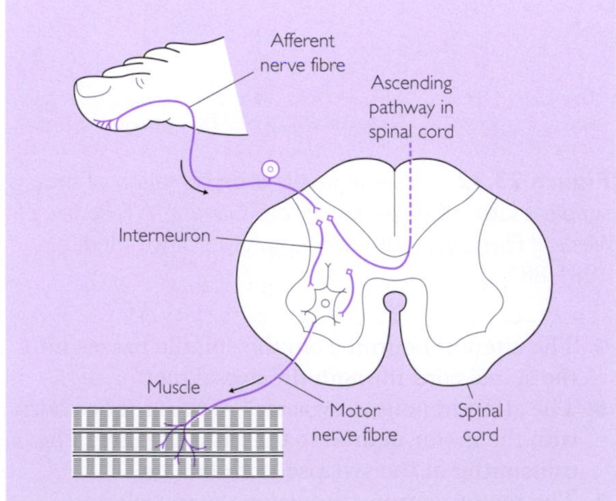


**Figure 23.35** The withdrawal or flexor reflex. This is a polysynaptic reflex, which has a complex response relying on inputs and modulation from other levels of the spinal cord.

| Table 23.3 Characteristics of lower and upper motor neuron lesions | | |
|---|---|---|
| **Clinical feature** | **Lower motor neuron lesion** | **Upper motor neuron lesion** |
| Muscle bulk | Reduced | Normal |
| Fasciculation | Usually present | Absent |
| Tremor | Absent | Absent |
| Tone | Reduced | Increased (spastic) |
| Power | Reduced | Usually reduced |
| Coordination | Impaired with severe weakness | Sometimes impaired |
| Reflexes | Reduced or absent | Increased |
| Plantar reflexes | Flexor | Extensor |
| Gait | Stepping | Spastic or hemiplegic |

reflexes in all limbs. This can be accompanied by bursts of pain sensation. Reflex contractions of the full bladder and rectum are usually maintained after spinal cord transection, although the bladder does not usually empty fully. There is an irradiation of stimuli from one reflex centre to another, and in chronic spinal transection a mass reflex can be initiated by minor stimuli. In a mass reflex, voiding of the bladder and rectum, sweating, blood pressure swings, and pallor can all occur. A modified mass reflex is used by some paraplegic patients to restore some bladder and bowel control.

Transection of tracts of the spinal cord and medulla above the pons leads to a spastic rigidity as a result of diffuse facilitation of spinal cord reflexes and increased γ-efferent discharge. This is called *decerebrate rigidity* because the influence of the cerebrum (the forebrain, see Chapter 22, Table 22.2) is absent. Muscle tonus is modulated by inputs from the motor cortex, basal ganglia, cerebellum, the reticular-activating system, and the vestibular system. When these are lost, the balance shifts to facilitation rather than inhibition, especially of the extensor muscles.

Decerebrate rigidity is usually incompatible with recovery and the damage to the cord that produces it often progresses to brain-stem death. When fully developed, there is internal rotation and hyperextension of all limbs, with hyperextension of the neck and spine, and absent righting reflexes. Similar posturing, which is shown in Figure 23.36, may be seen clinically as part of the coning process.

*Decorticate rigidity* occurs with lesions of the cortex that leave the basal ganglia and brain stem intact. Decorticate rigidity occurs because the area of cortex that inhibits the γ-efferent discharge via the reticular-activating system is lost. In this instance, lower limb extension, internal rotation, and plantar flexion are combined with moderate upper limb flexion (Figure 23.36). Passive rotation of the head to one side causes extension of the ipsilateral arm, with full flexion of the contralateral arm, due to intact tonic neck reflexes. Also, the contralateral leg may flex. This type of rigidity is seen in the hemiplegic side of a person who has had a cerebrovascular accident (CVA) involving the internal capsule, the site of 60% of CVAs.

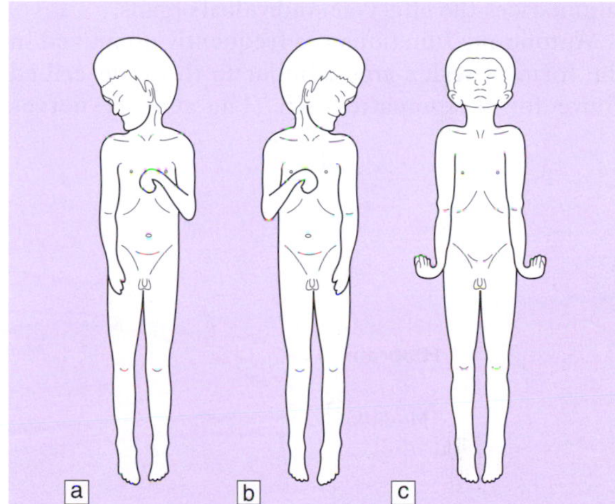


**Figure 23.36** Decorticate and decerebrate rigidity. (a, b) The tonic neck reflex patterns produced by turning of the head to the right or left in decorticate rigidity. (c) True decerebrate rigidity with extensor spasms in all limbs. (Adapted from Ganong WF. *Review of Medical Physiology*, 10th edn. Los Altos: Lange Medical, 1981, 161.)

## THE AUTONOMIC NERVOUS SYSTEM (ANS)

### Comparison with the somatic PNS

The unconscious, involuntary control of body functions is achieved through the efferent nerves of the ANS (see Chapter 22, Figure 22.1). There is integration with the motor and sensory systems. Higher centres can influence control and some individuals have trained themselves to alter autonomically mediated function such as heart rate. The somatic efferent and autonomic systems are compared in Table 23.4.

### Structure of the ANS

The system is divided into two parts: sympathetic and parasympathetic. The actions of the two parts are

**Table 23.4 Comparison of somatic efferent and autonomic nervous systems**

| Component | Somatic efferent | Autonomic |
|---|---|---|
| Effector organs | Skeletal muscles | Ganglia, glands, and cardiac and smooth muscle |
| Type of control | Usually voluntary, occasionally reflex | Totally involuntary, many reflexes |
| Nerve connections | One neuron extends from spinal cord to skeletal muscle | Efferent neuron from spinal cord goes to ganglion Effector organ activated by postganglionic neuron |
| Mode of action | Always excitatory | Excitatory or inhibitory depending on whether parasympathetic or sympathetic |
| Neurotransmitters | Acetylcholine | Acetylcholine or norepinephrine |

antagonistic but complementary. Many organs receive innervation from both systems.

The efferent autonomic pathways are shown in diagrammatic form in Figure 23.37, and Table 23.5 summarizes the effects on individual organs.

Autonomic functions are frequently organized in the form of reflex arcs, similar to those described above for the somatic PNS. The sensory nerves usually travel towards the spinal cord with the autonomic efferent nerves. Nuclei or centres in the brain stem and spinal cord integrate the incoming information and send efferent fibres out to supply the organs involved. The autonomic outflow is often described in detail, but it should be remembered that this is only the efferent limb of these complex reflexes.

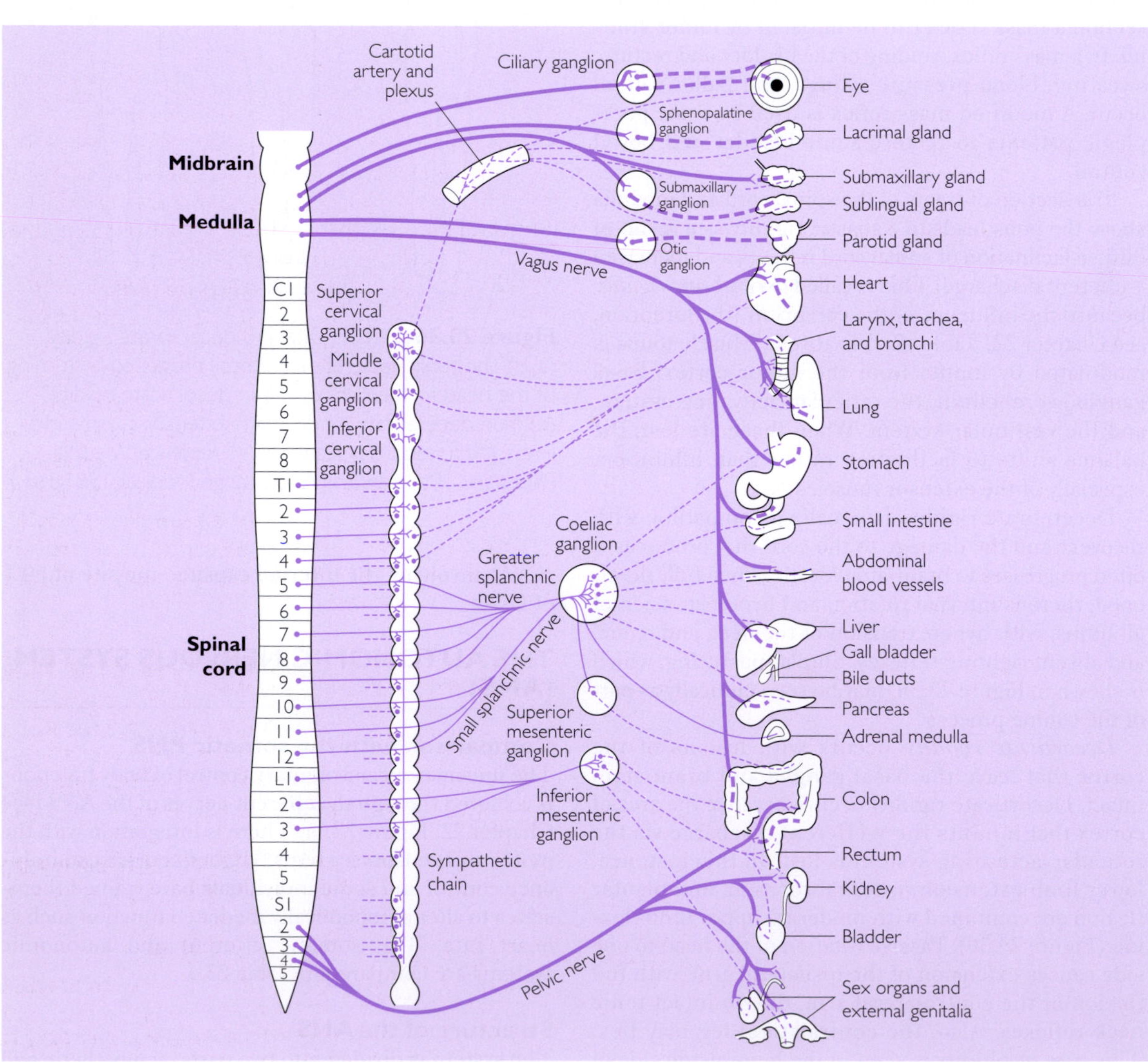


**Figure 23.37** Diagrammatic representation of sympathetic (—) and parasympathetic (**—**) pathways.

| Table 23.5 Summary of sympathetic and parasympathetic effects on various organs | | |
|---|---|---|
| **Sympathetic effect** | **Organ** | **Parasympathetic effect** |
| Dilate pupil<br>Relax ciliary muscle (far vision) | Eye | Constrict pupil<br>Constrict ciliary muscle (near vision) |
| Increase rate<br>Increase force of contraction<br>Coronaries dilated via β, and constricted via α | Heart | Decrease rate<br>Decrease force of contraction, especially the atria |
| Constrict (α effect), in all but skeletal muscle where dilatation occurs (β effect) | Blood vessels | None |
| Bronchi dilated, pulmonary circulation mild constriction | Lungs | Constricted |
| Decrease peristalsis and tone, increase sphincter tone | Stomach | Increase peristalsis and tone, relax sphincters |
| Glucose release, gallbladder and ducts relaxed | Liver and gallbladder | Slight increase in glycogen synthesis, constriction of the biliary tract |
| Detrusor muscle relaxed<br>Trigone excited | Bladder | Detrusor excited<br>Trigone relaxed |
| Copious sweating<br>Vasoconstriction and scant secretion | Glands: sweat and salivary | No effect on sweating<br>Copious secretion from all glands except pancreas |
| Secretion increased | Adrenal medulla | No effect |

The general structure of the ANS is similar in principle for both divisions but with significant differences. The outflow of both systems consists of a preganglionic neuron arising centrally and synapsing in the autonomic ganglion, and a postganglionic neuron that passes from the ganglion to the organ that it innervates. In general, the postganglionic neurons are long in the sympathetic system, arising from the sympathetic chain alongside the spinal cord and travelling to the organs that they innervate. In the parasympathetic system, the postganglionic neurons are short, because the parasympathetic ganglia are sited close to the organs that they innervate. The two divisions are compared in Table 23.6.

The parasympathetic outflow is divided into the cranial and sacral outflow (Figure 23.37). Preganglionic fibres arise from the brain stem and sacral outflow, and are myelinated B fibres. The cranial parasympathetic outflow is in cranial nerves III, VII, IX, and X. The preganglionic fibres end in ganglia, producing short postganglionic neurons that supply their effector organs.

Sympathetic nerves arise from the thoracolumbar outflow (Figure 23.37). The preganglionic fibres arise from the lateral horn of the spinal cord and the ganglia are arranged in a paravertebral chain either side of the spinal cord, at the dermatomal levels in which outflow occurs, entering via the white rami communicantes (Figure 23.38). This gives rise to long postganglionic fibres in the sympathetic division. Postganglionic fibres may travel up or down one or two levels in the chain before exiting via the grey rami communicantes to the effector organ via the spinal nerve. A proportion of fibres passes through the ganglia and synapses at ganglia

| Table 23.6 Structural features of sympathetic and parasympathetic divisions | |
|---|---|
| **Sympathetic** | **Parasympathetic** |
| Forms thoracolumbar outflow | Forms craniosacral outflow |
| Contains sympathetic trunk and prevertebral ganglia | Contains terminal ganglia |
| Ganglia are close to the CNS and distant from visceral effectors | Ganglia are near or on visceral effectors |
| Each preganglionic fibre synapses with many postganglionic neurons that pass to many visceral effectors | Each preganglionic fibre usually synapses with four or five postganglionic neurons that pass to a single visceral effector |
| Distributed throughout the body, including the skin | Distribution limited primarily to head and viscera of thorax, abdomen, and pelvis |

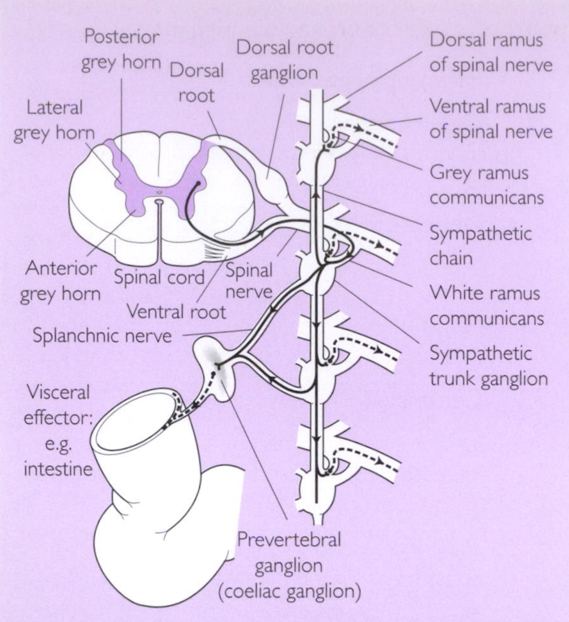


**Figure 23.38** The pattern of distribution of sympathetic nerves as they leave the spinal cord and form the sympathetic chain.

closer to the organ innervated. The postganglionic sympathetic supply to the head originates in the superior, middle, and stellate ganglia which are the cephalad extension of the sympathetic chain (Figure 23.37).

The adrenal medulla is a specialized ganglion that receives efferent inputs, which it translates into hormonal release of epinephrine and norepinephrine into the bloodstream in the ratio 30 : 70. These hormones then achieve their effect on distant adrenoceptors after distribution by the bloodstream. Norepinephrine has a predominant $\alpha$ action, whereas epinephrine has an approximately equal $\alpha$ and $\beta$ action.

## Transmitters in the ANS

These were outlined earlier in general terms in 'Postsynaptic receptors' and are summarized in Figure 23.12.

### *Acetylcholine*

Acetylcholine is the transmitter at all autonomic ganglia, and at postganglionic synapses in the parasympathetic system. The effect produced by acetylcholine is determined by the nature of the postsynaptic receptor with which it interacts. Transmission is nicotinic at ganglia and muscarinic at effector organs. In contrast, in the somatic system, receptors in the end-plates of skeletal muscle are nicotinic, but are a different subset of receptors from those in autonomic ganglia.

Acetylcholine is a postsynaptic transmitter in the sympathetic nervous system in only two sites, both of which are muscarinic:

1. receptors on sweat glands;
2. receptors that vasodilate skeletal muscle blood vessels.

### *Norepinephrine*

Norepinephrine is the transmitter at postganglionic sympathetic nerve endings, except for those to the sweat glands which are cholinergic and act on muscarinic receptors. The effect of the norepinephrine released is, as for acetylcholine, determined by the type of postsynaptic receptor. The $\alpha$ and $\beta$ classification has been described briefly above in 'Postsynaptic receptors'. The first subclassification came with $\beta_1$- and $\beta_2$-adrenoceptors:

- $\beta_1$-adrenoceptors are located in the heart and in the smooth muscle of the intestine, and at these sites epinephrine and norepinephrine have equipotent effects.
- $\beta_2$-adrenoceptors are found in bronchial, vascular, and uterine smooth muscle and are far more sensitive to the effects of circulating epinephrine than to norepinephrine, i.e. they behave as 'hormonal' rather than as 'transmitter' receptors.

$\alpha$- and $\beta$-adrenoceptors occur not only in the membranes of postsynaptic structures, but also in presynaptic endings. This is shown diagrammatically in Figure 23.39. In noradrenergic neurons, there are presynaptic receptors of the $\alpha_2$ type. Some of the norepinephrine released at synaptic junctions diffuses to the presynaptic $\alpha_2$-adrenoceptors, preventing excessive or prolonged release of norepinephrine. There is also strong evidence for the existence of presynaptic $\beta$-adrenoceptors which facilitate norepinephrine release.

In general, the stimulation of the $\alpha$-adrenoceptor results in an increased permeability to sodium followed by a depolarization; for this reason they are usually excitatory. Conversely $\beta$ stimulation results in an outward movement of potassium and an inward movement of chloride, which produces hyperpolarization. Thus, as described earlier, $\beta$ stimulation is usually inhibitory, with the important exception of the heart, where $\beta$ stimulation is excitatory. Most effector organs have either $\alpha$ or $\beta$ innervation, but some contain both. The effects of sympathetic stimulation are longer lasting than parasympathetic, because of the augmentation effect of blood-borne norepinephrine and epinephrine from the adrenal medulla. After acting on visceral

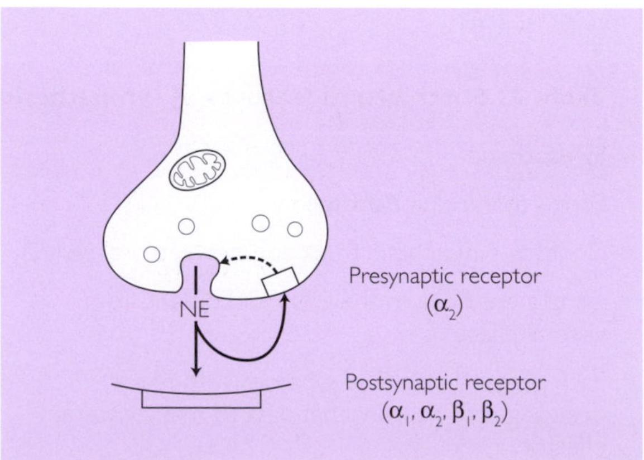


**Figure 23.39** A presynaptic receptor which responds to the quantity of norepinephrine (NE) in the synaptic cleft.

receptors, if not metabolized locally, both are inactivated by enzymes in the liver. Their breakdown pathways are shown in Figure 23.40.

Table 23.7 summarizes the classification and actions of adrenoceptors.

Subtyping of the α- and β-adrenoceptors and cloning of the receptors has led to a further, more detailed understanding of the action of these receptors (see Chapter 22, Table 22.8). The most recent analytical methods have brought the current total to nine: three subtypes each of $\alpha_1$- and $\alpha_2$-adrenoceptors and three of the β-adrenoceptor.

All adrenoceptors act via second-messenger systems. The receptors are on the cell surface, and are linked via G proteins (see Chapter 69). Each type of adrenoceptor preferentially couples to a different major subfamily of G proteins. Each of these can, in turn, link to numerous effector molecules, although most target cells have preferred linkages. β-Adrenoceptor actions have been evaluated in the most detail. All three subtypes activate adenylyl cyclase and increase cAMP via a stimulatory G protein. The biological effects are to stimulate the myocardium by increasing intracellular calcium, and to relax smooth muscle, possibly by phosphorylation of myosin light chain kinase to an inactive form.

α-Adrenoceptor activation is less well understood than β-adrenoceptor activation. The final common pathway of α-adrenoceptor activation is a rise in the cytosolic calcium ion concentration. In general, this is not accompanied by a rise in cAMP, but there is a rise in cytosolic inositol triphosphate ($IP_3$) and diacylglycerol (DAG). This releases sequestered calcium from intracellular stores, and in addition calcium channels are opened to allow calcium to enter from the extracellular fluid. $IP_3$ and DAG activate protein kinases which may regulate long-term α-adrenoceptor sensitivity. Cyclic AMP decreases in concentration during $\alpha_2$-adrenoceptor activation. Independent of this action $\alpha_2$-adrenoceptors also open potassium channels and close calcium channels.

Given the widespread expression of adrenoceptors and their role in regulating a wide variety of events, it is not surprising that alterations in these receptors might be present in several clinical settings or induced by therapy. A summary of the possible alterations is given in Table 23.8.

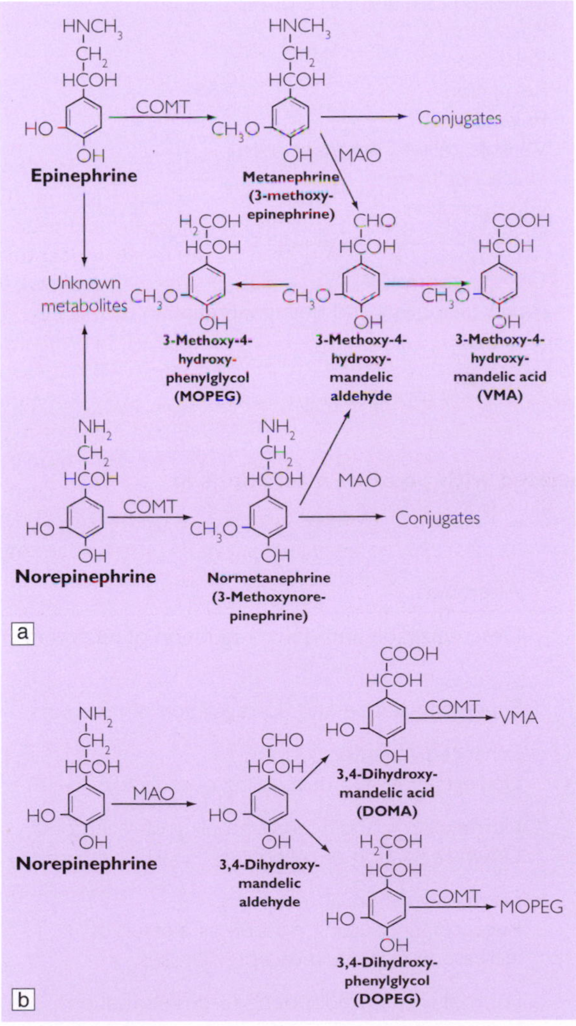

**Figure 23.40** The breakdown of epinephrine and norepinephrine. (a) The breakdown at the main site of catabolism in the liver. The conjugates are mostly glucuronides and sulphates. (b) The catabolism of norepinephrine in noradrenergic nerve endings. COMT, catechol-*O*-methyltransferase; MAO, monoamine oxidase; VMA, vanillyl mandelic acid.

## The ANS and the heart

The heart has an intrinsic rate, determined by the sinoatrial node, of about 100–120 beats/min. Changes from this rate are a result of the balance between the sympathetic and parasympathetic activity. Sympathetic activity increases the rate and force of myocardial contraction. At rest, vagal inhibition outweighs sympathetic stimulation and the normal heart rate is 70–80 beats/min. Vagal acetylcholine acts on $M_2$-receptors which activate a G protein and produce an inhibition of the cAMP second-messenger system. This results in hyperpolarization of the pacemaker cells and decreases their rate of spontaneous depolarization. High levels of vagal stimulation can produce profound bradycardia and even asystole. Vagal activity decreases the force of contraction of the atria, but the effect on the ventricle is very small.

Sympathetic stimulation releases norepinephrine which combines with $\beta_1$-adrenoceptors and acts via a G-protein link to increase cAMP in the cell; this lowers the threshold to depolarization of the cardiac pacemaker cells and increases the automaticity and heart rate. The length of time for depolarization is decreased, and there is a linear relationship between the frequency of stimulation of the nerve and the pulse interval. Sympathetic stimulation also increases the force of contraction of the myocardium via $\beta_2$-adrenoceptors. These receptors use a similar G protein/cAMP mechanism. The right cardiac sympathetic nerves increase heart rate more than the left.

## The ANS and the peripheral vasculature

Blood vessels receive innervation from sympathetic fibres, stimulation of which produces vasoconstriction via an $\alpha_1$-adrenoceptor. The arteriolar smooth muscle receives most of the innervation. There is an intrinsic level of activity in these sympathetic nerves that controls the diameter of the vessels – in the absence of

**Table 23.7 Classification and actions of adrenergic receptors**

| Receptor type | Site | Effect of stimulation |
|---|---|---|
| $\alpha_1$ | Vascular smooth muscle<br>Bladder smooth muscle (sphincter)<br>Radial muscle of iris<br>Intestinal smooth muscle<br>Uterus<br>Salivary glands<br>Liver<br>Pancreas | Contraction<br>Contraction<br>Contraction<br>Relaxation, but contraction of sphincters<br>Variable<br>Viscous secretions<br>Glycogenolysis<br>Decreased secretion of enzymes, insulin, and glucagon |
| $\alpha_2$ | Presynaptic membranes of adrenergic synapses<br>Postsynaptic membranes<br>Platelets | Reduced release of norepinephrine<br>Smooth muscle contraction<br>Aggregation |
| $\beta_1$ | Heart<br>Adipose tissue<br>Juxtaglomerular apparatus | Increased rate and force of contraction<br>Breakdown of stored triglycerides to fatty acids<br>Increased renin secretion |
| $\beta_2$ | Heart (33% of number of $\beta_1$-receptors)<br>Vascular smooth muscle (muscle beds)<br>Bronchial smooth muscle<br>Intestinal smooth muscle<br>Bladder sphincter<br>Uterus<br>Salivary glands<br>Liver<br>Pancreas | Increased rate and force of contraction<br>Relaxation<br>Relaxation<br>Relaxation<br>Relaxation<br>Variable; relaxes pregnant uterus<br>Watery secretion<br>Glycogenolysis<br>Increased insulin and glucagon secretion |
| $\beta_3$ | Omentum and brown fat<br>Gall bladder | Obesity control?<br>Promote lipolysis and heat generation in brown fat |

**Table 23.8 Clinical conditions and therapies associated with possible alterations in adrenoceptors**

| Clinical condition | Receptor type | Alteration |
|---|---|---|
| Adrenergic-agonist treatment, phaeochromocytoma | $\alpha$, $\beta$ | Desensitization and down-regulation of receptors |
| Antagonist withdrawal syndrome | $\alpha$, ?$\beta$ | Supersensitization and up-regulation of receptors |
| Myocardial ischaemia | $\alpha_1$<br>$\beta$ | Enhanced receptor coupling<br>Up-regulation and uncoupling of receptors |
| Hypertension | $\alpha$<br>$\beta$ | Up-regulation and altered coupling of receptors<br>Down-regulation of receptors |
| Congestive heart failure | $\beta_1$<br>$\beta_2$ | Down-regulation of receptors<br>Receptor uncoupling, possibly as a result of increase in G protein receptor kinases |
| Asthma | $\beta_2$ | Polymorphism predisposing to desensitization |
| Morbid obesity | $\beta_3$ | Polymorphism with ? decreased activity |

this sympathetic traffic there is profound vasodilatation as the vessel returns to its maximum diameter. This intrinsic activity is referred to as sympathetic *tone* and provides the peripheral vascular resistance, which influences blood pressure. Constriction of the capacitance vessels increases both venous return and cardiac output. Only small increases in sympathetic activity cause a relatively profound constriction of the capacitance system.

Vasoconstriction is mediated largely by norepinephrine, but sympathetic terminals also release neuropeptides, particularly neuropeptide Y, and purines, particularly ATP. Vascular smooth muscle expresses receptors for neuropeptides including neuropeptide $Y_1$-receptors and purine receptors of the type $P_{2x}$, and these agonists contribute to the vasoconstrictor effect of sympathetic stimulation.

The *vasomotor centre* in the medulla controls the level of activity in sympathetic neurons. The vasoconstrictor nerves are the efferent arm of a reflex arc (involving the baroreceptors) which maintains the blood pressure. Baroreceptors are stretch receptors in the carotid sinuses and aortic arch, which are stimulated by an increase in transmural pressure resulting from a greater volume of blood passing through the vessel. The sensory arm of this reflex travels in the glossopharyngeal and vagal nerves. The fibres relay in the nucleus of the tractus solitarius, where they release glutamate. An inhibitory pathway passes from this nucleus to the vasomotor area where GABAergic neurons inhibit the impulses in the vasoconstrictor nerves, leading to peripheral vasodilatation and a reduced venous return. This is the mechanism by which blood pressure is maintained. There is a phasic activity in this reflex arc during the cardiac cycle.

## THE PHARMACOLOGY OF THE ANS

The ANS presents numerous opportunities for pharmacological intervention. As a result of these opportunities, the effects of drugs can be quite specific, or very general. Drugs acting at autonomic ganglia can have varying effects in specific organs, depending on the balance of the effect on the sympathetic and parasympathetic systems. Specific agonists or antagonists for end-organ receptors can produce a very well-defined action.

As a general principle, where organs are innervated by both sympathetic and parasympathetic systems, a given effect (for example, increasing heart rate) can be achieved either by stimulating one system, for example with a sympathetic agonist, or by blocking the other system, for example with a muscarinic antagonist. In the parasympathetic system, it is preferable to refer to those drugs that antagonize acetylcholine at the muscarinic receptor as muscarinic antagonists, rather than anticholinergics or cholinergic antagonists, because acetylcholine has other actions as well and the term 'muscarinic antagonist' is more precise.

As described earlier, in whole or in part, enzymes terminate the action of neurotransmitters. Drugs that combine with these enzymes to block their actions prolong the action of the neurotransmitter and increase its effect. Where action is terminated by reuptake into nerve terminals, blocking of uptake mechanisms can potentiate the neurotransmitter's effects.

### Drugs acting at sympathetic and parasympathetic ganglia

All postsynaptic receptors in ganglia are nicotinic. The action of acetylcholine in sympathetic and parasympathetic ganglia can be antagonized by ganglion-blocking drugs. They are competitive antagonists at the postsynaptic nicotinic receptors, and are based on hexamethonium. These drugs were originally introduced for the treatment of essential hypertension, but the extensive effects of ganglion blockade on the whole autonomic system produced a large number of unacceptable side effects. The only drug in this class in current use is trimetaphan.

Trimetaphan is a sulphonium compound with several different actions. The competitive antagonism of acetylcholine in the ganglia is only one of the mechanisms by which it reduces blood pressure. In addition, it releases histamine from mast cells and has a direct vasodilator action on blood vessels, reducing both arteriolar and venous tone. The reduction in blood pressure results in a reflex tachycardia. It may sensitize the myocardium to catecholamines. Trimetaphan is unpredictable in its use: the histamine release can cause oedema and bronchospasm; the fall in blood pressure may be dramatic in susceptible patients; on the other hand acute tolerance can occur. The histamine effects can prolong the hypotension. The general effects on the ANS can result in paralytic ileus and urinary retention. Splanchnic and renal blood flow are decreased and cerebral blood flow is mildly reduced. The pupils are dilated and this effect persists after stopping the drug. Trimetaphan also has a mild anticholinergic action at the nicotinic receptors in the neuromuscular junction. It can potentiate the neuromuscular blocking drugs and, in high doses, causes ventilatory insufficiency. It is largely excreted unchanged in the urine.

### Drugs acting at parasympathetic effector organs

Muscarinic receptors are found on all effector organs innervated by parasympathetic postganglionic axons.

#### *Muscarinic agonists*

Directly acting muscarinic agonists fall into two chemical categories: the esters of choline and the alkaloids, based on muscarine. The alkaloids related to muscarine are well absorbed, with muscarine being the toxic ingredient of some poisonous mushrooms. Pilocarpine is the only alkaloid in clinical use.

Four choline esters are used: methacholine, carbamic acid, carbachol, and bethanechol. They are all quaternary amines, ionized at physiological pH and are poorly absorbed from the gastrointestinal tract. All are resistant to hydrolysis by acetylcholinesterase and can, in addition, have some action at the nicotinic receptor.

This group of drugs has two major therapeutic uses: in ophthalmology and in the management of some gastrointestinal and urinary tract conditions.

Use in ophthalmology is in the management of closed-angle glaucoma. The constriction of the pupil opens the flow of aqueous humour from the eye and lowers intraocular pressure. Methacholine, carbachol, and pilocarpine are used for this purpose. Pilocarpine is also used in open-angle glaucoma. They are administered as eye drops, or as a plastic film reservoir placed in the conjunctival sac.

In the gastrointestinal and genitourinary tracts, the drugs can be used to counteract atony of the bladder and to increase intestinal motility. Bethanecol is the only drug used for this purpose. Overdose with these drugs can produce nausea, vomiting, diarrhoea, salivation, sweating, cutaneous vasodilatation, and bronchospasm.

### The anticholinesterases

The effects of stimulating muscarinic receptors can be produced by improving the action of acetylcholine released from the preganglionic fibres through blockade of the enzyme acetylcholinesterase, which is responsible for its breakdown (see above). Drugs that do this are called anticholinesterases.

Acetylcholinesterase is a protein of molecular weight 320 000 daltons, present in high concentrations in cholinergic synapses. It hydrolyses acetylcholine in two steps. Initially acetylcholine binds to the enzyme at the active site and is hydrolysed to free choline and acetylated enzyme. Then, the covalent acetyl enzyme bond is split, regenerating the enzyme. The whole process takes 150 ms.

The primary therapeutic action of anticholinesterases is to enhance the nicotinic actions of acetylcholine on skeletal muscle. This is either to treat the condition myasthenia gravis or to reverse the effects of competitive neuromuscular blocking agents.

Anticholinesterases fall into three chemical categories and their uses and actions are summarized in Table 23.9.

The organophosphates bind covalently with acetylcholinesterase and are very long acting, because new enzyme has to be synthesized. These compounds are used as insecticides and chemical warfare agents.

The two groups of drugs in therapeutic use differ in their interaction with the enzyme. Edrophonium binds reversibly with the active site, and the enzyme–drug complex is unstable and short-lived. The carbamates undergo a two-stage interaction with the enzyme analogous to that of acetylcholine, producing an intermediate carbamyl–enzyme complex that is resistant to hydrolysis, and the second step is prolonged from 30 min to 6 h.

These drugs all have a quaternary charged group in the molecule. This results in generally poor absorption, and little distribution to the CNS. Physostigmine is the exception with good oral absorption and some central toxic effects. They are metabolized by non-specific esterases, but metabolism and excretion do not influence the duration of action, which is determined by the interaction of the drug with acetylcholinesterase.

Tacrine is another drug with anticholinesterase activity, which was originally introduced with the intention of prolonging the action of suxamethonium. This use was not practical because of the complexity of prolonged depolarizing block. It has since been reintroduced because of its central action where the potentiation of CNS acetylcholine seems to produce some improvement in Alzheimer's disease.

### Muscarinic antagonists

*Atropa belladonna*, the deadly nightshade plant, and *Hyoscymas niger*, the henbane plant, are sources of the naturally occurring antimuscarinic drugs. Tinctures of deadly nightshade were instilled into the eye to produce wide pupils as a fashion among women (belladonna) in the Middle Ages. Presumably these women suffered an inability to focus or accommodate as a result of their pursuit of beauty, further adding to the illusion of vulnerability and fragility, then seen as attractive features of a woman. The active drugs, atropine and hyoscine (scopolamine), are isomeric compounds: atropine is presented as a racemic mixture and hyoscine occurs naturally as the *laevo*-isomer.

Atropine and hyoscine are both absorbed from the gastrointestinal tract. They both enter the CNS and have toxic effects. Hyoscine is sedative in its action. Atropine has been used as a central antimuscarinic in the treatment of Parkinson's disease. These drugs are hydrolysed in the liver and tissues, and some is excreted in the urine unchanged.

The mode of action of these drugs is a competitive antagonism at muscarinic receptors. Atropine is non-selective for muscarinic receptors, but has greater potency in the salivary glands, bronchial tree, and sweat glands. None of the clinically available antimuscarine drugs is selective. The side effects of these drugs relate to this lack of specificity and can be predicted.

In the cardiovascular system, the sinoatrial node is slowed by vagal action. Central stimulation by atropine of the vagus causes initial bradycardia, followed by a tachycardia as vagal blockade allows unopposed sympathetic action. The atrioventricular node is also under muscarinic control and high doses of atropine prolong the PR interval. Blood vessels do not receive significant parasympathetic innervation; however, muscarinic receptors that respond to circulating agonists occur on endothelial cells and are involved in the release of nitric oxide and vasodilatation. These receptors are blocked by antimuscarinic drugs.

**Table 23.9 The anticholinesterases**

| Class | Uses | Duration |
|---|---|---|
| *Alcohols* | | |
| Edrophonium | Myasthenia gravis | 5–15 min |
| *Carbamates* | | |
| Neostigmine | Reversal of neuromuscular block | 0.5–2 hours |
| Physostigmine | Myasthenia gravis | 0.5–2 hours |
| Pyridostigmine | Myasthenia gravis | 3–6 hours |
| *Organophosphates* | Insecticides | Many hours |

In the respiratory tract, there is reduction of secretion and bronchodilatation. The antimuscarinic agents are of use in some patients with asthma and chronic obstructive airway disease. Salivation is blocked, but gastrin secretion less so. Muscarinic block reduces gastrointestinal motility, but does not abolish it completely; tone is lost and propulsive movements are reduced. Secretion of gastric acid is reduced but not abolished. The smooth muscle of the bladder is also relaxed and can result in urinary retention. Mild bladder spasm can be treated with antimuscarinic drugs.

A summary of antimuscarinic drugs and their range of therapeutic uses is found in Table 23.10.

### Drugs acting at sympathetic effector organs

The main transmitter at sympathetic effector organs is norepinephrine. As described earlier, there are two exceptions to this: the sweat glands and the vasodilator fibres on blood vessels in skeletal muscle. In both cases these nerves are cholinergic with muscarinic properties.

Generally, stimulation of the sympathetic nervous system ultimately results in the release of norepinephrine, and its interaction with postsynaptic adrenoceptors. In addition, the release of epinephrine from the adrenal cortex activates these adrenoceptors. Drugs that mimic the actions of epinephrine and norepinephrine are called sympathomimetic agents. The effects of sympathomimetic drugs are wide-ranging; the drugs are subclassified into those with direct action on the postsynaptic adrenoceptor, and those whose action is indirect either by releasing norepinephrine from the nerve ending or preventing its reuptake into the presynaptic nerve.

#### *Selective sympathomimetic drugs*

Epinephrine and norepinephrine are used therapeutically for their inotropic effect. They have similar potencies at the $\beta_1$-adrenoceptor in the heart, and at $\alpha$-adrenoceptors but they differ in their effects on $\beta_2$-adrenoceptors. Epinephrine activates $\beta_2$-adrenoceptors and causes dilatation in the blood vessels of the skeletal muscle, producing a fall in the peripheral vascular resistance. Norepinephrine has relatively less effect at the $\beta_2$-adrenoceptors and increases peripheral vascular resistance and systolic and diastolic pressure. Compensatory vagal effects reduce the chronotropic effects of norepinephrine. These drugs have very short plasma half-lives and must be given by infusion for therapeutic effect.

Isoprenaline (isoproterenol) is a potent $\beta$-adrenoceptor agonist with very little effect at $\alpha$-adrenoceptors. As a result it is chronotropic and inotropic, as well as being a potent vasodilator. Isoprenaline therefore produces an increase in cardiac output with a fall in diastolic and mean arterial pressure. Its strong $\beta$-adrenoceptor agonist action has led to its use in the treatment of asthma, where it is a potent bronchodilator. However, its use in asthma has been limited by its tendency to produce cardiac arrhythmias and has been superseded by the development of the specific $\beta_2$ agonists. A simplified summary of the effects of these drugs is given in Table 23.11.

Dopamine and dobutamine are drugs that act at dopamine receptors, but also at higher doses they will react with the adrenoceptors. $\beta_1$-Adrenoceptors in the heart are activated by dopamine at lower doses, but at higher doses $\alpha$-adrenoceptors are also activated leading to vasoconstriction. Dobutamine is relatively selective for $\beta_1$-adrenoceptors but can also have an $\alpha$ effect at very high doses.

#### *Non-selective sympathomimetic drugs*

Ephedrine is the most commonly used non-selective sympathomimetic in anaesthetic practice. It occurs in a number of plants, and has been in use for over 2000 years. It was introduced into Western medicine from China at the beginning of the twentieth century, and has been in use ever since as an orally active sympathomimetic drug for the treatment of nasal decongestion. It has a high oral bioavailability and a long duration of action. It is used parenterally as a pressor agent. It has two modes of action: it has a direct effect at the adrenoceptors and it releases norepinephrine from the sympathetic terminals. Its actions are non-specific, and it

**Table 23.10 Antimuscarinic drugs and their therapeutic uses**

| Drug | Uses |
|---|---|
| Atropine | Antisialogogue, antivagal, bronchodilator, reduces gastric acid |
| Hyoscine | Antisialogogue, antiemetic, amnesic |
| Homatropine | Mydriasis |
| Glycopyrrolate | Antisialogogue, antivagal |
| Propantheline | Reduction of gastrointestinal motility |
| Pirenzepine | Reduction of gastric acid secretion |
| Ipratropium | Bronchodilator |
| Benztropine | Anti-parkinsonian |

**Table 23.11 A comparison of the $\alpha$ and $\beta$ effects of sympathomimetic drugs**

| Drug | $\alpha_1$ effect | $\alpha_2$ effect | $\beta_1$ effect | $\beta_2$ effect |
|---|---|---|---|---|
| Dopamine | ++ | + | ++ | |
| Norepinephrine | +++ | ++ | + | |
| Epinephrine | ++ | ++ | ++ | ++ |
| Isoprenaline | | | +++ | +++ |
| Salbutamol | | | + | +++ |
| Dobutamine | + | + | +++ | |
| Methoxamine | +++ | | | |
| Ephedrine | ++ | + | ++ | + |

The shaded cells show indirect action. Dopamine acts directly and indirectly.

produces peripheral vasoconstriction and increased cardiac output.

The amphetamine group of drugs have clinical actions similar to ephedrine, but enter the CNS readily and have a marked stimulatory effect. These drugs have been used in the past as appetite suppressants, but currently their only therapeutic use is in the management of some hyperactive children. Their peripheral actions are brought about as a result of norepinephrine release.

Cocaine has a sympathomimetic action as a result of its ability to prevent the reuptake of norepinephrine into the sympathetic nerve terminal. It has a significant abuse potential, but has been used therapeutically as a local anaesthetic.

### Receptor-specific adrenoceptor agonists

#### Specific α agonists

The α-adrenoceptor agonists – metaraminol, phenylephrine, and methoxamine – are relatively selective for $\alpha_1$-adrenoceptors. They have a longer duration of action than epinephrine and norepinephrine, and can be used to raise blood pressure. Phenylephrine is used as a nasal decongestant and has been used in combination with local anaesthetics as a vasoconstrictor.

The $\alpha_2$-adrenoceptor agonist clonidine is not highly selective for the $\alpha_2$-adrenoceptor, and as such has some mixed effects. It is an interesting drug which has been used to reduce blood pressure, as an adjunct to anaesthesia, and in the treatment of chronic pain. $\alpha_2$-Adrenoceptors in the CNS are presynaptic and the stimulation of these receptors reduces the release of norepinephrine. Norepinephrine is involved in the control of the vasomotor centre, in the maintenance of mood, and in the pain pathway, both centrally and in the spinal cord. Prolonged use of clonidine followed by acute withdrawal can precipitate a hypertensive crisis. This sometimes severe complication, combined with its mixed $\alpha_1/\alpha_2$-adrenoceptor activity, has led to a decline in its use as an antihypertensive. Dexmetomidine is a more selective $\alpha_2$-adrenoceptor agonist licensed for veterinary anaesthesia, but not for human use.

The ergot alkaloids have a very high affinity for the α-adrenoceptor with partial agonist actions. They produce vasoconstriction and in long-term use can produce vascular insufficiency in the extremities. Their use in migraine is probably attributable to their interaction with 5HT (serotonin) receptors, not the α effect.

#### Specific β agonists

Selective $\beta_2$-adrenoceptor agonists have been developed for the management of asthma. Salbutamol, terbutaline, fenoterol, reproterol, and rimiterol have all been used. The bronchodilatation is produced by increasing intracellular cAMP and sequestration of intracellular calcium. All these drugs are only relatively selective and in high doses may show $\beta_1$ actions and unacceptable cardiovascular side effects.

$\beta_2$-Adrenoceptor agonists produce a relaxation of uterine smooth muscle and infusions of salbutamol are used for the management of premature labour.

### Sympathetic adrenoceptor antagonists

#### α-Adrenoceptor antagonists

α-Adrenoceptor antagonists have been used in the control of blood pressure, but their use is limited by the resulting reflex tachycardia. More effective antihypertensive drugs have been developed and the remaining use of α-adrenoceptor antagonists is in the management of phaeochromocytoma.

Phentolamine is an imidazoline derivative, and it acts as a competitive antagonist at all α-adrenoceptors. It is equally potent at $\alpha_1$- and $\alpha_2$-adrenoceptors, but it also has 5HT antagonistic properties and is an agonist at muscarinic, $H_1$-, and $H_2$-receptors. It is poorly absorbed from the gastrointestinal tract and, because of its wide range of actions, it has many unwanted effects. Its principal action is to produce hypotension, although it also has a positive inotropic action probably as a result of $\alpha_2$ blockade, increasing norepinephrine release. It has been used in the acute management of hypertension, for producing deliberate hypotension during anaesthesia, and in the pharmacological management of the perioperative period for removal of phaeochromocytoma.

Tolazoline is similar in its spectrum of activity to phentolamine, and has better oral absorption. It is occasionally used in peripheral vascular disease

Phenoxybenzamine is more selective for $\alpha_1$-adrenoceptors, binds covalently with the receptor, and has a long duration of action (up to 48 hours). Its therapeutic effects relate to α blockade, but it has pharmacological actions at acetylcholine, 5HT, and histamine receptors. It is absorbed orally and is used in the preoperative preparation of patients with a phaeochromocytoma. Occasionally, it may be used in the management of hypertensive crisis.

Prazosin is the most selective of the α-antagonists, having a higher affinity for $\alpha_1$-adrenoceptors. It causes less tachycardia as a result and has both arteriolar and venodilator actions. It has an oral bioavailability of 50% and a half-life of 3 hours.

The α-adrenoceptor antagonists have largely fallen out of use in the management of hypertension, because of unacceptable side effects. Patients taking these drugs may suffer from nasal congestion, gastrointestinal irregularities, and urinary tract symptoms, all of which make compliance by the patient low. Their use is now limited to acute management of hypertensive crisis, and even in this situation better drugs are now available.

#### Mixed α- and β-adrenoceptor antagonists

Labetalol is a drug with both α-blocking and β-blocking properties. It is a racemic mixture of two pairs of isomers with different affinities for the α- and β-adrenoceptors. When given intravenously, it is seven times more active at the β-adrenoceptor than at the $\alpha_1$-adrenoceptor. When used for the control of blood pressure perioperatively, the duration of the α action is less than that of the β action. Doses up to 200 mg by intermittent injection or infusion have been used, although sensitivity to the drug should be tested by starting with 5-mg doses. It has been used in the control of blood pressure in pre-eclampsia. It is relatively lipid insoluble, so it does not cross the placenta, but the slow elimination from the maternal circulation allows equilibrium such that the fetal : maternal ratio at delivery is 0.5.

*β-Adrenoceptor antagonists*

β-Adrenoceptor antagonists are competitive antagonists at the β-adrenoceptors. They have varying degrees of specificity for $\beta_1$- and $\beta_2$-adrenoceptors. Some of the drugs in this class are also partial agonists, some have local anaesthetic membrane-stabilizing effects, and there is a great variation in their pharmacokinetic characteristics.

They are largely well absorbed, but many of the drugs undergo extensive first-pass metabolism in the liver, giving them a low oral bioavailability. Some of the newer drugs in this class are resistant to first-pass metabolism. They are rapidly distributed and have large volumes of distribution, entering the CNS and having half-lives of the order of 2–5 hours. Esmolol is the exception. It is rapidly hydrolysed by plasma esterases and has a half-life of only 10 min. The clinical effects of these drugs often persist long after their pharmacokinetic half-lives. Table 23.12 outlines the characteristics of some commonly used β-adrenoceptor antagonists.

β-Adrenoceptor antagonists are used to lower blood pressure, via actions on the heart, blood vessels, and the renin–angiotensin system; some may have a central action. They are also used to reduce the frequency of angina, by reducing myocardial work, and for preventing and treating tachyarrhythmias by increasing the atrioventricular nodal refractory period. Long-term use after myocardial infarction increases survival. They have been used in the management of obstructive cardiomyopathy, to control systolic pressure in dissecting aneurysm of the thoracic aorta, and for the cardiac complications of thyrotoxicosis.

The major disadvantage of the non-selective β-adrenoceptor antagonists is the effect of blockade of $\beta_2$-adrenoceptors in the lungs. This may lead to an increase in airway resistance, particularly in patients with asthma. No currently available drug is completely free of $\beta_2$-adrenoceptor antagonistic activity, so these drugs are avoided in patients with asthma.

β-Adrenoceptor antagonists inhibit sympathetic stimulation of lipolysis, and have complex effects on carbohydrate metabolism, partially inhibiting gluconeogenesis in the liver. They should be used with caution in patients with insulin-dependent diabetes.

## FURTHER READING


Bradley PB. *Introduction to Neuropharmacology*. Bristol: Wright, 1989.

Calvey TN, Williams NE. *Principles and Practice of Pharmacology for Anaesthetists*, 3rd edn. Oxford: Blackwell Scientific, 1997.

Ganong WF. *Review of Medical Physiology*, 18th edn. Stamford, CA: Appleton & Lange, 1997.


**Table 23.12 Characteristics of some commonly used β-adrenoceptor antagonists**

| Drug | Selectivity | Partial agonist activity | Lipid solubility | Half-life (h) | Bioavailability (%) |
|---|---|---|---|---|---|
| Acebutolol | $\beta_1$ | Yes | Low | 3–5 | 50 |
| Atenolol | $\beta_1$ | No | Low | 6–9 | 40 |
| Esmolol | $\beta_1$ | No | Low | 0.2 | 100 |
| Labetalol | None | Yes | Moderate | 5 | 30 |
| Metoprolol | $\beta_1$ | No | Moderate | 3–4 | 50 |
| Nadolol | None | No | Low | 14–24 | 33 |
| Pindolol | None | Yes | Moderate | 3–4 | > 90 |
| Propranolol | None | No | High | 3–6 | 30 |
| Sotalol | None | No | Low | 12 | 90 |
| Timolol | None | No | Moderate | 4–5 | 50 |

# Chapter 24 Muscle and the neuro-muscular junction

N.J.N. Harper

## THE NEUROMUSCULAR JUNCTION

The neuromuscular junction is the site of a specialized nicotinic cholinergic synapse. The arrival of an action potential at the motor nerve terminal causes the release into the junctional cleft of a large quantity of acetylcholine, greatly in excess of that required to generate an action potential in the postjunctional muscle membrane. The fundamental differences between transmission at the neuromuscular junction and transmission at a nerve-to-nerve synapse are shown in Table 24.1.

### Synthesis of acetylcholine

Acetylcholine is synthesized in the nerve terminal by the acetylation of choline, catalysed by choline-*O*-acetyltransferase (choline acetylase). Choline is actively transported into the axoplasm from the extracellular fluid (including the synaptic cleft). Acetylcholine synthesis is an energy-consuming process; the rate of synthesis is related to the rate of firing of the motor nerve. It is probable that choline uptake and choline acetylase activity are modulated by intracellular sodium concentration.

### Release of acetylcholine

A single motor nerve impulse releases the contents of approximately 100 vesicles, each of which contains about 10 000 molecules of acetylcholine.

The excess of acetylcholine released ensures a safety margin of approximately tenfold. The release of acetylcholine is described as 'quantal' and a quantum is taken to be the contents of one vesicle. The 'quantal content' of a particular end-plate potential describes the number of vesicles that were expended in its production.

At rest, a few quanta are released at random intervals and each results in a miniature end-plate potential (MEPP), which is insufficient to depolarize the postjunctional membrane to threshold. The MEPPs do not summate and do not result in an action potential in the muscle membrane (Table 24.1).

There is a small, non-vesicular leakage of acetylcholine when the nerve terminal is depolarized, but the importance of this phenomenon in neuromuscular transmission is minor.

Approximately 50% of the acetylcholine present in the nerve terminal is encapsulated in vesicles. A small proportion of the vesicles (1%) is situated close to the synaptic border at the active zones in stores that are readily releasable. The remainder of the vesicles (99%) are held in a large reserve store in which the individual vesicles are anchored to the cytoskeleton by synapsin 1, a phosphoprotein. The active zones are positioned directly over the crests of the folds in the postjunctional muscle membrane which carry the cholinoceptors (Figure 24.1a).

The mechanisms that lead to the release of acetylcholine from the motor nerve terminal are as follows:

1. The motor nerve action potential arrives at the motor nerve terminal as a wave of depolarization.
2. Voltage-gated calcium channels open in the nerve membrane, allowing an influx of calcium ions into the nerve terminal along their concentration gradient.
3. The high intracellular concentration of calcium triggers the release of acetylcholine from the readily releasable pool into the synaptic cleft and also mobilizes vesicles from the reserve pool (Figure 24.1a):
   (a) calcium binds with synaptotagmin in the membranes of the vesicles which are close to the nerve terminal membrane;
   (b) activated synaptotagmin binds to docking proteins (syntaxins) in the nerve terminal membrane;

**Table 24.1 Differences between the graded postsynaptic potentials of a neuronal synapse and the all-or-none transmission of the neuromuscular junction**

| Synaptic junction | Neuromuscular junction |
|---|---|
| Multiple excitatory postsynaptic potentials summate until a threshold is reached | An excess of acetylcholine is released |
| Postsynaptic potentials can be excitatory or inhibitory<br>Inhibitory postsynaptic potentials hyperpolarize the postsynaptic membrane | Every motor nerve action potential (AP) leads to a muscle membrane AP |
| | All postjunctional potentials are excitatory |

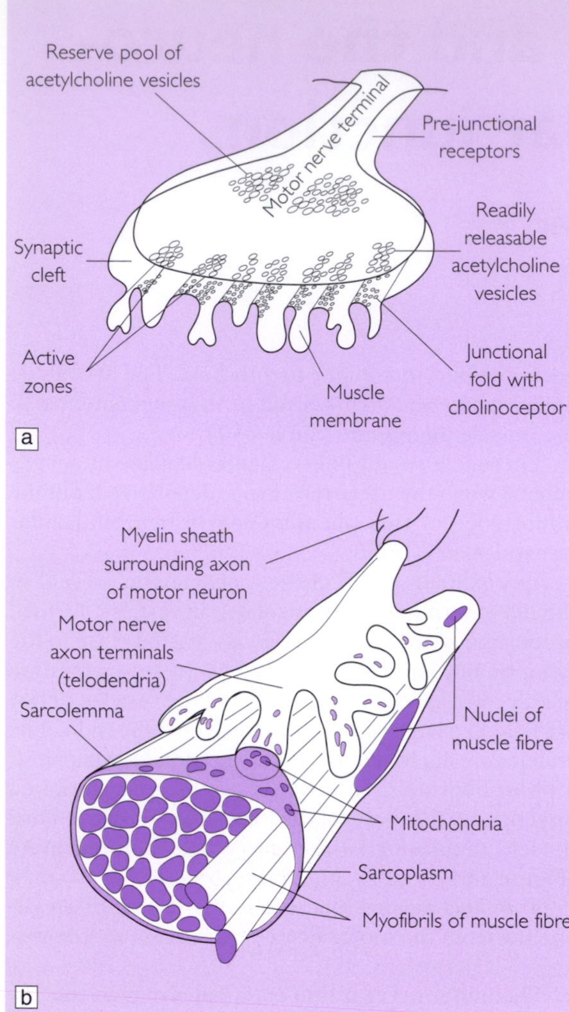


**Figure 24.1** The neuromuscular junction showing a single end-plate. (a) A close-up of a motor nerve terminal. Acetylcholine is contained in membrane-bound vesicles: the majority are held in a reserve pool and a minority are positioned over active zones in the nerve terminal membrane, in the readily releasable pool. Most nicotinic cholinergic receptors (postjunctional) are grouped along the crests of long folds in the muscle membrane. A smaller number (prejunctional receptors) are situated on the nerve terminal membrane and axon. (b) The motor nerve applied to a muscle fibre.

   (c) a pore opens in the terminal membrane, releasing acetylcholine into the junctional cleft. The membrane of the vesicle contains a further two proteins which facilitate these processes: synaptophysin and synaptobrevin. Synaptobrevin is the site of action of botulinum toxin which blocks neuromuscular transmission by inhibiting the release of acetylcholine from the motor nerve terminal.
4. The rise in intracellular calcium also mobilizes vesicles from the reserve pool to maintain the response to prolonged nerve activity. The process of mobilization is as follows:
   (a) intracellular calcium combines with calmodulin to activate protein kinase II (PK);
   (b) PK reduces the binding capacity of synapsin 1 (which anchors the vesicles to the cytoskeleton);
   (c) vesicles are released into the axoplasm and migrate to the active zones.
5. The vesicles undergo a recycling process:
   (a) docking with the membrane of the nerve terminal at the active zones;
   (b) fusion with the membrane;
   (c) release of acetylcholine via a fusion pore;
   (d) re-formation of the vesicle;
   (e) re-filling of the vesicle with acetylcholine.
6. Calcium ions are removed from the motor nerve terminal via a $Ca^{2+}/Na^{+}$ antiport, restoring the calcium ion concentration to the resting state.

### Prejunctional cholinoceptors and positive feedback

The axonal membrane of the motor nerve terminal carries many kinds of surface receptors including nicotinic cholinergic, muscarinic cholinergic, adrenergic, dopaminergic, and GABA (γ-aminobutyrate) receptors. The nicotinic cholinergic receptors on its surface provide a positive-feedback mechanism for the release of acetylcholine from the nerve terminal. Acetylcholine released from the nerve into the synaptic cleft interacts with nicotinic cholinergic receptors on the nerve membrane, facilitating the mobilization and release of further acetylcholine. It is not clear whether calcium or sodium channels are predominantly responsible. It is probable that this mechanism operates only during periods of rapid motor nerve activity when the demand for acetylcholine is highest. Competitive blockade of these prejunctional receptors is thought to be responsible for train-of-four, double burst, and tetanic fade. The action of catecholamines on prejunctional adrenergic receptors may be responsible for enhancing acetylcholine release during times of physiological stress. This effect can be antagonized by α-adrenoceptor blocking agents.

### The fate of acetylcholine after its release

Acetylcholine released into the synaptic cleft is immediately at the mercy of acetylcholinesterase situated on the basement membrane and in the junctional folds. The life of a molecule of acetylcholine is probably only 100 μs, during which time it may occupy a receptor site on a single occasion. Despite this high attrition rate, neuromuscular transmission is protected by the considerable excess of acetylcholine molecules released by each motor nerve impulse. Acetylcholinesterase contains an anionic site, which binds to the quaternary ammonium group of the acetylcholine molecule, and an esteratic site, which binds to the opposite end of the acetylcholine molecule. Acetylcholine is cleaved at its ester linkage to release choline and acetate.

### Generation of the muscle resting membrane potential

The muscle cytoplasm has a resting potential of approximately −90 mV in relation to the extracellular fluid. This is the result of a small excess of negative ions within the cell. The membrane is relatively impermeable to cations and is more permeable to potassium than to sodium (Figure 24.2). The $Na^{+}/K^{+}$ ATPase pump extrudes three sodium ions in exchange for moving two potassium ions into the cell, which contributes to the electrical gradient (see Chapter 19). This pump comprises an α subunit, through which sodium and potassium transport occurs, and a β subunit. Several isoforms of each subunit type occur: the $\alpha_2$ subunit is found in skeletal and cardiac muscle; $\beta_2$ subunits are found in fast glycolytic muscle fibres.

### The acetylcholine receptor

The nicotinic acetylcholine receptor comprises five protein subunits which form a channel (ionophore) that passes through the membrane (Figures 24.2 and 24.3). The subunits are encoded by four separate genes and their half-life is approximately one week. At birth, the human receptor has two α, one β, one γ, and one δ subunit. The γ subunit is substituted by an ε unit during the first few months of life, and the receptor then assumes its mature form. As the receptor is a dynamic entity, its constitution can revert at any time in response to an appropriate stimulus: for example, after an extensive burn injury.

When each of the α subunits is occupied by a molecule of acetylcholine the ion channel opens for approximately 1 ms. It is probable that the binding of acetylcholine to one α subunit positively influences the probability of a second molecule binding to its partner. The ion channel has a much larger internal diameter than the specific sodium and potassium channels found in muscle and nerve membranes, and it is also permeable to small anions in addition to cations.

Although the concentration gradient for potassium ions (151 mmol) is greater than for sodium ions (133 mmol), the flux of sodium ions out of the muscle cell is greater than the inward flux of potassium when the receptor channel opens (see Chapter 19). This is explained by the considerably greater voltage gradient for sodium. The equilibrium potential for sodium (+65 mV) is considerably further away from the resting membrane potential (–90 mV) than the equilibrium potential for potassium (–95 mV) (Table 24.2). The considerable net influx of sodium ions depolarizes the muscle membrane.

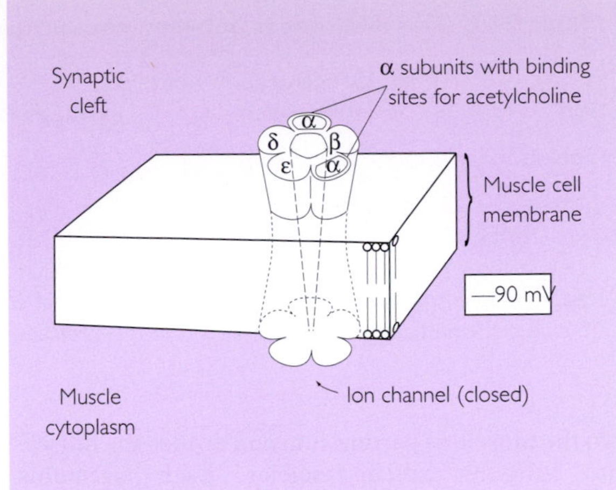


**Figure 24.3** The nicotinic cholinoceptor pierces the cell membrane. The mature receptor comprises five subunits: two α, one β, one γ, and one ε subunit. When receptors on both of the α subunits are occupied by acetylcholine, the ion channel opens and sodium ions flood into the muscle cell, causing depolarization. In the fetus (and after a major burn injury), the ε subunit may be substituted by a γ subunit.

When the motor nerve is quiescent, small numbers of vesicles release their acetylcholine at random intervals. The resulting change in end-plate potential is less than 1 mV (MEPP), and they do not summate to reach the threshold for an action potential in contrast to the excitatory postsynaptic potentials which occur in nerve-to-nerve transmission (see Table 24.1). Only when a nerve impulse arrives at the motor nerve terminal is sufficient acetylcholine released into the junctional cleft to generate an action potential in the muscle membrane. Less than 25% of the acetylcholine released is actually required to reach the threshold for a muscle action potential.

The action potential spreads outwards from the motor end-plate, which is usually near the middle of the muscle, in all directions over the surface of the muscle fibres. The duration of contraction of the muscle fibres (75–100 ms) is considerably greater than the duration of the action potential (5 ms). Unlike the nerve action potential there is no after-hyperpolarization in the muscle membrane.

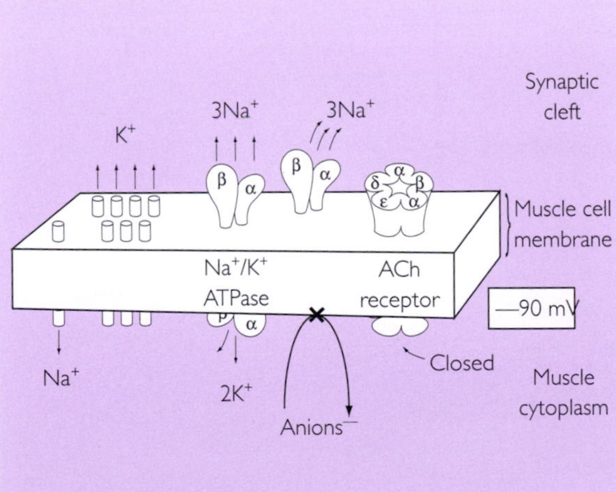


**Figure 24.2** Generation of the muscle resting membrane potential. The resting potential (–90 mV) is the result of several mechanisms. The membrane is relatively impermeable to anions. The $Na^+/K^+$ ATPase channels exchange three sodium ($Na^+$) ions for two potassium ($K^+$) ions, which more than compensates for the leakage of $K^+$ out of the cell via a larger number of ion-specific channels so that (1) $K^+$ accumulates within the cell and (2) the inside of the cell becomes negatively charged. The electrochemical gradients for $Na^+$ and $K^+$ are shown in Table 24.2. ACh, acetylcholine.

## MUSCLE AND THE CONTRACTILE PROCESS

### The structure of skeletal muscle

The structure of skeletal muscle is shown in Figure 24.4. The entire muscle is wrapped in a connective tissue layer called the epimysium, which invaginates

**Table 24.2 The differences between sodium and potassium in skeletal muscle**

| Ion | Concentration (mmol/L) Intracellular | Extracellular | Concentration gradient | Equilibrium potential (mV) |
|---|---|---|---|---|
| Sodium | 12 | 145 | 133 | +65 |
| Potassium | 155 | 4 | 151 | –95 |

Despite the greater concentration gradient for potassium, the equilibrium potential for sodium is further away from the resting muscle membrane potential (–90 mV) than that of potassium. The net effect is an influx of sodium ions into the muscle cell when acetylcholine binds to the receptor and its ion channel opens.

into the muscle as perimysium and divides the muscle into subunits called fascicles. Each fasciculus comprises groups of muscle fibres bundled together and separated by invaginations of perimysium called endomysium. The muscle fibre is the fundamental cell and has many hundreds of nuclei. Each fibre is 10–100 μm in diameter. It may stretch the full length of the muscle or may extend only part of the muscle length. Muscle fibres may be oriented along the axis or at an angle to the axis of the muscle. At each end of the muscle, the connective tissue layers condense to form tendons or aponeuroses.

The internal structure of a muscle fibre is shown in Figure 24.5. The surface of each muscle fibre is covered by a cell membrane, the sarcolemma. Packed in the cytoplasm of the fibre, running from one end to the other, there are bundles of myofibrils composed of interdigitating thin filaments (actin + tropomyosin + troponin) and thick filaments (myosin), together with two tubular conducting systems and mitochondria.

Inside the sarcolemma (Figure 24.5) two distinct systems of tubes conduct ions and electrical charge into and between the myofibrils. Each myofibril is surrounded by the sarcoplasmic reticulum, a network of interconnecting tubes that runs over the surface of the myofibrils. At intervals along the length of the myofibril, the tubes of the sarcoplasmic reticulum coalesce in terminal cisternae which form incomplete septa through which the thick and thin filaments pass.

Separate from the sarcoplasmic reticulum, small tubules invaginate into the substance of the fibre from the sarcolemma and form plates of interconnecting tubules at regular intervals at right angles to the axis of the fibre (the T system). The interior of the T system is in continuity with the extracellular fluid. The terminal cisternae of the sarcoplasmic reticulum are in close contact with the T system. Thus, both the terminal cisternae of the sarcoplasmic reticulum and the T system form partial septa at the same regular intervals along the muscle fibre. A single T system is sandwiched between a terminal cisterna of the sarcoplasmic reticulum on each side; this arrangement is known as a triad.

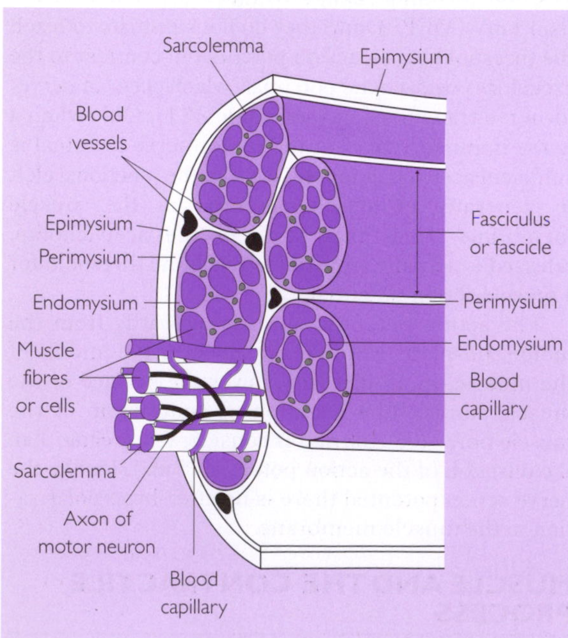


**Figure 24.4** The structure of skeletal muscle. (Adapted from Tortora GT and Anagnostrakos NP. *Principles of Anatomy and Physiology* 5th edn. Harper and Row, New York, 1987: 196.)

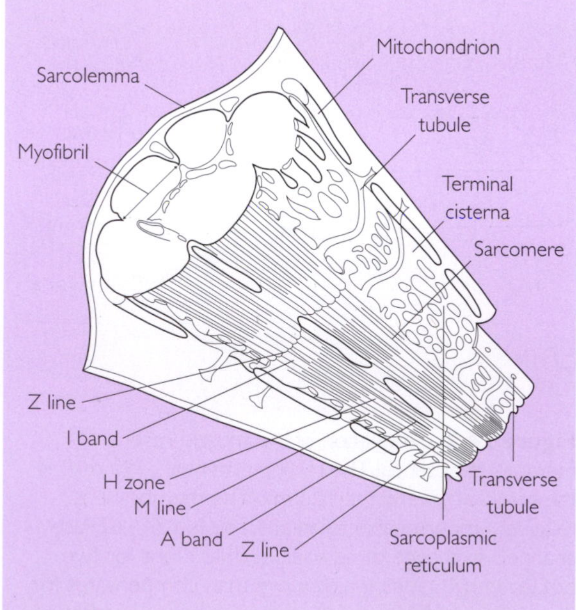


**Figure 24.5** The internal structure of a muscle fibre. (Adapted from Tortora GT and Anagnostrakos NP. *Principles of Anatomy and Physiology* 5th edn. Harper and Row, New York, 1987: 197.)

Under the microscope, the pattern of thick and thin filaments repeats at regular intervals along the myofibril related to the configuration of the thick and thin filaments: one unit of this pattern is termed a sarcomere. A sarcomere comprises a Z line at each end and an M line in the middle (Figure 24.6). Attached to each Z line, pointing inwards towards the middle of the sarcomere, are the thin filaments of actin. Attached to the M line, extending outwards left and right, are the thick myosin filaments. Confusingly, the dark appearance of the myosin filaments is termed the 'A band'.

***Thick filaments***

Each thick filament is made up of approximately 200 myosin molecules, which are hockey-stick like with a globular head and a long tail. They are arranged in bundles with the heads protruding from the bundle at intervals (Figure 24.7). Each myosin head carries two binding sites: an actin binding site and a myosin ATPase site. The heads point outwards from the centre of the thick filaments. When cross-bridges form between myosin and actin, movement of the myosin heads pulls the thin filaments towards the centre of the thick filaments and the myofibril shortens. The cross-bridges act independently and the cycle of attachment, movement, release, and reattachment occurs many times during a single muscle contraction. This process is analogous to hauling a rope hand over hand. At any one time, about 50% of the myosin heads are attached to myosin and contributing to muscle contraction.

***Thin filaments***

The thin filaments are composed of two, intertwined, helical chains of actin molecules which carry myosin-binding sites. Thinner chains of tropomyosin run alongside the actin and carry, at intervals, globular molecules of troponin (Figure 24.8). In the resting state, tropomyosin interferes with the interaction between myosin and actin by interposing between their binding sites. Tropomyosin is held in place by troponin which 'spot-welds' it to actin at intervals (Figure 24.8).

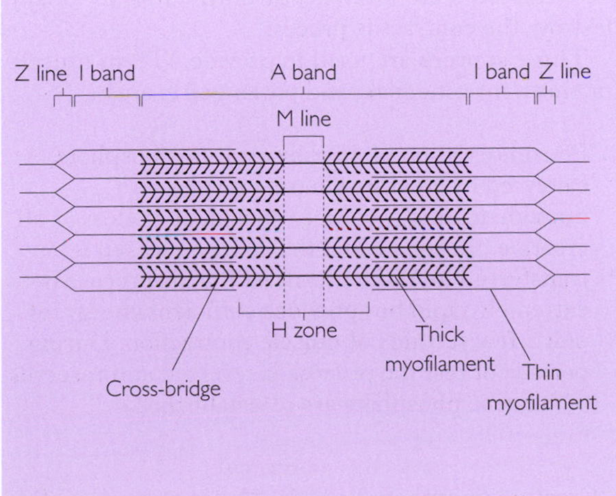


**Figure 24.6** The structure of a sarcomere.

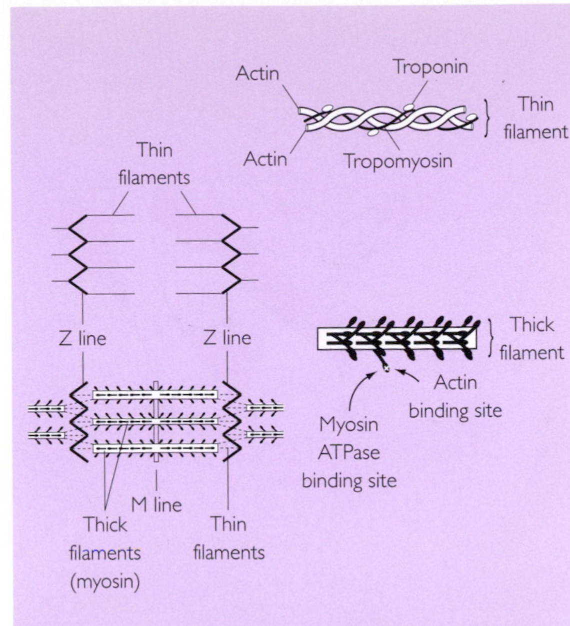


**Figure 24.7** The arrangement of thin (actin) fibres and thick (myosin) fibres which make up the myofibril. The thin filaments are attached at their ends to the Z lines. The portion of the myofibril between two Z lines is a sarcomere. The globular heads of the myosin filaments point away from the M line to which they are attached. During the contractile process, specific receptors on the myosin heads interact with specific receptors on the actin filaments to form cross-bridges. Inward movement of the myosin heads pulls together the thin filaments; the Z lines are drawn inwards and the length of the muscle is reduced. The lengths of the thin and thick filaments do not change during muscle contraction.

## Excitation–contraction coupling

The process that leads from the generation of an action potential in the membrane of the muscle to contraction of the muscle is known as excitation–contraction coupling:

1. The action potential is conducted rapidly over the exterior surface of the muscle plasma membrane and into the substance of the muscle fibre via the T tubules.
2. The T tubules conduct the action potential to the sarcoplasmic reticulum, and a proportion of the voltage-gated calcium channels in the lateral sacs open. Calcium ions diffuse into the cytosol of the myofibrils.
3. The calcium ions released from the sarcoplasmic reticulum interact with the remaining closed calcium channels and rapidly enhance further release of calcium (positive feedback).
4. Calcium ions bind to troponin causing the release of the blocking effect of tropomyosin on the interaction between actin and the myosin cross-bridges.
5. Actin-binding sites on the previously energized myosin (raised to a high energy state by the hydrolysis of myosin-bound ATP at the end of the previous bind–release cycle) interact with corresponding sites on the thin filaments (actin).

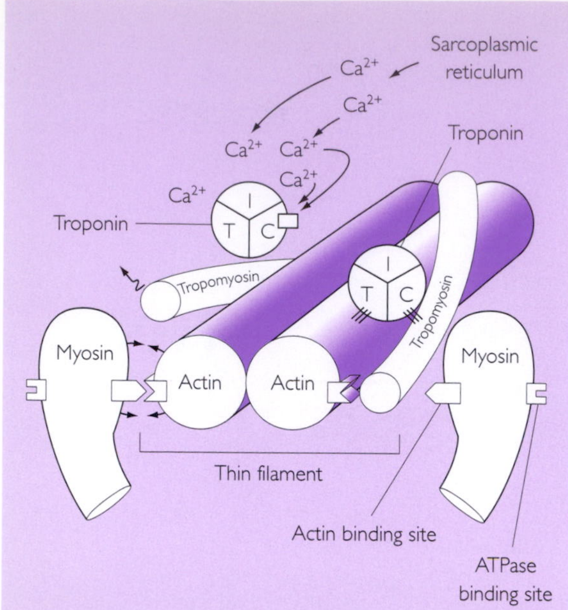


**Figure 24.8** In the resting state, the specific binding sites on the myosin heads are prevented from interacting with actin by the interposition of long tropomyosin molecules, which are held in position at intervals by globular troponin molecules. When an action potential spreads throughout the sarcoplasmic reticulum, calcium ions are released, which bind to receptors on troponin and release tropomyosin, permitting myosin and actin to interact. Troponin has three subunits: T, C, and I.

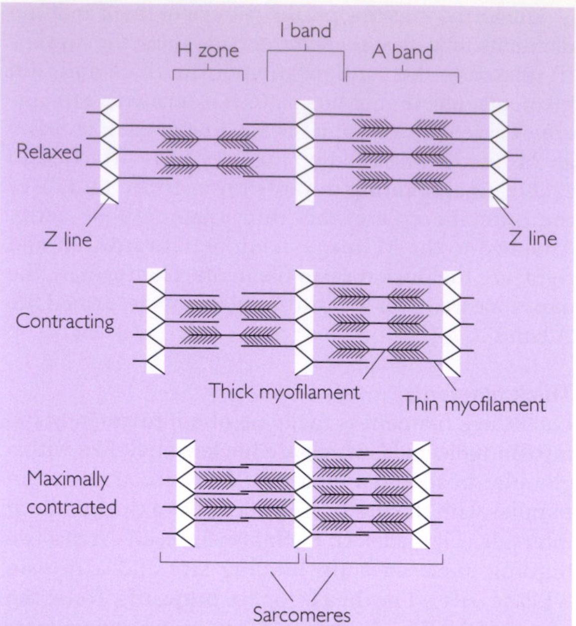


**Figure 24.9** The effect of contraction and relaxation on a sarcomere.

6. The process of actin–myosin binding releases the stored energy from myosin which results in movement of the bound cross-bridge and muscle contraction as the Z lines are pulled towards each other.
7. Calcium ions, which by now are present in the cytosol in high concentrations, bind to low-affinity sites situated on the calcium channels of the sarcoplasmic reticulum, causing their closure and halting any further release of calcium from the sarcoplasmic reticulum.
8. The primary active transport proteins ($Ca^{2+}$ ATPases) begin to pump calcium ions back into the lumen of the sarcoplasmic reticulum from the cytosol. This process requires ATP. The cytosolic levels of calcium remain high for some time and the muscle remains in a contracted state for about 100 ms. The contractile process does not have a refractory period. Further action potentials can cause enhanced muscle contraction by releasing more calcium ions from the sarcoplasmic reticulum.
9. The bond between actin and myosin is released when ATP binds to specific sites on the myosin cross-bridges. The binding of ATP to these sites decreases the affinity of myosin for actin (allosteric regulation).
10. After the cross-bridges are released, the ATP bound to myosin is hydrolysed by ATPase present on the myosin, with the release of energy. It is this important process that energizes myosin in anticipation of the next muscle contraction.
11. The muscle relaxes.
12. Falling cytosolic calcium concentrations cause dissociation of calcium ions from previously occupied sites on troponin, changing its configuration so that it is once more able to prevent the interaction of actin and myosin, by holding tropomyosin in a position where it covers the binding sites on the thin filaments.

The effect of contraction and relaxation on a sarcomere is shown in Figure 24.9.

### Source of energy for muscle contraction

Muscle contraction and relaxation are crucially dependent on the availability of large quantities of ATP. The importance of ATP in the process of muscle relaxation is exemplified in rigor mortis, when muscles remain in a contracted state after death until autolysis finally destroys the contractile process.

Three sources are used to provide ATP in muscle for short, intermediate, and prolonged exercise:

1. Phosphorylation of ADP by creatine phosphate, catalysed by creatine kinase, provides an immediate energy source. Phosphate is cleaved off creatine phosphate and the energy released is transferred to ADP to form ATP. This process is extremely rapid but provides sufficient energy for only a few seconds of muscle contraction. During periods of rest the process is reversed and reserves of creatine phosphate are re-established.

$$\text{Creatine phosphate} + \text{ADP} \underset{\text{Rest}}{\overset{\text{Exercise}}{\rightleftarrows}} \text{Creatine} + \text{ATP.}$$

2. During moderate exercise, ATP is provided by oxidative phosphorylation. For the first 5–10 min, the substrate for oxidative phosphorylation is muscle glycogen. Subsequently, blood-borne glucose becomes more important, supported after the first 30 min by fatty acids.
3. During strenuous and prolonged exercise, the supply of oxygen becomes rate-limiting for oxidative phosphorylation and the glycolytic pathway predominates. The glycolytic pathway does not require oxygen and yields only two molecules of ATP (+ two molecules of pyruvate) per molecule of glucose consumed. The first reaction in the glycolytic pathway produces glucose 6-phosphate, which is augmented from muscle glycogen. By this time, conditions are increasingly anaerobic and glycolysis becomes increasingly important. The pyruvate formed by glycolysis cannot enter the (aerobic) citrate cycle and it is converted to lactate and hydrogen ions in large quantities. The citrate cycle is intramitochondrial and muscles having few mitochondria rely totally on their cytosolic glycolytic enzymes with consequent high production of lactate.

When muscle activity ceases, the deficiency of creatine phosphate and glycogen must be restored. This process consumes an increased amount of oxygen for some time after the start of the rest period (oxygen debt).

### Muscle fatigue

Continuous activation of a muscle eventually results in a decrease of the force of contraction. This is most marked when the motor nerve activity is at a high frequency. The mechanism is different from the tetanic fade seen during non-depolarizing neuromuscular blockade because fatigue is also observed when the postjunctional muscle membrane is stimulated at high frequencies. Several mechanisms are involved in the development of muscle fatigue:

- depletion of muscle glycogen;
- rise in the concentration of hydrogen ions and inorganic phosphate, leading to inhibition of the cross-bridge cycle;
- decreased release of calcium ions from the sarcoplasmic reticulum. This may be the result of failure of conduction of the action potential from the plasma membrane along the T tubule, or failure of the calcium channels to open as a result of the accumulation of potassium and depletion of sodium in the T tubule.

## THE CONTROL OF MUSCLE CONTRACTION

### The motor unit

A motor neuron, together with all the muscle fibres that it stimulates, form a single motor unit. The number of muscle fibres in a single motor unit varies considerably according to the intended function of each muscle:

- Muscles that control precise movements, for example the extrinsic eye muscles, have fewer than 10 fibres in each motor unit.
- Muscles responsible for gross movements, for example the biceps brachii and gastrocnemius, have 500–1000 fibres per motor unit.
- The muscles of posture may have up to 2000 fibres in each motor unit.

As a consequence, the force generated by each motor unit is inversely related to the precision of control. The total tension in a muscle can be adjusted from moment to moment by varying the number of motor units activated at any one time. Resting muscle tone is the result of activation of a proportion of the motor units available for contraction.

### Types of muscle fibre

Three types of muscle fibre are found in the adult: slow oxidative, fast oxidative, and fast glycolytic. Slow fibres are also known as type I fibres and fast fibres as type II (Table 24.3). All the muscle fibres of a single motor

**Table 24.3 Characteristics of the three types of muscle fibre found in an adult**

| Fibre type | Slow oxidative (type I) | Fast oxidative (type IIa) | Fast glycolytic (type IIb) |
|---|---|---|---|
| Colour | Red | Red | White |
| Primary source of ATP | Oxidative phosphorylation | Oxidative phosphorylation | Glycolysis |
| Mitochondria, capillaries and myoglobin | +++ | +++ | + |
| Glycogen and glycolytic enzymes | + | ++ | +++ |
| Fatiguabililty | + | ++ | +++ |
| Contraction velocity | + | +++ | +++ |
| Fibre diameter, motor unit size and diameter of motor neurone | + | ++ | +++ |

Fast glycolytic fibres have a high conduction velocity, generate high forces, but fatigue rapidly. During prolonged muscle activity, the greater share of the work is performed by the fatigue-resistant oxidative fibres.

unit are of the same type. Most muscles contain a mixture of the three fibre types. Muscles of posture, which are fatigue resistant, have a predominance of slow oxidative fibres. Muscles that are able to produce large forces for a brief period of time have a larger proportion of fast glycolytic fibres.

Oxidative fibres (red fibres) are rich in mitochondria, capillaries, and myoglobin. They have a high capacity for intramitochondrial oxidative phosphorylation of glycogen, glucose, and fatty acids. Myoglobin has a high affinity for oxygen and very little oxygen will dissociate until the arterial oxygen tension ($P\text{O}_2$) is below 2.7 kPa (20 mmHg).

Glycolytic fibres (white fibres) contain few mitochondria but the cytosol is rich in glycolytic enzymes and stores of glycogen. There are few capillaries and little myoglobin. The oxygen consumption of these fibres is considerably less than that of oxidative fibres. Glycolytic fibres are generally larger in diameter than oxidative fibres and develop more contractile force per fibre over a shorter period of time (Figure 24.10).

### Control of muscle tension

The tension generated in a muscle is dependent on:

- the frequency of action potentials;
- the number of active motor units;
- the number of fibres per motor unit;
- fibre diameter;
- initial fibre length.

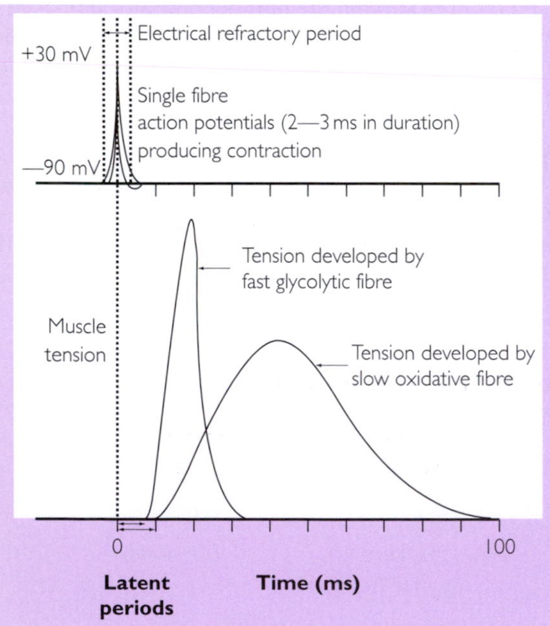


**Figure 24.10** The time course of a single fibre action potential and the ensuing contraction. Summation can take place because, although there is a brief electrical refractory period, there is no mechanical refractory period. The latent period between the action potential and the start of muscle contraction represents excitation–contraction coupling. Fast glycolytic fibres develop a greater tension than slow oxidative fibres over a shorter period of time. Slow oxidative fibres have a smaller diameter and are recruited first during a normal muscle contraction.

The maximal force of contraction is proportional to fibre diameter. Fast glycolytic fibres have the largest diameter and can generate the greatest tension, albeit for a short period of time.

### Recruitment

Recruitment provides the most important means of fine control of muscle tension. During the process of a sustained whole-muscle contraction, there is an increase in the number of motor units that are active at any one time. This process is known as recruitment; its function is to utilize the different types of muscle fibre in the most energy-efficient way. Only enough muscle fibres are recruited to perform the task in hand. Small-diameter motor neurons are activated initially. As a result of their smaller surface area, a given number of sodium ions entering their axoplasm will generate a greater depolarization. Small-diameter neurons supply small-diameter, slow, oxidative fibres which consequently are the first to contract. As greater demands are put on the muscle via increased motor nerve activity, the fast oxidative and, subsequently, the fast glycolytic fibres are brought to bear. The powerful fast glycolytic fibres are the first to fatigue so that they are useful only for short, strenuous activity, for example, lifting a heavy weight. During prolonged muscle activity, the greater share of the work is performed by fatigue-resistant oxidative fibres.

### Summation

A second action potential occurring during muscle fibre contraction results in an increased isometric tension of the whole motor unit (summation). This phenomenon can occur because:

- the duration of an action potential and its refractory period is considerable shorter than the duration of contraction of a single muscle fibre;
- the muscle fibre does not have a mechanical refractory period (Figure 24.10).

The absolute refractory period of a nerve refers to the period of time during which the nerve cannot generate a second action potential, even with a very strong stimulus. It corresponds roughly to the period of sodium-permeability changes. The absolute refractory period of large fibres is 0.4 ms and for small fibres it is 4 ms. It corresponds to the main 'spike' of the action potential from the time the firing level is reached. The relative refractory period refers to the period of time during which a second action potential can be initiated, but only with a stronger than normal stimulus. It corresponds roughly to the period of increased potassium permeability.

### Tetanus

If a continuous train of action potentials occurs at a high frequency, there is insufficient time for muscle fibre relaxation and a fused, continuous contraction results (tetanus). If the frequency is increased further, the tetanic tension also increases until it reaches a maximum which is approximately five times that of a single, isometric twitch. During maximal tetanic contraction the successive action potentials release sufficient calcium ions to saturate the capacity of the sarcoplasmic reticulum to reacquire it. These observations apply equally to the physiological situation and to the administration of external nerve stimulation during neuromuscular monitoring.

### The effects of nerve activity on muscle structure

The architecture of muscle is constantly changing and is crucially dependent on continuing motor innervation. The distinctive 'fast' or 'slow' characteristics of muscle fibres appear to be governed by their motor neurons. A slow muscle fibre can be converted experimentally to a fast fibre by attaching a regenerating nerve fibre previously cut from a fast fibre. The pattern of electrical excitation of a muscle appears to govern the expression of the 10 different isoforms of the myosin heavy chains.

Denervation produces muscle atrophy in which the denervated muscle fibres become smaller in diameter. In addition, γ-substituted cholinoceptors appear over large areas of the postjunctional muscle membrane. These receptors contain a γ, or fetal-type, subunit which replaces the normal, adult ε type (see Figure 24.3). This mechanism is partially responsible for the phenomenon of denervation hypersensitivity in which the muscle becomes extremely sensitive to acetylcholine.

### Exercise

Exercise does not change the number of muscle fibres. Low-intensity, prolonged exercise (aerobic exercise) influences the fast and slow oxidative fibres, which develop greater numbers of mitochondria and capillaries. High-intensity, short-duration exercise – for example, weight training – recruits fast glycolytic fibres; there is increased synthesis of actin, myosin, and glycolytic enzymes, and an increase in the diameter of the muscle fibres (hypertrophy).

### Local modulation of muscle activity

The many motor nerves that supply a muscle comprise the motor neuron pool for that muscle. Their cell bodies are located in the ventral horn of the spinal cord or in the brain stem. Synaptic communication is via interneurons which may be short or may extend for long distances in the brain stem and spinal cord. The functions of this system vary from reflexly dropping a hot object to unconsciously adjusting the force applied in lifting an unexpectedly heavy object, to manually moving an object over a precise distance. This level of control requires continuous monitoring of:

- absolute muscle length;
- changes in muscle length;
- changes in muscle tension.

#### *Muscle length*

Absolute muscle length and changes in muscle length are monitored by the muscle spindles, which function as encapsulated stretch transducers embedded in the muscle connected in parallel with the muscle fibres. Each spindle contains up to 10 modified muscle fibres (intrafusal fibres) which are either nuclear bag type or nuclear chain type. In each spindle, there are typically two nuclear bag fibres and eight nuclear chain fibres (Figure 24.11). Extrafusal fibres, which make up the bulk of the muscle, receive α motor neurons and intrafusal fibres receive smaller γ motor neurons.

The function of this system is primarily to maintain the desired muscle length irrespective of the load on the muscle. An example would be maintaining the position of a jug held in the hand while it is filled from a tap. The mechanism is as follows:

1. as the weight of the jug increases, the flexors of the arm tend to be stretched slightly;
2. the muscle spindles within the flexors are also stretched;
3. the frequency of firing in the spindle afferents increases;
4. connections within the spinal cord enhance the activity of the motor neuron pool in the anterior horn;
5. there is an increased α efferent discharge to the flexors which support the increased weight of the jug.

This feedback loop has a frequency of oscillation of approximately 10 Hz (physiological tremor). Primary endings on the nuclear bag fibres cause an increase in afferent discharge only during the process of stretching (dynamic response), whereas those of the nuclear

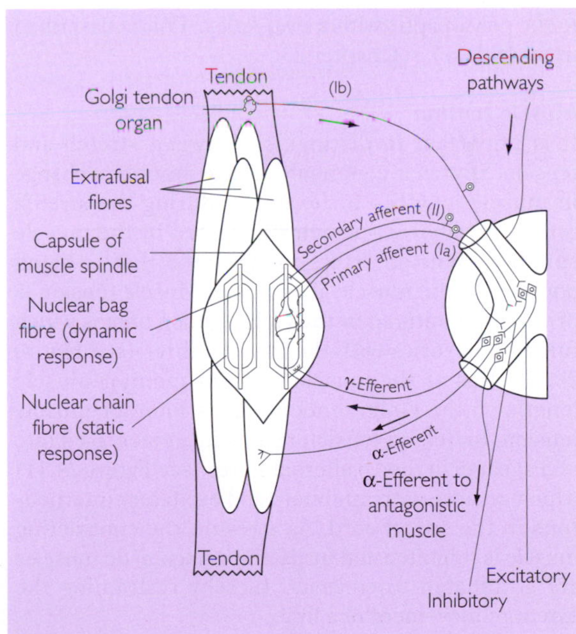


**Figure 24.11** Diagrammatic representation of the interaction between intrafusal and extrafusal muscle fibres. Extrafusal fibres (innervated by α-efferent neurons) are normal muscle fibres responsible for the primary process of muscle contraction. The intrafusal fibres (nuclear bag fibres and nuclear chain fibres) are supplied by γ-efferent fibres, and inform the motor nerve pool in the ventral horn of the spinal cord about their dynamic and static status via primary afferent and secondary afferent fibres. The stretch reflex results from monosynaptic communication between primary afferent and α-efferent neurons.

chain fibres result in a discharge frequency that is proportional to the length of the fibre (static response).

The amplitude of this feedback mechanism can be modulated within fine limits and extremely rapidly by stimulation of the γ-efferent system. This varies the contraction of the intrafusal fibres and hence the degree to which the specialized primary afferent nerve endings are stretched within the spindle. It functions as follows:

- the rate of γ-efferent discharge increases;
- the end portions of the intrafusal fibres contract;
- the annulospiral endings within the nuclear bag portions are stretched;
- the primary afferent fibres increase their rate of firing;
- within the spinal cord, there is an increase in the activity of the motor neuron pool;
- contraction of the extrafusal fibres is augmented via increased α-efferent discharge.

γ-Efferent discharge is controlled in several ways. It is normally linked to α-efferent discharge so that extrafusal fibres and intrafusal fibres contract simultaneously (co-activation). In addition, descending pathways modulate γ discharge as a result of a variety of inputs, including pain, anxiety, and primary afferent discharge from other muscles. Muscle tone is largely governed by the state of γ-efferent discharge.

Sudden, forceful stretching of a muscle results in the stretch reflex, which is monosynaptic, in contrast to the polysynaptic withdrawal reflex. This is described in more detail in Chapter 23.

#### *Muscle tension*

It is important to distinguish between stretch and tension. Stretch is commonly used to describe a change in muscle length – for example, during the stretch reflex (see above) – which is detected by the muscle spindles. Tension refers to the force that is being opposed by the muscle at any time. Muscle tension is primarily monitored by the Golgi tendon organs which function in series with the muscle fibres (see Figure 24.11). Just as the muscle spindles monitor muscle length, so the Golgi tendon organs monitor muscle tension. Increased tension results in an increased rate of discharge in the 1b afferent fibres (see Figure 24.11) which synapse with inhibitory and excitatory interneurons in the spinal cord. As a result, the contracting muscle is inhibited and ipsilateral antagonistic muscles are stimulated to contract, thereby restraining the extent of movement of a limb.

## CARDIAC MUSCLE

Cardiac muscle is striated but differs from skeletal muscle in its structural, electrical, and mechanical properties. Cardiac muscle fibres are relatively short and interconnect in networks via Y-shaped branches (see Chapter 20). The fibres join at intercalated discs, which anchor the extreme ends of the myofibrils and contain gap junctions that facilitate electrical conduction between fibres. In common with skeletal muscle, cardiac muscle fibres contain myofibrils into which are packed thin (actin) and thick (myosin) fibres. M lines and Z lines represent the attachments of thick and thin fibres respectively.

The cardiac conduction system contains muscle fibres with characteristics that permit the spontaneous generation of action potentials which is central to the rhythmicity of the heart. The morphology of action potentials in the heart is shown in Figure 24.12.

### Generation of action potentials

In common with skeletal muscle, the cardiac cell membrane is considerably more permeable to potassium than to sodium. The electrical events that are responsible for the initiation and maintenance of an action potential in the conducting system are different from those in the vast majority of the contractile cardiac muscle (non-pacemaker) cells.

#### *Non-pacemaker (cardiac muscle) cells*

Transient opening of voltage-gated sodium channels initiates the muscle action potential in a similar way to that in skeletal muscle (Figure 24.13b). The cardiac muscle action potential lasts a third of a second, in comparison with less than 10 ms in a skeletal muscle fibre (Figure 24.13a, c). This is the result of prolonged opening of voltage-gated calcium channels, which permit a large influx of calcium ions throughout the plateau phase (phase 2) (Figure 24.13b). The permeability of the membrane to potassium falls during the plateau phase of the action potential, and then increases above resting levels as potassium channels open during phase 3 and 4, permitting potassium to leave the muscle fibre and re-establishing the resting membrane potential.

#### *Pacemaker cells*

The resting membrane potential in these cells gradually falls, i.e. depolarizes, during diastole until the threshold for an action potential is reached (see Figure 24.13d). This is known as a pre-potential or pacemaker potential. At the end of the previous action potential, the permeability to potassium reduces and the number of potassium ions leaving the cell declines progressively,

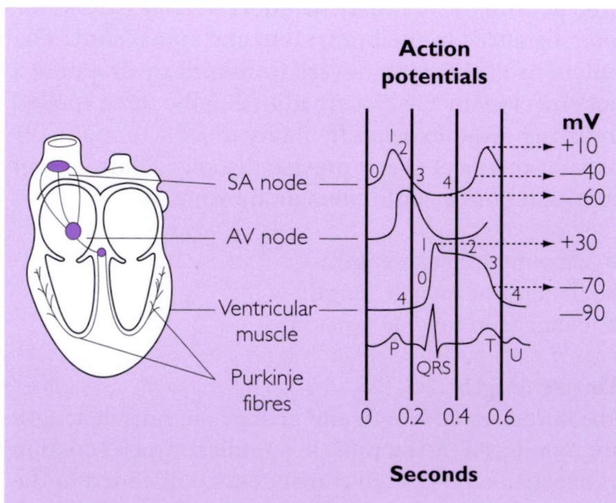


**Figure 24.12** The variation in the morphology of the action potential in the human heart. SA, sinoatrial node; AV, atrioventricular node.

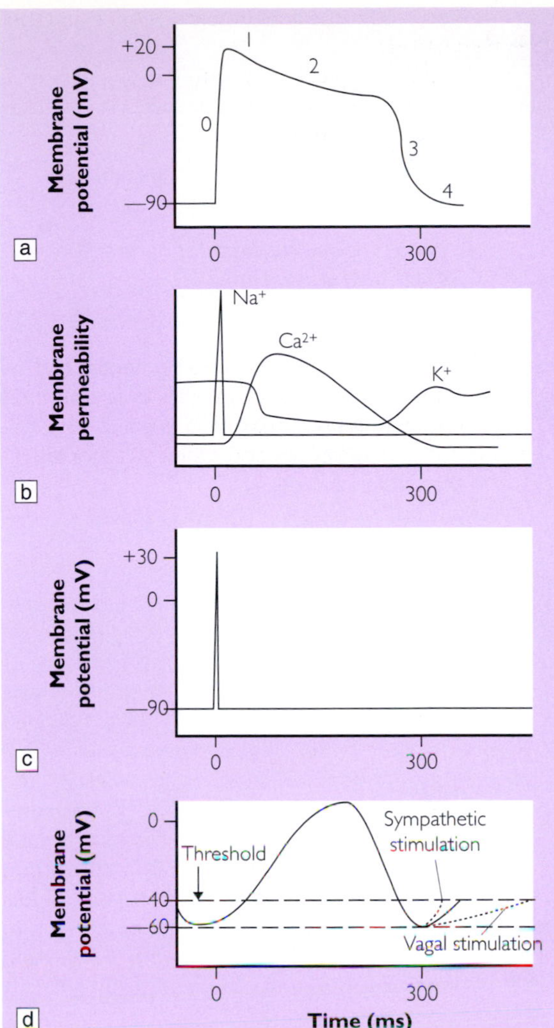


**Figure 24.13** The action potential in cardiac non-pacemaker (muscle) fibres (a, b) and pacemaker cells (c) and skeletal muscle (d).

initiating a slow process of depolarization. Transient (T) voltage-gated calcium channels open, permitting rapid influx of calcium ions and causing further depolarization. These mechanisms are opposed by vagal stimulation. The action of acetylcholine at muscarinic ($M_2$) receptors causes specific potassium channels to open, delaying the opening of calcium channels and prolonging the pre-potential (Figure 24.13d).

The ionic fluxes responsible for the action potential are different from those in non-pacemaker cells. Sodium channels do not play a part and the rise time is much slower (Figure 24.13d). The rise and decline of the action potential are almost entirely the result of opening and closing of long-lasting (L) calcium channels. Sympathetic stimulation accelerates the onset of the action potential by facilitating the early opening of the L calcium channels via an increase in intracellular cAMP.

Because of its importance, a comparison of the differences between cardiac and skeletal muscle action potentials and contraction is shown in Figure 24.14 and summarized in Table 24.4. Further details of cardiac muscle can be found in Chapter 20.

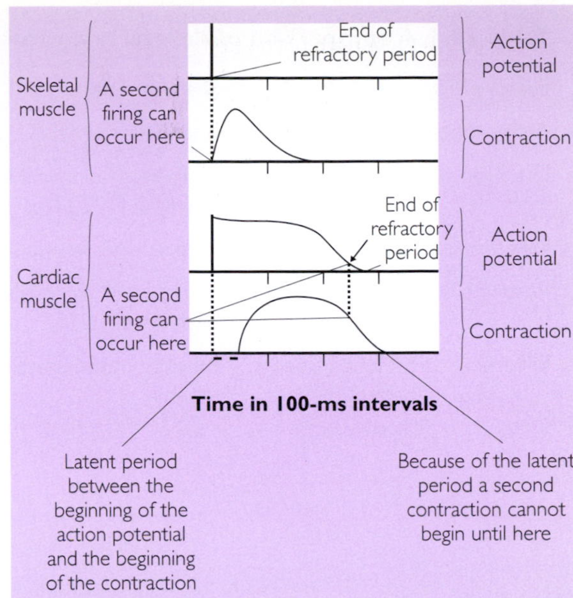


**Figure 24.14** A diagrammatic comparison of the contractile properties of skeletal and cardiac muscle.

## DISORDERS OF SKELETAL MUSCLE

### Malignant hyperthermia

Malignant hyperthermia (MH) is a potentially fatal inherited disorder of muscle which affects approximately 1 in 10 000 to 1 in 20 000 of the population. The inheritance pattern is autosomal dominant. When an MH-susceptible individual is exposed to a trigger agent, a clinical picture of excessive carbon dioxide production, metabolic acidosis, tachycardia, hyperkalaemia, muscle rigidity, and hyperthermia may develop. Trigger agents are suxamethonium or anaesthetic vapours. Two calcium channel abnormalities are thought to be responsible for the greatly increased intracellular calcium ion concentration seen in MH. These abnormalities are located at (1) the ryanodine receptor calcium channel and (2) the dihydropyridine receptor calcium channel in the T tubule.

Both these receptors play a role in excitation–contraction coupling (see above). In MH, large amounts of ATP are expended in an attempt to pump the excess calcium out of the cytosol. When ATP is exhausted, the architecture of the muscle cell starts to disintegrate and large quantities of potassium ions, myoglobin, and creatine kinase are released. Renal failure and disseminated intravascular coagulopathy may accompany MH. Management includes withdrawal of the trigger agent, hyperventilation with oxygen, administration of dantrolene, active cooling, treatment of acidosis and hyperkalaemia, and renal support. The clinical implications and management of MH are described in Chapter 13.

### Myotonia congenita

This inherited disorder in which muscle is excessively excitable appears to be associated with a mutation in the gene that codes for chloride channels in the muscle membrane. The exact normal function of chloride channels in the muscle membrane is unclear.

**Table 24.4 A comparison of skeletal and cardiac muscle**

| Feature | Skeletal muscle | Cardiac muscle |
|---|---|---|
| Action potential | Brief, approximately 1 ms | Long, 200–500 ms |
| Duration of contraction | Lasts much longer than action potential (> 200 ms) | Repolarization does not occur until after contraction completed |
| Initiation of contraction | Requires nerve impulse | No nerve impulse required for contraction |
| Resting potential | Stable, remains constant in healthy cell | Unstable, drifts towards zero |
| Differences from cell to cell | All cells in one muscle function similarly | Rate of drift, duration of action potential, and duration of the contraction differ in cardiac fibres from different regions<br>The drift is fastest and the other two shortest in the sinoatrial node |

## FURTHER READING

Booij LHDJ, ed. *Neuromuscular Transmission. Fundamentals of Anaesthesia and Acute Medicine Series*. London: BMJ Publishing Group, 1996.

Ganong WF. *Review of Medical Physiology*, 18th edn. Stamford, CA: Appleton & Lange, 1997.

Pollard BJ. Nerves, muscles and the electromyogram. *Curr Anaesth Crit Care* 1998;**9**:110–16.

# Chapter 25 The renal system

K.-L. Kong

## RENAL PHYSIOLOGY

The kidneys perform several important physiological functions. They:

- excrete the waste products of metabolism, drugs, and drug metabolites;
- conserve essential body nutrients such as amino acids and glucose;
- regulate the volume and composition of extracellular fluid;
- play an essential role in acid–base balance;
- perform endocrine functions, secreting renin, erythropoietin, kinins, and prostaglandins.

### Functional anatomy

The gross morphological anatomy of the kidney is shown in Figure 25.1. They are retroperitoneal organs, each approximately 12 cm long and 150 g in weight, which lie between vertebrae T12 and L3. The basic functional unit of the kidney is the nephron (Figure 25.2), comprising the glomerulus from which fluid is filtered and its renal tubule in which the filtered fluid is converted into urine. The glomerulus is formed by a tuft of capillaries invaginating into the dilated, blind end of the tubules known as Bowman's capsule (Figure 25.3). These capillaries are supplied by an afferent arteriole and drained by an efferent arteriole. There are about 1.3 million nephrons in each human kidney.

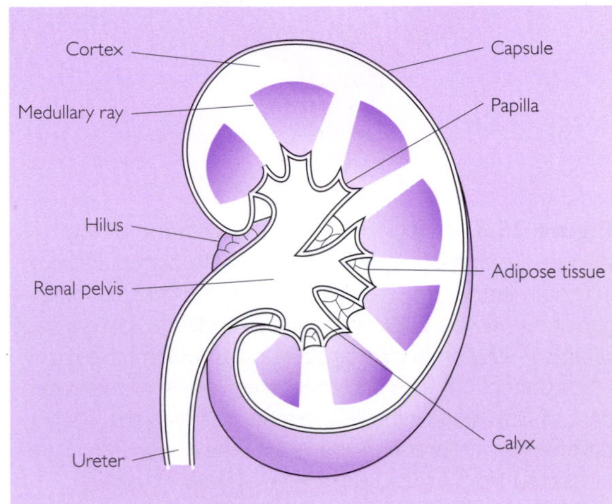


**Figure 25.1** The gross morphological anatomy of the kidney shown in longitudinal section. The vascular supply has been removed for clarity.

The glomerular filtrate formed in Bowman's capsule drains into the proximal tubule which is made up of convoluted and straight segments. Filtrate then enters the thin segment of the descending limb of the loop of Henle. Those nephrons in the outer portions of the renal cortex (cortical nephrons) have short loops of Henle, whereas those in the juxtamedullary region of the cortex (juxtamedullary nephrons) have long loops extending down to the medullary pyramids. In humans, 85% of nephrons are cortical and 15% juxtamedullary. The thin descending limb of the loop of Henle drains into the thin ascending limb (not found in cortical nephrons) and then into the thick segment of the ascending limb. From the loop of Henle, filtrate enters the distal convoluted tubule and then into a collecting duct. Collecting ducts pass through the renal cortex and medulla to empty into the renal pelvis at the apices of the medullary pyramids.

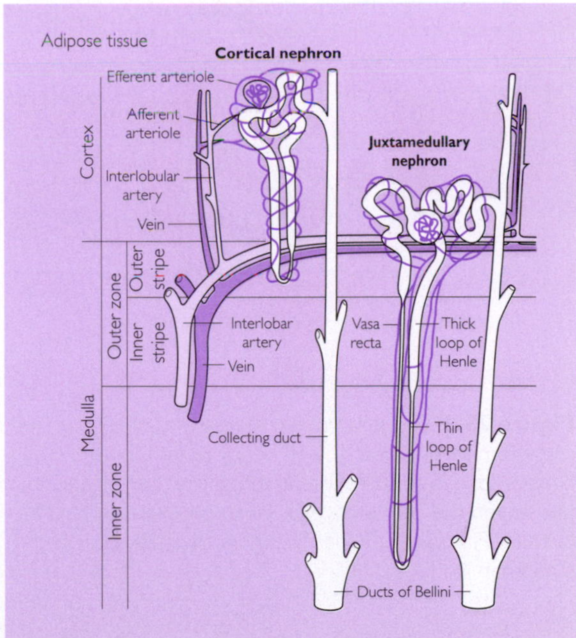


**Figure 25.2** Cortical (short looped) and juxtamedullary (long looped) nephrons showing differences in the blood supply to the two nephron types. (Adapted from Pitts RF. *Physiology of the Kidney and Body Fluids*, 3rd edn. Chicago: Yearbook Medical Publishers, 1974.)

Where the distal tubule passes through the angle between the afferent and efferent arterioles, the tubular epithelium is modified histologically to form the macula densa. Here, the walls of the afferent arterioles contain the renin-secreting juxtaglomerular cells. These cells, together with the macula densa and the granulated lacis cells near them, are collectively known as the juxtaglomerular apparatus (Figure 25.4).

### Renal circulation

In a resting adult, the kidneys receive 1.2–1.3 litres of blood per minute, or just under 25% of the cardiac

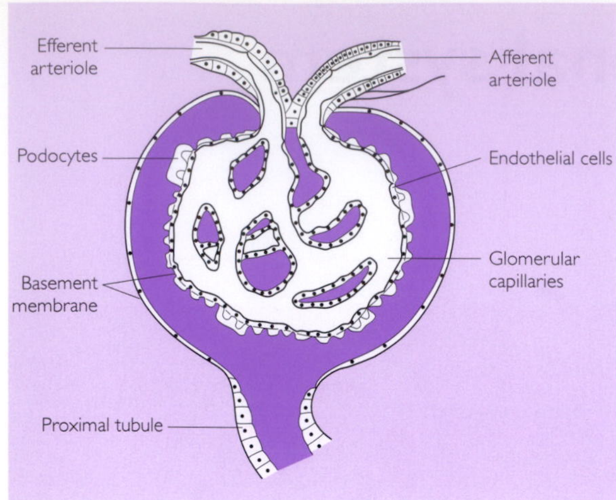


**Figure 25.3** A diagrammatic representation of the glomerulus and Bowman's capsule. In life, as the afferent arteriole enters Bowman's capsule it branches to form about six vessels. Each of these subdivides to form a knot of about 40 glomerular capillary loops, which have many interconnections. The basement membrane of the outer part of Bowman's capsule is continuous with the basement membrane of the rest of the nephron. (Adapted from Lote CJ. *Principles of Renal Physiology*, 3rd edn. London: Chapman & Hall, 1994: 34.)

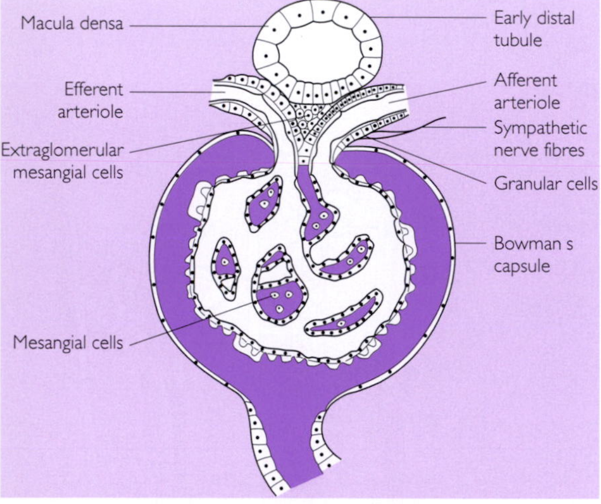


**Figure 25.4** A diagrammatic representation of the juxtaglomerular apparatus. The early distal tubule is closely applied to the afferent and efferent arterioles. In this region the cells show specialization. (Adapted from Lote CJ. *Principles of Renal Physiology*, 3rd edn. London: Chapman & Hall, 1994: 29.)

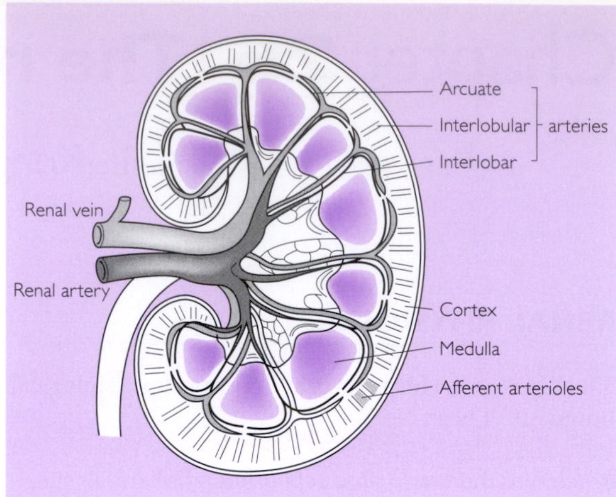


**Figure 25.5** A longitudinal section of the kidney showing the arrangement of the major blood vessels.

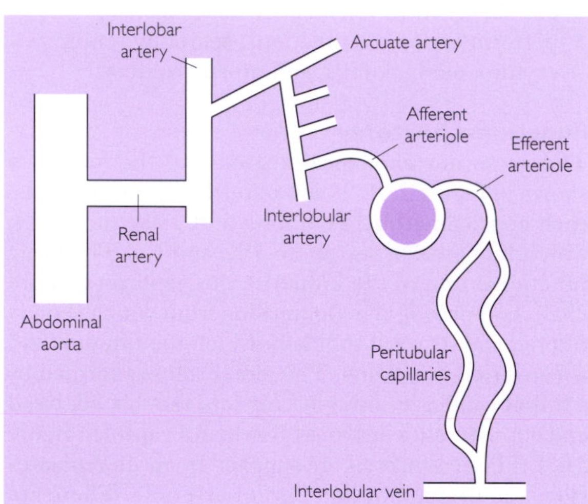


**Figure 25.6** A schematic representation of the renal circulation.

output. On the basis of flow per unit mass of tissue, this is 10 times the coronary and cerebral blood flow, and five times the flow to exercising muscle. The renal cortex receives about 75% of the renal blood flow. Arterial blood is supplied to the kidney by a renal artery or by multiple renal arteries (33% of subjects) from the abdominal aorta. The renal arteries divide into interlobar arteries, which in turn divide into arcuate and then interlobular arteries. This arrangement is shown morphologically in Figure 25.5 and diagrammatically in Figure 25.6. Afferent arterioles that supply blood to the glomeruli are short, straight branches of the interlobular arteries. The efferent arterioles break up into peritubular capillaries, which supply the renal tubules and collecting ducts before draining into the interlobular veins. Efferent arterioles from the juxtamedullary nephrons may, in addition, form hairpin loops (vasa recta) which dip into the medullary pyramids alongside the loops of Henle before returning to the renal cortex to empty into the veins. These peritubular capillaries play an important role in the reabsorption of fluid from the renal tubules. The vasa recta are particularly important in the formation of a concentrated urine (see 'osmotic gradients and the countercurrent mechanism').

The blood going to the kidney is not equally distributed: 90% goes to the cortex, which is perfused at 500 ml/min per 100 g tissue. The outer medulla has a blood flow of 100 ml/min per 100 g tissue and the inner medulla 20 ml/min per 100 g tissue. This makes the inner medulla highly susceptible to hypoxic

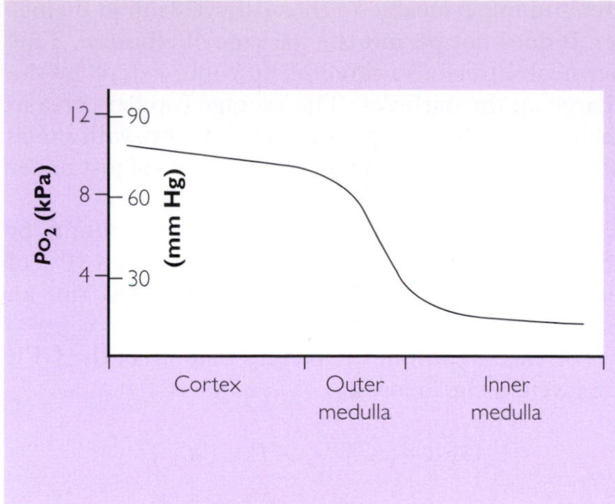


**Figure 25.7** The partial pressure of oxygen ($Po_2$ plotted from the cortex to the medulla. This shows the effect of the countercurrent exchange of oxygen in the vasa recta on the oxygen tension in the inner medulla. (Adapted from Lote CJ. *Curr Anaesth Crit Care* 1992;3:1–4.)

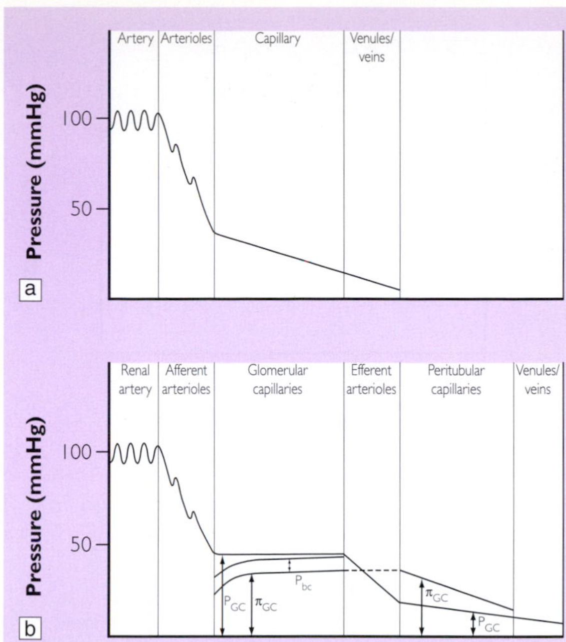


**Figure 25.8** A comparison between (a) a typical non-renal vascular bed and (b) a renal vascular bed. Note that the glomerular capillary hydrostatic pressure ($P_{GC}$) is controlled by both the afferent and the efferent arterioles and falls very little along the length of the capillary. ($\pi_{GC}$ is the osmotic pressure of the plasma in the glomerular capillaries; $P_{bc}$ is the hydrostatic pressure in the Bowman's capsule. (Adapted from Lote CJ. *Principles of Renal Physiology*, 3rd edn. London: Chapman and Hall, 1994.)

damage from falls in renal blood flow. The partial pressure of oxygen in the kidney is shown in Figure 25.7.

***Autoregulation of renal blood flow***

Renal blood flow (RBF) is determined by renal perfusion pressure and renal vascular resistance. The fall in blood pressure through the renal vasculature differs from that in other organs and is shown in Figure 25.8. The fundamental difference is the presence of afferent and efferent arterioles on either side of the glomerulus, which control the glomerular capillary pressure. Intrinsic and neurohumoral dilators and constrictors acting on these arterioles are summarized in Figure 25.9. Angiotensin II exerts a selective constrictor effect on the efferent arterioles. Prostaglandins increase RBF by causing renal vasodilatation. Atrial natriuretic peptide (ANP) causes afferent vasodilatation but efferent vasoconstriction, thus maintaining urine output in conditions of reduced blood flow. In addition, catecholamines constrict the renal vessels, particularly the interlobular arteries and afferent arterioles. Similarly, stimulation of the sympathetic noradrenergic nerves to the kidney causes a decrease in RBF mediated via $\alpha_1$- and postsynaptic $\alpha_2$-adrenoceptors.

Renal arterial autoregulation maintains RBF over a wide range of arterial pressures (Figure 25.10). RBF and glomerular filtration rate (GFR) remain relatively constant between mean arterial pressures of 80 and 180 mmHg. At and below a mean arterial pressure of 50 mmHg the decrease in RBF becomes highly significant. Renal autoregulation is an intrinsic phenomenon and is present in denervated kidneys. Two intrarenal mechanisms are responsible for autoregulation:

1. a direct contractile response of the smooth muscle of the afferent arteriole to stretch (the myogenic theory);
2. tubuloglomerular feedback (see later).

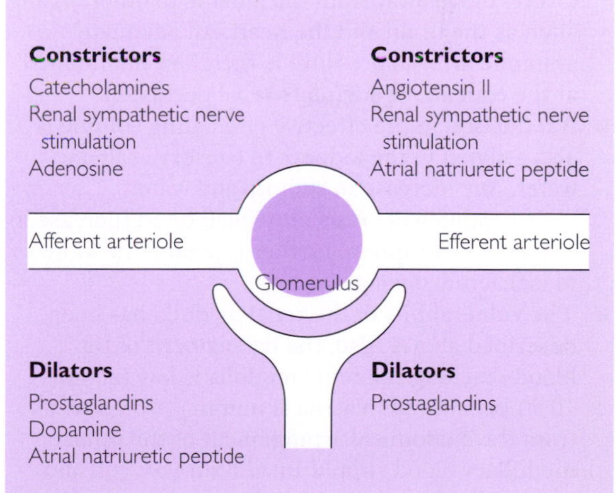


**Figure 25.9** Important modulators of renal vascular resistance.

***Renal oxygen consumption***

Although the kidneys have a high oxygen consumption, the arteriovenous oxygen difference across the kidney is small because of their enormous blood supply. About 80% of renal oxygen consumption is utilized to drive the $Na^+/K^+$ ATPase responsible for sodium reabsorption in the nephron. The higher the RBF, the greater the volume of filtrate produced and the higher the oxygen consumption necessary for

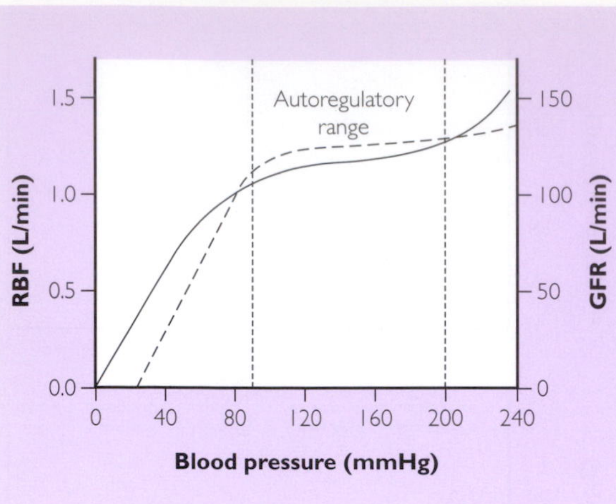


**Figure 25.10** The autoregulation of renal blood flow (RBF; solid line) and glomerular filtration rate (GFR; dashed line).

solute reabsorption from the renal tubules. Thus, renal oxygen consumption tends to vary linearly with RBF.

***Vulnerability of the kidneys to ischaemic damage***

Although the kidneys have a high supply of blood and oxygen, they are nevertheless vulnerable to ischaemic damage for the following reasons:

- The kidneys play a major role in the regulation of the systemic arterial pressure. When the effective circulating volume falls, sympathetic stimulation results in renal vasoconstriction which diverts blood away from the kidneys to other organs such as the brain and the heart. An adequate systemic arterial pressure is therefore maintained at the expense of adequate renal perfusion.
- A reduction in the effective circulating volume is also a signal to the kidneys to conserve salt and water. Any increase in sodium and water reabsorption will be accompanied by an increase in oxygen consumption, further exposing the kidneys to ischaemic damage.
- The vulnerability of the renal medulla has been described above. Also, the haematocrit of the blood reaching the renal medulla is low (about 10%) because of 'plasma skimming' which results from the anatomical arrangement of the renal medullary blood supply. In addition, oxygen and carbon dioxide take part in the countercurrent exchange mechanism in the vasa recta. The result is that the cells of the renal papilla are subjected to an environment of poor oxygen delivery, poor carbon dioxide removal, and high osmolality.

## Glomerular filtration

Glomerular filtration is the process by which fluid, solutes, and other substances move from the glomerular capillaries into Bowman's capsule. The glomerulus is approximately 200 μm in diameter. The blood is separated from the capsular space by capillary and tubular epithelium. Functionally, the glomerulus is permeable to neutral substances up to 4 nm in diameter and impermeable to those above 8 nm in diameter. It does not permit the passage of albumin. This permeability is also affected to some extent by the charge on the particles. The average capillary area in each glomerulus is approximately 0.4 $mm^2$, with a total filtration area for both kidneys in humans of just under 1 $m^2$.

The GFR in humans is about 125 ml/min or 180 L/day. This makes the GFR approximately 10% of the blood flow and 20% of the plasma flow (for an assumed haematocrit of 0.45).

For each nephron, the factors that affect the GFR are given by the following:

$$\text{GFR} = K_f\,[P_{GC} - P_{bc} - \pi_{GC}]$$

where $K_f$ is the glomerular ultrafiltration coefficient (the product of the glomerular capillary wall permeability and the effective filtration surface area), $P_{GC}$ is the mean hydrostatic pressure in the glomerular capillaries, $P_{bc}$ is the mean hydrostatic pressure in the Bowman's capsule, and $\pi_{GC}$ is the osmotic pressure of the plasma in the glomerular capillaries.

The glomerular capillary membrane is very many times more permeable than that of tissue capillaries. Whether a substance is filtered or not depends on its molecular size and electrical charge. Smaller substances are more likely to be filtered than larger substances, positively charged substances are more likely to be filtered than neutral substances, and neutral substances are more easily filtered than negatively charged ones.

***Glomerular filtration pressure***

The capillary hydrostatic pressure causes filtration of fluid from the glomerulus into Bowman's capsule, and this depends on an adequate renal perfusion pressure of about 60 mmHg. This is necessary to overcome the hydrostatic pressure in Bowman's capsule (about 18 mmHg) and plasma oncotic pressure. As blood passes through the glomerular capillaries, plasma protein concentration rises as a result of loss of fluid into Bowman's capsule. Thus, the plasma oncotic pressure rises from about 28 to 36 mmHg. The glomerular filtration pressure is the difference between these two sets of opposing pressures. Changes in the glomerular capillary hydrostatic pressure (caused by changes in systemic arterial pressure, or afferent or efferent arteriolar constriction), changes in hydrostatic pressure in Bowman's capsule, or changes in plasma proteins will have predictable effects on the net glomerular filtration pressure.

## Renal tubular function

The amount of any substance that is filtered is the product of the GFR and the plasma concentration of the substance. In addition, substances may be secreted into or reabsorbed from the tubular lumen. This is shown diagrammatically in Figure 25.11. Transport mechanisms include endocytosis, passive or facilitated diffusion down chemical or electrical gradients, or active transport against such gradients. Active transport systems have a maximal rate or transport maximum for a particular substance, above which the mechanism is saturated. Examples of substances that

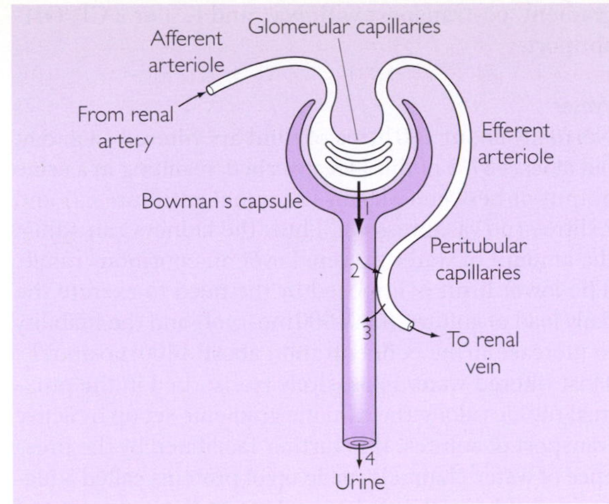


**Figure 25.11** A diagrammatic representation to illustrate the terminology of renal function. (1) Filtration that occurs at the glomerulus (2) is reabsorption and (3) is secretion that occurs along the nephron and collecting duct. (4) Urine that is excreted via the bladder. (Adapted from Lote CJ. *Principles of Renal Physiology,* 3rd edn. London: Chapman & Hall, 1994: 47.)

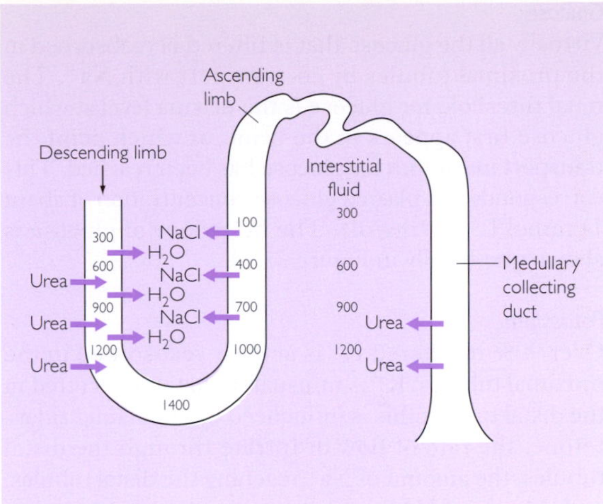


**Figure 25.12** Changes in the filtrate and interstitial osmolality brought about by the countercurrent mechanism. (Adapted from Vander AJ. *Renal Physiology,* 5th edn. New York: McGraw-Hill, 1995.)

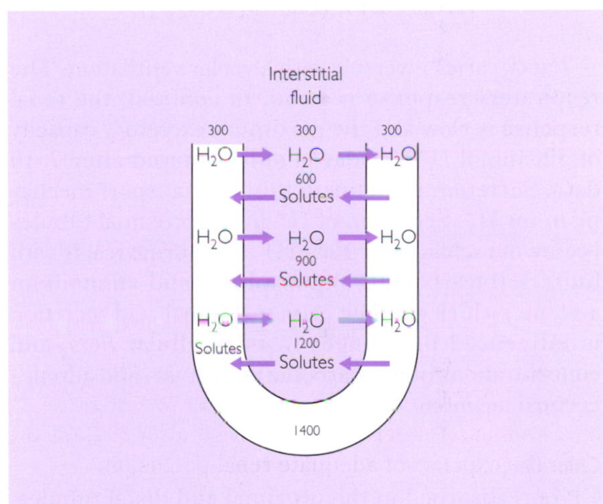


**Figure 25.13** The countercurrent exchange of water and solutes (sodium and urea) in the vasa recta.

are actively absorbed from the tubular lumen are $Na^+$, $Cl^-$, $K^+$, $Ca^{2+}$, and $PO_4^{2-}$ ions. Glucose and amino acids are absorbed from the lumen by secondary active transport, sharing a common carrier with sodium; the energy for the active transport is provided by the $Na^+/K^+$ ATPase which pumps the $Na^+$ out of the cell. $H^+$ and $K^+$ are examples of substances that are actively secreted into the tubular lumen. Their specific behaviour is described later.

#### *Osmotic gradients and the countercurrent mechanism*

The ability of the kidneys to produce a concentrated urine depends on the maintenance of a gradient of increasing osmolality along the medullary pyramids. This is brought about by the long loops of Henle of juxtaglomerular nephrons, which act as countercurrent multipliers, and their accompanying vasa recta, which act as countercurrent exchangers. The descending limb of the loop of Henle is relatively impermeable to solute but highly permeable to water. Water moves out of the tubule, and the concentration of $Na^+$ in the tubule rises as it extends deep into the medulla. In contrast, the ascending limb is impermeable to water so $Na^+$ is transported passively and actively out of the tubular fluid into the interstitium. In addition, urea enters the descending limb of the loop of Henle, increasing the osmolality of the tubular fluid in the medulla. Urea also diffuses freely from the inner medullary portion of the collecting ducts into the interstitium, maintaining the high osmolality of the medullary pyramids (Figure 25.12).

The osmotic gradient is maintained by the countercurrent exchangers (vasa recta) through the trapping of $Na^+$ and urea in the medullary pyramids. These solutes diffuse out of the vessels conducting blood towards the cortex and into the vessels descending into the pyramids. Conversely, water diffuses out of the descending vessels and into the ascending vessels (Figure 25.13). Energy is required for the countercurrent multiplier whereas countercurrent exchange in the vasa recta is a passive process.

#### *Reabsorption and secretion of specific substances*

*Sodium*

About 26 000 mmol of $Na^+$ are filtered each day. For a urinary $Na^+$ output of only 100–200 mmol/day to be achieved, 99% or more of the filtered load must be reabsorbed. Sodium is actively transported out of all parts of the renal tubule except the thin portions of the loop of Henle. In the thick portion of the ascending limb of the loop of Henle, $Na^+$ is co-transported from the lumen into the tubular epithelial cells with $K^+$ and $Cl^-$ and is then actively transported into the lateral intercellular spaces. About 80% of the $Na^+$ filtered is reabsorbed with $Cl^-$, 18.5% is reabsorbed while reabsorbing $HCO_3^-$, and very small amounts are reabsorbed in association with $H^+$ or $K^+$ secretion.

*Glucose*

Virtually all the glucose that is filtered is reabsorbed in the proximal tubules by co-transport with $Na^+$. The renal threshold for glucose is the plasma level at which glucose first appears in the urine, at which point the transport maximum for glucose has been reached. This corresponds to a plasma glucose concentration of about 11 mmol/L (200 mg/dl). The behaviour of glucose is shown graphically in Figure 25.14.

*Potassium*

Over 90% of filtered $K^+$ is actively reabsorbed in the proximal tubules. $K^+$ is unusual in that it is secreted in the distal tubule; this is influenced by circulating aldosterone, the rate of flow of filtrate through the distal tubules, the amount of $Na^+$ reaching the distal tubules, and the rate of $H^+$ secretion.

*Hydrogen*

$H^+$ homoeostasis is regulated by the body's respiratory and renal systems. The arterial $H^+$ activity can be represented by the Henderson equation (see Chapter 26):

$$[H^+] = 24 \times (Pa\text{CO}_2/[\text{HCO}_3^-]).$$

$Pa\text{CO}_2$ varies inversely with alveolar ventilation. The respiratory response is rapid. In contrast, the renal response is slow and the maximum excretory capacity of 300 mmol $H^+$ per day is only achieved after 7–10 days. Secretion is the main tubular transport mechanism for $H^+$. Secretion of $H^+$ in the proximal tubules occurs in exchange for $Na^+$. $H^+$ in the urine reacts with buffers (bicarbonate, diphosphate, and ammonium systems) which are then excreted. Renal acid secretion is influenced by changes in intracellular $P\text{CO}_2$ and concentrations of $K^+$, carbonic anhydrase, and adrenocortical hormone.

*Chloride*

$Cl^-$ is reabsorbed in the proximal and distal tubules, loop of Henle, and collecting ducts. This occurs by passive diffusion down a concentration or electrical gradient, co-transport with $Na^+$ and $K^+$, or a $Cl^-/OH^-$ antiport.

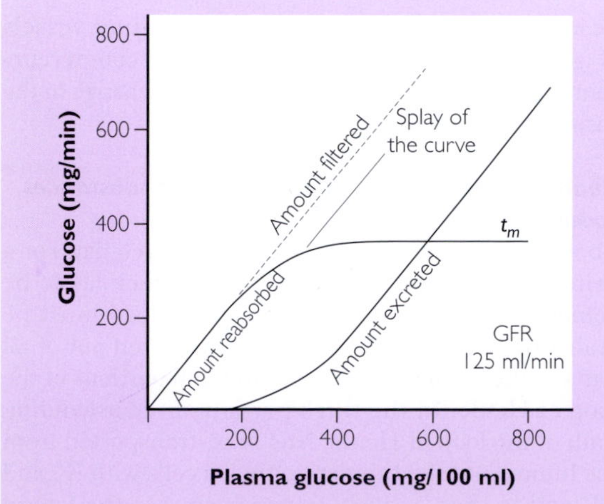


**Figure 25.14** The interrelationship of the plasma glucose concentration, the amount of glucose filtered, the amount reabsorbed, and the amount excreted. GFR, glomerular filtration rate; $t_m$, transport maximum.

*Water*

Normally about 180 litres of fluid are filtered each day, but at least 87% of this is reabsorbed, resulting in a urine output of between 500 ml (maximal antidiuresis) and 23 litres (no vasopressin). Thus, the kidneys can adjust the amount of water excreted over an enormous range. The lower limit is imposed by the need to excrete the daily load of solutes (600–900 mosmol) and the inability to increase urine concentration above 1400 mosmol/L. Most filtered water is passively reabsorbed in the proximal tubules along the osmotic gradients set up by active transport of solutes. It is further facilitated by the presence of water channels made up of proteins called aquaporin-1. These channels supplement the movement of water by simple diffusion. (Other members of this family are aquaporin-2 found in the cells of the collecting ducts, aquaporin-3 found in collecting duct membranes, aquaporin-4 found in the brain, and aquaporin-5 found in salivary and lacrimal glands.) Reabsorption of water continues along the loop of Henle (about 20% of the total), the distal tubules (about 5% of the total), and the collecting ducts, largely under the influence of the countercurrent mechanism, and the effects of antidiuretic hormone (ADH), ANP, and the renin–angiotensin–aldosterone system.

As described earlier, only 15% of the nephrons in humans are of the juxtamedullary type with long loops of Henle that pass through the medulla. The other 85% (see Figure 25.2) are cortical nephrons with short loops. The nephrons with short loops are unable to produce very hypertonic conditions. However, the collecting tubules of all nephrons pass through the medulla and are able to use the hypertonicity of the medulla to produce concentrated urine.

### *The changes in composition of the filtrate through the kidney*

The handling of individual substances and the production of hyperosmolar conditions have already been described. As an aid to understanding, this brief section considers the composition and volume of the filtrate as it flows through a juxtamedullary nephron. By comparing the nephron contents with the processes described immediately above, a more integrated picture emerges. In all these examples the nephron is represented linearly, as if it were stretched out.

The behaviour of water and the urine osmolarity are shown in Figure 25.15. It can be clearly seen from Figure 25.15a that 70% of the water is reabsorbed by the time the filtrate reaches the loop of Henle. The subsequent effect of ADH is shown in the cortical and medullary collecting ducts where the urine volume can vary from below 0.5% of the original filtered volume (< 0.5 L/day) to 13% (> 23 L/day). The changes in osmolarity as the filtrate moves through the nephron are shown in Figure 25.15b. It can be seen that the filtrate always changes from being iso-osmolar with plasma in the proximal tubule, through a peak of 1400 mosmol at the tip of the loop of Henle, to being hypo-osmolar in the upper part of the thick ascending loop of Henle. The final urine osmolarity is then determined by the action of ADH which produces a range

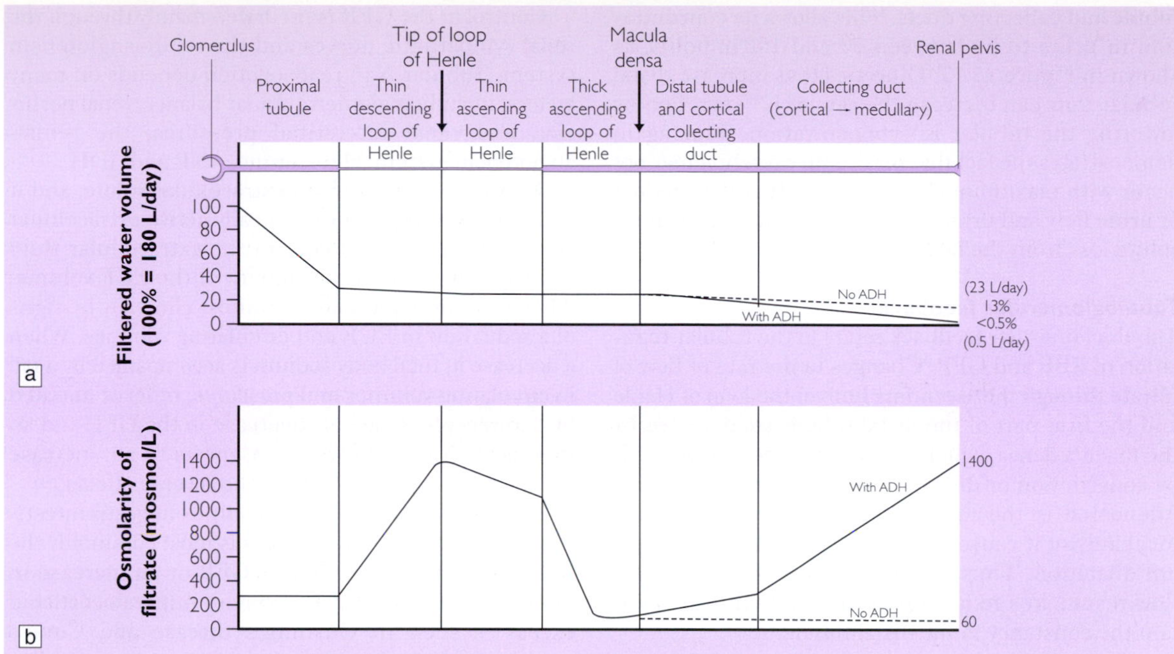


**Figure 25.15** The volume and osmolarity of the glomerular filtrate as it moves through the nephron. The nephron is represented linearly at the top of the graph with the changes plotted at corresponding points below. (a) The filtered water volume assuming that the volume is 100% to start with. (b) The osmolarity of the filtrate. In (a), 100% filtered water volume is 180 L/day. ADH, antidiuretic hormone. (See text for details.)

from 60 to 1400 mosmol secondary to the movement of water shown in Figure 25.15a.

The behaviour of $Na^+$ in many ways follows the concentration gradients similar to those of osmolarity (Figure 25.16a). The action of ADH can change the final $Na^+$ concentration from about 50 to 500 mmol/L secondary to the movement of water (Figure 25.16a and see Figure 25.15). The actual effect that this 10-fold concentration range has on the overall sodium balance of the body is, however, very much smaller. As can be seen in Figure 25.16b, the vast amount of $Na^+$ filtered (> 98%) is reabsorbed by the time the ADH can have its effect. Consequently, ADH is affecting, on average, only 1% of the total filtered $Na^+$.

Potassium is unusual in that it is secreted, possibly passively by electrochemical gradients, in the late distal

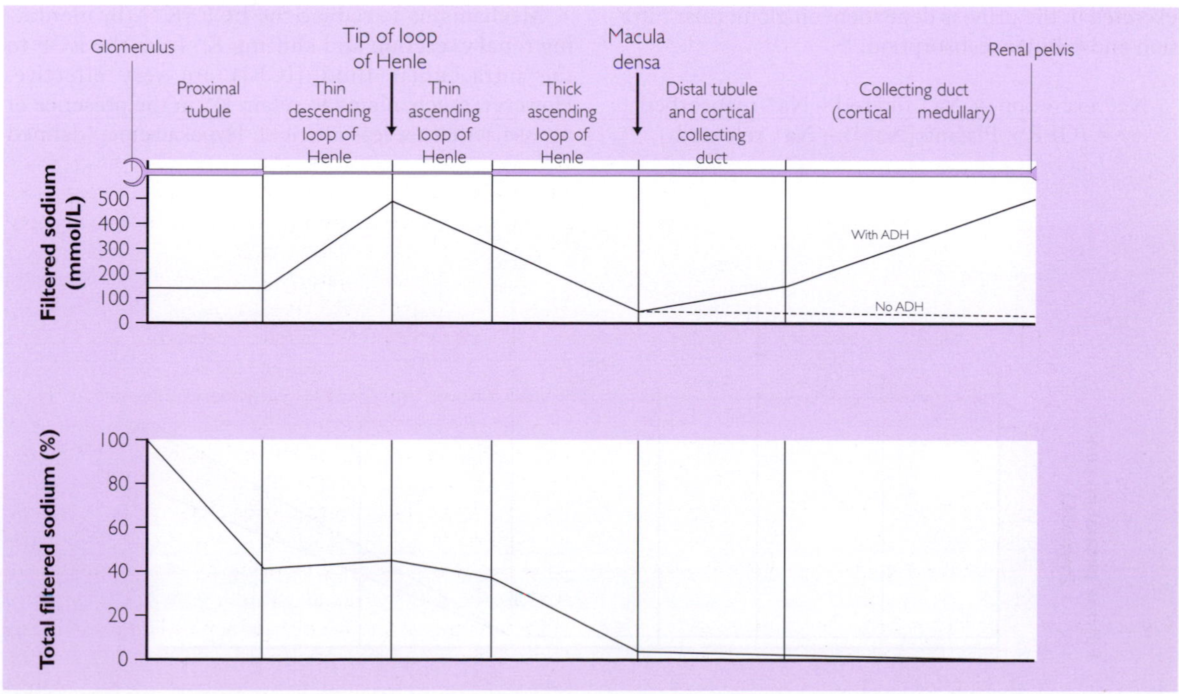


**Figure 25.16** The changes in the concentration of sodium in the filtrate and the total filtered sodium.

tubule and collecting ducts. This allows its concentration in urine to lie between 70 and 100 mmol/L, as shown in Figure 25.17. Diuretics that increase distal tubular flow can increase the rate of $K^+$ secretion by lowering the tubular $K^+$ concentration. This again demonstrates the fact that maximum excretion may not occur with maximum concentration. It is the product of urine flow and urine concentration that determines solute loss from the body.

### *Tubuloglomerular feedback*

Tubuloglomerular feedback refers to the tubular regulation of RBF and GFR. Changes in the rate of flow of filtrate through the ascending limb of the loop of Henle and the first part of the distal tubule are detected by the macula densa, which feeds back to adjust the GFR by constriction or dilatation of the afferent arteriole. Adenosine is the major mediator in this feedback mechanism; it causes afferent constriction but efferent dilatation. Thus, an increase in RBF and filtrate flow results in a reduction in RBF and GFR to maintain the constancy in the distal tubule.

### *Glomerulotubular balance*

This refers to the ability of the proximal tubule to reabsorb a constant fraction of the amount of substance filtered rather than a constant amount. This proportionality in reabsorption is especially important in the case of $Na^+$ where there may be large variations in the amount of $Na^+$ filtered in the glomeruli. The mechanisms responsible for glomerulotubular balance are completely intrarenal and are not under external neural or hormonal control.

## Homoeostatic functions and hormonal effects

### *Sodium homoeostasis*

Body sodium content is regulated by the balance between intake (in the diet) and output (mainly in the urine but also in sweat and faeces). The amount of $Na^+$ excreted in the urine is dependent on glomerular filtration and tubular reabsorption:

$$\begin{aligned} Na^+ \text{ excretion} &= Na^+ \text{ filtered} - Na^+ \text{ reabsorbed} \\ &= (\text{GFR} \times \text{Plasma } [Na^+]) - Na^+ \text{ released.} \end{aligned}$$

Control of the GFR is mediated mainly through the renal sympathetic nerves and the renin–angiotensin system. Tubular $Na^+$ reabsorption depends on many factors, including glomerulotubular balance, renal perfusion and renal interstitial pressures, the renin–angiotensin system, aldosterone, ANP, and ADH.

As $Na^+$ is essentially an extracellular solute, and it is the most important osmotically active extracellular solute, the amount of $Na^+$ in the extracellular fluid (ECF) is the major determinant of the ECF volume. Thus sodium depletion is manifest clinically by signs of a reduction in ECF and circulating volumes. When a decrease in total body sodium is accompanied by a fall in circulating volumes and pressures, reflexes initiated by baroreceptors cause a decrease in the GFR and an increase in $Na^+$ reabsorption. Conversely, any increase in total body sodium will have the reverse effects.

A net sodium deficit may result from gastrointestinal or renal loss. Sodium excess is most commonly the result of either a decrease in GFR or an increase in mineralocorticoid activity. Primary mineralocorticoid excess is seen in Cushing's disease and Conn's syndrome. Mineralocorticoid activity may be secondarily elevated in conditions that result in stimulation of the renin–angiotensin system, such as in cardiac failure, liver disease, or nephrotic syndrome.

### *Potassium homoeostasis*

About 90% of total body potassium is intracellular, and $K^+$ is the principal intracellular cation. Maintenance of total body potassium depends on the balance between dietary intake (normally 50–150 mmol/day) and urinary loss (normally 30–150 mmol/day). Aldosterone increases the secretion of $K^+$ in the distal tubules and collecting ducts. $K^+$ secretion is also enhanced by alkalosis and increased concentrations of $Na^+$ in the tubular filtrate. Intracellular $K^+$ concentration ($[K^+]$) is regulated by the $Na^+/K^+$ pump. The other important determinant is the pH: acidosis promotes a shift of $K^+$ into cells and alkalosis promotes the reverse shift.

Mechanisms to reduce the ECF $[K^+]$ (by increasing renal excretion and shifting $K^+$ from the ECF to the intracellular fluid [ICF]) are very effective. However, mechanisms to retain $K^+$ in the presence of hypokalaemia are less efficient. Hypokalaemia (defined

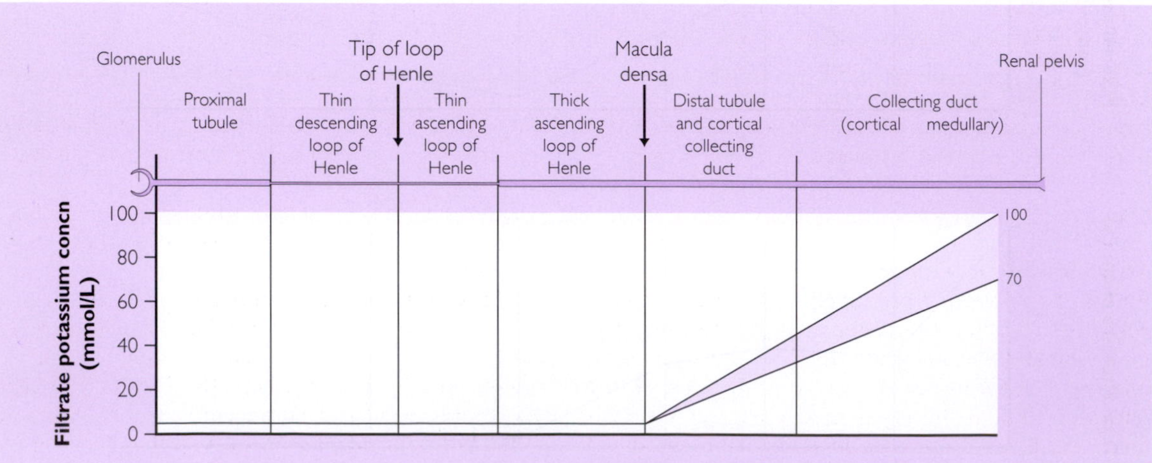


**Figure 25.17** The changes in the filtrate potassium concentration as it passes down the nephron.

as serum potassium < 3.5 mmol/L) is caused by decreased oral intake, increased renal or gastrointestinal losses, or a shift of $K^+$ from the ECF into the ICF. Hyperkalaemia (defined as serum potassium > 5.5 mmol/L) may be the result of excessive intake, renal failure, severe tissue damage, or a shift of $K^+$ from the ICF into the ECF.

#### *Antidiuretic hormone*

ADH or vasopressin is produced in the posterior pituitary. Its principal physiological effect is water retention by the kidneys. Both an increase in plasma osmotic pressure and a decrease in ECF volume are potent stimuli for its release. Other stimuli, such as pain and surgical stress, and drugs such as morphine also increase the release of ADH. ADH increases the permeability of the collecting ducts to water. This is effected by the insertion of protein water channels known as aquaporin-2. These are stored in endosomes inside the cell, and ADH causes their rapid translocation to the luminal membranes. When antidiuresis is maximal, water moves from the cortical and medullary collecting ducts into the renal interstitium, leading to the production of a highly concentrated urine. In the absence of ADH, the collecting duct epithelium is relatively impermeable to water, and the tubular fluid remains hypotonic, leading to the production of large volumes of dilute urine. In humans, the urine osmolality may be as high as 1400 mosmol/L or as low as 30 mosmol/L.

The syndrome of inappropriate ADH secretion is a condition where there is an increased level of ADH secretion in the absence of the usual osmotic or volume stimuli for ADH secretion (such as hypovolaemia and hypotension). Urinary sodium excretion exceeds 20 mmol/L and urine osmolality exceeds plasma osmolality, resulting in hypotonic hyponatraemia. Causes include ADH-producing tumours such as small-cell bronchogenic carcinoma, and central nervous system disorders such as head injuries.

#### *Water balance*

Total body water is kept constant by altering the intake and excretion of water. Intake is controlled by thirst, and excretion by the renal action of ADH, both being closely linked to the osmolality of the ECF. Plasma osmolalities of about 280 mosmol/L produce maximal suppression of ADH secretion and maximal urinary dilution. The osmotic threshold for ADH release therefore determines the lower limit of plasma osmolality. Maximum ADH secretion occurs at plasma osmolalities of about 295 mosmol/L. At these osmolalities, the thirst sensation is also stimulated which initiates drinking; this is more important in preventing dehydration than the effects of ADH.

#### *Atrial natriuretic peptide*

ANP is a polypeptide produced by the atrial muscle cells of the heart. Its secretion is increased when $Na^+$ intake is increased and when the ECF compartment is increased. ANP increases $Na^+$ excretion and urine output, although the exact mechanism of action is uncertain. It also lowers the blood pressure, produces vasodilatation of vascular smooth muscle, and inhibits the secretion of aldosterone, renin, and ADH.

#### *The renin–angiotensin–aldosterone system*

Renin, a proteolytic enzyme, is produced by the juxtaglomerular cells of the afferent arterioles of the kidneys. Renin secretion is increased by stimuli that decrease the ECF volume and blood pressure, or increase sympathetic output. Thus, factors that increase renin release include:

- decreased right atrial pressure;
- decreased renal perfusion pressure;
- increased sympathetic activity via renal nerve stimulation;
- increased circulating catecholamines via $\beta_1$-adrenoceptor stimulation;
- decreased delivery of filtered tubular $Na^+$ to the macula densa.

Renin release is inhibited by the following:

- increased $Na^+$ and $Cl^-$ reabsorption across the macula densa;
- ANP;
- angiotensin II;
- vasopressin.

Renin has a half-life in the circulation of 80 minutes and it converts angiotensinogen (a circulating $\alpha_2$-globulin formed in the liver) into angiotensin I (a decapeptide). Angiotensin I is rapidly converted into angiotensin II (an octapeptide) by pulmonary angiotensin-converting enzyme (ACE). Although most of this reaction occurs during the passage of the blood through the lungs, ACE is present in all epithelial cells. The metabolic pathway is shown schematically in Figure 25.18.

Angiotensin II is destroyed rapidly, its half-life in humans being only 1–2 minutes. The enzymes that destroy angiotensin II are lumped together under the term 'angiotensinase'. They include an aminopeptidase which produces a fragment with physiological activity called angiotensin III. Angiotensin II is the major mediator of the renin–angiotensin system and plays a predominant role in the long-term regulation of fluid volume homoeostasis and blood pressure. It acts via:

- the vascular smooth muscle, causing arteriolar vasoconstriction;
- the central and peripheral nervous system, facilitating sympathetic activity;
- the adrenal cortex, increasing secretion of aldosterone, leading to sodium and water reabsorption;
- the brain, increasing ADH secretion and inducing a dipsogenic effect leading to water retention.

Angiotensin III has the same mineralocorticoid activity as angiotensin II, but only 40% of its pressor activity.

Aldosterone is the principal mineralocorticoid secreted by the adrenal cortex (see Chapter 29). The main stimuli for its release are renin acting via angiotensin II, a rise in plasma [$K^+$] or a fall in plasma [$Na^+$], and circulating adrenocorticotrophic hormone. In the kidneys, aldosterone acts on the distal tubules and collecting ducts where increased amounts of $Na^+$ are exchanged for $K^+$ and $H^+$. As $Na^+$ reabsorption is

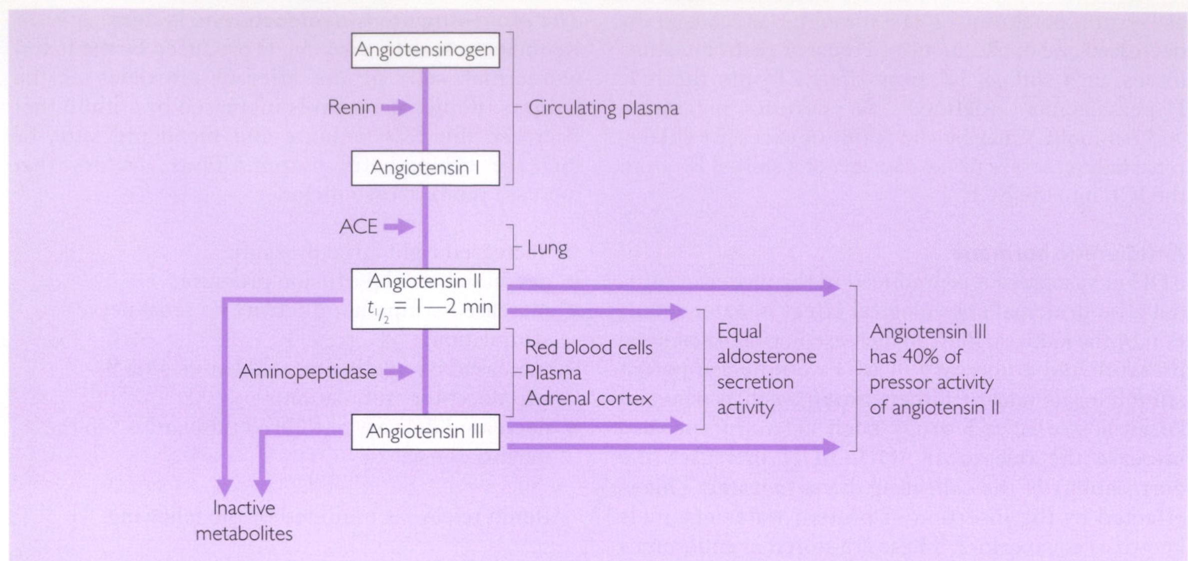


**Figure 25.18** The metabolic pathway of angiotensin formation and breakdown. ACE, angiotensin-converting enzyme.

accompanied by water reabsorption, the net result is an increase in ECF volume, a $K^+$ diuresis, and an increase in urine acidity.

### *Prostaglandins*

Many of the prostaglandins produced by the vascular endothelium and tubular epithelial cells of the kidneys are vasodilators. Production of these vasodilator prostaglandins such as $PGE_2$ and prostacyclin ($PGI_2$) is stimulated by increased renal nerve activity and angiotensin II. Vasodilator prostaglandins therefore play a renal protective role by maintaining RBF and GFR during times of stress.

### *Kinins*

Two vasodilator peptides, bradykinin and lysyl-bradykinin, are produced in the kidneys. These kinins are produced from precursor proteins called kininogens. Cells of the distal renal tubules secrete proteases called kallikreins which convert kininogens to kinins. Although bradykinin can exert potent effects on the renal vasculature, its precise physiological function in the kidneys is unclear.

### *Erythropoietin*

Erythropoietin is a glycoprotein produced primarily in the endothelial cells of the peritubular capillaries in the renal cortex. The remaining 15% is produced in the liver. Erythropoietin increases the number of stem cells in the bone marrow that are converted to red blood cell precursors and to mature erythrocytes. With anaemia or hypoxia, renal synthesis and secretion of erythropoietin can increase rapidly by 100-fold or more. Erythropoietin secretion is also increased by catecholamines and adenosine, and the alkalosis that develops at high altitude. The feedback loop can, however, be interrupted at any point – by renal disease, structural damage of the marrow, or iron, vitamin, or mineral deficiency. For example, iron deficiency from any cause will suppress the bone marrow response to high concentrations of erythropoietin.

The gene for erythropoietin has been cloned, and recombinant erythropoietin is available for clinical use such as for the treatment of anaemia associated with chronic renal failure.

## Physiological responses

### *Effects of hypovolaemia*

In mild hypovolaemia, glomerular filtration is maintained by a reduction in afferent arteriolar tone mediated by prostaglandins and ANP. Renal hypoperfusion also stimulates the release of renin from the juxtaglomerular cells, leading to the formation of angiotensin II. The potent vasoconstrictor effect of angiotensin II helps to maintain the systemic blood pressure. It also preferentially constricts efferent arterioles, maintaining the GFR. Aldosterone production is stimulated by angiotensin II, leading to increased $Na^+$ and water reabsorption, increased ECF volume, and venous return. As more severe hypovolaemia and hypotension develop, more profound systemic vasoconstriction is produced by the effects of sympathetic stimulation, catecholamines, and the renin–angiotensin system. The result is a progressive reduction in RBF and glomerular filtration, leading to prerenal uraemia and ultimately acute renal failure.

### *Changes in osmolality*

The plasma osmolality is maintained within a narrow normal range between 280 and 295 mosmol/L by a well-characterized negative feedback loop based on the function of the vasopressin-secreting and thirst mechanisms. An increase in plasma osmolality stimulates thirst, promoting increased water intake. This increase in plasma osmolality also stimulates the release of ADH in the posterior pituitary gland, leading to water retention.

## Measurement of renal blood flow

RBF is usually measured by the application of the Fick principle. As the kidneys filter plasma, the renal plasma flow (RPF) is estimated by measuring the amount of substance excreted per unit time divided by the renal arteriovenous difference. The RBF is then calculated from the equation:

$$\text{RBF} = \text{RPF}/(1 - \text{haematocrit}).$$

Any excreted substance can be used, provided that it is not metabolized, stored, or produced by the kidney, and it does not affect RBF. An infusion of *p*-aminohippuric acid is often used to measure RBF, although its clearance is only about 90%. Normal RBF in a resting adult is 1.2–1.3 L/min.

### Measurement of the GFR

Any substance that is freely filtered (i.e. not bound to plasma proteins), not reabsorbed or secreted by the renal tubules, and not metabolized or stored in the kidneys can be used to measure the GFR:

$$\text{GFR} = U_x V / P_x$$

where $U_x$ is the concentration of substance x in the urine, $V$ is the urine flow per unit time and $P_x$ is the arterial plasma concentration of x. This calculated value is also called the clearance of x. Inulin, a polymer of fructose with a molecular weight of about 5200, is commonly used to measure the GFR. In clinical practice, the clearance of creatinine is often used as an estimate of the GFR, although some creatinine is secreted and some reabsorbed in the renal tubules.

### Renal function tests

Baseline renal function is measured by standard laboratory tests of the GFR and of renal tubular function (Table 25.1). GFR is the most frequently used index of renal function, although most diseases affecting the kidney interfere with both GFR and renal tubular function. However, most renal function tests are insensitive measurements, and significant renal disease can be present despite normal laboratory values. For example, at least half of normal renal function may be lost before tests of GFR show abnormal results. Moreover, clinical evidence of renal failure is not seen until more than 75% of nephrons are non-functional. Trends are more useful than isolated measurements in evaluating renal function.

Creatinine clearance is a reliable clinical estimate of GFR, independent of the patient's age and whether a steady state is present. Highly significant renal dysfunction is present when creatinine clearance values are less than 25 ml/min. In these patients, the doses of drugs that depend on renal excretion, such as non-depolarizing neuromuscular blocking agents, should be decreased, and electrolyte and water replacement must be carefully monitored. Patients with a creatinine clearance of less than 10 ml/min are practically anephric and will require dialysis for water and electrolyte homoeostasis.

Analysis of a patient's urinary profile may help to distinguish between prerenal and renal causes of perioperative oliguria (a urine output of $< 0.5$ ml/kg/per h) (Table 25.2).

The renal response of a healthy kidney to poor perfusion is the excretion of small volumes of highly concentrated urine that is low in $Na^+$ because of maximum tubular reabsorption. In addition, the urine : plasma urea ratio is high. Once acute renal failure is established, the urine excreted (usually of small volume) is iso-osmotic with plasma with a high $[Na^+]$. The urine : plasma urea ratio is low.

**Table 25.1 Renal function tests**

| Glomerular filtration rate | Renal tubular function |
|---|---|
| Blood urea nitrogen | Urine specific gravity |
| Plasma creatinine | Urine osmolality |
| Creatinine clearance | |

## RENAL PHARMACOLOGY

### Renal protective drugs

The mainstay of preservation of renal function is to keep the patient well hydrated with a satisfactory perfusion pressure. Hypovolaemia, hypotension, and hypoxaemia are very damaging to the kidneys. Some renal protective drugs may prevent or delay the development of acute renal failure (ARF), or limit renal damage and hasten recovery in ARF.

#### *Diuretics*

Diuretics are drugs that increase the rate of urine flow. However, clinically useful diuretics also increase the rate of $Na^+$ excretion and may also modify the renal

**Table 25.2 Urinary profiles in pre-renal and intrinsic renal failure**

| Index | Pre-renal (normal kidney) | Renal (intrinsic failure) |
|---|---|---|
| Osmolality (mosmol/kg) | High (> 500) | Low (< 290) |
| Sodium content (mmol/L) | Low (< 10–20) | High (> 40) |
| Urine : plasma urea ratio | High (20) | Low (10) |
| Urine : plasma creatinine ratio | High (40) | Low (10) |
| Urine specific gravity | High (1.02) | Fixed (1.01–1.02) |
| Urine microscopy | Normal | Tubular cells, cell casts, granular casts |

handling of other cations ($K^+$, $H^+$, $Ca^{2+}$, and $Mg^{2+}$) and anions ($Cl^-$, $HCO_3^-$, and $H_2PO_4^-$). In addition, diuretics may indirectly alter renal haemodynamics. Figure 25.19 shows the sites of action of clinically useful diuretics on the nephron. Diuretics can also be classified according to their mechanism of action.

Carbonic anhydrase inhibitors (such as acetazolamide) potently inhibit both membrane-bound and cytoplasmic forms of the enzyme in the proximal tubular epithelial cells. Carbonic anhydrase catalyses the reaction between $CO_2$ and $H_2O$, facilitating secretion of $H^+$ and reabsorption of $HCO_3^-$ and $Na^+$. Thus, acetazolamide increases the excretion of $HCO_3^-$, $Na^+$, and water. As a result of increased $Na^+$ delivery to the distal tubules and the decreased amount of available $H^+$ for exchange with $Na^+$, $K^+$ loss is increased.

Osmotic diuretics (such as mannitol) are agents that are freely filtered at the glomerulus, undergo limited reabsorption by the renal tubule, and are relatively inert pharmacologically. They act in both the proximal tubule and the loop of Henle, increasing the excretion of water and $Na^+$.

Inhibitors of the $Na^+/K^+/2Cl^-$ symport (such as frusemide (furosemide), ethacrynic acid, and bumetanide), also called loop diuretics, act on the thick ascending limb of the loop of Henle. These diuretics are highly efficacious because the thick ascending limb has a great reabsorptive capacity and about 25% of the filtered load is normally reabsorbed by the thick ascending limb. By blocking the $Na^+/K^+/2Cl^-$ symport, loop diuretics cause a profound increase in the urinary excretion of $Na^+$ and $Cl^-$, and impair the generation of a hypertonic medullary interstitium, thereby weakening the kidney's ability to concentrate urine. As the thick ascending limb is also part of the diluting segment, loop diuretics also impair the kidney's ability to excrete a dilute urine. The increased delivery of $Na^+$ to the distal tubules increases urinary excretion of $K^+$.

The thiazide diuretics are inhibitors of the $Na^+/Cl^-$ symport; they act mainly on the distal convoluted tubules, increasing $Na^+$ and $Cl^-$ excretion. They also increase $K^+$ excretion as a result of increased delivery of $Na^+$ to the distal tubule. Thiazides are only moderately efficacious (maximum excretion of filtered $Na^+$ load is only 5%) because about 90% of the filtered load is already reabsorbed before reaching the distal convoluted tubules.

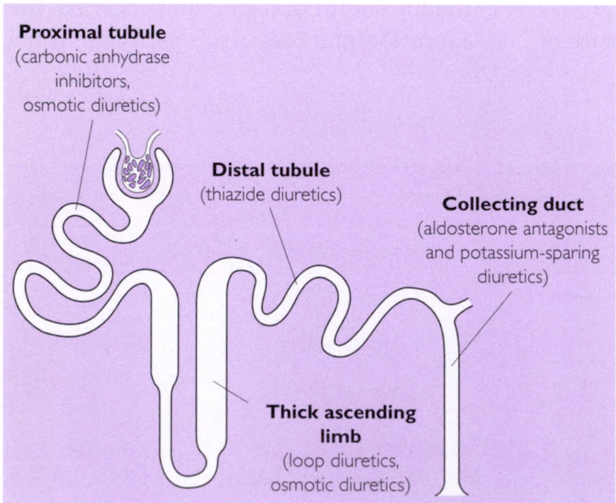


**Figure 25.19** A schematic representation of the nephron, indicating the sites of action of diuretics.

Potassium-sparing diuretics are diuretics that also have an anti-kaluretic action. Triamterene and amiloride act by blocking $Na^+$ channels in the principal cells of the late distal tubule and collecting duct. As the late distal tubule and collecting duct have a limited capacity to reabsorb solutes, these diuretics produce only a modest increase in the excretion rates of $Na^+$ and $Cl^-$. By blocking $Na^+$ reabsorption in these parts of the nephron, triamterene and amiloride also oppose the normal secretion of cations such as $K^+$ and $H^+$ in exchange for $Na^+$. Mineralocorticoids (such as aldosterone) cause salt and water retention and increase the excretion of $K^+$ and $H^+$ by binding to specific mineralocorticoid receptors. Spironolactone competitively inhibits the binding of aldosterone to cytoplasmic receptors in the cells of the late distal tubule and collecting duct. Its effects are very similar to those of triamterene and amiloride. However, its clinical efficacy is a function of the endogenous levels of aldosterone: the higher the levels of endogenous aldosterone, the greater the diuretic effects of spironolactone.

Proprietary preparations of diuretics with potassium such as Burinex K and Lasix+K are available although they are not always ideal. The amount of $K^+$ in these preparations may not be sufficient for those patients who require $K^+$ supplements, and may be a danger to those at risk of developing hyperkalaemia.

### *Diuretics and renal failure*

The use of osmotic diuretics such as mannitol in major vascular surgery, in situations of high pigment excretion (haemoglobinuria, myoglobinuria), and in jaundiced patients has been shown to be beneficial as a prophylaxis against ARF. Mannitol is completely filtered at the glomerulus and none of it is subsequently reabsorbed from the renal tubules. As a result, mannitol increases the osmolarity of renal tubular fluid and prevents reabsorption of water. Sodium is diluted in this retained water in the renal tubules, leading to less sodium reabsorption. As a result of this osmotic effect in the renal tubular fluid, there is an osmotic diuretic effect with urinary excretion of water, $Na^+$, $Cl^-$, and $HCO_3^-$ ions.

Potent loop diuretics such as frusemide may prevent or delay the progression of prerenal failure to ARF. They produce an increase in RBF and the GFR (by increasing intrarenal prostaglandin production), and decrease the oxygen-requiring function of the tubules by inhibiting $Na^+/K^+/2Cl^-$ transport in the thick ascending limb of the loop of Henle. However, frusemide itself can be nephrotoxic and, once renal failure is established, there is no evidence that diuretics influence morbidity or mortality.

Clinical management of renal impairment is described in Chapter 59.

### *Dopamine*

Low dose dopamine at 1–3 μg/kg per min may help to preserve renal perfusion.

At such dosage, dopamine predominantly stimulates dopaminergic $DA_1$ and $DA_2$-receptors, which are associated with a marked increase in RBF and sodium excretion. Increasing the infusion rate will, in a dose-dependent manner, also stimulate $\beta_1$- and $\alpha$-adrenoceptors. Several mechanisms have been advanced to explain the diuretic effects of dopamine:

- a selective increase in RBF, associated with a reduction in renal vascular resistance mediated via $DA_1$- and $DA_2$-receptors;
- an increase in RBF secondary to increases in cardiac output and blood pressure;
- an inhibitory effect on proximal tubular sodium reabsorption.

Although dopamine is widely used to prevent progression from oliguria to ARF, there has been no properly controlled study to demonstrate that renal dose dopamine (up to 5 µg/kg per min) improves outcome in patients with impending or established renal failure.

Dopexamine, a $DA_1$- and $\beta_2$-receptor agonist, may offer the same beneficial effects as renal dose dopamine.

#### *Inotropes*

Renal perfusion will be poor at mean arterial pressures of less than 60 mmHg. When adequate filling volumes and pressures have been achieved, inotropes may then be required to maintain adequate perfusion pressure, RBF, and GFR. In critically ill patients, dobutamine (a $\beta_1$- and $\beta_2$-adrenoceptor agonist) has been shown to increase the cardiac output and mean arterial pressure, leading to a significant increase in creatinine clearance.

### Renal excretion and biotransformation of drugs

The kidneys play a crucial role in the excretion of uncharged molecules and of water-soluble drugs and their metabolites which have low molecular weights (below 400 Da). The kidneys also have a role in drug biotransformation. In addition to the fluorinated inhalational anaesthetics, other drugs such as paracetamol, salicylates, morphine, pethidine, and isoprenaline (isoproterenol) are also metabolized in the kidneys.

#### *Excretion of drugs*

Net drug excretion depends on the interaction between:

- filtration in the glomerulus;
- secretion in the proximal tubule;
- reabsorption, mainly in the distal tubule.

These processes are shown diagrammatically in Figure 25.20.

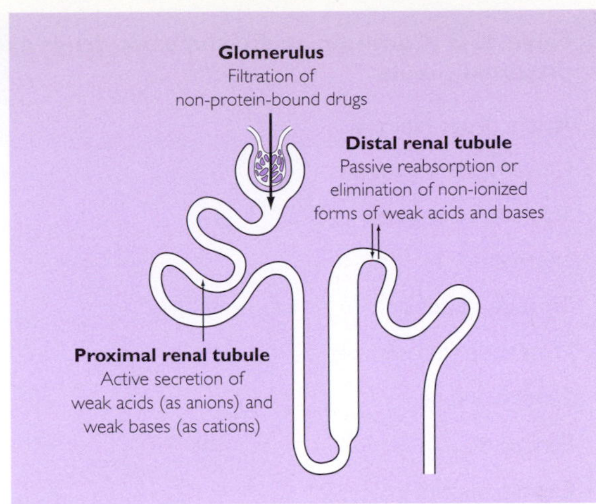


**Figure 25.20** Processes controlling renal elimination of drugs by glomerular filtration, proximal tubular secretion, and distal tubular reabsorption. In the distal tubule, weak acids and weak bases may be reabsorbed or excreted into urine, depending on their $pK_a$ values and the pH gradient between the urine and the cell. (Adapted from Calvey TN and Williams NE. *Principles and Practice of Pharmacology for Anaesthetists*, 3rd edn. Oxford: Blackwell Scientific, 1997.)

##### *Glomerular filtration*

Only the free or unbound fraction of a drug in plasma water is filtered into the tubule. The lower the protein binding, the greater the delivery (see Chapter 20, Table 19.20). However, because the time that plasma spends in the glomerulus is long compared with the dissociation time of reversible binding to protein, significant amounts of protein-bound drugs may still be delivered into the filtrate. Filtration is also the main route of excretion for uncharged molecules with a molecular weight of less than 50 000 Da (e.g. mannitol). The cut-off in molecular weight is related to the size of the pores, which are about 7.5 nm in diameter.

##### *Proximal tubular secretion*

Proximal tubular secretion occurs by active transport, often against a considerable concentration gradient (see Chapter 19, Figures 19.14 and 19.15). A considerable number of drugs are excreted by this mechanism (Table 25.3).

There are separate carrier mechanisms for acidic and basic drugs. Each type of drug may compete with a similar drug for receptor occupancy on the carrier. This can have clinical importance, e.g. thiazide diuretics compete with urate and can precipitate gout. Protein binding does not appear to reduce the effectiveness of secretion in the proximal tubule, again probably because of the rapid release of free drug into the plasma from the protein because it is taken up by the carrier system (see Chapter 19, Figure 19.13).

##### *Tubular reabsorption*

Reabsorption of drugs can be active but is mainly passive. The reabsorption of water and electrolytes (described above) creates a drug concentration gradient. Some passive reabsorption occurs for almost all substances that are filtered.

Active reabsorption of a limited number of drug metabolites occurs in the proximal tubule, together with pinocytosis of aminoglycosides. The main site of reabsorption is the distal tubule.

In the distal tubule, uncharged molecules, which were previously filtered and secreted into the tubule, may be reabsorbed into the cells of the tubule walls. The degree of ionization depends on the relationship

**Table 25.3 Common acidic and basic drugs excreted into the urine by active transport in the proximal tubule**

| Acidic drugs (anions) | Basic drugs (cations) |
|---|---|
| Glucuronide conjugates | Choline |
| Sulphate conjugates | Dopamine |
| Salicylates | Histamine |
| Thiazide diuretics | Lignocaine (lidocaine) |
| Frusemide (furosemide) | Morphine |
| Spironolactone | Neostigmine |
| Penicillins | Serotonin |
| Cephalosporins | Epinephrine (adrenaline) |
| Sulphonamides | Norepinephrine (noradrenaline) |

to the drug's $pK_a$ and the pH (see Chapter 19, Table 19.19).

In summary, for an acidic drug A and a basic drug B associating with a hydrogen ion, their dissociation can be expressed as:

$$AH \rightleftharpoons A^- + H^+$$

and

$$BH^+ \rightleftharpoons B + H^+.$$

This results in the pair of equations:

$$pK_a - pH = \log[AH]/[A^-]$$

and

$$pK_a - pH = \log[BH^+]/[B].$$

Consequently, the pH of the urine is fundamental in controlling the degree of reabsorption of the drug because an abundance of ionic species 'traps' the molecule in the tubule. This relationship is summarized in Table 25.4.

This pH dependence of drug elimination is made use of therapeutically on occasion, e.g. forced alkaline diuresis for salicylate poisoning.

### *Biotransformation of drugs*

The kidney possesses 10–20% of the microsomal mixed function oxidase activity of the liver. Some drugs are therefore metabolized in both sites. The highest concentrations of these enzymes are found in the proximal renal tubules of the cortex, but two important enzymes, prostaglandin endoperoxide synthase and fatty acid cyclo-oxygenase, are in the medulla. Examples of substances undergoing biotransformation in the kidney are listed in Table 25.5.

## Perioperative drugs and renal function

### *Inhalational agents*

There is no evidence that the choice of general anaesthesia or a regional technique itself makes any difference to postoperative renal function in patients at risk. Certain inhalational anaesthetic agents have, however, been implicated in the development of postoperative renal failure. Renal toxicity associated with methoxyflurane anaesthesia results from the biotransformation of this agent in high doses to fluoride ions, producing high-output renal failure. The degree of renal impairment is related to the total dose of methoxyflurane. The onset of subclinical renal toxicity usually occurs with 2.5 MAC hours, which corresponds to a serum fluoride concentration slightly above 50 μmol/L (MAC is the minimum alveolar concentration). Between 2.5 and 5.0 MAC hours, the serum fluoride concentration reaches 50–120 μmol/L and is associated with a mild clinical toxicity. More than 6.0 MAC hours of exposure produces overt clinical toxicity with severe polyuria, dehydration, thirst, and weight loss.

The other fluorinated methylethyl ether anaesthetics are also capable of liberating free fluoride ions

**Table 25.4 The relationship of the acidity of the urine to the degree of ionization of weakly acidic and basic drugs**

| Drug type | Plasma pH (7.4) | Acid urine | Alkaline urine |
|---|---|---|---|
| Acidic drug | Ionized [$A^-$] | Un-ionized [A] | Ionized [$A^-$] |
| Basic drug | Un-ionized [B] | Ionized [$BH^+$] | Un-ionized [B] |

**Table 25.5 Examples of substances undergoing biotransformation in the kidney**

| Metabolic reaction | Substrate |
|---|---|
| Hydroxylation | Insulin<br>Angiotensin I and II<br>Glucagon<br>Gastrin<br>Secretin<br>Vasopressin<br>Calcitonin<br>Oxytocin |
| Glucuronidation | Morphine<br>Paracetamol (acetominophen) |
| Glycine conjugation | Salicylates |
| Oxidation | Pethidine |
| Catechol-*O*-methyl transfer | Isoprenaline (isoproterenol) |

during their biotransformation. Enflurane will generate modest amounts of fluoride, but not to the level seen with methoxyflurane, a reflection of its stronger carbon–fluorine bonds and a lower lipid solubility, and because only about 2% of an absorbed dose undergoes biotransformation. Nevertheless, an inorganic fluoride level of 33 μmol/L after 6 hours of anaesthesia has been reported. Certain subpopulations of patients are at increased risk. These are patients undergoing prolonged anaesthesia, severely obese patients, patients who have been taking enzyme-inducing drugs (such as isoniazid), those with pre-existing renal dysfunction, and those receiving other nephrotoxic drugs. Enflurane is relatively contraindicated in these patients.

Only 0.2% of absorbed isoflurane is biotransformed. Serum fluoride levels rarely exceed 5 μmol/L. When used in subanaesthetic concentrations for prolonged sedation of mechanically ventilated patients in the intensive care unit (ICU), higher concentrations of inorganic fluoride have been reported. No renal dysfunction has, however, been attributed to fluoride ion nephropathy after isoflurane administration.

Desflurane is similarly thought to be safe in patients with impaired renal function because even a smaller proportion of desflurane undergoes biotransformation.

The situation is quite different with sevoflurane. About 5% of sevoflurane is biotransformed and inorganic fluoride concentrations of between 20 and 90 μmol/L have been measured after more than 7 MAC hours of anaesthesia. However, many patients with both normal and impaired renal function have been anaesthetized with sevoflurane with no deleterious effects on postoperative renal function. Some important differences in the metabolism of sevoflurane and methoxyflurane have been put forward to explain the observed differences in outcome. For example, sevoflurane metabolism occurs mainly in the liver and very little metabolism takes place in the kidneys. Serum inorganic fluoride concentrations are elevated for up to 12 hours after sevoflurane anaesthesia, whereas levels remain elevated for days in the case of methoxyflurane.

Another study found that some healthy patients anaesthetized with sevoflurane developed inorganic fluoride concentrations greater than 50 μmol/L. In these patients, urinary concentrating ability was impaired and there was also some evidence of acute injury to the proximal renal tubule, as indicated by an increase in the urinary excretion of *N*-acetyl-β-glucosaminidase.

Nephrotoxicity may also be mediated by another mechanism in addition to fluoride ion toxicity. Degradation of sevoflurane in soda lime leads to the formation of fluoromethyl-2,2-difluoro-1-vinyl ether (commonly known as Compound A), which has been shown to be nephrotoxic in rats. Although the applicability of this finding in humans is unknown, based on the potential for nephrotoxicity, sevoflurane should be used with caution in patients at risk of developing renal dysfunction until more information is available.

### Non-steroidal anti-inflammatory drugs

Both hypoxia and ischaemia are potent stimuli for renal prostaglandin synthesis. Free arachidonic acid is metabolized via three routes: lipo-oxygenase, cyclo-oxygenase, or mono-oxygenase enzyme systems. The major cyclo-oxygenase products, especially $PGE_2$ and $PGI_2$, have important vasodilatory properties and play an important role in maintaining RBF and GFR when the renal circulation is compromised. In addition, $PGE_2$ also reduces active sodium reabsorption in the thick ascending limb of the loop of Henle and the collecting duct, and hence reduces the oxygen consumption of the cells at these sites. Non-steroidal anti-inflammatory drugs that are cyclo-oxygenase inhibitors are therefore contraindicated in patients with impaired renal function because they cause marked decreases in RBF and GFR in these patients.

### Antibiotics and chemotherapeutic agents

Aminoglycosides are poorly lipid-soluble drugs that are rapidly bactericidal for aerobic Gram-negative bacteria by inhibiting protein synthesis in bacterial ribosomes. Aminoglycosides are nephrotoxic, and alter both the structure and function of renal proximal tubular cells. The toxic effects are attributed to the accumulation and avid retention of aminoglycosides in proximal tubule cells in the renal cortex. This correlates with the potential for these drugs to cause nephrotoxicity. Up to 25% of patients who receive an aminoglycoside for more than a few days will develop mild renal impairment, which is almost always reversible. The incidence of nephrotoxicity depends on the specific drug, duration of treatment, total dosage, dosing schedule, and presence of any predisposing factors such as advanced age and pre-existing renal disease. Neomycin is the most nephrotoxic of the aminoglycosides and streptomycin the least nephrotoxic.

Vancomycin, a glycopeptide antibiotic, is active against Gram-positive bacteria and is particularly useful in infections caused by methicillin-resistant staphylococci. Vancomycin has serious nephrotoxic potential especially when used concurrently with other nephrotoxic drugs such as aminoglycosides, or in patients with impaired renal function. It should be reserved for treatment of serious infections.

Tetracyclines are broad-spectrum antibiotics active against aerobic and anaerobic Gram-positive and Gram-negative bacteria. They are particularly useful in diseases caused by rickettsiae, mycoplasmas, and chlamydiae. Degraded tetracycline has a toxic effect on proximal renal tubules producing a Fanconi-like syndrome with polydipsia, polyuria, acidosis, glycosuria, and aminoaciduria.

Cyclosporin, a cyclic polypeptide, is an important drug used in immunosuppression therapy for the prevention and treatment of transplant rejection. Renal toxicity is a major adverse effect and may occur in as many as 75% of patients treated.

## Renal failure and drug handling

Renal impairment affects the way in which drugs are handled as a result of alterations in plasma protein binding, changes in cellular metabolism, and changes in drug and metabolite elimination. This can give rise to problems for several reasons.

### *Failure to excrete a drug or its metabolites may produce toxicity*

Filtration and secretion functions of the kidneys both decrease as renal failure progresses. For those drugs or their metabolites that are eliminated through the kidneys, there is a curvilinear relationship between the GFR and the drug's elimination half-life. With progressive deterioration in renal function and reduction in creatinine clearance, the half-life gradually increases until a creatinine clearance of about 20–25 ml/min is reached. Beyond this, the half-life increases dramatically with any further impairment in renal function.

Most non-depolarizing neuromuscular blocking agents undergo renal excretion and must be used with caution in patients with renal impairment. With pancuronium and *d*-tubocurarine, the amount of drug excreted in the biliary system is increased in renal impairment, although dosage reduction is still necessary. A suitable neuromuscular blocking agent for patients with renal failure is atracurium, which undergoes breakdown by three separate mechanisms: Hofmann degradation, ester hydrolysis, and organ-dependent clearance. Onset times, duration of action, and recovery profiles are unaltered in patients with renal failure. The breakdown products of atracurium include laudanosine. Convulsions have been reported in the dog when laudanosine concentrations exceed 17 µg/ml. Laudanosine is excreted through the kidneys and may accumulate in patients with renal failure. A *cis–cis* isomer of atracurium, cisatracurium, has been shown to be two and a half to three times more potent than atracurium. When cisatracurium and atracurium infusions were compared for the paralysis of critically ill patients undergoing mechanical ventilation in the intensive care unit, plasma laudanosine concentrations in the cisatracurium group were about a third to a quarter of those in the atracurium group. Cisatracurium may well be the neuromuscular blocking agent of choice in patients with renal failure.

The newer neuromuscular blocking agent, mivacurium, is metabolized by plasma and tissue esterases. Its duration of effect is only slightly prolonged in patients with renal failure and it is another suitable neuromuscular blocking agent for these patients.

The opioid analgesics, morphine, pethidine, fentanyl, and alfentanil, are largely metabolized in the liver (to the extent of 90–95%). Their kinetics are therefore unaltered in patients with renal impairment. However metabolites of morphine (morphine-3 and -6-glucuronides) and pethidine (norpethidine) are dependent on normal renal function for elimination. Morphine-6-glucuronide has potent analgesic properties and prolonged and pronounced ventilatory depression has been observed after morphine administration in patients with impaired renal function. Norpethidine is less analgesic than the parent drug, but has a greater convulsant activity. Central nervous excitatory side effects have been attributed to the accumulation of norpethidine.

Antibiotics such as the aminoglycosides are excreted almost entirely by glomerular filtration. It is essential to reduce the maintenance dose of these drugs in patients with impaired renal failure to reduce the incidence of toxicity, especially ototoxicity and nephrotoxicity.

### *Increased sensitivity to some drugs*

Although drug elimination may be unaltered, there may be increased sensitivity to drugs as a result of an increase in free drug fraction or an increase in the volume of drug distribution. Several mechanisms may account for this:

- reduced drug binding as a result of hypoalbuminaemia from increased excretion (as in the nephrotic syndrome) or decreased synthesis;
- alteration in the structure and affinity of drug-binding sites as a result of uraemia;
- increase in free drug fraction caused by competition for binding sites between drugs and their metabolites and accumulated endogenous and exogenous substrates.

The commonly used intravenous induction agents (thiopentone [thiopental], etomidate, propofol, midazolam) are highly protein bound. The free unbound fraction of these agents will be increased in patients with renal failure, although total drug clearance is either unaltered or increased. Thus, although it may not be necessary to decrease the actual induction dose, the rate of administration should be decreased to minimize the effects of any relative overdosage of free drug to the heart, kidneys, liver, and brain.

Increased cerebral sensitivity to anxiolytics, hypnotics, antipsychotics, and opioid analgesics in patients with impaired renal function is well recognized. These drugs should be used in small incremental doses, titrating drug dosage to effect.

### *Many side effects of drugs are tolerated poorly by patients in renal failure*

Antihypertensives such as β-adrenoceptors, ACE inhibitors, ganglion blockers, hydralazine, and diazoxide predispose to exaggerated falls in blood pressure, postural hypotension, and reduction in RBF, and may cause further deterioration in renal function.

Similarly, in patients with renal failure, the compensatory response to hypoglycaemia is impaired and dose

**Table 25.6 Degree of renal impairment according to the glomerular filtration rate (GFR) and serum creatinine**

| Degree of renal impairment | GFR (ml/min) | Serum creatinine (μmol/L) |
|---|---|---|
| Mild | 20–50 | 150–300 |
| Moderate | 10–20 | 300–700 |
| Severe | < 10 | > 700 |

Reproduced with permission from the British National Formulary (BNF). For information of dosage adjustment of individual drugs, refer to Appendix 3 in the BNF – *Renal impairment.*

reduction may be required with insulin and oral hypoglycaemics. The risk of bleeding is increased with heparin, the risk of metabolic acidosis is increased with acetazolamide, and that of hyperkalaemia is increased with potassium-sparing diuretics.

#### *Some drugs become less effective or cease to be effective when renal function is impaired*

The effectiveness of drugs that depend on normal renal function to exert their effects will be compromised in renal impairment. Such drugs include nalidixic acid, nitrofurantoin, probenecid, sulphinpyrazone, and desmopressin.

### Drug dosage adjustment in renal impairment

For drugs with no dose-related side effects or only minor ones, it is not necessary to modify the dose regimen precisely as a simple dose-reduction schedule is adequate. The drug dose can be decreased or the interval between doses increased. In these circumstances it may be important to give a loading dose in order to rapidly achieve steady-state plasma concentrations.

A dose regimen based on GFR is recommended for more toxic drugs with a small safety margin. Creatinine clearance is a useful measure of the GFR (see earlier). The serum creatinine concentration offers an approximate guide to renal function (Table 25.6) but is, however, dependent on the patient's age, weight, and sex.

For drugs with efficacies and toxicities critically related to plasma drug concentrations, dose regimens must, whenever possible, be adjusted according to plasma concentration and clinical response.

Many critically ill patients undergoing treatment in intensive care or high dependency care units have impairment of renal function and/or are on renal replacement therapy. Appropriate adjustments must be made in most drug prescriptions in these patients. The problem is particularly challenging in patients receiving peritoneal dialysis, haemodialysis, haemofiltration, or haemodiafiltration. Many factors affect the removal of drugs in these patients. They include patient factors (such as age and concomitant disease states), drug properties (such as volume of distribution, protein binding, electrical charge, molecular weight, and water solubility), the type of renal replacement therapy used, the duration of therapy, and the type of membrane used. Dosing guidelines are available for the commonly used antibiotics in patients on renal replacement therapy, although little or no information is available for many other drugs. In many cases, drug dosage has to be titrated to desired clinical or physiological response. However, for potentially toxic drugs, there is no substitute for careful monitoring of plasma drug concentrations.

## FURTHER READING


Boyd AH, Eastwood NB, Parker CJR, Hunter JM. Comparison of the pharmacodynamics and pharmacokinetics of an infusion of cisatracurium (51W89) or atracurium in critically ill patients undergoing mechanical ventilation in an intensive therapy unit. *Br J Anaesth* 1996;**76**:382–8.

Duke GL, Briedis JH, Weaver RA. Renal support in critically ill patients: Low-dose dopamine or low-dose dobutamine? *Crit Care Med* 1994;**22**:1919–25.

Ganong WF. *Review of Medical Physiology*, 18th edn. Stamford, CA: Appleton & Lange, 1997.

Guyton AC. *Textbook of Medical Physiology*, 7th edn. Philadelphia: WB Saunders, 1986.

Higuchi H, Sumikura H, Sumita S, Arimura S, Takamatsu F, Kanno M, Satoh T. Renal function in patients with high serum fluoride concentrations after prolonged sevoflurane anesthesia. *Anesthesiology* 1995;**83**:449–58.

Kharasch ED. Biotransformation of sevoflurane. *Anesth Analg* 1995;**81**:527–38.

Kong KL, Tyler JE, Willatts SM, Prys-Roberts C. Isoflurane sedation for patients undergoing mechanical ventilation: metabolism to inorganic fluoride and renal effects. *Br J Anaesth* 1990;**64**:159–62.

Lote CJ. Renal physiology and acute renal failure. *Curr Anaesth Crit Care* 1992;**3**:124–32.

Sear JW, Hand CW, Moore RA, McQuay HJ. Studies on morphine disposition: influence of renal failure on the kinetics of morphine and its metabolites. *Br J Anaesth* 1989;**62**:28–32.

Vander AJ. *Renal Physiology*, 5th edn. New York: McGraw-Hill, 1995.

# Chapter 26 Acid–base balance

J.W. Freeman

It may never be possible to obtain a complete understanding of acid–base balance, but we frequently make decisions on ill-understood and possibly erroneous mathematical formulae, based on complicated physiochemical concepts that most of us don't comprehend. There is a multiplicity of so-called 'simple' diagrams, tables, and jargon, which have evolved in an attempt to make sense of this vital homoeostatic mechanism. Unfortunately, they do not always achieve this aim and may at times enhance the confusion.

Numerical values of blood gas analysis frequently have no absolute meaning and should never be obtained and then used in isolation. Trends of analyses are much more significant and must always be interpreted in relationship to the patient and the relevant history.

This chapter attempts to help unravel some of these difficulties by explaining the basic concepts and terminology, and then using them to identify and treat common clinical conditions.

## TERMINOLOGY/GLOSSARY OF ABBREVIATIONS

Most of the difficulty in understanding acid–base balance stems from the unfamiliar terminology that is often employed. An inability to comprehend the meaning of these simple terms will obviously contribute to the confusion when trying to grasp the concepts and their relevance to abnormalities of the homoeostatic mechanism. The presence of several different systems of measurement, especially for pressure and concentration, continue to complicate the situation and it is unlikely that this will be resolved in the near future. The way that we measure acidity and alkalinity and express these states still has no uniformity throughout the world, which also exacerbates the problem.

The definitions and glossary (Table 26.1) will help with some of the common difficulties in the field of acid–base balance and should be used in the reading of this chapter.

### Acids

The acidity of a substance is its ability to ionize to form hydrogen ions. In 1964 the New York Academy of Sciences defined an acid as a proton donor and a base as a proton acceptor:

$$HA \rightleftharpoons H^+ + A^-.$$

Acidity is usually expressed in hydrogen ion concentration $[H^+]$ in units of nanomoles per litre (nmol/L) or as the negative logarithm of the hydrogen ion concentration (pH). The use of $[H^+]$ as a measurement has been criticized because its range in aqueous bodily fluids is extremely large. The exponential arithmetic of $[H^+]$, as described by Sorensen in 1909, may have some advantages in this context and its use is preferred by some workers. He described acid concentration in the terms of the seventh puissance (power) of hydrogen and this was later expressed by Karl Hasselbalch as its negative logarithm or pH. The pH notation is, however, one further source of confusion because, as the acidity increases, the pH decreases. To reduce the level of confusion, it is best to avoid the expressions of 'increase' or 'decrease' when referring to hydrogen changes but instead to use 'acid change' and 'alkaline change'.

The use of pH has the opposite effect to that of $[H^+]$ in that it can make the reader mistakenly believe that the body actually works within a very narrow range of acid–base homoeostatic control. This could not be further from the truth because, when the pH changes by only 0.3 unit from 7.4 to 7.1, the $[H^+]$ actually doubles from 40 to 80 nmol/L (Table 26.2 and Figure 26.1).

### Bases

A base is a substance that can accept hydrogen ions and by doing so reduces the $[H^+]$ and thus the acidity of a solution. It is defined as a proton acceptor. As referred to later in the text, a base deficit (or a minus base excess) is a situation where there is a deficit of base in a system leading to a degree of acidosis.

Neutrality is when there is neither base deficit nor excess. This situation exists with water when there are equal numbers of hydrogen ($H^+$) ions and hydroxyl ions ($OH^-$). Water is more ionized at body temperature than at room temperature and is neutral at a pH of 6.8 rather than 7.0 (the average pH of the intracellular fluid). The pH of blood is, however, 7.4 which is 0.6 pH unit above neutrality and is therefore alkaline in comparison.

### Buffers

Buffers are substances that, by their presence in solution, increase the amount of acid or base that has to be added to cause a unit change in $[H^+]$. They bring about this change by having the ability to absorb or release $H^+$ as an acid or base is added. Free acids within the body are scarce because they have a tendency to bond to weak or strong bases and are therefore disposed of.

For the equation:

$$HA \rightleftharpoons H^+ + A^-$$

where HA is the undissociated acid and $A^-$ the anion, the equation shifts to the left when acid is added, and to the right when a base is added. The changes in $[H^+]$ are thus minimized.

The pH change in such a balanced system can be described by the Henderson–Hasselbalch equation:

**Table 26.1 Glossary**

| Symbol | Factor |
|---|---|
| DA–a$O_2$ | Alveolar–arterial oxygen difference |
| BTPS | Body temperature and pressure |
| Ca$O_2$ | Arterial oxygen content |
| Cc′$O_2$ | End-capillary oxygen content |
| Cv$O_2$ | Oxygen content of mixed venous blood |
| DL | Diffusing capacity of the lung |
| D$O_2$ | Oxygen delivery |
| Fi$O_2$ | Fraction of inspired oxygen |
| [$H^+$] | Hydrogen ion concentration |
| Hb | Deoxyhaemoglobin |
| Hb$O_2$ | Oxyhaemoglobin |
| Pa | Arterial partial pressure |
| PA | Alveolar pressure |
| Patm | Atmospheric pressure |
| Pa$CO_2$ | Arterial carbon dioxide tension |
| PA$CO_2$ | Alveolar carbon dioxide tension |
| Pa$O_2$ | Arterial oxygen tension |
| PA$O_2$ | Alveolar oxygen tension |
| Pb | Barometric pressure |
| P$CO_2$ | Partial pressure of carbon dioxide |
| P$O_2$ | Partial pressure of oxygen |
| pH | Negative logarithm of the hydrogen ion concentration |
| P$H_2O$ | Water vapour pressure |
| P$N_2$ | Partial pressure of nitrogen |
| P$O_2$ | Partial pressure of oxygen |
| Pt$O_2$ | Tissue oxygen tension |
| P$\bar{V}CO_2$ | Average carbon dioxide tension in mixed venous blood |
| P$\bar{V}O_2$ | Average oxygen tension in mixed venous blood |
| Qc | Capillary perfusion |
| $\dot{Q}$s | Shunt flow |
| $\dot{Q}$T | Total blood flow |
| RQ | Respiratory quotient |
| Sa$O_2$ | Arterial oxygen saturation |
| RQE | Respiratory quotient exchange |
| $\dot{V}$a | Alveolar ventilation |
| Vd | Dead space |
| $\dot{V}O_2$ | Oxygen consumption |
| $\dot{V}CO_2$ | Carbon dioxide production |
| $V_T$ | Tidal volume |
| $\dot{V}/\dot{Q}$ | Ventilation–perfusion ratio |

**Table 26.2 Correlation of pH with hydrogen ion concentration (nmol/L)**

| pH | $H^+$ | pH | $H^+$ |
|---|---|---|---|
| 7.00 | 100 | 7.35 | 45 |
| 7.05 | 89 | 7.40 | 40 |
| 7.10 | 79 | 7.45 | 35 |
| 7.15 | 71 | 7.50 | 32 |
| 7.20 | 63 | 7.55 | 28 |
| 7.25 | 56 | 7.60 | 25 |
| 7.30 | 50 | 7.65 | 22 |

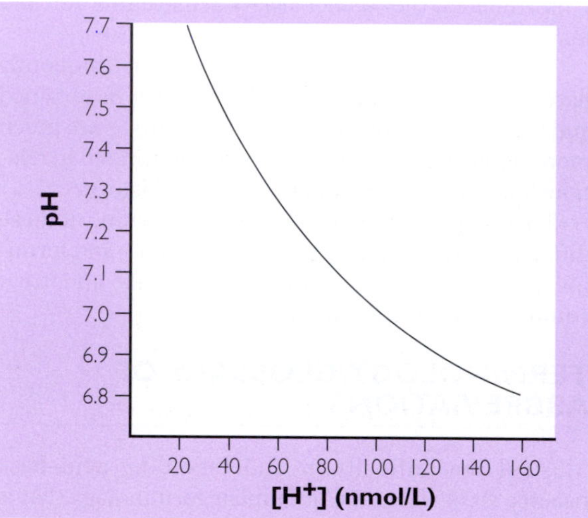


**Figure 26.1** Relationship between hydrogen ion concentration ([$H^+$]) and pH.

$$\text{pH} = \text{p}K + \log \frac{[A^-]}{[HA]}$$

When the pH equals the p*K* (the negative logarithm of the dissociation constant) of the buffer system, maximal buffering occurs because HA and $A^-$ will be at equal concentrations. Applied to the body with the carbonic acid/bicarbonate system this can be further expressed as:

$$H^+ + HCO_3^- \rightarrow H_2CO_3 \rightarrow H_2O + CO_2$$

where:

$$\text{pH} = \text{p}K + \log \frac{[HCO_3^-]}{[CO_2]}$$

$CO_2$ is then eliminated either by the lungs or by one of three separate renal routes.

Each system will have a p*K* value at which its buffering capacity is maximal. Most buffering occurs within ± 1 pH unit of the p*K* value of the system. Figure 26.2 shows the buffer curve for the bicarbonate system which is most effective at a p*K* of 6.2.

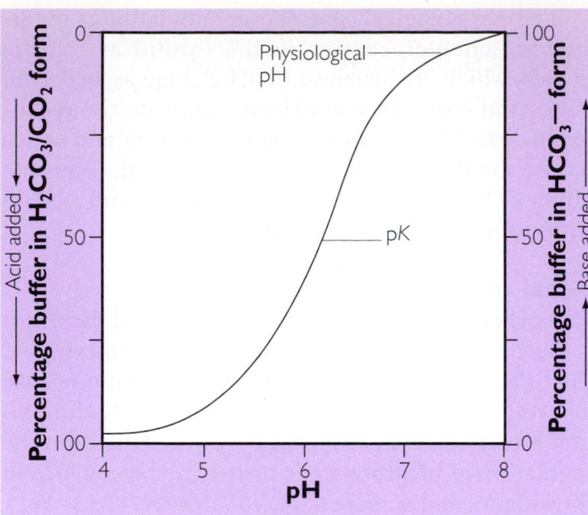


**Figure 26.2** The buffer reaction curve for the bicarbonate system.

## SOURCES OF ACIDS, BASES, AND BUFFERS

The main sources of acids and bases that find their way into the body are from food, metabolic processes, and extraneous administration in the course of medication or poisons. Food normally constitutes a minimal loading of both acids and bases, although certain fruits can be very acidic. The major component of acid–base loading is from normal metabolism and the most important potentially acidic substance is $CO_2$. This is further supplemented by lesser amounts of sulphuric, phosphoric, and lactic acids, again mostly as a product of metabolic processes. In certain conditions, the production of lactic acid may reach toxic levels and have negative effects on normal homoeostatic mechanisms and organ performance. This can occur with other acids when they are inadvertently or even deliberately administered, e.g. salicylic acid (aspirin).

The buffer systems of the body are present throughout our body fluids with some having more buffering power than others. Those of the blood are best understood and the most important of these are the bicarbonate/carbonic acid system, the dihydrogen phosphate/monohydrogen phosphate system and the proteins normally present in both plasma and red blood cells.

## REGULATION

The regulation of acid–base balance within the body is achieved by numerous processes and this non-reliance on a single system probably indicates how important the maintenance of homoeostasis is for the continuation of normal metabolic function. The three main regulatory systems are the buffers, the respiratory system and the renal system.

### Buffer systems

Buffer systems exist within the body to resist the excessive build-up of acids and bases, and there are several significant blood buffers that are well understood.

In the plasma component of blood, there are three main buffering systems; in order of significance they are the carbonic acid and sodium bicarbonate system (65%), the plasma proteins (5%), and the acid and alkaline phosphates (1%). Each of these systems exists as a buffer pair.

#### *Carbonic acid (free acid) and sodium bicarbonate*

$$\text{Ratio of } \frac{1}{20} = \frac{H_2CO_3}{NaHCO_3}$$

#### *Plasma proteins*

$$\frac{\text{H protein}}{\text{Na proteinate}}$$

The buffering ratio is $^1/_4$–$^1/_{10}$, depending on the protein concentration. This system has one-sixth of the buffering capacity of haemoglobin (Hb).

#### *Acid and alkaline phosphates*

$$\text{Ratio of } \frac{1}{4} = \frac{NaH_2PO_4}{Na_2HPO_4}$$

Within the red blood cells there are a further two additional buffering systems, one of which makes a very significant contribution to the total buffering ability of blood. They are the oxyhaemoglobin and reduced Hb system (29%), and a small contribution from the potassium salts of phosphoric acid.

#### *Oxyhaemoglobin and reduced haemoglobin*

Deoxygenated Hb is a better buffer than oxyHb. An explanation for this is that oxygenation of the iron alters its electronic structure in such a way that the molecule has a reduced affinity for $H^+$ ions on the imidazole nitrogen, and $H^+$ ions can dissociate more easily. On reduction this process reverses and the $H^+$ ions can recombine (Figure 26.3).

This works well in the body because Hb releases its oxygen in the tissues, which are rich in $H^+$ from metabolic processes. Its $H^+$ affinity increases; it binds the excess $H^+$ ions and then carries them to the lungs. On oxygenation, the affinity of the Hb molecules reduces and it releases the $H^+$ ions. This is the reverse process of that for the carriage of oxygen.

The dissociation of histidine residues from Hb gives the molecule six times the buffering power of the plasma proteins.

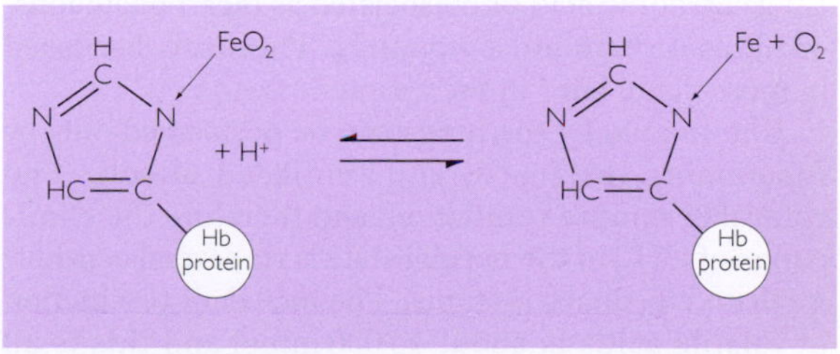

**Figure 26.3** The reaction shown is driven to the right in an acid environment. The imidazole group of the histidine molecule of haemoglobin acts as a buffer and binds hydrogen ions. In doing this, the haemoglobin becomes more acidic and less able to bind oxygen, which is subsequently released.

***Potassium salts of phosphoric acid***

$$\frac{\text{Acid potassium phosphate}}{\text{Alkaline potassium phosphate}} = \frac{KH_2PO_4}{K_2HCO_3}$$

As with other buffer systems, this one consists of a weak acid and its conjugate base, or a weak base and its conjugate acid. The mechanism of dissociation of carbonic acid to evolve $CO_2$ and effectively buffer added acid to the system is well understood, and is the most effective method employed by the body. Acids that can be buffered in this way are described as 'volatile acids' because they can dissociate to free $CO_2$ which can be removed by the lungs.

The concentration of bicarbonate and carbonic acid within the body is fixed by tight homoeostatic control mechanisms and it is in this way that the dissociation of the system can be manipulated and the pH of blood held within a narrow range. The kidneys control the bicarbonate concentration between 24 and 28 mmol/L, and the carbonic acid concentration is controlled by the respiratory system and evolution of $CO_2$. Within a system that constitutes 65% of the buffering control of the body, if anything affects either the renal bicarbonate control or respiratory evolution of $CO_2$, then it will markedly change the acid–base balance. This is why renal disease or disorders of gaseous respiratory exchange are complicated by severe derangements of acid–base balance.

### Respiratory regulation

The respiratory regulation of acid–base balance is mediated by the balance of $CO_2$ production and its elimination from the lungs. In a normal healthy state, the lungs are able to deal with large variations in $CO_2$ production and this is achieved simply by altering the body's minute ventilation. In diseased states, this can be seriously affected by altered diffusion kinetics, pulmonary–capillary blocks, and altered lung and chest wall mechanics.

$CO_2$ is produced primarily in the mitochondria as a major end-product of the metabolic process. The partial pressure of $CO_2$ in arterial blood ($Pa\text{CO}_2$) is determined by the balance between production ($\dot{V}\text{CO}_2$) and elimination by alveolar ventilation ($\dot{V}\text{A}$). Increased $\dot{V}\text{CO}_2$ results from increased metabolic rate and originates from the mitochondria. This occurs secondary to increased physical activity, elevation of the body temperature, hormonal effects, etc., and results in a build-up of $H^+$ at a cellular level. Once buffered, these are carried in the blood to the lungs to be eliminated as $CO_2$. Carriage in the blood is by one of three ways: (1) in physical solution, (2) as carbonic acid or dissociated as bicarbonate ions, or (3) as carbamino compounds. These are discussed in more detail later in the chapter.

Elimination by the lungs can be performed only by functioning, perfused, and ventilated alveoli. The control of minute ventilation, and therefore the elimination of $CO_2$, in the normal state is via several centrally mediated feedback systems. The total daily production of volatile acids is about 13 000 mmol and this is all removed by the lungs. Any central derangement in respiratory drive or alteration in lung function will rapidly lead to a rise or fall in $Pa\text{CO}_2$, with a resultant alteration in acid–base status. Doubling of the alveolar ventilation will halve the $Pa\text{CO}_2$, whereas halving the ventilation will double the $Pa\text{CO}_2$.

The physiological control over ventilation is mediated via chemoreceptors in the carotid and aortic bodies, which are sensitive to pH change as well as to $Pa\text{CO}_2$ and $Pa\text{O}_2$. An acid pH will stimulate the receptors to drive the minute ventilation centrally and hence reduce the $Pa\text{CO}_2$; an alkaline pH will have the opposite effect. This reflex is exceedingly rapid and occurs within seconds of a pH change.

### Renal regulation

The pH of arterial blood can be maintained if the major buffering system in the body functions properly, and the $Pa\text{CO}_2$ and bicarbonate concentrations are controlled. As described, the control of $CO_2$ elimination is both rapid and controllable by the lungs, but the regulation of bicarbonate is primarily the concern of the kidneys and is more liable to variation.

The kidneys help control acid–base homoeostasis by several mechanisms. Primarily, they control the rate of water loss from the body, but in doing so they are able to regulate the excretion of individual ions and therefore maintain normal electrolyte levels within the body. The ability to vary the acidity or alkalinity of the urine is paramount in the homoeostasis of acid–base balance. The renal tubules have the ability to secrete $H^+$ ions directly into the urine, but in doing so each ion secreted leaves one $OH^-$ ion within the renal tubular cells. In an attempt to neutralize this increasing pH the reaction:

$$CO_2 + H_2O \rightarrow HCO_3^- + H^+$$

is driven to the right in the cells. The $H^+$ is obtained from the blood but the process of intracellular neutralization results in a byproduct increase of bicarbonate ions, which are then added to the blood and act as the body's buffer generation. In an attempt to maintain electrical neutrality within the renal tubules, there has to be retention of a cation for every $H^+$ secreted, and normally this is mediated by sodium ion ($Na^+$) retention, although it may involve potassium ions in the presence of profound acidosis or hyponatraemia. Acids excreted via the kidneys rather than the lungs are called titratable acids and the main buffer for $H^+$ ion by this route is phosphate:

$$H_2PO_4^- \rightleftharpoons HPO_4^{2-} + H^+$$

Sodium ions ($Na^+$) and phosphate ions ($HPO_4^{2-}$) are filtered at the glomerulus and are initially present in a similar concentration as in the plasma. To maintain normal homoeostasis, it is essential that $Na^+$ is conserved, and to maintain electrical neutrality $H^+$ is substituted in the renal tubule (Figure 26.4).

Using the Henderson–Hasselbalch equation for the dissociation of the phosphate buffer pair and substituting the known parameters of p$K$ of 6.8 and a pH of plasma of 7.4, the ratio of the buffer and its weak diphosphate acid can be found:

$$\text{pH} = \text{p}K + \log\frac{[HPO_4^{2-}]}{[H_2PO_4^-]}$$

Substitution gives:

$$7.4 = 6.8 + \log\frac{[HPO_4^{2-}]}{[H_2PO_4^-]}$$

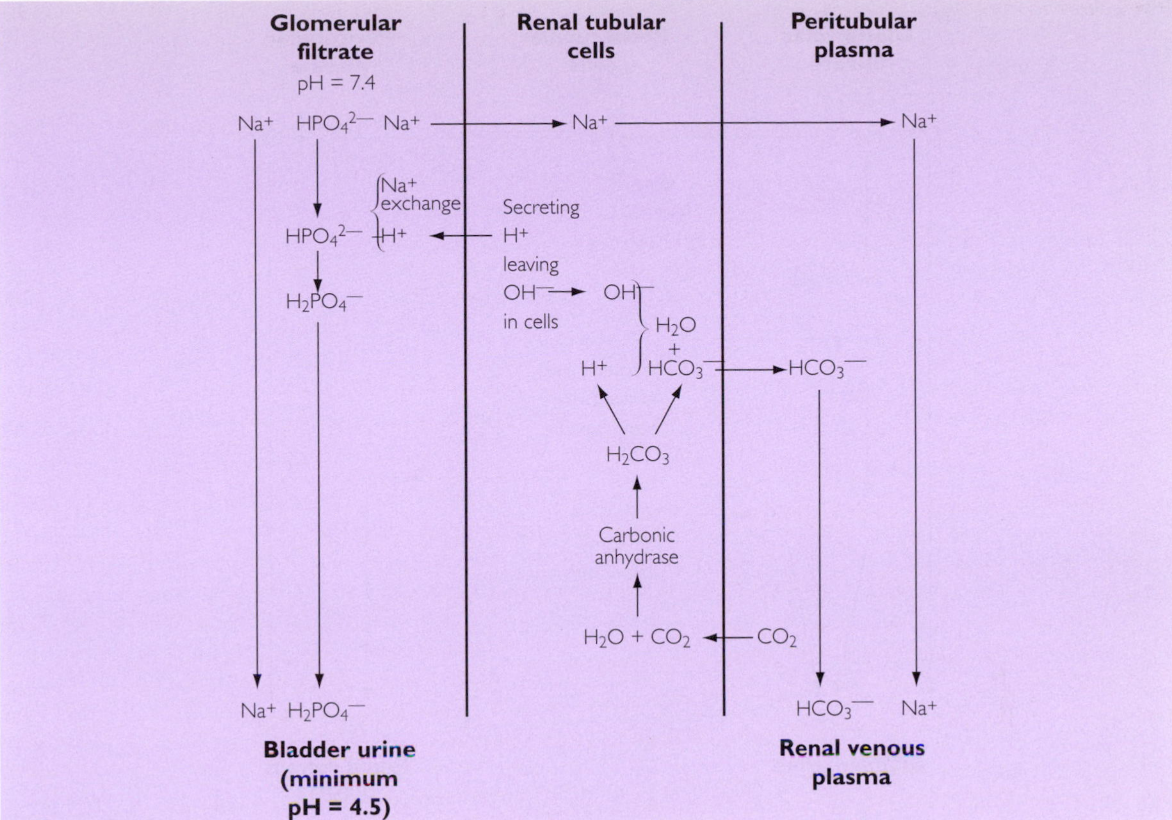


**Figure 26.4** Schematic representation of the phosphate buffering of urine and conservation of sodium.

therefore:

$$\frac{[HPO_4^{2-}]}{[H_2PO_4^-]} = \text{antilog } 0.6 = 4.$$

This means there is four times more dibasic phosphate than monobasic form in the glomerular filtrate, and for every five ions of this pair excreted there will be a net negative charge of nine. If this were to be balanced, then nine $Na^+$ would have to follow and be lost from the plasma. In an attempt to prevent this, $H^+$ is substituted to a variable extent to maintain normal acid–base balance.

The kidneys are able to excrete a urine with a maximum acidity of pH 4.5, which has a $[H^+]$ of 0.00003 mol/L. This is approximately 800 times more acidic than plasma and indicates the amazing power of the homoeostatic mechanism.

Another way in which $H^+$ can also be excreted and $Na^+$ conserved is by the formation of ammonia ($NH_3$) in the renal cells from glutamine and some amino acids. The $NH_3$ then diffuses into the renal tubules where it reacts with $H^+$ to form ammonium ions ($NH_4^+$). The binding of $H^+$ occurs in the glomerular filtrate and so attempts to buffer the acid urine; in this way the body is able to reduce the acidity of the urine excreted (Figure 26.5).

The bicarbonate ion concentration of the glomerular filtrate is similar to that of plasma and, in an attempt to conserve this valuable buffer, it is necessary for it to be reabsorbed in the renal tubules. This is facilitated by the bicarbonate buffering the secreted $H^+$ in the tubule to form carbonic acid, which is dehydrated to form water and $CO_2$. The $P\text{CO}_2$ of the tubular urine rises and most diffuses through the cell wall back into the plasma. Under the influence of carbonic anhydrase, the $CO_2$ is rehydrated and bicarbonate is reformed and conserved (Figure 26.6). The reciprocating anion for bicarbonate in this system is chloride ($Cl^-$) and, when plasma bicarbonate concentration is low, $Cl^-$ is preferentially excreted. When the bicarbonate concentration is high then $Cl^-$ is conserved.

## OXYGEN AND CARBON DIOXIDE CARRIAGE

As described under the section on regulation, acid–base balance is intimately connected to oxygen and $CO_2$ carriage within the blood because they are both affected by the buffering capacity of haemoglobin and the carbonic acid–bicarbonate system within the erythrocyte.

Oxygen is carried both in simple solution and by combination with Hb. It initially diffuses from the lungs down a concentration gradient to the plasma where it becomes dissolved; the amount carried is directly proportional to the $P\text{O}_2$. At normal barometric pressure and body temperature (BTPS), 0.023 ml of oxygen will be carried per millilitre of blood. This equates to a total of 3 ml/L or a total of approximately 15 ml for an adult, assuming that the $P\text{aO}_2$ is 13.3 kPa (100 mmHg). The mixed venous oxygen pressure ($P\text{vO}_2$) remains about 5.3 kPa (40 mmHg) which equates to about 1 ml/L of oxygen. Therefore, to supply the normal resting requirement of oxygen to maintain basal metabolic requirements of 250 ml/min, the

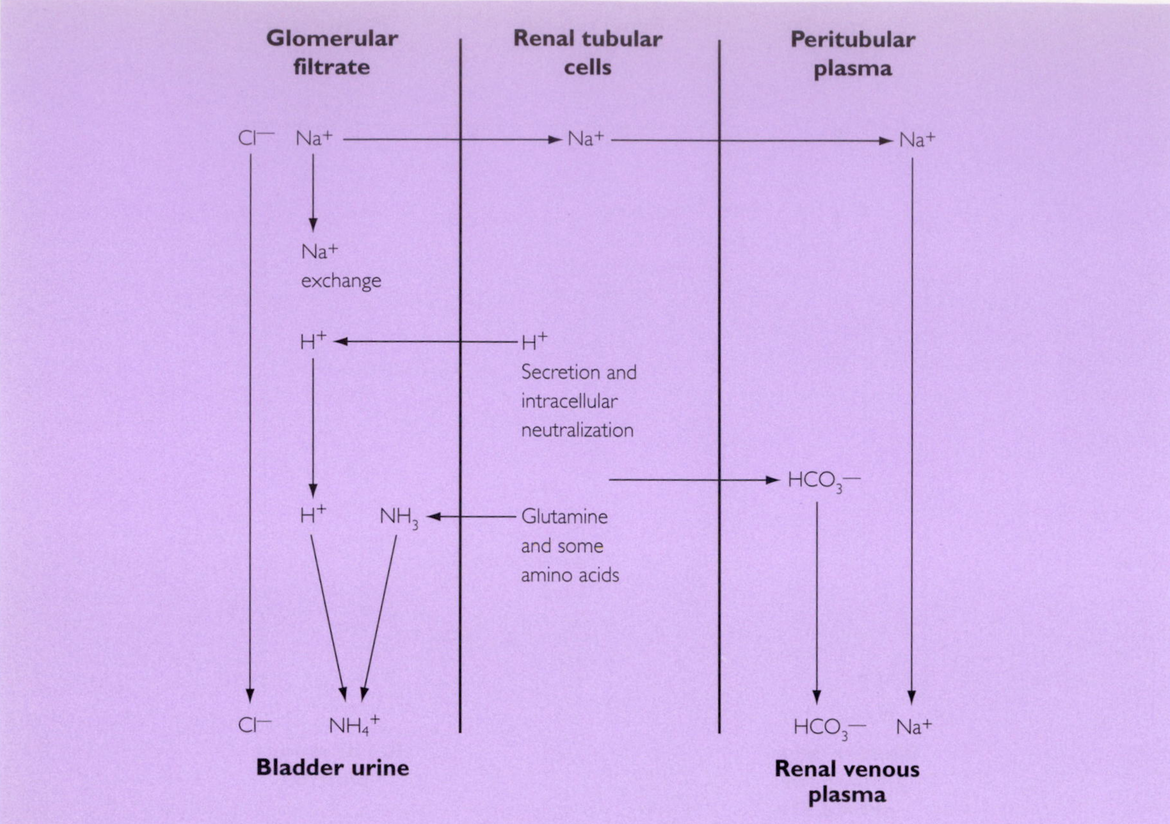


**Figure 26.5** Schematic representation of renal excretion of ammonium ions.

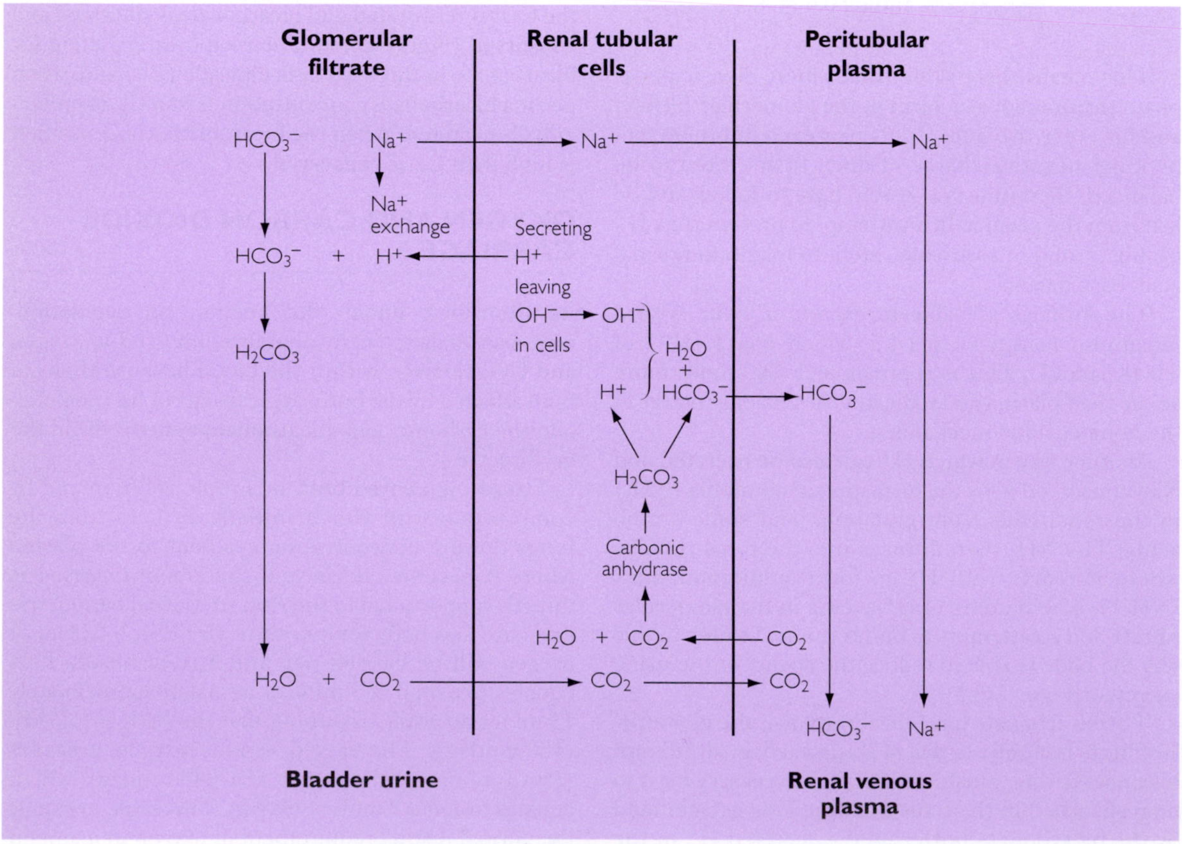

Glomerular filtrate | Renal tubular cells | Peritubular plasma

$HCO_3^-$ $Na^+$ → $Na^+$ → $Na^+$

$Na^+$ exchange

Secreting

$HCO_3^-$ + $H^+$ ← $H^+$

leaving

$OH^-$ → $OH^-$

in cells

$H_2O$ + $HCO_3^-$ → $HCO_3^-$

$H_2CO_3$

$H^+$

$H_2CO_3$

Carbonic anhydrase

$H_2O$ + $CO_2$ ← $CO_2$

$H_2O$ + $CO_2$ → $CO_2$ → $CO_2$

$HCO_3^-$ $Na^+$

Bladder urine | Renal venous plasma

**Figure 26.6** Schematic representation of the renal re-absorption of bicarbonate by the secretion of hydrogen ions.

cardiac output would have to be 125 L/min. This obviously is not possible and so another method of oxygen carriage other than in pure solution has to be used.

Hb has a great affinity for oxygen and can carry large volumes bound to the iron component. One mole of Hb (66 800 g) can combine with four moles (128 g) of oxygen:

$$4O_2 + Hb = Hb(O_2)_4$$

One mole of oxygen at STP occupies 22 400 ml and so, under the same conditions, 1 mol Hb can carry 89 600 ml oxygen. By calculation 1 g Hb can carry 1.34 ml and, as there are 150 g Hb per litre of blood, when fully saturated with oxygen each litre can carry approximately 200 ml. We know that the $P\text{vo}_2$ is around 40 mmHg because Hb does not give all its oxygen up to the tissues as a result of its sigmoid dissociation curve. This equates to about 30% remaining bound to the Hb, despite the right shift in the dissociation curve brought about by carriage of $CO_2$ and the resultant acidification of the imidazole radicals of the histidine molecule of Hb (see 'Buffers' and Figure 26.3).

The volume of oxygen available for use is equivalent to about 120–140 ml/L and so a normal cardiac output of 5 L/min in adults is sufficient to deliver up to 700 ml, which far exceeds the basal requirements. This is the body's minute oxygen delivery or $D\text{o}_2$. The body's oxygen consumption or $\dot{V}\text{o}_2$ can, however, equal or exceed delivery in certain circumstances, such as decreased cardiac output states and profound anaemia, or because of increased utilization as seen in sepsis. Oxygen carriage is seriously jeopardized in severe acidosis because the dissociation curve is shifted to the right and, although the Hb will give up its oxygen to the tissues more easily, it may not carry as much.

$CO_2$ carriage is less well evolved in one sense because there is no complex molecular binding system as there is for oxygen. There is, however, a very efficient enzymatic buffering reaction, which is able to carry large volumes away from the tissues and deliver the $CO_2$ to the lungs.

The $CO_2$ passes into the blood again down a diffusion gradient from the acidotic tissues. On entering the blood it has one of three possible routes to follow:

- Most diffuses into the erythrocytes.
- Some (a very small percentage) combines with amino groups on plasma proteins to form carbamino compounds:

$$R\text{-}NH_2 + CO_2 \rightleftharpoons R\text{-}NHCOO^- + H^+.$$

- Some dissolves in the plasma:

$$CO_2 + H_2O \rightleftharpoons H_2CO_3 \rightleftharpoons H^+ + HCO_3^-$$

This reaction is way to the left, with the ratio of $CO_2 : H_2CO_3$ being 1000 : 1.

Most of the $CO_2$ enters the erythrocyte by the first route. Here it forms carbamino compounds with the Hb, which is a very rapid reaction and is enhanced when the Hb is in the reduced form. The rest is dissolved in the intracellular fluid, as it is in the plasma. The difference between this reaction and that previously described is that the equilibrium is pulled to the right by an enzymatic process and the two resulting ions are quickly removed: $H^+$ by the efficient Hb buffer system and bicarbonate diffuses into the plasma down a concentration gradient (Figure 26.7).

The diffusion of bicarbonate ions out of the red cell disturbs the electrical equilibrium and neutrality is maintained by the shift of $Cl^-$ ions into the cell. The reverse of these events occurs when the erythrocyte reaches the alveolus and $CO_2$ is evolved.

## ASSESSMENT OF ACID–BASE DISORDERS

To assess acid–base status it is essential to have a reproducible measuring system that can be utilized to calculate, either directly or indirectly, the $[H^+]$ within the blood. Modern blood gas machines are just more automated versions of the old manual devices, used to measure $[H^+]$ by a glass electrode, which behaves as though it is permeable to $H^+$ so deriving a pH value. The $P\text{co}_2$ is measured by a Severinghaus electrode which is a modified glass electrode with a $CO_2$-permeable membrane. All the other measurements are derived indirectly by extrapolation from pH and standard $CO_2$ curves. The best known of these is the Siggaard-Andersen nomogram (Figure 26.8).

This nomogram is a graphic representation of the Henderson–Hasselbalch equation in which the pH is plotted against log $P\text{aco}_2$. Lines can be plotted showing the changes in pH that occur when a sample with a normal Hb concentration is equilibrated with various concentrations of $CO_2$. It is obtained by taking an arterial blood sample, equilibrating it with two gas mixtures of known $CO_2$ concentration, and then measuring the pH. This will give two points that can be plotted on the nomogram by a straight line, which is called the 'buffer line'. The pH of the patient's blood is also measured and plotted along the buffer line. Using this method, the $CO_2$ of the sample can be interpolated from the nomogram. The standard bicarbonate value can be obtained from the point where the plotted buffer line crosses the horizontal bicarbonate line, which will be at a $P\text{co}_2$ of 5.3 kPa (40 mmHg). The standard bicarbonate by definition is the concentra-

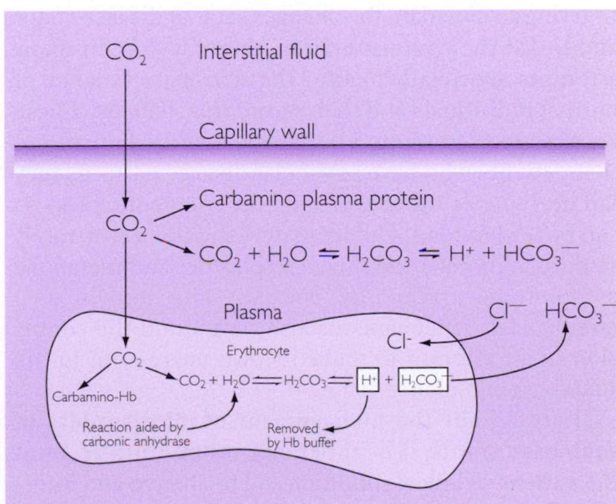


**Figure 26.7** Schematic representation of the fate of carbon dioxide on entering the blood from the tissues.

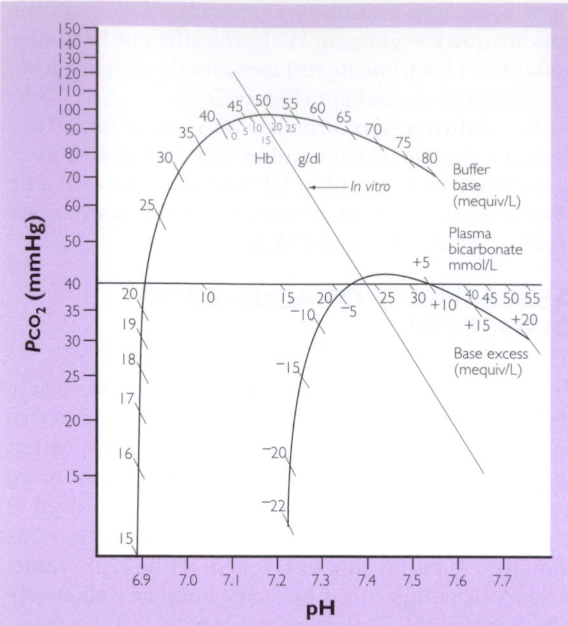


**Figure 26.8** The Siggaard-Andersen nomogram.

tion of bicarbonate in plasma after it has been equilibrated with $CO_2$ at 5.3 kPa (40 mmHg) at 37°C.

Errors will occur if the Hb concentration is out of the normal range; standard correction lines are plotted on the nomogram to help reduce this effect.

The base excess is the base concentration of whole blood when measured by titration against a strong acid to standard end-points. It is, by definition, the number of millimoles of acid required to titrate 1 litre of blood to a pH of 7.4 at a temperature of 37°C, while the $P\text{CO}_2$ is held at 5.3 kPa (40 mmHg). This value can also be derived from the standard curves of the Siggaard-Andersen nomogram. Base excess is changed only by fixed acids and so it measures the true non-respiratory acid–base status. It is an attempt to quantify the excess or deficit of bicarbonate in the system.

## CLINICAL ASPECTS

In trying to elucidate the changes seen in disease states and to aid their interpretation, there have been many attempts artificially to alter the acid–base balance of normal individuals and then record the changes. These results are then plotted to provide standard curves so that patients who have particular disease patterns may fall into one or other area, and the metabolic process can be understood. Unfortunately, the process is rarely so pure in disease and mixed respiratory and metabolic components frequently coexist. The body's own homoeostatic mechanisms also compound the confusion in an attempt to make its own correction to the acid–base imbalance.

Throughout the management of all disorders of acid–base status, it is imperative to take into account the patient's clinical condition and to analyse and interpret all the results together. Never view the values in isolation and always review the trends rather than a 'snap-shot' result.

### Artificial changes in acid–base balance

Artificial changes in acid–base balance can be induced by the ingestion of certain pure preparations such as ammonium chloride, which produces a metabolic acidosis, and sodium bicarbonate, which produces a type of metabolic alkalosis. The observation of changes in $P\text{aCO}_2$ and pH are useful in understanding the compensatory mechanisms in the normal state.

This is also helpful when trying to understand the mechanisms of severe toxin ingestion as seen in salicylate poisoning. In this situation the metabolic acidosis is out of keeping with the acid load, but this is because the compound has a direct stimulant effect on the metabolic rate, further increasing the acidosis and production of fixed acids. Salicylates also have a direct effect on the medulla, causing a centrally mediated hyperventilation out of step with the metabolic acidosis and the 'compensatory' respiratory alkalosis is more dramatic than one would expect. The spectrum of responses seen in different people is also wide. The use of standard nomograms and plots can be of some use in trying to establish where the patient lies in his or her disease state. Classic examples are the Goldberg plot and the Fleney acid–base diagram. These plot observed relationships between $P\text{aCO}_2$ and pH, in a variety of acute and chronic respiratory and metabolic disorders, in order to build up a so-called 'acid–base map' (Figures 26.9 and 26.10).

### Hypoxia

Hypoxia is the reduction of oxygen availability for tissue respiration and can result from several causes. Classically divided into hypoxic hypoxia (hypoxaemia), anaemic hypoxia, stagnant hypoxia, and histotoxic hypoxia, the effect of all causes is that there will be a relative deficit of cellular oxygen, with a resultant increase in anaerobic respiration and acidosis. The loss of aerobic metabolism in the cytochrome oxidase

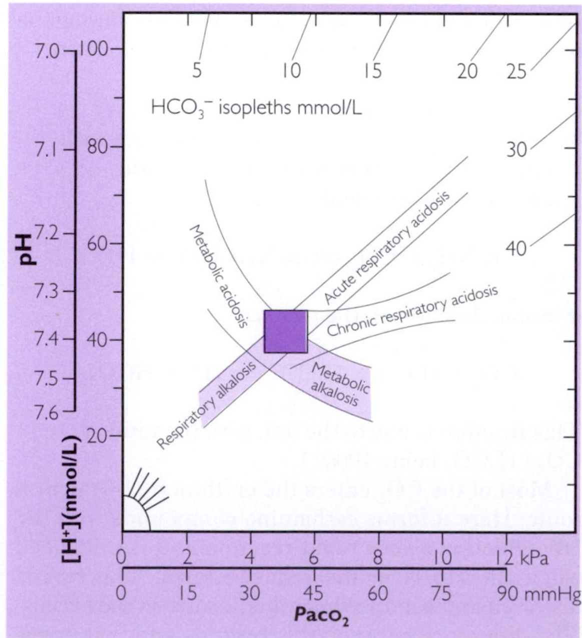


**Figure 26.9** The Fleney acid–base diagram.

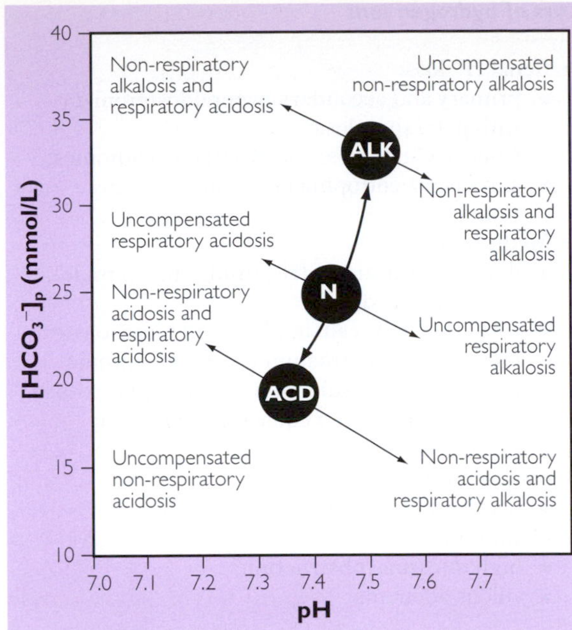


**Figure 26.10** The relationship of bicarbonate and pH to the status of respiratory and non-respiratory acidosis and alkalosis. (Modified from Davenport HW. *The ABC of Acid–Base Chemistry*. Chicago: University of Chicago Press, 1965.)

system leads to a build-up of lactic acid which, if not cleared, has a negative effect on many body systems. The increasing acidaemia causes a right shift in the oxygen dissociation curve and compounds oxygen uptake and delivery to the tissues.

### Hypercapnia

An increase of $CO_2$ above 6 kPa (45 mmHg) is considered to be pathological in most circumstances and is the result of such causes as increased production, reduced alveolar ventilation ($\dot{V}$A), a $\dot{V}/\dot{Q}$ mismatch or shunt, or increased inspired $CO_2$. The derangement affects most body systems because a respiratory acidosis occurs, leading to increased respiratory drive, a right shift in the oxygen dissociation curve, increased sympathetic activity with a tachycardia, and centrally mediated narcosis. Compensatory mechanisms, apart from increased respiratory drive, include renal conservation of bicarbonate and potassium ions and preferential excretion of $H^+$ ions. These renal processes are relatively slow and will not compensate for acute $CO_2$ retention.

The respiratory effects on acid–base balance relate mainly to the retention or over-ventilation of $CO_2$. The common causes of the resultant respiratory acidosis include the following:

- chronic obstructive airway disease (COAD);
- respiratory centre depression, either primarily neurological or secondary to opioid analgesics, or during spontaneous breathing maintained with volatile anaesthetic agents;
- impaired neuromuscular function such as paralysis, incomplete reversal of neuromuscular blockade postoperatively, and myasthenia gravis;
- increased inhalation of inspired $CO_2$;
- increased $CO_2$ production as in fever;
- restrictive chest wall or lung disease;
- acute lung injury.

Typical blood gases in the acute patient are given in Table 26.3, together with those in chronic disease states, where one would expect to see further renal compensation. Any treatment in the first instance is purely symptomatic, but the only effective therapy would be one aimed at treating the underlying cause. Ventilation to normality will only exchange the respiratory acidosis for one of metabolic alkalosis.

Respiratory alkalosis is a high pH associated with a low measured $P$aCO$_2$. Common causes include:

- hysterical hyperventilation;
- compensation for underlying metabolic acidosis;
- neurological ones such as head injury or encephalitis;
- some interstitial lung diseases stimulating ventilation;
- early pulmonary oedema;
- hepatic failure (secondary effects).

Compensatory changes occur with time but are too slow to keep up with acute respiratory alkalosis. In chronic respiratory alkalosis, there is a rise in 2,3-diphosphoglycerate (2,3-DPG) which binds strongly to the β chains of deoxygenated Hb, inhibits oxygen binding, and shifts the oxygen dissociation curve to the right. This counteracts the early left shift changes in the dissociation curve with its resultant increased oxygen affinity seen as a result of a rise in pH.

### Metabolic acidosis

Metabolic or non-respiratory acidosis occurs when abnormal amounts of non-carbonic acid are formed and not adequately buffered. It can also occur in the presence of abnormal loss of base. The pH is disproportionately low for the measured $P$aCO$_2$. The following are some of the most common causes:

- increased acid production:
  - ketone bodies in diabetes mellitus;
  - lactate from shock or excessive exercise;
- acid ingestion (salicylate overdose);
- failure of excretion of $H^+$:
  - renal failure;
  - distal tubular acidosis;
  - carbonic anhydrase inhibitors (acetazolamide);

**Table 26.3 Blood gases (breathing air) in acute and chronic respiratory disease and in metabolic alkalosis**

| | Acute disease | Chronic disease | Metabolic alkalosis[a] |
|---|---|---|---|
| pH | 7.2 | 7.3 | > 7.44 |
| PaCO$_2$ (kPa) | 9.5 | 8.0 | > 6.0 |
| PaO$_2$ (kPa) | 9.5 | 9.5 | |
| $HCO_3^-$ (mmol/L) | 29 | 35 | > 32 |

- loss of bicarbonate:
  - diarrhoea;
  - gastrointestinal fistulae (pancreatic, biliary);
  - proximal renal tubular acidosis;
  - ureteroenterostomy;
  - cholestyramine.

The clinical effects of metabolic acidosis are as for respiratory acidosis and include:

- decreased cardiac output;
- pulmonary hypertension;
- cardiac arrhythmias;
- oliguria;
- increased circulating catecholamines;
- changes in mentation.

Treatment of metabolic acidosis is aimed at reducing the problems from chronic disease, as well as trying to treat the underlying condition.

Sodium bicarbonate therapy, although frequently given in the past, is reserved for severe conditions (pH $< 7.1$) because its use is not without risk. The 8.4% formulation has 1 mmol/ml of sodium and bicarbonate. There is a potential danger of sodium overload and precipitating heart failure. The solution is also hypertonic and must be given centrally to avoid tissue damage.

Acute alteration in acid–base balance with such drastic therapy as 8.4% sodium bicarbonate is useful in emergency situations but in chronic disease there are other consequences to consider. An increase in 2,3-DPG in chronic alkalosis results in a right shift of the oxygen dissociation curve. This will be further enhanced by sodium bicarbonate therapy and, although potentially beneficial in the normal individual, this may have negative effects in the diseased state. Treatment also produces a rise in $CO_2$ production and it is imperative that the patient is able to excrete this via the lungs.

If bicarbonate has to be used, the intravenous infusion dose (in mmol) can be calculated from the following formula:

$$0.33 \times \text{base excess} \times \text{body weight (kg)}$$

Half of this dose is given initially and the blood gas analysis performed and further treatment reassessed.

Other agents that can be used include sodium dichloroacetate, Carbicarb (sodium bicarbonate and carbonate in equimolar concentrations) and THAM (2-amino-2-hydroxymethyl-1,3-propanediol). This last agent is a non-sodium-containing buffer which has the benefit of avoiding a sodium load.

### Metabolic alkalosis

The diagnosis of a metabolic alkalosis is one of an inappropriately high pH for the measured arterial $P\text{CO}_2$ and occurs as a result of either an excessive production or administration of base or an abnormal loss of non-carbonic acid.

Typical blood gas findings are shown in Table 26.3. The following are the main causes.

#### *Loss of hydrogen ions*

- Renal $H^+$ loss:
  - primary and secondary hyperaldosteronism with potassium loss;
  - Conn's, Cushing's, and Bartter's syndromes;
  - adrenocorticotrophic hormone-secreting tumour.
- Medication:
  - diuretics: thiazides, frusemide (furosemide), ethacrynic acid;
  - corticosteroids causing $Na^+$ and bicarbonate retention and potassium excretion; chronic hypokalaemia results in preferential $H^+$ loss in the renal tubules to conserve potassium;
  - carbenoxolone.
- Gastrointestinal:
  - nasogastric suction;
  - vomiting;
  - high intestinal obstruction;
  - villous adenoma.

#### *Alkali gain*

- Iatrogenic milk alkali syndrome.
- Chronic administration of $NaHCO_3$ and other antacids.
- Metabolic conversion of organic acid ions to bicarbonate:
  - citrate: this used to be seen frequently with the conversion of citrate from stored blood in massive transfusion. The reduction in citrate use has reduced its occurrence, although fresh frozen plasma, cryoprecipitate and platelets are still suspended in citrate-phosphate-dextrose (CPD) solution and have a high citrate load if given in massive transfusion states;
  - lactate: large volume replacement with Ringer's lactate solution provides a high lactate load which can lead to a mild-to-moderate alkalosis.

#### *Miscellaneous*

- Dehydration.
- Sepsis.

The main clinical effects of metabolic alkalosis confine themselves to the central nervous system. Mentation is frequently obtunded and confusional states are common. Paraesthesia can also be seen, as can tetany, and these are mediated by the reduction in free ionized calcium concentration secondary to the altered protein binding.

Treatment is aimed at restoring the normal acid–base status, but as alkalosis can occasionally be life threatening it may be necessary to treat urgently. This is specifically the case when there is a profound secondary hypokalaemia, which occurs as a result of the body's homoeostatic mechanism to conserve $H^+$ ions.

Therapy is mainly directed at restoring the normal internal milieu including the extracellular fluid volume. This can be done by infusing almost any colloid or crystalloid, but avoid lactate-containing fluids and CPD blood unless indicated. It is important to give chloride if at all possible and therefore, unless there is any contraindication, it is probably best to administer sodium chloride. Hypokalaemia needs to be corrected as a priority and, in chronic alkalosis, it may take a large dose to do so because the extracellular and intracellular reserves are replaced. It may be advisable to treat with potassium-sparing diuretics if indicated. Spironolactone can be administered to help conserve potassium by restricting renal tubular loss.

More drastic measures can be taken, such as the use of acetazolamide to inhibit carbonic anhydrase or the direct acidification of blood by the administration of hydrogen chloride, ammonium chloride, lysine or arginine hydrochloride.

## LACTIC ACIDOSIS

Lactic acidosis is described as a metabolic acidosis accompanied by raised plasma lactate levels usually over the normally accepted limit of 0.8–2 mmol/L. There is a simultaneous increase in lactate and $[H^+]$ ions in this condition and they reflect a relative imbalance between oxygen requirement and supply to the cells. Nearly all organs manufacture some lactate from cellular metabolism as a by-product of the citrate cycle, but it is readily cleared in the normal state by the liver and rarely causes a problem. It is only over recent years that we have been able to measure lactate directly; previously it could only be implied indirectly by measuring the anion gap. Unfortunately, the relationship between the lactate level and the anion gap has been found to be quite weak.

The classification of lactic acidosis as described by Cohen and Woods has stood for some time, but it is probably now outdated. In their classification they described two types: type A and type B.

### *Type A lactic acidosis*

This relates to tissue hypoxia and causes include:

- exercise;
- shock;
- hypoxia;
- anaemia.

### *Type B lactic acidosis*

This includes all other causes including:

- drugs: phenformin, ethanol, paracetamol;
- intravenous feeding with excessive sorbitol or fructose;
- diabetes mellitus;
- renal failure;
- liver disease;
- infection: sepsis;
- leukaemia;
- lymphoma;
- thiamine deficiency;
- hereditary: glucose-6-phosphate deficiency.

The most common cause of acute type B lactic acidosis was biguanide therapy for diabetes, but this is now exceedingly rare. It is also quite probable on reflection that all of the other causes of type B fall into the hypoxic or metabolic categories of type A lactic acidosis. The relationship between cellular metabolism, tissue hypoxia, and lactate levels is also not that clear because lactate can rise as a result of reduced breakdown and clearance by the liver.

Treatment of lactic acidosis, as with other causes of acidotic states, should be directed at the underlying cause, and adequate provision and delivery of oxygen to the tissues is paramount. Intensive cardiopulmonary resuscitation to optimize $D\text{O}_2$ has been shown to be effective, as have measures to improve fluid status and treat underlying sepsis.

Alkalinization with sodium bicarbonate has been the mainstay of therapy, but it is really only a holding measure while the underlying condition is being treated. Isotonic sodium bicarbonate (1.4%) should be used to bring the pH back towards normal over 6–12 hours. Amine buffers, insulin and glucose infusions, and stimulation of pyruvate dehydrogenase with sodium dichloroacetate have all been used to treat this condition.

## ANION GAP

For normal homoeostasis, the electrical neutrality of the body must be maintained throughout all tissues and fluids. For this to occur, the number of anions in the body must always be balanced by the number of cations. Most of the cations can easily be measured and in plasma the major contribution to the cation charge is that of the $Na^+$ ion. It is not so easy to count the anion charge because a significant contribution is made by the proteins and this cannot be easily measured. For this reason there is an acceptable and predictable gap in the charge equation when balancing out the major players. Normally sodium and potassium contribute the cation component and chloride and bicarbonate the anion component:

$$\text{Anion gap} = (Na^+ + K^+) - (Cl^- + HCO_3^-)$$

When calculated there is a difference of between 10 and 16 and this is termed the anion gap. In disease states and acid–base imbalance, there is a tendency for this gap to widen, signifying other major contributors to the equation.

Causes of increased anion gap include:

- uraemic acidosis;
- ketoacidosis;
- salicylate poisoning;
- lactic acidosis;
- toxicity:
  - methanol;
  - ethylene glycol;
  - paraldehyde;
- dehydration;
- therapy with sodium salts of strong acids:
  - sodium lactate;
  - carbenicillin.

Causes of a low anion gap include:

- dilutional states;
- hypoalbuminaemia;
- hypernatraemia;
- hypomagnesaemia;

- hypercalcaemia;
- paraproteinaemia.

## HAEMODILUTION

Massive transfusion states have already been implicated for their contribution to acid–base imbalance. As well as the obvious direct effects of administration of acids or alkalis, there are the more subtle effects of dilution of the normal homoeostatic mechanisms present in the blood and plasma. A relative anaemia can be tolerated with ease by most individuals and, in fact, is of benefit to a certain point because of the lowering of viscosity and increased rheology. $D\text{O}_2$ is thought to be best at a haematocrit of 28–33%. However, in acute haemodilution states, the sensitive equilibrium between the plasma proteins, Hb, enzymatic processes, and buffering power are all disturbed.

We have already discovered the magnitude of the buffering capacity of the erythrocyte and Hb, and the way that this is affected in hypoxic states, poor flow, and alterations in acid–base balance. Although it is acceptable to a point that acute profound anaemia is experienced in massive blood loss and electively during some types of surgery, it is imperative to realize the consequences that this may have on the body's homoeostatic mechanisms. Haemodilution, as its name implies, reduces all components of the intravascular compartment and with this the reserve the body may have to resist major changes in acid–base status. The reduction in plasma proteins will alter the ability to buffer $H^+$, as will the loss in Hb. This effect is compounded by the transfusion of acidic blood with low 2,3-DPG levels, such that there will be a left shift in the oxygen dissociation curve. A low Hb will also reduce the body's ability to buffer $H^+$ or carry $CO_2$ from the tissues. In the 'normal' individual, the reserve is probably sufficient to cope with these changes but, in disease states, where there may be coexistent pulmonary or cardiac disease, then $D\text{O}_2$ and acid–base homeostasis may be compromised.

## SURGERY

Just as disease states can have a significant effect on acid–base balance, there are many other ways that we can influence the normal homoeostatic mechanisms in relatively fit individuals. Haemodilution and transfusion are two significant insults inflicted on the surgical patient, but they are also compounded by altered haemodynamics induced by anaesthesia and surgery, as well as other serious alterations in physiology. The surgical patient frequently arrives in the operating room starved and relatively hypovolaemic. Tissue perfusion has already been compromised and peripheral shutdown with areas of relative hypoxaemia may already exist. Further reduction in $D\text{O}_2$ on induction of anaesthesia aggravates the impending problem.

Improved oxygenation on ventilation and volume expansion with an intravenous infusion help to rectify the situation transiently, but this is soon offset by loss of smooth muscle vascular control induced by opioids. The patient sinks further into a state of tissue hypo-perfusion. The surgical insult imparted by laparotomy and manipulation of the bowels and mesentery induces a third-space effect with further volume depletion. The mesenteric blood flow is compromised and the liver, kidneys, and bowel suffer a mild hypotensive insult. Loss of renal blood flow now reduces the body's ability to control one of its main routes of $H^+$ ion excretion. The other, namely the lungs, is no longer under the control of the hypothalamus but at the mercy of the anaesthetist. A fixed minute volume removes the flexibility to control $CO_2$ excretion. Liver hypoperfusion reduces its ability to metabolize lactate and other metabolic byproducts, which could further contribute to acid–base imbalance. Hypothermia ensues and metabolic processes are slowed, and oxygen dissociation impaired.

All of these events happen every day in the patients for whom we are responsible. Their own sensitive homoeostatic mechanisms are rendered inoperative and they rely on the coarse manipulations that, at best, we administer in an attempt to maintain control. An understanding of the way that these systems operate and interact may help us to direct better placed therapy in the clinical environment and to improve the outcome of those in our care.

## SUMMARY

- The body's buffer systems are set up primarily to neutralize acids.
- Alkalosis is tolerated poorly.
- Patients with anaemia, low plasma proteins, and decreased muscle mass have a reduced buffering capacity and are very likely to have wide pH swings when ill or injured.
- Patients suffering from shock, sepsis, or trauma who are not hyperventilating have an increased risk of developing respiratory failure. This is made worse by parenteral nutrition.
- Biological systems react primarily to the rate of change of electrolytes and not to the absolute levels. Sudden changes, even to correct severely abnormal values, may be deleterious.
- Abnormalities should be treated at approximately the same rate as that at which they developed. If their duration is unknown, only half the deficit should be corrected and repeated results obtained.
- A rise in pH of 0.1 is associated with a corresponding fall of about 0.5 mmol/L in plasma potassium. The reverse is also true.
- A 10 mmHg increase or decrease in $P\text{CO}_2$ (i.e. 1.35 kPa) causes an opposite change of approximately 0.1 in pH (i.e. $[H^+]$ 9 mmol/L) at normal levels of around pH 7.4 ($[H^+]$ 40 mmol/L).
- Plasma chloride and bicarbonate concentrations tend to move in opposite directions. In metabolic alkalosis, chloride falls and bicarbonate rises. In metabolic acidosis, however, the bicarbonate falls, but the chloride seldom rises much above normal.
- A $P\text{CO}_2$ below 20–25 mmHg (2.7–3.3 kPa) may seriously interfere with cerebral perfusion and function.
- In patients with metabolic acidosis, the reduced $P\text{O}_2$ and the increased $P\text{CO}_2$ resulting from compensatory hypoventilation may cause an erroneous diagnosis of pulmonary insufficiency.
- Treatment of metabolic acidosis should be directed initially and primarily to the underlying

cause of the impaired cell metabolism. Base deficits persisting after such therapy may then be corrected with bicarbonate.

- It is essential to proceed slowly to correct severe chronic respiratory acidosis. Too rapid correction may cause sudden, severe, combined metabolic and respiratory alkalosis, and may result in seizures, severe cardiac arrhythmias, or death.
- In patients with chronic hypercapnia, administration of high concentrations of oxygen may severely depress or arrest ventilation, and may cause further hypercapnia and death.
- Patients with apparently excessive hyperventilation may be cautiously sedated. They may become severely lethargic after the cycle of hyperventilation and respiratory alkalosis has been broken.
- An acid urine despite the presence of an alkalosis in the blood is evidence of hypokalaemia or total body potassium deficit until proven otherwise.

## FURTHER READING


Bowe EA, Klein EF. Acid base, blood gas, electrolytes. In: Barash J, ed. *Clinical Anaesthesia*. New York: Lippincott, 1989: 669–706.

Breyer MD, Jacobson HR. The diagnosis and treatment of disorders of acid base balance. In: Kelly W, ed. *Textbook of Internal Medicine*. Philadelphia: Lippincott, 1988: 922.

Davenport HW. *The ABC of Acid–Base Chemistry*. Chicago: The University of Chicago Press, 1965.

Donaldson MDJ, Seamn MJ, Park GR. Review article. Massive blood transfusion. *Br J Anaesth* 1992;**69**:621–30.

Fowler NO, Holmes JC. Blood viscosity and cardiac output in the acute experimental anaemia. *J Appl Physiol* 1973:**36**:453–6.

Isbister JP. Blood transfusion, blood products and autologous transfusion. *Curr Opin Anaesthesiol* 1992;**5**:263–71.

Willatts SM. Acid base balance. In: Willatt SM, ed. *Lecture Notes on Fluid and Electrolyte Balance.* London: Blackwell Scientific Publications, 1982: 234–57.

# Chapter 27 The gastrointestinal tract

L. Bromley, J.W. Sear, and G.M. Cooper

## GENERAL FUNCTION

The gastrointestinal (GI) tract is the boundary between the external and the internal environments where food is prepared for passage to the internal environment. Nutrients are propelled and mixed by the musculature of the GI tract and broken down into smaller units (digestion) that are absorbed through the intestinal tract mucosa into the lymph or portal blood. The absorption process takes place by diffusion, carrier transport, or endocytosis.

Digestion begins in the mouth, where the large food particles are reduced in size, mixed with saliva, and converted into a semifluid mass. Swallowing transfers the chewed food to the oesophagus. The food passes through the oesophagus to the stomach, where it is mixed with gastric juice and liquefied. This liquefied food passes through the pyloric sphincter into the duodenum. Exocrine secretions from the intestinal cells and digestive juices from the pancreas and gallbladder are added to the intestinal contents in the duodenum. Bile produced by the liver aids digestion of fats as well as removing bilirubin. The liver plays a key role in the metabolism of carbohydrates, fats, proteins, and hormones (see Chapter 28). The pancreas contributes bicarbonate and digestive enzymes in addition to its endocrine function. A number of GI hormones that contribute to the regulation of digestion are primarily produced in the upper part of the small intestine, the lower stomach, and in the pancreas.

Most of the absorption of the digested food takes place in the small intestine. The fluid balance of the GI tract is summarized in Figure 27.1. About 2 litres of water (much contained in food) are ingested each day and approximately 7 litres of various secretions enter the GI tract. Nearly all of this is absorbed. About 2 litres of water passes to the colon, of which 90% is absorbed. The contents of the large intestine, faeces, consist mainly of unabsorbable vegetable matter, desquamated cells, and bacteria.

The time required for passage of food through the different parts of the GI tract varies between individuals and also depends on the composition of the food. Mean passage times are illustrated in Figure 27.2. Of particular relevance to anaesthetists is the fact that (normally) 50% of the water entering the stomach has left it in 10–20 min whereas the time for solids is anything from 1 to 4 hours. Carbohydrates are emptied more easily than proteins and fats linger the longest. Thus, in normal circumstances, there is a need to allow longer for fatty meals to be absorbed and 2 hours' starvation after ingesting clear fluids should be ample. Nevertheless, it must be remembered that pain and

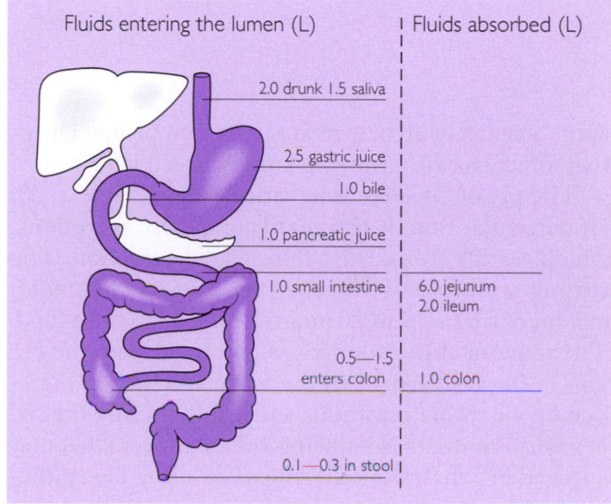


**Figure 27.1** Daily fluid balance of the gastrointestinal tract.

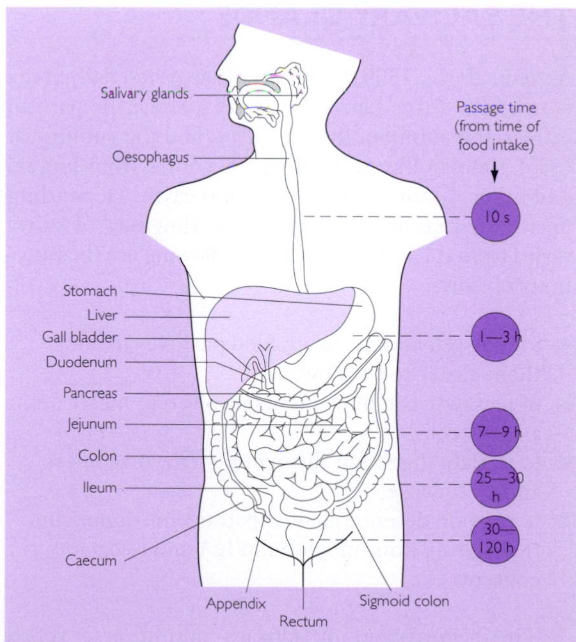


**Figure 27.2** Passage time of food in the gastrointestinal tract. (From Despopoulos A and Silbernagl S, eds. *Color Atlas of Physiology*, 4th edn. New York: Thième Medical Publishers, 1991.)

**Table 27.1 The pH of gastrointestinal secretions**

| Secretion | pH |
|---|---|
| Saliva | 6–7 |
| Gastric fluid | 1.0–3.5 |
| Bile | 7–8 |
| Pancreatic fluid | 8.0–8.3 |
| Small intestine | 6.5–7.5 |
| Colon | 7.5–8.0 |

apprehension or anxiety retard gastric emptying. Drugs that affect gastric emptying are discussed later.

The pH of GI secretions varies widely (Table 27.1). Of particular note is the acidity of gastric secretions, which results from hydrochloric acid secretion. The resting secretion of hydrogen ($H^+$) ions of 2 mmol/h can increase to up to 20 mmol/h on ingestion of food. The mucosa of the stomach is protected from the $H^+$ ions in the gastric juice by the active secretion of bicarbonate ions which, without noticeably altering the pH of gastric contents, adequately buffer any acid that may succeed in penetrating the mucus covering the epithelium.

The physiology of the individual parts of the GI tract and pharmacology related to each organ are considered together.

## THE SALIVARY GLANDS

As seen above, 1500 ml of saliva is secreted daily. This is from the three pairs of salivary glands: the parotid (20%), the submandibular (70%), and the sublingual (5%) glands. The remaining 5% comes from lingual and other minor glands in the oral cavity. Depending on the degree of stimulation, the flow rate of saliva varies from 0.1 to 4 ml/min. The following are the functions of saliva:

- to moisten and lubricate food particles making them easier to swallow;
- to facilitate the movements involved in mastication and speech;
- to initiate digestion through the enzymes lipase and $\alpha$-amylase;
- to provide defence against pathogenic organisms through its immunoglobulin IgA and lysozyme content.

The stimulation of salivary output is a reflex response set off by taste, smell, and touch receptors, as well as by chewing. Secretion of watery saliva is controlled by the parasympathetic nervous system. The parotid gland is innervated by the glossopharyngeal nerve, and the submandibular and sublingual glands by the facial nerve. The salivary glands also receive a sympathetic innervation, stimulation of which produces a viscous secretion. The reason for two different sorts of salivary secretion is not known.

### The antimuscarinic drugs

This group of drugs acts as competitive antagonists of acetylcholine at muscarinic receptors throughout the autonomic nervous system (see also Chapter 23). Muscarinic cholinergic receptors are examples of G-protein-coupled receptors (see Chapter 23) that also depend on second-messenger coupling. Differences in action of antimuscarinic drugs are related to the subclasses of muscarinic receptors present in different parts of the GI tract. $M_3$-receptors control salivary and bronchial secretions, and are inhibited by lower doses of anticholinergic drugs than are needed to inhibit the $M_2$-receptors that regulate acetylcholine effects on the heart and eye.

Larger doses of anticholinergic drugs inhibit cholinergic control of the GI and genitourinary tracts, thus decreasing tone and motility of the intestine and inhibiting micturition. Even larger doses of anticholinergic drugs are required to inhibit gastric secretion of $H^+$ ions through the $M_1$-receptor. Therefore, a dose of anticholinergic drug that inhibits gastric secretion of $H^+$ ions invariably affects salivary secretion, heart rate, oculomotor accommodation, and micturition. Thus atropine, hyoscine, and glycopyrrolate act on $M_1$-, $M_2$-, and $M_3$-receptors. At present the only selective muscarinic blocker available is pirenzepine which acts on $M_1$-receptors to prevent gastric $H^+$ secretion. A selective $M_2$-receptor blocker would be useful to prevent the bradycardia caused by parasympathetic stimulation, but as yet none is available.

#### *Atropine*

This naturally occurring alkaloid is extracted from the plant *Atropa belladonna*, the deadly nightshade. Its onset of action when given intravenously is very rapid, and by intramuscular injection is within 10–15 min. Of the amount given orally 60–70% is absorbed from the small intestine. Atropine is a tertiary amine that crosses the blood–brain barrier. It has a short duration of action of only 1–1.5 hours. It is extensively metabolized by liver esterases, with very little of the unchanged drug appearing in the urine. Table 27.2 summarizes the comparative effects of the antimuscarinic drugs.

#### *Hyoscine*

Hyoscine is also a naturally occurring alkaloid which is found in *Hyoscimus niger*, the henbane plant. It is also a tertiary amine, and has more pronounced central effects. Its duration of action is short, of the order of 1 hour. Its terminal half-life is 2 hours. It is well absorbed from the GI tract, and can be given transdermally, this use being primarily for its antiemetic effect (see 'Antiemetic drugs'). It undergoes extensive liver esterase metabolism, only 1% appearing unchanged in the urine.

#### *Glycopyrrolate*

This drug, by contrast, is an ionized semisynthetic quaternary amine and does not readily cross the blood–brain barrier. It can be given by intramuscular and intravenous routes. It is largely excreted unchanged in the urine with a terminal half-life of 75 minutes. Its antisialagogue action is long, more than 6 hours, and its antisialagogue potency is about five times that of atropine.

**Table 27.2 Comparative effects of antimuscarinic drugs (in usual clinical dose)**

| Effect | Atropine | Hyoscine | Glycopyrrolate |
|---|---|---|---|
| Sedation | + | +++ | 0 |
| Antisialogogue | + | ++ | +++ |
| Antiemetic | + | +++ | 0 |
| Increase in heart rate | +++ | + | ++ |
| Smooth muscle relaxation | ++ | + | ++ |
| Effect on eye (mydriasis) | + | +++ | 0 |
| Reduced gastric H+ secretion | + | + | + |
| Amnesia | + | ++ | 0 |

0 = no effect, + mild, ++ moderate, +++ marked.

## THE OESOPHAGUS

The oesophagus is 25–30 cm in length, which fact is useful to know when inserting a nasogastric tube. If more than this has been introduced and no aspirate is obtained, it is likely that the tube has kinked or curled somewhere en route. The oesophagus passes through the chest behind the heart (see Chapter 6). Although dysphagia usually points to oesophageal or nervous system pathology, it should also be remembered that mediastinal masses (e.g. an enlarged left atrium) can cause subjective difficulty in swallowing. The musculature at the upper third of the oesophagus is striated and the remainder is smooth muscle.

Progressive peristaltic pressure waves pass from the upper oesophagus down the oesophageal body to the lower oesophageal sphincter (LOS) and are initiated by swallowing (primary peristalsis) or distension secondary to physiological gastro-oesophageal reflux (secondary peristalsis). Non-propulsive waves in the lower oesophagus (tertiary peristalsis) may be seen in oesophageal motility disorders.

The LOS, which permits the passage of food from the oesophagus to the stomach, is a physiological (not an anatomical) sphincter at the cardia composed of smooth muscle. This normally prevents the gastric contents from refluxing into the oesophagus. Its barrier function is supported by the skeletal muscle at the hiatus in the diaphragm and by the angle of insertion of the oesophagus with the stomach. The LOS relaxes at the end of a peristaltic pressure wave. The only other physiological situation of physiological relaxation is during vomiting.

Various drugs affect LOS function (Table 27.3). It should be borne in mind that the drugs have greater effect on a normal LOS than on one damaged in the course of gastro-oesophageal reflux disease.

**Table 27.3 Drugs that affect lower oesophageal sphincter tone**

| Increase | Decrease |
|---|---|
| Anticholinesterases<br>Neostigmine<br>Edrophonium | Antimuscarinics<br>Atropine<br>Glycopyrrolate |
| Cholinergics | Volatile anaesthetic agents |
| Suxamethonium | Sodium nitroprusside |
| Pancuronium | Thiopentone (thiopental) |
| Histamine | β-Adrenoceptor agonists |
| α-Adrenoceptor agonists | Dopamine |
| Metoclopramide | Opioids |
| Domperidone | Peppermint oil |
| Antacids | |
| Ergometrine | |
| Cisapride | |

The LOS is affected pathologically by achalasia. In this disorder, oesophageal peristalsis is absent and the LOS pressure fails to relax in response to swallowing. Treatment is aimed at reducing LOS pressure by dilatation with large diameter balloons or surgical myotomy. Anaesthetists should be aware that food may persist in the oesophagus.

Cricoid pressure decreases LOS pressure, presumably as a result of stimulation of mechanoreceptors in the pharynx from external pressure on the cricoid cartilage. In patients with a hiatus hernia, part of the stomach herniates into the chest. This may promote gastro-oesophageal reflux by trapping gastric acid in the hernial sac, which may then flow back into the oesophagus when the LOS relaxes during swallowing.

The pressure in the lumen at the gastro-oesophageal junction (at the LOS) is a measure of the strength of the antireflux barrier. This is normally between 10 and 30 mmHg at the end of expiration. Opposing this is the pressure within the stomach, which is normally above 7 mmHg. These pressures can be measured by either static or ambulatory oesophageal manometry. The difference between the LOS tone pressure and the intragastric pressure is known as the barrier pressure. Thus, factors that increase intragastric pressure (e.g. a large meal, pregnancy, pyloric stenosis) or decrease LOS will predispose to reflux. In a person who is supine, gastric contents may reflux into the pharynx. If the larynx is open there is a danger of aspiration of gastric contents into the trachea.

## THE STOMACH

### Gastric acid secretion

The stomach stores and processes food for digestion. As shown earlier (see Figure 27.1) about 2.5 litres of gastric juice are secreted daily, the main components of which are hydrochloric acid, pepsinogens, mucus, and intrinsic factor. Hydrochloric acid kills bacteria, aids protein digestion, provides the necessary pH for pepsin to start protein digestion, and stimulates the flow of bile and pancreatic juice.

Secretion of hydrochloric acid is dependent on stimulation of the parietal cell membrane by histamine (via $H_2$-receptors), acetylcholine (via $M_1$-receptors), and gastrin. All these receptors increase the transport of $H^+$ into the gastric lumen under the influence of carbonic anhydrase and a $H^+/K^+$ adenosine triphosphatase (ATPase)-driven proton pump.

Peptic ulceration commonly involves the stomach, duodenum, and lower oesophagus. Healing can be promoted by general measures, stopping smoking and taking antacids, and by antisecretory drug treatment, but relapse is common when treatment is stopped. The previously held belief that ulcers were caused by excessive gastric acid secretion led to development of drugs that raise the pH of gastric contents (see below). It has, however, recently been appreciated that nearly all duodenal ulcers and most gastric ulcers not associated with non-steroidal anti-inflammatory drugs (NSAIDs) are caused by *Helicobacter pylori*. Long-term healing of duodenal and gastric ulcers can be achieved by eradicating *H. pylori* with triple therapy for one week (e.g. amoxycillin + metronidazole + omeprazole).

The role of NSAIDs in the aetiology of peptic ulceration is also important; although the overall incidence of peptic ulceration has declined over the past 20 years, its incidence has increased in middle-aged and elderly people through NSAID usage. These drugs inhibit prostaglandin synthesis, and result in the impaired secretion of mucin and bicarbonate, as well as impaired wound healing. The prostaglandin $E_1$ analogue misoprostol reduces the incidence of gastric ulceration in those patients taking NSAIDs.

The need to raise the pH of the gastric contents is usually more acute in anaesthetic practice than required by a gastroenterologist, and the drugs that have been developed do not necessarily serve that purpose ideally. The avoidance of pulmonary aspiration of gastric contents is the prime objective of the use of these drugs in anaesthesia. To achieve this objective, ideally reduction of the volume of the stomach contents as well as raising the pH are required. In experimental studies, a volume of less than 25 ml and a pH above 2.5 have been taken as the criteria to achieve, although the actual clinical relevance is arguable. It is important to understand that drugs will not affect the volume of the stomach contents or the pH at the time of administering the drug. The full stomach needs to be dealt with by other means. The pH of gastric contents can be raised by chemical neutralization with alkaline agents.

### The alkalis

There are a number of alkaline solutions available for antacid action, but in anaesthetic practice the most commonly used drug is sodium citrate. This is given in a 0.3 mol/L solution in a dose of up to 30 ml, immediately before induction of anaesthesia. It has the advantage of acting rapidly, although it has little buffering capacity. Sodium citrate does not produce carbon dioxide like the bicarbonate alkalis, and it is not particulate like the aluminium salts, both of which have been shown to contribute to an increased risk of complications from aspiration.

### Drugs that raise gastric pH

The pharmacological approach to the reduction of gastric acid secretion is based on the physiological understanding of the mechanism of secretion. Thus drugs can be divided into those with an antivagal action or an anti-gastrin action, and those that antagonize the paracrine modulators of secretion.

### Antivagal drugs

The vagus affects gastric acid secretion by two mechanisms. It has a direct action on the parietal cell via $M_1$-muscarinic receptors on the surface of the cell. It also stimulates the secretion of gastrin from the antrum of the stomach, a hormone released in response to food entering the stomach.

Atropine, hyoscine, and glycopyrrolate antagonize acetylcholine and prevent stimulation of the $M_1$-receptor. However, antivagal drugs cannot completely abolish the production of gastric acid because acetylcholine is only one of the modifiers of $H^+/K^+$ ATPase activity. Of the other two mediators, gastrin secretion is reduced by antimuscarinic drugs, but histamine is unaffected.

### Histamine $H_2$-receptor antagonists

Histamine acts at the $H_2$-receptors on the parietal cell surface to activate a G protein that stimulates adenylyl cyclase. This increases cyclic AMP and increases the activity of the $H^+/K^+$ ATPase proton pump. The $H_2$ antagonists are competitive antagonists at this receptor, and cause a dose-related reduction in gastric acid secretion. They also reduce the total volume of the gastric contents. A reflex rise in gastrin occurs.

The $H_2$ antagonists are chemically related to histamine in structure. They are well absorbed orally, although the concomitant use of antacids can reduce their absorption by up to 30%. Examples are shown in Table 27.4.

Many millions of people throughout the world have taken $H_2$ antagonists, particularly cimetidine, which is available across the counter in many countries. As a result, remarkably few unwanted effects have been recorded. These consist principally of effects on the central nervous system (CNS), the cerebrovascular system (CVS), and the liver.

#### *CNS effects*

Cimetidine can cause headache, dizziness, sleepiness, and less commonly delirium and confusion. There are also reports of hallucinations. These effects do not occur with ranitidine or the newer drugs that do not cross the blood–brain barrier.

**Table 27.4 $H_2$ antagonists and their pharmacological properties**

| Drug | Protein binding (%) | Relative potency | $t_{1/2}$ (hours) | Metabolism (%) |
|---|---|---|---|---|
| Cimetidine | 20 | 1 | 1.5–2 | 30–40 |
| Ranitidine | 15 | 4–10 | 1.6–2.5 | 10 |
| Famotidine | 15–20 | 20–50 | 3.0 | Minimal |
| Nizatidine | 35 | 4–10 | 1.3–1.6 | Minimal |

#### *CVS effects*

These are seen when using infusions of the drug. They are produced by actions at the $H_2$-receptors in the atria. Cimetidine occasionally causes bradyarrhythmias whereas ranitidine has a slight inotropic effect, as a result of an action on sympathetic presynaptic receptors.

#### *Hepatic effects*

These drugs bind to cytochrome P450 in liver microsomal enzymes to varying degrees, cimetidine being the most marked, ranitidine five- to tenfold less, and famotidine and nizatidine insignificantly. The binding of cimetidine produces enzyme inhibition, but its binding characteristics vary with different isoenzymes, so its effects on the metabolism of other drugs varies. Benzodiazepines, theophylline, and dobutamine are significantly affected.

In addition, cimetidine, and to a lesser extent ranitidine, interfere with active renal tubular secretion of procainamide and metformin.

### The proton pump inhibitors

These drugs bind covalently with the enzyme $H^+/K^+$ ATPase on the gastric surface of the parietal cell. This blocks gastric acid secretion from all stimuli in a dose-dependent manner, with the maximal effect after 5 days.

Omeprazole is the original drug in this group. It is a substituted benzimidazole prodrug which, after conversion to the active form, becomes trapped in the parietal cell. Although it is widely distributed, this trapping effect tends to concentrate the drug preferentially in the parietal cells. The covalent binding with the enzyme results in a very long duration of action, of the order of 24 hours. Any free drug is rapidly metabolized with a plasma half-life of 1.5 hours. The reduction in gastric acid produces a reflex increase in gastrin production.

Lansoprazole and pantoprazole are two newer proton pump inhibitors that share the same mechanism of action, but differ in their pharmacokinetics. They are better absorbed and have a greater bioavailability. Lansoprazole is said to have significant antibacterial effect on *H. pylori*.

### Gastric motility

The rate of normal gastric emptying and physiological factors influencing it have been mentioned (see also Figure 27.2). The motor function of the stomach is controlled by cholinergic mechanisms via the myenteric plexus. A number of drugs are said to be prokinetic, i.e. they promote normal gastric motility in an onward direction. Largely, these actions are bought about by increasing acetylcholine, but 5-hydroxytryptamine (5HT; serotonin) is probably also involved. $5HT_4$-receptors are present in the wall of the gut and are stimulated by its distension.

#### *Drugs that increase gastric motility*

*Metoclopramide*

Metoclopramide is used principally as an antiemetic (see below), but it also promotes gastric motility, and increases LOS tone. It can be given orally, intramuscularly, or intravenously, and accelerates gastric clearance of liquids and solids. It does not affect gastric acid secretion. Its actions include release of acetylcholine from nerve endings in the myenteric plexus, sensitizing neurons to the action of acetylcholine and as a dopamine antagonist. In high doses, it is also a $5HT_4$ antagonist, although at low doses it has a partial agonist action at this receptor. Its prokinetic actions are probably accounted for by its cholinergic actions, although the partial agonist action at $5HT_4$-receptors may also be involved.

The major disadvantage of metoclopramide as a prokinetic agent is its central effect. The drug crosses the blood–brain barrier and is capable of producing significant dysphoric and parkinsonian, unwanted effects as a result of its antidopaminergic action.

*Cisapride*

Cisapride is an orally administered prokinetic agent. It is used for the treatment of reflux oesophagitis, but its action extends to the entire length of the gut. It increases motility and aids gastric emptying, as well as raising LOS tone. It does not cross the blood–brain barrier, and therefore has no central effects.

Concomitant administration of cisapride with drugs that inhibit its metabolism can raise plasma cisapride concentrations, which may result in QT prolongation and serious ventricular arrhythmias. Such drugs include clarithromycin, erythromycin, fluconazole, and ketoconazole.

Cisapride is highly protein bound in the plasma and has a half-life of 10 hours.

#### *Drugs that reduce gastric motility*

*Antimuscarinic drugs*

Atropine and hyoscine have been used to reduce intestinal spasm through their anticholinergic action. The acceptability of these drugs for this purpose is low because of the incidence of dry mouth.

A number of homologues of atropine and hyoscine are in use: homatropine, hyoscine-*n*-butylbromide, and propantheline as a gastrointestinal antispasmodic during endoscopy.

Pirenzepine is related to the tricyclic antidepressant drugs and selectively blocks muscarinic $M_1$-receptors as discussed earlier. The drug is not used in anaesthetic practice because it lowers the oesophageal sphincter tone and barrier pressure.

### Gastric absorption

The villous structure characteristic of absorptive membranes is absent and therefore the stomach is a poor absorptive area. As a result, only highly lipid-soluble liquids, such as alcohol, and some drugs, such as aspirin, can be significantly absorbed from the stomach.

## NAUSEA AND VOMITING

### Physiology

#### *Definitions*

Nausea is an unpleasant, but not painful, sensation referred to the pharynx and upper abdomen, associated with the desire to vomit. Vomiting is the forceful expulsion of upper GI contents through the mouth. Retching involves the same muscle groups, but does not result in expulsion of gastric contents and usually, but not always, precedes it. Vomiting must not be confused with gastro-oesophageal reflux or regurgitation, which is a passive process dependent on gravity and does not involve the same pattern of muscle activity.

It is likely that the vomiting reflex evolved as a protective reflex against the ingestion of toxic substances. Poisons are not always detected by sight, taste, or smell and therefore may be eaten inadvertently. Once contaminated food has been swallowed, it can be ejected rapidly only by vomiting. Toxins are identified as such by detectors before absorption in the lumen of the upper GI tract and in the circulation after absorption. These detectors then set up a series of events which causes:

- nausea to prevent further ingestion of poisonous substance;
- gastric relaxation to reduce gastric emptying;
- retching and vomiting to eject the poison from the body.

In this sense, nausea and vomiting would be seen as beneficial, but in anaesthetic practice it is more often seen as an unpleasant sequel of surgery and anaesthesia.

The accompanying symptoms of nausea, which are salivation, pallor, lacrimation, tachycardia, and cold sweating, are mediated via the sympathetic nervous system. It is thought that the vomiting centre (see below) activates sympathetic efferents in the hypothalamus to trigger these effects.

The process of vomiting involves the following sequence:

- increased salivation;
- deepened breathing;
- closure of the glottis;
- breath held in midinspiration;
- contraction of abdominal muscles;
- relaxation of oesophageal sphincters;
- gastric contents expelled.

In addition to the unpleasantness there are adverse physiological effects of vomiting, which are summarized in Table 27.5. The importance of these effects and their occurrence depends on the severity of symptoms and the general condition of the patient (see also Chapter 1).

The control of vomiting is quite complex and involves a wide variety of afferent inputs. The control of vomiting is shown in the schematic diagram of Figure 27.3. From this it can be appreciated that there are many influences on the occurrence of postoperative nausea and vomiting.

The vomiting centre is in the medulla close to the fourth ventricle. It is stimulated by sensory afferents in

**Table 27.5 The adverse physiological effects of postoperative nausea and vomiting**

| System | Effect |
|---|---|
| Cardiovascular system | As in Valsalva manoeuvre during vomiting (see Chapter 19)<br>Hypotension and bradycardia (vagal response)<br>May cause myocardial ischaemia |
| Respiratory system | Aspiration of gastric contents if larynx incompetent<br>Hypoxia during breath-holding while retching<br>Rib fracture if severe retching |
| GI tract | Oesophageal tear or rupture<br>Dehydration if prolonged<br>Metabolic alkalosis through loss of gastric acid<br>Loss of sodium and potassium |
| General | Muscular strain<br>Fatigue<br>Wound disruption (abdominal, eye, plastic surgery wounds)<br>Bruising of face and upper body<br>Psychological aversion to anaesthesia |

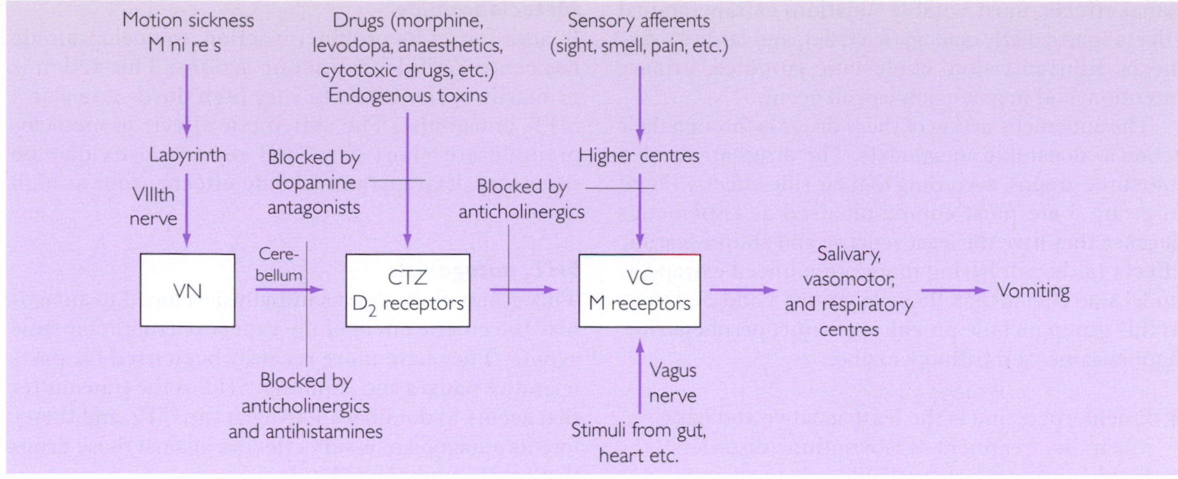


**Figure 27.3** Schematic diagram of the control of vomiting, showing influences on the vomiting centre (VC) and the chemoreceptor trigger zone (CTZ). VN, vestibular nucleus.

the cerebral cortex, vagally mediated stimuli from the GI tract, the heart, or pelvic organs and from the chemoreceptor trigger zone (CTZ). The CTZ is an area situated in the area postrema of the medulla, on the lateral walls of the fourth ventricle. It lies outside the blood–brain barrier, unlike the vomiting centre which is within it. Chemoreceptor cells within the CTZ are thus directly exposed to blood-borne chemicals and therefore able to respond rapidly. The CTZ is stimulated by dopamine, norepinephrine (noradrenaline), acetylcholine, 5HT, and opioid receptor agonists. Stimulation of the CTZ stimulates the vomiting centre, which initiates vomiting.

## The pharmacology of antiemetic drugs (Table 27.6)

As shown in Figure 27.3, the possible triggers to postoperative nausea and vomiting are numerous. The drugs used to control nausea and vomiting come from a number of different families, as might be expected from the numbers of transmitter substances involved in the physiology of this reflex response. It is also not surprising that a single therapeutic approach to the treatment of postoperative vomiting is frequently unsuccessful.

### *The anticholinergics*

Hyoscine is the most potent of the anticholinergic drugs in use for its antiemetic action. The input of the vestibular apparatus to the CTZ is a cholinergic pathway, and for this reason hyoscine is most effective against motion sickness. Its use as a premedicant contributes to the prevention of postoperative nausea and vomiting and, as it is often combined with an opioid, it offsets some of the emetic effect of these drugs. However, its action is not sufficient to control established postoperative nausea and vomiting.

### *The phenothiazines*

This group of drugs is used primarily for their antipsychotic effect, antiemetic effects being an additional action. A number are sufficiently potent antiemetics to be used for that purpose in the postoperative period. As a result of their profound effect on neurotransmitters, they can inevitably produce a wide variety of addi-

**Table 27.6 Antiemetic drugs and their specificity for different receptors**

| | Dopamine | Cholinergic $M_3$ | Histamine $H_1$ | $5HT_3$ |
|---|---|---|---|---|
| Location of receptors | CTZ and vomiting centre | Gut wall, CTZ, and vomiting centre | CTZ and vomiting centre | Gut wall, CTZ, and vomiting centre |
| Anticholinergics | | +++++ | + | |
| Phenothiazines | ++++ | ++ | +++ | + |
| Butyrophenones | ++++ | | + | + |
| Antihistamines | ++ | ++ | +++ | |
| Metoclopramide | +++ | | + | ++ |
| $5HT_3$ antagonists | | | | ++++ |

CTZ, chemoreceptor trigger zone.

tional effects, most notably sedation, extrapyramidal effects (particularly oculogyric crisis), and tardive dyskinesia. Blurred vision, cholestatic jaundice, urinary retention, and hypotension can all occur.

The antiemetic action of these drugs is through their action as dopamine antagonists. The drugs are divided into three groups, according to their side effects. Those in group 3 are most commonly used as antiemetics because they have the least sedative and antimuscarinic effects (although having more pronounced extrapyramidal side effects than those in groups 1 and 2). Drugs in this group include prochlorperazine, perphenazine, fluphenazine, and trifluoperazine:

- Prochlorperazine is the least sedative and has a role in the treatment of labyrinthine disorders.
- Perphenazine is now available only in an oral formulation, which may be given as a premedicant. It produces sedation and was commonly associated with oculogyric crisis.
- Chlorpromazine was originally introduced as an adjunct to anaesthesia for its antiemetic effects. It is now rarely used for this purpose and is primarily an antipsychotic drug.
- Promethazine has both antihistaminic and antidopaminergic actions. It is markedly sedative, the effect lasting longer than the antiemetic effect.

### The butyrophenones

Droperidol is the only drug in this group in use in anaesthesia. It has anti-dopaminergic and anti-GABA (γ-aminobutyrate) actions, its antiemetic effects being related to the former site of activity. It is less sedative than the phenothiazines. It has been used in combination with opioids in patient-controlled analgesia systems, and has been shown to reduce the incidence of nausea and vomiting seen with that technique. It is used in prophylaxis in particularly vulnerable patients. Its side effects include sedation and dysphoria. It is metabolized in the liver and has a plasma half-life of 2 hours.

### The antihistamines

$H_2$-Receptors are found in both the CTZ and the vomiting centre. In addition, they are concentrated in the nucleus tractus solitarus, which processes incoming sensory information likely to cause emesis. Most antihistaminic drugs with an antiemetic action work on the CTZ.

Cyclizine has both antihistaminic and antimuscarinic effects. It is less sedative than the other antihistaminic drugs, and has the best side effect profile of the commonly used antiemetics. It is, however, only moderately efficacious in reducing nausea and vomiting, and is unlikely to be sufficient to prevent nausea and vomiting in those patients who are particularly vulnerable. It is prepared in combination with morphine (Cyclimorph), but, as its duration of action is longer than that of morphine, repeat doses can lead to accumulation of cyclazine and sedation. This has led to a decline in the use of Cyclimorph.

Cinnarizine and chlorpheniramine are both antihistamines that have some antiemetic effects, but they are not in routine use in the perioperative period.

### Metoclopramide

In addition to its prokinetic action, metoclopramide has central antidopaminergic actions. This action is primarily at the CTZ. In very high doses it is also a $5HT_3$ antagonist. The antiemetic effects of metoclopramide are short-lived and repeat doses may be necessary. Extrapyramidal side effects occur at high doses.

### $5HT_3$ antagonists

This group of drugs was initially developed to antagonize the emetic effect of the cancer chemotherapeutic agents. They have more recently been used for postoperative nausea and vomiting. 5HT is the transmitter that seems to dominate activity at the CTZ and therefore its antagonism is very effective against those drugs that act through the CTZ.

Opioids also have a significant direct effect on the vomiting centre, making postoperative nausea and vomiting more resistant to the effect of the $5HT_3$ antagonists.

$5HT_3$-receptors occur in the wall of the gut, and are the receptors in the myenteric plexus that instigate vagal input to the midbrain. They are stimulated by distension of the gut wall and $5HT_3$ antagonists also produce antiemesis by this route.

Ondansetron was the first of these drugs to be introduced clinically and is licensed for use in postoperative nausea and vomiting. The drug is metabolized in the liver and has the shortest half-life of the drugs in the group. Side effects include headaches, dizziness, and fatigue, and there may be elevation of the liver enzymes during treatment.

Granisetron and tropisetron have been licensed for perioperative use and are similar in their action to ondansetron, although they have longer half-lives. The major advantage of this group of drugs is the absence of sedative and extrapyramidal effects.

## INTESTINAL FUNCTION

In the small intestine, the intestinal contents are mixed with the secretions of the mucosal cells and with pancreatic juice and bile. Digestion, which begins in the mouth and stomach, is completed in the lumen and mucosal cells of the small intestine, and the products of digestion are absorbed. The site of absorption of various substances is given in Table 27.7. The importance of these should be related to differing pathologies (e.g. someone with a short small bowel may have difficulty absorbing water-soluble vitamins, protein, and amino acids).

By referring also to Figure 27.1, the possible amount of dehydration can be estimated (see also Chapters 42 and 61). Loss of gut contents (e.g. through vomiting, by gastric aspiration, diarrhoea, or fistulae) may lead to dehydration and significant electrolyte losses whereas loss of gastric contents will result in a metabolic alkalosis (see Chapter 26); the loss of intestinal secretions will cause a metabolic acidosis.

Jejunal transport of foodstuffs and fluids occurs rapidly, and most of the nutrients are absorbed in this region. This results in the intestinal contents remaining isotonic. In contrast, ileal transport is slower, and the gut contents are hypertonic. Bile salts and the

| Table 27.7 Site of absorption of products of digestion | | | | |
|---|---|---|---|---|
| Substance | Duodenum | Jejunum | Ileum | Colon |
| Glucose | ++ | +++ | ++ | 0 |
| Amino acids | ++ | +++ | ++ | 0 |
| Fatty acids | +++ | ++ | + | 0 |
| Bile salts | 0 | + | +++ | 0 |
| Water-soluble vitamins | +++ | ++ | 0 | 0 |
| Vitamin B12 | 0 | + | +++ | 0 |
| Sodium | +++ | ++ | +++ | +++ |
| Potassium | 0 | 0 | + | ++ |
| Hydrogen | 0 | + | ++ | ++ |
| Chloride | +++ | ++ | + | 0 |
| Calcium | +++ | ++ | + | ? |

From Stoelting RK. *Pharmacology and Physiology in Anaesthetic Practice*, 3rd edn. Philadelphia: Lippincott-Raven, 1997, 745.

intrinsic factor–vitamin B12 complex are also absorbed in the terminal ileum.

***Blood supply***

The intestines are supplied by a series of parallel circulations from branches of the superior and inferior mesenteric arteries. There are extensive anastomoses between these vessels, but blockage of a large intestinal artery still leads to infarction of the bowel. The blood flow to the mucosa is greater than that to the rest of the intestinal wall, and it responds to changes in metabolic activity. Thus, blood flow to the small intestine doubles after a meal, and the increase lasts up to 3 hours. The intestinal circulation is capable of extensive autoregulation, i.e. it is independent of systemic blood pressure.

Venous blood containing substances absorbed from the intestine is drained to the liver via the portal vein (see Chapter 28). Most of the fatty components are taken up by the intestinal lymphatics, thus bypassing the liver to reach the general circulation.

## DRUG ABSORPTION

Many drugs are given orally. This is a convenient and economical route because the formulation does not have to be sterile and administration does not require skilled help. Absorption of drugs from the GI tract depends on the pharmaceutical properties of an individual drug, as well as the motility of the gut and any drug interaction that may affect absorption.

Drugs can be formulated as liquids or tablets. Liquids may be of three types:

- *Mixtures* which are made up of either solutions or suspensions of the drug in water. A suspending agent such as methylcellulose may also be present in suspensions.
- *Emulsions* which are oil-in-water preparations into which a suspension of drug is dissolved.
- *Elixirs* which are alcoholic solutions in which drugs are dissolved.

In general, a tablet is made up of the drug as a granular powder, together with a number of materials known collectively as 'excipients'. Excipients may include:

- a diluent (e.g. 'Fuller's Earth', calcium sulphate, lactose) to increase the volume of the active drug;
- binders (e.g. methylcellulose) to hold the contents of the tablet together;
- disintegrating agents (e.g. starch, sodium bicarbonate) to facilitate breakdown in the stomach or upper GI tract. Before a drug can be absorbed it must enter solution. When the preparation is taken in solid tablet form, disintegration is an essential preliminary stage. The tablet may be formulated so as to disintegrate or even effervesce in contact with water, thus facilitating dissolution by breaking the active compound into fine particles.
- Lubricants aid drug passage down the oesophagus and along the GI tract. Drugs may be contained in capsules (e.g. gelatine) which protect the patient from an unpleasant taste but which dissolve readily to release the drug in the stomach.
- Enteric-coated capsules resist the acid medium of the stomach and release drug in the upper jejunum whose contents are alkaline. The purpose of such a formulation may be to protect the stomach from irritants, or to protect drugs such as penicillin from destruction by a strongly acid environment.

Factors that influence the uptake and availability of orally administered drugs are summarized in Figure 27.4. and detailed below.

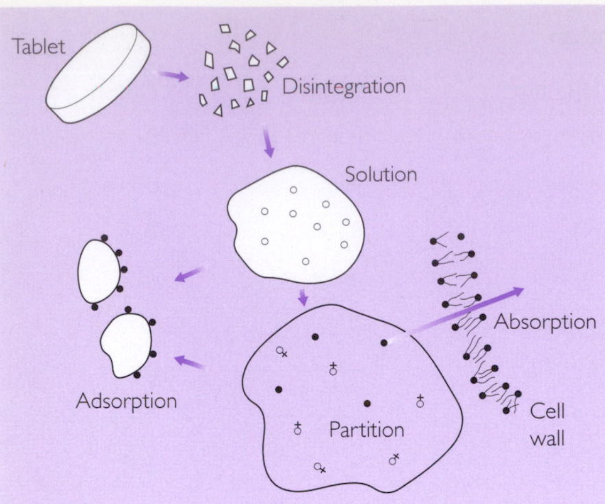


**Figure 27.4** Factors affecting the uptake and availability of orally administered drugs.

***Factors influencing dissolution***

- Surface area of drug particles: smaller particles have a greater surface area : mass ratio and a faster speed of dissolution.
- Solubility in the diffusion layer: different salts of a drug differ in their water solubility. Highly soluble salts have an increased dissolution rate compared with that of the drug formulated as a free acidic or basic form.
- Crystalline formation aids dissolution.
- Crystal hydration: anhydrous salts of drugs are more readily soluble in water.
- Influence of excipients: the addition of water-repellent lubricants (such as magnesium stearate) will decrease the rate of dissolution, whereas water-attracting compounds (e.g. sodium lauryl sulphate) will increase the rate of tablet breakdown.

Examples of drugs in which alterations in the formulation may significantly alter the bioavailability include digoxin, chloramphenicol, and paracetamol.

Drugs are absorbed from the GI tract by the following means:

- Aqueous diffusion is the mode of absorption for low-molecular-weight drugs such as ethyl alcohol. This is only a minor route for fully ionized drugs which are absorbed slowly and incompletely.
- Pinocytosis is the route of absorption of high-molecular-weight drugs, or drugs existing as polyaggregates, such as the complex of intrinsic factor and vitamin B12.
- Co-absorption with fats is important for lipid-soluble drugs. This may be enhanced if the drug is formulated in liposomes.
- Active transport is an important route for drugs that are similar in structure to naturally occurring compounds. Examples include L-dopa and α-methyldopa, which are absorbed via the amino acid transport system, and 5-fluorouracil and 5-bromouracil which are absorbed by the active transport pyrimidine uptake system.

***Factors within the GI tract affecting absorption***

*The acidity of GI contents*

In the acidic environment of the stomach, the ionization of acidic drugs is reduced, and hence they are well absorbed. At higher pH, the increased ionization will decrease drug absorption. Similarly, the higher pH of the intestines will aid the absorption of basic drugs.

*Absorptive area*

The area for drug absorption is normally about $200\,m^2$, and this receives about 10% of the cardiac output. The area for absorption will obviously be reduced after intestinal resections.

*Concentration of the drug*

In the presence of high drug concentrations, diffusion gradients will be greater.

*Gastrointestinal secretions*

Gastric acid causes hydrolysis of drugs that are formulated as esters (e.g. procaine), as well as activating some prodrugs (e.g. chlorazepate to nordiazepam). Gastric and intestinal enzymes also destroy polypeptide drugs such as insulin and oxytocin.

*Gastrointestinal bacteria*

These important organisms play a role in drug metabolism and absorption. For example, hydrolysis of biliary excreted phase II glucuronides may lead to re-formation of active parent compounds, which can then be reabsorbed resulting in enterohepatic recirculation. Like the intestinal secretions, these bacteria may convert a prodrug into an active compound (e.g. anthraquinone purgatives; cyclamates to cyclohexamines).

*Metabolism during absorption*

Many of the enzymes necessary for drug metabolism are contained in the cells of the intestinal epithelium. Biodegradation therefore occurs during absorption and hence the oral bioavailablity may be reduced. This applies to the sulphate conjugation of isoprenaline (isoproterenol) and chlorpromazine, and to a lesser extent the oestrogens, L-dopa, and α-methyldopa; the decarboxylation of L-dopa by amino acid decarboxylase; and the hydrolysis of glyceryl trinitrate, and to a lesser extent of pethidine and pentazocine.

*Clearance after absorption*

High drug clearance rates lead to low plasma concentrations, and hence an increased drug absorption as a result of the maintenance of the concentration gradient; similarly, increased binding of drugs to plasma proteins and other acute phase proteins will lower the free drug concentration and hence increase facilitated transport.

*Presence of food*

A fatty meal in the stomach will adsorb lipid-soluble drugs and slow their absorption, as well as delaying their progress into the small intestine.

*Gastrointestinal motility*

Drugs such as opioids, antimuscarinics, and alcohol delay gastric emptying, and hence slow the passage of drug into the small intestine, so absorption is delayed. As seen above, other drugs (e.g. cisapride and metoclopramide) increase the rate of gastric emptying and hence absorption of other drugs.

## FURTHER READING


Ganong WF. *Review of Medical Physiology*, 18th edn. Stamford, CA: Appleton & Lange, 1997.

Hindle AT. 5HT3 receptor antagonists. *Curr Anaesth Crit Care* 1995;**6**:242–9.

Souhami RL, Moxham J, eds. *Textbook of Medicine*, 2nd edn. Edinburgh: Churchill Livingstone, 1994.

Watcha MF, White PF. Antiemetics. In: Frink EJ, Brown BR, eds. *New Pharmacological Vistas. Baillière's Clin Anaesthesiol* 1995;**9**:119–36.

# Chapter 28 The liver

J.W. Sear and P. Hutton

## FUNCTIONS OF THE LIVER

The liver is a complex biochemical factory, the main functions of which can be summarized as listed below.

### Intermediary metabolism

It is the site of a great deal of carbohydrate, protein, nucleic acid, fat, mineral, and vitamin metabolism.

### Processing of newly absorbed nutrients

The portal system carries the products of digestion to the liver for processing. Depending on the body's needs, the liver can convert excess monosaccharides into glycogen or fat, both of which can be stored, or it can convert glycogen, fat, and protein into glucose.

### Storage

The liver stores glycogen, copper, iron, and vitamins A, B12, D, E, and K.

### Manufacture of bile

This is essential for the digestion of fats and the elimination of a wide variety of endogenous substances and drugs.

### Excretion and detoxification

Bile carries with it bile salts, cholesterol and cholic acid, and the breakdown products of bilirubin, toxins, and drugs. The liver is also the location of the urea cycle and the management of nitrogenous wastes (e.g. ammonia).

### Manufacture

The liver manufactures, in addition to the substances listed above, albumin and most of the other plasma proteins.

### Haematological and immunological functions

The liver produces blood in the embryo and in some disease states. In the adult, it produces fibrinogen, prothrombin, and heparin. The Kupffer reticulo-endothelial cells phagocytose worn-out red and white blood cells.

## ANATOMY

### Macroscopic

The liver is the largest organ in the adult body, weighing 1.2–2.0 kg. It is divided into right and left lobes, the left being the smaller and constituting approximately one-sixth of the whole. It is related superiorly to the diaphragm, which separates it from the pleura, lungs, pericardium, and heart. Its posteroinferior (visceral) surface abuts the abdominal oesophagus, the stomach, duodenum, hepatic flexure of the colon, and the right kidney and suprarenal gland. Anteriorly, it is covered by the lower ribs and anterior abdominal wall. These relationships are shown in Figure 28.1 which demonstrates the topographical anatomy of the liver.

The biliary system arises from a condensation of fine bile capillaries, which originate in the liver lobules. The right and left hepatic ducts fuse in the porta hepatis to form the common hepatic duct. This in turn joins with the cystic duct, which drains the gallbladder to form the common bile duct (CBD). The CBD is formed 2.5 cm above the duodenum; it passes behind this to open at a papilla on its medial aspect. For part of its course, the CBD lies behind or within the head of the pancreas. The usual arrangement is shown in Figure 28.2 but variations are common.

### Microstructure

The liver architecture is traditionally referred to as being arranged in polyhedral hepatic lobules (Figure 28.3). In histological section, these appear to be hexagonal and measure approximately 1 mm across. Each has a small centrilobular vein (which is a tributary of the hepatic vein) running down its central axis, which drains the surrounding sinusoids into the inferior vena cava. The sinusoids of each lobule are fed from the surrounding portal triads, each of which contains a

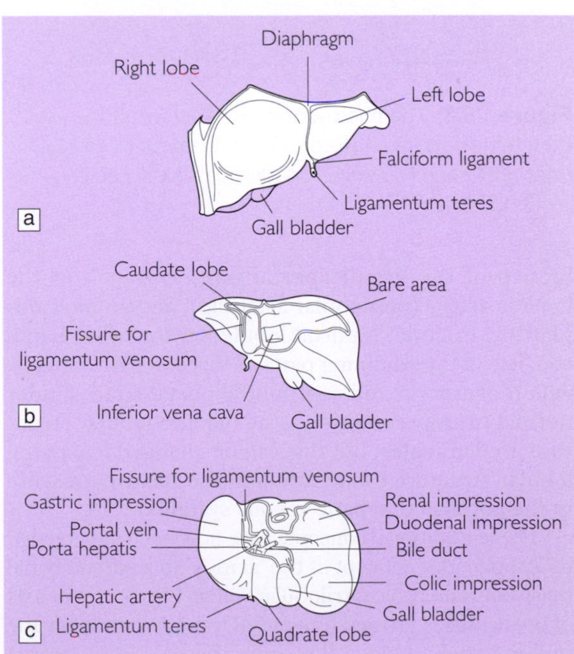


**Figure 28.1** The topographical anatomy of the liver: (a) anterior aspect, (b) posterior aspect, (c) inferior aspect.

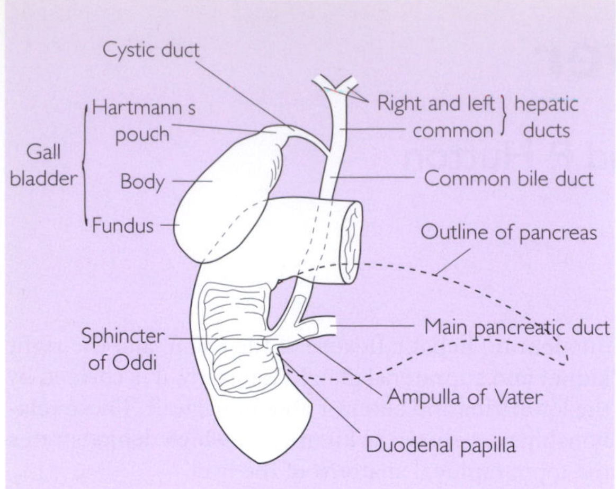


**Figure 28.2** The interrelationships of the gall bladder, bile ducts, duodenum, and pancreas.

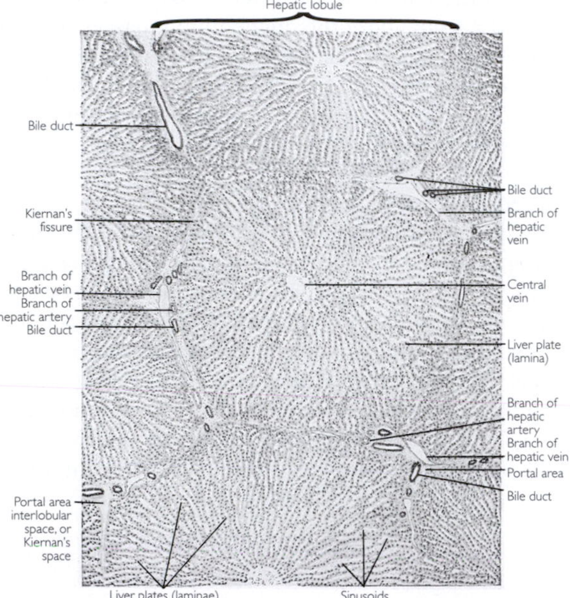


**Figure 28.3** The microscopic architecture of the liver. (See text for details.) (Reproduced from Di Fiore MSH, *Atlas of Human Histology*. Philadelphia: Lea & Febiger, 1973: 155.)

branch of the hepatic portal vein, a branch of the hepatic artery (perilobular arteriole), and an interlobular bile ductule. A portal lobule, on the other hand, consists of the adjoining parts of three hepatic lobules, which centre on and surround a portal triad. Under normal healthy conditions, the hepatic lobular structure predominates, but this can be changed to a portal lobular structure by alteration in the relative pressure in the portal and hepatic venous systems.

These traditional concepts have now been superseded by Rappaport's concept of the 'acinus' in a parenchymal mass between two centrilobular veins. The centre or axis of the acinus is formed by a portal triad. Functionally the unit is based on blood flow from these vessels towards each of the centrilobular veins – giving rise to a non-uniformity of hepatocyte function. There is a progressive decrease in oxygen saturation within the sinusoids as blood passes from the inflow to the efflux vessels; there are three functionally separate zones:

1. Zone 1: periportal hepatocytes receiving blood with the highest oxygen saturation, and showing the highest metabolic activity. The cells contain high activities of the transaminase enzymes, and are thought to be mainly involved in protein anabolism and catabolism.
2. Zone 3: centrilobular hepatocytes receiving blood with a lower oxygen saturation. The cells are the site of drug biotransformation and have high cytochrome P450 contents.
3. Zone 2: cells intermediate to the other two zones, in both blood oxygen saturation and enzyme activities.

In normal liver, there is no basement membrane throughout the length of the sinusoids, aiding solute transfer. There is, however, separation of the sinusoids and the plates of hepatocytes by the perisinusoidal space of Disse, which becomes distended under conditions of anoxia by plasma fluid, which permeates through from the sinusoids. In addition, the hepatocytes have high contents of smooth and rough endoplasmic reticulum. (The former is the site of protein synthesis; the latter is associated with drug biotransformation – see Chapter 19.) There are also the peroxisomes – small structures contiguous with the two types of endoplasmic reticulum, the function of which is not well understood, although they are the site of catalase storage, and ω-oxidation of fatty acids. Microtubules are also present in the hepatocyte cytoplasm, and are probably involved in bile secretion.

There are two additional groups of cells. The first is the Kupffer cells, which are mobile macrophages of the reticuloendothelial system that can phagocytose bacteria, viruses, foreign particles, and denatured proteins passing through the liver from the gastrointestinal tract via the portal vessels. They also scavenge ferritin and haemosiderin (breakdown substances from red blood cells). In addition, they may have a role in the metabolism of drugs and intermediary metabolites (such as glutamine) and the production of immunoregulatory cytokines. The second group of cells are the Pitt cells (mobile lymphocytes), which are attached to the endothelium and appear to have a role in the defence against infection and tumour cells.

## ENZYME ACTIVITY AND REGENERATION

The size, glycogen content, and protein content of the liver are affected by nutritional status. Maintenance of an animal on a high protein diet for 2–3 days will increase the activity of the enzymes involved in amino acid catabolism and gluconeogenesis. The converse will occur in animals fed on high carbohydrate diets. After hepatectomy, regeneration occurs at 50–100 g/day. The factors responsible for growth are not clear, but may include induction of liver enzymes, and humoral factors.

Liver regeneration is probably controlled by four cytokines, which facilitate both cellular differentiation and tissue hyperplasia. The cytokines are a heterogeneous collection of proteins that act via cell surface receptors to regulate and modify cell growth, maturation, and repair. They are derived from activated leukocytes (in particular monocytes), and also from activated fibroblasts and endothelial cells. The cytokines are synthesized as required and do not appear to be stored before release.

All of the liver growth factors are normally totally cleared during a single passage through the liver, and so have little systemic metabolic effect. However, after liver resection, there appears to be inadequate hepatic clearance by the remaining tissue of these growth factors, which can therefore initiate cell differentiation and growth elsewhere in the body.

## LIVER INNERVATION AND BLOOD FLOW

### Innervation

The nerve supply to the liver comes from the hepatic plexus which enters via the porta hepatis. The hepatic plexus is derived from branches of the coeliac plexus, the right and left vagus nerves, and the right phrenic nerve. It has afferent and efferent sympathetic and parasympathetic functions. The termination of many fibres is not known with certainty, but some control the gallbladder and sphincter of Oddi.

### The blood supply and its control

#### *Supply*

The liver requires 1–1.5 ml/kg per min oxygen to meet its basal needs, and this equates to a total liver blood flow of 1100–1800 ml/min (which is 25–30% of the resting cardiac output). The blood supply arises principally from two origins – the hepatic artery and the portal venous system. There is also input from collateral vessels of the azygous system, the retroperitoneal anastomoses, and the inferior rectal veins.

*Hepatic artery*

This delivers about 30% of the total hepatic blood flow (350–530 ml/min), but about 40–55% of the total hepatic oxygen supply. The pressure in the hepatic artery is 40–70 mmHg, with a further drop to the arteriolar system (at 30–35 mmHg). The arterial blood is 98% oxygen saturated, and its flow is controlled by sphincteric mechanisms (see below).

*Hepatic portal vein*

This arises from a confluence of splenic, superior mesenteric, left and right gastric, cystic, and paraumbilical veins, and enters the liver via the porta hepatis. It supplies 70% of total liver blood flow, and 50–60% of basal oxygen supply. The oxygen saturation of portal venous blood is between 60% and 75%, depending on the minute-by-minute activity of the gastrointestinal tract. Hepatic vein oxygen partial pressure (about 6.7 kPa or 50 mmHg) is higher than true mixed venous $P\text{O}_2$ because of mesenteric arterial shunting. Blood velocity in the portal vein is slow (about 9 cm/s), and is half that of the hepatic artery. The pressure in the portal venous system is 5–10 mmHg.

The portal vein is a valveless system and resistance to flow is 6–10% of that seen in the hepatic artery. Flow is solely dependent on the pressure gradient within the venous system. It is influenced by a number of external factors – controlled respiration, increased intra-abdominal pressure, gravity, and gut wall activity. During exercise, there is a marked decrease in portal flow produced by the generalized splanchnic vasoconstriction.

Hepatic venous pressures can be measured by the following techniques:

- percutaneous splenic puncture – the pressure equates well with that in the portal vein;
- wedged hepatic vein pressure;
- direct portal vein cannulation.

#### *Control*

This is broadly divided into factors that alter blood flow and drugs that affect hepatic flow, listed in Table 28.1.

**Table 28.1 Factors influencing hepatic blood flow**

| Increased liver blood flow | Decreased liver blood flow |
|---|---|
| Hypercapnia | Hypocapnia<br>? Hypoxia |
| Acute hepatitis: viral and alcoholic | Chronic cirrhosis |
| Food and digestion | Surgery (packs, compression, etc.) |
| Glucagon | IPPV and PEEP |
| | Acute haemorrhage |
| **Drugs** | |
| β-Adrenoceptor agonists | α-Adrenoceptor agonists |
| Phenobarbitone | β-Adrenoceptor antagonists |
| Any other enzyme inducer (e.g. rifampicin, phenytoin) | Cimetidine (ranitidine) |
| | Pitressin |
| | Anaesthetics: both volatile and intravenous |

IPPV, intermittent positive pressure ventilation; PEEP, positive end-expiratory pressure.

*Intrinsic control*

*Intrinsic pressure–flow regulation*

Over the range of normal physiological blood pressure, the hepatic artery is able to constrict in response to increased blood pressure and to dilate in response to a fall in blood pressure. Autoregulation of arterial flow occurs down to systolic arterial pressures of about 80 mmHg; below that, flow and pressure are interdependent, although the significance of this mechanism in humans is uncertain.

*Hepatic arteriovenous reciprocity*

Decreases in portal blood flow reduce hepatic arterial vascular resistance, and hence increase arterial flow, and vice versa. However, changes in arterial flow do not cause reciprocal responses of the same magnitude in the portal venous system. The mechanism for this regulation of flow (the so-called 'hepatic arterial buffer response') is controlled by the intrahepatic production of adenosine, with the subsequent wash-out or build-up of this dilator.

*Extrinsic control*

Intermittent positive pressure ventilation with large tidal volumes decreases splanchnic blood flow, as well as increasing resistance to hepatic vein and portal vein flow. As the reduction in portal venous flow is not accompanied by a reciprocal increase in hepatic artery flow, effective total liver blood flow decreases. These changes are independent of changes in pH or carbon dioxide partial pressure ($Pa\text{CO}_2$). As a result of the decrease in flow, oxygen delivery to the liver falls. However, extraction increases to maintain oxygen supply. This is in contrast to the fall in oxygen supply to the remainder of the splanchnic bed. Positive end-expiratory pressure also decreases hepatic blood flow, secondary to the decrease in cardiac output and the increase in intrathoracic pressure which impedes venous return.

Acute haemorrhage leads to a greater reduction in portal venous flow than in arterial flow. However, oxygen supply is initially maintained by increased extraction. In addition, the liver functions as a vascular reservoir, containing up to 25–30 ml blood/100 g tissue (approximately 10–15% of blood volume). If the circulating blood volume falls, as in haemorrhage, sympathetic stimulation can result in changes of the liver blood volume, and about 50% of the reservoir blood can be mobilized into the systemic circulation.

Hormonal effects on blood flow are through vasoconstriction or vasodilatation. The hepatic artery has $\alpha$- and $\beta$-adrenoceptors, but the portal vein has only $\alpha$-adrenoceptors. Thus, epinephrine (adrenaline) and angiotensin cause vasoconstriction of both inflow systems, whereas glucagon acts as a dose-related vasodilator. Vasopressin has both properties – it is a dilator to the portal vein and a constrictor to the hepatic artery. Dopamine has little effect on blood flow.

Anaesthetic agents have complex and different actions on liver blood flow:

- Spinal and epidural anaesthesia cause a reduction in total liver blood flow which parallels the decrease in mean arterial pressure – mainly through a decrease in portal venous flow.
- Volatile agents (such as halothane and enflurane) cause dose-related decreases in arterial, portal venous, and total hepatic blood flow, whereas isoflurane, sevoflurane, and desflurane are all associated with a better preservation of hepatic arterial flow (probably through less effect on the arterial buffer response mechanism).
- Intravenous anaesthetics (such as etomidate, thiopentone [thiopental], and propofol) all produce a dose-related fall in total liver blood flow; only ketamine is associated with no significant reduction in liver blood flow.

Hypercapnia causes vasodilatation of vascular beds as a direct effect of carbon dioxide together with systemic sympathoadrenal stimulation. The net effect is to increase portal flow while producing little change in the hepatic artery flow. Hypocapnia can reduce total hepatic flow by over 30% through the reverse mechanism.

The response of the circulation to hypoxia is inconsistent in that the true effect of hypoxia is to depress the cardiac output but, indirectly, the hypoxia-mediated release of catecholamines does the opposite. The literature is inconclusive on the overall effect.

## Measuring liver blood flow

Total hepatic blood supply and the separate components of arterial and portal flow can be determined by either direct (invasive) or indirect (semi-invasive) methods.

### *Direct methods*

These include application of electromagnetic flow probes or thermodilution techniques during laparotomy. The latter approach has only limited application in anaesthetized humans, but has been used extensively in animals.

### *Indirect methods*

These are based on uptake of a marker substance by the liver and knowing or determining the hepatic extraction ratio. One important consideration in these methods is the need for hepatic vein cannulation. The principal properties of any marker are that it must be metabolized or excreted solely by the liver. Marker substances include indocyanine green (ICG), bromsulphthalein (BSP), and radiolabelled colloidal suspensions such as $^{131}$I-labelled albumin. However, BSP may undergo enterohepatic recirculation, so most clinicians use ICG, which is eliminated solely by the liver without recirculation and has an extraction ratio of about 74% in normal volunteers. Use of peripheral venous rather than hepatic vein sampling will provide an approximate estimate of liver blood flow, but will result in an overestimation of the extraction ratio.

Three techniques can be used to estimate liver blood flow from markers.

*Continuous infusion of markers*

A continuous infusion of ICG, preceded by a loading dose of 0.5 mg/kg, is administered for about 20 min until steady-state conditions are reached. Blood samples are taken simultaneously from the hepatic vein and any peripheral artery and analysed for ICG:

$$\text{Clearance} = (\text{infusion rate}) / Ca \quad (1)$$

where $Ca$ is the arterial concentration of ICG.

$$\text{Extraction ratio} = \frac{(Ca - Cv)}{Ca} \quad (2)$$

where $Cv$ is the hepatic vein concentration.

$$\text{Hepatic blood flow} = \frac{\text{Clearance}}{\text{Extraction ratio}} \quad (3)$$

The concept of clearance and its relationship to flow is discussed in Chapter 19.

*Single bolus injection of a marker*
ICG (0.5 mg/kg) is injected intravenously, and venous samples collected from the contralateral limb vein every 2 min for 14 min. The decay profiles of concentration–time are analysed by non-linear regression analysis. Clearance is derived as:

$$\text{Average clearance} = \frac{\text{Dose}}{\text{AUC}}$$

where AUC is the area under the concentration–time curve extrapolated to infinity (see Chapter 19 for derivation). The extraction ratio for ICG is assumed to be 0.74, and then equation (3) is used to derive liver blood flow. Alternatively, clearance may be calculated from pharmacokinetic models as described in Chapter 19.

*Uptake and wash-out methods*
The Kupffer cells remove colloidal particles entering the liver; this is utilized in studying the rates of clearance of radiolabelled colloidal particles ($^{99m}$Tc-labelled sulphur colloid particles, $^{198}$Au-labelled colloid, or $^{131}$I-labelled denatured albumin) from the circulation, and equating this with liver blood flow. The usual sampling method is placement of a gamma-camera over the liver with the counting of isotope accumulation. The area under the initial exponential phase is a measure of liver blood flow. This technique has the advantage of not requiring hepatic vein cannulation. Using the colloidal gold technique, estimated liver blood flow before anaesthesia is reported to be about 1700 ml/min. It is reduced by 16% during halothane anaesthesia alone, and by 24% and 58%, respectively, during body surface and upper abdominal surgery.

Alternatively, blood flow can be similarly determined non-invasively by the uptake of radioactive inhaled xenon, measured by a surface gamma-counter. This method suffers from several drawbacks, including a variability of the partition coefficient for xenon between different hepatic tissues. This renders it inaccurate in patients with fatty liver or cirrhosis.

A method suitable only for fatal animal experiments is the injection of radioactive microspheres into the hepatic artery or portal vein. After death, the liver is excised and the radioactivity (or other marker) measured.

## INTERMEDIARY METABOLISM IN THE LIVER

The liver is the main site of carbohydrate, lipid, and protein metabolism. Some of the more important of these biochemical functions are listed in Table 28.2.

### Carbohydrate metabolism

After dietary ingestion, carbohydrates are broken down into mono- and disaccharides by salivary ptyalin and pancreatic amylase. Disaccharides are further cleaved to hexoses by enzymes (maltase, lactase, sucrase) in the intestinal mucosal cells. Uptake into the portal venous system is an energy-dependent process. Hepatic uptake is not energy dependent, or specifically facilitated by the action of insulin as in most other tissues of the body. Rather, the action of glucokinase, converting glucose to glucose 6-phosphate, maintains a low intracellular glucose concentration, so allowing the continued uptake by diffusion.

The old concept that dietary glucose served as precursor for glycogen and fat is probably incorrect in humans. Glycogen arises mainly from three-carbon

**Table 28.2 Important biochemical functions of the liver involved in intermediary metabolism**

| Biochemical group | Anabolic and catabolic reactions |
|---|---|
| Carbohydrate metabolism | Synthesis and storage of glycogen and the regulation of blood glucose<br>Oxidation of carbohydrate<br>Conversion of carbohydrate to fat |
| Lipid metabolism | Synthesis of fatty acids and phospholipids<br>Oxidation of lipids<br>Regulation of blood lipids |
| Protein metabolism | Deamination of amino acids and the synthesis of urea<br>Oxidation of the carbon skeleton of amino acids<br>Synthesis of plasma proteins, including those associated with blood clotting<br>Synthesis of non-essential amino acids |
| Nucleic acid metabolism | Synthesis of purine and pyrimidine nucleotides<br>Degradation of purines and pyrimidines |

compounds (such as lactate) and fructose (via triose phosphates); the former are also better substrates for lipogenesis. In humans, 70–90% of glucose is initially processed extrasplanchnically. This indirect and apparently inefficient pathway for glucose disposition has been termed the 'glucose paradox' (Figure 28.4). Overall, 50% of dietary glucose is metabolized to carbon dioxide and water by glycolysis, 30–40% to fatty acids, and about 10% to glycogen (glycogenesis). Gluconeogenesis is inhibited in the carbohydrate-fed state.

Glycolysis produces acetyl-CoA as substrate for lipogenesis, and subsequent esterification with glycerol 3-phosphate to triglyceride (see later). In the fed state, the liver stores about 75 g of glycogen to provide glucose and hence ATP by glycolysis during starvation.

The breakdown of glucose to pyruvate and its incorporation into the tricarboxylic acid cycle as acetyl-CoA produces 38 molecules of ATP per molecule of glucose. This compares with 156 molecules of ATP per molecule by β-oxidation of a $C_{16}$ fatty acid. Under anaerobic conditions, when pyruvate is converted to lactate, net ATP synthesis is only two molecules per molecule of glucose. The major metabolic pathways of carbohydrate metabolism are summarized in Figure 28.5.

During starvation, the body utilizes about 180 g glucose per 24 hours, with energy provided by fatty acid oxidation and ketone-body formation. The liver is the sole source of the latter under physiological conditions. Short-term glucose provision is by glycogenolysis, whereas gluconeogenesis is of importance after medium-term food deprivation. Eventually, hepatic ketogenesis provides alternative energy sources (ketone bodies) during long-term starvation.

The liver also deals with products of partial glucose metabolism in other tissues. These products are carried to the liver (and also the kidney) where they are resynthesized to glucose. A good example of this is lactate formed by the oxidation of glucose in skeletal muscle and by erythrocytes which, after transfer to the liver, re-forms glucose that again becomes available via the circulation for oxidation in the tissues. This process, known as the Cori or lactic acid cycle, is shown in Figure 28.6.

The regulation of carbohydrate metabolism is by both hormonal and non-hormonal mechanisms. With feeding, insulin release (see Chapter 29) increases in response to the rise in portal blood sugar. This increases glucose phosphorylation, activates glycogen synthase, increases glycolysis, increases pyruvate dehydrogenase activity (with increased formation of acetyl-CoA), and inhibits both glycogenolysis and gluconeogenesis. During fasting, glucagon has the major 'hepatic effects', increasing both glycogenolysis and gluconeogenesis, and aiding the hepatic uptake of gluconeogenic amino acids. Increases in cortisol concentration influence the metabolism of amino acids, which are released into the blood after peripheral tissue proteolysis. Both epinephrine and norepinephrine (noradrenaline) increase hepatic gluconeogenesis and glycogenolysis.

Another important synthetic function of the liver is the formation of NADPH by the pentose phosphate pathway. Here glucose 6-phosphate is reduced with synthesis of two NADPH per molecule of glucose and the five-carbon sugar, ribose 5-phosphate. NADPH plays an important role in microsomal and mitochon-

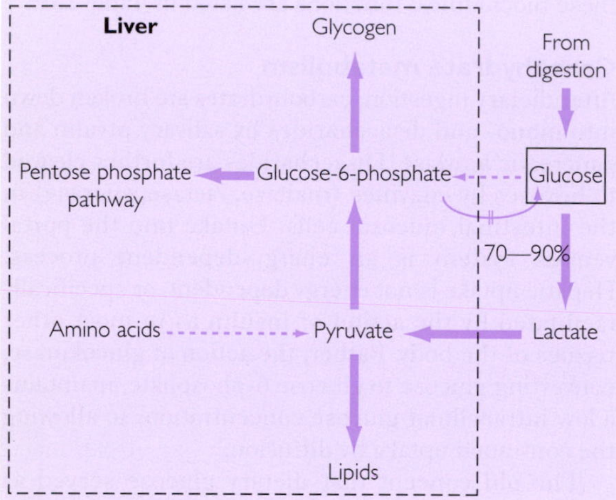

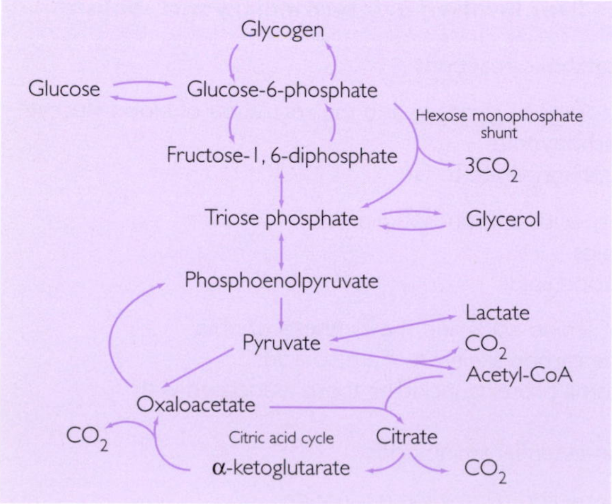

**Figure 28.4** The paradoxical uptake of glucose into the liver via metabolic intermediates such as lactate.

Glycogen
Glucose
Glucose-6-phosphate
Hexose monophosphate shunt
Fructose-1, 6-diphosphate
$3CO_2$
Triose phosphate
Glycerol
Phosphoenolpyruvate
Lactate
Pyruvate
$CO_2$
Acetyl-CoA
Oxaloacetate
$CO_2$
Citric acid cycle
Citrate
α-ketoglutarate
$CO_2$

**Figure 28.5** The major metabolic pathways for carbohydrate metabolism.

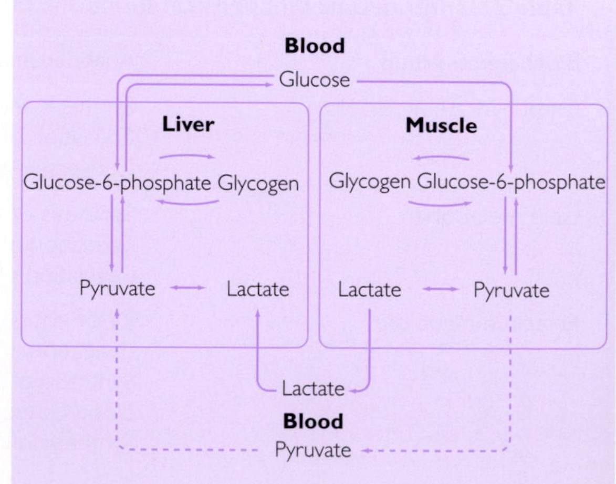


**Figure 28.6** The lactic acid or Cori cycle.

drial hydroxylation of steroid hormones and many drugs and xenobiotics, and provides reducing power for hepatic lipogenesis.

## Lipid metabolism

The liver has two main roles in lipid metabolism:

1. Synthesis of fatty acids and cholesterol (and other compounds based on the cyclopentanoperhydrophenanthrene nucleus), then conversion of fatty acids into triacylglycerol and very-low-density lipoproteins (VLDLs) (a transportable form of triacylglycerol);
2. Partial oxidation of fatty acids to ketone bodies.

### *Fat digestion and absorption*

Most fat is ingested as triglycerides (esters of fatty acids and glycerol). The short-chain fatty acids are water soluble, and can be absorbed by diffusion into the portal venous system. However, water-insoluble triglycerides must undergo initial emulsification in the stomach and then digestion in the duodenum by lipases. Pancreatic lipase splits off fatty acids in both α and β positions of the triglyceride molecule, leaving a monoacylglycerol. Intestinal lipase only degrades triglycerides in the β position, leaving diacylglycerol. Lipase activity is maximal in the presence of bile acids, and a protein cofactor co-lipase.

The lipases produce a mixture of fatty acids and acylglycerides, which are water insoluble. However, bile acids act in a detergent-like manner on the fats – producing polymolecular aggregates (micelles), which are taken up into the intestinal cell by pinocytosis. In the cell, triglycerides are re-formed by mechanisms that are poorly understood, and then pass, together with cholesterol and some phospholipids, as particles of about 1 μm diameter (chylomicrons) into the lacteal vessels.

### *Anabolic processes*

VLDLs are produced by the combination of fatty acyl-CoA with glycerol 3-phosphate to form triacylglycerol, which then interacts with one or more apoproteins to form lipoproteins that pass out of the liver into the circulation. VLDLs are broken down in adipose tissue by lipoprotein lipase to fatty acids. The different apoproteins are also synthesized in the liver. As well as forming VLDLs, they activate enzymes (e.g. lipoprotein lipase) and interact with specific endothelial wall receptors.

### *Catabolic processes*

The diet contains mainly saturated fatty acids (e.g. $C_{16}$: palmitic; $C_{18}$: stearic), together with some unsaturated fatty acids (e.g. oleic, linoleic, and linolenic acids). β-oxidation occurs in the mitochondria, which are readily permeable to short-chain fatty acids. However, long-chain fatty acids require the carrier molecule, carnitine, to facilitate uptake. Degradation of fatty acids produces one molecule of NADH, one reduced molecule of FAD, and one acetyl-CoA molecule for shortening of the fatty acid by two carbons, giving rise to 17 molecules of ATP. Branched-chain (α- and β-fatty acids) and the unsaturated fatty acids are degraded by the same pathways. The end product of β-oxidation is

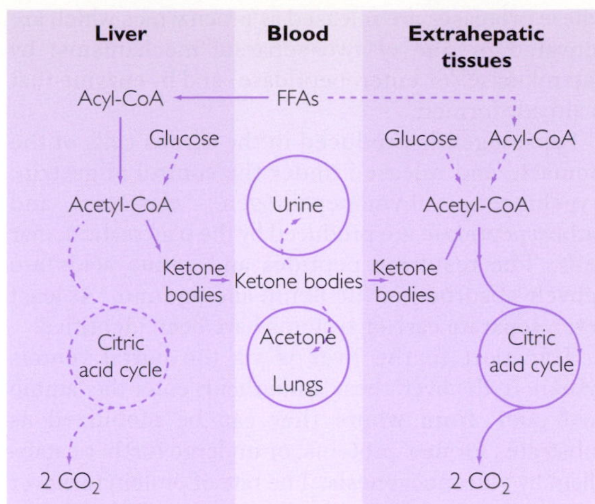


**Figure 28.7** The formation, utilization, and excretion of ketone bodies, showing the relationship of the liver, blood, and extrahepatic tissues. The main pathways are indicated by the solid arrows. FFAs, free fatty acids.

acetyl-CoA, which is either incorporated into the tricarboxylic acid cycle as citrate after combination with oxaloacetate or used to synthesize ketone bodies. This sequence of reactions is shown in Figure 28.7.

Falls in blood glucose and insulin concentrations stimulate lipolysis and increase fatty acid flux to the liver. Under conditions of excess acetyl-CoA, or a relative shortage of oxaloacetate, acetoacetate, β-hydroxybutyrate, and acetone (known collectively as ketone bodies) are formed. The β-hydroxybutyrate : acetoacetate ratio in the blood is normally between 3 : 1 and 6 : 1. Ketone-body formation is controlled by several factors: fasting, starvation, and insulin activity. Insulin reduces ketone body formation by inhibiting lipolysis and stimulating esterification of fatty acids. Although the liver cannot utilize ketone bodies as an energy source, under aerobic conditions they can be utilized by muscle, heart tissue, kidney, brain, and intestinal cells.

## Protein metabolism

The liver has a central role in protein catabolism and anabolism, as well as maintaining normal plasma amino acid concentrations. Amino acid metabolism also occurs in intestinal cells, muscle, and fatty tissues. If an animal is fed on a minimal protein diet, such that nitrogen balance is just maintained, the activity of the key enzymes responsible for degradation of the essential amino acids (leucine, valine, isoleucine, methionine, threonine, lysine, phenylalanine, tryptophan, histidine, and arginine) and the aminotransferase enzymes of catabolism is low. This regulates against a high rate of degradation. If, however, intake is greater than requirement, the activity of these enzymes increases.

### *Catabolic processes*

Dietary proteins are broken down in the gastrointestinal tract by four different enzymes:

- pepsin – released in the stomach;
- trypsin, elastase, and carboxypeptidase – released in the ileum.

These proteases are released as proenzymes which are activated by one of two separate mechanisms: by enterokinase (or enteropeptidase) and by enzyme that is already formed.

Pepsinogen is produced in the serous cells of the stomach, and released under the control of gastrin; trypsinogen, chymopepsinogen, elastase, and carboxypeptidase are produced by the pancreatic acinar cells. The resulting peptides and amino acids are actively absorbed in the ileum and jejunum. At least seven separate carrier systems have been identified.

Transport to the liver is via the portal venous system. In the liver, these amino acids enter the 'amino acid pool' from where they can be mobilized as substrates for new proteins, or undergo further catabolism by gluconeogenesis. The rate of protein turnover varies between different tissues – from about 10 days for liver and plasma proteins, 180 days for muscle proteins, 5–7 days for proteins of the gut mucosal cells, to only a few minutes for many hormones and enzymes.

Amino acid biodegradation produces carbon skeletons that enter the tricarboxylic acid cycle. These include acetyl-CoA, 2-oxoglutarate, succinyl-CoA, oxaloacetate, and fumarate. The following are the main pathways of breakdown:

- transamination;
- deamination;
- other fates including decarboxylation to primary amines, oxidative deamination to keto acids, side-chain modification, and polymerization.

Some amino acids are degraded mainly in the liver (arginine, histidine, lysine, methionine, threonine, phenylalanine, and tryptophan), whereas aspartic acid, glutamic acid and glutamine, glycine, proline, and alanine are metabolized in both hepatic and muscle tissue.

### Anabolic processes

The liver synthesizes a number of important proteins (or protein groups). However, synthesis expends energy. Six molecules of ATP are needed for the addition of a single amino acid to a peptide chain. The products of anabolism are listed below.

#### *Plasma proteins*

The plasma proteins manufactured in the liver are albumin, prealbumin, and globulins.

Albumin is synthesized only in the liver, at a rate of about 200 mg/kg body weight per day. Simultaneously, about 4% of the total body pool of 3.5–5 g/kg undergoes breakdown. Albumin is found in the vascular compartment and extracellular fluids. Synthesis is regulated by a number of factors, including nutritional status, hormonal balance, and plasma oncotic pressure. Albumin's main functions are maintenance of the plasma oncotic pressure, and as a carrier molecule for hormones, bilirubin, and drugs. In chronic liver disease plasma albumin concentrations correlate well with prognosis (as a marker of hepatic synthetic activity), but, because of its long half-life (about 20 days), albumin is a poor marker of acute liver damage.

Prealbumin has a shorter half-life (1.5 days) and may be a useful prognosticator of acute liver disease.

The liver synthesizes $\alpha_1$-, $\alpha_2$-, and $\beta$-globulins, but not $\gamma$-globulins. Globulins have transport and binding functions (e.g. transferrin, transcobalamin, haptoglobin, ceruloplasmin, and transcortin). Globulins also make up the complement proteins.

#### *Clotting factors*

Most of these, including the vitamin-K-dependent factors (factors II, VII, IX, and X), are synthesized in the liver. They have half-lives ranging from 1.5–6 hours (factor VII and proconvertin) to 28 days (factor II and prothrombin). As factor VII has a short half-life, it is a useful guide to hepatic synthetic function – by measurement of either the plasma concentration or its activity as the prothrombin time (see Chapter 31). The liver also synthesizes antithrombin III, a glycoprotein. If its activity falls, there is an increased tendency to thrombosis.

Vitamin-K-dependent factor deficiency occurs in both parenchymal and cholestatic liver disease; however, the aetiologies are different. In parenchymal disease, there is vitamin K availability but an inability of the hepatocyte to synthesize protein; in cholestatic disease, absence of gastrointestinal bile reduces vitamin K absorption.

#### *Other proteins*

The liver synthesizes other nitrogen-containing compounds: the purine and pyrimidine bases (adenine and guanine; thymidine, cytosine, and uracil, respectively), and nicotinamide. The purine nucleotides are formed from D-ribose 5-phosphate (a product of the pentose phosphate pathway) via inosinic acid, and the pyrimidines from carbamoyl phosphate via oritidine 5-phosphate. Breakdown of nucleic acids produces uric acid, urea, and ammonia. The balance between protein synthesis and degradation is related to dietary intake and nutritional status, and is also influenced by hormones and intermediary metabolites (see Chapter 29).

## Urea synthesis

A moderately active man consuming about 100 g of protein per day as part of a balanced diet must excrete approximately 16.5 g of nitrogen daily. Of this, 95% is eliminated by the kidneys and the remaining 5% in the stool. The major pathway of nitrogen excretion in humans (80–90%) is as urea synthesized in the liver, released into the blood, and cleared by the kidney (see Chapter 25). In the healthy adult, about 30 g of urea will be produced daily from a 100-g protein diet.

Ammonia is the nitrogenous end-product of amino-acid degradation, and is normally present in concentrations between 12 and 55 μmol/L. The overall flow of nitrogen in amino-acid catabolism is shown in Figure 28.8. Ammonia is eliminated as urea after synthesis in the liver by the ornithine or urea cycle. It is toxic in elevated concentrations (> 1 μg/ml, equivalent to about 70 μmol/L). Urea formation is energy dependent, utilizing three ATP molecules per molecule synthesized.

Two alternative, but quantitatively less important, routes for elimination of ammonia are also present. These are by combination with 2-oxoglutarate to form glutamate and glutamine, and by renal excretion of ammonia (a weak base) by non-ionic diffusion.

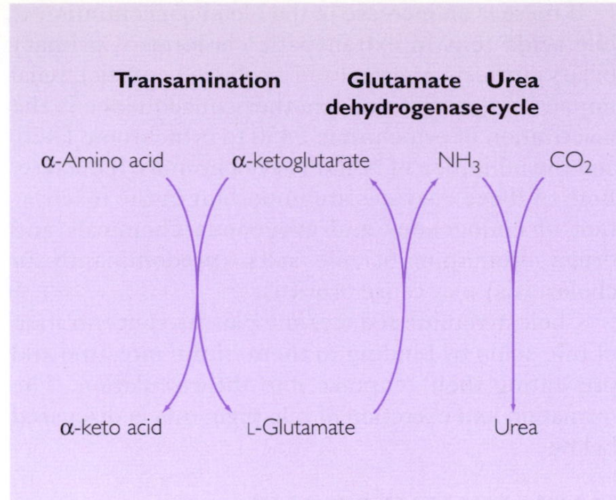


**Figure 28.8** The stages in the transfer of nitrogen from amino acids to urea. Although the reactions shown are reversible, they are represented as being unidirectional to emphasize the direction of metabolic flow in human amino acid catabolism.

### Integrated metabolic activity

The regulation of intermediary metabolism is under a complex control system, involving hormones, metabolic intermediates, physical activity, and dietary intake. These determine whether the body is in the absorptive or fasting state. The major intermediate metabolic pathways and their directions are compared in Figure 28.9.

## PRODUCTION AND COMPOSITION OF BILE

Approximately 500–1000 ml of bile is formed each day by the hepatocytes and secreted into the biliary canaliculi (see Figure 28.3). When the gallbladder is functioning normally, between meals, the sphincter of Oddi (see Figure 28.2) prevents entry of the bile into the duodenum and re-routes it into the gallbladder which usually has a capacity of up to 50 ml. When food enters the duodenum, cholecystokinin is released from the mucosal cells and enters the circulation. This subsequently causes relaxation of the sphincter of Oddi and contraction of the gallbladder. Many adults have a gallbladder that is non-functional and it can be removed without loss of digestive function.

The bile, which is alkaline, contains two classes of substances:

1. Those that are present in the same concentrations as in plasma (e.g. sodium, potassium, chloride, glucose), excluding plasma proteins, i.e. an ultrafiltrate of the blood.
2. Those that are found in much higher concentrations than in plasma (e.g. bile salts, bile pigments, some drugs), i.e. they are actively secreted.

Bile has the following functions:

- emulsification of fats;
- neutralization of acid;
- excretion of toxins, drugs, bile pigments, inorganic compounds;
- the excretion of cholesterol both directly and by conversion to bile acids.

The concentrations of substances in newly formed bile are very different from those that are delivered into the duodenum, especially if the gallbladder is working normally. This is because of the absorption of water and electrolytes (but not bile acids, bile pigments, or cholesterol) during storage in the gallbladder and biliary system. The composition of hepatic duct and gallbladder bile is given in Table 28.3.

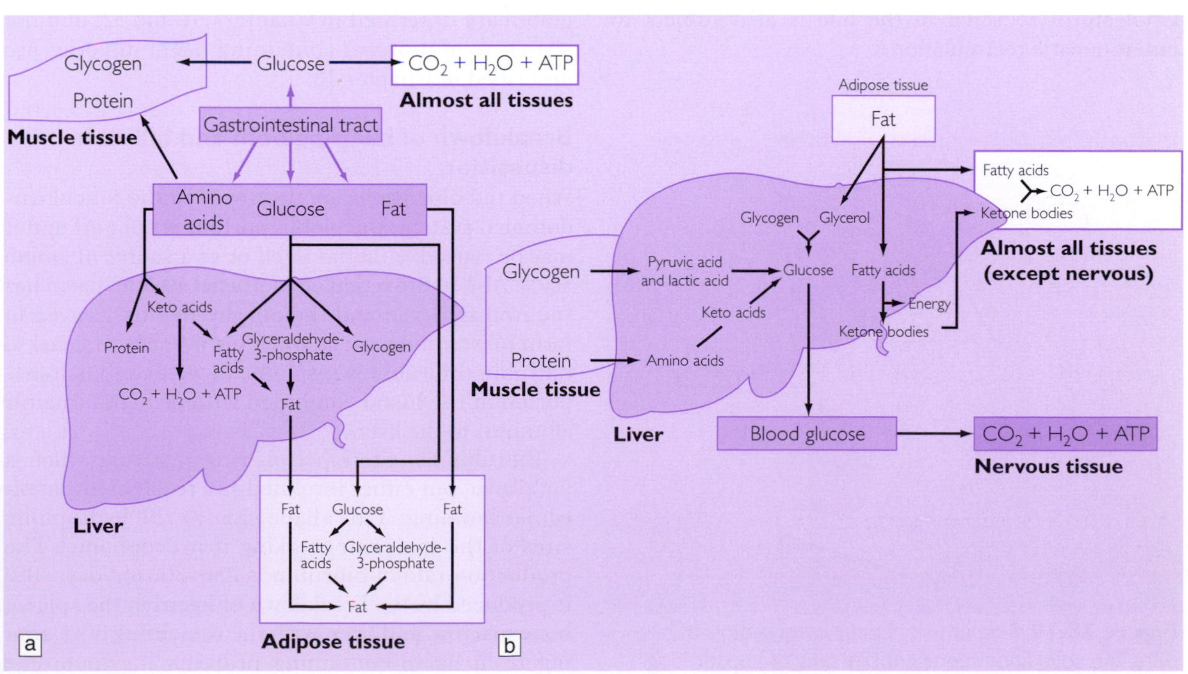


**Figure 28.9** The regulation of intermediary metabolism in (a) the absorptive state and (b) the postabsorptive or fasting state.

**Table 28.3 The composition of hepatic duct and gallbladder bile**

| Component | Hepatic duct bile (%) | Gallbladder bile (%) |
|---|---|---|
| Water | 97 | 85 |
| Salts of bile acids | 0.7 | 9 |
| Bile pigments | 0.2 | 3 |
| Cholesterol | 0.06 | 0.3 |
| Inorganic salts | 0.8 | 0.6 |
| Fatty acids and fat | 0.2 | 0.3 |
| Lecithin | 0.1 | 1.8 |
| Alkaline phosphatase | Trace | Trace |

Alkaline phosphatase is made by osteoblasts and removed from the plasma by the liver.

The two main bile acids manufactured in the liver are cholic acid (50%) and chenodeoxycholic acid (30%), with manufacture of smaller quantities of deoxycholic acid (15%) and lithocholic acid (5%) by bacteria in the gut. The bile acids may be thought of as the end-points of cholesterol breakdown in the body. They are synthesized from cholesterol but the tissues cannot break down the steroid nucleus. Consequently, measurement of the output of bile acids is a way of estimating the amount of cholesterol being processed. Once produced in the liver cells, the bile acids are conjugated to glycholic acid (67%) and taurocholic acid (33%) which, in the alkaline bile, form sodium and potassium salts.

Of the bile salts 90–95% are absorbed from the terminal ileum by active transport. They are then transported back to the liver and reprocessed (Figure 28.10). The bile salt pool recycles five to eight times per day. Cholesterol secreted in the bile is also subject to enterohepatic recirculation.

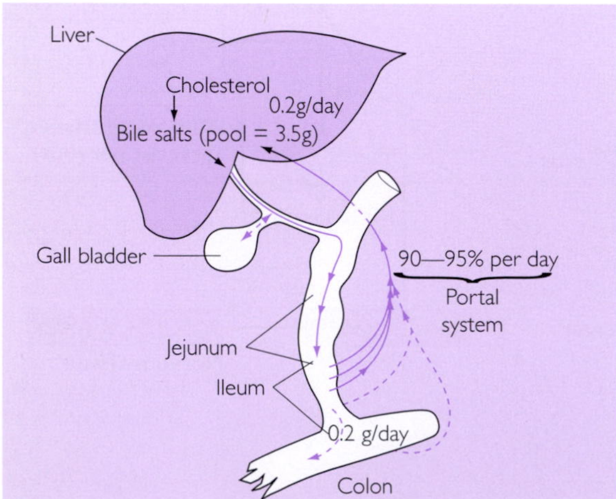


**Figure 28.10** The enterohepatic recirculation of bile salts. The solid lines represent bile salts of hepatic origin and the dashed lines bile salts resulting from bacterial action.

If there is an increase in the blood concentration of bile acids (e.g. in extrahepatic cholestasis, primary biliary cirrhosis, and viral and alcoholic hepatitis), renal impairment may occur. Another consequence is the inactivation of cytochrome P450 to cytochrome P420, and the inhibition of NADPH cytochrome c reductase. Both of these enzymes are important in the inactivation of endogenous and exogenous chemicals and drugs. Retention of bile salts (predominantly in cholestasis) may cause pruritus.

Cholestyramine reduces the plasma concentration of bile acids by binding to them in the intestine and preventing their reuptake into the circulation. The formation and excretion of bile pigments is discussed below.

## HAEM SYNTHESIS AND BREAKDOWN, AND BILIRUBIN DISPOSITION

### Synthesis of haemoglobin

Haemoglobin, myoglobin, and the various haem enzymes (cytochromes, peroxidase, catalase) are all tetrapyrrole ring compounds. The enzymes involved in haem synthesis are located in the liver, bone marrow, intestinal mucosal cells, kidney, and nucleated red cells.

The condensation of succinyl-CoA and glycine forms δ-aminolaevulinic acid (δALA). This occurs in the mitochondria, the δALA then passing to the cytosol where other enzymes are responsible for the condensation of two molecules of δALA to form porphobilinogen (PBG). Four PBG molecules then condense to form two molecules of uroporphyrinogen and co-proporphyrinogen III (CP-III). The further oxidation of CP-III and incorporation of iron into the tetrapyrrole ring structure results in haem (Figure 28.11). Haem then binds with globin to form haemoglobin. The formation of haem is under feedback control from protohaemin IX, an intermediate compound in the synthetic process. Species of haemoglobin are described in Chapters 31 and 52, and the structure of proteins containing haem moieties are described in Chapter 18.

### Breakdown of haemoglobin and bilirubin disposition

When red blood cells are destroyed in the reticuloendothelial system, the globin portion is split off and it may be reused, either as itself or as a source of amino acids. Also in the reticuloendothelial system, haem has the iron removed and the porphyrin ring cleaved to form biliverdin by oxidation. This is easily reduced to bilirubin. Bilirubin is insoluble in water and is transported in the blood combined with proteins (mainly albumin) to the liver.

Bilirubin has a tetrapyrrole ring structure which is not planar, but rather involuted as a result of intramolecular bonding. This shape shields the hydrophilic sites of the molecule, making it hydrophobic. The production rate of bilirubin is 250–300 mg/day; 70% is produced by the breakdown of haem in the spleen, bone marrow, and liver, with the remaining 30% arising from haem-containing proteins – cytochrome P450 and catalase. Under normal conditions, bilirubin formation and clearance rates are equal, and the

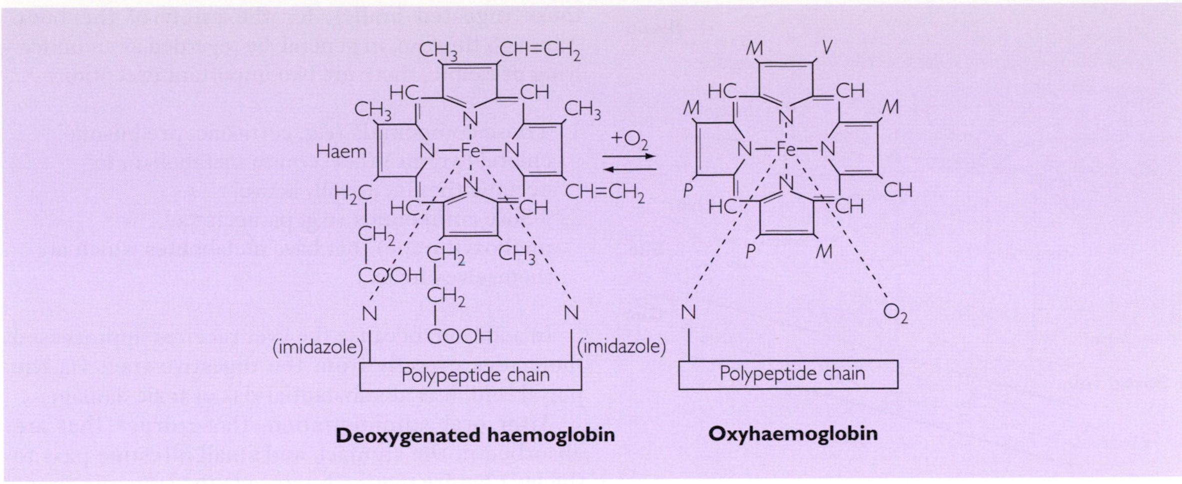


**Figure 28.11** The structure of haem and its attachment to its polypeptide chain in the reduced and oxygenated state.

plasma bilirubin concentration will be 0.3–1.0 mg/dl (5–19 μmol/L). Increased production above the handling capacity of the liver or decreased clearance results in jaundice. High bilirubin concentrations are usually well tolerated, but can cause pruritus, kernicterus in the newborn, and occasionally renal damage.

Albumin has at least two large-capacity binding sites used by bilirubin, and some free bilirubin is also present in plasma (< 0.2%). Saturation of albumin binding sites may occur at concentrations more than 300–350 mg/L, unbound bilirubin being precipitated. Some drugs compete for the same albumin binding sites (e.g. salicylates, non-steroidal anti-inflammatory drugs, diuretics, and some sulphonamides). There is a second, non-dissociable form of albumin-bound bilirubin (δ-bilirubin) found in some hepatobiliary diseases, which cannot undergo liver uptake and excretion, and has a longer plasma half-time (12–14 days).

It is unclear how bilirubin separates from albumin and passes into the cell. There is a non-specific anionic binding site on the membrane, and a high-capacity carrier-mediated transport system. About 30% of bilirubin refluxes back into the plasma. Once in the hepatocyte, bilirubin attaches to a second carrier system, which on the endoplasmic reticulum binds bilirubin to the glucuronic acid. The reaction is catalysed by the enzyme UDPG transferase, with the resultant conjugates being more polar and water soluble and therefore excretable in the bile (Figure 28.12).

The transferase enzymes are inducible by drugs (e.g. phenobarbitone [phenobarbital], ethanol, phenytoin, rifampicin, and the polychlorobiphenyls). In the Crigler–Najjar syndrome, and the Gunn river rat, the transferase is deficient. Enzyme inhibition may occur (at least *in vitro*) by drugs (e.g. novobiocin, chloramphenicol, and high concentrations of diethyl ether).

Bilirubin is actively excreted into the biliary tract, mainly as the diglucuronide (> 80%). The carrier system is separate from those involved in bile acid secretion, and can be induced by phenobarbitone and

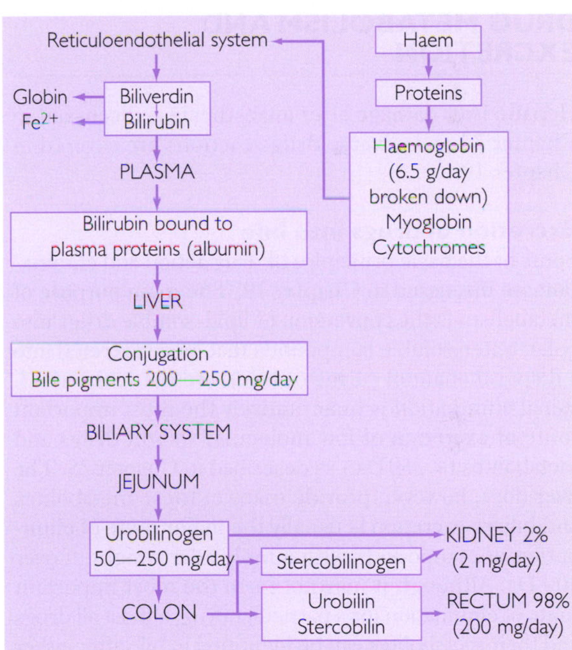


**Figure 28.12** The pathway of haemoglobin conversion to bilirubin, and the subsequent conjugation and excretion of bilirubin.

amplified by spironolactone. Disturbances of bilirubin excretion are seen in many of the parenchymal liver diseases (hepatitis, cirrhosis, intrahepatic cholestasis), and in the Dubin–Johnson syndrome.

Once excreted into the gastrointestinal tract, conjugated bilirubin is reduced to urobilinogens, which can then undergo reabsorption in the terminal ileum and colon (up to 20%) if deconjugation has taken place through the activity of β-glucuronidases in the intestinal flora. Further bacterial action results in the formation of stercobilinogen and stercobilin. This process is summarized in Figure 28.13.

In health, most of the breakdown products leave in the stool via the rectum; 1–2% of water-soluble products (mainly urobilinogen) are excreted by the kidney.

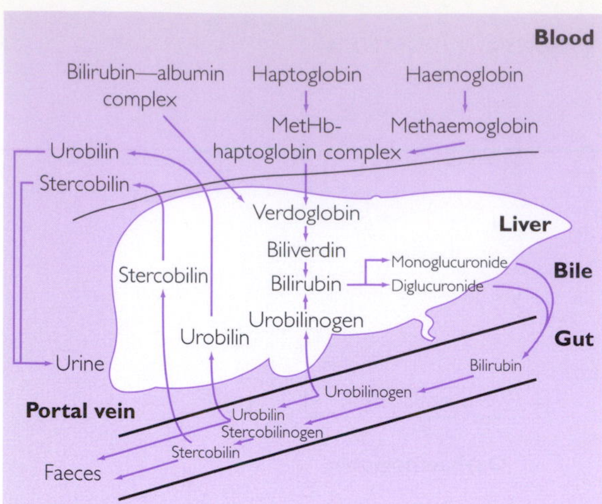


**Figure 28.13** A summary of bilirubin metabolism and excretion. (Adapted from Sear JW. *Curr Anaesth Crit Care* 1990;1:196.)

## DRUG METABOLISM AND EXCRETION

Hepatic liver damage after anaesthesia is discussed in Chapter 33 and adverse drug reactions are covered in Chapter 19.

### Excretion of drugs into bile

Some of the basic principles of drug action and elimination are discussed in Chapter 19. The main purpose of metabolism is the conversion of lipid-soluble drugs into polar, water-soluble compounds that, once excreted into a disposal channel (urine or bile), are not reabsorbed. Renal elimination is quantitatively the most important route of excretion of low molecular weight drugs and metabolites (< 350 Da,) as described in Chapter 25. The liver does, however, provide many of these metabolites and biliary excretion is usually the major route of elimination of compounds with a molecular weight of over 400 Da. Although it may not form the most important route of elimination for a particular drug, almost all drugs and their metabolites can be identified in bile after either oral or parenteral administration.

High molecular weight anions (including glucuronide and sulphate conjugates) and cations (including quaternary amines) are actively transported by separate systems from the hepatocyte to the biliary canaliculus. Examples of such drugs are given in Table 28.4.

Biliary secretion is not particularly specific and similar drugs and endogenous compounds compete for the same transport mechanisms. Active transport can work against a concentration gradient of 100 or more. This is put to good use in prescribing certain antibiotics (e.g. ampicillin) for biliary infections.

Some compounds present in the bile as glucuronide conjugates may be hydrolysed in the intestine by bacteria, only to be reabsorbed by enterohepatic circulation. Many steroid drugs (e.g. oral contraceptives) undergo extensive enterohepatic recirculation.

### Oral drugs and the first-pass effect

A primary function of the liver is the deactivation of exogenous and endogenous compounds (particularly those ingested orally), for the safety of the body. Although this can, in general, be regarded as an underlying principle, there are two important exceptions:

1. Those compounds (e.g. cortisone, prednisone, chloral hydrate) that require metabolism to become therapeutically active.
2. Those compounds (e.g. paracetamol, methoxyflurane) that have metabolites which are themselves toxic.

In addition, because the liver receives unprocessed molecules directly from the digestive tract via the portal vein, it is at substantial risk of toxic damage.

After oral administration, those drugs that are absorbed in the stomach and small intestine pass to the liver before they gain access to the systemic circulation. In so doing, only a proportion of the absorbed drug may reach its intended site of action. This phenomenon is called first-pass metabolism. The effect of first-pass metabolism depends on the clearance and extraction ratio (ER) of the drug (see later). To be effective, drugs given orally must have a low ER and a limited first-pass effect. An unexpectedly high first-pass effect in patients with induced enzymes (see later) can explain a lack of response to normal oral doses.

The liver microstructure with the hepatic sinusoids (see Figure 28.3) is ideally designed to allow the free distribution of blood proteins. It enables protein-bound drugs to come into direct contact with hepatocyte membranes. Conventionally, the metabolic processes that occur in the liver are divided into two groups: phase 1 and phase 2 reactions.

#### *Phase 1 reactions*

Phase 1 reactions alter the existing functional groups of a drug molecule to increase the water solubility or hydrophilicity. The reaction can be oxidation (most common), hydrolysis (much less common,) or reduction (rare). Oxidation covers a number of reactions such as:

- hydroxylation (addition of -OH group);
- dealkylation (removal of $CH_3$- or $C_2H_5$- group);
- *N*-oxidation (N to N-O) and *S*-oxidation;
- *O*-dealkylation ($C_2H_5O$- to -OH) and *N*-dealkylation;
- dehalogenation and desulphuration.

Most of these reactions occur on the smooth endoplasmic reticulum (the microsomal fraction) and are catalysed by cytochrome P450, which is also called the mixed-function oxidase system. The term P450 comes from the wavelength (450 nm) at which the reduced enzyme absorbs light. Many different forms of cytochrome P450 (isoenzymes) have been identified and each person is considered to have his or her own cytochrome P450 'fingerprint' derived from a combination of genetic and environmental factors. Although most phase 1 reactions utilize P450, some do not. Indeed, in some circumstances, phase 1-type reactions may occur in the plasma. Examples of phase 1 reactions in the liver are given in Table 28.5.

**Table 28.4 Acidic (anionic) and basic (cationic) drugs secreted into the bile by hepatocytes**

| Acidic drugs | Basic drugs |
|---|---|
| Glucuronide conjugates of many drugs | Pancuronium |
| Sulphate conjugates of many drugs | Vecuronium |
| Radiographic contrast media | Tubocurarine |
| Ampicillin and amoxycillin | Glycopyrrolate |
| Rifampicin | |
| Cephaloridine | |
| Bromosulphophthalein | |
| Probenecid | |

**Table 28.5 Examples of phase I reactions**

| Reaction type | Site | Enzyme system | Example of substrate |
|---|---|---|---|
| Oxidation | Hepatic ER<br>Mitochondria<br>Hepatic cell cytoplasm | Cytochrome P450<br>Monoamine oxidase<br>Alcohol dehydrogenase | Thiopentone<br>Dopamine<br>Alcohol |
| Hydrolysis | Hepatic ER<br>Hepatic cell cytoplasm | Esterase<br>Amidase | Pethidine<br>Lignocaine (lidocaine) |
| Reduction | Hepatic ER<br>Hepatic cell cytoplasm | Cytochrome P450<br>Alcohol dehydrogenase | Azoreduction (e.g. prontasil)<br>Chloral hydrate |

ER, endoplasmic reticulum.
Adapted in part from Calvey TN and Williams NE. *Principles and Practice of Pharmacology for Anaesthetists*, 3rd edn. Oxford: Blackwell Scientific, 1996.

***Phase 2 reactions***

These are reactions that combine unchanged drugs or the products of phase 1 reactions with other chemical groups to increase water solubility. Some drugs only undergo phase 2 reactions. Phase 2 reactions are also used to render lipid-soluble endogenous ligands (e.g. bilirubin, cholesterol) more water soluble.

Quantitatively, the most important reaction is glucuronide conjugation. Other reactions involve sulphate, acetate, glycine, or methyl groups. Examples are given in Table 28.6.

### Enzyme induction and inhibition

The activity of many enzymes, and particularly microsomal enzymes, can be enhanced by the repeated use of certain drugs or substances. Induction usually takes place over days or weeks. In contrast, many drugs can also inhibit the action of enzymes, both competitively and non-competitively. Examples of such drugs are given in Table 28.7. Note that some drugs can act as both inducers and competitive inhibitors. Enzyme induction can occur in the healthy liver and in one with mild-to-moderate cirrhosis.

**Table 28.6 Examples of phase 2 reactions**

| Reaction type | Site | Enzyme system | Substrate |
|---|---|---|---|
| Glucuronidation | Hepatic ER | Glucuronyl transferase | Morphine |
| Sulphation | Hepatocyte cytoplasm | Sulphalanase | Minoxidil |
| Acetylation | Kupffer cells | Acetyl transferase | Sulphonamides |
| Glycine | Hepatocyte cytoplasm | Glycyl transferase | Salicylic acid |
| Methylation | Hepatocyte cytoplasm | Methyltransferase | Norepinephrine (noradrenaline) |

ER, endoplasmic reticulum.

**Table 28.7 Examples of drugs that induce or inhibit microsomal enzymes (acting on one or more isoenzymes of cytochrome P450)**

| Enzyme inducers | | Enzyme inhibitors | |
|---|---|---|---|
| Drug class | Examples | Drug class | Examples |
| Barbiturates | Phenobarbitone<br>Thiopentone | Monoamine oxidase inhibitors | Phenelzine<br>Tranylcypromine |
| Anticonvulsants | Phenytoin<br>Carbamazepine | Antiarrhythmics | Amiodarone<br>Verapamil<br>Diltiazem |
| Steroids | Glucocorticoids<br>Androgens<br>Cortisone | Anti-histamines | Cimetidine |
| Recreational drugs | Alcohol<br>Tobacco<br>Cannabis | Cytotoxic drugs | Cyclophosphamide |
| Hormone analogues | Oral contraceptive | Anti-inflammatory drugs | Phenylbutazone |
| Antibiotics and antifungals | Rifampicin<br>Griseofulvin | Anti-urate | Allopurinol |
| | | Antibiotics | Metronidazole<br>Chloramphenicol<br>Ciprofloxacin<br>Sulphonamides |

Adapted in part from Calvey TN and Williams NE. *Principles and Practice of Pharmacology for Anaesthetists*, 3rd edn. Oxford: Blackwell Scientific, 1996.

### Clearance, extraction ratio, and protein binding

Clearance and the ER have been defined and discussed in principle in Chapter 19. In summary, clearance is the volume of blood from which the drug is removed per unit time or, alternatively, the rate of drug elimination per unit concentration. The ER is the fraction of drug extracted from each unit volume of perfusing blood per unit time.

The other factors that determine the extraction of drugs from the liver are the activity of enzyme systems (the lower the Michaelis constant or $K_m$ [see Chapter 19], the greater the rate of reaction per unit concentration of drug), the fraction of free drug in the plasma, and the rate at which the drug is presented to the liver.

When the ER is very high, because the hepatic vein concentration will be almost zero, clearance approaches liver blood flow. Under these conditions, the liver has excess metabolic capacity for the drug and the clearance is almost totally dependent on liver blood flow. In summary, the liver will almost immediately metabolize all the drug presented to it.

When the ER is low, there are two possible mechanisms:

1. The enzyme simply has a low efficiency (high $K_m$), and consumes drug at a low rate. Only a small fraction of the drug presented to the liver will be metabolized. Perfusion is therefore no longer the limiting factor.
2. The enzyme may have high efficiency (low $K_m$), but there may be few enzyme-binding sites available. Consequently, the enzyme will be working well up on its saturation curve and operating at, or close to, zero-order kinetics (see Chapter 19). It will then be insensitive to changes in the amount of substrate presented to it.

This concept can be put to use to classifying drugs into two major types:

1. Flow-limited drugs with an ER > 0.7 whose clearance is dependent on liver blood flow;
2. Capacity-limited drugs with ER < 0.3 whose clearance is dependent on the rate of hepatic metabolism. They are called 'capacity limited' because the ER is limited by the capacity of the liver to metabolize that particular drug.

Between these two arbitrarily selected values of ER will be drugs that have a mixture of the two properties. These three classes of drug are shown grouped in Figure 28.14 and a selection of examples is given in Table 28.8.

Drug metabolism is also affected by protein binding because it is only the unbound drug fraction that is available to enter cells. However (see Chapter 19), the ratio of the unbound to the bound fraction is constant and, as free drug is taken up and metabolized, the ratio is immediately re-established. Consequently, protein binding does not prevent the metabolism of those drugs that have a high ER; their clearance is still limited by the rate at which the drug is presented to the liver. On the other hand, those drugs with a low ER can be affected by protein binding. If their enzyme system is fully occupied, and it is being shared with other

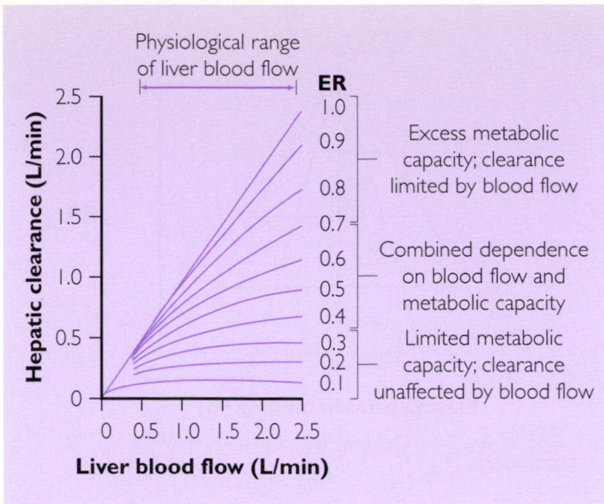


**Figure 28.14** The relationship between liver blood flow and total hepatic clearance for drugs with varying extraction ratios (ER). The normal physiological range of liver blood flow is shown. (Adapted from Wilkinson GR and Shand DG. *Clin Pharmacol Ther* 1975;18:377.)

ligands, increasing the concentration of free drug will improve the competition for enzyme-binding sites and the concentration gradient across the hepatocyte membrane. This will be much more relevant to highly bound drugs than to those that are poorly bound. A reduction in binding from, say, 95% to 90% will double the concentration of free drug, whereas a reduction from 15% to 10% has a much less proportionate effect. This means that drugs with a low ER can be further divided into binding-sensitive and binding-insensitive groups (Table 28.8). Drugs that are highly bound are also more sensitive to being displaced by competing ligands from their binding sites on the protein itself. The interrelationship of ER and protein binding is presented graphically in Figures 28.15 and 28.16. On both these figures, the position of some common drugs has been superimposed.

## CLINICAL BIOCHEMISTRY OF LIVER DISEASE

Biochemical measurements for both screening and identification of the type of liver disease have five main aims:

- detecting intrinsic hepatocellular damage;
- detecting cholestasis;
- detecting and differentiating between the types and causes of jaundice;
- assessing the synthetic functions of the liver;
- diagnosis of primary carcinoma.

The way these are carried out and applied in clinical practice is described in Chapter 58.

**Table 28.8 Effect of extraction ratio (ER) and protein binding on elimination of drugs by the liver**

| Drug | Approximate ER | Protein binding (%) | Metabolic consequences |
|---|---|---|---|
| **Flow-limited drugs** | | | |
| Labetalol | 0.85 | 40 | Changes in liver blood flow associated with liver disease affect these drugs |
| Verapamil | 0.80 | 92 | The shunting of blood that bypasses the liver has important effects on bioavailability. |
| Morphine | 0.75 | 35 | |
| Propranolol | 0.65 | 95 | |
| Lignocaine (lidocaine) | 0.60 | 65 | |
| **Flow- and capacity-sensitive drugs** | | | |
| Metoprolol | 0.56 | 10 | Changes in both liver blood flow and free fraction of drug in the blood may be important for this class of drugs |
| Methohexitone | 0.53 | 70 | |
| Pethidine | 0.50 | 70 | |
| Paracetamol | 0.30 | 20 | |
| Chlorpromazine | 0.30 | 95 | |
| Ranitidine | 0.28 | 15 | |
| **Capacity-limited, binding-sensitive drugs** | | | |
| Diphenylhydantoin | 0.03 | 92 | This class of drugs will be considerably influenced by changes in protein binding |
| Chlordiazepoxide | 0.02 | 96 | |
| Diazepam | 0.02 | 97 | |
| Warfarin | 0.005 | 99 | |
| **Capacity-limited, binding-insensitive drugs** | | | |
| Hexobarbitone | 0.15 | 47 | This class of drugs will not be influenced much by changes in protein binding |
| Antipyrine | 0.05 | 10 | |
| Theophylline | 0.05 | 62 | |
| Caffeine | 0.04 | 31 | |

Adapted from Eagle CJ and Strunin L. *Curr Anaesth Crit Care* 1990;1:204.

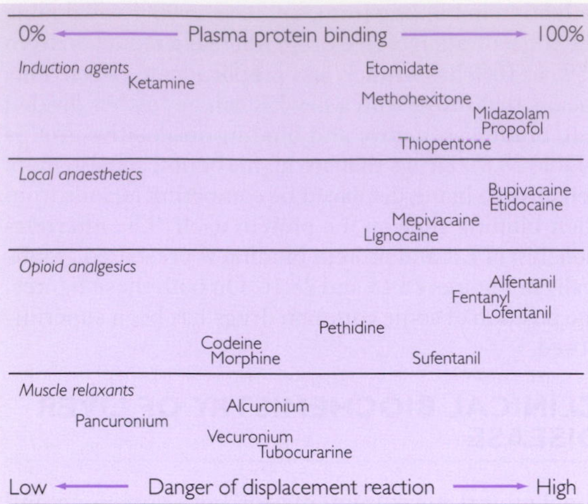


**Figure 28.15** The plasma protein binding of some drugs used in anaesthesia. (Adapted from Jorm CM and Stamford SA. *Ballière's Clin Anaesthesiol* 1992;6:751; Wood M. *Anaesth Analg* 1986;65:786.)

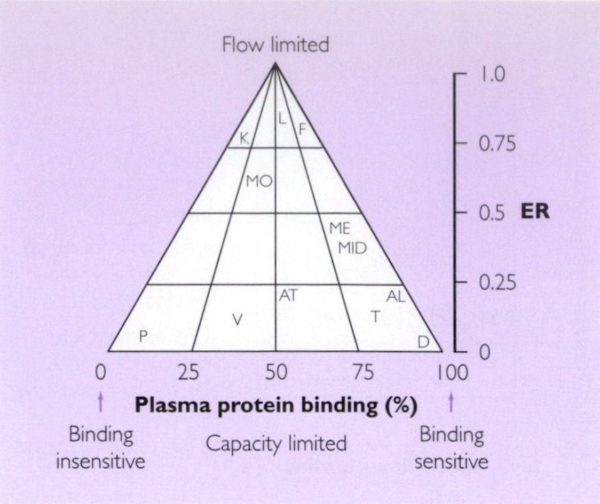


**Figure 28.16** The relationship between flow-limited and capacity-limited drug metabolism and the hepatic extraction ratio. This diagram is often referred to as Blaschke's triangle. Examples of anaesthetic drugs have been placed in their appropriate positions. AL, alfentanil; AT, atracurium; D, diazepam; ER, extraction ratio; F, fentanyl; K, ketamine; L, lignocaine (lidocaine); MID, midazolam; ME, methohexitone; MO, morphine; P, pancuronium; T, thiopentone; V, vecuronium. (Adapted from Blaschke TF. *Clin Pharmacokin* 1977;2:32; data from Hull CJ. *Pharmacokinetics for Anaesthesia*. Oxford: Butterworth– Heinemann, 1991:129.)

## FURTHER READING

Ganong WF. *Review of Medical Physiology*, 18th edn. Stamford, CA: Appleton & Lange, 1997.

Sear JW. Hepatic physiology. *Curr Anaesth Crit Care* 1990;**1**:196–203.

Sear JW. Anatomy and physiology of the liver. *Baillière's Clin Anaesthesiol* 1992;**6**:697–727.

# Chapter 29 Endocrine systems

J.W. Sear and P. Hutton

## GENERAL PRINCIPLES

### Definitions and the scope of modern endocrinology

Endocrinology is the study of the actions of hormones and the glands in which they are synthesized. The historical definition of a hormone is a chemical messenger released into the bloodstream and acting on a distant target organ. This definition is, however, now far too restrictive, because chemical messengers released by endocrine glands may act as circulating hormones, local regulators or neurotransmitters, or any combination of these functions. The boundaries of endocrinology are therefore now very blurred, particularly where it touches subjects such as prostaglandin and histamine release.

This chapter is written primarily for anaesthetists, so the approach taken is directed towards complementing those aspects of endocrinology that underpin clinical practice. To this end, a mixture of the classic and modern approaches is taken. Little consideration is given to the testis, ovary, and gut hormones. The hormone changes of pregnancy are described in Chapter 30, and the perioperative management of endocrine disorders is discussed in Chapters 55 and 56. Although it is not an absolute rule, unrecognized endocrine dysfunction is unlikely if:

- there is a normal blood glucose estimation and/or no glycosuria;
- body weight is unchanged from the normal for that person;
- blood pressure and heart rate are normal;
- there is no recent history of endocrine-related medication;
- sexual function and body hair are normal.

The endocrine system acts in close cooperation with vegetative centres in the brain and with the autonomic nervous system in regulating nutrition, metabolism, growth, development, and maturation. It also allows the organism to adapt to changes in its surroundings and has a major role in maintaining the 'milieu interieur'. Most of these principally 'automatic or subconscious' functions are subject to central control by the hypothalamus, which is itself influenced by higher centres of the brain.

In the hypothalamus, electric (neural) stimuli are converted into chemical (hormonal) signals. Special nerve cells within the hypothalamus, called neuroendocrine cells, synthesize hormones that are released in response to stimulation and are carried in the blood to their target. Substances released at other nerve endings (e.g. acetylcholine, γ-aminobutyric acid [GABA]) have only to traverse the synaptic cleft and are known as transmitters. Again, this distinction becomes blurred in the case of catecholamines, which act both locally as transmitters and through the circulation as hormones.

The endocrine system used to be regarded as being specialized for the slow, chronic transmission of signals, using the circulatory system to cover the large distances within the body. Although it is never as rapid as the nervous system, the action of local hormones nevertheless does not fit well into this traditional picture. As those hormones released into the bloodstream circulate more or less together, there has to be some way of ensuring that the hormone and its specific target cells recognize one another. For this purpose the target cell is equipped with specific binding sites (receptors) for the hormone in question. The affinities of these receptors for the hormone has to be extremely high because the hormone concentrations amount to only $10^{-8}$–$10^{-12}$ mol/L.

Endocrinology suffers from a complex nomenclature with different names for the same substance. There is now an accepted international classification. This is given in Appendix 29.1 to which reference can be made while reading the chapter.

### The organization of endocrine systems

There are usually three types of hormone action defined:

1. that on a distant cell via the bloodstream (haemocrine), the classic definition;
2. that on neighbouring cells (paracrine), e.g. angiotensin II, bradykinin, histamine, serotonin, and prostaglandins;
3. that on the cell secreting it (autocrine), e.g. interleukin 2.

The classic blood-borne system is shown diagrammatically in Figure 29.1. Details of the various pathways are given later. The actions of the paracrine and autocrine systems are described in the text as they occur.

### Types of hormone

Three types of hormones are characteristically described:

1. amines (e.g. catecholamines, thyroid hormones);
2. steroids (e.g. glucocorticoids, mineralocorticoids, sex hormones);
3. polypeptides (which covers all other hormones).

However, in addition to these three traditional classes of hormone at least one other group must be added:

4. the fatty acid derivatives.

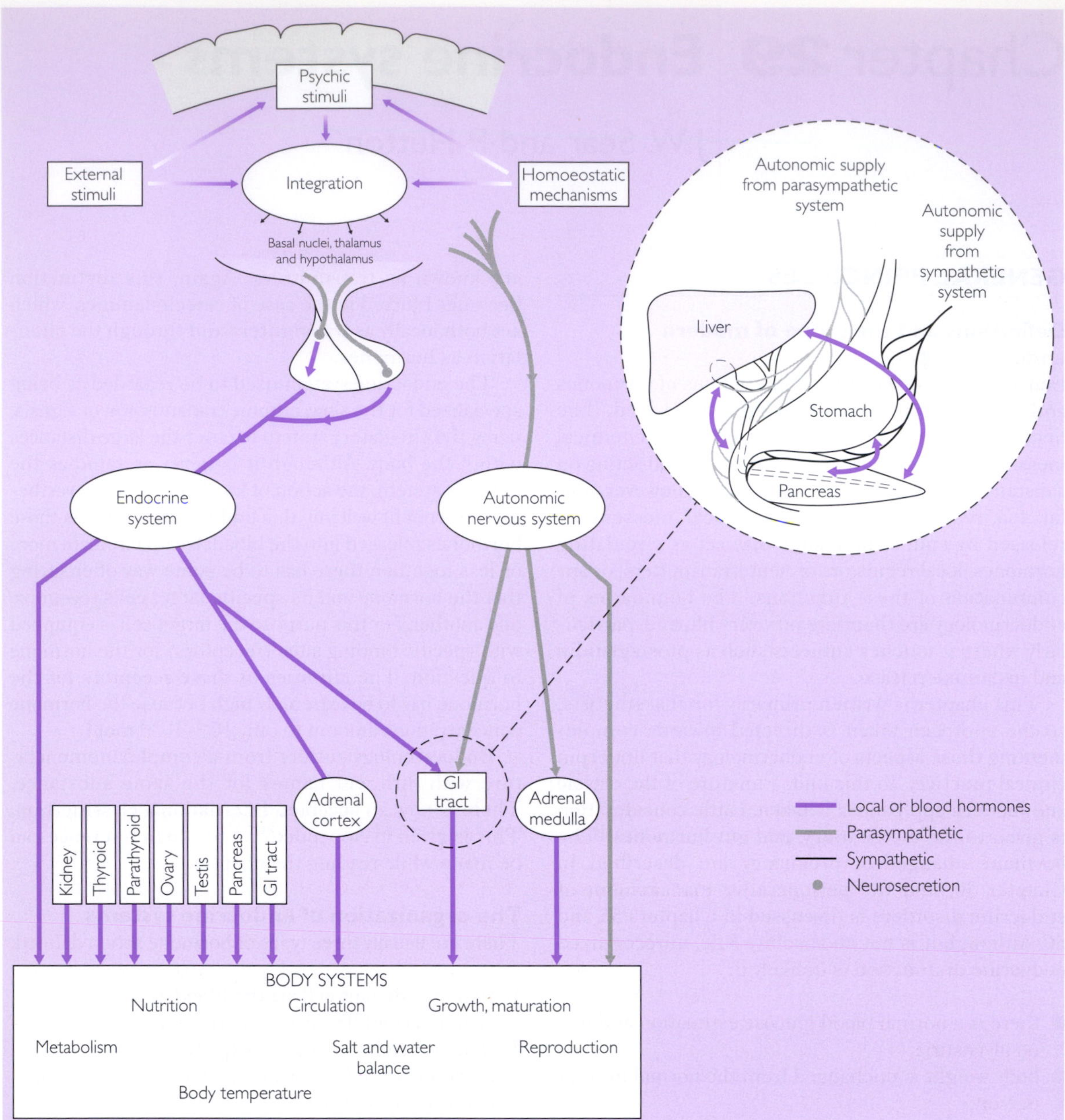


**Figure 29.1** The organization of the endocrine system showing its interrelationship with the nervous system. GI, gastrointestinal.

***Amines***

These are synthesized from the amino acid tyrosine, and serve as the circulating messengers of sympathetic nervous system activation. Other amine hormones include thyroxine, dopamine, serotonin (5-hydroxytryptamine), and histamine.

Once synthesized, amine hormones are either stored in follicles (as in the case of the thyroid hormones) or as secretory granules (e.g. as with the catecholamines). After release into the circulation, they may bind to plasma proteins (e.g. the binding of thyroid hormones to plasma globulins). There is also conversion of some of these active hormones into equally, more, or less active forms at sites distant from their site of origin. The best examples of this are the conversion of thyroxine into the more active triiodothyronine ($T_3$) – by deiodination or inactivation into the reverse molecule, reverse triiodothyronine ($rT_3$).

***Steroids***

The synthesis of these hormones occurs in the mitochondria of adrenal and gonadal cells by a series of hydroxylation reactions that depend on cytochrome P450. Unlike the polypeptides, they are usually produced and secreted to demand, with cell stimulation leading to synthesis and direct release of the hormones. Once released, these hydrophobic steroid hormones are bound to proteins in the blood, some of which are specific transport proteins. Examples are transcortin for cortisol and progesterone, or the globulin that binds the sex hormones, testosterone and oestrogen.

***Polypeptides***

Polypeptide hormones often contain associated carbohydrate residues, and are then termed 'glycoproteins'. Synthesis is usually as a larger protein which is inactive, and which then undergoes cleavage to produce active hormone or hormones. There may even be a precursor of the prohormone (termed a 'pre-prohormone'), e.g. pre-proglucagon in the pancreas is processed into glucagon, which acts to inhibit insulin release and increase the blood sugar.

Polypeptide hormones are stored in secretory granules in the cytoplasm of the secreting cell to prevent their degradation by proteolytic enzymes. They are released from cells by exocytosis (see Chapter 18) whereby the granules fuse with the cell membrane and the contents are subsequently released directly into the circulation.

#### Fatty acid derivatives

Fatty acid derivatives include the prostaglandins and leukotrienes which are synthesized from arachidonic acid. These hormones are involved predominantly in paracrine control of a wide range of biological functions such as intrarenal blood flow, endothelial stimulation of platelet activation, and the blood clotting cascade.

A summary of the types of hormone is given in Table 29.1.

### Receptors and the cellular transmission of hormone signals

Hormones, as humoral signal or messenger substances (first messenger), reach their respective target cells via the extracellular route. For hormones other than the lipophilic ones, the outer surface of the target cell membrane possesses hormone receptors that are specific for each hormone and bind it with high affinity. As far as is known, these receptors are peptide chains (around 50 000 Da) that penetrate the cell membrane many times in a zig-zag manner (Figure 29.2). In contrast to this, lipophilic hormones enter the cell and bind to specific cytoplasmic binding proteins.

After binding to a receptor, hormones produce their effects by three general mechanisms:

1. directly by cell membrane effects;
2. by intracellular effects mediated by a second messenger;
3. intracellularly by effects on protein synthesis.

As the specificity of the hormone action is provided by the receptors on or within the target cell, different hormones can employ the same second messenger. In addition, the concentration of second messenger in the cell can be raised by one hormone but lowered by another. The action of G proteins and other receptor systems is described in Chapter 69, to which reference should be made for an understanding of the following mechanisms.

#### Direct cell membrane effects

These directly alter the permeability of the cell membrane to ion channels and ion pumps ($K^+$, $Ca^{2+}$) via $G_s$, $G_i$, and other G proteins ($G_o$, $G_k$) without the intervention of adenylyl cyclase or other second messengers. The onset of effect by this route is rapid, and may be mediated via tyrosine kinases attached to the receptor. Examples of hormonal effect mediated this way are those seen after insulin, insulin growth factor 1, epidermal growth factor, growth hormone, and prolactin. The insulin receptor is shown in Chapter 19, Figure 19.36.

#### Intracellular effects mediated by second messengers

These hormones bind to plasma membrane receptors, and cause intracellular effects via second messenger activation.

##### *For a cAMP-mediated cell response*

For such a response, the membrane of the target cell must contain, in addition to the receptor, stimulating or inhibiting guanyl nucleotide-regulatory proteins, $G_s$ (stimulatory) or $G_i$ (inhibitory) or both. They are made up of the three subunits: $\alpha_s$ (stimulating) or $\alpha_i$ (inhibiting), $\beta$, and $\gamma$. At rest, $\alpha$ is bound to guanosine diphosphate (GDP). If the hormone reacts with the receptor (in the presence of $Mg^{2+}$), $\alpha_s$-GTP (guanosine triphosphate) or $\alpha_i$-GTP is formed, of which the former activates the adenylyl cyclase on the inside of the membrane (i.e. cAMP rises), whereas $\alpha_i$-GTP inhibits it (cAMP drops). Some of the reactions characterized by this mechanism are shown in Table 29.2.

Cyclic AMP activates protein kinase A which phosphorylates proteins (mostly enzymes or membrane proteins, including the receptor itself). The specific cell response depends on the nature of the phosphorylated protein, which in turn is determined by the particular protein kinase present in the target cell.

To switch off the chain of signals, $\alpha$-GTP is reconverted by the hormone-activated GTPase to $\alpha$-GDP, which eventually joins up again with $\beta$–$\gamma$ to form G-GDP (see Chapter 19). Further, cAMP is inactivated by a phosphodiesterase to 5′-AMP, and also the previously phosphorylated proteins can be dephosphorylated by phosphatases. Inhibition of the reaction cAMP $\rightarrow$ 5′-AMP (e.g. by theophylline or caffeine) prolongs the life of cAMP and also, therefore the hormone action.

Cholera toxin blocks the GTPase, thus cutting out its 'turning off' effect on the adenylyl cyclase, and the cellular cAMP concentration rises to extremely high values in intestinal cells. Pertussis toxin inhibits the $G_i$ protein, deinhibiting its effect on adenylyl cyclase, and thus also causing a rise in cAMP in the cell.

##### *Other second messengers*

For other secondary messengers, including cGMP (cyclic guanosine monophosphate), inositol-1,4,5-trisphosphate ($IP_3$), and 1,2-diacylglycerol (DAG), after extracellular hormone receptor binding and the action of G proteins ($G_p$ and others), phospholipase C on the inside of the cell membrane is activated. This enzyme splits the phosphatidylinositol-4,5-bisphosphate of the cell membrane into $IP_3$ and DAG, which as parallel second messengers have different effects. The effect of DAG persists considerably longer than that of $IP_3$ because the $Ca^{2+}$ set free by the latter (see below) is immediately pumped out.

The lipophilic DAG remains in the cell membrane where it activates protein kinase C; this also phosphorylates and activates the carrier protein for the $Na^+/H^+$ exchange. One of the results of this is a rise in intracellular pH, which is another important signal for many other cell processes.

**Table 29.1 A simple classification of some common hormones**

| Polypeptides | Glycoproteins | Steroids | Amines (tyrosine derivatives) | Arachidonic acid derivatives | Indole (tryptophan derivatives) | Histidine derivatives |
|---|---|---|---|---|---|---|
| Insulin | Erythropoietin | Corticosteroids | Thyroxine | Prostaglandins | Serotonin (5HT) | Histamine |
| Glucagon | FSH | Aldosterone | Triiodothyronine | Leukotrienes | | |
| Somatostatin | LH | Vitamin D | Epinephrine | | | |
| PTH | TSH | Oestrogens | Norepinephrine | | | |
| Calcitonin | | Progesterone | PIH (dopamine) | | | |
| Somatomedins | | Testosterone | | | | |
| Vasopressin | | Androgens | | | | |
| Oxytocin | | | | | | |
| Corticotrophin | | | | | | |
| MSH | | | | | | |
| Somatotrophin | | | | | | |
| Prolactin | | | | | | |
| FSH-RH<br>LH-RH | | | | | | |
| TRH | | | | | | |
| Somatostatin | | | | | | |
| SRH | | | | | | |
| MRH | | | | | | |
| MIH | | | | | | |
| CRH | | | | | | |

For synonyms and explanation of terms and abbreviations, see Appendix 29.1.

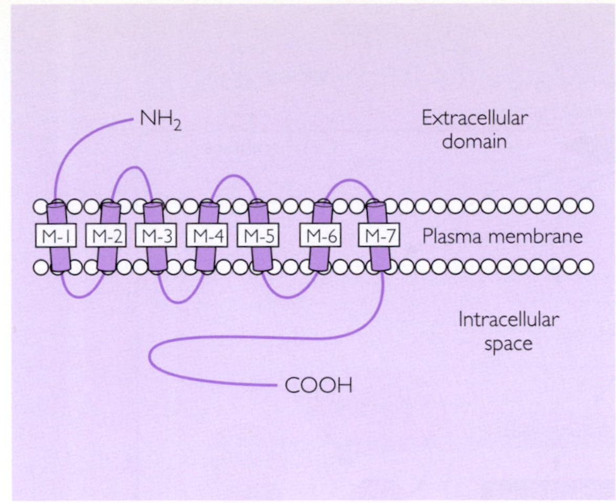


**Figure 29.2** A peptide chain repeatedly crossing the plasma membrane to act as a receptor for adrenergic hormones. The receptor is G protein linked to a second messenger. (Adapted from Insel PA. *N Engl J Med* 1996;334:580.)

| **Table 29.3 Hormone and receptor type regulated by IP$_3$ and DAG** |
|---|
| Epinephrine ($\alpha_1$-adrenoceptors) |
| Acetylcholine ($M_1$-receptors) |
| 5-Hydroxytryptamine (serotonin) (5HT$_1$-receptors) |
| Thyroliberin ? TRH |
| Cholecystokinin |
| Gastrin ? LH-RH FSH-RH |
| Adiuretin (VP$_1$-receptors) |
| Histamine ($H_1$-receptors) |
| Thromboxane |

TRH, thyroid-releasing hormone. LH-RH, luteinizing hormone releasing hormone; FSH-RH, follicle stimulating hormone releasing hormone; VP, vasopressin

Most of the IP$_3$ reaches the cell's stores of calcium on the endoplasmic reticulum via the cytoplasm, so that the calcium can now, as a third messenger, influence numerous cell functions. Examples of hormones working via IP$_3$ and DAG are given in Table 29.3 and their intracellular modes of action are shown in Figure 29.3.

***Intracellular effects mediated by effects on protein synthesis***

The steroid hormones (see Table 29.1) and the lipid-soluble thyroid hormones (in contrast to the hydrophilic hormones) pass through the cell membrane relatively easily on account of their fat solu-

**Table 29.2 Hormones acting via G proteins which increase or decrease cAMP**

| Hormones acting via G$_s$, and increasing cAMP | Hormones acting via G$_i$ and decreasing cAMP |
|---|---|
| Glucagon | Acetylcholine ($M_2$-receptors) |
| Vasoactive intestinal polypeptide | Somatostatin |
| Oxytocin | Opioids |
| Adenosine ($A_2$-receptors) | Adenosine ($A_1$-receptors) |
| 5-Hydroxytryptamine (serotonin) (5HT$_2$-receptors) | 5-Hydroxytryptamine (serotonin) (5HT$_{1a}$-receptors) |
| Secretin | Angiotensin II |
| PGI$_2$ | Dopamine ($D_2$-receptors) |
| PGE$_2$ | Epinephrine ($\alpha_2$-adrenoceptors) |
| Histamine ($H_2$-receptors) | |
| Dopamine ($D_1$-receptors) | |
| Adiuretin (VP$_2$-receptors) | |
| LH and FSH | |
| TSH | |
| Corticotrophin | |
| Epinephrine ($\beta_1$- and $\beta_2$-adrenoceptors) | |
| Corticoliberin | |
| Somatoliberin | |

For synonyms and explanation of terms and abbreviations, see Appendix 29.1.

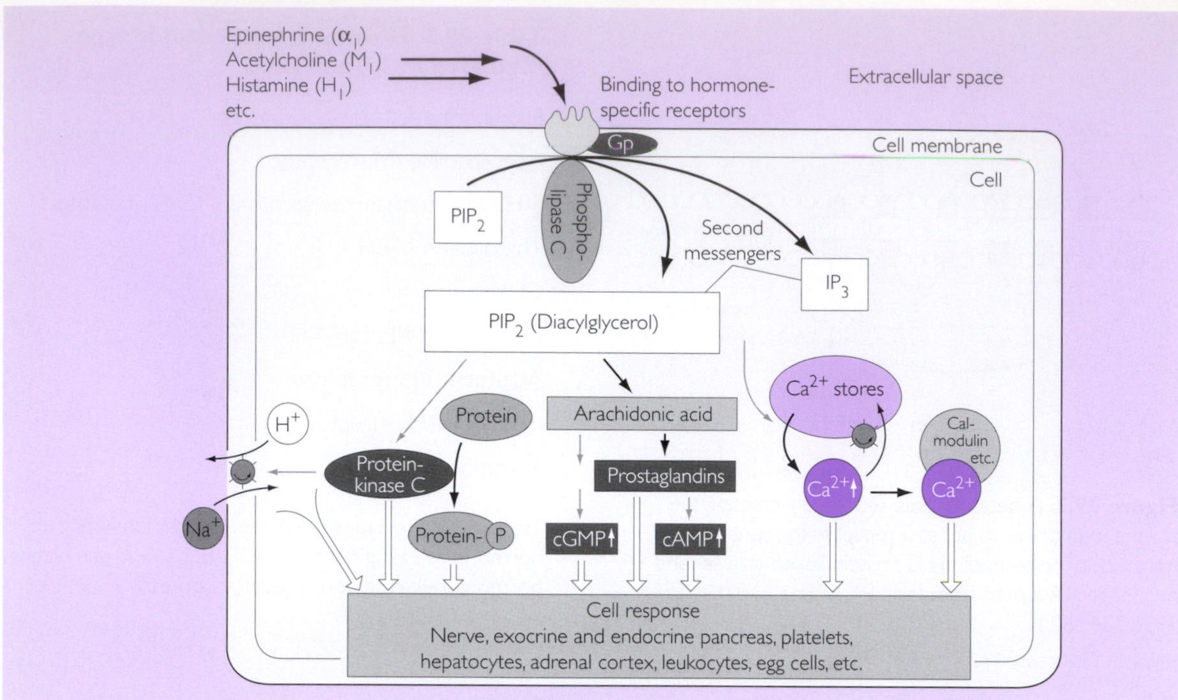


**Figure 29.3** The mode of action of hormones acting via inositol-1,4,5-trisphosphate ($IP_3$) and diacylglycerol. $PIP_2$, phosphoinositide 4,5-bisphosphate.

bility. Inside their respective target cells, they find their own specific cytoplasmic binding protein ('receptor' protein) to which they attach. This hormone–receptor binding is essential for hormonal activity because neither of the partners on its own has an effect.

For some hormones (e.g. oestradiol) there is more than one receptor protein in the target cell; other cells may have receptors for several hormones (e.g. for oestradiol and progesterone). The concentration of the receptor protein is variable. Oestradiol, for example, can increase the number of progesterone receptors in progesterone target cells.

After its formation, the hormone–receptor protein complex passes into the cell nucleus (translocation), where, after binding to nuclear receptors, it stimulates increased production of mRNA (see Chapter 19 for further details of this process). This is summarized schematically in Figure 29.4.

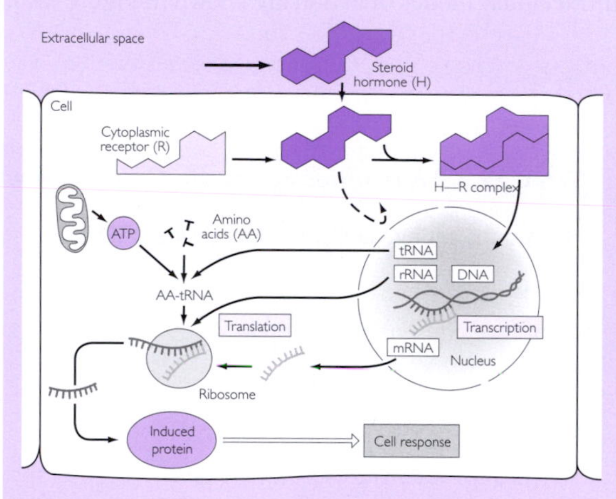


**Figure 29.4** The mechanism of action of steroid hormones.

The mRNA-producing or 'structural genes' of a chromosome are 'switched' on and off by what is termed an 'operator gene'. A repressor, formed by a so-called regulator gene, switches the operator gene to 'off'. The probable effect of the hormone is to inactivate this repressor. This consequently 'switches on' the operator gene, i.e. more mRNA is produced. The mRNA leaves the cell nucleus and migrates to the ribsomes, the site of protein synthesis. Here, the increased number of templates (mRNA) makes increased copying (translation) of proteins possible. The increased number of proteins resulting from this synthesis then produce the actual cell response.

Cholesterol is the source of all steroid hormones. It is formed in the liver and endocrine glands via a number of intermediate steps from acetyl-CoA. Although the placenta can synthesize steroid hormones, it cannot form cholesterol, and therefore must take it up from the blood. Steroid hormones are stored only in small quantities at their site of production (adrenal cortex, testes, ovaries), which means that they have to be synthesized from cellular reserves of cholesterol when needed.

### Feedback control systems

Like any control system, the endocrine system is subject to feedback control. It uses four methods: three of these are of the normal negative type (high concentration of end-product reduces the production) and one is of the positive feedback type (hormone production stimulates its own increased production). Positive feedback is the exception rather than the rule. Their actions can be classified as follows.

### *Direct negative feedback*

This is very straightforward: presence of the product directly reduces the continued action of the hormone. The best example of this is the relationship between glucose and insulin.

### *Indirect negative feedback*

This is the control of hormone output by the effects of the level of hormone on both the stimulating hormone from the anterior pituitary and the releasing factor from the hypothalamus (see later). A good example is the secretion of glucocorticoids by the adrenal cortex. This is shown diagrammatically in Figure 29.5.

### *Intracellular negative feedback*

This is effected by intrinsic metabolic feedback loops within the cells of the endocrine gland, whereby the product inhibits is own synthesis. An example of this is organic iodine in the thyroid gland inhibiting thyroid hormone synthesis.

### *Positive feedback*

Some hormones can, in certain circumstances, stimulate their own secretion. This is seen in the ovulatory cycle where the surge in luteinizing hormone (LH) that precedes ovulation is contributed to by the LH itself. Any positive feedback loop is, by definition, 'run-away' and unstable, and hence, once a preset level has been reached, secondary mechanisms have to switch production off.

Not only do the trophic hormones govern the formation and release of the hormone end-product, they also influence the growth of the peripheral endocrine gland from which the hormone end-product is released. If the concentration of the hormone end-product in the blood is still too low despite maximal synthesis and release, the gland's cells multiply and hypertrophy until there is a sufficient feedback effect from the hormone end-product. Such a compensatory hypertrophy also takes place when part of an endocrine gland is removed operatively, as in unilateral adrenalectomy. The remaining gland increases in size and function until the original rate of secretion is restored.

When a hormone (e.g. cortisone) is given as chronic medication, it causes a reduction in secretion of the corresponding trophic hormone (e.g. corticotrophin, also know as adrenocorticotropic hormone [ACTH], in the same way as the natural hormone. Consequently, the endocrine gland atrophies.

Rebound is a phenomenon observed when hormonal medication is stopped. During this period of 'rebound', the balance of the feedback system has not fully recovered and the trophic hormone (in the above example, corticotrophin) is temporarily released in hypernormal quantities, as shown in Figure 29.6.

## The hypothalamus and pituitary

The pituitary gland weighs less than 1 gram and yet it is one of the most important controlling organs of the body. Embryologically, it has two quite different ectodermal origins. The neurohypophysis begins as a downgrowth from the hypothalamus; the adenohypophysis originates as an upward growth from the roof of the mouth known as Rathke's pouch. When the two meet, they fuse and the pouch loses its connection with the mouth. The part of the pouch that fuses with the neurohypophysis is called the pars intermedius or intermediate lobe. On either side of this boundary are the anterior (adenohypophysis) and posterior (neurohypophysis) lobes. The process of formation is shown in Figure 29.7.

There are a number of different cell types in the anterior pituitary, each of which synthesize and release separate secretions:

- somatotrophs (which synthesize and release growth hormone) account for about 50% of the total cell mass;
- lactotrophs (which synthesize prolactin) make up 20% of the cells;
- corticotrophs synthesize the pro-peptide pro-opiomelanocortin;
- gonadotrophs produce follicle-stimulating hormone and LH;
- thyrotrophs are the least abundant of the cells, and are responsible for synthesis and release of thyroid-stimulating hormone (TSH).

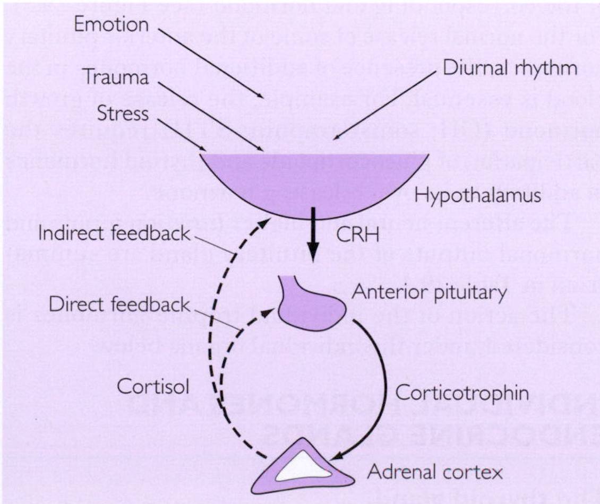


**Figure 29.5** Hormonal feedback from the adrenal cortex showing both direct and indirect negative feedback control. CRH, corticotrophin-releasing hormone.

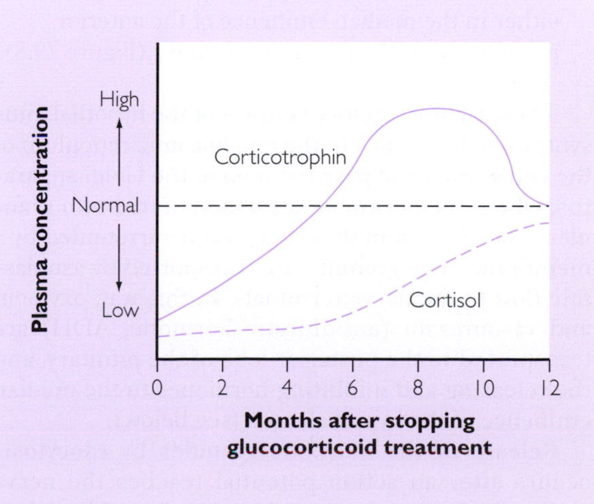


**Figure 29.6** The pattern of corticotrophin and cortisol secretion after stopping glucocorticoid treatment.

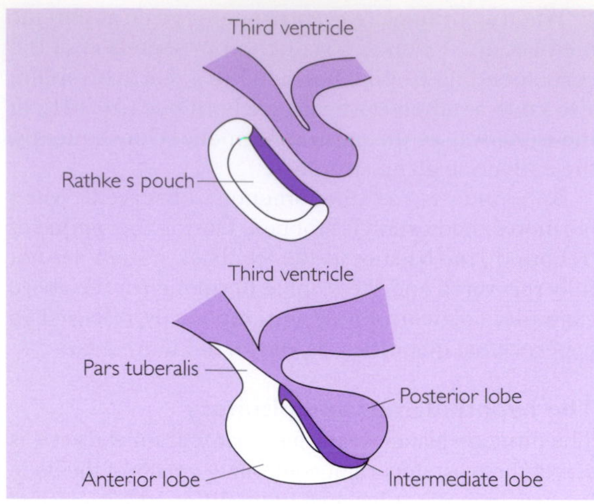


**Figure 29.7** A diagrammatic representation of the formation of the pituitary gland.

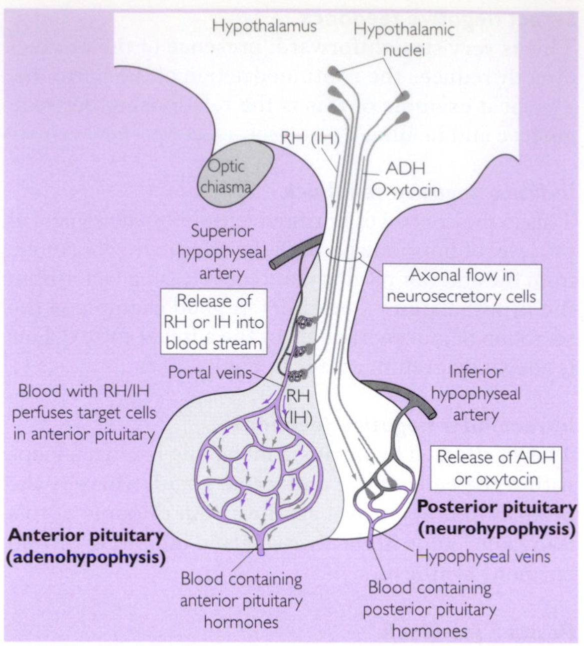


**Figure 29.8** A diagrammatic representation of the pituitary gland showing its central neuronal connections, the neurosecretory neurons, and the release of hormones into the blood. RH releasing hormone; IH, inhibitory hormone; ADH, antidiuretic hormone.

The hypothalamus receives many processed inputs from a number of defined nuclei. These inputs can be physiological or from feedback mechanisms (see Figure 29.5). The hypothalamus is also intimately connected with the limbic system, the reticular formation, and (via the thalamic nuclei) the cerebral cortex. The hormone balance is thus concerned not only with purely vegetative regulation (energy and water balance, circulation, respiration), but also with the sleeping–waking (circadian) rhythm and with psychic–emotional factors. Stress situations can, for example, be the reason for the absence of menstrual bleeding, or the production of urine.

All these factors are integrated to control the release of short peptide hormones called releasing and inhibiting factors (Figure 29.8) from specialized neurons, which travel from the hypothalamus to the pituitary gland. These neurons have two unique properties:

1. They synthesize and secrete peptides as their main function.
2. Although these neurons may form conventional synapses through collateral branches, their function is 'neurosecretion into the vasculature' through neuronal endings on capillary networks either in the median eminence of the anterior pituitary, or in the posterior pituitary (Figure 29.8).

These neurosecretory neurons of the hypothalamus synthesize hormones in the endoplasmic reticulum of the cell's soma and pass them on to the Golgi apparatus, where the hormones are incorporated into granules (100–300 nm in diameter), each surrounded by a membrane. The granules are transported by axoplasmic flow to the nerve terminals. In this way, oxytocin and vasopressin (antidiuretic hormone; ADH) are transported to the posterior lobe of the pituitary, and the releasing and inhibiting hormones to the median eminence of the hypothalamus (see below).

Release of the hormone granules by exocytosis occurs after an action potential reaches the nerve ending. This is accompanied by an influx of $Ca^{2+}$ into the nerve ending, as in the release of neurotransmitters. The action potential in neurosecretory nerves lasts up to 10 times longer than in other nerves, to allow sustained release of the hormone.

The hormones of the posterior lobe of the pituitary, i.e. vasopressin and oxytocin, are released from the neurosecretory nerves directly into the systemic circulation. The releasing and inhibiting hormones for the anterior lobe of the pituitary are secreted from the neurosecretory neurons of the hypothalamus into a kind of portal blood system, or 'short-cut' to the vascular network of the anterior pituitary (Figure 29.8). Here they bring about secretion (via second messengers, see above) of the trophic hormones of the anterior pituitary into the general circulation. Regulation of the secretion of releasing and inhibiting hormones is accomplished by feedback via the plasma concentration of the trophic anterior pituitary hormone and/or of the corresponding end hormone (see Figure 29.5). For the normal release of some of the anterior pituitary hormones, the presence of additional hormones in the blood is essential. For example, the release of growth hormone (GH; somatotrophin; STH) requires the participation of glucocorticoids and thyroid hormones in addition to its own releasing hormone.

The afferent neural and higher function inputs and hormonal outputs of the pituitary gland are summarized in Table 29.4.

The action of the individual trophic hormones is considered under the individual organs below.

## INDIVIDUAL HORMONES AND ENDOCRINE GLANDS

### The thyroid gland

#### *Hormone synthesis*

The thyroid gland is made up of two lobes joined at the level of the second and third tracheal cartilages, and is

**Table 29.4 Afferent neural and higher function inputs and hormonal outputs of the pituitary gland**

| Afferent inputs | Neural integrating areas | Part of pituitary involved | Composition and destination of neurosecretion | Resulting action | Final target organ |
|---|---|---|---|---|---|
| Osmoreceptors/volume receptors/thirst | SON and PVN | Posterior lobe | Vasopressin secreted into systemic circulation | Acts directly | Kidneys, peripheral vasculature |
| Touch receptors (breast/uterus/ genitalia) | SON and PVN | Posterior lobe | Oxytocin secreted into systemic circulation | Acts directly | Ejection of milk from mammary glands<br>Acts on uterus |
| Touch receptors (breast/others) | Arcuate nucleus | Median eminence/portal system/anterior lobe | PRF and PIF released into portal circulation | PRL secreted into systemic circulation | Stimulates secretion of milk<br>Affects maternal behaviour |
| Temperature/?seasonal/ ? other receptors | DMN | Median eminence/portal system/anterior lobe | TRH causes release into portal circulation | TSH secreted into systemic circulation | Thyroid gland produces thyroxine with widespread action in many tissues |
| Sexual stimulation/stress/ menstrual cycle | PO area | Median eminence/portal system/anterior lobe | LH-RH and FSH-RH released into portal circulation | LH and FSH secreted into systemic circulation | Gonads secrete testosterone, oestrogens, and gestogens |
| Diurnal rhythm/emotion/ stress/infection | SChN, limbic system, reticular formation | Median eminence/portal system/anterior lobe | CRH released into portal circulation | Corticotrophin secreted into systemic circulation | Acts on adrenal cortex to produce corticosteroids |
| Unknown inputs | PVN and arcuate N | Median eminence/portal system/anterior lobe | GHRH and GHIH released into portal circulation | GH secreted into systemic circulation | Controls skeletal growth and maturation |

Hormonal feedback mechanisms (see Figure 29.5) are not included in this table.

SON, supraoptic nucleus; PVN, paraventricular nucleus; DMN, dorsomedial nucleus; PO area, preoptic area; SChN, suprachiasmatic nucleus; TRH, thyrotrophin-releasing hormone; CRH, corticotrophin-releasing hormone; LH-RH, luteinizing hormone releasing hormone; FSH-RH, follicle stimulating hormone releasing hormone; PIF, prolactin-inhibiting factor; PRF, prolactin-releasing factor; GHRH, growth hormone releasing factor; GHIH, growth hormone-inhibiting factor; TSH, thyroid-stimulating hormone; β-LPH, β-lipotrophin; LH, luteinizing hormone; FSH, follicle-stimulating hormone; PRL, prolactin; GH, growth hormone.

ensheathed by the pretracheal fascia. Blood supply to the thyroid gland is via the superior and inferior thyroid arteries, whereas venous drainage is through superior, middle, and inferior thyroid veins, which arise from a venous plexus on the surface of the gland. Its anatomical position is shown in Chapter 6, Figures 6.10 and 6.15, and its histological appearance when active and inactive is shown in Figure 29.9.

The glandular tissue contains two types of cells:

1. follicular cells which secrete $T_3$ and thyroxine ($T_4$), the latter being considered by many to be a pro-hormone for $T_3$;
2. parafollicular cells which secret thyrocalcitonin

Thyroid hormone synthesis occurs in the colloid of the thyroid gland (Figure 29.9) through the iodination of tyrosine. Dietary iodine is converted to iodide before absorption into the bloodstream, and this is then actively transported into the follicular cells and concentrated in the colloid. Thyroglobulin is a glycoprotein synthesized by the thyroid cells from amino acids (including tyrosine) to which carbohydrate groups are added. Thyroglobulin is then released into the colloid and iodinated to form iodothyroglobulin, which is taken up into the follicular cells and broken down enzymatically to release $T_3$ and $T_4$. Excess iodide in the body will lead to decreased $T_4$ production. Thyroxine biosynthesis in the colloid of the thyroid cell is shown schematically in Figure 29.10.

The main output from the gland is $T_4$ with a smaller amount of $T_3$. The ratio of $T_3$ and $T_4$ in plasma is 1 : 100. Most of the daily production of $T_3$ occurs by a second route – namely the mono-deiodination of $T_4$ in peripheral tissues. The release of $T_4$ is the feedback controller for the secretion of TSH and thyroid-releasing hormone by the anterior pituitary and hypothalamus, respectively.

### *Hormone transport*

$T_3$ and $T_4$ are transported in the blood bound to plasma proteins, albumin, thyroxine-binding globulin (TBG), prealbumin, and globulin. Only 0.02% of $T_4$ is unbound, and a slightly greater amount of $T_3$ (0.2%). Most of the

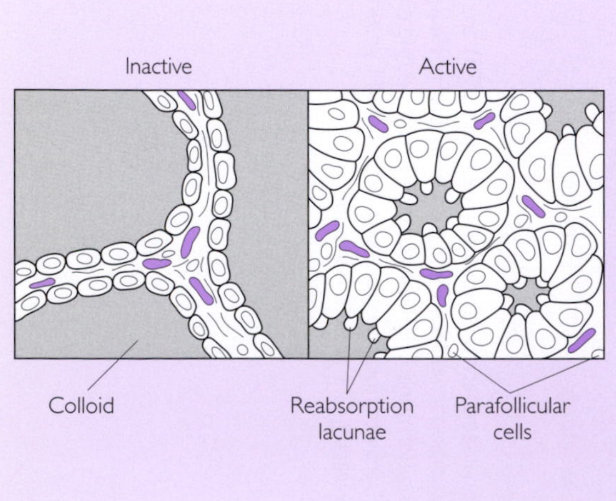


**Figure 29.9** The histology of the thyroid gland during active and inactive phases.

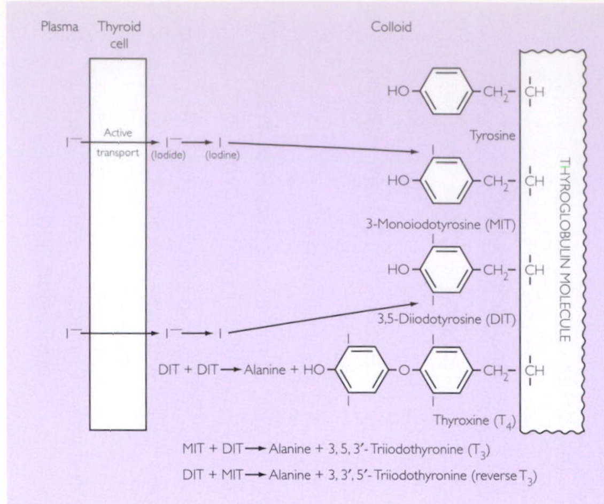


**Figure 29.10** An outline of thyroxine biosynthesis in the colloid of the thyroid cell. The molecules are bound by peptide linkages to the thyroglobulin.

circulating $T_4$ is bound to TBG, and alterations of this and the other binding proteins will alter the total thyroid hormone concentration rather than the free (unbound) hormone. As already mentioned, $T_3$ is more biologically active, with $T_4$ considered to be the 'prohormone'. About 33% of $T_4$ is converted to $T_3$, and another 45% to $rT_3$, i.e. the amount of $T_4$ in the body is about 20% of that synthesized and secreted. The half-life of $T_4$ is 6–7 days, whereas that of $T_3$ is shorter.

### *Mechanism of action of thyroid hormones*

$T_3$ interacts with a nuclear $T_3$ receptor located in the non-histone proteins of the chromatin in the cell nucleus. After binding, there is DNA transcription, with new mRNA and protein synthesis. The affinity of the nuclear receptors for $T_4$ is 10 times less than for $T_3$. Under the influence of $T_3$ the number of mitochondria and their cristae increase, which is the basis of the increased metabolic activity brought about by $T_3$ and its precursor $T_4$. $T_3$, like the catecholamines, stimulates oxygen utilization and energy turnover, and thus increases heat production. $T_3$ is important in thermoregulation.

### *Effects of the thyroid hormones*

These are listed in Table 29.5.

## The parathyroid glands

In humans there are usually four parathyroid glands, two in the superior and two in the inferior poles of the thyroid (Figure 29.11). The abundant chief cells, which have a clear cytoplasm, secrete parathyroid hormone (PTH) and are important in calcium metabolism. The other cell type, the oxyphil cell, has no known function.

Calcium is an important intracellular and extracellular cation which is key in the control of cellular depolarization of nerve and muscle. The resting intracellular calcium concentration is about 10 nmol/L, whereas the extracellular concentration is between 2.2 and 2.5 mmol/L. Of this extracellular calcium, 40% is free or ionized, 40–50% of the protein is bound to albumin, and the remainder is complexed to phosphate and bicarbonate. The ionized serum calcium is therefore

| Table 29.5 The actions of thyroid hormones |
|---|
| Calorigenic effect to increase the metabolic rate; this is mediated through the action of catecholamines, and does not reflect an uncoupling of mitochondria; the increased metabolic effect is found in most tissues except: adult brain, testes, uterus, lymph nodes, spleen, and anterior pituitary |
| Increased urinary nitrogen excretion secondary to increased protein catabolism |
| Increased body temperature |
| Carotenaemia (caused by stimulation of the conversion of carotene to vitamin A) |
| Milk secretion |
| Increased central nervous system activity |
| Increased numbers of cardiac β-adrenoceptors |
| Increased carbohydrate absorption from the intestinal tract |
| Decreased circulating cholesterol |
| Increased tissue growth and maturation |
| Increased red blood cell 2,3-diphosphoglycerate |

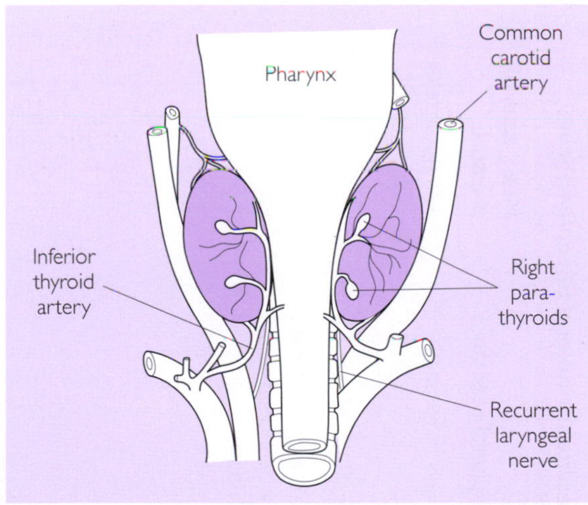


**Figure 29.11** The anatomy of the human parathyroid glands viewed from behind.

influenced by the total calcium concentration and by the serum albumin.

Normal homoeostasis of calcium concentration is under the control of two separate factors:

- circulating PTH levels;
- activated vitamin D.

Both act to increase the plasma calcium concentration but with different associated actions. Vitamin D causes increases in both calcium and phosphate simultaneously, whereas PTH (which is a peptide made up of 84 amino acids) causes a fall in phosphate concentration.

Calcitonin, secreted by the C cells of the thyroid gland, also lowers serum calcium and phosphate levels by inhibiting bone resorption, although its physiological role is uncertain. Although calcitonin may be relevant to skeletal development, there is general agreement that it is relatively inactive in adults.

PTH is secreted directly into the circulation in response to a fall in serum calcium and then cleaved into a number of fragments, most of which have no biological activity. The half-life of active PTH is less than 20 min. Both a pre-pro-PTH and a pre-PTH have been identified as intracellular precursors.

In the presence of a low calcium (or high phosphate), as PTH levels increase, this, in turn, leads to:

- mobilization of calcium from bone (and stimulation of new bone formation and bone resorption);
- increased renal calcium reabsorption (with associated increased phosphate loss);
- activation of the renal enzyme 1α-hydroxylase, which is responsible for the hydroxylation of vitamin D (from 1α- to 1α,25-dihydroxycholecalciferol). By this particular action it indirectly increases calcium absorption from the gut (see below).

The metabolism of vitamin D, the other hormone important in calcium metabolism, is depicted in Figure 29.12. Vitamin D is essential for normal bone formation and lack of it results in rickets or osteomalacia. 1α,25-Dihydroxycholecalciferol increases plasma calcium by increasing intestinal absorption of calcium and mobilizing calcium from bone. In addition to these two main influences on plasma calcium:

- GH increases calcium excretion in the urine, but increases its uptake in the intestine, resulting in a net positive calcium balance.
- Glucocorticoids decrease absorption of calcium and phosphate from the intestine, increase the renal excretion of both, and reduce the protein matrix of bone.

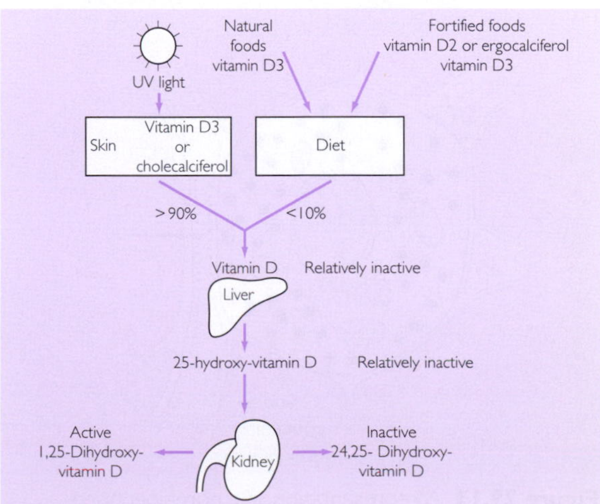


**Figure 29.12** Vitamin D metabolism. Under normal circumstances the major source of vitamin D is the action of sunlight on the skin.

## The adrenal medulla

The adrenal glands lie on either side of the body above the kidneys. They have two functionally separate regions: the medulla and the cortex. Their blood supply is derived from the inferior mesenteric arteries, the renal arteries, and the aorta. Venous drainage goes centrally through the medulla to the adrenal vein. The left adrenal vein drains into the left renal vein whereas the right drains directly into the inferior vena cava. This anatomical difference is relevant in the use of blood sampling of the outflow from the glands for the diagnosis of endocrine tumours.

The adrenal medulla constitutes about 28% of the whole gland, and is responsible for the synthesis and excretion of catecholamines. These are synthesized from tyrosine with the conversion of the amino acid to 3,4-dihydroxyphenylalanine (dopa) in the neuronal cytoplasm. The enzyme involved in this rate-limiting step is tyrosine hydroxylase. Dopa is then decarboxylated to dopamine, which is transported to storage granules where it is either stored unchanged or hydroxylated to norepinephrine (noradrenaline). A catecholamine-secreting cell is shown diagrammatically in Figure 29.13. Norepinephrine leaves the granules to be converted to epinephrine (adrenaline) by phenylethanolamine-*N*-methyltransferase. This enzyme exists only in the adrenal medulla, and is dependent for its action on a high concentration of glucocorticoids. This biochemical pathway is described in more detail in Chapter 23.

The output from the medulla is mainly epinephrine (80–90%), with a smaller fraction (10–20%) of norepinephrine. The medulla also produces enkephalins and dopamine. In many respects, the gland acts as a sympathetic ganglion – being purely secretory but with no postganglionic cells. The medulla has no parasympathetic innervation.

The action of the catecholamines is terminated by both neural reuptake and biotransformation through the action of the enzymes monoamine oxidase (a mitochondrial enzyme) and the circulating catechol-*O*-methyltransferase. The actions of the two catecholamines are compared in Table 29.6 and Figure 29.14.

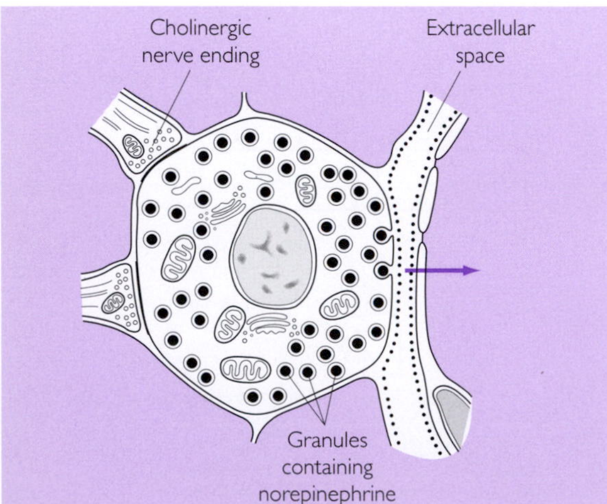


**Figure 29.13** A representation of a norepinephrine-secreting cell of the adrenal medulla. The granules containing norepinephrine are released by exocytosis. This is shown by the arrow.

**Table 29.6 A comparison of the effects of epinephrine and norepinephrine**

| | Cardiac output | Peripheral resistance | Mean arterial pressure | Free fatty acid mobilization | Stimulation of central nervous system | Increased heat production | Increase in blood glucose |
|---|---|---|---|---|---|---|---|
| Norepinephrine | Decreased at low dose, may be increased at high dose | Always increased | Always increased | ++++ | ++++ | +++ | + |
| Epinephrine | Always increased | Decreased at low dose<br>May be increased at high dose | ± at low dose<br>Increased at high dose | +++ | ++++ | ++++ | ++++ |

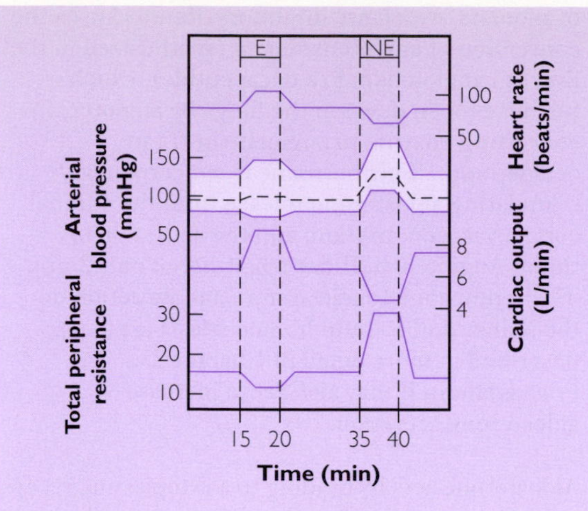


**Figure 29.14** A comparison of the actions of epinephrine (adrenaline, E) and norepinephrine (noradrenaline, NE) when administered by infusion in the physiological dose range. At high dose levels, epinephrine (because of a combination of the increasing cardiac output and its α vasoconstrictor properties) will also produce a rise in the diastolic blood pressure. (Adapted from Barcroft H and Swan HJC. *Sympathetic Control of Human Blood Vessels.* London: Arnold, 1953.)

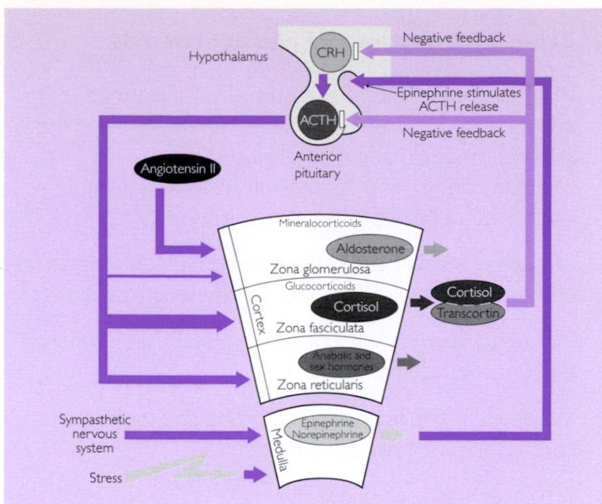


**Figure 29.15** A diagrammatic representation of the cross-section of the adrenal gland together with its trophic and feedback mechanisms. CRH, corticotrophin-releasing hormone; ACTH, corticotrophin.

Further details of the receptors and actions of catecholamines are given in Chapter 23.

## The adrenal cortex

The adrenal cortex constitutes about 70% of the adrenal gland and is made up of three layers, which are distinct with regard to histology, cellular organization, and their relationship to blood supply. From the outside inwards these layers are as follows:

- The zona glomerulosa comprises about 15% of the gland, and is the main site of mineralocorticoid production. The major mineralocorticoid is aldosterone (95%) with the balance being made up by corticosterone and deoxycorticosterone.
- The zona fasciculata is the major part of the gland (50%), and the major site of glucocorticoid production (mainly cortisol and to a much lesser extent cortisone).
- The zona reticularis (7%) is the site of both anabolic and sex hormone synthesis.

The adrenal gland is shown in diagrammatic cross-section in Figure 29.15.

The hormones are transported bound to plasma proteins. Cortisol binds avidly to an $\alpha_2$-globulin (transcortin), and to a lesser extent to corticosteroid-binding globulin. Small amounts are even carried bound to albumin. Aldosterone has a lower protein binding, and hence a shorter half-life (20 min compared with 80–110 min for cortisol).

### *Glucocorticoids*

The control of the synthesis and release of glucocorticoids is almost entirely by corticotrophin which is released from the anterior pituitary. This is a polypeptide made up of 39 amino acids, which also acts to increase androgen synthesis and secretion by the adrenal cortex. It may also be involved in aldosterone release (see below) but this is less substantiated. Corticotrophin is itself under the control of the hypothalamic corticotrophin-releasing hormone (CRH; see above and Figure 29.5). The anterior pituitary can secrete only small quantities of corticotrophin in the absence of CRH.

Corticotrophin release is under three separate controls:

- circadian rhythm – high in the early hours and morning, low in the evening;
- the response to stress (both psychological and physiological);
- negative feedback (see earlier), where corticotrophin release is inhibited by the presence of high circulating concentrations of the glucocorticoids (see Figure 29.5).

Of the endogenous glucocorticoids, cortisol accounts for about 95% of all activity, with the remainder being the result of corticosterone and a very small amount being provided by cortisone. Cortisol is essential for life. Basal cortisol production is about 20 mg/day, but this can increase up to 150–300 mg/day. The main physiological effects of glucocorticoids are given in Table 29.7.

Receptor proteins for glucocorticoids have been found in nearly every organ. Clearly, the (essential) glucocorticoids have a wide variety of effects.

Cortisol acts by binding to stereospecific intracellular cytosol receptors. The ligand–receptor complex stimulates specific mRNA production, which modulates the production of regulatory proteins. The plasma half-life of cortisol is 80–110 min, but the intracellular receptor changes are of longer duration – such that the plasma half-life grossly underestimates the duration of cortisol's physiological effects.

Cortisol production above 30 mg/day is thought of as being supraphysiological. Under these circumstances,

**Table 29.7 Actions of glucocorticoids**

| |
|---|
| Maintenance of blood pressure (by facilitating the conversion of norepinephrine to epinephrine in the adrenal medulla) and by activation of phenylethanolamine-*N*-methyltransferase, which converts norepinephrine to epinephrine |
| Hyperglycaemia caused by increased gluconeogenesis, and an inhibition of peripheral glucose utilization |
| Increased lipolysis with raised levels of triacylglycerol and ketone bodies |
| Increased protein catabolism producing hyperglycaemia and increased urea excretion |
| Increased vascular reactivity |
| Central nervous system effects (slow EEG waves, personality change with adrenal insufficiency) |
| Decreased circulating eosinophils, basophils, and lymphocytes; increased neutrophils, platelets, and red blood cells (these effects are probably mediated through the action of cytokines) |
| Retention of sodium and excretion of potassium (although predominantly mineralocorticoid effects) both facilitated by cortisol |
| Anti-inflammatory and antiallergy effects (especially in the presence of high plasma concentrations) |
| Production of gastric juice enhanced |
| Secretion increased as a result of physiological or psychological stress |

cortisol can exhibit mineralocorticoid effects (such as water retention, loss of potassium and hydrogen, and increase in serum bicarbonate).

### *Mineralocorticoids*

The main mineralocorticoid is aldosterone. Its major action is to promote sodium reabsorption in the distal convoluted tubules and collecting ducts of the kidney. However, it also has other effects – including sodium reabsorption in sweat glands, salivary glands, and the colon. This reabsorption of sodium involves an active ion exchange for potassium or hydrogen. The latter exchange increases the acidity of the urine.

The control of aldosterone release is complex:

- Plasma sodium and potassium concentrations have a direct effect.
- Corticotrophin (from the hypothalamus) has a permissive effect on its production.
- The most important control mechanism is the renin–angiotensin system. This has a role in blood pressure homoeostasis. Either low sodium delivery to the macula densa or reduced perfusion to the juxtaglomerular apparatus (JGA) will lead to the release of renin (a proteolytic enzyme) from the granular cells of the JGA. Other factors include β-agonists which stimulate renin release, and α-agonists, which are inhibitory. Renin causes the conversion of angiotensinogen (synthesized in the liver) to angiotensin I (a decapeptide), which is further broken down in the lungs by angiotensin-converting enzyme to angiotensin II (an octapeptide). This hormone is concerned with stimulating aldosterone release from the adrenal cortex, vasoconstriction, and the sensation of thirst. Angiotensin II has a half-life of only 2 min. The renin–angiotensin system and its action on the kidney and sodium homoeostasis are described in more detail in Chapter 25.
- Prostaglandin E may also act to increase aldosterone secretion.

Aldosterone acts by binding to a cytoplasmic receptor, which then migrates to the cell nucleus, where the complex causes increased DNA transcription with increased mRNA and protein synthesis.

Mineralocorticoid secretion is stimulated by:

- high serum potassium concentration;
- the renin–angiotensin system;
- secondary aldosteronism (in congestive cardiac failure, cirrhosis, nephrosis);
- low sodium intake;
- surgery;
- anxiety;
- physical trauma;
- haemorrhage.

Aldosterone is not the only hormone involved in sodium homoeostasis – glucocorticoids also have an effect on electrolyte and water balance, although this is a less important control mechanism.

## Growth hormone

Human GH stimulates growth of all tissues in the body and invokes intense metabolic effects. Excess secretion results in gigantism and acromegaly. The metabolic effects of GH include:

- increased rates of protein synthesis (anabolic effect);
- increased mobilization of free fatty acids (ketogenic effect);
- direct antagonism of glucose (diabetogenic effect);
- initiation of bone and soft tissue synthesis.

GH is released in a pulsatile fashion with peaks every 3–4 hours; the greatest peaks occurring during sleep. Other stimuli for GH release include hypoglycaemia and the consumption of a high protein meal.

The function of the somatotrophs in the anterior pituitary cells is influenced by two diametrically opposing factors: GH-releasing hormone (GHRH) and GH-inhibiting factor (GHIF, also known as somatostatin). GHRH stimulates the somatotrophs both to synthesize and to release GH, the latter being mediated through a cAMP mechanism. GHRH release is also potentiated by a high circulating level of two other hormones of the glucagon-secreting family (namely vasoactive intestinal peptide and gastric inhibitory peptide). GHIF is synthesized by cells both in the hypothalamus and elsewhere in the brain.

The control of the GH system is by two feedback mechanisms: GH suppresses the activity of the somatotroph to produce more GH. This may be through activation of GHIF. The second control loop involves the production of somatomedins (particularly in the liver). These hormones mediate some of the metabolic effects of GH, and may stimulate somatostatin release.

### The gut

Gastrointestinal hormones are complex in that many were postulated to exist before they were identified, usually by radioimmunoassay. Furthermore, when doses outside the physiological range are given, there is considerable overlap in their action. A summary of their actions is given in Table 29.8.

### The kidney

The kidney is relevant to hormone actions in the following ways:

- It responds to the action of mineralocorticoids (and to a much lesser extent of glucocorticoids) in the control of electrolytes (see above and Chapter 25).
- The cells of the JGA secrete renin (see above and Chapter 25).
- More than 90% of the production of erythropoietin comes from the glomeruli; the rest comes from the liver. The stimulus is cellular oxygen deficiency.
- The kidney produces prostaglandins (see later).
- The kidney is involved in the modification of vitamin D (see above).
- The cells of the distal tubule and collecting duct are sensitive to vasopressin and play a crucial role in the control of body water. This is described below.

#### *Vasopressin*

Vasopressin is a peptide made up of nine amino acids; it has a short half-life of 18 min and is synthesized by the cells of the supraoptic and paraventricular nuclei, and stored in the posterior pituitary (see above and Figure 29.8).

There are two types of vasopressin receptors:

1. Stimulation of the $V_1$-receptor leads to constriction of arteriolar smooth muscle, release of corticotrophin, and contraction of uterine smooth muscle and mammary myoepithelial cells.
2. Activation of the $V_2$-receptor leads to increased reabsorption of water in the renal collecting ducts. This latter action occurs in response to two

**Table 29.8 A summary of the actions of gastrointestinal hormones**

| Hormone | Actions |
|---|---|
| Gastrin | Secreted by the glands of the antral mucosa and possibly the duodenum<br>Its principal physiological actions are stimulation of gastric acid and pepsin secretion, and stimulation of the growth of the gastric mucosa |
| Glucagon | Secreted by the A cells of the mucosa of the stomach and duodenum<br>Glucagon from the gastrointestinal tract may play a role in hyperglycaemia of diabetes |
| Glucagon-like immunoreactivity | Function unknown |
| Secretin | Secreted by cells in mucosa of small intestine<br>Causes secretion of watery, alkaline pancreatic juice |
| Cholecystokinin | Also called pancreozymin<br>Causes contraction of gallbladder and secretion of pancreatic juice rich in enzymes |
| Gastric inhibitory peptide (GIP) | Secretion stimulated by glucose and fat in the duodenum; inhibits gastric secretion and motility<br>May be the physiological β-cell-stimulating hormone of the gastrointestinal tract |
| Motilin | Stimulates gastric acid secretion |
| Vasoactive intestinal peptide (VIP) | Stimulates intestinal secretion of electrolytes and water<br>In high concentrations can dilate peripheral blood vessels<br>VIPomas occur |
| Substance P | Not been proved to enter circulation but increases motility of small intestine |
| Somatostatin | Secreted mainly into gastric lumen rather than blood<br>Inhibits secretion of gastrin, VIP, GIP, secretin, and motilin |
| Bombesin | Increases gastric secretion<br>May be neurotransmitter for vagally mediated increases in gastrin secretion |
| Neurotensin, enkephalins, serotonin | Function unknown in gastrointestinal tract |

separate 'afferent systems' – namely the osmoreceptors of the anterior hypothalamus, and the volume and pressure receptors of the right atria, left atria, and pulmonary blood vessels; and the carotid sinus and aortic arch (see Chapter 25).

Vasopressin secretion is also influenced by other factors. Secretion is increased by:

- pain, emotion, stress, exercise;
- drugs – morphine, nicotine, barbiturates, chlorpropamide, clofibrate, and carbamazepine;
- angiotensin II.

Secretion is decreased by alcohol.

Thus, the actions of vasopressin can be summarized as an antidiuretic effect – the magnitude of which is influenced by both the existing plasma osmolality and the state of volaemia of the individual – and vasoconstriction, leading to an increase in blood pressure

## The pancreas and control of blood glucose

The pancreas has both an exocrine and an endocrine function. Only the latter will be considered here. The hormone-producing cells are in the islets of Langerhans and are of three types:

- A or α cells which comprise 25% of the total and produce glucagon;
- B or β cells which comprise 60% of the total and produce insulin;
- D or δ cells which comprise 10% of the total and produce somatostatin.

In addition, pancreatic polypeptide is released from the islets of the head of the pancreas. It has no definite function in mammals. The three major hormones influence one another locally at the production stage and may function together as a form of paracrine control unit. Their effects on one another are summarized in Figure 29.16.

The chief functions of the pancreatic hormones are:

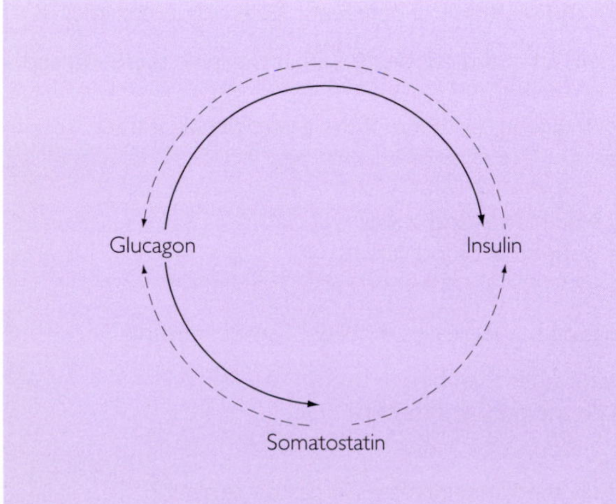


**Figure 29.16** The effect of glucagon, insulin, and somatostatin on each other. Solid arrows indicate stimulation, dashed arrows inhibition.

- to bring about the storage, in the form of glycogen and fat, of the nutrients taken up in the food (via insulin);
- to remobilize the energy reserves during the phase of hunger or during work, in stress situations, and so on (via glucagon and catecholamines);
- to keep the blood sugar level as near to constant as possible;
- to promote growth.

Intermediate carbohydrate metabolism has been considered previously in Chapters 18 and 28. Reference should be made to these for an explanation of glucose metabolism and its transport between different organ systems. The clinical features of diabetes mellitus and the actions of various insulins are described in Chapter 55.

### *Insulin*

Insulin is a polypeptide synthesized as a single chain called pre-proinsulin on the endoplasmic reticulum of the B cells. It is converted to proinsulin. Insulin-containing granules are formed and expelled when required by exocytosis (see Chapter 18, Figure 18.48). Insulin works on an insulin receptor of a specific cell surface glycoprotein (of molecular weight 300 000 Da) which has been described earlier (see Chapter 19).

The insulin content of the pancreas is roughly 6–10 mg, of which about 2 mg (50 units) is released daily. The half-life of insulin is 5–20 min. It is mainly broken down in the liver and kidneys. The factors that stimulate and inhibit the release of insulin are given in Table 29.9. In health, by far the most important on a daily basis is the level of blood glucose. Blood glucose and insulin levels parallel each other with great precision.

Insulin is an anabolic hormone that has widespread intracellular effects. It controls blood glucose by promoting facilitated diffusion (see Chapter 18) into cells. Its principal actions are listed in Table 29.10 and, very importantly, it also promotes growth. Reference should also be made to Figure 19.36.

It is clear from Table 29.10 that insulin is a hormone of energy storage which is antigluconeogenic and glycogenic. The administration of exogenous insulin in a healthy person reduces endogenous production.

### *Glucagon*

Glucagon is a peptide hormone of 29 amino acids, produced in the A cells of the pancreas from proglucagon. Like insulin (see above) it is stored in granules and released by exocytosis.

The main stimulators and inhibitors of glucagon release are given in Table 29.11.

The main effect of glucagon is antagonistic to that of insulin and consists of raising the blood sugar level, thus ensuring an adequate supply of glucose throughout the organism. The ways in which this is accomplished are:

- by increased glycogenolysis (liver, not muscle);
- increased gluconeogenesis from lactate, amino acids (catabolism), and glycerol (lipolysis).

**Table 29.9 Factors affecting insulin secretion**

| Stimulate secretion | Inhibit secretion |
|---|---|
| Serum glucose is the chief stimulator | Epinephrine is a potent inhibitor *in vivo* |
| Glucagon | Somatostatin |
| Selective β-adrenoceptor agonists | Selective β-adrenoceptor antagonists |
| Amino acids | Selective α-adrenoceptor agonists |
| β-Keto (fatty) acids | Thiazide diuretics |
| Theophylline | Phenytoin |
| Sulphonylureas | Diazoxide |
| Acetylcholine | Atropine |
| Vagus stimulation | Stimulation of sympathetic nerves |
| Other gastrointestinal tract hormones (see above) | |

**Table 29.10 The principal actions of insulin on fat, muscle, and liver**

| Adipose tissue | Skeletal muscle | Liver |
|---|---|---|
| Increased glucose entry | Increased glucose entry | Increased protein synthesis |
| Increased fatty acid synthesis | Increased glycogen synthesis | Increased lipid synthesis |
| Increased triglyceride deposition | Increased amino acid uptake | Increased glycogen synthesis |
| Increased potassium uptake | Increased potassium uptake | Decreased ketogenesis |
| Activation of lipoprotein lipase | Increased ketone uptake | Decreased cAMP |
| Inhibition of hormone-sensitive lipase | Increased protein synthesis on ribosomes | |
| | Decreased protein catabolism | |
| | Retention of gluconeogenic amino acids | |

**Table 29.11 Stimulators and inhibitors of glucagon release**

| Stimulators | Inhibitors |
|---|---|
| Hypoglycaemia and low free fatty acids | High serum glucose |
| Hunger | Somatostatin |
| Amino acids | Free fatty acids |
| Infections and other stresses | Ketones |
| Exercise | Insulin |
| Selective β-adrenoceptor agonists | Selective α-adrenoceptor agonists |
| Cholecystokinin, gastrin | |

The interrelationship of insulin and glucagon with fat, muscle, and the liver is summarized diagrammatically in Figure 29.17.

A rise in concentration of amino acids in the plasma leads to the release of more insulin (see above) and, if additional glucose is not available, hypoglycaemia would result. This is prevented, however, because the amino acids also stimulate the release of glucagon, which elevates the blood sugar. Additionally, however, glucagon increases gluconeogenesis from (particularly excess) amino acids, i.e. the latter are to some extent channelled into energy metabolism. Therefore, if a

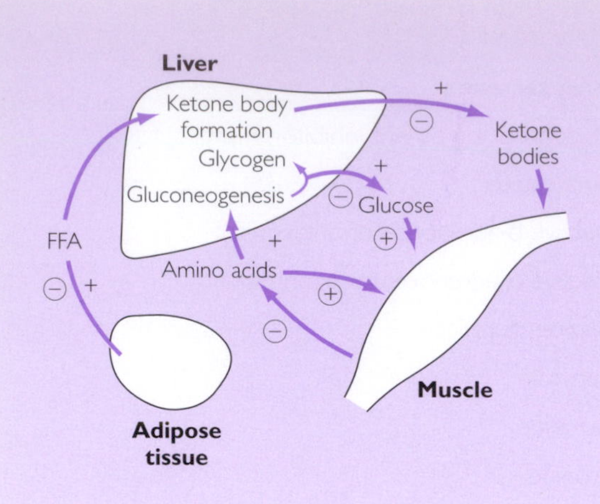


**Figure 29.17** The interrelationships of insulin and glucagon on fat, muscle, and liver. ⊕ increased by insulin; ⊖ decreased by insulin; + increased by glucagon; FFA, free fatty acid. (Adapted from Gerich JE *et al. New Engl J Med* 1975;292:985.)

patient is given an infusion of amino acids with the object of building up protein, it is essential to provide glucose simultaneously in order to prevent the oxidation of the amino acids.

Glucagon secretion is also inhibited by free fatty acids and ketones. However, this inhibition can be overridden, because plasma glucagon levels are high in diabetic ketoacidosis.

#### *Somatostatin*

Somatostatin is an inhibitor of insulin and glucagon release (paracrine action) and decreases the rate of assimilation of all nutrients from the gastrointestinal tract. Somatostatin release is stimulated by high plasma levels of glucose, amino acids, and fatty acids. It is inhibited by catecholamines. Somatostatin also has an endocrine inhibitory effect on motility and secretion in the gastrointestinal tract. Thus, it is probably part of a feedback loop preventing a rapid overload of nutrients. Somatostatin may also act as an anti-obesity hormone.

### Endocrine regulation of blood sugar levels

The level of serum glucose in health is kept between tight limits and below the renal threshold (see Chapter 25). The major players in this are insulin, glucagon, and somatostatin, in that order. Their actions are as described above.

The actual molar ratio of insulin to glucagon at any particular time will depend on the varying stimuli and the conditions that preceded them. For example, on a balanced diet between meals the insulin to glucagon ratio will be approximately 2.5; during starvation, it may be 0.5, and during an infusion of glucose it could be 25.

Many other hormones also have important roles. Insulin and glucagon respond to their effects primarily through the resulting blood glucose concentration. The major hormones that perturb the system are catecholamines, thyroid hormone, glucocorticoids, and growth hormone. Their effects have been detailed earlier but the key points are given below for convenience.

#### *Catecholamines*

β-Adrenoceptor stimulation stimulates glycogenolysis in the liver with the release of glucose into the circulation. Simultaneously, in muscle, glycolysis results in the formation of lactate which enters the circulation and is taken into the liver as part of the Cori cycle (see Chapter 28). This then acts a substrate for the formation of liver glycogen. Therefore the response to an injection of epinephrine is an initial glycogenolysis followed by a rise in hepatic glycogen. The series of events is shown in Figure 29.18.

#### *Thyroid hormone*

Thyrotoxicosis aggravates clinical diabetes mellitus. Thyroid hormone both increases the uptake of glucose from the intestine and depletes liver glycogen. If the pancreatic reserve is low, thyrotoxicosis may lead to B-cell exhaustion because it also accelerates the breakdown of insulin.

#### *Glucocorticoids*

Glucocorticoids are gluconeogenic in a permissive way; their actions have been listed above. In summary, protein catabolism is increased with increased gluconeogenesis in the liver, increased hepatic glycogenesis and ketogenesis, and a decrease in the peripheral glucose utilization.

#### *Growth hormone*

Of patients with GH-secreting tumours, 25% are diabetic; GH treatment reduces insulin responsiveness. GH mobilizes free fatty acids from fat, decreases glucose uptake into some tissues, and increases hepatic glucose output. The hyperglycaemia that this produces may eventually exhaust the B cells. All these conflicting effects on blood glucose levels are summarized in Figure 29.19.

### Prostaglandins

These are lipid acids, derived from a common precursor, the fatty acid arachidonic acid, which act as local

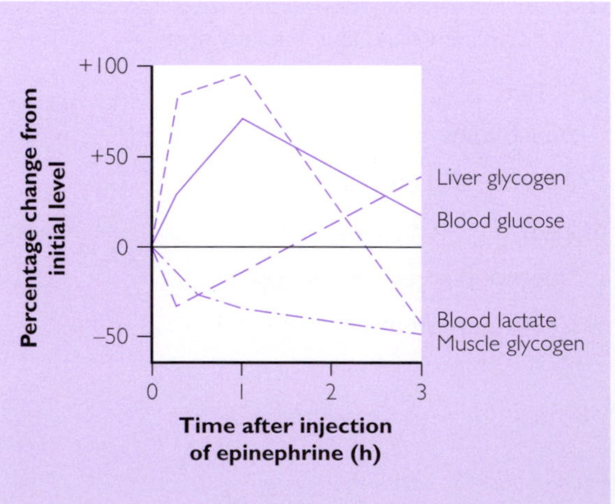


**Figure 29.18** The effect of epinephrine on tissue glycogen, blood glucose, and blood lactate levels in experimental rats. (Adapted from Russell JA. In: Ruch T and Paton HD, eds. *Physiology and Biophysics*, 19th edn, Vol 3. Philadelphia: Saunders, 1966: 1142.)

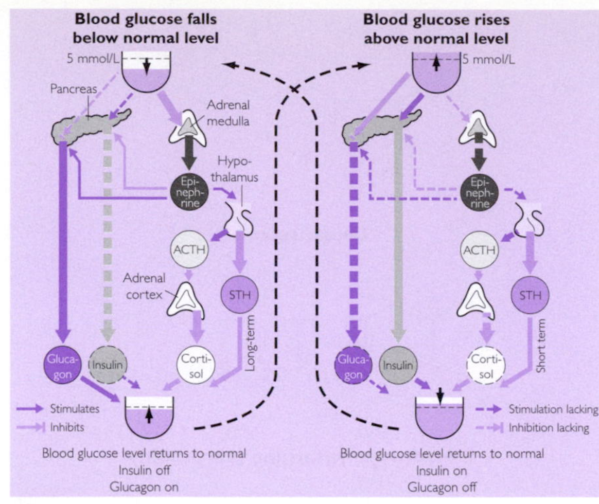


**Figure 29.19** Hormonal control and the conflicting factors involved in determining and controlling the blood glucose level. ACTH, adrenocorticotrophic hormone (corticotrophin); STH, somatotrophin.

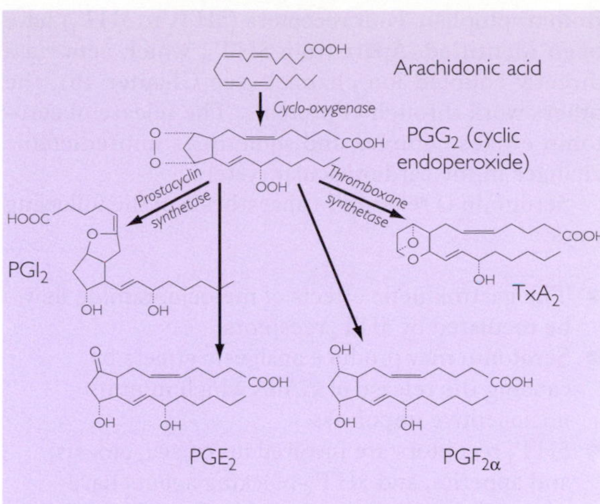


**Figure 29.20** The conversion of arachidonic acid via cyclic endoperoxidase into prostaglandins ($PGE_2$ and $PGF_{2\alpha}$), thromboxane ($TxA_2$), and prostacyclin ($PGI_2$).

hormones. They are synthesized and released as required rather than being stored in intracellular granules. Their synthesis takes place in two stages (Figure 29.20):

1. Cyclo-oxygenase catalyses the formation of cyclic endoperoxides. Cyclo-oxygenase is inhibited by aspirin and other non-steroidal anti-inflammatory drugs.
2. Tissue-specific enzymes lead to the formation of prostaglandins, prostacyclin ($PGI_2$), or thromboxane ($TxA_2$) depending on the exact requirement.

The classification of prostaglandins is confusing, not least because their early classification into the E and F series was based on their solubility in ether. The number of double bonds in the side chains is indicated by subscript numbers.

Some typical effects of prostaglandins are:

- bronchial muscle: $PGF_{2\alpha}$ contracts, $PGE_2$ relaxes;
- gastrointestinal secretion: $PGE_2$ usually inhibits;
- uterus: $PGE_2$ and $PGF_{2\alpha}$ contract;
- kidney: $PGE_2$ and $PGI_2$ provoke vasodilatation, natriuresis, etc.;
- pain: $PGE_2$ and $PGI_2$ sensitize nociceptive nerve endings (inflammation);
- platelets: $TxA_2$ causes aggregation, $PGI_2$ inhibits.

An alternative pathway from arachidonic acid catalysed by lipoxygenases leads to the formation of leukotrienes.

## Histamine and serotonin

### *Histamine*

Histamine (which acts as a local hormone and/or neurotransmitter) is manufactured from histidine by the action of histidine decarboxylase; this utilizes vitamin B6 as a cofactor (Figure 29.21). Histamine is present in the gastric mucosa, lungs, and skin, as well as being stored in mast cells and blood platelets. Histamine has three receptor types, called $H_1$, $H_2$, and $H_3$. They are distributed widely within the nervous system and throughout the body.

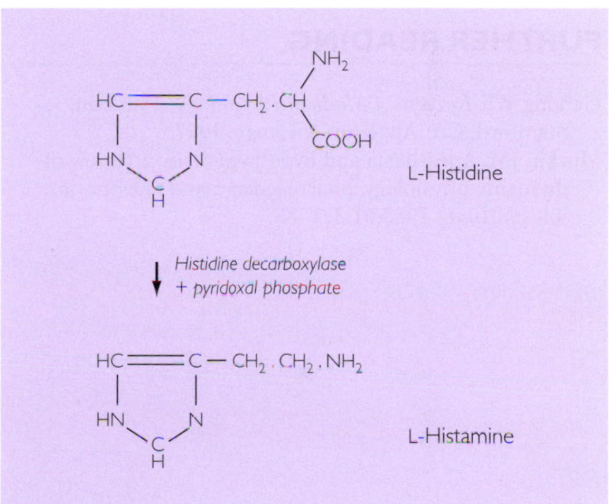


**Figure 29.21** The synthesis of histamine from histidine.

The importance to anaesthesia is as follows: $H_1$ receptors mediate the contraction of smooth muscle in the respiratory and gastrointestinal tracts and via release of nitric oxide (NO) cause a potent increase in gastric secretion. These actions are blocked by histamine ($H_2$) receptor blockers such as cimetidine and ranitidine.

The third type of receptor ($H_3$) has been proposed to exist in the CNS and is thought to inhibit the release of histamine.

Histamine released from mast cells can be part of an anaphylactic or anaphylactoid process (see Chapter 13), producing widespread vasodilatation and life-threatening hypotension. A drug that prophylactically prevents the release of histamine from mast cells is disodium cromoglycate.

### *Serotonin*

Serotonin is an indole present in many neurons in the CNS and is also found in platelets, mast cells, and the enterochromaffin cells of the gut. It is manufactured from tryptophan. Four receptors ($5HT_1$ to $5HT_4$) have been identified. Apart from $5HT_3$, which acts via a directly coupled ion channel (see Chapter 18), the others work through G proteins. The release of serotonin evokes complex and sometimes unpredictable changes in the cardiovascular system.

Serotonin is relevant in anaesthesia in the following ways:

- The gastrokinetic effects of metoclopramide may be mediated by $5HT_4$ receptors.
- Serotonin may produce analgesic effects by causing the release of GABA which inhibits nocioceptive impulses.
- $5HT_3$ receptors are involved in nausea, emesis, and appetite, and $5HT_3$-blocking agents have provided a new generation of antiemetic drugs (see Chapter 27). These are structurally similar to serotonin and one of them, ondansetron, is shown for comparison in Figure 29.22.
- Serotonin-secreting tumours can provide several intraoperative cardiovascular problems.

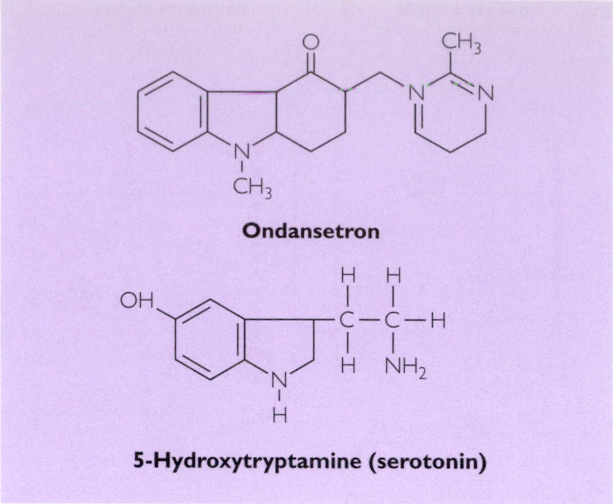

**Figure 29.22** The structure of ondansetron compared with that of serotonin.

## FURTHER READING


Ganong WF. *Review of Medical Physiology*, 18th edn. Stamford, CA: Appleton & Lange, 1997.

Murkin JM. Anesthesia and hypothyroidism: a review of thyroxine physiology, pharmacology, and anesthesia. *Anesth Analg* 1982;**61**:371–83.

## APPENDIX 29.1 THE NOMENCLATURE OF HORMONES

| Recommended name[a] | Other names | Abbreviations |
|---|---|---|
| **Hypothalamus[b]** | | |
| Corticoliberin | Corticotrophin RF | CRF, CRH, ACTH-RH |
| Gonadoliberin | Follicle-stimulating hormone RH[c]<br>= luteinizing hormone RH[c] | FSH-RH, FSH-RF<br>LH-RH, LH-RF |
| Melanostatin | Melanotrophin release-IF | MIH, MIF |
| Melanoliberin | Melanotrophin RH | MRH, MRF |
| Prolactostatin | Prolactin release IF (= dopamine) | PIH, PIF |
| Somatostatin[d] | Somatotrophin (or growth hormone) release-IH | STS, SIH, GH-IH |
| Somatoliberin | Somatotrophin (or growth hormone) RH | SRH, SRF, GH-RH |
| Thyroliberin | Thyrotrophin RH | TRH, TRF |
| **Anterior lobe of pituitary[e]** | | |
| Corticotrophin | Adrenocorticotrophic hormone | ACTH |
| Follitrophin | Follicle-stimulating hormone | FSH |
| Lutrophin | Luteinizing hormone or interstitial cell-stimulating hormone | LH<br>ICSH |
| Melanotrophin | Melanocyte-stimulating hormone | MSH |
| Somatotrophin | Growth hormone | STH, GH |
| Thyrotrophin | Thyroid-stimulating hormone | TSH |
| Prolactin | Luteotrophic or mammatrophic hormone | PRL, LTH |
| **Posterior lobe of pituitary** | | |
| Oxytocic or oxytocin | | |
| Vasopressin,<br>antidiuretic hormone, adiuretin | | ADH, AVP |

[a]Most names are recommended by IUPAC–IUB Commission on Biochemical Nomenclature, 1974.
[b]The ending -liberin is used for releasing hormones (RH) or factors (RF). The ending -statin is used for release-inhibiting hormones (IH) or factors (IF).
[c]The releasing hormones for LH and FSH are identical.
[d]Also released by the pancreas and other gastrointestinal organs.
[e]The ending -trophin is used for anterior pituitary hormones.

# Chapter 30 Pregnancy and fetal physiology

A.D. Wilkey and J.P. Millns

The anaesthetic management of the pregnant woman is important to all anaesthetists in training. Practical aspects of the care of the pregnant woman are described in Chapter 45. Optimal management requires an understanding of the underlying physiological changes in the mother and fetus. This chapter separates these into maternal physiology, the placenta, and fetal development.

## MATERNAL PHYSIOLOGY

The body undergoes major physiological changes during pregnancy. These changes may be seen as promoting the healthy growth and delivery of the baby, as well as being partly the result of that process. For an anaesthetist, a thorough knowledge of these alterations is vital, because they will have implications for the care of the mother and, in particular, safe conduct of regional and general anaesthesia.

Hormonal changes that occur after ovulation and that are maintained in the early phase of pregnancy prepare the body for the needs of the developing fetus and placenta.

We shall consider the physiology of each body system in turn.

### Respiratory system

#### *Anatomical considerations*

Blood flow to the mucosal membranes increases and they become congested. This may be exacerbated by concurrent upper respiratory tract infection, fluid overload, or pre-eclampsia. Epistaxis may be precipitated by the use of nasal tubes/airways or nasogastric tubes.

#### *Ventilatory changes*

Progesterone has a fundamental role in initiating ventilatory changes seen in early pregnancy. It is secreted in increasing amounts during the second part of the menstrual cycle, but levels remain elevated after conception as a result of release from the corpus luteum. The hormone stimulates respiration and enhances the response of the respiratory centre to carbon dioxide. As a consequence, even by the end of the first trimester, maternal $Pa\text{CO}_2$ may be reduced to 4 kPa (32 mm Hg). The drop in $Pa\text{CO}_2$ is the result of an increase in minute ventilation caused by an increase in tidal volume and, to a lesser extent, respiratory rate. The lowered $Pa\text{CO}_2$ in the mother is beneficial to the fetus with respect to excretion of its own carbon dioxide. However, if maternal enzyme systems are not to be disadvantaged by the development of respiratory alkalosis, then compensation must occur. This is effected by renal excretion of bicarbonate, which allows the maternal arterial pH to return towards normal.

Arterial $P\text{O}_2$ rises slightly in the mother. Some decrease may be seen as pregnancy advances, especially if the mother is lying supine. Here, the effect of reduced cardiac output may be exaggerated by encroachment of closing capacity on functional residual capacity (FRC.)

The elevated pH and reduced $Pa\text{CO}_2$ would suggest that the oxyhaemoglobin dissociation curve (ODC) in the mother would shift to the left. In theory, this would disadvantage the fetus because the mother's haemoglobin would retain oxygen more avidly. In fact, the mother's ODC is shifted to the right, favouring the delivery of oxygen to the fetus, due to a rise in red cell 2,3-diphosphoglycerate.

#### *Volume changes*

The stimulant effect of progesterone increases tidal volume by about 40%. Expiratory reserve volume diminishes by 20% and, in parallel, FRC is reduced by 20%, mainly as a result of the presence of the enlarged uterus. This means not only that the composition of alveolar gas can be altered quicker, but also that any oxygen reservoir in the lungs is reduced compared with the non-pregnant state (Figure 30.1).

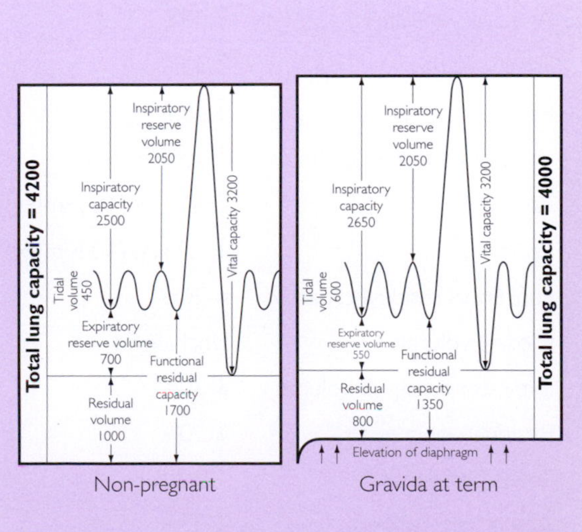


**Figure 30.1** Changes in pulmonary volumes in a pregnant woman at term (right) compared with a non-pregnant woman (left). All volumes are in millilitres. (Adapted from Bonica JJ. *Principles and Practice of Obstetric Analgesia and Anesthesia*. Philadelphia: Davis, 1967.)

Inspiratory reserve volume stays the same, so inspiratory capacity rises slightly. This implies that vital capacity stays the same, although its components change, as indicated above. Forced expiratory volume in one second and peak expiratory flow rate are unaffected.

Although lung compliance does not change, total compliance drops as a result of a fall in chest wall compliance of about 30%. The transverse and anteroposterior diameters of the thorax increase early in pregnancy. Oxygen requirements increase by 20% at term from about 250 ml/min to 300 ml/min. When this fact is linked to a reduction in FRC, then it is obvious that a pregnant mother rendered apnoeic at term will desaturate more quickly than her non-pregnant counterpart. Multiple pregnancy and morbid obesity exacerbate the fall even more alarmingly.

Volume changes are summarized in Table 30.1 and their relevance to anaesthesia in Table 30.2.

## Cardiovascular system

### *Anatomical considerations*

The heart enlarges as a result of increases in myocardial thickness and chamber size. Elevation of the diaphragm shifts the position of the heart, the apex beat moving upwards and laterally.

Auscultation of the heart may reveal several changes:

1 The first sound is frequently split.
2 A systolic ejection murmur is common in association with a third heart sound. This reflects increased blood flow and vasodilatation.

**Table 30.1 Respiratory changes in pregnancy**

| Variable | Change |
|---|---|
| Minute ventilation | ↑ 50%; 300% in labour |
| Alveolar ventilation | ↑ 70% |
| Tidal volume | ↑ 40% |
| Respiratory rate | ↑ 15% |
| Oxygen consumption | ↑ 20% |
| $PaO_2$ | ↑ 1.3 kPa (10 mmHg) |
| $PaCO_2$ | ↓ 1.3 kPa (10 mmHg) |
| Functional residual capacity | ↓ 20% |
| Closing volume | Unchanged |
| Expiratory reserve volume | ↓ 20% |
| Residual volume | ↓ 20% |
| Total compliance | ↓ 30% |
| Airway resistance | ↓ 35% |
| Vital capacity and $FEV_1$ | Unchanged |

$FEV_1$, forced expiratory volume in one second.
Adapted from Cheek TG and Gutsche BB. In: Shnider SM and Levinson G, eds. *Anesthesia for Obstetrics*, 3rd edn. Baltimore: Williams & Wilkins, 1993:3.

Electrocardiography may show left axis deviation, flattened or inverted T waves, and, occasionally, ST depression.

The chest radiograph shows increased vascularity.

### *Blood volume*

Total blood volume increases by about 40% during pregnancy, although this change is complete by around 32 weeks' gestation. It comes about as a result of a marked rise in plasma volume (about 45%) coupled with a 20% rise in red cell volume. Haemoglobin concentration thus falls from about 14 g/dl to 12 g/dl. Blood viscosity is reduced, which aids peripheral blood flow. Normal blood volume status is reached at 10–14 days *post partum*.

### *Haemodynamic changes*

The increase in blood volume is associated with an increase in cardiac output (Figure 30.2), so that beyond the second trimester cardiac output is 40% above pre-pregnancy values. This occurs as a result of a 15% increase in heart rate and a 30% increase in stroke volume. Early studies on changes in cardiac output pointed to a fall in cardiac output during the final trimester. This is not the case; it would seem that observations did not take account of aortocaval compression. Cardiac output increases further during labour, but is at its peak immediately *post partum* as a result of autotransfusion from the involuting uterus. This is the most critical time for mothers with limited cardiac reserve. Normal values are seen again by 2 weeks after delivery. Thus, despite a fall in haemoglobin concentration, oxygen delivery to the tissues is more than maintained by an increase in cardiac output.

Although circulating volume increases, the central venous pressure and pulmonary artery wedge pressure do not rise. The vascular system becomes dilated as a result of the effect of progesterone and prostacyclin. This aids oxygen delivery and heat dissipation. Vasodilatation and the presence of the developing low-resistance placental vascular bed gives rise to a fall in systemic vascular resistance.

As pregnancy proceeds, the enlarging uterus produces increased venous pressure and stasis in the leg veins. When coupled to the increased thrombotic tendency (discussed below) there is an increased likelihood of deep venous thrombosis and subsequent pulmonary embolism. This remains a potent cause of maternal mortality.

Systolic blood pressure falls during the second trimester, rising again towards term. Diastolic blood pressure, similarly, is at its lowest in mid-pregnancy and is affected more than systolic pressure. From 20 weeks' gestation, particularly in the presence of polyhydramnios or multiple pregnancy, blood pressure may be recorded as low in the supine mother as a result of aortocaval compression. In this situation, venous return and cardiac output are reduced because of compression of the inferior vena cava. Many mothers will compensate for this by vasoconstriction, but at term about 15% feel faint when lying flat. It should be remembered that, whether or not the mother feels fine, venous compression will adversely affect placental perfusion, particularly if there is aortic compression as well, with consequent reduction in uterine arterial pressure. The haemodynamic changes of pregnancy are summarized in Table 30.3.

**Table 30.2 Respiratory changes: anaesthetic significance**

| |
|---|
| A. Airway management is more challenging |
| 1. Weight gain and breast engorgement hinder laryngoscopy |
| 2. Swollen mucosa bleeds easily; avoid intranasal manipulation |
| 3. Use smaller endotracheal tube (6–7 mm) |
| B. Response to volatile anaesthetic agents |
| 1. MAC decreased |
| 2. Decreased FRC results in faster induction with insoluble agents |
| 3. Increased minute ventilation speeds induction with soluble agents |
| 4. Rapid overdose with loss of airway reflexes |
| C. Greater risk of hypoxaemia |
| 1. Decreased FRC means less oxygen reserve |
| 2. Increased oxygen consumption |
| 3. Rapid airway obstruction |
| D. Excessive mechanical hyperventilation ($P_{ETCO_2}$ < 3.2 kPa [24 mmHg]) may reduce maternal cardiac output and uterine blood flow |
| E. Maternal and fetal hypoxaemia is associated with pain-induced hyper- and hypoventilation; can be avoided with effective analgesia |

FRC, functional residual capacity; MAC, minimum alveolar concentration; $P_{ETCO_2}$, partial pressure of end-tidal $CO_2$; Adapted from Cheek TG and Gutsche BB. In: Shnider SM and Levinson G, eds. *Anesthesia for Obstetrics*, 3rd edn. Baltimore: Williams & Wilkins, 1993: 6.

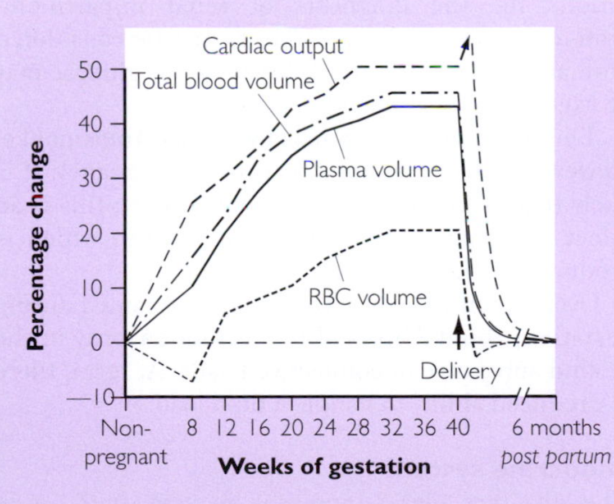


**Figure 30.2** Changes in cardiac output, total blood volume, plasma volume, and red blood cell (RBC) volume in the mother during pregnancy. Note that, in early pregnancy, the RBC volume tends to decrease before it starts increasing and that the increase in plasma volume is greater than the increase in RBC volume, thereby reducing the haematocrit. (Adapted from Bonica JJ. *Obstetric Analgesia and Anesthesia*, 2nd edn. Amsterdam: WFSA, 1980.)

**Table 30.3 Cardiovascular changes in pregnancy**

| Variable | Change |
|---|---|
| Blood volume | ↑ 35% |
| Plasma volume | ↑ 45% |
| Cardiac output | ↑ 40%<br>↑ over 200% in labour |
| Peripheral resistance | ↓ 15% |
| Blood pressure | ↓ especially diastolic |
| Femoral venous pressure | ↑ 15 mmHg |
| Central venous pressure | Unchanged |
| Organ blood flow | ↑ particularly uterus, kidney, skin |
| Coagulability of blood | ↑ especially factors VII, VIII, X, and XII |
| Aortocaval compression | By gravid uterus decreases utero-placental blood flow |

Adapted from Cheek TG and Gutsche BB. In: Shnider SM and Levinson G, eds. *Anesthesia for Obstetrics*, 3rd edn. Baltimore: Williams & Wilkins, 1993:7.

### Haematology

Red cell volume increases by 20%, although haematocrit falls. The mean corpuscular volume increases slightly. Provided that there is adequate iron intake, mean corpuscular haemoglobin concentration remains constant.

Lymphocyte count remains the same, although cell-mediated immunity is suppressed. Raised cortisol and oestrogen levels stimulate neutrophil production. Counts as high as $20 \times 10^9$/L may be seen normally and are even higher values in labour.

Platelet concentration may decrease slightly towards term, although function is maintained. Blood becomes hypercoagulable. This assists the body to cope with the sudden separation of the placenta at parturition, when haemorrhage may be severe.

Fibrinogen levels rise from about 2.5 g/L to 5 g/L. In addition, concentrations of factors II, VII, VIII, and IX show particular increases. Bleeding time, prothrombin time, and partial thromboplastin time do not alter from the non-pregnant state.

Plasminogen levels stay the same, but plasminogen activator activity decreases and, together with increases in antiplasmin and macroglobulin, this leads to reduced fibrinolytic activity.

### Gastrointestinal system

The question of whether or not gastric acid production is increased by the action of placental-derived gastrin is debatable. However, lower oesophageal sphincter tone is reduced by the action of progesterone and the gravid uterus alters the position of the gastro-oesophageal angle and increases intragastric pressure. All of this means that acid reflux is common in pregnancy.

The traditional view was that gastric motility is reduced in late pregnancy and gastric emptying time was prolonged. Recent research suggests that emptying time does not increase until labour is under way. Pain, anxiety, and, in particular, the use of opioids for pain relief will all increase gastric emptying time. This returns to normal by the second postpartum day, assuming that the effect of drugs given to the mother has receded.

Intestinal motility is reduced and constipation becomes a common complaint.

### The liver

Hepatic blood flow does not alter. Serum bilirubin concentration stays the same, but small elevations in serum aspartate aminotransferase and alanine aminotransferase concentrations may occur normally. The placenta produces alkaline phosphatase, which is usually the explanation for a raised plasma level being recorded.

Of particular interest to anaesthetists is the fact that serum cholinesterase concentration is reduced by about 25% at term, 33% at 3 days post partum, and returns to normal over the following 6 weeks. However, in the patient with normal cholinesterase, this does not produce a clinically relevant prolongation of the effect of suxamethonium. Total protein and albumin concentrations fall and as a result plasma oncotic pressure is reduced.

Pregnancy leads to an increase in lipolysis, with a rise in circulating fats. Fatty acid metabolism is enhanced and serum ketone levels rise. Ketonuria is common in labour.

### Nervous system

The increased concentrations of progesterone and endogenous opioids (β-endorphin especially) are the most likely explanation for the observed reduction in minimum alveolar concentration for volatile anaesthetic agents.

Less local anaesthetic is required to produce the same effect in pregnancy when compared with the non-pregnant state. In part, this arises as a result of engorgement of the epidural veins caused by aortocaval compression or during the pushing phase of labour; this leads to a reduction in the volume available for spread of local anaesthetics within the vertebral canal. In addition, nerve tissue is rendered more sensitive to a specific concentration of local anaesthetic, an effect mediated via increased oestrogen and progesterone.

### Urinary system

#### *Anatomical considerations*

Progesterone produces dilatation of the renal tract and ureteric dilatation may be increased by uterine pressure at the pelvic brim.

#### *Renal function*

There is an enormous increase in renal blood flow and glomerular filtration rate (GFR) by the end of the first trimester – of the order of 50%. Tubular reabsorption of sodium and water increases in line with this, to maintain homoeostasis; in fact, some 900 mmol extra sodium are retained during the course of the pregnancy. The absolute plasma sodium concentration falls slightly.

Plasma renin, angiotensin, and aldosterone values are raised. Aldosterone and deoxycorticosterone, which are produced in much greater quantities during pregnancy, contribute to the increase in sodium reabsorption.

The increase in GFR leads to increased clearance of urea and creatinine with lower plasma concentrations becoming the norm in pregnancy – this has implications for the diagnosis of renal impairment. Proteinuria up to 0.3 g in 24 hours may be considered normal. Similarly, the renal threshold for glucose may be exceeded and glycosuria occur.

The serum osmolality falls by about 10 mosmol/kg. However, polyuria is not a feature of pregnancy. It is likely that osmoreceptor threshold is reset; this is an effect of human chorionic gonadotrophin which is produced by the placenta.

Overall, some 6–8 litres of water are retained during gestation; about 2 litres of this is hidden away in the ground substance of connective tissue. At term, there is a reduced ability to handle a fluid load.

### Endocrine system

The pituitary gland increases in size, with more prolactin-producing cells apparent. Corticotrophin and cortisol levels increase. The increase in steroid hormones, together with the production of placental lactogen, which is similar in structure to growth hormone, favour hyperglycaemia.

Thyroxine-binding globulin concentration is increased. This is associated with increased thyroxine and triiodothyronine. However, the free thyroxine index remains in the normal range. There may be slight thyroid enlargement.

## THE PLACENTA

### Formation

The outer layer of cells in the blastocyst becomes the trophoblast, which is responsible for embryo nutrition.

The primitive trophoblast erodes the decidual surface by enzymatic action and penetrates maternal sinusoids, to allow the blastocyst to lie in a pool of blood. The trophoblastic cells proliferate to form branched extensions called villi. This allows an increase in surface area for gas and nutrient exchange. It also helps to anchor the blastocyst in the decidua. The trophoblast then differentiates into two layers:

1. Outer syncytiotrophoblast: this is multinuclear with no distinct cell boundaries.
2. Inner cytotrophoblast: this is a single layer of cuboidal cells.

On the deep decidual surface (decidua basalis) of the blastocyst the villi continue to proliferate and enlarge to form the chorion frondosum. This is where the placenta forms. Maternal and fetal blood are therefore separated by several layers (Figure 30.3).

After 16 weeks' gestation, the cytotrophoblast regresses and the syncytiotrophoblast reduces as pregnancy advances. The mesoderm also reduces, so that at term the barrier between the two circulations is about 0.002 mm. This is still thicker than the alveolar membrane! Fully developed, the placenta is a disc, about 3 cm thick and tapering at the edges. It weighs about 500 g. The umbilical cord has within it two arteries, returning blood from the fetus to the placenta, and one vein, carrying oxygenated blood to the fetus. Blood flow through the placenta is shown in Figure 30.4.

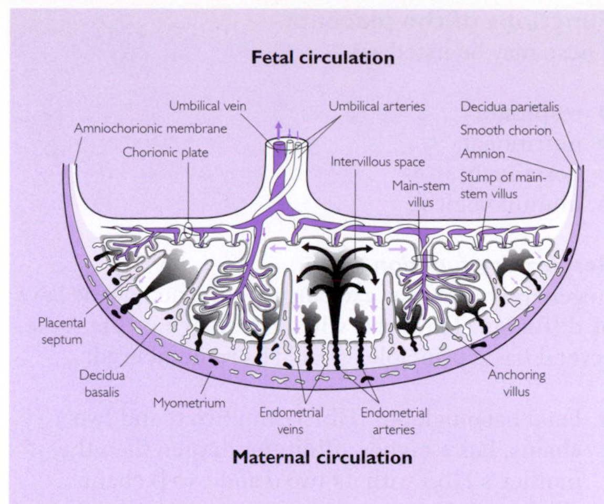


**Figure 30.4** Schematic representation of blood flow through the placenta. Note that the cotyledons (15–30 in number) are formed by placental septa arising from the decidua basalis. The placenta is essentially a large volume of sinusoids of maternal blood into which fetal villi project. In the diagram, alternate cotyledons show the maternal blood supply (arising from spiral arteries and returning via the endometrial veins) and the fetal villi. These of course both exist in each cotyledon, and gas and substance exchange occurs between them. (Adapted from Moore KL. The fetal membranes and the placenta. In: *The Developing Human: Clinically Oriented Embryology*, 3rd edn. Philadelphia: Saunders, 1982.)

## Blood supply to the placenta

### *From the mother*

During pregnancy, uterine blood flow increases from about 50 ml/min to about 700 ml/min. About 80% of this is distributed to the placenta. Blood enters the intervillous space from some 100 spiral arteries. These arteries lose their smooth muscle as the placenta forms, which means that they have lowered resistance to flow. They either spurt blood directly into the intervillous space or around the villi, depending on their relative positions.

Autoregulation is not a feature of uterine blood flow. Alpha-adrenoceptors are found in uterine vessels, which makes them susceptible to endogenous and exogenous catecholamine effects.

The fundamental relationship between uterine blood flow (UBF) and perfusion pressure is:

$$\text{UBF} \propto \frac{(\text{UAP} - \text{UVP})}{\text{UVR}}$$

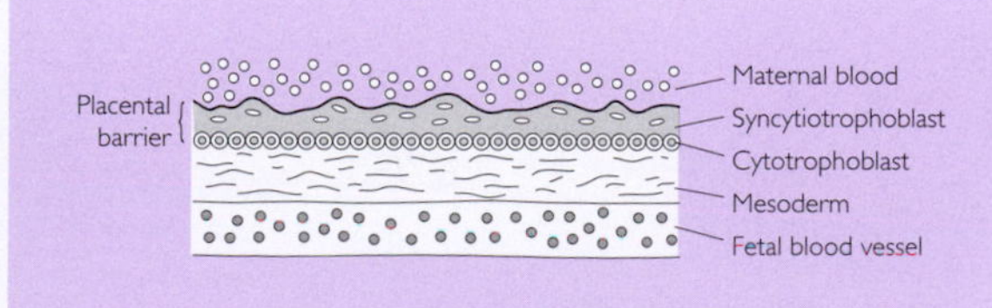


**Figure 30.3** The interface between maternal and fetal blood. (Adapted from Garrey MM *et al. Obstetrics Illustrated*, 2nd edn. Edinburgh: Churchill Livingstone, 1974: 17.)

where UAP is the uterine arterial pressure, UVP the uterine venous pressure, and UVR the uterine vascular resistance.

Consequently, uterine blood flow may be adversely affected by the following:

- reduced maternal blood pressure:
  - aortocaval compression;
  - haemorrhage;
  - vasodilatation after regional blockade;
- increased uterine venous pressure:
  - contractions;
  - aortocaval compression;
- increased uterine vascular resistance:
  - pre-eclampsia;
  - increased myometrial tone, e.g. from overstimulation with oxytocin;
  - catecholamine action.

### *From the fetus*

Two arteries pass to the placenta which carry 40–50% of the fetal cardiac output. This amounts to about 250 ml/min. On the fetal side of the placenta, the villous vessels possess both α- and β-adrenoceptors.

For optimal transfer of gases to occur, both the placental and the umbilical circulation are important. Oxygen delivery to the fetus is dependent on umbilical blood flow, umbilical venous oxygen content and tension. Factors that reduce intervillous blood flow on the mother's side reduce the mean umbilical venous oxygen content. The fetus compensates for hypoxaemia in several ways, including perfusing vital organs preferentially.

## Functions of the placenta

These may be listed as:

- respiratory;
- nutritional;
- hormonal;
- immunological.

### *Respiratory function*

In general terms, gas exchange is governed by the laws of diffusion. However, when considering this topic, several basic principles should be remembered:

- Fetal haemoglobin (HbF), with two α and two γ chains, has a higher affinity for oxygen than the mother's HbA with its two α and two β chains (Figure 30.5).
- Gas exchange across the placenta is *flow-limited* despite the diffusion gradients that operate.
- Subtle changes in carbon dioxide and pH levels alter the positions of the two ODCs at various key points to promote gas exchange.

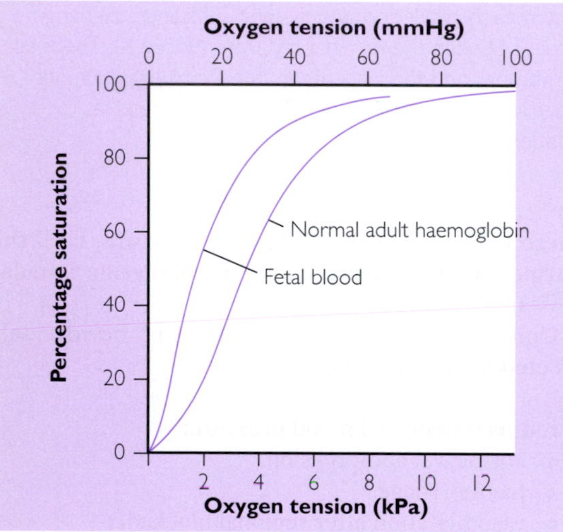


**Figure 30.5** The oxyhaemoglobin dissociation curves of fetal and adult blood. (Adapted from Nunn JF. *Applied Respiratory Physiology*, 2nd edn. London: Butterworths, 1977: 403.)

It is probably easiest to consider first the point in the cycle where fetal blood gives up carbon dioxide. As blood enters the intervillous space from the umbilical artery, diffusion of carbon dioxide into the mother's blood shifts her own ODC to the right and promotes oxygen release (the Bohr effect).

Offloading of carbon dioxide shifts the fetal ODC to the left and increases its own affinity for oxygen (the double Bohr effect). As a result of the action of the Haldane effect, oxygenated fetal haemoglobin releases carbon dioxide and the mother's reduced haemoglobin binds carbon dioxide with greater affinity (the double Haldane effect). The gas tensions of maternal and fetal blood across the placenta at term are given in Table 30.4.

### *Nutritional function*

The placenta is freely permeable to water, sodium, potassium, and chloride, the last by simple diffusion. Active transport mechanisms are involved in the transfer of calcium, iron, iodide, and some other ions where they are concentrated in the fetus.

Carbohydrates cross the placenta by facilitated diffusion. Amino acids require active transfer mechanisms, but the placenta is relatively impermeable to polypeptides.

Fetal fat is derived from free fatty acids transferred across by simple diffusion and acetate. Cholesterol crosses slowly. It is needed for fetoplacental steroid hormone production.

### *Hormonal function*

The syncytiotrophoblast is the site of production of hormones. The major hormones produced are discussed below.

#### *Human chorionic gonadotrophin*

Human chorionic gonadotrophin is detectable in maternal serum only 1 day after ovum implantation. Its levels peak at about 10 weeks. It functions to prolong the life of the corpus luteum; this allows adequate progesterone and oestrogen levels to be maintained, so enabling the pregnancy to continue until placental steroidogenesis takes over. Its presence at an early stage is the basis of detecting pregnancy using a urine test.

**Table 30.4 The approximate gas tensions of maternal and fetal blood across the placenta at term (the values for a non-pregnant woman are given for comparison)**

| Variable | Non-pregnant | Pregnant, term | Fetus (umbilical vein) | Fetus (umbilical artery) |
|---|---|---|---|---|
| $Po_2$ (kPa/mmHg) | 13.3/100 | 14.7/110 | 4/30 | 2.4/18 |
| Haemoglobin saturation (%) | 95–100 | 98–100 | 80 | 60 |
| $Pco_2$ (kPa/mmHg) | 5.3/40 | 4/30 | 5.3/40 | 6.7/50 |
| pH | 7.4 | 7.4 | 7.35 | 7.28 |
| Bicarbonate (mmol/L) | 24 | 20 | 20 | 22 |

Data adapted from Shnider SM and Gregory GA. In: Shnider SM and Levinson G, eds. *Anesthesia for Obstetrics*, 3rd edn. Baltimore: Williams & Wilkins, 1993: 696.

*Oestrogens*
Their main function appears to be the stimulation of growth of the uterus and its blood supply.

*Progesterone*
This initiates early physiological changes, as discussed previously. However, in association with oestrogens it stimulates fetal genital and breast development and growth of the decidual vascular bed.

*Human placental lactogen*
This hormone has an anti-insulin effect, preventing glucose uptake by maternal tissues. It also increases lipolysis and inhibits gluconeogenesis.

### *Immunological effects*

A unique situation exists in pregnancy, where a genetically dissimilar fetus develops in the mother without rejection. Although maternal T-cell immunity is suppressed a little in pregnancy, it is likely that the placenta has a major role to play, either by action of trophoblastic hormones or by production of chemicals that mask antigens. The mechanisms have not been fully elucidated.

### Principles of drug transfer across the placenta

As well as nutritional substances, drugs, in order to reach the fetus from the mother, must cross what is in effect a lipid membrane – the syncytiotrophoblast. However, whereas nutritional substrates have a variety of mechanisms to assist their passage, drugs must cross by passive diffusion; their transport is thus governed by Fick's law of diffusion.

Lipophilic molecules with molecular weights up to 1000 Da diffuse readily across the placenta. This is, therefore, a group that includes commonly used anaesthetic drugs, e.g. induction agents and volatile anaesthetics. Hydrophilic molecules diffuse easily only up to a molecular weight of about 100 Da.

The rate of transfer of lipophilic substances is dependent on the rate at which they are delivered to the placenta (flow-dependent transfer). Factors that reduce placental blood flow will reduce transfer of these substances. The diffusion gradient also governs transfer. The gradient is dependent on maternal factors such as the administration rate and distribution volume, as well as on the degree of protein binding and ionization on either side of the membrane.

The pH will affect the degree of ionization. The degree of ionization of basic drugs, e.g. pethidine (meperidine) and local anaesthetics, is greater on the fetal side and that of acidic drugs is greater in the mother. The pH also affects protein binding, altering the proportion of unbound, potentially transferable drug.

Similarly, where protein concentration falls, the proportion of unbound drug increases.

For substances with poor lipid solubility, placental transfer is permeability dependent. This is dictated by the transplacental concentration gradient, membrane thickness and area available for transfer. Permeability is inversely proportional to molecular weight.

## FETAL DEVELOPMENT

Fertilization of the oocyte occurs in the outer part of the fallopian tube approximately 14 days before the next expected menstrual period. Within a few hours of fertilization, the oocyte undergoes the first cell division and then rapidly undergoes further division forming, at about 3 days, a solid sphere of cells called the morula. The inner cell mass of the morula eventually gives rise to the embryo, although the outer cells form the trophoblast which contributes to the placenta.

The fertilized oocyte is propelled into the uterine cavity after 3–4 days and comes to lie in the folds of the secretory endothelium (Figure 30.6). The blastocyst, as it is now called, undergoes further differentiation. The trophoblast adheres to and invades the endometrium, thereby developing a supply of oxygen and nutrients. The inner cell mass has, by day 16, produced a three-layer germ disc composed of ectoderm, mesoderm, and endoderm, and further tissue and organ differentiation occur from these layers. All the major organs are formed during weeks 3 to 8. The subsequent fetal period until birth entails maturation of the tissues and rapid growth.

The fetal heartbeat is seen on ultrasound scan from week 6 and is heard by ultrasonography from week 10. Fetal movements are first felt during the fifth month. The duration of pregnancy is 40 weeks after the start of the last menstrual period or 38 weeks from fertilization.

### Teratogenesis

Major structural abnormalities occur in 4–6% of infants, with a further 15% showing minor anomalies. In most cases, the cause is unknown but about 15% are genetic factors, 10% environmental factors, and 20–25% are a combination of these.

A number of environmental factors have been identified including infections, radiation, and chemical

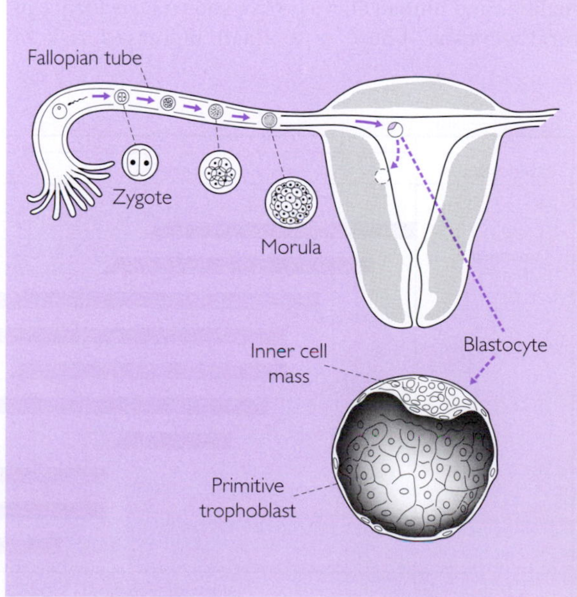


**Figure 30.6** The early development of the embryo.

agents. The effect that they produce will depend on the amount of exposure, genetic susceptibility, and the developmental stage of the embryo. During the preimplantation and early embryonic stages, strong influences may kill the embryo and lead to miscarriage. Major malformations are most likely to arise during the stage of organogenesis, from weeks 3 to 8, different anomalies arising depending on the exact timing of the insult (Figure 30.7).

Teratogenic infectious agents include rubella, cytomegalovirus, herpes simplex, and varicella. Other viral agents have been implicated. Radiation is a well-known teratogen, and protection of the fetus during radiography is routinely undertaken. Maternal pyrexia has been associated with anencephaly, and hypoxia has been shown to induce malformations in experimental animals, although women with congenital cyanotic heart disease or living at altitude do not show this effect.

The risk of teratogenicity from drugs has been well recognized since the limb abnormalities that arose after use of thalidomide in 1961.

During pregnancy, anticonvulsant drugs, e.g. phenytoin and sodium valproate, may cause a variety of abnormalities and their use must be balanced against the risks from poorly controlled epilepsy. Warfarin may cause central nervous system defects and a change to the non-teratogenic heparin is usually made. Angiotensin-converting enzyme inhibitors may cause growth retardation, renal dysfunction, and fetal death and are contraindicated. There is conflicting evidence concerning the phenothiazines and benzodiazepines, but increased incidence of cleft lip and other abnormalities has been reported.

Local and general anaesthetic agents are probably free from any major teratogenic effect. Most concern has centred on nitrous oxide. There is a mechanism for teratogenic activity through the temporary inhibition of methionine synthetase, affecting folate metabolism and hence the conversion of uridine to thymidine, therefore interfering with DNA synthesis. However, in animal studies, only extreme conditions produce abnormalities and human surveys have shown no evidence of teratogenesis. There is a small increased risk of miscarriage after chronic exposure to nitrous oxide. It is difficult to separate the effect of anaesthesia from the surgery and the underlying condition.

Overall, it is best to avoid all drugs during early pregnancy and surgery should, if possible, be delayed until after the first trimester or, ideally, until after delivery.

## Fetal circulation

The rather complex arrangement of the circulation in the fetus has the overall effect of supplying relatively highly saturated blood to the brain and heart and less well saturated blood to the lower body (Figure 30.8).

The two umbilical arteries branch off the common iliac arteries and deliver poorly saturated blood to the placenta. As placental gas exchange is a relatively inefficient process, the blood leaving the placenta in the umbilical vein is only 80% saturated ($P\text{O}_2$ 4 kPa [32 mmHg]). Most of this blood bypasses the liver through the ductus venosus and enters the inferior vena cava (IVC) where the $P\text{O}_2$ is further depressed by some mixing with portal and systemic venous blood (saturation or $S\text{O}_2$ of 67%). The bulk of flow from the IVC passes through the right atrium and directly into the left atrium via the foramen ovale, and hence to the left ventricle and ascending aorta ($S\text{O}_2$ 62%), where it preferentially enters the cerebral and coronary vessels because of the effect of flow through the ductus arteriosus distally. Blood from the head and upper limbs returning in the superior vena cava mixes with a small portion of IVC blood, passes into the right ventricle and hence into the pulmonary artery. As a result of high pulmonary vascular resistance in the collapsed fetal lungs, pulmonary artery pressure is slightly higher than arterial pressure, and most of the pulmonary arterial blood is diverted through the ductus arteriosus ($S\text{O}_2$ 52%) and down the descending aorta ($S\text{O}_2$ 58%). The fetal lungs receive only 15% of the cardiac output. This arrangement is shown diagrammatically in Figure 30.9.

## Changes at birth

At birth, the placenta separates from the uterus, causing hypoxia and hypercapnia in the infant and stimulating its first gasps. Expansion of the lungs and the subsequent increase in $P\text{O}_2$, lower the pulmonary

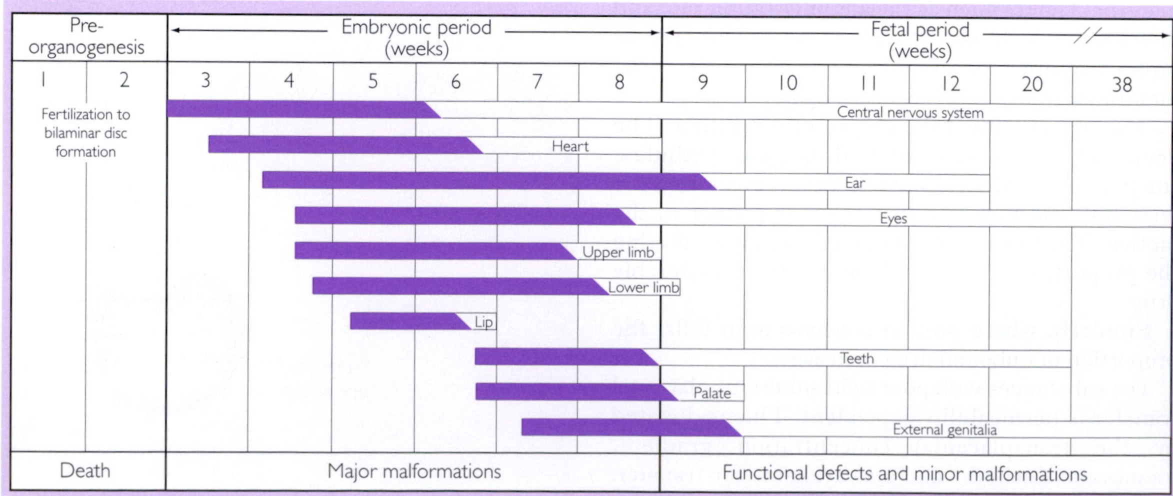


**Figure 30.7** The susceptibility to teratogenesis for organ systems. The coloured bar denotes highly suspicious periods.

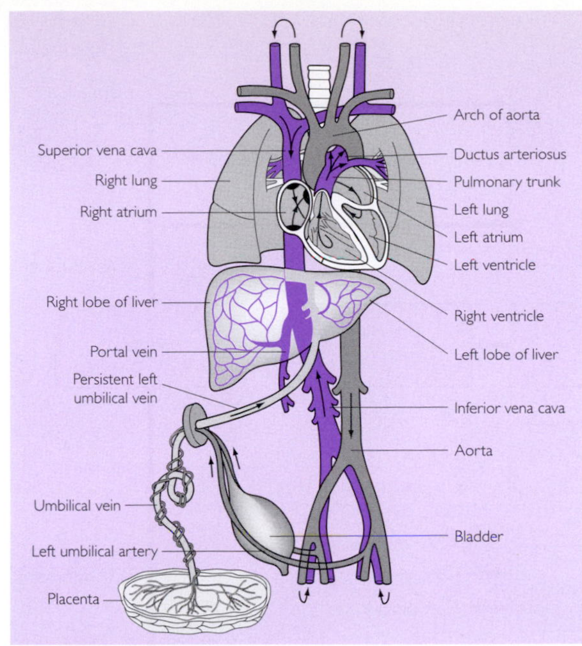


**Figure 30.8** The fetal circulation. (Adapted from Warwick R and Williams PL. *Gray's Anatomy*, 35th edn. London: Longman, 1973: 613.)

vascular resistance to less than 20% of the *in utero* value. The flap-like foramen ovale closes as a result of the increase in pulmonary venous return to the left atrium, and a drop in right atrial pressure secondary to the loss of umbilical vein flow into the IVC.

Systemic vascular resistance increases as a result of loss of placental circulation. Blood flow through the ductus arteriosus initially reverses and then ceases when the vessel constricts as a result of increased $PO_2$, reduced prostacyclin levels, and bradykinin released from the lung. The ductus arteriosus is effectively functionally closed between 10 and 24 hours. The adult pattern of circulation consequently becomes established, as shown in Figure 30.10. By comparing Figures 30.9 and 30.10 it is easy to see the effect of a patent foramen ovale (atrial septal defect) and a patent ductus arteriosus on pulmonary and systemic blood flow. The fetal circulation also explains why single ventricle or common outlet defects are compatible with normal fetal growth but may be incompatible with extra-uterine life. Clinical aspects of persistent fetal circulation are described in Chapter 51.

40% saturated
Brain, upper body
62% saturated
Superior vena cava
Coronary circulation
$^2/_3$ flow in aorta
Foramen ovale
Left atrium
Left ventricle
Aorta
Right atrium
Right ventricle
Pulmonary veins
$^1/_3$ flow in aorta
62% saturated
Inferior vena cava
Lungs (high resistance to blood flow)
Ductus arteriosus
52% saturated
58% saturated
67% saturated
Pulmonary trunk
Ductus venosus
Liver
Body
Major arteries
Single umbilical vein
80% saturated
Placenta
Two umbilical arteries
Oxygen
Carbon dioxide

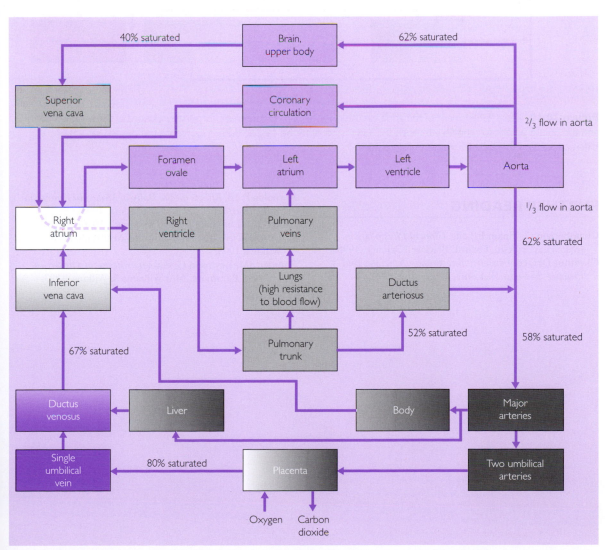

**Figure 30.9** Diagrammatic representation of the fetal circulation showing oxygen saturations. The flow through the lungs is less than 15% of the cardiac output.

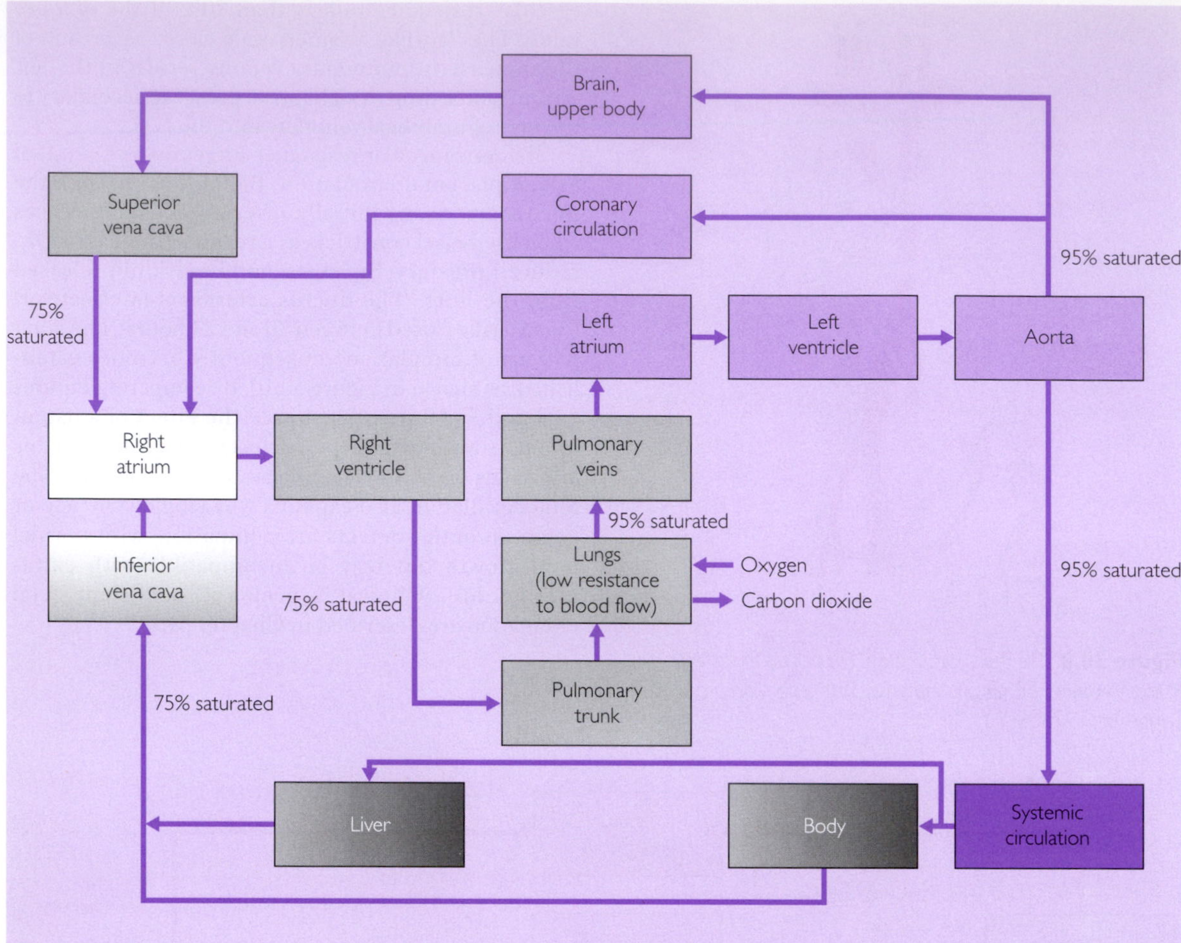


**Figure 30.10** The establishment of the adult circulation shown in diagrammatic form After closure of the foramen ovale and the ductus arteriosus, the flow through the lungs is equal to the cardiac output. Compare the oxygen saturations at different parts of the vascular tree with Figure 30.9.

## FURTHER READING

Chamberlain G, Pipkin FP, eds. *Clinical Physiology in Obstetrics*, 3rd edn. Oxford: Blackwell Science, 1998.

Chestnut DH, ed. *Obstetric Anesthesia: Principles and Practice* 2nd edn. St Louis, MI: Mosby, 1999.

Reynolds F, ed. *Effects on the Baby of Maternal Analgesia and Anaesthesia.* London: Saunders, 1993.

Sadler TW, Langman J, eds. *Langman's Medical Embryology*, 7th edn. Baltimore, MA: Williams & Wilkins, 1995.

Shnider SM, Levinson G, eds. *Anesthesia for Obstetrics*, 3rd edn. Baltimore, MA: Williams & Wilkins, 1993.

# Chapter 31 Blood and its constituents

C.S. Reilly

## THE FUNCTIONS AND COMPOSITION OF BLOOD

### Functions

The supply of blood to the tissues is fundamental to their survival and function. Blood therefore fulfils a number of essential functions which can best be classified under the headings: transport, homoeostasis, and defence.

#### *Transport*

Transport is the most obvious function and involves the supply of nutrients required from normal cell function and repair (oxygen, glucose, proteins, etc.) and removal of waste products for excretion ($CO_2$, lactate, urea, etc.). In addition to this role, blood transports the chemicals and cells involved in homoeostasis and defence to their sites of action.

#### *Homoeostasis*

The homoeostatic functions of the blood are diverse and include roles in: pH buffering, fluid and electrolyte balance, temperature regulation, and hormonal responses. These are considered in other chapters.

#### *Defence*

The defence functions centre around the role of cells and chemicals in the immune system, coagulation, and the repair of damaged vessels and tissues.

It is clear that there is considerable overlap between these functions. For example, chemicals released into the blood locally in response to tissue damage result in the transport of cellular defences to that area.

### Composition

The total blood volume in adults is around 70 ml/kg (5 L in a 70-kg adult) but is nearer 80 ml/kg in infants. Plasma constitutes approximately 55% of this volume, and cellular elements 45%. A bar chart showing proportionate components is shown in Figure 31.1.

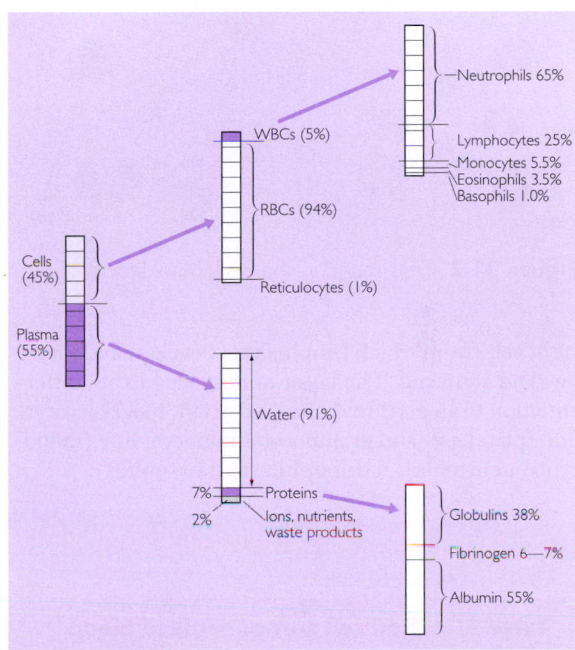


**Figure 31.1** The components of blood. RBCs, red blood cells; WBCs, white blood cells.

#### *Plasma*

Plasma is a colloidal solution which is over 90% water (by weight). Proteins account for a further 7% (by weight) with almost 60% of this being albumin, nearly 40% globulins, and the remainder fibrinogen. As well as being a major component of colloid osmotic pressure, albumin acts as a buffer and as a carrier protein for drugs and hormones. The globulins can be subclassified into $\alpha_1$ and $\alpha_2$ (acute phase reaction proteins), $\beta$ (lipoproteins and complement), and $\gamma$ (immunoglobulins), and have a wide range of functions including antibody synthesis, complement, and transport proteins. Transport globulins may be specific (e.g. transferrin for iron) or non-specific (e.g. $\alpha_1$-acid glycoprotein which binds a wide range of drugs). The remaining 2–3% of plasma is formed from the ions, nutrients, gases, and waste products.

#### *Cellular elements and their production*

Around 95% of the volume of cells is erthyrocytes and the remaining 5% is white cells. Cells in the peripheral blood are shown in Figure 31.2.

Normal haematological values for red blood cells and reticulocytes are given in Table 31.1.

White blood cells comprise five different types: neutrophils, lymphocytes, monocytes, eosinophils, and basophils. The relative proportions of these, together with the normal platelet count are given in Table 31.2.

The structure and functions of red and white blood cells are described later.

All cell types (white and red) are thought to arise from a common pluripotent stem cell, as shown in Figure 31.3. Through a series of differentiations and divisions the stem cell first gives rise to a lymphoid

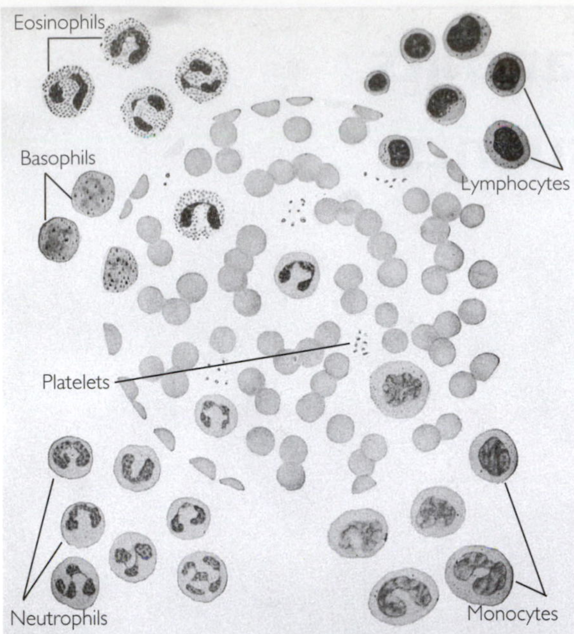


**Figure 31.2** Cells found in the peripheral blood.

stem cell (from which lymphocytes develop) and mixed myeloid stem cell. The latter undergoes further differentiation to an erythroid line (red cells), megakaryocyte line (platelets), and granulocyte/monocyte line (monocytes, neutrophils, eosinophils, and basophils).

This process is under the control of a number of glycoprotein growth factors. The activity and release of these factors may be specific or generalized. An example of a specific response is erythropoietin released from the kidney in response to hypoxaemia. That of a more generalized response is the inflammatory process in which white-cell production is stimulated by a number of factors, including the interleukins (mainly Il-1 and Il-6) and tumour necrosis factor. This in turn results in an increase in granulocyte–macrophage colony-stimulating factor (GM-CSF).

## RED BLOOD CELLS

### Structure

The mature red cell (see Table 31.1 and Figure 31.2) is a biconcave disc, 6.5–8.5 μm in diameter and 1.5–2.5 μm thick, with a volume of 75–95 fl. This shape provides a large surface area and is also able to undergo reversible deformation, an essential property for a cell that has to pass through capillary beds of less than 4 μm in diameter. The structure of the cell membrane and cellular metabolism maintain this flexibility.

The red-cell membrane is a lipid bilayer that contains 50% protein, 40% lipid (mainly phospholipid), and 10% carbohydrate. There is a matrix of structural and contractile proteins (spectrin, actin) on the inner surface of the membrane, which is important in the maintenance of cell shape. Abnormalities in these proteins may explain the defect found in spherocytosis.

**Table 31.1 Red cell components of blood**

| Component | Women | Men |
|---|---|---|
| Haemoglobin (g/100 ml) | 14.0 (2.0) | 15.0 (2.0) |
| Red cell count ($\times 10^{12}$/L) | 4.3 (0.5) | 5.0 (0.5) |
| Packed cell volume (vol/vol) | 0.41 (0.04) | 0.45 (0.05) |
| Mean cell volume (fl) | 92 (10) | 92 (10) |
| Mean cell haemoglobin (pg) | 29.5 (2.5) | 29.5 (2.5) |
| Reticulocytes (L) | 0.5–2.0<br>(25–85 $\times 10^9$/L) | 0.5–2.0<br>(25–85 $\times 10^9$/L) |

Values in parentheses are 2SD.

**Table 31.2 White cell components of blood**

| | Normal range ($\times 10^6$/ml) | Percentage of total white blood cells |
|---|---|---|
| Neutrophils | 1.7–6.5 | 60–70 |
| Lymphocytes | 1.0–3.0 | 20–30 |
| Monocytes | 0.25–1.0 | 2–6 |
| Eosinophils | 0–0.4 | 1–4 |
| Basophils | 0–0.1 | 0.5–1 |
| Platelets | 140–370 | – |

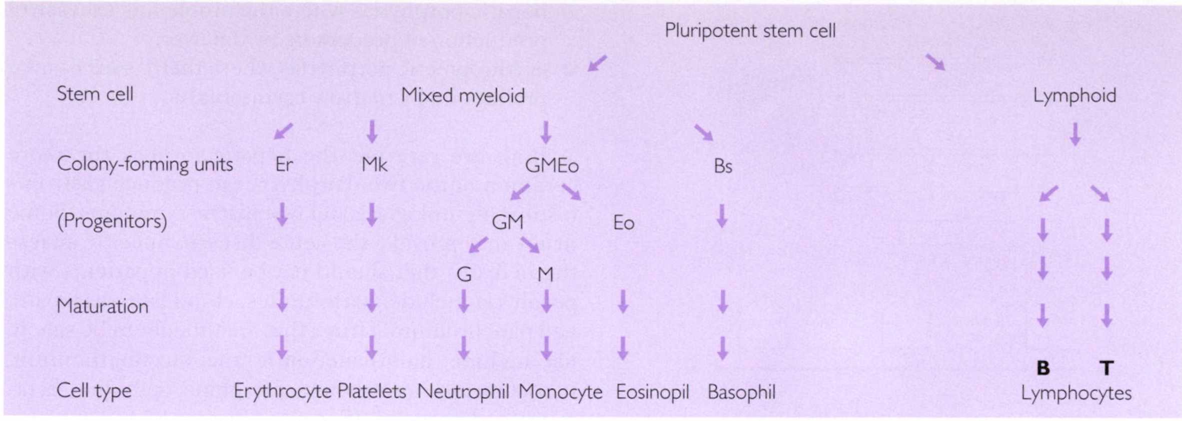


**Figure 31.3** The maturation of blood cells from a common stem cell. Er, erythroid; Mk, megakaryocyte; GMEo, granulocyte, monocyte, and eosinophil; GM, granulocyte and monocyte; Eo, eosinophil; Bs, basophil; G, granulocyte; M, monocyte.

The carbohydrates are on the outer surface of the membrane in the form of glycoproteins and glycolipids, where they are responsible for the antigenic identity of the cell. The ABO system is considered in more detail later and in Chapter 18.

The red cell requires energy to maintain its shape and to maintain the iron in haemoglobin in a reduced (ferrous) state. The cell is therefore capable of producing ATP via the Embden–Meyerhof pathway, and NADPH by the hexose monophosphate shunt.

### Erythropoiesis and the lifespan of the red cell

The development of an erythrocyte from a dedicated stem cell (proerythroblast) occurs within the bone marrow, takes around 7 days, and involves four cell divisions, i.e. 16 cells from one proerythroblast. After the final division, the cells evolve through the reticulocyte stage, where they lose their nucleus, to form mature red cells following their release into the circulation.

Normally, less than 2% of circulating red cells are at the reticulocyte stage, but this proportion may be higher if production has been increased in response to major blood loss or chronic anaemia. The normal daily turnover (i.e. destruction and production) of red cells is around 1% of the total within the circulation ($25 \times 10^{12}$). This process is controlled by the polypeptide hormone erythropoietin, which is secreted from the juxtaglomerular apparatus of the nephron in response to hypoxaemia (anaemic or hypoxic). After an increase in erythropoietin secretion, increased marrow cellularity will occur in 2–3 days and an increased reticulocyte count in 5–7 days.

On average the red cell is in the circulation for up to 120 days. During this time it is subjected to repeated deformation and may be exposed to toxins. These factors result in damage to the cell, loss of function, and the inability to maintain its shape. Abnormally shaped cells are sequestered in the spleen and, to a lesser extent, the liver, where they are broken down for excretion or recycling. The lifespan of red cells may be reduced in the event of physical (e.g. burns) or chemical (e.g. drug-induced) injury.

### Haemoglobin

In parallel to the maturation process described above for the red cell, haemoglobin is produced within the cell. The haemoglobin molecule consists of four polypeptide (globin) chains and four haem subunits. Haem is synthesized in bone marrow erythroblasts in a process that starts with succinyl-CoA and glycine, and results in the production of the functional subunit porphobilinogen. Subsequently, four of these subunits are linked to make a ring centred round an iron atom to form the haem moiety. The globin chains are covalently bound to the haem molecule. Each haemoglobin molecule can carry four oxygen atoms – one bound to each haem moiety. Haemoglobin forms 33% of the mass of a red cell.

Normal adult haemoglobin (HbA) consists of two $\alpha$ and two $\beta$ chains. The globin chains are synthesized within the cell microsomes and consist of 141 ($\alpha$ chain) or 146 ($\beta$ chain) amino acids. Fetal haemoglobin (HbF) has two $\alpha$ and two $\gamma$ chains. A normal variant which is found in small quantities in adult blood ($HbA_2$) contains two $\alpha$ and two $\delta$ chains. The construction of the haemoglobin molecule and its binding to the haem moiety are shown diagrammatically in Figure 31.4. The effect of different types of haemoglobin on the oxygen dissociation curve is shown in Figure 31.5.

A number of factors influence the binding of oxygen to haemoglobin. A major factor is 2,3-diphosphoglycerate (2,3-DPG) which is produced by red cell glycolysis. In the deoxygenated state, 2,3-DPG binds between the $\beta$ chains maintaining low oxygen affinity. Exposure to increased oxygen tension leads to binding of the first oxygen atom to an $\alpha$ chain. This in turn leads to a conformational change which moves the $\beta$ chains closer to each other, preventing 2,3-DPG binding, thus facilitating further oxygen uptake. This explains, in part, the lower sigmoid section of the oxyhaemoglobin dissociation curve. An increase in 2,3-DPG has the effect of stabilizing the deoxystate and shifting the dissociation curve to the right.

Chemical toxicity can also produce effects on haemoglobin's ability to bind oxygen. Methaemoglobin, where the iron atom is in the ferric ($Fe^{3+}$) rather than the ferrous ($Fe^{2+}$) state, cannot bind oxygen. Methaemoglobin normally represents less than 1% of

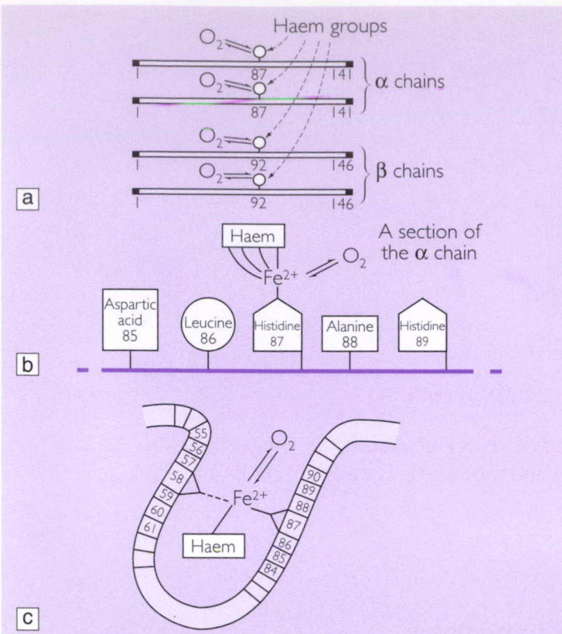


**Figure 31.4** The haem moiety in the haemoglobin molecule. (a) The pairs of α and β chains which together make up a haemoglobin molecule with the sites of attachment of the haem groups; (b) the attachment of the haem group to the α chain; (c) the crevice that contains the haem group.

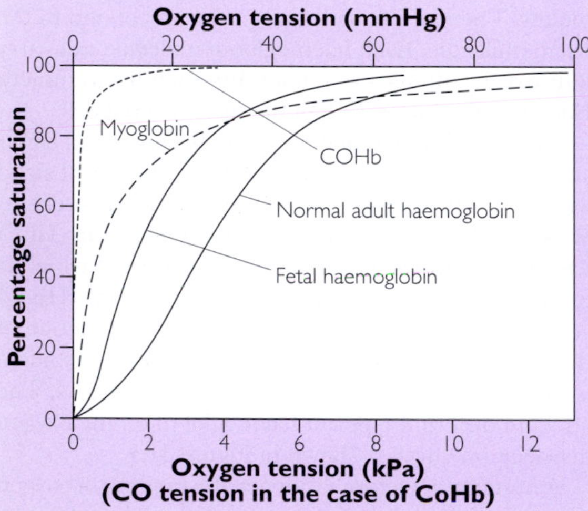


**Figure 31.5** Oxygen dissociation curves of a variety of haemoglobins. COHb, carboxyhaemoglobin. (Adapted from Nunn JF. *Applied Respiratory Physiology*, 2nd edn. London: Butterworths, 1977: 403.)

the total and a significant effect is found at concentrations greater than 10%. Carboxyhaemoglobin is formed when carbon monoxide (CO) binds to haemoglobin. As CO has an affinity 250 times that of oxygen for haemoglobin, its uptake is preferential and difficult to reverse. Carboxyhaemoglobin is normally less than 1% but may be greater than 10% in heavy smokers.

Excessive production of porphobilinogen is the primary defect in the porphyrias. These can be classified as:

- hepatic porphyrias where the problem is excessive production of precursors by the liver;
- erythropoietic porphyrias where there is excessive production by marrow erythroblasts.

Both are rare but the hepatic form is the more common of the two. Porphyria can produce gastrointestinal, neurological, and psychiatric symptoms. Some drugs may provoke the acute disease. Specific anaesthetic drugs that should not be used in patients with porphyria include: barbiturates, etomidate, diazepam, and pancuronium. Drugs that are thought to be safe to use include: halothane, enflurane, suxamethonium, tubocurarine, neostigmine, morphine, pethidine, ketamine, and propofol. (See also Chapter 87.)

### Haemoglobinopathies

Abnormalities of haemoglobin production are known as haemoglobinopathies and can be broadly classified into production of abnormal chains (e.g. sickle cell) and of abnormal quantities of normal chains (e.g. thalassaemia).

A large number of abnormal globin chains have been described (> 150) but the majority are extremely rare. The more common ones are HbS (sickle haemoglobin), HbC, HbD, and HbE. These forms interfere with oxygen carriage and are therefore of interest to the anaesthetist. The abnormalities are inherited through autosomal recessive genes and can manifest as a milder (heterozygous) or more severe (homozygous) form. They demonstrate discrete geographical distribution with HbS, the most widespread, being found in equatorial Africa, the West Indies, Middle East, Greece, and southern India. HbC is found in West Africa, HbD in North India, and HbE in southeast Asia. More than one defect may be found in an individual, such as HbSC and HbS-thalassaemia.

The defect in HbS is an abnormality in the β chain (valine replaces glutamic acid at position 6) which produces binding between chains when the haemoglobin is in the deoxygenated state. This leads to a conformation change in the cell (sickling), which is initially reversible but which quickly becomes irreversible, leading to cell destruction. The cells of a homozygous individual (HbSS which causes sickle-cell disease) are more vulnerable to deoxygenation than those of a heterozygote (HbSA, the sickle-cell trait). The critical oxygen tensions for conformational change are 5.3 kPa and 2.7 kPa, respectively. These values are, however, only approximate and sickling could occur at higher oxygen tensions in the presence of acidosis. Clinical management is discussed in Chapter 52.

An imbalance in the amount of the two haemoglobin chain types occurs in the thalassaemias. In β-thalassaemia there is an underproduction of β chains relative to the number of α chains, although the chains are almost always of a normal structure. The imbalance leads to the formation of unstable complexes in the cell, which precipitate, leading to cell destruction. Beta-thalassaemia is the form most frequently encountered in the UK and is most common around the Mediterranean. In its more severe (homozygous) form it presents in childhood with anaemia, hepatosplenomegaly, and bony abnormalities.

## WHITE BLOOD CELLS

White cells (leukocytes) (see Table 31.2 and Figure 31.2) have important roles in homoeostasis and the defence of the body. The cells are in general motile and can leave the circulation by passing between endothelial cells and entering the tissues. They enter the tissues in response to chemicals (chemotaxis) released locally by, for example, an inflammatory response.

White cells can be classified in several ways and this is a potential source of confusion. The most appropriate classification is based on their origin, which has the added advantage of coinciding with a functional classification. Thus, the myeloid cells – neutrophils, basophils, eosinophils, and monocytes – which arise from the mixed myeloid stem cell, are all phagocytic in action. The lymphoid cells – T and B lymphocytes – arise from a lymphoid stem cell and have an immunological role.

Histological classification groups the cells into granulocytes (neutrophils, basophils, and eosinophils) and agranulocytes (lymphocytes and monocytes). This is less useful now that the functions of cell types are more clearly defined.

### Neutrophils

Neutrophils are the most common white cell, representing 60–70% of the total. Their microscopic appearance shows a dense nucleus with two to five lobes (polymorphonuclear) and a granular cytoplasm. The role of neutrophils is to seek out and phagocytose bacteria and other foreign material. Neutrophils develop in the bone marrow in a process similar to that described above for red cells, involving a stem cell, serial divisions, and then maturation. This process takes 6–10 days and is controlled by a number of factors including interleukins and GM-CSF. After release from the bone marrow, neutrophils spend 5–10 hours in the circulation before entering the tissues to act as phagocytes, where they usually survive for less than 5 days.

The function of neutrophils can be divided into three phases: chemotaxis, phagocytosis, and digestion. Chemotaxis involves the movement of the cell into the site of infection, inflammation, or damage in response to chemicals released by that damage or by complement components. The neutrophil phagocytoses material identified as foreign, which has been tagged (opsonized) with immunoglobulins or complement. Neutrophils can kill and digest bacteria and cells using superoxide, hydrogen peroxide, and lysosomal enzymes.

### Monocytes

Monocytes are the largest of the white cells and represent 2–6% of the total population. Macrophages are derived from them. Microscopically monocytes have a large oval nucleus and are relatively agranular. Monocytes originate from the same precursor as neutrophils and share some of the same growth factors. However, they spend a shorter period of their growth in the bone marrow and, after 1–3 days in the circulation, enter the tissues to complete their maturation.

Once in the tissues, monocytes take on functions specific to that tissue. These include: Kupffer cells in the liver, macrophages in the lung, spleen, and bone marrow, microglia in the brain, and mesangial cells in the kidney. Monocytes have a key role in defence and are responsible for recruitment and activation of cells involved in the inflammatory and immune responses. This is done by secretion of chemotactic agents and growth-stimulating factors. They are also capable of identifying foreign antigens and presenting them to lymphocytes to initiate an immune response (see below).

### Eosinophils

Eosinophils normally represent 1–4% of all white cells, are slightly larger than neutrophils, and have a bi-lobed nucleus and a granular cytoplasm, which is red in the presence of the acidic stain eosin. The pattern of development is similar to that of neutrophils but with a longer period within the circulation.

Eosinophils migrate into tissues and appear to have their main role in areas of local antigen–antibody responses and in defence against parasitic infections. They migrate to sites of inflammation by chemotaxis and act to reduce inflammation. They are often found in the tissues in conjunction with mast cells.

### Basophils

Basophils are the least common of the white cells and usually represent less than 1% of the total. They are of a similar size to eosinophils, but the cytoplasm contains many dense basic-staining granules which contain histamine and heparin. Basophils are capable of migration into tissues where they become mast cells.

Their main action is in hypersensitivity reactions. They have immunoglobulin IgE receptors which, when triggered, cause degranulation of the cell, releasing the histamine and heparin. These components of the inflammatory response act to increase blood flow to the area and therefore to enhance defence.

### Lymphocytes

Lymphocytes represent 20–30% of the total white cells. They derive from the lymphoid stem cell and are classified as B and T cells. This terminology originated from early experiments on the development of immunity in chickens. Both cell types originate in the bone marrow but mature differently. B cells were dependent for their development on the bursa of Fabricius (found in chickens) whereas T cells required modification by the thymus.

These cell types correlate with the two major types of immunological reaction:

- B cells are responsible for the synthesis and release of free antibody into the blood and other body fluids – *humoral immunity*.
- T cells become 'sensitized' lymphocytes which develop antibody-like molecules on their surface – *cell-mediated immunity*.

The development of both cell types and the relationship between them is shown in Figure 31.6. The equivalent of the bursa in humans is probably distributed across lymphoid tissue associated with the gut and respiratory tract such as the tonsils, the appendix, Peyer's patches, and lymph nodes.

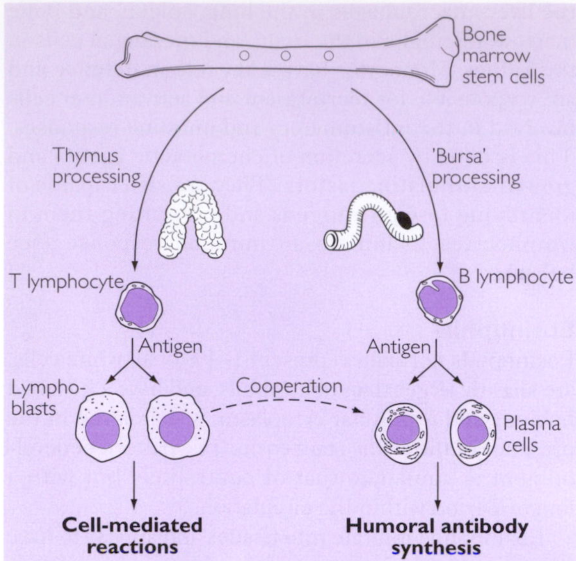


**Figure 31.6** The development of B and T lymphocytes. (Adapted from Roitt I. *Essential Immunology*, 2nd edn. Oxford: Blackwell Scientific Publications, 1974: 48.)

B cells are concerned with humoral immunity, i.e. they secrete antibody for defence against bacteria and toxins within blood and tissues. They are capable of producing a highly specific response based on cell surface receptors, which identify specific hostile antigens and initiate secretion of an immunoglobin specific to that antigen. After activation this mechanism can initiate proliferation of B cells that secrete the specific immunoglobulin. This would be noted as a raised lymphocyte count during a bacterial infection

T cells are concerned with cell-mediated immunity, i.e. a cellular response against intracellular infection (bacterial, viral, etc.) or 'foreign' cells (tumour, transplant, etc.). They act by destroying the infected cell and producing specific immunoglobulins. T cells can be further classified by their function into:

- inducer and suppressor T cells which regulate B-cell production and function;
- killer cells which destroy cells that they recognize as foreign;
- memory cells which store the information about previous antigen–antibody responses and can proliferate immediately if the body is re-exposed to the antigen.

## PLATELETS

Platelets are derived from fragmentation of megakaryocytes which arise from the myeloid stem cell. The megakaryocytes develop in the bone marrow over a period of around 10 days, during which time there are serial intracellular nuclear divisions and the development of cytoplasmic granules. The granules coalesce with the membrane to release the platelets (around 4000/cell). The platelets are about 2 μm in diameter and are present in the circulation and spleen for 7–10 days. The surface of the platelet contains glycoproteins involved in adhesion and the interior contains mitochondria, glycogen, and granules containing chemicals involved in platelet activation and haemostasis. The role of platelets in haemostasis is described below. Platelets are also known as thrombocytes and lack of them is called thrombocytopenia.

## HAEMOSTASIS AND CLOTTING

Injury resulting in loss of integrity of a blood vessel evokes the haemostatic mechanism which has three components: vascular spasm, platelet adhesion, and coagulation.

### Vascular spasm

Vascular spasm occurs in both arterial and venous vessels as a result of smooth-muscle contraction in response to neural and chemical stimuli. Thromboxane $A_2$, which is released from cell membranes and platelets, is a potent vasoconstrictor involved in the process.

### Platelet adhesion

Simultaneous with the vascular response, platelets are activated by exposure of endothelial connective tissue and go through a sequence involving adhesion, chemical release, and aggregation; this results in the formation of a platelet plug. Glycoproteins on the platelet surface membrane adhere to the exposed collagen. This is facilitated by the presence of von Willebrand's factor. Platelet prostaglandin synthesis is also stimulated. After adhesion, platelets release ADP and thromboxane. This encourages further platelet adhesion to the site and enlargement of the adherent platelets. This sequence, which is enhanced by thrombin, continues until there is a sufficient platelet plug to block the leaking vessel. This is then reinforced by fibrin. Platelet adhesion will arrest bleeding from capillaries, pin pricks, and small holes. This mechanism is independent of the coagulation cascade described below and the bleeding time can be normal in patients with major coagulopathies, e.g. haemophilia.

### Coagulation

Coagulation describes a sequence of chemical steps that result in the formation of a blood clot. Once the process is initiated, there is a cascade of events via two activating pathways. These are:

- an extrinsic pathway which is activated by substances normally found outside the vascular system (e.g. connective tissue);
- an intrinsic pathway activated by substances present within the system.

Both these pathways eventually converge on to the following four steps:

1. Prothrombin activator is produced.
2. Prothrombin activator converts prothrombin to thrombin.
3. Thrombin converts fibrinogen to fibrin.
4. Finally, the fibrin threads are stabilized by factor XIII.

It can be seen that the final common pathway involves the activation of thrombin which in turn leads to the production of fibrin. Fibrin is a long polypeptide chain which forms the matrix for the blood clot. A detailed description of the cascade is beyond the scope of this book but the sequence is summarized in Figure 31.7 and synonyms for the numbered coagulation factors are given in Table 31.3.

The coagulation cascade may be altered by a number of factors including congenital or acquired deficiencies, and anticoagulants. Congenital deficiencies have been described for most of the clotting factors but the majority are extremely rare. The most common are haemophilia (factor VIII deficiency), Christmas disease (factor IX deficiency), and von Willebrand's disease (low factor VIII and impaired platelet adhesiveness). Acquired disorders are more common and include: deficiencies in the factors requiring vitamin K for synthesis (factors II, VII, IX, and X) as a result of malabsorption or liver disease, disseminated intravascular coagulation, and massive blood transfusion.

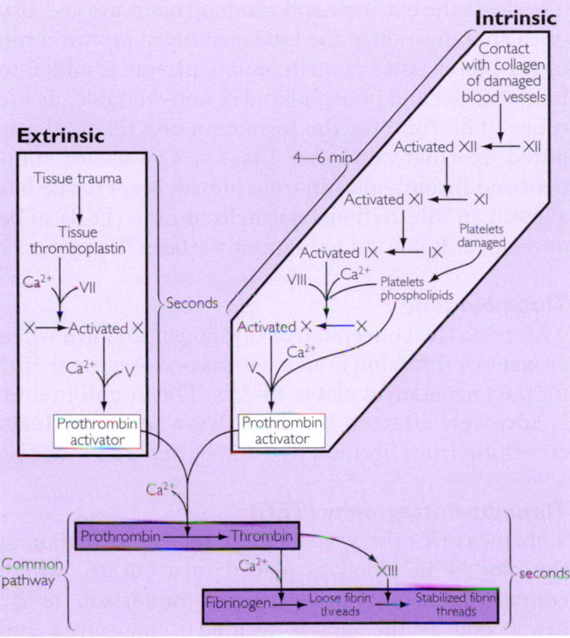


**Figure 31.7** The blood clotting cascade.

Of the commonly used anticoagulants:

- Warfarin acts on the liver where it competes with vitamin K in the synthesis of factors II, VII, IX, and X. This results in these factors lacking an essential carboxyl moiety, which renders them ineffective.
- Heparin potentiates the action of antithrombin III and in so doing inhibits the effects of factors IX, X, XI, and XII. It also affects thrombin and inhibits platelet aggregation by fibrin.

Parallel to the sequence controlling formation of a blood clot, is a feedback system that controls lysis of the clot. The presence of factor XII activates the proenzyme plasminogen to form plasmin, which in turn breaks fibrin into fragments. Plasminogen can also be activated therapeutically by streptokinase.

## Clotting tests

### *Bleeding time*

The bleeding time is defined as the time between the infliction of a standard incision and the moment at which bleeding stops, i.e. when a platelet plug forms. The most reliable method uses a spring-loaded blade to inflict one or two standard incisions on the volar surface of the forearm while a blood pressure cuff is inflated around the upper arm to 40 mmHg. The incision is dabbed with filter paper every 30 s until the

**Table 31.3 International nomenclature of clotting factors and other names in common use**

| Factor number | Name(s) |
|---|---|
| I | Fibrinogen |
| II | Prothrombin |
| III | Tissue thromboplastin |
| IV | Calcium ions |
| V | Proaccelerin, accelerator globulin, prothrombokinase |
| VI | An unused number |
| VII | Prothrombinogen, serum prothrombin conversion accelerator (SPCA) |
| VIII | Antihaemophilic factor |
| IX | Christmas factor |
| X | Stuart or Stuart–Prower factor |
| XI | Plasma thromboplastin antecedent |
| XII | Hageman factor or glass factor |
| XIII | Fibrin or clot-stabilizing factor |

bleeding stops. A normal value lies between 2 and 9 min. The test does, however, suffer from poor reliability and reproducibility, and is of questionable value other than as a gross indicator of platelet effectiveness.

***Platelet count***

This is a quantitative test only and does not measure platelet function. If the platelets are normal, spontaneous bleeding rarely occurs unless the platelet count is decreased to less than 30–50 × $10^6$/ml. The platelet count can be decreased by the presence of foreign surfaces (e.g. filters, cardiopulmonary bypass equipment), blood dyscrasias, bone marrow failure, immune destruction, renal failure, hepatic failure, pre-eclampsia, and drugs. The platelets that do exist may not function normally. A list of drugs that induce platelet dysfunction is given in Table 31.4.

***Whole blood clotting time (WBCT)***

This is the original bedside test of the intrinsic and common pathways. It uses the spontaneous coagulation occurring in a glass tube without the presence of tissue activators, and has long since been superseded by other tests. It is nevertheless very useful at times when it is unclear why a patient will not stop bleeding and an immediate confirmation of a coagulopathy is required. The WBCT can be estimated by putting 10 ml of blood into a plain glass tube, putting the tube into a water bath at 37°C and agitating it once or twice every minute. The blood should clot in 8–12 min. It is, however, a rather inexact test and can give normal results with borderline coagulation factor levels. On the other hand, if the WBCT is significantly prolonged, a coagulopathy is extremely likely.

***Activated clotting time (ACT)***

This, as its name suggests, is a form of accelerated WBCT which measures the intrinsic and common pathways. Whole blood is put into a tube containing diatomaceous earth (celite) and a magnet. The tube is placed within a temperature-controlled device which rotates the tube and records when the magnet is incorporated into clot. The normal value is 90–140 s. It is used to measure heparin effectiveness.

***Activated partial thromboplastin time (APTT) and partial thromboplastin time with kaolin (PTTK)***

These also test the intrinsic and common pathways. Phospholipid and kaolin are added to plasma from centrifuged blood and the clotting time measured similarly to the ACT. The combination of additives speeds up the process and normal values (check with the manufacturer's information) are usually less than 40 s.

***Prothrombin time***

This tests the extrinsic and common pathways and also gives an indication of the total quantity of prothrombin in the blood. After centrifugation, plasma is added to brain extract and phospholipid in non-wettable plastic tubes. The time for the formation of a fibrin clot is noted. Normal values are 10–15 s. The use of standardized thromboplastin from human brain tissue has allowed an international normalized ratio (INR) to be developed. It is used to monitor warfarin therapy

***Thrombin time***

This tests the conversion of fibrinogen to fibrin when exogenous thrombin is added to plasma. A normal time for the formation of clot is 10–15 s. The thrombin time is adversely affected by fibrin degradation products (resulting from fibrinolysis), and by heparin.

***Thromboelastography (TEG)***

This measures the speed and method of formation of the clot. The blood is placed in a cuvette which contains an oscillating drum, and the torsion on the drum axle as the clot is formed is measured and displayed on a graph. Its use in intraoperative monitoring has yet to be determined but it appears to be gaining favour. The characteristic features of the TEG trace are shown in Figure 31.8.

The effect of warfarin, heparin, and some clinical disorders on the common tests of coagulation are summarized in Table 31.5.

**Table 31.4 Drugs that induce platelet dysfunction**

| Table 31.4 Drugs that induce platelet dysfunction |
|---|
| Anti-inflammatory drugs: aspirin, ibuprofen, indomethacin |
| Antibiotics: ampicillin, gentamicin, cephalosporins |
| Cardiovascular drugs: dipyramidole, hydralazine, propranolol |
| Diuretics: acetazolamide |
| Heparin |
| Protamine |
| Psychotropic agents: amitriptyline, diazepam, chlorpromazine |
| Respiratory drugs: aminophylline, theophylline |
| Miscellaneous: alcohol, caffeine, hydrocortisone |
| Blood transfusion |

## CROSS-MATCHING AND BLOOD PRODUCTS

### Cross-matching

The scientific basis of blood transfusion was developed during the 1940s. The determinants of the safety of blood transfusion are the compatibility of the genetic profile of antigens and antibodies of the donor and recipient. A large number of antigens have been described for red cells, but the ABO and rhesus status are of greatest clinical relevance.

The antigens are glycoproteins or lipoproteins attached to the cell surface. There are three antigen types: A, B, and none (O), which are inherited. This gives rise to only four phenotypes because the O is not expressed as an antigen. The phenotypes (and genotypes) of the four groups are: A (AA, AO), B (BB, BO), AB (AB), and O (OO), and are present in around 40%, 10%, 3%, and 46% of the UK population, respectively. Individuals of any group will possess naturally occur-

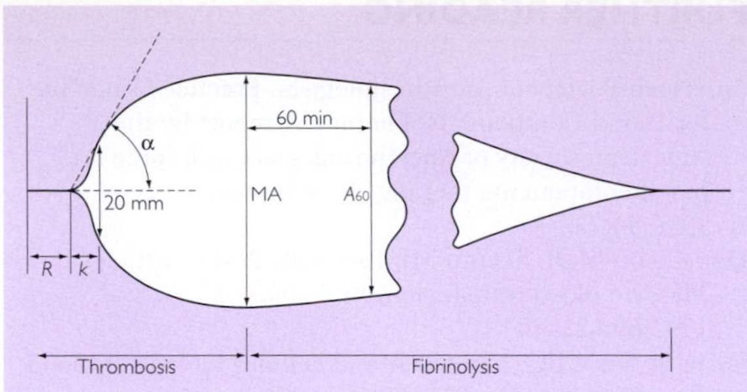


**Figure 31.8** A characteristic thromboelastography (TEG) trace with standard measurements. *R*, reaction time; normal range 6–8 min; time taken from starting TEG to trace reaching an amplitude of 2 mm; represents rate of fibrin formation. *k*, clot formation time; normal range 3–6 min; measure from *R* to the point where the trace reaches 20 mm. *R* + *k*, coagulation time; normal range 10–12 min. α, alpha angle; normal range 50–60°; the angle formed by the slope of the TEG trace from the *R* to the *k* value. MA, maximum amplitude; normal range 50–60 mm; the greatest amplitude on the trace; reflects clot strength. $A_{60}$, amplitude 60 min after MA is reached; normal range MA – 5 mm. This is a measure of clot retraction or lysis. (Adapted from Mallett SV and Cox DJA. *Br J Anaesth* 1992;69:307.)

ring antibodies (IgM) to the antigen(s) of other groups. Thus, group A will have anti-B antibodies, group B anti-A antibodies, group O both anti-A and anti-B antibodies, and group AB no antibodies to A or B. Transfusion of incompatible blood, e.g. group A donor to a group B recipient, will result in a severe haemolytic reaction.

Blood grouping includes the rhesus status of the patient. The rhesus (or more accurately the D) antigen is present in about 80% of the population, i.e. Rh positive (Rh+ve). Unlike ABO groupings, antibodies to D (anti-D) rarely occur naturally in Rh-negative individuals and are acquired only on exposure to Rh-positive blood. Rhesus incompatibility is a potential cause of haemolytic disease of the newborn. This occurs when a Rh-negative mother has a Rh-positive fetus. Leakage of fetal Rh-positive red cells into the maternal circulation causes the mother to develop anti-D antibodies. These antibodies may then cross the placenta to enter the fetal circulation and produce haemolysis. This can be prevented by giving the mother anti-D immunoglobulin (IgM), which attaches to any fetal red cells in the maternal circulation and prevents a maternal immune response (see also Chapter 45).

An antigen–antibody reaction is the basis of cross-matching for transfusion compatibility. Presenting antigen A with antibody A *in vitro* will result in clumping (agglutination) of the red cells. The recipient's blood is tested against standard solutions of antigens and antibodies, and against potential donor blood for agglutination reactions. The clinical implications of red cell antigens and blood product antibodies are described in Chapter 14.

### Blood products

Blood donated for subsequent transfusion can be stored for up to 5 weeks in the presence of additives that maintain red cells: 2,3-DPG and ATP. Increasingly, donated blood is fractionated on collection into its constituent parts to allow a greater range of use. Thus, collected blood is separated into cellular and plasma components which are both then subdivided to more specific products (Figure 31.9). The main components and their uses are given in Table 31.6. The clinical management of blood loss is described in Chapter 14.

**Table 31.5 Effect of various disorders of coagulation on tests of coagulation**

| Category | Disorder | PT | ACT/APTT | TT | FDPs | Platelets | Fibrinogen |
|---|---|---|---|---|---|---|---|
| Therapeutic | Heparin therapy | ↑ | ↑↑ | ↑↑ | → | →[a] | → |
| | Warfarin therapy | ↑↑ | ↑ | → | → | → | → |
| Acquired | Massive blood replacement | ↑ | ↑ | ↑ | → | ↓ | → |
| | DIC[b] | ↑ | ↑ | ↑↑ | ↑ | ↓ | ↓ |
| | Thrombocytopenia | → | → | → | → | ↓ | → |
| | Hepatic failure | ↑ | ↑ | ↑/→ | → | ↓/→ | ↓/→ |
| | Primary fibrinolysis | ↑ | ↑ | ↑ | ↑ | → | ↓ |
| Congenital | Haemophilia | → | ↑ | → | → | → | → |
| | Christmas disease | → | ↑ | → | → | → | → |
| | von Willebrand's | → | ↑/→ | → | → | → | → |

PT, prothrombin time; ACT, activated clotting time; APPT, activated partial thromboplastin time; TT, thrombin time; FDPs, fibrin degradation products. ↑, increase; ↓, decrease; →, no change.

[a]Thrombocytopenia may complicate heparin therapy after several days.

[b]DIC (disseminated intravascular coagulation) may complicate hepatic failure and massive blood transfusion.

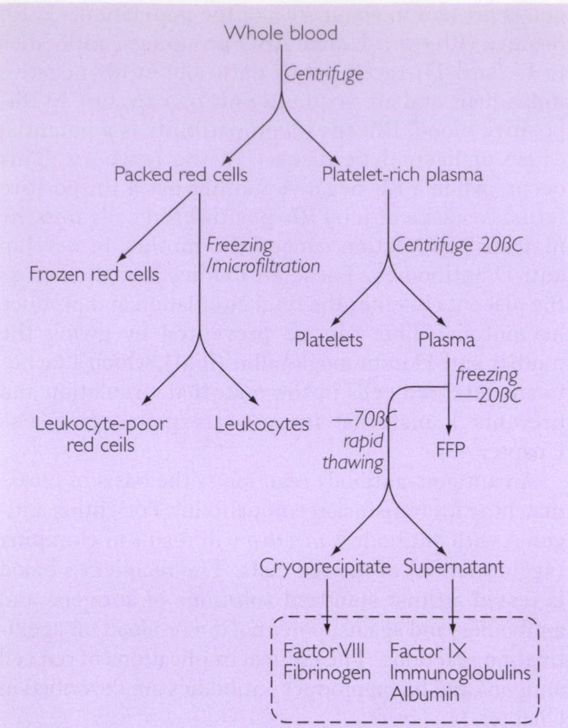


**Figure 31.9** The fractionation of blood into its components. The products enclosed by the dotted line are obtained from pooled plasma. FFP, fresh frozen plasma.

## FURTHER READING

American Society of Anesthesiologists. Practice Guidelines for Blood Components Therapy. A report by the American society of Anesthesiologists task force on blood components therapy. *Anesthesiology* 1996;**84**:732–47.

Donaldson MDJ, Seamn MJ, Park GR. Review article. Massive blood transfusion. *Br J Anaesth* 1992;**69**:621–30.

Furie B, Furie BC. Molecular and cellular biology of blood coagulation. *N Engl Med J* 1992;**326**:800–6.

Ganong WF. *Review of Medical Physiology*, 18th edn. Stamford, CA: Appleton & Lange, 1997.

Goodnough LT. The role of recombinant growth factors in transfusion. *Br J Anaesth* 1993;**70**:80–6.

McClelland B, ed. *Handbook of Transfusion Medicine*, 2nd edn. London: HMSO, 1996

**Table 31.6 Available blood products and their uses**

| Blood product | | Indication |
|---|---|---|
| Cells | Whole blood (not usually available) | Major acute blood loss |
| | Packed red cells | Anaemia, blood loss |
| | Granulocyte concentrate | Severe neutropenia |
| | Platelet concentrate | Thrombocytopenia, massive replacement, chemotherapy |
| Plasma | Fresh frozen plasma | Massive replacement, DIC |
| | Cryoprecipitate | Clotting factor deficiencies |
| | Freeze-dried factors | Factor VIII for haemophilia, factor IX for Christmas disease |
| | Immunoglobulins | Hypogammaglobulinaemia |
| | Albumin 4.5% | Volume replacement in shock |
| | Albumin 20% | Severe hypoalbuminaemia |

DIC, disseminated intravascular coagulation.

# Chapter 32 Intravenous induction agents

G.M. Cooper and J.W. Sear

Intravenous induction agents are substances that can produce unconsciousness in one arm–brain circulation time when given in appropriate dosage. They are used for the following purposes:

- to induce anaesthesia before maintenance with other agents;
- as the sole agent for short operations;
- to maintain anaesthesia after induction by intravenous infusion;
- to provide sedation (e.g. as an adjunct to regional anaesthesia; on an intensive care unit [ICU]).

Several classifications have been used for intravenous induction agents, but probably the simplest is that based on their chemical types:

- barbiturates;
- imidazoles;
- hindered phenols;
- phencyclidines;
- steroids.

Drugs from all these groups have been used in clinical anaesthetic practice. Some are not currently used, mostly because of allergic reactions or other adverse effects. However, their properties are included here as the search continues for their replacement, by pharmacological manipulation of the parent substances. Other agents used historically, such as propanidid, are not discussed. Other substances that can induce anaesthesia, but are not used for this purpose, such as local anaesthetics, alcohol, and magnesium sulphate, are not included in this chapter. Benzodiazepines are sometimes used to induce anaesthesia, but do not produce rapid loss of consciousness in therapeutic doses. They are considered in Chapter 22.

## MECHANISM OF ACTION

Understanding of the mechanisms of anaesthesia is progressing but still rudimentary. The rapid onset of anaesthesia after administration of an induction agent suggests that it acts on receptors and presynthesized molecules, rather than being dependent on the initiation of transcription and translocation of proteins. To have an effect on a neuron the anaesthetic must first cross the blood–brain barrier, and then the phospholipid plasma membrane of the neuron, or initiate a transmembrane signal.

Although the exact site of action is uncertain, there is growing evidence that many intravenous induction agents are able to interact with the benzodiazepine receptor–γ-aminobutyric acid ($GABA_A$) receptor–chloride channel complex, as well as with acetylcholine receptors and voltage-dependent sodium channels. The barbiturates, etomidate, propofol, and the benzodiazepines all modulate the binding of ligands to the GABA receptor. By acting on the $GABA_A$ channel, they increase chloride conductance. This receptor is a pentameric structure that spans the membrane. The two α subunits appear necessary for the binding of benzodiazepines, with the barbiturates and steroid hypnotic agents acting at a different site. Barbiturates also prolong the duration of the inhibitory postsynaptic potential. Ketamine has a separate site of action – the *N*-methyl-D-aspartate (NMDA) receptor, where it acts as a non-competitive antagonist to the influx of $Na^+$ and $Ca^{2+}$, and the efflux of $K^+$ ions. The actions and properties of receptors are described in Chapter 19 and the mechanism of action of all anaesthetic agents is considered in more detail in Chapter 72.

## PROPERTIES OF AN IDEAL INTRAVENOUS INDUCTION AGENT

The desirable properties of a perfect intravenous induction agent are given in Table 32.1. In addition to these properties, low production cost would be advantageous! Needless to say, currently none of the available agents fully meets these requirements.

The efficacy and duration of an intravenous induction agent depend largely on its physicochemical and pharmacological properties. All intravenous anaesthetics must be administered in aqueous solution or as an oil or emulsion which is readily miscible with plasma. They also need to be partially non-ionized and lipid soluble in plasma at pH 7.4 in order to cross the blood–brain barrier. These conflicting requirements are usually resolved by the use of alkaline solutions or by giving water-soluble drugs in water-miscible oils and emulsions. Consequently, bases, buffers, or solubilizing agents are frequently added to solutions of anaesthetic agents. Some agents (e.g. thiopentone [thiopental], midazolam) undergo isomeric change to more lipid-soluble compounds after injection (see later and Chapter 19).

## CHARACTERISTICS OF THE INDUCTION PROCESS

### Induction by bolus dose

Whatever the mechanism of action of the intravenous induction agent, the subsequent pharmacodynamic

**Table 32.1 The desirable properties of an ideal induction agent**

| Physical properties | Pharmacological properties |
|---|---|
| Water soluble | Induction of anaesthesia in one arm–brain circulation time |
| Stable in solution | Minimal myocardial depression |
| Long shelf-life | No vasodilatation |
| No pain on intravenous injection | Minimal respiratory depression |
| Not irritant when injected subcutaneously | Does not release histamine |
| Has a low incidence of thrombophlebitis | Does not cause hypersensitivity reactions |
| The amount required for induction is contained in a small volume of isotonic solution | Metabolized to pharmacologically inactive compounds |
| Causes pain when injected into an artery | Does not cause myoneural blockade |
| | Has no emetic effects |
| | Does not cause excitation, e.g. coughing, hiccough, involuntary movement |
| | Does not cause emergence nightmares |
| | Recovery is 'clear-headed' |
| | Does not cause adrenocortical suppression |

duration of effect of the drug depends on its pharmacokinetic properties and the patient's individual response. The principles of pharmacodynamics and pharmacokinetics after bolus dosage are described in Chapter 19. After a single induction dose, the serum concentration initially falls rapidly and then more slowly (Figure 32.1). The initial rapid fall is the result of redistribution of the drug from the blood, initially to well-perfused compartments and subsequently to less well-perfused compartments. The division of body compartments based on differential perfusion rates is shown in Table 32.2.

The movement of drug from compartment to compartment during the distribution phase (Figure 32.1) occurs under the influence of passive forces such as diffusion gradients, percentage of free drug, and degree of ionization (see Chapter 19). As such, the early fall in serum level is relatively predictable. After a normal bolus dose of induction agent, the patient awakens during this early distribution phase, producing reliable wake-up times.

In contrast, the later part of the curve (Figure 32.1) falls because of metabolism and elimination. This carries much more interpatient variability, the serum concentration at a given time sometimes varying by a factor of 10 from one person to another. This has two important consequences:

- Although predictable for populations, elimination kinetics, half-lives, and clearance (see Chapter 19) are difficult to predict for individuals. It is difficult to know when the agent will be completely cleared from the body.
- When intravenous induction agents are used for the maintenance of anaesthesia by infusion (see later under 'Total intravenous anaesthesia'), the fall in serum concentration after stopping the infusion depends greatly on metabolism and elimination, and the predictability in wake-up times is lost.

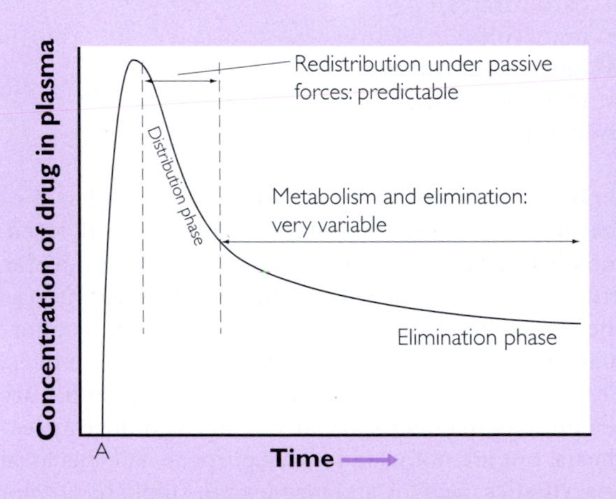


**Figure 32.1** Plasma concentration of an intravenous induction agent after administration at point A.

Although not an induction agent, the concept is well illustrated by the behaviour of a single 500 µg intravenous bolus of fentanyl. This dose is sufficiently large that its analgesic effect is terminated by metabolism and elimination rather than by redistribution. Reilly in 1985 concluded that, after a 500 µg bolus dose of fentanyl, 'the patient's plasma fentanyl concentration will fall below analgesic concentrations somewhere

**Table 32.2 Tissue compartments with differential perfusion rates**

| Perfusion group | Tissues | Percentage body mass | Percentage cardiac output | Blood flow (L/100 kg tissue per min) |
|---|---|---|---|---|
| High (vessel rich) | Brain, heart, liver, kidney | 9 | 75 | 75 |
| Medium | Skeletal muscle (resting) | 50 | 18 | 3.5 |
| Low | Fat | 19 | 5 | 2.5 |

Adapted from Ghoneim MM and Spector R. Pharmacokinetics of drugs administered intravenously. In: Scurr C and Feldman S, eds. *Scientific Foundations of Anaesthesia*, 3rd edn. London: Heinemann Medical, 1982.

between 13 min and 6 h later'. This contrasts sharply with the reliably short duration of action of a much smaller dose (e.g. 50 µg) to provide analgesia for a procedure such as dilatation and curettage.

The distribution of thiopentone into the compartments listed in Table 32.1 after an intravenous bolus injection was graphically illustrated in 1960 by Price. His results are presented in an amended form in Figure 32.2. Although there may be disagreement in some publications concerning the exact numerical proportions of the distributed dose, the central message is clear and unambiguous.

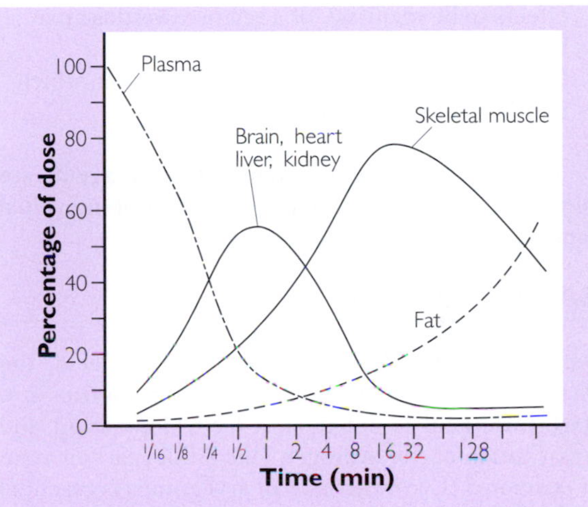


**Figure 32.2** The estimated distribution of thiopentone in various tissues after intravenous bolus injection. (Adapted from Price HL. *Anesthesiology* 1960;21:40.)

### Induction by infusion

Instead of using bolus doses, hypnosis can be induced using rapid infusions. This, in general, produces a longer induction time but fewer adverse effects. Induction by infusion is not suitable for patients in danger of aspiration.

One of the most interesting aspects of infusion induction is the insight it gives into the biophase (see Chapter 19) and the mode of drug action. The results of inducing anaesthesia by propofol at infusion rates of 50, 100, and 200 mg/min are shown in Figure 32.3. Here it can be seen that, as the rate of delivery increases, although the time to unconsciousness falls, the dose necessary to produce unconsciousness increases. In fact, at 50 mg/min it takes only about 50% of the dose required at 200 mg/min to produce unconsciousness. This is because there is a time delay (hysteresis, see Chapter 19) for the injected propofol to reach its site of action. The consequences of this in clinical practice are obvious: when administering bolus doses it is very easy to overdose the patient, especially if they have a very slow circulation time. Minimizing the side effects means giving the minimum dose, and this means giving it slowly.

Induction by infusion is very relevant to total intravenous anaesthesia (TIVA) (see below). It is particularly helpful with TIVA because it automatically partly 'fills up' the peripheral compartments during induction, making subsequent predictions of serum concentrations easier.

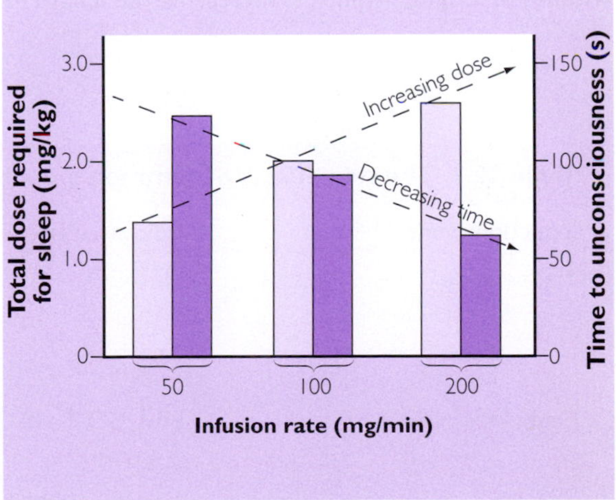


**Figure 32.3** The dependence of induction dose and time to unconsciousness on the infusion rate of propofol. ■, Total dose for sleep; ■, time to unconsciousness. (Adapted from Stokes MA and Hutton P. *Anesth Analg* 1991;72:578.)

### Side effects of induction

In general, all intravenous agents have a number of similar side effects on body organs and tissues. These include:

1. CNS depression, leading to reductions in cerebral metabolism, cerebral blood flow, and hence intracranial pressure. Many of the intravenous induction agents are also anticonvulsant (thiopentone, midazolam, diazepam, and possibly propofol). Following CNS depression, there is a reduction in $\alpha$ band activity of the EEG, and an increase of $\delta$ and $\theta$ activity.

2. Cardiovascular depression caused by a central action on the vasomotor centre in the brain stem, and also direct depression of myocardial contractility. These actions lead to a decrease in arterial blood pressure and cardiac output, and possibly some effects on systemic vascular resistance – although this may occur secondary to ventilatory depression and the increase in arterial carbon dioxide tension. These cardiovascular effects may be exaggerated in patients with hypovolaemia or a fixed cardiac output. The onset of action of an induction agent is also delayed in patients with a low cardiac output, and hence it is necessary to wait a sufficient length of time for the effects to be manifest, or a relative overdose may be given.
3. Centrally mediated respiratory depression, which may be accompanied by apnoea.

The side effects of common induction agents are summarized in Table 32.3; the properties of individual agents are described below.

## BARBITURATES

Barbiturates are derivatives of barbituric acid, the structural formula of which is shown in Figure 32.4. Barbituric acid is not itself a CNS depressant and substitution of the hydrogen ions on the carbon atom at position 5 (C-5) with alkyl or aryl groups is essential for hypnotic activity. A phenyl group on C-5 or one of the nitrogen atoms of the barbituric acid ring confers anticonvulsant activity on the compound, such as found in phenobarbitone (phenobarbital). Thus, hypnotic and anticonvulsant properties are relatively independent and phenobarbitone may be used as an anticonvulsant without producing hypnosis. Increasing the length of one or other of the alkyl side chains at C-5 increases hypnotic potency but, if the side chains are increased to more than five or six carbons, hypnotic activity is reduced and convulsant properties may result.

Compounds having a barbituric acid ring (oxygen at C-2) are oxybarbiturates, whereas those in which the oxygen at C-2 is replaced by sulphur are called thiobarbiturates. This substitution usually results in a lipid-soluble, rapidly acting hypnotic drug, which can be used as an intravenous induction agent. Thiopentone is the thio analogue of pentobarbitone. Introducing a methyl (-$CH_3$) or an ethyl (-$C_2H_5$) group on the nitrogen at position 1 of the barbituric ring also produces rapidly acting compounds, and a high incidence of excitatory phenomena, such as involuntary movement, hypertonus, and tremor. Methohexitone (methohexital) is an oxybarbiturate whose rapidity of action is the result of methylation at position 1 on the barbituric acid ring. The only two barbiturates used as induction agents are thiopentone and methohexitone. Their structural formulae are shown in Figure 32.5.

Barbiturates are not readily soluble in water, except in alkaline solutions. In aqueous conditions, their solubility is dependent on isomerism from the *keto* to the *enol* form (tautomerism), and their presence as weak acids (Figure 32.6).

Isomerism from the *keto* to the *enol* form is pH dependent, and occurs readily in alkaline solutions. The water solubility of sodium salts of barbituric acid relies on the presence of the *enol* form and its subsequent ionization in alkaline solution. The isomerism of thiopentone in relation to membrane penetration is discussed in Chapter 19.

Barbiturates have depressant effects on cellular function in general, but cells in the CNS are particularly sensitive.

**Table 32.3 The side effects of common induction agents**

| Induction agent | Cardiovascular effects | Other effects |
|---|---|---|
| Thiopentone | ↓ BP, ↓ CO | Arterial and extravascular complications<br>Laryngospasm and bronchospasm<br>Enzyme induction<br>Anti-analgesic |
| Methohexitone | ↓ BP, ↓ CO, ↑ HR | Pain on injection<br>Excitatory effects<br>Muscle movements<br>Irritable respiratory tract |
| Etomidate | Minimal | Pain on injection<br>Excitatory effects<br>Adrenocortical suppression |
| Propofol | ↓ BP, ↓ CO | Occasional pain on injection<br>Marked apnoea |
| Ketamine | ↑ BP, ↑ CO, ↑ HR | Analgesia<br>↑ ICP<br>Dysphoria |

BP, blood pressure; CO, cardiac output; HR, heart rate; ICP, intracranial pressure.

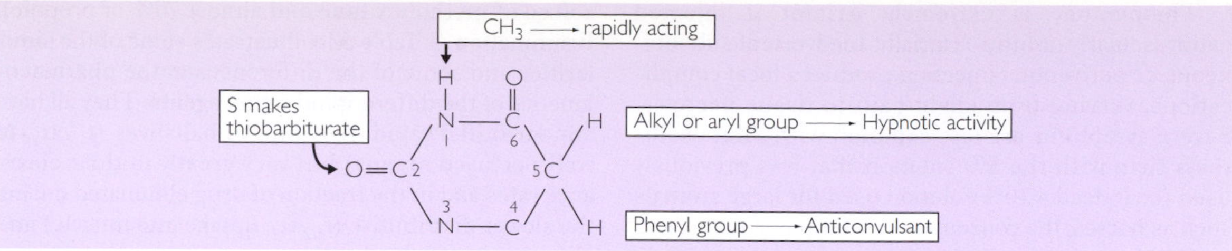


**Figure 32.4** The structural formula of barbituric acid. The *keto* form that is shown can convert to the *enol* form by transition of the hydrogens at positions 1 or 3 in the ring to oxygen at position 2. The effect of substitutions in various positions is illustrated.

**Figure 32.5** Structural formulae of (a) thiopentone and (b) methohexitone.

**Figure 32.6** The *keto–enol* tautomerization of thiopentone.

## Thiopentone

Thiopentone was synthesized in 1932 and first used as an induction agent in 1934.

The sodium salt of thiopentone is a pale-yellow powder with a bitter taste. The solution commonly used to induce anaesthesia (2.5% w/v) has a pH of 10.5 which renders it bacteriostatic.

Thiopentone powder is stored in nitrogen to prevent chemical reaction with atmospheric carbon dioxide, and mixed with 6% anhydrous sodium carbonate. This produces free hydroxyl ions in solution, and it is added to prevent precipitation of the insoluble free acid. Solutions of thiopentone may remain stable at room temperature for up to 2 weeks (and longer at 4°C), although they should not normally be used more than 48 h after their preparation. Solutions must always be discarded if they are cloudy. Thiopentone should not be mixed with oxidizing agents, acidic solutions, or drugs normally administered as sulphates, chlorides, or hydrochlorides. This means that intravenous saline or flush solution should be given after thiopentone and before, for example, vecuronium or calcium chloride to prevent precipitation.

The effects of thiopentone on the CNS are closely related to the dose and rate with which it is given. The rapid loss of consciousness (one arm–brain circulation time of approximately 30 s) after a normal induction dose of 3–5 mg/kg is a result of the high blood flow to the brain (25% of the cardiac output) and because thiopentone in the blood is highly lipid soluble, with more than 90% of the drug in cerebral capillaries crossing the blood–brain barrier. Induction of anaesthesia is smooth and is rarely associated with involuntary movements or pain on injection. Awakening usually occurs 5–10 min after a single dose. Thiopentone is anticonvulsant and is a suitable drug for the treatment of status epilepticus. It has a more rapid onset of action than diazepam, which can be a considerable advantage. It should be used only if personnel and equipment are available to manage the airway.

Thiopentone (and other barbiturates) is also sometimes used to protect the brain from the effects of hypoxia after stroke and head injury. The haemodynamic effects of thiopentone may reduce cerebral blood flow, but cerebral perfusion pressure may be improved because the depression of cerebral metabolism reduces cerebral oedema and intracranial pressure. Meticulous care of the airway, cardiovascular parameters, and intracranial pressures is essential. The balance of oxygen supply and demand is discussed in Chapter 22.

There is a dose-related depression of the respiratory centre, decreasing the responsiveness to $CO_2$ and hypoxia. Apnoea is common. As with any induction agent, it is important always to have facilities available for oxygenation by artificial ventilation. The loss of airway reflexes, which accompanies any induction agent, contraindicates their use in patients who have airway obstruction (or potential obstruction). Laryngospasm is readily precipitated by the presence of secretions or an airway in the mouth, or by early surgical stimulation. Thiopentone does not have analgesic properties, and in fact decreases the pain threshold.

Transient urticarial responses after thiopentone are not uncommon. These are usually related to histamine release from mast cells and may be associated with raised plasma histamine concentrations. Anaphylactic responses are rare (see Table 32.5) but can be profound and are associated with a high mortality.

Thiopentone is extremely irritant if injected extravascularly or intra-arterially. Inadvertent subcutaneous or perivenous injection produces local complications, varying from slight pain to tissue necrosis. Severe symptoms are less common with dilute solutions than with the 5% solution that was previously used (or indeed a 10% solution used for large animals such as horses, the concentrated solution being needed so that the induction dose can be contained in a single syringe). This local tissue irritation is probably caused by precipitation of non-ionized thiopental acid at the pH of extracellular fluid, rather than simply as a result of its alkalinity, because it is not observed as frequently with extravascular methohexitone which is slightly more alkaline. Dispersal of the thiopentone by local injection of hyaluronidase is helpful.

Accidental intra-arterial injection of thiopentone causes immediate, intense pain, usually followed by arterial spasm, blanching of the limb, loss of peripheral (radial) pulses, and later oedema and gangrene. This last complication is the result of the deposition of thiopentone crystals in the small arterioles, causing a chemical arteritis and release of norepinephrine (noradrenaline). Urgent treatment is necessary. It is most important not to remove the needle but to use it to inject saline as a diluent, a vasodilator (e.g. papaverine 40 mg or tolazoline 40 mg) to reduce arterial spasm, and heparin to reduce subsequent thrombosis. Brachial plexus or stellate ganglion block may be advantageous for pain relief, and sympathetic blockade to increase regional blood flow. This subject is also discussed under 'Induction of anaesthesia' in Chapter 2.

Care is always needed with the administration of thiopentone, taking account of the longer time needed for its effects to be seen in low cardiac output states. The recommended dose of 3–5 mg/kg may need to be reduced considerably in elderly, debilitated, and hypovolaemic patients. It has a low therapeutic index ($LD_{50} : ED_{50}$ being about 4). At pH 7.4, 75–80% of thiopentone is bound to plasma albumin, and 61% of the non-protein-bound fraction is ionized. The kinetics of thiopentone and other intravenous induction agents are shown in Table 32.4. (See Chapter 19 for explanation of $t_{1/2}$, etc.)

At the time of awakening after an induction dose, only 18% of the injected dose of thiopentone will have undergone metabolism, compared with about 38% of a dose of methohexitone and almost 70% of propofol. Examination of Table 32.4 illustrates some of the similarities and some of the differences in the pharmacokinetics of the different induction agents. They all have similar initial rapid distribution half-lives ($t_{1/2}\ \alpha_1$, to well-perfused organs) but vary greatly in their clearance rates and in the fraction of drug eliminated during the slower distributive ($t_{1/2}\ \alpha_2$, uptake into muscle) and elimination ($t_{1/2}\ \beta$) phases.

The clearance of thiopentone is approximately 10–20% of liver blood flow. This is consistent with capacity-limited elimination by the liver and is sensitive to changes in plasma protein binding. Thiopentone is metabolized in the liver (and possibly by other tissues) to thiopentone carboxylic acid, hydroxythiopentone, and pentobarbitone. Less than 1% is eliminated unchanged in the urine. Thus, metabolism is entirely responsible for its elimination from the body. This slow elimination of thiopentone of about 10–15% per hour necessitates care in the prolonged recovery, with warnings not to drive or operate machinery within 24 hours of its administration. Patients should be also be warned of the synergistic effects of thiopentone with other sedative drugs and alcohol.

All barbiturates are contraindicated in patients with acute intermittent porphyria and porphyria variegata. In these conditions, thiopentone increases the synthesis of cytochrome P450 from haem, and thus induces the enzyme δ-aminolaevulinic acid (δALA) synthetase. This enzyme is crucial in porphyrin synthesis and its induction increases synthesis of porphobilinogen and other porphyrins, which can cause progressive demyelination and neuropathy, muscle weakness, abdominal pain, and psychiatric sequelae. The precipitation of an acute porphyria can be fatal and therefore barbiturates must be avoided. The importance of recognizing acute porphyria as a cause of abdominal pain is emphasized in Chapter 61.

### Methohexitone

Methohexitone was first used in 1957. It is presented as a white powder with 6% anhydrous sodium carbonate. The chemical formula is given in Figure 32.5. Of the four possible optically active isomers of the compound, a racemic mixture of two of these stereoisomers is used in clinical anaesthesia. The drug is usually prepared as a 1% solution with a pH of about 11.

**Table 32.4 Pharmacokinetic properties of intravenous induction agents**

| Agent | $t_{1/2}\ \alpha_1$ (min) | $t_{1/2}\ \alpha_2$ (min) | $t_{1/2}\ \beta$ (h) | Clearance (ml/min per kg) | Volume of distribution (L/kg) |
|---|---|---|---|---|---|
| Thiopentone | 2–7 | 30–60 | 5–11 | 1.4–5.7 | 1–4 |
| Methohexitone | 6 | 2–58 | 1.6–4 | 10–13 | 1.2–2.2 |
| Etomidate | 1–3 | 12–29 | 1–1.5 | 10–24 | 2.2–4.3 |
| Propofol | 1–4 | 5–69 | 5–11 | 21–29 | 3.3–5.7 |
| Ketamine | 1–3 | 8–18 | 1.5–3 | 17–20 | 2.9–3.1 |

Adapted from Calvey LN and Williams NE. *Principles and Practice of Pharmacology for Anaesthetists*, 3rd edn. Oxford: Blackwell Scientific, 1997.

Aqueous solutions maintained at room temperature have a shelf-life of at least 6 weeks. If dextrose or saline is used instead of water, solutions may become unstable within 24 hours. Like thiopentone, solutions of methohexitone are bacteriostatic as a result of their alkalinity.

The usual induction dose of methohexitone is 1–2 mg/kg. Onset of action is rapid because of its high lipid solubility and the extensive blood supply to the brain. In most respects it has similar effects to thiopentone. The important differences are highlighted below:

- There is less danger of tissue damage and vascular complications from extravenous injection. This may be partly related to the lower concentration of drug in solution.
- Pain on intravenous injection is more common, especially when the veins are small. The reason for this is not known.
- Excitatory side effects such as involuntary muscle movements, tremor, hypertonus, coughing, and hiccoughing are much more common, occurring in up to 80% of patients.
- Methohexitone can precipitate convulsive activity in those with an abnormal EEG and people with known epilepsy. Its use in the latter patients is controversial, but it is considered to be the drug of choice for electroconvulsive therapy, where the aim is to produce a modified convulsion.
- Methohexitone is considered to produce less hypotension than thiopentone, and it may induce more tachycardia.
- Complete recovery is significantly quicker after methohexitone than after equipotent doses of thiopentone. Similarly, when given by intermittent injection or by infusion, methohexitone is less likely to accumulate. This is because of the shorter terminal half-life. Clearance of methohexitone is approximately 50% of liver blood flow, and the relatively high extraction ratio is consistent with flow-limited hepatic elimination.
- Although hypersensitivity reactions are more common than with thiopentone (Table 32.5), they are less serious. Facial and periorbital oedema have been reported but no deaths.
- Methohexitone is metabolized to hydroxymethohexitone which probably has no hypnotic activity. This is eliminated as the glucuronide metabolite in the urine. Only trace amounts of methohexitone are excreted unchanged in bile and urine.

## IMIDAZOLES: ETOMIDATE

Etomidate was first introduced in 1973. An imidazole is a five-membered ring of three carbon atoms and two nitrogen atoms. The carboxylated derivative is etomidate whose structural formula is shown in Figure 32.7. Although the sulphate is freely soluble in water, it is presented in 35% propylene glycol which improves the stability of the solution. It is prepared as a 0.2% solution (2 mg/ml) which has a pH of 8.1. The normal induction dose is 0.3 mg/kg; 75% is bound to plasma proteins after injection.

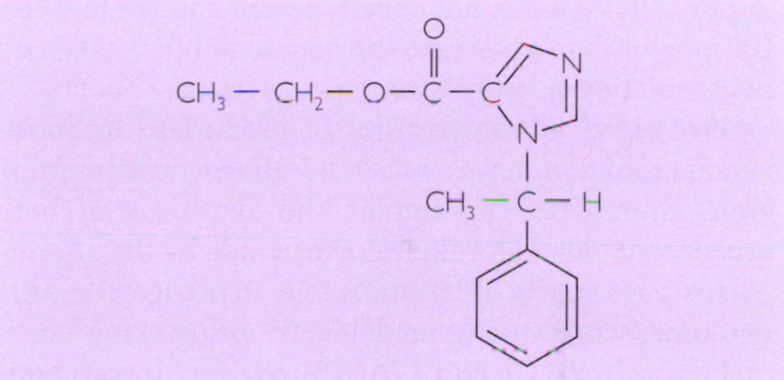

**Figure 32.7** Structural formula of etomidate.

**Table 32.5 Incidence of hypersensitivity reactions to intravenous induction agents and other drugs**

| Drug | Incidence |
|---|---|
| Thiopentone | 1 in 14 000–1 in 20 000 |
| Methohexitone | 1 in 1600–1 in 7000 |
| Propofol (Cremophor formulation) | 1 in 1131 |
| Propofol (emulsion formulation) | 1 in 80 000–1 in 100 000 |
| Etomidate | 1 in 50 000–1 in 450 000 |
| Ketamine | 2 cases |
| Althesin (in Cremophor) | 1 in 400–1 in 1100 |
| Neuromuscular blocking agents | 1 in 5000 |
| Penicillin | 1 in 2500–1 in 10 000 |
| Dextran | 1 in 3000 |
| Gelatins | 1 in 900 |
| Hydroxyethyl starch | 1 in 1200 |

The most significant advantage is its relatively high safety margin. The $LD_{50} : ED_{50}$ is approximately 30 compared with only 4 for thiopentone. Etomidate has little or no effect on the cardiovascular system, causing only mild decreases in peripheral vascular resistance and blood pressure.

Etomidate does not release histamine. It is probably the only intravenous induction agent to have this property. Hypersensitivity reactions are uncommon (Table 32.5). It causes only transient and minimal respiratory depression and no inhibition of the hypoxic pulmonary vasoconstrictor reflex. Thus, etomidate offers advantages during induction of anaesthesia in patients with poor cardiac reserve and hypovolaemia. Experimental studies have shown that a continuous infusion of etomidate increases levels of δALA synthetase, which calls into question its suitability for patients with porphyria (see above and Chapter 87).

Etomidate is not without side effects and these have limited the use of this agent in anaesthetic practice. It causes pain on injection (especially when administered into small vessels on the dorsum of the hand) in up to 50% of patients, which is probably caused by the propylene glycol. Its use is also associated with a high incidence of nausea and vomiting, and excitatory movements. These limit its usefulness in day-case surgery, despite the relatively rapid metabolism by non-specific hepatic esterases. Haemolysis has also been noted, although it is not usually severe enough to cause haemoglobinuria because the haemoglobin is taken up by circulating haptoglobin.

Prolonged administration of etomidate by intravenous infusion may result in adrenocortical suppression. Etomidate can impair the synthesis of both glucocorticoids and mineralocorticoids by the adrenal cortex. As a result of its imidazole structure, the drug combines with cytochrome P450, resulting in inhibition of 11β-hydroxylase and 17α-hydroxylase. Intravenous infusion for sedation on the ICU has been implicated as increasing mortality. Etomidate is contraindicated for administration by continuous infusion.

## HINDERED PHENOLS: PROPOFOL

Propofol (2,6-diisopropylphenol) is a chemically inert phenolic compound with anaesthetic properties; the structural formula is shown in Figure 32.8. It was first used in 1977 and was introduced into clinical practice in 1986. It was originally formulated in Cremophor-EL, but was reformulated before commercial release because of fears of hypersensitivity reactions similar to those seen with alphaxalone (Althesin) (see below), which was also solubilized in this agent. It is now presented as a 1% oil–water emulsion containing 10% soya bean oil, 1.2% egg phosphatide, and 2.25% glycerol. Both 1% and 2% concentrations are also available in pre-filled syringes for use in TIVA. Propofol is not bacteriostatic: contamination has occurred during infusion which has been implicated in causing septicaemia and therefore particular care is required in its preparation. This is especially important when propofol is used for TIVA.

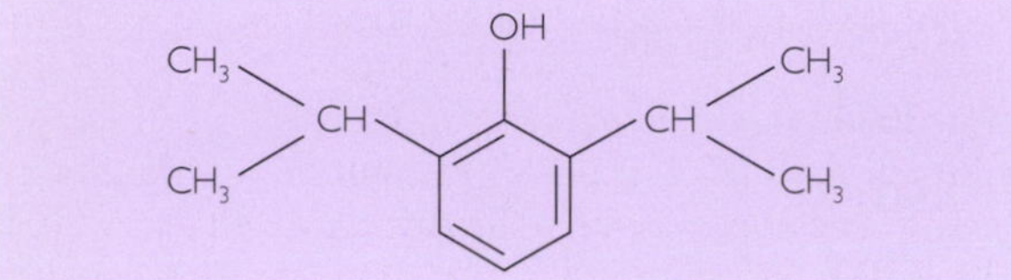

**Figure 32.8** Structural formula of propofol.

The normal induction dose of 1.5–2.5 mg/kg produces rapid loss of consciousness as a result of the immediate uptake of the lipid-soluble drug into the brain. Of the drug 98% is protein bound after intravenous administration. After redistribution of the drug, recovery of full consciousness is rapid and the patient is clear-headed. Propofol is mainly dependent on hepatic metabolism to the glucuronide metabolites of 2,6-diisopropylphenol and 2,6-diisopropylquinol which are subsequently excreted in the urine. The clearance of the drug is high (see Table 32.4) which accounts partly for the quality of recovery.

Postoperative nausea and vomiting are extremely uncommon. This probable antiemetic property and the rapid clear-headed recovery make propofol especially popular for day-case surgery. Pain on injection is common, especially when injected into small veins on the dorsum of the hand. The mechanism is obscure and thrombophlebitic sequelae are rare. Prior injection of, or mixing with, lignocaine (lidocaine) can reduce the pain.

The safety margin of propofol is less than that with etomidate but greater than with the barbiturates. This is true with regard to both unwanted side effects and hypersensitivity reactions (Table 32.5). Relative hypotension is common and is probably caused by decreased systemic vascular resistance. There is also probably direct myocardial depression and a reduction in cardiac output. The heart rate does not increase and indeed there is frequently a bradycardia. This has been suggested to result from a resetting of the baroreflex. There is also a greater reduction of the pressor response to laryngoscopy after propofol than after thiopentone.

Respiratory side effects are uncommon, apart from respiratory depression. Apnoea is usually transient, but is more prolonged at higher doses and if given with other ventilatory depressants such as opioids. Upper airway reflexes are obtunded more readily than after thiopentone, allowing instrumentation or manipulation of the airway. Propofol is the induction agent of choice for inserting a laryngeal mask airway.

Excitatory side effects, including myoclonus, opisthotonos, and convulsions, have been associated with the use of propofol. Its use in people with epilepsy is controversial, but is probably best avoided because thiopentone or diazepam is likely to be more suitable.

Propofol is not licensed for children under the age of 3 years. Some of the advantages of the drug (such as the ability to insert a laryngeal mask airway before deepening anaesthesia with a volatile agent) are lost in children who waken too rapidly because of the rapid redistribution caused by the high cardiac output. Unexpected deaths have been reported in children who have had long-term sedation with propofol while in intensive care. Increasing metabolic acidosis, bradycardia, and progressive myocardial failure were the presenting symptoms. The aetiology is obscure, although both the drug itself and the lipid content of the solvent have been implicated.

Propofol is suitable for TIVA because significant accumulation of the drug does not occur after bolus doses or a continuous infusion. Studies have shown that propofol concentrations of 4–6 μg/ml in the plasma provide anaesthesia in the presence of either nitrous oxide or an opioid infusion. Without the use of nitrous oxide, in healthy patients, plasma concentrations of 6–8 μg/ml may be required. It is not possible to measure actual plasma concentrations during anaesthesia, but technology now available computes an estimated concentration. This takes into account the age and weight of the patient and the amount of propofol given over a given time. At awakening, the plasma concentration of propofol is 1.0–1.5 μg/ml. Nevertheless, there is a wide variability in the therapeutic drug concentration window (which is related to age, general health, and type of surgery) and intersubject kinetics, and therefore propofol dosing has to be titrated to effect, in a manner similar to that of adjusting vapour concentrations.

Propofol infusions decrease clearance of flow-dependent and capacity-limited drugs by dose-related reductions in liver blood flow and decreases in the hepatic extraction ratio. This will be of greater relevance during sedation on intensive care than during anaesthesia. Also of relevance is that propofol contains 900 cal/L, which is the same energy content as 10% fat emulsion.

Provided that care is used to avoid overdosage and, hence, excessive hypotension, infusions of propofol can be particularly useful in patients with ischaemic heart disease. This is because the slower heart rates associated with this technique reduce myocardial work and hence oxygen requirements.

## PHENCYCLIDINES: KETAMINE

Ketamine hydrochloride was first used in 1965. It is a phencyclidine ('angel dust') derivative that is less likely to cause hallucinations. The structural formula is shown in Figure 32.9. Although it does not usually cause unconsciousness in one arm–brain circulation time, it is commonly classed as an induction agent. It is presented as a racemic mixture (see Chapter 19 for definitions of isomerism), the two stereoisomers $R(-)$ and $S(+)$ having different potencies, but similar kinetics. $S(+)$ ketamine is 3.4 times more potent than $R(-)$ ketamine in terms of anaesthesia, and is a better analgesic but causes more psychic emergent reactions. $S(+)$ ketamine has been isolated and is currently being evaluated as a sole agent.

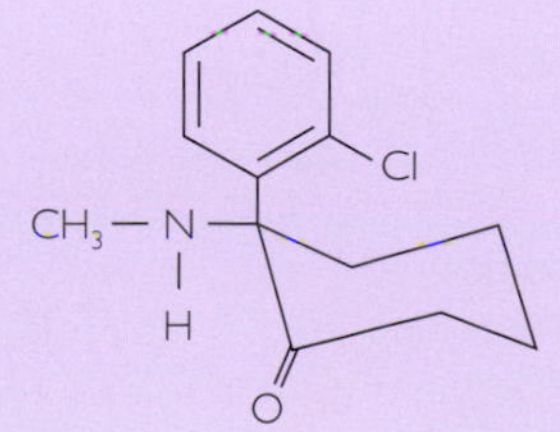

**Figure 32.9** Structural formula of ketamine.

Ketamine hydrochloride is freely soluble in water, forming an acidic solution of pH 3.5–5.5. It is presented in 10, 50, and 100 mg/ml solutions. The two stronger solutions contain benzethonium chloride 0.01% as a preservative.

Ketamine differs from other induction agents in several respects:

- It is almost devoid of hypnotic properties but produces a state of dissociative anaesthesia: patients do not close their eyes or lose the eyelash reflex as they do with thiopentone.
- It has profound analgesic properties. These are thought to result from effects on the spinoreticular tracts which are concerned with the perception of pain or to the binding of ketamine by opioid receptors (particularly μ-receptors).
- The onset of CNS effects may take up to 90 s to become apparent after intravenous administration (induction dose 1–2 mg/kg). Effects last for 5–10 min.
- It can be given intramuscularly (dose 10 mg/kg) where the onset of effect may take up to 8 min and last for 20–30 min.
- It has local anaesthetic properties. It has been used for spinal and extradural anaesthesia, in doses of up to 50 mg, for chronic pain conditions, and for control of postoperative pain.
- Excessive salivation occurs; atropine is required to control this.
- Ketamine invariably produces tachycardia, increases cardiac output, and raises plasma norepinephrine. Systolic and diastolic blood pressures are increased, as is pulmonary vascular resistance. The positive inotropic effects are the result of indirect activation of β-adrenoceptors by inhibition of norepinephrine re-uptake. If the agent is applied to the isolated heart, ketamine is like all other induction agents in that it causes a negative inotropic effect, and also acts as a peripheral vasodilator.
- Cerebral blood flow, cerebral oxygen consumption, and intracranial pressure are all increased.
- Respiratory activity is little affected in normal dosage.
- It is a bronchodilator.
- Emergence phenomena frequently occur. These range from vivid dreams and visual images to hallucinations and delirium, which may continue for up to 24 hours after its administration. These sequelae can be very unpleasant and are thought to be caused by misperception or misinterpretation of sensory information. Emergence phenomena can be significantly modified by premedication with a benzodiazepine.

The elimination of ketamine depends on the mixed-function oxidase system associated with the smooth endoplasmic reticulum. Its main metabolite, norketamine, has some hypnotic activity, with a potency of around 30% of that of the parent drug, and a longer elimination half-life. Both ketamine and norketamine may be metabolized further to hydroxylated derivatives. These are subsequently conjugated and eliminated in the urine as glucuronides. Hence, the efficacy of ketamine may be enhanced in patients with renal impairment.

The adverse effects of ketamine on the cardiovascular system and CNS mean that ketamine has only a limited place in anaesthetic practice. It is contraindicated as an induction agent in patients with a history of cerebrovascular disease, hypertension, ischaemic or valvular heart disease, or psychotic illness, and in the presence of increased intracranial or intraocular pressure. In paediatric practice, it is a useful agent when venepuncture is difficult or poorly tolerated or for repeated procedures. In adults, the indications are less well defined. It is often used in shocked patients, or for repeat anaesthesia such as needed for burns dressings. It can be given by infusion for maintenance of anaesthesia and, in emergency situations, it can be given satisfactorily via the intraosseous route (see Chapter 78).

A summary of the metabolic breakdown products of the common induction agents is given in Table 32.6.

## STEROIDS

The hypnotic properties of steroids were identified in 1941 by Selye who showed reversible unconsciousness in rats after injection of large quantities of several steroid hormones into the peritoneum. In 1955 hydroxydione was introduced into clinical practice. Although this had a wider safety margin than thiopentone, there was a delay in onset of action, the duration of action was rather too long, and there was an unacceptably high incidence of thrombophlebitis. Hydroxydione enjoyed only a short popularity as a non-barbiturate alternative to thiopentone, but was rapidly abandoned because of the adverse properties mentioned.

A number of other steroids were studied but it was some time before it was appreciated that rapid induction and high potency were associated with the presence of a free hydroxy group in the steroid molecule. Attempts to achieve solubility of such steroids by esterification, however, produced compounds with reduced potency or increased induction time.

Continuing research revealed that alphaxalone showed promise as an anaesthetic, having a rapid onset of action, high potency, and a wide safety margin. Problems of solubility were not entirely solved by the use of the non-ionic surface active agent, Cremophor-EL (polyoxyethylated castor oil). Addition of a small amount of another steroid, alphadolone, increased the solubility of alphaxalone in Cremophor-EL more than threefold. Alphadolone has anaesthetic properties similar to those of alphaxalone, but it is half as potent and was merely additive as a hypnotic. This mixture was known in the UK as Althesin and in some other countries as Alfathesin.

Althesin possessed many of the properties of an ideal anaesthetic agent, having a rapid, consistent action with only a few extraneous muscle movements. The quality of recovery was particularly good. It was introduced in 1971 and withdrawn from clinical practice in 1984 because of hypersensitivity reactions to the solubilizing agent, Cremophor-EL. Although (see Table 32.5) this occurred in 1 in 1000 administrations, reported deaths were few. It is of interest that 50% of dogs exhibited allergic reactions to Althesin, yet it is still available in veterinary practice!

The search for a water-soluble steroid continued, and minaxolone underwent clinical trials in 1978–9. It was withdrawn after 1250 administrations, for toxicological reasons. Although minaxolone had a rapid onset of action, the required induction dose was not as predictable as with other agents. There was a high incidence of excitatory effects and a long awakening time, with subsequently good quality of recovery.

The steroid metabolite of progesterone, pregnanelone, formulated in a soya bean emulsion, underwent clinical trials in the early 1990s. It produced a smooth rapid induction of anaesthesia with cardiovascular stability. The adverse effects found in the 2100 patients and volunteers included involuntary muscle

**Table 32.6 Metabolites of common induction agents**

| Induction agent | Metabolites |
|---|---|
| Thiopentone | Thiopentone carboxylic acid<br>Hydroxythiopentone<br>Pentobarbitone |
| Methohexitone | Hydroxymethohexitone<br>Hydroxymethohexitone glucuronide |
| Etomidate | Ethyl alcohol<br>Imidazole derivative of carboxylic acid |
| Propofol | Diisopropylphenol glucuronide<br>Diisopropylquinol glucuronide |
| Ketamine | Norketamine<br>Hydroxynorketamine<br>Hydroxyketamine glucuronide<br>Hydroxynorketamine glucuronide |

Adapted from Calvey LN and Williams NE. *Principles and Practice of Pharmacology for Anaesthetists*, 3rd edn. Oxford: Blackwell Scientific, 1997.

movements, rash, urticaria, and convulsions (similar incidence to that seen with propofol) and prompted clinical trials to cease; hence this drug did not reach the market.

Thus, currently, there are no steroid anaesthetic agents used. It is nevertheless likely that the search will continue for a suitable water-soluble steroid without adverse side effects. When it is found, comparison with the above agents is inevitable.

## HYPERSENSITIVITY REACTIONS

As the overall process of anaesthesia has become safer, the relative importance of hypersensitivity or anaphylactic reactions has increased. The incidence of such adverse events to intravenous agents is between 1 : 5000 and 1 : 20 000. It is not possible to give a more precise figure because anaesthetic techniques inevitably involve some polypharmacy and the role of other drugs (e.g. neuromuscular blocking agents or colloid infusions) may be difficult to determine. The incidence associated with individual induction agents is given in Table 32.5. Allergic reactions to some other drugs are also included for comparison.

Hypersensitivity reactions to intravenous induction agents may include bronchospasm, hypotension, peripheral vascular collapse, erythema, urticaria, oedema, and abdominal pain. The clinical course of the reaction is variable: vasodilatation may occur immediately after injection, rapidly followed by bronchospasm and cyanosis, with an impalpable pulse and unrecordable blood pressure. The ECG usually shows a tachycardia. Localized or generalized oedema may subsequently develop. Occasionally, reactions to intravenous induction agents may develop over 10–90 min in which case their clinical manifestations are usually relatively benign and their cause may not be recognized.

Many of the presenting symptoms are similar to those induced by histamine. Other mediators implicated include bradykinin, leukotrienes, prostaglandins, and 5-hydroxytryptamine (serotonin). The mechanisms involved may be one of four types:

1. A type I hypersensitivity reaction depends on previous exposure and sensitization to the intravenous induction agent and formation of IgE antibodies. The antibodies bind to mast cells and basophils; subsequent exposure to the agent results in an antigen–antibody reaction on the mast cell membrane and disruption of its cytoplasmic granules, which release histamine and other vasoactive amines.
2. Occasionally, a type II hypersensitivity reaction has been reported. IgG or IgM antibodies bind to an antigen on the cell surface which then activates the classic complement pathway. C4 and C3 are consumed, activating the remaining complement proteins, and cell lysis occurs and some C3a (anaphylatoxin) is formed. This reaction has been identified after a hypersensitivity reaction to propofol.
3. An anaphylactoid response that does not require prior exposure to the drug involves the alternative complement pathway. In this reaction, a larger proportion of C3 is converted to C3a and C5a. Many of the reactions to Althesin involved this mechanism.
4. A direct action of the drug on circulating basophil and mast cells can result in the release of histamine, which appears to be related to the dose and speed of injection of the drug. Previous exposure to the drug is not a feature and the systemic manifestations are usually mild. This reaction may be regarded as anaphylactoid or a direct pharmacological effect of the drug concerned. The severity of such a reaction will be reduced by slow administration of a moderate dose of an induction agent.

Treatment of hypersensitivity reactions is discussed in Chapter 13.

## TOTAL INTRAVENOUS ANAESTHESIA

TIVA is an anaesthetic technique that employs only intravenous agents and does not involve inhalational agents. Drugs are usually given by infusion to achieve hypnosis, analgesia, and, where required, muscle relaxation. The patient breathes, or is ventilated with, oxygen or oxygen-enriched air. The advantages of TIVA are summarized in Table 32.7.

However, there are certain constraints and some disadvantages of TIVA, which are summarized in Table 32.8. Although any intravenous anaesthetic agent may be used for TIVA, drugs most suited for delivery by infusion are those with a rapid offset of action once the infusion is stopped. The longer the infusion of drug is continued, the longer it takes to eliminate the drug. Drugs that have suitable pharmacokinetics include propofol, alfentanil, remifentanil, atracurium, vecuronium, and mivacurium. It is also possible to use methohexitone satisfactorily from knowledge of its pharmacokinetics. However, the development of well-publicized schemes for both manual administration and target-controlled infusions specifically for propofol (in addition to the clinical advantages of this drug) have enhanced the popularity of propofol for this purpose. Etomidate was also used for TIVA (more commonly sedation), but discovery of the effect on steroid synthesis led to its discontinuation.

The administration of volatile agents via the lungs is, in fact, an infusion-like process but it differs considerably from an infusion of an intravenous anaesthetic agent. The uptake characteristics of volatile agents and their distribution in the body are well understood, and they can be actively eliminated by continued ventilation of the lungs with the agent switched off. Very importantly, their concentration in expired air can be monitored in real time. In contrast, during TIVA, delivery must be matched to the size of the patient and the distribution of the drug; the elimination varies from patient to patient. In addition, the serum concentration cannot be monitored in real time and there is no way to accelerate the termination of the drug once administered.

To compare the properties of volatile agents, the concept of MAC (the minimum alveolar concentration to prevent movement in 50% of the population to a standard incision) was introduced. An analogous concept, MIR, was introduced for intravenous agents

**Table 32.7 Advantages of total intravenous anaesthesia**

| |
|---|
| Anaesthesia possible when access to airway limited (e.g. bronchoscopy) |
| Avoids environmental pollution (greenhouse effect; effects on operating room staff) |
| Minimal cardiovascular depression possible with suitable choice of agents |
| High inspired oxygen concentrations easily possible, e.g. for one-lung anaesthesia |
| Possible to avoid depressant effect of nitrous oxide on bone marrow |
| Avoids gas expansion with nitrous oxide (e.g. pneumothorax, bowel, middle ear) |
| Avoids adverse effects of volatile agents (e.g. halothane hepatitis) |
| Safe in malignant hyperpyrexia |
| Potentially less postoperative nausea and vomiting |

**Table 32.8 Constraints and disadvantages of total intravenous anaesthesia (TIVA)**

| |
|---|
| Drugs with suitable pharmacokinetics must be used |
| Preferably no active breakdown products |
| Secure, independent venous access is essential |
| Care needed to avoid interrupting administration by inflation of blood pressure cuff |
| Equipment for accurate delivery is required |
| Agents and equipment are expensive |
| Precise pharmacokinetic data for the patient population must be available |
| Cardiovascular, renal, or hepatic impairment may affect drug disposition |
| Concurrent administration of other drugs may affect pharmacokinetics of TIVA |
| Depth of anaesthesia not measurable; awareness of concern, partly because of individual variability |
| Feedback mechanism of increased ventilation to enhance volatile agent uptake absent |

being given by infusion. The MIR is the minimum infusion rate of an intravenous anaesthetic that prevents movement in response to an initial, standardized, skin incision in 50% of patients. It assumes that the serum concentration of the drug is constant and that the infusion rate equals the elimination and/or breakdown of the drug.

Although, in theory, MAC and MIR should be equivalent, in practice there are differences. It is more difficult to secure proper steady-state conditions using an intravenous infusion, the variability in MIR is greater for intravenous agents, and for some intravenous agents clearance can vary with infusion rate. Furthermore, the relationship between blood concentration and brain concentration depends on the degree of ionization and protein binding of the drug. Despite these apparent drawbacks, TIVA can be very successful and its popularity is again increasing, possibly because of pre-programmed, computer-driven syringes (see Figure 32.10).

The simplest form of TIVA is when a bolus dose is given for induction and then followed by a steady infusion. The change in serum concentration follows the pattern shown in Figure 32.11. This can clearly result

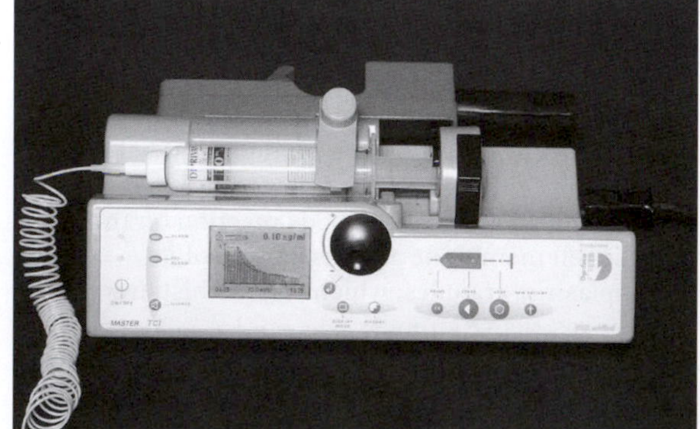

**Figure 32.10** A target-controlled infusion syringe used for the delivery of propofol. The pattern of delivery is shown on the screen.

in a period of awareness early on or, on the other hand, relative overdosage with time. As a result of the uptake kinetics of intravenous agents, the infusion rate needs to be continuously changed exponentially to maintain a steady serum concentration as peripheral compart-

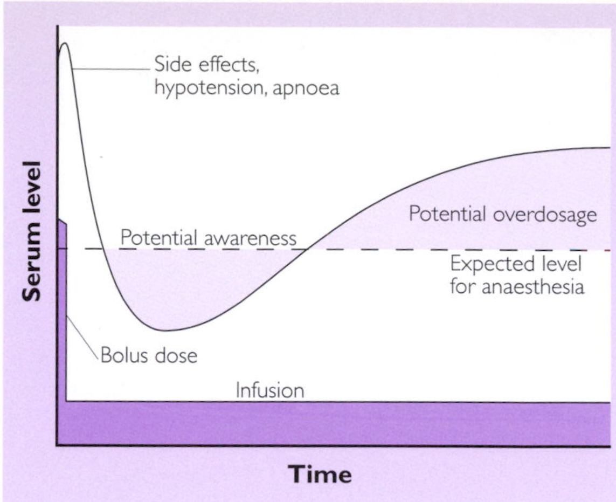


**Figure 32.11** Constant rate infusion after intravenous bolus induction dose.

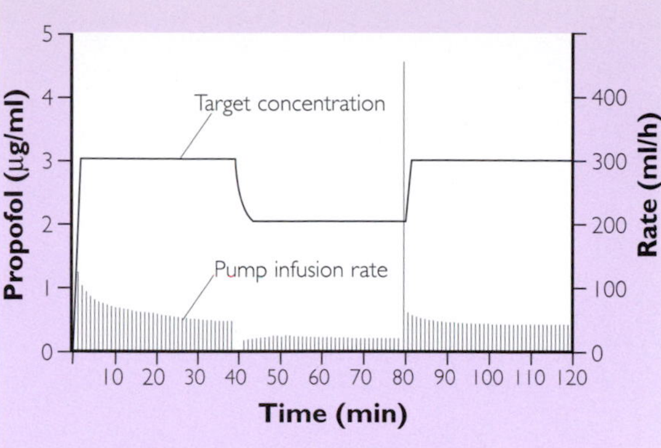


**Figure 32.13** Blood concentrations of propofol and infusion rates given by a computer-controlled system to achieve different target concentrations. Note the initial fast infusion rate, decreasing exponentially to achieve a steady target concentration. When a lower target concentration is selected, the pump stops infusing and resumes at a slower infusion rate. It increases again when a higher target concentration is desired. (Adapted from White PF and Kenny G. In: Nimmo W, Rowbotham DJ, and Smith G, eds. *Anaesthesia*, 2nd edn. Oxford: Blackwell Scientific Publications, 1994: 106.)

ments are filled up and metabolism and elimination begin. This can be done by changing the infusion rate manually (Figure 32.12) or by using a pre-programmed chip built into a programmable syringe pump. Such a device (e.g. the Diprifusor) needs to have a 'chip' whose properties reflect the kinetics of the population being anaesthetized. There would, for instance, be differing requirements for the young and elderly patient.

Use of this type of technology allows a predicted serum concentration to be dialled in, together with the patient's body weight, and the pump does the rest! An example of the changes in infusion rate required to achieve a step variation in serum concentration is shown in Figure 32.13. It should be noted that increases in serum concentration can be achieved quickly by the pump infusing: falls rely on the patient metabolizing and redistributing the drug. With practice, the use of such devices can become similar to turning a knob on a vaporizer, the serum concentration being set in the same way as the inspired percentage by assessing the patient's physiological responses to surgery. In addition to predicting serum concentration, some of these pumps also predict time to wakening. Such pumps are also used to provide sedation with target concentrations of 1–1.5 µg/ml propofol.

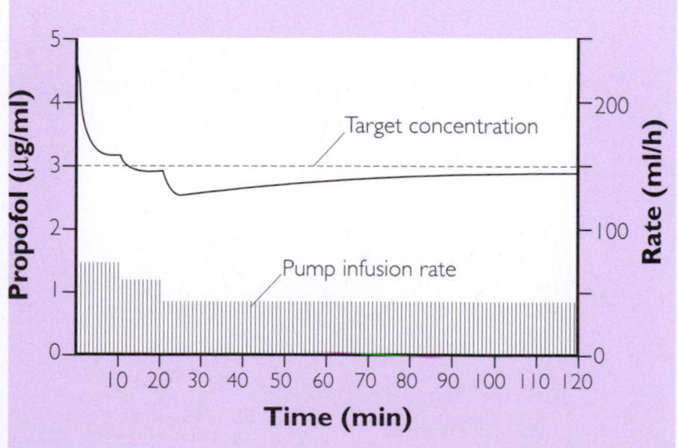


**Figure 32.12** Blood concentration of propofol predicted from multistep manual infusion. (Adapted from Roberts *et al*. *Anaesthesia* 1988;43:S14; and redrawn from White PF and Kenny G. In: Nimmo W, Rowbotham DJ, and Smith G, eds. *Anaesthesia*, 2nd edn. Oxford: Blackwell Scientific Publications, 1994: 106.)

## FURTHER READING


Biebuyck JF, Gouldson R, Nathanson M, White PF, Smith I. Propofol: an update on its use. *Anesthesiology* 1994;**81**:1005–43.

Calvey TN, Williams NE. *Principles and Practice of Pharmacology for Anaesthetists*, 3rd edn. Oxford: Blackwell Scientific, 1997.

Dundee JW, Bryant AM. *Intravenous Anaesthesia*, 2nd edn. Edinburgh: Churchill Livingstone, 1988.

Articles in: Dundee JW, Sear JW, eds. *Intravenous Anaesthesia – What is New?* In: *Baillière's Clin Anaesthesiol* 1991;**5**:267–474.

Hartmannsgruber MWB, Schulte-Steinberg H, Conzen P, Doenicke A. New intravenous induction agents. In: Frink EJ, Brown BR, eds. *Baillière's Clin Anaesthesiol* 1995;**9**:51–66.

Hull CJ. *Pharmacokinetics for Anaesthesia*. Oxford: Butterworth-Heinemann, 1991.

McKinnon RP, Wildsmith JAW. Histaminoid reactions in anaesthesia. *Br J Anaesth* 1995;**74**:217–28.

Articles in: Mirakhur RK, ed. Target controlled intravenous anaesthesia using 'Diprifusor'. *Anaesthesia* 1998;**53**:1S–86S.

Myles PS, Hendrata M, Bennett AM, Langley M, Buckland MR. Postoperative nausea and vomiting. Propofol or thiopentone: Does choice of induction agent affect outcome? *Anaesth Intensive Care* 1996;**24**:355–9.

Oye I. Ketamine analgesia. NMDA receptors and the gates of perception. *Acta Anaesthesiol Scand* 1998;**42**:747–9.

Articles in: White PF, ed. *Kinetics of Anaesthetic Drugs in Clinical Anaesthesiology*. In: *Baillière's Clin Anaesthesiol* 1991;**5**.

Sutcliffe NP, Murdoch JAC, Kenny GNC. Pharmacodynamics of anaesthetic agents. *Curr Anaesth Crit Care* 1997;**8**:207–13.

# Chapter 33 Inhalational anaesthetic agents

T. Gallacher and P. Hutton

## THE QUEST FOR THE IDEAL INHALATIONAL AGENT

Inhalational agents to deaden pain and produce unconsciousness were introduced into medical practice in the 1840s and today they continue to be the most popular drugs for maintenance anaesthesia. Over the past 150 years at least 18 compounds have been introduced into clinical practice (Figure 33.1), of which six remain in use (Table 33.1).

The regular introduction of new compounds attests to the fact that each was an attempt to improve on the shortcomings of those that existed. What therefore are the desirable properties that were being sought? These are listed in Table 33.2. Later, when individual agents are being described they can be compared against this checklist of ideal properties.

During the search for better inhalational agents, many compounds were investigated, most of which were discarded because of unwanted side effects. Such compounds have nevertheless led to a better understanding of structure–activity relationships, which are summarized in Table 33.3. These are analogous to changes in the barbituric acid ring resulting in the different properties of intravenous induction agents (see Chapter 32).

It is likely that no more new inhalational agents will be introduced into clinical practice. At least one major company has taken the policy decision that future work to refine the already highly acceptable agents will not be cost-effective. The possible exception might be xenon, which is now being produced in large quantities as a result of the decommissioning of nuclear power stations.

The technique of gaseous induction of anaesthesia is discussed in Chapter 2 and maintenance in Chapter 3. Vaporizer design and the production of accurate concentrations is described in Chapter 8.

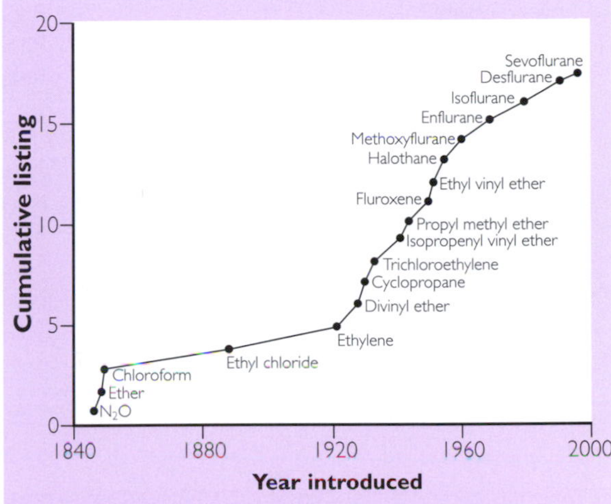


**Figure 33.1** Timeline of inhalational anaesthetics introduced into clinical practice since the early use of nitrous oxide ($N_2O$) in 1844. (Adapted from US data supplied by Anaquest, New Jersey, USA, 1993.)

**Table 33.1 Inhalational agents still in current use**

| Agent | Year of introduction |
|---|---|
| Nitrous oxide | 1844 |
| Halothane | 1956 |
| Enflurane | 1966 |
| Isoflurane | 1971 |
| Sevoflurane | 1990 |
| Desflurane | 1992 |

## DEFINITIONS AND PHYSICOCHEMICAL PROPERTIES

With the exception of nitrous oxide ($N_2O$), all inhalational agents in current use are halogenated organic compounds, as shown in Figure 33.2. In precise terminology, all inhaled anaesthetic agents are vapours rather than gases. This is because they are used in clinical practice at temperatures below their critical temperature, which is the one above which a gas cannot be liquefied solely by increasing the pressure (see Chapter 37). $N_2O$ (which is usually referred to as a gas) has a critical temperature of 36.5°C, which strictly means that it is inhaled as a vapour and exhaled as a gas!

The physical principles related to gases, liquids, and vaporization are discussed in more detail in Chapters 8, 37, and 38. A brief resumé is given here to aid understanding of the behavioural characteristics of inhalational agents.

### Partial pressure

A partial pressure is the pressure exerted by each component of a gas mixture. Dalton's law states that

**Table 33.2 The properties of an ideal inhalational agent**

| Characteristic | Requirements |
|---|---|
| Molecular stability | Stable to light, alkali, and soda lime<br>Safe in closed circle system<br>Not corrosive<br>Long shelf-life in all storage conditions<br>No requirement for preservatives<br>Non-flammable or -explosive<br>Not metabolized |
| Potent | Allows use in high concentration of oxygen<br>Allows use as sole agent |
| Low solubility | Rapid rise in alveolar concentration<br>Rapid induction and recovery<br>Ready adjustment of depth of anaesthesia |
| Not pungent | Permits smooth induction by inhalation |
| Anaesthetic specific effects | Analgesia, amnesia, hypnosis<br>No CNS excitation<br>No cardiovascular or respiratory effects<br>No adverse drug interactions<br>No organ-specific toxicity |

Adapted from Jones RM. *Br J Anaesth* 1990;65:527–36.

**Table 33.3 Structure–activity relationships of inhalational agents**

| Molecular characteristic | Result |
|---|---|
| Increasing halogenation of hydrocarbons and ethers | Increasing potency<br>Increasing arrhythmogenesis: F < Cl < Br < I<br>Full halogenation usually convulsant |
| Increasing fluorination of ethers | Partial fluorination causes convulsant action<br>Full fluorination decreases potency<br>Increasing stability, less flammable |
| Class of halogenated ether | Methyl ethyl ethers more potent, stable, and better anaesthetics than diethyl ethers<br>Vinyl ethers tend to be unstable and toxic<br>Thioethers: unpleasant odour, potent, and toxic |
| Chirality (see Chapter 19) | Ethers containing an asymmetric carbon atom are good anaesthetics (i.e. –CHFCl, –CHFBr, –CHClBr, and –CFClBr) |

Adapted from Cousins M and Seaton H. Volatile anaesthetic agents and their delivery systems. In: Healy TEJ and Cohen PJ, eds. *A Practice of Anaesthesia*, 6th edn. London: Edward Arnold, 1995.

the total pressure exerted by a mixture of gases is the sum of the partial pressures of each of its component gases. In other words, the total pressure is the sum of the pressures exerted by each gas if it alone occupied the volume of the gas mixture.

For a gas dissolved in a liquid, the term 'tension' is often used instead of partial pressure. The partial pressure of a gas in solution is the pressure of the same gas in the gaseous state above the liquid when it is in equilibrium with it. Note that this is not the same as the volume of gas or number of molecules of the gas that are dissolved in the liquid. The volume or mass of dissolved gas will depend on how soluble the gas is in that particular liquid. Solubility is discussed later, but an example of its sometimes surprising effects is demonstrated in Figure 33.3. In this figure, water is in equilibrium with air (assumed to be a two-gas mixture) in a closed container. The partial pressures (tensions) of oxygen and nitrogen in the two phases will be equal, as shown on the left-hand side of the figure. The mole fractions of the two gases in the air will be 21% and 79%, as shown in the upper right-hand bar graph. If,

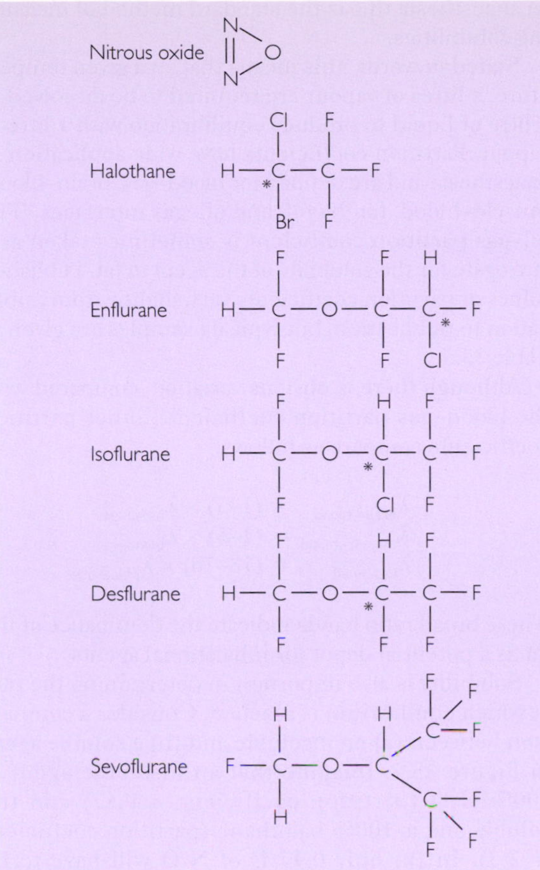


**Figure 33.2** The structural formulae of inhalational anaesthetic agents in current use. The presence of a chiral carbon atom is shown by an asterisk (*).

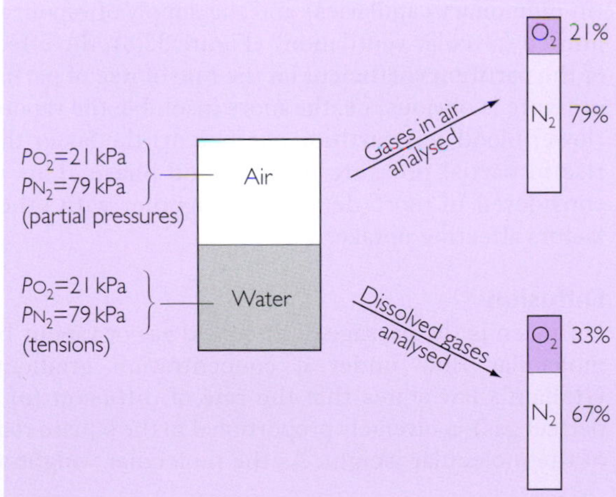


**Figure 33.3** The gaseous content of air (assumed to be 21% oxygen and 79% nitrogen) and water in equilibrium with it at 20°C.

however, the water is separated off and boiled, and the expelled gases analysed, it will be found that the mole fractions of the two gases will be different: oxygen 33% and nitrogen 67%. The reason for this is that they have different solubilities (see later and Table 33.5). The important message is that, in a liquid phase in equilibrium with a gaseous phase, the mole fractions of individual dissolved gases will not necessarily be in the same ratio as those in the gaseous phase.

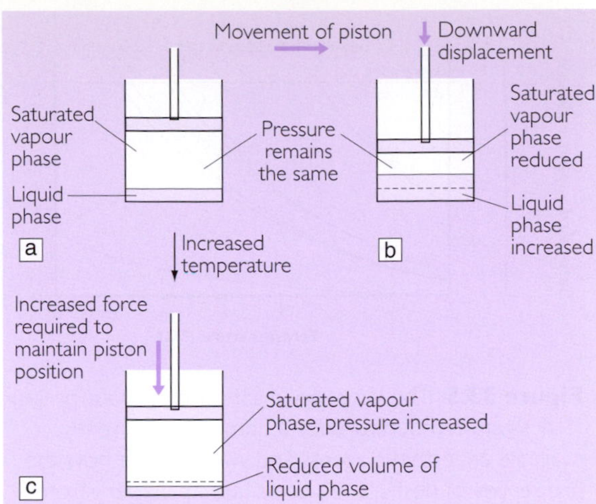


**Figure 33.4** Properties of saturated vapours. (See text for details.)

### Saturated vapour pressure

The saturated vapour pressure (SVP) is the pressure of a vapour that exists in equilibrium with its own liquid. This has a unique property. If the temperature is kept constant and the piston is pushed downwards from (a) to (b) in Figure 33.4, the pressure $P$ does not rise. Instead, more vapour condenses and the vapour pressure remains constant. The vapour pressure of a saturated vapour is therefore independent of its volume. If, however, the temperature is changed, the kinetic velocity of the molecules increases, more molecules evaporate, and they exchange more momentum with the piston (Figure 33.4c). Greater force is therefore required to maintain the position of the piston. The SVP is consequently highly dependent on temperature, and typical SVP curves are shown in Figure 33.5. More details of properties of vapours can be found in Chapter 37. Saturated vapour pressures for agents in common use are given in Table 33.4.

### Saturation

Saturation is measured as percentage volume per volume (%v/v). This means that in, say, a 2% concentration of halothane in oxygen there are 2 moles of halothane in 100 moles of mixture. Alternatively, it can be equivalently stated that the mole ratio of halothane : oxygen is 2 : 98. As the mole ratio is equal to the ratio of the volumes of the individual components under the same conditions of temperature and pressure, (v/v) is often written instead of (mol/mol). This, alternatively stated, means that a 2% halothane in oxygen mixture has 2 volumes of halothane per 100 volumes of the mixture.

### Solubility

Solubility is a term with a number of meanings but in this chapter it is meant to mean a measure of the extent to which one substance dissolves in another. There are two absolute measurements of solubility: the Bunsen and Oswald solubility coefficients, which measure the volume (or mass) of gas dissolving in a unit volume of

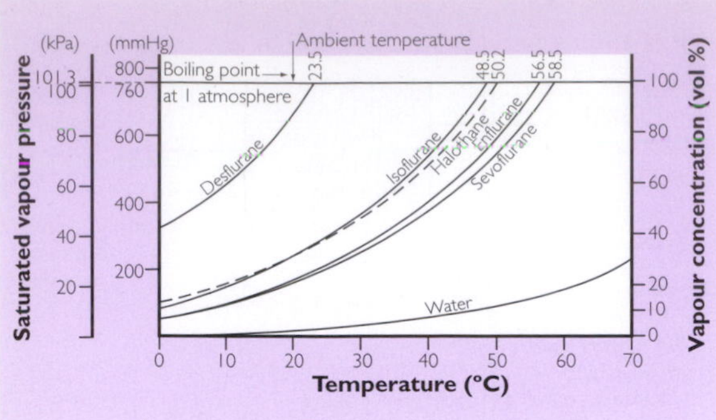


**Figure 33.5** The variation in saturated vapour pressure (SVP) with temperature for a number of currently available anaesthetic agents and water. Note how the properties of desflurane necessitate its delivery from a pressure-balanced, heated vaporizer instead of one of conventional design. At ambient temperature, the SVP of water is so low that for it to humidify air effectively or carry drugs by the inhalational route it has to be either heated or nebulized. (Data on sevoflurane from Abbott Laboratories; on desflurane from Susay SR *et al. Anesth Analg* 1996;83:864; on isoflurane, halothane, enflurane, and water from Rodgers RC and Hill GE. *Br J Anaesth* 1978;50:415.)

liquid at a specified temperature. In anaesthesia, because of its usefulness in clinical practice, it is far more convenient to describe solubility at a specified temperature in terms of partition coefficients, which are given the Greek letter lambda (λ) to represent them.

A partition coefficient can be understood as follows. Figure 33.6 shows a 2-litre container half filled with 1 litre of liquid. Vapour is introduced and flows through the container until the liquid is saturated with the vapour (Figure 33.6a). The container valves are then closed, the liquid removed, and the vapour extracted from the liquid. The corresponding comparative volumes of vapour, under the same conditions of temperature and pressure, will be (for instance) as shown in Figure 33.6b. The liquid–gas partition coefficient can then be determined from:

$$\lambda = \frac{\text{Volume of vapour extracted from liquid phase}}{\text{Volume of vapour in gas phase}} = \frac{x\text{ litres}}{1\text{ litre}}$$

giving:

$$\text{Partition coefficient } (\lambda) = x.$$

In anaesthesia this is the standard method of measuring solubilities.

Stated in words, this means that, at a given temperature, x litres of vapour are required to be dissolved in 1 litre of liquid to produce equilibration with 1 litre of vapour. Partition coefficients have wide application in anaesthesia and are defined for blood–gas, brain–blood, muscle–blood, fat–blood, and oil–gas interfaces. The oil–gas partition coefficient is sometimes taken as a surrogate for the solubility of the agent in fat. Published values of partition coefficients vary slightly from publication to publication, but typical examples are given in Table 33.5.

Although there is obvious variation, compared with the blood–gas partition coefficients, other partition coefficients compare as follows:

$$\lambda_{\text{brain–blood}} = (1\text{–}3) \times \lambda_{\text{blood–gas}}$$
$$\lambda_{\text{muscle–blood}} = (1\text{–}5) \times \lambda_{\text{blood–gas}}$$
$$\lambda_{\text{fat–blood}} = (18\text{–}70) \times \lambda_{\text{blood–gas}}$$

These broad ratio bands indicate the dominance of the fat as a potential depot for inhalational agents.

Solubility is also important in determining the rate at which equilibrium is reached. Consider a comparison between (a) an insoluble and (b) a soluble agent in Figure 33.7. Imagine that an insoluble agent is 100% $N_2O$ (partition coefficient = 0.47) and the soluble one is 100% halothane (partition coefficient = 2.3). In (a) only 0.47 L of $N_2O$ will have to be dissolved in blood to come into equilibrium with the vapour; the uptake curve is shown. In (b), 2.3 L of halothane must be taken up to achieve the same equilibrium state. The accompanying uptake curve is also shown.

If, as in life, the blood is flowing past the interface (in pulmonary capillaries) and the supply of vapour is limited (alveolar ventilation) (Figure 33.8), the effect of the partition coefficient on the rate of rise of partial pressure is obvious, i.e. the more insoluble the vapour (lower blood–gas partition coefficient) the faster the rise in partial pressure in the liquid phase. This is considered in more detail later together with other factors affecting uptake.

## Diffusion

Diffusion is the passage of dissolved gas or vapour by molecular flow under a concentration gradient. Graham's law states that the rate of diffusion (of a perfect gas) is inversely proportional to the square root of the molecular weight. As the molecular weight of

**Table 33.4 Some physical properties of inhalational anaesthetic agents**

| Physical property | Nitrous oxide | Desflurane | Isoflurane | Halothane | Enflurane | Sevoflurane |
|---|---|---|---|---|---|---|
| Boiling point (°C) at atmospheric pressure | −88 | 23.5 | 48.5 | 50.2 | 56.5 | 58.5 |
| Molecular weight | 44 | 168 | 184 | 197 | 184 | 200 |
| Saturated vapour pressure at 20°C (kPa) | 5200 | 89.2 | 32.5 | 32.1 | 23.3 | 22.7 |

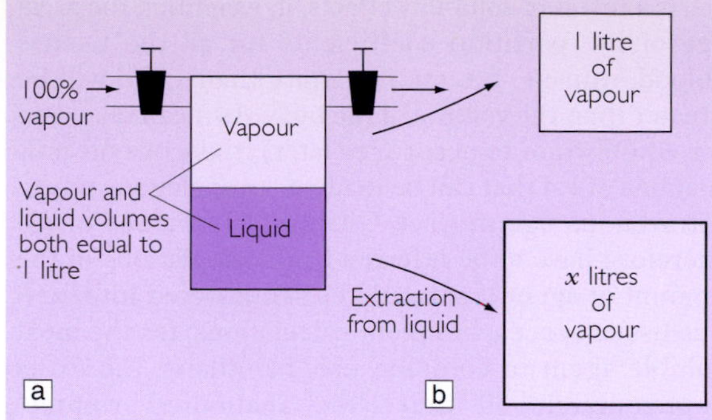


**Figure 33.6** A diagrammatic representation of the derivation of the partition coefficient.

oxygen is 32 and that of carbon dioxide is 44, this would predict that:

$$\frac{\text{Rate of diffusion of } O_2}{\text{Rate of diffusion of } CO_2} = \frac{\sqrt{44}}{\sqrt{32}}$$

$$= 1.17$$

This suggests that oxygen will diffuse 17% faster than carbon dioxide and this is true in a pure gas mixture. In clinical practice, however, the nature of the membrane exerts a much more important effect on the rate of movement of substances across it (often still termed the 'rate of diffusion') because it is the uptake of a substance into the membrane that determines the rise in partial pressure, which allows diffusion to occur. Consequently, the rate of diffusion is more closely related to the absorption of the agent into the tissues than to its molecular weight. This is why carbon dioxide 'diffuses' 20 times faster than oxygen and $N_2O$ 14 times faster than oxygen. These results can be predicted from a consideration of the partition coefficients in Table 33.5.

Having pointed out the importance of the membrane in differential rates of diffusion, when compared with most drugs, all the respiratory gases ($O_2$, $CO_2$, $N_2$), $N_2O$, and volatile agents pass rapidly through physiological membranes. Equilibrium between alveolar and end-capillary gas tensions is virtually complete at all times during induction, maintenance, and recovery from anaesthesia. Uptake from the lungs is blood-flow limited, not diffusion limited. Examples of when the speed of diffusion becomes important are found when normal physiology is disturbed. If pulmonary oedema develops, the distance from the alveoli to the capillary blood increases. Under these conditions, it is much easier to maintain normocapnia than it is to prevent hypoxia; one of the reasons for this is that carbon dioxide transfers 20 times more rapidly than oxygen and hence is less affected by the pathology.

Also, were it not for rapid diffusion through membranes, effective intracellular diffusion of $O_2$ and $CO_2$ between the mitochondria and the perfusing capillary would not be possible and, accordingly, nor would human life. In addition, the low blood–gas partition coefficients of $O_2$, $CO_2$, and $N_2$ (see Table 33.5) ensure

**Table 33.5 Typical values of partition coefficients for respiratory gases, tracer gases, and anaesthetic agents at 37°C (arranged in order of blood–gas solubility)**

| Agent | Blood–gas | Brain–blood | Muscle–blood | Fat–blood | Oil–gas |
|---|---|---|---|---|---|
| Helium[a] | 0.009 | | | | |
| Nitrogen[a] | 0.014 | | | | |
| Carbon monoxide[a] | 0.024 | | | | |
| Oxygen[a] | 0.026 | | | | |
| Xenon | 0.17 | 1.0 | 0.73 | 7.94 | 1.9 |
| Desflurane | 0.42 | 1.3 | 2.3 | 30.0 | 18.7 |
| Nitrous oxide | 0.47 | 1.1 | 1.2 | 2.3 | 1.4 |
| Sevoflurane | 0.68 | 1.7 | 3.6 | 55.0 | 42.0 |
| Carbon dioxide[a] | 0.82 | | | | |
| Isoflurane | 1.4 | 1.6 | 3.4 | 52.0 | 91.0 |
| Enflurane | 1.9 | 1.4 | 1.7 | 36.0 | 96.0 |
| Halothane | 2.3 | 2.0 | 4.0 | 62.0 | 224.0 |

[a]These are partition coefficients for water–gas, not blood–gas. Empty cells indicate that no data could be found.
The data in this table have been derived from interpolation of tables in: Garside JE and Phillips RF. *A Textbook of Pure and Applied Chemistry*, 2nd edn. London: Pitman, 1962: 167–8; Eger EI. The uptake and distribution of inhalational anaesthetic agents. In: Nunn JF, Utting JE, eds. *General Anaesthesia*, 4th edn. London: Butterworths, 1980: 67–97; Katoh T, Ikeda K. *Anesthesiology* 1987;66:301–3; Malviva S and Lerman J. *Anesthesiology* 1990;72:793–6; Terrell RC. *Br J Anaesth* 1984;56:3–7s; Yasuda N *et al. Anesth Analg* 1990;70:S444; Eger EI. Uptake, distribution and elimination of inhaled anaesthetics. In: Scurr C and Feldman S, eds. *Scientific Foundations of Anaesthesia*, 3rd edn. London: Heinemann, 1982: 468; Manufacturers' Data Sheets.

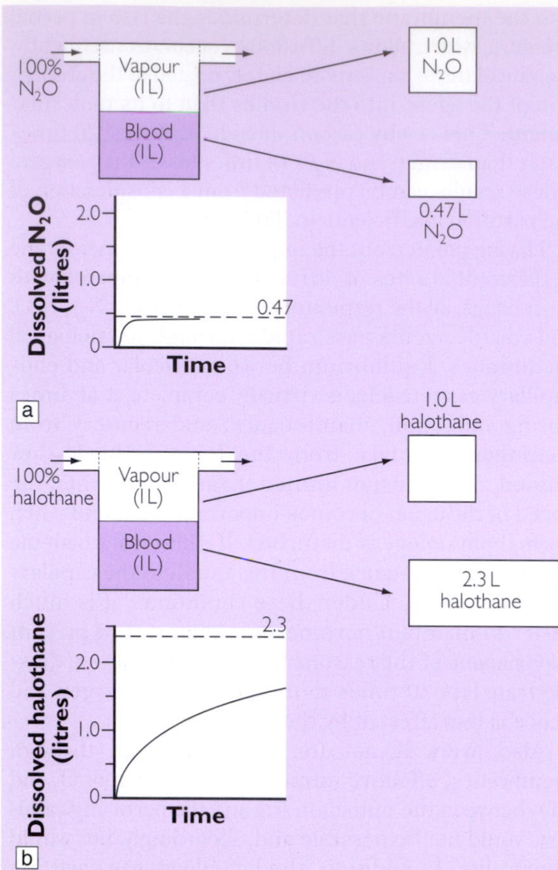


**Figure 33.7** A comparison of the uptake properties of (a) $N_2O$ and (b) halothane.

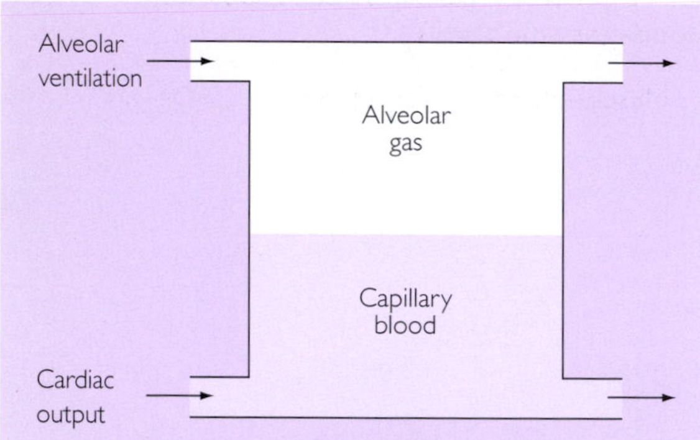


**Figure 33.8** A diagrammatic representation of the interface between alveolar ventilation and the circulating blood.

a rapid rise in the partial pressure within the liquid phase with the immediate generation of effective gradients for passive transport.

### Distribution volume

The distribution volume ($Vd$) for volatile agents is exactly analogous to that for intravenous agents (Chapters 19 and 32). If $x$ g of agent were administered, equilibrium between compartments occurred, the lungs were ignored, and there was no metabolism or elimination, $Vd$ would be given by:

$$\text{Dose administered/Blood concentration.}$$

As a result of solubility effects, if, weighting the average of the partition coefficients for all the tissues (blood, muscle, fat, etc.) as more than 1, $Vd$ will be greater than the volume of the body. As it can take days for equilibrium to occur (see later), there are no estimations of $Vd$ that can be made in an analogous way to intravenous agents (see Chapter 19). Values of $Vd$ therefore have to be inferred from calculations of the amount of agent that would be sequestered into various tissue spaces. From our calculations, for the most soluble agent in common use, halothane, the $Vd$ is approximately 30 times the anatomical volume, compared with approximately 1.5 times for $N_2O$. The main cause of this variation is the difference in tissue and particularly fat solubilities.

## POTENCY AND MINIMUM ALVEOLAR CONCENTRATION

Potency is a loose term with connotations of power, efficacy, and strength. For anaesthetic agents it has a strict definition in relationship to the clinical effectiveness of a specified alveolar concentration, which is usually abbreviated to MAC (minimum alveolar concentration).

### Definition of MAC

MAC is the minimum alveolar concentration of an anaesthetic at 1 atmosphere pressure under steady-state conditions that prevents reflex movement in 50% of the population in response to a standard noxious stimulus. The stimulus is usually an abdominal skin incision, but tetanic stimulation with a peripheral nerve stimulator has also been used. It was originally defined for oxygen–air mixtures but has also been obtained for $N_2O$–$O_2$ mixtures. Opioids and other analgesics present at the time of measurement also modify its value. Typical values for MAC are given in Table 33.6.

MAC is in effect the $ED_{50}$ (see Chapter 19) of the inhaled agent, i.e. half the patients will be adequately anaesthetized and half not. The $ED_{95}$ is probably a more useful measure and in data published to date has always been less than 1.5 MAC. ($ED_{50}$ is the dose required to produce 50% of the maximum response and $ED_{95}$ is that required to produce 95% of the maximum response.) The full explanation of $ED_{50}$ and $ED_{95}$ as pharmacological concepts is given in Chapter 19, Figure 19.20. In some of the published literature, the $ED_{50}$ and $ED_{95}$ are called the $AD_{50}$ and $AD_{95}$ when applied to volatile agents. An example of the type of plot used to determine the $ED_{50}$ and $ED_{95}$ for sevoflurane in oxygen and $N_2O$ is shown in Figure 33.9. Examples of the $ED_{50}$ and $ED_{95}$ for some inhalational and intravenous agents and their confidence limits are given in Table 33.7. This table is not complete for all the agents in current use, but represents the information that could be found in the current literature. The intravenous equivalent of MAC is the minimum infusion rate (MIR) defined in the same way in response to a standard incision. (See Chapter 19 for details of this.)

### MAC and solubility

Following the work of Meyer and Overton at the turn of the century (1900, not 2000!), it has been known that the potency of anaesthetic agents is closely related to

**Table 33.6 MAC values and oil–gas partition coefficients for inhaled anaesthetic agents**

| Physical property | Nitrous oxide | Halothane | Enflurane | Isoflurane | Desflurane | Sevoflurane |
|---|---|---|---|---|---|---|
| MAC in oxygen–air (% v/v) | 104 | 0.75 | 1.63 | 1.17 | 6.6 | 1.8 |
| MAC in oxygen–70% nitrous oxide (% v/v) | 34 | 0.26 | 0.57 | 0.41 | 2.3 | 0.62 |
| Oil–gas partition coefficient[a] | 1.4 | 224 | 98 | 95 | 26 | 80 |
| MAC in oxygen × oil–gas partition coefficient | 145.6 | 168 | 159.7 | 111.2 | 171.6 | 144 |

[a]The oil–gas coefficient varies depending on the oil used (e.g. olive or corn, etc.).
Data from same sources as Tables 33.5 and 33.7.

their solubility in olive oil. Since that time many correlations have been made between lipid solubility and measures of anaesthetic potency. The relationship between the oil–gas partition coefficient and the MAC is shown in Figure 33.10. which plots the numerical data in Table 33.6. It can be seen to be an inverse relationship when plotted on logarithmic scales. The potency of a new agent could therefore be predicted from its oil–gas solubility. In Figure 33.10, $N_2O$ is omitted and methoxyflurane (a highly soluble agent, now withdrawn) is included to demonstrate a convenient working range for the relationship.

Although the lipid solubility has been shown to be robust in terms of prediction, there are now much more sophisticated theories on the mechanism of action of anaesthetics (see Chapter 72). Some authors have emphasized the inverse relationship to the extent of saying that the product of the MAC and oil–gas partition coefficient produces a constant product of 140. How closely this ideal is approached can be judged from the last line in Table 33.6. The other major limitation of the theory is that it does not explain why many other fat-soluble compounds with similar oil–gas solubilities do not have any anaesthetic activity.

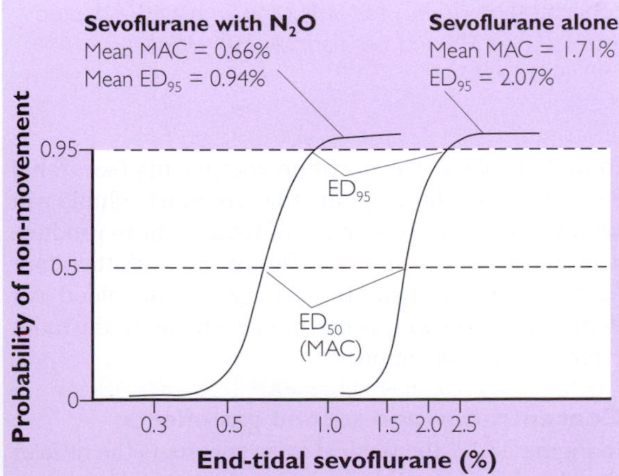


**Figure 33.9** The probability of non-movement to a standard surgical stimulus at different levels of end-tidal sevoflurane with and without nitrous oxide ($N_2O$). Note that $N_2O$ displaces the probability curve laterally and slightly alters its gradient. For definitions of MAC, $ED_{50}$, and $ED_{95}$ see the text. (Adapted from Katoh T and Ikeda K. *Anesthesiology* 1987;66:301.)

### Factors affecting MAC

Many physiological and pharmacological variables influence MAC, including age, premedication, metabolic status, and concomitant drug therapy.

Some drugs, such as opioids and alcohol, have different effects in different circumstances. Acute ingestion lowers MAC as a result of their sedative affects, whereas chronic intake, by altering resting cellular physiology, leads to an increased anaesthetic requirement. Conversely, the acute stimulant effect of amphetamine raises MAC whereas chronic usage lowers it.

Pregnancy and old age also reduce MAC. Children have a higher MAC which decreases from a peak at about 6–12 months of age to reach that of an adult in their early teens (Figure 33.11; see also Chapter 42, Figure 42.10).

In critically ill patients, the MAC is often markedly reduced as a result of the lowering effects of hypoxia, hypotension, and acidosis which often occur in these patients. The MAC is also dependent on body temperature, with pyrexia raising and hypothermia lowering it. Likewise, disturbances of sodium balance alter the MAC, with hyponatraemia lowering it and hypernatraemia having the opposite effect. Factors that are known to alter MAC are summarized in Table 33.8.

The sex of the patient or the duration of anaesthesia does not affect the MAC.

## UPTAKE AND DISTRIBUTION

### Initial uptake

When a steady concentration of anaesthetic agent is introduced into the inspired gas, it enters the alveoli and is taken up by the blood. As it is taken up, the concentration in the blood rises and that in the alveoli falls. When this blood perfuses the body, the anaesthetic agent begins to enter the tissues and, on arrival in the pulmonary arteries, the venous blood has an anaesthetic tension considerably less than when it previously left the lungs. While this delivery in the tissues has been occurring, the alveolar concentration

**Table 33.7 Mean values and confidence intervals for the MAC and minimum infusion rate (MIR) ($ED_{50}$), and $ED_{95}$ of some inhalational and intravenous agents**

| Agent | MAC or MIR ($ED_{50}$) in oxygen–air | 95% confidence limits of $ED_{50}$ | $ED_{95}$ | $ED_{50}$ : $ED_{95}$ |
|---|---|---|---|---|
| Halothane | 0.75 | 0.5–1.1 | 0.9 | 1.2 |
| Isoflurane | 1.17 | 1.1–1.7 | 1.63 | 1.4 |
| Enflurane | 1.63 | 0.9–1.75 | 1.88 | 1.4 |
| Sevoflurane | 1.8 | | 2.1 | 1.2 |
| Desflurane | 6.6 | | | |
| Propofol | 130.0 | 105–170 | 350 | 2.7 |
| Methohexitone | 66.0 | 25–109 | 81 | 1.2 |

The MAC is given in % (v/v) and the MIR in μg/kg per min. Confidence limits vary widely in the literature. Data derived from the same sources as Tables 33.5 and 33.6 and, in addition, from Sear JW *et al. Anaesthesia* 1983;38:931; Turtle MJ *et al. Br J Anaesth* 1987;59:283; de Jong RH *et al. Anesthesiology* 1975;42,384; Leslie K and Crankshaw DP. *Br J Anaesth* 1990;64:734; Katoh T and Ikeda K. *Anesthesiology* 1987;66:301.

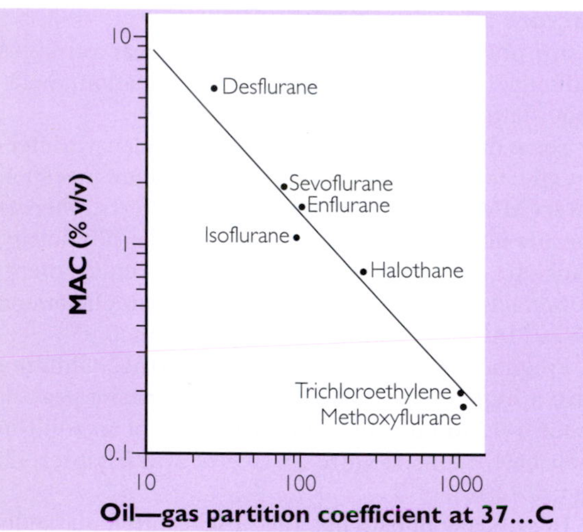


**Figure 33.10** The relationship between the oil–gas partition coefficient and the minimum alveolar concentration (MAC) for different anaesthetic agents.

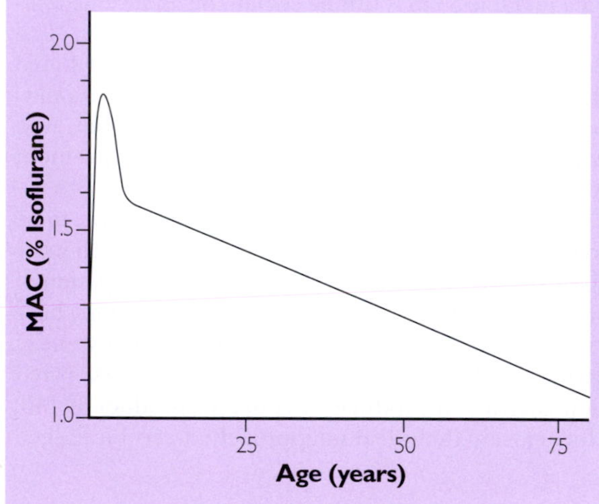


**Figure 33.11** The variation of minimum alveolar concentration (MAC) for isoflurane with age. (Adapted from Le Dez KM and Lerman J. *Anesthesiology* 1987;67:301.)

will have been increased by continued alveolar ventilation with fresh gas. In its next passage through the lung, anaesthetic agent will again be taken up by the blood, but less rapidly than on the first pass. Gradually, over time, the body will become more saturated with anaesthetic agent, less will be extracted from the lungs, and eventually, when there is complete saturation, the alveolar concentration will equal the inspired concentration. At each stage, the end-capillary tension of the agent can be approximated by the partial pressure of the agent in the alveolar plateau of the expired gas.

In this way, the rise in alveolar tension of the anaesthetic agent can be plotted with time to observe how it approaches the inspired tension. This is demonstrated in Figure 33.12. It can be seen that all the curves rise steeply initially, and then progressively less so with time in an exponential fashion (see Chapter 37). The differences between their rates of rise are to be expected from their blood–gas partition coefficients (see Table 33.5), because those agents that are most soluble will require the greatest delivery of total agent to produce a given partial pressure (see Figure 33.7). We therefore find that the less soluble an agent is in blood (as defined by its blood–gas partition coefficient), the more rapid its onset of action.

### Concentration and second gas effects

In Figure 33.12, the vertical axis represents the ratio of the alveolar to the inspired partial pressure of agent. Consequently, if the initial inspired partial pressure was doubled or trebled, so would each of the alveolar partial pressures at the same time after start of administration. Thus the system is a linear, first-order, exponential, wash-in process (see Chapter 37). This has been confirmed in practice for most agents inhaled at concentrations of less than 10%.

| Table 33.8 Physiological and pharmacological variables that alter MAC | |
|---|---|
| Variables that increase MAC | Variables that decrease MAC |
| **Physiological** | |
| Hyperthermia (> 40°C) ↑ | Hypothermia (< 30°C) ↓↓ |
| Hyperthyroidism ↑ | Hypothyroidism ↓ |
| Infants ↑ | Pre-term babies and neonates ↓ |
| Children ↑ | Old age ↓ |
| Anxiety ? ↑ | Pregnancy ↓ |
| Hypernatraemia ? ↑ | Hyponatraemia ? ↓ |
| | Hypotension (including induced) ↓ |
| | Hypoxia (< 5 kPa) ↓ |
| | Metabolic acidosis ↓ |
| | Hypo-osmolality ↓ |
| **Pharmacological** | |
| High catecholamines ↑ | Low catecholamines ↓ |
| Acute amphetamine intake ↑↑↑ | Chronic amphetamine abuse ↓ |
| Chronic ethanol abuse ↑ | Acute ethanol intake ↓ to ↓↓ |
| Chronic opioid abuse ↑ | Acute opioid use ↓ to ↓↓ |
| | Benzodiazepines ↓ |
| | Clonidine ↓ |
| | Chlorpromazine ↓ |
| | Barbiturates ↓ to ↓↓ |
| | Lithium ↓ |

This table is adapted in part from Calvey TN and Williams NE. *Principles and Practice of Pharmacology for Anaesthetists*, 3rd edn. Oxford: Blackwell Science, 1997: 245.↑ or ↓ = 0–30% change; ↑↑ to ↓↓ = 30–60% change; ↑↑↑ = > 60% change.

There is, however, one important exception to this – high concentrations of $N_2O$. At inspired concentrations greater than 20%, the rate of rise at which the alveolar concentration (FA) approaches the inspired concentration (FI) is greater the higher the inspired concentration. In other words, the time taken for the alveolar concentration to reach 50% of the inspired value (50% *FA*/*FI*) will be less with 70% $N_2O$ than with 20% $N_2O$. This is a phenomenon known as the concentration effect and is shown in Figure 33.13.

The reason for this concentration effect is that, at high concentrations, the actual volume of $N_2O$ taken up into the lungs is such that more gas is drawn into the alveoli from the respiratory bronchioles under passive transport processes. This has the action of increasing the effective alveolar ventilation and, with it, the rate of rise of alveolar partial pressure. It might be argued that this would be countered by the elution of nitrogen into the alveoli to replace the $N_2O$ taken up. The solubility of nitrogen compared with $N_2O$ (see Table 33.5) is, however, 30 times less, so it does little to offset the uptake of the $N_2O$.

A consequence of the rapid absorption of $N_2O$ secondary to a high administered concentration is that the rapid uptake of $N_2O$ from the alveolus has the effect of increasing the alveolar delivery of the other co-administered gases. Consequently, the rate of delivery of a volatile agent in the inspired gas mixture is correspondingly increased, causing a more rapid approach to the inspired concentration. This is known as the second gas effect and is also shown in Figure 33.13.

### Distribution

Inhaled anaesthetics are distributed from the lungs to the body tissues in an analogous way to the redistribution of an intravenous dose of drug from the venous blood. Thus, the body can be approximated to a number of groups of tissues with similar solubilities (and hence a similar capacity for storage) with differing blood supplies carrying the anaesthetic to and from them. This is summarized in Table 33.9.

It should be noted that, although Table 33.9 suggests well-defined anatomical regions, these really represent mathematically conceptualized compartments rather than true physiological groupings. This point is discussed in more detail in Chapter 19. It is, nevertheless, an instructive way of interpreting uptake and distribution phenomena.

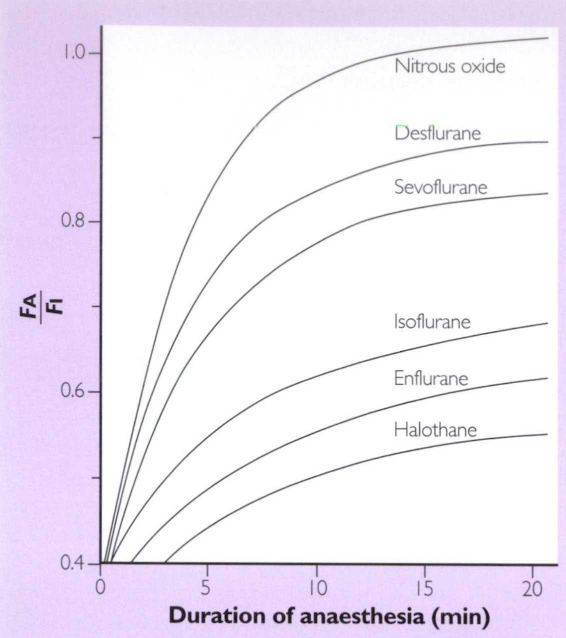


**Figure 33.12** The approach of the fractional alveolar concentration (*F*A) to the fractional inspired vapour concentration (*F*I) with time for inhalational agents in current use. Note that the less soluble the agent (i.e. the lower the blood–gas partition coefficient), the faster the rise in this ratio to its asymptotic value of unity.

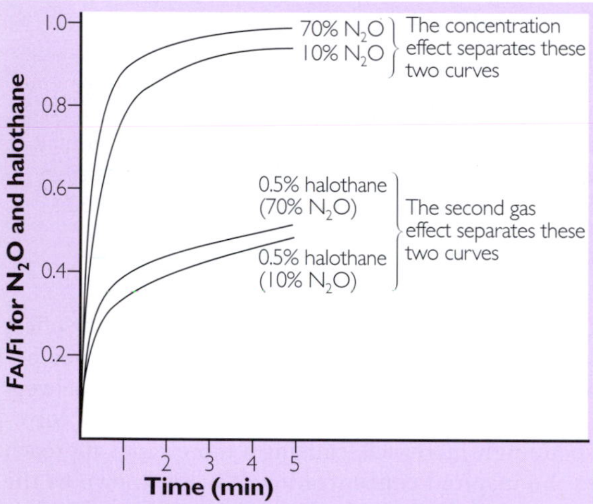


**Figure 33.13** A demonstration of the concentration and second gas effects. See text for details. (Adapted from Epstein RM *et al. Anesthesiology* 1964;25:364.)

The visceral compartment, which includes brain, heart, liver, and kidneys, has a good blood supply but a small storage capacity for anaesthetic. Muscle is a large tissue and therefore it has a medium-to-large storage capacity related to this mass, and fat, although being only a small (large in some cases!) mass of tissue, has a large storage capacity because anaesthetics are very soluble in fat. Fat, however, has the poorest blood supply of the three compartments and so accumulation of anaesthetic takes place only slowly despite the potential size of the depot. These concepts are represented graphically in Figure 33.14.

An intuitive way of representing the significance of factors can be understood by considering an analogy developed by Mapleson, based on water tanks. The flow of water through the pipes to the tanks has been shown in practice, as well as in theory, to behave very similarly to the uptake and distribution of inhaled anaesthetics (Figure 33.15).

In this analogy, the water corresponds to the anaesthetic, the water tanks represent the anaesthetic storage capacity of the compartments, and the pipes represent the ability of the blood to supply that compartment. The level of water in the tanks is analogous to the partial pressure of anaesthetic agent in that tissue compartment. The mouth tank represents the inspired partial pressure in the anaesthetic breathing system, and the pipe between the mouth and lungs allows for the effects of ventilation. As this can be variable, there is a tap controlling the flow of water from the mouth to the lungs.

In the visceral compartment (see Table 33.9), the water level will quickly reach the same level as that in the lung tank because it has a large pipe and a relatively low volume. The result in practice is that the partial pressures of agent in the lung and vessel-rich viscera rapidly reach equilibration. The depth of anaesthesia is determined by the partial pressure of anaesthetic in the brain (which is the same as the other components of the visceral compartment) and is proportional to the height of water in the visceral tank for a given agent, i.e. in this schematic representation the higher the water level in the visceral tank, the deeper the level of anaesthesia.

On the other hand, water will fill the muscle and fat tanks more slowly as a result of the small pipes and the large tank volumes, and it will be a long time before the levels in these tanks reach the same levels as in the lung tank. In the case of inhaled anaesthetic agents, the partial pressure of the agent in both muscle and fat will be below the level of that in the alveolus during the

**Table 33.9 Blood supply and volume of tissue compartments and their storage capacity for inhalational agents**

| Tissue compartment | Relative blood supply | Tissue volume | Storage capacity |
|---|---|---|---|
| Viscera: heart brain, kidneys, liver | Good | Small | Small |
| Muscle | Moderate | Large | Medium to large |
| Fat | Poor | Small to large | Very large |

course of the anaesthetic, even if the anaesthetic is continued for several hours. This can also be appreciated from a consideration of Figure 33.14.

Metabolism would be represented by a hole in the tank of a size proportional to the rate of metabolism although, as modern agents are not metabolized to any clinically significant degree (with the exception of halothane – see later), this is ignored in the model.

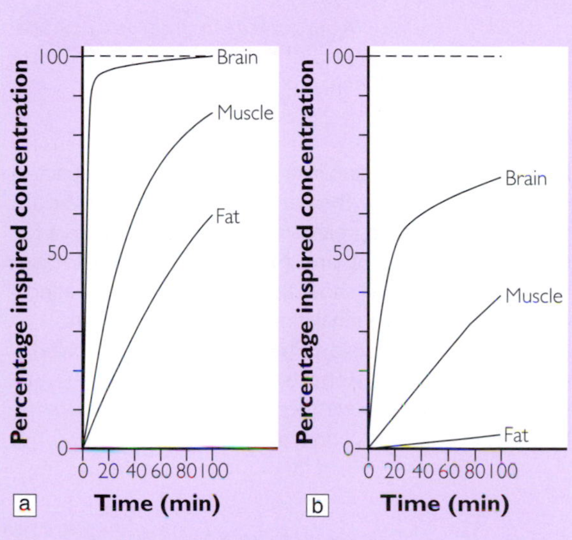


**Figure 33.14** The uptake characteristics of (a) nitrous oxide (the most insoluble agent in current use) and (b) halothane (the most soluble agent in current use). The curves show the variability in the rate of rise of partial pressure in brain, muscle, and fat. (Adapted from Eger EI. Applications of a mathematical model of gas uptake. In: Papper EM and Kits RJ, eds. *Uptake and Distribution of Anaesthetic Agents*. New York: McGraw Hill, 1963.)

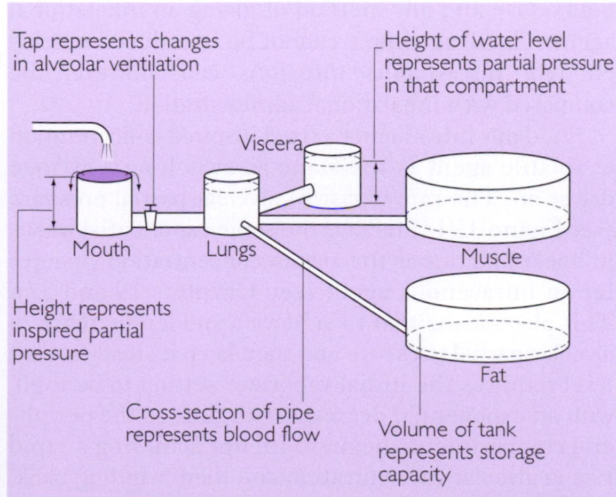


**Figure 33.15** The water tank analogy for the distribution of inhaled anaesthetic agents. (Adapted from Mapleson WW. Pharmacokinetics of inhaled anaesthetics. In: Prys-Roberts C and Hug CC, eds. *Pharmacokinetics of Anaesthesia*. Oxford: Blackwell Scientific Publications, 1984: 89.)

Accepting this as the basic model of inhaled anaesthetic uptake by the body, some of the components of the system will now be examined more closely to determine how they affect its performance and the manner in which they are altered under special circumstances.

### *Varying the inspired concentration*

For agents in clinical use, there is rapid equilibration between the lung and visceral compartments as a result of the excellent blood supply. This is depicted by the large pipe connecting the two (see Figure 33.15) and is also apparent in Figure 33.14. Let us first consider the situation where the level in the mouth tank is reduced in size as shown in Figure 33.16. Here there is a lower water level in the lungs and viscera when these two reach their equilibrium. The pressure of water in the system is reduced because the height of the water in the mouth tank (the partial pressure) has been reduced but the pipe sizes remain the same. Although the driving pressure is reduced, we do not need to fill the visceral tank to the same height to reach equilibrium so the time to reach equilibrium is approximately the same.

The exceptions to this are the concentration and second gas effects mentioned above.

### *Effects of ventilation*

Now consider the effects of adjusting the tap in the pipe between the mouth and lung tanks (see Figure 33.15), while replacing any water lost from the mouth tank with water from our water source, i.e. keep the mouth tank level unchanged. As the tap is opened, the flow of water from the mouth to the lung compartments increases and so the rate of rise of water in the lung tank also increases. Similarly, as the tap is partially closed, the water flow and the rate of rise of the water level will decrease.

Thus, increases in minute volume allow more anaesthetic to enter the lungs more quickly and, conversely when the minute volume falls, the passage of inhaled anaesthetic to the lungs is reduced. Consequently, increases in minute volume produce an increase in the rate of rise of partial pressure of the agent in the lung (which rapidly equilibrates with the brain) and low minute volumes will slow this rate of rise. Increasing

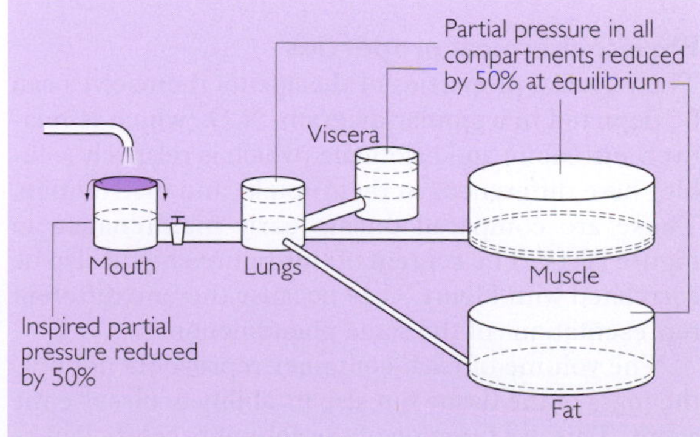


**Figure 33.16** The water tank model showing the effect of reducing the inspired partial pressure by 50%. The level at 50% reduction in the fat compartment is not shown for clarity.

minute volume will thus reduce the induction time of a gaseous induction technique, whereas hypoventilation and breath-holding (common during gaseous induction, see Chapter 2) result in an increased induction time.

### *Effect of cardiac output*

Variation in the sizes of the pipes leading from the lung tank to the visceral, muscle, and fat tanks represents changes in the blood flow to the various compartments (see Figure 33.15). The total of their individual increases represents an increase in cardiac output.

As cardiac output increases, the outflow of water from the lung tank will be increased, whereas the inflow to the lung tank is constant. Therefore, the balance is to produce a slower rate of rise in the lung tank. The visceral tank will be at the same level as the lung tank, although the level will be reached much more quickly as a result of the larger pipe connecting the two, but again the rate of rise of the visceral tank will be reduced in line with that of the lung tank. Consequently, and paradoxically, a rise in cardiac output in the presence of constant ventilation increases the time of induction. This can be appreciated by a simple numerical model.

If we assume that 10 ml of agent A (an imaginary inhaled anaesthetic) dissolves in 100 ml of blood, then a cardiac output of 5 L/min will remove 500 ml/min from the lungs and carry it to the tissues. However, a cardiac output of 10 L/min will remove 1000 ml/min of agent A from the lungs. This reduces the rate of rise of the alveolar level of agent A and hence the brain level, because these two are in rapid equilibrium, and so slows the rate at which we achieve our desired brain partial pressure.

With low cardiac output states, the reverse situation occurs. The removal of agent from the lungs is reduced while ventilation maintains the supply of agent. The net result is that the lung concentration rises more quickly. As a result of autoregulation, blood flow to the brain is preserved at the expense of that to other organs, so equilibration occurs rapidly.

Thus, with inhaled agents, we have observed that high-output states are associated with a slow induction of anaesthesia whereas low-output states accelerate induction. Note the difference with an intravenous induction agent when anaesthesia occurs more rapidly in the presence of a high cardiac output.

## Physicochemical properties

The physical properties of the agents themselves can be depicted in a similar diagram. $N_2O$ (which is relatively insoluble) and halothane (which is relatively soluble) have differences in their uptake and distribution. These are compared during early maintenance in Figure 33.17. The content of this figure should also be correlated with Figure 33.14 because they are different representations of the same phenomenon.

The volume of each container represents not only the mass of the tissue but also its ability to dissolve the agent. This is a function of the solubility coefficient as explained earlier in the chapter. The higher the oil–gas solubility coefficient, the larger the fat tank. A low blood–gas coefficient means that very little drug will be carried off by the blood from the lungs so lung partial pressures will rise quickly. This is represented by small pipes. Agents that are highly soluble in blood will be carried away more readily from the lungs by blood, as represented by an increase in the diameter of the pipes connecting the tanks. These analogies are clearly seen in Figure 33.17 by comparing the drawings for $N_2O$ and halothane.

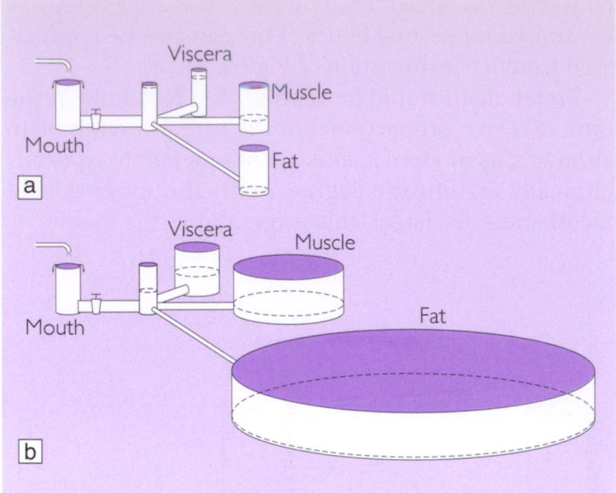


**Figure 33.17** The application of the water compartment model to show the partial pressures in the various compartments during early maintenance anaesthesia for (a) $N_2O$ and (b) halothane. Nitrous oxide and halothane have been chosen to show the range of solubility effects in currently available inhalational anaesthetic agents. (Adapted from Mapleson. Pharmacokinetics of inhaled anaesthetics. In: Prys-Roberts C and Hug CC, eds. *Pharmacokinetics of Anaesthesia*. Oxford: Blackwell Scientific Publications, 1984: 89.)

## Comparison of the pharmacokinetics of volatile and intravenous agents

There is no direct analogy between an intravenous bolus dose and any method of giving an inhalational agent. The drug simply cannot be introduced quickly enough. Intravenous infusions can, however, be compared with inhalational administration.

Suddenly introducing a fixed inspired concentration of volatile agent is the same as switching a syringe driver on. The rate of rise of alveolar partial pressure (see Figure 33.12) follows the same exponential wash-in linear kinetics as the serum concentration changes for an intravenous agent (see Chapters 19 and 32). This also means that to achieve a sudden increase in alveolar partial pressure and then keep it steady at that level requires the initial vaporizer setting to be high, with an exponential decrease with time as the peripheral compartments begin to fill up. Achieving a rapid rise in alveolar concentration and then 'winding back' is called using 'over-pressure'.

Figure 33.18 shows a three-stage decreasing vaporizer setting regimen that is designed rapidly to achieve and then maintain the same alveolar partial pressure. This should be compared with the three-stage infusion pump regimen shown in Figure 32.12. The similarity is obvious.

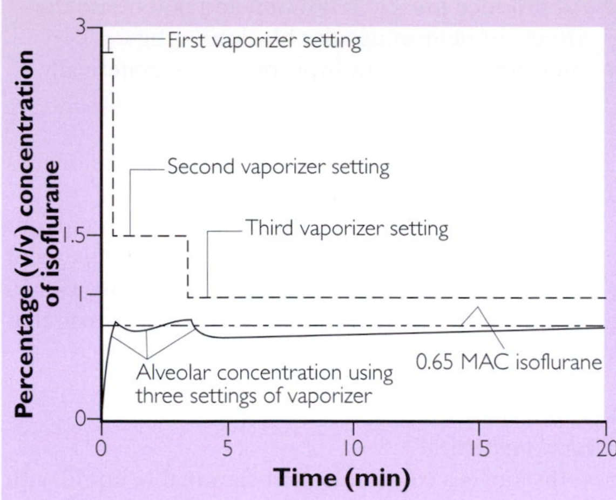


**Figure 33.18** The use of a three-stage vaporizer setting regimen to produce a rapid increase of the alveolar concentration and then to maintain it at a constant level using isoflurane in 70% nitrous oxide. See text for details. (Adapted from Mapleson WW. Pharmacokinetics of inhalational anaesthetics. In: Nunn JF, Utting JE, Brown BR, eds. *General Anaesthesia*, 5th edn. London: Butterworths, 1989: 44.)

## INDIVIDUAL AGENTS

### Nitrous oxide

#### *History*

$N_2O$ was discovered by Joseph Priestley in 1772, but its usefulness to medical science did not become apparent until 1844 when Horace Wells, a Connecticut dentist, noticed that it was a very potent analgesic.

Before this time and continuing for some years after, $N_2O$ was also what would be termed today a 'recreational drug', with the affluent in society gathering for so-called 'laughing gas' parties. It was at a lecture-demonstration of these effects that Wells made his now famous observation that a member of the audience who had inhaled $N_2O$ gashed his leg badly and seemed oblivious to the pain that he must have experienced. Wells attributed the analgesia to the effect of the inhaled $N_2O$, and subsequently successfully utilized $N_2O$ to alleviate the pain of dental extraction.

However, Wells' demonstration of $N_2O$ to a group of medical students at the Massachusetts General Hospital was a failure, with the patient screaming in pain as the tooth was extracted. Unfortunately, $N_2O$ fell into disrepute for some time, with first ether and then chloroform being preferred. However, $N_2O$ remains the only nineteenth-century anaesthetic agent still commonly used today.

#### *Synthesis*

$N_2O$ is synthesized from the thermal decomposition of ammonium nitrate at around 250°C:

$$NH_4NO_3 + \text{Heat} \rightarrow N_2O + 2H_2O.$$

After purification, the resulting product is usually 99.5% $N_2O$; traces of higher oxides of nitrogen, carbon dioxide, carbon monoxide, and water account for the other 0.5% of the mixture.

#### *Clinical effects*

$N_2O$ is a sweet-smelling, non-irritant, colourless gas. With an MAC value of 104, and the need to supply oxygen, it is insufficient to provide anaesthesia as a sole agent. $N_2O$ is relatively insoluble, does not undergo metabolism in the body, and is excreted unchanged. This does not mean, however, that the body is ever completely saturated with $N_2O$ and uptake ceases. In totally closed circuit anaesthesia, after the initial uptake kinetics have been satisfied, there is still a need to continue supplying it at approximately 100 ml/min (Figure 33.19). This is presumably to counter losses into spaces such as the gastrointestinal tract and evaporation from the skin.

#### *Analgesia*

$N_2O$ has long been recognized as a potent analgesic at subanaesthetic doses and evidence is now emerging of a likely mechanism for this effect. The major inhibitory neurotransmitter in mammalian brains is γ-aminobutyric acid (GABA) whereas the major excitatory transmitter is glutamate. GABA functions by activating fast neurotransmitter-gated receptors, allowing the influx of chloride ions and thus hyperpolarizing the cell. Glutamate is the transmitter at the *N*-methyl-D-aspartate (NMDA) receptor, having an excitatory effect on its target cell. Many inhalational and intravenous anaesthetics (with the notable exception of ketamine) potentiate the action of GABA at its receptor, thereby inhibiting synaptic transmission, while having little or no effect on NMDA receptors. It had been assumed that $N_2O$ had similar effects. However, it has recently been discovered that $N_2O$ antagonizes the NMDA receptor, but has no effect at GABA receptors.

NMDA receptors are involved in the processes of memory, learning, and pain perception and this may go some way to explain the analgesic effects of $N_2O$, which may occur via blockade of spinal cord NMDA receptors. Other NMDA antagonists such as ketamine are known for their analgesic and psychotomimetic properties – possibly accounting for the euphoric effects that made $N_2O$ so popular in the nineteenth century.

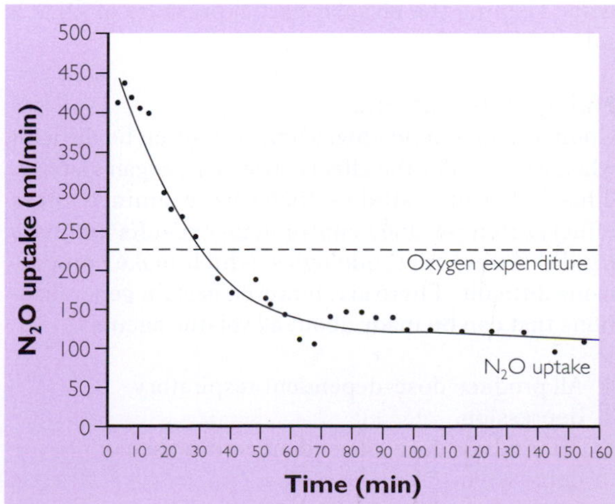


**Figure 33.19** The uptake of nitrous oxide ($N_2O$) from a totally closed circuit with time. (Adapted from Barton F and Nunn JF. *Br J Anaesth* 1975;47:350.)

Cell death after head trauma and hypoxia is mediated via NMDA receptors and NMDA antagonists afford protection to the cells following such insults. $N_2O$ has a similar neuroprotective effect, but unfortunately, like other NMDA antagonists, it also produces a neurotoxicity of its own, thus limiting its potential for use as a neuroprotectant after an insult.

The NMDA-mediated neurotoxicity is obtunded by concurrent GABA stimulation – as occurs with administration of inhalational and intravenous anaesthetics. It is therefore hypothetically possible (although experimentally or clinically unproven) that the co-administration of other anaesthetics with $N_2O$ protects against the potential neurotoxic effects of $N_2O$ mediated via NMDA antagonism.

### *Diffusion hypoxia*

In 1955 Fink, a New York anaesthetist, was the first to explain a then well-recognized phenomenon in which patients became cyanosed in the recovery area after anaesthesia involving $N_2O$ and oxygen, despite seemingly adequate ventilation.

$N_2O$ is administered in high concentrations during anaesthesia, often as high as 70% in oxygen. It is, however, 35 times more soluble than nitrogen and 20 times more soluble than oxygen in blood. This is discussed above in the 'concentration effect'. At the end of the anaesthetic administration, when the inspired gases are changed from a $N_2O/O_2$ mixture to a $N_2/O_2$ mixture, 20 times more $N_2O$ diffuses from the blood into the alveoli than $O_2$ diffuses into the blood. This results in a reduction in the partial pressure of $O_2$ because of dilution by the $N_2O$ being excreted into the alveoli. If the patient is allowed to breathe room air ($F\text{IO}_2$ of 0.21), the partial pressure of $O_2$ in the alveoli will fall below normal levels, leading to arterial hypoxaemia.

To overcome this, and thereby avoid arterial hypoxaemia, we can administer higher inspired concentrations of $O_2$ in the recovery period to increase the partial pressure of $O_2$ in the alveoli. An alternative approach is to stop $N_2O$ administration before the end of the anaesthetic (while maintaining anaesthesia with another agent) and revert to a high concentration of $O_2$ in air (or 100% $O_2$) to allow the wash-out of $N_2O$, while keeping the alveolar partial pressure of $O_2$ at a safe level.

## Halogenated agents

Comparison of individual agents can often be difficult when we consider the effects on specific organ systems. This is because studies that have examined these effects often produce contradictory results and have used different methodologies, which make comparisons difficult. There are, however, certain generalizations that can be made about all volatile agents:

- All produce dose-dependent respiratory depression.
- All produce dose-dependent cardiovascular depression.
- All produce dose-dependent narcosis.
- All have the potential to increase intracranial pressure (ICP).
- All relax uterine smooth muscle.
- All produce muscle relaxation and potentiate the effects of neuromuscular blocking drugs.
- All trigger malignant hyperpyrexia in genetically susceptible patients.

The degree to which each of these effects occurs differs from agent to agent.

Each of the volatile halogenated agents in current use is described below. All are preservative free, except halothane, which contains thymol 0.01%. They can all be used safely with soda lime; the breakdown that occurs with sevoflurane is discussed later.

### *Sevoflurane*

#### *Physical properties*

Sevoflurane is a colourless, non-flammable liquid with a mild ethereal odour which is well tolerated when inhaled. It has an MAC value of 1.8, and, as a result of its low blood–gas solubility of 0.68, the alveolar concentration approaches inspired concentration relatively rapidly, causing a rapid onset of anaesthesia during inhalational induction (see Figure 33.12). About 5% of the administered dose is metabolized by the liver.

#### *Neurological effects*

As with other inhalational anaesthetics, sevoflurane produces a dose-dependent increase in cerebral blood flow (CBF) and ICP. However, under hypocapnic conditions in both humans and animals, 1 MAC does not produce a rise in ICP. The responsiveness of cerebral vasculature to changes in $CO_2$ is maintained under sevoflurane anaesthesia; however, this is greatly diminished by the concomitant administration of $N_2O$. The cerebral metabolic rate of $O_2$ consumption ($\text{CMRO}_2$) is reduced but, unlike isoflurane and desflurane, autoregulation (the process of maintaining CBF constant over a wide range of cerebral perfusion pressures – see Chapter 22) is preserved.

#### *Cardiovascular effects*

Sevoflurane does not sensitize the myocardium to the effects of endogenous or exogenous catecholamines, and its administration does not result in tachycardia as is the case with isoflurane and desflurane. It depresses cardiac output and systemic vascular resistance (SVR) in a similar dose-dependent fashion to isoflurane, and appears to produce vasodilatation by a direct action on vascular smooth muscle. It has minimal effect on coronary vasculature and does not produce 'coronary steal'. Liver blood flow is preserved to the same degree as with isoflurane and significantly better than with either halothane or enflurane.

#### *Respiratory effects*

As with all inhalational anaesthetics, sevoflurane produces a dose-dependent increase in respiratory rate and a decrease in tidal volume, resulting in an overall decrease in minute volume which in turn causes a rise in arterial partial pressure of carbon dioxide. At concentrations greater than 1 MAC, this is more pronounced than that resulting from either halothane or enflurane. It does not produce airway irritation and is likely to become the agent of choice for inhalational induction. It is a bronchodilator, inhibits hypoxic pulmonary vasoconstriction, produces a degree of muscle relaxation, and enhances the effects of neuromuscular blocking drugs.

Its relative insolubility makes sevoflurane a good agent for day-case anaesthesia.

### Desflurane

#### Physical properties

Desflurane is a halogenated ether, structurally related to isoflurane and enflurane. Compared with the other volatile anaesthetics, it is very insoluble, with a blood–gas partition coefficient of 0.42 and an oil–gas partition coefficient of 18.7. As a result of the low oil–gas partition coefficient, its potency is low, with an MAC value of 6. However, its low solubility in blood means that the onset of anaesthesia and recovery are rapid. It approaches the speed of $N_2O$ during induction and is approximately 2–2.5 times faster than either halothane or isoflurane.

Desflurane is not degraded by carbon dioxide absorbers at temperatures below 60°C. Although it can be degraded to produce carbon monoxide at clinical temperatures, this breakdown is attenuated by the water content encountered in absorbers during clinical use. Only 0.02% of the administered dose is metabolized and increases in inorganic fluoride concentrations are not seen.

Conventional vaporizers are not designed to work with volatile agents at or near their boiling points because of the steep nature of the temperature/vapour pressure curve. The temperature of a desflurane vaporizer has to be above the boiling point (it is actually at 39°C, achieved by electrical heating), which produces a gas under pressure. This is then pressure-reduced and in effect injected into the fresh gas flow.

#### Neurological effects

There is a dose-dependent increase in CBF and a decrease in cerebrovascular resistance and $CMRO_2$. At 1 MAC this results in a rise in ICP. The cerebral vascular response to carbon dioxide is maintained. It impairs cerebral autoregulation, which is almost absent at levels of 1.5 MAC.

#### Cardiovascular effects

Cardiovascular function is depressed with central venous pressure and heart rate increasing, whereas SVR, contractility, and mean arterial pressure (MAP) decrease. Despite a decrease in stroke volume, cardiac output is maintained as a result of the tachycardia produced. These effects are maximal in the first 90 min or so of anaesthesia and during prolonged anaesthesia – lasting several hours – the effects are reduced, indicating the development of a degree of cardiovascular tolerance.

When large increases in concentration are made quickly on the first commencement of the agent, there can often be an initial phase of sympathetic stimulation resulting in hypertension and tachycardia.

Desflurane does not reduce hepatic arterial blood flow, although it slightly reduces portal venous blood flow, and it does not sensitize the heart to catecholamines.

#### Respiratory effects

As with all inhalational anaesthetics, there is a decrease in minute volume and tidal volume with an accompanying increase in respiratory rate, and the response to carbon dioxide is obtunded. At concentrations of 1 MAC it is a respiratory irritant, resulting in a high incidence of breath-holding and laryngospasm. There are often excessive secretions and apnoea and coughing are common.

#### Clinical use

In both adults and children, there is a high incidence of reflex airway irritation, which limits the use of desflurane for inhalational induction despite its highly desirable pharmacokinetic profile. A gradual increase in the inspired concentration reduces these respiratory problems, as can prior administration of fentanyl or midazolam.

The rapid recovery characteristics (which are significantly faster than for other inhalational anaesthetics but not for propofol) make it a suitable drug for use in ambulatory (day-case) anaesthesia.

Its use is not recommended for induction in children because of its respiratory effects.

### Isoflurane

#### Physical properties

Isoflurane has been available in the UK since 1983, and is a non-flammable, stable, volatile anaesthetic which has a somewhat pungent odour. It is stable in light, does not attack metals, and is not degraded by soda lime. It has a similar vapour pressure to halothane and so, although not to be recommended, it could be used in the same type of vaporizer as halothane.

It has a low blood–gas solubility of 1.4 and a MAC of 1.15; as such it should produce a rapid induction of anaesthesia. However, as a result of its respiratory irritant effects in clinical practice, this is often not the case because of the incidence of coughing and breath-holding.

Only 0.2% of the administered dose is metabolized and the resultant nephrotoxic inorganic fluoride ion concentrations are very low and clinically insignificant, even after prolonged anaesthesia.

It shows no spontaneous degradation even after 5 years on the shelf.

#### Neurological effects

In concentrations of less than 1 MAC, isoflurane does not significantly increase CBF and reduces $CMRO_2$. Vasoconstriction in response to hypocapnia is preserved, as is cerebral autoregulation. These properties mean that isoflurane produces a minimal rise (if any) in ICP during anaesthesia. It does not, unlike enflurane, affect either cerebrospinal fluid (CSF) production or reabsorption which also contributes to the minimal rise in ICP.

#### Cardiovascular effects

There is depression of myocardial contractility in a dose-dependent manner but this effect is less *in vivo* than that seen *in vitro*. This is probably the result of a direct β-adrenergic effect, a view supported by the tachycardia and vasodilatation that are also seen. Systemic arterial pressure falls as a result of a drop in peripheral vascular resistance, whereas cardiac output is maintained.

Isoflurane is a coronary vasodilator and there is some concern over the possibility of 'coronary steal' in patients with ischaemic heart disease. If the patient has a diseased coronary artery that is unable to dilate, and the other coronary arteries dilate and thus reduce their perfusion pressure, there is a possibility that blood will be diverted from the area of supply of the diseased artery to that of the healthy vasodilated arteries, resulting in local ischaemia or infarction. This has been demonstrated to occur in some studies but not in others, and so it must remain an area of controversy. Nevertheless, isoflurane should be used with care in patients with ischaemic heart disease, and efforts should be made to maintain mean arterial pressure (MAP) (avoiding hypertension) and prevent excessive tachycardia.

Isoflurane obtunds the pulmonary vasoconstrictive response to hypoxia, although probably not to a clinically significant extent, and it does not sensitize the heart to catecholamines.

As with all inhalational anaesthetics, there is an additive myocardial depressant effect with calcium channel blockers, but as isoflurane produces the least myocardial depression it provides the largest margin of safety.

Reduction in liver blood flow is less than that seen with halothane or enflurane.

*Respiratory effects*

There is the same qualitative reduction in minute ventilation as with the other volatile anaesthetics. Quantitatively, however, this is less than that for enflurane and greater than that for halothane at equipotent concentrations. As with the other volatile agents, this respiratory depression can be partially offset by surgical stimulus, but in the absence of stimulus apnoea usually occurs at concentrations of 2 MAC with all agents.

Isoflurane is a bronchodilator with a similar quantitative effect to halothane.

*Clinical use*

Isoflurane is a good, general purpose agent. The minimal effect on ICP and CBF means that isoflurane has become a popular agent for use in neuroanaesthesia. Likewise, despite the risk of coronary steal, the ability of isoflurane to preserve cardiac output has meant that it has found popularity in anaesthesia for patients with pre-existing cardiovascular disease. Its pungent odour makes it less than ideal (despite its relatively low blood–gas solubility) for use in inhalational inductions.

### Enflurane

*Physical properties*

Enflurane is a clear, colourless, non-flammable, ether anaesthetic, which has been available in the UK since 1978. It does not corrode metal and requires no preservative. Isoflurane and enflurane are structural isomers and, as for isoflurane, enflurane is not significantly degraded by soda lime. It has a relatively pleasant odour, a blood–gas solubility of 1.91, and an MAC of 1.7. About 2% of the administered dose undergoes metabolism.

*Neurological effects*

CBF increases less than with halothane, and in some studies enflurane has been shown to produce only a small rise compared with awake levels. It has, however, been consistently shown to produce a dose-related decrease in $CMRO_2$. Under enflurane anaesthesia at low MAC, hypocapnia causes a decrease in CBF as a result of an increase in vascular resistance, so carbon dioxide responsiveness is maintained. In concentrations of less than 2% and during controlled ventilation, enflurane has little effect on the ICP.

Epileptiform activity on the EEG has been reported and this activity is made worse by increasing doses of enflurane and by hypocapnia. The changes are reversible with hypercapnia.

*Cardiovascular effects*

In humans *in vivo*, contrary to *in vitro* findings, enflurane produces less myocardial depression than halothane, although more than that seen with isoflurane. There are dose-dependent decreases in both SVR and MAP with an increase in preload – which results in an increase in myocardial oxygen demand. Enflurane would, however, appear to cause less vasodilatation than does isoflurane.

There is no sensitization of the myocardium to effects of catecholamines, but at higher concentrations enflurane often produces a nodal rhythm as a result of prolongation of the atrioventricular node conduction time. The incidence of potentially serious arrhythmias is less than that seen with halothane.

*Respiratory effects*

As with other volatile agents, enflurane produces respiratory depression, although compared with other agents it produces more respiratory depression at equipotent concentrations. It reduces the ventilatory response to carbon dioxide and hypoxia, is a bronchodilator, and is well tolerated during inhalational induction.

*Clinical use*

Enflurane is widely used in anaesthetic practice. It is well tolerated during inhalational induction, and has less arrhythmic potential than halothane, although in this situation it would seem likely that sevoflurane will become the drug of choice.

It should not be used in patients with epilepsy, nor should it be used in situations where hyperventilation resulting in hypocapnia is likely to be employed, because hypocapnia, even in normal individuals, results in epileptiform EEG changes.

### Halothane

*Physical properties*

This was the first halogenated ether anaesthetic, introduced in the late 1950s; it is a colourless, non-flammable liquid with a similar vapour pressure to isoflurane. It spontaneously degrades in light and has to be kept in a darkened bottle with the addition of a preservative (thymol 0.01%) to prevent the generation of bromide ions.

Its blood–gas partition coefficient is 2.4 and its MAC 0.75. The relatively pleasant odour means that it does not irritate the airway. Of the administered dose 20% is metabolized; the issue of the potential resultant hepatotoxicity is discussed later.

*Neurological effects*

$CMRO_2$ is reduced and there is an increase in CBF which seems to be greater than that produced by either enflurane or isoflurane. The vasoconstrictive response to carbon dioxide is maintained; however, autoregulation becomes obtunded. On balance, halothane is likely to produce a greater rise in ICP than other volatile anaesthetics.

*Cardiovascular effects*

During anaesthesia, MAP is reduced as a result of myocardial depression in the form of a reduced cardiac output and stroke volume, with a concomitant rise in preload. In contrast to other inhalational agents, the drop in MAP is predominantly from myocardial depression rather than vasodilatation – although this also occurs to a lesser degree.

Halothane has lost favour with many anaesthetists in modern practice because of the high incidence of arrhythmias. Not only are relatively minor arrhythmias, such as nodal rhythm (common with many volatile agents), associated more frequently with halothane, but so also are potentially more dangerous ventricular arrhythmias such as ventricular bigeminy.

In addition, the presence of endogenous or exogenous catecholamines increases the frequency of these arrhythmias, as does hypercapnia and acidosis.

*Respiratory effects*

Tidal volume is reduced and respiratory rate increased with an overall reduction in minute volume. The respiratory depression is less than with enflurane, but probably greater than with isoflurane. Halothane is a non-irritant bronchodilator, which is well tolerated during inhalational induction.

*Clinical uses*

Halothane is declining in use as newer agents with improved safety properties are reducing in relative cost. This is primarily because of concerns over the arrhythmogenic potential of halothane and fears surrounding its potential hepatotoxicity.

Local anaesthetic solutions containing epinephrine (adrenaline) are commonly used for infiltration of the surgical field. Halothane is not the preferred drug if this is the case, because of the potential for arrhythmias and the availability of suitable alternative inhalational agents. Halothane is, however, still used commonly, particularly for inhalational induction during which it is well tolerated. In the absence of hypercapnia (e.g. during controlled ventilation) and with no underlying acidosis, halothane is still a safe anaesthetic agent, as proven by the large numbers of patients safely anaesthetized over almost 40 years.

The clinical properties of inhalational agents currently in use are given in Table 33.10.

## ELIMINATION AND METABOLISM

Inhalational agents are unusual in that their route of elimination is mainly through their route of introduction i.e. via the lungs. This means that their rate of removal is very dependent on alveolar ventilation and cardiac output as for their uptake but in reverse. Comparative early and late wash-out curves for volatile anaesthetic agents are shown in Figures 33.20 and 33.21. It should, however, be noted that the longer the period of administration, the longer the time of elimination.

Although the lungs are the major source of elimination, metabolism still occurs, principally in the liver. Metabolism can be estimated either by measuring metabolites or by comparison of the amount of inhaled anaesthetic with that exhaled (mass balance). These methods give different results, as shown in Table 33.11. This is not surprising because recovery of metabolites will underestimate the magnitude of metabolism unless the recovery is complete.

From such comparisons, it is probably reasonable to conclude that alveolar ventilation is almost totally responsible for the elimination of $N_2O$, desflurane, and isoflurane, principally responsible for the elimination of sevoflurane and enflurane, and 50–80% responsible for the elimination of halothane.

## TOXICITY

### Nitrous oxide

The toxic effects of $N_2O$ are a function of the duration and the concentration of the exposure. They have been measured in both animal and human studies. The potential species variability makes it difficult to extrapolate from animal studies to humans, and so the issue of toxicity remains controversial.

Haematological and neurological toxicity have been observed in humans. In animals $N_2O$ has been shown to be teratogenic; however, it must be stressed that $N_2O$ has *never* been shown to be teratogenic in humans (see also Chapter 45). There have been suggestions that $N_2O$ may reduce fertility in dental assistants repeatedly exposed to high levels.

$N_2O$ exerts its toxic effects on the blood via inhibition of the derived coenzymes of cobalamin (commonly known as vitamin B12). Cobalamin is synthesized by only a few micro-organisms, but is essential for metabolism in all animals. Humans obtain their cobalamin from meat in the diet and it is absorbed as a complex in the small intestine after combination with intrinsic factor – a small glycoprotein secreted by the stomach.

$N_2O$ oxidizes the cobalt ion in vitamin B12 from the monovalent to the divalent form, and thereby inhibits the action of methionine synthase. In the cytosol of mammalian cells, methyltetrahydrofolate is converted to tetrahydrofolate through removal of a methyl group by methylcobalamin. Methionine synthase (known more correctly as homocysteine methyl transferase) then catalyses the subsequent transfer of this methyl group to homocysteine, to produce methionine, as shown in Figure 33.22. Recovery of methionine synthase activity requires synthesis of new enzyme and this needs 3–4 days in humans. This effect, the net result of which is megaloblastic anaemia, is of importance if the duration of $N_2O$ anaesthesia exceeds 8 hours.

Inhibition of methionine synthase (in animals as well as in humans) also blocks transmethylation, thus preventing methionine or tetrahydrofolate production, or both. This is important because methionine is the

**Table 33.10 Clinical properties of inhalational anaesthetics in current use**

| Properties | Nitrous oxide | Halothane | Enflurane | Isoflurane | Desflurane | Sevoflurane |
|---|---|---|---|---|---|---|
| Onset/offset of action | Extremely rapid | Less rapid | Rapid | Rapid | Extremely rapid | Extremely rapid |
| Analgesic properties | Marked | Poor | Moderate | Moderate | Moderate | Moderate |
| Effect on respiration | Non-irritant<br>Respiratory rate ↑<br>Tidal volume ↓<br>$Pa_{CO_2}$ normal<br>Enters body cavities and air-filled spaces | Non-irritant<br>Respiratory rate ↑<br>Tidal volume ↓↓<br>$Pa_{CO_2}$ ↑ | Non-irritant<br>Respiratory rate ↑<br>Tidal volume ↓↓<br>$Pa_{CO_2}$ ↑↑ | Slightly irritant<br>Respiratory rate ↑<br>Tidal volume ↓↓<br>$Pa_{CO_2}$ ↑ | Pungent and irritant<br>Respiratory rate ↑<br>Tidal volume ↓↓<br>$Pa_{CO_2}$ ↑ | Non-irritant<br>Respiratory rate ↑<br>Tidal volume ↓↓<br>$Pa_{CO_2}$ ↑ |
| Effect on cardiovascular system | Little or no effect<br>Cardiac sensitivity to catecholamines ↑/↓ | Heart rate ↓↓<br>Blood pressure ↓↓<br>Cardiac output ↓↓<br>Peripheral resistance ↓<br>Cardiac sensitivity to catecholamines ↑↑↑ | Heart rate ↑<br>Blood pressure ↓↓<br>Cardiac output ↓<br>Peripheral resistance ↓<br>Cardiac sensitivity to catecholamines ↑ | Heart rate ↑↑<br>Blood pressure ↓↓<br>Cardiac output ↓<br>Peripheral resistance ↓↓<br>Cardiac sensitivity to catecholamines ↑<br>Coronary steal at high MAC ? | Heart rate ↑<br>Blood pressure ↓↓<br>Cardiac output ↓<br>Peripheral resistance ↓↓<br>Cardiac sensitivity to catecholamines ↑<br>Coronary steal at high MAC ? | Heart rate ↑/↓<br>Blood pressure ↓↓<br>Cardiac output ↓ (slight)<br>Peripheral resistance ↓<br>Cardiac sensitivity to catecholamines ↑<br>Coronary steal at high MAC ? |
| Effects on EEG | None | Decreased voltage<br>Burst suppression | Changes similar to grand mal or focal seizure activity and muscle twitching | Decreased voltage<br>Burst suppression | Decreased voltage<br>Burst suppression | Decreased voltage<br>Burst suppression |
| Cerebral blood flow | ↑ | ↑↑↑ | ↑ | ↑ | ↑ | ↑ |
| Potentiation of non-depolarizng neuromuscular blockade | None | Moderate | Marked | Marked | Marked | Marked |
| Effect on uterus | None | Slight relaxation | Slight relaxation | Slight relaxation | Slight relaxation | Slight relaxation |
| Metabolism (%) | Minimal | 15–45 | 2–3 | 0.2 | 0.02 | 3–5 |
| Fluoride production | None | Minimal | Significant | Minimal | Minimal | Significant |

cont'd

**Table 33.10 Clinical properties of inhalational anaesthetics in current use (cont.)**

| Properties | Nitrous oxide | Halothane | Enflurane | Isoflurane | Desflurane | Sevoflurane |
|---|---|---|---|---|---|---|
| Toxicity and hypersensitivity reactions | Inactivation of vitamin B12<br>Neutropenia | Hepatic damage types I (?20%) and II (very rare) | Hepatic damage (extremely rare)<br>Renal toxicity? (see text for details) | None | None | Renal toxicity? (see text for details) |

↑ or ↓ = minimal change; ↑↑ or ↓↓ = moderate change; ↑↑↑ = marked change; ↑/↓ = no change.
Adapted from Calvey TN, Williams NE. *Principles and Practice of Pharmacology for Anaesthetists*, 3rd edn. Oxford: Blackwell Science, 1997: 256–7.

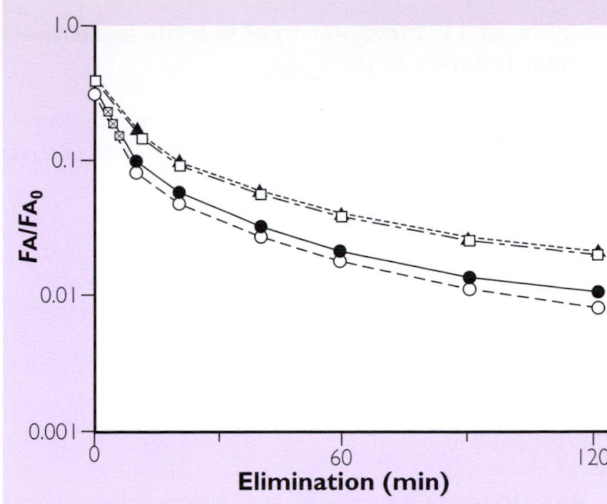


**Figure 33.20** Early wash-out curves for a number of volatile anaesthetic agents. The vertical axis shows the ratio of the end-tidal anaesthetic concentration (*F*A) to its value immediately before the beginning of elimination (*F*$A_0$), i.e. the axis represents FA/F$A_0$). (⊠ nitrous oxide; ▲, halothane; □, isoflurane; ●, sevoflurane; ○, desflurane). (Adapted from Yasuda N *et al. Anesth Analg* 1991;72:316.)

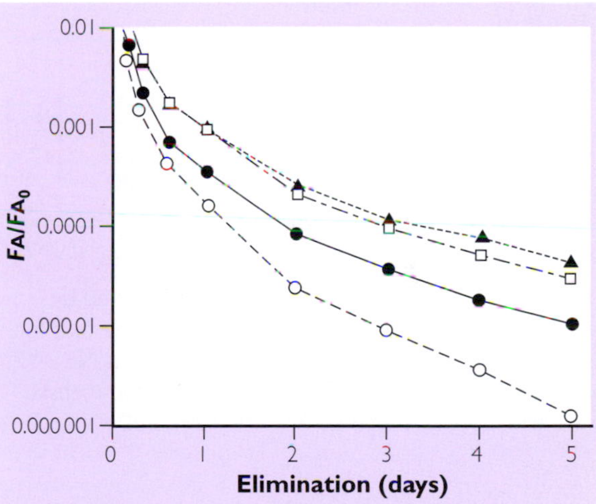


**Figure 33.21** Late wash-out curves for a variety of inhalational anaesthetic agents. The vertical scale is derived in the same way as in Figure 33.20. (▲, halothane; □, isoflurane; ●, sevoflurane; ○, desflurane). (Adapted from Yasuda N *et al. Anesth Analg* 1991;72:316.)

precursor of *S*-adenosylmethionine – the methyl donor for a large number of methylation reactions, including protein synthesis, the conversion of norepinephrine (noradrenaline) to epinephrine, arachidonic acid formation, and myelination.

In addition, methionine synthase catalyses the conversion of methyltetrahydrofolate to tetrahydrofolate, which, after a series of intermediate steps, is involved in the synthesis of deoxythymidine – an essential component of DNA. Prolonged exposure to $N_2O$ may thus cause agranulocytosis and bone marrow aplasia.

**Table 33.11 Metabolism of volatile anaesthetic agents as measured by metabolite recovery and mass balance studies**

| Agent | Magnitude of metabolism<br>Metabolite recovery (%) | Mass balance studies (%) |
|---|---|---|
| Nitrous oxide | 0.004 | |
| Desflurane | 0.02 | |
| Isoflurane | 0.2 | |
| Enflurane | 3.0 | 8.5 |
| Sevoflurane | 5.0 | |
| Halothane | 15–20 | 46.0 |

Adapted from Carpenter RL *et al. Anesthesiology* 1986;65:201.

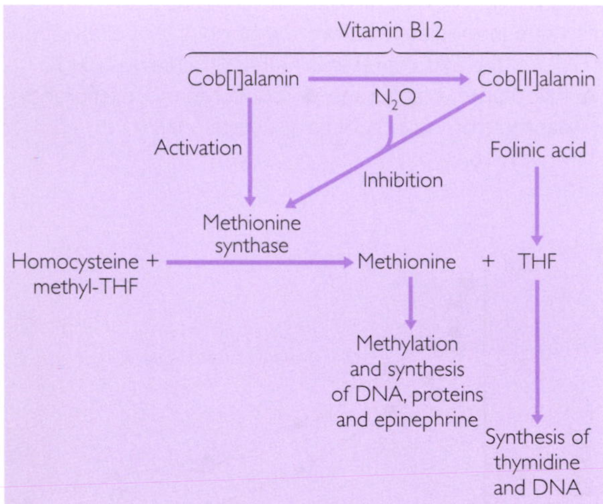


**Figure 33.22** The metabolic pathways affected by nitrous oxide ($N_2O$). THF, tetrahydrofolate. See text for details. (Adapted from Calvey TN and Williams NE. *Principles and Practice of Pharmacology for Anaesthetists,* 3rd edn. Oxford: Blackwell Science, 1997: 260.)

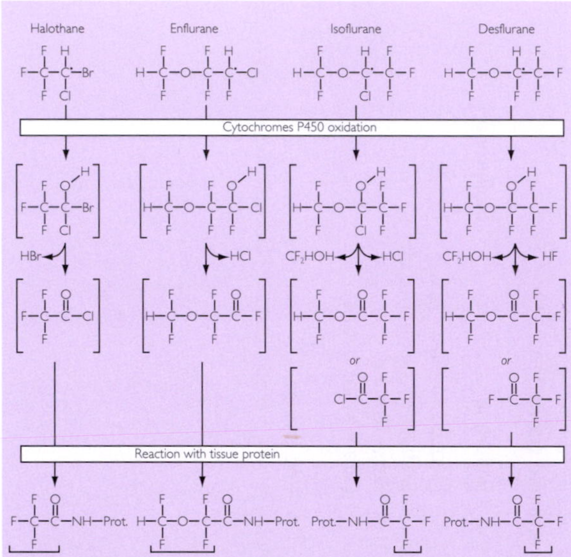


**Figure 33.23** Pathways for the oxidative metabolism of some fluorinated inhalational anaesthetics by cytochrome P450 enzymes to form acetylated protein adducts. Note that sevoflurane is unable to follow a similar metabolic pathway. See text for details. (Adapted from Martin JZ *et al. Anesthesiology* 1995;83:1125.)

## Halogenated anaesthetics

### *Malignant hyperpyrexia*

All halogenated anaesthetic agents have been reported to be triggers for malignant hyperpyrexia. For the management of this see Chapter 13.

### *Metabolism*

The halogenated anaesthetics are all metabolized by oxidative enzymes, but the extent of their metabolism varies considerably, with the newer agents undergoing significantly less metabolism than the older ones. Metabolism is by cytochrome P450 enzymes present in the endoplasmic reticulum of liver (see Chapter 28) and to a much lesser degree by enzymatic breakdown in renal proximal tubular cells (see Chapter 25). Metabolism results in the production of:

- acetylated protein products after oxidation (Figure 33.23);
- free halide ions namely, $F^-$, $Cl^-$, and $Br^-$. The C–F bond is the most stable with C–Cl being more stable than C–Br.

### *Renal effects*

The fluoride ions resulting from metabolism are nephrotoxic at plasma concentrations of 50–90 μmol/L or greater. Methoxyflurane was withdrawn because of its high metabolism and generation of fluoride ions which are highly nephrotoxic (Figure 33.24). After methoxyflurane anaesthesia, some patients developed high-output renal failure which often went unnoticed because there was no oliguria. This occurred because inorganic fluoride ions produce resistance to the action of antidiuretic hormone (vasopressin) in the distal convoluted tubule of the kidney. This led to the concept of the maximum number of tolerable MAC hours of anaesthesia at a given MAC.

Of the halogenated agents in current use, sevoflurane has the greatest production of fluoride ions and is

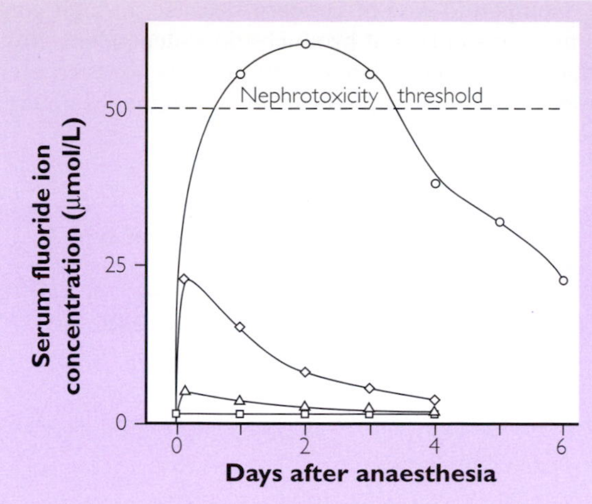


**Figure 33.24** The level of fluoride ions following anaesthesia with a number of halogenated inhalational anaesthetics (○, methoxyflurane; ◇, enflurane; △, isoflurane; □, halothane). (Data supplied by Anaquest, New Jersey, USA, 1993.)

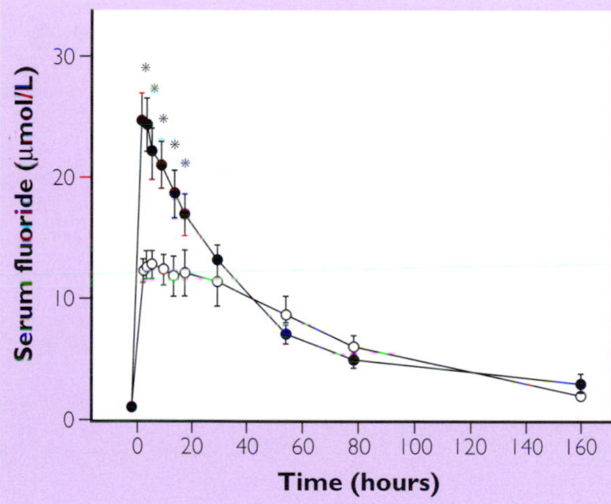


**Figure 33.25** Plasma fluoride concentrations resulting from sevoflurane (●) ($n = 21$) and enflurane (○) (n = 20) anaesthesia; * designates a statistically significant difference. (Adapted from Conzen PF *et al.* *Anesth Analg* 1995;81:569.)

shown compared with enflurane in Figure 33.25. Despite this, there are, as far as the authors know, no reports of it affecting renal concentrating ability in healthy patients and volunteers. Although theoretically it should perhaps be avoided in those with renal failure, again there are no confirmed reports that contraindicate its use.

#### *Liver dysfunction*

Halothane was introduced into the UK in 1956 and in 1958 reports of massive hepatic necrosis after halothane anaesthesia began to appear in the US literature. This prompted the National Academy of Sciences in the USA to commission The National Halothane Study. This retrospectively examined more than 850 000 general anaesthetics over a 4-year period from 1959 to 1962 inclusive. This sample included 250 000 anaesthetics when halothane had been administered.

The study was unable to demonstrate clearly an association between halothane and massive hepatic necrosis, and in fact concluded that the risks of hepatic necrosis were outweighed by the improved safety of halothane in relation to other anaesthetic agents in common use at the time. However, there were seven cases of unexplained postoperative hepatic necrosis where halothane had been administered, which meant that the existence of halothane-induced massive hepatic necrosis could not be refuted; it could merely be accepted that, if it existed, it was very rare, and of the order of 1 in 37 000. Since this study, so-called 'halothane hepatitis' and other forms of liver damage have been extensively investigated by many researchers worldwide. There are now consistent findings which are generally accepted.

There appear to be two distinct forms of liver dysfunction after halothane exposure:

- Type I in which there is a rise in liver enzymes including serum aspartate aminotransferase (up to three times normal). It occurs within the first two postoperative weeks in 20% of patients and is very much more common in patients who have received halothane.
- Type II, very rare, idiosyncratic, massive hepatic necrosis.

Type I hepatitis is thought to result from the toxic effects of the anaesthetic molecule either directly or after covalent bonding with critical cellular structural proteins or enzyme systems. It may be secondary to intraoperative reductions in liver blood flow or localized hypoxia.

Type II reactions are almost entirely limited to halothane, although there have been isolated reports after enflurane, isoflurane, desflurane, and sevoflurane. However, these are limited to individual case reports and their rarity precludes the drawing of definitive conclusions about the potential for massive hepatic necrosis with these agents. If it exists, the risk is very, very small.

Type II hepatitis was originally thought to be triggered by reductive metabolites, but is now regarded as being most probably caused by an oxidative pathway (see Figure 33.23). In susceptible patients a trifluoroacetylated product binds to liver proteins and produces an immune reaction. The trifluoroacetyl oxidative metabolite is present in up to 75% of affected patients, but not in patients with other forms of hepatitis, or in control patients who have received halothane but have not developed hepatitis. When idiosyncratic reactions occur, the reactive intermediaries may act as haptens, combining with cellular macromolecules, rendering them antigenic, and leading to immunological destruction of the cell (Figure 33.26). It should perhaps be noted that sevoflurane cannot undergo the formation of trifluoroacetylated products and would therefore not be expected to produce immune-mediated toxicity by this method.

Risk factors for type II halothane hepatitis, its clinical features, and the guidelines for avoiding repeat

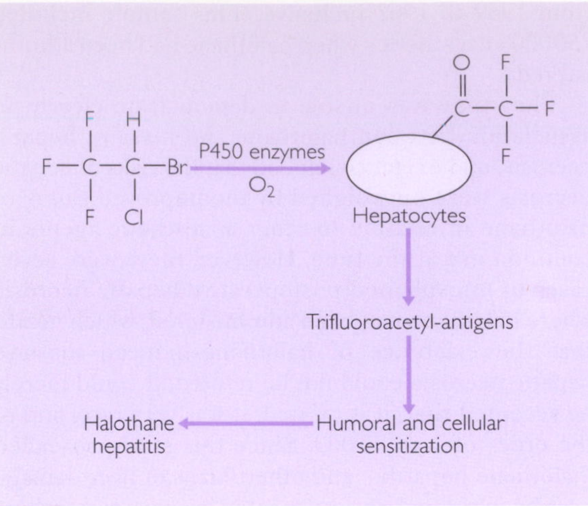


**Figure 33.26** The generation of halothane hepatitis from humoral and cellular sensitization. See text for details. (Adapted from Njoku D *et al. Anesth Analg* 1997;84:173.)

halothane anaesthesia are given in Tables 33.12, 33.13, and 33.14, respectively.

***Sevoflurane and compound A***

When sevoflurane breaks down in the presence of the strong bases found in carbon dioxide absorbers, it forms a variety of products, the principal one of which is compound A (Figure 33.27). Compound A is a vinyl ether which is also present in sevoflurane as an impurity of the manufacturing process at a level of approximately 1 part per million. Both barium hydroxide (Baralyme) and sodium hydroxide (soda lime)-based absorbers produce it, but the degradation of sevoflurane to compound A is four to five times faster in the former than in the latter. The rate of production increases as the sevoflurane concentration increases and as the absorber temperature rises, but decreases as the absorber becomes wet.

**Table 33.12 Risk factors for type II halothane hepatitis**

| Degree of risk | Factor |
|---|---|
| High | Recent previous exposure |
| | Previous adverse reaction |
| Uncertain | Obesity |
| | Female |
| | Drug allergy |
| | Lymphocyte sensitivity to phenytoin |
| | Familial history of halothane hepatitis |

Adapted from Neuberger J. Halothane and the implications of hepatitis. In: Kaufman L, ed. *Anaesthesia Review*, Vol 8. London: Churchill Livingstone, 1991: 179.

Compound A is of concern because, in high concentrations in rats, it produces dose-dependent proximal tubular renal damage. In humans however, even under low-flow anaesthesia, sevoflurane has never been shown to produce renal damage.

**Table 33.13 The clinical features of type II halothane hepatitis**

| Feature | Incidence |
|---|---|
| Female : male ratio | 1.6 : 1 |
| Previous exposure (%) | 78 |
| Autoantibodies (%) | 29 |
| Eosinophilia (%) | 21 |
| Drug allergy (%) | 15 |

Adapted from Neuberger J. Halothane and the implications of hepatitis. In: Kaufman L, ed. *Anaesthesia Review*, Vol 8. London: Churchill Livingstone, 1991: 179.

**Table 33.14 Halothane exposure guidelines from the Committee on the Safety of Medicines (UK)**

| Avoid halothane exposure if: |
|---|
| Previous exposure within 3 months |
| Previous adverse reaction to halothane |
| Family history of adverse reaction to halothane |
| Adverse reaction to another halogenated hydrocarbon anaesthetic |
| Pre-existing liver disease |

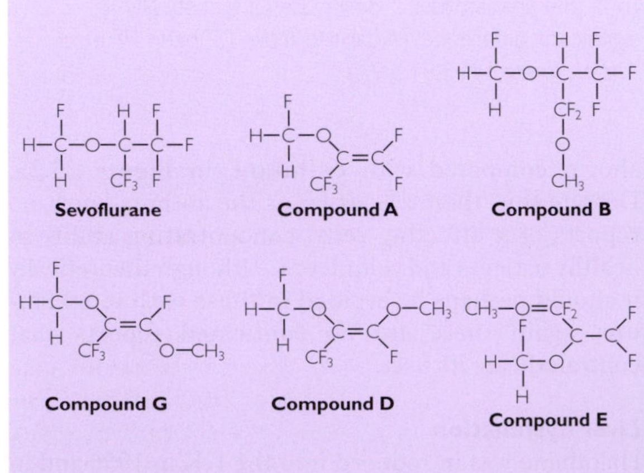


**Figure 33.27** The breakdown products of sevoflurane on exposure to a strong base at 60°C or above. The principal product is compound A.

## FURTHER READING


Biebuyck JF, Eger II EI. New inhaled anesthetics. *Anesthesiology* 1994;**80**:906–22.

Brown BR, Frink EJ. Sevoflurane: an update. In: Frink EJ, Brown BR, eds. *New Pharmacological Vistas. Baillière's Clin Anaesthesiol* 1995;**9**:1–14.

Calvey TN, Williams NE. *Principles and Practice of Pharmacology for Anaesthetists*, 3rd edn. Oxford: Blackwell Scientific, 1997.

Dale O. Drug interactions in anaesthesia: focus on desflurane and sevoflurane. In: Frink EJ, Brown BR, eds. *New Pharmacological Vistas. Baillière's Clin Anaesthesiol* 1995;**9**:105–117.

Elliott RH, Strunin L. Hepatotoxicity of volatile anaesthetics. *Br J Anaesth* 1993;**70**:339–48.

Hayashi Y, Kagawa K. Dysrhythmogenicity of anaesthetics. *Curr Anaesth Crit Care* 1998;**9**:312–17.

Hull CJ. *Pharmacokinetics for Anaesthesia*. Oxford: Butterworth-Heinemann, 1991.

Weisz MT, Jones RM. Desflurane: an update. In: Frink EJ, Brown BR, eds. *New Pharmacological Vistas. Baillière's Clin Anaesthesiol* 1995;**9**:15–36.

Articles in: White PF, ed. *Kinetics of Anaesthetic Drugs in Clinical Anaesthesiology*. Baillière's Clin Anaesthesiol, 1991;**5**:3–256.

# Chapter 34 Opioids, non-steroidal anti-inflammatory drugs, and other analgesics

D.J. Rowbotham

## OPIOID ANALGESICS

### Definitions

A clear understanding of some definitions is important in opioid pharmacology. An opioid is any drug acting at the opioid receptor. An opiate is a naturally occurring opioid derived from opium (from the Greek *opion*, poppy juice), e.g. morphine, codeine, papaverine. The term narcotic is derived from the Greek *narco* (to be numb) and is used often in a legal sense to describe a drug of addiction.

Potency and efficacy are specific pharmacological definitions and often confused, especially when describing the clinical use of opioids. Potency is defined as the dose required to produce 50% of the maximum response ($ED_{50}$) and efficacy describes the magnitude of the maximum response. For example, morphine has the same efficacy as fentanyl (both can cause respiratory arrest) but fentanyl is more potent (lower $ED_{50}$) (Figure 34.1). Conversely, buprenorphine is more potent than morphine (typical dose 0.3 – 0.6 mg i.m.) but has less efficacy (inferior analgesia). Opioids and their antagonists are subject to competitive behaviour. For ease of reference, the effect of a competitive antagonist on the dose – response curve is shown in Figure 34.2 and that of a non-competitive antagonist in Figure 34.3.

Tolerance, dependence, and addiction are important pharmacological phenomena. Tolerance describes the requirement to administer increasing doses of opioid in order to obtain the same effect. Dependence is a state in which an abstinence syndrome may occur after either abrupt withdrawal or reduction in dose of an opioid agonist or during the administration of an opioid antagonist. Tolerance and/or dependence do not necessarily infer addiction. Addiction is defined as a behavioural pattern of drug use, characterized by compulsive self-administration on a continuous or periodic basis in order to experience its psychic effects and sometimes to avoid discomfort of its absence; supplies are often secured by deceptive or illegal means. Addiction is extremely rare in patients receiving opioids for postoperative and chronic pain relief, but tolerance and dependence may occur during prolonged administration.

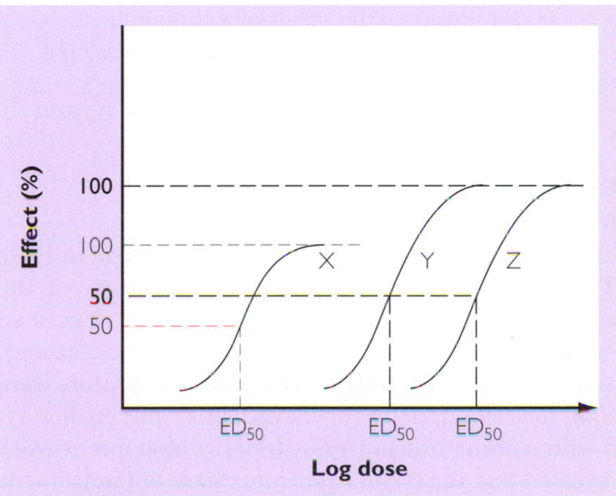


**Figure 34.1** Efficacy and potency of opioids. Opioids Y and Z have the same efficacy, i.e. the maximum effect of both drugs is the same. However, Z is less potent than Y because a greater dose is required to produce 50% of the maximum response, i.e. the $ED_{50}$ of Y is lower than that of Z. The efficacy of opioid X is less than that of Y and Z because the maximum effect is less. However, it is more potent, i.e. the $ED_{50}$ is less than that of Y and Z. In this example, X could be buprenorphine, Y fentanyl, and Z morphine.

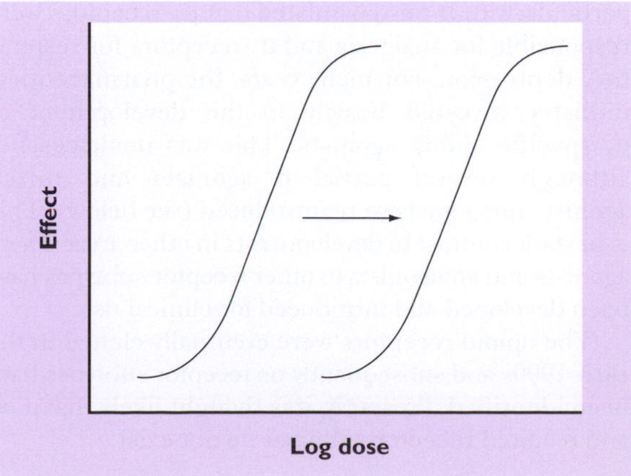


**Figure 34.2** Effect of a competitive antagonist on the dose–response curve.

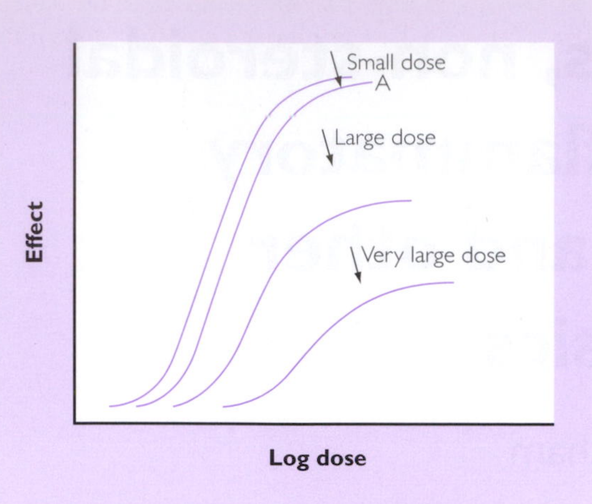


**Figure 34.3** Effect of increasing doses of a non-competitive antagonist. A *small* dose often produces a curve (A) similar to the effect of a competitive antagonist because, at low concentrations, not all the receptors will be occupied.

## Receptors

### *Mu, kappa, and delta receptors*

Opioid receptors were first classified by Martin in 1976. This classification was based on the nature of the agonists acting at the receptor. Three were described originally: mu (μ, morphine), kappa (κ, ketocyclazone), and sigma (σ, SKF10047). Two further receptors were soon described; delta (δ, enkephalins) and epsilon (ε, β-endorphins but not morphine). Subsequent work revealed that the σ and ε receptors were not in fact true opioid receptors. Therefore, three opioid receptors were recognized: μ, δ, and κ.

All three receptors are linked to potassium and calcium channels (see below) and can also inhibit the action of adenylyl cyclase. Naloxone is an antagonist at each receptor. Stimulation of the μ-receptor causes all of the classic opioid effects (see below), but all three receptors are thought to be responsible for analgesia. The κ-receptor is responsible for dysphoria and the role of the κ- and δ-receptor in respiratory depression is not certain.

Pharmacological experimentation has suggested the possibility of receptor subtypes for the opioid receptors, particularly μ. It was postulated that $\mu_1$-receptors were responsible for analgesia and $\mu_2$-receptors for respiratory depression. For many years, the pharmaceutical industry invested heavily in the development of $\mu_1$-specific opioid agonists. This was unsuccessful, although several partial μ agonists and mixed agonist–antagonists were introduced (see below). This is in stark contrast to developments in other areas where agonists and antagonists to other receptor subtypes have been developed and introduced for clinical use.

The opioid receptors were eventually cloned in the early 1990s and subsequently no receptor subtypes have been identified. Presently, it is thought likely that μ, κ, and δ opioid receptor subtypes do not exist.

### *Reclassification of opioid receptors*

The opioid receptors have now been classified according to their structure and it is likely that this classification will be adopted generally (Table 34.1). The orphan (ORL1) receptor is described below.

### *Natural ligands*

The natural ligands acting at opioid receptors are shown in Table 34.2. It has been known for some time that the ligands at the δ- and κ-receptors are the enkephalins and dynorphins, respectively, but there has been some debate as to the nature of the natural ligand at the μ-receptor. The endorphins have affinity for this receptor but are not very selective. Recently, highly specific agonists at the μ-receptor have been described in animals and humans. They consist of four amino acids and are known as endomorphin I and II.

### *Mechanism of action*

Two main mechanisms of action are postulated at spinal and supraspinal sites: inhibition of excitatory neurotransmitter release from presynaptic terminals, and hyperpolarization of postsynaptic membranes, decreasing the response of pain pathways to nociceptive stimuli. In the spinal cord, opioid receptors are found at the terminal zones of C fibres, primarily in lamina I and the substantia gelatinosa (see Chapter 23 for details of these structures and pathways). Although δ-receptors are classically considered to be spinal, μ-receptors still predominate (e.g. in the rat 70% μ, 24% δ, and 6% κ). Stimulation of the presynaptic μ- and δ-receptors is associated with hyperpolarization of the terminal and reduced neurotransmitter release. This results primarily from inhibition of voltage-gated calcium channels. Postsynaptic membranes contain opioid receptors that are linked to potassium channels. Stimulation of the receptor enhances the outward flow of potassium through these channels, stabilizing the membrane, which becomes less likely to respond to

**Table 34.1 Nomenclature of opioid receptors**

| New | Conventional |
|---|---|
| OP1 | delta (δ) |
| OP2 | kappa (κ) |
| OP3 | mu (μ) |
| ORL1 | orphan |

ORL, opioid receptor like.

**Table 34.2 Natural opioid ligands**

| Receptor | Ligand |
|---|---|
| μ (OP3) | Endomorphins I and II |
| κ (OP2) | Dynorphins |
| δ (OP1) | Enkephalins |
| Orphan (ORL1) | Orphanin FQ |

neurotransmitters. Opioid receptors can also be linked by an inhibitory G protein to adenylyl cyclase.

### *Orphan (ORL1) receptor*

The δ opioid receptor was the first to be cloned and subsequent use of nucleic acid probes on this receptor led to the cloning not only of the μ- and κ-receptors, but also of a new opioid-like receptor. This was called the orphan receptor because there was no known ligand when it was cloned. However, the ligand was soon discovered simultaneously by two groups who named the agonist 'orphanin' and 'nociceptin'. The latter name reflected initial experiments suggesting that stimulation of the orphan receptor was associated with pain behaviour in animals. However, these early experiments were flawed and it is currently thought that agonists at this receptor cause analgesia at the spinal level. However, there may be an anti-opioid action centrally.

The receptor is now termed 'opioid receptor-like type 1' (ORL1) and its ligand orphanin FQ. The receptor functions in similar ways to the other opioid receptors, e.g. it enhances outward potassium flow from the cell and inhibits voltage-gated calcium channels. Early work suggests that this receptor is widespread and it may be that drugs of clinical significance acting at this receptor will be available eventually.

## Classification and action of opioids

### *Classification*

Opioid drugs can be classified in a number of ways (Table 34.3). Traditionally, opioids have been classified as strong, intermediate, and weak, according to their perceived analgesic properties. However, this classification is misleading, because it implies that 'weak' opioids, e.g. codeine, are less hazardous. Codeine is simply less potent than morphine, i.e. a greater dose is required for the same effect. It can still lead to respiratory depression if given in a sufficient dose. Partial μ agonists (less efficacy than morphine) or mixed agonist–antagonist opioids (e.g. antagonist at the μ-receptor but agonist at the κ-receptor) are often referred to as 'intermediate' opioids, and pure opioid agonists (e.g. morphine, pethidine, fentanyl, alfentanil, sufentanil, etc.) are described as 'strong'.

Opioids can be classified according to their structure (Table 34.3): the morphinans (e.g. morphine) (Figure 34.4), phenylpiperidines (e.g. pethidine, fentanyl) (Figure 34.5), and diphenylpropylamines (e.g. methadone, dextropropoxyphene) (Figure 34.6). The phenylpiperidines and diphenylpropylamines are derived structurally from the morphinans. Remifentanil is a phenylpiperidine (fentanyl) derivative but, uniquely, it is also an ester.

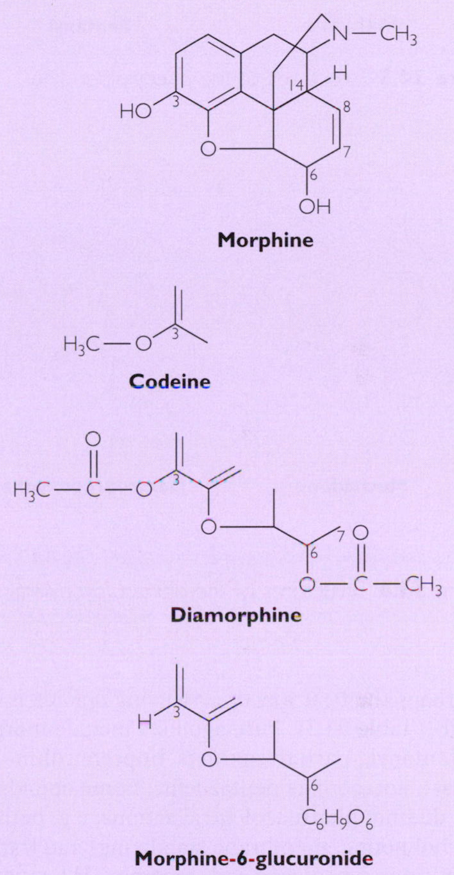

**Figure 34.4** The chemical structure of morphine and its derivatives.

**Table 34.3 Classification of opioid drugs**

| Traditional | Structural | Functional |
|---|---|---|
| **Strong** | **Morphinans** | **Pure agonists** |
| Morphine, fentanyl | Morphine, codeine | Morphine, fentanyl |
| **Intermediate** | **Phenylpiperidines** | **Partial agonists** |
| Partial agonists,<br>mixed agonist–antagonist | Pethidine, fentanyl | Buprenorphine |
| **Weak** | **Diphenylpropylamines** | **Agonist/antagonist** |
| Codeine | Methadone, dextropropoxyphene | Pentazocine |
| | **Esters** | **Mixed action** |
| | Remifentanil | Pethidine, tramadol |

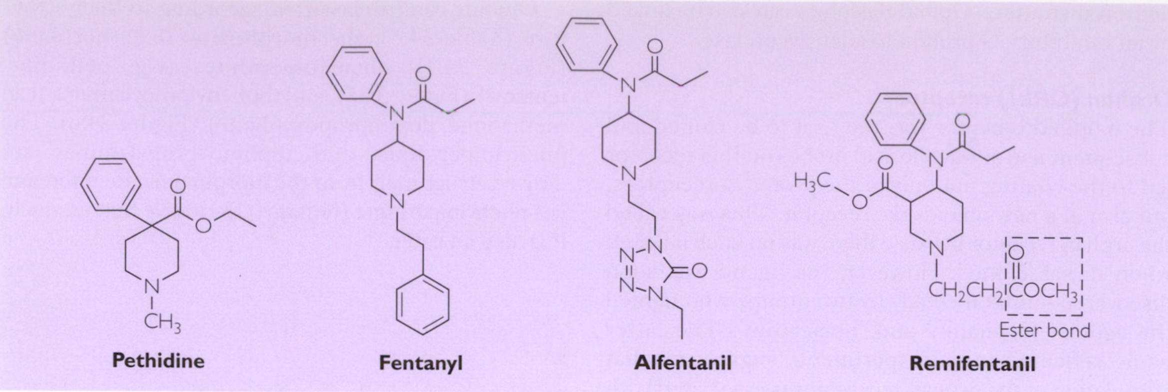


**Figure 34.5** Structures of the phenylpiperidines.

Methadone

Dextropropoxyphene

**Figure 34.6** Structures of the diphenylpropylamines.

Perhaps the best way of classifying opioids is functionally (Table 34.3). Pure agonists include morphine and fentanyl, partial agonists buprenorphine, and agonist- antagonists pentazocine. Some opioids have other distinct pharmacological actions, e.g. pethidine (anticholinergic, membrane stabilizing) and tramadol (inhibits norepinephrine and serotonin/5HT reuptake).

### Pharmacodynamics of opioids

These are summarized in Table 34.4. Individual opioids have very similar physiological effects and any significant differences are usually the result of pharmacokinetics or active metabolites. The pharmacodynamic phenomena of tolerance, dependence, and addiction have been described (see above).

Central nervous system effects include analgesia, sedation, respiratory depression, miosis, and nausea and vomiting. Opioids stimulate the chemoreceptor trigger zone in the area postrema of the medulla, causing nausea; effects on the gastrointestinal tract may also contribute to this. Euphoria is often reported but dysphoria may occur.

Inhibition of the brain-stem respiratory centre causes respiratory depression; rate and tidal volume are reduced. There may be periods of prolonged apnoea and upper respiratory tract obstruction, particularly during sleep. The carbon dioxide response curve is shifted to the right and the slope is decreased (Figure 34.7). In addition, opioids inhibit the respiratory response to hypoxia.

**Table 34.4 Opioid pharmacodynamics**

| Central nervous system |
|---|
| Analgesia<br>Sedation<br>Nausea and vomiting<br>Miosis<br>Euphoria<br>Dysphoria |
| **Respiratory** |
| Central depression – decrease rate and tidal volume<br>Right shift of $CO_2$ response curve<br>Upper respiratory tract obstruction<br>Decreased response to hypoxia |
| **Cerebrovascular system** |
| Hypotension |
| Bradycardia |
| **Gastrointestinal tract** |
| Reduced gastric emptying<br>Increased intestinal tone<br>Decreased intestinal propulsive contractions<br>Increased tone of sphincter of Oddi |
| **Urogenital tract** |
| Inhibition of voiding reflex<br>Increased detrusor muscle tone |
| **Miscellaneous** |
| Muscle rigidity<br>Histamine release (incidence varies)<br>Pruritus (spinal administration) |

Significant cardiovascular effects are most often observed after intravenous administration. Bradycardia is common. Sympathetic tone is reduced and this may result in hypotension, particularly if cardiovascular stability is dependent on a high sympathetic tone, or in patients with poor cardiac reserve. This is especially so if there is enhanced sympathetic activity because of pain or previous loss of circulating fluid volume.

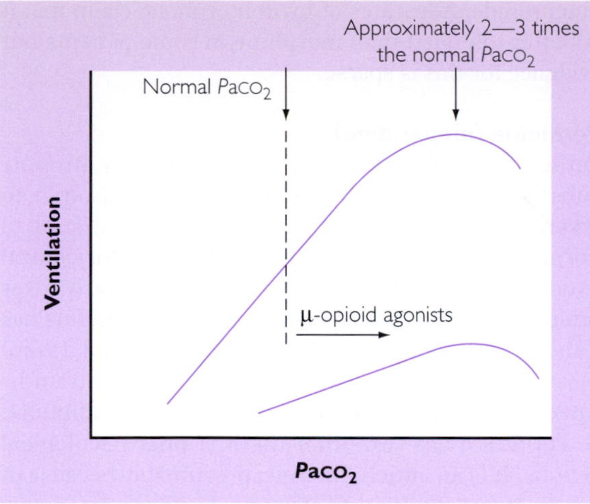


**Figure 34.7** Effect of μ-opioid agonists on the $CO_2$ response curve.

Gastric emptying is reduced significantly by opioids, intestinal tone is increased, and propulsive contractions are reduced. This leads to delayed drug absorption and constipation. There are multiple opioid receptors in the GI tract; poorly absorbed opioid antagonists can prevent constipation. Opioids constrict the sphincter of Oddi, increasing pressure within the biliary tract. Inhibition of the voiding reflex and increased tone in the detrusor and external sphincter of the bladder may cause urinary retention.

Local histamine release is often seen (flushing, pruritus), particularly with morphine and pethidine, and after administration of large intravenous doses. Pruritus is also common with spinal administration. This is not likely to be caused by histamine release because it is reversed by naloxone.

Rapid intravenous administration of large doses of opioids can cause muscular rigidity. The precise cause of this is uncertain but it can be treated by administration of neuromuscular blocking drugs.

### Pharmacokinetics of opioids

There are important pharmacokinetic differences between opioids, often the most important factor in the clinical choice of drug. Pharmacokinetic values of commonly used opioids are summarized in Table 34.5. Many of the opioids used in anaesthesia have extremely poor bioavailability, e.g. fentanyl. However, some are used effectively when given orally; their bioavailabilities are shown in Table 34.6.

Most opioids have a relatively large volume of distribution with the exception of alfentanil and remifentanil. Remifentanil has the combination of rapid clearance and a small volume of distribution; this results in a very short half-life. Methadone has a low clearance and a prolonged half-life. This enables once- or twice-daily administration - a distinct advantage over other opioids.

Opioids have a narrow therapeutic index and the pharmacokinetic values described here represent only average values. *There is enormous interpatient variability. Consequently, for safe and effective use, it is important to titrate opioid dose to effect.*

### Individual opioids

#### *Papaveretum*

Papaveretum is a mixture of opium alkaloids, the principal constituents of which are morphine (50%), codeine, papaverine, and noscapine. Noscapine may be teratogenic, and is no longer a component of commercially available papaveretum in the UK.

**Table 34.5 Approximate pharmacokinetic values of commonly used opioids**

| | Volume of distribution (L/kg) | Clearance (ml/min per kg) | Elimination half-life (h) |
|---|---|---|---|
| Alfentanil | 0.8 | 6 | 1.6 |
| Codeine | 2.6 | 11 | 2.9 |
| Fentanyl | 4.0 | 13 | 3.5 |
| Hydromorphone | 4.1 | 22 | 3.1 |
| Methadone | 3.8 | 1.4 | 35 |
| Morphine | 3.5 | 15 | 3 |
| Nalbuphine | 3.8 | 22 | 2.3 |
| Oxycodone | 2.6 | 9.7 | 3.7 |
| Pentazocine | 7.1 | 17 | 4.6 |
| Pethidine | 4.0 | 12 | 4 |
| Remifentanil | 0.4 | 40 | 0.1 |
| Sufentanil | 1.7 | 12.7 | 2.7 |
| Tramadol | 2.9 | 6 | 7 |

| Table 34.6 Approximate bioavailabilities (%) of commonly used opioids | |
|---|---|
| Codeine | 50 |
| Hydromorphone | 25 |
| Methadone | 92 |
| Morphine | 25 |
| Nalbuphine | 16 |
| Oxycodone | 60 |
| Pentazocine | 47 |
| Pethidine | 52 |
| Tramadol | 75 |

### *Morphine*

Morphine (Morpheus, Greek god of dreams) was first isolated from opium in 1806 and synthesized in 1952. Raw opium (extract of the poppy *Papaver somniferum*) consists of over 25 alkaloids (morphine 9–17%). Oral bioavailability is approximately 25% and metabolism occurs through hepatic conjugation to produce morphine 6-glucuronide (M6G) and morphine 3-glucuronide (M3G) which are excreted in the urine. Small amounts of normorphine are produced by demethylation. M6G is an agonist at the μ-receptor and more potent than morphine; it accumulates in renal failure. M3G is probably inactive.

### *Diamorphine (3,6-diacetylmorphine, heroin)*

Diamorphine is a semi-synthetic compound with no activity at the μ-receptor. It is converted rapidly to the active metabolite 6-monoacetylmorphine, which is metabolized further to morphine. There are no significant differences in the pharmacodynamics of diamorphine and morphine, despite the common belief that diamorphine is associated with more euphoria and less nausea and vomiting.

### *Codeine (3-methoxymorphine)*

Codeine (bioavailability approximately 50%, half-life 3 h) is metabolized in the liver primarily by glucuronidation, but also by *N*-demethylation (norcodeine) and *O*-demethylation (morphine). About 10% is converted to morphine by the polymorphic CYP2D6 enzyme, and this is likely to be responsible for analgesia because codeine itself has a low affinity for opioid receptors. The CYP2D6 enzyme is absent in some individuals (e.g. 7% of the white population) suggesting that these patients derive no benefit from codeine.

### *Hydromorphone*

Hydromorphone is a semi-synthetic opioid used primarily for the treatment of pain in cancer. It is approximately six times more potent than morphine, but has a similar duration of action. In contrast to morphine, the 6-glucuronide metabolite is not produced in any significant amount; the major metabolite is hydromorphone 3-glucuronide. Advocates of hydromorphone claim that it is better tolerated than morphine in some patients but evidence for this is sparse.

### *Pethidine (meperidine)*

Pethidine was discovered during a search for atropine substitutes in 1939. It is metabolized by hydrolysis to several inactive compounds and by *N*-demethylation to norpethidine. Norpethidine is responsible for central excitation, including convulsions, particularly after prolonged and high-dose administration. Pethidine has a shorter duration of action than morphine and its oral bioavailability is approximately 50%. It is contraindicated in patients taking monoamine oxidase inhibitors.

Pethidine has two other distinct pharmacological actions. It is an anticholinergic, presumably because of its structural similarity to atropine. Furthermore, pethidine has a local anaesthetic effect and indeed intrathecal pethidine has been used to provide local anaesthesia for procedures such as prostatectomy.

### *Fentanyl*

Fentanyl is approximately 100 times more potent than morphine and is the parent compound for several other opioids, e.g. alfentanil, remifentanil, sufentanil, and lofentanil. Metabolism is by *N*-dealkylation to the inactive norfentanyl and then to other inactive compounds, which are excreted in urine. It was one of the first opioids developed specifically for use in anaesthesia because of its relatively rapid but short duration of action. It is very lipid soluble and fentanyl can be given transdermally for the management of chronic pain.

### *Alfentanil*

Alfentanil is less potent than fentanyl but its half-life is shorter. It is the relatively small volume of distribution that gives alfentanil its shorter half-life despite the fact that the clearance of fentanyl is more rapid. In spite of being less lipid soluble than fentanyl, alfentanil has a more rapid onset because, at pH 7.4, 89% of the unbound drug in plasma is un-ionized, thus generating a large concentration gradient for diffusion across the blood–brain barrier. Alfentanil is metabolized by *N*-dealkylation and *O*-demethylation to inactive metabolites.

Although the half-life of alfentanil after bolus administration is short, the drug accumulates during infusion and the plasma half-life increases with duration of infusion (see below).

### *Sufentanil*

Sufentanil is more potent than remifentanil and its half-life is between that of alfentanil and fentanyl (see Table 34.5). Although used extensively elsewhere, it is not available in the UK.

### *Remifentanil*

Remifentanil is a fentanyl derivative with an ester bond that is broken down by tissue esterases. Consequently, remifentanil has a short and predictable half-life which is not affected by hepatic or renal function. Furthermore, the pharmacokinetics are not affected by plasma cholinesterase (butyrylcholinesterase or pseudocholinesterase) deficiency. The main metabolic product of ester hydrolysis is a carboxylic acid derivative which is excreted by the kidneys (elimination half-life of approximately 100 min). Although its elimination is delayed in renal failure, significant pharmacological effects are unlikely because its potency relative to remifentanil is only 0.1–0.3%.

Context-sensitive half-time is defined as the time for the plasma or effector-site concentration of a drug to fall by 50%, after terminating an intravenous infusion designed to maintain a constant plasma concentration. Context refers to duration of infusion. This is constant with remifentanil, i.e. no matter how long the drug is infused, the half-life will remain the same (about 5 min). This is in contrast to alfentanil and fentanyl where half-life is prolonged significantly depending on duration of infusion (Figure 34.8). This is because alfentanil accumulates in the tissues and moves back into the plasma for some time after the cessation of the infusion. Remifentanil does not accumulate and is metabolized in the tissues.

#### *Methadone*

Methadone is a synthetic opioid with a high oral bioavailability (see Table 34.6). The duration of action of a single dose is similar to that of morphine but this is entirely the result of redistribution. Significant accumulation occurs and the elimination half-life of methadone is 20–45 h. In fact, on oral administration, a steady-state plasma concentration may not be reached for 10 days. Therefore, a once-daily dosage is possible when the steady state has been reached – an advantage not just for chronic pain but also for the management of opioid abusers. There is some suggestion that analgesic efficacy is greater than that of morphine, particularly for cancer pain, and it may be that methadone also acts at the *N*-methyl-D-aspartate (NMDA)-receptor. The latter is involved intimately in pain transmission in the spinal cord and the phenomenon of wind-up.

#### *Tramadol*

Tramadol is a mixture of two stereoisomers and a centrally acting analgesic with relatively weak μ-opioid receptor activity. However, it also inhibits norepinephrine (noradrenaline) and serotonin uptake. It is extensively metabolized by *O*- and *N*-demethylation, glucuronidation, and sulphation. *O*-Desmethyltramadol production is dependent on the enzyme CYP2D6 and is an active μ agonist, with more receptor affinity than the parent molecule. Advantages over traditional opioids are reduced likelihood of tolerance and addiction, and minimum respiratory depression, but opioid-induced side effects do occur, e.g. nausea, constipation.

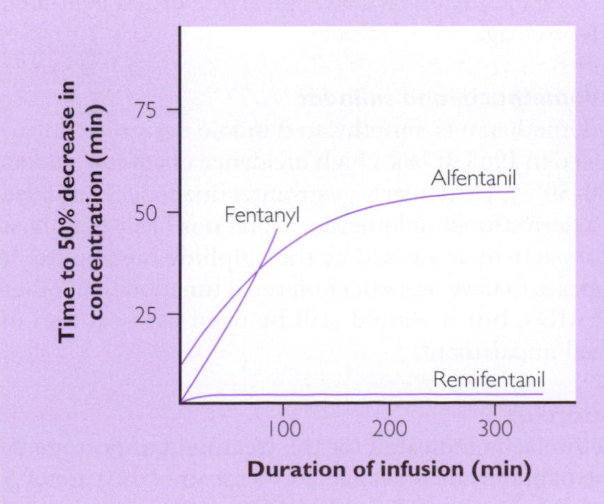


**Figure 34.8** Effect of duration of infusion on plasma half-life. (From Egan DT. *Clin Pharmacokinet* 1995;29:67.)

#### *Buprenorphine*

Buprenorphine is a partial μ agonist. However, it is 30 times more potent than morphine and, despite being only a partial agonist, its receptor affinity is high, and it associates with and dissociates from the receptor very slowly. Thus, peak effect may take 3 hours, with a duration of action of 10 hours. In theory, a partial agonist may stimulate the receptor sufficiently to produce analgesia, but not enough for respiratory depression and with less potential for abuse. However, respiratory depression can occur and, if it does, may be difficult to reverse with naloxone alone because of the receptor kinetics. It is accepted generally that buprenorphine is not as effective as morphine. Furthermore, it is not devoid of other opioid-like effects such as constipation and nausea and vomiting. The partial agonist may give rise to withdrawal symptoms in patients taking morphine.

#### *Mixed agonist–antagonist opioids*

Drugs in this class of opioids include pentazocine, butorphanol, and nalbuphine. They are antagonistic at the μ-receptor and may cause withdrawal symptoms in patients tolerant to other opioids. It is thought that the analgesic activity of the agonist–antagonists arises from κ-receptor activation. In terms of analgesia, they are not as efficacious as pure μ agonists but have less effect on respiratory function, and there is less risk of abuse. However, dysphoria and nausea are relatively common side effects.

## NON-STEROIDAL ANTI-INFLAMMATORY DRUGS

### General properties

#### *Mechanism of action*

Non-steroidal anti-inflammatory drugs (NSAIDs) inhibit prostaglandin synthesis from arachidonic acid by inhibiting the enzyme cyclo-oxygenase (COX) (Figure 34.9). This action leads to the analgesic, antiplatelet, antipyretic, and anti-inflammatory effects of NSAIDs. Classically, it has been thought that the analgesic properties of NSAIDs are the result of this peripheral action, but there is now considerable evidence implicating an important central mechanism.

COX exists in two isoforms: COX I and COX II. COX I is important in the regulation of prostaglandin synthesis in the gastric mucosa and renal vascular bed and thromboxane $A_2$ in platelets. It is the inhibition of this enzyme that is responsible for side effects such as gastrointestinal ulceration, impaired renal function, and bleeding.

COX II is produced in cells involved in the process of inflammation, e.g. endothelial cells, fibroblasts, and macrophages. All NSAIDs available at the time of writing inhibit both forms of the enzyme, although some

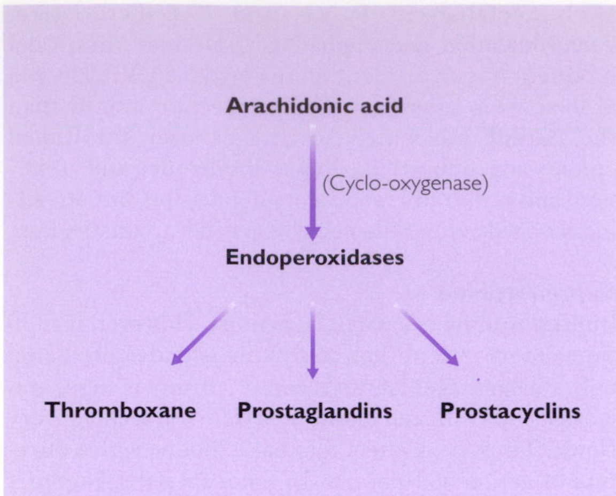


**Figure 34.9** Prostaglandin synthesis. NSAIDs inhibit cyclo-oxygenase.

have relative selectivity for COX II. There are several NSAIDs under development that inhibit only COX II. In theory, these drugs should be effective analgesics with no gastrointestinal side effects. Work so far indicates that this is indeed the case. COX II is not only produced in cells at the site of inflammation. It is present in the brain and its expression can be induced by electroconvulsive therapy. COX II is also present in the kidney and may play a role in the renal response to sodium and volume depletion.

### *Pharmacokinetics of NSAIDs*

Relative differences in efficacy and particularly side effects of conventional NSAIDs may be the result of the intrinsic activity of each drug against COX I and COX II. However, most differences are in the pharmacokinetics.

NSAIDs are rapidly and almost completely absorbed after oral administration with a short $t_{max}$ and are highly bound to albumin in plasma (often > 95%). They all have a low volume of distribution and most have short half-lives (2–3 h). However, some have long half-lives (particularly the oxicams) and several are available in slow-release formulations.

Biotransformation, conjugation, and renal excretion is the usual metabolic pathway. The commonly used NSAIDs produce inactive metabolites. However, active metabolites are associated with some (e.g. phenylbutazone, fenbufen, nabumetone, sulindac). Piroxicam undergoes enterohepatic circulation.

### *Side effects*

Gastric mucosal damage is relatively common and may or may not be associated with epigastric pain, nausea, and vomiting. Parenteral administration is not devoid of this side effect. The risk increases with dose, age, smoking, alcohol, and other drugs, e.g. corticosteroids and warfarin. Reduced production of thromboxane $A_2$ leads to inhibition of platelet aggregation and increased surgical blood loss in some studies. Prostaglandins play an important role in renal perfusion and NSAIDs may cause impaired renal perfusion and function, particularly in elderly people and during hypovolaemia, heart failure, and concomitant administration of diuretics.

### *Drug interactions*

There are several important potential interactions with NSAIDs and this is often the result of extensive binding to plasma albumin sites. The likelihood of each interaction depends on the type of NSAID. NSAIDs displace warfarin and, combined with antiplatelet activity, there is a real danger of bleeding. Other important drug interactions include: lithium, tolbutamide, phenytoin, methotrexate, antihypertensives, and anti-cardiac failure therapy (Table 34.7). Situations in which NSAIDs should be used with caution are given in Table 34.8 and those where they should be avoided in Table 34.9.

## Specific NSAIDs

Only the commonly used NSAIDs are described. In general, they are all very similar (if not COX II specific) and any differences are usually caused by the pharmacokinetics.

### *Salicylates*

Aspirin (acetylsalicylic acid) is hydrolysed to salicylic acid (half-life 2–3 h). This short half-life is dose dependent (rate-limiting hepatic conjugation) and can be increased to as much as 30 h. There is a relatively high incidence of side effects at moderate-to-high doses and, because of the association with Reye's syndrome, aspirin is contraindicated in children.

Diflunisal (difluorophenyl derivative of salicylic acid) is better tolerated than aspirin. It is more potent with a longer duration of action and it is metabolized to salicylic acid.

### *Diclofenac*

Diclofenac is a phenylacetic acid derivative. It is absorbed rapidly but its bioavailability is only about 50% because of the first-pass effect. Its terminal half-life is approximately 2 h and it is metabolized almost completely by conjugation to at least four metabolites. It is available in various oral formulations and as rectal and intramuscular preparations. The latter is associated with a high incidence of pain at the injection site.

### *Propionic acid derivatives*

Drugs in this class, e.g. ibuprofen, ketoprofen, fenoprofen, naproxen, and fenbufen, are used widely. They have very similar pharmacological properties. Fenbufen is a prodrug.

### *Indomethacin and sulindac*

Indomethacin is a methylated indole derivative, introduced in 1963. It has a high incidence of adverse effects (30–50%), particularly gastrointestinal ones. Sulindac is a derivative of indomethacin and it is likely that most of its activity is caused by the sulphide metabolite. It appears to have less effect on renal function than other NSAIDs, but it should still be used with caution in renal impairment.

### *Ketorolac*

Ketorolac is indicated for the treatment of postoperative pain only. It is available as a racemic mixture of *S* and *R* ketorolac hydrochloride for intramuscular and intravenous administration. The *S* form is biologically active. It is highly protein bound (99%) with a termi-

**Table 34.7 Potential drug interactions with NSAIDs[a]**

| Drug | Effect |
|---|---|
| Warfarin | ↑ warfarin effect |
| Hypertensive and cardiac failure treatment | ↓ effectiveness, $Na^+$, and water retention |
| ACE inhibitors and $K^+$-sparing diuretics | Hypokalaemia |
| Tolbutamide | ↑ hypoglycaemia |
| Phenytoin | ↑ free phenytoin concentration, ↓ metabolism |
| Methotrexate | ↑ plasma methotrexate |
| Lithium | ↓ lithium clearance, ↑ plasma lithium |

[a]Likelihood depends on type of NSAID.
ACE, angiotensin-converting enzyme.

**Table 34.8 Situations where NSAIDs should be used with caution**

| |
|---|
| Elderly people |
| Diabetes |
| Asthma |
| Widespread vascular disease |
| Cardiac, hepatobiliary, major vascular surgery |
| Concomitant administration of: |
| Angiotensin-converting enzyme inhibitors |
| Potassium-sparing diuretics |
| β-Adrenergic blockers |
| Cyclosporin |
| Methotrexate |

From Royal College of Anaesthetists Working Party. *Evidence-based Guidelines on the Perioperative Use of Non-steroidal Anti-inflammatory* Drugs. London: Royal College of Anaesthetists, 1998.

**Table 34.9 Situations where NSAIDs should be avoided**

| |
|---|
| Past history of gastrointestinal bleeding or peptic ulceration |
| Aspirin-sensitive asthma |
| Renal impairment |
| Hypovolaemia |
| Hyperkalaemia |
| Circulatory failure |
| Severe liver dysfunction |
| Uncontrolled hypertension |
| Pre-eclamptic toxaemia |
| Systemic inflammatory response syndrome |

From Royal College of Anaesthetists Working Party. *Evidence-based Guidelines on the Perioperative Use of Non-steroidal Anti-inflammatory Drugs*. London: Royal College of Anaesthetists, 1998.

nal half-life of about 5 h. This is increased significantly in elderly people (about 7 h) and in renal impairment (about 10 h). Metabolism is primarily by hydroxylation and conjugation in the liver. Maximum plasma concentration after intramuscular administration is achieved by about 1 h.

### *Oxicams*

Piroxicam is well absorbed after oral administration with a terminal half-life of about 50 h. Metabolism is by hydroxylation and conjugation and less than 5% is excreted unchanged. Nabumetone is a prodrug; 30% is converted to the active metabolite 6-methoxy-2-naphthylacetic acid (6MNA); 6MNA is more than 99% bound to plasma proteins and its half-life is about 25 h. Tenoxicam is well absorbed after oral administration, has a prolonged half-life (about 72 h) and is cleared almost completely by metabolism.

## OTHER ANALGESICS

### Paracetamol (acetaminophen)

The mechanism of action of paracetamol (active derivative of phenacetin) still has to be elucidated, but it may inhibit brain prostaglandin synthesis. It has no significant effect on peripheral COX and therefore has no anti-inflammatory activity; it does not cause gastric ulceration and bleeding. Paracetamol is rapidly and almost completely absorbed after oral administration with a plasma half-life of 2–3 h. It is metabolized in the liver, chiefly by conjugation. In contrast to the NSAIDs, plasma protein binding is only 20–50% and, at recommended doses, side effects are rare.

Paracetamol may cause fatal hepatic necrosis if taken in overdose. In patients with induced enzymes, toxicity can occur from inadvertent overdosage from self-medication. A highly reactive metabolite

(*N*-acetyl-benzoquinoneimine) is formed during normal metabolism, but this immediately reacts with the sulphydryl groups in glutathione to form a non-toxic compound. Glutathione is easily depleted and, if large amounts of paracetamol are metabolized, the toxic metabolite accumulates, causing hepatic necrosis. Hepatotoxicity may occur after a single dose of 10–15 g, or even less when there is pre-existing liver disease. Despite this, paracetamol is a relatively safe and effective analgesic, and it can be particularly effective when used in combination with other analgesics.

## Analgesic adjuvants

Some drugs have significant analgesic properties in particular situations, but are not classified as analgesics. These are often termed 'analgesic adjuvants' and are used particularly in chronic pain syndromes.

### *Antidepressants*

Antidepressants in small doses are prescribed frequently in the chronic pain clinic, particularly for neuropathic pain. They have specific analgesic effects independent of any antidepressant action. Amitriptyline is used most commonly, but others include desipramine, imipramine, nortriptyline, and doxepin. Tricyclic antidepressants inhibit the reuptake of monoamine neurotransmitters from the synaptic cleft into the presynaptic terminal This facilitates noradrenergic and serotonergic transmission. Desipramine is a more potent inhibitor of norepinephrine reuptake compared with amitriptyline but has less effect on serotonin.

The tricyclic antidepressants are rapidly absorbed from the gastrointestinal tract, highly protein bound, and undergo extensive first-pass metabolism in the liver. Metabolism involves methylation, *N*-oxidation, hydroxylation, and glucuronidation, and active metabolites may be produced. Nortriptyline (a metabolite of amitriptyline) is more potent than its parent molecule at inhibiting norepinephrine reuptake. An important pharmacokinetic feature is the very large volume of distribution (about 10–50 L/kg) leading to prolonged half-lives (e.g. $t_{1/2}$ of amitriptyline is approximately 20 h).

Side effects include drowsiness (this often limits therapy), dry mouth, constipation, blurred vision, urinary retention (anticholinergic action), agitation, and confusion. Arrhythmias are not common but, after overdose, anticholinergic (tachyarrhythmias) or quinidine-like (conduction impairment) effects can be life threatening.

### *Anticonvulsants*

Many drugs of this type inhibit sodium channels and stabilize neuronal membranes. Carbamazepine probably inhibits high-frequency neural discharges with no effect on normal conduction. It is effective particularly in neuropathic pain, e.g. trigeminal neuralgia. Bioavailability is 85–100%, plasma protein binding 75%, and an active metabolite (10,11-epoxide) is formed. Carbamazepine is often very effective, but treatment is limited by side effects, e.g. gastrointestinal upset, headaches, confusion, visual disturbances, rash, leukopenia, agranulocytosis, and aplastic anaemia.

Sodium valproate is well absorbed after oral administration, and is metabolized extensively in the liver by conjugation and oxidation to form several metabolites, some of which are potent anticonvulsants. It is 90% protein bound and better tolerated than carbamazepine. However, side effects include gastrointestinal upset, rashes, ataxia, tremor, and thrombocytopenia. Fatal liver dysfunction has been reported, particularly in children aged under 3 years on multiple anticonvulsant therapy.

Gabapentin has been used recently for the treatment of neuropathic pain but its mechanism of action is unknown. It is related structurally to $\gamma$-aminobutyric acid (GABA), but it does not interact with GABA receptors. Gabapentin is virtually unbound to plasma proteins ($< 3\%$), is not metabolized, and is excreted unchanged by the kidneys (half-life about 6 h).

### *Antiarrhythmics*

Lignocaine (lidocaine) infusion and oral mexiletine are occasionally used for the treatment of neuropathic pain. Mexiletine is a class Ib antiarrhythmic agent with a structure similar to lignocaine, but it can be taken orally (bioavailability 85%). It has no active metabolites and the terminal half-life is 6–12 h. In practice, its use is limited significantly by relatively frequent and troublesome side effects, e.g. nausea, gastrointestinal upset, dizziness, palpitations, and several others.

## Capsaicin

Capsaicin is the active ingredient of red chilli peppers and is often effective, when applied as a cream, for some types of neuropathic pain, e.g. postherpetic neuralgia and diabetic neuropathy. Its mechanism of action is as yet uncertain. It stimulates selectively polynodal nociceptors (C and A$\delta$ fibres) and it has been postulated that this depletes stores of neurotransmitters such as substance P. Capsaicin has recently been shown to activate non-selective cation currents in the dorsal root ganglion neurons.

Initially, application of the cream may be associated with a burning sensation or even pain. However, repeated application is associated with desensitization and inhibition of C-fibre conduction. Maximum effects may not be observed for 6–8 weeks and treatment may be limited by the unpleasant sensation on initial application.

# FURTHER READING


Burkle H, Dunbar S, Vanaken H. Remifentanil – a novel, short-acting mu-opioid. *Anesth Analg* 1996;**83**:646–51.

Dhawan BN, Cesselin F, Raghubir R, Reisine T, Bradley PB, Portoghese PS, Hamon M. International Union of Pharmacology. 12. Classification of opioid receptors. *Pharmacol Rev* 1996;**48**:567–92.

Eggars KA, Power I. Tramadol. *Br J Anaesth* 1995;**74**: 247–9.

Fainsinger R, Schoeller T, Bruera E. Methadone in the management of cancer pain – a review. *Pain* 1993;**52**: 137–47.

Henderson G, McKnight AT. The orphan opioid receptor and its endogenous ligand – nociceptin/orphanin FQ. *Trends Pharmacol Sci* 1997;**18**:293–300.

McQuay H, Carroll D, Jadad R, Wiffen P, Moore A. Anticonvulsant drugs for management of pain: a systematic review. *BMJ* 1995;**311**:1047–52.

Meunier JC. Nociceptin/orphanin FQ and the opioid receptor-like ORL1 receptor. *Eur J Pharmacol* 1997;**340**: 1–15.

Ripamonti C, Zecca E, Bruera E. An update on the clinical use of methadone for cancer pain. *Pain* 1997;**70**: 109–115.

Royal College of Anaesthetists Working Party. *Evidence Based Guidelines on the Perioperative Use of Non-steroidal Anti-inflammatory Drugs*. London: Royal College of Anaesthetists, 1998.

Satoh M, Minami M. Molecular pharmacology of the opioid receptors. *Pharmacol Ther* 1995;**68**:343–64.

Thompson JP, Rowbotham DJ. Remifentanil – an opioid for the 21st century. *Br J Anaesth* 1996;**76**:341–3.

Winter J, Bevan S, Campbell EA. Capsaicin and pain mechanisms. *Br J Anaesth* 1995;**75**:157–68.

Yaksh TL. Pharmacology and mechanisms of opioid analgesic activity. *Acta Anaesthesiol Scand* 1997;**41**:94–111.

# Chapter 35 Neuromuscular blocking and reversal agents

J.M. Hunter

## HISTORY OF NEUROMUSCULAR BLOCKING AGENTS

Neuromuscular blocking agents were first used in clinical surgery in 1942. Griffith and Johnson in Montrèal, Canada, gave 'Intocostrin' to a patient undergoing an appendicectomy. Until that time, muscle relaxation was achieved during surgery by the use of deep anaesthesia with potent inhalational agents such as ether. There were many disadvantages to deep inhalational anaesthesia: recovery from sleep was slow, risking aspiration of stomach contents; cardiac arrhythmias were common, risking myocardial ischaemia and even death; and, in addition, surgical conditions were not ideal, especially for upper abdominal or thoracic procedures.

It was known that some natural products, used by South American Indians as arrow poisons, killed prey by paralysing voluntary muscle. These poisons were derived from the bark of the creeping plant, *Chondrodendron tomentosum*, and were known to be a mixture of curariform alkaloids. The natural product was known as Intocostrin. As with all natural products, the potency of this mixture was variable and difficult to define. Thus, although Intocostrin was used by Griffith and Johnson, attempts were made to obtain a purified extract of this mixture. In 1946, J. Halton and T. C. Gray in Liverpool were the first to administer the single extract, *d*-tubocurarine, to anaesthetized patients in the UK. They used small doses of the drug and only rarely antagonized residual neuromuscular block at the end of surgery. Such practice became increasingly popular, but problems were encountered with the new technique. These were of two types: one was a pharmacological reaction to tubocurarine; this was usually cardiovascular in nature. Tubocurarine causes histamine release, which can cause a drop in blood pressure and a tachycardia. In large doses, the drug has ganglion-blocking effects. Tubocurarine is a long-acting agent which is excreted mainly in the urine; its effect can be prolonged in patients with any degree of renal dysfunction.

The second problem with this new technique was probably caused by inadequate artificial ventilation and incomplete reversal of residual neuromuscular block. It took a decade for anaesthetists to realize that it was essential to take over ventilation fully during surgery, even if only a small dose of relaxant had been given, and to reverse residual block at the end of the procedure. As a result of these complications, the use of neuromuscular blocking drugs fell into some disrepute.

In 1954, Beecher and Todd realized that the number of anaesthetic deaths was increasing and this was thought to be caused by the new technique. The search began for an ideal neuromuscular blocking drug which was free of the side effects of tubocurarine.

## DEPOLARIZING NEUROMUSCULAR BLOCKING DRUGS

### Suxamethonium (succinylcholine)

This neuromuscular blocking drug became available in 1951. Suxamethonium is a quaternary amine, with a structure equivalent to two molecules of acetylcholine (Figure 35.1). It initially acts in the same way as acetylcholine: it stimulates the postsynaptic nicotinic receptor, opening the ion channel, which allows the passage of an ion current. Thus, suxamethonium initially stimulates a muscle contraction known as a 'fasciculation'. Suxamethonium remains at the nicotinic receptor for much longer than acetylcholine, however. The neuro-

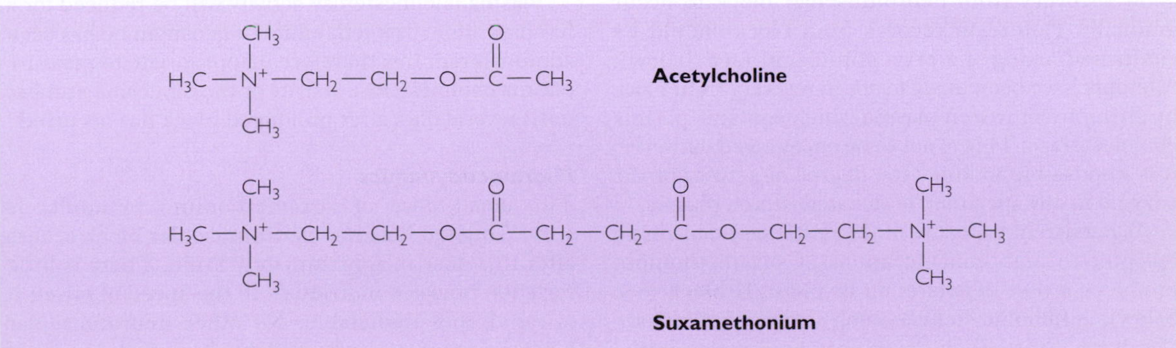

$$H_3C-\underset{\underset{CH_3}{|}}{\overset{\overset{CH_3}{|}}{N^+}}-CH_2-CH_2-O-\overset{\overset{O}{||}}{C}-CH_3$$

**Acetylcholine**

$$H_3C-\underset{\underset{CH_3}{|}}{\overset{\overset{CH_3}{|}}{N^+}}-CH_2-CH_2-O-\overset{\overset{O}{||}}{C}-CH_2-CH_2-\overset{\overset{O}{||}}{C}-O-CH_2-CH_2-\underset{\underset{CH_3}{|}}{\overset{\overset{CH_3}{|}}{N^+}}-CH_3$$

**Suxamethonium**

**Figure 35.1** The structures of acetylcholine and suxamethonium.

transmitter is broken down in milliseconds, but suxamethonium remains attached to the postsynaptic receptor for a few minutes, only diffusing away down a concentration gradient as the plasma concentration falls. Suxamethonium is not metabolized at the neuromuscular junction. While the drug is attached to the nicotinic receptor, the ion channel cannot close and the muscle becomes flaccid.

### Metabolism

Suxamethonium is broken down in the plasma by the enzyme, plasma cholinesterase (once known as pseudocholinesterase), first to succinyl monocholine and then to choline and succinic acid. Succinyl monocholine has about one-twentieth of the neuromuscular blocking potency of the parent compound. Only a very small percentage of suxamethonium is excreted in the urine, less than 10% in 24 h. Plasma cholinesterase is synthesized in the liver. The activity of this enzyme can be reduced by either inherited or acquired factors.

#### *Inherited factors*

Plasma cholinesterase is a glycoprotein; its structure has now been fully annotated. Only a small part of the enzyme contributes to the metabolism of suxamethonium. The reason for its physiological existence is not known. If the amino acid sequence of the active moiety is altered by a mutation in one of the genes controlling its synthesis, then the ability of the enzyme to metabolize suxamethonium is impaired.

The genes controlling the synthesis of plasma cholinesterase are inherited in an autosomal recessive manner. About 14 different mutations of the relevant genes have now been identified. The most common is the normal configuration, designated the usual $E_u$ gene, followed by the atypical gene, designated $E_a$. Other abnormal genes include the fluoride gene ($E_f$), the silent gene ($E_s$), and many other, even rarer, mutations. If one abnormal gene is inherited with a normal gene, e.g. $E_uE_a$, or $E_uE_f$, then the duration of action of suxamethonium will be increased by about 30 min; it will be of little clinical concern. But if the patient is homozygous for atypical cholinesterase – $E_aE_a$ – then the duration of effect of suxamethonium will be markedly prolonged, by up to a few hours (Table 35.1). This prolongation is not in itself life threatening, but artificial ventilation and anaesthesia must be continued until recovery from block has occurred. In such circumstances, metabolism of suxamethonium by other non-specific plasma esterases, and urinary excretion, allow recovery from neuromuscular block to occur gradually. Failure to recover from block should be confirmed using a nerve stimulator (see below). Attempts have been made to speed recovery from block by giving fresh frozen plasma which contains plasma cholinesterase. This is not to be encouraged, however; it is impossible to know the degree of activity of the enzyme in any specimen of donated, stored plasma.

As persistent exposure of the postsynaptic nicotinic receptor to high concentrations of suxamethonium produces a non-depolarizing or phase II block (see below), anticholinesterases such as neostigmine have also been given. Such drugs may produce an initial recovery, followed by an increase in the degree of a block, and are not recommended.

#### *Dibucaine number*

Confirmation that the patient has genetically abnormal plasma cholinesterase is obtained by measurement of the dibucaine number. This *in vitro* test (described by Kalow and Genest in 1957) measures the percentage inhibition by the local anaesthetic, dibucaine, of the light-producing interaction between the substrate, benzoylcholine, and plasma cholinesterase. In the presence of normal plasma cholinesterase, dibucaine significantly inhibits this light-producing reaction, and the normal homozygote ($E_uE_u$) will have a high dibucaine number – around 80, which is a measure of the percentage inhibition. In the presence of atypical cholinesterase however, the inhibition will be less; if the patient is heterozygous for atypical cholinesterase ($E_uE_a$) it will be about 60, but, if the patient is a homozygote for atypical cholinesterase ($E_aE_a$), the dibucaine number will only be 20. Addition of fluoride instead of dibucaine will detect the presence of the abnormal fluoride gene. If the gene is silent, no inhibition occurs with either dibucaine or fluoride. In such patients, the duration of action of suxamethonium is prolonged for several hours (Table 35.1). Patients known to have genetically abnormal plasma cholinesterase should carry some form of identity card or bracelet.

#### *Acquired factors*

Plasma cholinesterase activity can be reduced by decreased synthesis of the enzyme, by increased breakdown, or by competitive blocking of its action. In each instance, the plasma cholinesterase is of normal chemical structure.

Decreased synthesis of plasma cholinesterase occurs in the presence of severe liver disease, such as carcinomatosis or hepatic cirrhosis. It also occurs if metabolic factors such as hypothyroidism reduce the rate of enzyme synthesis. Increased breakdown of the enzyme occurs with technical procedures such as the use of any form of extracorporeal circulation, e.g. haemodialysis or plasmapheresis. Other drugs also metabolized by plasma cholinesterase (e.g. ester local anaesthetics, esmolol, trimetaphan, mivacurium, and etomidate) can slow the rate of metabolism of suxamethonium. Plasma cholinesterase activity may be reduced during pregnancy, partly because of haemodilution, but also because of the impairment of enzyme synthesis by high circulating levels of oestrogens. In all these instances, the duration of action of suxamethonium will be increased only by minutes, not hours.

Plasma cholinesterase activity will be reduced for a few days after suxamethonium or neostigmine has been administered. It is therefore inappropriate to measure plasma cholinesterase activity or the dibucaine number until several days after prolonged block has occurred.

### Pharmacodynamics

The usual dose of suxamethonium in adults is 1.0–1.5 mg/kg. Maximal neuromuscular block occurs after this dose in approximately 1 min. There is little variation between individuals in the speed of onset; it is rapid and predictable. No other neuromuscular blocking agent currently available has a faster onset of action than suxamethonium. It is therefore the ideal neuromuscular blocking drug to use if it is essential to

**Table 35.1 The genotypes of plasma cholinesterase and the response to suxamethonium**

| Genotype | Incidence | DN | FN | Response |
|---|---|---|---|---|
| $E_u E_u$ | 96% | 80 | 61 | Normal |
| $E_u E_a$ | 1 in 25 | 62 | 50 | Slightly prolonged |
| $E_a E_a$ | 1 in 2000 | 21 | 19 | Prolonged |
| $E_f E_f$ | 1 in 154000 | 67 | 36 | Moderately prolonged |
| $E_s E_s$ | 1 in 100000 | – | – | Very prolonged |
| $E_u E_f$ | 1 in 200 | 74 | 52 | Slightly prolonged |
| $E_u E_s$ | 1 in 190 | 80 | 61 | Slightly prolonged |
| $E_a E_f$ | 1 in 20000 | 53 | 33 | Moderately prolonged |
| $E_a E_s$ | 1 in 29000 | 21 | 19 | Very prolonged |
| $E_f E_s$ | 1 in 150000 | 67 | 36 | Moderately prolonged |

From Whittaker M. *Anaesthesia* 1980;35:174–97.
DN, dibucaine number; FN, fluoride number.
Normal range (DN, FN) = 77–83, 55–67; heterozygote = 54–70, 39–57; homozygote = 18–28, 18–28.

insert a tracheal tube rapidly as, for instance, when the stomach is full.

The duration of action of suxamethonium is longer than is often appreciated. Full recovery of the twitch or train-of-four (TOF) response (see below) takes about 12 min after suxamethonium 1.0 mg/kg. Recovery of the TOF to 10% takes 4–5 min, by which time some respiratory effort may be detectable. Another dose of suxamethonium, or a non-depolarizing neuromuscular blocking drug, should not be given until some recovery from block has been detected by either clinical means or neuromuscular monitoring. Otherwise, it is impossible to know whether prolonged neuromuscular block, either from an acquired or inherited cause, has occurred.

Suxamethonium potentiates the duration of action of any non-depolarizing neuromuscular blocking agent administered immediately after it.

### Side effects of suxamethonium

Suxamethonium has many side effects, related in part to its structural similarity to acetylcholine.

#### *Cardiovascular*

As with acetylcholine, suxamethonium can cause a vagal effect, leading to sinus bradycardia or bradyarrhythmias. This is more common in patients with a high vagal tone, such as children and physically fit individuals. The effect is also more common if repeated doses of suxamethonium are given, a technique for which, with the modern non-depolarizing agents now available, there is no indication.

#### *Histamine release*

Quaternary amines tend to stimulate histamine release from mast cells. Suxamethonium is recognized to produce such a response, and to stimulate anaphylactoid reactions more frequently than any other neuromuscular blocking drug. Such histamine release can also cause bronchospasm.

#### *Hyperkalaemia*

The initial muscle contraction caused by suxamethonium can cause a rise in extracellular potassium concentration; after suxamethonium 1.0 mg/kg, the plasma potassium concentration rises by about 0.5 mmol/L during halothane anaesthesia. The increase is less when more modern inhalational agents are used. The increase is not exaggerated in patients with renal disease, although, as these patients may already have an elevated serum potassium, such an increase may be sufficient to cause cardiac arrhythmias.

In patients with thermal injury, the increase in plasma potassium may be more marked. This effect starts within a few days of the insult, as the damaged muscles become swollen, and continues until healing is complete. A similar, albeit less exaggerated response can occur after a severe crush injury. Cardiac arrest has been described after the use of suxamethonium in a patient with thermal injury; the plasma potassium level was 13 mmol/L.

#### *Muscle pains*

These are thought to result from the initial contractions, or fasciculations, caused by suxamethonium. They are more common in healthy patients with a significant muscle mass, and in those who become ambulant within a few hours of anaesthesia. The pains occur in the large muscle masses across the back and in the thighs.

#### *Increased intraocular and intracranial pressure*

The initial voluntary muscle contraction produced by suxamethonium in the external ocular muscles is thought to contribute to the increase in intraocular pressure caused by this drug. The fine muscle fibres in the internal ocular muscles are also thought to undergo a tonic contracture in response to suxamethonium. The increase in intraocular pressure lasts for the same period as the neuromuscular block. Concern has often been expressed that the increase in intraocular pressure may cause expulsion of intraocular contents if suxamethonium is given to a patient with a penetrating eye injury, but the evidence for this is poor.

Intracranial pressure may also increase after administration of suxamethonium. If a further increase is thought to be contraindicated, suxamethonium should be avoided in neurosurgical procedures. In both these circumstances, avoidance of the increase in pressure induced by suxamethonium must be balanced against the increased risk of aspiration of stomach contents if the drug is not used; the latter may well be of more importance.

*Increased intragastric pressure*

Suxamethonium causes an increase in intragastric pressure but, in the presence of an intact lower oesophageal sphincter, the increase is insufficient to overcome lower oesophageal sphincter tone. Thus regurgitation does not occur. In the presence of an incompetent lower oesophageal sphincter, however, passive regurgitation may occur after administration of suxamethonium, with the risk of aspiration of stomach contents.

*Malignant hyperthermia*

Suxamethonium is one of the trigger agents for malignant hyperthermia (see Chapter 13). It should be avoided in patients susceptible to this condition.

*Muscle disorders*

Patients with muscular dystrophy may have an altered response to suxamethonium. A myotonic contracture may occur, especially in the masseter muscles, threatening the safety of the airway by preventing tracheal intubation. This contracture may cause an elevation in serum potassium sufficient to cause cardiac arrhythmias and even cardiac arrest. It is accompanied by an increase in plasma creatine kinase levels (see Chapter 24). These responses may be accompanied by a hyperpyrexia, which is thought to be distinct from malignant hyperthermia.

Patients with any form of myotonic dystrophy may produce a similar response to suxamethonium. Paraplegic patients and those undergoing prolonged artificial ventilation in an intensive care unit may suffer an exaggerated hyperkalaemic response after suxamethonium which, on occasion, is sufficient to cause cardiac arrest.

## NON-DEPOLARIZING NEUROMUSCULAR BLOCKING DRUGS

Non-depolarizing neuromuscular blocking drugs act by competing with acetylcholine at the postsynaptic nicotinic receptor. They do not initially stimulate the receptor, and thus no initial contraction is seen before relaxation. As a result, some of the side effects of suxamethonium are avoided. As with suxamethonium, however, non-depolarizing drugs possess at least one quaternary ammonium radical which clings to the α-subunit of the postsynaptic receptor to prevent access by acetylcholine. If the drug possesses two, rather than one, quaternary ammonium radicals ($^{+}N(CH_3)_3$), it is likely to be a more potent drug.

Potency of neuromuscular blocking drugs is measured in terms of the effective dose known to produce a given degree of neuromuscular block. For instance, the $ED_{95}$ is the effective dose required to produce 95% depression of the twitch response. It is usual to give at least two times the $ED_{95}$ ($2 \times ED_{95}$) to ensure adequate conditions for intubation in all patients.

In an attempt to produce a neuromuscular blocking drug that is free of the side effects of tubocurarine, the next non-depolarizing agent to become available was the trisquaternary amine, gallamine.

### Gallamine triethiodide

This drug was first used in the UK in 1951. It only rarely produces histamine release, but gallamine has even greater cardiovascular effects than tubocurarine. It produces marked vagolytic and sympathomimetic effects, leading to tachycardia and hypertension. This trisquaternary amine is excreted unchanged in the urine. It may have an altered effect in any patient with acute or chronic renal dysfunction. There have been reports of a dose of gallamine persisting for up to 5 days in patients with chronic renal failure. It would now be culpable to use gallamine in such circumstances.

***Pre-curarizing doses of non-depolarizing neuromuscular blocking drugs***

The muscle pains produced by suxamethonium can be obtunded by the use of a small dose of a non-depolarizing agent, given 2–3 min before suxamethonium. The response is variable depending on the drug used, the dose administered, and the time interval, but gallamine has been shown to be more efficacious in this respect than any other agent. It is the only remaining indication for the drug.

### Alcuronium chloride

This semi-synthetic derivative of strychnine is similar in structure to tubocurarine. It produces about one-third of the histamine release of tubocurarine, but it does have a slight vagolytic effect. It is excreted almost entirely in the urine. It has a duration of action almost as long as tubocurarine. With the advent of atracurium and vecuronium, this drug was used less frequently and has now been withdrawn, but for many years it was the most popular non-depolarizing agent available in the UK.

Further development of new neuromuscular blocking drugs has been aimed at producing an agent that is free of the side effects of suxamethonium, but that has as rapid an onset of action. Non-depolarizing drugs developed since gallamine and tubocurarine have been of two main chemical groups: the aminosteroids and the benzylisoquinoliniums.

### Aminosteroid compounds

***Pancuronium***

In 1964, this was the first aminosteroidal, non-depolarizing, neuromuscular blocking drug to become available. Pancuronium is a bisquaternary aminosteroid which does not possess the histamine-releasing properties of tubocurarine, but is as long acting. As with tubocurarine, it takes at least 3 min to have an effect, and has a clinical duration of action of about 45 min.

Pancuronium is excreted unchanged in the urine. It is also metabolized in the liver by de-acetylation at the C-3 and C-17 positions on the steroid nucleus to produce 3-desacetyl-, 17-desacetyl-, and 3,17-desacetylpancuronium (Figure 35.2). These metabolites are glucuronidated in the liver to make them water soluble, and then excreted in the urine. The 3-desacetyl metabolite has about 50% of the neuromuscular blocking properties of pancuronium; it may accumulate and contribute to prolonged neuromuscular block if pancuronium is given in excessive dosage, especially to patients with renal dysfunction.

Pancuronium has vagolytic and sympathomimetic properties which may cause tachycardia. The usual dose range in adults is 0.08–0.1 mg/kg.

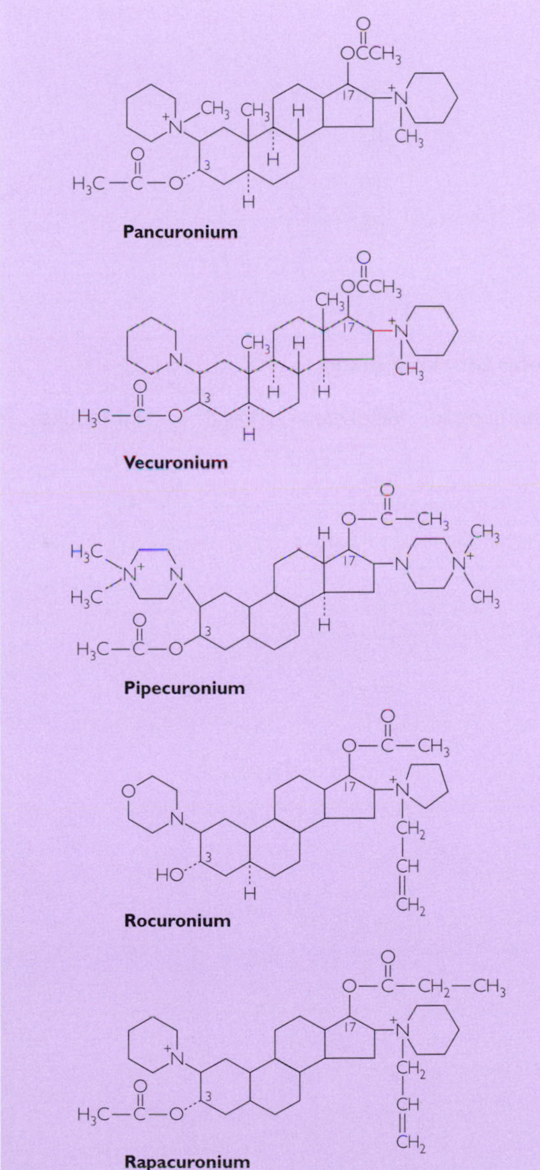


**Figure 35.2** The structure of the aminosteroid non-depolarizing neuromuscular blocking drugs. An acetyl group is sometimes present at the C-3 and C-17 positions. If present, this is removed in the first stage of metabolism of aminosteroids and replaced by a hydrogen ion.

### *Vecuronium*

In an attempt to overcome the cardiovascular effects of pancuronium and to shorten its duration of action, vecuronium was synthesized. It became available in 1982. This is a monoquaternary amine, although under acidotic conditions the second nitrogen attached to the steroid ring may become positively charged (Figure 35.2b), increasing the potency of the drug. Vecuronium has a slightly more rapid onset of action than pancuronium (about 2.5 min) and a clinical duration of 25–30 min. It is free of the cardiovascular effects of pancuronium, but this allows the unmitigated vagal effects of other drugs, such as the opioids or halothane, to become manifest. Thus bradycardia may be seen when vecuronium is used.

Vecuronium is excreted to a lesser extent than pancuronium in the urine (25–30% compared with 60% in 24 h), but it undergoes similar hepatic metabolism. It also has an active 3-desacetyl metabolite which is excreted in the urine and can contribute to neuromuscular block.

The drug is provided as a powder, for preparation immediately before use.

### *Rocuronium*

In an attempt to produce a non-depolarizing aminosteroid with an onset of action as rapid as suxamethonium, rocuronium was developed. This drug, in a $2 \times ED_{95}$ dose (0.6 mg/kg), produces maximum neuromuscular block in about 75 s (Table 35.2), but the effect is more variable than that of suxamethonium. Nevertheless, rocuronium has the most rapid onset of action of any non-depolarizing agent yet available. It should be used in a large dose, e.g. 0.9 mg/kg ($4 \times ED_{95}$), when a very rapid onset of action is essential but suxamethonium is contraindicated, such as the repair of an open eye injury in a patient with a full stomach. However, the drug in this dosage has a duration of effect as long as that of pancuronium. In equipotent doses, rocuronium has a similar duration of action to vecuronium (Table 35.2).

As rocuronium does not have an acetyl group at the C-3 position (Figure 35.2), it does not possess an active 3-desacetyl metabolite. The 17-desacetyl metabolite of rocuronium is thought, from animal studies, to possess only one-twentieth of the neuromuscular blocking properties of the parent drug. This may prove to be an advantage of rocuronium over the older aminosteroid agents.

Rocuronium may have a slight vagolytic effect (Table 35.3). This is not as marked as with pancuronium, but the heart rate when using rocuronium will be noticeably higher than with vecuronium. The drug is available in solution.

### *Pipecuronium*

This aminosteroid has been available in the USA and parts of Europe, although not in the UK, since 1991. It has an onset and duration of action as long as those of pancuronium (see Table 35.2), but is free from cardiovascular effects (Table 35.3). It is a bisquaternary aminosteroid that is metabolized in the liver and excreted in the urine. It probably has an active metabolite.

### *Rapacuronium (Org 9487)*

This aminosteroid is undergoing clinical trials in Europe. It has a similar onset of action to rocuronium but a shorter duration of effect (see Table 35.2). It is

**Table 35.2 Time to onset of maximum block after approximately 2 × $ED_{95}$ of several non-depolarizing neuromuscular blocking drugs compared with suxamethonium. Time to 25% recovery of the first twitch of the train of four ($T_1/T_0$), when neuromuscular block produced by non-depolarizing drugs can be safely antagonized, is also given.**

| | Maximum block (min) | 25% recovery, $T_1/T_0$ (min) |
|---|---|---|
| Suxamethonium (1.0 mg/kg) | 1.1 | 8.0 |
| **Aminosteroids** | | |
| Pancuronium (0.1 mg/kg) | 2.9 | 86 |
| Vecuronium (0.1 mg/kg) | 2.4 | 44 |
| Pipecuronium (0.15 mg/kg) | 2.5 | 95 |
| Rocuronium (0.6 mg/kg) | 1.25 | 43 |
| Rapacuronium (1.5 mg/kg) | 1.1 | 19 |
| **Benzylisoquinoliniums** | | |
| Tubocurarine (0.6 mg/kg) | 3.4 | 55 |
| Atracurium (0.5 mg/kg) | 2.4 | 38 |
| Doxacurium (0.05 mg/kg) | 5.9 | 83 |
| Mivacurium (0.15 mg/kg) | 1.8 | 16 |
| Cisatracurium (0.1 mg/kg) | 4.0 | 46 |

**Table 35.3 The cardiovascular effects of neuromuscular blocking drugs**

| Neuromuscular blocking drug | Ganglion block | Sympathomimetic | Vagolytic | Vagal | Histamine |
|---|---|---|---|---|---|
| Suxamethonium | – | – | – | ++ | ++ |
| Gallamine | – | +++ | +++ | – | + |
| Alcuronium | – | – | + | – | + |
| **Aminosteroids** | | | | | |
| Pancuronium | – | ++ | ++ | – | – |
| Vecuronium | – | – | – | – | – |
| Pipecuronium | – | – | – | – | – |
| Rocuronium | – | – | + | – | – |
| Rapacuronium | – | – | + | – | + |
| **Benzylisoquinoliniums** | | | | | |
| Tubocurarine | + | – | – | – | +++ |
| Atracurium | – | – | – | – | + |
| Doxacurium | – | – | – | – | – |
| Mivacurium | – | – | – | – | ++ |
| Cisatracurium | – | – | – | – | – |

the first aminosteroid that has been reported occasionally to release histamine and induce bronchospasm. As it has an acetyl group at the C-3 position, it has an active metabolite (Org 9488).

This drug is presented as a powder for preparation immediately before use. Sales of the drug in the US have recently been suspended by the manufacturer following reports of episodes of severe bronchospasm in five children.

### Benzylisoquinolinium compounds

These are derived from tubocurarine. Benzylisoquinoliniums consist of long carbon chains connecting two charged nitrogen radicals. In the case of tubocurarine, the carbon chain is linked into a circle, with nitrogen atoms equidistant in the loop. The charged quaternary nitrogen radicals are spaced at a distance of 1.4 nm, the same distance as that between the two α-subunits of the postsynaptic nicotinic receptor (see Chapter 23). Slim carbon chains are more vulnerable to breakdown in the plasma than a bulky steroid nucleus. But benzylisoquinolinium compounds are more likely to release histamine than aminosteroids.

It was realized that all quaternary ammonium compounds undergo spontaneous degradation at certain temperatures and pH – a process known as Hofmann degradation or elimination. An attempt was therefore made by a pharmaceutical chemist at Strathclyde University in Glasgow, Professor John Stenlake, to produce a neuromuscular blocking agent that broke down spontaneously at body temperature and pH. Thus atracurium was synthesized – a major development in its time. It is also metabolized by non-specific esterases in the plasma, but not by plasma cholinesterase. About 10% of a dose is excreted unchanged in the urine over 24 h.

### *Atracurium besylate*

This drug is a mixture of 10 stereoisomers and geometric isomers. It has four isomeric or asymmetrical sites: two at each end of the carbon chain and one on the benzyl ring at the adjacent carbon atom to the charged nitrogen at each end of the chain (Figure 35.3). The bond attaching the methyl group to that asymmetrical carbon or nitrogen can be placed either anteriorly (►) or posteriorly (⦙⦙⦙) at each end of the chain. Thus 16 potential isomers of atracurium exist, although four are mirror images of each other, reducing the number of *cis* or *trans* and *R* or *S* isomers to 10.

Atracurium does release histamine, but only to about one-third of the extent of that caused by tubocurarine. The localized cutaneous response may spread over the body and be accompanied by hypotension and tachycardia. It is possible to reduce this effect by premedication with $H_1$- and $H_2$-receptor-blocking drugs.

Atracurium $2 \times ED_{95}$ (0.45 mg/kg) has a more rapid onset of action than tubocurarine (see Table 35.2), and a clinical duration of about 35 min. Its effect is unaltered in the presence of renal or hepatic disease, making it the neuromuscular blocking drug of choice in patients with any degree of organ dysfunction, and in elderly people, whose organ function may be impaired.

### *Laudanosine*

Hofmann degradation of atracurium occurs at the site in the molecule where the carbon chain is linked to the quaternary nitrogen (Figure 35.4). One molecule of laudanosine is produced by Hofmann degradation of one molecule of atracurium. Ester hydrolysis occurs at the double bond in the carbon chain, producing mono-

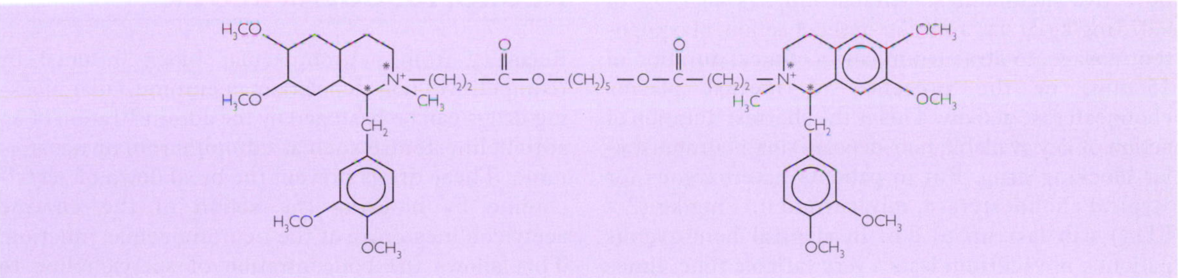

**Figure 35.3** The isomeric structure of atracurium besylate; * denotes the four isomeric sites.

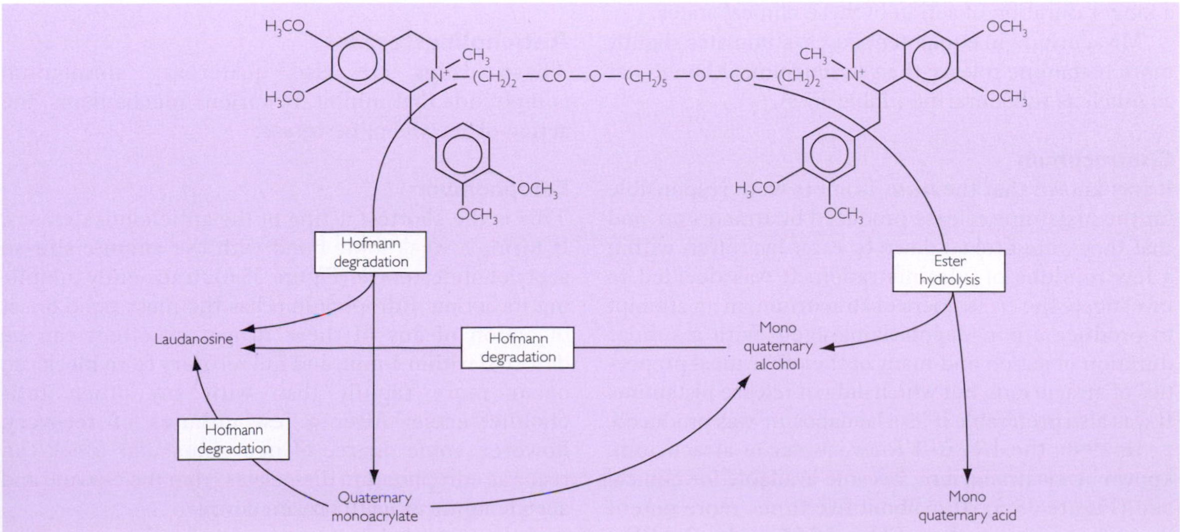


**Figure 35.4** The routes of metabolism of atracurium besylate, by Hofmann degradation and ester hydrolysis, to produce two molecules of laudanosine.

quaternary alcohol and acid (Figure 35.4). Monoquaternary alcohol undergoes Hofmann degradation to produce a second molecule of laudanosine from one molecule of atracurium.

Laudanosine is a product of many naturally occurring opioids. It is known to produce cerebral irritation in animals. The peak plasma laudanosine concentration in adults after a bolus dose of atracurium 0.5 mg/kg is around 0.3 μg/ml; the plasma concentration that causes cerebral irritation in dogs is about 14.0 μg/ml and epileptic fits occur in this species at 17.0 μg/ml. There is no evidence of such plasma laudanosine concentrations being reached in anaesthetized patients in the operating room, and there have been no reports of convulsions from laudanosine when atracurium is used in such circumstances.

Laudanosine is excreted in the urine and also undergoes metabolism in the liver. Plasma laudanosine levels will therefore be higher when atracurium is given to patients with renal or hepatic disease, and when atracurium is given by continuous infusion for many hours. Plasma laudanosine levels of about 5.0 μg/ml have been reported in critically ill patients, with multisystem organ failure, who are undergoing artificial ventilation in an intensive care unit; no adverse effects were noted. The plasma levels were higher in the patients with acute renal or hepatic failure.

#### *Mivacurium*

This benzylisoquinolinium compound is broken down, as is suxamethonium, by plasma cholinesterase. It has no active metabolites. Mivacurium has an $ED_{95}$ of 0.075 mg/kg. It has a similar onset of action, in equipotent dosage, to atracurium, and a clinical duration of 15 min, in the presence of normal plasma cholinesterase activity. This is the shortest duration of action of any available non-depolarizing neuromuscular blocking drug. But in patients heterozygous for atypical cholinesterase, mivacurium 0.15 mg/kg (2 × $ED_{95}$) can last up to 2 h. In atypical homozygous patients, mivacurium lasts a very variable time; times of up to 8 h have been reported. As plasma cholinesterase activity may be reduced in patients with cirrhosis or chronic renal failure, mivacurium may have a longer duration of action in these clinical states.

Mivacurium, in equipotent doses, stimulates slightly more histamine release than atracurium, although not as much as tubocurarine (Table 35.3).

#### *Cisatracurium*

It was known that the *trans* isomers were responsible for the histamine release produced by atracurium, and that they were broken down by ester hydrolysis within a few minutes of administration. It was decided to investigate the *cis* isomers of atracurium, in an attempt to produce a non-depolarizing agent with a similar duration of action and many of the other ideal properties of atracurium, but which did not release histamine. It was also preferable if less laudanosine was produced.

In 1996, the 1*R cis*–1′*R cis* isomer of atracurium, known as cisatracurium, became available for clinical use (Figure 35.5). It is about five times more potent than atracurium, with an $ED_{95}$ of 0.05 mg/kg; 2 × $ED_{95}$ (0.1 mg/kg) has a slightly longer onset of action than an equipotent dose of atracurium, at about 4 min (see Table 35.2); its duration of effect is similar to, or perhaps slightly longer than, the parent compound. As yet there have been no reports of adverse cardiovascular effects from cisatracurium.

As a result of its stereochemistry, cisatracurium undergoes more Hofmann degradation and less ester hydrolysis than atracurium. As it is a more potent compound, requiring a smaller dose to produce the same degree of block, less laudanosine is produced. After a bolus dose of cisatracurium of 0.1 mg/kg to healthy adults, the peak plasma laudanosine concentration is around 0.03 μg/ml – 10 times lower than after atracurium. The maximum plasma laudanosine levels reported in critically ill patients given a continuous infusion of cisatracurium are about 1.0 μg/ml – much less than after atracurium. Cisatracurium is a safer drug than atracurium to use in the critically ill patient.

#### *Doxacurium*

This benzylisoquinolinium became available in the USA in 1991, but is not sold in the UK. It was the first benzylisoquinolinium compound that had no adverse cardiovascular effects (see Table 35.3), but it does *not* undergo plasma breakdown. As with tubocurarine, it is excreted mainly unchanged in the urine. It is a very potent drug ($ED_{95}$ = 0.025 mg/kg) with a long and variable onset of action and duration of effect (see Table 35.2). Its effect is prolonged in patients with renal failure.

## ANTAGONISM OF RESIDUAL NEUROMUSCULAR BLOCK

Recovery from neuromuscular block induced by (competitive) non-depolarizing neuromuscular blocking drugs can be hastened by the administration of an anticholinesterase such as edrophonium or neostigmine. These drugs prevent the breakdown of acetylcholine by blocking the action of the enzyme acetylcholinesterase at the neuromuscular junction. This allows the concentration of acetylcholine to increase and compete with the falling concentration of neuromuscular blocking drug, overcoming residual block.

### Anticholinesterases

These drugs are also quaternary ammonium compounds that inhibit, by various mechanisms, the action of acetylcholinesterase.

#### *Edrophonium*

This is the shortest acting of the anticholinesterases. It forms a weak ionic bond with the anionic site on acetylcholinesterase (Figure 35.6), transiently inhibiting its action. Edrophonium has the most rapid onset of action of any of these drugs; its effect can be detected within 1 min, and full recovery from block can occur more rapidly than with any other anticholinesterase. After a few minutes of recovery, however, some degree of neuromuscular block can recur as edrophonium dissociates from the enzyme and acetylcholine is again broken down.

A dose of edrophonium is used to diagnose myasthenia gravis – the Tensilon test. This disease is caused by an antibody-mediated decrease in acetylcholine

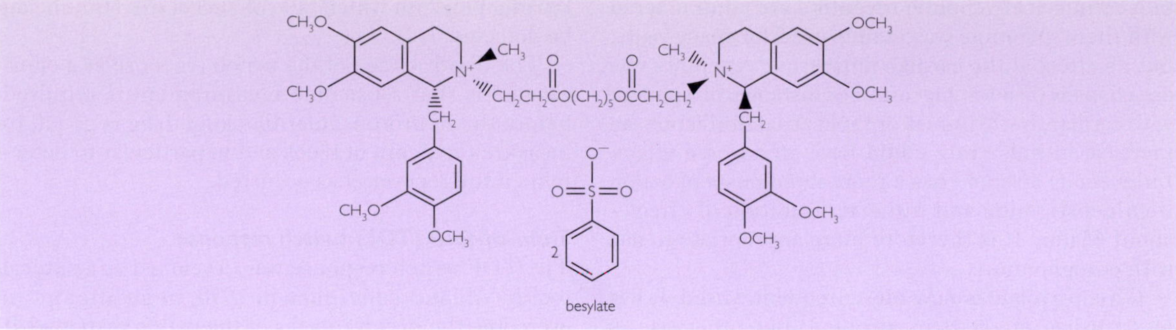

**Figure 35.5** The structure of cisatracurium besylate. The solid arrows denote the forward direction of the bond; the broken arrows denote the backward direction of the bond.

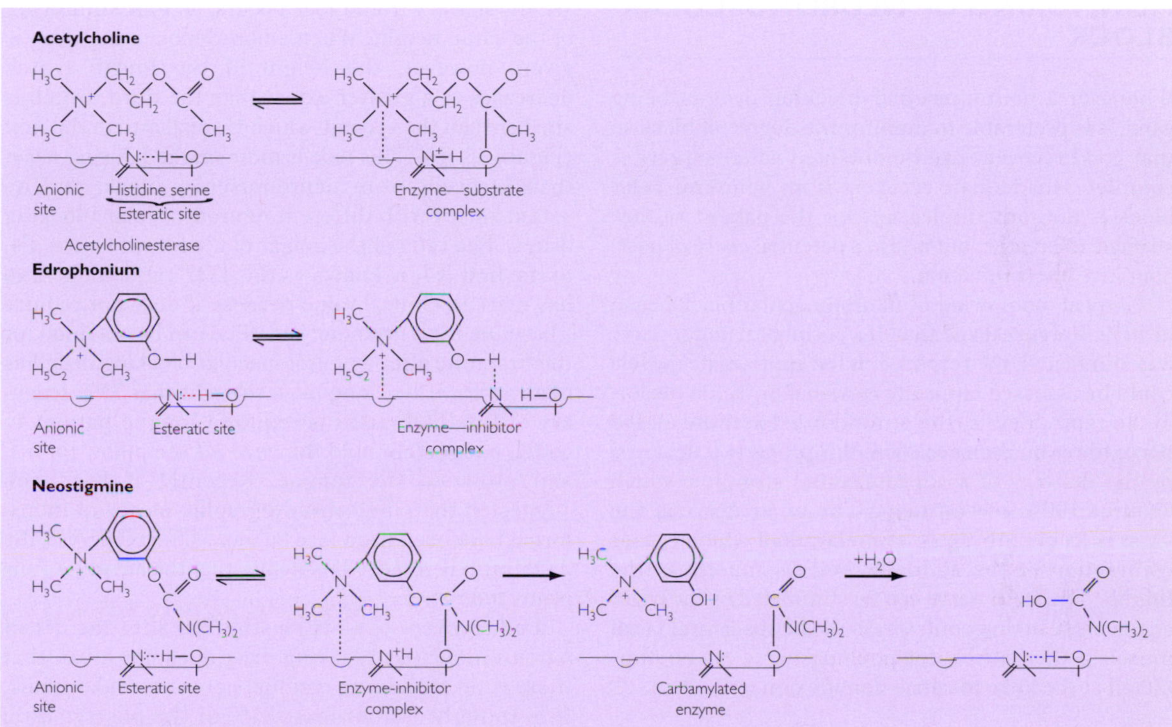


**Figure 35.6** The interaction of acetylcholine, edrophonium, and neostigmine with the anionic and esteratic sites on the enzyme, acetylcholinesterase.

release at the neuromuscular junction. Administration of an anticholinesterase therefore results in a transient increase in neuromuscular transmission and increased muscle power.

### *Neostigmine*

This anticholinesterase forms a double bond with the esteratic site on the enzyme. Its effect takes a little longer than edrophonium to commence. Full recovery from block after administration of neostigmine takes up to 7 min, and is more sustained than after edrophonium.

Edrophonium and neostigmine are water soluble, ionized compounds, which are mainly excreted unchanged in the urine.

### *Pyridostigmine*

This anticholinesterase has a longer onset of action and duration of effect than neostigmine. It is not used in anaesthetic practice but is given orally as treatment for patients with myasthenia gravis.

### *Physostigmine*

This anticholinesterase is a tertiary amine. It is more lipid soluble than edrophonium and neostigmine, and can therefore cross the blood–brain barrier, producing cerebral effects such as sedation and confusion. It is rarely used in anaesthetic practice.

### *Organophosphorus compounds*

These anticholinesterases bind irreversibly to acetylcholinesterase, destroying the esteratic receptor site. New enzyme must be synthesized before recovery from their effect can occur. These agents are used in chemical warfare, e.g. phosgene nerve gas.

As anticholinesterases also have a muscarinic effect, anticholinergic agents that have an effect only at the muscarinic acetylcholine receptors are administered with them. Atropine was mainly used for many years, but its effect at the cardiac muscarinic receptors was occasionally disadvantageous. For instance, in a patient with cardiac dysrhythmias or rapid atrial fibrillation, an increase in pulse rate could have an adverse effect. Intravenous atropine has a more rapid onset of action than neostigmine and a shorter duration of effect – about 45 min. It is therefore more appropriate to use with edrophonium.

Glycopyrrolate is now more frequently used. It has less cardiac effect than atropine, but otherwise is equally effective. Glycopyrrolate has an onset of action more similar to that of neostigmine, thus reducing the initial tachycardia that can be produced by atropine.

## MONITORING OF NEUROMUSCULAR BLOCK

Whenever a neuromuscular blocking drug is being used, it is preferable to monitor the degree of block so that good recovery can be obtained when surgery is complete. Inadequate recovery from neuromuscular block is not only unpleasant for the patient as they struggle to breathe, but is also a potential cause of postoperative chest infection.

Clinical monitoring of neuromuscular block began in 1959. It was realized that, if a peripheral motor nerve was stimulated, the response in the appropriate muscle could be assessed clinically, by visual or tactile means. To be reproducible, the stimuli must activate all the nerve fibres on each occasion; this property is achieved by the delivery of a supramaximal stimulus, which ensures 100% recruitment. The ulnar nerve at the wrist is frequently used, stimulation of which causes contraction of the adductor pollicis muscle in the thumb. The facial nerve can be stimulated by the trigor of the ear, causing contraction of the ipsilateral facial muscles. Alternatively, the popliteal nerve can be stimulated at the knee to cause dorsiflexion of the foot.

### Modes of stimulation

Single 'twitch' stimuli given at 0.1–2.0 Hz have the benefit of being tolerated by the conscious patient. There is no residual effect if twitch stimuli have been applied during anaesthesia; no pain is experienced postoperatively. If the patient is given a small dose of a depolarizing agent, the height of a twitch stimulus decreases. If successive twitch stimuli are applied, e.g. every second, the height of successive twitch stimuli after a small dose of suxamethonium will be similar. This is known as Phase I block. If a larger dose of suxamethonium is given, the twitch response disappears completely, only to return gradually as the effect of the suxamethonium wears off and recovery from block occurs.

If a small dose of a non-depolarizing agent is given, the twitch height falls but successive twitch responses at, for example, 0.5-s intervals, sequentially decrease in amplitude; this is known as 'decrement' or 'fade' of the twitch response (Phase II block). If a larger dose of non-depolarizing agent is given, the twitch is ablated. If repeated doses or an infusion of suxamethonium are given, then the twitch response may change from a Phase I, depolarizing block, to a Phase II, non-depolarizing block, in which fade of successive stimuli can be detected.

The disadvantage of the twitch response as a clinical tool is that a baseline measurement is required before the neuromuscular blocking drug is given, to measure the depth of block and in particular to determine if full recovery has occurred.

#### *Train-of-four (TOF) twitch response*

The TOF twitch response was developed as a clinical tool by Ali and colleagues in 1970, in an attempt to overcome the disadvantages of the twitch response. It consists of four stimuli each of 2 Hz, in total of 2 s duration, with a 10-s interval between trains (Figure 35.7a). In the presence of a depolarizing agent, the height of all four stimuli is reduced to the same degree. When recovery from block occurs, all four stimuli are of the same height. When a non-depolarizing drug is given, however, the height of the fourth twitch decreases to a greater extent than the third, which is smaller than the second, which is smaller than the first (Figure 35.7b). This fade is more marked during onset than recovery from neuromuscular block, and its extent varies with different neuromuscular blocking drugs. The ratio of the height of the fourth twitch T4, to the first T1, is known as the TOF ratio. This ratio has marked clinical value because it does not require a baseline measurement; the value can be obtained for the first time after a neuromuscular blocking drug has been given. It has long been thought that 75% recovery of the TOF ratio is required for the patient to cough adequately, hold the head off the pillow for 5 s, and protrude the tongue. Recently, it has been suggested that, if electromyographic means of monitoring have been used (see below), 90% recovery of the TOF ratio is required to ensure that the airway is fully protected.

Full recovery of a twitch stimulus after the use of a neuromuscular blocking drug does not mean that there is no remaining residual neuromuscular block. It is thought that at least 75% of the postsynaptic nicotinic receptors must be occupied by a non-depolarizing agent before any degree of neuromuscular block is detectable; only 20% of these receptors need to be occupied by suxamethonium to detect an effect.

As it is difficult to detect fade of the TOF ratio visually or by tactile means when it is greater than 0.4, more sensitive methods of clinically detecting minimal residual block were sought.

#### *Double-burst stimulation*

The double-burst stimulation (DBS) consists of two or three bursts of 50 Hz tetanus every 20 ms, separated by a 750-s interval (Figure 35.7c). More marked fade will be detectable during the later stages of recovery with this monitoring method than with TOF stimulation (Figure 35.7d).

#### *Tetanic stimuli*

These can detect lesser degrees of block than twitch stimuli. Stimuli of 100 Hz are even more sensitive than those of 50 Hz. Fade of a tetanic response can be detected when full recovery of the twitch response has

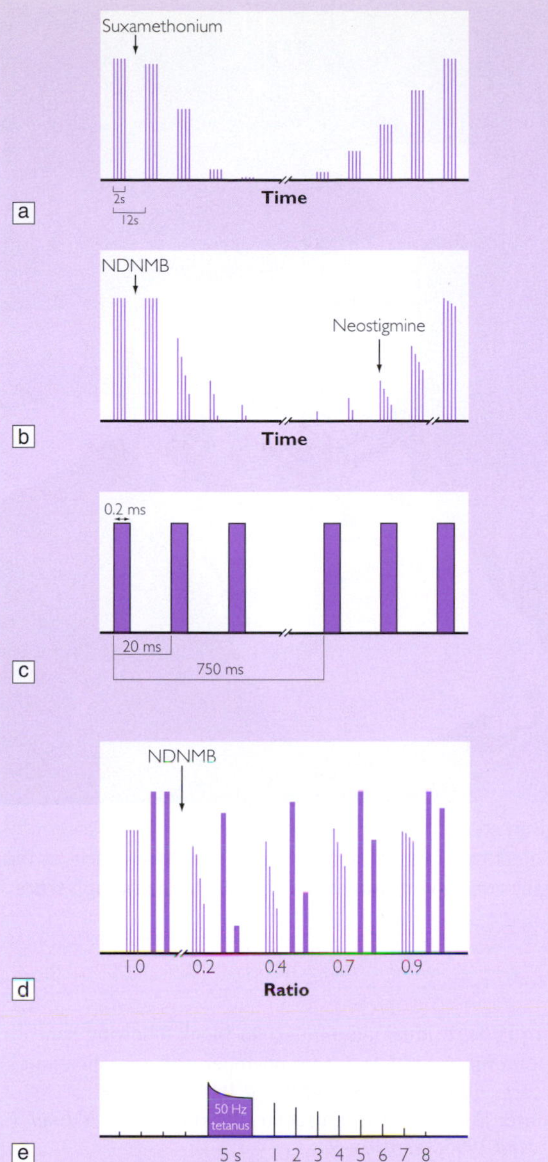


**Figure 35.7** The effect of (a) suxamethonium and (b) a non-depolarizing neuromuscular blocking drug (NDNMB) on the train-of-four (TOF) response. Note the fade of the TOF response during onset and recovery from block when a non-depolarizing drug is used. (c) Double-burst stimulation (DBS) consists of two or three tetanic bursts every 20 ms, delivered at 750-ms intervals. (d) The fade of DBS is more exaggerated than the fade of the TOF after an NDNMB, especially during the later stages of recovery. (e) Single-twitch stimuli every 1 s produce very little response when a large dose of an NDNMB has been given. After tetanic stimulation for 5 s at 50 Hz, the reintroduction of a twitch stimulus produces a greater response, which gradually disappears if successive twitch stimuli are applied. This is known as post-tetanic facilitation. The number of recordable twitch stimuli after a tetanic burst is known as the post-tetanic count.

been demonstrated after the use of a non-depolarizing drug. The disadvantage of tetanic stimulation is that it is unbearably painful in the conscious state and, even if applied during anaesthesia, some residual discomfort can be experienced on awakening.

#### *Post-tetanic facilitation*

This occurs when, after a run of 1-s twitch stimuli for at least 5 s with no recovery from block, a 5-s tetanic stimulus of at least 50 Hz is given, followed by another run of twitch stimuli at 1-s intervals. The presynaptic mobilization of acetylcholine produced by the tetanic stimulus causes a transient recovery from block, which disappears after a few seconds (Figure 35.7e). The number of twitch stimuli detectable after the run of tetanus is called the post-tetanic count.

### Monitoring equipment

If neuromuscular monitoring is being used in clinical practice, it is not necessary to measure the response accurately. But if clinical research is being carried out in which it is required to measure accurately various pharmacodynamic variables, such as time to onset of maximal block, or time to full recovery from block, then an accurate method of measuring the response is required. Two methods are mainly used: mechanography and electromyography (EMG).

#### *Mechanomyography*

The force of isometric contraction, usually of the thumb, is measured using a strain gauge transducer. The hand and arm must be immobilized and a preload tension of more than 200 g applied to the thumb. A control response should be obtained for at least 3 min before a neuromuscular blocking drug is given. The Myograph and Myotest are examples of this type of monitoring method.

#### *Electromyography*

The EMG response is measured as a waveform from an active electrode placed over the belly of the stimulated muscle. A reference electrode is placed over the insertion of the muscle and a ground electrode between the recording and stimulating electrodes (Figure 35.8). The height of the EMG response or the area under the response curve can then be measured.

The Datex Relaxograph is an example of a clinical tool that utilizes this form of neuromuscular monitoring. The benefits of the Datex Relaxograph for clinical research are, however, limited because significant baseline shift occurs with this instrument during the monitoring period. The phenomenon can be difficult to eradicate.

#### *Acceleromyography*

This has recently been developed on the basis of Newton's law – for a constant mass, force is directly proportional to acceleration. This technique monitors the rate of acceleration of the thumb in response to electrical stimulation of the ulnar nerve using a piezoelectric wafer or small aluminium rod with electrodes on both sides. The TOFguard is one commercially available acceleromyograph. It is a useful instrument for recording the TOF response in clinical situations when standard techniques would be difficult to instigate, such as long-term monitoring in the intensive care unit, or monitoring during radiological procedures. Although improved by splinting of the arm and

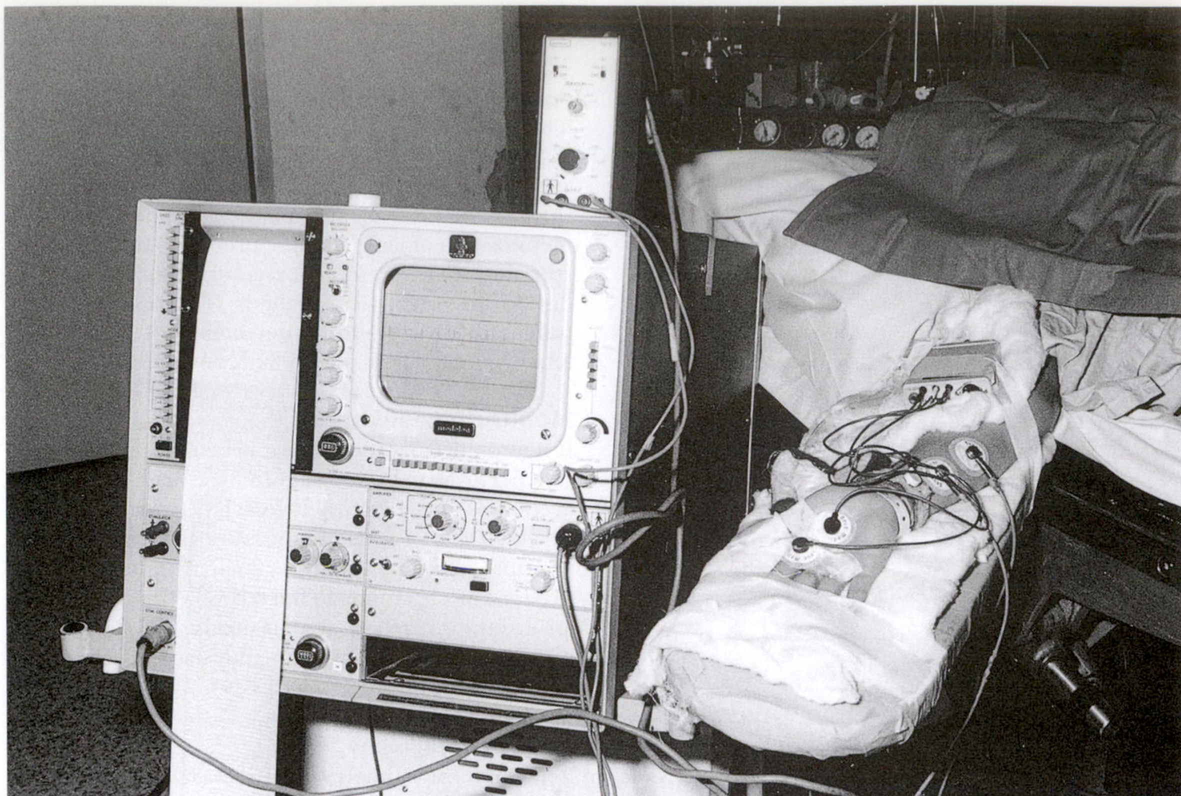

**Figure 35.8** An electromyograph (MS6) in use during a research study. The stimulating electrodes can be seen placed over the ulnar nerve in the forearm, with the reference electrode placed at the insertion of the muscle at the base of the hand, and the recording electrode placed most distally over the muscle belly. The electromyograph trace is recorded on light-sensitive paper.

wrist, the accuracy of the TOF guard is insufficient to use it during clinical research.

Monitoring of neuromuscular transmission has been reviewed by Viby-Mogensen (1982), Ali and Savarese (1976), and Beemer and Goonetilleke (1996) (see Further reading).

## FURTHER READING


Ali HH, Utting JE, Gray TC. Stimulus frequency in the detection of neuromuscular block in humans. *Br J Anaesth* 1970;**42**:967 – 78.

Ali HH, Savarese JJ. Monitoring of neuromuscular function. *Anesthesiology* 1976;**45**:216 - 49.

Beecher HK, Todd DP. A study of the deaths associated with anaesthesia and surgery. *Ann Surg* 1954;**140**:2 - 34.

Beemer GH, Goonetilleke PH. Monitoring neuromuscular transmission. *Curr Anaesth Crit Care* 1996;**7**:101 – 6.

Berg H. Is residual neuromuscular block following pancuronium a risk factor for postoperative complications? *Acta Anaesthesiol Scand Suppl* 1997;**41**:156 - 8.

Hunter JM. New neuromuscular blocking drugs. *N Engl J Med* 1995;**332**:1691 – 9.

Kalow W, Genest K. A method of detection of atypical forms of human pseudocholinesterase. *Can J Biochem Physiol* 1957;**35**:339 - 46.

Pantuck EJ. Plasma cholinesterase: gene and variations. *Anesth Analg* 1993;**77**:380 - 6.

Stenlake JB, Waigh RD, Urwin J, Dewar GH, Coker GG. Atracurium: conception and inception. *Br J Anaesth* 1983;**55**:3S - 10S.

Viby-Mogensen J. Clinical assessment of neuromuscular transmission. *Br J Anaesth* 1982;**54**:209 - 23.

Whittaker M. Plasma cholinesterase variants and anaesthesia. *Anaesthesia* 1980;**35**:174 - 97.

# Chapter 36 Local anaesthetics

L. Bromley

General anaesthesia produces reversible loss of sensation in the whole central nervous system (CNS). Local anaesthesia produces a reversible loss of sensation in a specific area of the body. This is bought about by reversibly preventing the conduction of action potentials in sensory nerves supplying the specified area. This largely involves the peripheral nervous system, although the spinal action of some local anaesthetic agents is probably more complex.

The action of these drugs is sometimes described as 'membrane stabilizing' and a wide variety of different classes of drugs can reduce the conduction of action potentials in excitable tissue. For this reason, some drugs that are primarily used for other therapeutic purposes may also have local anaesthetic properties (Table 36.1), and the drugs that are used as local anaesthetics also have other uses, e.g. as antiarrhythmic drugs.

The first drug to be used as a local anaesthetic was the naturally occurring alkaloid, cocaine. This drug is extracted from the coca plant (*Erythroxylon coca*) which grows in the foot hills of the Andes. The plant is still used to produce a tea-like drink, or the leaves may be chewed as a remedy for altitude sickness. The stimulant effect of the drug alleviates the depressive effects of the hypoxia at such altitudes, although it carries some risk; those who have chewed the leaves observe the local anaesthetic effects in the resulting numbness of the oral mucosa. The plant was brought to Europe in the nineteenth century, and the active drug isolated and studied in Germany. It was used as a mood-enhancing drug among the intelligentsia; Conan Doyle was familiar with its use, as were several other literary figures in Britain. Sigmund Freud was the first to use it clinically; he attempted to wean a morphine-addicted patient using cocaine, but this resulted only in the patient becoming addicted to cocaine instead. Koller, an ophthalmologist, was the first to use cocaine as a local anaesthetic; initially, it was used for surface anaesthesia, but it was rapidly taken up for infiltration and spinal anaesthesia. By the end of the nineteenth century, the addictive nature of cocaine was well known and the search started for other molecules that would provide local anaesthesia without its disadvantages.

The search for better local anaesthetics initially produced a number of drugs that were chemically related, all having an ester linkage in their structure. Of this group only three drugs are still in use. Most of the currently used local anaesthetic agents have an amide linkage, and the first of these to be introduced was lignocaine (lidocaine). Lignocaine was synthesized in 1943 and has been the basis for a series of other drugs, of which the most widely used are bupivacaine, prilocaine, and the new drug ropivacaine.

## PHYSICAL AND CHEMICAL PROPERTIES

Most of the currently used local anaesthetic agents are insoluble in water, but their hydrochloride salts are very soluble. The dilute solution is therefore acidic (pH 4.0–5.5). They are very stable and have a long shelf-life. The amide local anaesthetics are heat stable and can be sterilized by autoclaving; the esters were liable to breakdown at high temperatures, one of the disadvantages that has led to the decline in their use (Table 36.2).

Chemically, the drugs have a common structural form. This consists of a lipophilic group, an intermediate chain and a hydrophilic group (Figure 36.1).

The relationship between the physiochemical properties and the pharmacological action of local anaesthetics has been well defined by the development of the different drugs (Figure 36.2).

### Duration of action

Duration of action is influenced by three properties of the drug: the physical shape of the molecule, as

| Table 36.1 Drugs that have local anaesthetic properties in addition to their primary use |
|---|
| Anticonvulsants |
| Antiarrhythmics |
| β-blockers |
| Opioids |
| Antihistamines |
| Barbiturates |

| Table 36.2 Ester local anaesthetics |
|---|
| Relatively unstable in solution |
| Hydrolysed by plasma and tissue esterases |
| Metabolite *p*-aminobenzoate associated with hypersensitivity and allergic reactions |
| Not heat stable |
| Now largely superseded |

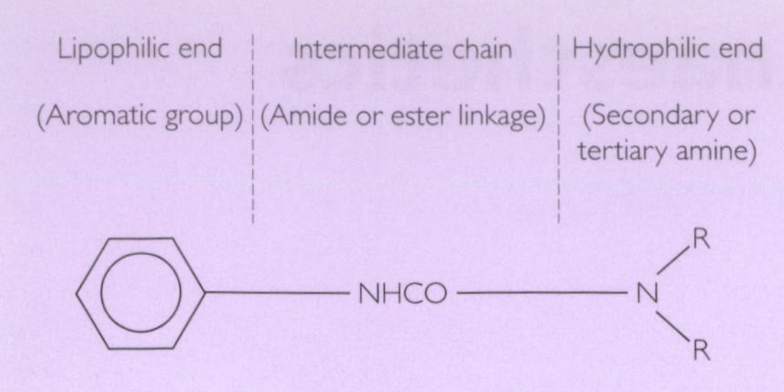


**Figure 36.1** The basic structure of local anaesthetics.

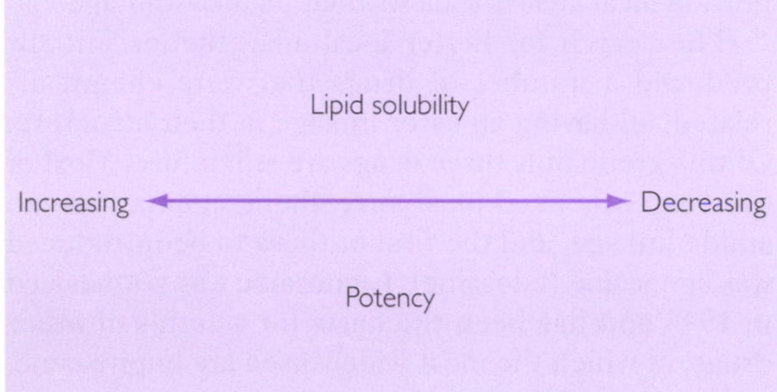


**Figure 36.2** Potency and lipid solubility.

influenced by the length of the intermediate chain, can alter the duration of action. In addition, the degree of plasma and tissue protein binding will influence duration, because the drug will interact with the tissue for a greater time if it binds extensively (Figure 36.3).

### Onset of action

The rapidity of onset is determined by the dissociation constant of the drug ($pK_a$).

The chemical definition of an acid is a moiety that accepts protons, and a base is a moiety that donates protons. Most drugs are weak acids or weak bases. Local anaesthetics are basic drugs, and to understand the effect of dissociation on onset of action it is necessary to understand the relationship between the $pK_a$ of the drug molecule and the pH of the solution in which the drug is dissolved.

In general:

$$HA \rightleftharpoons H^+ + A^-.$$

All electrolytes are ionized in solution, the position of the equilibrium depending on the pH of the solution and the $pK_a$ of the molecule.

$$K_a = \frac{[H^+][A^-](\text{ionized})}{[HA](\text{un-ionized})}$$

$$pKa = -\log_{10} K_a.$$

Therefore the $pK_a$ is $-\log_{10}$ of the equilibrium constant of the reaction:

$$HA \rightleftharpoons H^+ + A^-.$$

The scale for $pK_a$ is very wide; acids have low numbers and bases high numbers.

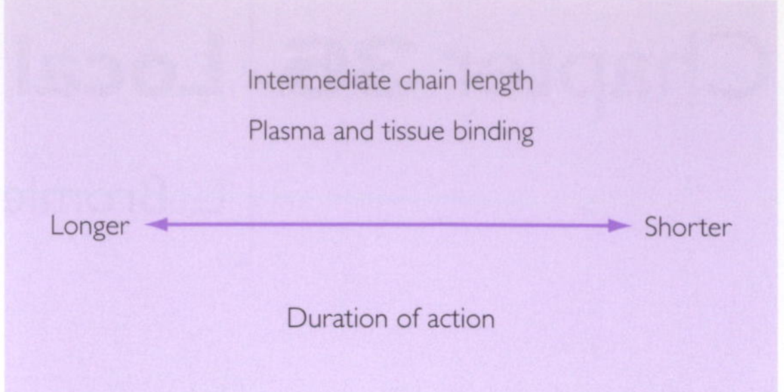


**Figure 36.3** Binding, chain length, and duration of action.

Now, pH is the $\log_{10}$ of the hydrogen ion concentration ($H_3O^+$), so in a weak solution:

$$K_a = \frac{[H_3O^+][A^-]}{[HA]}$$

Taking logs of each side:

$$\log_{10} K_a = \log_{10} [H_3O^+] + \log_{10} [A^-] - \log_{10} [HA]$$

so:

$$\log_{10} K_a - \log_{10} [H_3O^+] = \log_{10} [A^-] - \log_{10} [HA].$$

As $\log_{10} [H_3O^+]$ is by definition the pH, and $\log_{10} K_a$ is by definition the $pK_a$ we can rewrite this as:

$$pK_a - pH = \log_{10} [A^-] - \log_{10} [HA].$$

To do a bit of mathematical rearrangement we can say that:

$$pH - pK_a = \log (\text{ionized/un-ionized}).$$

Therefore for a base, lowering the pH will increase the ionization of the drug and vice versa. Also it can be seen that, when pH = $pK_a$, the ratio will be 50 : 50, i.e. the $pK_a$ is the pH at which the drug is 50% ionized.

Figures 36.4 and 36.5 show the pH and ionization for an acid and base respectively and the $pK_a$ values are shown in Table 36.3.

At physiological pH, the local anaesthetics are present in both the ionized and the un-ionized form, with more in the former than in the latter. As the pH becomes more acidotic in the tissues, the equilibrium moves to increase ionization, and in infected tissues where the pH can be very acidic indeed the ionization

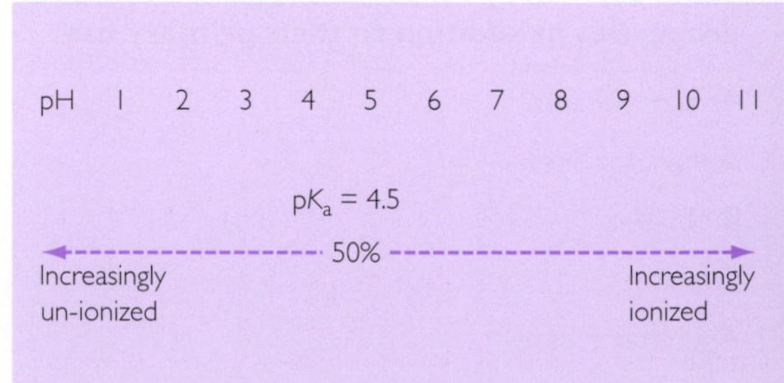


**Figure 36.4** Ionization and pH for an acid.

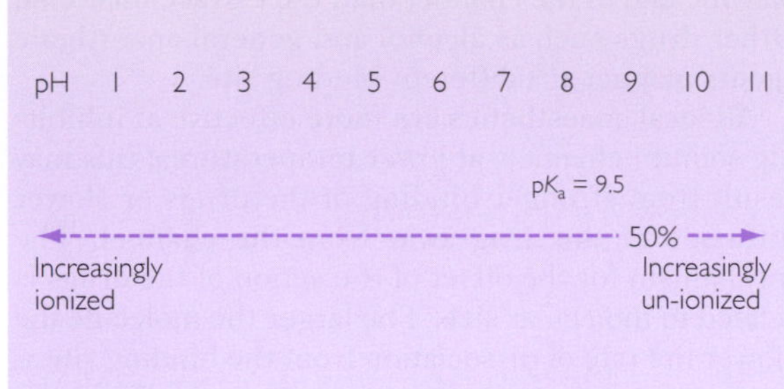


**Figure 36.5** Ionization and pH for a base.

| **Table 36.3 The pK$_a$ values of local anaesthetics** | |
|---|---|
| **Esters** | |
| Amethocaine | 8.5 |
| Procaine | 8.9 |
| **Amides** | |
| Mepivacaine | 7.6 |
| Etidocaine | 7.7 |
| Lignocaine | 7.7 |
| Prilocaine | 7.7 |
| Bupivacaine | 8.1 |
| Ropivacaine | 8.1 |

may be almost total. This is important for onset of action because it is only the un-ionized form of the drug that can diffuse across the nerve membrane to reach the site of action of the drug.

## MECHANISM OF ACTION

Local anaesthetics block impulses by inhibiting individual sodium channels in the nerve membrane and thus reducing the inward sodium current of the nerve fibre.

### The membrane

The resting membrane potential is maintained by a membrane-bound enzyme, $Na^+/K^+$ ATPase. This pumps out three sodium ions for every two potassium ions that it pumps in. The resting membrane potential is –50 to –90 mV, with the interior of the cell negative with respect to the outside (Figure 36.6).

### The sodium channel

The sodium channels are voltage gated. Gating refers to the movements of the channel molecules that underlie the transitions between conducting and non-conducting forms. During an action potential, the voltage-gated sodium channels open briefly, allowing a small quantity of $Na^+$ to enter the cell; this depolarizes the membrane. The sodium channels close spontaneously. A slow developing outward current then develops, which is made up of $K^+$ flowing through voltage-gated potassium channels. A local ionic current in the cytoplasm helps to propagate the wave of depolarization throughout the cell's excitable membrane.

The sodium channel itself is made up of proteins within the membrane. There is a large hydrophobic region which is arranged as an α helix which spans the membrane and is interspersed with the hydrophilic regions that line the pore. The glycoprotein has the role of acting like an enzyme to catalyse the passage of ions through the otherwise highly resistant membrane. A channel is open when the energy barrier is low enough for the ions to flow through. The lining of the channel pore can be rearranged to alter the energy barrier. Gating currents are caused by movements of electrically charged regions of the channel macromolecule, and are minuscule compared with the size of the inflowing current when the channel opens. These gating currents have been studied electrophysiologically and there is an 'on' gating current transiently moving outwards at the beginning of depolarization, and an 'off' gating current immediately after repolarization.

The channel has multiple sites, which can bind to other molecules. Six different binding sites have been identified for toxins derived from different animals. Tetrodotoxin from the Japanese puffer fish, saxitoxins from dinoflagellates that contaminate shellfish, and some types of scorpion venom all bind to sodium channels. These toxins bind at the extracellular surface of the channel, using a different mechanism from local anaesthetics.

There are two non-conducting forms in which the sodium channel can exist: a resting form, from which it can move to an activated form and produce an 'on' gating current, and an inactive form. The inactive form has an 'immobilized' gate which cannot be activated until it returns to the resting form (Figure 36.7).

An open channel can move to one of two states: closed or inactivated. If the membrane is depolarized for a long time, a move to the deactivated state is favoured. Recovery from the inactive state requires prolonged repolarization.

### Interaction of drugs with the sodium channel

Local anaesthetic drugs can potentially bind with the channel in any of the forms in which it exists. The local anaesthetic drug interacts with the channel from the intracellular surface of the membrane; it must cross the membrane and enter the cell before it binds with

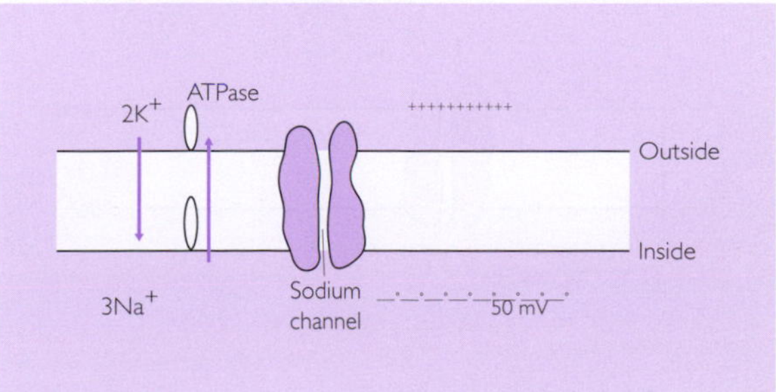


**Figure 36.6** Sodium channels in the cell membrane.

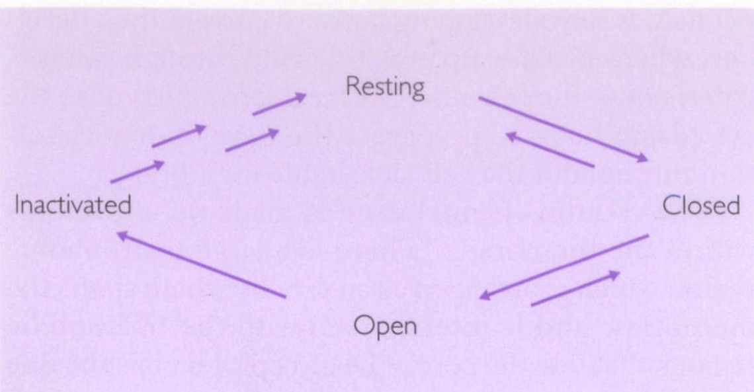


**Figure 36.7** Active and inactive states of the sodium channel.

the channel. Although the drug passes through the membrane most rapidly in its un-ionized form, it must dissociate into the ionized form to interact with the channel. The ionized form enters the sodium channel from the cytoplasm via the 'hydrophilic pathway'. The action of the drug is to interfere with the conformational changes in the channel, which occur during activation. These events happen as the channel moves from the closed resting state to the open state. The drugs do not 'block' the channel in a physical sense; rather they prevent movement to an open, conducting form.

Local anaesthetic drugs can inhibit sodium currents in two different ways. If the nerve is conducting few impulses a 'tonic' block is produced; as the frequency of impulses increases a 'phasic' block is produced. These different types of inhibition are proposed as the result of binding with different forms of the channel, phasic block being associated with a block of the open form of the channel. With repeated depolarizations, an increasing fraction of the available sodium channels becomes blocked. This is sometimes referred to as use-dependent block (Figure 36.8).

This type of block, which depends on the local anaesthetic drug being present in the ionized form, is probably the major mechanism of action for this class of drugs. However, some local anaesthetics are not ionized at the pH of the inside of the cell, e.g. benzocaine and benzyl alcohol, and a second mechanism is proposed for these and tertiary amine local anaesthetics. These molecules alter the configuration of the channel via a 'hydrophobic pathway', bringing about their action while dissolved in the membrane. These drugs act at the same binding site as the ionized drugs, but reach that site by a different pathway. Evidence suggests that this binding site is nearer to the cytoplasmic end of the channel than the extracellular end. Other drugs such as alcohol and general anaesthetic agents may act at a different binding site.

All local anaesthetics are more effective at inhibiting sodium channels at lower temperatures; this may result from stronger binding of the drugs or slower diffusion of the drug away from the channel. The mechanism for the offset of the action of the drugs is related to molecular size. The larger the molecule the slower the rate of dissociation from the binding site.

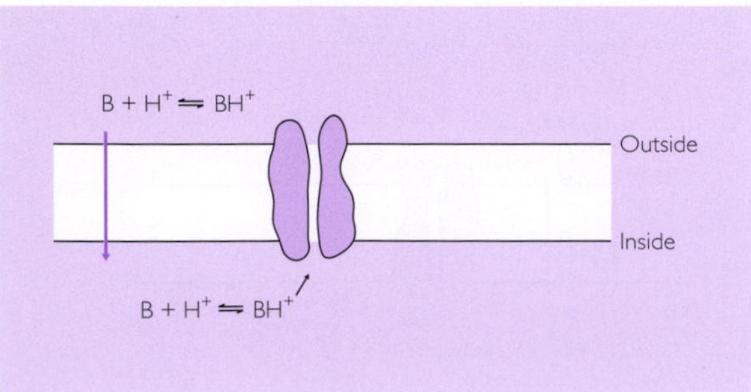


**Figure 36.8** Interaction of drugs with the sodium channel.

### Actions on whole nerves

The action of local anaesthetics on individual sodium channels has been studied in depth, and accounts for the structure–activity relationship observed with different drugs. There are some considerations that must be taken into account when considering the action of the drugs on whole nerve trunks rather than on individual sodium channels. In a mixed nerve, there are fibres of different diameter, which subserve different functions. As nerve diameter increases, the degree of myelinization of the nerve increases. Myelinization is the result of the spiral wrapping of the nerve by the membranes and cytoplasm of a Schwann cell. A number of individual Schwann cells wrap around the axon of a peripheral nerve along its length; at the junctions between the cells, there is an area of lower electrical resistance called the nodes of Ranvier. The internodal distance depends on the diameter of the fibre and the size of the Schwann cells. Conduction along myelinated fibres is from one node of Ranvier to the next, rather than sequentially along the membrane as in unmyelinated fibres – called saltatory conduction. This confers an advantage of greater speed of conduction (Figure 36.9).

To produce a block of this type of nerve, the local anaesthetic must be given in sufficient dosage to block at least three consecutive nodes of Ranvier.

Sensory nerves, and particularly those conducting pain, are of two types: the smallest fibres or C fibres, and Aδ fibres. C fibres are unmyelinated, the lack of a myelin sheath allowing penetration of the nerve more easily by the local anaesthetic drug; motor fibres are, however, of the largest type, all myelinated, and the local anaesthetic can act only at the nodes of Ranvier because the myelin constitutes a block to the diffusion of the

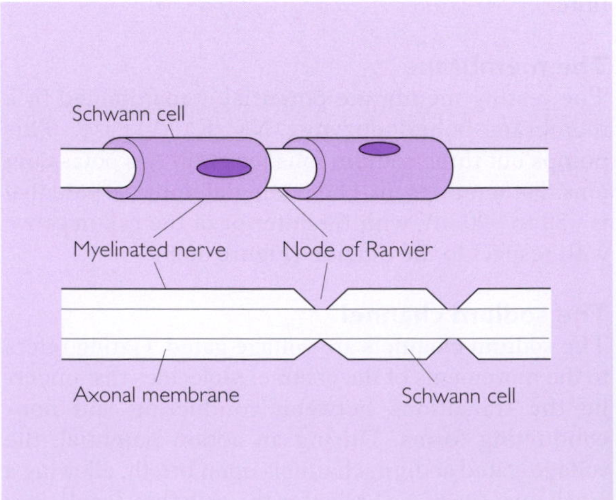


**Figure 36.9** Conduction along myelinated fibres.

drug. This results in a differential sensitivity of these fibres to local anaesthetic action (Table 36.4).

This accounts for the differentiation in sensory and motor block seen in local anaesthetic use. It may not be as marked as might be expected because of the arrangement of fibres in large nerves, where motor fibres are often arranged circumferentially and are therefore exposed to the drug first. However, in general, there is a tendency to separation of the intensity of block, which is particularly useful in the use of these drugs for postoperative analgesia

### Spinal and epidural actions of local anaesthetics

The mechanism of action of the local anaesthetics in the spinal cord is more complex than just producing a block of action potentials in nerves leaving the cord. Local anaesthetics affect many other proteins associated with the cell membrane as well as the sodium channel. Adenylyl cyclase, guanylyl cyclase, calmodulin-sensitive proteins, and the $Na^+/K^+$ ATPase and $Ca^{2+}/Mg^{2+}$ ATPase systems are all modified by local anaesthetics. In addition to these, phospholipase $A_2$ and phospholipase C are inhibited, producing an extensive effect on second messenger systems.

Synaptic transmission in the spinal cord may be inhibited by modification of postsynaptic receptors and blockade of presynaptic calcium channels, reducing transmitter release. This may account for the observation that epidural analgesia with low-dose infusions of local anaesthetic may be effective despite the absence of a clear segmental sensory block of cold sensation.

### Pharmacokinetics

The pharmacokinetic properties of local anaesthetic agents are summarized in Table 36.5.

#### *Absorption*

Local anaesthetics are well absorbed from their site of injection, as they are able to cross lipid membranes, both into the axon and into other body compartments. The amount of absorption, and the rate of absorption, depend on the individual drug, the site of injection, particularly the vascularity of the area, and the surface area available for absorption. Thus some sites may produce significant plasma levels of the local anaesthetic, and others negligible levels (Figure 36.10).

It is clear therefore that the same dose of local anaesthetic may have different toxicities depending on the site of use. The plasma level after injection is further influenced by the presence or absence of a vasoconstrictor. This may be an intrinsic effect of the drug, as with cocaine, or an added substance specifically there to vasoconstrict. Cocaine produces vasoconstriction by its action on sympathetic nerve terminals. It blocks the uptake mechanism for the return of norepinephrine (noradrenaline) to the nerve terminal after the nerve ending has discharged in response to an action potential. Specifically it blocks the enzyme system known as uptake I. As a result, the amount of norepinephrine in the synaptic cleft is increased, producing a generalized increase in sympathetic activity. This accounts for a number of the pharmacological effects of cocaine, including the precipitation of myocardial infarction in some subjects, and the

**Table 36.4 Differential sensitivity of nerve fibres to lignocaine**

| | Fibre | Sensitivity |
|---|---|---|
| Most sensitive | C fibres | Pain and temperature |
| | B fibres | Sympathetic vasoconstrictor fibres |
| | Aδ fibres | 'Slow' pain fibres |
| | Aγ fibres | Muscle spindles |
| | Aβ fibres | Motor and pressure |
| Least sensitive | Aα fibres | Large motor and proprioception |

**Table 36.5 Pharmacokinetic properties of local anaesthetic agents**

| | Terminal half-life (min) | Clearance (L/min) | Apparent volume of distribution (L) | Plasma protein binding (%) | Maximum recommended dose |
|---|---|---|---|---|---|
| Lignocaine | 100 | 1 | 92 | 64 | 200 mg |
| Prilocaine | 100 | 2.4 | 191 | 50 | 400 mg |
| Bupivacaine | 180 | 0.6 | 73 | 95 | 2 mg/kg |
| Ropivacaine | 111 | 0.82 | 59 | 94 | Maximum bolus 250 mg |

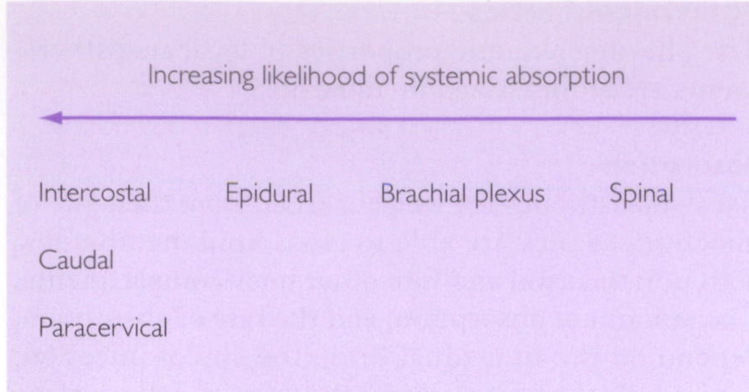


**Figure 36.10** The toxicity of local anaesthetic agents depends on the site of injection.

ischaemic damage to the nasal septum, which results from long-term nasal inhalation of cocaine, as a result of local vasoconstriction.

### *Added vasoconstrictors*

Vascular smooth muscle has a biphasic response to the other local anaesthetic agents, with a vasodilator action prominent (Figure 36.11).

To overcome this effect and to reduce the absorption from highly vascular sites, local anaesthetics are frequently presented combined with epinephrine (adrenaline). The addition of epinephrine reduces the peak plasma concentration by 50% when used in intercostal nerve blocks. Addition of epinephrine to cocaine solutions for topical use in nasal surgery can reduce the absorption tenfold, although it carries the potential disadvantage of increasing the incidence of cardiac arrhythmias. Epinephrine remains the most commonly used vasoconstrictor, despite efforts to popularize phenylephrine, norepinephrine, octapressin, and felypressin (vasopressin analogues). Doses of epinephrine in excess of 200 μg using a concentration of 5 μg/ml solution (1 in 200 000) confer no advantage and carry a risk of unwanted effects. Evidence suggests that neither bupivacaine nor ropivacaine have their maximal plasma concentration reduced by the addition of epinephrine.

## Distribution

Initial rapid distribution with a half-life of 1–3 min is followed by a slower decline in plasma concentration as the drug is increasingly metabolized and excreted. The curve may be bi- or triexponential. As a result of rapid metabolism by tissue and plasma esterases, the ester local anaesthetics have a short terminal half-life of about 10 min. By contrast, the amides have a longer terminal half-life: 100 min for lignocaine, 111 min for ropivacaine, and 180 min for bupivacaine.

Protein binding does not occur with the ester local anaesthetics, and varies for the amides. The binding is principally with $\alpha_1$-acid glycoprotein (Figure 36.12).

The extent of plasma protein binding is readily reversible and does not seem to affect uptake into other tissues. Changes in concentration in $\alpha_1$-acid glycoprotein occur at the extremes of age, in pregnancy, renal disease, malignancy, and myocardial infarction, and after surgery. Protein binding is increased and the free portion of the drug is reduced. This has implications for placental transfer: highly bound drugs cross the placenta less than those with a larger plasma concentration of the free drug. Thus, less bupivacaine appears in the umbilical veins than with lignocaine and prilocaine. However, there is less $\alpha_1$-acid glycoprotein in the fetal circulation, so that the proportion of free drug in the fetus is greater. Lignocaine, given in repeated doses in labour, can produce toxicity in the newborn – the 'floppy baby' syndrome. Bupivacaine, and by implication ropivacaine, produce minimal neurobehavioural effects in the newborn.

## Metabolism and excretion

The metabolism of local anaesthetic agents does not take place in the neuronal tissue. In the case of ester local anaesthetics, they are metabolized by esterases that are widespread throughout the body. In plasma they are specifically metabolized by plasma cholinesterases. Procaine and its derivatives are metabolized to *p*-aminobenzoic acid and diethylaminoethanol. Cocaine, alone among the esters, is metabolized in the liver.

Amide local anaesthetics are metabolized principally in the liver. The amide linkage is hydrolysed by microsomal enzymes: the mixed function oxidases, cytochrome P450, and amidases in the hepatocytes. The metabolites of the amides are pharmacologically active, the main metabolite of lignocaine (monoethylglycinexylidide or MEGX) being associated with CNS effects. Prilocaine is metabolized to *o*-toluidine and then to hydroxytoluidine (Figure 36.13).

The hepatic extraction of these drugs varies from moderate to high, so the metabolism of the amides is dependent on hepatic blood flow. Prilocaine has a clearance that exceeds liver blood flow, which suggests that it is also metabolized elsewhere, the most likely site being the lung. The metabolism of these drugs is

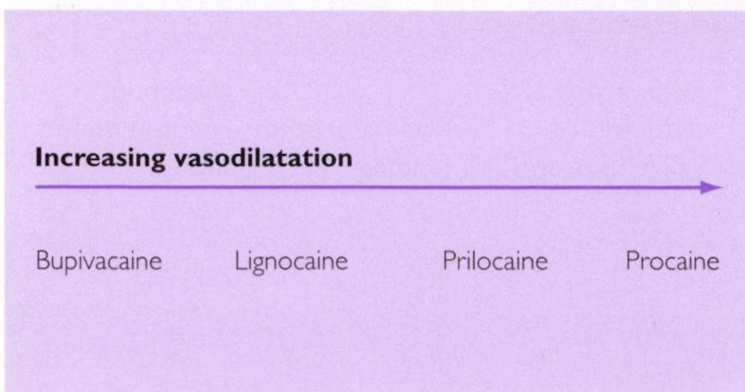


**Figure 36.11** Action of local anaesthetics on vascular smooth muscle.

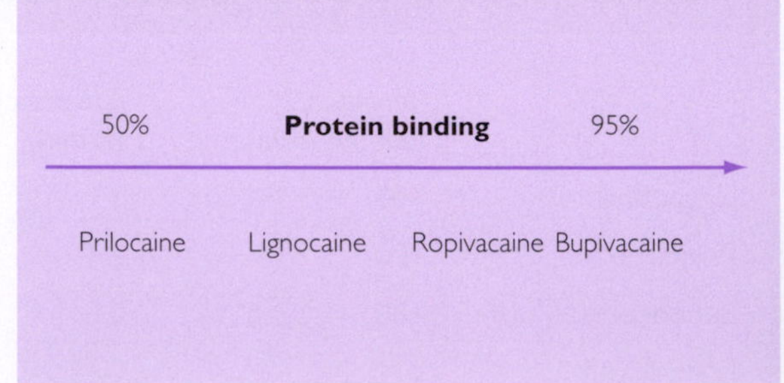


**Figure 36.12** Protein binding of local anaesthetic agents.

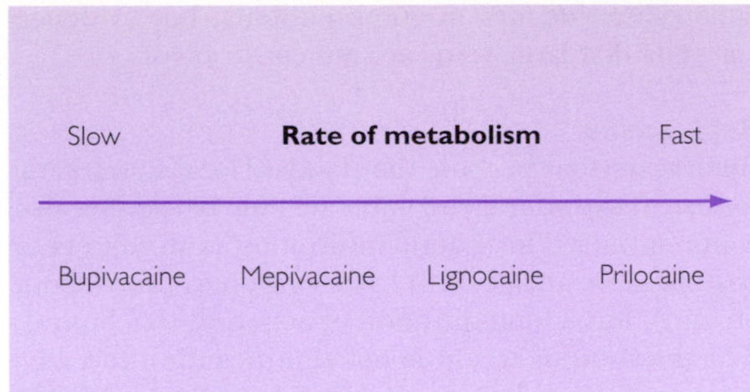


**Figure 36.13** The rate of metabolism of amide local anaesthetic agents.

therefore slowed in cardiac failure and in liver disease, which may result in toxicity. Neonates have a decreased clearance and increased half-life for amines.

Renal disease can produce a build-up of the polar metabolites, but has little or no effect on the half-life of the parent drug. Renal excretion of the unaltered drug is minimal. The metabolites are highly water soluble and are excreted in the urine.

## TOXICITY

Toxicity is related to absolute or relative overdose. Overdose results from a large dose reaching the vascular system; this may be related to regional anaesthesia or inadvertent intra-arterial injection. The onset of symptoms is related to the rate of injection as well as the total dose. With slow injection there may be early signs of CNS toxicity before major toxic effects are seen.

### CNS toxicity

The local anaesthetics readily cross the blood–brain barrier and have a biphasic effect on the CNS. Small doses of lignocaine have an anticonvulsant effect, and have been used for this purpose in neurosurgery. Larger doses produce CNS excitation by depressing cortical inhibitory pathways, allowing unopposed activity of the excitatory components. There is a transitory phase of unbalanced excitation followed by generalized CNS depression. As the plasma concentration rises, the patient experiences perioral tingling and numbness, light-headedness, visual disturbances, confusion, tremors, and restlessness. Grand mal convulsions, coma, and respiratory arrest occur as the plasma concentration reaches the order of 2 μg/ml for bupivacaine and ropivacaine and 9 μg/ml for lignocaine. At these plasma levels cardiotoxicity is imminent. If the overdose occurs very rapidly, there may be no early signs and the first sign of overdose will be convulsions, followed immediately by cardiac arrest.

### Cardiac toxicity

Cardiac toxicity is related to the action on the cardiac action potential. The action of local anaesthetics on cardiac sodium channels appears to differ from the action on those in nerves. The cardiac action potential is characterized by long depolarization periods, which induce the transition of the channels to the slow inactivated form; this recovers to an activated form in tens to hundreds of milliseconds. The antiarrhythmic effect of a drug such as lignocaine relates to its high affinity with this slow inactivated form of the channel. Bupivacaine appears to bind only to this form and to dissociate from it slowly, accounting for its greater cardiac toxicity. This results in a decrease in the maximum rise of phase 0 of the cardiac action potential. The maximal rate of rise ($V_{max}$) is depressed by all local anaesthetics in a dose-dependent manner (Figure 36.14).

This effect on sodium channels is stereospecific: $S(-)$ bupivacaine has a lower binding affinity than the $R(+)$ enantiomer; ropivacaine, which is in the form of an $S$ enantiomer only, has significantly less cardiotoxicity.

In addition to the effect on sodium channels, local anaesthetics also have a broad, non-selective action in reducing the amplitude of potassium and calcium currents. Effects described in the spinal cord on second messenger systems may also be seen in the heart. Cardiac slowing, and prolongation of the PR interval and the QRS interval allows re-entry arrhythmias and ultimately ventricular fibrillation. These effects are potentiated by hypoxia, acidosis, and hyperkalaemia.

Cardiac muscle is more resistant than brain to the effect of overdose by local anaesthetics. The plasma concentration to produce cardiac collapse is seven times that needed to produce CNS toxicity for lignocaine and four times that for bupivacaine; ropivacaine appears to be intermediate between the two.

Pregnancy has been shown to exacerbate the cardiotoxic effect of bupivacaine, but not of lignocaine or ropivacaine.

### Other adverse effects

#### *Allergy*

Allergy to local anaesthetic drugs is very rare. The metabolites of the esters have been implicated in promoting skin rashes and occasionally anaphylactic reactions have occurred. *p*-Aminobenzoic acid is said to act as a hapten and promote antibody production. Preservatives added to local anaesthetic solutions have been implicated in allergic reactions.

#### *Drug interaction*

*p*-Aminobenzoic acid can antagonize the effects of sulphonamides. Sulphonamides prevent the incorporation of *p*-aminobenzoic acid into the folic acid nucleus. The presence of a very high concentration of *p*-aminobenzoic acid antagonizes their effect.

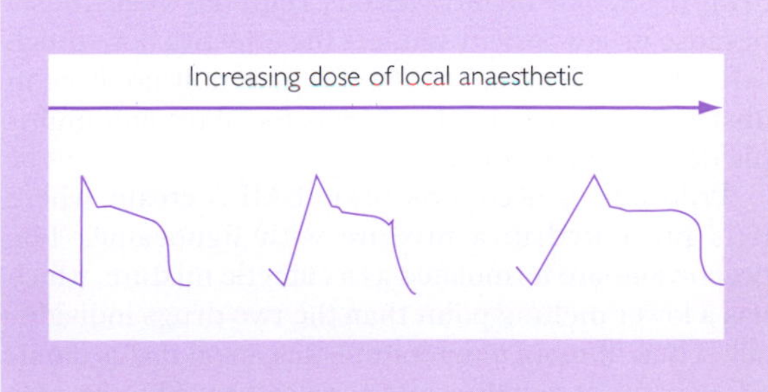


**Figure 36.14** Dose-dependent depression of $V_{max}$ in phase 0 of the cardiac action potential.

Drugs that reduce liver blood flow decrease the clearance of amide local anaesthetics, e.g. propranolol, and general anaesthetics. Liver enzymes can be inhibited by many drugs, thereby decreasing clearance of amides. Common examples are barbiturates, phenytoin, and cimetidine.

Verapamil displaces amides from their protein-binding sites and raises the unbound fraction of the drug. Epinephrine can increase the clearance of amides by altering cardiovascular dynamics.

#### *Methaemoglobinaemia*

Prilocaine is metabolized to 6-hydroxytoluidine which induces methaemoglobinaemia. This can be reversed by administering methylene blue 5 mg/kg. Neonates are particularly vulnerable to the effects of methaemoglobinaemia, because they lack sufficient of the enzyme in their erythrocytes to reduce the methaemoglobin back to haemoglobin. This may be clinically significant when using EMLA cream (a eutectic mixture of lignocaine and prilocaine) in very small children who have a high surface-area-to-volume ratio and can absorb significant quantities of the drug. Children may also lick the cream off and swallow it.

## INDIVIDUAL LOCAL ANAESTHETIC AGENTS

### The amides

#### *Lignocaine*

Since its introduction in the 1940s, lignocaine has become the most commonly used agent for local infiltration, topical anaesthesia, and peripheral nerve blocks. It has a rapid onset, its duration of action is moderate (1–2 hours) and its potency four times that of procaine. It has relatively low toxicity.

Lignocaine is a class Ib antiarrhythmic drug used to treat ventricular arrhythmias. It has been used parenterally as an anticonvulsant, an analgesic, and specifically by infusion in the management of neuropathic pain. It is commonly added to intravenous drugs such as propofol and methohexitone (methohexital) to reduce pain on injection. Lignocaine has also been said to have antithrombotic, anti-inflammatory, and antimicrobial activity.

#### *Prilocaine*

The major advantage of prilocaine is its reduced risk of toxicity compared with the other agents. It has a rapid onset, similar potency to lignocaine, but a duration of action that is longer than that of lignocaine but shorter than that of bupivacaine. It has become the drug of choice in intravenous regional anaesthesia because its low toxicity renders the effective dose much safer than with other agents. It is generally not used in obstetrics because its duration is too short and multiple doses are required.

Prilocaine is used topically in EMLA cream, where it is presented in a mixture with lignocaine. The proportions are formulated as a eutectic mixture, which has a lower melting point than the two drugs individually. Thus, at room temperature, it is an oil that is emulsified in water and presented as a cream. The cream is applied under an occlusive dressing and produces good surface anaesthesia in 60 min. Local small vessel vasoconstriction occurs in some patients, but evidence suggests that large veins are not constricted.

#### *Bupivacaine*

Bupivacaine has become the standard local anaesthetic for use in extradural and subarachnoid block. It is also commonly used for wound infiltration as an adjunct to postoperative analgesia. It has a long onset time (about 20 min), but a long duration of action (3 to 5 hours). The duration of action is not significantly altered by vasoconstrictors, because it depends on the high binding affinity of bupivacaine for tissues rather than its diffusion characteristics.

Low-dose infusions of bupivacaine combined with opioids have been used to extend analgesia into the postoperative period. The combination of these drugs can be shown pharmacologically to be synergistic. This allows low doses to be used and reduces the risk of toxicity.

Bupivacaine toxicity is related to its tissue-binding affinity. It produces arrhythmias by the same mechanism as the other local anaesthetics, but resuscitation is less successful than for other local anaesthetics as a result of the difficulty of displacing the drug from the myocardium. Bupivacaine has been separated into its enantiomers and the S enantiomer, marketed as Levo Bupivacaine, is claimed to be a less toxic alternative.

#### *Ropivacaine*

This drug, closely chemically related to bupivacaine, is prepared as the *S* enantiomer only. Its development has been primarily to produce a drug with a lower toxicity than bupivacaine, but similar therapeutic actions. Its lipid solubility is intermediate between that of lignocaine and that of bupivacaine; it is marginally less protein bound and has the same $pK_a$. It is less toxic to the cardiovascular system than bupivacaine, and is unaffected by pregnancy; although it produces some arrhythmias, it is less likely to produce ventricular fibrillation. There has been a suggestion that there is a difference in the degree of motor and sensory block with ropivacaine compared with bupivacaine. Extradural analgesia with bupivacaine is associated with motor block as the dose increases. Ropivacaine is associated with a less intense and shorter duration of motor block than bupivacaine.

### The esters

#### *Cocaine*

Cocaine is used for topical analgesia in ear, nose, and throat (ENT) surgery. Its addictive properties and its cardiovascular stimulation make it unsuitable for other use. It is prepared in solution for application to the nasal mucosa as an adjunct to nasal surgery. For topical anaesthesia it may be used as a paste applied to the nose before examination and surgical drainage of the sinuses. Cocaine was introduced into ENT practice by Moffat, who described a method of producing anaesthesia of the nasal mucosa. The vasoconstrictor effect of cocaine was supplemented by the addition of epinephrine. This solution, or some variant of it, has been used to produce good operating conditions for nasal surgery under general anaesthesia. The potential interaction between cocaine and epinephrine and anaesthetic agents does not appear to result in clinically significant morbidity. A potentially safer combination would be to combine lignocaine and a vasopressin analogue; however, tradition among ENT surgeons results in the continued use of cocaine.

### *Amethocaine*

Amethocaine is the most potent and longest acting of the esters. It is also the most toxic. In the UK, its use is restricted to topical anaesthesia. It has been introduced as a gel for dermal anaesthesia, where it has the advantage of a fast onset of action of 30–45 min. It is associated with small vessel vasodilatation, producing a reddening of the skin, but has little effect on the diameter of the larger skin vessels.

## FURTHER READING


Butterworth JF, Strichartz G. Molecular mechanisms of local anaesthetics: a review. *Anesthesiology* 1990;**72**:711–34

Calvey TN, Williams NE. *Principles and Practice of Pharmacology for Anaesthetists*, 3rd edn. Oxford: Blackwell Scientific, 1997.

Hull CJ. *Pharmacokinetics for Anaesthesia*. Oxford: Butterworth-Heinemann, 1991.

McClure JH. Ropivacaine. *Br J Anaesth* 1996;**76**:300–7.

Reynolds JEF. Local anaesthetics. In: *Martindale the Extra Pharmacopoeia*, 30th edn. London: Pharmaceutical Press, 1993: 995–1018.

Richards A, McConachie I. The pharmacology of local anaesthetics. *Curr Anaesth Crit Care* 1995;**6**:41–7.

Articles in: White PF, ed. *Kinetics of Anaesthetic Drugs in Clinical Anaesthesiology. Baillière's Clin Anaesthesiol,* 1991;5.

Chapter **37**

# Principles of physics and clinical measurement I: units, measurement, gases, vapours, and flows

D. Cochrane, K. Burchett, C.J. Vallis, and P. Hutton

## UNITS OF MEASUREMENT AND SIMPLE MECHANICS

The Système International d'Unites (or SI units) is the internationally recognized system of units of measurement.

The advantages are:

- a decimal system based on unchanging, fundamental, and reproducible properties of nature, independent of the pull of the Earth's gravity;
- a link between physics, medicine, and engineering in common units of measurement;
- derived units are built up from fundamental units, usually in unitary proportions;
- all derived units mean the same from whichever branch of science they come. Thus a joule, a unit of energy that combines dimensions of mass, time, and length, is the same, whether it refers to a unit of electrical, mechanical, or heat energy.

### Fundamental or base units

There are seven fundamental SI units. Any unit not in the list defined in Table 37.1 is either a derived unit or not an SI unit at all.

The SI practice is to use the basic unit or multiples of $10^3$ or $10^{-3}$ in expressing numerical values. Thus length is expressed in metres $10^1$, millimetres $10^{-3}$, and kilometres $10^3$. Other examples are given in Table 37.2.

The particular multiple chosen should avoid decimal notation where possible. There is then less likely to be confusion when, for example, the dose of a drug is expressed as 50 µg rather than 0.05 mg, or worse still 0.00005 g.

The litre is an oddity. It is not an SI unit but is retained for general use. The proper SI unit, the cubic metre, is rather large and the equivalent of the litre, the millicubic metre, is rather a mouthful (1 cubic metre or $m^3 = 10^3$ litres).

### Derived units

#### *Force*

Our sensation of weight is that resulting from the attraction of gravity acting on a mass, this force being proportional to the size of the mass. Gallileo showed that weights of different mass, simultaneously dropped off the Leaning Tower of Pisa, hit the ground at the same time. This was repeated by the 'guinea and feather' experiment of Isaac Newton. These results imply that, irrespective of mass, the acceleration is the same. This constant acceleration, known as the acceleration caused by gravity, is 9.81 metres per second per second ($m/s^2$), although it varies slightly at different latitudes. It is given the symbol **g**.

Force is that property which, when applied to a mass, causes acceleration or a change in the direction of motion. Our traditional units of force, the kilogram-weight or pound-weight, are equal to a force of gravitational attraction on a mass of one kilogram or one pound. This is hardly appropriate in the era of space travel. The SI unit of force is the newton (N) which is independent of gravity.

> A newton is that force which, if applied to mass of 1 kg, gives it an acceleration of 1 $m/s^2$ along the line of the applied force, i.e. $F = m \times a$.

#### *Work and energy*

When a force moves its point of application in the line of the direction of the force, it is said to do work:

$$\text{Work} = \text{Force} \times \text{Distance}$$

and is therefore measured in (newton × metres) or joules.

In Figure 37.1, if friction is ignored, a relatively small force, $f$, can be used to get the ball up a long ramp $D$, or a larger force, $F$, can lift it vertically up a smaller distance $d$. The work done is the same. In Figure 37.1:

$$F \times d = f \times D.$$

When the ball is at the top of the slope it has potential energy and can roll down. While it is moving it possesses kinetic energy. The potential energy (mg × $d$) is the product of its weight (mass × **g**) and the vertical displacement ($d$).

**Table 37.1 Fundamental SI units**

| Quantity | Unit (abbreviation) | Description |
|---|---|---|
| Length | Metre (m) | Based on the wavelength of specified emissions from the krypton-86 atom |
| Time | Second (s) | Based on timed events related to the atoms of caesium-133 |
| Mass | Kilogram (kg) | A kilogram is equal in mass to the prototype standard piece of metal alloy held in France |
| Electric current | Ampere (A) | An ampere is defined as the current that flows down two parallel wires of infinite length and negligible thickness 1 m apart to produce a force between them of $2 \times 10^{-7}$ N per m of length |
| Temperature | Kelvin (K, not °K) | A kelvin is 1/273.16 of the thermodynamic temperature of the triple point of water where the vapour liquid and solid phases are in equilibrium<br>°C or Celsius, although not an SI unit, is still allowable to express difference in temperature because 1°C= 1 K in magnitude<br>0°C = +273.15 K, therefore K = °C + 273.15<br>The triple point of water is therefore 0.01°C |
| Number of particles | Mole (mol) | A mole is the number of unitary particles (these must be specified, e.g. atoms, ions, molecules) as there are atoms in 0.012 kg (12 g) of carbon-12 |
| Luminosity | Candela (cd) | This is derived from comparison with the luminous intensity emitted from the body of freezing platinum under specified conditions |

**Table 37.2 Multipliers used in SI practice**

| Multiplier | Power of 10 | Symbol | Example |
|---|---|---|---|
| Pico | $10^{-12}$ | p | Picofarads, a measurement of capacitance |
| Nano | $10^{-9}$ | n | Nanomoles, a number of hydrogen ions |
| Micro | $10^{-6}$ | μ | Micrograms, drug dose |
| Milli | $10^{-3}$ | m | Milliamps, current to cause ventricular fibrillation |
| Kilo | $10^{3}$ | k | Kilopascals, pressure |
| Mega | $10^{6}$ | M | Megawatts, the power from an electricity generator |
| Giga | $10^{9}$ | G | Gigabytes, as in computer memory |

Energy is the capacity to do work and it is measured in the same units: joules or N·m.

Energy can be considered as stored work. Potential energy can be stored in many forms, e.g. a wound-up spring, a kilogram of carbohydrate, a pressurized cylinder, a battery, a tank full of hot water. No matter how the energy is stored or converted from one form to another, the units used are the same and equivalent, i.e. joules. Potential energy is usually easily converted into kinetic energy, e.g. free-wheeling a bicycle down a hill or opening a cylinder of gas.

Energy, like matter, cannot be created or destroyed, it can only be changed from one form to another (laws of conservation of mass and energy).

When work is done to produce heat, e.g. by friction, by using electricity, or by burning coal, the ratio of the work done to the heat produced is always the same. This is the first law of thermodynamics and follows on from the above.

When a body is moving, it possesses kinetic energy and work is done or energy is lost as the body comes to rest. The formula for kinetic energy is $\frac{1}{2}mv^2$ ($m$, mass; $v$, velocity). Velocity plays the proportionately

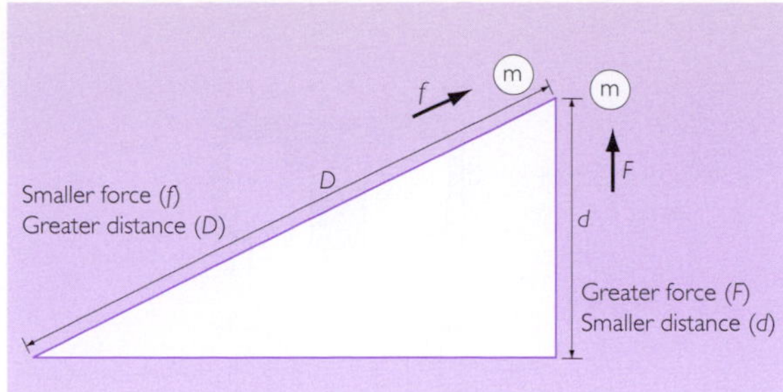


**Figure 37.1** The concept of work. The work done to get the mass to the top of a slope equals force × distance and is given in newton metres (N•m) or joules (J). At the top of the hill it has the same stored potential energy however it got there. This can be converted into kinetic energy when the mass rolls down again.

greater part in this equation, which is why a high-velocity bullet of relatively little mass is so destructive.

Cardiac work is estimated as:

$$\text{Mean arterial pressure} \times \text{Stroke volume}.$$

Mean arterial pressure has the units of force/area and stroke volume has the units of area × length. This gives cardiac work the units of force × length, i.e. N·m = joules = work.

### Power

Power is the rate at which energy is used up, often in doing work. It is measured in watts, which are equal to joules per second (J/s) or newton metres per second (N·m/s).

Step aerobics provides a familiar idea of the difference between work and power. The same work is done by getting up on the step no matter how long it takes. Power is the rate at which you get up on the step.

In a similar manner, the work done by electricity is the energy needed to move a charge against a voltage ($V$). Current ($I$) is charge per second, so electrical power is ($V \times I$), measured in joules/s or watts.

### Pressure

Pressure is force per unit area:

$$\text{Pressure} = \frac{(\text{Total force}, F)}{(\text{Total area}, A)}$$

Force is measured in newtons and area in square metres. The force of 1 N applied to an area of 1 $m^2$ is one pascal (Pa).

All traditional units of pressure measured the force of gravity acting on a mass, and hence there was kilogram-weight per square centimetre (kg/$cm^2$) or pounds-weight per square inch (p.s.i.) or millimetres of mercury (mmHg). A newton, in gravitational terms, exerts the same force as the gravitational pull on 102 g (i.e. a small apple). This, applied over 1 $m^2$, is such a small pressure that kilopascals (kPa) are used in medicine, and megapascals (MPa) in engineering. The bar, although not an SI unit, is an approved unit of pressure, equal to 100 kPa. It is approximately equal to the atmospheric pressure at sea level (Figure 37.2).

$$1\,\text{bar} = 100\,\text{kPa} = \text{approximately } 760\,\text{mmHg} = \text{approximately } 1000\,\text{cmH}_2\text{O}.$$

The last two, being gravitational units, are not approved, but are still widely used. Pressure in a liquid can be measured in terms of height because, for a given density, the weight or force applied by the fluid is proportional to its volume, and volume is height × area. If a larger diameter tube is used, both the area and the volume increase but, because the increased force is now applied over a proportionately larger area, the pressure at a given depth remains unchanged (Figure 37.3).

The principle of pressure being a distribution of force over area is immediately understood if one imagines a person wearing skis or stiletto heels ($P = F/A$). The dangers of localized pressure damage to skin or nerves during anaesthesia is well recognized by anaesthetists.

The other side of the equation ($F = P \times A$) is not so readily apparent. The children's 'bouncy castle', where a simple blower producing a relatively low pressure over a large surface area of plastic supports the weight of the structure and that of the children, is an example of the principle.

To apply pressure there must be resistance and, as fluids (liquids, gases, and vapours) are compressed, the container provides the resistance. Because fluids flow under pressure gradients:

> If pressure is applied to a fluid in a closed container, it is transmitted equally to all parts of the fluid and acts equally in all directions

Figures 37.4, 37.5, and 37.6 show practical examples of the relationship of pressures, forces, and areas. Laplace's law (Figure 37.7), which originally related to the pressure inside a soap bubble, states that the pressure inside the bubble ($P$) is given by $P = 2T/R$, where $T$ is the tension in the wall and $R$ the radius of the sphere.

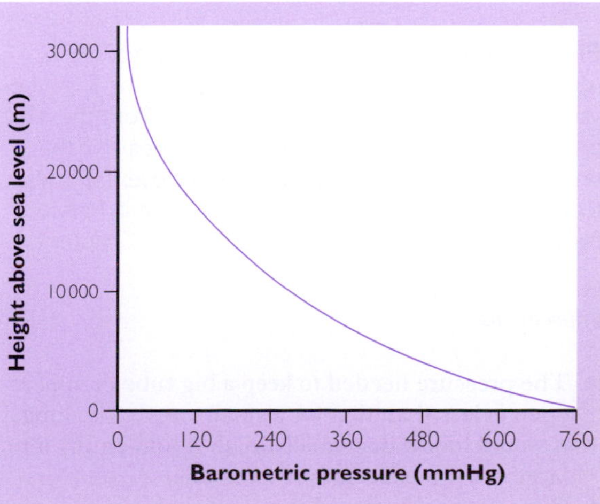


**Figure 37.2** The change in atmospheric pressure with altitude. The relationship is exponential.

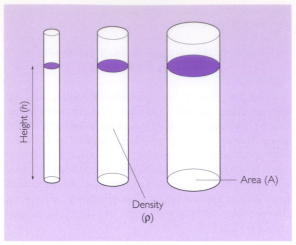

**Figure 37.3** The measurement of pressure with fluid columns. Pressure is independent of the volume supported. The height of column supported by any given pressure is dependent on the density of the liquid. As mercury is 13.6 times denser than water, 1 mmHg equals 1.36 $cmH_2O$. Force on base area = mass of fluid × g = volume of fluid × density (ρ) × g = $A \times h \times \rho \times g$. Pressure on base = force on base area/base area = $(A \times h \times \rho \times g)/A = h\rho g$ = depth × density × g. Therefore pressure at a given depth in a liquid is independent of volume.

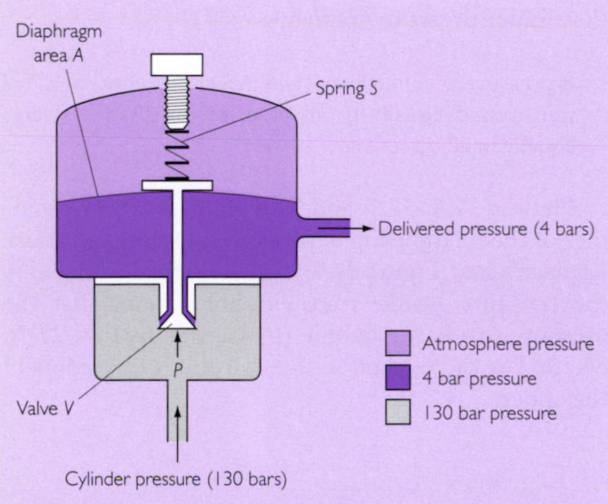


**Figure 37.4** The balance of forces in a pressure regulator. The force applied by the large spring *S* on the valve *V* is matched by an equivalent force from the 4 bar pressure applied to the diaphragm with area *A*. If the pressure exceeds 4 bar, the valve *V* will close; if it is less than 4 bar the force of the spring will open it. Pressure regulators are considered in more detail in Chapter 8.

*Implications*

- The pressure needed to keep a big tube or sphere open is less than that for a small one. In the lung, it would follow that small alveoli would empty into large ones. Surfactant prevents this.
- Once a vessel is closed down, a much greater pressure is needed to open it than to keep it open before it collapses.

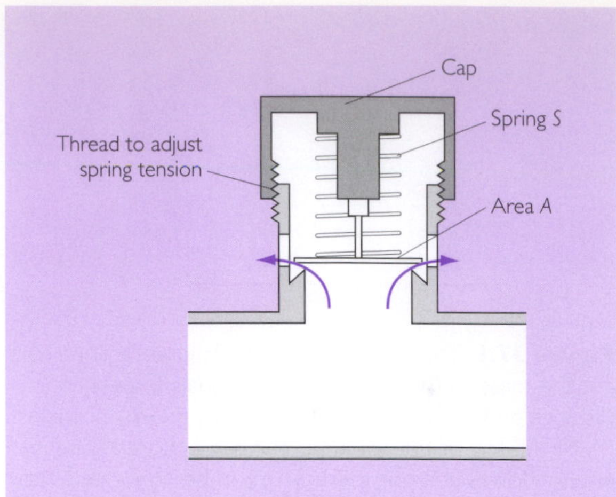


**Figure 37.5** This is a diagrammatic representation of the commonly used spill valve or adjustable pressure-release valve. The thread on the cap allows adjustment of the force the spring *S* applies to the valve of area A. The strength of the spring is chosen so that when the cap is unscrewed the valve lifts easily during spontaneous expiration but, when the cap is partially screwed down, there is sufficient resistance in the valve to allow hand ventilation from a reservoir bag.

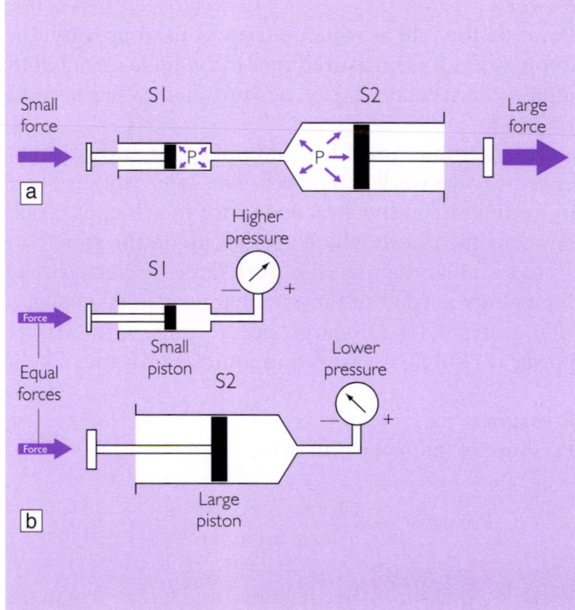


**Figure 37.6** The pressure in a fluid and the force on a piston. In (a) the force applied to the area of the piston of the small syringe (S1) is transmitted as fluid pressure which is exerted in all directions and is applied to the larger area of the piston in S2, thus producing a larger net force on the piston. This is the principle of the hydraulic jack. The plunger moves a greater distance in S1 than the piston in S2 moves forwards (work = force × distance). In (b) equal forces applied to pistons of different sizes produce different pressures. The pressures are determined by the area over which the forces are applied.

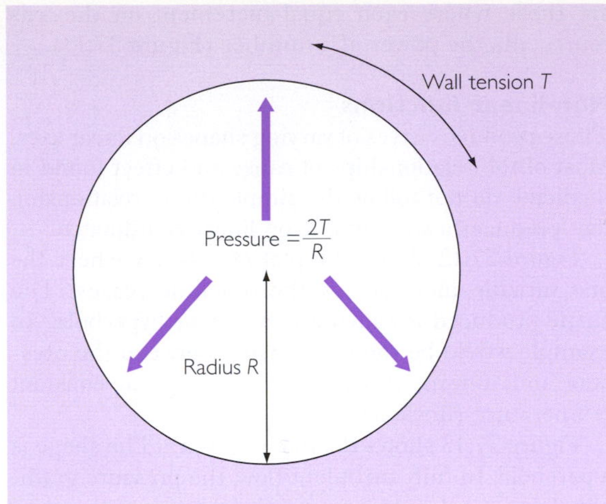


**Figure 37.7** Laplace's law for a bubble with free inner and outer surfaces.

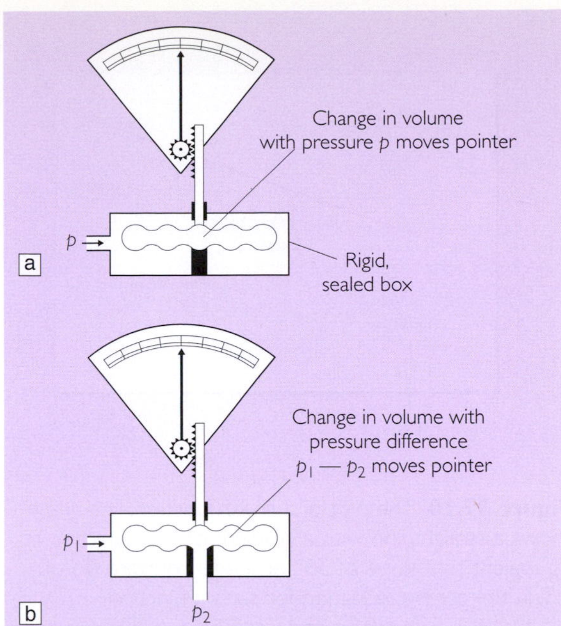


**Figure 37.9** The principle of the aneroid gauge. (a) Total or partial evacuation: the gauge can be calibrated for negative as well as positive gauge pressures, i.e. it is capable of measuring absolute pressures. (b) Response to pressure differences between the inside ($p_2$) and outside ($p_1$); its measuring range will depend on the inner pressure.

Gauge pressure means the pressure *above* atmospheric pressure. Absolute pressure *includes* atmospheric pressure. The pressure in a full oxygen cylinder can be quoted as 137 bar gauge pressure or 138 bar absolute pressure. Negative pressure (properly called subatmospheric pressure) always refers to gauge pressure because negative absolute pressures do not exist.

The devices used to measure pressure depend on the magnitude of the pressure under consideration. All require atmospheric pressure to be known to measure absolute values. Fluid columns and pressure transducers can be used either above or below atmospheric pressure. Although there are some exceptions, Bourdon gauges are usually used above atmospheric pressure and aneroid gauges below it. Examples of Bourdon and aneroid gauges are given in Figures 37.8 and 37.9.

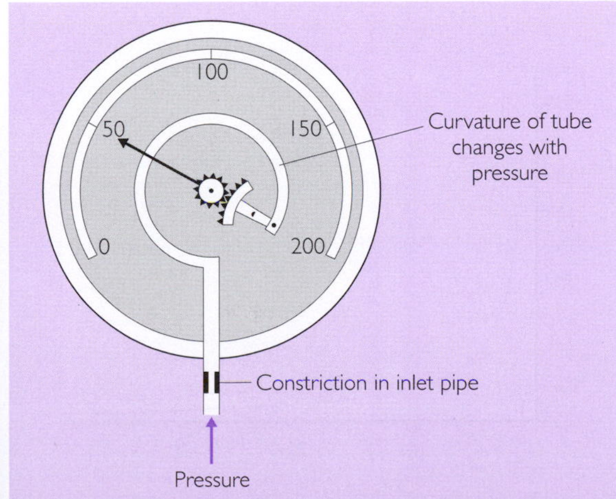


**Figure 37.8** The principle of the Bourdon gauge which measures pressures greater than 1 bar. Note the constriction in the inlet to prevent sudden pressure changes being transmitted directly to the hollow coil.

## MATHEMATICAL RELATIONSHIPS RELEVANT TO BASIC SCIENCES

The concepts of cause and effect and proportionality are fundamental to anaesthesia. These relationships can be represented in graphical form. Conventionally, *cause*, the independent variable, is plotted on the $x$ or horizontal axis and *effect*, the dependent variable, on the $y$ or vertical axis.

### Linear functions

These produce straight-line graphs on linear axes (Figure 37.10).

The familiar concept of a hill with a one in two gradient means that, for every 2 m of horizontal displacement, there is a vertical displacement of 1 m. The slope of the hill is 30°; the tangent of 30° (opposite/adjacent) is $^1/_2$ or 0.5. Thus, the precise relationship between the horizontal and the vertical variables of this gradient can be expressed as a 1 in 2, 30°, or 0.5 slope. If the slope is over 90°, this is a negative or downhill slope. In the example of Figure 37.10:

$$\begin{matrix}\text{Vertical} \\ \text{displacement}\end{matrix} = \begin{matrix}\text{0.5 horizontal} \\ \text{displacement or } y\end{matrix} = 0.5(x)$$

The value 0.5 is the fixed proportionality factor or *function* relating changes in $y$ to changes in $x$. The general equation for this linear plot is therefore $y = f(x)$ where $f(x) = 0.5x$. This means that $y$ is a function of $0.5x$ (not $x^2$, $x^3$, $\sqrt{x}$, or $\log x$ for instance). If our gradient started 4 m above sea level (Figure 37.10) and our vertical measurements were taken from sea level, then our formula would be:

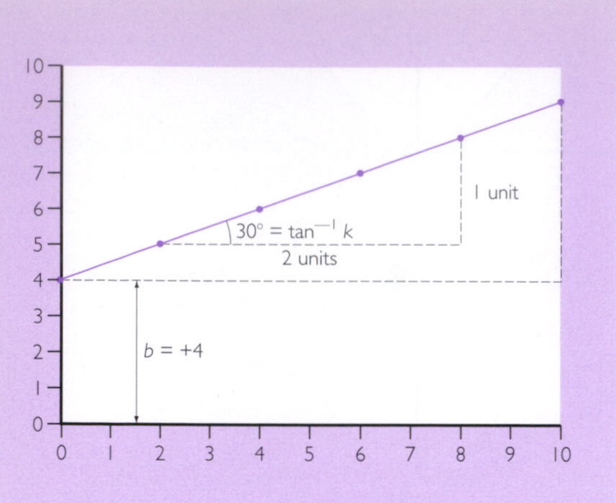


**Figure 37.10** The plot of a linear function. The graph shows a straight line with a gradient of 1 : 2, which is equivalent to a slope of 30° or a rate constant ($k$) of 0.5. In the general equation for such a function $y = f(x) + b$, $f(x) = 0.5x$, and $y = 0.5x + b$; when $x = 0$, $y = b = 4$, therefore, $y = 0.5x + 4$.

$$y = f(x) + 4, \text{ or, in general terms, } y = f(x) + b.$$

Here, the slope of the line is unchanged, but when $x$ is zero, $y$ is 4. ($f$ and $b$ are constants for this particular relationship and are termed 'parameters' because they are not true or immutable constants, such as π or e.) In mathematical terms:

$$y = f(x) + b \text{ where } f(x) = ax$$

is therefore the equation of a linear plot with gradient $a$ and intercept $b$; $b$ could be zero or any number, positive or negative. Examples of linear functions include:

- pressure gradient against flow (in conditions of laminar flow);
- lung volume against inflation pressure (over the normal working range);
- oxygen consumption against carbon dioxide output.

The slopes of these lines represent resistance, compliance, and the respiratory quotient, respectively.

The corollary is that, where one variable is plotted against another and the predicted relationship is not found, then either:

- the relationship has changed, as in the upper and lower ends of the lung compliance curve; or
- it is not there in the first place, such as the failure to get a 'best-fit' line in simple linear regression in statistics.

Where the variable $y$ is plotted against time (time is always on the $x$ axis), the slope represents the rate of change of the variable $y$, with time. The slope, usually designated $k$, becomes the rate constant.

Where a graph encompasses a very wide range of values, logarithmic coordinates can be used for either or *both* the $x$ and $y$ axes. Logarithmic scales are those where each equal increment on the axis represents the power of a number (Figure 37.11).

### Non-linear functions

These produce curves of varying shapes on linear axes. Most of the relationships of cause and effect found in medicine do not follow the simple direct relationship that produces a straight line on linear coordinates.

Figure 37.12 shows the plot of $y = 1/x$ where the one variable increases as the other decreases. The shape produced is called a rectangular hyperbola. An example would be the relationship between the pressure and volume of a fixed mass of gas at constant temperature (Boyle's law).

Figure 37.13 shows the plot of $y = x^2$. The shape is a parabola. In fully turbulent flow, the pressure gradient down a tube varies with the square of the flow. Note that because $(-x)^2$ results in a positive value of $y$, the curve never crosses the $x$ axis. This plot is *not* that of an exponential function, although it has a superficial resemblance to it.

#### *Power functions and logarithms*

The word logarithm comes from the Greek *logos*, reckoning, *arithmos*, number. A logarithmic scale has

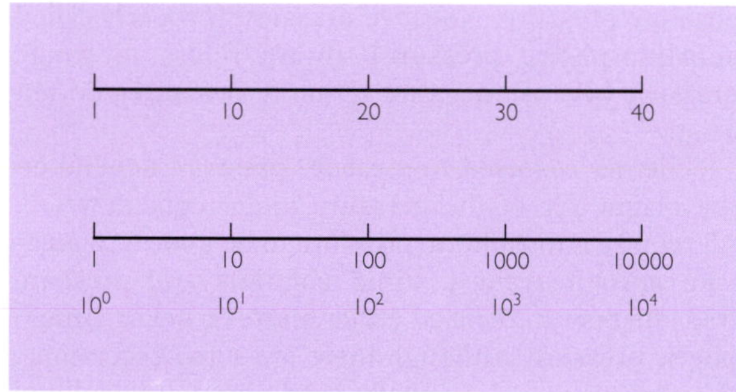


**Figure 37.11** Linear (top) and logarithmic (bottom) scales. Note on the logarithmic scale that equal increments imply that the value has increased by a factor (or power) of 10.

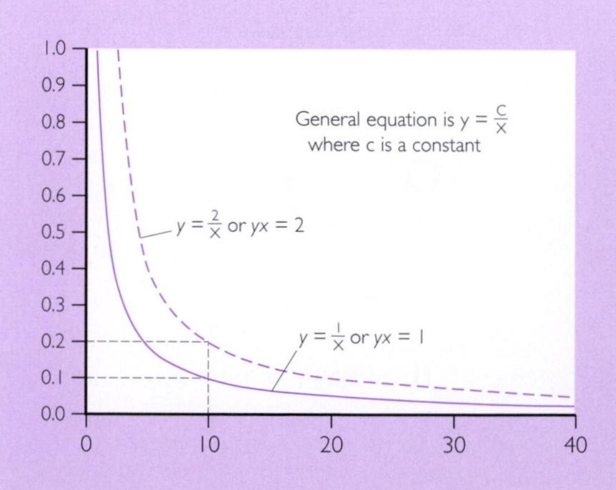


**Figure 37.12** The plot of an inverse function is a hyperbola. The solid line shows the relationship for $yx = 1$ and the dotted line for $yx = 2$. The general equation is $y = c/x$, where $c$ is a constant.

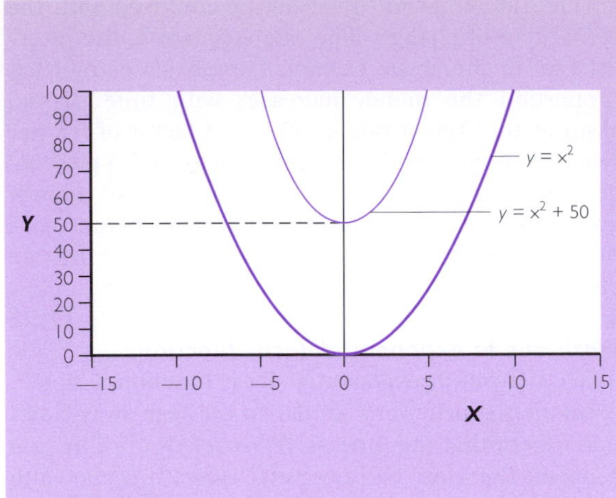


**Figure 37.13** The graph of $y = x^2$ and $y = x^2 + 50$, Note that, as $(-x)^2$ is always positive, the graph never has negative values of $y$.

already been shown in Figure 37.11: 10, 100, 1000, 10 000, 100 000, expressed as $10^1$, $10^2$, $10^3$, $10^4$, $10^5$, is a familiar concept; 2, 4, 6, 8, 16, 32, expressed as $2^1$, $2^2$, $2^3$, $2^4$, $2^5$ is a little less so, as we are conditioned to count in units of 10. The 3 in $10^3$ or $2^3$, known as the *index* or *exponent*, signifies the number of 10s that must be multiplied together in the first example and 2s in the second to give the arithmetic number. The index or exponent is also called the power of, as in 10 to the power of one, two, three, and so on.

$$10\,000 \times 100 = 1\,000\,000$$

can be expressed as:

$$10^4 \times 10^2 = 10^6.$$

Large numbers can therefore be multiplied or divided by each other by *adding* or *subtracting* the exponents of the two numbers. This was the driving force behind the invention of logarithms. The power of a number specifies how many of the given number must be multiplied together. The more general term 'logarithm' specifies how many of a specific number, called the *base*, must be multiplied together to produce the given number.

An example of this is as follows. The equation $\log_{10} (10\,000) = 4$ is derived as follows. As the base in this case is 10, four 10s have to be multiplied together to produce the number 10 000; 4 is the logarithm of 10 000 and 10 000 is the anti-log of 4. Where no base is specified it is assumed to be base 10.

Note that $10^1 = 10$, and $10^0 = 1$. There is no log of zero, which is why logarithmic scales never start or end at zero.

Although log to the base 10 is the most frequently used, other bases can be used. $\text{Log}_2 (64) = 6$, which means that six 2s have to be multiplied together to produce 64. This is used in binary arithmetic, which forms the basis of computer functions.

Logarithms are important in medicine. The whole concept of pH is based on logarithms, a pH of 7 signifying a hydrogen ion concentration of $10^{-7}$ moles per litre. The response of most sense organs obeys the Weber–Fechner law which states: equal increments in the *logarithm* of the signal produce equal increments in sensation. Thus, audiograms are expressed in decibels or dB, the bel being the log of the ratio of two different sound intensities. The ear requires a tenfold increase in sound intensity to register one increment of increase in loudness. The dose–response curve of many drugs follows the same principle. The effect of using a logarithmic scale, such as pH or dB, is to linearize the effect of the changes in the value, with respect to the effectiveness of the variable.

In $\log_e (n)$, the logarithm of e means the number of numbers having the value e that must be multiplied together to produce the number $n$. Logarithms to the base e are known as natural logarithms. The non-terminating constant e has a value of 2.71828…, abbreviated to 2.7183. This and π are the most important constants in mathematics.

## EXPONENTIAL EQUATIONS

The equation $y = x^2$ has a fixed exponent, i.e. 2. On the other hand, $y = k^x$ has a variable exponent $x$. The latter is an exponential function. There are many processes in physics and biology that grow or decay at a rate that is proportional to how far the process has already gone, or how far it still has to go. These processes are known as *natural exponential functions* because the rate at which they change is proportional to an exponent of the power of e, as in $e^x$ where $x$ is measured in periods of time. There are three main forms of exponential behaviour: the tear-away function, the wash-out function, and the wash-in function.

### *Tear-away function*

The tear-away function is described by $y = e^{kx}$ or $e^{kt}$ when time is the independent variable. Examples are compound interest and the growth of bacteria.

The increase in money, invested at compound interest, illustrates both an exponential tear-away function and the nature of e. Consider a sum of £1.00 invested at compound interest of 100% per year. The final sum after one year would be £2.00. If, however, the interest is calculated and added twice per year, the total sum would be £2.25 (£1.50 = sum after 6 months. £1.50 + £0.75 is the sum after the second 6 months).

If the interest is calculated 10, 100, 1000, or 10 000 times in one year you would get £2.5937, £2.7048, £2.7169, and £2.7181, respectively. An infinite number of calculations would give the number £2.7183. In other words, your original sum has increased by 2.7183 times, or by a factor of e, the base of natural or naperian logrithms. The ratio final sum/original sum = e.

If you doubled the interest rate, the increase would be 7.3892 times = $e^2$. To calculate for several years the exponent is simply multiplied by the number of time periods.

Thus, the ratio of the new to the starting value is equal to $e^{kt}$, where $k$ is the interest rate and $t$ the number of time periods over which the interest rate applies. The general formula for exponential functions of this type is therefore $y = e^{kt}$ (Figure 37.14a).

If each side of the equation is multiplied by $\log_e$, which is conventionally abbreviated to ln (for natural logarithm) then $[\ln y] = [\ln e^{kt}]$. But $kt$ is the power to which e must be raised to produce $e^{kt}$, i.e. it is its log, so the equation can be written as $[\ln y] = kt$. This resembles the equation of a linear function and, provided the $y$ axis is plotted on a logarithmic scale, the result will be a straight line graph (Figure 37.14b). Certain important observations can be deduced from these graphs.

- In exponential change, the time taken to change by a factor of $e^1$ or 2.7183 is a single time period known as a time constant and given the Greek letter tau, $\tau$; $e^2$ takes two time constants, $e^3$ three time constants, etc. On the natural logarithm scale $e^1$ is 1, $e^3$ is 3, and so on.
- If the rate constant ($k$) doubles, the change of e will happen in half the time, or, if halved, in double the time; $k$ is therefore the reciprocal of the time constant: $k = L/\tau$.
- The process of extrapolation and interpolation can be usefully applied to exponential graphs because, if the starting value is known and either the rate or the time constants are known, then the values at other times can be calculated. Extrapolation measures the predicted value beyond two known values on a graph and interpolation of the predicted value between known values.

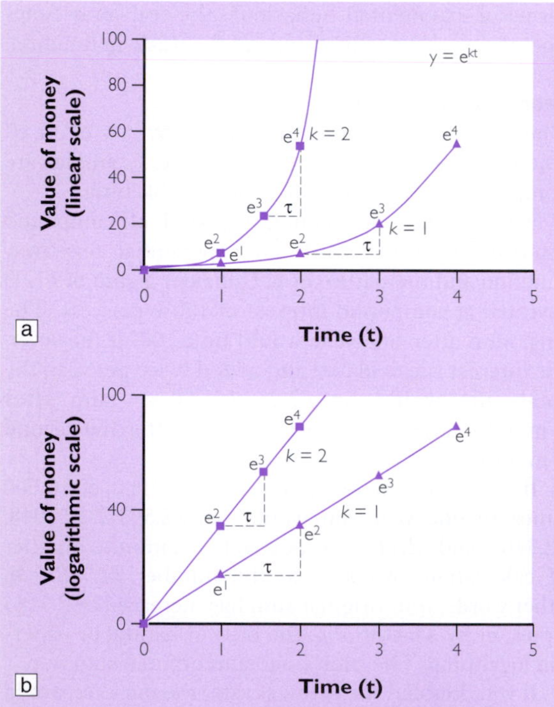


**Figure 37.14** Tear-away exponential functions with the general equation $y = e^{kt}$. (a) A linear plot of two functions with different rate constants of 1 and 2. (b) This shows (a) re-plotted on a semi-logarithmic scale linearizes the graphical relationship. Note that the value of $\tau$ for the two relationships is different. (See text for explanation.)

The rate constant must not be confused with the actual rate of change. The rate constant $k$, the interest rate in the above example, simply states by what proportion the money increases with time. If you assume an interest rate of 50% or a factor of 0.5 per year, the money will increase by a factor of 0.5 per year *at the present amount of money*. As the money increases, the actual rate of change also increases proportionately and does not remain fixed like the rate constant.

### *Wash-out or exponential decay function*

The wash-out or exponential decay function, $y = e^{-kt}$, is mathematically very similar to the tear-away function except that the process *decreases* by $e^{kt}$. The rate constant therefore has a negative value. It is shown in Figure 37.15.

Consider removing blood continuously from a patient, while at the same time infusing equal volumes of plasma substitute. Initially, whole blood would be removed from the patient, but, as the process proceeds, the number of red blood cells per volume removed decreases as the blood becomes more and more diluted. The rate of removal of red blood cells is therefore proportional to the magnitude of their concentration in the blood at any one time. The volume exchange rate constitutes the rate constant $k$, because a fixed proportion of the, albeit decreasing, remaining red blood cells is being removed per unit of time.

The wash-out of indicators such as cold saline in the measurement of cardiac output is analogous to the above example. The volume of blood flowing out of the heart removes the indicator and that flowing in to the heart dilutes the indicator. The exponential decay of the concentration of the indicator, measured as temperature, can be plotted as a straight line on a semi-logarithmic plot and is extrapolated through any secondary hump on the plot caused by re-circulation (see Figure 37.22).

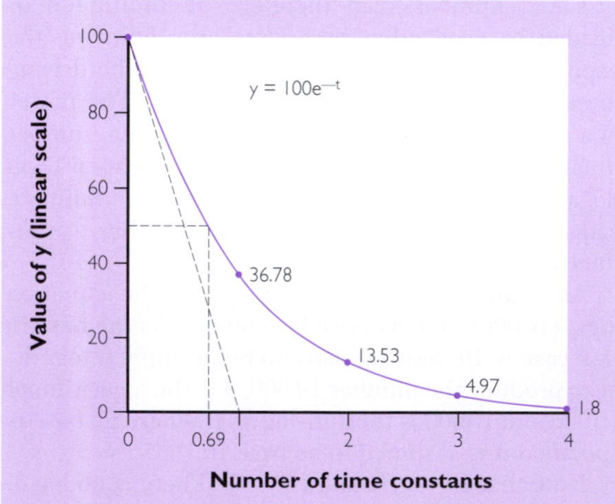


**Figure 37.15** An exponential decay function plotted on linear axes. The horizontal axis is numbered in time constants. Note that the value of the function reduces by a half in 0.69 time constants. This value of time for which the value of the function halves is known as the half-life. General equation is $y = ce^{-kt}$, where $c$ is a constant = 100 and $k$ = 1 in this case. The time constant $\tau = 1/k$.

Exponential decay curves are very important in pharmacokinetics. Consider the elimination of a drug from the plasma, where its concentration ($C$) decreases with time, as $dC/dt = -kC^n$, where d stands for a very small change. This equation states that the concentration falls with time, according to a proportionality factor $k$, or $-k$, as it is decreasing. The rate of fall, $dC/dt$, is also affected by the concentration of the drug at any one time and depends on whether the $n$, as in $C^n$, is 0 or 1. If it is 0, $C^0 = 1$, and the rate of fall will be independent of the concentration. If $n$ is 1, $C^1 = C$, and the rate of fall will decrease according to the magnitude of the concentration at any one time – hence the terms zero- ($n = 0$) and first-order ($n = 1$) kinetics. First-order kinetic reactions, when integrated, behave as exponential wash-out curves. More details of these are given in Chapter 19. Most drugs that do not saturate their enzyme systems are eliminated by first-order kinetics.

The elimination of alcohol from the blood is, however, an example of zero-order kinetics, because the enzyme systems involved in its metabolism are soon saturated and the concentration no longer becomes a factor in the rate of elimination. Without this particular pharmacological feature, it would be much more difficult to become inebriated.

Other examples of exponential decay are the decay of radioactivity, the discharging of a capacitor, or the emptying of a lung, and the exponential decay of drugs from different compartments of the body with time.

Figures 37.15 and 37.16 show typical exponential decays plotted against time constant and half-life, respectively. Important features to note from these graphs are:

- The ratio of the final to the original value of $y$ is 1/e or 1/2.7183 of the previous value for each time constant; $(100 \times 1)/2.7183 = 36.8\%$; 1/e is in turn applied to the 36.8% producing 13.5%. After three time constants, $1/e^3$, only 5% remains and the process can be judged to be almost complete. In theory the graph never reaches zero.
- If the original rate of decay continued unchanged, the $y$ variable would reach zero in one time constant.
- The time taken for the process to decay by 50%, i.e. starting value/new value = 0.5, is 0.693 of a time constant (0.693 is the natural logarithm of 2). This is known as the half-life, $t_{1/2}$. After five half-lives, the process has decayed to 3.125% of its original value, and is assumed in most practical applications to be complete (Figure 37.16a).

An example of exponential decay is passive exhalation. The initial flow of gas from a lung breathing out through the resistance of the airways is proportional to the product of the compliance $C$ of the lung and the airway resistance $R$. The time constant in numerical terms is:

$$C \times R = (0.05\,\text{L/cmH}_2\text{O}) \times (6\,\text{cmH}_2\text{O/L per s}) = 0.3\text{ s}.$$

After three time constants (0.9 s), 95% of the expiration will have occurred, although individual lung units may have different time constants.

***The wash-in or rising exponential decay function***

The wash-in or rising exponential decay function, $y = 1 - e^{-kt}$, is basically the wash-out graph inverted with the variable $y$ rising exponentially, at an ever-decreasing rate, to a final value called the asymptote (Figure 37.17). The concepts of half-life, time constant, and rate constant are applied in a similar manner to the wash-in plot. Examples are the increase in volume of the lung when connected to a constant pressure ventilator, the flow of current into a capacitor from a constant voltage source, and the rise in drug concentration to a final level from a continuous infusion.

Figure 37.18 shows the wash-in and wash-out curves after a continuous infusion of a drug and its elimination. If the elimination $t_{1/2}$ is known for a wash-in curve, then the time taken to achieve a steady level in the plasma will, for practical purposes, be equal to $5 \times t_{1/2}$.

## Rotation and oscillation

***The sine wave function (y = sin x)***

The sine of an angle in a right-angled triangle is the ratio of the opposite ÷ the hypotenuse (Figure 37.19a).

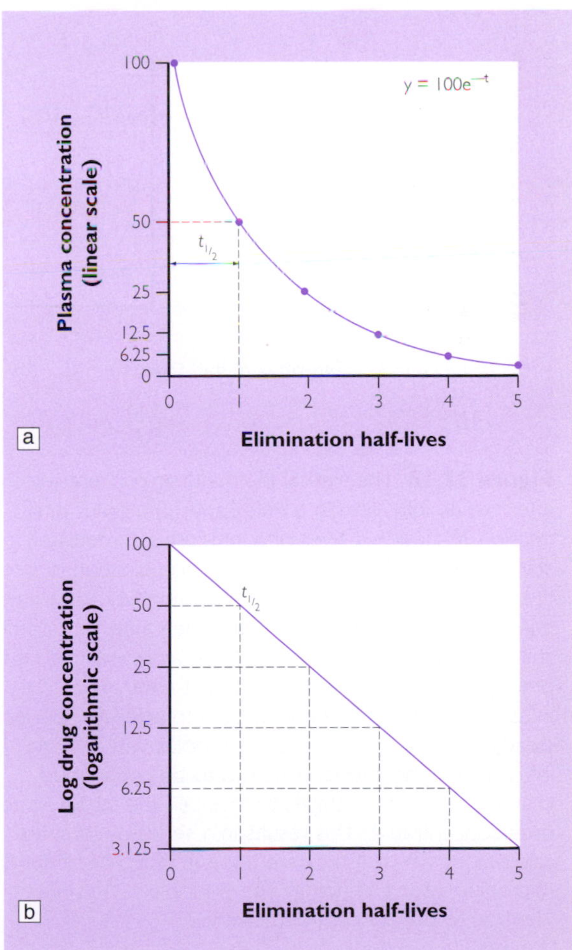


**Figure 37.16** Exponential wash-out curves plotted with elimination half-lives on the horizontal axis. This behaviour represents first-order pharmacokinetics. The plasma concentration on (a) a linear scale and (b) a logarithmic scale. $y = 100e^{-kt}$; $k = 1$ and the time constant $\tau = 1/k$.

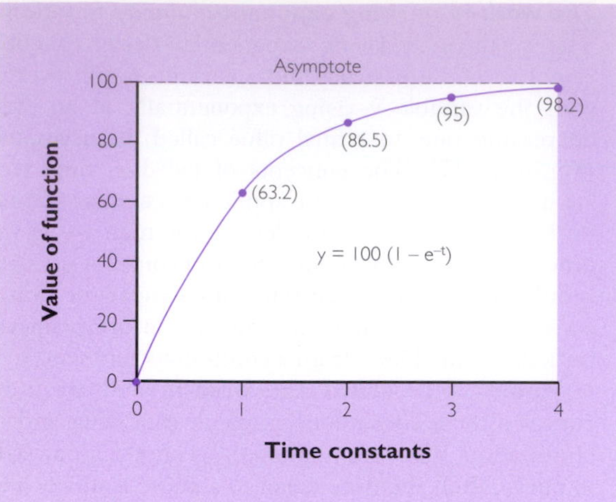


**Figure 37.17** A wash-in function of the general type $y = c(1 - e^{-kt})$, where $c$ (constant) = 100 and $k = 1$ in this case. The variable $y$ rises to a final value at infinite time called the asymptote. The proportionate progression to this asymptote is indicated by the numerical data on the graph.

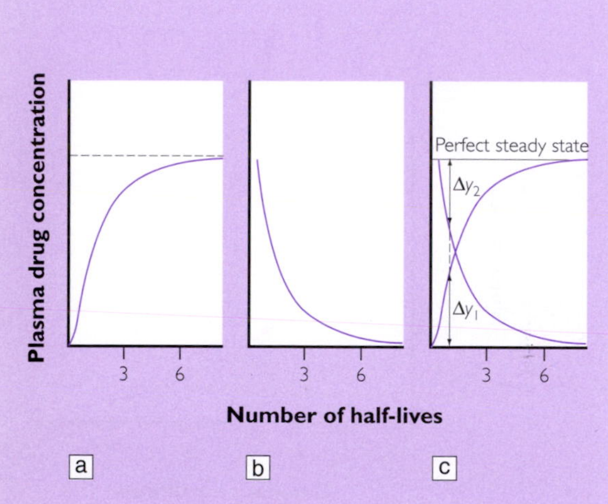


**Figure 37.18** Theoretical plasma drug concentrations after: (a) an infusion, (b) a bolus, and (c) a bolus plus infusion. If a bolus is given and infusion is immediately started, the resultant drug level is a combination of both. If, as shown in (c), the rise in the infusion ($\Delta y_1$) is always equal to the fall in the bolus ($\Delta y_2$), then a perfect steady-state serum concentration would be achieved. In clinical practice this is the objective of target-controlled drug infusions. It is not, however, possible to achieve a perfect steady state by combining a single bolus with a single infusion, and the infusion rate has to be continuously changed in the early stages to maintain the steady-state drug concentration. This results in a series of complex calculations which, if they are done in real time, require microprocessor technology. The principle is, however, identical to the concept demonstrated.

Consider the vertical displacement of a bicycle pedal from the horizontal, at point P (Figure 37.19b). The vertical displacement is 0 and the sine of the angle θ is also 0. The vertical displacement (A) progressively increases as the chain wheel rotates until it reaches its maximum at the top, i.e. 90° to the horizontal. Here the vertical displacement is equal to that of length of the pedal and the sine of the angle is 1. As the pedal starts its way down again, the sine of the angle decreases until it again reaches 0, when the pedal is again horizontal. The process is repeated below the horizontal where the sine of the angle now has a negative value. The hypotenuse of the triangle is the radius of the circle, which is constant. The amplitude of vertical displacement of the pedal (A) therefore varies with the sine of the angle of rotation from the horizontal and is independent of the length of the radius. At all times (Figure 37.19b), vertical displacement (A) $= R \times \sin \theta$.

If the sine of the angle displaced is plotted on the $y$ axis and time on the $x$ axis, the familiar sine wave results (Figure 37.19c, see below). Oscillating systems such as the displacement of a pendulum and a weight on a spring also vary in a sinusoidal fashion.

As an example, Figure 37.19c shows the typical sine wave of mains electricity voltage, produced from a rotating generator at the power station. The following are points to note:

- Time on the $x$ axis can be measured in degrees or time if the rotation is at constant velocity.
- One full rotation of 360° is a *cycle* and the number of cycles per second is the frequency measured in hertz. The *frequency* varies inversely with the wavelength. Sine waves with a frequency that is a multiple of the *fundamental* frequency are known as *harmonics*.
- The relationship of one sine wave of identical behaviour with time, but starting at a different point on the cycle, is said to be out of phase with the other. The phase difference is measured in degrees (Figure 37.19d).
- When two or more sine waves are added together, the result is an arithmetic mean of the values at any one time on the $y$ axis. Thus, two identical waves which are 180° out of phase will cancel each other out. The mean value of a single sine wave is also zero. Use is made of this principle in the technique of signal averaging, which can be used to clean up noisy signals that have positive and negative components.
- Complex waveforms can be produced from simple sine waves and their harmonics (Figure 37.20). The converse is also true, and any complex waveform can be broken down and analysed as a fundamental frequency and multiples of it. This is the process known as Fourier analysis. In clinical measurement, faithful reproduction of a frequency range between the fundamental and the eighth to tenth harmonic is sufficient for practical purposes. This range of frequencies is known as the *band width*. Fourier reconstruction of a typical arterial pressure wave is shown in Figure 37.21.

### Slopes, differentials, and integrals

The slope of a straight-line graph is a constant and signifies the predictable relationship between the variable $y$ and the variable $x$ (see above). In many complex functions, the result is a curve. In such functions, the inability to produce a slope by taking large increments of $y$ and dividing them by large incre-

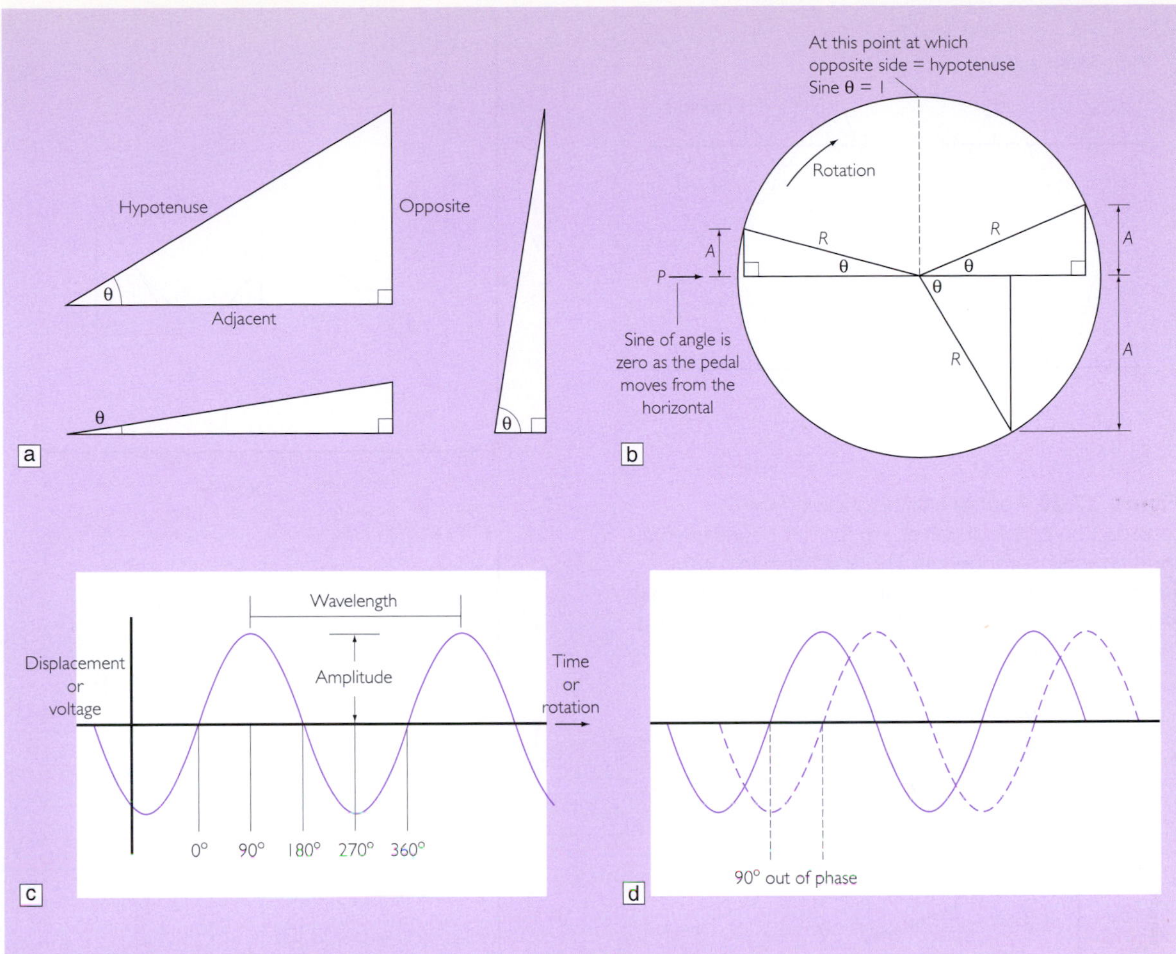


**Figure 37.19** Examples of the sine of an angle and its application. (a) In a right-angled triangle, the sine of an angle is given by the ratio of the length of the opposite side to the hypotenuse. Note that, as the angle gets bigger and approaches 90°, the length of the opposite side approaches the length of the hypotenuse and hence the sine approaches the value 1. As the angle reduces to zero the reverse effect occurs and the sine of the angle approaches zero. Sin θ = (Length opposite)/(Length of hypotenuse). (b) The rotational behaviour of a bicycle pedal. See text for details. (c) The sine of $x$ plotted out with time or rotation of the function. (d) Two sine waves separated from each other in time, i.e. they are out of phase.

ments of $x$ is surmounted by taking very small increments instead. The process is known as *differentiation* and the shorthand is $dy/dx$, or $dy/dt$ if time is on the $x$ axis.

If a sufficiently small segment of the curve is taken, it is effectively straight and a tangent is drawn at this point. The tangent gives the slope of the graph. The relationship is for this point only (Figure 37.22a).

In integration the symbol $\int$ has a similar meaning to $\Sigma$ in statistics. It means sum the following numbers. In the case of $\int y dx$, it says sum the values of $y$ multiplied by small increments of $x$. Integration can be done graphically, by dividing the area under the curve into small segments, calculating the area of each, and adding them together, ignoring the small error caused by the segments that are not rectangles (Figure 37.22b). The smaller the segment, the smaller the error.

In both differentiation and integration, the calculation of infinitesimally small gradients and areas can be done mathematically with calculus, if the curve can be described by a mathematical equation. The most convenient solution for clinical use is to differentiate or integrate in real time, using dedicated electronic circuits. Differentiating circuits can give a false picture with high-frequency noisy signals, because the steep gradients inherent in the noise will 'fool' the system. Integrating circuits, on the other hand, will tend to average out the noisy signals and not materially affect the result. An example of the use of integration in anaesthetic practice is shown in Figure 37.23.

## PRINCIPLES OF MAKING MEASUREMENTS

Scientific instruments are extensions of the senses. They enable the user to measure physical and chemical quantities that the unaided senses can estimate only in relative terms or are unable to perceive at all. To make the best use of the extra information they provide, and to avoid the possibility of error in the interpretation of the information, it is essential to have some understanding of how the instrument works, as well as its limitations.

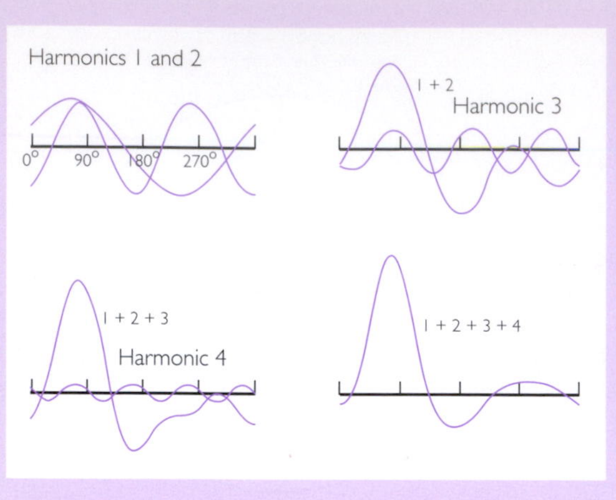


**Figure 37.20** Fourier analysis showing the construction of a final waveform from the fundamental and harmonic components. The first harmonic is the fundamental wave with the same frequency as the final waveform. (Adapted from McDonald DA. *Blood Flow in Arteries*. London: Arnold, 1960.)

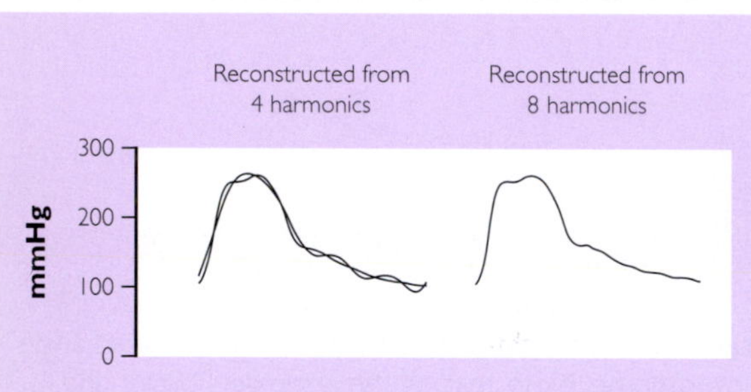


**Figure 37.21** The reconstruction of an arterial pressure wave using Fourier analysis. The left-hand wave shows the reconstruction using four harmonics and the right-hand wave using eight harmonics. It can be seen that, as the number of harmonics increases, so does the closer approximation of the reconstructed wave to the original. (Adapted from Prys-Roberts C. Invasive monitoring of the circulation. In: Saidman LJ and Ty Smith N, eds. *Monitoring in Anesthesia*, 2nd edn. Stoneham, USA: Butterworth, 1984: 89.)

The person who listens to a recording of an orchestral concert on a hi-fi system expects to hear a faithful reproduction of the original sound. They would be well aware that the reproduction is only as good as the weakest link in the chain and a poor recording cannot be restored, even by the most sophisticated playback system. There must be no reverberations in the concert hall, nor should the furniture in the room resonate at certain frequencies. When the volume is turned up, the amplification of the flutes should rise in equal proportion to that of the double bass. Extraneous noise, say from the traffic outside, should not be of such a level as to be detectable. The sound should also not be distorted and the amplifier should not drain power from the motor thus slowing it down. Identical demands are made of devices used in clinical measurement.

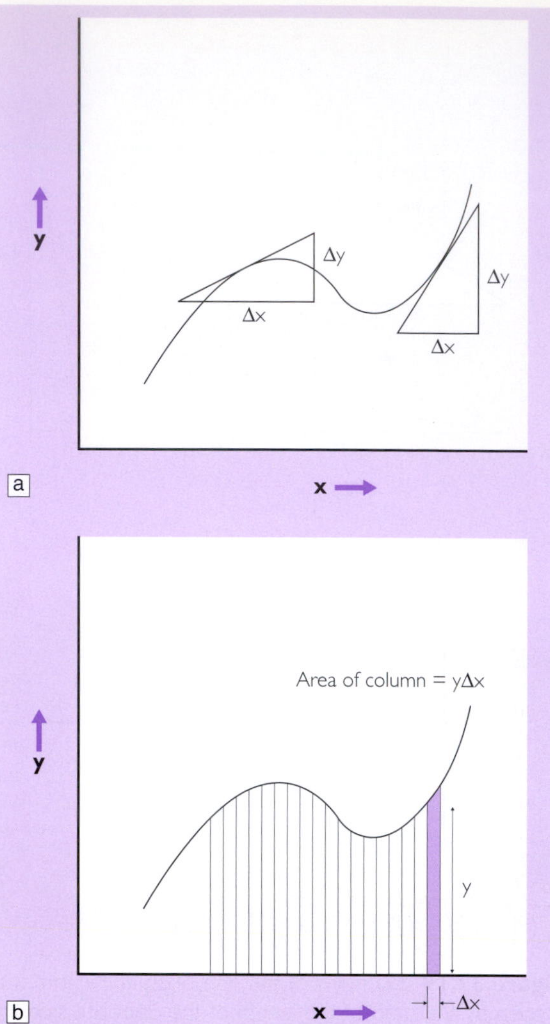


**Figure 37.22** The principles of (a) differentiation, which gives the gradient or rate of change of a function, and of (b) integration, which measures the area under the function.

### Interference by the measuring system itself

The measuring device should not draw energy from or interfere with the measured quantity in such a way as to affect the measurement materially. A mercury thermometer used on a very small piece of tissue would, in making its measurement, draw off heat and cool it down, thus introducing errors. In a flow-measuring device (Figure 37.24a), whether for current or gas flow, the device such as in a pneumotachograph should have *low-input impedance,* where its resistance to flow does not materially alter the flow being measured. Similarly, an electronic device, measuring the potential difference between resistances (or a pressure transducer in fluids), should not provide a significant alternative pathway for the current (or flow) (Figure 37.24b). It should provide *high-input impedance* to the current.

Input and output impedances should also be matched to minimize energy transfer. A cyclist wishing to transfer power to the wheels of his cycle must engage an appropriate gear so that the impedance to the movement of the pedals matches his optimal effort. Similar considerations apply to electronic devices where impedance matching is essential for accurate measurement.

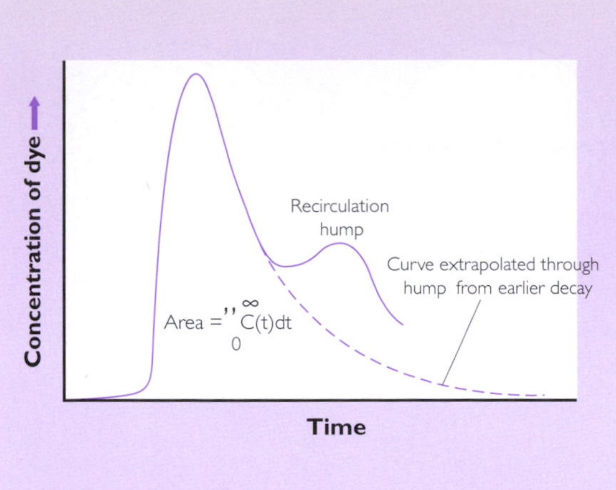


**Figure 37.23** A practical application of integration and extrapolation in a dye or thermal dilution curve. The decay of the concentration curve can be shown to be an exponential wash-out function (it produces a straight line on a semi-logarithmic plot), so its decay to 'zero concentration' can be extrapolated mathematically through the recirculation hump. The area under the concentration or temperature curve divided by time represents the mean concentration of indicator over time. Knowing the injected volume and indicator concentration then allows the cardiac output to be calculated from: Cardiac output = Quantity of dye/($\int C(t)dt$), where $C(t)$ = concentration at time $t$. An analogous expression can be derived for temperature changes instead of dye concentration.

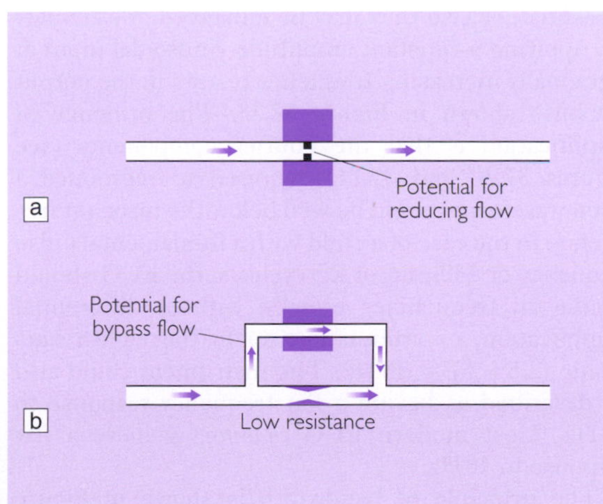


**Figure 37.24** The effect of a measuring device on the measurement itself. (a) A flow or current measuring device should have very-low-input impedance. If such a device has a high-input impedance it significantly changes the flow, which itself is trying to measure. (b) A pressure- or voltage-measuring device should have a high-input impedance. If this has a low-input impedance it provides a low-resistance bypass, thereby reducing the flow through the main passage. When this occurs, the pressure or voltage measured is significantly altered by the presence of the device itself.

### Zero stability

This is the ability to maintain a zero reading on a display unit, when the input signal is zero. It is commonly termed 'baseline drift' in pressure and ECG recordings when zero stability fails. Drift is eliminated by electronic circuits that respond only to fluctuating changes (e.g. pulsatile pressure) and not to slow changes in signals (e.g. temperature variations in electrical components). This is less of a problem with modern transistor circuits.

### Accuracy, sensitivity, bias, precision, and gain

- Accuracy is the amount by which a reading differs from a known correct value.
- Sensitivity is the smallest change in the measured quantity that an instrument can reliably detect. The sensitivity of an instrument will generally be higher than its accuracy. An ordinary moving coil galvanometer will typically have a rated accuracy of ±1% of full-scale deflection, but many will reliably indicate a change in current of 0.1%. Incorrect calibration of a pressure transducer will render the system inaccurate, without necessarily affecting the sensitivity at all.
- Bias is an offset from the true reading.
- Precision describes the repeatability of the same measurement, i.e. whenever measured, the reading is the same.

The terms accuracy, precision, and bias are often used interchangeably and incorrectly. Figure 37.25 illustrates the differences between them and defines their meaning.

- Gain is the ratio of the amplitude of the input to the output signals.

Gain can often be adjusted in a measuring system. The simplest example of this would be in a lever system, where a small movement at one end produces a larger movement of a pointer at the other. By moving the fulcrum, the gain of the system can be altered. In electronic systems, one or more gain controls sets the input : output ratio, which should remain constant and at a level that allows ample reserve for a particular function.

### Zero offset, linearity, and gain

The ideal relationship between signal input to display output in a measuring system is that of a linear function (see 'Mathematical relationships'). Even in non-linear relationships, a linear graph can be produced with a suitable modification of scales. The essence of amplitude stability is that this relationship should be maintained throughout the range of measurement.

Figure 37.26 shows the effect of altering the zero offset (bias) and the gain and linearity of a measuring system. The most commonly used application of these principles is in pressure transducers.

### Hysteresis

Certain processes display a difference in the cause–effect relationship, depending on whether the signal is rising or falling in value. This can be thought

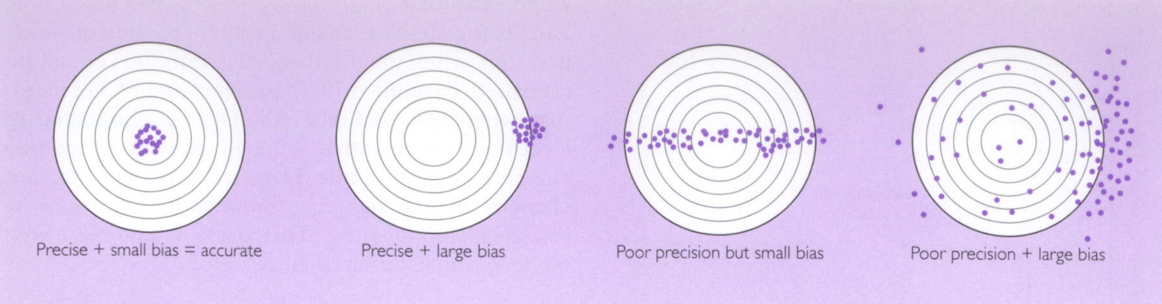


**Figure 37.25** Demonstrations of accuracy, precision, and bias. (Courtesy of Dr TH Clutton-Brock.)

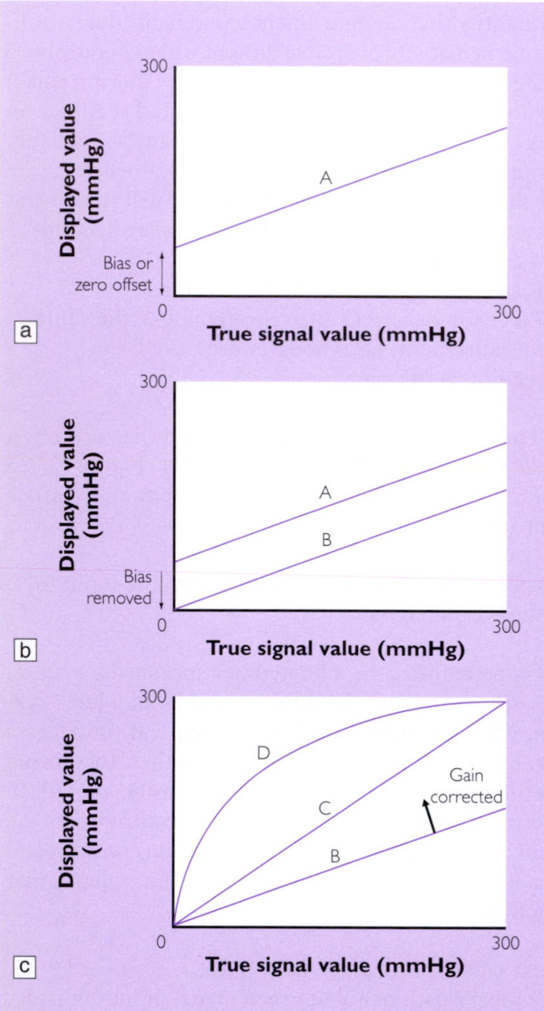


**Figure 37.26** Bias, linearity, and gain in a pressure monitoring system. (a) A bias with a zero input signal not corresponding to a zero displayed value. Zero calibration is therefore required. The input : output relationship is, however, linear. (b) The system has now been zeroed by moving line A to line B by providing an electrical offset. The gain is, however, still incorrect because a true signal value of 300 mmHg is not displayed as such. (c) Here the system has been calibrated by altering the gain of the amplifier to move line B to line C. For obvious reasons zeroing always precedes calibration. Line D shows why a two-point calibration (zero and one other point) is justified only if the system has a linear response.

of as an effect of friction in the system. The elliptical shape of the static compliance curve of the lung is such an example. Thermistors also display hysteresis which can be a cause of non-linearity. The effect is shown in Figure 37.27. Drug action can also be subject to hysteresis depending on whether the serum level is rising or falling (see Chapter 19, Figures 19.44 and 19.45).

### Resonance, attenuation, and phase distortion

In the section on mathematical relationships, it was noted that even complex waveforms could be effectively reproduced by the addition of a series of sine waves from the fundamental to the eighth to tenth harmonic. The person trying to get maximum height from a garden swing knows that she must adjust her efforts according to the natural frequency of the swing. Measuring and transmission systems, likewise, have their own inherent resonant frequency and this frequency should be well outside the range of any of the component frequencies of the waveform to be measured, or else they may be enhanced or attenuated. Applying a constant amplitude sinusoidal input at a gradually increasing frequency results in the output response shown in Figure 37.28. The principle of amplification is that the Fourier components (see Figures 37.20 and 37.21) required to reproduce a given waveform should be well below the resonant frequency. In the case of a child with a fundamental pulse frequency of 150/min or 2.5 cycles/s, the ECG should handle all frequencies equally, without differential amplification, or attenuation up to the eighth harmonic ($2.5 \times 8$) = 20 Hz. The instrument could also be described as having a flat frequency response to 20 Hz. Most modern ECG *monitors* achieve a flat response to 40 Hz.

The principle of bandwidth is shown in Figure 37.29. It is the frequency range over which the amplifier will faithfully reproduce the input signal. In the example given, the amplifier will function perfectly from 0.14 to 50 Hz. At 0.05 Hz and 100 Hz, the amplitude of the output signal will be reduced by 3 decibels. The decibel (defined in the logarithms section) measures the logarithm of the ratio of the amplitude of the output signal to that which would be achieved by a perfect amplifier.

The sharper the gradient on a waveform, the higher the frequency the bandwidth has to be to reproduce it faithfully. Square waves (such as in ST segments)

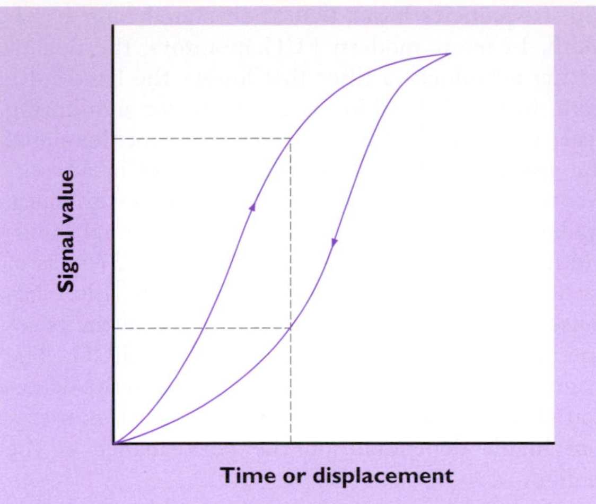


**Figure 37.27** A signal that shows hysteresis. Note that at a measured time or displacement the signal value recorded depends on whether the signal is increasing or decreasing at that point in time. Hysteresis normally involves the absorption of energy, e.g. by friction, or losses in a magnetic core.

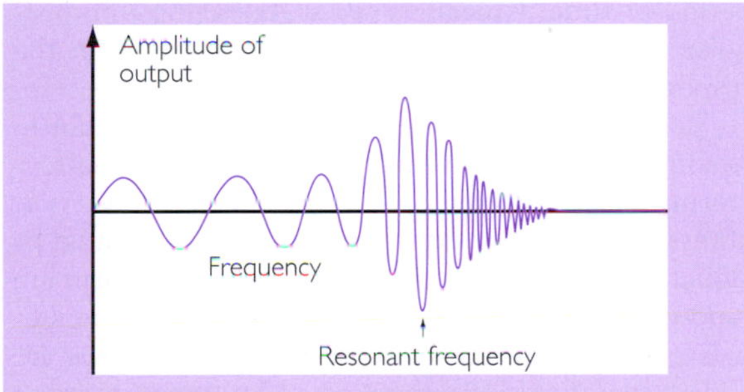


**Figure 37.28** Resonance occurring in the output signal as the exciting frequency of a system increases.

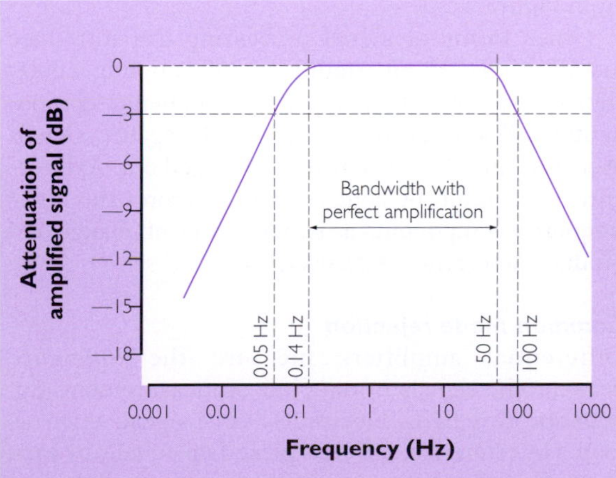


**Figure 37.29** The bandwidth of an amplifier. The attenuation on the vertical scale relates to the reduction in the amplified signal coming out of the amplifier, compared with what it should be. An attenuation of zero is therefore perfect amplification. See text for details.

require a particularly high bandwidth for faithful reproduction. If this is not provided, the amplifier can distort the input signal. *Diagnostic* ECG recorders require a wide bandwidth of approximately 0.05–75 Hz.

Not only must signals of different frequencies be amplified equally, they must also maintain their spatial relationships, otherwise they become *out of phase* with each other. A different waveform to the original will then result. Failure in both of these aspects will result in phase and amplitude distortion (see Figure 37.30 and later under 'Filters').

### Noise

Noise is any unwanted signal that tends to obscure the measured quantity. It may appear at source, e.g. from a shivering patient with an ECG, or be introduced along the way, e.g. from 50 Hz mains interference transmitted from fluorescent lighting, or high-frequency interference from the diathermy (Figure

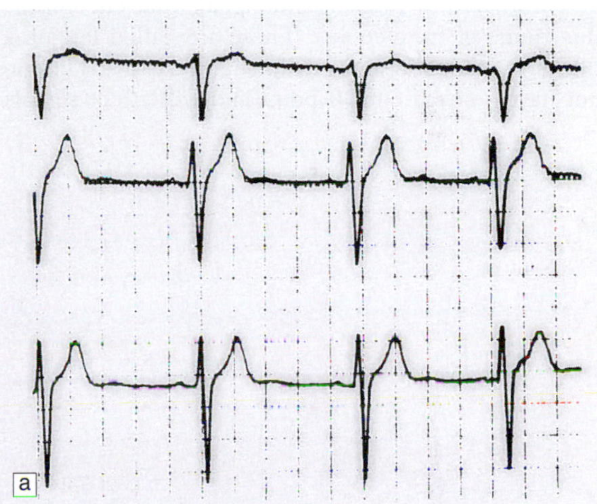


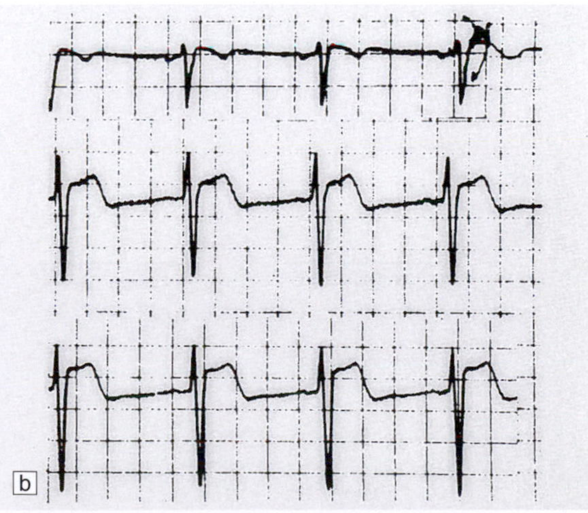


**Figure 37.30** A demonstration of signal distortion by faulty amplification. An ECG from a patient has been processed through two different amplifiers. (a) The true ECG; (b) the distorted ECG with apparent ST segment changes suggestive of ischaemia. The distortion is the result of a combination of bandwidth and phase change problems. (Adapted from Tayler DI and Vincent R. *Br Heart J* 1985;54:121.)

37.31). Sometimes, the signals, such as evoked cortical potentials, swim in a sea of extraneous signals of a greater order of magnitude than the signal itself, and specialized techniques have to be used to extract the desired information.

Noise is reduced or eliminated by various electronic processes. Many methods of noise reduction can alter the signal to a clinically significant extent, thus some knowledge of their mechanism is obligatory. Noise reduction includes the use of:

- filters;
- signal averaging;
- common mode rejection.

Filters, by definition, remove something from the signal. They are effective when the noise is produced from signals outside the bandwidth necessary for faithful reproduction of the measured quantity. Their principle is shown in Figure 37.32. Thus interference from 50 Hz mains and 1 MHz diathermy signals can be eliminated by filtering out signals that encompass this range of frequencies. These are called low-pass filters as they allow lower frequencies to pass. They do not have a sharp cut-off point and will affect signals with frequencies lower than their stated filter bandwidth. In many modern ECG monitors, the default setting introduces a filter that lowers the bandwidth from 40 to 20 Hz. This is adequate for monitoring heart rate and rhythm, but it can corrupt the signal and give false information where changes in ST segments are being monitored. Square waves with sharp gradients and flat sections need a much larger bandwidth to be reproduced accurately. Figure 37.30 is of particular relevance to anaesthetists. The filter has caused phase distortion with corruption of the baseline, T waves, and ST segments of the ECG. The diagnostic value of filtered ECG signals, in the detection of morphological changes in the heart, is therefore highly dependent on the performance of the monitor.

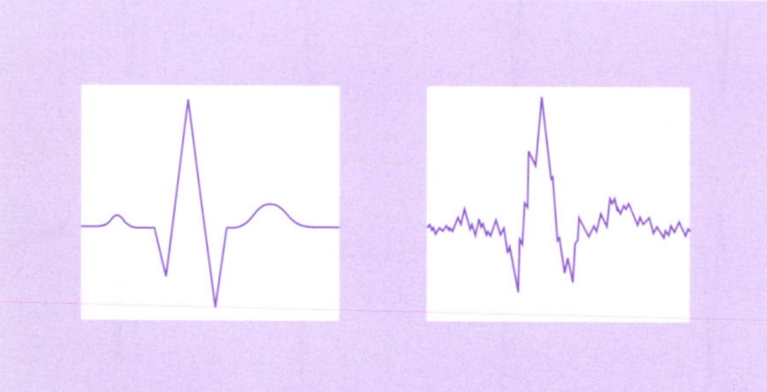

**Figure 37.31** The effect of noise distorting an ECG signal.

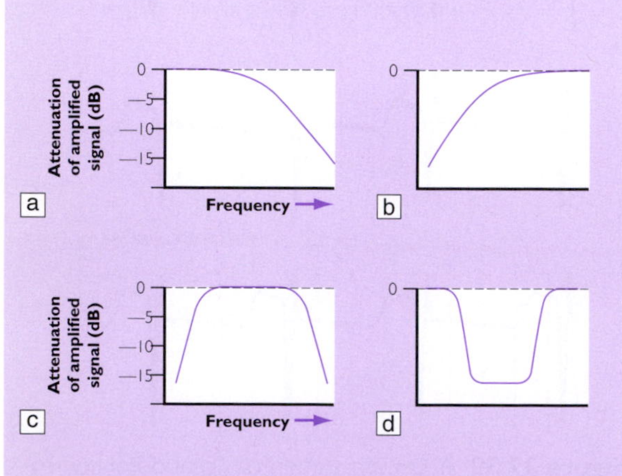


**Figure 37.32** Principles of electronic filters. When the attenuation of the amplified signal is zero, the amplifier is working perfectly. Zero attenuation of the amplified signal means that there is always a constant ratio between the input and output signals. (a) Low-pass filter; (b) high-pass filter; (c) band-pass filter; (d) band-stop filter.

A favourable scenario is thus one where there is a *high signal-to-noise ratio*. The anaesthetist recognizes this by using ECG monitoring leads (such as lead II or CM5) which lie parallel to the electrical axis of the normal heart, or over the most powerful myocardium, and so produce the greatest possible signal.

## Signal averaging

This is seen in its simplest form in the pulse oximeter where several pulses are averaged together over a period of time, typically 5–10 s. Averaging improves noise rejection at the expense of an increase in the response time.

Monitoring an evoked cortical potential is akin to looking for a ripple evoked by a stone thrown into a stormy sea. Provided, however, the evoked event always occurs in the same spot, it can be extracted by signal averaging, because the effects of the storm are random and sum to zero. In clinical devices the signals produced by 400 or more evoked responses are added together and averaged. The random noise diminishes with an increasing number of signals because the mean of positive and negative deflections of equal value is zero. The evoked potentials, however, are in phase with each other and a peak emerges from the averaged-out noise. This principle is demonstrated in Figure 37.33.

Other forms of signal processing can introduce modifications. An integrating circuit sampling a noisy signal with lots of spikes (high-frequency components) will sum all the positive and negative signals over time and the noise will be averaged out. A differentiating circuit, by contrast, will interpret the high-frequency components as sudden rates of change and produce an erroneous answer.

### *Common mode rejection*

Differential amplifiers measure the *difference* between the signals from points of measurement, e.g. between two ECG electrodes. Any signal, such as mains interference, which is picked up equally by each electrode will not register a difference and will thus be rejected. The ability of the amplifier to do this is measured by its *common mode rejection ratio.* If, however, the contact resistance between the electrode and the skin differs significantly for each electrode, the mains interference will be differentially picked up and amplified. Most noisy ECG traces can be improved by lowering the skin and electrode resistance or by

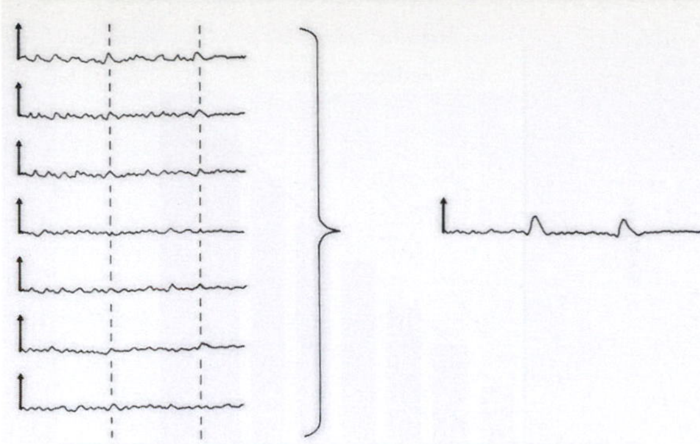

**Figure 37.33** The principle of measurement of evoked potentials using signal averaging. The stimulus represented by the solid arrow is applied regularly and the evoked potentials resulting from each stimulus are summed together. The background noise averages to zero and genuine recurrent evoked signals emerge as peaks.

degreasing and abrading the skin, thus ensuring good electrical contact. In EEG recordings the potential difference between the skin and the electrode (the junction potential) can be larger than the microvolt differences in the EEG signal itself. Specialized very-low-resistance electrodes, not subjected to movement which pierces the skin, are therefore required.

## PHYSICS OF GASES AND VAPOURS

### Kinetic theory of matter and the gas laws

A basic knowledge of the kinetic theory of matter greatly simplifies understanding of the physics of gases and vapours.

All matter is made up of particles, atoms, or molecules, which are in a state of motion, the velocity of this motion increasing with temperature. Temperature is the manifestation of the violence of this motion. The existence of molecular motion is exemplified by the fact that ammonia poured out the front of a lecture theatre will soon be smelt by those at the back, even in still air. The molecules of ammonia blast their way through the air molecules with individual mean velocities equal to that achieved by Concorde.

In solids, attractive forces that fall off rapidly with distance (van der Waals' forces) bind the molecules together, although they still vibrate, e.g. like a clock spring oscillating around a fixed point. In liquids, although the intermolecular attraction is appreciable, it is not sufficient to prevent the particles moving among themselves. It is, however, still large enough to give the liquid a definite surface and volume, and to generate the effect measured as 'surface tension'. In gases, the molecules are so separated from each other that they can move quite freely and behave as if the intermolecular forces did not exist. In a perfect gas, most of the volume is empty space, but, as the molecules are compressed or their energy is diminished by cooling, they occupy a larger percentage of the volume and the gas liquefies and becomes incompressible.

In ice, the intermolecular attractive forces predominate. As the kinetic energy and dispersive tendencies of the molecules are increased by raising the temperature, the ice turns to liquid and then to a gas or vapour. If the vapour is compressed or its temperature lowered, thus increasing the effect of intermolecular attraction, then the process is reversed. If, however, the temperature is so high that the dispersive forces are too great, then no matter how great the pressure applied, the gas cannot be liquefied. This temperature is known as the critical temperature.

> The critical temperature is that temperature above which a gas cannot be liquefied, no matter how much pressure is applied.

> The critical pressure is the pressure needed to liquefy the gas at the critical temperature.

By convention, although the physical states are identical, a gaseous substance is termed 'a gas' when it is above its critical temperature and 'a vapour' when it is below it. At room temperature, oxygen is a gas (critical temperature −118°C). Nitrous oxide ($N_2O$) is a vapour (critical temperature +36.5°C) when inhaled at 20°C, but is defined as a gas when exhaled at 37°C. This is shown in Figure 37.34.

The pressure in a gas is proportional to the violence and number of collisions the molecules have with their container per second. (In physics this is known as change in momentum with time.) Temperature is the manifestation of the average kinetic energy or $^1/_2\, mv^2$ (where $m$, mass of each molecule, $v$, root mean square velocity of the molecules). Concentrating the gas in a smaller volume increases the rate of collisions with the container and increases the pressure.

Increasing the temperature increases the average velocity of the molecules, and thus the number of collisions per second, as well as increasing the violence of these collisions. The relationships between pressure, volume, and the temperature of a gas are defined in Boyle's and Charles' laws.

Boyle's law describes to the relationship between the pressure and volume of a fixed mass of a perfect gas at constant temperature, hydrogen coming closest to the ideal (Figure 37.35). The shape of the relation-

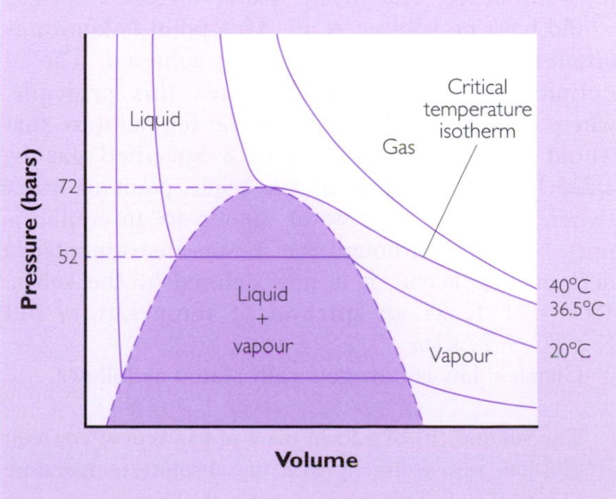


**Figure 37.34** The phase diagram for nitrous oxide close to the critical point with some isothermals superimposed.

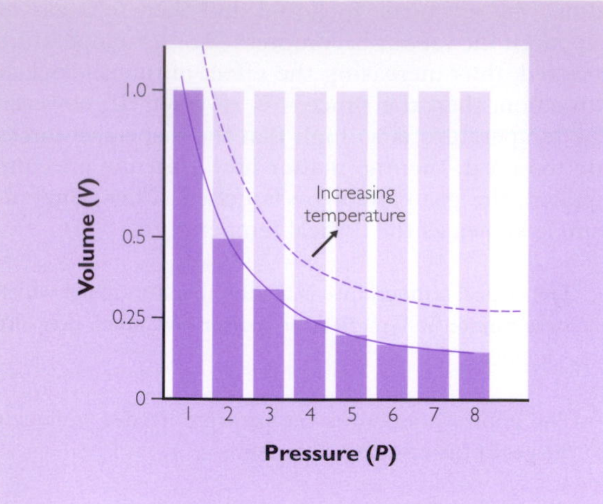


**Figure 37.35** A graphical illustration of Boyle's law: at a constant temperature, $P \propto 1/V$ or $PV$ = constant. The relationship between volume and pressure is a rectangular hyperbola. The dotted line represents what would happen to the same mass of gas if the volume–pressure relationship were recorded at a higher temperature.

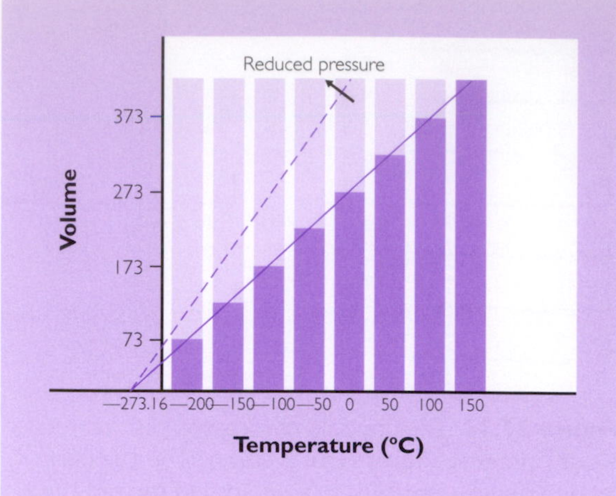


**Figure 37.36** A graphical representation of Charles' law: gas expands at 1/273 of its volume at 0°C, per degree at a constant pressure ($V \propto T$). It can be seen that there is a direct linear relationship between volume and temperature which intersects the axis at −273.16°C. If the same mass of gas had its volume varied with temperature at a reduced pressure, then the relationship would move to the position shown by the dotted line.

ship is a rectangular hyperbola (see earlier for mathematical details). It applies less accurately as gases approach their critical temperature and pressure, when intermolecular forces become important (see Figure 37.34).

Note that Boyle's law only applies to a fixed mass of gas. If the volume is kept constant and the pressure changes because gas is lost, then the pressure in the cylinder is proportional to the remaining gas, providing the temperature is the same (i.e. Boyle's law does not apply). This is the principle of using a pressure gauge to measure the contents of an oxygen cylinder. The relationship between pressure gauge readings and cylinder contents is considered in detail for all anaesthetic gases in Chapter 8.

Charles found that, if a gas was kept at a constant pressure, its volume would vary by a constant amount per °C change in temperature (Figure 37.36). This volume change was 1/273.16 of its volume at the melting point of ice. This meant that at −273.16°C the gas would have no volume at all. This point is known as *absolute zero* and has never been achieved. The SI definition of temperature utilizes this principle, where the kelvin (K *not* °K) is the temperature that would change the volume of a specified gas by 1/273.16 of its volume at the triple point of water (where ice, water and water vapour are in equilibrium). Note that although the °C was instrumental in defining the kelvin, it is now defined *by* the kelvin. 1°C = 1 K as an interval of temperature, but K = °C + 273.16.

Charles' law is now generally stated as follows.

> The volume ($V$) of a fixed mass of gas kept at constant pressure varies directly with the absolute temperature ($T$), or $V \propto T$. This graph is a straight line.

Combining these laws gives the universal gas law which states:

$$P \times \frac{V}{T}$$

is a constant for a fixed mass of gas. This can be written as:

$$\frac{PV}{T} = \text{constant} = nR$$

Or, more familiarly, as:

$$PV = nRT$$

the usual form of the universal gas equation, where $n$ is the number of moles (see below) of a gas and $R$ the universal gas constant, which is the same for all gases.

From this equation it can be seen that, for a fixed mass of gas, if the volume is kept constant then the pressure varies directly with the absolute temperature ($P/T$ = constant). This is sometimes referred to as Gay-Lussac's law, although the relationship was first discovered by Amontons in 1702. He is sadly now forgotten, but Charles, Boyle, and Gay-Lussac are not. The universal gas equation assumes that the gas is behaving as a perfect gas and that intermolecular forces are small.

Kinetic theory also assumes that the volume of the gas particles themselves is small, and that attraction and repulsion between them is negligible. When these assumptions do not apply (close to liquefaction), then, as can be seen in Figure 37.34, the perfect gas equation ceases to describe the relationship between $PV$ and $T$.

As the molecules move closer together, because of either increasing pressure or reducing temperature, their actual volume and intermolecular forces become important. Generally, molecules at close distances attract each other and these are the cohesive forces that keep liquids and solids together. However, as the intermolecular distances continue to reduce even further and approach approximately the diameter of a molecule, short-range repulsive forces develop. The intermolecular distance represents the equilibrium position between these attractive and repulsive forces with minimum potential energy. This is shown in Figure 37.37.

### Moles and the quantity of matter

A mole is the measure of the number of molecules of a substance (element or compound). A gram molecular weight is the quantity of an element or compound that has a weight, in grams, numerically equal to the element or compound's molecular weight. The terms 'molecular weight' and 'gram molecular weight' are used whether the molecule is that of an element, e.g. $O_2$, or of a compound, e.g. $CO_2$. It therefore follows that the gram molecular weights of different substances contain the same number of molecules: 6.023 × $10^{23}$ molecules. This number is called Avogadro's number; the quantity of substance that contains Avogadro's number of molecules is called a mole (abbreviation mol). The universal gas constant ($R$), is the same for 1 mol of any perfect gas.

> Avogadro's law states that equal volumes of all gases under the same conditions of temperature and pressure contain the same number of molecules. At STP (standard temperature and pressure = 0°C and 101.3 kPa) the molecular weight of a gas expressed in grams has a volume of 22.4 litres.

### Diffusion

If two gases at the same pressure and with identical temperatures (and hence equal values for $^1/_2mv^2$) have different molecular weights, it follows that the gas with the heavier molecules will have lower molecular velocities. It is the molecular velocity that determines the speed of diffusion of a gas, so high-density gases diffuse slowly and low-density gases diffuse rapidly. This phenomenon is described by Graham's law.

> Graham's law of diffusion states that the rate of diffusion of a gas is proportional to 1/√density.

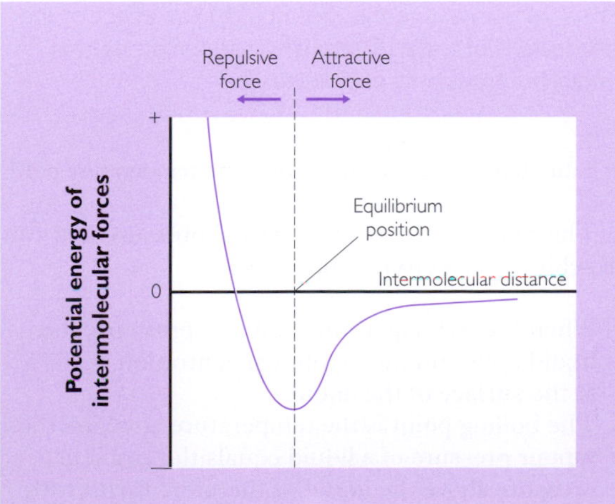


**Figure 37.37** The determination of intermolecular distance by the balance of attractive and repulsive forces.

### Partial pressures

When there is a mixture of two gases in a container, under kinetic theory the volume occupied by both gases is the same and equal to the volume of the container. Assume that the volume of the container is 1 litre and the total number of moles is 1, 80% of the molecules being $N_2$ and 20% being $O_2$. Note that both nitrogen and oxygen occupy the whole of the 1-litre volume. Then, applying the universal gas equation:

For nitrogen, $PV = nRT$

$$P_{N_2} \times 1 = 0.8 \times R \times T \qquad (1)$$

For oxygen, $PV = nRT$

$$P_{O_2} \times 1 = 0.2 \times R \times T \qquad (2)$$

For the mixture of gases (total 1 mol), $PV = nRT$

$$P_{total} \times 1 = 1 \times R \times T = RT \qquad (3)$$

Adding together equations (1) and (2) gives:

$$P_{N_2} + P_{O_2} = 0.8\ \mathrm{RT} + 0.2\ \mathrm{RT} = RT$$

Comparing this with equation (3) results in:

$$P_{N_2} + P_{O_2} = P_{total}.$$

This principle of adding the component pressures to give the total gas mixture pressure is called Dalton's law. The ratio of partial pressure is in proportion to the mole fraction of the components.

> Dalton's law says, in effect, that the total pressure exerted by a mixture of gases is the sum of the pressures that each would exert by itself in the volume of the container, provided that there is no chemical reaction.

This means that the partial pressure of a gas is the fractional concentration multiplied by total pressure, or:

$$\text{Fractional concentration} = \frac{\text{partial pressure}}{\text{total pressure}}$$

If the total pressure is 137 bar, a fractional concentration of 0.1 or 10% would be 13.7 bar. To prepare a 10% $CO_2$ in $O_2$ mixture, the manufacturer fills the cylinder with pure $CO_2$ to a pressure of 13.7 bar, then continues with $O_2$ to 137 bar total cylinder pressure.

### Calculation of vapour concentration: application of partial pressures and gas laws

The saturated vapour pressure of a volatile agent (SVP, see below) is a partial pressure (albeit the maximum that can be achieved at a given temperature), and this formula is used in calculating the saturation concentration of a vapour, e.g. the SVP for isoflurane at 20°C is 250 mmHg. If ambient pressure is 760 mmHg, then the maximum possible concentration of isoflurane is calculated from:

$$\frac{250}{760} = \begin{matrix}\text{Fractional concentration}\\ \text{of isoflurane}\end{matrix} = 0.33 \text{ or } 33\%.$$

If the SVP is given in kPa, the calculation becomes even simpler, because, if the ambient pressure is taken to be 100 kPa, the SVP and the saturation concentration have, for practical purposes, the same value.

The method used by Joseph Clover over 150 years ago to prepare a known concentration of chloroform illustrates the practical application of the above laws. Clover is shown in Figure 37.38. The leather bag over Clover's shoulder had a known volume of 40 litres and he put into it a known quantity of chloroform to produce a predictable vapour mixture. A modern calculation for producing 1% vol/vol concentration of isoflurane goes as follows:

- 185 g (molecular weight = 184.5) of isoflurane vaporized at STP (0°C, 1 bar) would have a volume of 22.4 litres (Avogadro's law).
- At 20°C its volume would increase to 24 litres, i.e. by 1/273 of its volume at 0°C for every °C rise in temperature (Charles' law).
- 1 g of isoflurane would produce 24/185 = 130 ml of saturated vapour at 20°C.
- The density of liquid isoflurane is 1.5 g/ml (density = mass/volume) thus: 1 ml of liquid isoflurane will produce 130 × 1.5 = 195 ml of isoflurane vapour; 2 ml of liquid isoflurane (producing 390 mls) vaporized into a 40-litre bag of gas at 20°C will therefore provide approximately 1% vol/vol concentration.

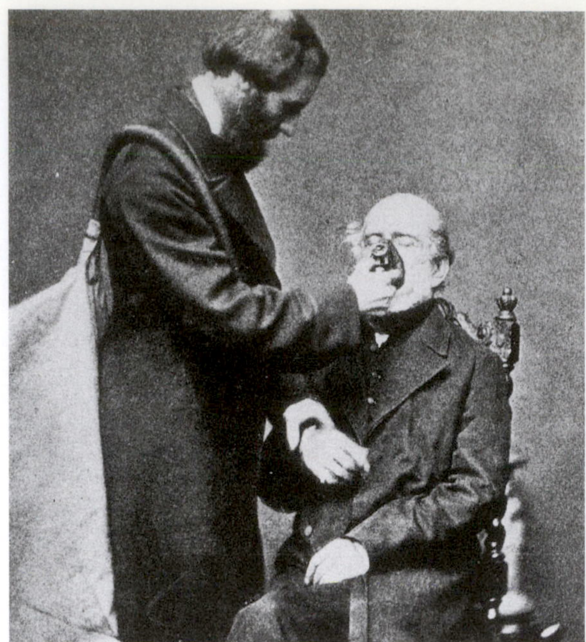

**Figure 37.38** Joseph Clover using prepared concentrations of chloroform delivered from the large bag that is slung over his shoulder.

## Saturated vapour pressure

The experiment by Torricelli in 1643 (Figure 37.39) illustrates the concept of saturated vapours. The pressure exerted by the column of mercury at area A is matched by the atmospheric pressure applied through the mercury bath on the same area (Figure 37.39a). When a drop of water is introduced in the vacuum, it vaporizes, exerting vapour pressure. Introducing more water increases the vapour pressure until a point is reached where the pressure no longer increases. The vapour is now saturated (Figure 37.39b) and a water droplet remains.

The effect of water vapour is to provide a pressure above the mercury where previously there was a vacuum. This pressure presses onto the mercury column so that less mercury can be supported by the same atmospheric pressure and the meniscus falls (Figure 37.39b). The difference in mercury levels is a measure of the SVP of water at the given temperature when there is a liquid remaining that is not evaporated.

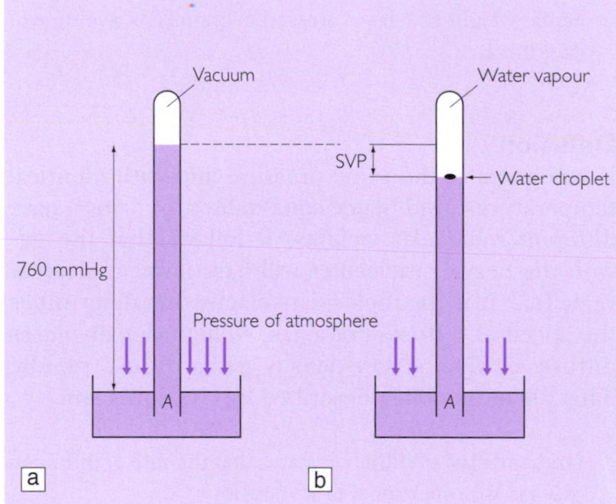


**Figure 37.39** The effect of saturated vapour pressure (SVP) on a torricellian vacuum. (a) The column height with a vacuum above the mercury; (b) the effect of the introduction of water. A saturated vapour is one that is in equilibrium with its own liquid.

> A saturated vapour is one that is in equilibrium with its own liquid.

Saturation means that the number of molecules entering the vapour phase is matched by the number re-entering the liquid phase. If the kinetic energy of the molecules is increased by raising the temperature, more molecules leave the liquid (to exert vapour pressure) until a new equilibrium is reached and the SVP rises. If the ambient pressure increases, *the SVP of the liquid is unchanged, although it forms a smaller proportion of the total pressure*. Thus the *concentration* of the vapour changes with ambient pressure, but:

> Saturated vapour pressure varies with temperature only!

The SVP is the maximum partial pressure that can be achieved at a given temperature:

- When the SVP equals the ambient pressure, the liquid boils and the vapour concentration is 100% at the surface of the liquid.
- The boiling point is the temperature at which the vapour pressure of a liquid equals the ambient pressure above the liquid. It therefore varies with the ambient pressure. This makes it difficult to make a decent cup of tea at high altitude without using a pressure cooker.

- Vaporization occurs on the surface of the liquid. At the boiling point it also occurs within the body of the liquid.

Although the SVP is only dependent on temperature, it has a non-linear relationship with it. This is shown in Figure 37.40. For comparison, this figure includes $N_2O$, the volatile agents, and water. Across this wide spectrum, note how those agents that can be administered from conventional vaporizers (isoflurane, halothane, enflurane, and sevoflurane) are grouped together. The triple points of water and $N_2O$ where gas, liquid, and solid exist simultaneously in equilibrium are marked. At the freezing point of water, the SVP is not zero, but 4.6 mmHg. The SVP at the triple point is sometimes called the sublimation pressure. The SVP curves for the volatile agents stop at 0°C because of the lack of published experimental data below this level.

#### *Implications for the anaesthetist*

At altitude, at a given temperature, SVP does not change, but the ambient pressure decreases. Although the partial pressure of the vapour does not change, its proportion of the ambient pressure is now greater. The percentage output (fractional concentration) therefore rises. Anaesthetic action depends, however, on partial pressure, not fractional concentration, so no adjustment to the vaporizer is required.

The boiling point of desflurane is just above room temperature so very little heat is required to raise it to its boiling point (i.e. 100% saturation) in its vaporizing chamber.

At high pressures water boils at a temperature greater than 100°C. This is made use of in autoclaves and pressure cookers.

### Adiabatic and isothermal changes

Adiabatic changes are those in which no heat leaves or enters the system. When work is done on gas in order to compress it, or the gas is allowed to expand and there is no heat loss, the compression or expansion is said to be adiabatic in nature, i.e. the energy changes are being kept within the system. There is an accompanying change in the gas temperature. If the concentration or expansion is performed sufficiently slowly, heat can be conducted through the wall of the containing vessel without a measurable change in the temperature. This is defined as an isothermal change and is a condition of Boyle's law. The compression ignition diesel engine provides an example of an adiabatic change.

### Latent heat

The molecules of a liquid do not all have the same velocity. Some of the more vigorous molecules escape from the liquid into the vapour phase so the average kinetic energy of the remaining molecules decreases. Thus, there is a cooling effect from evaporation on the remaining liquid. Heat can be applied to the liquid to maintain or increase vaporization by ensuring the continued supply of high-energy molecules. The additional heat required to convert a given mass of liquid into vapour at the same temperature is *the latent heat of vaporization*. The latent heat of vaporization varies with the temperature of the liquid and this must be specified.

To change a solid into a liquid the same principle applies. This is the *latent heat of fusion*. The reverse also applies and heat is given out when the conversion from vapour to liquid or from liquid to solid takes place. This effect is shown in principle in Figure 37.41.

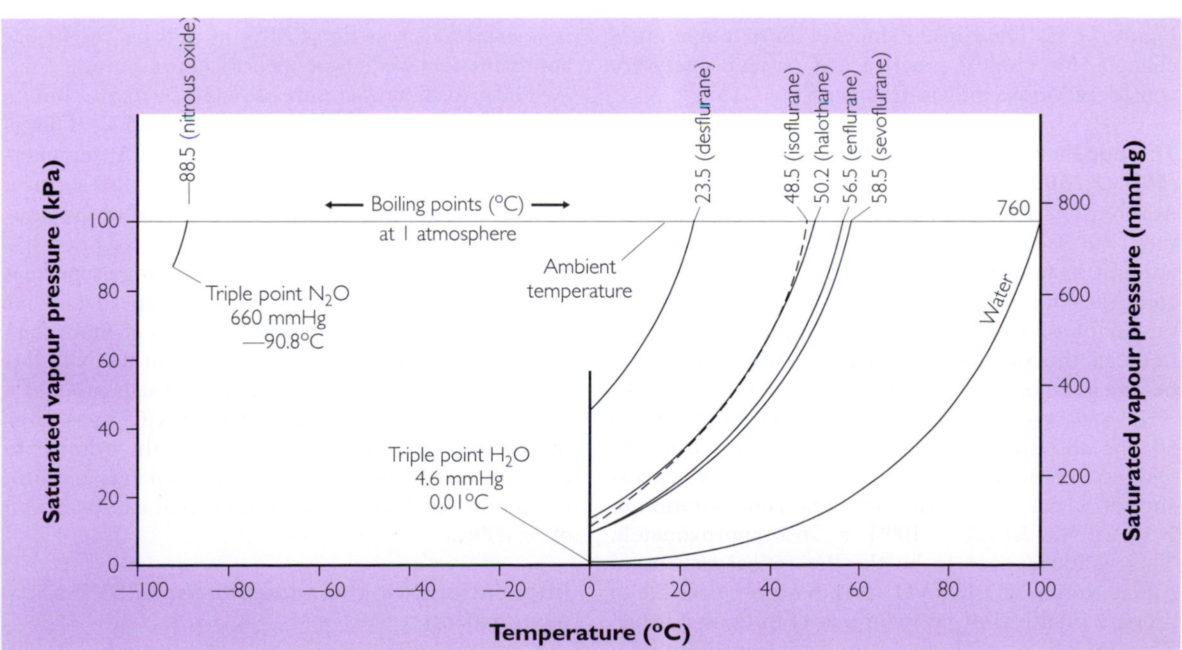


**Figure 37.40** The relationship of saturated vapour pressure (SVP) and temperature. (Data on nitrous oxide ($N_2O$) from Grant WJ. *Medical Gases*. Aylesbury, UK: HM & M Publishers, 1978; on sevoflurane from Abbott Laboratories; on desflurane from Susay SR *et al. Anesth Analg* 1996;83:864; on isoflurane, halothane, enflurane, and water from Rodgers RC and Hill GE. *Br J Anaesth* 1978;50:415.)

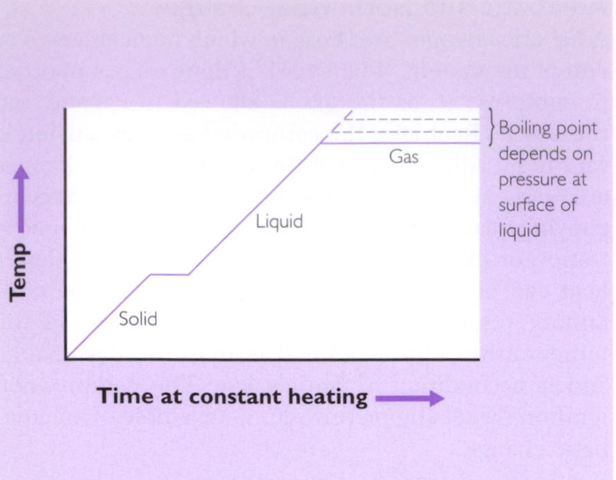


**Figure 37.41** The principle of latent heat. The specific latent heat is the heat required to convert 1 kg of a substance from one phase to the other at a given temperature. Units are J/kg. When constant heating is applied to water in the solid state, the temperature rises linearly, except at the melting and boiling points where heat energy is absorbed to effect a change in state without a rise in temperature. When the water reaches its boiling point, provided that the container is not enclosed, the temperature will not rise further as it will continue to evaporate.

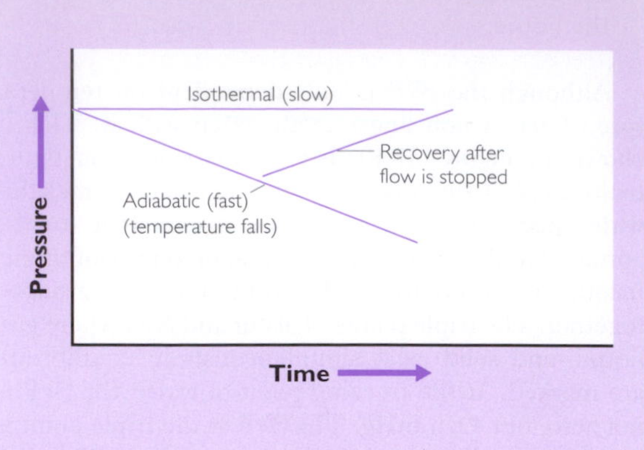


**Figure 37.42** Diagrammatic demonstration of the effects of fast and slow emptying on the pressure in a nitrous oxide ($N_2O$) cylinder that contains liquid $N_2O$. At fast rates of emptying, heat is drawn from the cylinder contents to provide the latent heat of vaporization. The pressure in the cylinder falls as a result of the decrease of the saturated vapour pressure of $N_2O$ secondary to the fall in temperature. When the cylinder is turned off, it regains its original temperature and pressure, with heat conducted from the surroundings. At slow rates of emptying, the cylinder is able to maintain its temperature and pressure as heat flows in from ambient sources. The effect of these changes in temperature on clinical anaesthesia is discussed in more detail in Chapter 8.

The specific latent heat is the heat required to convert 1 kg of a substance from one phase to another at a given temperature. The units are J/kg.

### The behaviour of nitrous oxide

The properties of $N_2O$ close to the critical point are given in Figure 37.34. The emptying of an $N_2O$ cylinder is a good example of evaporative temperature change. The effect is shown diagrammatically in Figure 37.42. The consequences of these temperature changes for clinical practice and patient safety are considered more fully in Chapter 8.

#### *The peculiar properties of Entonox ($50\%\ O_2 : 50\%\ N_2O$)*

At room temperature, i.e. below the critical temperature, the SVP of $N_2O$ is approximately 50 bar. If an attempt is made to raise its pressure above this by compression, more $N_2O$ will condense from the vapour phase and the pressure will remain the same until all the vapour is condensed. After this it will behave as an incompressible liquid (see Figure 37.34).

If such a cylinder is filled with gaseous $N_2O$ to 50 bar and then with $O_2$ to 138 bar, according to Dalton's law of partial pressures $N_2O$ will exert a pressure of 50 bar and $O_2$ the rest. The concentration of $N_2O$ will be $50/138 \times 100\% = 36\%$ approximately. This would appear to be the theoretical maximum concentration of $N_2O$ in $O_2$. It is, however, possible to prepare mixtures of up to 70% $N_2O$ in $O_2$ at 138 bar. This is only possible because of molecular interactions between $O_2$ and $N_2O$ that are peculiar to them.

Entonox is manufactured by introducing an appropriate amount of liquid $N_2O$ into a cylinder, inverting it and then bubbling $O_2$ through it. Some of the $O_2$ dissolves in the $N_2O$, while the rest carries up droplets into the gas above. Eventually all the liquid $N_2O$ is carried into the gaseous phase to produce a 50% mixture of $O_2$ and $N_2O$. The physical property that allows this to occur is known as the *Poynting effect*. The 50% $N_2O$ now exerts a pressure of 50% of 138 bar = 70 bar approximately, well above its critical pressure.

The critical temperature of $N_2O$ is +36.5°C, but its interaction with oxygen lowers it to −5.5°C. This is known as the *pseudocritical temperature*. At temperatures below −6°C, liquefaction of $N_2O$ takes place. This is sometimes termed 'lamination' or 'separation'. Under these conditions, the liquid $N_2O$ now has about 20% $O_2$ dissolved in it, with a varying proportion of $N_2O$ in the $O_2$-rich gas above. If the supernatant gas is drawn off it has an $O_2$ concentration of more than 50%. As this is used up, $O_2$ dissolved in the $N_2O$ liquid will come out of solution and eventually produce a hypoxic mixture. In large cylinders of $N_2O$, a gas withdrawal tube extends to the bottom of the cylinder to ensure that, in the event of *lamination* (separation), the minimum concentration of $O_2$ that can be drawn off is 20%.

### Implications for the anaesthetist of SVP and evaporation

- Vaporizers cool so SVP and output decrease unless compensating mechanisms are present.
- $N_2O$ cylinders cool as they empty, SVP decreases. Gauge pressure decreases (see later and Chapter 8).

- Liquid oxygen in its vacuum-insulated evaporator must be kept below its critical temperature of –118°C. In practice it is kept at –160°C. No amount of insulation will keep it at this level indefinitely; it must be cooled. This is done by vaporization, i.e. by using it (see later and Chapter 8).
- Wet drapes increase evaporative heat loss from the patient.
- Vaporization of water from the respiratory tract to humidify inspired dry gas is associated with significant heat loss.
- Steam causes more thermal damage than water at the same temperature.

## DYNAMICS OF FLUIDS: FACTORS AFFECTING FLOW

### Viscosity

Viscosity is the property of a fluid that tends to prevent it from flowing when it is subjected to an applied force. The tenacity with which a moving layer or *lamina* drags adjacent layers with it determines its viscosity. Laminar or streamline flow can be likened to a pack of cards, where the top card is pushed along its long axis (Figure 37.43). The rest of the cards move by friction, but at different velocities. To keep the cards moving requires a continuous application of the applied force (Figure 37.43a).

Just as in the definition of pressure, the effect on the fluid depends on the area over which the force is applied. The force per unit area is termed 'the shear stress' and is measured on the SI system in pascals (newtons per square metre). Viscosity is a measure of how effectively the force applied on a liquid surface is able to get the layers below to drag one another along. It is defined for a given liquid by the coefficient of viscosity (μ) which is the ratio of the shear stress (τ) applied to the rate of shear it produces (Figure 37.43b).

It is easier to turn this definition round and say that the coefficient of viscosity (μ) is the shear stress (force per unit area) that has to be applied to keep layers 1 metre apart moving with a relative velocity of 1 m/s.

For those who prefer to interpret things mathematically, the derivation of this relationship and the consequent system of units is given below. If preferred it can be skipped without loss of understanding and would not be expected to be reproduced in examinations.

With reference to Figure 37.43b, the behaviour of the fluid is described mathematically as:

$$\tau = \frac{\mu(V_1 - V_2)}{x} \text{ or } \frac{\mu(dV)}{dx}$$

or, rearranging:

$$\mu = \frac{(\tau x)}{(V_1 - V_2)} \text{ or } \frac{\tau}{(dV/dx)}.$$

μ is thus a derived SI unit with SI components of:

$$\mu = (N/m^2)(m/m \text{ per s}) = (N{\cdot}s)/m^2 = Pa{\cdot}s.$$

The unit of viscosity often used in practice is the poise (after Poiseuille) which is the c.g.s. equivalent. They are related such that 1 Pa·s = 10 poise.

A newtonian fluid is one in which the shear stress is directly proportional to the rate of shear, irrespective of the applied force. Alternatively, this means that the coefficient of viscosity is independent of $dV/dx$, the velocity gradient through the fluid. The coefficient of viscosity changes with temperature, falling as temperature increases in liquids and rising in gases.

Saline and plasma behave as newtonian fluids with viscosities of 1 and 1.1–1.6 centipoise (cp), respectively. Blood is distinctly non-newtonian, with a viscosity very dependent on shear rate. These features are shown in Figure 37.44. The viscosity of blood falls as the shear rate rises because of the decrease in clumping of the erythrocytes. One of the major effects, at a given shear rate, on the viscosity is the haematocrit. The relative viscosity of blood with respect to plasma as the haematocrit rises is shown in Figure 37.45.

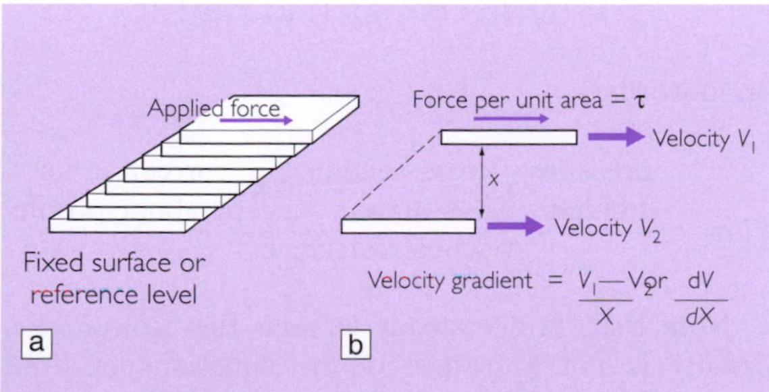


**Figure 37.43** A demonstration of the effect of viscosity. (a) The applied force on the upper layer gradually drags the layers below it along with it. (b) The definition of the velocity gradient in the liquid resulting from an applied shearing force. x is distance within the liquid. See text for explanation.

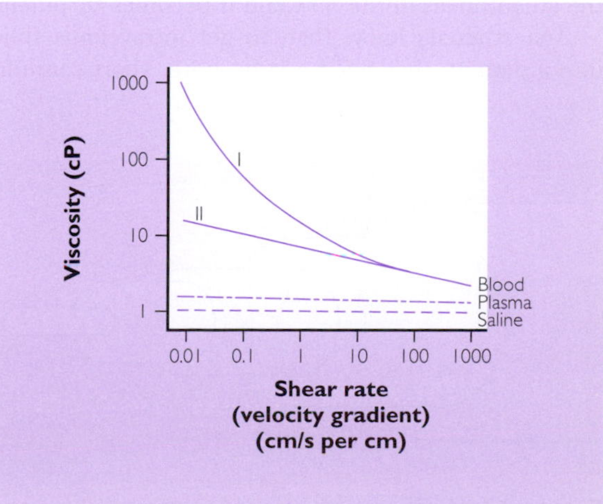


**Figure 37.44** The variability in viscosity with shear rate. I, whole blood; II, defibrinated blood.

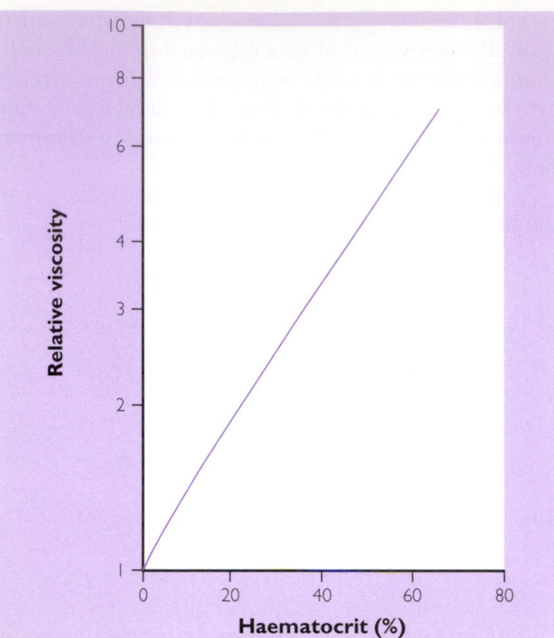


**Figure 37.45** The variability in relative viscosity of blood with increasing haematocrit at a fixed shear rate. The relative viscosity on the vertical axis is the ratio of the viscosity of blood to that of plasma. (Adapted from Whitmore RL. *The Rheology of the Circulation*. Oxford: Pergamon Press, 1968: 71.)

## Pipe flow

### *Laminar flow*

Molecules of a fluid flowing close to the side of a tube keep colliding with it and are subject to 'drag'. This slows them down. These molecules in turn affect flow in the adjacent layer. This process continues until there is a gradation of velocities, maximal along the central axis of the tube, reducing to zero next to the walls. This type of 'onion skin' movement is shown in Figure 37.46. When particle velocities are plotted across a cross-section, the result is called a velocity profile. In laminar flow, the cross-sectional profile is parabolic. Laminar flow will prevail unless the velocity of flow becomes so great that the layers break up, or rough edges or sudden changes in direction disrupt the smoothness of the flow and it becomes turbulent.

Anaesthetists know that, to get intravenous fluid into a patient, they need a large-bore, short cannula, using a bag containing the least viscous fluid, which is then pressurized, i.e.

$$\text{Flow} \propto \frac{\text{cross-sectional area}}{\text{viscosity}} \times \frac{\text{pressure drop}}{\text{length}}$$

This is a sort of hydraulic Ohm's law where:

$$\begin{array}{l}\text{Current (flow} \\ \text{per unit area)}\end{array} = \frac{\text{voltage (pressure gradient)}}{\text{resistance (viscous effects)}}$$

Similarly, pneumotachographs measure flow by measuring pressure difference across a fixed resistance.

This principle, expressed in the form of an equation for laminar flow, is Poiseuille's law. In laminar flow, because of the parabolic velocity profile (see Figure 37.48), the greater proportion of the flow occurs down the axis of the tube. This makes the flow proportional to the fourth power of the radius, rather than the radius squared. Trainees need to understand the underlying principles of Poiseuille's equation and to describe its component terms. They would not be expected to derive it from the equations of motion of a fluid, so the calculation below could be skipped if preferred.

Included for the sake of completeness and for the mathematically inclined, Poiseuille's equation is derived as follows. The velocity profile is obtained by integrating the equation derived earlier, $\tau = \mu(\mathrm{d}V/\mathrm{d}x)$, across the pipe cross-section. This produces the equation of the velocity profile as:

$$V = \frac{(\Delta p)}{L} \frac{([r_o^2 - r^2])}{4\mu}$$

where $(\Delta p/l)$ is the pressure gradient down the pipe, $r_o$ is the radius of the pipe, and $V$ is the velocity at radius $r$. It can be seen that when $r = r_o$ (at the pipe surface), $V = 0$, and on the centre line ($r = 0$) $V$ is maximum.

If the velocity profile is further integrated up across the pipe cross-section to obtain flow ($\dot{Q}$):

$$\dot{Q} = (\Delta p/l)(\pi r_o^4/8\mu).$$

This is known as Poiseuille's equation.

Rearranging the expression for comparison with earlier equations, this becomes

$$\dot{Q} = (\Delta p/l) \times (\pi r_o^2) \times (1/\mu) \times (r_o^2/8)$$

or, in words:

$$\text{Flow} = \frac{\begin{array}{c}\text{pressure} \\ \text{gradient}\end{array} \times \begin{array}{c}\text{cross-sectional} \\ \text{area}\end{array} \times \begin{array}{c}\text{correction for} \\ \text{parabolic profile}\end{array}}{\text{viscous resistance}}$$

Note that, under steady laminar flow conditions, density is not a feature of the equations of fluid motion. It would be if the fluid were accelerating or decelerating.

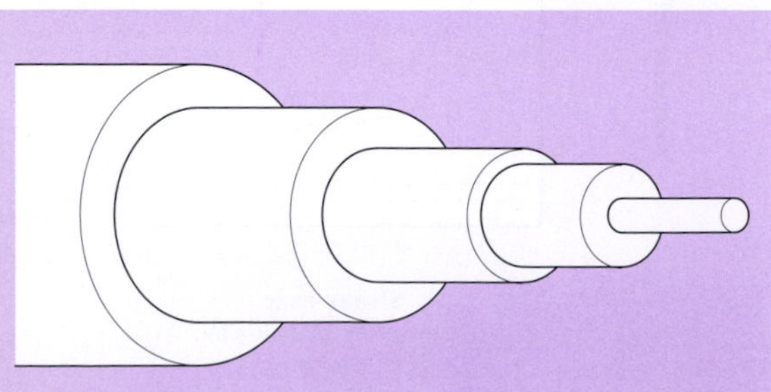

**Figure 37.46** The development of a laminar flow profile. Note how the 'onion skin' movement of adjacent layers gradually elongates the envelope of velocities.

## Flow at the entrance to a pipe

Velocity profiles are not always parabolic as they are in well-established laminar flow in a circular pipe. At the entrance to a pipe leading from a tank, initially all the molecules enter with the same velocity. As the fluid moves along the pipe, the layers drag on one another until the familiar parabolic profile eventually emerges. This is shown in Figure 37.47. The distance over which the ideal parabolic profile develops is called the 'entrance length' and is typically over 20 pipe diameters in length. The flow pattern is further complicated in the arteries because the flow is not steady but pulsatile. Consequently, although Poiseuille's equation provides a good theoretical model for understanding of the importance of tube diameter and pressure gradient as determinants of flow, it is a poor numerical approximation to the actual events occurring in the arterial tree and airways.

### Turbulent flow

As the pressure gradient down a pipe increases, laminar flow continues to prevail, with the central velocities steadily increasing, making the velocity profile more and more pointed. In specially set-up conditions, the velocities can increase to very high levels by this mechanism. However, in practical systems the flow is not perfect and it is subject to disturbances from rough edges and surface irregularities. At low flows, the effect of viscosity immediately contains these disturbances, which try to push molecules from one layer to another, and laminar flow is preserved. As the flow increases, the effect of disturbances produces particles of much greater momentum trying to cross the parallel laminar flow layers. A point occurs when these transverse effects can no longer be suppressed by viscous forces and there is then a transfer of molecules from streamline to streamline across the cross-section of the pipe. The flow has now become turbulent. This transfer of molecules of different kinetic energies results in collisions, which tend to reduce the differences in velocities between adjacent layers. Consequently, at these higher flows the velocity profile changes from parabolic to flatter, sometimes termed 'plug flow'. This is shown in Figure 37.48. Physical comparisons of laminar flow and turbulent flow down a pipe and round a cylinder are shown in Figure 37.49.

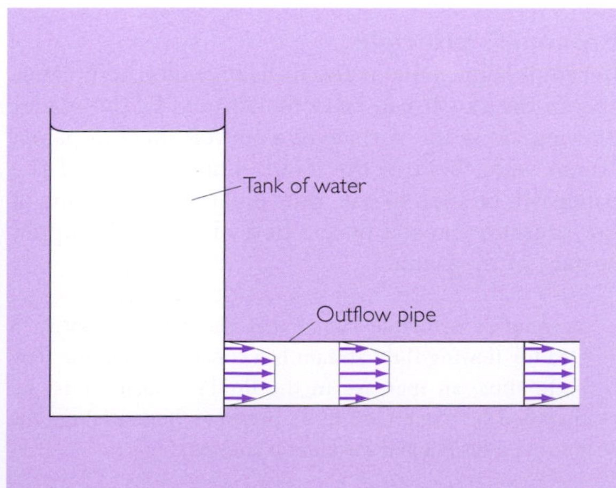


**Figure 37.47** The change in the velocity profile at the entrance to a pipe as water flows into it from a tank. (Adapted from Prandtl L and Tietjens OG. *Applied Hydro- and Aeromechanics.* New York: Dover Publications Inc., 1957: 26.)

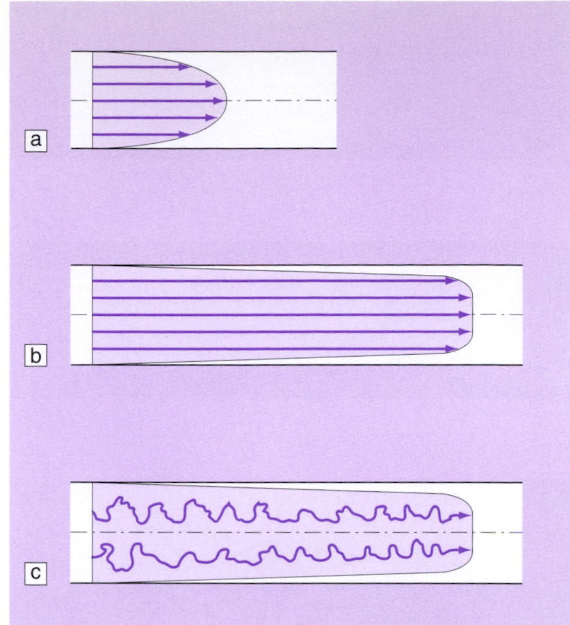


**Figure 37.48** A comparison of (a) laminar and (b, c) turbulent flow. (b) The velocity profile and (c) the path of individual particles. (a) Laminar flow: parabolic velocity profile with all particles moving parallel to each other along a streamline. (b) Turbulent flow: flat-ended velocity profiles producing 'plug flow'. The streamlines represent mean longitudinal velocity, not true particle paths. (c) Turbulent flow: actual path is as shown. At any one time, a given particle has a transverse and longitudinal velocity. The transverse velocity promotes momentum transfer between adjacent fluid layers and tends to equalize the velocities across the cross-section. The ratio between the transverse and longitudinal velocities is used to measure the intensity or 'strength' of the turbulence.

Turbulence, the phenomenon of energy transfer between adjacent layers, was investigated by Reynolds, and the point at which it occurs is predicted by a dimensionless ratio called the Reynolds' number (Re). It is defined as:

$$\text{Re} = (v\rho d)/\mu = \frac{(\text{Mean velocity} \times \text{density} \times \text{diameter})}{\text{viscosity}}$$

Transition from laminar to turbulent flow occurs at the critical Re of between 2000 and 2500. Note that, in turbulent flow (unlike steady laminar flow), the density of the fluid (ρ) as well as the viscosity becomes important. This is because the development of turbulence depends on momentum transfer.

Once turbulence has occurred, there is no single equation that will predict the relationship between pressure drop and flow, except to say that they are non-linearly related and the pressure drop required is much greater than in laminar flow. Several equations have been proposed for given circumstances. A common one is that the pressure drop is proportional to the square of the velocity. These features are shown diagrammatically in Figure 37.50.

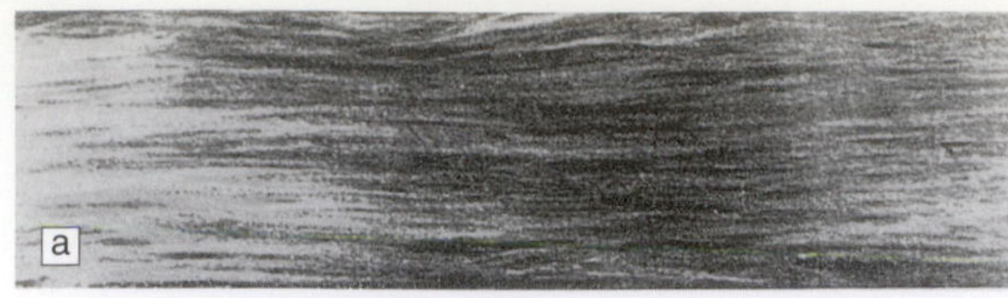


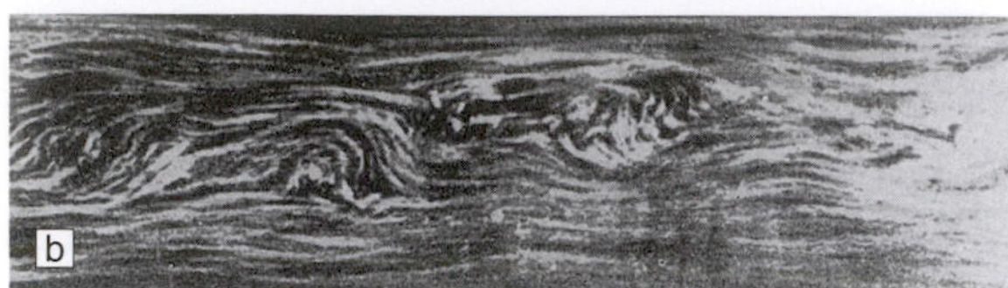


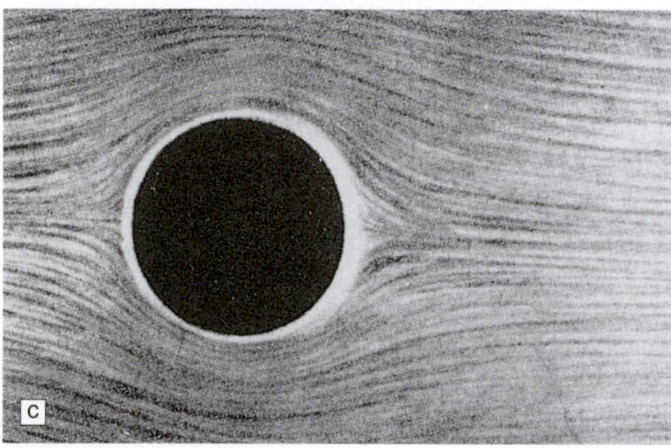


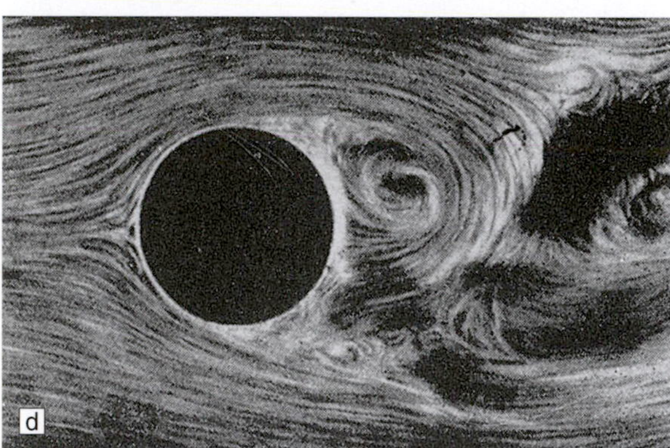


**Figure 37.49** A comparison of (a) laminar and (b) turbulent flow in an open channel, and (c) laminar and (d) turbulent flow around a vertical cylinder. (Adapted from Schlichting H. *Boundary Layer Theory* 6th edn. New York: McGraw-Hill, 1968, pp. 409 and 524.)

Although, in most textbooks the critical Reynolds' number is described as the number over which turbulence will occur, it is more strictly defined as the number below which viscous forces predominate to ensure laminar flow. This is why, under special circumstances, turbulence free flow can be preserved to very high Reynolds' numbers.

Note that a rise in temperature (or pressure) *increases* the viscosity of gases and *decreases* that of liquids (treacle flows with heat).

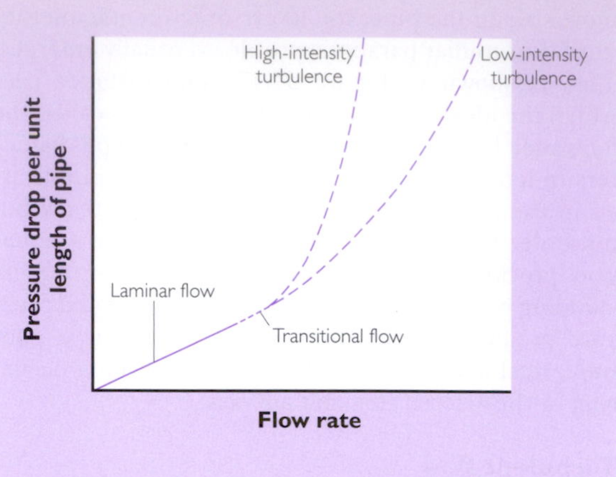


**Figure 37.50** The relationship of pressure drop to flow rate for laminar and turbulent flow. Initially, under laminar flow conditions, the pressure drop is proportional to the flow rate and the gradient is determined by the viscosity of the fluid. When turbulence occurs, the density of the fluid and factors such as pipe roughness become important. The effect of differing intensities of turbulence is shown diagrammatically.

***Anaesthetic implications***

- The best conditions for the rapid transfusion of blood require a short wide-bore cannula and a pressurized blood bag.
- Avoid small endotracheal tubes and sharp bends, e.g. right-angled connectors.
- Dead space in airways is less than predicted (particularly at low tidal volumes) as a result of axial flow.
- Murmurs and bruits in heart and blood vessels are often caused by turbulent flow.
- The turbulent resistance across an airway stenosis (e.g. caused by a tumour) can be alleviated by low-density inspired gases such as helium and oxygen mixtures.

## Bernoulli's principle

Bernoulli's principle is the basis on which aeroplanes stay in the sky. It can be demonstrated by the reader blowing along the surface of a curved sheet of paper, 10 cm wide, held in the hand. The free end of the paper will be seen to *rise*, thus illustrating the zone of low pressure caused by the flow of air on the upper surface of the paper.

> Bernoulli's principle states that the total energy in a steadily flowing fluid stream is a constant along the flow path; thus, an increase in the fluid's velocity must be matched by a decrease in its pressure (potential energy has been exchanged for kinetic energy).

This is another example of the law of conservation of energy. Bernoulli's principle applied to frictionless pipe flow is illustrated in Figure 37.51.

The application of Bernouilli's principle to the flow over an aerofoil, which provides the lift for an aeroplane, is demonstrated diagrammatically in Figure

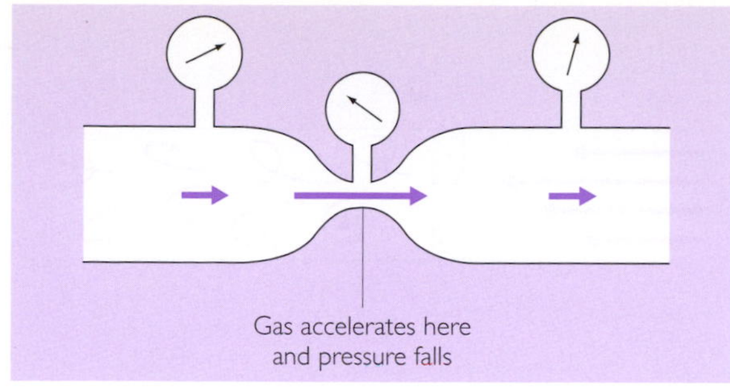


**Figure 37.51** Bernoulli's principle applied to pipe flow.

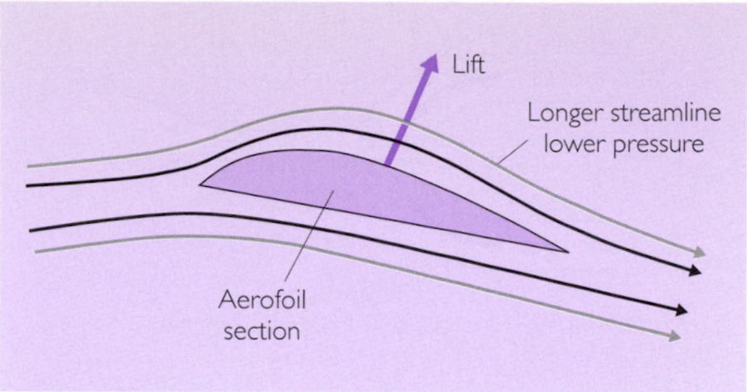

**Figure 37.52** The generation of lift across an aerofoil section.

37.52. The lift is caused by the differential velocities above and below the aircraft wing and depends on the maintenance of proper streamline flow around the aerofoil. Stalling is when the onset of turbulence in the boundary layer immediately adjacent to the wing destroys this differential. An example of the growth of disturbances along a flat plate as the fluid velocity increases, which would cause stalling, is shown in Figure 37.53.

Figure 37.54 shows how a Venturi utilizes Bernoulli's principle to generate significant subatmospheric pressures and entrainment of fluid. The jet of gas emerging from the nozzle expends energy to attain increased velocity with consequent loss of pressure. This low-pressure region entrains air from the side channels, which causes an increase in the net flow, deceleration of the jet, and partial restitution of the pressure. *It is a feature of Venturis that, provided the flow through the jet is adequate (above a preset minimum), and the dimensions of the device do not alter, then the entrainment ratio of driving gas to entrained gas is constant.*

This principle is used in anaesthesia in high-flow oxygen entrainment masks (Figure 37.55). In such a mask the entrainment ratio is determined by the nozzle and the inlet holes for the air. The system produces a fixed concentration so long as the recommended minimum driving flow is set or exceeded. Such masks are shown in physical form in Chapter 6.

Of clinical significance is that a particular Venturi system produces a *fixed* concentration of oxygen over wide limits of flows of the driving oxygen. A 60% Ventimask will produce 60% oxygen whether you use 5 or 15 litres of driving oxygen. The recommended oxygen flow setting ensures that the oxygen plus the entrained air produces *total* gas flow at the patient's face at least equal to the peak inspiratory flow (30 litres), so that the patient does not take in air from the atmosphere. A 60% mask requires 15 litres of oxygen (1 : 1 oxygen : air ratio). A 30% mask requires 4 litres of oxygen (1 : 7 oxygen : air ratio) in order to exceed the 30-litre peak inspiratory flow.

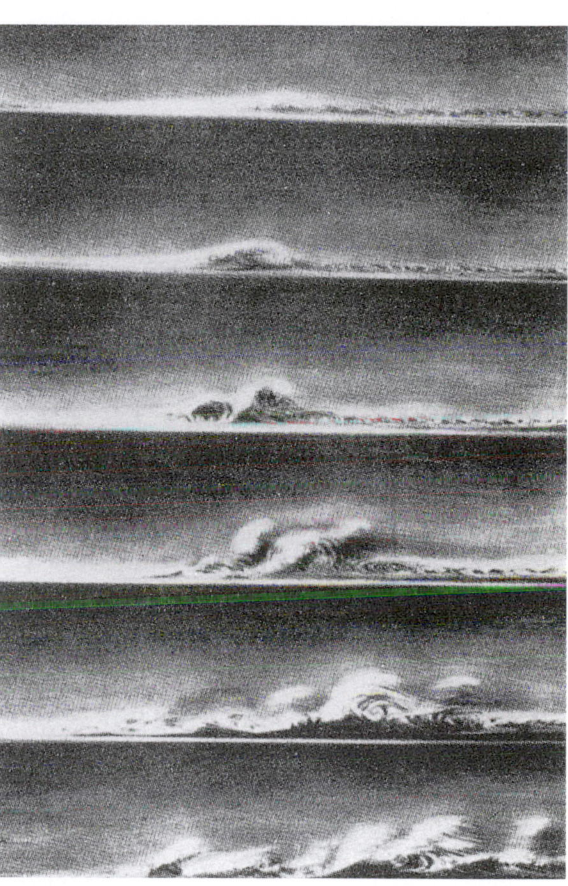

**Figure 37.53** The growth of disturbances along a flat plate as the fluid velocity increases. The velocity is least in the top frame and greatest in the bottom. (Adapted from Schlichting H. *Boundary Layer Theory* 6th edn. New York: McGraw-Hill, 1968, 457.)

### *Practical applications of Venturis in anaesthesia*

- Some portable ventilators use Venturis in the 'airmix' mode to produce given $F_{IO_2}$.
- Some portable and anaesthetics suckers use 4 bar oxygen driving gas to produce a vacuum.
- The reservoir bag of a Bain circuit often collapses if you use a poorly fitting mask. The flow of gas leaving the orifice of the inner tube generates a subatmospheric pressure, which entrains gas from the outer tube. The rapid collapse of the reservoir bag, when the oxygen flush is used, tests and confirms the integrity of the inner tube.
- The Sanders injector: when fired into a rigid bronchoscope, oxygen at 4 bar pressure entrains ambient air and the resulting mixture is used to inflate the lungs. The entrainment ratio decreases as inflation proceeds as a result of back pressure in the bronchoscope (see Chapter 6).

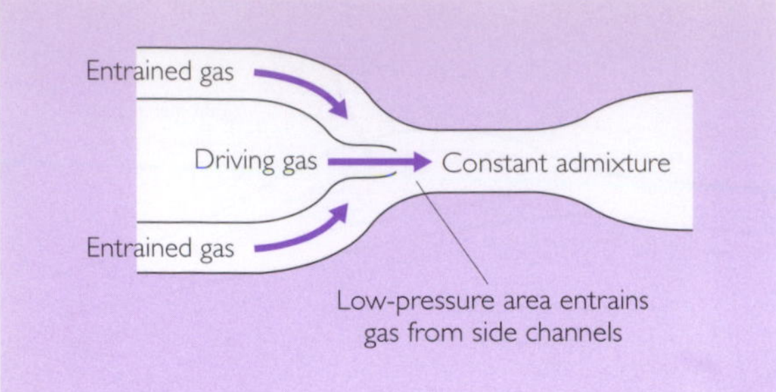


**Figure 37.54** The entrainment of gas by high-pressure driving gas expanding through a nozzle.

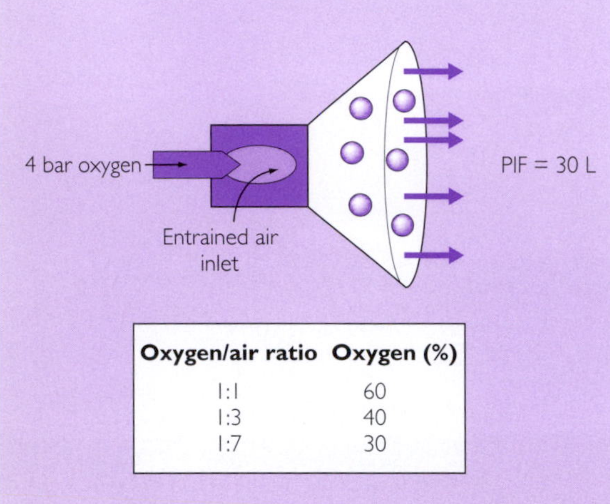


| Oxygen/air ratio | Oxygen (%) |
|---|---|
| 1:1 | 60 |
| 1:3 | 40 |
| 1:7 | 30 |

**Figure 37.55** A diagrammatic representation of a high-airflow entrainment mask. Venturi masks have a fixed entrainment ratio. (PIF, peak inspiratory flow) See text for details.

## Flow of fluids through an orifice

When a laminar fluid flow emerges from an orifice, the disruption of the fluid stream produces turbulent flow as shown diagrammatically in Figure 37.56. Experimentally it is found that:

Flow rate ($F$) $\propto$ √(Difference in pressure across the orifice, [$\Delta P$])
$\propto$ 1√(Density of fluid, ρ)
$\propto$ Area of the orifice ($A$).

Combining these gives the flow rate ($F$) through the orifice as:

$$F \propto \frac{A\sqrt{(\Delta P)}}{\sqrt{\rho}}$$

This relationship has obvious implications for the design of rotameters. Another practical application is the use of helium in upper airway obstruction, where there is an orifice-like opening for the air to pass through. The densities of nitrogen and helium are very different, being 1.2 and 0.16, respectively. This means that if helium is substituted for nitrogen and the inspiratory force is the same, the ratio of inspired flows will be:

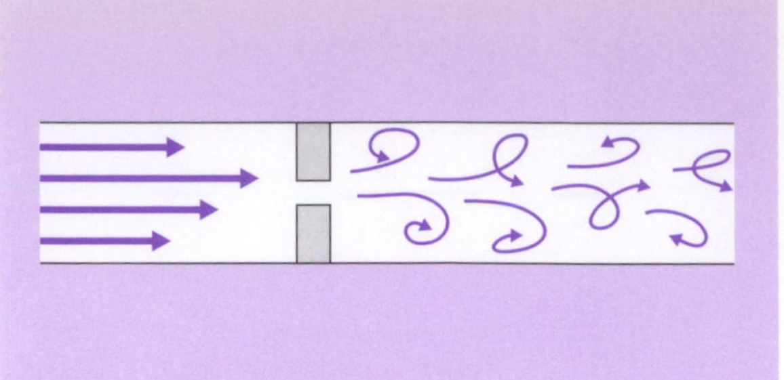

**Figure 37.56** A diagrammatic representation of flow through an orifice.

$$\frac{\sqrt{1.2}}{\sqrt{0.16}} = 2.73.$$

This is the theoretical basis for the use of oxygen/helium mixtures in upper airway obstruction.

## The Coanda effect

When a fast-moving, turbulent airstream emerges from a nozzle, there is a fall in pressure and it entrains surrounding air (Figure 37.57a). If a wall is placed close to the jet (Figure 37.57b), then an area of low pressure develops close to the wall, because little if any air is entrained on this side. The jet is pulled over to the wall, trapping a small separation bubble. Coanda discovered this effect in an unfortunate way in 1910. He used a mica baffle to shield his wooden plane from the jet engine powering it. This served only to channel the exhaust flames on to the fuselage, causing him to crash into a building, surviving to tell the tale. He subsequently investigated the cause of this – thus great discoveries are often made. The Coanda effect applies to fluids whether they are gases or liquids.

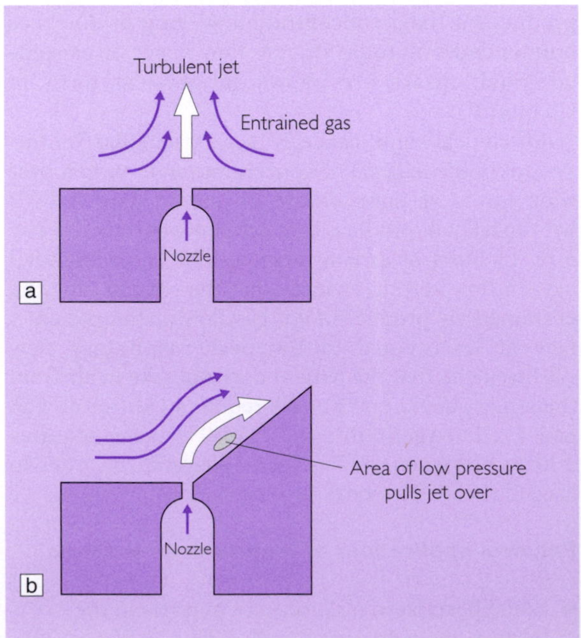


**Figure 37.57** (a) The formation of a turbulent jet and (b) its adherence to the wall.

Figure 37.58a shows a nozzle where the jet of fluid leads into a Y junction. The jet has, as it were, to choose which road to take and, once chosen, continues to stick to one or other of the channels. It does not, however, need much persuading to flip from one channel to the other by a relatively small pneumatic force applied at right angles to the airstream, as shown in Figure 37.58b. This either/or (bistable) circuit is the basis of binary computer function; some fluid logic circuits are built on this principle.

## MEASUREMENT OF VOLUME AND FLOW

### Units

The SI unit of volume is the cubic metre ($m^3$). The volume of fluid passing a point in a unit of time is the flow. The unit of time is the second (s) so the SI unit of flow is cubic metres per second ($m^3/s$). However, in clinical anaesthesia, it is more usual to measure volume in millilitres (ml) or litres (L) and time in minutes (min).

In physiological equations volume is often represented as $V$, and flow rate, the rate of change of volume with time, $dV/dt$, is sometimes represented as $\dot{V}$ or $Q$.

### Measurement of gas flow

#### *Rotameter flowmeters*

The most frequently used device to measure gas flow on an anaesthesia machine is the variable orifice constant pressure device usually referred to by its original trade name of Rotameter (Figure 37.59). The reading is taken at the top of the bobbin.

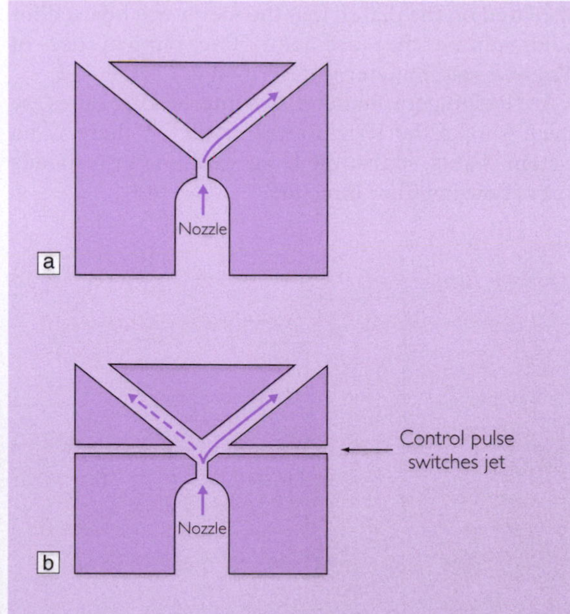


**Figure 37.58** A diagrammatic representation of the ability to switch a jet from one channel to another using a control pulse. Once the jet is going down one of the two exit channels (a) it is perfectly stable but can be sucked across to the other one by negative pressure applied close to the throat (b). See text for details.

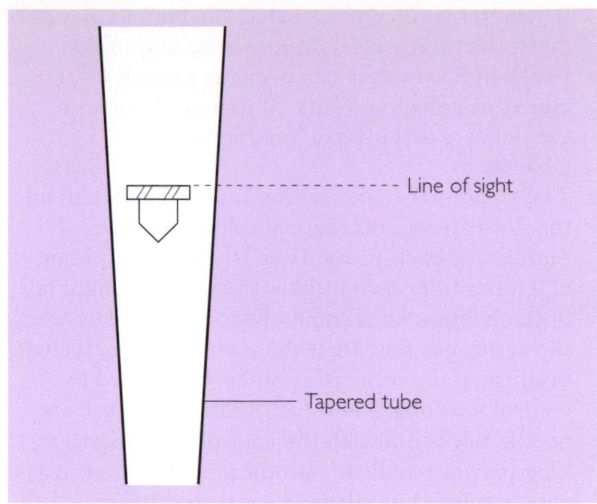


**Figure 37.59** A diagrammatic representation of a rotameter flowmeter.

The flowmeter has a slightly tapered glass tube, wider at the top than the bottom. Gas flows upwards through the tube, supporting a bobbin. Small grooves are cut at an angle in the upper flange of the bobbin so that it rotates in the centre of the gas flow. At low gas flows, the bobbin is at the lower end of the glass tube, and there is only a narrow gap around it. The width of the gap is small compared with the length of the bobbin, so the gas flow is assumed to be largely laminar and dependent on the viscosity of the gas (see 'Pipe flow' for an analogy). At higher gas flows, the bobbin rises into the upper, wider part of the tube, where the gap around it is larger in comparison to its length. It thus corresponds more to an orifice. Flow through an orifice is turbulent and depends on density rather than viscosity. The weight of the bobbin is of course constant; thus, the pressure drop across it that is needed to keep it suspended in one position in the tube is always the same. Hence, the flowmeter is termed a 'variable orifice, constant-pressure device'.

In the flowmeter there is thus both turbulent and laminar flow, with the flow being predominantly laminar at low flows and becoming mainly turbulent at higher flows. This means that each flowmeter is calibrated for one particular gas at one particular temperature at a given downstream pressure. Erroneous readings will ensue if other gases are used. Other sources of error include the following:

- The bobbin can touch the wall of the tube because of tilting, dust particles, or static electricity. The anaesthetist may be alerted to this by the bobbin not spinning. Modern flowmeters are made of conducting glass or incorporate a conducting strip to reduce static changes. The needle valves below the flowmeter, which control the gas flow, incorporate a dust filter.
- In some flowmeters used on wards or for transportation, the bobbin is a simple sphere. Sighting is usually at the middle of the sphere, which is less accurate than the top of a bobbin, though sufficient for most situations. If the

flowmeter is tilted or inverted, the bobbin may roll down the tubing even if there is no flow of gas.

- Leaks in flowmeters can occur as a result of cracks or defective joints. This may also cause the delivery of a hypoxic mixture (see Chapter 8).
- The rotameter scale reading is very dependent on the downstream pressure at calibration. Significant back-pressure caused by the addition of a humidifier or ventilator may cause a slight fall in the bobbin, i.e. a small under-reading. However, the actual gas flow (mass/s) is virtually unaffected because of the properties of the valves used to control flow of gas into the flowmeter. These are needle valves in which the control knob moves a long narrow needle or spindle in and out of the gas supply tube, thus allowing gas flow. The gas velocity around the spindle is very high (sonic), and mass flow (but not recorded volume flow) is relatively unaffected by, for example, the small upstream pressure increase when attaching a humidifier. Scale reading changes caused by downstream pressure and resistance changes may therefore occur in the presence of constant gas delivery.
- At low gas flows, as may be found when using a circle system, accurate setting of gas flow may be difficult. This problem is commonly overcome by using two flowmeters together, one for low flows up to 1 litre, and the other for higher flows (see Chapter 8).
- At high flows, the bobbin at the top of the tube may 'disappear' and be missed by the anaesthetist on cursory inspection of the flowmeter. This is a particular potential hazard where the $N_2O$ is not interconnected with oxygen to prevent hypoxic mixtures, or where a carbon dioxide flowmeter is fitted.

The safety and practical use of rotameter flowmeters is described in Chapter 8, together with methods of avoiding hypoxic gas mixtures.

#### *Pressure-compensated flowmeters*

Where there is a significant and variable downstream resistance to flow, such as caused by the connection of narrow-bore oxygen tubing, pressure-compensated bobbin flowmeters are used. These are of the type invariably found in recovery rooms, on the wards, or connected to oxygen cylinders. The needle valve is on the outlet of the flowmeter and not at the inlet, as in rotameters. The changes in downstream resistance do not affect the reading, because they are negligible compared with the resistance across the controlling needle valve. Such flowmeters are calibrated at a pressure of 400 kPa. A practical problem in having the needle valve downstream of the bobbin is that, should the plastic housing be broken, then an unrestricted issue of gas at 4 bar will result! An alternative system for delivering stepped increases of up to three or more known flows of gas is increasingly used in oxygen therapy equipment. The output from the regulator is connected to one of a number of fixed diameter orifices, each calibrated to give flows of sufficient accuracy for their purpose.

#### *Other types of inspired gas flowmeters*

Another type of flowmeter is the Coxeter, shown in Figure 37.60. This flowmeter has parallel sides, the gas pushing the bobbin up the tubing and escaping through small holes in the walls of the tube. The gas rises until there are sufficient holes exposed for it to escape. The precision of flow measurement depends on the number of holes, a large number of small holes giving more precise measurements than the coarser measurement obtained with a smaller number of large holes. This type of flowmeter is now largely of historical interest for anaesthesia machines, but may occasionally still be seen in other situations.

The bubble flowmeter has a tube of a design not unlike the Coxeter flowmeter. The gas flow to be measured passes down a tube immersed in water, escapes through holes in the side, and bubbles up through the water. As gas flow increases, the level of water in the tube is pushed down, allowing more holes for the gas to escape.

Whereas flowmeters measure constant flow, the flow produced by patients and ventilators is continually changing. Different types of instrument are therefore required for use within the patient circuit or for investigation of patients on the ward.

### Rotor meters

In these meters the flowing gas turns a rotor or vane which is usually connected to a dial by mechanical connection through a geared system or is sensed electrically (Figure 37.61).

In a Wright's respirometer, a single vane is caused to rotate in one direction only by a flow of gas directed by angled silts. Gas flow in the reverse direction causes no rotation. The speed of rotation of the vane is determined by the velocity of the gases passing through the meter. This is related to volume, which is displayed on the dial so that the meter can be used for tidal volume measurement. The clinical use of Wright's respirometer is described in Chapter 12.

In the Drager volumeter, two interlocking vanes are used. Unlike the Wright's respirometer, there is no system of slits, so that the Drager volumeter responds to gas flow in either direction.

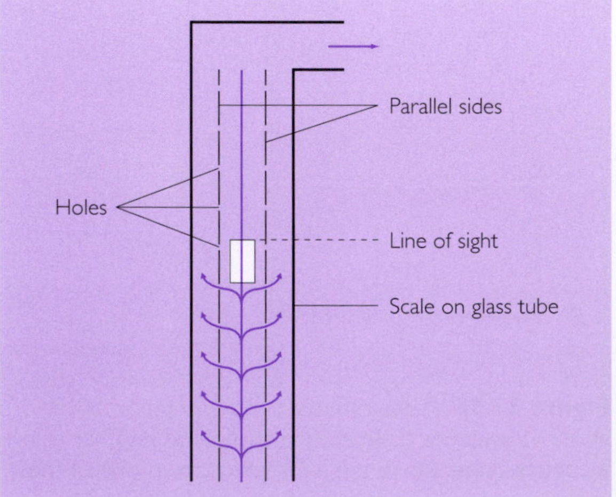


**Figure 37.60** A diagrammatic representation of a Coxeter flowmeter.

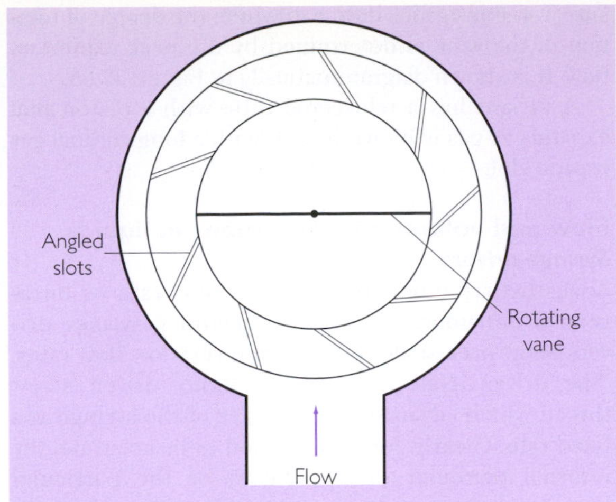


**Figure 37.61** A diagrammatic representation of a vane-driven rotor meter similar in mechanism to the Wright's respirometer.

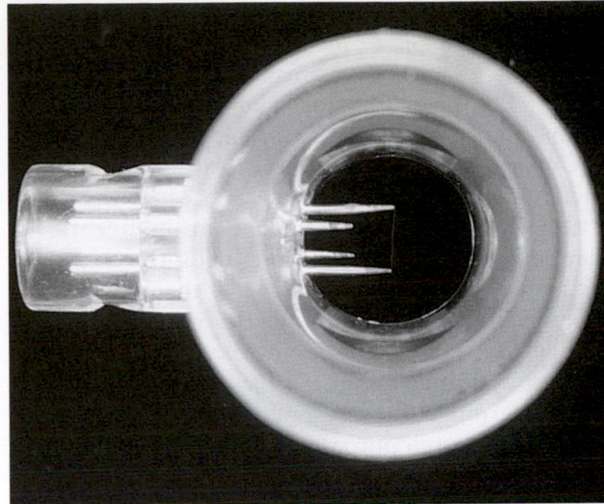

**Figure 37.62** An example of a hot wire anemometer used to measure the expiratory flow in a ventilator.

Problems and disadvantages of rotor meters include:

- Inertia and friction: this produces falsely low readings at low flows. To reduce these errors the vanes are mounted on low-friction jewelled bearings (which are not indestructible should the meter be dropped!). A low-flow version of Wright's respirometer, designed for paediatric work, is available.
- Collection of moisture and other foreign material: this leads to falsely low readings.
- Overshoot: at the end of a period of high flow, the vane continues to rotate for a short time after flow has stopped, giving falsely high readings.
- This type of meter is calibrated to be used for short periods for tidal volume measurements. They are inaccurate if used for long periods, for example for continuous measurement on the intensive care unit (ICU).
- Mechanically geared devices do not give an electrical output for recording. Electronic flowmeters are available for this purpose in which a photoelectric cell detects interruptions to a beam of light by the spinning vane. Such a meter is shown in Chapter 12.

### Heated wire sensors

A heated wire is placed in the flow of gas. As the gas is cooler than the wire, the wire will be cooled, which reduces its electrical resistance. The change in resistance is calibrated against flow. These devices are in increasingly common use, both on anaesthetic circuits and in ICUs where they are suitable for continuous use. Inaccuracy may arise if the wire becomes coated with foreign material and because calibration of the wires is non-linear. The temperature decrease depends on the thermal conductivity of the gas being measured, which may become a source of inaccuracy in a few circumstances, for example with helium. An example of a hot wire anemometer is given in Figure 37.62.

### Pneumotachographs

In anaesthesia, pneumotachographs are used mainly for research purposes where a continuous recording of the patient's airflow is required. By electronic integration, pneumotachographs can indicate volumes as well as flows. Clinically they are found in some ICU ventilators.

They are based on differential pressure measurements when the flow is restricted or made laminar by a long narrow tube or driven through an orifice. Two types are shown diagrammatically in Figure 37.63: the greater the flow rate, the greater the pressure drop between $P_1$ and $P_2$. A satisfactory device for clinical use has a linear relationship between the pressure drop and the flow.

In pneumotachographs, the actual resistance to flow is designed to be low and the effect on the actual flow rate is usually negligible for practical purposes. It

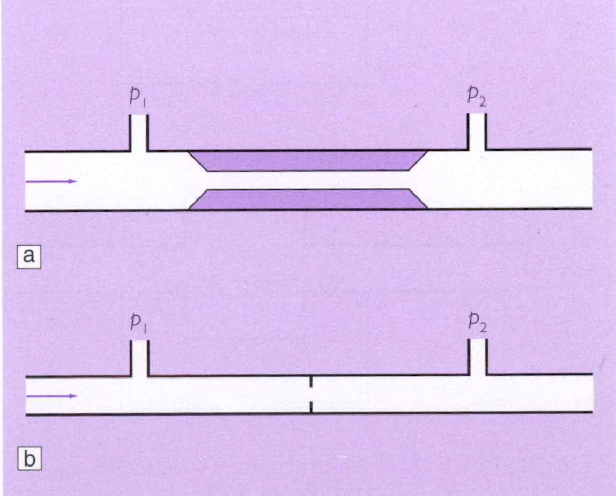


**Figure 37.63** The principle of flow measurement in a pneumotachograph. (a) The concept of a long thin tube to linearize the flow; (b) the concept of an orificial flowmeter. The difference between $p_1$ (the upstream pressure) and $p_2$ (the downstream pressure) is used to measure flow rate.

is usually either a gauze screen as in, for example, the Seimens Servo or, as in the Fleisch pneumotachograph, a large number of small parallel tubes (Figure 37.64). The pressure drop across the resistance is normally measured by an electronic transducer.

Outside the calibration range, the response of pneumotachographs is non-linear because the properties of the gas flow change at higher flows. Electronic circuitry can compensate for this and make the response linear, but this will be the case only for one specific gas mixture. If the gas composition changes (for example, changing $F_{IO_2}$ from 0.35 to 1 at the end of a procedure), the flow measurement may become erroneous by several percent, a significant factor for research purposes.

As would be expected, pneumotachographs become seriously impaired if they become contaminated with secretions or condensed water. Heating the gauze screen or tubes reduces the latter problem.

### Peak flow measurement

This can be done using a Wright peak flowmeter, a convenient and hence frequently used hand-held device, which is available in two forms. In its original form the patient blows into the instrument, causing a vane to rotate against the resistance of a spring. The vane is connected to a pointer on the instrument dial, and a ratchet brake mechanism allows the vane and pointer to move forwards, but not to fall back. As the vane moves around the inside of the instrument, a slot of gradually increasing width is revealed, allowing the gas to escape. As the resistance to the movement of the vane by the spring is constant, but the size of the slot for the gas to escape is variable, the meter is in effect a constant-pressure, variable-orifice device in which the degree of rotation of the vane is determined by the peak expiratory flow. It is shown diagrammatically in Figure 37.65.

A variant has a telescopic tube with a piston that expands as gas is blown into it, with a longitudinal gas escape slot.

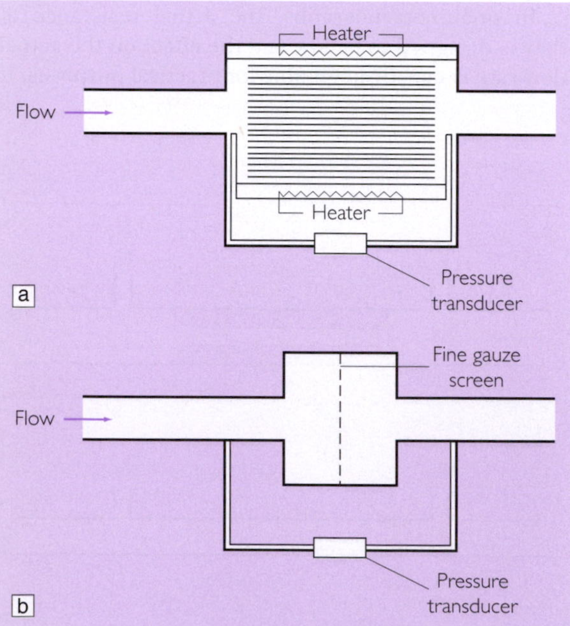


**Figure 37.64** A diagram of practical flowmeters based on the principle shown in Figure 37.63. (a) A Fleisch pneumotachograph that linearizes the flow with a series of small parallel-sided tubes ; (b) a Siemens (gauze) pneumotachograph that measures the pressure drop across a fine gauze screen acting as multiple orifices.

### Flow and volume measurement in liquids

#### *Syringe drivers*

Anaesthetists often measure the flow rate of intravenous infusions. For greatest accuracy, syringe drivers allow precise delivery of even very low flow rates. The driver itself is usually a motor-driven screw thread which advances the plunger of the syringe at a fixed rate. Clearly, for this method to be accurate, the internal diameter of the barrel of the particular syringe in use must be known to the syringe driver. It is usual for some sort of over-pressure alarm to be incorporated, otherwise large volumes of fluid may be forced through an extravasated cannula. The advantage of syringe drivers is that they are independent of the characteristics of the fluid being delivered. Microprocessor-controlled syringe pumps are used for relatively simple operations, such as patient-controlled analgesia, and for more complex uses, such as target-controlled infusion systems (see Chapter 32).

#### *Drop counters*

A beam of light is passed through the drip chamber of an intravenous giving set, and is interrupted by the drops of fluid. A photodetector on the other side of the chamber is used to count the number of drops (usually about 20/ml). If an assumption is made about the volume of each drop, this can be used to calculate flow and control the infusion. However, variations in surface tension between different liquids and within the same liquid at different temperatures make this an unreliable method if precise control is needed. Other intravenous infusion controllers use giving sets incorporating a cassette, which is loaded into a motorized infusion pump; this gives greater accuracy and removes the problems caused by varying surface tensions mentioned above.

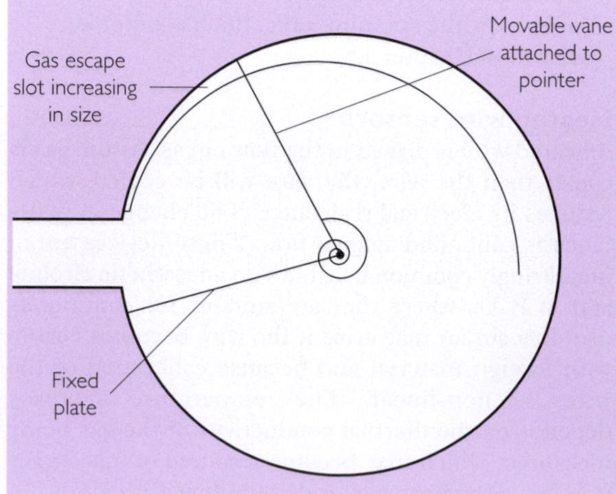


**Figure 37.65** The principle of a Wright's peak flowmeter.

## Measurement of blood flow

### *Cardiac output by dye or thermal dilution*

This has been described earlier and is shown in Figure 37.23.

### *Ultrasonic (Doppler) flowmeters*

Ultrasonography is sound outside the range of normal hearing (over 20 kHz) and the ultrasonography used medically is of frequencies up to 100 times higher than this. Ultrasonography is used both for imaging of body structures and for measuring flow. When used for imaging, use is made of the fact that ultrasound will pass through body tissue until it meets an interface between structures of different density. Some of the sound will be reflected back whereas some will be refracted forwards. This principle, used in echocardiography, is shown in Figure 37.66. The proportions of sound reflected and refracted depend on the angle of incidence of the sound, and the difference in density of the two materials at the interface.

When used as a flowmeter, ultrasound is directed towards a blood vessel from a probe held against the skin, and acoustically coupled to it by gel. Sound that strikes moving red blood cells will be reflected back at a higher frequency than that which is reflected from stationary tissue (Figure 37.67). The faster the red blood cells are moving towards the probe, the greater the frequency rise, the greater the flow velocity. Velocity readings can be accurately converted into flow measurements only when the cross-sectional area of the pipe is known, the velocity profile is square, and the angle of incidence is known. Doppler probes have one crystal, which acts as both a transmitter of pulsed sounds and their receiver, or use separate transmitter and receiving crystals continuously.

A simple Doppler probe will give information about flow velocity. Pulsed Dopplers may be used to assess vessel diameter as well as flow velocity. In this case, flow may then be calculated. Some machines display different flow rates and directions in different colours. By positioning the probe in the suprasternal notch, and looking at blood flow in the aortic arch, non-invasive estimations of cardiac output may be made, although accuracy depends on correctly assessing aortic root diameter and the assumptions made about the velocity profile.

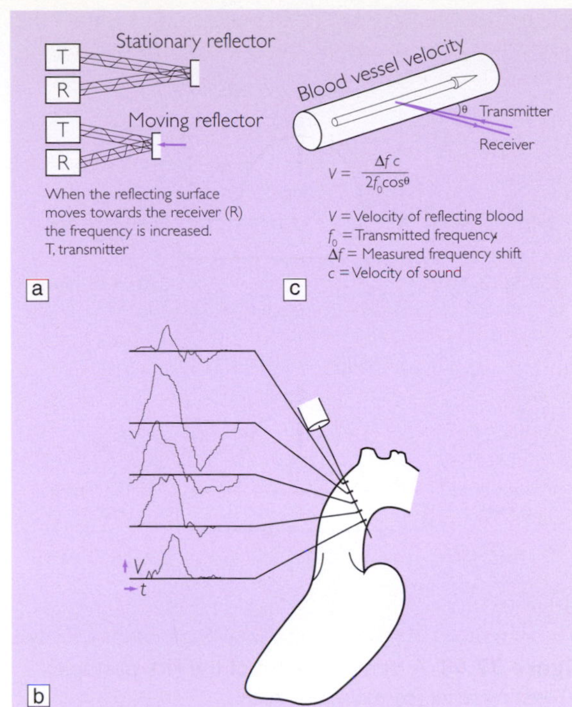


**Figure 37.67** The principle of Doppler flow measurement. (a) The generation of a Doppler shift by a moving surface; (b) the application of this principle to velocity measurements; (c) the dependence of the velocity measurements with time at various points on the aortic cross-section. This clearly shows the inaccuracies that would result in multiplying a single signal by the cross-sectional area to obtain flow. (See Chapter 12 and Hutton P and Prys-Roberts C, eds. *Monitoring in Anaesthesia and Intensive Care*. London: Saunders, 1994: 180.)

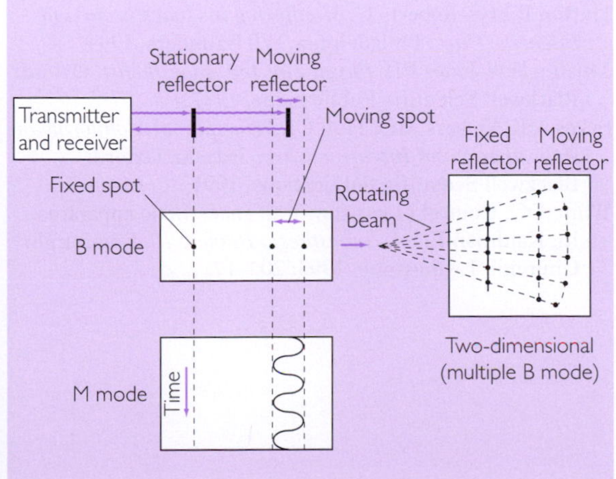


**Figure 37.66** A diagrammatic representation of echocardiography. (Adapted from Durkin M. Echocardiography. In: Hutton P and Prys-Roberts C, eds. *Monitoring in Anaesthesia and Intensive Care*. London: Saunders, 1994: 91.)

Transoesophageal imaging ultrasonography may have a future in intraoperative monitoring for ischaemia, because abnormal ventricular wall movement may be detectable before ST changes on the ECG become apparent. As the density difference between blood and air is large, bubbles in the blood give an intense reflection. Because of this, ultrasonography is the 'gold standard' for detection of an air embolism.

### *The Fick principle*

This is included for its historical importance and basic methodology. It is an uptake method which is demonstrated in Figure 37.68.

Figure 37.68a shows the normal or resting situation. The uptake of oxygen per litre of blood is 50 ml. As 250 ml of oxygen is taken up per minute, the flow through the lungs (i.e. the cardiac output) is

$$250 \frac{\text{mlO}_2}{\text{min}} \div \frac{50\ \text{mlO}_2}{\text{litres}} = 5\ \text{L/min}$$

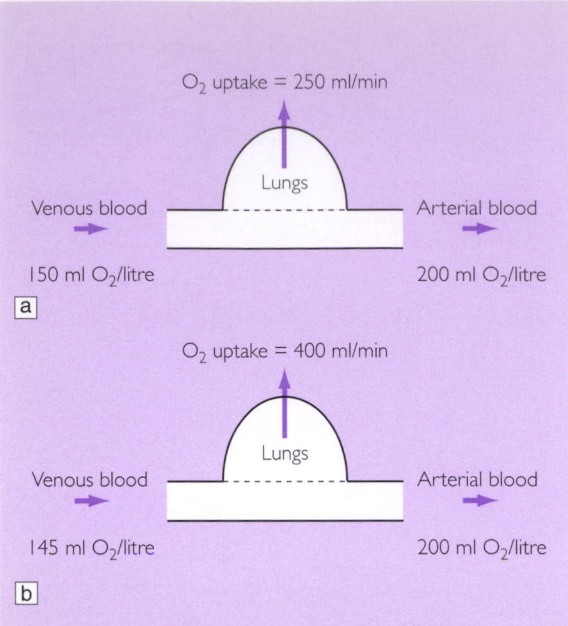


**Figure 37.68** A demonstration of the Fick principle: (a) resting man; (b) exercising man.

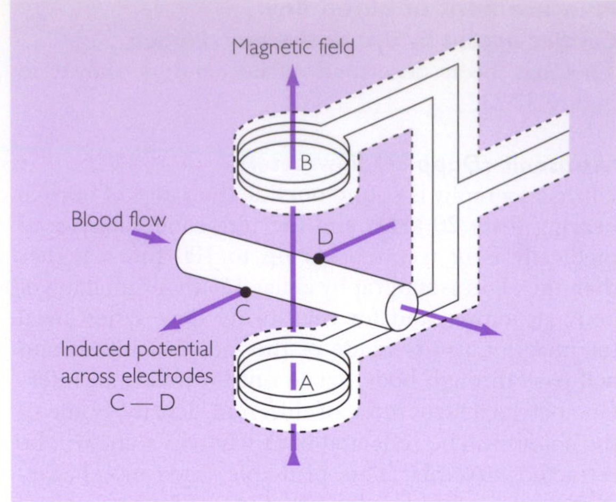


**Figure 37.69** The principle of the electromagnetic flowmeter.

Figure 37.68b shows the situation during exercise. Blood returns with more oxygen extracted from it and the oxygen uptake has risen to 400 ml/mm. By analogous calculations to the above, the flow through the lung is $400 \div (200 - 145) = 7.3$ L/min.

In summary, therefore, the Fick principle involves the measurement of the uptake of the substance and its input and output concentrations. It can be applied to the measurement of cardiac output, brain–blood flow, and the measurement of blood flow through individual organs. The marker or tracer substance used in the calculations can be a physiological compound (as illustrated), a chemical compound, a dye, or radioactivity.

### *Electromagnetic flowmeters*

These utilize electromagnetic induction as first described by Faraday. A conductor (blood in this case) moves through a magnetic field (the north and south pole of a magnet, on either side of the blood vessel [A and B]). An electrical current is generated at right angles to both the blood flow and the magnetic field. Electrodes on opposite sides of the vessel (C and D) measure the induced potential, as shown in Figure 37.69. Given that the magnetic field is constant, this potential is proportional to the average velocity. This method can be used experimentally, where vessels can be exposed or in certain limited clinical situations, but is not in widespread use. In practice, an alternating rather than a steady magnetic field is used and the alternating component of the potential is measured. This improves the stability of the measured value.

## FURTHER READING


Al-Shaikh B, Stacey S. *Essentials of Anaesthetic Equipment*. Edinburgh: Churchill Livingstone, 1995.

Cruickshank S. *Mathematics and Statistics in Anaesthesia*. Oxford: Oxford University Press, 1998.

Davis PD, Parbrook GD, Kenny GNC. *Basic Physics and Measurement in Anaesthesia*, 4th edn. Oxford: Butterworth-Heinemann, 1995.

Davey A, Moyle JTB, Ward CS. *Anaesthetic Equipment*, 3rd edn. Philadelphia: WB Saunders, 1994.

Dorsch JA, Dorsch SE. *Understanding Anaesthesia Equipment*, 3rd edn. Baltimore, MA: Williams & Wilkins, 1994.

Gardner MC, Adams AP. Anaesthetic vaporizers: design and function. *Curr Anaesth Crit Care* 1996;**7**:315–21.

Geddes LA. *Handbook of Blood Pressure Measurement*. Clifton NJ: Humana Press, 1991.

Hutton P, Prys-Roberts C. *Monitoring in Anaesthesia and Intensive Care*. Philadelphia: WB Saunders, 1994.

Mushin WW, Jones PL. *Physics for the Anaesthetist*. Oxford: Blackwell Scientific Publications, 1987.

Sykes MK, Vickers MD, Hull CJ. *Principles of Monitoring in Anaesthesia and Intensive Care*, 3rd edn. Oxford: Blackwell Scientific Publications, 1991.

White DC. Control of gas flow into anaesthetic apparatus. In: Kaufman L, ed. *Anaesthesia Review 10*. Edinburgh: Churchill Livingstone, 1993: 203–17.

# Chapter 38 Principles of physics and clinical measurement II: heat, humidity, colligative properties, and electricity

C.J. Vallis, D. Cochrane, K. Burchett, and P. Hutton

## HEAT TRANSFER AND TEMPERATURE MEASUREMENT

### Heat transfer

The anaesthetist has a vital role in the maintenance of a patient's body temperature and the manipulation of thermal balance. Some knowledge of the physics of heat transfer is therefore obligatory.

Temperature measures the average level of the kinetic energy of the molecules of a substance (see Chapter 37), whereas heat content relates to the total amount of energy. Thus an iceberg will contain much more heat energy than a litre of boiling water, although their temperatures are quite different.

Heat flows from high levels of thermal potential (high temperature) to low levels of thermal potential (low temperature). Newton's law of cooling, an example of this principle, describes the flow of heat from a hot body as follows.

> The rate of heat loss from a body to its surroundings is proportional to its excess temperature over the surroundings.

This transfer of heat is analogous to high and low electrical potentials being required for the transfer of electric current, which is independent of the quantity of charge at each electrode. A small battery connected to a large battery will discharge into it if the former is at a higher voltage.

Heat is transferred from one body to another by conduction, convection, or radiation and may also be lost by the process of evaporation:

- conduction: no movement of medium;
- convection: requires movement of fluid medium;
- radiation: needs no intervening medium;
- evaporation: requires change in state from liquid to gas.

### Conduction

Heat is transmitted by conduction when it passes, by molecular transfer, down a temperature gradient, from the hotter to the colder parts of a substance. The image of a poker, red hot at one end and the other end held by the hand, instantly conveys this concept. In metals and other good conductors of heat, the energy transfer is effected by free electrons, whereas in insulating materials it is transmitted by molecular vibrations. The ability to transfer heat is known as the *thermal conductivity*. It relates the amount of heat energy, in joules, that will pass down a conductor per unit temperature gradient.

The principle of conduction is shown in Figure 38.1 which also gives the definition of thermal conductivity ($k$). When two 'real' conductors are brought together there is, at intermolecular level, imperfect matching of the two surfaces. This leads to a reduction in conductivity at the interface, known as 'contact

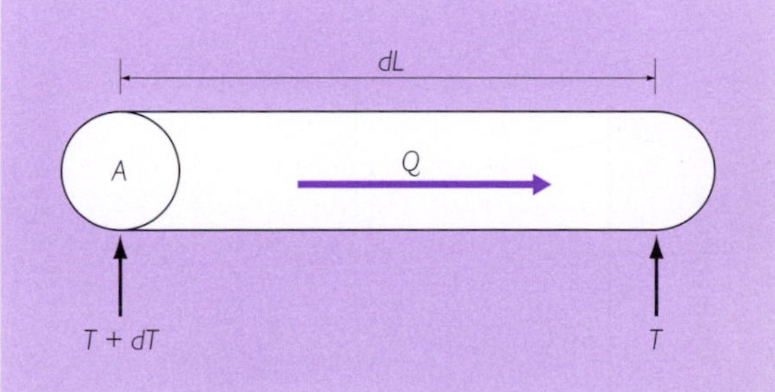


**Figure 38.1** The process of conduction. Heat flows down a temperature gradient and the rate of transfer of energy, $Q$, is determined by the equation $Q = kA(dT/dL)$, where $k$ is the thermal conductivity, $A$ the cross-sectional area, $T$ the temperature and $L$ the length. The thermal conductivity is high for good conductors of electricity and low for insulators.

resistance' (Figure 38.2). This is very important in practice when surface heating and cooling are being used.

## Convection

Convection is the process of heat transfer that occurs when fluids (gases or liquids) are heated in one place, flow to another, and then transfer their heat to a second cooler surface. The actual process of heating the fluid at the fluid/solid interface is by conduction. Convection cannot take place in solids.

### *Natural convection*

Natural convection depends on gravity. When the fluid particles immediately adjacent to the hot surface have been heated, they expand, their density falls, and buoyancy effects cause them to move away. They are replaced by more of the original cooler fluid and the process repeats itself. This process of buoyancy, being responsible for movement of fluid, is termed 'natural convection'. It is dependent on the orientation of the hot surfaces to the vertical. An example is the heating of water in a kettle on a hot ring. The kettle base is heated by conduction but the heat is transferred through the water by natural convection. Another example is the transfer of heat to room air by the misnamed central heating radiator. This process is shown diagrammatically in Figure 38.3.

### *Forced convection*

Forced convection requires forced movement of fluid. It occurs when heated fluid particles immediately adjacent to the hot surface are blown or driven away and do not depend on buoyancy changes for movement. This is far more efficient than natural convection. Turbulent flow, which presents a constantly changing supply of cold fluid because of its transverse velocities and eddies (see Chapter 37), is more efficient than laminar flow in extracting heat from a surface. The effects of forced convection are seen with

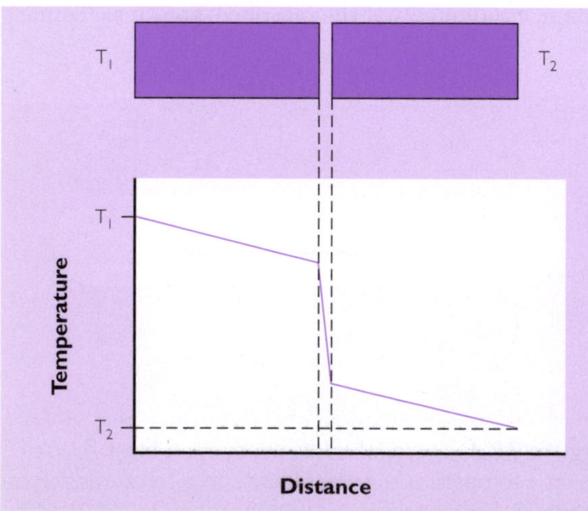


**Figure 38.2** The effect of contact resistance on the temperature gradient. The temperature falls steadily along each of the two metal bars as shown, but where they are in contact there is a sudden fall in temperature. This is caused by imperfect matching of the adjoining surfaces at the molecular level.

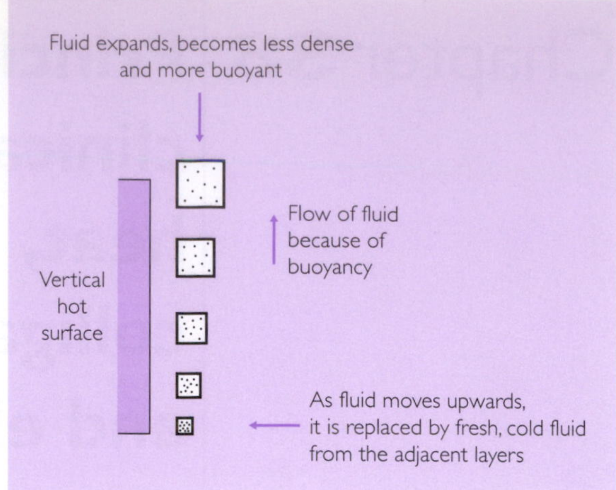


**Figure 38.3** The process of natural convection. This is illustrated here by considering the fluid motion adjacent to a vertical hot surface.

draughts in the operating room and the chill factor in exposure incidents. The difference in efficiency between forced and natural convection is illustrated by the car radiator. While the car is moving at speed, the turbulent airflow across the radiator cools the circulating water. When the car is stationary, with the engine running, the thermostatically controlled fan will cut in to continue the forced convection, because the alternative natural convection will be insufficient to keep the water cool. The transfer of heat around the body by the heart or cardiac bypass pump is another example of forced convection. The same effect in reverse produces the 'chill factor' from cold winds.

## Radiation

During radiation, heat is transmitted by electromagnetic radiation and there is no contact between the emitter and the absorber. *Radiation from a body depends only on its absolute temperature*. Radiation will pass through a vacuum but it is absorbed by gases, liquids, and solids. The principle is illustrated in Figure 38.4.

The most efficient absorber possible is one that absorbs all the electromagnetic radiation that falls on it and is given the name *black body*. Bodies that are good absorbers are also good emitters of radiation. Human skin is an almost perfect black body in thermodynamic terms.

> Boltzmann's law states that the total emissive power of a body is proportional to the fourth power of the absolute temperature, the constant of proportionality being the Stefan-Boltzmann's constant.

The transfer of heat by radiation obviously depends on whether the relevant surfaces can 'see' each other and the angle that they make with each other, because electromagnetic radiation travels in straight lines. The heat transfer from a hot body in a totally closed environment, the simplest situation, is shown in Figure 38.5. A curled up baby will radiate much less than one spread out because the surface area is proportionally reduced.

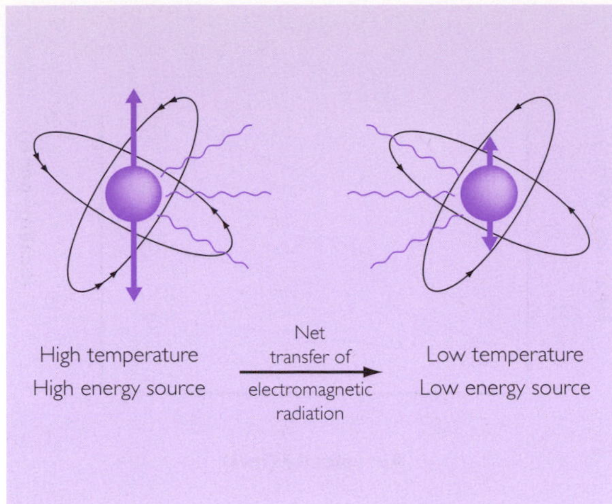


**Figure 38.4** The concept of heat transfer by radiation.

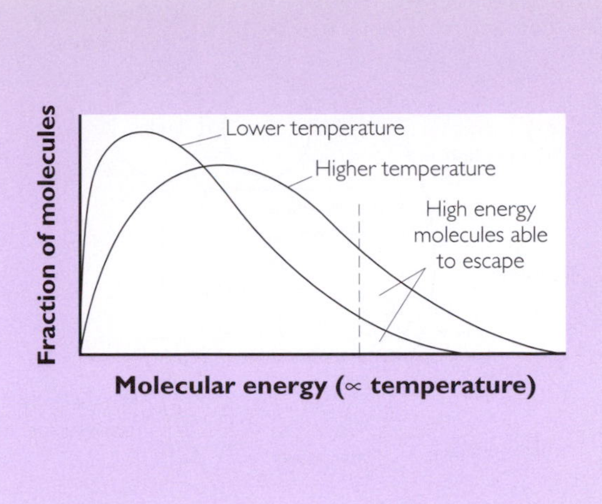


**Figure 38.6** The process of evaporation. When high-energy molecules are lost, the average energy (and hence the temperature) of the remaining liquid falls.

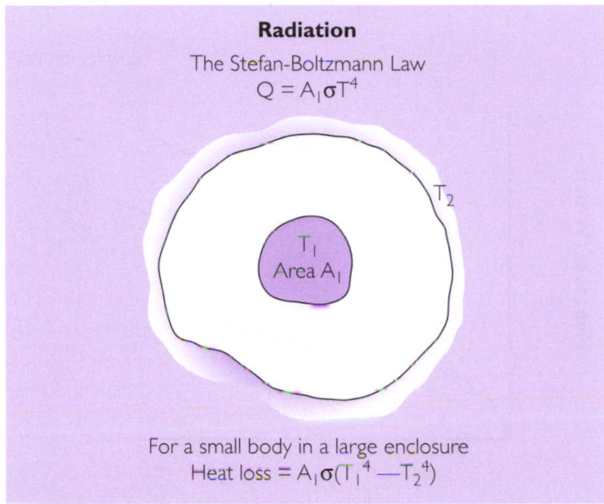


**Figure 38.5** Heat transfer from a hot body in a totally closed environment. $\sigma$ is the Stefan-Boltzmann constant.

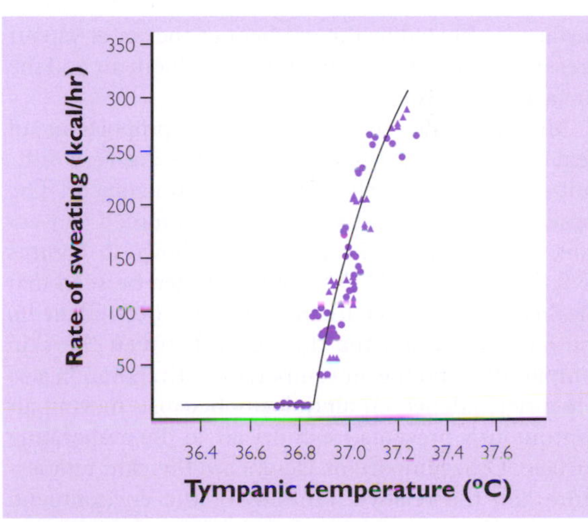


**Figure 38.7** The production of sweat and its relationship to the tympanic temperature. (Adapted from Benzinger TH. *Phys Rev* 1969;671.)

### Evaporation

Evaporation and vapour pressure have been considered in Chapter 37 in relationship to kinetic theory. The principle is shown again diagrammatically in Figure 38.6, where the high-energy molecules leave the liquid and the remaining liquid cools down. The importance of surface evaporation is that it can be turned on and off by the secretion of sweat. This is the main active way of adjusting the body's heat loss and is used to keep the core temperature constant. As shown in Figure 38.7, the rate of sweat production is exquisitely sensitive to body temperature. Sweating is 'turned on' at a tympanic temperature of just over 38.6°C. Sweating can increase the heat loss tenfold as a result of increasing the amount of moisture available for evaporation at the skin.

### Heat loss from the body

Heat loss occurs by all of the four mechanisms described above. Forced convection brings warm blood to the surface; the heat is conducted through the skin to the surroundings. The surrounding air is then replaced by colder air as a result of convection currents, i.e. draughts. Heat is lost or gained by radiation depending on whether the skin's temperature is higher or lower than that of the surroundings. The humidification and heating of respiratory gases and evaporation of water from the skin are also significant sources of heat loss. These principles are summarized in Figure 38.8.

The exact proportion of heat loss attributable to each modality depends on the circumstances. Respiratory losses can increase substantially in cold weather, because not only is the air colder, but it also contains less water vapour, so that in addition to having to heat the air there is increased loss from evaporation in producing fully saturated gases at 37°C. This is one of the disadvantages of inhaling completely dry anaesthetic gases. Each litre of dry inspired air at 20°C requires 64 joules to raise its temperature to 37°C and fully saturate it with water vapour. During surgery, the heat lost by evaporation from the body

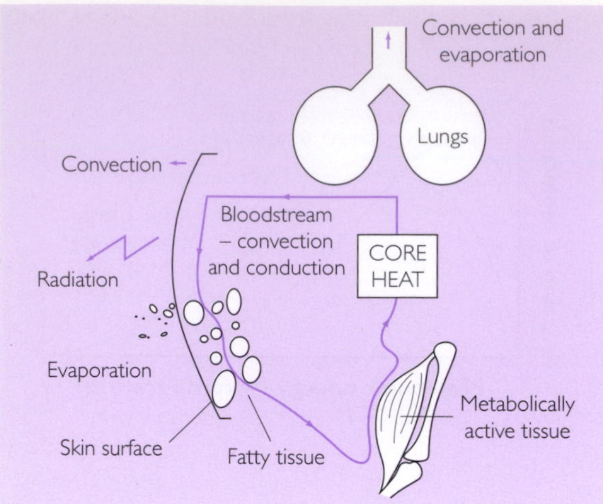


**Figure 38.8** Sources of heat loss and gain. (Adapted from Holdcroft A. *Body Temperature Control*. London: Baillière Tindall, 1980: 4.)

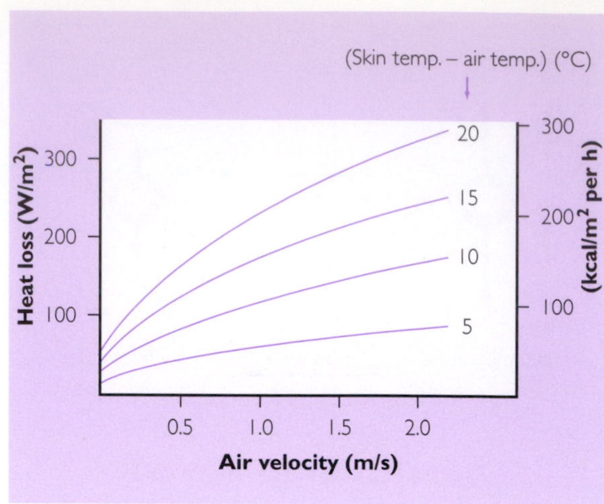


**Figure 38.9** Heat losses from forced convection. (Derived from the work of Colin J and Houdas Y. J *Appl Physiol* 1967;22:31.)

surface is affected by the gradient of the water vapour pressure between the skin and the ambient air and the surface area of moist skin exposed.

Measurements to determine the proportions of heat loss resulting from each modality are very difficult except in very well controlled circumstances. The losses in watts per square metre from forced convection, evaporation, and radiation are shown in Figures 38.9, 38.10, and 38.11 respectively. It can be seen that the losses from forced convection are dependent on the air velocity and the difference between the skin temperature and the air temperature. Evaporation also has a dependence on air velocity because moving air continuously presents fresh dry air to the evaporating surface. Other important factors are the skin temperature and the relative humidity of the environment. Radiation losses are dependent solely on the temperature of the skin and the enclosure wall.

The proportionate heat losses from a supine man in a total body calorimeter (where there is no forced convection) as the temperature of the calorimeter is changed are shown in Figure 38.12. These experiments were done over 60 years ago and have never been repeated. Note how much each component can change, depending on the environmental temperature. In everyday practice, the effect of forced convection from draughts (omitted from Figure 38.12) can be substantial. During surgery, a great deal of heat loss can be reduced by covering the patient with a waterproof surface which protects from draughts and prevents evaporation to the atmosphere. This is shown diagrammatically in Figure 38.13.

A *neutral environment* is one in which the patient loses heat at the rate that it is produced by metabolism and received from other sources. It is of greatest relevance to pre-term babies and neonates who have poorly developed homoeostatic mechanisms. The optimum environmental temperature to keep the body temperature constant changes daily as their metabolism and physiology develop. A comparison of pre-term and full-term babies is shown in Figure 38.14.

Heat output is often represented by the symbol $Q$. In an adult the basal output of heat, generated mainly

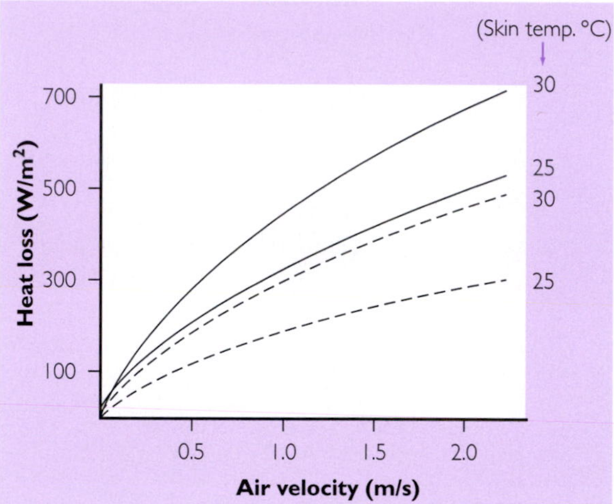


**Figure 38.10** Evaporative heat losses from surface water (– dry air; - - - 50% relative humidity; constant ambient temperature of 22°C). (Derived from Clifford J, Kerslake D, Waddell JL. *J Physiol* 1959;147:253.)

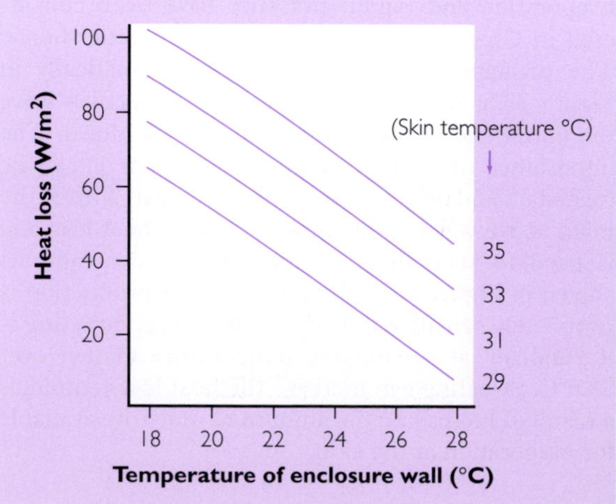


**Figure 38.11** Human heat loss by radiation. (Calculated assuming the human to be a perfect black body.)

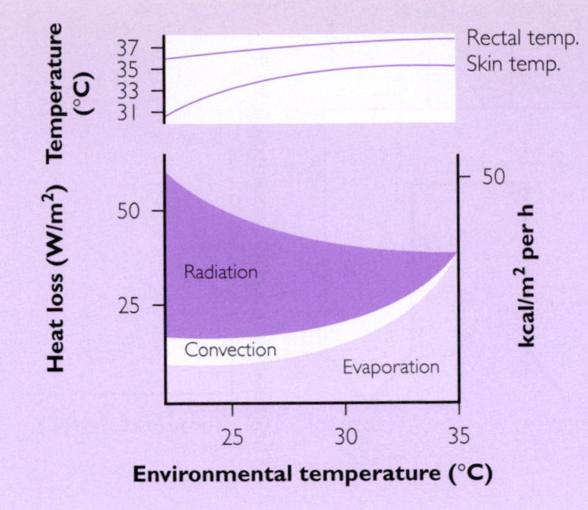


**Figure 38.12** Heat loss from a man in a calorimeter. (Derived from the work of Hardy JD and Dubois EF. *J Nutr* 1938;15:477.)

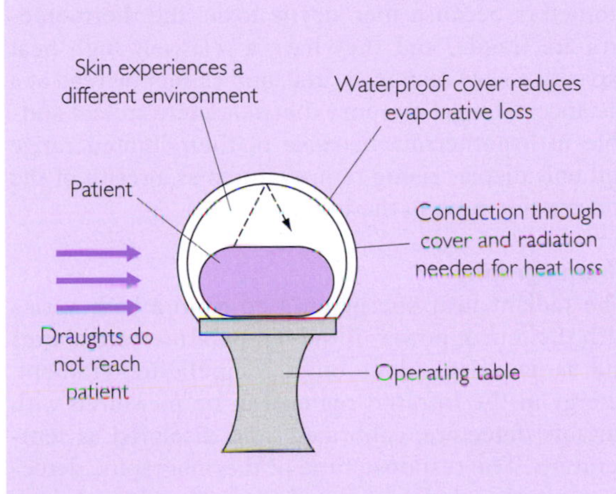


**Figure 38.13** Covering a patient with a waterproof surface reduces heat loss.

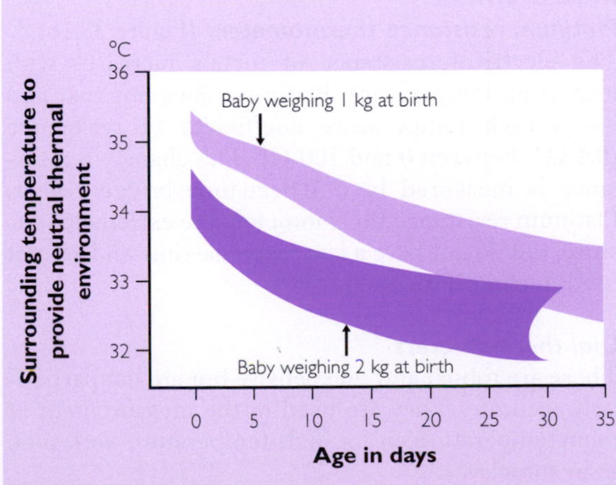


**Figure 38.14** The neutral environment required for pre-term and full-term babies. (Adapted from Hey EN and Katz G. *Arch Dis Child* 1970;45:328.)

from skeletal muscle and hepatic metabolism, is about 80 W ($Q_{metab}$). Whether a person's body temperature rises or falls depends on this metabolic activity and the balance of heat transfer to and from the environment. The heat balance ($Q_{bal}$) is given by:

$$Q_{bal} = Q_{metab} - (Q_{conv} + Q_{cond} + Q_{rad} + Q_{evap}).$$

If this balance is positive, the body temperature will rise and homoeostatic mechanisms will try to increase the heat loss; if it is negative the reverse will occur.

## Heat capacity

It requires less heat to warm up a given volume of air than to warm the same volume of water to the same temperature. This is because water and air have different *heat capacities*. The heat capacity of an object is the product of the mass and the specific heat capacity (i.e. heat capacity per unit mass) of that substance.

The units of specific heat capacity can be derived from SI units. Taking the definition:

> The specific heat capacity is the amount of heat required (in joules) to raise the temperature of 1 kilogram of a substance by a temperature of 1 K,

the units of specific heat capacity are therefore J/kg per K or, alternatively, J/kg per °C.

The mean specific heat capacity of tissues of the human body, including blood, is 3.5 kJ/kg per °C. The heat capacity of a 70-kg person is therefore:

$$70 \times 3.5 = 245\,\text{kJ/°C}.$$

The total heat energy at 37°C over that at 20°C is $245 \times (37 - 20) = 4165$ kJ. This is the order of magnitude of heat input that may be required at the end of cardiopulmonary bypass.

When transfusing cold blood it is easy to calculate that replacing 2 litres of blood at 37°C with an equivalent amount at 4°C involves the loss of 231 kJ of heat. This is approximately the amount of heat required to change the temperature of a 70-kg person by 1°C.

Gases tend to be measured in volumes at a given temperature and pressure and so are their specific heat capacities. The specific heat for room air is 1.2 J/L per °C. In terms of mass, it would be 1.0 kJ/kg per °C. This has important clinical implications:

- The heat from the body needed to raise the temperature of inspired air *per se* is small. A minute volume of 6 litres of air heated from 20 to 37°C needs 122 J/min or 2 W (1 W = 1 J/s). To this must be added the energy to raise the relative humidity to 100% at 37°C which is over three times as much (see above).
- Hot gases, as they lose heat, cool extremely rapidly. Thus, hot gases very rarely cause thermal burns of the lower respiratory tract because heat is lost in the upper airways, trachea and major bronchi.

## Clinical measurement of temperature

Temperature is a measure of the thermal potential or 'hotness' of a body, and two bodies are said to be at the same temperature when they are brought into thermal contact and no net heat transfer occurs between them. Reference temperatures are defined by reproducible thermal phenomena, such as melting, freezing, and boiling. The International Temperature Scale (which is developed from the thermodynamic scale based on the constant volume hydrogen thermometer as described by Charles' law) has well defined points between −182.9°C and 1060°C which can be reproduced easily, e.g. ice point = 0°C, silver point = 960°C. These are interpolated by straight lines, and extrapolation downwards defines absolute zero as −273.15°C or 0 K.

The constant volume hydrogen thermometer sets the reference standard for the measurement of temperature as described by Charles' law. Changes in the physical properties of other substances with temperature are used in practical thermometry.

In clinical anaesthesia and critical care four types of thermometer are in common use:

- thermistors;
- thermocouples;
- liquid expansion thermometers;
- thermography.

### *Thermistors*

These are semi-conductors whose electrical resistance varies exponentially (positively or negatively) with temperature, depending on the type. They are manufactured from heavy-metal oxides, are cheap to make, and may be smaller than a grain of rice, so that their response time can be extremely fast. Their resistance change is of the order of 5% per °C, and their range of temperature is more than adequate for clinical measurement. If subjected to high temperatures, i.e. heat sterilization, their calibration may be altered.

Thermistors are also subject to ageing and hysteresis. They are used in all types of temperature probes and in thermodilution pulmonary artery catheters.

### *Thermocouples*

If two dissimilar metals are joined to make an electrical circuit (Figure 38.15) and the junctions are maintained at different temperatures, a voltage is produced across the junctions that is proportional to the temperature difference. This is known as the Seebeck effect. Metals commonly used are iron or copper and an alloy of copper and nickel (constantin). One of the junctions, the reference junction, should be either kept at a constant low temperature, or subject to electronic compensation. The output is extremely small, 40 μV/°C. Thermocouples cannot be made as small as thermistors so their response time is slower but, as the output is a linear function of the temperature in °C, simpler electronic circuits are required. They are now commonly used in nursing practice with hand-held recorders and disposable probes.

### *Liquid expansion thermometers*

The linear increase in the volume of liquids and metals with temperature provides a convenient method of temperature measurement. The three most common substances in use are alcohol, water, and mercury. Mercury is used in clinical thermometers. However,

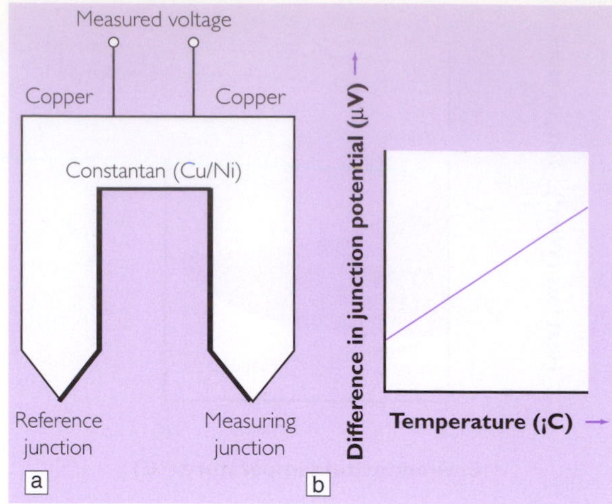


**Figure 38.15** (a) The principle of the thermocouple. (b) The output is directly proportional to the difference in temperature between the two junctions.

these are rapidly being superseded by electrical thermometers because mercury is toxic, the thermometers are fragile, and they have a relatively high heat capacity, a slow response time, and cannot be read at a distance. Clinical mercury thermometers are not suitable in hypothermia because of their limited range and only display rising temperatures as a result of the constriction next to the bulb.

### *Thermography*

The radiant heat energy emitted from a body varies with the fourth power of the temperature (see above) and is not dependent on a temperature gradient. Energy in the infrared region can be measured with suitable detectors, calibrated, and displayed as temperature. The response time of thermographic detectors is extremely fast, as can be seen in infrared video imaging. In medicine, only surface temperatures can be measured, but using the tympanic membrane gives access to core temperatures. Their use in clinical practice is increasing.

## Other methods of temperature measurement

***Platinum resistance thermometers*** (Figure 38.16)

The electrical resistance of metals increases with increasing temperature. Platinum does not rust and has a high temperature coefficient of resistance (0.4 Ω/V between 0 and 100°C). The change in resistance is measured by a Wheatstone bridge circuit. Platinum resistance thermometers are extremely sensitive, but do not have a fast response time and are not used in clinical medicine.

### *Dial thermometers*

These are robust and inexpensive but are not particularly accurate. They are used in the measurement of room temperature, or for high-temperature work such as in autoclaves.

#### *The Bourdon gauge*

This gauge (Figure 38.17) responds to the change of pressure which follows the changes in temperatures

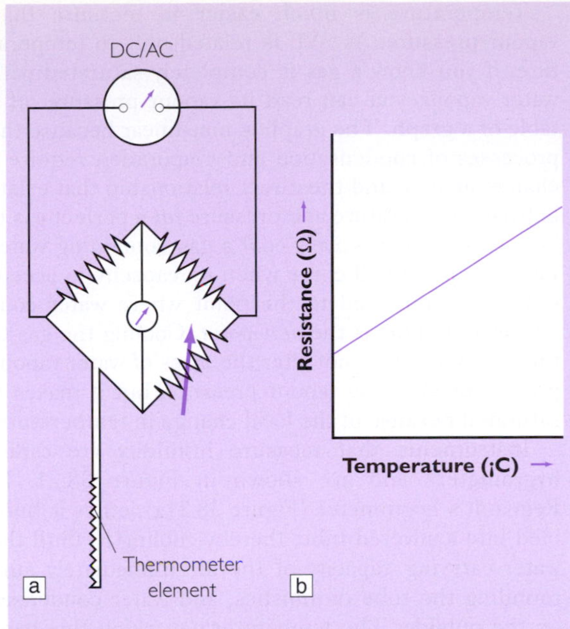


**Figure 38.16** (a) The platinum resistance thermometer in a Wheatstone bridge circuit. (b) The change in resistance with temperature.

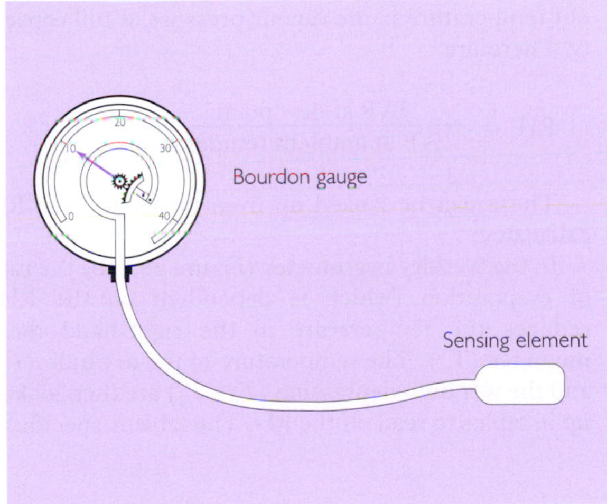


**Figure 38.17** A Bourdon gauge thermometer.

of the gas or vapour contained in the Bourdon tube. The curved tube straightens out with increasing pressure of the gas, this pressure being displayed as temperature on a scale. They are reliable, but not used when precision is required. They are found in humidifiers, water baths, autoclaves, and refrigerators.

*The bimetallic strip*
This type (Figure 38.18) has a coil of two metal bands of different temperature coefficients of linear expansion, bonded together. One end is fixed and the other is attached via a mechanical linkage to a pointer that moves over a scale. The differential expansion of the two metals with changes in temperature causes the coil to bend further. The bimetallic strip principle is used in thermostats, fire alarms, and temperature-compensating elements in vaporizers.

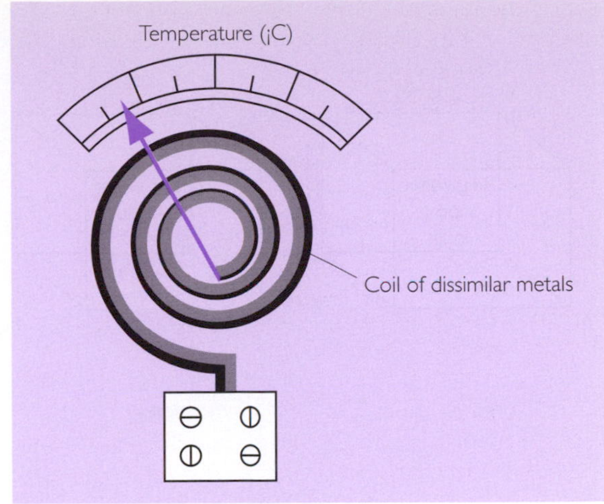


**Figure 38.18** A bimetallic strip thermometer.

***Liquid crystal thermometers***
These are strips of transparent plastic impregnated with crystals that change colour with temperature. Although suitable as room and desk thermometers, their use as a clinical instrument has proved disappointing, mainly because their physical form lends itself to measuring surface temperatures only. They are not particularly sensitive, 0.3°C being the minimum detected temperature change.

## HUMIDITY AND HYGROMETRY

The importance of humidity in the heat balance of the body (see earlier) and the functioning of the airways is of particular relevance to the anaesthetist. The use of dry anaesthetic gases and the bypassing of the natural humidifying processes of the nose and upper airways carries certain penalties. An informed assessment of the various humidifiers available requires a knowledge of the physics of humidity. The clinical relevance of humidity and humidifiers is given in Chapter 8.

Absolute humidity measures the concentration of water vapour in air in the same way as density is measured in mass/volume. The usual units of measurement (which are numerically equivalent) are g water per $m^3$ air or mg/L. There is a maximum value to absolute humidity, beyond which condensation occurs. This maximum value of 100% saturation depends on the temperature (Figure 38.19). At 100% saturation, the water vapour pressure is the saturated water vapour pressure (SVP, see Chapter 37) at that temperature.

Relative humidity is a ratio, expressed as a percentage in the same way as percentage saturation of oxyhaemoglobin is a ratio, and relates the amount of water vapour present to the amount that could be carried at full capacity, i.e. when saturated. It is defined as:

$$\frac{\text{Mass of water present per unit volume}}{\text{Mass present at full capacity per unit volume}} \times 100\%$$

Absolute humidity describes the water concentration in a gas; relative humidity (RH) tells you whether

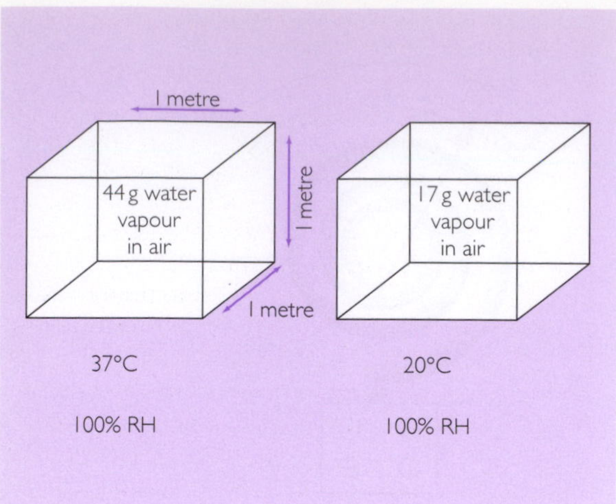


**Figure 38.19** The concept of absolute humidity. The maximum carrying capacity of a gas varies with temperature. At full saturation air can carry 44 g of water vapour at 37°C and 17 g of water vapour at 20°C. If fully saturated air at 37°C lost half its water vapour, its relative humidity (RH) would be 50% but it would still contain more water vapour than air fully saturated at 20°C.

it can accept any more. The capacity of gases to take on more water vapour increases with temperature. At 37°C air can accept 44 g/m$^3$ but at 20°C it can accept only 17 g/m$^3$. The RH in each case is 100% but their absolute humidities are 44 and 17 g/m$^3$ respectively (see Figure 38.19).

The vapour pressure of water at 100% and 50% RH and its variation with temperature is shown in Figure 38.20.

Vapour pressure is *approximately* proportional to the mass of water vapour present and relative humidity can therefore be expressed as:

$$\frac{\text{Vapour pressure of water as measured}}{\text{Vapour pressure at full capacity (i.e. saturated)}} \times 100\%$$

Temperature is much easier to measure than vapour pressure. As SVP is related only to temperature, if you know a gas is completely saturated with water vapour, you can read its vapour pressure off a table or a graph. The graph is non-linear because the processes of condensation and evaporation require a change in state and the direct relationship that exists between temperature and pressure for a perfect gas is lost. If you progressively cool a gas containing water vapour, a point will come when its capacity to accept water is diminished to the point where water condenses out. This is the *dew point*. Cooling the gas to the dew point does not alter the mass of water vapour present or alter the vapour pressure, but it makes it saturated because of the local change in temperature.

Instruments that measure humidity are called hygrometers and are shown in Figure 38.21. In Regnault's hygrometer (Figure 38.21a), ether is bubbled into a silvered tube, thereby cooling it, until the water-carrying capacity of the air immediately surrounding the tube diminishes, and water condenses on the outside. The temperature at which this happens is the *dew point*. The temperature at the dew point determines the SVP at this temperature and this is equal to the vapour pressure of the water at ambient temperature (which will have an RH $<$ 100%). If the RH were 100%, water would be condensing on all surfaces in the local environment. The SVP at the ambient temperature is the vapour pressure at full capacity. Therefore:

$$\text{RH} = \frac{\text{SVP at dew point}}{\text{SVP at ambient temperature}} \times 100\%$$

These can be looked up from tables and the RH calculated.

In the wet/dry hygrometer (Figure 38.21b) the rate of evaporation (which is dependent on the RH) reduces the temperature in the right-hand thermometer ($T_w$). The temperature of the dry bulb ($T_d$) and the wet bulb depression ($T_d - T_w$) are then looked up in tables to read off the RH. The table is specific to

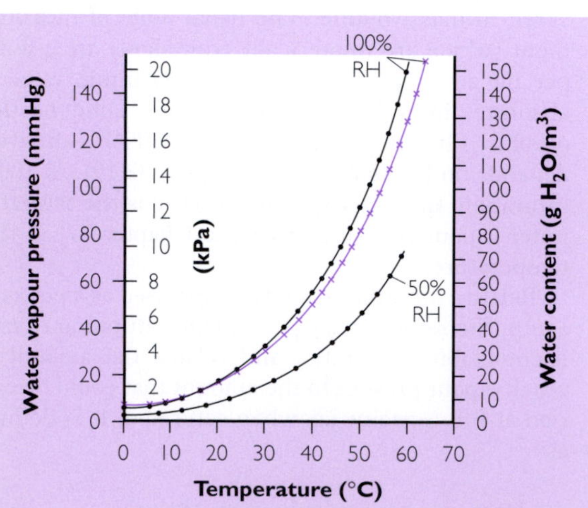


**Figure 38.20** Water vapour pressure (•–•) and water content (x - - x) curves for air which is fully saturated (relative humidity [RH] = 100%) and water vapour pressure for air that is half-saturated (RH = 50%).

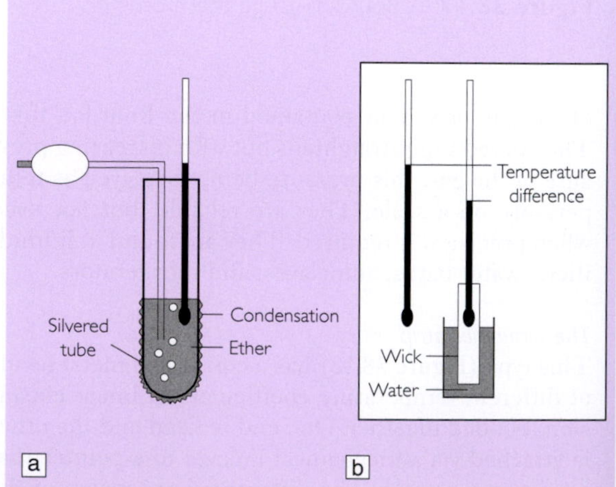


**Figure 38.21** Types of hygrometer. (a) Regnault's dew point hygrometer: the silver tube fogs at the dew point. (b) A wet and dry bulb hygrometer: the difference in temperature results from the cooling effect of evaporation.

the model in use (some of which are designed to be whirled around) but a typical set of figures is given in Table 38.1.

Other methods of measuring humidity are:

- desaturation of air by passing it over hygroscopic substances – measures the change in weight;
- lengthening of horse hair as it absorbs moisture (range 15–85% RH);
- electrical methods:
  - resistive sensors: thin films of aluminium oxide or lithium chloride are formed into electrical resistors whose resistance varies with RH. They are small and accurate, and have a fast response time;
  - capacitance sensors: hygroscopic substances are incorporated as the dielectric (the 'filling' in the sandwich) of a capacitor whose capacitance varies with humidity, with similar advantages to resistive sensors;
- colour-change indicators: certain salts change colour at high RH;
- mass spectrometer (very temperamental!).

#### *Anaesthetic implications*

- Operating room environment should be 50–70%. RH – too high, sweaty; too low, promotes the build-up of static electricity, with the possibility of sparks and explosions.
- Bone dry anaesthetic gases inhibit columnar ciliary activity of respiratory passages and produce inspissated secretions.
- There is significant heat loss from heating and humidifying bone dry anaesthetic gases.

## COLLIGATIVE PROPERTIES OF SOLUTIONS

Colligative properties are those that depend on the *number* of particles present and not on their size or nature. When a solute is dissolved in a pure solvent, the following properties of the solvent are changed.

- The freezing point is lowered.
- The vapour pressure is lowered.
- The boiling point is increased.
- The osmotic pressure is increased.

### Temperature and vapour-pressure effects

Figure 38.22 illustrates the changes in dynamic equilibrium induced in a solvent by the addition of solute. The effect of adding salt means that the concentration of water molecules is now less than that of pure water. The rate at which the molecules move from the ice to the water will initially be unaltered, but that from the water to ice will be less. The melting ice will absorb the latent heat of fusion from the system and the temperature of the solution will fall. The lower temperature has a greater effect on the rate of molecules leaving the ice than on that of those leaving the solution, so that a new dynamic equilibrium state is reached between ice and solution, at a lower temperature. The new dynamic equilibrium at the liquid vapour interface also results in a lower vapour pressure for a given

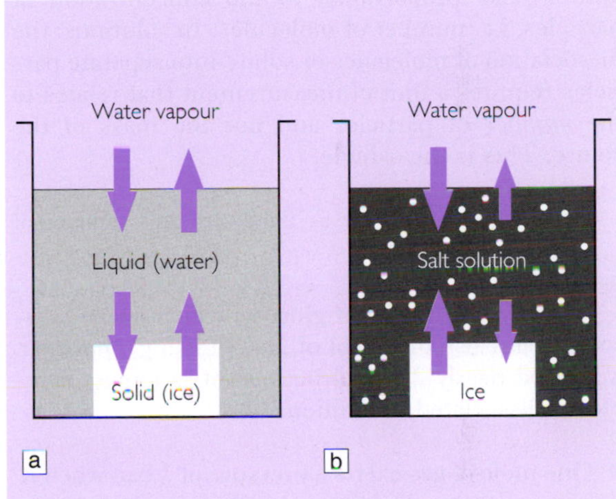


**Figure 38.22** (a) Ice in pure water at the triple point of water, 0.01°C, where there is a dynamic equilibrium between the vapour, liquid, and solid phases of water; (b) the effect of adding salt to the water. The change in arrow size indicates the colligative effect.

**Table 38.1 An example of a table supplied with a wet and dry bulb hygrometer**

| Wet bulb depression ($T_d$ - $T_w$) (°C) | Relative humidity (%) when dry bulb temperature ($T_d$) is: 10°C | 20°C | 30°C | 40°C |
|---|---|---|---|---|
| 1 | 88 | 91 | 93 | 94 |
| 2 | 77 | 83 | 86 | 88 |
| 3 | 66 | 74 | 79 | 82 |
| 4 | 55 | 66 | 73 | 77 |
| 6 | 34 | 51 | 61 | 67 |
| 8 | 15 | 37 | 50 | 57 |
| 10 | – | 24 | 39 | 48 |

Adapted from Mushin WW and Jones PL. *Physics for the Anaesthetist*, 4th edn. Oxford: Blackwell Scientific, 1987: 128.

temperature. This results in an increase in the temperature needed to boil the water, in order to make the vapour pressure increase to be equal to that of the atmosphere.

Raoult's law states that the depression of the freezing point or lowering of vapour pressure of a solvent is proportional to the molar concentration of solute.

### Osmosis

The addition of solute particles to one side of a semi-permeable membrane is shown in Figure 38.23. The particles of solute are contained in a separate compartment by a membrane that is permeable to the water but not to the solute. The dynamic equilibrium now favours a net diffusion of water molecules from the less to the more concentrated solution. This process is known as osmosis. The osmotic pressure exerted by solute particles dissolved in a dilute solution is equal to that exerted by the molecules of a gas occupying the same volume as the solvent. In gases, at a given temperature, pressure is also proportional to the concentration of particles, i.e. number of molecules. In solutions, the dissociation of molecules of solute into separate particles requires a unit of measurement that relates to the *number* of particles and not the mass of the solute. This is the osmole.

One osmole is defined as the Avogadro's number of particles ($6.02 \times 10^{23}$).

Thus 1 mol (180 g) of glucose, which doesn't dissociate, is 1 osmol; 1 mol of NaCl (58.5 g), however, would be nearly 2 osmol because it is almost completely dissociated in solution.

- One mole of gas exerts a pressure of 1 bar, when it is contained in 22.4 litres at 0°C (Avogadro's law).
- One osmole of solute exerts an osmotic pressure of 1 bar when dissolved in 22.4 litres of solvent or 22.4 bar when dissolved in 1 litre of solvent at 0°C.

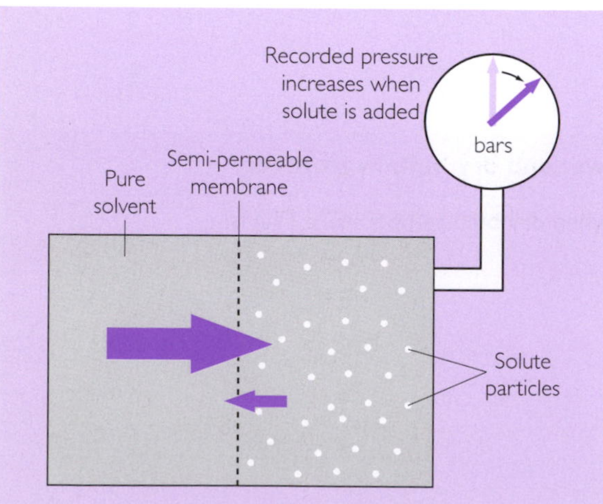


**Figure 38.23** The addition of particles of solute to one side of a semi-permeable membrane. As the water phase moves across the membrane, the pressure on the side containing the solute rises.

- At a given temperature, the osmotic pressure is proportional to the solute concentration (compare Boyle's law where pressure is proportional to the reciprocal of volume).
- At a given solute concentration, the osmotic pressure is proportional to the absolute temperature (compare with Charles' law where pressure is proportional to temperature).

The concentration of particles is measured as either osmolarity or osmolality.

Osmolality is the number of osmoles of solute particles per **kilogram** of solvent (not temperature dependent): 1 milliosmole (mosmol) = $10^{-3}$ osmol.

This is the unit of measurement used in clinical chemistry. The solvent is invariably water.

Osmolarity is the number of osmoles of solute particles per **litre** of solvent, again usually water.

The volume of solvent varies with temperature, but the difference between the two units, in aqueous solutions, is clinically insignificant.

As shown in Figure 38.23, osmotic pressure depends on the relative concentration of particles across a semi-permeable membrane. As the cell wall acts as a semi-permeable membrane to many substances, the transmembrane osmotic pressure difference is of great clinical significance. It is salutary to remember that, if red blood cells (RBCs) (300 mosmol/kg) are placed in pure water instead of extracellular fluid (ECF), the transmural pressure difference is of the order of 7 bar (over three times the pressure in car tyres). It is not surprising that the cells burst. The clinical relevance of avoiding sudden changes in osmolality in the body is obvious, particularly in the brain enclosed in the rigid skull.

It is, however, the *difference* in osmotic pressure across membranes that is important in the body. The osmolality of ECF is, as for the RBC, of the order of 300 mosmol/kg (285–295) and this is almost entirely attributable to crystalloids. The plasma osmolality is however always slightly higher than that of the interstitial fluid as a result of the *difference* in protein (mainly albumin) concentration. The basement membrane of the capillary acts as a semi-permeable membrane and is relatively impervious to protein. This produces a colloid osmotic (oncotic) pressure (COP) difference of 25 mmHg and is largely responsible for 'holding' water within the plasma compartment. (See also Chapter 19, Figures 19.1 and 19.9.)

The osmotic composition of two commonly used physiological fluids are as follows:

- 'isotonic' glucose 5.0% = 50 g/L = 55/180 mol/L = 278 mosmol/kg;
- 'isotonic' NaCl 0.9% = 9.0 g/L = 9.0/58.4 × 1.86* mol/L = 286 mosmol/kg. (*NaCl dissociates into 1.86 particles.)

Any additional solute dissolved in these solutions will, by definition, produce a hypertonic solution, e.g. dextran in 0.9% NaCl.

### *Clinical indications for the measurement of osmolality*

Providing that there are no unmeasured osmotically active particles present, the osmolality of the blood can be estimated from the plasma electrolytes, with a fair degree of accuracy, from the formula:

$$\underset{\text{(mmol/L)}}{2[\text{Na}^+] + [\text{Urea}] + [\text{Glucose}]} = \underset{\text{(mosmol/kg)}}{\text{Osmolality}}.$$

The concentration of sodium ions makes up most of the osmolality in the ECF. The concentration of potassium is ignored in this formula, as $2Na^+$ is an overestimate, the sodium chloride being only 93% dissociated.

When unmeasured substances are present in significant quantities, e.g. ethanol or mannitol, there is a difference between the estimated and the measured osmolality. This is known as the *osmolar gap*. A blood alcohol of 100 mg% will increase the measured osmolality by 20 mosmol/kg and provides a quick way of estimating blood alcohol concentrations.

The main indication for osmometry is in the determination of renal concentrating and diluting power. It is not possible to estimate easily the osmolality of urine because many of its constituents are not routinely measured and the pH of urine is subject to wide variation. The pH affects the degree of dissociation of weak electrolytes, such as phosphate, so affecting the osmolality. Because of this, the specific gravity of urine is a more useful indicator of solute concentration, as shown in Table 38.2. The osmolality of urine can range from 40 to 1400 mosmol/kg. Normal ranges are not given because a given value may be appropriate in certain circumstances and not in others.

### *Laboratory measurement of osmolality*

In theory, any of the colligative properties of solutes could be used as a basis for the measurement of osmolality. Vapour pressure osmometers are no longer popular, partly because the change of vapour pressure varies with temperature. These constraints do not apply in osmometers that depend on the depression of freezing point with osmolality.

In aqueous solutions, the freezing point of the sample will decrease by 1.86°C for every osmole of solute per kilogram of solvent. When solutions are cooled rapidly to below their freezing temperature, however, they have a tendency to remain in the liquid state, unless agitated. This effect is known as supercooling and is used in osmometry.

Figure 38.24 shows the principle of action of a freezing-point osmometer. Plasma or urine is placed in the sample chamber of the instrument and its temperature measured with a very sensitive thermistor. The sample is made to cool rapidly by the Peltier effect (which is the absorption of heat at a junction of two different metals when an electric circuit is applied, i.e. the reverse of the thermocouple) until it reaches 0°C, when the rate of cooling is made to slow until the temperature eventually reaches −7°C when it is supercooled. Then a mechanical pulse induces the sample to freeze and raises its temperature until the sample reaches its actual freezing point. Then the temperature plateaus. Thermal equilibrium is achieved and the plateau temperature is measured. From it is calculated and displayed the osmolality in milliosmoles per kilogram.

These instruments are now largely automated and can routinely determine differences of 2 mosmol/kg.

**Table 38.2 Relationship between urine specific gravity and osmolality**

| Specific gravity (g/ml) | Osmolality (mosmol/kg) |
|---|---|
| 1.010 | 350 |
| 1.020 | 700 |
| 1.030 | 1050 |

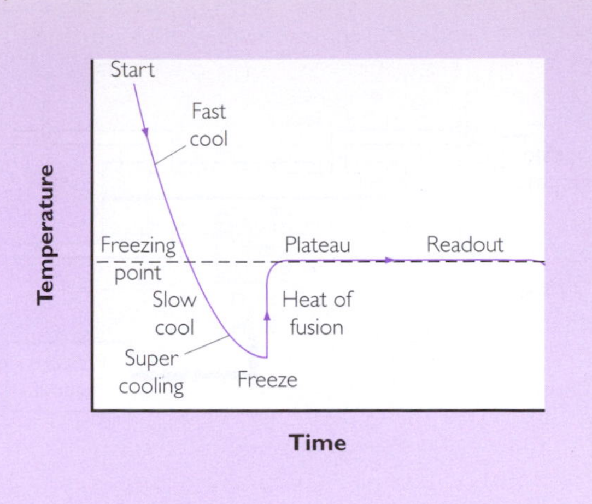


**Figure 38.24** Freezing-point osmometry. The path of the changes in temperature shows the method of operation of the osmometer. See text for details.

### *Measurement of colloid osmotic (oncotic) pressure*

COP is the transmembrane pressure attributable to molecules of molecular weight 30 000 or more. Albumin is the main component. Direct measurement of COP is more accurate than predictions made from serum protein measurements because the relationship between COP and albumin concentrations is not a linear one and plasma expanders such as dextrans can exert two to eight times the COP for a given concentration (weight/volume) than albumin. A knowledge of the COP is useful in the assessment of abnormalities of water balance and serum protein concentrations which, in severe cases, can lead to pulmonary oedema.

The method of measurement of COP is shown in Figure 38.25. Isotonic saline is introduced on either side of the semi-permeable membrane which is impermeable to particles of molecular weight 30 000 or more. The pressure transducer is zeroed and the protein-containing samples introduced into the upper chamber. There is a net transfer of fluid from the lower to the upper chamber, and the negative pressure measured by the transducer is the COP pressure. Less than 500 µl are required and the instruments can achieve a precision of 0.5 mmHg in less than 1 min.

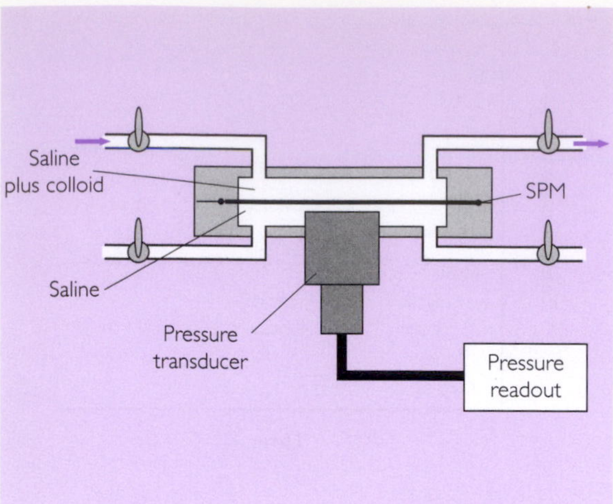


**Figure 38.25** The measurement of colloid osmotic pressure. SPM, semi-permeable membrane.

## BASIC CONCEPTS IN ELECTRICITY

### Current, potential difference, and charge

Routine anaesthesia practice requires the use of electronic equipment. Such equipment can be represented either by a 'black box' diagram, which simply describes its input–output characteristics, or by a circuit diagram, which identifies the way the internal circuitry is laid out and the components it contains. Examples of such components are shown in Figure 38.26. This section will examine the basic concepts of electricity and describe the function and use of common circuit components.

Electric current is the passage of electrons along a conductor as they jump from one atom to the next. A reasonable analogy is ball bearings rolling down an inclined tube. The number of ball bearings moving past a point on the tube (equivalent to the current) will depend on the difference in height between the two ends of the tube (comparable to potential difference or voltage), the diameter of the tube (conductance), and any constrictions in the tube (resistance).

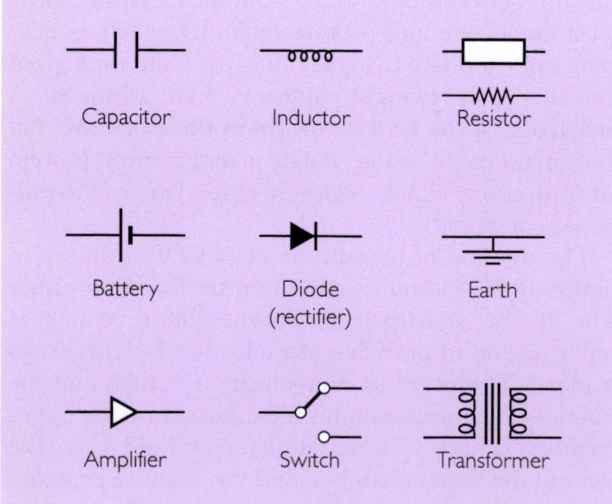


**Figure 38.26** Internationally agreed symbols used to represent common electrical circuit components.

The larger the difference in the height and/or the wider the tube, the greater the number of ball bearings that will roll through the tube each second.

The term 'current' relates to the passage of electricity along a conductor, and is measured in the fundamental SI unit, the ampere (A). The SI unit of quantity of electricity is the coulomb (C), 1 coulomb being equivalent to $6.24 \times 10^{18}$ electrons; 1 A flows when 1 C passes a fixed point per second. The difference in electrical pressure between two points of a circuit is the potential difference (or electromotive force [EMF]) and is measured in volts (V). Conductance is the ease with which a conductor allows electricity to pass (measured in siemens), but the quantity more commonly measured is resistance, this being the reciprocal of conductance, and is measured in ohms (Ω).

### Resistance

When a potential difference is applied between two points on a conductor, a current will flow. The relationship between the current and the potential difference is given by Ohm's law, which states that, provided the physical condition remains constant (e.g. temperature, magnetic field, light intensity), the current flow through a conductor is proportional to the potential difference across it. The constant of proportionality is the resistance.

This can be expressed mathematically as:

$$R = \frac{V}{I}$$

where $I$ is current (amperes), $V$ is the potential difference (volts), and $R$ is a constant with the dimensions of resistance. The formula can be rearranged to give the more familiar:

$$V = IR$$

This relationship is shown graphically in Figure 38.27.

The practical application of the interrelationship of resistance and potential difference is readily understood by anyone who turns on a water tap. Decreasing the resistance (opening the tap) increases the flow of water. A variation in the potential difference (water pressure) will alter the flow for a given position of the tap.

Applying Ohm's law to resistors in series and in parallel to calculate the equivalent single resistance, which would have the same effect as the original combination, shows that:

- In series, resistances are additive and the total resistance is higher:

$$R_{total} = R_1 + R_2 + R_3.$$

- In parallel, resistances allow the current to pass via a variety of routes and the total resistance is lower than their summated values. If two resistances of equal value are placed in parallel, their net resistance is a half of each of their individual resistances. Mathematically, for the general case:

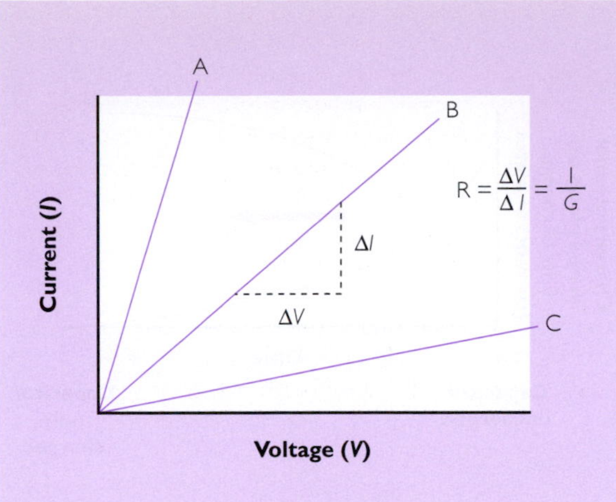


**Figure 38.27** The relationship between the voltage applied to a resistor and the current through it. Resistor B shows the way in which the resistance ($R$) is calculated as the ratio of the change in voltage ($\Delta V$) divided by the change in current ($\Delta I$). The reciprocal of this relationship is the conductance which is given the symbol $G$. Resistor A has a lower resistance than that of B because a greater current flows for the same applied voltage. Resistor C has a higher resistance than resistor B because less current flows for the same applied voltage.

$$\frac{1}{R_{total}} = \frac{1}{R_1} + \frac{1}{R_2} + \frac{1}{R_3}$$

These properties are demonstrated in Figure 38.28.

Resistors present the same obstruction to the passage of current, whether the voltage is steady or fluctuating, i.e. their properties are the same for alternating current (AC) as for direct current (DC), and the change in voltage is always in phase with the change in current. (See Chapter 37 and Figure 37.19 for an explanation of 'phase'.)

Many instruments in medical practice (e.g. thermometry by thermistor or resistance thermometer [see Figure 38.16], or pressure via a strain gauge) depend on something physical causing an alteration in resistance. This change in resistance can then be calibrated for the parameter being measured (e.g. a change of 10 Ω equals a temperature change of 1°C).

A Wheatstone bridge circuit (Figure 38.29) is designed to measure accurately small changes in resistance. Some current will pass through the galvanometer and cause it to move, unless points X and Y are exactly equipotent, and this will only occur if the ratio of resistances, $R_A : R_B$, is the same as $R_C : R_D$ (the system is then said to be balanced).

If three of these four values are known, the fourth can be found from:

$$\frac{R_A}{R_B} = \frac{R_C}{R_D}$$

when the circuit is balanced and the galvanometer has zero deflection.

This system is more sensitive than just using an ammeter to measure the current across a resistor and applying Ohm's law, because a small change in current would be reflected by a similarly small change in needle deflection of the ammeter, and this is difficult to measure accurately. The galvanometer, on the other hand, reflects the potential difference between X and Y (Figure 38.29) and when balanced does not carry any energizing current. The galvanometer is therefore very sensitive and can detect very small changes in potential difference and hence, indirectly, in resistance.

### Power

Electrical power is the rate of doing work, and this may be movement, heat production, or both. Energy is measured in joules (J). One joule/second or watt (W) is the power dissipated when 1 A of current is driven by a potential difference of 1 V, i.e.

$$W = VI$$

and, since:

$$V = IR \text{ (Ohm's law; see below)}$$

$$W = I^2R.$$

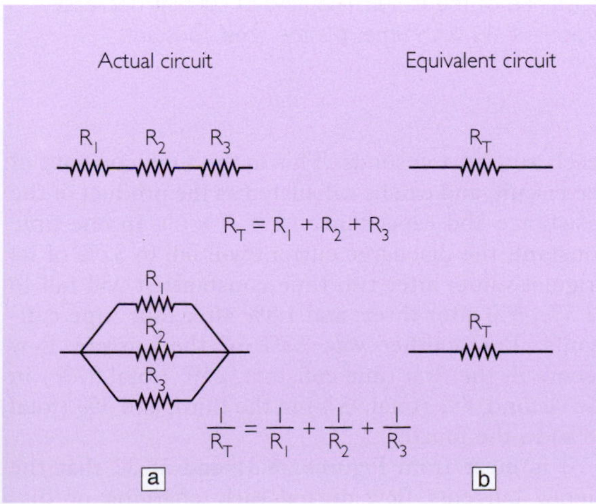


**Figure 38.28** Resistors in (a) series and (b) parallel.

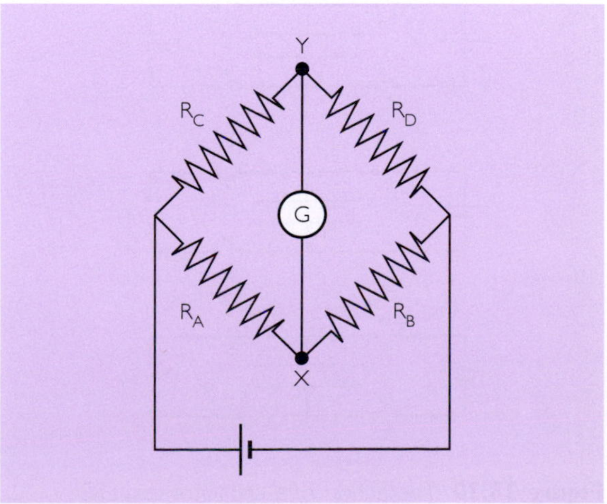


**Figure 38.29** A Wheatstone bridge circuit. At balance (zero deflection on the galvanometer): $R_A/R_B = R_C/R_D$.

## Capacitance

A capacitor is a device that stores charge. It consists of two or more plates of conducting material arranged to be very close, but not touching, and separated by an insulator (dielectric) which may be air (Figure 38.30).

In Figure 38.30a, the capacitor is uncharged. When switches $S_1$ and $S_2$ are closed (Figure 38.30b), electrons flow from the battery to the capacitor plates until the capacitor plates have a potential difference between them equal to that of the battery. If $S_1$ and $S_2$ are again opened, the charge on the capacitor plates is stored for future use. When $S_3$ and $S_4$ are closed (Figure 38.30c), the capacitor discharges through the attached device.

The capacitor plates, when charged, have a potential difference between them and, like a battery, store energy. This is given by the formula:

$$J = \frac{1}{2} C \times V^2$$

where J is the energy, V the potential difference between plates, and C the capacitance.

The capacitance depends on the physical size and proximity of the plates, and the nature and thickness of the substance between them. The unit of capacitance is the farad (F): 1 C of electricity (e.g. 1 A flowing for 1 s) will charge a 1-F capacitor to a potential of 1 V. In practice, 1 F is very large, so the more usual units are microfarads ($\mu F = 10^{-6}$ F) or picofarads (pF $= 10^{-12}$ F).

The rate of charging (and discharging) a capacitor is exponential. The properties of exponentials are dealt with on page 661. Initially, the current flow is high, but, as the charge on the plates builds up, the potential difference between it and the battery decreases, and the electron flow diminishes. When the capacitor is fully charged, no current flows (Figure 38.31).

As shown in Figure 38.32, the reverse occurs when the capacitor is discharged through a load (resistance). If the initial discharge current rate were continued and did not decline progressively, it would reach zero in τ seconds. This is the time constant of the circuit, and can be calculated as the product of the resistance and capacitance ($\tau = R \times C$). In one time constant, the discharge current will fall to 37% of its original value; after two time constants it will fall to 13.5%, 5% after three, and 1.8% after four time constants. Put another way, 63% of the current flow occurs in the first time constant, 24% (total 87%) in the second, 8% (total 95%) in the third, and 3% (total 98%) in the fourth.

It is clear from Figures 38.31 and 38.32 that the higher currents flow during early charging or discharging and, consequently, the more rapidly the capacitor is charged and discharged, the greater the

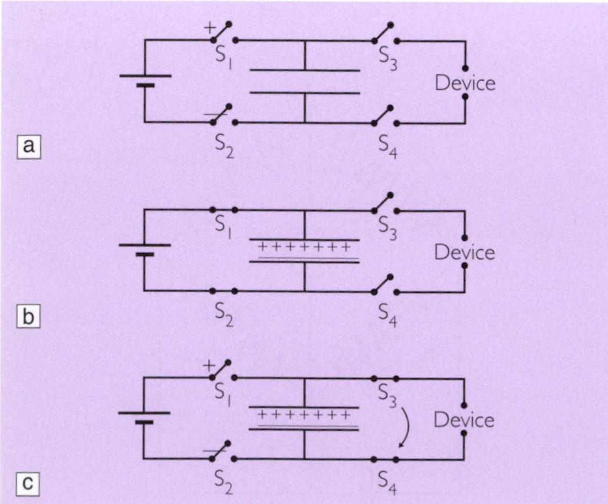


**Figure 38.30** The action of a capacitor in a DC circuit. See text for details. The arrow in (c) shows the flow of current.

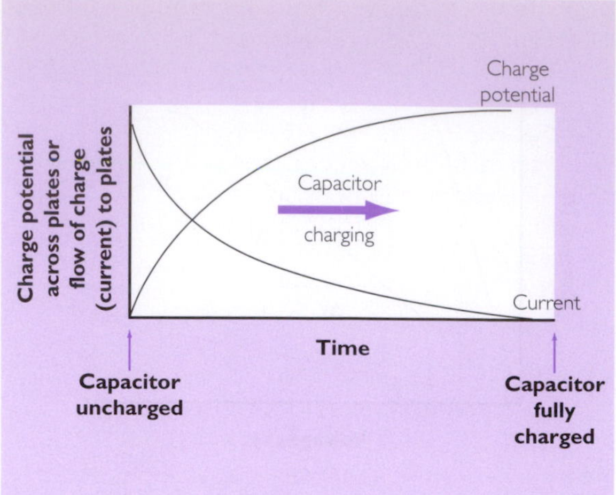


**Figure 38.31** Current and charge potential changes across a capacitor's plates as the capacitor is charged. This diagram represents the behaviour of voltage and current on the capacitor plates in Figure 38.30b when switches S1 and S2 are closed.

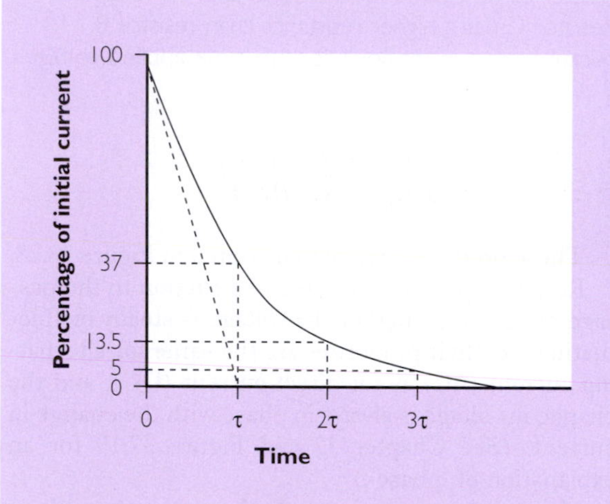


**Figure 38.32** The relationship of current to time when a capacitor is discharged. The pattern of current flow shown here is similar to that which would occur in Figure 38.30c when switches S3 and S4 are closed. The initial value of the current is determined by the resistance of the circuit. The flow of current decreases exponentially with time. τ is the time constant.

currents that will flow. This is a very important phenomenon because it means that a capacitor will behave very differently in response to DC and AC.

Whereas a capacitor will resist DC (once charged, no current will flow), it will conduct AC with increasing ease as the frequency increases. This is shown diagrammatically in Figure 38.33. The opposition to the transmission of AC by a capacitor is called reactance, and can be expressed as:

$$X_c \text{ (reactance)} = 1/(2\pi fC)\ \Omega$$

where $f$ is the frequency (Hz).

When capacitors are connected together, the final capacitance depends upon the configuration. If capacitors $C_1$, $C_2$, and $C_3$ are connected in parallel, it is as if they were one large capacitor and, the total capacity is the sum of the individual capacities:

$$C_{total} = C_1 + C_2 + C_3$$

but, when connected in series, the reciprocals are added:

$$\frac{1}{C_{total}} = \frac{1}{C_1} + \frac{1}{C_2} + \frac{1}{C_3}.$$

Note that this is the reverse of the relationship for resistances shown in Figure 38.28. The proof of this relationship, deduced from circuit equations, can be found in more specialized texts.

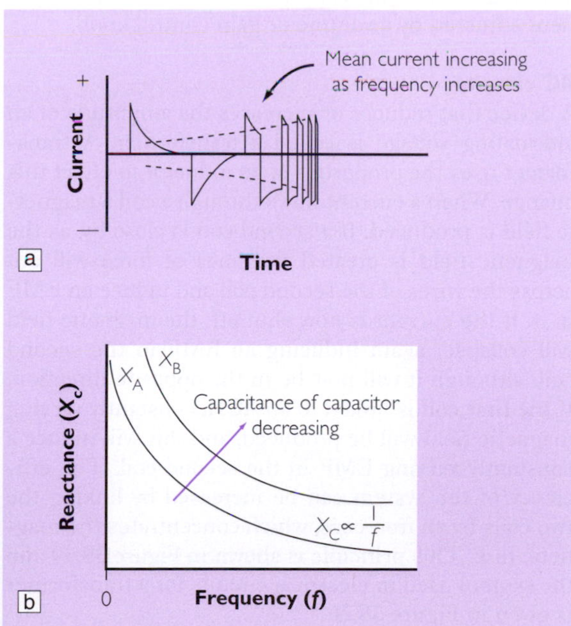


**Figure 38.33** (a) Diagrammatic representation of the gradually increasing current that is passed through a capacitor as the frequency increases. The relationship that produces this is shown in (b) where it can be seen that, as the frequency increases, the reactance falls. The reactance of a capacitor ($X_C$) is directly proportional to the reciprocal of frequency ($f$). $X_B$ is the reactance of a capacitor with a lower capacitance than that of $X_A$. See text for further details.

In medical practice, capacitors are found as circuit components in monitoring equipment; they are used to store energy in defibrillators and they protect against electrical shock during diathermy. These properties are demonstrated in Chapter 39.

### Inductance

An inductor is essentially a coil of wire. If a current is switched on (or suddenly increased), a change in the magnetic field around the coil is produced by the flow of this current. As this magnetic field change cuts across the loops of the coil it induces an EMF in the coil which opposes the current that produced it. This is called the back EMF. As the magnetic field becomes constant this back EMF rapidly diminishes, so that the current flows at a level determined by the pure resistivity of the inductor. If the current is now switched off (or suddenly reduced) the magnetic field will collapse and the movement of charge will again induce an EMF in the coil – but this time it will induce a current that flows in the same direction as the original current until all the magnetic field change has disappeared.

In circuit equations inductance is usually given the symbol $L$ and the unit that quantifies inductance is the henry (H). When a current through a coil changes at the rate of 1 A/s, a 1 H coil will induce a back EMF of 1 V. The magnitude of the inductance depends on the number of turns in the coil, its diameter, length, cross-sectional area, and the material around which it is wound. The energy (J) stored in an inductor that will be released when the current is switched off is given by the formula:

$$J = \tfrac{1}{2} L \times I^2.$$

The voltage change across, and current changes through, an inductor are exponential in an equivalent fashion to the current in a capacitor, but the time constant is now $L/R$. This is shown in Figure 38.34.

Inductors offer little opposition to the passage of DC because once the back EMF has dissipated, current will flow as if the inductor were a simple resistor. With AC, however, the effect of the back EMF will be significant. The higher the frequency, the greater the effect. The reactance of an inductance ($X_L$) increases linearly with frequency according to the relationship:

$$X_L = 2\pi fL$$

as shown in Figure 38.35.

Like ohmic resistances, inductances in series are additive, but in parallel it is the reciprocals that are additive:

$$L_{total} = L_1 + L_2 + L_3 \text{ (series)}$$

$$\frac{1}{L_{total}} = \frac{1}{L_1} + \frac{1}{L_2} + \frac{1}{L_3} \text{ (parallel)}.$$

### Circuits combining resistance, capacitance, and inductance

The properties of resistors, capacitors, and inductors are compared in Table 38.3.

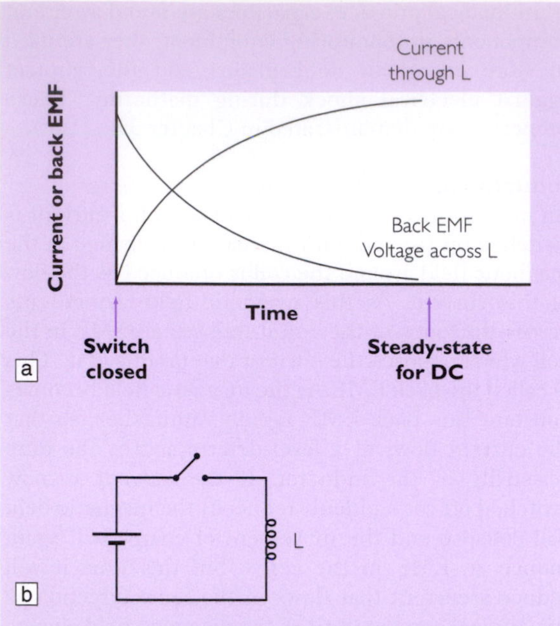


**Figure 38.34** The behaviour of an inductor as a voltage is applied. (a) The relationship between the current through and back electromotive force (EMF) across the inductor with time as the switch is closed in circuit (b).

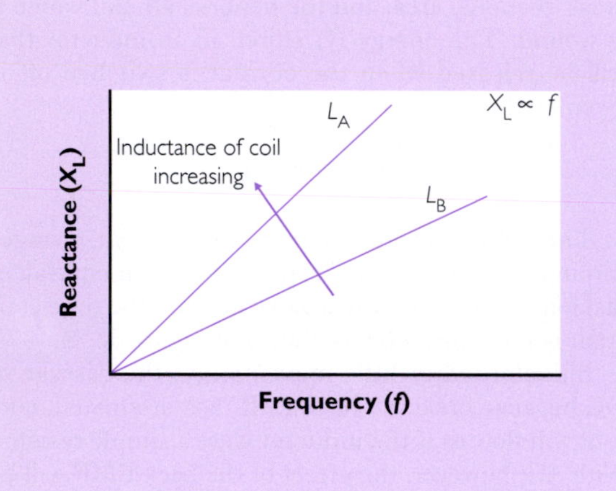


**Figure 38.35** The relationship between the reactance of an inductor and the frequency of the applied voltage. Inductor $L_A$ will have a reactance in henrys, which is greater than that of $L_B$. The reactance of an inductor ($X_L$) is directly proportional to the frequency ($f$).

In summary, capacitors block DC flow, but pass AC with increasing ease as the frequency increases; inductors pass DC, but block AC more effectively as the frequency increases. The resistance of a resistor to the flow of AC does not vary with the frequency. As many circuits have, or behave as if they have, a combination of resistors, capacitors, and inductors, the ability of the system to pass a current is complex and partly depends on the frequency of the current flowing. In these circumstances, the term 'impedance' is used in preference to resistance. The unit of impedance is still the ohm, but is often indicated by the symbol Z and is sometimes given at a specified frequency.

Figure 38.36 shows a circuit that includes an inductance, a capacitor, and a resistance in series with a source of AC. As the frequency increases, the reactance of the capacitor will fall, but that of the inductor will rise. At the frequency $f_R$, the sum of $X_c$ and $X_L$ is at a minimum. This is the resonant frequency of the circuit, and current flow will be at a maximum. The value of this maximum current is also very dependent on resistance $R$, whose properties are independent of the frequency. At all other frequencies the total reactance will be higher and will reduce current flow. This is the basis of a 'band-pass' filter. If a variable capacitor is used, the circuit can be tuned to a desired resonant frequency, as in a radio receiver.

If the inductance and capacitor are placed in parallel (Figure 38.37), the effect of the resonance is to increase the reactance greatly so that a 'band-reject' or 'band-stop' filter is formed. Filters are commonly used in measuring equipment to select frequencies of interest and reject areas of interference. More details of the behaviour of filters and amplifiers can be found in Chapter 37, Figures 37.29 and 37.32.

## Reducing and increasing voltages: transformers

### *DC circuits*

A device that reduces the voltage applied across a load or device is known as a potential divider. It is shown diagrammatically in Figure 38.38. Application of Ohm's law to the circuit produces the equations given in Figure 38.38. Practical devices can have a series of resistors, which allows a variety of output voltages. The variable resistor shown in Figure 38.38b (often known as a rheostat) is frequently used as the component adjusted by a volume or gain control knob.

### *AC circuits*

A device that reduces or increases the amplitude of an alternating voltage is called a transformer. A transformer uses the properties of an inductor to effect this change. When a current flows through a coil a magnetic field is produced. If a second coil is close by, as the magnetic field is created the lines of force will cut across the wires of the second coil and induce an EMF in it. If the current is now shut off, the magnetic field will collapse, again inducing an EMF in the second coil, although it will now be in the opposite direction. If the first coil is linked to an AC, a constantly varying magnetic field will be produced, and this will induce a constantly varying EMF in the second coil. The efficiency of the system can be increased by linking the two coils by an iron core, which concentrates the magnetic flux. This principle is shown in Figure 38.39 and the symbol used in electrical circuits for a transformer is given in Figure 38.26.

The ratio of the EMFs in the two coils will be the same as the ratio of the number of turns in each coil (i.e. if the first coil has twice as many turns as the second coil, the EMF produced in the second coil will be half that of the first).

This can be written mathematically as (Figure 38.39):

$$\frac{V_1}{V_2} = \frac{N_1}{N_2}$$

**Table 38.3 A comparison of the properties of resistors, capacitors, and inductors**

| | | urrent | Alternating current | | |
|---|---|---|---|---|---|
| **Circuit component** | | **Immediately after switch closure** | **At steady state** | **Low frequency** | **High frequency** |
| Resistor | | Constant resistance | Constant resistance | Constant resistance | Constant resistance |
| Capacitor | Charge potential across plates | Low charge potential across plates | Maximum charge potential across plates | High charge potential across plates | Low charge potential across plates |
| | Current flow | Maximum current flow | Zero current flow | High resistance to current flow | Low resistance to current flow |
| Inductor | Back EMF | Maximum back EMF | Zero back EMF | Low back EMF | High back EMF |
| | Current flow | Low current flow | Maximum current flow | Low resistance to current flow | High resistance to current flow |

See Figures 38.30–35 for a graphic representation.

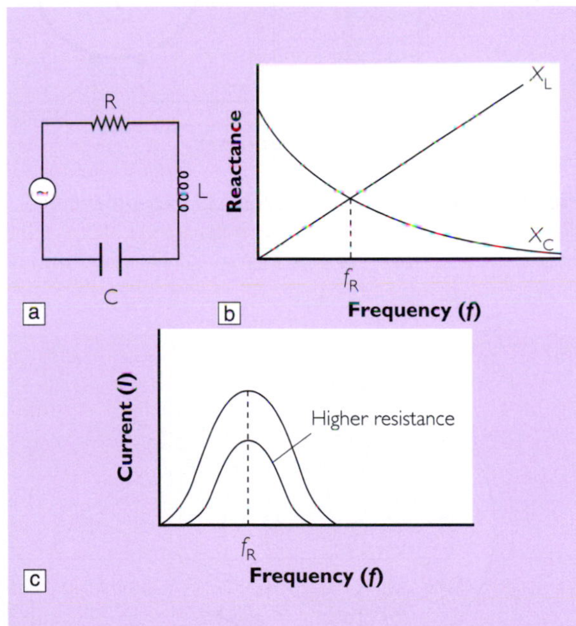


**Figure 38.36** The principle of a band-pass filter: (a) a series RLC circuit powered by an alternating current; (b) the relationship between the reactances of the capacitor ($X_C$)and inductor ($X_L$) with current. Frequency $f_R$ where the sum of $X_C$ and $X_L$ is at a minimum is the resonant frequency of the circuit. (c) The relationship between the current in the circuit and the exciting frequency. It can be seen that the maximum current occurs at the resonant frequency of the circuit. The effect of increasing the value of *R* is shown.

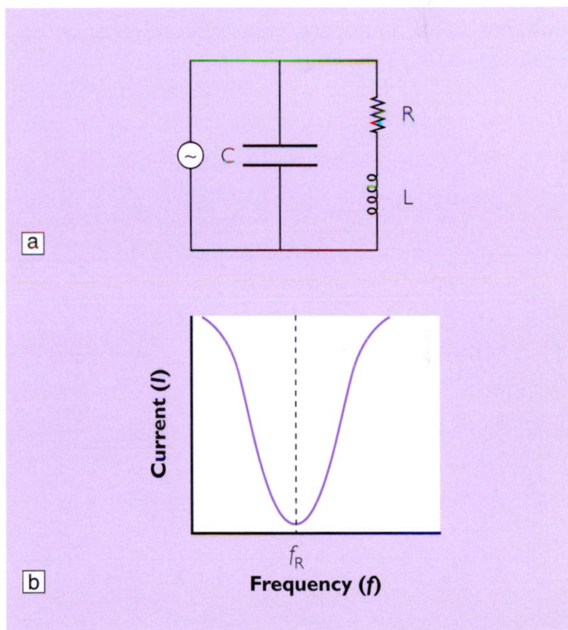


**Figure 38.37** The principle of a band-stop or band-reject filter. (a) The circuit layout and (b) the current resulting as the frequency is varied. At $f_R$, the resistance to current flow is maximum and on either side of this value the impedance to current flow reduces.

where $V_1$ is the primary voltage, $V_2$ the secondary (induced) voltage, $N_1$ the number of turns in the primary coil, and $N_2$ the number of turns in the secondary coil.

A step-up transformer (as shown in Figure 38.39) is one in which the secondary winding has more turns than the primary winding, i.e. $N_2 > N_1$. In this case the output voltage will be of a greater amplitude than the input. A step-down transformer ($N_1 > N_2$) behaves in the reverse manner.

Transformers are used in many pieces of electrical equipment to reduce the voltage from mains value to the few volts needed by most circuit components. As there is no physical connection between the two coils, they can be used to isolate one electrical circuit from another (see later). They are also used to increase the

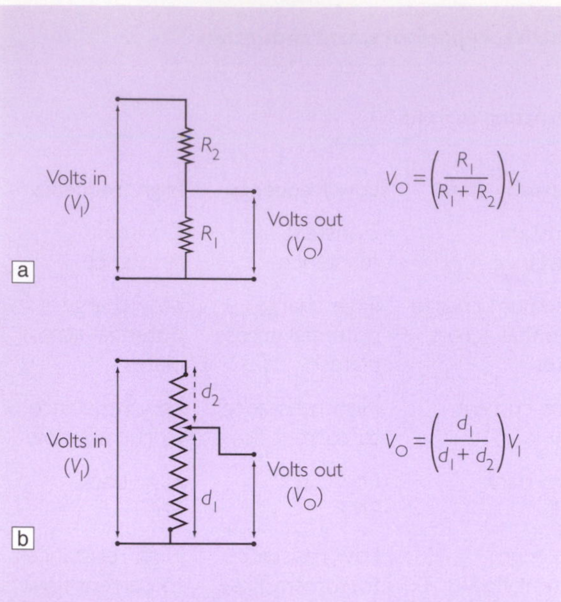


**Figure 38.38** The principle of the potential divider. (a) A potential divider with fixed resistances $R_1$ and $R_2$. (b) A potential divider with a slider that moves across a resistance coil; $d_1$ and $d_2$ are linear measurements of the resistance coil.

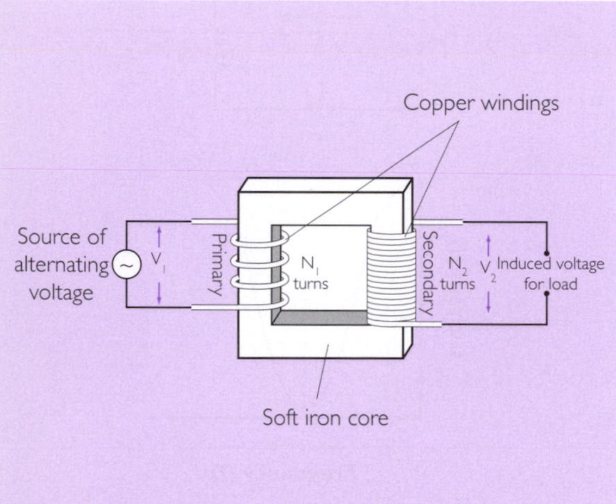


**Figure 38.39** The principle of mutual inductance as used in a transformer.

voltage at power stations to several thousand volts for more efficient, long-distance, electrical power transmission.

## Alternating currents and power supplies

### *Generation of AC*

Alternating electrical voltages and currents are produced for mains electrical supplies. The reason for this is because AC is easier to generate than DC supplies. The basic principle relies on the generation of an EMF when a magnetic field changes within a coil of wire. This effect was first demonstrated by Faraday in 1831, as shown in Figure 38.40. As the north pole of the magnet moves downwards, the galvanometer deflects to the right and, as it moves upwards, it deflects to the left.

In a commercial generator, there are three sets of windings and a magnetic field that rotates. This is shown diagrammatically in Figure 38.41a. The three sets of windings are separated from each other by 120°C and each has an EMF produced in it as the magnetic rotor rotates. The output from each of these coils is sinusoidal and for one rotation of the coil there are three equally spaced sine waves per cycle. This is shown in Figure 38.41b. The frequency of the sine waves is equal to the revolutions per unit time of the

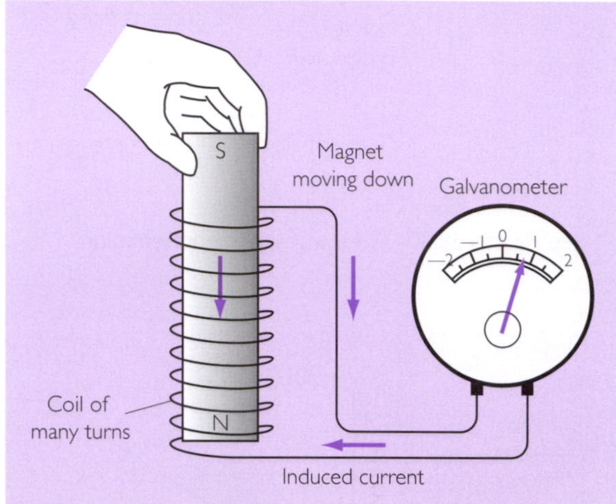


**Figure 38.40** A diagram of Faraday's experimental discovery of induced electric currents.

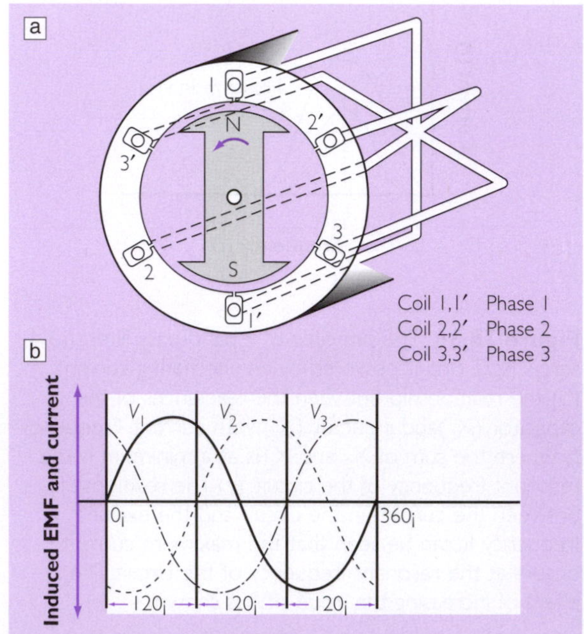


**Figure 38.41** The generation of electrical current from a three-phase alternator. (a) A diagrammatic representation of the alternator showing the relationship of the rotating poles and the windings. (b) The phase relationship between the voltage outputs of each of the three windings. $V_1$ is produced by coil 1, $V_2$ by coil 2, $V_3$ by coil 3.

rotor. In the UK, the rotor rotates at 50 cycles/s and in the US at 60 cyles/s. Depending on the design of the generator, it will produce a voltage of between 2.5 and 10 kV.

As the transmission of electrical energy is more efficient at higher voltages (the current is lower and losses from heating are much reduced), the main electrical supply plant uses step-up transformers to produce high voltages for distribution, which subsequently have to be reduced for practical usage. The principle of this is shown in Figure 38.42. The power cables transmit three-phase power (see Figure 38.41b) at voltages of between about 130 and 400 kV. The exact voltage at any one time is managed by national or regional 'grids'. These transmission voltages are then 'stepped down' by transformers close to the consumers' property. Each large building or road is supplied from one of the three phases from the transformer. Some industrial installations actually take three-phase power for supplying heavy machinery, but this does not occur in domestic or hospital installations.

### *Use of AC*

The voltage at the line and neutral pins of an alternating supply varies as shown in Figure 38.43. Axes are given for both UK and US supplies. It can be seen that the peak voltages given do not relate to those of 240 V and 120 V, respectively, normally quoted. This is because the quoted voltage is the constant value that would have the same power dissipation as the curves shown in Figure 38.43. The explanation of this is as follows.

It was shown earlier that the power dissipated in a resistor is equal to $I^2R$. When AC flows through a resistor, power is lost regardless of the direction of the current. Figure 38.44 shows the graphical relationship between $I$ and $I^2$. The power dissipated over one cycle is equal to the area under the graph, shown shaded, multiplied by the resistance of the circuit, i.e. $\int I^2R\,dt$. If this power had been dissipated by a constant current of $I_{RMS}$ it can be shown mathematically that:

$$I_{RMS} = 0.71 \times \text{peak current}$$

This equivalent power current is called the RMS current because it is the square root of the average value of $I^2$ taken over a complete cycle. RMS stands for root mean square (current). As $I$ is related linearly to $V$ by $R$, the term RMS voltage is also used. Similarly:

$$V_{RMS} = 0.71 \times \text{Peak voltage.}$$

This, by consideration of Figure 38.43, makes the RMS voltage in the UK:

$$V_{RMS} = 0.71 \times 340 = 240\ \text{V}$$

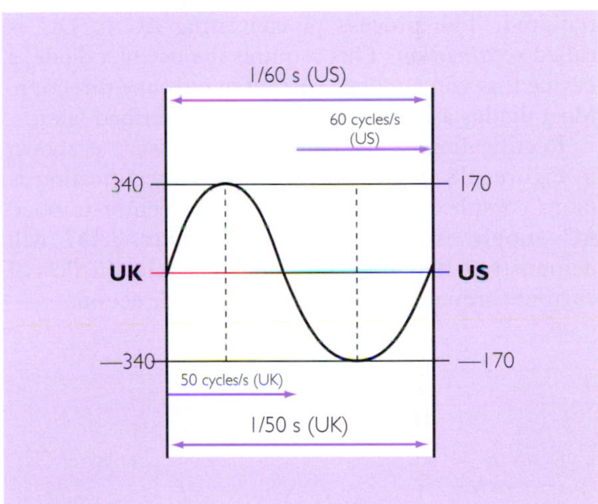


**Figure 38.43** The mains voltages produced at plug sockets in the UK and US.

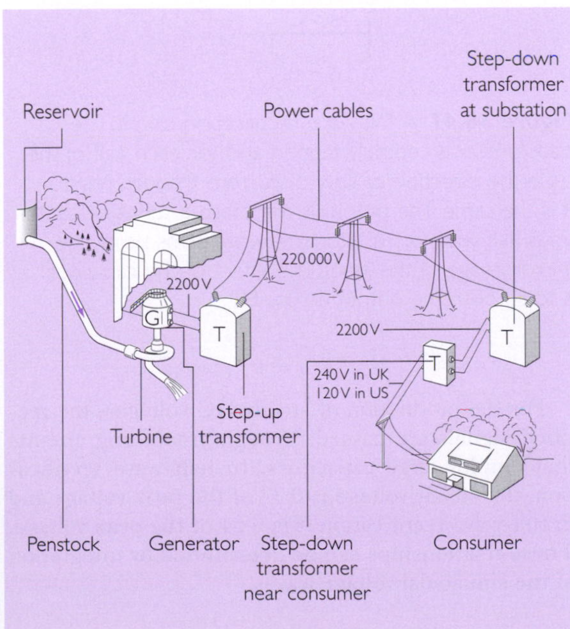


**Figure 38.42** A diagrammatic representation of a hydroelectric scheme used to produce domestic power.

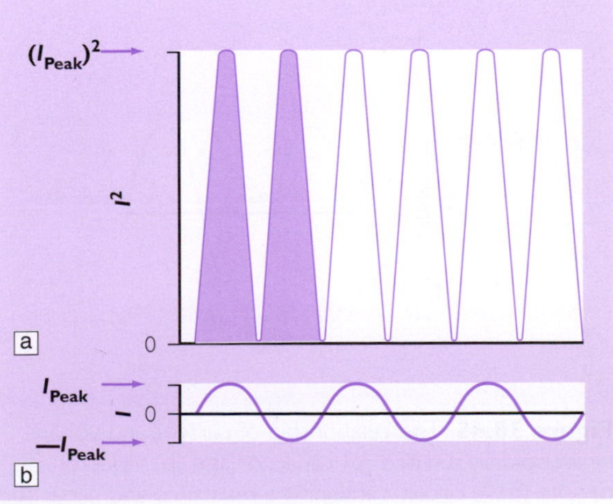


**Figure 38.44** The relationship between $I$, the current in a resistor, and $I^2$. The shaded section shows the graph of $I^2$ over a full cycle.

and in the US:

$$V_{RMS} = 0.71 \times 170 = 120 \text{ V.}$$

### *Phase relationships*

An AC voltage or current is continuously switching direction. The effect of changing voltages and the rate at which they change has been considered earlier (see Table 38.3). It can be seen from Figures 38.30–35 that, in an inductor and capacitor, the maximum current flow does not coincide in time with the maximum voltage or back EMF. Consequently, the current through and voltage across a capacitor and inductor are not in phase with each other.

The relationship of voltage to current in a capacitor and inductor is shown in Figure 38.45. In a capacitor, the current leads the voltage by 90° and, in an inductor, the current lags behind the voltage by 90°. These phase differences can be important in the design of amplifiers as described in Chapter 37.

### *Rectification*

AC flows both ways but for many applications DC is required. The process of converting AC to DC is called *rectification*. This requires the use of a diode, a device that will conduct current in only one direction. Most diodes are transistors and are described later.

Rectification can be half wave or full wave as shown in Figures 38.46 and 38.47. Full-wave rectification is more complex because it requires a centre-trapped AC supply. A consideration of Figure 38.47 will demonstrate that, for each half of the cycle, the flow of current through $R$ will be in the same direction.

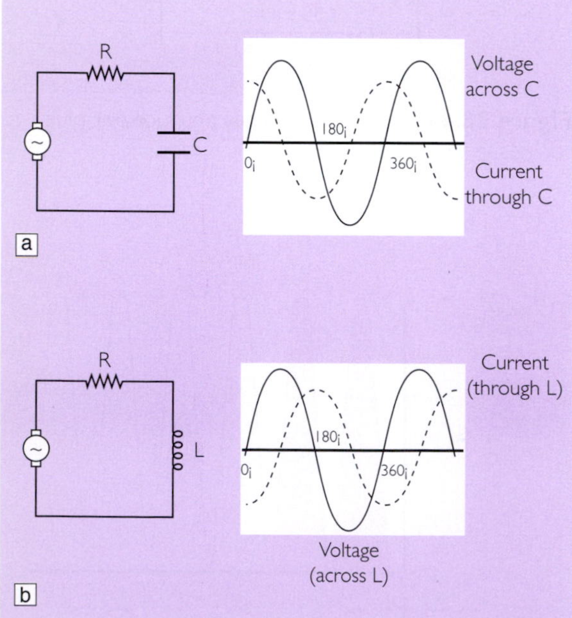


**Figure 38.45** The relationship of current and voltage in sinusoidally excited (a) capacitor and (b) inductor circuits. (a) A circuit containing a resistance and capacitor with the associated voltage and current changes; (b) a circuit containing a resistance and inductor together with the associated current and voltage changes.

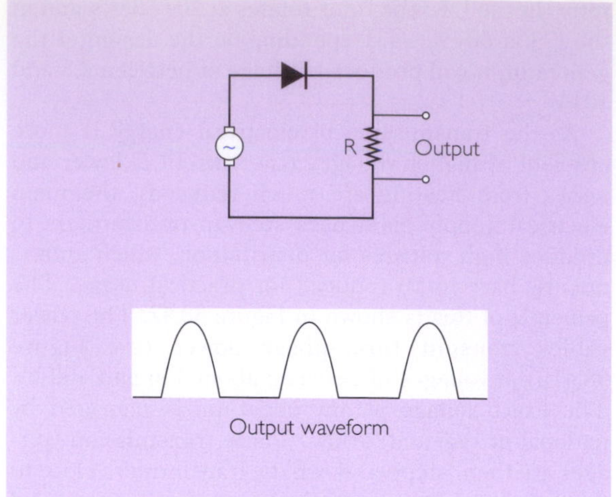


**Figure 38.46** Half-wave rectification. The diode conducts only when the input voltage is positive and hence a series of half-wave forms appears on the output.

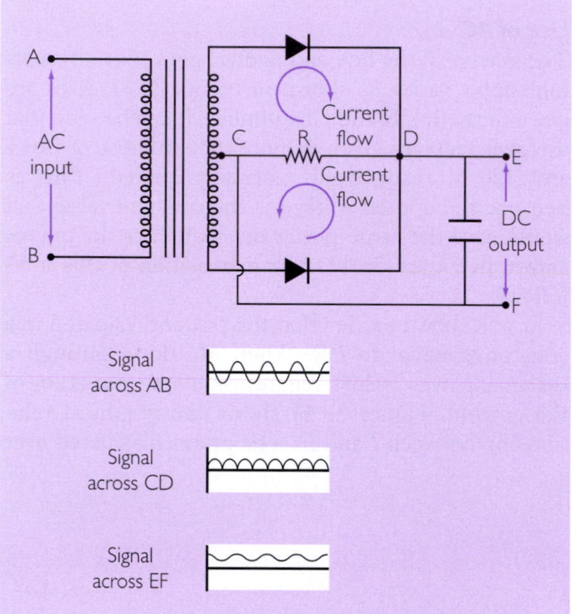


**Figure 38.47** A full-wave rectification circuit. The transformer is centrally tapped and for each half of the cycle the direction of flow of current through resistor R is the same. The output is therefore a series of continuous half waveforms, alternate waveforms being the mirror image of the input. The effect of the capacitor is to smooth the output across EF.

For the production of steady DC voltages, the rectified signals are passed through smoothing circuits that employ large capacitors. In half-wave rectification, the steady voltage is 0.32 of the peak voltage and in full-wave rectification it is 0.64 of the peak voltage. These relationships can be determined by integration of the sinusoidal voltage waves.

### Transistors

Transistor is a word derived from the 'transfer of resistance'. Transistors were developed in 1948 by

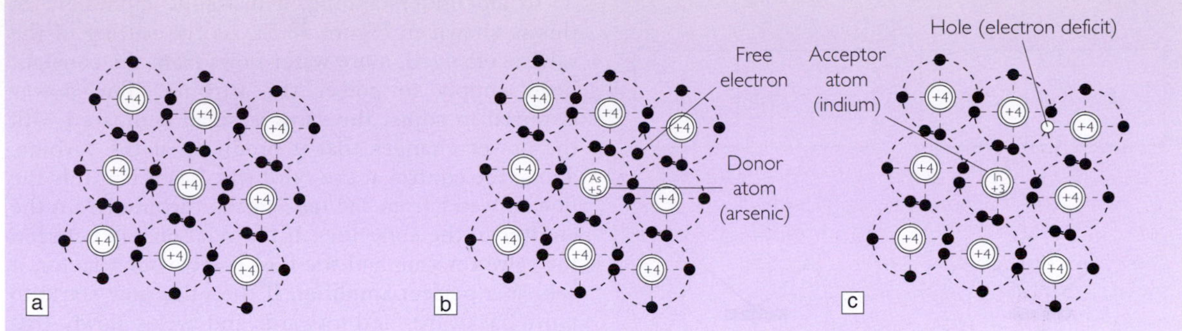


**Figure 38.48** The crystal structure of semi-conductors. (a) The representation of a germanium or silicone crystal. (b) An *n*-type semi-conductor with an arsenic donor; (c) a *p*-type semi-conductor with an indium acceptor.

Shockley, Bardeen, and Brattain and rely on a group of substances called *semi-conductors*. Semi-conductors, as their name suggests, can, depending on the conditions, act as conductors or insulators. The main semi-conductors are germanium and silicon. They have four valency electrons in their outer ring and form a regular lattice structure as shown in Figure 38.48a. Each valency electron is covalently bonded with that of another atom. The three-dimensional structure is represented two dimensionally in Figure 38.48. In this perfect state (Figure 38.48a), the semi-conductors possess insulating properties because there are no free electrons.

If, however, impurities are introduced that have either five valency electrons in their outer shell (arsenic, antimony, phosphorus) or three valency electrons in their outer shell (indium, boron, aluminium), this equilibrium is upset. A five-valency inclusion is shown in Figure 38.48b; this is called an *n*-type semi-conductor. Four of the valency atoms will bind to the lattice and the fifth will be available to act as a current carrier. As the impurity atom now only has four electrons, it is a positive ion, although the crystal as a whole remains neutral because of the free electrons.

When a three-valency inclusion is added, it accepts an electron and creates a deficit or 'hole' in an adjacent electron shell. This is shown in Figure 38.48c and is known as a *p*-type semi-conductor. By analogy to the above, there is now a negative impurity ion but the lattice, which remains electrically neutral, has a freely movable 'hole' or positive charge.

When *p*- and *n*-type semi-conductors are combined, they possess properties that can be used to make diodes and amplifiers. When *p*- and *n*-type materials are fused, there is some mixing of impurities at the interface, which opposes the drift of holes and electrons across it. This is called the *junction barrier* and has to be overcome by a small potential difference before electrons can move across it.

The behaviour of a *pn* junction is shown in Figure 38.49. If terminal A is made progressively more positive with respect to terminal B, holes will be attracted from *p* to *n* and electrons from *n* to *p*. Once the barrier potential difference has been overcome, a current will flow across the *pn* junction as shown. If, however, the reverse voltage is applied, the holes and electrons will be held in position and no current will flow. These two situations are called *forward* and *reverse biasing*, respectively, as shown in Figure 38.49. The *pn* junction thus acts as a diode over the normal working range, shown as Range 1 in Figure 38.49.

If the reverse voltage is increased to much higher levels, the covalent bonds are broken, which produces many carriers and at this reverse breakdown voltage an avalanche effect occurs. Some diodes, called *Zener* diodes, are specially designed to work like this (Range 2, Figure 38.49). They act principally as constant voltage sources because they allow the passage of wide variations of current for negligible changes in voltage.

For the purposes of amplification, semi-conductors are sandwiched into layers of *pnp* or *npn* construction. Their symbols are shown in Figure 38.50. There are a large number of ways in which transistors can be used, but only one will be described. The

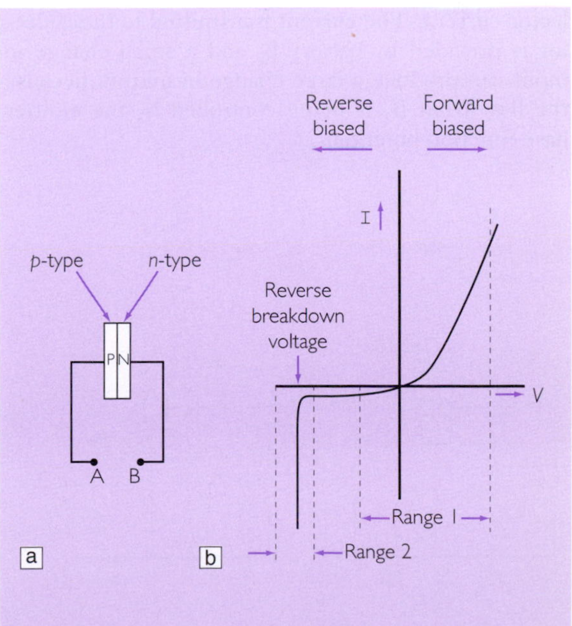


**Figure 38.49** (a) A diagrammatic representation of a *pn* junction and (b) its electrical characteristics. The junction is forward biased when terminal A is positive with respect to terminal B. There is great variability in performance characteristics depending on the exact transistors being considered.

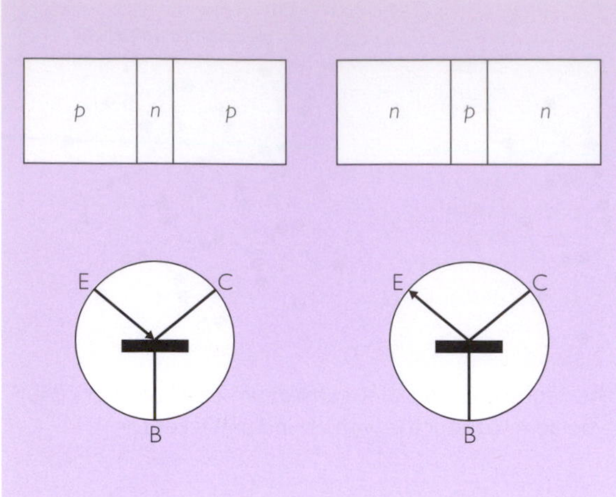


**Figure 38.50** The representation of *pnp* and *npn* transistors in electrical circuits. The emitter (E) is shown as an arrow indicating the direction of current flow (opposite to the direction of electron flow). C represents the collector towards which the current flows and B represents the base, which controls the flow of current from the emitter to the collector.

details of others can be found in more specialized texts. The one described is a *pnp* transistor arranged as a common emitter, which is a frequently used amplification method. This is shown in Figure 38.51. Battery $B_1$ encourages holes to drift from the *p*-type emitter to the *n*-type base. During their drift through the base, because of the polarity of the *p*-type collector provided by battery $B_2$, the majority of the holes will flow across the base on to the collector. Consequently, variations in the base current at the input allow corresponding changes to occur in the collector current. The current transmitted to the collector is provided by battery $B_2$ and a small change in input can produce a large change in output, because the flow from $B_2$ is being controlled by the emitter base junction potential.

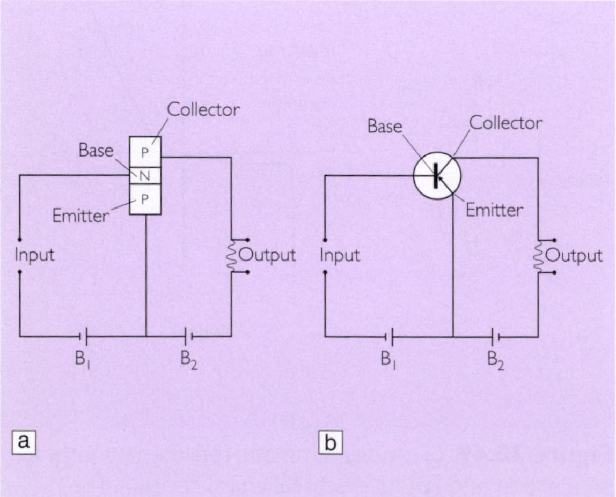


**Figure 38.51** (a) A common emitter circuit made from a *pnp* transistor and (b) shown as a circuit diagram.

To aid understanding, a hydraulic equivalent of this is shown in Figure 38.52. As the setting of the valve is changed, more water flows from the constant head supply to power the turbine. The power required to adjust the valve is small compared with the power changes that it produces at the turbine. Thus, the control at the valve (the base) controls the flow of water from the tank to the turbine (from the emitter to the collector). If the relationship between the valve rotation and the flow is a constant factor, it acts as a perfect amplifier. If the valve now starts to move backwards and forwards and cycles slowly, this constant of proportionality between the valve position and turbine output will probably remain. If, however, the frequency increases it may not, and under these conditions the amplifier is at the limit of its frequency response. This concept of frequency dependence of amplifying circuits was considered earlier under 'Principles of measurement' in Chapter 37, Figures 37.29 and 37.32.

Two other important analogies can be drawn from Figure 38.51:

- If the flow through the valve is greater than that from the tap, the pressure head of water will change as the water level falls. Linearity will be lost because the power rating of the source is too low for the load.
- The flow of water (current) from emitter to collector goes through the resistance of the transistor. The transistor will therefore heat up and its properties will be changed. Consequently, transistors, if they conduct substantial current, have to be cooled by fans or mounted on finned metal bases with a high thermal capacity.

Examples of the physical form of transistors are shown in Figure 38.53.

Operational amplifiers have a large number of transistors combined into a single 'black box', designed to reduce the problems of non-linearity and temperature instability associated with single transistors. Amplifiers will not respond to all input frequencies equally, and the range of frequencies over which

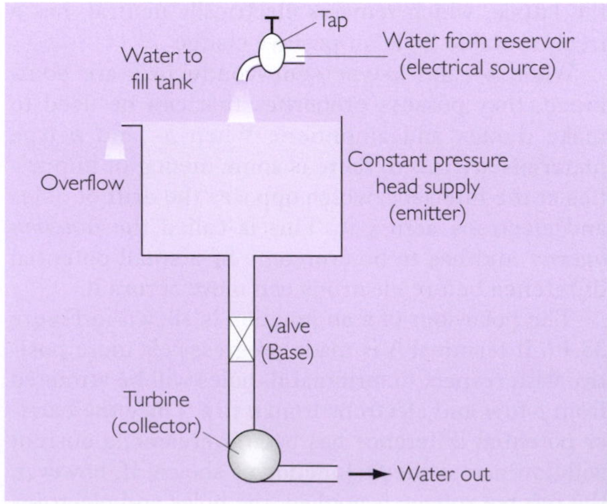


**Figure 38.52** A hydraulic equivalent of a *pnp* common emitter circuit. See text for details.

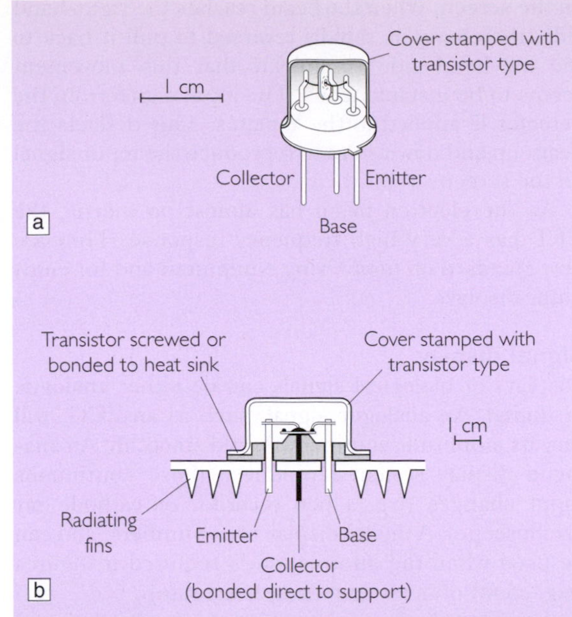


**Figure 38.53** Examples of germanium transistors. (a) A conventional low-power germanium alloy transistor, which would be mounted in a printed circuit board and (b) a cross-section of a germanium alloy power transistor mounted on a set of heat-radiating fins.

amplification is reasonably constant is called the *band width* of the amplifier (see Chapter 37, Figures 37.29 and 37.32). The correct band width should be chosen to match the input frequency:

- For an ECG, the frequency range will be 0.5–100 Hz.
- For an EEG, the frequency range will be 1–70 Hz.
- For an EMG, the frequency range will be 5–1000 Hz.

The input signal voltage from many biological sources is small, and may be distorted by interference currents produced by either inductance or capacitance from nearby mains cables.

To reduce this mains interference (50 Hz in the UK; 60 Hz in the US) to an ECG signal, a differential amplifier is used (one that measures the difference in potential between two sources – in this case two ECG electrodes). Any mains interference will then appear at both electrodes in phase at the same time and, as only the difference between the electrodes is amplified, will not be seen in the amplified signal. The ability to ignore interference common to both inputs is known as the common mode rejection ratio. For an ECG amplifier this should be at least 1000 : 1 – which means that a signal applied simultaneously at both inputs needs to be 1000 times larger than a signal applied between them to distort the output. (See also Chapter 37).

Interference from muscle activity may swamp the small EEG signal, but, because such interference is of a much higher frequency than the EEG, its effect can be greatly reduced by filtering out the high-frequency response of the amplifier.

The amplifier should be matched to the voltage range of the input signal. For example, the input signal for an EEG is about 50 μV, whereas the ECG input is about 1 mV. The ratio of output power to input power is the gain of the amplifier, and is measured in bels; 1 bel (B) is a power gain of × 10, and 2 B is a gain of × 100. As a bel is a large unit, it is more common to use the decibel (dB), 1 B being 10 dB.

### Recorders

Most recorders used for relatively slow analogue signals are based on galvanometers. This is a coil of wire suspended between the two poles of a magnet and, when a current passes through the coil, a magnetic field is induced, which reacts with that of the magnet to try to rotate the coil, the force being proportional to the current. A needle attached to the coil will then follow the changes in current, and a permanent record is made by, for example, inking the end of the pointer and allowing it to write on a moving roll of paper, or using a heated stylus to mark heat-sensitive paper. Other methods include the use of an ink jet, or replacing the pointer with a mirror and shining light onto photosensitive paper.

Although widely used, these types of recorders have several shortcomings. The inertia of the needle (which is increased by the bulky heated stylus or inking mechanism) limits the speed at which it can respond to signal changes and produces a slope instead of a square wave (Figure 38.54a). The maximum frequency response of a heated stylus instrument is about 80 Hz (just satisfactory for ECG recordings). As a mirror can be very light and have much less inertia, photographic recorders can reproduce frequencies of 200 Hz. Ink-jet recorders can handle up to 500 Hz, but are more expensive and much more temperamental.

Another disadvantage of the simpler moving-pointer recorders is that the arm moves in an arc, not a straight line, which means that the height of the deflection is not directly proportional to the current (Figure 38.54b).

Sine distortion can be reduced by increasing the length of the recorder arm, because this decreases the angle $A$ for the same amount of deflection. Unfortunately, this also increases the inertia of the system. The arc also causes a timing error related to the cosine of angle $A$. Using paper with a curved vertical axis compensates for the timing error. If the heated stylus is elongated into a bar and the paper rides over a knife edge, the effective length of the recorder arm increases as angle $A$ increases, so that vertical lines remain straight (Figure 38.54c).

For the display of signals of higher frequency, a cathode ray tube (CRT) is needed. A hot wire (cathode) produces a stream of electrons, which are focused into a beam and accelerated onto a phosphorescent screen where it produces a spot of light. The beam passes between two sets of plates which can be electrostatically charged. The negatively charged cathode ray will be deflected away from the negatively charged plate and towards the positively charged one, the amount of deflection being proportional to the charge. Plates mounted in the $y$ axis will deflect the beam up or down, whereas those set in the $x$ axis

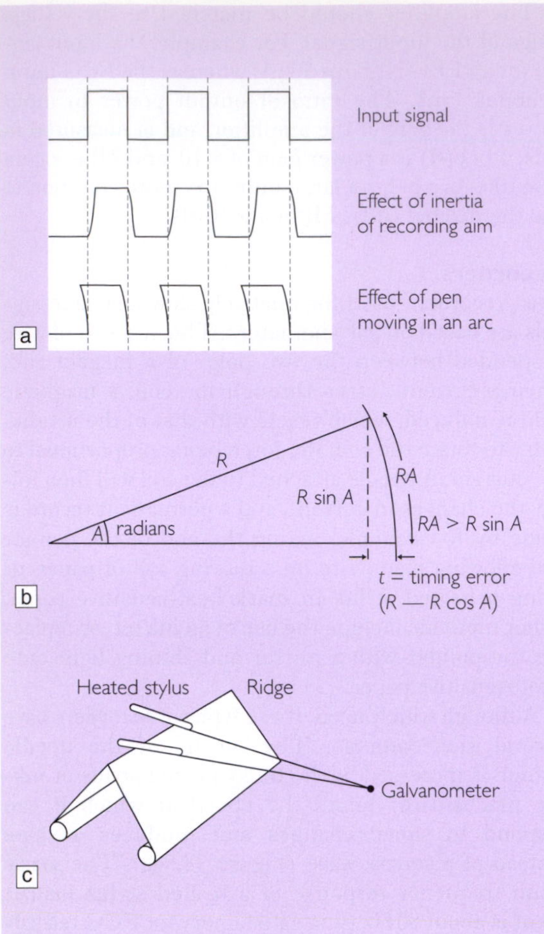


**Figure 38.54** Methods of making a recording. (a) The effect of inertia and sine distortion on the recorded signal; (b) the effect of elongating the stylus from the point into a bar and moving the paper over a ridge as shown in (c) to reduce sine distortion.

move the beam from side to side (Figure 38.55). (Larger CRTs use electromagnets instead of plates.) The charge on the X plates is varied to move the beam steadily from left to right, producing a horizontal line on the screen. When the beam reaches the right-hand side, the charge is rapidly reversed to pull it back to the left-hand side so quickly that this movement seems to be instantaneous. The input signal from the detector is applied to the Y plates. This deflects the beam up and down so as to reproduce the input signal on the screen.

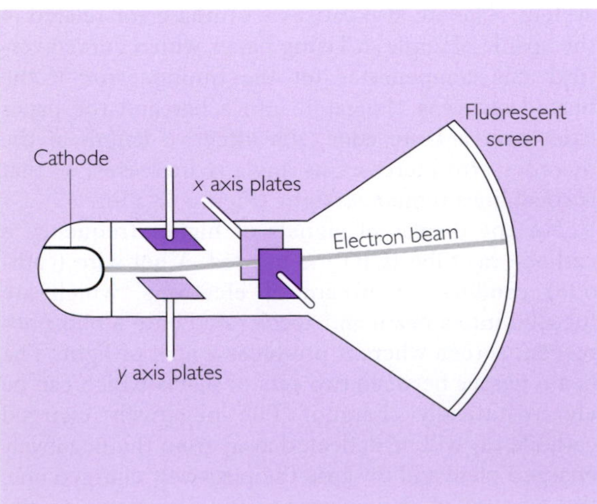


**Figure 38.55** The principle of the cathode ray oscilloscope.

As the electron beam has almost no inertia, the CRT has a very high frequency response. They are now standard on monitoring equipment and for computer displays.

### Signal display

Displays of biological signals can be either analogue or digital. An analogue signal, such as an ECG, will vary its amplitude continuously and smoothly. An analogue display system reproduces those continuous input changes (e.g. a pen recorder or cathode ray oscilloscope). A digital display uses numbers, and can be used when the information is required in figures (e.g. count of nerve impulses, heart rate).

Alternatively, an analogue input may be digitized (i.e. turned into numbers) for storage or processing by microcomputers. To do this, the amplitude of the analogue input is regularly sampled and measured, the resulting series of numbers giving an approximation of the original signal. The detail of reproduction will depend on the sampling frequency and the accuracy of the heights of the bars from which the curve is reconstructed, as shown in Figure 38.56.

To process signals digitally in a computer, a binary counting system is used. Unlike the familiar decimal system in which there are ten digits (0–9), a binary system uses only two (0 and 1), and can therefore correspond electronically to one of two stable and unique states – a switch can be either on or off, a transistor

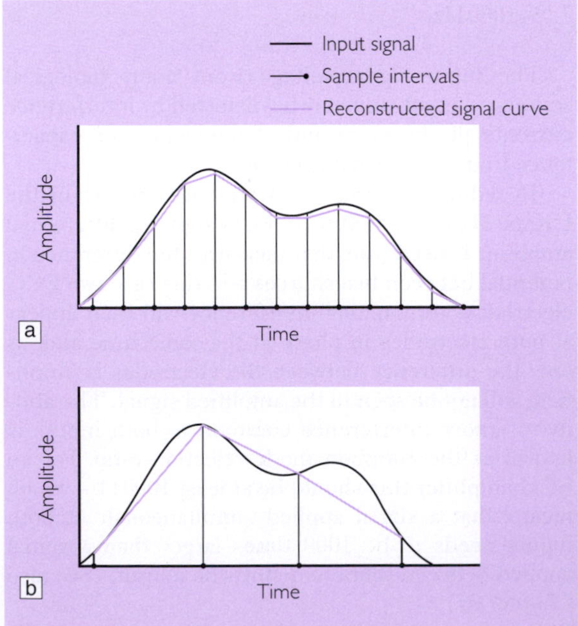


**Figure 38.56** The effect of the sampling time interval on the quality of the reconstructed signal. The frequency of sampling in (a) is greater than in (b) with improved reconstruction of the original waveform.

**Table 38.4 Decimal and binary equivalents**

| Decimal number | $2^3$ (8) | $2^2$ (4) | $2^1$ (2) | $2^0$ (1) |
|---|---|---|---|---|
| 0 | 0 | 0 | 0 | 0 |
| 1 | 0 | 0 | 0 | 1 |
| 2 | 0 | 0 | 1 | 0 |
| 3 | 0 | 0 | 1 | 1 |
| 4 | 0 | 1 | 0 | 0 |
| 5 | 0 | 1 | 0 | 1 |
| 6 | 0 | 1 | 1 | 0 |
| 7 | 0 | 1 | 1 | 1 |
| 8 | 1 | 0 | 0 | 0 |
| 9 | 1 | 0 | 0 | 1 |
| 10 | 1 | 0 | 1 | 0 |

either conducting or non-conducting etc. Table 38.4 shows the relationship between binary and decimal numbers up to 10. Reading from right to left, the ones and zeroes in each column indicate whether or not the number contains 1, 2, 4, and 8 and so on, doubling for each shift to the left. The binary number 1111 will therefore be 8 + 4 + 2 + 1 = 15, and 0110 is 0 + 4 + 2 + 0 = 6. Each binary digit (0 or 1) is called a bit.

The accuracy of reproduction depends on the number of bytes that represent the reading. An 8-bit byte will resolve to an accuracy of 0.4% full-scale deflection and a 12-bit byte to 0.2%. A system that handles 100 bytes per second (100 baud) is adequate for most monitoring purposes.

### The piezo-electric effect

Crystals of quartz and certain other salts and, more recently, certain ceramic materials containing lead compounds, when heated in a magnetic field, their component molecules line up as a series of parallel magnets pointing in the same direction. The magnetic orientation is maintained after cooling when the crystal is cut obliquely to the magnetic fields. If two faces of the crystal are compressed or stretched (Figure 38.57), the magnetic dipoles oscillate and during the movement an electrical potential is produced across the faces which is proportional to the applied force. Conversely, when a voltage is applied across two of the faces, it produces movement between them. Many common items use the piezo-electric effect (from the Greek *piezein* to press) to produce electricity. Crystal microphones, crystal pick-up heads in record players, and non-battery-powered gas lighters transform mechanical movement into electrical energy.

Piezo-electric crystals can be induced to vibrate and produce ultrasound by applying a high-frequency alternating voltage across them. Conversely, the crystal will receive ultrasound and produce an alternating voltage.

The piezo-electric effect is used in ultrasonography and measurement as both a transmitter and receiver of ultrasound. Medical uses of ultrasonography include lithotripsy, cavitating ultrasonic aspirators (as used in neurological and ophthalmic surgery), ultrasonic nebulizers, and cleaners. The piezo-electric effect is also used in force transducers and as part of a stable resonant circuit in digital watches.

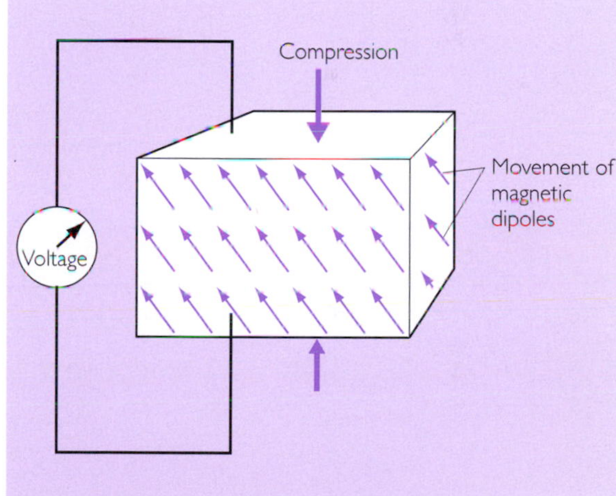


**Figure 38.57** The piezo-electric effect.

## FURTHER READING

Al-Shaikh B, Stacey S. *Essentials of Anaesthetic Equipment*. Edinburgh: Churchill Livingstone, 1995.

Davey A, Moyle JTB, Ward CS. *Anaesthetic Equipment*, 3rd edn. Philadelphia: WB Saunders.

Davis PD, Parbrook GD, Kenny GNC. *Basic Physics and Measurement in Anaesthesia*, 4th edn. Oxford: Butterworth-Heinemann, 1995.

Dorsch JA, Dorsch SE. *Understanding Anaesthesia Equipment*, 3rd edn. Baltimore, MA: Williams & Wilkins, 1994.

Geddes LA. *Handbook of Blood Pressure Measurement*. Clifton, NJ: Humana Press, 1991.

Hutton P, Prys-Roberts C. *Monitoring in Anaesthesia and Intensive Care*. Philadelphia: WB Saunders, 1994.
Mushin WW, Jones PL. *Physics for the Anaesthetist*. Oxford: Blackwell Scientific Publications, 1987.
Sykes MK, Vickers MD, Hull CJ. *Principles of Monitoring in Anaesthesia and Intensive Care*, 3rd edn. Oxford: Blackwell Scientific Publications, 1991.

# Chapter 39 Principles of physics and clinical measurement III: applied clinical measurement and safety

K. Burchett, C.J. Vallis, D. Cochrane, and P. Hutton

## LUNG FUNCTION TESTS

Lung function tests are used to measure the extent and nature of any pulmonary disorders. Basic clinical assessments not involving complex apparatus can be used as a screening process, but are imprecise and non-specific. They include the ability to walk up one or two flights of stairs, breath-hold for 30 seconds, or blow out a lighted match held 15 cm (6 in) in front of the patient's open mouth (Snider test). Failure to do the latter is presumed to indicate a forced expiratory volume (FEV) in 1 second ($FEV_1$) of less than 1 litre.

### Component lung volumes

Static lung volumes can be measured using a Benedict Roth spirometer (Figure 39.1). A neutrally buoyant bell moves up and down with the patient's respiration, and the movement is recorded on a calibrated rotating drum. This apparatus can measure tidal volume (quiet breathing) and vital capacity (VC; maximal inspiration followed by maximal expiration), and from these inspiratory and expiratory reserve volumes can be calculated. In lung function terminology a 'capacity' is the sum of at least two 'volumes'. A 'volume' cannot be further subdivided. Measurement of func-

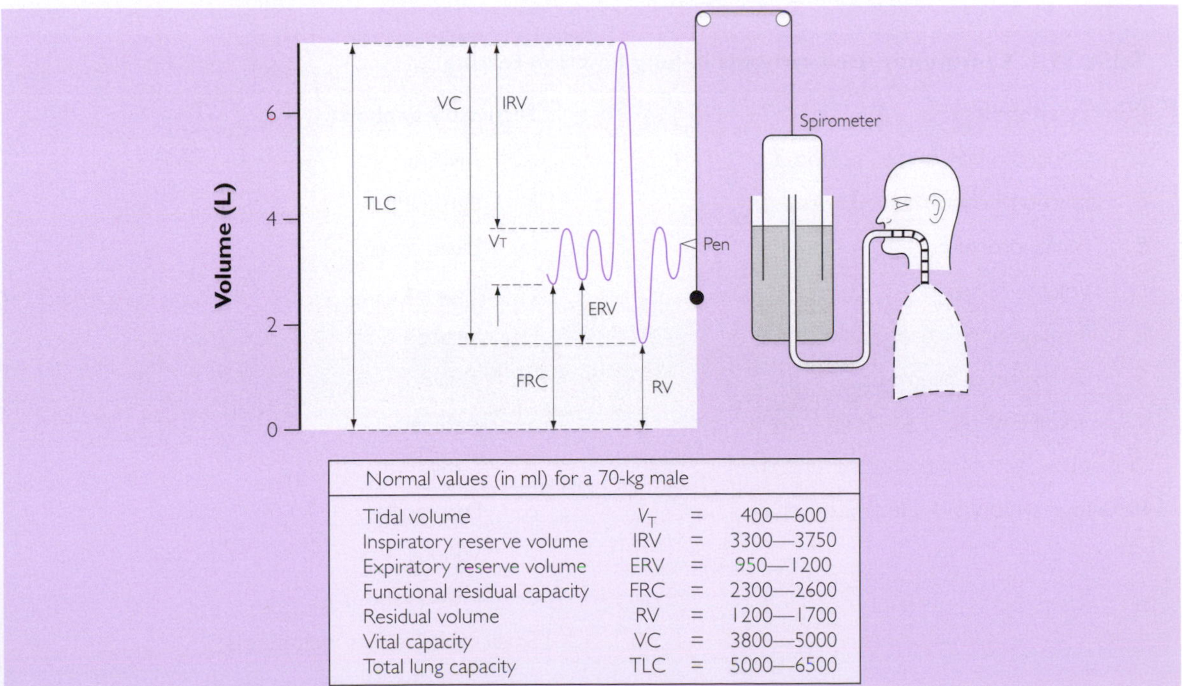


| Normal values (in ml) for a 70-kg male | | | |
|---|---|---|---|
| Tidal volume | $V_T$ | = | 400—600 |
| Inspiratory reserve volume | IRV | = | 3300—3750 |
| Expiratory reserve volume | ERV | = | 950—1200 |
| Functional residual capacity | FRC | = | 2300—2600 |
| Residual volume | RV | = | 1200—1700 |
| Vital capacity | VC | = | 3800—5000 |
| Total lung capacity | TLC | = | 5000—6500 |

**Figure 39.1** Lung volumes as measured using a spirometer. Residual volume and functional residual capacity cannot be measured with a spirometer. Values for individual subjects should be obtained from standard tables because they depend on sex, age, and body size.

tional residual capacity requires helium dilution, nitrogen wash-out, or body plethysmography, but is essential if residual volume and total lung capacity are to be calculated.

Commonly used symbols in lung function testing are given in Table 39.1. Primary symbols describe a measurement and secondary symbols indicate where it is from.

### $FEV_1$ and flow measurements

Water-containing spirometers are not suitable for routine day-to-day clinical use. Dry spirometers such as the Vitalograph are more portable (Figure 39.2). The patient blows gas into the empty bellows, which are connected to a pen moving over a chart. As soon as the pen moves as a result of the expansion of the bellows, the motor-driven chart starts to move, and hence a graph can be plotted of FEV against time. A Vitalograph chart with a series of readings is shown in Figure 39.3. The $FEV_1$ is the volume recorded after 1 second, and the FEV is the maximum volume reached. This is often slightly less than the VC measured during slow expiration with a wet spirometer. In normal health, the $FEV_1$ : FVC% is 80% or over (FVC is the forced VC). Care should be taken when looking at the results. One scale is calibrated at ambient temperature and pressure saturated (ATPS) whereas the other scale is corrected for body temperature and pressure saturated (BTPS).

When taking the reading for VC, the BTPS scale should strictly be used, but when calculating the $FEV_1$ : VC ratio, the scale does not matter as long as the volume at 1 second and the total expired volume are taken from the same scale.

Peak expiratory flow rate (PEFR) can be calculated from the initital gradient of this trace, but is generally more easily measured using a peak flowmeter or gauge. This is described in Chapter 37, Figure 37.65.

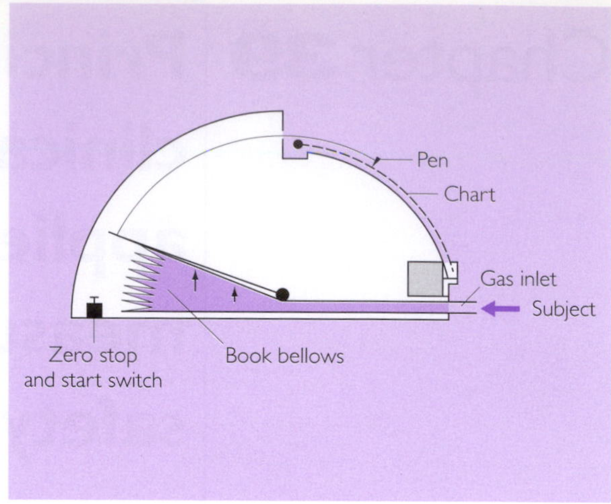


**Figure 39.2** A diagrammatic representation of the Vitalograph dry gas spirometer.

Lung function tests will help to distinguish between two main disease states: restrictive and obstructive lung disease. In restrictive disease (such as pulmonary fibrosis), both the FVC and $FEV_1$ are reduced, but the $FEV_1$ : FVC% is normal or high. In obstructive conditions such as asthma or chronic obstructive airway disease (COAD), the FVC is reduced but the $FEV_1$ is reduced even more, producing a low $FEV_1$ : FVC ratio. Mixed patterns are frequently seen. The PEFR is always decreased in obstructive disease, but may

**Table 39.1 Commonly used symbols in lung function testing**

| Primary symbols | | Secondary symbols | |
|---|---|---|---|
| *C* | Concentration of gas in blood | A | Alveolar |
| *F* | Fractional concentration in dry gas | B | Barometric |
| *P* | Partial pressure | D | Dead space |
| *Q* | Volume of blood | E | Expired |
| *R* | Respiratory exchange ratio | I | Inspired |
| *S* | Saturation of haemoglobin with $O_2$ | T | Tidal |
| *V* | Volume of gas | a | Arterial |
| Dot above symbol indicates 'per unit time' | | c | Capillary |
| Bar above symbol indicates 'mean value' | | c′ | End-capillary |
| | | v | Venous |
| | | $\bar{v}$ | Mixed venous |
| | | Small capital letters indicate gas | |
| | | Lower case letters indicate liquid | |

A secondary symbol normally follows a primary symbol as a subscript but may stay on the line, although the case is preserved, e.g. $PAO_2$ represents the partial pressure (*P*) of oxygen ($O_2$) in the alveoli (A).

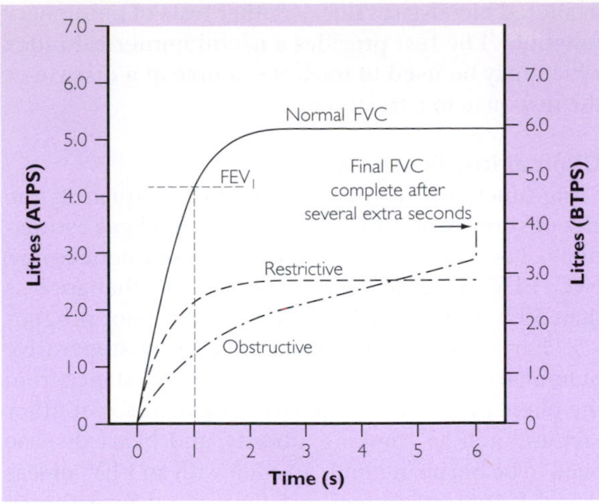


**Figure 39.3** A Vitalograph chart showing different patterns of expiration. ATPS, ambient temperature and pressure saturated; BTPS, body temperature and pressure saturated.

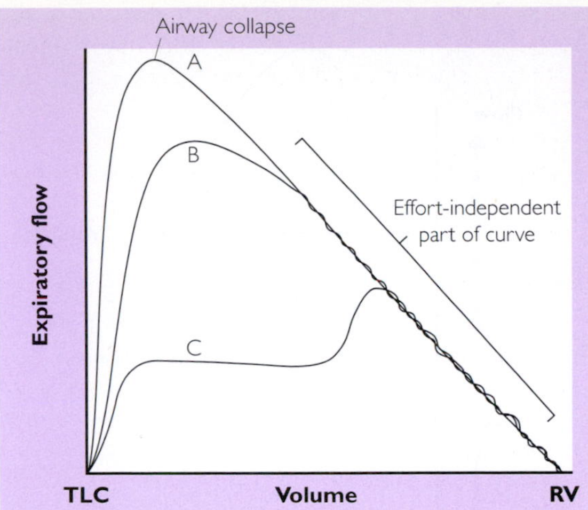


**Figure 39.4** Expiratory flow–volume curves: the descending part of the curves follows airway collapse. The expiration then becomes effort independent and all the curves therefore overlap. (A) Maximal forced expiration from TLC in normal lungs; (B) submaximal expiration; and (C) slow initial expiration which is later forced. TLC, total lung capacity; RV, residual volume.

improve with bronchodilators. The PEFR is usually normal in restrictive states if the reduced lung volume is taken into account. Common findings in obstructive and restrictive lung disease are given in Table 39.2.

Flow–volume curves derived from pneumotachograph studies (see Chapter 37, Figure 37.64) can also be used to investigate obstructive and restrictive patterns. To obtain these, instantaneous expiratory airflow is plotted against lung volume during a forced expiration. Initially, the flow rate will be high, but after a relatively small amount of gas has been exhaled the flow rate declines over the remainder of the expiration. This is because flow is limited by airway compression, and is determined by the resistance of the airways proximal to the collapse, and to the elastic recoil of the lungs. No matter how the subject breathes out (forced expiration throughout or only at the end), they will not penetrate the envelope, and will end up on the effort-independent part of the curve (Figure 39.4). Flow–volume loops of a whole respiratory cycle also produce characteristic shapes. Figure 39.5 shows a maximum inspiration from RV to TLC followed by a maximum expiration from TLC to RV for normal lungs, lungs with COAD and lungs with restrictive illness. In obstructive lung disease the flow rate is very low with a rapid decline just after the point of maximum flow, giving a scooped-out appearance.

### Diffusing capacity

Another test of lung function is to measure the ability of gas to diffuse across the alveolar wall into the capillary. The diffusing capacity of the lungs ($D_L$) is defined as:

$$D_L = \frac{\text{Net rate of gas transfer (ml/min or L/min)}}{\text{Partial pressure gradient between alveolus and pulmonary capillary (kPa or mmHg)}}$$

The diffusion of carbon monoxide (CO) has been studied in detail and is used as a pulmonary function test. The affinity of CO for haemoglobin is so high that, for all practical purposes, the gas tension of CO in pulmonary capillary blood is effectively zero, irrespec-

**Table 39.2 Summary of common findings in restrictive and obstructive lung conditions**

| Measurement | Restrictive | Obstructive |
|---|---|---|
| $FEV_1$ | Low | Very low |
| FVC | Low | Low |
| $FEV_1$/FVC% | Normal | Low |
| FRC | Low | High |
| TLC | Low | Normal or increased |
| PEFR | Normal for lung volume | Low |

$FEV_1$, forced expiratory volume in 1 s; FVC, forced vital capacity; FRC, functional residual capacity; TLC, total lung capacity; PEFR, peak expiratory flow rate.

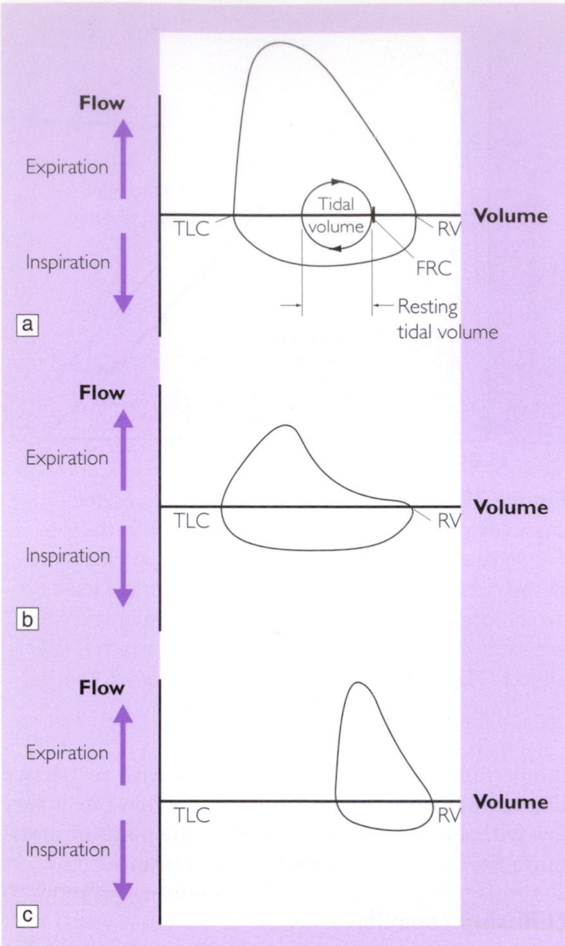


**Figure 39.5** Idealized flow–volume loops. (a) A normal lung; (b) a lung with obstructive disease; and (c) a lung with restrictive disease. RV, residual volume; TLC, total lung capacity; FRC, functional residual capacity.

tive of the rate of uptake. The formula for the calculation of $D\text{L}$ for CO ($D\text{LCO}$) therefore becomes:

$$D\text{LCO} = \frac{\text{CO uptake}}{P\text{ACO}}$$

where $P\text{ACO}$ is the alveolar partial pressure of CO.

CO uptake can be measured by the single-breath or steady-state methods. Using the single-breath method, the rate of disappearance of CO from alveolar gas during a 10-s breath-hold is measured with an infrared analyser. An adjustment has to be made because the alveolar concentration is not constant throughout the 10 s. A steady state can be reached by allowing the patient to breathe a low concentration of CO (0.1%) for 30 s, then measuring the constant rate of disappearance. The normal value at rest is around 25 ml/min per mmHg, and may be high in exercise or where there is increased pulmonary blood flow as in left-to-right shunts. A low transfer factor is more likely to result from ventilation/perfusion mismatch than from diffusion impairment.

Despite the factors that affect the determination of $D\text{LCO}$, it remains a useful and sensitive test. It can show changes in lung function well before these are reflected in altered blood-gas values or other tests of pulmonary function. The test provides a useful numerical index which may be used to track the course of a disease or the response to a treatment.

### Clinical implications

Lung function tests may be used to help quantify the risk of surgery in addition to arterial blood gas estimations. For patients scheduled for pneumonectomy, FVC, $FEV_1$ : FVC, and gas transfer values that are less than 50% of predicted values indicate a poor prognosis. For other surgery, the risk of postoperative pulmonary complications declines as the distance from the chest to the site of operation increases, but other factors such as smoking, obesity, and heart disease need to be borne in mind. An adult with an $FEV_1$ of less than 1 L indicates a high risk for general anaesthesia, and the possible need for postoperative ventilation. The interpretation of blood gas results is described in Chapters 26 and 54.

## PRINCIPLES OF CAPNOGRAPHY AND AGENT MONITORING

Instruments for the measurement of anaesthetic gases and vapours have been available for many years, but it is only with the introduction of microprocessor technology that reliable and robust instruments suitable for routine clinical use have been developed. The most relevant techniques of expired gas and vapour analysis are:

- absorption spectrometry;
- photoacoustic measurement;
- Raman scattering;
- mass spectrometry;
- refractometry;
- physical methods based on solubility.

By far the most common method in clinical use is absorption spectrometry. As a result of its importance, this is dealt with individually and the other methods are grouped together later.

### Absorption spectrometry

When a white light is viewed through a spectroscope, it appears as a continuous band of colour (the spectrum) from red to violet. If the light is first passed through an absorbing medium, the spectrum no longer appears as a continuous band, but shows certain regions that are diminished in intensity or absent altogether. This is known as an absorption spectrum. Its character depends on the absorption of light energy of specific wavelengths, which, in turn, depends on the nature of the absorbing medium. The absorption band widths of gases are much narrower than those of liquids.

Instruments that measure the absorption of light are known as spectrometers. Spectrometry is applicable outside the visible spectrum and absorption of X-rays and ultraviolet and infrared light is used in chemical analysis. Absorption of energy from radio and microwaves is the underlying principle in magnetic resonance imaging and spectroscopes.

Gases and vapours that have two or more different atoms in the molecule absorb light in the infrared region. These include $CO_2$, nitrous oxide ($N_2O$), water, and volatile anaesthetic agents. Infrared light is detected by its thermal effects on gases or on semiconductor photodetectors. Its spectrum occupies the interval between visible light and radio waves and extends from approximately 0.8 to 100 µm. Oxygen [$O_2$], by contrast, does not absorb infrared radiation but has paramagnetic properties. Nitrogen has neither of these properties.

The basic elements of an infrared analyser, using $CO_2$ measurement as an example, are shown in Figure 39.6. The absorption of the infrared light is governed by the Beer–Lambert law (see Figure 39.21); it is proportional to the concentration of the absorbing gas in the sample chamber when the chamber is of a known fixed length.

### Capnography

#### The normal capnograph

A capnometer makes use of infrared absorption to measure $CO_2$ in inspired and expired gases. It provides numerical information about the levels of $CO_2$. A capnograph displays such information as a waveform. Instruments that do not display a waveform are unsuitable for clinical use.

A normal capnograph record is shown in Figure 39.7. Exhalation begins at point 1, but there is no initial rise in expired $CO_2$ as anatomical dead space gases are exhaled first. Between points 2 and 3, there is a sharp rise in $CO_2$ as alveolar gas begins to be exhaled. Between points 3 and 4, there is a plateau when alveolar gas alone is sampled. The maximum level of exhaled $CO_2$ at point 4 is called 'end-tidal' $CO_2$. The symbol for this is given as $P_{E'}CO_2$ or $P_{ET}CO_2$. After this, there is a sharp fall to point 5 as inspiration begins again.

The plateau, between points 3 and 4, is never quite horizontal but rises slowly. This is the result of different alveolar units emptying at different rates, i.e. they have different time constants. Those with the longest time constants provide more time for the unloading of $CO_2$ into the alveoli. This can be demonstrated by taking a deep breath and then expiring slowly over 20 s or so, sampling the breath with a capnograph. The expired concentration of $CO_2$ rises continuously and will eventually reach a level approaching venous $CO_2$.

Further examples of the clinical use of capnography are given in Chapter 12.

#### Measuring $CO_2$ in expired air

To perform an analysis, patient gas is sampled by one of two methods: (1) side stream; (2) main stream. The most common method is side-stream sampling where a sample is aspirated from the breathing circuit and measured by a sensor in the capnometer. In main-stream sampling, the sensor is in the anaesthetic circuit itself.

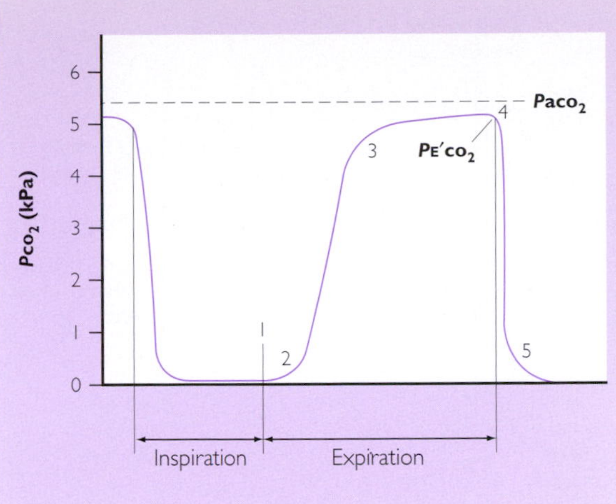


**Figure 39.7** The capnograph record from a healthy patient. Note the end-tidal $CO_2$ at point 4 is less than 0.5 kPa below the arterial $CO_2$ level. $P\text{CO}_2$, partial pressure of $CO_2$; $P\text{aCO}_2$, arterial partial pressure of $CO_2$. (See text for details.)

In side-stream analysis, about 100–200 ml/min of gas is aspirated by a fine tube from the patient's airway, filtered and dried. It then passes to a measuring chamber within the instrument. The chamber has a volume of only a few millilitres, and filters ensure that only infrared light of the appropriate wavelength is passed through it. Sapphire glass is used for the measuring chamber because ordinary glass absorbs infrared light. An infrared detector measures the light transmitted through the chamber – the greater the level of $CO_2$ the less light will be transmitted. The prototype Luft-type detector unit, which gave capnography the potential to be a clinical monitor, is shown in Figure 39.8. In this device, that proportion of the infrared light not absorbed by the sample heats up absorbent gas in the detector, causing it to expand and contract alternately with the intermittent pulses of infrared light that emerge from the chopper. The amplitude of diaphragm excursion will therefore vary inversely with the concentration of $CO_2$. The use of a reference chamber is discussed later.

In side-stream analysers there is a delay while the gas is conducted to the measuring chamber(s). This

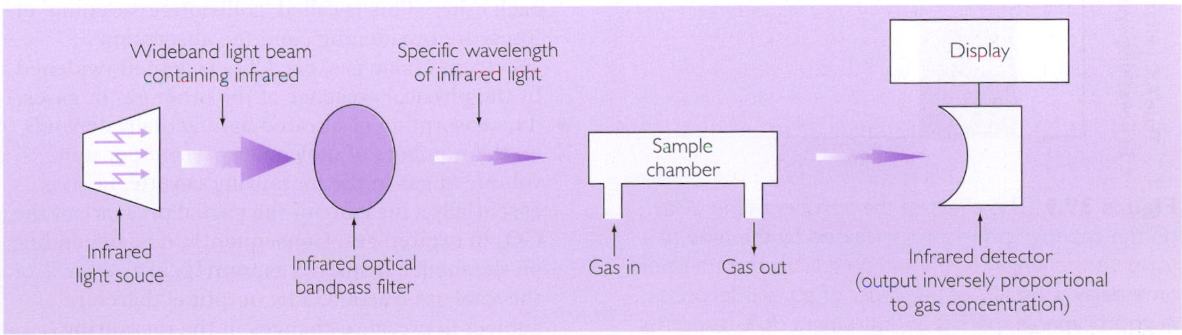


**Figure 39.6** The basic components of an infrared analyser.

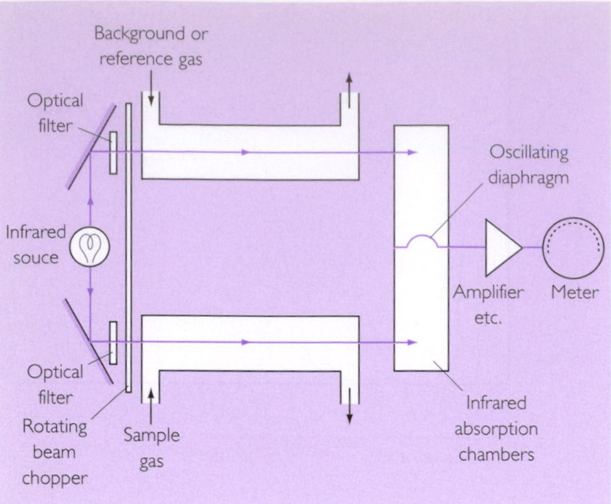


**Figure 39.8** The principle of the Luft-type carbon dioxide detector.

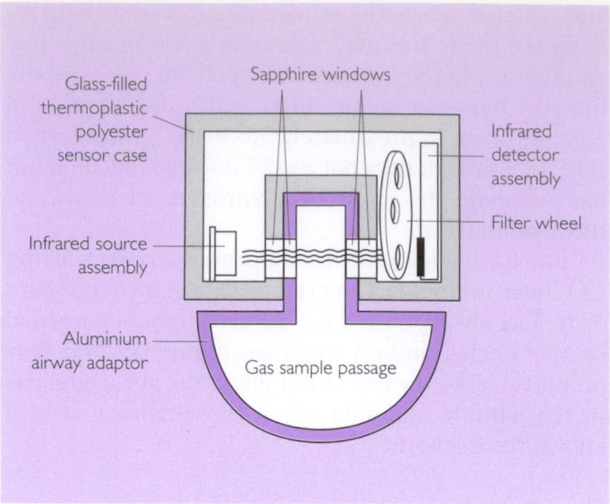

**Figure 39.10** A mainstream capnograph cuvette.

can result in the capnometer giving an expired reading during inspiration (Figure 39.9). In very low flow circle systems, allowance must be made for the loss of the volume of aspirated gas, unless it is returned to the circle. The principal advantages of the side-stream system are that they are robust and frequent zeroing is performed automatically by switching the aspirating pump to entrain room air. In some side-stream analysers, the aspirated sample can, in addition, be passed to a whole series of other sensors for the analysis of other gases and vapours.

In main-stream analysis, measurement takes place in the main flow. The measuring unit contains a small chamber, with windows on either side, again made of sapphire glass, as shown in Figure 39.10. The analyser, with its infrared source and detector, clips over the chamber. It obviously measures $CO_2$ in humid gas. The potential drawback of a main-stream analysis system is the lack of a reference chamber, so that the signal may be prone to drift. Some models are unsuitable for use with rebreathing circuits because they zero on inspired gas. The chamber and analyser also add to the bulk of the circuit. However, the advantage of having the measuring chamber in the main-stream gas flow is that the measurement is not delayed.

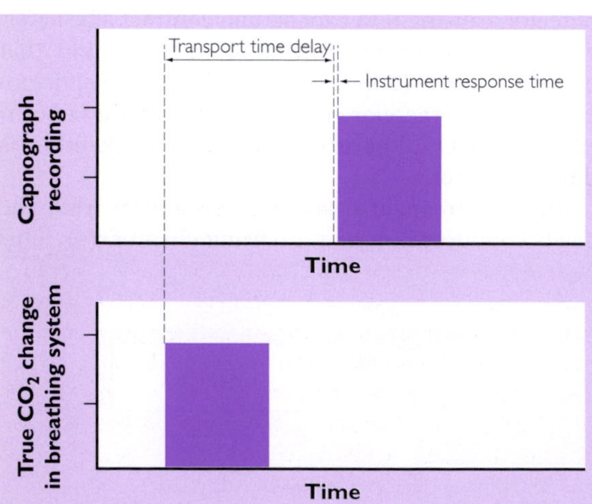


**Figure 39.9** The effect of the transport time delay on the capnograph recording caused by the time to traverse the length of the sampling tube. The transport time delay is usually of the order of several seconds. A good capnograph has an instrument 95% response time of under 100 ms.

*Sources of error and their correction*

Infrared $CO_2$ analysis has several sources of error. The following are four principal ones:

- Variations in the intensity and temperature of the infrared source.
- There is cross-sensitivity from overlap of the absorption bands of $CO_2$ with those of the unwanted components of the sample. Other gases and vapours that have dissimilar atoms such as $N_2O$, CO, and volatile agents, also absorb infrared light and have complex absorption patterns over a wide band with the potential for interference. The principal absorption bands of $CO_2$, $N_2O$, and CO centre around 4.3, 4.5, and 4.7 μm, respectively. Those for halogenated anaesthetic agents centre around 3.3 μm. The absorption spectra for $CO_2$ and $N_2O$ are shown in Figure 39.11. It is clear that if an instrument is calibrated on pure $CO_2$ and then $N_2O$ is added to the gas mixture, it will read falsely high unless measures are taken to prevent this.
- When different molecules are present in a gas mixture they absorb from, and transmit energy to, each other. This is called 'collision broadening' or 'pressure broadening', and the absorption spectrum of one gas, e.g. $CO_2$, is actually widened by the physical presence of the other gas or gases.
- The absorption of infrared light actually depends on the numbers of molecules present per unit volume of gas in the measuring cuvette, i.e. it is essentially a measure of the partial pressure of the $CO_2$ in expired gas. Consequently, it is, depending on the model, displayed as mmHg, kPa, or vol% of the total gas fraction. The output is therefore subject to pressure changes in the measuring cuvette. These occur mainly from atmospheric

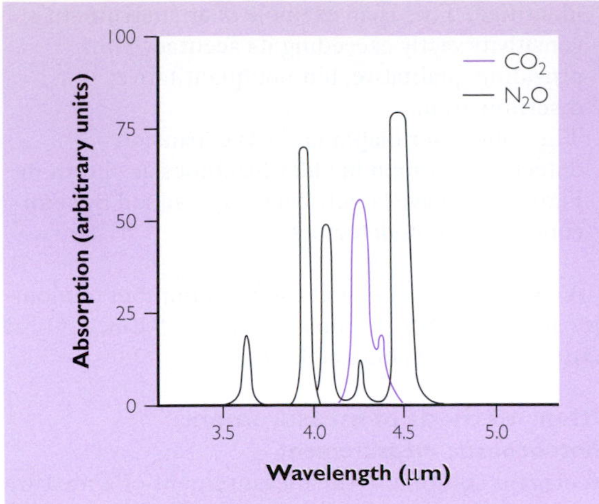


**Figure 39.11** The absorption spectra for carbon dioxide ($CO_2$) and nitrous oxide ($N_2O$). (Adapted from McPeak H *et al. Anaesthesia* 1988;43:1035.)

pressure changes and the effect of ventilators. Atmospheric pressure at sea level varies from approximately 960 to 1020 millibars and the pressure in a ventilated breathing system typically varies by up to 30 mmHg.

The ways in which these sources of error can be compensated for or eliminated are improving all the time and vary from one manufacturer to another. Methods that have been applied are as follows:

- The stability of the infrared sources has been improved.
- Many instruments use light from a single source, which passes through a second chamber containing a known concentration of $CO_2$. This acts as a reference and compensates for variations in intensity. The level of $CO_2$ is thus proportional to the difference in absorption between the two chambers rather than the absolute level in only one.
- Optical filters are now produced with very narrow band widths. Several different ones can be used simultaneously, together with microprocessor technology to produce data on the presence of $CO_2$, $N_2O$, and anaesthetic agents.
- The aspirating pump must apply constant suction to the chamber, which is measured by a differential pressure transducer. Some analysers automatically detect blockages (from kinks, sputum, or condensation) or increased resistance in the sampling lines, and flush them out. Others have sampling tubes made of a special material that is impermeable to gases but absorbs water vapour and transmits it to the atmosphere.
- Zero drift is minimized by the use of a beam chopper (a wheel rotating at approximately 300 Hz) which provides an intermittent beam for analysis. A series of pulses rather than a constant signal enables the instrument to be set up to respond only to measurement of rapid changes in absorption and not to slow baseline drift.
- The effect of $N_2O$ is minimized in a number of ways. Old machines assumed, if used, that its concentration would be 70% and usually there was a $N_2O$ 'compensation' button, which could be pressed to offset the effect electronically. Nowadays, a number of gas analysers analyse for $O_2$, $N_2O$, and $CO_2$, and use software to make an appropriate compensation. For research work it is necessary to test any machine against a known $CO_2$-containing calibration gas in the range 4–5%.
- The effect of barometric pressure is small but some instruments include a barometer and electronic circuitry which makes the necessary correction.

In summary, modern instruments do, for clinical purposes, process a satisfactory degree of accuracy, which is usually about ±0.1% in the range 0–10% $CO_2$. For the way in which a particular instrument functions and for its own performance curves, the manufacturer's literature should be consulted.

#### *Clinical applications of capnography*

The response time of a capnograph is very short compared with the length of the respiratory cycle. Even with side-stream analysis, the delay in displaying a change in $CO_2$ concentration is only a few seconds. Thus, the capnograph is still a rapidly responding monitor compared with many others.

A sudden drop in end-tidal $CO_2$ to zero or near zero is an indication to search immediately for the cause. Equipment problems associated with this event include ventilator malfunction, a disconnection in the breathing circuit, or an obstructed endotracheal tube. It is also possible that, particularly if the patient has been moved on the table, the endotracheal tube has become misplaced and is in the oesophagus. Problems such as these will be detected rapidly and well before the pulse oximeter has registered a change.

A significant drop in end-tidal $CO_2$ over a period of 10 or so breaths usually gives warning of a major problem with the patient's cardiovascular or respiratory systems. This may be sudden decompensation and/or hypotension associated with massive blood loss, complete circulatory arrest, or air or other pulmonary embolism. Further consideration of this is given in Chapter 12.

It is important to remember that capnometry, like other forms of monitoring, is an aid to the evaluation of the patient and is not an end in itself. A major change in the indicated readings is an indication to check the patient, not the monitor. Thus, in the serious situations described above, the patient should be clinically evaluated immediately, with auscultation of the chest, observation for cyanosis, and pulse and blood pressure measurements. (In other words a rapid check of ABC.) When this is complete and the patient's condition is found to be satisfactory, it is only then possible to assume that the problem with unexpected readings may lie with the caponometer.

### Measuring volatile anaesthetic agents

The principle of measurement of $N_2O$ and the halogenated hydrocarbons by absorption spectrometry is identical to that described for $CO_2$ above. $N_2O$ and the volatile agents have their own identifying absorption spectra and can be distinguished from each other by the use of appropriate filters which provide specific wavelengths of infrared light. Absorption spectra for halothane, enflurane, and isoflurane are shown in Figure 39.12. (Note that Figure 39.12 plots transmittance whereas Figure 39.11 plots absorbance.) Figure 39.12 shows the most commonly used part of the absorption spectrum, but for volatile agents there are also peaks from 7 to 15 µm. The main practical problem is that the commonly used halogenated volatile agents absorb infrared at virtually identical wavelengths, albeit to a different extent. The instrument must therefore be calibrated for a specific agent. A typical arrangement is as follows:

- One infrared filter with a narrow band pass centring at 3.3 µm is used for detection of anaesthetic agent.
- The filter characteristics for each of the five possible anaesthetic agents is established during production and is permanently stored in the machine's memory.
- Only one anaesthetic agent can be used at a time and the machine must be informed of the identity of the agent, either automatically or manually. (A patient induced with sevoflurane and maintained with isoflurane will initially exhale a mixture of agents, causing inaccuracies of measurement.)
- Automatic agent identification is incorporated into some machines. The narrow-band infrared source emerging from the sample chamber is passed through filters with even narrower bandwidths, specific to the absorption response of the agents concerned, and then passed to infrared detectors. The filter/detector pair specific to the anaesthetic agent in the sample cell will have a reduced output compared with the others, enabling it to be identified. This is an example of an instrument's sensitivity vastly exceeding its accuracy, thus providing qualitative, but not quantitative, discrimination.
- The condenser diaphragm gas expansion detectors common in older machines as shown in Figure 39.8 have largely been superseded by semi-conductor photodetectors.

A common arrangement used in a number of monitors is for $N_2O$ to be measured at 3.9 µm, $CO_2$ at 4.3 µm, and the vapours at 3.3 µm.

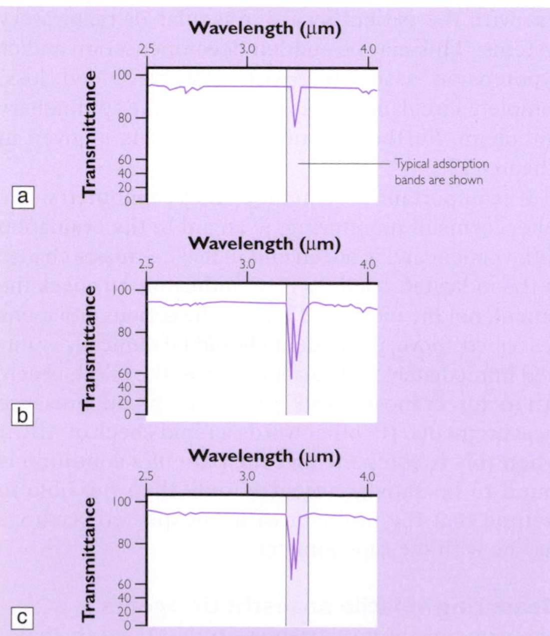


**Figure 39.12** The absorption spectra for volatile anaesthetic agents: (a) halothane; (b) enflurane; and (c) isoflurane. (Adapted from McPeak H *et al.* *Anaesthesia* 1988;43:1035.)

## Other methods of measurement

### *Photoacoustic measurement*

An elegant solution to the measurement of a mixture of gases and vapours in a single chamber is that applied in the Bruel and Kjaer monitor.

A wide-band infrared source is pulsed by the interposition of a rotating disc containing apertures in the form of slits. Three distinct pulsed frequencies in the sonic range are achieved by having three concentric rings of slits, with each ring containing a different number of apertures. Each of the three resulting pulsed wide-band infrared emissions are transmitted though a separate, narrow-band, optical filter at a wavelength specific to the principal absorption bands of $CO_2$, $N_2O$, and anaesthetic agents. The pulsed infrared light causes expansion and contraction by intermittent heating and cooling of the different component gases and vapours. As the three distinct infrared sources are pulsed at different frequencies, vibration *frequency* now becomes the discriminator between $CO_2$, $N_2O$, and anaesthetic agents. The *amplitude* of vibration at a particular frequency will vary with the concentration of the vapour. The principle is shown in Figure 39.13. $O_2$ is not able to absorb infrared light, but as a result of its paramagnetic properties it is made to vibrate at its own identifiable frequency by a varying electromagnetic field. This principle of measurement is described later.

A microphone measures the amplitude and vibration frequency of the sound waves produced in the mixture of gases and vapours. The signals are processed in a manner similar to that found in the graphic equalizer of domestic sound systems, which are able to separate out different frequency bands and their amplitudes. The frequency identifies a specific gas or vapour, and the amplitude at that frequency is inversely proportional to its concentration.

### *Raman scattering*

When light is shone into a gas or vapour, a varying proportion will be reflected at the same frequency without loss of energy. This is known as Rayleigh scattering. A tiny proportion of this light (less than one millionth) loses energy to the vibrating molecules of gas/vapour and emerges at right angles to the beam at a lower frequency. This is known as the Raman effect. It was first observed in 1928 and has received more interest recently because of the advent of cheap, reliable lasers, sophisticated monochromators, and sensitive light detectors.

In commercially available instruments, molecules of gases or vapour are illuminated with argon laser light. This results in light of a different wavelength, i.e.

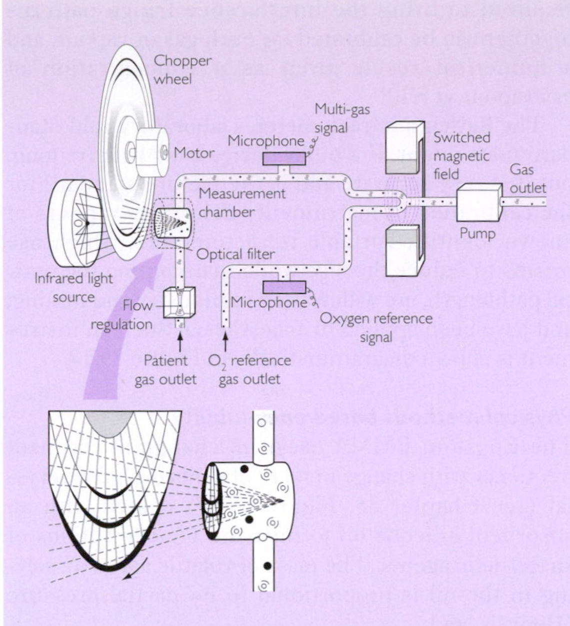


**Figure 39.13** Components of a photoacoustic spectrometer. (Adapted from Sykes MK, Vickers MD, Hull CJ. *Principles of Measurement and Monitoring in Anaesthesia and Intensive Care*. Oxford: Blackwell Scientific, 3rd edn 1991, 238.)

different colour, being emitted. The nature and amount of this emitted radiation are specific to the molecules concerned and to their concentration. Using suitable photodetectors, all anaesthetic gases and vapours can be measured in this way. The instruments can also measure and differentiate between the volatile anaesthetics. The principle of action is shown in Figure 39.14.

The response time of these instruments is suitable for clinical use and, as soon as a compact robust instrument with a stable laser source is produced, it will provide a viable alternative to absorption spectrometers.

### *Mass spectrometry*

The respiratory mass spectrometer has for many years provided the laboratory gold standard for measurement of respiratory gases. It is both specific and quantitative. Although the original research instrument has been developed to be much more user friendly, able to be used close to the patient as well as for multi-site time sharing, the rapid development of the instruments described above has meant that the mass spectrometer remains largely a research tool.

Mass spectrometers have three major components:

1. A vacuum pump continuously aspirates the sample gas through a capillary into the sample chamber.
2. A very high vacuum pump ($10^{-6}$ bar) draws a tiny proportion of the sample gas through a very small aperture (molecular leak) where it enters an ionization chamber. This is shown in Figure 39.15. The sample molecules are then ionized in an electric field. Ionization means that the molecules now possess an electrical charge and, because they are moving, they generate a magnetic field. They can therefore be attracted or repelled by another electromagnetic field. In the modern instruments the ions are accelerated to and fro by an oscillating electromagnetic field comprising direct and alternating current (DC and AC) components. This electronic gate is known as a quadrupole unit and is shown in Figure 39.16. It can be tuned so that only those ions travelling for a given distance in a given direction can get through the gate into the detector before the polarity of the magnetic field is reversed. The distance travelled by these ions in unit time is determined by their mass and the force of attraction of the electric charge. The ions are thus separated according to their mass : charge ratio.
3. The ions that get through the quadrupole are then collected on a detector. The signal is subsequently amplified and processed to give the desired information. The number of ions detected per unit time is a measure of the concentration of the

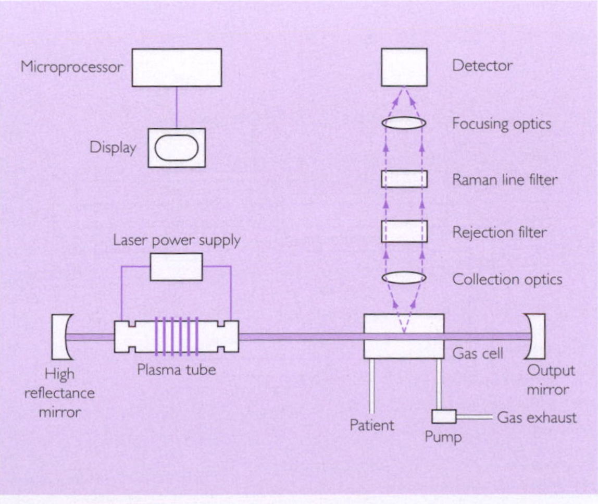

**Figure 39.14** The principle of Raman spectrometry. (Adapted from Westenskow DR *et al. Anesthesiology* 1989;70:350.)

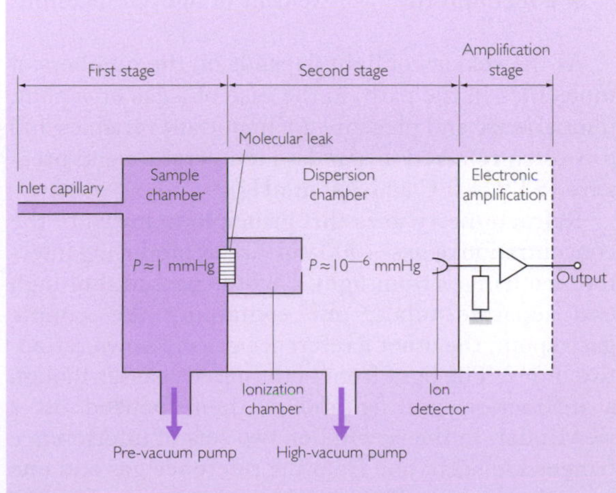


**Figure 39.15** Schematic diagram of a respiratory mass spectrometer. (Adapted from Scheid P. Respiratory mass spectrometry. In: *Measurements in Clinical Respiratory Physiology*. London: Academic Press, 1983: 131.)

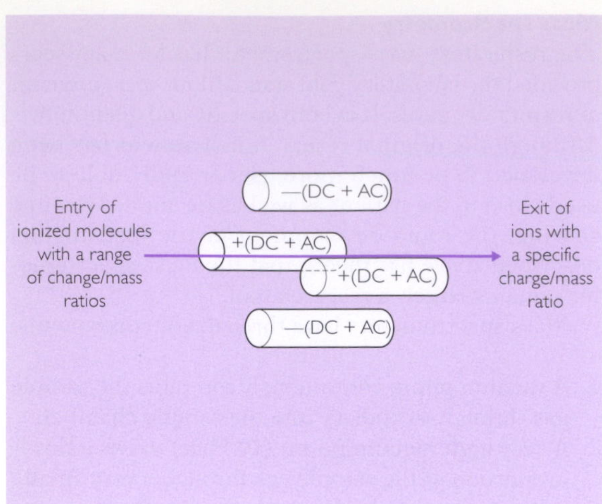


**Figure 39.16** Diagrammatic representation of a quadrupole unit. The quadrupole rods surround the ionization chamber in the second stage of Figure 39.15.

ions in the sample. The ion gate can be tuned to allow only one component through at a time, but this tuning can be altered rapidly to effectively allow simultaneous monitoring of several gases.

Each ionized expired or anaesthetic gas or vapour has a unique mass : charge ratio except $CO_2$ and $N_2O$, both with a mass : charge ratio of 44. They can, however, be distinguished from one another because the process of ionization causes fragmentation of the molecules into other molecular forms and elements. This fragmentation always produces the same proportion of a particular breakdown product which can be used as an indirect assay.

### *Refractometry*

Light travels fastest in a vacuum. When it passes through transparent physical matter it is slowed down, the degree of slowing being proportional to the number of molecules in its path.

$$\text{The refractive index of a medium } (\mu) = \frac{\text{Velocity of light in a vacuum.}}{\text{Velocity of light in medium}}$$

As the velocity of light depends on the numbers of molecules in the path, in the case of a gas or vapour, temperature and pressure are important variables and μ is often referred to standard temperature and pressure (STP = 0°C and 760 mmHg).

Refractometry uses this principle to measure the concentration of gases and vapours by producing interference fringes from light. Light is passed thorough two separate tubes, one containing the sample gas/vapour, the other a reference gas of known refractive index. The light from both sources passes though a diffraction grating and is then focused on a viewfinder. In the viewfinder, two sets of interference fringes are seen: one from the reference gas and one from the test gas. The fringes are displaced relative to each other if the gas compositions are different. A glass plate or prism, the effective thicknesses of which varies with rotation, is placed in the path of the beam from the sample. The rotation of the glass plate required to bring the interference fringe patterns together can be calibrated for each gas or vapour, and a numerical result given as a concentration of gas/vapour at STP.

The Rayleigh refractometer, a laboratory gold-standard instrument, is a bulky device over 1 metre long, but it is very accurate and is the factory standard for the calibration of instruments delivering vapours of known identity. Portable refractometers, which use prisms to reduce the size while maintaining the optical pathlength, are widely used in industry and mining, and have been applied to anaesthesia. Such an instrument is shown diagrammatically in Figure 39.17.

### *Physical methods based on solubility*

The Engstom EMMA uses the change in resonant frequency with change in mass of a piezo-electric crystal (see Chapter 38, Figure 38.57) coated with an absorbent silicone oil to measure concentrations of anaesthetic agents. The mass of volatile agent dissolving in the oil is proportional to its partial pressure (Henry's law).

A similar principle applies in the Drager Narkotest. The change in the elasticity of silicone rubber bands by the adsorption of anaesthetic agents is used as a crude method of measurement of the concentration of the agent.

Neither of these methods now meets contemporary standards of measurement.

## THE MEASUREMENT OF $Po_2$

### Paramagnetic $O_2$ analysis

$O_2$ is paramagnetic, which means that it is attracted to a magnetic field. This property is the result of unpaired electrons in the outer shell that are able to generate a magnetic field of their own. Nitrogen is a weakly diamagnetic gas, which is repelled by a magnetic field. This difference between nitrogen and $O_2$ is the basis of the action of the paramagnetic $O_2$ analyser (PMOA).

In the original PMOA there were two glass nitrogen-filled spheres arranged like a dumb-bell (Figure 39.18).

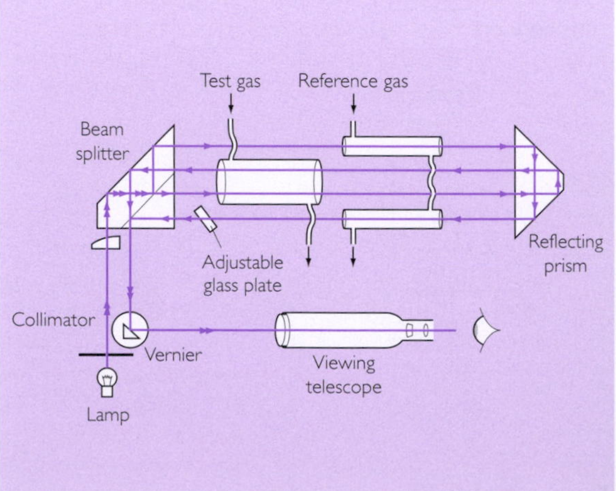


**Figure 39.17** Diagrammatic representation of a portable refractometer. (Adapted from Hulands GH and Nunn JF. *Br J Anaesth* 1970;42:1051.)

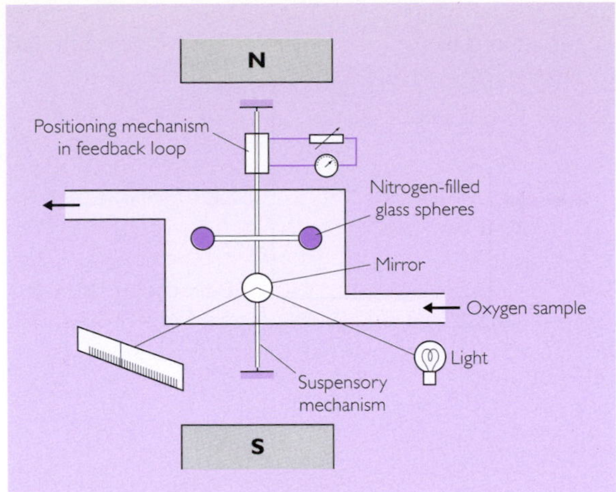


**Figure 39.18** Diagrammatic representation of a paramagnetic $O_2$ analyser. N, north pole; S, south pole.

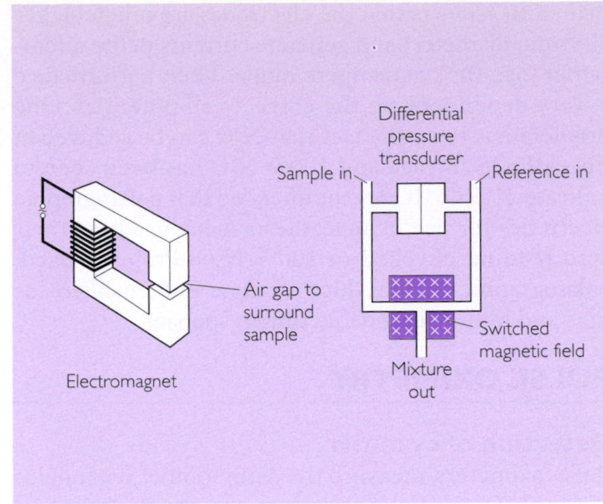


**Figure 39.19** Diagrammatic representation of a rapid paramagnetic $O_2$ analyser using an oscillating electromagnetic field. (Adapted from McPeak H *et al.* *Anaesthesia* 1988;43:1035.)

The dumb-bell was suspended in a gas-filled measuring cell between the poles of a strong magnet on a tensioned suspension. When $O_2$-containing gas is drawn through such a cell, the molecules of $O_2$ are attracted to the centre of the magnetic field and displace the glass spheres. The mirror on the suspension deflects, and its rotation can be calibrated against the partial pressure of $O_2$. The measurement can be made either by allowing the light beam to traverse a circumferential scale, or as shown in Figure 39.18, by using a feedback loop to keep the beam position constant. When this is done, the current (or voltage) in the feedback loop, which is required to prevent the movement of the beam by applying an adverse torque to the suspensory mechanism, becomes the measure of $O_2$ concentration.

The PMOA possesses an accuracy of approximately 0.1% $O_2$ which can be improved by the use of a digital voltmeter. It does, however, respond too slowly to follow breath-by-breath variations, the 95% response time being of the order of 1 min.

In more recent designs, the permanent magnet has been substituted by an electromagnet that cycles at approximately 110 Hz. The principle is shown diagrammatically in Figure 39.19. Background reference gas (usually atmospheric) and sampled gas are drawn through the oscillating magnetic field and very small (20–50 μbar) pressure fluctuations occur. These are transduced by a small microphone acting as a differential pressure transducer. The pressure differences measured are linearly related to the differential concentration of $O_2$.

The device is sensitive to changes in temperature and there is a small $N_2O$ effect (under-reading by approximately 1.5% with 100% $N_2O$). It is, however, very stable, has a practical extraction rate of 100 ml/min, and has a greatly improved 95% response time of 150 ms. This makes breath-by-breath analysis possible.

### Fuel cells

The principle of the fuel cell is that the current between an anode and cathode depends on the partial pressure of $O_2$ ($PO_2$) at the cathode. Fuel cells are used in anaesthesia and intensive care to measure inspired $O_2$ concentrations.

The cathode reaction is identical to that of a polarographic electrode:

$$O_2 + 4e^- + 2H_2O \rightarrow 4OH^-.$$

A typical cell is shown diagrammatically in Figure 39.20. There is surprisingly little literature on their performance. In general they have an accuracy of a few percent and are too slow for breath-by-breath analysis, a typical equilibration response to a step change in the partial pressure of $O_2$ being almost a minute. All fuel cells are temperature sensitive and compensation in the output signal may be provided by a thermistor. As the element is consumed in the reaction, a fuel cell's life is reduced by the measurement of high $PO_2$ values.

### Polarography

This is identical in principle to the method used for the determination of $PO_2$ in blood described later. The

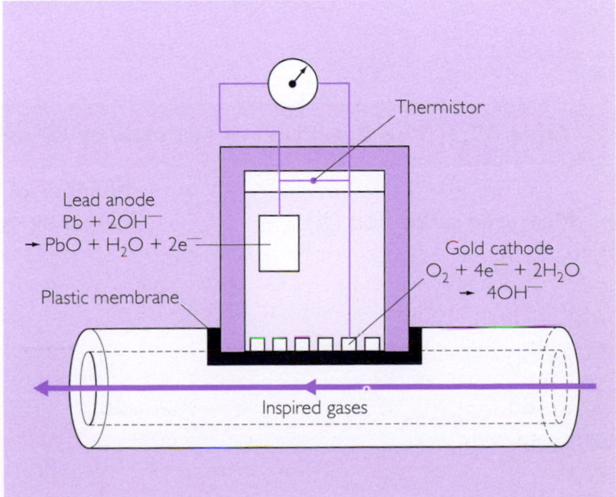


**Figure 39.20** A fuel cell for measuring the partial pressure of $O_2$.

main difference is that the electrodes are much bigger (1–2 mm diameter) and generate currents in the micro- rather than the nanoampere range. Their performance is very dependent on the correct cell potential. One problem has been the fact that $N_2O$ can be reduced at the cathode surface and 100% $N_2O$ has been seen to indicate 21% $O_2$. It is recommended that polarographic electrodes for use in anaesthesia machines have their zero reading checked in 100% $N_2O$. Properly used, polarographic cells produce accurate and reliable readings and have a reasonable time response.

## PULSE OXIMETRY

### Detection of cyanosis

Pulse oximeters measure the saturation of haemoglobin with $O_2$ and are therefore essentially 'cyanosis monitors'. Detecting cyanosis by eye has been proved many times to be unreliable. The fundamental work was done over 50 years ago by Comroe and Bothelho. They allowed 89 experienced observers, under ideal conditions, to indicate when cyanosis occurred in fit subjects made progressively hypoxic. The results are shown in Table 39.3.

It is clear from Table 39.3 that clinical observation is a 'soft' end-point, and explains why the use of pulse oximetry to measure oxygenation is now mandatory in many hospitals.

### Principle of action of oximeter probes

The principle of the pulse oximeter is based on the differential absorption of two different wavelengths of light by oxygenated and deoxygenated haemoglobin according to the Beer–Lambert law. If one imagines shining a light through a glass container full of coloured fluid, it becomes apparent that the amount of light transmitted through the container will depend on (Figure 39.21):

- the length of light path ($L$), i.e. the size of the container;
- the concentration of the dye or chromophore ($C$) (or in the case of blood haemoglobin);
- the specific absorption of the dye or chromophore for a particular wavelength of light (β).

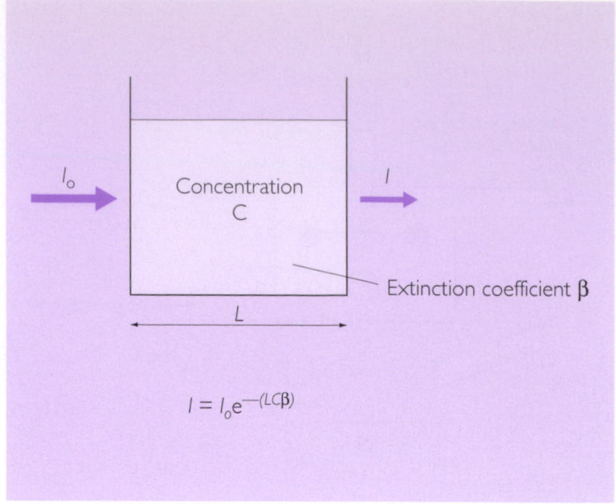


**Figure 39.21** The attenuation of incident light by the Beer–Lambert law.

$L$, $C$, and, β multiplied together represent the absorbance or optical density of the medium. β is known as the molecular extinction coefficient (also called the molar absorption coefficient) and is constant for a specific solute (chromophore) at a specific wavelength.

As the light passes through the medium, the probability of absorption depends on the probability of a collision between the light quanta and the chromophore. At any one section of the absorbing medium, the incidence of collisions is proportional to the number of light quanta, i.e. to the intensity of the light. Consequently, there is an exponential decay (see Chapter 37, Figure 37.15) in the number of quanta available for interaction as the light is transmitted through the chromophores of the absorbing medium. Combining the principle of absorption at a particular cross-section with the exponential decay results in the Beer–Lambert law where:

$$\text{Emergent light } (I) = \text{Incident light } (I_O) \times e^{-(LC\beta)}.$$

Taking logarithms gives:

$$\log (I_O/I) = LC\beta.$$

**Table 39.3 The detection of cyanosis by 89 experienced observers under ideal lighting conditions**

| Measured saturation (%) | Number of observers detecting cyanosis | Percentage of observers detecting cyanosis |
|---|---|---|
| 96–100 | 1 | 1.1 |
| 91–95 | 11 | 12.1 |
| 86–90 | 20 | 22.5 |
| 81–85 | 26 | 29.2 |
| 76–85 | 11 | 12.3 |
| < 75 | 20 | 22.5 |

Data from Comroe JH and Botelho S. *Am J Med Sci* 1947;214:1.

For this law to hold good, the light must be monochromatic, in a parallel beam, and directed perpendicularly to the chamber. There should be no scattering (reflection and refraction) of light. The term 'absorbance' and not 'absorption' is used because, strictly speaking, the light is absorbed and then much of it is re-transmitted by radiation.

In classic *in vitro* or bench oximetry, two or more lights of different wavelengths are shone through a cuvette containing the sample of blood. The length of the light path $L$ (the cuvette) and the concentration of haemoglobin are constant. The extinction coefficient β (Figure 39.22) will vary for the different wavelengths. This differential absorbance by the sample for light of different wavelengths is then used to compute the percentage of the species of haemoglobin present in the sample.

The pulse oximeter by contrast measures *changes* in the light coming out with each pulse. It is essentially a two-wavelength plethysmograph which assumes the presence of only two types of haemoglobin, i.e. oxygenated and reduced haemoglobin.

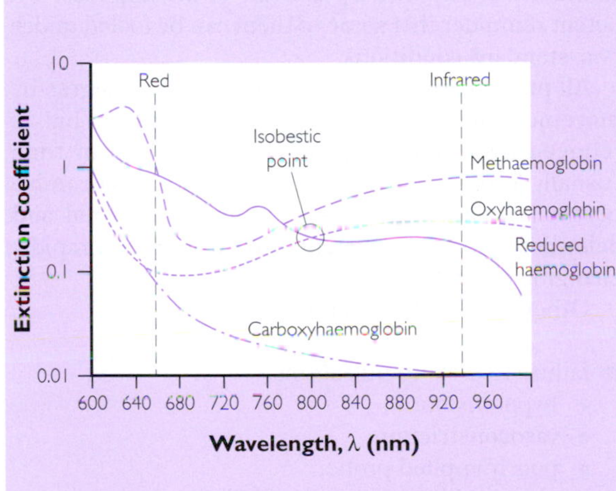


**Figure 39.22** Extinction coefficients for various types of haemoglobin. (Adapted from Tremper KK and Barker SJ. *Anesthesiology* 1989;70:98.)

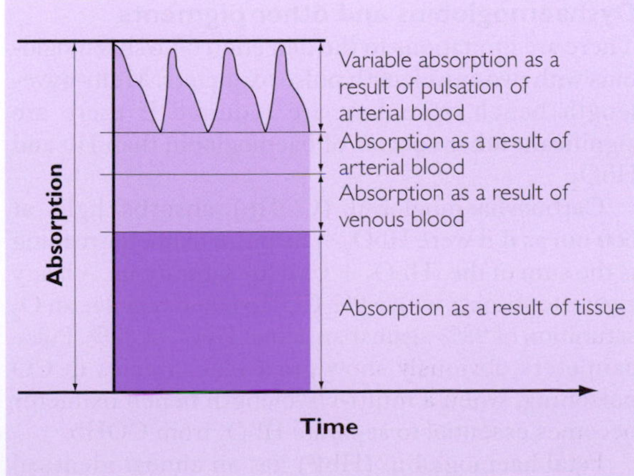


**Figure 39.23** The absorption of light through a finger between the emitter and receiver of a pulse oximeter plotted against time.

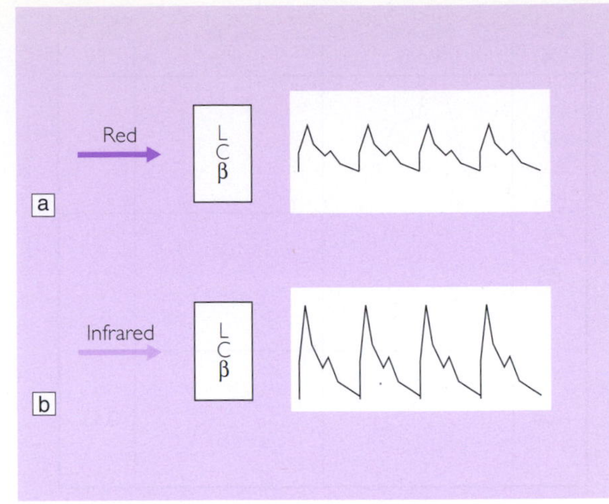


**Figure 39.24** The absorption by light of a single sample of haemoglobin in the (a) red and (b) infrared regions.

Figures 39.23 and 39.24 show the principle of action. Monochromatic lights of two different wavelengths are sequentially transmitted (but so rapidly that they are effectively simultaneous) and detected through a finger or other suitable appendage. The change in the transmitted light is processed and displayed as the familiar pulse plethysmographic waveform. For each light source, if the patient remains well oxygenated, the length of the light path, $L$, is the only factor that changes. $C$ and β, the other components of absorbance, are constant. The length of the light path is altered by the changes in the volume of the vascular bed with arterial pulsation. This effect is shown in Figure 39.16, where it can be seen that the variability resulting from arterial blood forms only a minor component in the full pattern of absorbance.

When the light of two wavelengths is shone through the tissues, the output is two pulsatile traces (Figure 39.24). The oximeter records a change in light transmission as a change in the pulse waveform amplitude of transmission, which decreases with increased volume of the vascular bed. The waveforms A and B (Figure 39.24) are identical to each other in every respect except amplitude. This difference in amplitude is the result of the difference in β, the extinction coefficient of the haemoglobin for the particular wavelength of light being used. The absorption of red and infrared light at different oxyhaemoglobin concentrations is shown in Figure 39.25 and the 'real-time' response of the pulse oximeter in Figure 39.26. The relative magnitude of each transmitted signal is determined by the extinction coefficient at the given wavelength.

The *ratio* of the amplitudes of the pulsatile components (Figure 39.26) is used to estimate the relative amounts of deoxy- and oxyhaemoglobin, from which the arterial saturation is computed. Most modern pulse oximeters have red: infrared absorbance ratios stored in a table. The computation is made, on an empirical basis, by calibration against healthy volunteers desaturated to an inspired $O_2$ concentration of approximately 15%.

In a pulse oximeter, the two light-emitting diodes (LEDs) – one emitting red (about 660 nm) and the

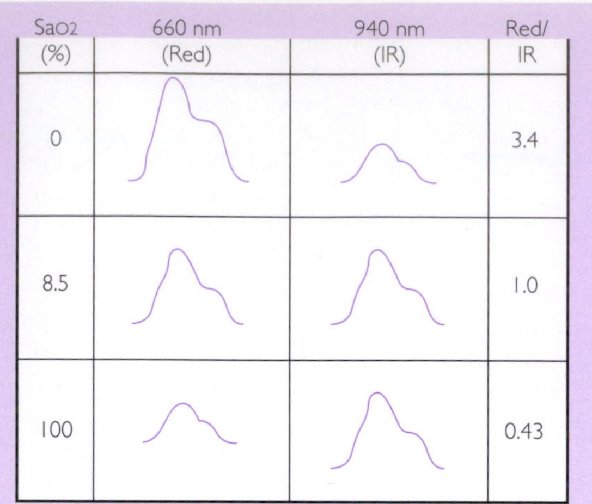

Sao2 (%)
660 nm (Red)
940 nm (IR)
Red/IR
0
3.4
8.5
1.0
100
0.43


**Figure 39.25** The absorption of red and infrared light at different oxyhaemoglobin concentrations. $SaO_2$, $O_2$ saturation; Red/IR, ratio of absorption in red and infrared regions. (Adapted from Hutton P and Fletcher R. Pulse oximetry. In: Hutton P, Prys-Roberts C, eds. *Monitoring in Anaesthesia and Intensive Care*. London: Saunders, 1994, 234.)

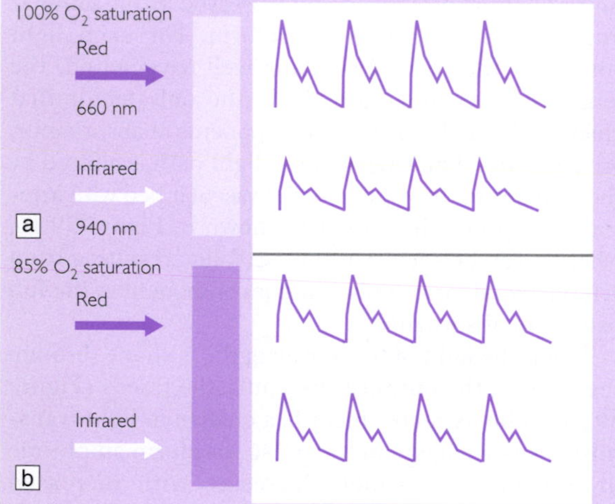


**Figure 39.26** The transmitted signals from the red and infrared wavelengths at $O_2$ saturations of (a) 100% and (b) 85%.

other infrared (about 940 nm) wavelength – are illuminated, in turn, at frequencies that vary with the manufacturer, but they may be as high as several hundred hertz. A third phase, with both LEDs switched off, permits the oximeter to detect and allow for extraneous and background light. The photodetector cannot distinguish between the different wavelengths, but it does not need to, because only the *ratio* of the amplitudes of changes in the light outputs for the two wavelengths is needed. By only measuring the pulsatile *changes* in the signal, the background absorption of light by fingernails, venous blood, tissue, bone, and melanin are eliminated (see Figure 39.23). The *changes* in light transmission are assumed to be caused by the influx of arterialized blood, not only because of increased volume but also because the erythrocytes expose more of their long axis and line up more perpendicularly to the light source with the increased velocity of arterial flow.

### Calibration

Microprocessors in pulse oximeters use an algorithm to compute arterial saturation, which contains various correction factors. It assumes that all pulsatile flow comes from the arterial system and that the only haemoglobin present is HbA, in either oxygenated or deoxygenated form. Some have a correction factor for CO, usually around 2%.

Oximeters are not calibrated in the laboratory. The validity of the algorithm is developed and tested on human volunteers breathing hypoxic mixtures of $O_2$ and nitrogen. Modern instruments have been demonstrated to be accurate with a standard error of 2% between 70% and 100% $O_2$ saturation. Below this, the accuracy decreases, but it would be unethical to subject humans to breathing more hypoxic mixtures of gases.

### Sources of inaccuracy

Pulse oximeters can suffer from optical illusions. The demonstration of an oximeter probe attached to a drip chamber of a saline infusion, with the saline showing a saturation of 85% and a pulse rate of the drip rate, is a potent reminder that some of them can be fooled under non-standard conditions.

All pulse oximeters are affected to some degree by movement artefact and signal variability. This is reduced by averaging signals over a period of time (usually 5–10 s). The averaging time is a compromise between having increased smoothing of the signal, and delay between the occurrence and display of a rapidly changing saturation.

Other causes of inaccuracy are:

- failure to pick up pulsations:
  - hypotension;
  - vasoconstriction;
  - poorly applied probe;
  - electrical interference, e.g. diathermy;
- increased scattering of light:
  - venous pulsations;
  - movement artefact;
  - bones and nails.

### Dyshaemoglobins and other pigments

There are limitations to the detection of dyshaemoglobins with two-wavelength pulse oximeters. Multi-wavelength bench oximeters are required if there are significant other species of haemoglobin than Hb and $HbO_2$.

Carboxyhaemoglobin (COHb) absorbs light at 660 nm as if it were $HbO_2$. The pulse oximeter reading is the sum of the ($HbO_2$ + COHb) saturations. A heavy cigarette smoker with a 9% COHb could register an $O_2$ saturation of 98% against an actual $HbO_2$ of 89%. Pulse oximeters obviously show great inaccuracies in CO poisoning, when a multi-wavelength bench oximeter becomes essential to separate $HbO_2$ from COHb.

Fetal haemoglobin (HbF) has an almost identical absorption spectrum to adult haemoglobin at the measured wavelengths, so the accuracy of the pulse oximeter in measuring saturation is essentially unaffected by the presence of HbF.

Methaemoglobin has identical absorptions at 660 and 940 nm. Pulse oximeters interpret this 1 : 1 absorption ratio as a saturation of 85% (see Figure 39.25).

Methylene blue and indocyanine green absorb light in the 660-nm bands. If either is injected into a patient the blood appears more blue and the oximeter will under-read. Bilirubin, which principally absorbs light in the green–yellow spectrum, has little detectable effect on the accuracy of pulse oximeters.

Skin pigmentation should, theoretically, not affect the accuracy of pulse oximetry, but the poorer signal-to-noise ratio, caused by decreased signal strength, has been shown to affect the accuracy of some pulse oximeters in some studies. Blue nail varnish can cause underestimation of $O_2$ saturations of up to 6%. Placing the probe on sideways may overcome this problem.

### Clinical pitfalls in pulse oximetry

The shape of the oxyhaemoglobin dissociation curve (see Chapters 21, 31 and 52) means that $PaO_2$ has to suffer a considerable fall to change the $O_2$ saturation. Depending on the state of the circulation, there can be a significant time lag, (usually > 20 s), before central changes in blood oxygenation are reflected in a peripheral probe. The ear-lobe probe gives earlier warning of changes in the $O_2$ saturation than the finger probe. The use of averaging and smoothing circuits can increase this lag time considerably. *For these reasons, the pulse oximeter must not be relied on to provide an early indication of the failure of the $O_2$ supply, as a disconnection monitor, or to confirm correct endotracheal intubation.* Furthermore, a patient breathing high inspired $O_2$ concentrations may take several minutes to desaturate centrally, even if apnoea occurs.

The pulse oximeter gives no indication of the adequacy of ventilation. With high inspired concentrations of $O_2$ it is possible to have satisfactory $O_2$ saturations in the presence of very high levels of $CO_2$. *Pulse oximetry alone is therefore a poor indicator of the bellows function of the lungs.*

The amplitude of the pulse waveform may not reflect the pulse volume because a number of commercial instruments automatically alter the height of the displayed pulse wave in order to fill the screen. *The displayed height of the wave may therefore not change in spite of significant changes in pulse volume.*

Many pulse oximeters have artefact recognition programmes. Although generally useful, these can sometimes mistakenly indicate a severe dysrhythmia or cardiac arrest as 'probe off patient'. *The rule is, as for capnography, if an abnormal reading is displayed, check the patient first and the instrument last.* There may be a fault in reality!

## MEASUREMENT OF pH AND DISSOLVED GASES IN BLOOD

During the past 30 years or so, the ability to measure pH and blood gas values accurately has been of enormous benefit in the understanding and treatment of various pathological processes.

Although differing methods of measuring pH and blood gases are available, this section concentrates on the electrochemical methods used by the machines commonly found in the clinical areas of hospitals, and which are used by anaesthetists in their day-to-day work. The interpretation of the results obtained is aided by a basic understanding of what these machines actually measure, how they do it, their limitations, and common sources of error. The blind acceptance of any monitoring equipment as a magic 'black box' that produces infallible results may result in inappropriate clinical action being taken.

### General principles

An electrochemical cell consists of two electrodes (Figures 39.27 and 39.28) which are made to interact with a specific substance in solution. The mechanism that ensures specificity of action is usually a membrane that is permeable to a selected ionic species. A signal is produced from the electrodes, which passes through a transducer to a signal processor. This, in turn, calculates the result in the desired form, and then displays or prints it.

Transducers may function in two ways. First, the transducer may simply measure the potential difference or voltage between the two electrodes ('potentiometric') (Figure 39.27). Alternatively, a voltage can be actively applied to the electrodes and the resultant current flow measured ('amperometric') (Figure 39.28).

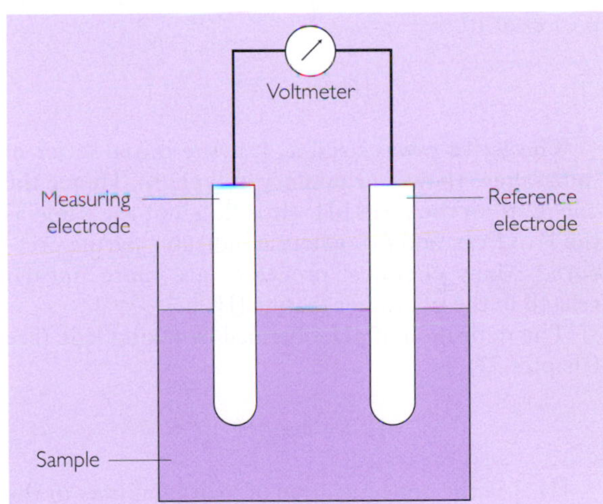


**Figure 39.27** The principle of the potentiometric cell.

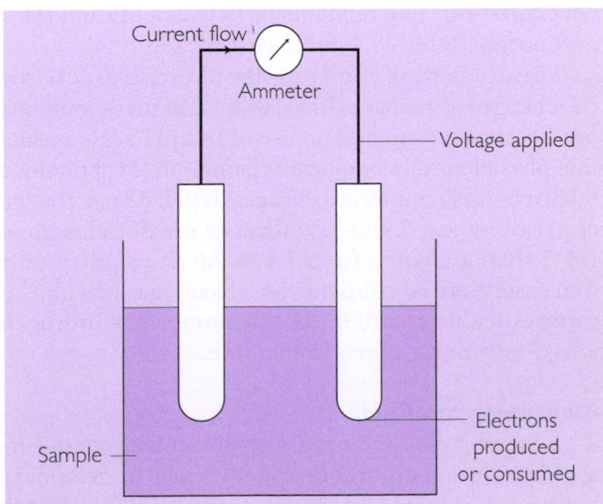


**Figure 39.28** The principle of the amperometric cell.

Strictly speaking, what is measured is the activity of an ion (i.e. the numbers of ions that are free to interact in a solution) rather than the concentration of the ion. In weak solutions (which are common in physiological fluids), the activity is nearly the same as concentration, but in concentrated solutions the activity is less than the concentration.

### Measurement of hydrogen ion concentration (pH)

Acidity is still usually expressed as pH, a scale that has some limitations. Acidity and the pH scale are therefore briefly discussed before describing the measurement of hydrogen ion concentration $[H^+]$.

#### *Definition*

An acid is defined as being capable of donating a hydrogen ion, and a base as being capable of accepting a hydrogen ion. The degree of acidity depends on the number of hydrogen ions present in solution, which in general can vary very widely, from small numbers present in low concentrations of weak acids (weak acids dissociate poorly) to high numbers in concentrated strong acids (strong acids are highly dissociated). To make the expression of this wide range of concentrations easier, a logarithmic scale is used. The scale was first developed by Sorenson, who described $[H^+]$ in terms of exponents, or powers of 10.

$$[H^+] = 10^{-p}.$$

The letter p was used as it is the initial letter of 'puissance' (power or potency in French). Hence the use of 'p' in the term pH. (It is thus not the same as the P in $P\text{CO}_2$ and $P\text{O}_2$ where it indicates partial pressure.) Many chemical processes are more linearly related to the pH rather than to $[H^+]$.

The definition of pH, obtained by taking logs (see Chapter 37), is:

$$\text{pH} = -\log_{10}[H^+].$$

$[H^+]$ is the concentration of hydrogen ions in the solution, or more precisely their activity. The use of a negative logarithmic scale means that there is a tenfold difference in $[H^+]$ for every full unit of pH change, and a lower pH value corresponds to a greater hydrogen ion concentration. The relationship between pH and $[H^+]$ is shown in Table 39.4 and Figure 39.29.

The necessity of employing the pH scale to describe the changes of acidity in blood acid–base measurements has been questioned. The use of the pH scale means that physiologically significant changes in $[H^+]$ produce relatively small numerical changes in pH. Also, a change of pH from, say, 7.4 to 7.2 reflects a greater change in $[H^+]$ than a change from 7.4 to 7.6. It requires only minor software adjustments for a blood–gas machine to express acidity as either pH or nanomoles of hydrogen ions. Many now will read either unit.

#### *Measurement of pH*

The sensing electrode has a very thin hydrogen-ion-specific glass membrane, which forms the boundary between the inside of the electrode and the sample (Figure 39.30). Inside the electrode there is a buffer solution that holds the inner $[H^+]$ fixed. If the hydrogen ions in the sample are of a different concentration, a difference in potential develops across the membrane. The membrane is hydrogen ion specific, so the presence of other ions has no effect, the size of the potential difference depending only on the $[H^+]$ in the sample. The circuit is completed via a reference elec-

**Table 39.4 The relationship between pH and hydrogen ion concentration $[H^+]$**

| pH | $[H^+]$ (nmol/L) |
|---|---|
| 6.0 | 1000 |
| 7.0 | 100 |
| 7.2 | 63 |
| 7.4 | 40 |
| 7.6 | 25 |
| 8.0 | 10 |

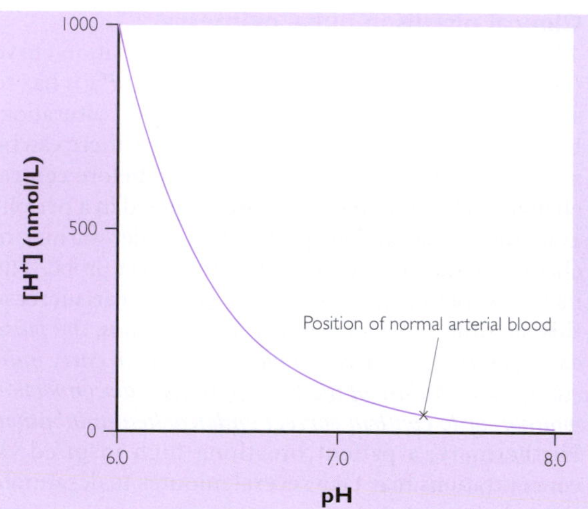


**Figure 39.29** The relationship between pH and hydrogen ion concentration $[H^+]$.

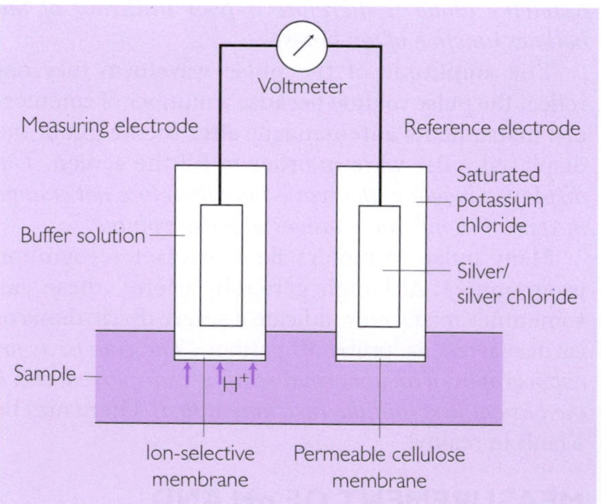


**Figure 39.30** The principle of the pH electrode.

trode, which contains a saturated potassium chloride (KCl) solution. In this system, there is no actual flow of hydrogen ions into the measuring cell, so there is no actual flow of current. It is the potential difference, or voltage, that is measured. The whole electrode assembly is kept constant at 37°C.

Thus, the only variable potential developed in this system is at the hydrogen-ion-specific membrane. The potential, $V$, is given by the Nernst equation:

$$V = K \log [H^+]$$

where $K = (R \times T \times 2.3)/(Z \times F)$, and R is the ideal gas constant, $T$ the absolute temperature, $Z$ the valency (1 for hydrogen), and $F$ the Faraday constant.

At a body temperature of 37°C, $K = 0.061$. A difference in pH between the electrodes of 0.1 will therefore produce a potential difference of 6 mV. Calibration of pH electrodes is by the use of standard test solutions spanning the physiological range.

In a modern blood–gas machine, the appearance of the pH electrode will be similar to that shown in Figure 39.31.

The reference electrode used on modern machines contains a silver/silver chloride wire surrounded by saturated potassium chloride (Figure 39.32). The solution is kept fully saturated by the presence of a block of solid KCl in the electrode. As the KCl is saturated, its concentration does not alter, and the electrical potential is constant. Blood-gas machines usually use a single reference cell. It is used as the reference cell for both the pH and $CO_2$ sensors, and also with other sensors that may be present on the same machine. Sensors for ions such as sodium, potassium and calcium are very similar to the pH sensor described above. Changing the composition of the electrode membrane makes it specifically permeable to different ions.

### *Other methods of estimating pH*

*Dyes*

Indicator dyes and papers have been in use for many years, and still have use in such situations as confirming nasogastric tube placement. The accuracy of dyes may be improved by using light absorption techniques.

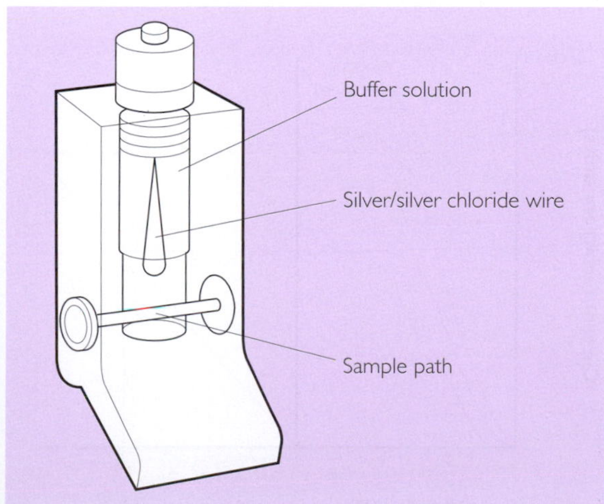


**Figure 39.31** The physical form of a modern pH electrode. (Courtesy of Chiron Diagnostics, Emeryville, CA, USA.)

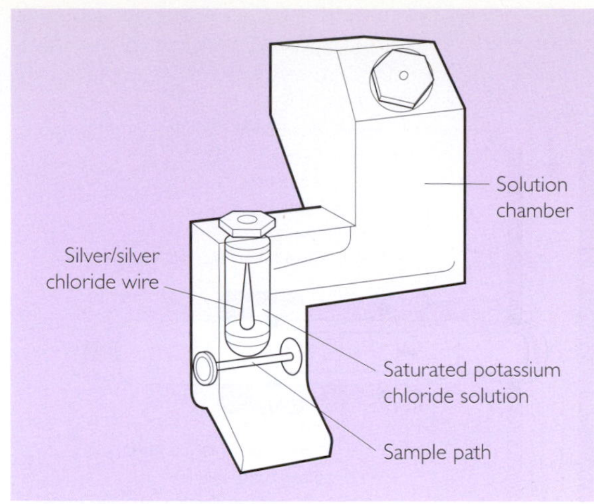


**Figure 39.32** The physical form of a modern reference electrode. (Courtesy of Chiron Diagnostics, Emeryville, CA, USA.)

Although this may apply to clear solutions, however, it is difficult to apply to blood.

*Indirect methods*

The pH can be calculated from a knowledge of the $P_{CO_2}$ and bicarbonate concentration using the Henderson–Hasselbach equation. In fact, in many blood–gas machines, bicarbonate is not measured, and it is more usual to turn the above situation around and calculate bicarbonate and other acid–base values from measured pH and $P_{CO_2}$ values (see below).

### Measurement of $P_{CO_2}$

The $CO_2$ electrode is a modified form of the pH electrode described above. $CO_2$ dissolved in the sample diffuses across a membrane permeable to the gas. It is shown in Figure 39.33. Inside the membrane is a solution of sodium bicarbonate and sodium chloride, where the following takes place:

$$CO_2 + H_2O \rightleftharpoons H_2CO_3 \rightleftharpoons H^+ + HCO_3^-.$$

The hydrogen ion formed by the reaction is then measured by an internal pH electrode, using the same reference electrode as the pH electrode described earlier. The potential difference reflects the pH change, which is related logarithmically to the $P_{CO_2}$ by the Henderson–Hasselbalch equation:

$$\mathrm{pH} = \mathrm{p}K + \log \frac{[HCO_3^-]}{[H_2CO_3]}$$

or, as the concentration of carbonic acid ($[H_2CO_3]$) is directly proportional to the partial pressure of $CO_2$ in solution:

$$\mathrm{pH} = \mathrm{p}K + \log \frac{[HCO_3^-]}{0.03 \times P_{CO_2}}$$

when $P_{CO_2}$ is in mmHg. Replace 0.03 with 0.23 when $P_{CO_2}$ is in kPa. The Henderson–Hasselbalch equation is discussed in more detail in Chapter 26.

Inside the electrode, where the temperature is fixed and there are no other buffer systems present, the p$K$

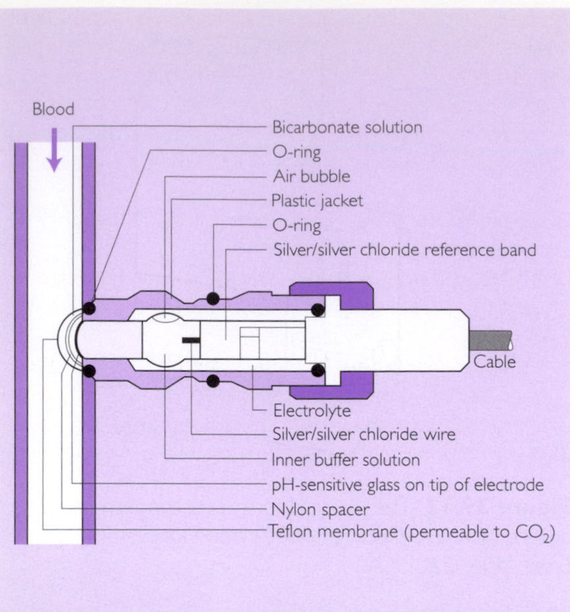


**Figure 39.33** A diagrammatic representation of the $PCO_2$ electrode.

is constant at 6.1, so the $PCO_2$ can be reliably calculated. It can be seen from the equations that the pH is related logarithmically to the $PCO_2$, so an anti-log amplification circuit is used to produce a linear relationship between signal and $PCO_2$.

$PCO_2$ electrodes are linear between about 1 kPa and 30 kPa. Their function depends on the integrity of the membrane, which is made from thin Teflon or silicone rubber. Speed of response declines if the membrane becomes coated with proteinaceous material; blood–gas machines automatically wash the electrodes at regular intervals. Calibration is from known gas concentrations, usually containing about 5% and 10% $CO_2$.

## Measurement of $PO_2$

The $O_2$ electrode (Clark's electrode) has a cathode that consists of a thin wire fused in a glass cylinder. The wire is usually platinum, although the other noble metals (gold or silver) may be used. A fixed voltage, usually of –0.6 V, is applied to this. Incorporated in the same unit is a reference anode, a silver/silver chloride wire in a solution of KCl and phosphate buffer. It is shown diagrammatically in Figure 39.34. $O_2$ diffuses onto the cathode through a Teflon or polypropylene membrane, where the voltage causes it to be reduced.

$$O_2 + 2H_2O + 4e^- \rightarrow 4\,OH^-.$$

The circuit is completed at the anode where the silver is oxidized. The reaction here is:

$$4Ag = 4Ag^+ + 4e^-$$
$$4Ag^+ + 4Cl^- = 4AgCl.$$

The $O_2$ electrode is amperometric, in that a current actually flows, and it is the amperage that is measured. For the current to be proportional to the $PO_2$, the electrode has to operate in its plateau region where all the

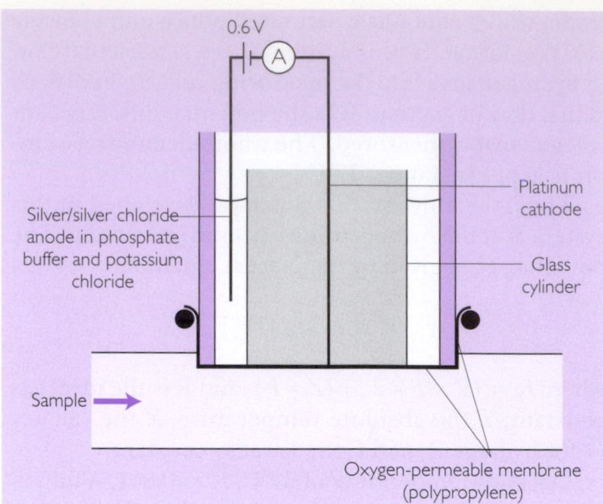


**Figure 39.34** A diagrammatic representation of an $O_2$ electrode.

$O_2$ at the membrane surface is measured, i.e. it is independent of the applied voltage. The principle of this is shown in Figure 39.35. Under these conditions, the rate of diffusion of the $O_2$ through the membrane, and hence the flow of current, is proportional to the $PO_2$, with a typical $PO_2$ of 13 kPa, producing a current of 1 nA.

The appearance of a modern $O_2$ electrode is shown in Figure 39.36. In an $O_2$ electrode, $O_2$ is actually consumed. To minimize this the cathode is made as small as possible. The consumption of $O_2$ by the cathode may cause a differential in readings between gas and liquid samples because, in liquids, the diffusion of $O_2$ to the cathode to replace that consumed is slower. Calibration is by known concentrations of gas spanning the physiological range of 0–20 kPa. A correction factor has to be applied when calibrating the blood–gas machine with liquids rather than with gases. Most blood–gas machines are not calibrated above 20 kPa.

## Sources of error in blood–gas machines

Despite the ease of use and accuracy of modern blood–gas machines, blood-gas analysis may be

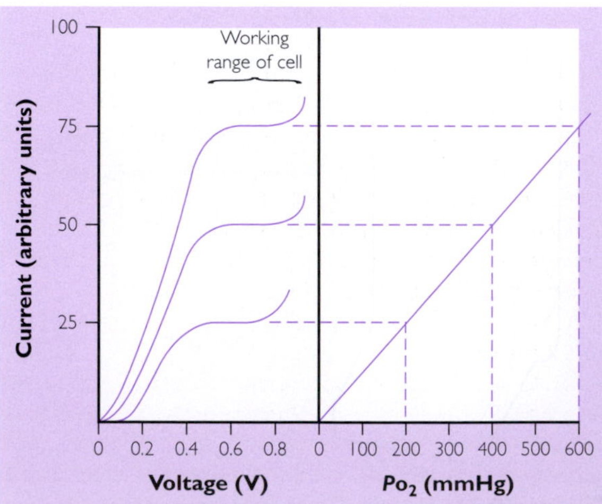


**Figure 39.35** The plateau region of an $O_2$ electrode and its relationship to the measured $PO_2$.

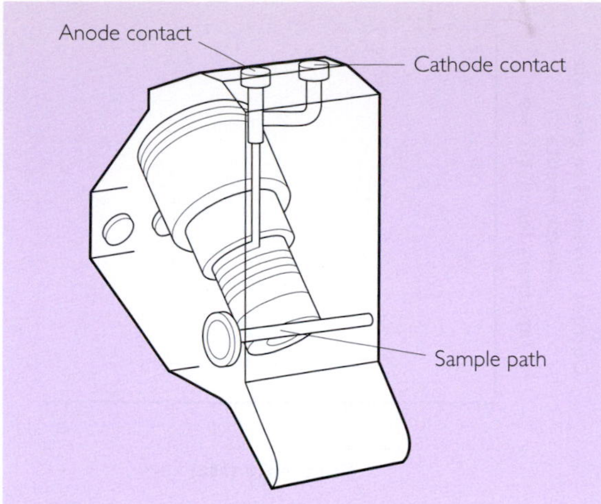


**Figure 39.36** The appearance of a modern $O_2$ electrode. (Courtesy of Chiron Diagnostics, Emeryville, CA, USA.)

erroneous. Clinical aspects are outside the scope of this chapter (see Chapter 26), but appropriate interpretation clearly depends on the knowledge of the source of the sample, whether arterial, venous, or mixed venous. The sample syringe should not contain excessive heparin or the pH result will be falsely low. The sample must be drawn anaerobically, and the syringe sealed, because air bubbles will affect the result. If the sample is not analysed immediately, metabolism will consume $O_2$ and produce $CO_2$ unless the syringe is kept on ice. (Although plastic is more permeable to $O_2$ than glass, in practice there is little difference between glass and plastic syringes.) Finally, electrode drift means that regular servicing and calibration of gas machines is essential.

The acid–base parameters measured by blood–gas machines are $P\text{CO}_2$, and pH. All other acid–base values given by the machine are calculated from these results. Bicarbonate is derived from the Henderson–Hasselbach equation described earlier. The accuracy of the bicarbonate estimation depends on the p$K$ having a value of 6.105. In fact, there is some variability from day to day, even in the same healthy individual, and p$K$ also varies with temperature and the effect of other organic buffering systems on the body. Hence, the true value of bicarbonate is known with less absolute reliability than the measured values of pH and $P\text{CO}_2$. The same applies to other variables such as base excess and standard bicarbonate, which are also calculated rather than actually measured (see Chapter 26).

Classically, measurements of pH, $P\text{CO}_2$, and $P\text{O}_2$ have been 'corrected' by the blood–gas machine if the patient's temperature differs from 37°C. It is now becoming more common not to correct acid–base values for temperature. The arguments are complex. The following is given as an example of one aspect of the problem.

In terms of acid–base, it should be noted that water has a pH of 7 only at 25°C. At lower temperatures, there is less dissociation into $H^+$ and $OH^-$. As the hydrogen activity is lower, the pH is raised. However, water is still neutral, because there are equal amounts of $H^+$ and $OH^-$ in solution. To correct the pH at low temperatures to 7 would imply a greater hydrogen ion activity, i.e. 'acidic water', which is clearly not the case. Maintenance of acid–base balance at different temperatures depends on a constant ratio between $H^+$ and $OH^-$, not on a constant pH. A full discussion of this complex area can be found in texts describing blood-gas management during cardiopulmonary bypass.

### Transcutaneous measurement of $P\text{CO}_2$ and $P\text{O}_2$ ($P\text{TCCO}_2$ and $P\text{TCO}_2$)

In the intensive care of babies, particularly neonates, transcutaneous measurement of $P\text{O}_2$ and $P\text{CO}_2$ is well established.

The electrode unit is approximately 1 cm in diameter and consists of concentric $P\text{CO}_2$ and $P\text{O}_2$ electrodes, which in principle function in the same way as those described earlier. In recent versions of the $P\text{CO}_2$ electrode, the fragile liquid-filled pH glass electrode is replaced with a pH-sensitive glass bonded to a ceramic material, which is more durable. The unit contains a heater that heats the patient's skin beneath it to 42–44°C, to 'arterialize' it, i.e. to cause vasodilatation and promote diffusion of gases through the skin. The electrode is held in close contract with the skin, and a contact gel or liquid excludes air. The skin surface $P\text{TCCO}_2$ and $P\text{TCO}_2$ differ from the true arterial values. However, they have a linear relationship that can be built into the calibration of the electrodes, so that the actual display approximates to the true arterial values.

The most suitable sites are on the chest below the clavicles or other central areas. The heated electrodes cause erythema, and the electrode site should be changed at least every 4 hours to prevent burns.

In practice, these electrodes function better on young patients with thinner skin than adults. Accuracy is impaired when the patient is vasoconstricted and hypoperfused. Regular comparison of their indicated values with true blood gases is desirable. However, they do have the great advantage of providing continuous measurement of trends. Furthermore, and importantly in neonates, the measurement of $P\text{TCO}_2$ detects hyperoxia, which pulse oximetry does not.

They have proved less satisfactory for use in anaesthesia, and there are other sources of inaccuracy. Halothane and $N_2O$ are reduced and produce falsely high readings of $P\text{TCO}_2$, and other volatiles have the same effect, although of lesser magnitude.

## ELECTRICAL SAFETY, DEFIBRILLATORS, AND PACEMAKERS

### Mains and earth

As described earlier in Chapter 38 (Figures 38.42 and 38.43), the mains supplies of electricity in the UK and the US use alternating currents of 50 Hz and 60 Hz respectively. This set frequency of current and voltage is a convenient time reference for fixed speed motors, machinery, and clocks. Alternating current enables the use of transformers to increase or decrease voltage. High voltages are used for long-distance transmission because it is more efficient (smaller current flow and heating effect), but is stepped down at the local substation because high voltages arc across switches more easily, and lower voltages are required for the domestic situation (Figure 39.37).

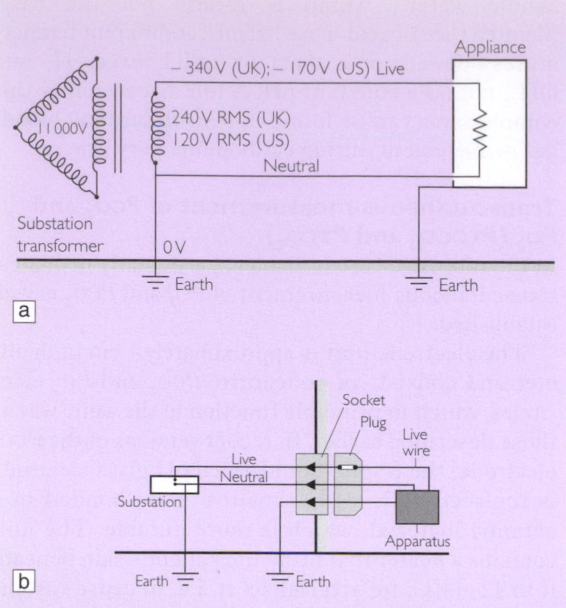


**Figure 39.37** The connection of a domestic appliance to the mains supply. (a) The schematic layout and (b) the physical distribution.

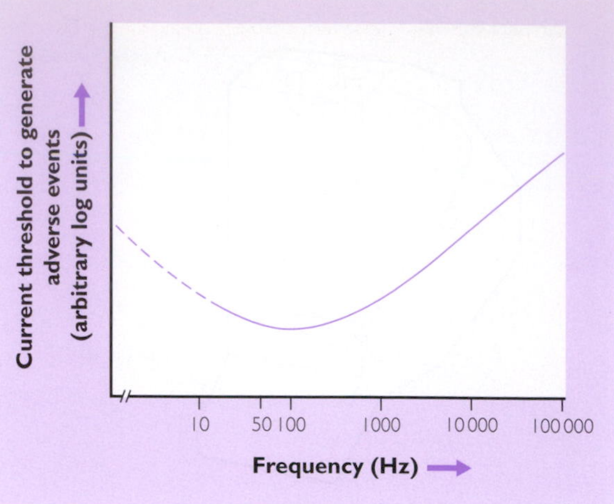


**Figure 39.38** The variation in the threshold for pathophysiological effects of electric current with frequency. Note that the threshold is lowest close to the mains frequency. (Adapted from Davey A, Moyle JTB, Ward CS. *Anaesthetic Equipment*, 3rd edn. London: Saunders, 1994, 336.)

Neither wire of the mains supply can truly be referred to as positive or negative. One of them is connected to earth at the generator and is called the neutral wire. Its potential stays almost at zero whereas that of the other 'live' wire varies sinusoidally (see Figure 38.43). An entirely separate earthing system (the normal earth) is used at the consumer site (Figure 39.37). Leakage currents resulting from capacitative coupling (the casing and the electrical elements act as plates of a capacitor) always occur and the low-resistance earth connection allows them to dissipate safely.

## Electric shock

The nature and extent of injuries following gross electrocution depend on:

- the voltage (usually the mains supply);
- the current (mA to A);
- the resistance of the pathway (skin, clothing);
- the duration of exposure (the threshold for fibrillation decreases as the period of current flow increases);
- the frequency of the current.

As shown in Figure 39.38, 50–60 Hz is particularly effective at producing cardiac problems. The risk of fibrillation diminishes as the frequency increases, and at 100 kHz or more, the frequency used in surgical diathermy, alternating currents have no fibrillating potential. Ventricular fibrillation (VF) can occur at a lower current in patients with myocardial disease or dysrhythmias. Note that it is current flow, not voltage, that kills. Many people receive shocks from static electricity with no ill effect.

The approximate thresholds for adverse effects are given in Table 39.5, and the effect of the magnitude and duration of the shock in Figure 39.39.

If the current flows through the body via two conductors (e.g. holding a live wire while touching a pipe connected to earth), the skin resistance will determine the amount of current. This can vary with the thickness of the skin and the degree of sweating from 1000 Ω up to 50 kΩ. Applying Ohm's law ($V = IR$), for a voltage of 240 V the current flowing may be as high as 240 mA (probably fatal) or as low as 4.5 mA (a painful shock, but unlikely to be fatal). If the current passes back to earth through high-resistance footwear, then the current flow could be even smaller.

## Protection against electric shock

The safety of medical electrical equipment is governed by the International Electrotechnical Standard 601 which, in the UK, corresponds to British Standard 5724. These standards classify equipment into three groups according to the means of protection against electrocution.

### *Class I*

Class I equipment has a connection from any conducting part that is accessible to the user (e.g. metal casing) to earth via the yellow and green wires of the mains supply. A fuse is also incorporated into the system (usually in the plug), so that, if a fault develops (e.g. a connection is made between the live supply and the casing [a short circuit]), a large current will flow, which melts the fuse and disconnects the equipment from the electrical supply (Figure 39.40).

Fuses are rated in amps (e.g. 3A, 5A, 13A) and the correct value as specified by the manufacturer must be used. The rating of a fuse does not indicate the current at which it will 'blow', but the maximum current it can survive for 1000 hours without deterioration.

### *Class II*

Class II equipment, also called double insulated, has all accessible parts protected by two layers of insulation (or reinforced insulation), so that there is no possibil-

**Table 39.5 Approximate response and thresholds for effects of a 50-Hz hand-held current**

| Total current flow (mA) | Effect |
|---|---|
| 0.5 | Perceptible shock (tingling) |
| 1–5 | Distinct shock, pain, mild muscle contraction |
| 5–15 | Sustained contraction, pain |
| 30 | 'No-let-go' threshold, increased cardiac output |
| 30–50 | Possible respiratory muscle paralysis, asphyxia |
| 100–150 | If current flow from hand to hand, current density through heart may provoke ventricular fibrillation |
| ≥ 1000 or greater | Tissue burning, cardiac standstill, severe burning |

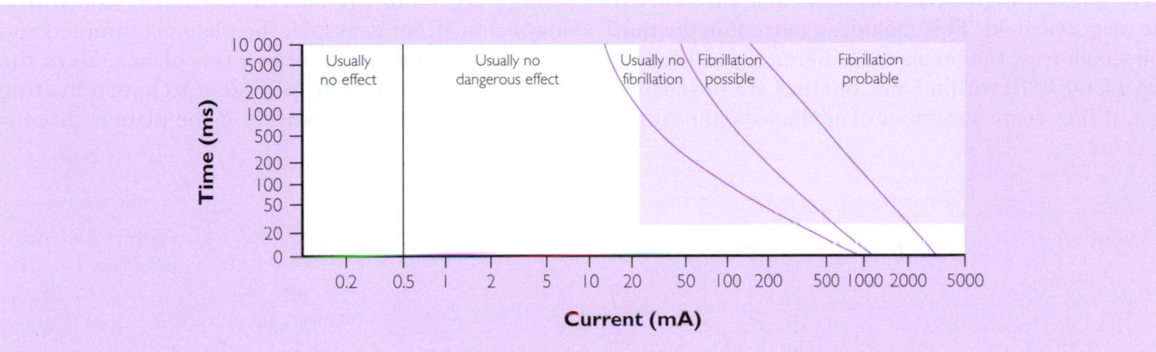


**Figure 39.39** The relationship between the time applied and current that produce a particular physiological effect from a mains supply. The shaded area represents the protection given by a current-operated earth leakage circuit breaker. Note that, in this instance, time is plotted vertically on a logarithmic scale. (Adapted from Davey A, Moyle JTB, Ward CS. *Anaesthetic Equipment*. London: Saunders, 1994, 331.)

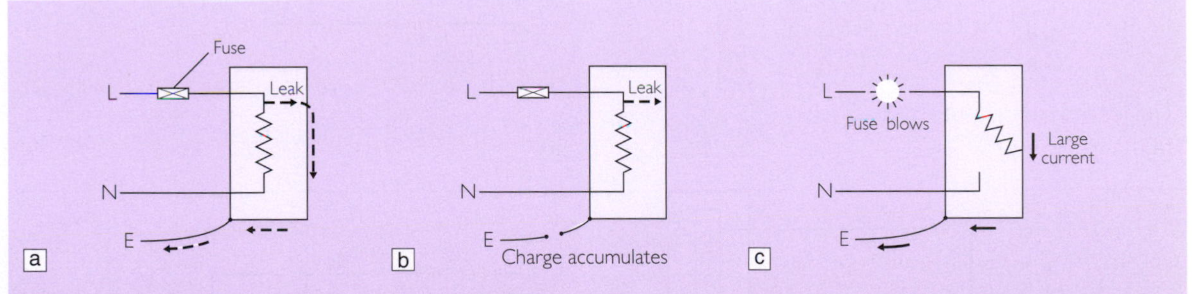


**Figure 39.40** (a) Class I equipment protected by an earth line and fuse. (b) Leakage currents caused by capacitative or inductive coupling normally dissipate via the earth line, but can accumulate to produce a small shock if the earth line is broken. (c) With an intact earth line, a major fault that allows the casing to become live will produce a large current flow down the earth linkage sufficient to blow the fuse in the live wire. L, live; N, neutral; E, earth.

ity of these parts becoming live if a fault occurs. A considerable amount of medical equipment is designed in this way. Earth wires are not needed for class II equipment.

### *Class III*

Class III is internally powered equipment which has its own power source, usually batteries. As a result of the low voltages used, the risk of a damaging shock is small.

### *Circuit breakers*

Improved protection from earth faults, especially if two faults develop, is provided by an earth leakage circuit breaker (ELCB). The essential feature for its action is a tripping coil which, when energized either directly or indirectly, releases a latching device that allows the circuit breaker to open and cut off the current to the faulty equipment. It will not operate when a short circuit occurs across live and neutral poles, or when a circuit is overloaded. For those faults, a fuse is still needed. It is important to stress that ELCBs provide protection only if a live conductor is touched when standing on, or in contact with, the ground or earthed metal. It does not prevent a fatal shock if both live and neutral conductors are touched when standing on an insulated surface. *Nothing can prevent a fatal shock in those circumstances.*

A voltage-operated ELCB (VOELCB) has a relay operating a circuit breaker connected between the earth conductor and the earth or neutral line. If the voltage between these two exceeds a predetermined level (say 40 V), the breaker is tripped (Figure 39.41). These will function in a single- or double-fault situation. An alternative is a current-operated ELCB (COELCB) (Figure 39.42). In normal operation, the current flowing in the live and neutral wires is the same and induces equal and opposite magnetic fluxes in the toroidal transformer. Leakage of current to earth (e.g. through a patient) leads to a difference in the magnetic field. This includes a current in the third coil which trips the breaker. A difference of 30 mA can trip a COELCB within 5 ms, but they are so sensitive that, if they serve a number of appliances, the sum of their leakage currents (each harmless in itself) may be sufficient to trip the system. Repeated false alarms have, unfortunately on occasions, encouraged staff to render ELCBs inoperative with tooth picks or sticking plaster. Their area of operation is shown in Figure 39.39.

### Diathermy

Surgical diathermy is used either to coagulate small blood vessels or to cut tissue by a local heating effect. A current of high frequency (1 MHz) passes through the body from the electrode in the surgeon's hand to the neutral or patient plate. The degree of burning produced depends on the current density, and as, at the cutting electrode, the current is channelled through a very small area, this is where heating and burning take place. No heating should occur at the patient plate because the current here flows through a large area, and the current density is low. Burns may occur if, for example, the plate is crumpled and skin contact occurs at only a few places. Here the current density may be sufficient to have a heating effect and burn. Alternatively, if the plate is discon-

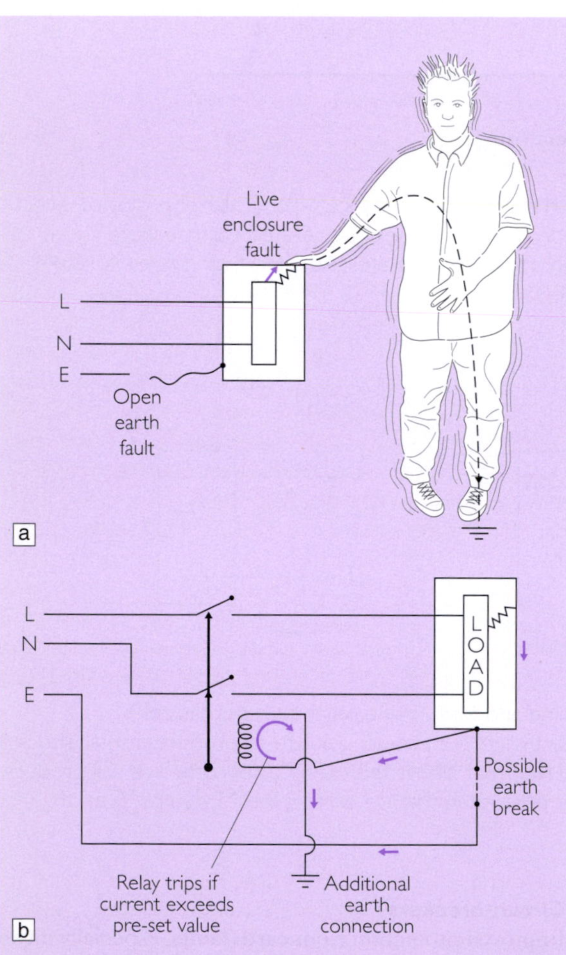


**Figure 39.41** A voltage-operated earth leakage circuit breaker (VOELCB) and a two-fault situation with a live casing and broken earth linkage. A VOELCB gives protection because the relay operating the circuit breaker is connected between the earth conductor and the earth or neutral line. (a) No VOELCB: shock occurs – current flows through human; (b) VOELCB fitted.

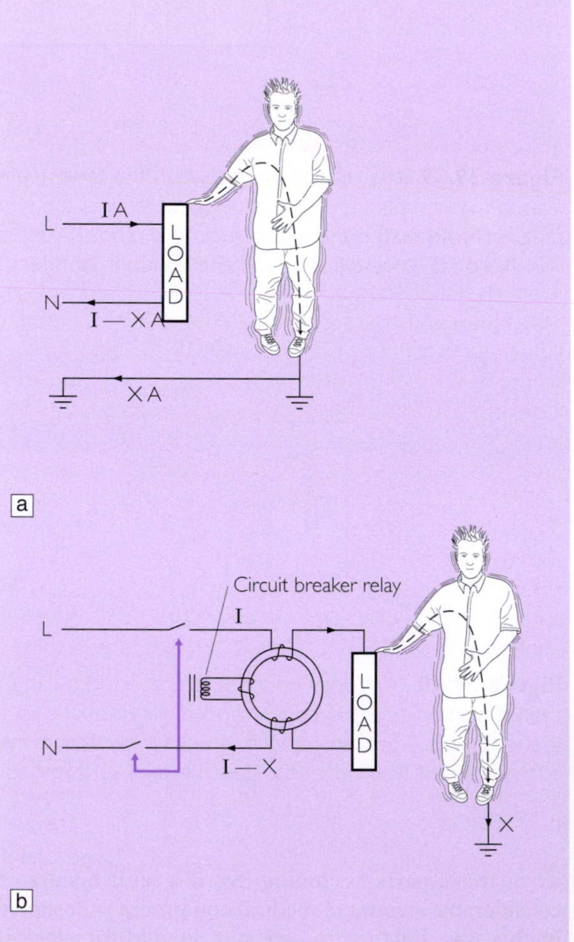


**Figure 39.42** A current-operated earth linkage circuit breaker (COELCB). A difference in current flow between the live and neutral lines (which will occur when there is flow through a person if a fault develops) trips the circuit breaker. (a) No circuit breaker: shock occurs; (b) difference between $I$ and $I - X$ trips the circuit breaker and switch.

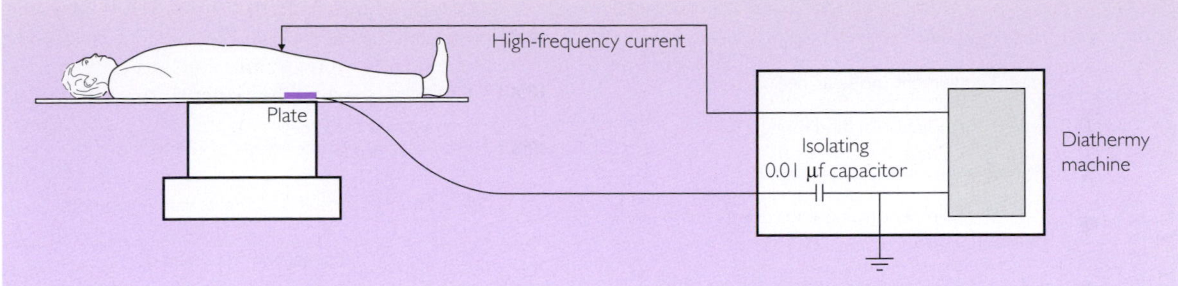


**Figure 39.43** The use of an isolating capacitor with a diathermy apparatus. The isolating capacitor in the diathermy machine allows high-frequency diathermy current to flow freely, but offers a high resistance to mains (50/60 Hz) current.

nected, the current may flow through any earthed object that is in contact with the patient (e.g. operating table, ECG electrode), producing a burn at that point.

Gross electrocution could occur through a diathermy plate that is connected directly to earth if the patient is touched by live, faulty equipment. If, however, an isolating capacitor is placed in the earth line, it will have a high impedance to low frequency mains current (50 Hz), but very low impedance to the high frequency diathermy current (1 MHz). A 0.01-μF capacitor will produce only 15 Ω impedance for the diathermy current (and so hardly affect its passage) but 300 000 Ω for mains frequency, allowing a current of only 0.8 mA to flow. The theory of this is summarized in Chapter 38, Figure 38.33 and Table 38.8, and the principle is shown in Figure 39.43.

### Floating circuits

An isolated or floating patient circuit is also known as an earth-free circuit, because those elements in contact with the patient have no connection to earth. In contrast to this, in old ECG monitors the neutral electrode on the patient was attached to the casing, and thus directly to earth. This increased the chance of electrocution if the patient accidentally came into contact with a mains source, and burns could be produced if the diathermy plate was faulty (Figure 39.44a). In modern apparatus, the neutral lead connects to the amplifier, which passes the signal to the rest of the equipment through a transformer. The patient is isolated from both the earth and the mains (Figure 39.44b).

The use of an isolated circuit is an additional method of classifying equipment, and is applied to the three classes described above. With such equipment, there is little chance of gross shock, but alternating currents can produce small currents by inductive and capacitative coupling.

### Leakage currents and permitted usage

Leakage currents can give rise to microshock (see below), and there are classifications according to maximum leakage currents permitted for particular applications. The highest standard is for equipment that may contact the heart directly. This is labelled CF. The C indicates cardiac use and the F denotes that it has a floating circuit. The leakage current through its intracardiac connection must be less than 50 μA, even if operating with a single fault.

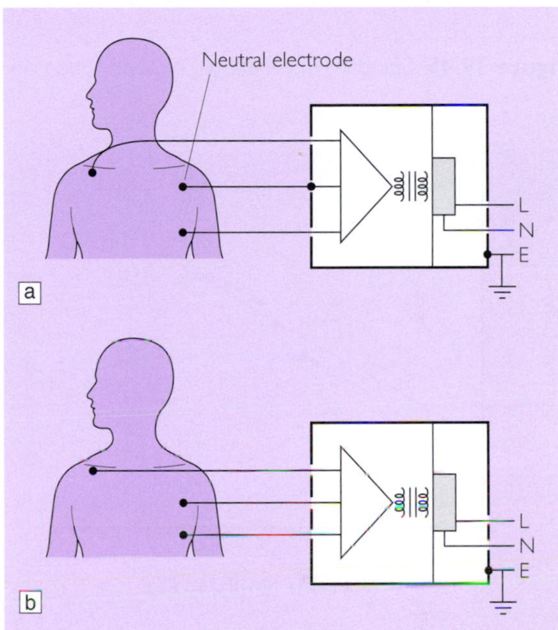


**Figure 39.44** An isolated or floating patient circuit. An earth-free floating circuit avoids the risk of electrocution from another source through the electrode connected to the monitor case. (a) Neutral electrode connected to earthed casing: danger of shock; (b) floating circuit: no possibility of shock.

Type B equipment (or BF if it has a floating circuit) is permitted a current leakage of 500 μA under single fault conditions.

Figure 39.45 shows standard symbols relating to electrical safety, some of which indicate its permitted use (e.g. protected against dripping water).

### Microshock

VF can be induced if very small electric currents are applied directly to the heart (microshock). These can occur in specialist areas (cardiac catheter laboratories, intensive care units, operating rooms). They combine low voltage, low resistance, and low current, but high current density, to the myocardium. Microshock is not associated with burning or striated muscle contraction in other parts of the body. The threshold for producing VF depends on the site (ventricles are more susceptible than atria); it is proportional to surface area and decreases the longer the current passes. The

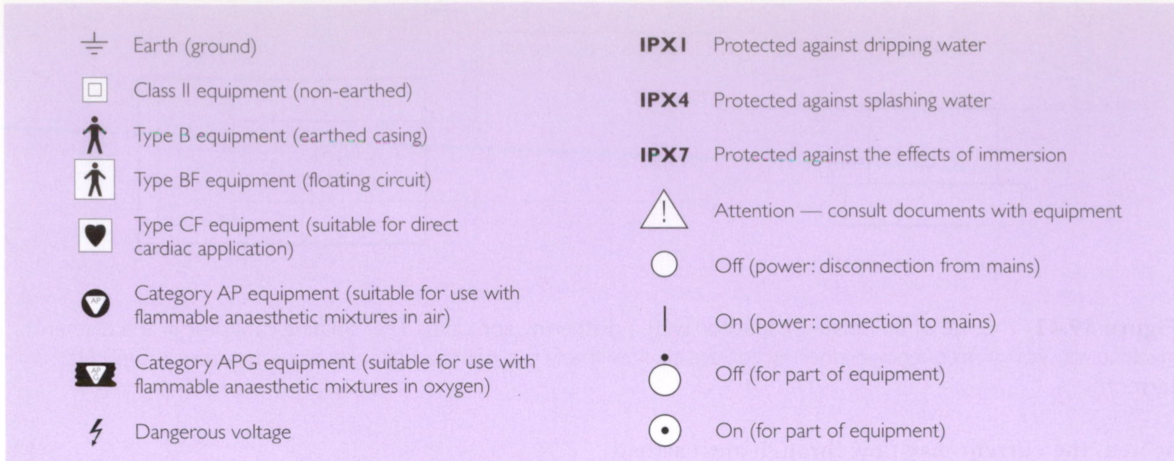


**Figure 39.45** Standard international symbols found on electrical equipment (IEC 1988).

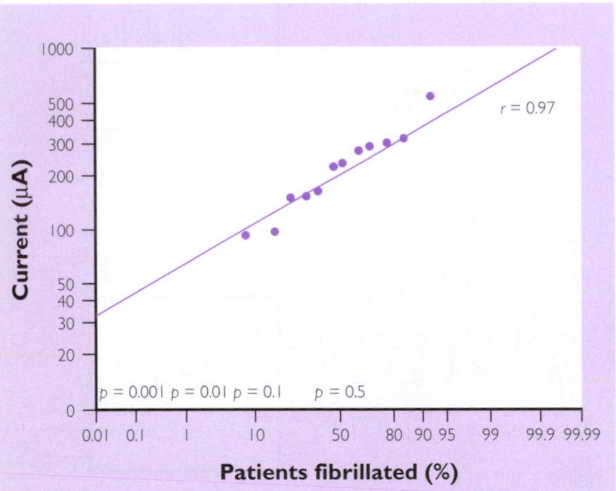


**Figure 39.46** The approximate current threshold for ventricular fibrillation in humans when applied from a 50 Hz source via a small ventricular endocardial electrode. The horizontal axis indicates the current at which the probability of any single patient fibrillating is 0.5 (50%), 0.1, 0.01, and 0.001. (Adapted from Watson AB, Wright JS, Loughman J. *Med J Aust* 1973;1:1179, and Hull CJ. *Br J Anaesth* 1978;50:647.)

**Figure 39.47** The risk of microshock from a central catheter. There is a risk of microshock because leakage current from the pump cannot dissipate to earth because its return line is broken. A small current flows along the saline-filled central catheter through the heart and back to earth via the ECG electrode and monitor. This would not occur if the ECG was of a floating circuit type.

threshold in humans is shown in Figure 39.46. As with gross electrocution, a frequency of 50 Hz is particularly good at inducing fibrillation. A current of less than 44 μA is unlikely to cause fibrillation; 65 μA gives rise to a 1% risk, which increases to 50% at 200 μA. As the currents required to produce microshock are so small, static build-up or leakage may be sufficient to produce problems. Figure 39.47 illustrates a situation where a central catheter is connected to an electrical device (e.g. a pump) that has developed a fault in its earth line. Capacitive or inductive coupling has produced a small leakage current, which can no longer dissipate to earth, and this could produce a microshock if the patient is now earthed. The current flowing through this person would be too small to be noticed by them, although its effect on the heart may be dramatic.

The risk of microshock can be minimized by staff awareness, using only CF-rated and, if possible, battery-operated equipment in the immediate vicinity of patients at risk, and ensuring that other electrical circuits that may come into contact with the patient are isolated from earth.

### Defibrillators

Electrical defibrillation is often the only effective way of terminating VF and restoring a normal cardiac rhythm. Defibrillation may be either external, with paddles applied to the chest wall, or internal, with paddles placed directly on the heart as during cardiac surgery. The current passed through the myocardium must be sufficient to ensure that all myocardial cells are depolarized simultaneously .

Defibrillators (Figure 39.48) have a power source, which is usually mains but may be battery. A variable transformer is used to select an appropriate voltage, and the secondary voltage must be converted to direct

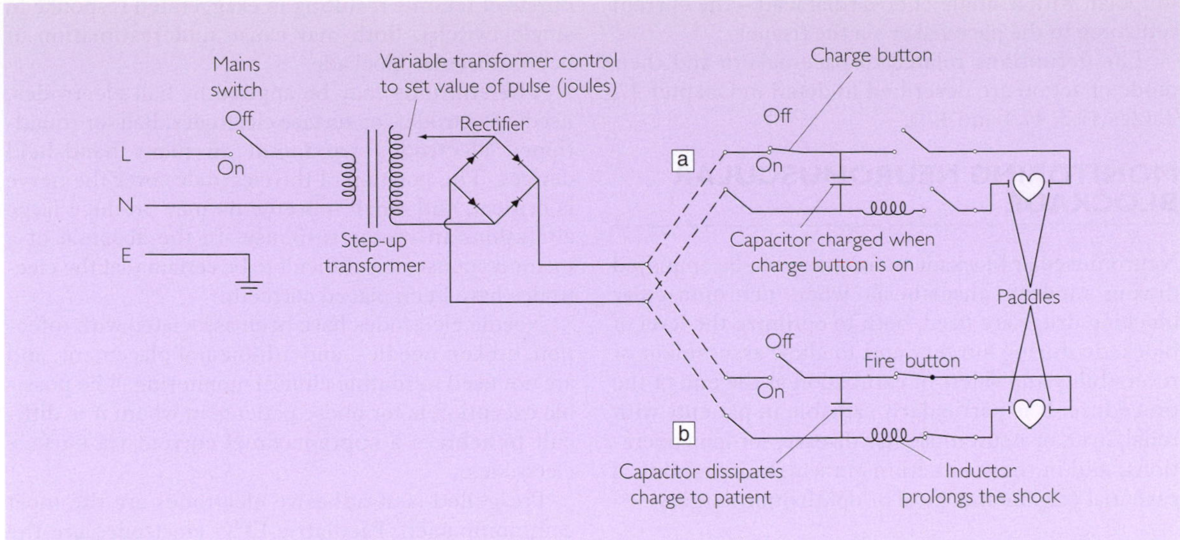


**Figure 39.48** A schematic layout of a defibrillator circuit. The paddles used are either internal or external types, and the charge is set appropriately for each of them. (a) The plates charging and (b) the defibrillator discharging through the heart.

current by means of a rectifier. When the charge button is pressed (A in Figure 39.48) the direct current voltage is applied across the capacitor.

A typical charge potential across the plates of a defibrillator might be 4000–6000 V when using external paddles. It is, however, usual to express the stored (or output) energy of the defibrillator in terms of units of energy (joules) rather than volts. For an adult, the energy available for internal paddles is typically up to 50 J and for external paddles typically up to 400 J.

Defibrillators have an inductance coil in the discharge path of the electrical current to the patient. This coil opposes any sudden change in current flow, as will happen when the discharge or 'fire' buttons (B in Figure 39.48) are depressed. This slows down the otherwise rapid discharge of the capacitor, and gives the shock its optimum duration of between 4 and 12 ms. Some of the energy of the pulse is absorbed by the inductor. It is modern practice to allow for this in the displayed energy of the defibrillator – the displayed energy being that which will be delivered to the paddles, not that stored on the capacitor.

Successful defibrillation depends on the discharged electrical energy passing through the patient's heart. Hence the importance of correct paddle position, with one paddle below the right clavicle and the other below the apex of the heart. Paddle positioning on the anterior and posterior chest walls is an alternative. Good contact with the skin must be made with jelly or gel pads. As much of the current traverses other structures such as the lungs, less than 10% of the current delivered from the paddles may actually pass through the heart.

In treating VF, the first external shock is 200 J (2 J/kg in children), which is a compromise. Too small a shock is less likely to be successful, whereas too high a shock will in itself cause damage to the myocardium. The second shock is the same nominal value but, because of the reduction in tissue resistance caused by the passage of the first shock, the transcardiac current is now higher. (See Chapter 13 for further clinical details of defibrillation.)

The average human transthoracic impedance is 70–80 Ω but in some cases it is higher. To avoid inappropriately low and therefore ineffective energies, some new defibrillators can automatically measure the impedance, and adjust the shock size accordingly in those patients with high impedance. Automatic implantable defibrillators are available for patients at high risk of dysrhythmias. New developments also include biphasic defibrillators because it appears that the defibrillation threshold is lower using biphasic waveforms.

### Pacemakers

As with defibrillation, a capacitatively held charge (although very much smaller) is delivered to the heart. Cardiac pacemakers can be temporary or permanent. Temporary pacemakers may be transvenous with a pacing wire inserted via a central vein. At the end of the wire are two electrodes, and a small current is passed, usually from the distal to the proximal electrode, stimulating nearby myocardium. The pulse has a total duration of under 100 ms, and the current is usually 1–2 mA but may be up to about 40 mA maximum. There is a danger of unintended microshock, as discussed earlier.

As a result of the difficulty in establishing transvenous pacing in an emergency, non-invasive temporary pacemakers have been developed with either transoesphageal pacing or completely external pacing via large adhesive electrodes attached to the front and back of the patient's chest. Temporary pacers can have an automatic function and monitor the patient's rate, stimulating the heart when the rate falls below a preselected level. The current generated is higher than transvenous wires, being up to 140 mA.

Permanent pacemakers involve the subcutaneous implantation of a pacemaker box, and are usually unipolar, with a single endocardial lead – the current returning to the pacemaker via the tissues.

The definitions related to pacemakers and their mode of action are described in detail in Chapter 47, Tables 47.3, 47.4 and 47.5.

## MONITORING NEUROMUSCULAR BLOCKADE

Neuromuscular blockade monitoring can be employed during modern anaesthesia when neuromuscular blocking drugs are used, both to optimize the level of blockade during surgery and to allow assessment of reversibility and safety of extubation at the end of the procedure. It is particularly valuable in patients with renal, liver, or neuromuscular disease, for long operations, and in those situations in which immobility is essential (e.g. neurological or ophthalmic surgery).

### Producing the stimulus

Routine, clinical, perioperative monitoring involves the supramaximal stimulation of an accessible peripheral motor nerve using a nerve stimulator and surface electrodes (see Chapters 24 and 35 for clinical applications).

The characteristics of an ideal neuromuscular stimulator are given in Table 39.6.

The stimulus should be a unipolar square wave, having a duration of between 0.1 and 0.3 ms (i.e. shorter than the refractory period of the neuromuscular junction). The current must be sufficient to activate all the nerve fibres in the underlying nerve (supramaximal stimulation). In 75% of patients, the supramaximal current will be in the range 15–40 mA for surface electrodes used over the ulnar nerve at the wrist. Obese patients may require 50–60 mA. Excessively high currents may produce 'overstimulation' – with direct muscle contraction or repetitive nerve firing (mini-bursts of tetanus resulting in exaggerated response to single twitch). Both may cause underestimation of neuromuscular blockade.

The stimulus may be applied by ball electrodes, needle electrodes, or surface electrodes. Ball- or round-tipped electrodes are found on many hand-held devices. The position of the electrodes over the nerve is critical, and small movements may produce large alterations in motor response. In the absence of a motor response, it is difficult to be certain that the electrodes have been placed correctly.

Needle electrodes have been associated with infection, broken needles, and intraneural placement, and are not used in routine clinical monitoring. The possible exception is for obese patients in whom it is difficult to achieve a supramaximal current via surface electrodes.

Pre-gelled, self-adhesive electrodes are the most commonly used. Paediatric ECG electrodes are the appropriate size for accurate anatomical placement and maintenance of current density. A large electrode surface area reduces current density and may result in submaximal stimulation if constant voltage stimulators are used. Most commercial stimulators are now the constant current variety, and are able to supply a preset current despite small changes in electrode impedance.

It is usual to connect the distal electrode to the negative terminal of the stimulator (i.e. proximal positive) because this minimizes the current required for supramaximal stimulation, although, if both electrodes are placed within a few centimetres of each other along the nerve, the polarity does not affect twitch response.

### Site of stimulation

Thumb adduction caused by contraction of adductor pollicis after stimulation of the ulnar nerve at the wrist is the most widely used and researched method of monitoring neuromuscular blockade. The first (distal)

| **Table 39.6 Characteristics of an ideal neuromuscular stimulator** |
|---|
| Constant current design |
| Adjustable current up to a 80 mA into 2.5 kΩ load |
| Unipolar square waves stimulus of 0.1–0.3 ms duration |
| Polarity of electrodes indicated |
| Current output display |
| Available stimulus patterns to include:<br>Single twitch<br>Train of four (TOF)<br>Tetanus 50 Hz<br>Double burst |
| Preset timing for repeat stimulations |
| Visual/audible warning during stimulation |
| Battery operated, with battery-condition indicator |
| Inexpensive and robust |
| Conforms to current electrical safety standards |

electrode is then placed 1 cm proximal to the proximal skin crease at the wrist, just to the radial side of the tendon of the flexor carpi ulnaris muscle. The second electrode is then positioned 2–3 cm proximal, along the line of the ulnar nerve. The ulnar nerve at this point is superficial, easy to stimulate, accessible in many anaesthetized patients, and always supplies the adductor pollicis. The muscle response is easily visible or measurable, is relatively immune from direct muscle stimulation, and gives good correlation with required levels of relaxation. Clinical experience is that full recovery of the adductor pollicis assures adequate respiratory muscle recovery. Relative to the adductor pollicis, the diaphragm and vocal cords are more resistant to neuromuscular blockade as is the abdominal musculature.

During some types of surgery, the facial nerve may be more accessible to the anaesthetist. Electrodes are placed over the main trunk of the facial nerve, or over one of its major divisions (e.g. the temporal branch supplying the orbicularis oculi and frontalis). The response most commonly seen with facial nerve stimulation is movement around the mouth and eyebrow. It must be remembered that the facial muscles are more resistant to neuromuscular blockade than the adductor pollicis, so that twitches may be seen around the eye when there is no response at the wrist. Direct muscle stimulation is also more likely at this site, so that either or both of these features may result in under-estimation of the degree of neuromuscular blockade.

If neither the ulnar nor the facial nerves are accessible, the lower limb may be used. The common peroneal nerve can be stimulated using electrodes placed at the neck of the fibula, leading to dorsiflexion of the toe and foot. Plantar flexion of the great toe (flexor hallucis brevis and abductor hallucis muscles) is seen after stimulation of the posterior tibial nerve behind the medial malleolus.

### Patterns of stimulation

Several stimulus patterns have been described in an attempt to monitor and quantify the changes in neuromuscular blockade that occur during surgery. One of the earliest forms of monitoring neuromuscular blockade used the response to single pulses in combination with tetanic stimulation at 50 Hz. Single twitches should be given no more frequently than at 2-s intervals to allow normal muscle function to return after each stimulus. Normal physiological firing rates producing maximal sustained force are of the order of 50 Hz. (Higher frequencies may produce fade in the absence of neuromuscular blockade.) In controls, a 5-s, 50-Hz tetanic stimulation produces little or no post-tetanic potentiation with subsequent single twitches (Figure 39.49a). Partial competitive (non-depolarizing) neuromuscular blockade produces a decrease in single twitch height, fade (progressive reduction of twitch height) during tetanic stimulation, with post-tetanic potentiation (increased twitch height) of the single response (Figure 39.49b). Depolarizing (non-competitive) neuromuscular blockade, however, produces depressed single twitch height but no fade during tetanic stimulation, and little or no post-tetanic potentiation (Figure 39.49c). Overdosage of depolarizing neuromuscular blocking drugs may produce a

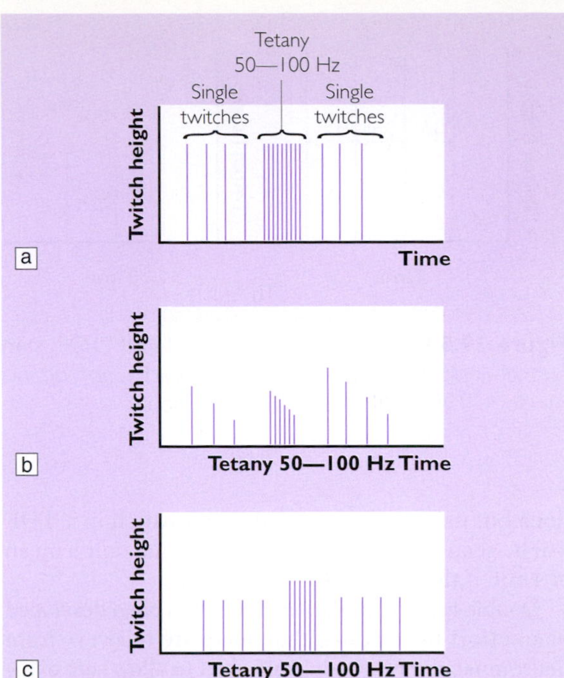


**Figure 39.49** The response to regular single twitches and tetanic stimulation of peripheral nerves in the presence of (a) normal unblocked nerve, (b) a partial non-depolarizing or competitive block showing fade and post-tetanic potentiation (PTP), and (c) a partial depolarizing block – no fade or PTP.

dual block, which has the characteristics of a block produced by non-depolarizing drugs. A 5-s tetanus may damage muscle, and should not be repeated more than once every 5–10 min, although a 1-s tetanus applied more frequently does not appear to cause obvious problems.

More information about the degree of non-depolarizing blockade can be obtained by using the train-of-four (TOF) stimulus pattern (Figure 39.50). This is the most commonly used form of neuromuscular block monitoring during surgery, and was introduced because it does not require reference to a control response. Four pulses are delivered at 0.5-s intervals (i.e. at 2 Hz). The last stimulus is therefore 1.5 s after the first. The number of palpable or visible twitches (depending on the stimulation site) is counted as a response (TOF count or TOFC). When four twitches are produced, and quantitative measurement of the response is possible, the ratio of the fourth to the first response gives the TOF ratio or TOFR.

If neuromuscular blockade is so dense that there is no response to single stimuli, TOF, or short tetanic stimulation, quantification of the degree of blockade may be possible using the post-tetanic count (PTC). After stimulation at 1 Hz for 1 min, a 50-Hz tetanus is applied for 5 s. After a 3-s pause, 1-Hz stimulation is restarted and a count made of the number of single twitches produced. The correlation between PTC and time to first TOF response is drug specific. Using pancuronium and tactile assessment, a PTC of 4 is associated with a mean wait of 20 min (95% confidence limits 4–36 min) before the first TOF reappearance, rising to 40 min if the PTC is 1. Under the same condi-

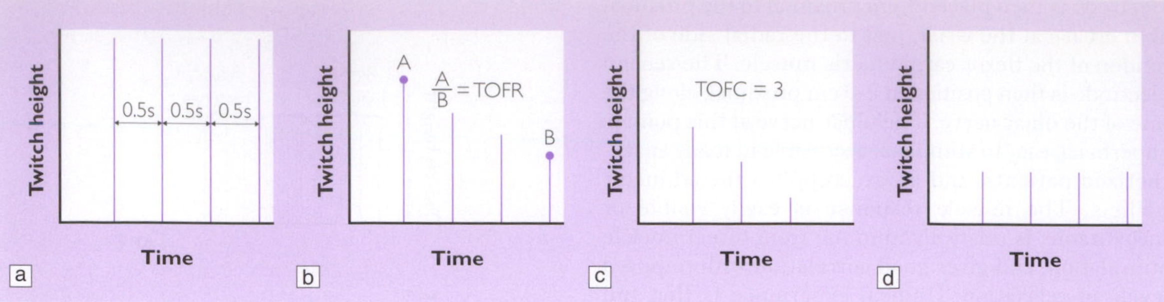


**Figure 39.50** The response to train-of-four (TOF) stimulation of a peripheral nerve is the response (a) from a normal unblocked nerve, (b, c) from a partial non-depolarizing or competitive block, and (d) from a partial depolarizing block. TOFR, TOF ratio; TOFC, TOF count.

tions but using atracurium, the first twitch in a TOF will be seen at 9 min after a PTC of 1, and only a mean of 4 min if the PTC is 4.

Double burst stimulation (DBS) has been developed in an effort to establish that adequate recovery from neuromuscular blockade, sufficient to allow safe extubation, has occurred without the need to measure the TOFR mechanically. The problem with TOF is that gauging the true relationship between the first and fourth response by feeling thumb movement is difficult, and most observers judge each response of the TOF to be equally strong when the mechanically measured TOFR is only 0.3–0.5. DBS consists of two short bursts of tetanus (three 50-Hz stimuli in each train) separated by 0.75 s. The response of the muscles to these bursts is perceived as two twitches, and if they feel equal, the measured TOFR will be greater than 0.5.

### Evaluation of responses

Visual observation of the presence or absence of a response is commonly used in clinical practice, and is all that is available when stimulating the facial nerve. The number of TOF or PTC twitches can be easily counted and appropriate adjustments made. Using vecuronium as the neuromuscular blocking agent, the first response to TOF is seen when mechanical measurements indicate a return to 8% of control values, a level associated with good surgical relaxation.

Tactile assessment of the force of contraction gives more reliable information about the degree of blockade and should be used in preference to visual monitoring. The thumb should be abducted in the same plane as the palm with a resting force of 2–300 g and the stimulus applied.

This subjective assessment tends to over-estimate the true TOFR, and a mechano- or electromyographic (e.g. Relaxograph, Datex) technique is essential for research work. They do, however, have to be set up with some care, occupy space, and often require the limb to be in an inconvenient position intraoperatively (see Chapter 35). This limits their applicability to routine anaesthesia and, for most applications, visual or tactile assessment is quite adequate.

### Interpretation

At induction, a TOFC of 1 usually allows enough relaxation for laryngoscopy and endotracheal intubation, but, to avoid any bucking or coughing, a PTC of 0–1 is needed. Good conditions for most abdominal surgery can be ensured with a TOFC of 1 (90–99% single twitch depression), which can be monitored every 5–15 min. A PTC of 9 is similar to a TOFC of 1.

Reversal of blockade should not be attempted if the TOFC is 0. A PTC can be used to estimate when a response will reappear. The TOFC should ideally be 3 before reversal, especially when using longer-acting drugs. A TOFR of 0.7–0.8 and a sustained response (no fade) to tetanic stimulation indicate safe clinical recovery of muscle function. If TOFR cannot be measured, DBS may be helpful, but does not rule out significant residual muscle paralysis. A sustained head lift for 5 s indicates a blockade of 30% and adequate function.

## PRESSURE TRANSDUCERS

Pressure is defined as force per unit area and is discussed in detail in Chapter 37, page 657. One standard atmosphere is 101.325 kPa or 760 mmHg. Pressures can be measured using liquid manometers, mechanical gauges or electronic devices. The movement of a flexible diaphragm caused by a pressure wave may be measured optically or electrically.

Electromechanical transducers employ many different systems to convert the movement of a diaphragm into an electrical signal that is proportional to the degree of movement. Wire strain gauges, single or double-bonded strain gauges, silicon strain gauges, capacitance (as in a condenser microphone), or inductance devices are all in use (Figure 39.51). Transducers are usually used for the direct measurement and display of arterial and venous pressure waves. Complex waveforms such as arterial pressures can be reduced by Fourier analysis to a set of sine and cosine waves of differing frequency, amplitude, and phase (see also Chapter 37, Figure 37.20). The fundamental frequency, or first harmonic, is the lowest frequency sine wave and for an arterial pressure trace is the same as the pulse rate. The second harmonic is a sine wave of twice the frequency of the fundamental, the third harmonic is a sine wave of three times the frequency, and so on. The lower harmonics tend to have the largest amplitudes and therefore the greatest impact on the shape of the final wave. An example of Fourier analysis is shown in Figure 39.52.

Fourier reconstructions that approximate to the original arterial pressure wave have been shown earlier in Chapter 37, Figure 37.21 . A very good approxima-

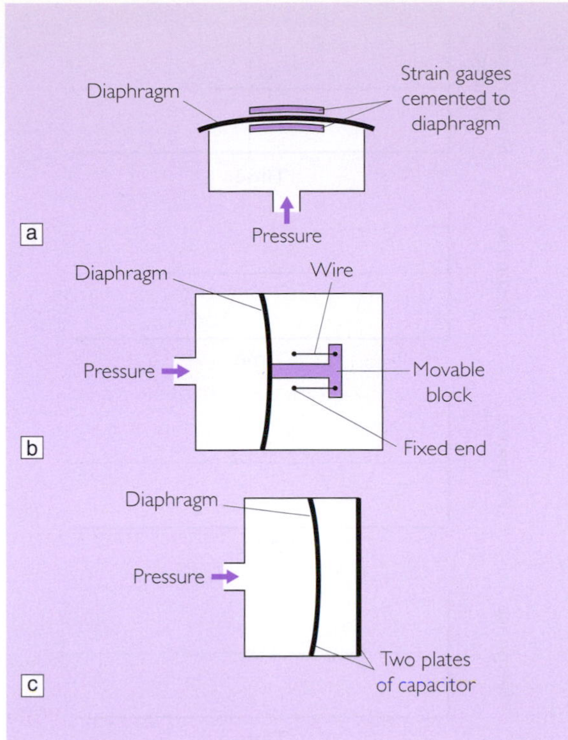


**Figure 39.51** Diagrammatic representation of pressure transducer mechanisms. (a) Bonded strain gauge: as the pressure increases the curvature of the diaphragm, one gauge is compressed and the other stretched, changing the resistance in opposite directions. The changes in resistance are calibrated to reflect changes in pressure. (b) Wire strain gauge: diaphragm movement stretches the wire, altering its resistance. (c) Capacitance pressure transducer: the diaphragm constitutes one plate of a capacitor, the other being fixed. As the diaphragm moves, the distance between the plates, and hence capacitance changes.

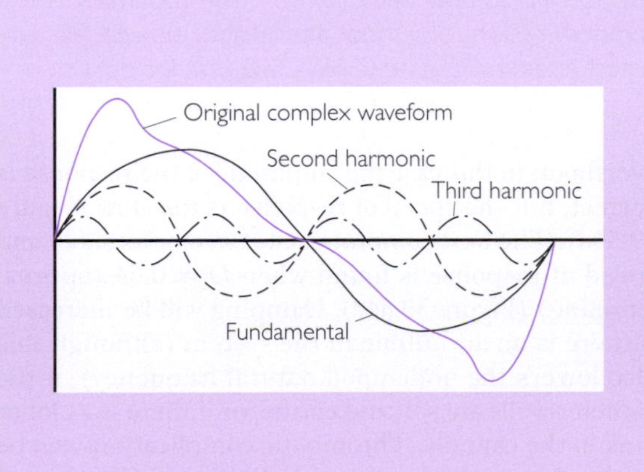


**Figure 39.52** Fourier analysis: the complex waveform is made by combining the first three harmonics. Fourier analysis reduces complex waves to its fundamental frequency and component harmonics, altering the amplitude and phase of each to reproduce the original complex waveform when added together. Compare with Figure 37.20 and 37.21 and accompanying text in Chapter 37.

tion to the arterial wave can be obtained from the first 8–10 harmonics. For a pulse rate of 70 beats/min, the tenth harmonic would have a frequency of (70 × 10)/60 = 11.7 Hz, rising to 30 Hz at 180 beats/min. A pressure transducer and amplifier should therefore be able to reproduce these frequencies accurately if the display is not to be distorted. To achieve this, the combination of transducer and coupling (catheter and tubing) should be designed to have a high resonant frequency and the right amount of damping. Everything that vibrates has a resonant frequency (undamped natural frequency), where a small input at that frequency will produce very large oscillations. For example, a pendulum can be made to swing large distances if it is pushed gently at the top of each swing (i.e. the driving frequency [push] coincides with the natural resonant frequency of the pendulum, which is determined by its length).

A flexible diaphragm behaves like a spring, and the undamped natural frequency ($f_o$) is described by the formula:

$$\frac{1}{2\pi}\sqrt{\frac{S}{M}}$$

where $S$ is the stiffness of the diaphragm and $M$ is the mass of moving fluid in the system – mainly that in the tubing. This mass will depend on the radius and the length of the tubing, and the density of the fluid.

A clinical transducer–catheter–amplifier measuring system under test is shown diagrammatically in Figure 39.53. As shown in Figure 39.53a, there is a common source of constant-amplitude, variable-frequency pressure waves. These are drawn in Figure 39.53b. The common source of pressure fluctuations is then applied to two measuring systems: a reference system and the clinical system under test. The reference system has a short, stiff, wide-bore catheter (the transducer is often tapped directly into the pressure chamber), and a transducer and amplifier with very high specification responses.

As the frequency of pressure fluctuations in chamber C increases, the output from the two systems will be as shown in Figure 39.53c. The transducer under test reproduces the correct signal at low frequencies but overshoots at the mid-range, which coincides with its resonant frequency. The signal becomes progressively damped at higher frequencies. The specification for each monitoring system needs to be checked in the manufacturer's handbook, but for pressure monitoring in adults it is often flat to around 20 Hz.

The resonant frequency will be highest when the transducer diaphragm is stiff and the tubing is short and wide. Attaching the transducer directly to the cannula minimizes tubing, but makes blood sampling difficult and is prone to movement artefact. Intra-arterial transducers are now available, but are expensive.

Stiffer diaphragms have a smaller movement for a given pressure change, and will therefore be less sensitive. This can, in part, be overcome by improving the quality (and price) of the amplifier, but in general a high-frequency response and high sensitivity are mutually exclusive characteristics. Although most pressure transducers in clinical use have undamped natural frequencies of 100 Hz or more, the addition of long, narrow tubing, three-way taps with narrow passages,

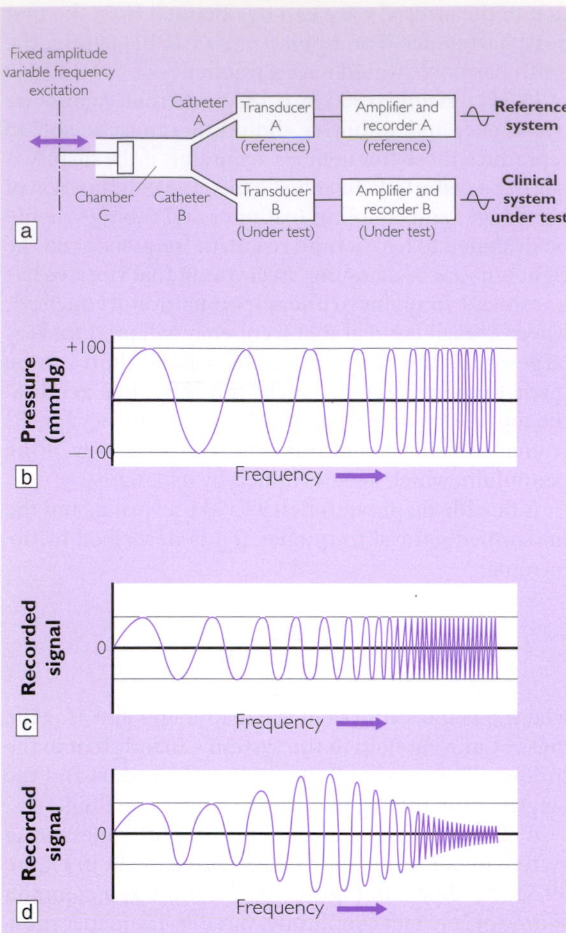


**Figure 39.53** (a) A diagrammatic representation of the method of testing a clinical catheter–transducer–amplifier system; (b) actual pressure swings in chamber C as frequency increases; (c) output from system A in volts; (d) output from system B in volts. See text for details.

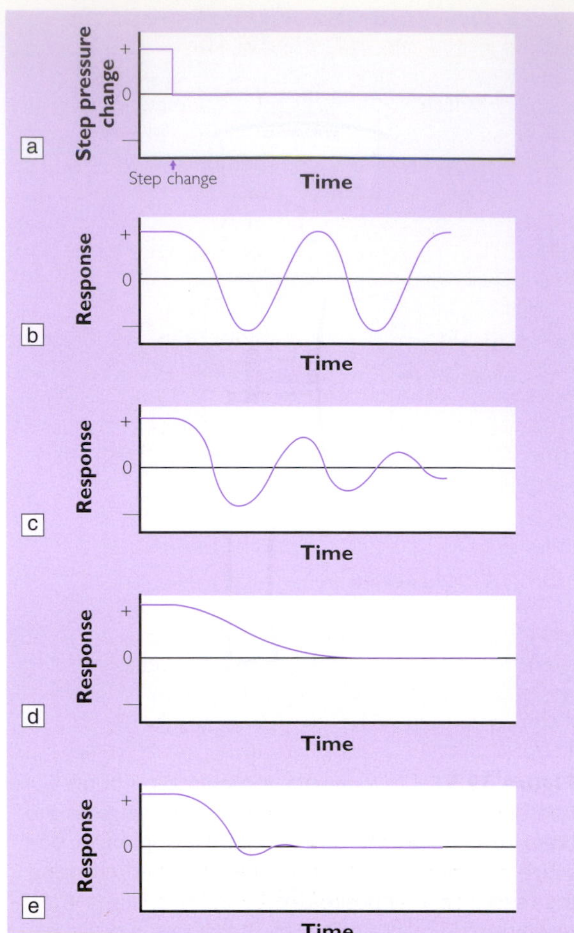


**Figure 39.54** The effect of different degrees of damping on the output of a pressure transducer system subjected to a single step change of pressure. (a) Single step change in pressure; (b) $D = 0$ (no damping) – the output overshoots, then oscillates at the system's natural undamped frequency; (c) $D = 0.2$ (minimal damping) – large overshoot followed by swings of decreasing amplitude; (d) $D = 1$ (critically damped) – no overshoot, but slow fall to new value; (e) $D = 0.64$ (optimally damped) – slight overshoot after slightly slowed fall; fastest attainment of new value. See text for details.

and the arterial cannula can markedly reduce this to levels close to the upper harmonics of the driving frequency, leading to distortion of the signal. This problem can be minimized by the correct amount of damping.

The effects of damping are shown in Figure 39.54, where a catheter transducer system is subjected to a single step change in pressure. Damping is a term that is easy to understand intuitively, but requires advanced mathematics to define precisely. The damping coefficient (D) can de derived from a complex logarithmic function of the ratio between successive amplitudes of response following a step input into the system. It can theoretically have values ranging from 0 to infinity. If there is no damping ($D = 0$), the system clearly overshoots, then oscillates continuously at the undamped natural frequency (Figure 39.54b). (Clearly this never happens in practice because friction and viscosity always cause some damping.) When there is minimal damping ($D = 0.2$), the signal oscillates at close to the undamped natural frequency, but the amplitude decreases with time (Figure 39.54c). Critical damping ($D = 1$) occurs when the signal falls but just fails to overshoot; in this case the amplitude of the response is correct, but the speed of response is too slow (Figure 39.54d). The best compromise between overshoot and speed of response is found when $D = 0.64$ (optimal damping) (Figure 39.54e). Damping will be increased if there is an air bubble in the system (although this also lowers the undamped natural frequency), if the catheter walls are soft and elastic, or if there is a clot or kink in the cannula. Thrombotic complications can be reduced by using small, parallel-sided Teflon cannulas, and a continuous slow-flush device.

Optimal damping also minimizes the problem of phase shift. The various harmonic components of a pressure wave will travel along a thin catheter at different velocities. As they then arrive at the transducer at different times, the recorded signal will be distorted in shape and amplitude. It so happens that, if the damping is optimal ($D = 0.64$), then all the harmonics will experience the same delay in time and, although the overall timing of the wave will be delayed, the composition and shape of the waveform will remain unchanged.

The American National Standards Institute demands an accuracy ±3% for disposable blood pressure transducers. Static calibration can be carried out with a mercury manometer attached to the transducer. Increments and decrements of 10 mmHg are applied across the physiological range to test for accuracy, linearity, and hysteresis.

In summary, for accurate waveform reproduction, the transducer/catheter system should have an adequate undamped natural frequency and the whole system should be optimally damped. Combinations of natural frequency and damping coefficient for adequate dynamic response are shown in Figure 39.55. In clinical practice, if there are no signs of resonance, the dicrotic notch can be seen and there is a good, sharp response to a flush, the system is likely to be functioning adequately.

Excess damping will occur if there are air bubbles or clots in the tubing, or if the catheter walls are soft. An overdamped system will produce a flattened trace, under-read the systolic pressure, and over-read the diastolic pressure (see Chapter 12, Figures 12.21–12.23). If the system has too low a resonant frequency, the trace will overshoot and oscillate, over-reading systolic pressure and under-reading diastolic pressure (Figure 39.56). Mean pressures remain unaltered. Further errors of recording and artefacts can be seen in Chapter 12, Figure 12.2, and Chapter 20, Figure 20.28.

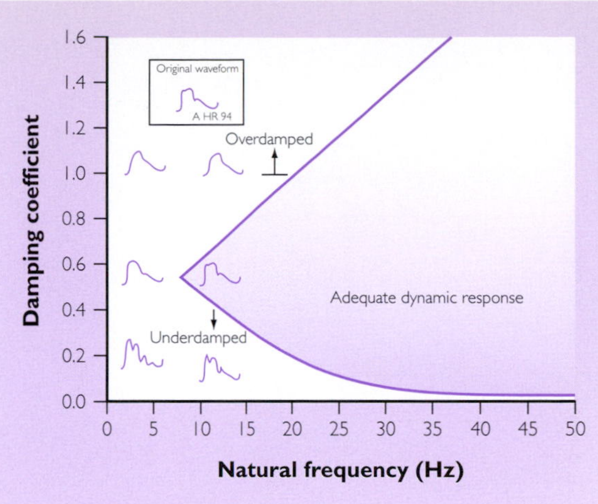


**Figure 39.55** The effect of combinations of natural frequency and damping coefficient on waveform reproduction. (Adapted from Gardner RM. *Anesthesiology* 1981;54:227.)

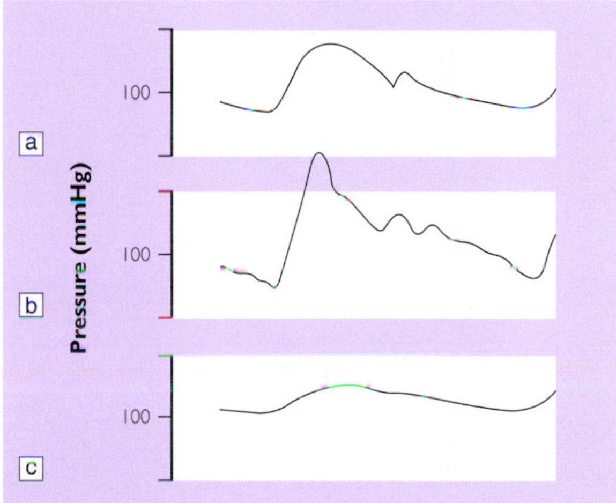


**Figure 39.56** Arterial waveform traces produced from systems that are (a) optimally damped, (b) under-damped, and (c) over-damped. (a) Accurate representation of input waveform and systolic and diastolic pressures; (b) resonance causes spiked trace which over-estimates systolic and under-estimates diastolic pressures; (c) waveform detail is lost, with under-estimation of systolic and over-estimation of diastolic pressures. The same mean pressure is given by all three traces.

## FURTHER READING


Al-Shaikh B, Stacey S. *Essentials of Anaesthetic Equipment*. Edinburgh: Churchill Livingstone, 1995.

Davey A, Moyle JTB, Ward CS. *Anaesthetic Equipment*, 3rd edn. Philadelphia: WB Saunders.

Davis PD, Parbrook GD, Kenny GNC. *Basic Physics and Measurement in Anaesthesia*, 4th edn. Oxford: Butterworth-Heinemann, 1995.

Dorsch JA, Dorsch SE. *Understanding Anaesthesia Equipment*, 3rd edn. Baltimore, MA: Williams & Wilkins, 1994.

Geddes LA. *Handbook of Blood Pressure Measurement*. Clifton, NJ: Humana Press, 1991.

Gravenstein JS, Paulus DA, Hayes TJ. *Gas Monitoring in Clinical Practice*, 2nd edn. Newton MA: Butterworth-Heinemann, 1995.

Hutton P, Prys-Roberts C. *Monitoring in Anaesthesia and Intensive Care*. Philadelphia: WB Saunders, 1994.

Lake CL. *Clinical Monitoring*. Philadelphia: WB Saunders, 1990.

Moyle JTB. Pulse oximetry. In: Hahn CEW, Adams AP, eds, *Principles and Practice Series*. London: BMJ Publishing Group, 1994.

Mushin WW, Jones PL. Physics for the Anaesthetist. Blackwell Scientific Publications, 1987.

O'Flaherty D. Capnography. In: Hahn CEW, Adams AP, eds, *Principles and Practice Series*. London: BMJ Publishing Group, 1994.

Sykes MK, Vickers MD, Hull CJ. *Principles of Monitoring in Anaesthesia and Intensive Care*, 3rd edn. Oxford: Blackwell Scientific Publications, 1991.

Figure 29.55 [illegible]

Figure 29.56 Arterial waveforms [illegible] optimally damped [illegible]

overall tuning of the wave will be delayed; the components and shape of the waveform will remain unchanged.

The American National Standards Institute demands an accuracy ±3% for disposable blood pressure transducers. Static calibration can be carried out with a mercury manometer attached to the transducer. Increments and decrements of 10 mmHg are applied across the physiological range to test for accuracy, linearity and hysteresis.

In summary, for accurate waveform reproduction, the transducer–catheter system should have an adequate undamped natural frequency and the whole system should be optimally damped. Combinations of natural frequency and damping coefficient for adequate dynamic response are shown in Figure 29.56. In clinical practice, [illegible] response [illegible] ing accurately.

Excess damping will occur if there are air bubbles or clots in the tubing, or if the catheter walls are soft. An overdamped system will produce a flattened trace, under-read the systolic pressure, and over-read the diastolic pressure (see Chapter 12, Figures 12.21–12.24). If the system has too low a resonant frequency, the trace will overshoot and oscillate, over-reading systolic pressure and under-reading diastolic pressure (Figure 29.55). Mean pressures remain unaltered. Further errors of recording and artefacts can be seen in Chapter 12, Figure 12.25, and Chapter 20, Figure 20.28.

## FURTHER READING


Al-Shaikh B, Stacey S. *Essentials of Anaesthetic Equipment*. Edinburgh: Churchill Livingstone, 1995.

Davey A, Moyle JTB, Ward CS. *Ward's Anaesthetic Equipment*, 3rd edn. Philadelphia: WB Saunders.

Davis PD, Parbrook GD, Kenny GNC. *Basic Physics and Measurement in Anaesthesia*, 4th edn. Oxford: Butterworth-Heinemann, 1995.

Dorsch JA, Dorsch SE. *Understanding Anesthesia Equipment*, 3rd edn. Baltimore, MD: Williams & Wilkins, 1994.

Geddes LA. *Handbook of Blood Pressure Measurement*. Clifton, NJ: Humana Press, 1991.

[illegible] Hines RL, [illegible]. [illegible] Philadelphia: [illegible]

Hutton P, Prys-Roberts C. *Monitoring in Anaesthesia and Intensive Care*. London: WB Saunders, 1994.

Lake CL. *Clinical Monitoring*. Philadelphia: WB Saunders, 1990.

Moyle JTB. Pulse Oximetry. In: Hahn CEW, Adams AP (eds). *Principles and Practice Series*. London: BMJ Publishing Group, 1994.

Mushin WW, Jones PL. *Physics for the Anaesthetist*. Blackwell Scientific Publications, 1987.

O'Flaherty D. Capnography. In: Hahn CEW, Adams AP (eds). *Principles and Practice Series*. London: BMJ Publishing Group, 1994.

Sykes MK, Vickers MD, Hull CJ. *Principles of Measurement and Monitoring in Anaesthesia and Intensive Care*, 3rd edn. Oxford: Blackwell Scientific Publications, 1991.

# Chapter 40 Statistical principles

D. Saunders

## RATIONALE AND AIMS

Anaesthetists will encounter statistics on at least three occasions during their working life. First, statistical knowledge will be tested in the Fellowship examinations, second during the design of curriculum-vitae- enhancing projects, and third when making a judgement on what is properly conducted experimentation when reading scientific journals. It is therefore essential that anaesthetists gain a feel for the nature and application of statistical principles. The acquisition of this is not easy. Statistics is essentially a practical subject, which may be compared with bicycle riding, not readily taught through books and classroom lectures. These difficulties may be overcome by hands-on workshop teaching, by gaining experience manipulating the data that are generated by research projects, and by being required to teach statistical principles to colleagues. It is perceived to be a subject requiring advanced mathematical skills; this is undoubtedly true if one is trying to prove the principles behind the subject. However, the possession of a sound knowledge of when and how to apply these principles allows a black-box approach to the subject and the mathematics required is reduced to that of simple arithmetic. The danger of this approach, however, is that misapplication of poorly understood statistics is ridden with pitfalls to trap the unwary and the advice of a competent statistician should be sought in all but the simplest of problems. Statistical packages for personal computers are tremendously useful, but if used without knowledge of statistical principles their output may be, at best, dubious.

It will be obvious that this chapter can scratch only the surface of statistical knowledge. However, the syllabuses for postgraduate examinations have been taken into account during its preparation. It should be borne in mind that, in an attempt to make the subject understandable, certain concepts have been simplified to the extent that a purist might point to inaccuracies in the text.

### What are statistics?

If a variable could be measured in the whole population, statistics would be unnecessary. The basis of statistics is that necessarily small samples are drawn from large populations and the statistics of the sample are used to estimate the parameters of the population. The predictive ability of this estimation is given limits by the rules of probability. Factors describing the mathematical nature of a population are known as parameters; those of the sample are termed 'statistics'. It is essential that the term 'parameter' is reserved for this definition and the term 'variable' used to describe an individual characteristic or reading. A single measurement of a variable is given the symbol $x$. Statistics may be defined as a mathematical manipulation of $x$ values (Figure 40.1). Later we shall see that the parameters of a normal distribution are its mean and standard deviation, the same terms as the statistics of a sample drawn from it.

### Why are they used?

The aims of statistics are twofold:

- to provide a convenient and conventional description of data: descriptive statistics;
- to make deductions and draw conclusions from that data: inferential statistics.

## DESCRIPTIVE STATISTICS AND THE TYPE OF DATA

### Scales of measurement

Identifying the nature of the data under consideration is the key that enables the occasional statistician to use the correct method of manipulating the data and ultimately to choose an appropriate test of significance.

### Categorical data

Categorical data do not take a numerical value. Frequently, the outcome of a clinical trial involves placing an individual or an event into one of two mutually exclusive categories, e.g. the patient was male/female or the patient did/did not vomit postoperatively. These are examples of two-category data. However, it is frequently possible to apportion these type of data into multiple categories, e.g. the patient was Welsh, Swiss, or Albanian. Audit data are frequently in this form: Box 177 was ticked – the patient is under the care of

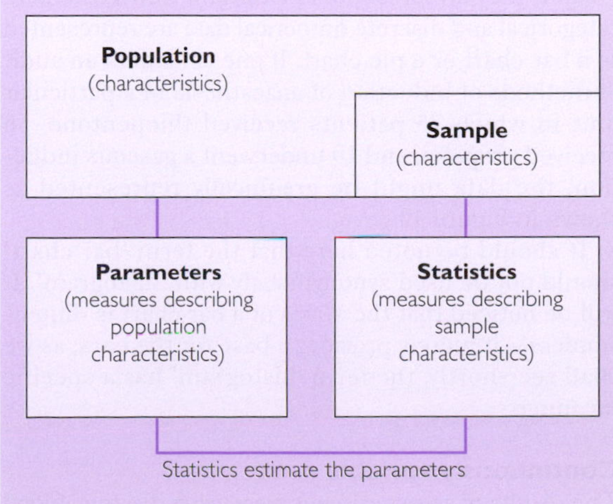


**Figure 40.1** The interrelationships of population, parameters, sample, and statistics

Dr Thompson. These type of data are referred to as nominal data.

### Numerical data

#### *Discrete (non-continuous) data*

If, in an undergraduate examination, three students are placed first, second, and third, it is possible to say that the first student has done better than the second and third. This is an example of ordinal data; this merely means that categorical data can be put into a meaningful order or ranked. It does not indicate that there is a significant difference between the students, by how much the first placed was better than the second, or indeed that any of them passed the examination. In anaesthesia, there is increasing use of scoring systems, e.g. the Malampatti scoring system of airway assessment. The fact that there are four scores (1, 2, 3, and 4) does not mean that a grade 2 is twice as difficult to intubate as grade 1. Another type of discrete data may have a numerical value that is an integer, e.g. 'three outpatient visits per year'. A frequently used example of discrete numerical data is the number of radioactive counts over a period of time. However, if the count rate is high the data tend to be treated as continuous data. Similarly heart rate, although an example of discrete numerical data (a fraction of a heartbeat is impossible), is similarly treated as continuous data.

#### *Continuous data*

Plasma sodium concentration, height, age, and an induction dose of thiopentone (thiopental) are all examples of continuously variable data. The number of decimal places to which they may be expressed is dependent on the particular measuring system. Incidentally, one should beware of spurious precision when dealing with these type of data – measuring serum pH to three places of decimals would suggest that the measuring system has the ability to detect a change of one part in 10 000.

## THE GRAPHICAL PRESENTATION OF DATA AND FREQUENCY DISTRIBUTIONS

### Categorical data

The implications of collected data are far easier to grasp if they are presented pictorially. Conventionally, categorical and discrete numerical data are represented as a bar chart or a pie chart. If one considers an audit of methods of induction of anaesthesia in a particular unit in which 75 patients received thiopentone, 56 received propofol, and 19 underwent a gaseous induction, the data might be graphically represented as shown in Figure 40.2.

It should be noted here that the term 'bar chart' should not be used synonymously with 'histogram'. It will be noticed that the $x$ axis of a bar chart is dimensionless – it merely provides a base for the bars; as we shall see shortly, the term 'histogram' has a specific meaning.

### Continuously variable data

The results of an experiment measuring diastolic blood pressure in a group of preoperative patients are shown in Table 40.1.

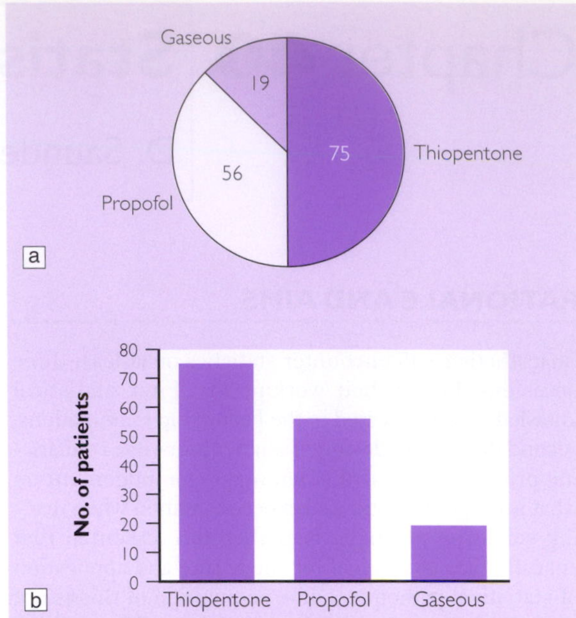


**Figure 40.2** Representation of non-parametric data: (a) a pie chart and (b) a bar chart.

By searching the data, it is possible to define the highest and the lowest values. This information is, however, more easily obtained if the data are presented in an array. This involves placing the data in numerical order (Table 40.2). This enables an assessment of the 'shape' of the data to be made, in which the relationship of individual observations to the rest of the data is noted. The progression of the data, discontinuities, and 'humps' may be studied. By noting the highest and lowest values in the array, a quantification of the range of variables in the array can be made. By summing the variables and dividing by the number of observations, the mean may be calculated:

$$\frac{\Sigma x}{n}$$

where $\Sigma$ is the sum of and $n$ the number of observations.

Continuous data may be displayed by grouping the data into discrete bands. Each observation in a particular group is then entered. This process is known as tallying (Figure 40.3a).

It will be seen that, if a tally is turned through 90°, a histogram will result (Figure 40.3b). If a large (theoretically infinite) number of observations were made, taking smaller and smaller bands, the jagged histogram would become a smooth curve which would represent the distribution of the population. The 'smoothness' of an experimentally derived curve depends on the number of observations in the sample.

### Types of distribution

#### *The normal or gaussian distribution*

This is a distribution in which most of the observations are grouped around the average value, and fewer and fewer individual measurements are found at the more extreme portions of the range. For example, most men

**Table 40.1 Diastolic blood pressure (mmHg) in 100 patients, measured using an automated method**

| | | | | | | | | | |
|---|---|---|---|---|---|---|---|---|---|
| 90 | 104 | 94 | 105 | 95 | 92 | 102 | 84 | 78 | 95 |
| 68 | 80 | 66 | 101 | 90 | 90 | 92 | 106 | 86 | 82 |
| 84 | 82 | 80 | 61 | 88 | 82 | 65 | 88 | 78 | 96 |
| 66 | 78 | 84 | 96 | 62 | 64 | 70 | 84 | 83 | 76 |
| 68 | 96 | 88 | 96 | 75 | 70 | 56 | 75 | 82 | 98 |
| 98 | 82 | 90 | 94 | 58 | 94 | 86 | 82 | 84 | 91 |
| 77 | 64 | 97 | 84 | 60 | 88 | 74 | 78 | 74 | 72 |
| 77 | 108 | 89 | 105 | 62 | 94 | 80 | 88 | 88 | 82 |
| 99 | 62 | 92 | 66 | 58 | 74 | 75 | 105 | 92 | 80 |
| 92 | 88 | 80 | 74 | 82 | 84 | 78 | 93 | 72 | 93 |

**Table 40.2 An array created from the data in Table 40.1**

| | | | | | | | | | |
|---|---|---|---|---|---|---|---|---|---|
| 56 | 58 | 58 | 60 | 61 | 62 | 62 | 62 | 64 | 64 |
| 65 | 66 | 66 | 66 | 68 | 68 | 70 | 70 | 72 | 72 |
| 74 | 74 | 74 | 74 | 75 | 75 | 75 | 76 | 77 | 77 |
| 78 | 78 | 78 | 78 | 78 | 80 | 80 | 80 | 80 | 80 |
| 82 | 82 | 82 | 82 | 82 | 82 | 82 | 82 | 83 | 84 |
| 84 | 84 | 84 | 84 | 84 | 84 | 86 | 86 | 88 | 88 |
| 88 | 88 | 88 | 88 | 88 | 89 | 90 | 90 | 90 | 90 |
| 91 | 92 | 92 | 92 | 92 | 92 | 93 | 93 | 94 | 94 |
| 94 | 94 | 95 | 95 | 96 | 96 | 96 | 96 | 97 | 98 |
| 98 | 99 | 101 | 102 | 104 | 105 | 105 | 105 | 106 | 108 |

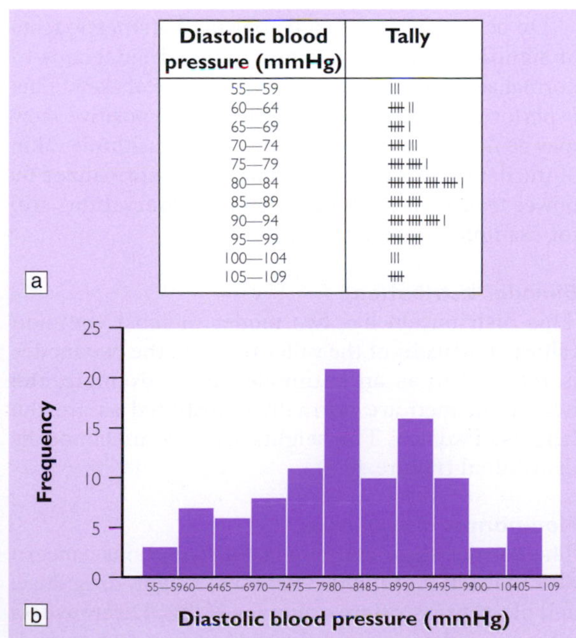

Diastolic blood pressure (mmHg)
Tally
55—59
60—64
65—69
70—74
75—79
80—84
85—89
90—94
95—99
100—104
105—109
a
Frequency
25
20
15
10
5
0
Diastolic blood pressure (mmHg)
b


**Figure 40.3** The data in Table 40.1, tallied (a) and as a histogram (b).

will be between 1.50 metres and 1.90 metres in height. There are unlikely to be many below 1.40 metres or above 2.00 metres.

The normal distribution (Figure 40.4) is a bell-shaped curve with a very specific formula. The position of the curve on the $x$ axis is governed by the value of $\mu$, the population mean. The breadth of the curve is described by $\sigma$, the population standard deviation. The two factors, $\mu$ and $\sigma$, are known as the population parameters and, if normal distribution is assumed, the data are said to be parametric, i.e. the parameters of the population are known.

It is very important to realize that populations have parameters whereas samples have statistics (Table 40.3).

*Measures of location of continuously variable distributions*

The terms 'mean', 'median', and 'mode' are called the measures of location of a population; the terms may also be used to describe a sample.

- The mean is the mathematical average of the individual observations.
- The median is the value of the middle observation in an array; for arrays containing an even number

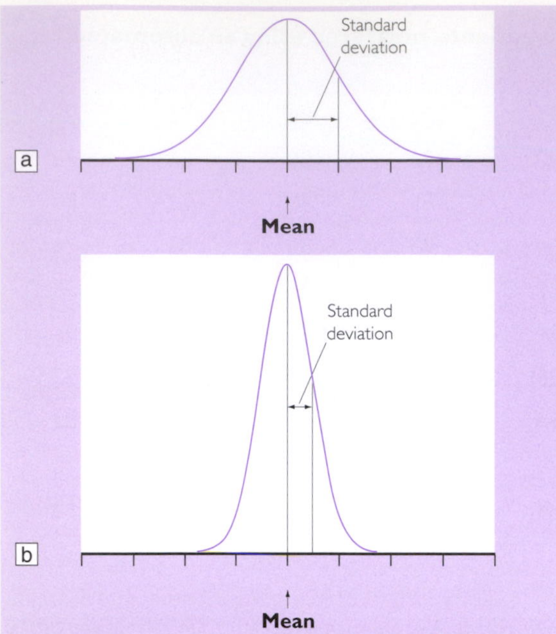


**Figure 40.4** Two normal distributions with widely differing standard deviations. The curve has a specific formula (based on its two parameters μ and σ) given by the formula:

$$y = \frac{1}{\sigma\hat{}2\pi} \cdot e^{\frac{1}{2}\left(\frac{x-\mu}{\sigma}\right)}$$

(Adapted from Moore DS. *Statistics: Concepts and Controversies*. San Francisco: WH Freeman, 1979.)

| **Table 40.3 Difference between parameters and statistics** | |
|---|---|
| Population | Sample |
| Parameters | Statistics |
| μ = mean | x̄ (x bar) = mean |
| σ = standard deviation | S = standard deviation |

of samples, the average of the two middle observations is made. The area under the population curve is divided into two equal portions by the median.

- The mode is the most commonly occurring value.

In a normal distribution the three measures of location are co-located (Figure 40.5a). If the three measures do not coexist, the distribution is said to be skewed. A positive skew exists if the tail of the distribution is found over the larger values (Figure 40.5b); in a negative skew, the tail is over the lower values (Figure 40.5c). It should be noted that, in a skewed distribution, the median is always found between the mode and the mean. In the data given in Table 40.1, the mean is 83.1 mmHg, the median 84 mmHg, and the mode 82 mmHg. The fact that the three values are numerically very close would make a normal distribution likely.

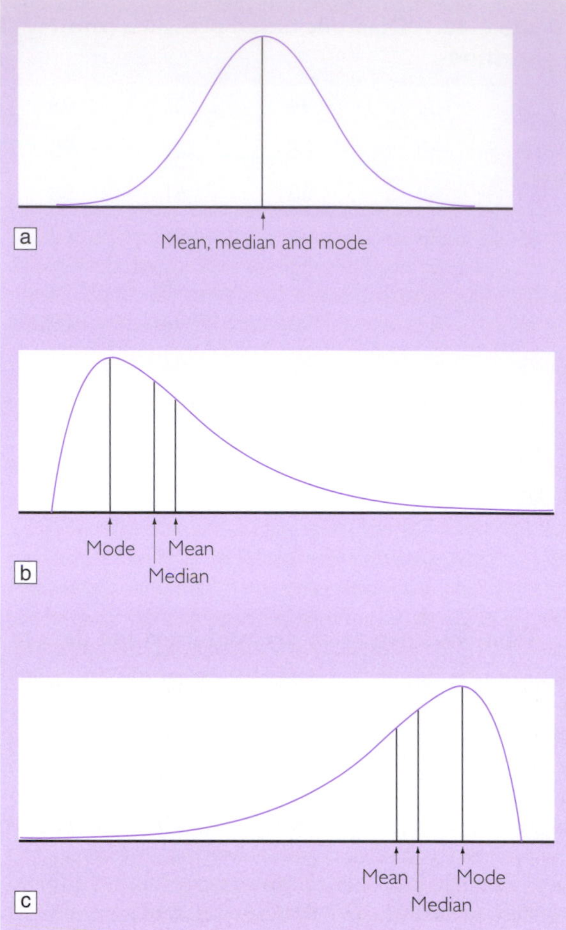


**Figure 40.5** (a) The mean, median, and mode of a normal distribution are identically positioned. In (b) a positively skewed and (c) a negatively skewed distribution, the median is located between the mode and the mean. (Adapted from Moore DS. *Statistics: Concepts and Controversies*. San Francisco: WH Freeman, 1979.)

On occasions (e.g. when applying parametric tests of significance), it is deemed to be advantageous to normalize the data, i.e. reduce the degree of skew. This is performed by transforming the data. A positive skew may be normalized by employing the logarithmic value of the data, and a negative skew may be normalized by power transformation in which the observations are, for example, squared or cubed.

### *Bimodal distribution*

This distribution has two modes or most common values. The nadir of the valley between the two modes is referred to as an antimode. As an example, the heights of men are normally distributed as are the heights of women. The heights of *people* are bimodally distributed (Figure 40.6).

### *Non-normal distributions*

The normal, skew, and bimodal distributions concern data that are continuously variable; height, drug dose, and blood pressure are examples of this. Discrete data – for example, yes/no or did/did not vomit – are dealt with under the title 'binomial distribution', a special case of polynomial distribution where only two cases

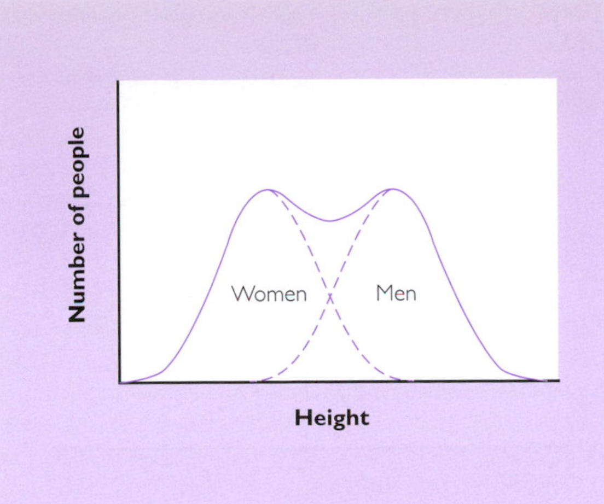


**Figure 40.6** A bimodal distribution. The heights of men are normally distributed as are those of women. The heights of *people* are bimodally distributed.

may exist. To satisfy a binomial distribution, experimental data must satisfy all of the following conditions:

- Successive observations are independent, i.e. the results of one observation do not depend on any other.
- For any measurement, the result must have one of two values (did/did not vomit).
- The chance of either of these values occurring does not vary from one observation to another. The chances are expressed in terms of $p$ and $q$. If the probability of a given event is $p$, the probability of an event not occurring is $1 - p = q$.

### Information available from distribution curves

In the example given in Table 40.1, two important statistics were defined: the mean and the range. However, two 'normal' curves may have the same mean, although one curve is tall and narrow and the other is low and wide (Figure 40.4). The mean value and the range give no information about the spread of observation around the mean, and it is necessary to compute a measure of this scatter if the nature of the data is to be described to another worker; this is the variance and standard deviation.

To obtain an average of how far the observations differ from the mean, each observation is subtracted from the mean value. The sum of all these values is obtained, ignoring the sign, and then divided by the number of observations. This value may be referred to as the mean absolute deviation.

$$\frac{\Sigma|x - \bar{x}|}{n} = \text{Mean absolute deviation} \qquad (1)$$

There are various reasons why this mathematically reasonable treatment of the data is less than ideal for our purposes, for example, it is not numerically independent of the value of the mean. For reasons that are outside the scope of this chapter, this objection is removed if the differences are squared before being summed.

$$\frac{\Sigma (x - \bar{x})^2}{n} = s^2 \text{ (variance)} \qquad (2)$$

This value $S^2$ is referred to as the variance. It has the advantage that all the values are positive and, second, the sum of the terms may be derived simply from a shorthand formula known as the sum of squares:

$$\Sigma (x - \bar{x})^2 = \Sigma x^2 - \frac{(\Sigma x)^2}{n} = \text{SS (sum of squares)} \qquad (3)$$

It can be seen that the calculation does not require the arithmetical value of the mean to be known and is therefore independent of it. It is the method of calculation that pocket calculators employ. In statistics, the variance is a very powerful factor because it may be mathematically manipulated. In descriptive statistics, however, the units are very large and are not the same as those observed in the experiment; the variance of time would be expressed as square hours – a tricky concept! To return to the units of observation, it is conventional to express the measure of dispersion as the square root of the variance – the standard deviation.

$$\sqrt{\frac{\Sigma (x - \bar{x})^2}{n}} = s \text{ (standard deviation)} \qquad (4)$$

This value is expressed as σ if the population standard deviation is being referred to or as $s$ if that of a sample.

It will have been noted that, on certain occasions, the sum of the squares of the difference is divided by $n - 1$ rather than by $n$; indeed some calculators allow a choice of the two to be made. Dividing by $n - 1$ acts to give a larger calculated value for variance; the scatter about the mean is overestimated. This manoeuvre allows the experimental sample standard deviation to be used to approximate the unknown population standard deviation. When $n$ is large (say > 30) this correction makes virtually no difference; indeed sample statistics for large samples may be used as population parameters with very little error being incurred.

### Confidence intervals

In any normal distribution, half the observations fall above the mean and half below. Sixty-eight percent of the observations fall within one standard deviation unit (sometimes referred to as $z$ units) either side of the mean. Half of these (34%) fall between the mean and +1 standard deviation unit and half between the mean and −1 standard deviation unit (34%). A further 28% fall between −2 and +2 standard deviations of the mean. Thus 96% of observations are found between two standard deviations of the mean. Ninety-five percent of observations fall between +1.96 and −1.96 standard deviations of the mean. Three standard deviations either side of the mean contain 99.7% of the population; thus a normal distribution is about six standard deviations wide (Figure 40.7).

This knowledge of the proportions of the normal distribution contained by multiples of standard deviation units allows a prediction of the results of a further single sample from the population. The standard deviation of the diastolic blood pressure data in Table 40.1 proved to be 12.4 mmHg. Thus, there is a 68% chance

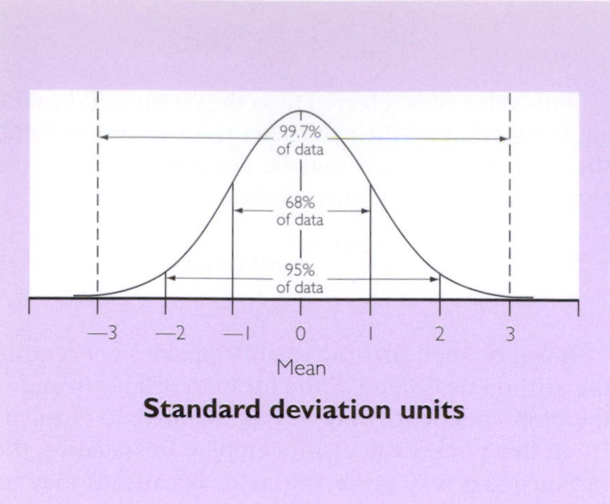


**Figure 40.7** The areas under a normally distributed curve bounded by standard deviation units. (Adapted from Moore DS. *Statistics: Concepts and Controversies*. San Francisco: WH Freeman, 1979.)

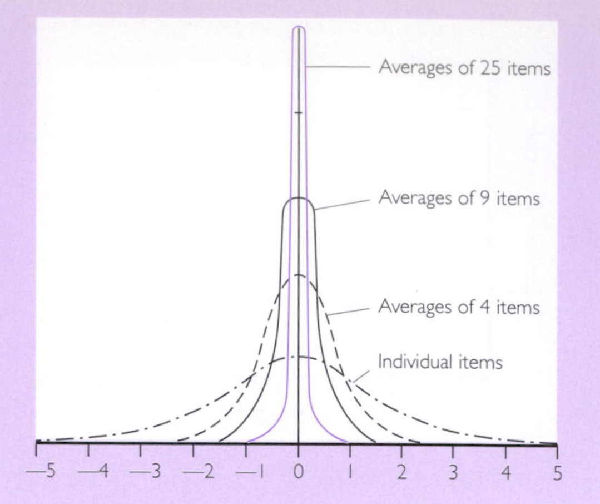


**Figure 40.8** The distribution for the averages of samples becomes more and more compact as the sample size increases, the standard deviation being inversely proportional to the square root of the number of items in the sample. Note that 0 on the horizontal scale is equal to the grand average value for the whole population. (Modified from Moroney MJ. *Facts from Figures*, 3rd edn. Basingstoke: Penguin Books, 1956.)

that the next patient will have diastolic blood pressure within 1 standard deviation of the mean (70.7–95.5 mmHg); 95% of the time the single reading will fall within 1.96 standard deviations of the mean (58.5–107.4 mmHg). In the latter case, a prediction is made at the 95% confidence limit and the range is referred to as the 95% confidence interval. It has to be accepted, however, that the observation will fall outside these limits five times out of each 100 samples.

### The standard error of the mean

The key concept to grasp when considering the standard error of the mean (SEM) is that, when the means of samples taken from a normal population are plotted, they too are normally distributed. The normal distribution that we have considered may be thought of as the frequency distribution of means of samples where the sample size is one (i.e. $n = 1$). Thus, in this instance, the mean value and the value itself are identical. If a sample size of 10 is now chosen and a large number (in theory infinity) of samples are made and plotted, a normal distribution will result in which the scatter about the mean is much reduced. As the sample size is increased to 100, the distribution becomes narrower again and so on, until the sample size is infinite and the distribution becomes a vertical straight line at the population mean. As the number of measurements in a single sample increases therefore, the resultant sample mean is likely to represent the 'true' mean more closely (Figure 40.8).

As the means are normally distributed, it follows that the distribution must have a standard deviation. It is this standard deviation that is referred to as the SEM. Put another way, the SEM is the standard deviation of a distribution of sample means at a particular sample size.

From this it follows that the variance of the mean of a sample from a population is equal to the population variance ($\sigma^2$) divided by the number in the sample:

$$\text{variance}\ (\bar{x}) = \frac{\sigma^2}{n} \qquad (5)$$

The standard deviation of the mean of a sample is equal to the square root of this value:

$$\text{SD}\ (\bar{x}) = \sqrt{\frac{\sigma^2}{n}} = \frac{\sigma}{\sqrt{n}} \simeq \frac{\text{SD}}{\sqrt{n}} \qquad (6)$$

Thus, the SEM of a sample may be calculated by dividing the sample standard deviation by the square root of the number of individuals in the sample.

From our knowledge of confidence limits, the SEM allows us to predict what would happen if a further single sample were drawn from the population. The sample mean would fall within 1 SEM either side of the population mean on 67% of occasions; 95% of the time it would be within 1.96 SEM. More importantly, we may be confident 95% of the time that the unknown population mean falls within the limits 1.96 either side of our sample mean. It has to be accepted, however, that 5% of the time this assumption will be wrong, the 'true' mean lying outside the 95% confidence limits.

In simple terms, the SEM is used as a tool for predicting how nearly the sample mean is likely to approximate to the true population mean.

### Graphical representation of errors

Error bars may be incorporated in bar charts (Figure 40.9a) or in plots representing the mean and its errors (Figure 40.9b). The inclusion of the standard error makes the assumption that the data are normally distributed. The representation of non-parametric data is shown in Figure 40.9c and d. The factor used to show the spread of data about the median is the interquartile range (IQR) and this represents the data limited by the 25% and 75% values in an array. The total range is also plotted. This is sometimes shown graphically as a lozenge, where the points of the lozenge represent the range, its shoulders the IQR, and the broad line towards the centre the median. More commonly, the relationship is given by a 'box-and-whisker' plot in which the range is given by the ends of the whiskers, the IQR by the vertical extremes of the box, and the median as a line within the box. A lozenge or box-and-whisker plot shows that the authors are treating the data non-parametrically.

## INFERENTIAL STATISTICS

### Probability

It has been demonstrated that, from a knowledge of the mean, variance (or standard deviation), and SEM of a sample, it is possible to estimate the population parameters within certain levels of probability. Probability is the key to the understanding of statistics; it is denoted by the letter $P$ and may assume a value from 0 (an event never occurs) to 1 (an event always occurs) (Figure 40.10).

Between the theoretical extremes of zero and unity, every value of probability is possible. The classic example of $P = 0.5$ is tossing a coin: the coin will land, on average, as a head half of the time. Experience tells us that five consecutive tosses of 'head' are in no way surprising; 20 successive 'heads' would make one suspicious. Thus, predicting with 95% confidence is in most respects analogous to $P = 0.05$. In other words, we allow ourselves to be incorrect 5% of the time. We accept that our prediction will be wrong once in 20 times that a sample is made, and that an individual measurement will not fall within the 95% confidence limits. Or, using the value of $P < 0.05$ as a significance level, once in 20 times a value of $P$ below 0.05 has no 'true' significance, the apparent significance being the result of chance. The value of $P = 0.05$ as the limit of significance has, over the years, achieved the status of a magic number; it is no such thing. The value is totally arbitrary and has arisen merely as a convention. It may be that, if resources were strictly limited, a significance level of $P < 0.1$ is justifiable or that, if a greater certainty is required, $P$ should be less than 0.01, i.e. we accept that our hypothesis will be incorrect once in 100 times. Over the last few years, the usefulness of hypothesis testing, requiring the probability to be less than a 'significant' value, has been questioned. An alternative approach involves the demonstration of confidence intervals, thereby providing readers with a method by which they can make up their own minds about the significance of any particular result. This will be dealt with later.

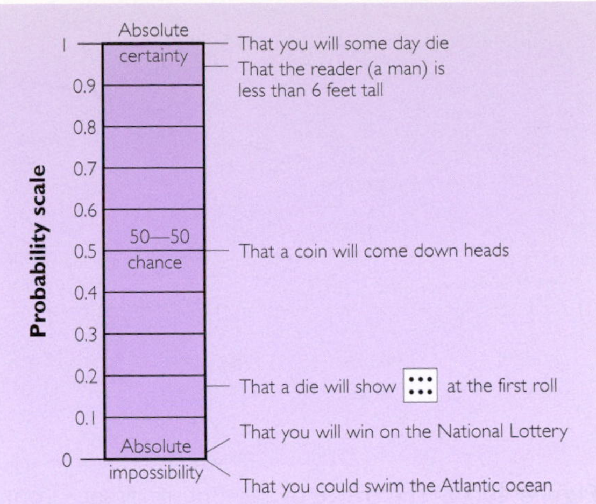


**Figure 40.10** The probability scale. (Modified from Moroney MJ. *Facts from Figures*, 3rd edn. Basingstoke: Penguin Books, 1956.)

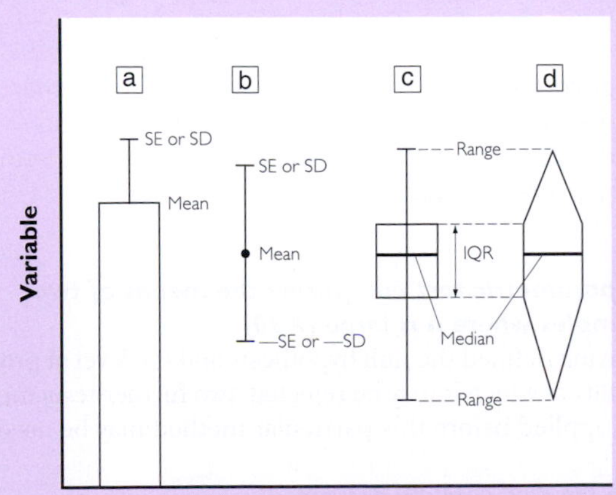


**Figure 40.9** Graphical representation of means and medians. (a) The standard error (SE) or standard deviation (SD) about a bar chart representing the mean of parametric data; (b) SE or SD about a mean represented by a point; (c) a box-and-whisker plot of non-parametric data; (d) a lozenge plot of the data in (c). IQR, interquartile range.

### Tests of statistical significance

Tests of statistical significance are used to test a chosen hypothesis (Figure 40.11). The choice of an appropriate test of significance is governed by the recognition of the type of data with which one is presented: the recognition of whether data are (1) continuous or non-continuous (discrete) and (2) parametric (the type of distribution is known) or non-parametric (also called distribution free). For each parametric test there is a choice of non-parametric tests.

Thus, comparing induction doses of thiopentone, it will be recognized that drug dose is a continuous variable. The decision has to be made whether a normal distribution may be assumed. Goodness of fit of data to a normal distribution may be judged using a probit plot, the details of which are outside the realm of this chapter. (See page 131 of Kirkwood in the Further reading for a simple explanation.) If the data are adjudged to be normally distributed, then the presence of a statistically significant difference between two samples may be detected by comparison of means using a Student $t$-test. If the data prove not to be normally distributed, even after transformation, or if no distribution is to be assumed, then a non-parametric test may be used, e.g. the comparison of medians by a Mann–Whitney $U$ test. A non-parametric test may be used if the data are normally distributed, but the ability to detect small differences will be reduced. If such data are proved to be significantly different using a non-parametric test, it will certainly be significant if a $t$-test

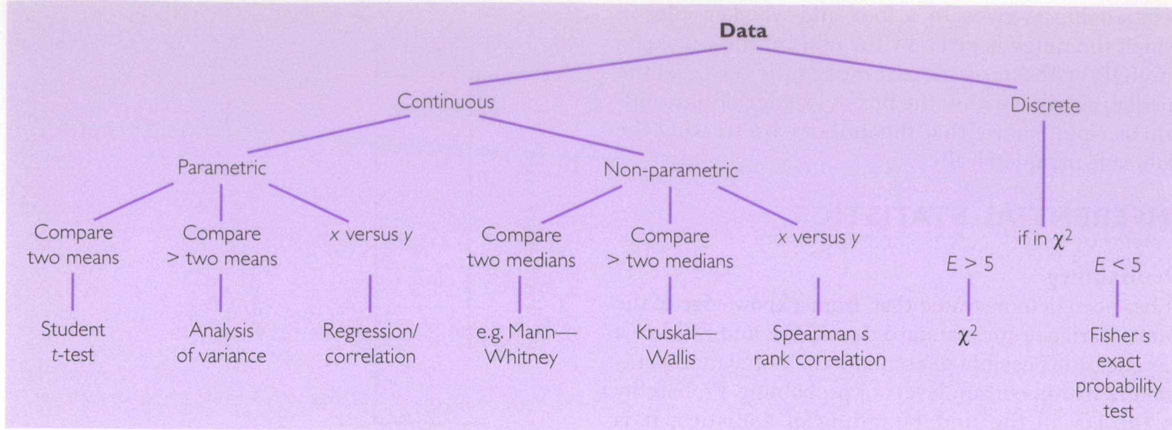


**Figure 40.11** The choice of a test of significance from knowledge of the type of data. E = expected value in $\chi^2$ test.

is used. There has recently been controversy over whether a parametric test may be used for the analysis of data from a visual analogue scale (VAS). The purists would say that these data are not normally distributed and a non-parametric test should be used. Care must be taken when comparing variables with a logarithmic relationship. Although it is acceptable to take a mean of hydrogen ion concentration, one should probably not do so for values of pH.

### *Before the start of any test of significance*

There are two tasks that must be performed before any test of significance is commenced.

#### *Define the null hypothesis*

At the start of a statistical investigation, it is assumed that there is no difference between the tests or samples being considered, e.g. there is no difference in the results from a standard method or from a new method. Or, there is no difference between two samples. In this case, it is assumed that both samples are drawn from the same population.

This assumption of identity is called the null hypothesis ($H_0$) (Figure 40.12). The alternative hypothesis would state that there is indeed a difference; the two samples were drawn from different populations. All tests of significance seek to disprove the null hypothesis at a level of probability. If a statistical significance can be shown between two groups, the null hypothesis may be rejected at that level of probability. If statistical significance is not detected at a level of probability, it is equivalent to a verdict of not proven; it may be that collection of further samples may lead to statistical significance. Conversely, statistical significance does not indicate clinical significance. In a large clinical trial, a difference in systolic blood pressure of 1 mmHg may prove highly significant statistically; clinically it is probably irrelevant.

#### *Define the level of probability at which $H_0$ is rejected*

As outlined above, statistical significance is assumed if the observed result could occur by chance less than one time in 20, i.e. $P < 0.05$. This particular level of probability is only a convention.

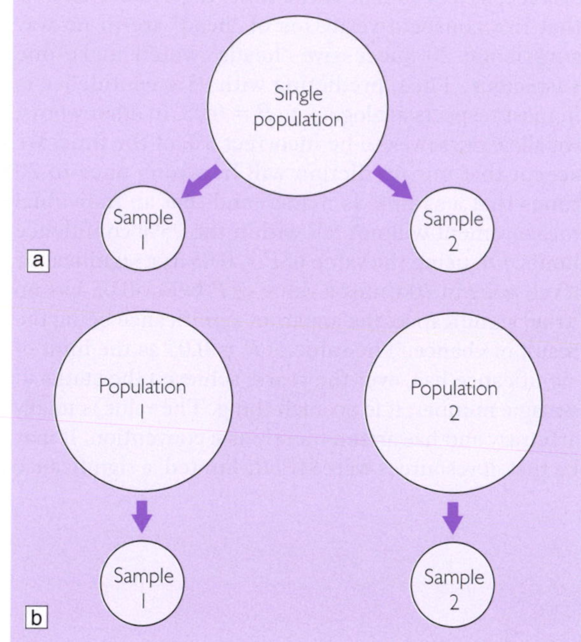


**Figure 40.12** (a) The null hypothesis which assumes that two samples are drawn from a single population, and (b) the alternative hypothesis that they come from two different populations.

### *A parametric test comparing the means of two samples where n is large (>30)*

Having defined the null hypothesis and the level of probability at which it may be rejected, two further tests must be applied before this particular method may be used.

#### *Are the data normally distributed?*

We have already considered the parameters of the normal distribution, transformations to 'normalize' data, and probit plots. These tests are fairly robust and, because of a mathematical relationship known as the central limit theorem, the means and variances of samples from moderately skewed distributions approach the population means and variance if the sample size is sufficiently large.

*Are the variances of the two samples sufficiently similar?*
It is possible to imagine two distribution curves with identical means, i.e. having the same locus on the abscissa ($x$ axis), but widely different standard deviations. Thus one curve may be tall and narrow and the other short and broad. If a comparison of means is performed, the result will indicate that there is no difference between the two samples drawn from obviously different populations. If one is uncertain about the similarity of the two sample variances, before embarking on this particular test a variance ratio test should be performed, which tests the significance of the difference between sample variances. This is referred to as the $F$ test.

$$F \text{ (variance ratio)} = \frac{\text{Greater estimate of the population variance}}{\text{Lesser estimate of population variance}}$$

The population referred to is the common population assumed by the null hypothesis. The value of $F$ is entered into the appropriate table.

A sample mean differs by more than twice its standard error from the population mean only once in 20 times. The differences between sample means are normally distributed and thus possess a standard error – the so-called standard error of the difference. As the population mean is unknown, it is necessary to assume that there is a 95% chance that one of the two sample means under comparison lies within 1.96 standard errors of it. If, now, the second sample mean lies within 1.96 of the population mean, the chances are, at the 95% level, that both samples have been drawn from the same population.

The variance of the sum or difference of two independent random variables is equal to the sum of their variances. Thus:

$$\text{var}(\bar{x}_1 - \bar{x}_2) = \frac{\sigma_1^2}{n_1} + \frac{\sigma_2^2}{n_2} \qquad (7)$$

where $\sigma_1$ and $\sigma_2$ are the population standard deviations and $n_1$ and $n_2$ the number of samples drawn from these populations.

Then the standard error of the difference:

$$\text{SE difference} = \sqrt{\frac{s_1^2}{N_1} + \frac{s_2^2}{N_2}} \qquad (8)$$

### An example

The mean value of diastolic blood pressures given in Table 40.1 is 83.1 mmHg and the calculated standard deviation 12.4 mmHg. Let us compare this sample with another sample of 100 measurements in which the mean pressure is 89.3 mmHg and the standard deviation 10.4 mmHg.

| | **Sample 1** | **Sample 2** |
|---|---|---|
| Mean | 83.1 mmHg | 89.3 mmHg |
| SD | 12.4 mmHg | 10.4 mmHg |
| $n$ | 100 | 100 |

First, it is necessary to apply the two universal tests, and assume that the data are normally distributed and the variances are not significantly different. We will set the level of probability at which the null hypothesis may be rejected at $P \leq 0.05$. Then:

Arithmetical difference between means (89.3 – 83.1) = 6.2 mmHg

$$\text{SE difference} = \sqrt{\frac{(10.4)^2}{100} + \frac{(12.4)^2}{100}} \qquad (9)$$

$$= 1.61 \text{ mmHg}$$

If we now calculate how many multiples of the standard error of the difference this represents, i.e.

$$Z = \frac{\text{Arithmetic difference between means}}{\text{SE difference}}$$

$$= \frac{6.2}{1.61}$$

$$= 3.9 \times \text{SE}.$$

If we consult Table 40.4, which relates the probability of a particular result occurring to multiples of standard deviations (or standard errors) for a normal distribution, we see that this figure is considerably in excess of the 1.96 standard deviation units necessary to reject the null hypothesis at the level of probability that was chosen. Indeed, the value is considerably above the 3.29 standard deviation units necessary to give a probability of 0.001 (that the result could be the result of chance once in 1000 times). Thus, we have demonstrated that the null hypothesis is extremely unlikely and that a statistical difference exists between our two samples at our chosen level of probability.

### A parametric test for small samples where n < 30

W.S. Gossett (who worked for Guiness, the brewers) modified the above test in 1908, publishing the work under the *nom de plume* 'Student'. Again, it is assumed that the two samples are drawn from populations that are normally distributed and the variances of which are similar. The level of probability at which the null hypothesis may be rejected is defined. The ratio calculated is very similar to that for large numbers, namely:

$$t = \frac{\text{Difference between sample means}}{\text{Estimated standard error of the difference}}$$

It will be noted that the ratio for large numbers was a Z ratio, i.e. a number of standard deviation units. For small sample numbers, the ratio is denoted the so-called Student '*t*'. The estimated standard error of the difference is calculated slightly differently, being that of the pooled data from the two samples. Student's contribution was to calculate frequency distributions for samples of specific sizes; $t$ tables are a numerical representation of these distributions (Figure 40.13).

The larger the sample size, the nearer the $t$ distribution approaches the normal distribution. It will be seen that $t$ distributions are wider than the normal distribution. In essence, this means that the value of $t$ for any comparison has to be greater than that necessary to achieve significance if the normal distribution can be assumed.

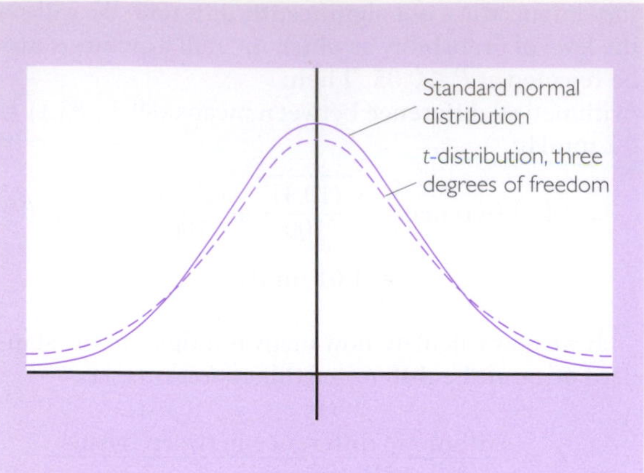


**Figure 40.13** The *t*-distributions are plotted at various degrees of freedom; the one for three degrees of freedom is shown. The *t*-distributions are wider than the normal distribution. (Adapted from Hayslett HT. *Statistics Made Simple*. London: WH Allen, 1968.)

### Degrees of freedom

In tests of samples from a continuously variable population, once the mean is specified arbitrary values may be ascribed to all but the final value, which is predetermined by the other values in the group and the mean. Thus, for a single sample the number of degrees of freedom is one less than the sample size ($n - 1$). For pairs of data the degree of freedom (df) is equal to the number of pairs minus one. For unpaired data such as those in the worked example above, the df is equal to $(n_1 - 1) + (n_2 - 1)$, in this case: $99 + 99 = 198$.

To test whether the calculated $t$ value is significant at any particular level of probability, the figure is taken into '$t$ tables' and compared with the number of degrees of freedom (Table 40.5).

The $t$ table is entered on the appropriate row on the vertical scale, which denotes the number of degrees of freedom. The calculated value of $t$ is compared with the critical value of $t$ in the column headed by the level of probability at which it has been decided that the null hypothesis may be rejected. If the calculated value of $t$ exceeds the critical value, there is said to be a difference in means at that level of probability. When the number of degrees of freedom is very large, the critical value of $t$ approaches 1.96, representing the normal distribution.

### Paired t-tests

A paired $t$-test compares the differences between the means of samples of paired data. For example, if a trial is made of a new antihypertensive agent and the pretreatment mean blood pressure is compared with the value after treatment, each subject has acted as their own control and the data are said to be paired.

#### *One- and two-tailed t-tests*

The above examples consider data in which a difference may occur in either direction: the mean of a second sample may have a value higher or lower than the first. This is said to be a two-tailed test. If it is predicted at the outset that a change may occur in only one direction, it is permissible to use a one-tailed test. The calculation of $t$ is very similar but, as the results are considered to be significant if the $t$ value is in the upper 5% (as opposed to 2.5%) of the distribution, the numerical value of $t$ required to achieve a particular level of significance is lower. Trials using one-tail testing must be carefully scrutinized to ensure that the original prediction of change in one direction only is valid.

#### *The comparison of several means*

Consider an experiment in which a variable is measured at a control time and at 5, 10, 15, and 20 min. Five means are obtained. It is not acceptable to compare the control mean with the mean at time 5 min, the mean at 10 min and the means at 15 and 20 min using separate $t$-tests, unless a correction is made or another method employed. The preferred method is to employ a one-way analysis of variance test. In this the variance within the individual groups is compared with the variance between the groups. Instead of comparing the means of the samples, therefore, the second sample

**Table 40.4 Probability related to multiples of standard deviations (or standard errors) for a normal distribution**

| Number of standard deviations | Probability of observation showing at least as large a deviation from the population mean |
|---|---|
| 0.674 | 0.50 |
| 1.0 | 0.317 |
| 1.645 | 0.10 |
| 1.960 | 0.05 |
| 2.0 | 0.046 |
| 2.576 | 0.01 |
| 3.0 | 0.0027 |
| 3.291 | 0.001 |

Adapted by permission of the author and publishers from Table 2.5 of *Statistical Methods in Medical Research*. Armitage P and Berry G. Oxford: Blackwell Scientific Publications, 1987.

**Table 40.5 An extract from t tables**

| Degrees of freedom (ν) | Probability of P ≥ 0.5 | 0.2 | 0.1 | 0.05 | 0.01 | 0.001 |
|---|---|---|---|---|---|---|
| 1 | 1.000 | 3.078 | 6.314 | 12.706 | 63.657 | 636.619 |
| 2 | 0.816 | 1.886 | 2.920 | 4.303 | 9.925 | 31.598 |
| 3 | 0.765 | 1.638 | 2.353 | 3.182 | 5.841 | 12.924 |
| 4 | 0.741 | 1.533 | 2.132 | 2.776 | 4.604 | 8.610 |
| 5 | 0.727 | 1.476 | 2.015 | 2.571 | 4.032 | 6.860 |
| 10 | 0.700 | 2.764 | 1.812 | 2.228 | 3.169 | 4.587 |
| 30 | 0.683 | 1.310 | 1.697 | 2.042 | 2.750 | 3.646 |
| 120 | 0.677 | 1.289 | 1.658 | 1.980 | 2.617 | 3.373 |
| ∞ | 0.674 | 1.282 | 1.645 | 1.960 | 2.576 | 3.291 |

Adapted with permission from Armitage P and Berry G. *Statistical Methods in Medical Research*. Oxford: Blackwell Scientific Publications 1987.

statistic typical of a distribution, the variance, is used. Once again the null hypothesis is defined, namely that none of the means differs significantly from any of the others and the level of probability at which the null hypothesis will be rejected is defined. An example of an analysis of variance is shown in Table 40.6.

**Table 40.6 Analysis of variance to compare systolic blood pressure measured on five separate occasions in 10 patients**

Systolic blood pressure (mmHg) during induction of anaesthesia

| Patient | Pre-induction | 1 min | 2 min | 5 min | 10 min |
|---|---|---|---|---|---|
| 1 | 160 | 84 | 108 | 140 | 145 |
| 2 | 135 | 128 | 112 | 128 | 135 |
| 3 | 145 | 114 | 123 | 138 | 143 |
| 4 | 142 | 126 | 132 | 122 | 178 |
| 5 | 176 | 127 | 140 | 167 | 158 |
| 6 | 128 | 98 | 128 | 134 | 141 |
| 7 | 172 | 108 | 165 | 140 | 136 |
| 8 | 145 | 112 | 129 | 127 | 134 |
| 9 | 137 | 84 | 112 | 133 | 141 |
| 10 | 161 | 80 | 142 | 171 | 156 |

| | Sum | Mean |
|---|---|---|
| Pre-induction | 1501 | 150.1 |
| 1 min | 1061 | 106.1 |
| 2 min | 1291 | 129.1 |
| 5 min | 1400 | 140.0 |
| 10 min | 1467 | 146.7 |

| | Sum of squares | df | Mean square | *F* | *P* |
|---|---|---|---|---|---|
| Between columns | 12581.2 | 4 | 3145.3 | 11.54 | < 0.0001 |
| Residual | 12264.8 | 45 | 272.6 | | |
| Total | 24846 | 49 | | | |

The variance is given by SS (the sum of squares) and the number of degrees of freedom by df. The mean square (MS) is calculated by dividing SS by df. The ratio $F$ is calculated by dividing the between-group MS by the within-group MS. If there is little difference between the individual samples, $F$ is close to unity. The probability of the result occurring is derived from tables in which $F$ is read against df. An analysis of variance test will indicate that the difference between the five means did not occur by chance at the 95% level; it will not indicate which mean varies from which. It is therefore necessary to perform a further test to show which means are different from which others. An example of such a test is Scheffé's test.

It is possible to use a $t$-test if there is a correction to the probability at which the null hypothesis is rejected. In the above example, in which five groups are compared, if the value of $P$ is set at 0.05, then tables are entered at the level $P/5$, i.e. $0.05/5 = 0.01$. Thus, although the $\alpha$ error (see below) is set at 5%, when comparing two of the means, it is necessary to achieve the critical value of $t$ at $P = 0.01$. This is called Bonferroni's correction.

The Kruskal–Wallis test is a non-parametric test equivalent to one-way analysis of variance.

## Errors in significance testing

Assuming that the correct test of significance has been applied to the measured data, it is necessary to assess whether the correct conclusions have been drawn from the calculated significance. To this end it is important to examine the conclusions for false positives and false negatives. This is performed by consideration of the errors inherent in statistical methods (Table 40.7).

There are two errors to be considered: type I and type II. The type I error is subject to manipulation and is set by the experimenter when defining the level at which the null hypothesis is to be rejected. If the probability is set at $P \leq 0.05$, it has to be accepted that the assumed significance of a difference is correct 95% of the times that we might repeat the test. However, 5% of the time we must accept that the conclusion we have drawn is a false positive, the numerical difference having occurred by chance.

The concept of a type II error is much more difficult to grasp. Florey (see Further reading) gives a readily understandable account. Briefly, if a sample is too small the trial may be declared not significant (NS) when, in fact, had the sample been larger a significant relationship may have been demonstrated: a false negative.

## Non-parametric tests for continuously variable data

So far, one of the criteria by which tests of significance for continuously variable data have been chosen has been that the data are normally distributed, approximate to normality, or capable of transformation to normality. If the parameters of the distribution are not known or are incapable of being transformed to acceptable normality, a non-parametric (distribution-free) series of tests may be performed. These tests require that the data can be ranked, i.e. ordinal data.

### *A distribution-free test for unpaired data: the Mann–Whitney test*

Consider the plasma potassium levels (mmol/L) in two groups of patients:

| Group A | Group B |
|---|---|
| 4.7 | 3.4 |
| 3.9 | 3.0 |
| 4.2 | 4.0 |
| 3.8 | 3.9 |
| 3.5 | 3.2 |
| 4.3 | 3.1 |
| 3.6 | 3.6 |
| 4.4 | 3.7 |

We do not know whether the data in this small sample are normally distributed. We define first the null hypothesis (i.e. all the observations have been made from a single population) and, second, the level of probability at which it will be rejected, say $P < 0.05$. The samples do not need to be of equal size. The combined data are ranked. If the data are tied, the ranks involved are summed and divided by the number involved in the tie (e.g. two values of 3.6 tied in rank 6; add 6 and 7 – the ranks involved – and divide by 2, the number of tied observations).

| Rank | | Rank | |
|---|---|---|---|
| 1 | 3.0 (B) | 9 | 3.8 (A) |
| 2 | 3.1 (B) | 10.5 | 3.9 (B) |
| 3 | 3.2 (B) | 10.5 | 3.9 (A) |
| 4 | 3.4 (B) | 12 | 4.0 (B) |
| 5 | 3.5 (A) | 13 | 4.2 (A) |
| 6.5 | 3.6 (B) | 14 | 4.3 (A) |
| 6.5 | 3.6 (A) | 15 | 4.4 (A) |
| 8 | 3.7 (B) | 16 | 4.7 (A) |

**Table 40.7 Errors in significance testing**

| Conclusion of test of significance | In reality $H_0$ true | In reality $H_0$ false |
|---|---|---|
| Reject $H_0$ | Type I error<br>($\alpha$ error)<br>False positive | Correct conclusion |
| $H_0$ **not** rejected | Correct conclusion | Type II error<br>($\beta$ error)<br>False negative |

$H_0$, null hypothesis

The rank values of groups A and B are then summed.

Rank sum group A = 89
Rank sum group B = 47.

The smaller of these two values is taken into Mann–Whitney tables along with the sample sizes $n_1$ and $n_2$. When $n_1 = 8$ and $n_2 = 8$, the critical range within which the smaller rank sum should lie, if the null hypothesis is not to be rejected at the chosen level of probability, is 49–87. Thus, as the value 47 falls outside this range the null hypothesis may be rejected.

Equivalent distribution-free tests that rely on the ability to rank the data are available for other parametric methods. For example, the non-parametric test that is the equivalent of a paired *t*-test is the Wilcoxon signed rank test.

## The parametric comparison of two continuous variables

### *Linear regression*

One might have formed the opinion that the weight of a patient governs the dose of an intravenous agent necessary to induce surgical anaesthesia: the greater the body weight the larger the dose required. It will be seen that both body weight and drug dose are continuous variables. If this opinion proves to be true, the two variables are said to be correlated. In this case the correlation would be positive: the greater the body weight the higher the drug dose. If one variable decreases as the other increases, they are said to be negatively correlated. Two caveats must be heeded. First, a mathematical correlation does not, of necessity, prove a causal relationship and, second, it is important not to extrapolate outside the measured range.

As with any test of significance, the null hypothesis is defined: body weight and induction dose are not related. The level of probability at which the null hypothesis is to be rejected is stated. Two further conditions must be met:

1. The values of $y$ at any particular value of $x$ should be normally distributed.
2. As we shall be examining linear regression, it is necessary that a straight-line relationship exists between the two variables. Mathematical tests for linearity exist, but a good idea of the degree of linearity may be obtained by plotting a scattergram. In this, the data are plotted and examined for patterns suggesting non-linearity. Transformation of relationships such as concentration–effect curves may be normalized by transforming the data – in the case of exponential data by taking the logarithmic values.

The position of the two variables on the axes is important. It is conventional to plot the independent variable on the $x$ axis (the abscissa) and the dependent variable on the $y$ axis (the ordinate). It is usually obvious which is the independent variable, e.g. time. In the example of drug dose and weight, weight is obviously the independent variable. In comparing standard and new measures of a variable, the standard method is placed on the $x$ axis. It is important to note that the regression analysis of $y$ on $x$ is different from that of $x$ on $y$.

The equation defining a straight line is $y = bx + a$ where $b$ is the slope of the line and $a$ is the intercept. To define the slope it is necessary to calculate a 'best-fit' for the data. This is achieved by performing a regression analysis. The slope of the line is called the regression coefficient ($b$) and is given by the formula:

$$\text{b (slope)} = \frac{\Sigma\,(x - \bar{x})\,(y - \bar{y})}{\Sigma\,(x - \bar{x})^2} \tag{10}$$

The intercept is not given directly by the formula, but, knowing that the coordinate (mean $x$, mean $y$) lies on the best-fit line, the slope may be placed accurately on the axes. It is possible to include confidence limits of the slope and we can test whether the slope we have measured differs from the line of identity or whether two measured slopes differ very significantly from each other by using a *t*-test where:

$$t = \frac{\text{Difference between slopes}}{\text{Standard error of the difference between slopes}}$$

### *Correlation*

The 'goodness of fit' of the individual data points to the regression line and hence the statistical validity of the relationship between $x$ and $y$ is given by the correlation coefficient $r$ (Figure 40.14),where:

$$r = \frac{\Sigma\,(x - \bar{x})\,(y - \bar{y})}{\sqrt{\Sigma\,(x - \bar{x})^2\,\Sigma\,(y - \bar{y})^2}} \tag{11}$$

If all the points lie on a positive slope $r = +1$. If all the points fall on a negative slope, $r = -1$. If no correlation exists, $r = 0$. The closer the correlation between the two variables, the further away from zero is the correlation coefficient. The statistical significance of the correlation may be calculated using a *t*-test where:

$$t = \sqrt{\frac{n - 2}{1 - r^2}} \tag{12}$$

A further way of demonstrating the goodness of fit of a relationship is by consideration of how much of the noted variation is the result of the variability of $y$ on $x$ in the chosen relationship. This is performed by calculation of the term $r^2$. Thus, although the slope may be statistically significant, a low value of $r^2$ indicates that the noted variability in $y$ is caused by factors other than the variations in the values of $x$.

### *Residuals*

The mathematical difference between an observation and the regression line is called a residual (Figure 40.15).

If the residuals of any comparison are plotted against the values of $x$, the relationship should be constant throughout the range of $x$ and no evidence of a curvilinear relationship should exist.

## Comparison between methods of clinical measurement

Frequently, one sees the results of the comparison between two methods of measuring a single variable.

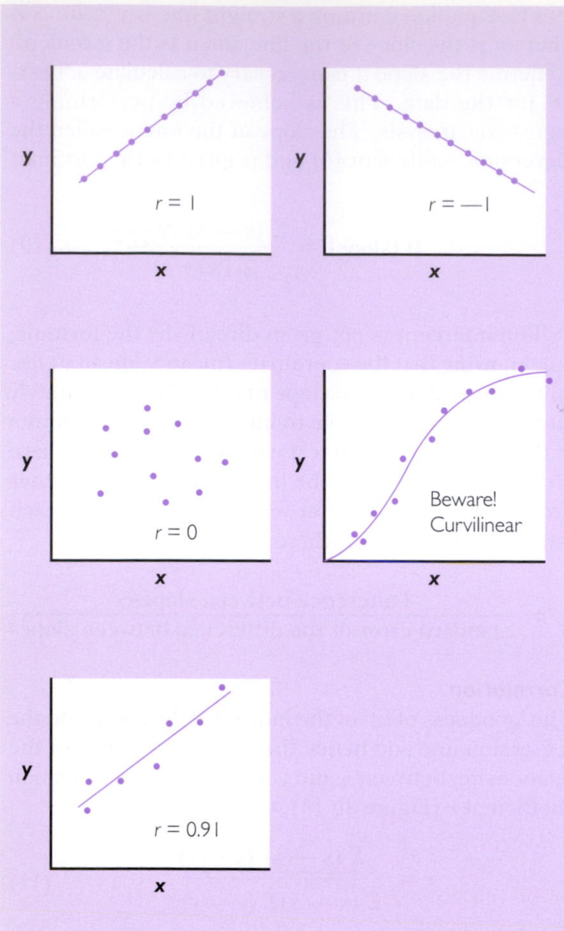


**Figure 40.14** The correlation coefficient, *r*.

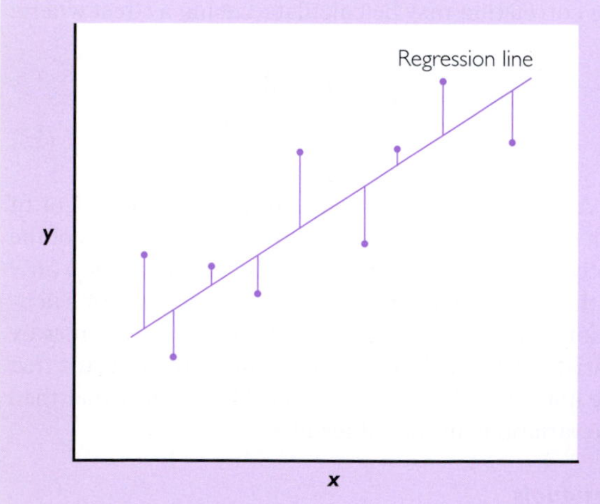


**Figure 40.15** Residuals represent the degree to which individual observations differ from their fitted values.

This is often expressed as a satisfactorily high value for *r*. Bland and Altman (see Figure 40.16), stating that the use of correlation was misleading, sought to establish a more specific measure for the comparison. The correlation coefficient may show perfect agreement ($r = 1$) not only if the points lie exactly on the line of identity but also if they are along any straight line. This

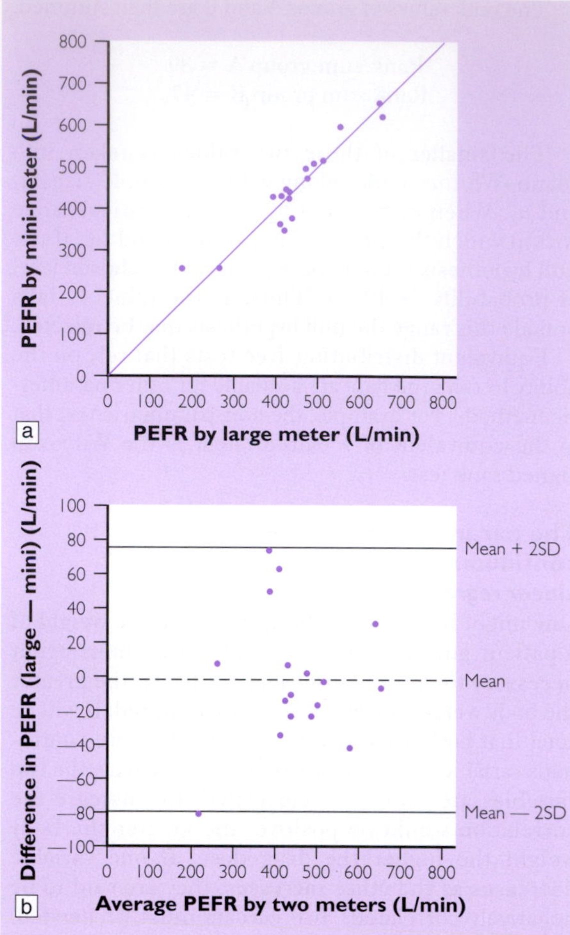


**Figure 40.16** Bland and Altman's comparison of methods: (a) a scattergram of the data with the line of identity (equality); (b) the 'Bland/Altman' plot. PEFR, peak expiratory flow rate. (Adapted from Bland JM and Altman DG. Statistical methods for assessing agreement between two methods of clinical measurement. *Lancet* 1986;i:307–10.)

is equivalent to a systematic error (bias). Although the correlation coefficient may be statistically significant, a high degree of scatter about the line may be seen in the scattergram; this represents a random error (see Figure 40.14).

The method of Bland and Altman consists of plotting the difference between the two readings against their mean (Figure 40.16b). Bias is shown by considering the relationship between the difference and the mean and, in the presence of constant bias, individual measurements may be corrected by subtracting or adding this amount. The degree of random error may be estimated by calculating an envelope defining the 95% confidence limits of the difference between the methods. In Figure 40.16b, using Bland and Altman's data, the limits of agreement are between –80 L/min and +75 L/min. This represents a large discrepancy between the methods, which is not obvious from the data in Figure 40.16a.

### Tests for the significance of discontinuous (discrete) data

In these tests the significance of the frequency of occurrence of categorical variables is investigated (Table 40.8).

**Table 40.8 2 × 2 contingency table of 'Novom' trial**

| Drug | Did vomit | Didn't vomit | Total |
|---|---|---|---|
| 'Novom' | 30 (39) | 70 (61) | 100 |
| Cyclizine | 48 (39) | 52 (61) | 100 |
| Total | 78 | 122 | 200 |

Values in parentheses are the expected values if there is no difference between the drugs.

Consider the data in Table 40.8. It is proposed that a new drug 'Novom' is effective in the treatment of postoperative nausea and vomiting. It is to be compared with cyclizine. The data satisfy the criteria for a binomial distribution, described earlier. The data is arranged into a 2 × 2 table (contingency table, Latin square). The null hypothesis is defined, i.e. cyclizine and Novom are equally effective in the treatment of nausea and vomiting. Statistical significance will be assumed at a probability of $P < 0.05$. The test chosen for this type of data is $\chi^2$ (chi-squared). The mathematics behind a $\chi^2$ relationship is beyond the scope of this chapter and, as long as the conditions for its use are satisfied, detailed knowledge of the distribution is unnecessary.

The formula for the calculation of $\chi^2$ is given by:

$$\chi^2 = \frac{\Sigma(\mathrm{O} - \mathrm{E})^2}{\mathrm{E}} \tag{13}$$

In each cell the number defining the frequency measured by the test is called the observed (O) value. The value for the expected (E) value is calculated in each cell by multiplying the total of the row by the total of the column, and dividing by the total number of observations (the law of multiplication). Thus, considering the top left box, the patients receiving Novom who subsequently vomited:

$$\mathrm{O} = 30$$

$$\mathrm{E} = \frac{\text{row total (100)} \times \text{column total (78)}}{\text{grand total (200)}}$$

$$= \frac{100 \times 78}{200}$$

$$= 39.$$

Thus $(\mathrm{O} - \mathrm{E})^2/\mathrm{E}$ for this box is $(30 - 39)^2/39 = 2.08$. The sum of the calculations from the four boxes is 6.82; this is the $\chi^2$ statistic. To determine whether a statistically significant difference exists in the data, it is necessary to enter tables defining the percentage points of the $\chi^2$ distribution. The value of $\chi^2$ is compared with the df in the contingency table.

### *Degrees of freedom for $\chi^2$*

When considering the number of df in the test, having given a number to one cell and having defined $\chi^2$, the values in the three remaining cells cannot be arbitrarily ascribed. In a 2 × 2 square there is therefore one df. To calculate the general case where more than two rows or columns exist:

$$\mathrm{df} = (\text{Number of rows} - 1) \times (\text{Number of columns} - 1).$$

Thus, in a 2 × 2 table, df = (2 – 1) × (2 – 1) = (1 × 1) = 1 df. If four columns existed, e.g. the four blood groups in the ABO system, and the presence or absence of a condition was investigated, four columns and two rows would exist. Thus df = (4 – 1) × (2 – 1) = (3 × 1) = 3.

In our trial of postoperative vomiting, the $\chi^2$ statistic 6.82 is thus examined when df = 1. We find from tables that $0.01 > P > 0.001$. Thus, the null hypothesis may be rejected; Novom appears to be more effective than cyclizine in the treatment of postoperative nausea and vomiting.

### *Yates' correction*

The $\chi^2$ distribution is continuous and, when dealing with a 2 × 2 table, it is being used to test binomial data and it is conventional to apply a correction. This consists of reducing by 0.5 the values in a 2 x 2 table that exceed the expected values, and increasing those that fall below it by the same amount. This is called Yates' correction. Its effect is to make significance at any particular level of probability more difficult to achieve and is now thought to overcompensate.

### *Small numbers*

If the expected (E) number in any cell should fall to five or less, the $\chi^2$ test should not be used. For a 2 × 2 table, Fisher described an exact probability test in which the probability of achieving the measured or a more extreme result by chance was defined (Table 40.9).

If the letters in the table denote the frequencies, then the exact probability is given by:

$$\text{Exact probability} = \frac{e! \times f! \times g! \times h!}{n! \times a! \times b! \times c! \times d!}$$

where $n!$ is the factorial value of $n$ (i.e. $n! = 1 \times 2 \times 3 \times 4 \times \ldots \times n$).

It is possible similarly to calculate the more extreme possibilities and to sum them to give the required probability. If writing a program to do the calculation, logarithms should be used to make it easier to handle the very large numbers generated by factorials.

**Table 40.9 Notation for a 2 × 2 contingency table – general case**

| Drug | Did vomit | Didn't vomit | Total |
|---|---|---|---|
| 'Novom' | *a* | *b* | *e* |
| Cyclizine | *c* | *d* | *f* |
| Total | *g* | *h* | *n* |

Adapted from Kirkwood BR. *Essentials of Medical Statistics*. Oxford: Blackwell, 1988.

### Sequential analysis

If data are binomially distributed, a simple method of comparison is possible in which no mathematical skills are required by the user. A sequential analysis chart is shown in Figure 40.17. This test is particularly useful for cross-over clinical trials or those involving matched pairs.

Consider a clinical trial in which two anaesthetic induction agents are being tested for patient satisfaction. A patient having received the two anaesthetic drugs would subsequently report whether drug A was preferable to drug B or vice versa. If drug A was preferred to drug B, a box would be filled on the vertical axis; if drug B was preferred, a box on the horizontal axis would be filled. The trial would continue until the line of filled boxes emerged from the chart indicating a preference for one or other of the drugs (in the example above, drug A is preferred) or no significant difference was expressed if the line emerged in between the two limbs of the chart. The charts are specific for various levels of probability; the less the probability the greater the number of boxes on the chart (Figure 40.17b).

## INTERPRETATION OF RESULTS AND CLINICAL RELEVANCE

When applying statistical tests it is important to remember that a statistical correlation does not, of necessity, imply a causal relationship between two variables. This may or may not be the case. A frequently quoted example is the apparent relationship between suffering from rheumatoid arthritis and having red hair. It may be that the actual correlation is between being Scottish and having rheumatoid arthritis, and our red-headed population may contain a large percentage of Scots. This is a specific example of a more general case when a third unseen variable links the two variables being tested. The passage of time is a common third variable. It is also important to remember that a high statistical significance does not necessarily indicate a high clinical significance.

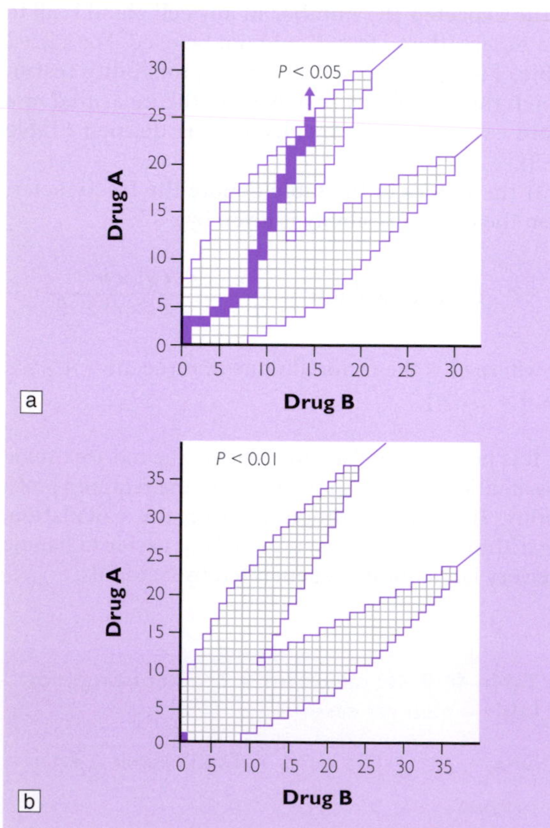


**Figure 40.17** Sequential analysis: the path emerges at the top right of the plot and, in this instance, drug A is better than drug B. (Adapted from Sykes MK, Vickers MD, and Hull CJ. *Principles of Clinical Measurement*. Oxford: Blackwell Scientific Publications, 1981.)

The expression $P$ = NS ('not significant') conveys very little information about the results of a trial; had one more measurement been made, $P$ might have equalled 0.05 and been considered significant. It may be that, under certain circumstances, $P = 0.1$ may be considered worthy of further investigation. The calculated probability delivered by most computerized statistical packages can be most useful when reporting clinical trials; the phrase 'not significant' should be avoided. In recent years the slavish attention to arbitrary levels of probability has been challenged and, largely through the work of Gardener and Altman (see Further reading), the concept of confidence intervals has been introduced. These values allow a reader to assess whether they consider a range of values or calculated differences to be clinically significant. A 95% confidence interval for a population mean from consideration of a single sample is calculated by multiplying the calculated sample standard error by the critical value of $t$, when the number of degrees of freedom are read against the chosen level of significance.

Thus, if the mean dose of an induction agent in a sample of 10 was 200 mg and the standard error of the mean was calculated to be 20 mg, the 95% confidence interval would be given by 2.26 (the critical value of $t$ for $P = 0.05$ and $(10 - 1) = 9$ df) multiplied by 20 (the SEM). Thus, the 95% confidence interval for the population mean would be 200 mg ± 45.2 mg i.e. 154.8–245.2. The reader could then decide whether this degree of uncertainty was acceptable when calculating a recommended drug dose. Similarly, the difference between the means of two samples may be given a confidence interval. Considering the recovery time from two inhalational agents, the measured difference for the two samples may be 5 min. When the 95% confidence interval is calculated, the range of difference if the experiment is repeated may be –2 (representing a difference in the other direction) to 12 min. The reader must decide whether this statistically significant difference is clinically important. The confidence interval is, of course, reduced if the sample size is increased. It is possible to calculate confidence intervals for all parametric and non-parametric tests.

## FURTHER READING

Altman DG. *Practical Statistics for Medical Research*. London: Chapman & Hall. 1991. (Arguably the most useful all-round book for amateur medical statisticians.)

Armitage P, Berry, G. *Statistical Methods in Medical Research*, 3rd edn. Oxford: Blackwell, 1994.

Florey C du V. Sample size for beginners. *Br Med J* 1993;**306**:1181–4.

Kirkwood BR. *Essentials of Medical Statistics.* Oxford: Blackwell, 1988.

Pipkin FB. *Medical Statistics Made Easy*. Edinburgh: Churchill Livingstone, 1984.

# Section 3

# The presenting patient

# Chapter 41 The assessment of anaesthetic risk and the fit patient

G.M. Cooper

## ASSESSMENT OF RISK

Patients present for many different surgical procedures in a wide variety of sizes, shapes, ages, ethnic origins, and degrees of fitness. This spectrum of possible combinations requires anaesthesia to be administered on an individual basis, making preoperative assessment a vital part of the process. The patient should be seen soon enough before surgery to allow time to organize any necessary investigations, and yet not so long that the medical and surgical conditions have changed significantly.

The time available for such preoperative assessment is frequently limited, especially for emergencies and when patients are admitted on the day of surgery. Relevant information is gained from:

- the patient;
- the medical admission notes;
- the drug chart;
- medical correspondence;
- liaising with the surgical team.

In principle, there are two general questions that should always be asked and answered:

1. Can the patient's physical condition be improved and, if so, is it necessary to do so?
2. When the patient has been optimized, do the anticipated benefits of surgery outweigh the combined risks of surgery and anaesthesia?

In this section of the book, specific problems pertinent to patient groups are highlighted and help answer the first question. In some conditions it may also be helpful to call on the expertise of the appropriate medical specialist. To answer the second question requires knowledge of the patient's physical state, their expectations, the likelihood of surgical success, and the physiological perturbations expected during surgery, as well as those inherent in the anaesthetic process. Risks and benefits for individuals are not easy to quantify numerically but may be described as minimal, moderate, or high. Sympathetic but honest discussion is needed when the risks are high and the benefits uncertain. A good yardstick to follow is whether surgery would be the option chosen for one's own relative in similar circumstances (assuming you wished the treatment to be a success!).

A system that attempts to categorize the physical state of patients, regardless of the type of medical disease, is that of the American Society of Anesthesiologists (ASA). The five categories are:

| | |
|---|---|
| ASA I | A normal healthy person |
| ASA II | A person with mild systemic disease with no functional limitation |
| ASA III | A person with severe systemic disease that has functional limitation but is not incapacitating |
| ASA IV | A person with incapacitating systemic disease that is a constant threat to life |
| ASA V | A moribund patient who is unlikely to survive 24 hours with or without an operation |

The letter E is added to each category if it is an 'emergency' procedure. These categories cannot predict individual outcome but the mortality rates after anaesthesia and surgery for elective and emergency operations correlate with each category. These are:

| | |
|---|---|
| ASA I | 0.1% |
| ASA II | 0.2% |
| ASA III | 1.8% |
| ASA IV | 7.8% |
| ASA V | 9.4% |

These need to be borne in mind and compared with an overall mortality rate of about 0.6% covering a broad range of surgical procedures in patients of all ages. The overall mortality attributable to anaesthesia itself is about 1 in 10 000. Factors that contribute to anaesthetic mortality include inadequate assessment of the patient before surgery, inadequate supervision and monitoring during surgery, and inadequate supervision and management after surgery.

Good communication between the anaesthetist and the patient is crucial and belies the common public misconception that anaesthetists have no need to talk to patients because they are asleep. In the often brief preoperative visit the anaesthetist needs to:

- gain rapport;
- elicit the relevant medical information;
- explain planned procedures;
- obtain consent for procedures such as local blocks and inserting suppositories;

- answer the patient's questions;
- engender confidence.

This requires more skill and knowledge than is required for traditional history taking and physical examination, and improves with practice. Communication skills are also particularly important when talking to patients and relatives in intensive care units (ICUs) and pain clinics. A further need for anaesthetists to communicate effectively is with surgeons and other members of the medical, nursing, and ancillary staff to ensure optimum patient care.

The management and problems of the fit patient outlined below are relevant as a basic standard of care for all patients.

## THE FIT PATIENT

Most patients presenting for elective surgery are apparently fit and healthy. It is therefore surprising that most standard texts do not discuss this group of patients who form the largest number in day-to-day practice. Just because they are fit does not mean that they do not have problems relevant to anaesthesia. Preoperative anxiety, for instance, may be just as common in fit patients as in those with concomitant disease. This section outlines routine practice and discusses controversies concerning anaesthesia and healthy patients. It will become apparent that frequently a degree of judgement needs to be exercised and that there are not always right and wrong answers, just decisions, all of which involve an element of risk. In the reality of the world in which we live, problems need to be solved expeditiously and pragmatically, bearing in mind the attendant risks and practicalities of individual decisions.

Like pornography, fitness is easier to recognize than it is to define. In the context of this section, it implies a person between the ages of 16 and 65 years, accepting that at the upper limit biological age is more important than chronological age, without any apparent medical problem. Questionnaires about general health have a useful part to play in providing information about known concurrent medical disease; an example is given in Chapter 46. The truly fit patient usually presents the fewest anaesthetic problems, but the greatest potential loss and the highest stakes if difficulties arise.

### Preoperative phase

#### History

In general the history gives a better guide to fitness than findings on examination. Even the patient who is known to be fit should always be asked certain questions. These are detailed below.

*Previous anaesthetics*

After introducing oneself as 'Doctor Gas', the anaesthetist, it is often helpful for the first question to be: 'Have you ever had an anaesthetic before?' Besides offering the chance to explore any difficulties that may have been encountered (e.g. unintentional awareness, postoperative nausea and vomiting, unplanned ICU admission, difficult intubation, etc.), it focuses the patient on why you are visiting and that you are a doctor fully involved in their care. When the patient has not previously had an anaesthetic, or only regional anaesthesia, enquiry should be made as to whether blood relatives have had serious problems with anaesthesia. This may elicit familial disorders such as malignant hyperpyrexia or suxamethonium apnoea. In addition, fears may be uncovered such as when a relative has died after surgery of a cause related, or unrelated, to anaesthesia. This introductory question also allows those with predetermined views (needle or mask phobias, preferred site of venous access, etc.) to air these, giving the anaesthetist the chance to think about whether it is appropriate to accede to them, while questioning further about general health.

*Relevant surgical problem*

Even though the operation should be 'listed', it is relevant, in most instances, for the anaesthetist to enquire about:

- the reason for proposed surgery;
- whether the condition has been causing distress;
- where a lesion (e.g. skin tumour, hernia, etc.) is situated (e.g. on the back, left or right inguinal, or umbilical region, etc.).

This helps gain rapport and understanding of the particular surgical requirements, and is a check on the surgical site and the patient's knowledge of what is going to happen to him or her.

*General health/intercurrent illness*

The fit patient will of course not admit to any concurrent medical illness and profess general good health; the reply should be judged in conjunction with the general demeanour (optimistic tone of voice or flat affect) and appearance. Lassitude and disinterest are abnormal and can be the presenting features of a variety of conditions (e.g. viral illness, depression, malignancy, renal failure, addiction). Further brief questioning makes sure that their exercise tolerance is equivalent to that of their peers.

If an intercurrent illness, such as an upper respiratory tract infection, is found, it is often a difficult decision as to whether to postpone elective surgery. This is especially so when the symptoms have just started and it is unclear how severe the illness will be. There is no doubt that it is best to perform any surgery when general health is optimal but, on the other hand, there is an understandable reluctance to waste an operating slot. The patient may have had a long wait for surgery and have made considerable arrangements at home and at work to enable surgery to occur. Individual judgement has to weigh up the likely risks against the patient's wishes: for example, in the presence of an upper respiratory tract infection, one view is to continue with surgery provided that the patient can breathe through the nose and is apyrexial (indicating lack of systemic illness). On the other hand, the presence of a productive cough before surgery would mitigate against elective abdominal surgery because of the increased likelihood of serious pulmonary complications, exacerbation of postoperative pain, and unnecessary stress on the wound.

*Drug history*

Even totally fit patients may be taking some medication of relevance. An obvious example is that of oral contraceptives, which may need to be discontinued before major surgery if the risk of thrombosis is considered to be greater than that resulting from possible pregnancy.

*Allergies*

The presence of any known allergies should always be ascertained. Antibiotics are of particular relevance because prophylaxis against infection is now common for many operations. It is worth noting that an egg allergy may contraindicate drugs solubilized in egg phosphatide, such as propofol. Food allergies may possibly, and unpredictably, give rise to anaphylactic reactions when blood is transfused, and are therefore very relevant. Latex allergy will require advance warning to operating room staff to provide alternative gloves. Many patients describe reactions to drugs 'which don't agree with me' and the nature of these should be elucidated. This often applies to analgesics where indigestion may have occurred after aspirin and other non-steroidal anti-inflammatory drugs, and antibiotics that have produced abdominal upset and opportunistic infection.

*Smoking*

The relevance of smoking relates in the long term to effects on health (e.g. ischaemic heart disease, lung cancer, etc.) and in the short term to the effect of carbon monoxide in cigarette smoke, which converts haemoglobin to carboxyhaemoglobin. In heavy cigarette smokers, this may reduce available oxygen by as much as 25%. The short half-life of carboxyhaemoglobin (4–6 h at rest: 10–12 h asleep) means that abstinence for 12 h will improve arterial oxygen content. Furthermore, the effect of smoking on the respiratory tract results in a sixfold increase in postoperative pulmonary complications. To reduce morbidity from this cause, it has been suggested that abstinence for at least 6 weeks is required. Although pragmatists will say that the committed smoker will not heed advice to stop smoking, it is fair to impart the information rather than pretend that there is no detriment. Nevertheless, the smoker who is nervous about surgery will probably continue to smoke whatever is said. Despite the hazards involved (including that of fires), current practice seems to be that abstinence is not normally strictly enforced.

*Alcohol intake*

High alcohol consumption is associated with relative resistance to anaesthesia and increased dosage requirements. Chronic alcohol abuse causes proliferation of the endoplasmic reticulum of the hepatocytes and induces enzymes in the microsomal oxidase system. High doses of sedatives and analgesics may have little effect on the alcoholic who is not currently drinking, but in combination with alcohol they may be dangerous because of competition for a common metabolic pathway. Delirium tremens, characterized by agitation, confusion, hallucinations, fever, and autonomic hyperactivity, occurs within 3–5 days of abstinence and has a 5–15% mortality rate. The obvious implication is that this may develop during the postoperative period. The anaesthetist should be aware that the stated alcohol intake might be under-estimated!

*Concerns/nervousness*

A high proportion of surgical patients are anxious about the forthcoming operation and/or anaesthetic. There is a significant inverse relationship between anxiety and smoothness of induction of anaesthesia. Venous access is also more difficult in the patient paralysed by fear. In addition to obvious humanitarian aspects, there are thus good reasons for allaying preoperative anxiety. This can often be effected by honest explanations of perioperative procedures and by reassurances about particular fears. Sometimes anxiety is only relieved at wakening after surgery and realizing that all is well. There is, however, a definite role for preoperative anxiolytic drugs for patients who continue to be unduly nervous despite explanations and reassurances. The benzodiazepines are the most popular and have the advantage of oral administration, low likelihood of adverse side effects, and choice of drug for desired duration of effect.

*Preoperative starvation*

Oral intake before surgery is restricted in order to reduce the likelihood of vomiting and aspirating gastric contents, which can cause either respiratory obstruction or pulmonary damage. It is essential to check when the patient last ate or drank. An unduly long duration of starvation may result in dehydration; equally, some patients may have 'slipped through the net' and eaten nearer the time of surgery than intended. The guidelines on the desired length of preoperative starvation have relaxed a little in recent years, but they are still subject to individual variation. There is evidence that clear fluids may be drunk with reasonable safety up to 2 h before surgery and that no solid food (which includes milky drinks) should be taken within 8 h of surgery. It is mandatory to enquire about the duration of starvation before emergency surgery, recognizing that the stomach may not have emptied because of pain (e.g. after an accident) or pathology (e.g. appendicitis).

### Examination

A complete physical examination of a patient who, as a result of questioning, appears to be fit is probably not cost- or time-effective, because of the low chance of finding an abnormality that would alter anaesthetic management. Nevertheless, there are certain aspects that should always be considered before dismissing full systematic examination as unnecessary; these are outlined here. In hospital practice, both for the experience of junior staff, by custom and practice, and for medicolegal reasons, patients receive a thorough examination. Therefore, there is an expectation that it will be done thoroughly, rather than miss an important finding. It is obvious that any examination relevant to the proposed operation (e.g. vaginal and abdominal examination for gynaecological conditions, neurological examination before craniotomy) should be performed on an awake, consenting patient before the operation and this is a responsibility of the surgical team. On many occasions we rely on results of examination conducted by others.

*General observation*

While taking the history the patient should be observed, looking for any outward signs of ill health or inconsistencies with the history given. At the same time, ease of breathing should be observed by seeing whether sentences can be completed without drawing breath or whether accessory muscles are being used. Sight of the patient walking in the ward is also useful because impairment will suggest the need for further direct questioning and examination. If there are no obvious veins seen on the back of the hand, more formal searching for possible venous access is useful. Any deviation from average build (e.g. fat or thin) should be noted. Any abnormalities deserve further relevant examination.

*Intubation/airway*

The likely ease of intubation should be considered in every patient even if it is planned to use a facemask, laryngeal mask airway, or regional anaesthesia. Anatomical features of difficult intubation include a small jaw with acute mandibular angles, limited mouth opening, a large tongue, limited neck movement, and a short muscular neck with full dentition. These are outlined in more detail in Chapter 7. If a difficult intubation is anticipated, as opposed to unexpected, the problem is half solved. Taking an estimate of 600 deaths annually (in the developed world) as a result of complications at the time of tracheal intubation, its importance in healthy patients is paramount.

The dentition must be examined. The presence of any loose teeth, dental caps or crowns, and dentures needs to be ascertained. When there are well-fitting dentures, the surgical procedure is short, and it is planned to manage the airway with a facemask, there are advantages in keeping the dentures in place because they help maintain facial structure and a good seal with a facemask.

*Blood pressure/heart rate*

These should be measured before surgery in all patients and they provide valuable baseline information even in the absence of abnormalities. The measurements can be done satisfactorily by nurses, but the anaesthetist should always note the result. Abnormalities in cardiovascular parameters may be very significant and may be present in otherwise apparently healthy people; a complete examination of the cardiovascular system is then necessary and further action should be taken to define the cause. An advantage of feeling the pulse oneself is assessing the regularity, or otherwise, which will not normally be commented on by nursing staff.

*Weight*

Knowledge of the patient's weight guides dose requirements of many drugs used in anaesthesia. It is also useful for assessing blood volume, ventilation requirements, and adequacy of urine output.

*Previous anaesthetic records*

It is helpful to look at previous anaesthetic records held within the notes in order to establish whether there were any difficulties in airway management or other complications. If the patient knows that there have been complications and the previous anaesthetic was undertaken in another hospital, it is important to establish exactly what the problem was and, wherever possible, to see the relevant records from that hospital.

*Temperature*

Measurement of the patient's temperature before surgery may detect unrecognized intercurrent infection. There is controversy over whether it is advisable to perform minor surgery in the presence of mild pyrexia where there is no obvious source of infection. One of the possible risks is that of a viral myocarditis with potentially fatal consequences. Thus one can understand a cautious attitude when surgery is not urgent.

***Investigations***

Preoperative investigations in healthy patients are performed either to screen for unsuspected pathology or to provide baseline information before major surgery. The most helpful factors in determining the need for specific investigations are a careful history and examination. Performing a battery of tests on healthy patients as a routine is costly and uninformative, and has little influence on decision-making. This does not mean that appropriate investigations should be omitted when there are clinical indications. It is self-evident that any investigations deemed necessary should be seen and acted on before surgery.

In general, routine screening for occult disease is of greatest value in elderly people, in whom the prevalence of unrecognized cardiovascular, pulmonary, and other organ system disease is high, and a positive test is more likely to represent true pathology than a false-positive result.

*Urinalysis*

The purpose of routine urinalysis is to detect undiagnosed diabetes mellitus or renal disease by the presence of glycosuria or proteinuria. It is a cheap non-invasive test which may pick up abnormalities in asymptomatic patients.

*Full blood count*

The key role of haemoglobin in oxygen transport, coupled with the low cost of a full blood count, make it easy to justify this routine measurement before surgery. Looking a little more critically, it may be argued that it is not essential for healthy young men undergoing minor surgery, where the likelihood of finding anaemia or needing blood transfusion is extremely low. However, routine haemoglobin estimation in fit premenopausal woman reveals anaemia frequently enough to suggest that it should be mandatory in this population. For patients undergoing major surgery, the baseline haemoglobin concentration affects the need for perioperative blood transfusion. Where malignant disease is suspected in an otherwise apparently fit person, the haemoglobin concentration may be low and needs to be measured. The low likelihood of finding anaemia in healthy children does not justify the distress caused by venepuncture in this group of patients.

If an abnormal result is detected, it is important that it is acted on. The type of anaemia should be determined from the blood film and further investigations made to determine the cause. In the presence of chronic anaemia, there is no justification in simply transfusing blood to achieve an acceptable haemoglobin concentration! Indeed, in some patients (e.g. in those with renal disease), it may cause added complications.

*Urea and electrolytes*
There should be no need to measure serum urea and electrolytes in fit patients undergoing elective surgery.

*Chest radiograph*
Although good at demonstrating structural abnormalities, the chest radiograph is a poor guide to pulmonary function, and has been an expensive and possibly detrimental routine investigation in the past. It should be reserved for detection of possible disease that may alter surgical management (e.g. the presence of primary or secondary malignancy in the lungs) or for baseline reference (e.g. before thoracic, cardiac, or major upper abdominal surgery). The Royal College of Radiologists has produced a booklet on who should have what.

*ECG*
In an otherwise fit patient, an ECG is routinely required for most surgery only in patients over the age of 60 years. See Chapter 47 for details of interpreting an ECG.

*Consent*
The consent form for surgery has been the subject of recent debate. There is no doubt that the patient should be aware of the nature of intended surgery and of its major attendant risks. Verbal consent is perfectly satisfactory, but written witnessed consent has the advantage of documenting that the patient acknowledged the explanations. It is a matter of course to document the failure rate and likely irreversibility of sterilization procedures, although for many other procedures there is debate over when less common, or less serious, complications should be detailed. There is no doubt that there is a tendency nowadays to be more detailed in itemizing possible complications.

Consent for surgery is invalid if obtained after the patient has received premedicant drugs. Traditionally, consent for anaesthesia has been given as a consequence of surgical consent. However, there is disquiet that the surgeon who obtains consent may be unaware of the hazards of anaesthesia for that particular patient, and indeed may be ignorant of whether regional or general anaesthesia is likely to be employed. It seems logical that the anaesthetist should obtain consent separately, although, currently, this does not happen. The detail required for such consent is also debated. Serious and common complications should be detailed and it is sensible to explain the method by which postoperative analgesia will be provided. However, should one detail each individual procedure such as venous cannulation, arterial cannulation, endotracheal intubation, laryngeal mask usage, administration of neuromuscular blockade drugs, intramuscular injections, rectal suppositories, and type of mechanical ventilation used? It is clear that each of these has possible side effects or complications and yet most patients would be overwhelmed if presented with such a daunting list of possible adverse events.

It seems sensible to answer specific questions honestly to the best of one's ability, without being alarmist. When asked about risks in general, one approach is to suggest that, although anaesthesia is not without risk even in the fit patient, it is probably less than the risk of an accident while driving to the hospital.

There is considerable debate about the validity of consent given for epidural analgesia in labour, when the patient is in considerable pain and may have received opioid analgesics. This is an example of when pragmatism is called into play, because it is impractical for all patients to anticipate the degree of analgesia required before the onset of labour and give consent prospectively.

*Preoperative preparation*
The operative site should be shaved and this is usually done on the ward. The patient dons a suitable clean hospital gown which allows access to the operative site. The nervous patient will benefit from the premedicant anxiolytic prescribed.

### Intraoperative phase

The anaesthetist has a duty to provide safe anaesthesia for all patients. There are certain provisions that must be made in order to do so:

- Suitable assistance must be available for the anaesthetist.
- The anaesthetic equipment used must be fully functional and safe, and a check made that it is so (see Chapter 12). When neuromuscular blocking agents are used, a self-inflating bag must be available for emergency use.
- Monitoring equipment must be used that warns of unsafe gas mixtures, inadequate blood oxygen saturation, inappropriate pulmonary ventilation, cardiac arrhythmias, and abnormalities in heart rate and blood pressure (see Chapter 12).
- The anaesthetist responsible must be suitably trained and kept up to date. A trainee must be supervised appropriately according to his or her experience.
- The anaesthetist must be physically capable of delivering a high-quality service. It is obvious that the anaesthetist with a broken arm cannot safely manage anaesthesia, but a more difficult area is where the anaesthetist is tired or weary, through overwork or other reasons.
- Techniques within the limits of currently accepted practice and technical capabilities of the individual should be used.
- An adequate written record of the anaesthetic procedure (see Chapter 12) should be made. This is particularly important for handing over a case to another anaesthetist, for recovery staff, as well as possible defence of medicolegal cases. It is also a useful reference for any subsequent anaesthetic procedures.
- Responsibilities should be limited to caring for a single patient at a time. The exception to this occurs at caesarean section, although the anaesthetist should not also be responsible for resuscitation of the neonate.
- The patient should be given undivided attention at all times, so that any physiological deviations from the norm can be corrected rapidly.
- Regional or general anaesthesia may be employed. Indwelling venous access is always advisable.
- Close attention must be paid to fluid replacement and postoperative needs (see Chapter 14).

- The provision of postoperative analgesia should be anticipated and prescribed (see Chapter 5).

### Postoperative phase

The early recovery period is a potentially dangerous time. Large surveys have shown that one in five patients develops a complication and that 40% of complications associated with anaesthesia occur at this time. Close monitoring immediately after surgery is therefore essential, to ensure that the benefits of good surgery and safe anaesthesia are not compromised by lack of attention in the postoperative period. The anaesthetist should ensure that the patient returns to the ward fully conscious, with good airway control, adequate ventilation, comfortable, and free from nausea and vomiting.

## FURTHER READING


Apfel CC, Greim CA, Haubitz I, Goepfert C, Usadel J, Sefrin P, Roewer N. A risk score to predict the probability of postoperative vomiting in adults. *Acta Anaesthesiol Scand* 1998;**42**:495–501.

Arvidsson S. Preparation of adult patients for anaesthesia and surgery. *Acta Anaesthesiol Scand* 1996;**40**:962–970.

Association of Anaesthetists of Great Britain and Ireland. *Information and Consent for Anaesthesia*. London: AAGBI, 1999.

Bell MDD, Bodenham AR. Problems and pitfalls of practical procedures: a medico-legal perspective. *Curr Anaesth Crit Care* 1998;**9**:278–89.

Bullingham A, Strunin L. Prevention of postoperative venous thromboembolism. *Br J Anaesth* 1995;**75**:622–30.

Eriksson LI, Sandin R. Fasting guidelines in different countries. *Acta Anaesthesiol Scand* 1996;**40**:971–4.

Forrest JB, Rehder K, Cahalan MK, Goldsmith CH. Multicenter study of general anesthesia. III. Predictors of severe perioperative adverse outcomes. *Anesthesiology* 1992;**76**:3–15.

McHardy FE, Chung F. Postoperative sore throat: cause, prevention and treatment. *Anaesthesia* 1999;**54**:444–53.

Maltby JR. Preoperative fasting. *Curr Anaesth Crit Care* 1996;**6**:276–80.

Pearce AC, Jones RM. Smoking and anesthesia: preoperative abstinence and perioperative morbidity. *Anesthesiology* 1984:**61**:576–84.

Prause G, Ratzenhofer-Komenda B, Smolle-Juettner F, *et al*. Operations on patients deemed 'unfit for operation and anaesthesia'. What are the consequences? *Acta Anaesthesiol Scand* 1998;**42**:316–22.

# Chapter 42 The paediatric patient

G.M. Cooper and C. Vallis

The principles of anaesthetizing children are no different from those in the adult. However, differences in anatomy, physiology, psychology, and pharmacology need to be understood to achieve the same goals. The special problems of neonatal anaesthesia are not dealt with here, although the spectrum of physiological change is included for completeness. Most, but not all, neonates will have surgery in specialized centres cared for by anaesthetists experienced in this field; many older children undergo uncomplicated eye, ENT, orthopaedic, or general surgical operations in general hospitals.

Neonates are babies under the age of 4 weeks. Infants are aged from 4 weeks to 1 year, and children are aged (in law) up to 16 years, although the physical disparity from adults reduces from puberty. There is obviously a gradation over the years in the differences between children and adults, and the rate of maturing varies between individuals – some people never seeming to make the transition to adult behaviour!

## ANATOMY AND PHYSIOLOGY

The most obvious difference between adults and children is that of size, although the difference is more than simply one of size. Appropriately sized equipment has to be selected for all procedures. The correct size may be estimated by formulae or guidelines involving the child's weight or age, and these parameters always need to be known.

### Respiratory system

In infants and young children, the head and tongue are relatively large, the nares are smaller, and the neck is shorter than in the adult. These factors predispose to upper airway obstruction, which may be worsened in the presence of hypertrophied adenoids and tonsils. The relatively large head resting on a pillow may cause the neck to be flexed too far and therefore the airway is often best managed in a neutral position. Over-extension of the head or pressure from the anaesthetist's fingers on the soft tissues under the jaw may worsen the airway. A correctly sized oral airway may be useful in an unconscious child. The correct size reaches roughly from the centre of the lips to the angle of the jaw when placed on the face (see Table 42.4 for guide to sizes). The wrong size will probably make the airway worse (Figure 42.1).

The vocal cords in the infant are more cephalad and are situated opposite C4 rather than opposite C6 in the adult. The epiglottis, which lies at a 45° angle to the vocal cords, is long, narrow, and U or V shaped, compared with the flat leaf-shape of the adult's. These factors mean that a straight-bladed laryngoscope is sometimes required to lift the epiglottis in order to visualize the infant's or young child's larynx.

Until puberty, the narrowest part of the upper airway is at the cricoid ring, just below the vocal cords (rather than at the cords as in an adult). An endotracheal tube that passes through the cords may wedge here. Pressure on the tracheal epithelial tissues from a tightly fitting tube, or from a cuff, may damage the epithelium and underlying soft tissues, causing oedema, raising airflow resistance, and producing extubation stridor. The change to a cuffed tube is usually made at about the age of 10 years. The probable appropriate size of the endotracheal tube is calculated from the formula:

$$\frac{\text{Age in years}}{4} + 4.$$

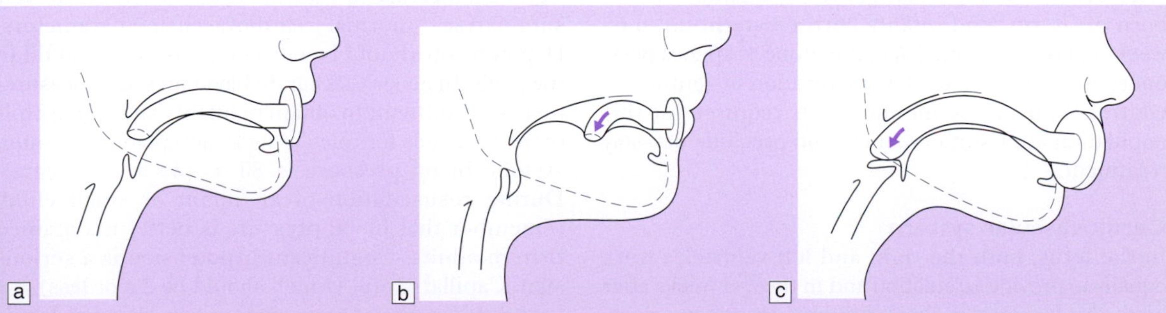


**Figure 42.1** The sizing of Guedel airways. (a) A correctly sized airway will reach roughly from the centre of the mouth to the angle of the jaw when laid over the patient's cheek. When the airway is too small, as in (b), or too large as in (c), it is more difficult to maintain an airway. (Adapted from *Advanced Paediatric Life Support: The Practical Approach*, 2nd edn. London: BMJ Books, 1997.)

Note that this formula does not apply to neonates or infants.

The trachea is relatively short (about 4 cm in a full-term neonate) and the bifurcation is at T2, rather than at T4 as in the adult. Hence endobronchial intubation occurs easily. This is especially so using preformed endotracheal tubes with the head flexed. Conversely, extension of the head may lead to accidental extubation. After intubation, or a change in the patient's position, the chest should be auscultated to check that the tube has been placed correctly. This should be done in both axillae rather than just on the anterior chest wall, or transmitted sounds may lead to erroneous conclusions.

Respiratory function at birth is immature: the number and structure of alveoli are underdeveloped, resulting in a small surface area for gas exchange. The functional residual capacity (FRC) is proportionately small. Oxygen consumption in a thermoneutral environment is about 7 ml/kg/min which is twice that of the adult. This is achieved by a higher ventilatory rate (30–40 breaths/min at birth, 24 breaths/min at 1 year) which also results in a higher dead space ventilation per minute. Tidal ventilation remains constant through life at 7 ml/kg. The energy required for normal breathing is adequately supplied, but increased airway resistance or other increases in the work of breathing mean that the spontaneously breathing anaesthetized baby tires easily. The breathing in neonates is primarily diaphragmatic because of the immature intercostal muscles and a very compliant chest wall, the cartilaginous ribs of which are placed horizontally (Figure 42.2). This mechanical disadvantage increases the neonate's and infant's susceptibility to ventilatory impairment. Thus intermittent positive pressure ventilation (IPPV) is required for all but the shortest procedures. Gastric distension may be caused by over-vigorous hand ventilation on a facemask, and should be relieved by passing a fine-bore gastric tube or suction catheter.

In young children and infants in particular, the chest wall is very compliant and cannot oppose the action of the diaphragm to maintain the FRC. There is also an increased tendency towards airway closure, so that the infant is predisposed to intrapulmonary shunting and hypoxia. When using IPPV, there are advantages to using relatively large chest excursions with modest positive end-expiratory pressure (PEEP) to maintain oxygenation.

Control of breathing is similar to that of the adult after the neonatal period. However, infants who are born pre-term (and infants born pre-term up to 60 weeks of postconceptual age) are prone to apnoea postoperatively because of slow maturation of ventilatory control. Thus, close monitoring is required for this population after surgery and would preclude day-stay treatment.

### Cardiovascular system

In the fetus, both the right and left ventricles work equally to provide circulation and in the 2–3 weeks after birth the foramen ovale and ductus arteriosus close, resulting in the adult circulation (see Chapter 30). The higher systemic pressure results in hypertrophy of the left ventricle, which attains relative adult proportions by 3–6 months.

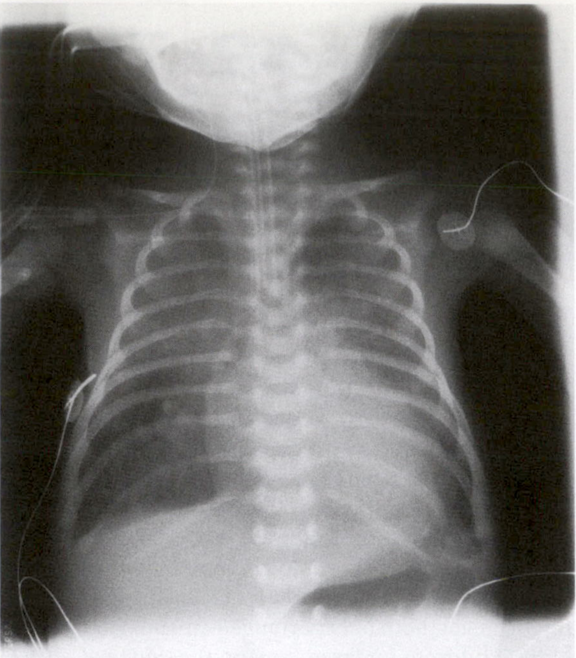

**Figure 42.2** A chest radiograph of a 3-week-old neonate recovering from respiratory distress syndrome. Note the horizontal ribs, the air bronchogram, and that the endotracheal tube is near the bifurcation of the trachea.

The cardiac output at birth is 200 ml/kg per min and this declines gradually to 100 ml/kg per min by puberty. Resting stroke volume in all ages is about 1 ml/kg. The cardiac output at younger ages is maintained by increases in heart rate. Conversely, bradycardia, especially in the newborn, implies reduced cardiac output. The normal heart rate in babies is 120–140 beats/min decreasing to 70–80 beats/min by adolescence. There is an increased sensitivity to vagal stimulation (the sympathetic nervous system is less well developed in infants) and bradycardias occur more readily. To maintain cardiac output, it is therefore important to rectify any bradycardia that may occur during anaesthesia, remembering that one of the most potent reasons for bradycardia is hypoxia.

Systolic blood pressure at birth is about 60 mmHg, and increases to 95 mmHg by 1 year. It remains at this value until the age of 6–7 years and thereafter there is a gradual increase to 120 mmHg at puberty. Table 42.1 summarizes normal cardiovascular parameters. Hypotension should be corrected just as it should in the adult. In general, accurate blood pressure measurements are difficult to obtain in infants and young children. A formula for calculating an acceptable minimum systolic blood pressure is 80 + (2 × age in years). During resuscitation of an infant or small child, remember that blood pressure is better maintained than in adults – significant hypotension is a serious sign. Capillary refill (which should be 2 s or less) is a useful sign to assist resuscitation (see later for details of measurement).

Subcutaneous fat often hides the veins on the backs of the hands in children aged 4–18 months. Small veins on the front of the wrist or scalp veins may be cannu-

**Table 42.1 Normal cardiovascular parameters in babies, infants, and children**

| Age | Systolic BP (mmHg) | Diastolic BP (mmHg) | Heart rate (beats/min) |
|---|---|---|---|
| Pre-term (1000 g) | 45 | 25 | 110–180 |
| Term | 60 | 35 | 100–180 |
| 1 week | 70 | 40 | 100–180 |
| 6 months | 90 | 50 | 80–130 |
| 2 years | 95 | 60 | 75–115 |
| 10 years | 105 | 65 | 70–110 |

When measuring the blood pressure (BP), it is important to use as big a cuff as will fit comfortably on the arm.
A narrow cuff will give falsely high readings. If a child seems to fall between two sizes, use the larger one. Automated BP machines may give an erroneously high figure on very small patients, especially neonates under 1500 g.
The systolic reading may be more reliable than the diastolic, as the fourth Korotkoff sounds are sometimes difficult to hear or, alternatively, audible down to zero.
Other indicators of circulatory adequacy include pulse volume, respiratory rate, mental status, and urine output.

lated to induce anaesthesia. The long saphenous vein found anterior to the medial malleolus of the ankle is a vein of constant position, which may be cannulated if other sites do not reveal palpable or visible veins.

## Blood

Blood volume is estimated at 100 ml/kg in the pre-term neonate, 80 ml/kg at full term, and 75 ml/kg at 2 years. Blood transfusion should be considered when there is a loss of 10% of the estimated blood volume, just as in the adult, and therefore blood loss should be carefully measured. Blood must always be warmed before transfusion, even if the volume is as little as 10 ml.

At birth the haemoglobin concentration is 16–18 g/dl, of which about 80% is fetal haemoglobin (HbF). The dissociation curve compared with adult haemoglobin (HbA) is shown in Figure 42.3. The greater affinity of HbF for oxygen is overcome in the tissues of the fetus because of low tissue oxygen tension ($PO_2$) and a metabolic acidosis. The acidosis aids oxygen delivery to the tissues by shifting the dissociation curve to the right. Alkalosis (e.g. caused by hyperventilation) reduces oxygen availability and hence should be avoided. Just as in adults, there are good reasons for ventilating to normocapnia (see below). The haemoglobin concentration decreases to about 10 g/dl by 3 months and reaches 12–14 g/dl by 1 year (Figure 42.4). Sickle haemoglobin (see Chapter 52), in those who have it, is produced at the same rate as HbA and sufficient amounts to produce a positive sickledex test may not be present until 3–4 months of age.

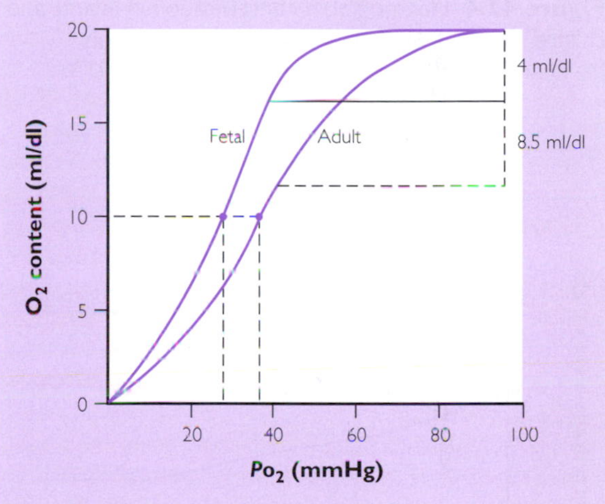


**Figure 42.3** Oxygen equilibration curves for fetal and adult haemoglobin. The $P_{50}$ (the partial pressure of oxygen [$Po_2$] at which saturation is 50%) of fetal haemoglobin is 27 mmHg (3.6 kPa) compared with 36 mmHg (4.8 kPa) for adult haemoglobin. Note that, as the oxygen tension decreases from 95 mmHg (12.7 kPa) in the arterial circulation to 40 mmHg (5.3 kPa) in the mixed venous circulation, twice as much oxygen is extracted from adult blood as from the fetal blood. This is because of differences in oxygen affinity between the two types of haemoglobin. (From Rudolph AM. *Pediatr Cardiol* 1983;4(S2):17.)

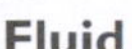

## Fluid

The neonate contains proportionately more water than its adult counterpart (75% compared with 65% body weight); this decreases over the first year. This occurs as a result of a larger extracellular fluid compartment (Figure 42.5).

Renal function at birth is immature, with an obligatory salt loss. There is a limited ability to conserve or excrete water, causing the neonate to be intolerant of dehydration and fluid overload. Although renal function is fully developed by 1 year, infants are less able to deal with fluid restriction because of their large body surface area : weight ratio.

Normal maintenance fluid requirements are shown in Table 42.2. These are guidelines; fluid administration should be titrated against the patient's physiological status and response to fluid administration, bearing in mind the pathological process (e.g. allow for preoperative deficiencies), the type of surgery (more in bowel surgery), and the environmental temperature (increased evaporative losses in warm surroundings).

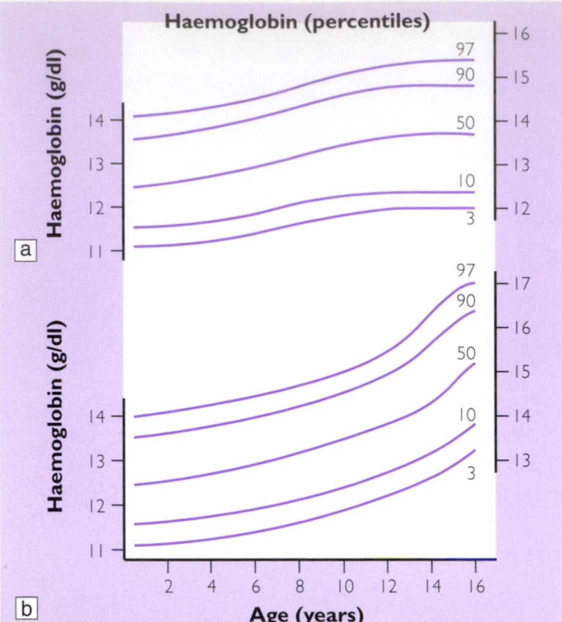


**Figure 42.4** Haemoglobin concentration in infants and children living at sea level: (a) girls; (b) boys. (From Dallman PR and Siimes MA. *J Pediatr* 1979;77:941.)

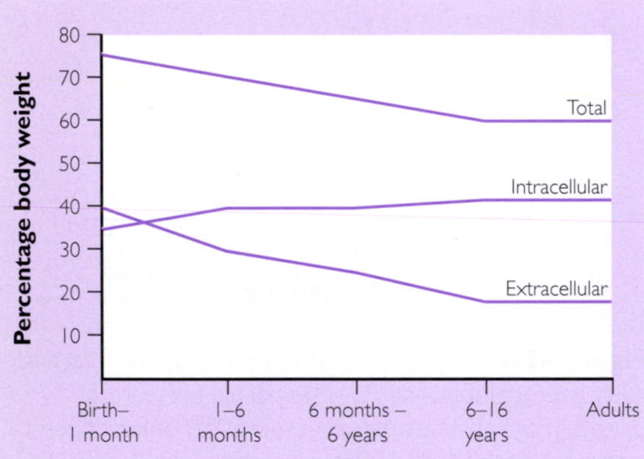


**Figure 42.5** Changes in body fluid composition (as percentage of body weight) with age. (From Bush GH. *Ann R Coll Surg* 1971;49:92–101.)

### *Fluid resuscitation*

A dehydrated child needs fluid in addition to the normal requirements outlined above. The extent of dehydration can be estimated clinically by feeling for a distinct demarcation line on the limbs, beyond which the skin is noticeably cooler. After reference to Figure 42.6, the fluid deficit can be estimated from the formula:

$$\begin{matrix}\text{Deficit} \\ \text{(in ml)}\end{matrix} = \%\ \text{dehydration} \times \frac{\text{weight}}{\text{in kg}} \times 10$$

Other physical signs, such as poor skin turgor, sunken fontanelle in babies, and possibly tachypnoea, tachycardia, and drowsiness, will be present. Urine output will be reduced.

If the child is not shocked, the extra fluid required can often be delivered over 24 h, as shown in the case history below. In severe dehydration such as seen in diabetic ketoacidosis, a 48 h period may be more appropriate. On the other hand, a child presenting for urgent surgery will require more rapid correction. Repeated clinical assessment and biochemical testing are required to assess the response to therapy.

> A 6-year-old child is cold below the knees and elbows. Body weight is 20 kg.
> Normal requirements are therefore 60 ml/h (4% dextrose/0.18% saline)
> Deficit = 10 × 20 × 10 = 2000 ml
> (given over 24 h = 2000 ÷ 24 = 83 ml/h)
> Total requirement = 60 + 83 = 143 ml/h

If a patient is shocked, with prolonged capillary refill (see box below for practical details), then *immediate* fluid resuscitation is required with boluses of 20 ml/kg, repeated as necessary.

> After pressure on a digit or a foot, capillary refill should occur within 2 s. The limb being tested should be lifted a little above the heart, to ensure that arteriolar capillary refill is measured (rather than venous). Slower refill indicates poor perfusion, and is a useful sign in resuscitation, particularly in sepsis. This test is quick to perform and record. However, the child should be warm for it to be a valid sign.

**Table 42.2 Maintenance fluid requirements in normal children**

| Body weight (kg) | Calorie needs per day | Fluid requirements per day | Fluid requirements per hour |
|---|---|---|---|
| < 10 | 100 cal/kg | 100 ml/kg | 4 ml/kg |
| 10–20 | 1000 cal + 50 cal/kg of body weight > 10 kg | 1000 ml + 50 ml/kg of body weight > 10 kg | 40 ml for first 10 kg + 2 ml/kg for body weight > 10 kg |
| > 20 | 1500 cal + 20 cal/kg of body weight > 20 kg | 1500 ml + 20 ml/kg of body weight > 20 kg | 60 ml for first 20 kg + 1 ml/kg for body weight > 20 kg |

A suitable fluid for maintenance in children is 4% dextrose/0.18% saline; 20 mmol/L KCl may be added for routine maintenance out of the operating room.

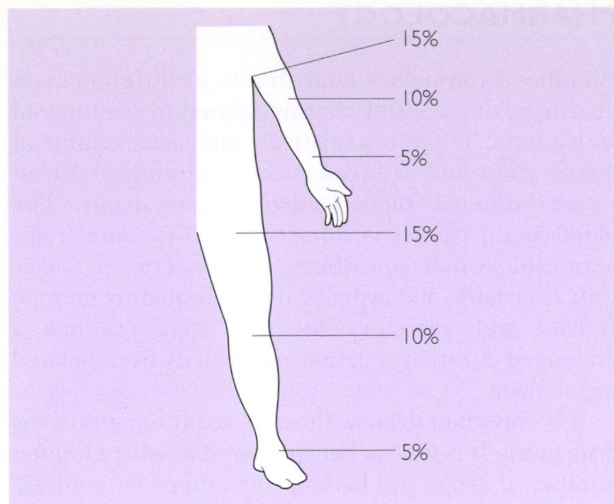


**Figure 42.6** Body outline showing the percentage dehydration present when the limb is felt to be noticeably colder beyond the demarcations indicated. (See text.)

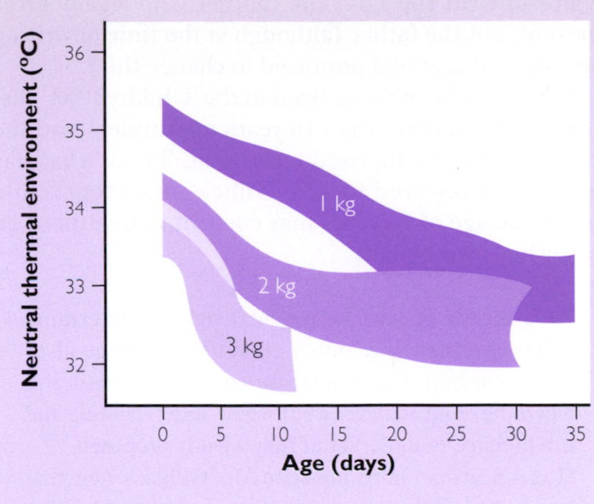


**Figure 42.7** The neutral thermal environment. (From Hey EN and Katz G. *Arch Child* 1970;45:328–34.)

Normal fluid requirements in childhood are 4% dextrose/0.18% saline, but gastrointestinal losses correspond more closely to 0.9% saline (physiological saline). In this situation, rather than give these fluids separately, it would be reasonable in the first instance to give the total requirement as half-physiological saline with dextrose. Urgent serum electrolyte estimation is needed to confirm this and may indicate the necessity to add some potassium.

### Metabolic rate

The metabolic rate in children is approximately twice that of adults. Newborn babies have relatively few carbohydrate reserves and are therefore prone to hypoglycaemia if fasted excessively before anaesthesia. Hypoglycaemia is defined as 1.6 mmol/L in the term newborn and 2.2 mmol/L in those older than 3 days.

### Temperature regulation

Small babies are vulnerable to heat loss because their thermoregulatory mechanism is immature, the surface area : weight ratio is large, they have less insulating subcutaneous fat, and there is poor cutaneous vasomotor control. The ability to shiver in response to cold is not yet developed and heat is produced by non-shivering thermogenesis from brown fat. This results in excessive oxygen consumption.

The control of brown-fat metabolism is compromised by general anaesthesia, and so it is important to maintain body temperature by other means. The operating room temperature needs to be kept warmer than is usual for adults, at about 25°C. However, further means are necessary to help maintain normal body temperature.

The large head of a baby is a particular source of heat loss and it should be covered while in the operating room and during transit. A fluid warmer should be used for blood and other cold fluids. Use of a humidifier to warm and humidify the otherwise cold and dry anaesthetic gases is very helpful in temperature maintenance.

An incubator is the best way to transport babies any distance. Different sizes and gestations need different incubator temperatures to maintain body temperature. It is no good simply putting the baby into a vaguely warm incubator and hoping for the best, especially for long journeys. Figure 42.7 shows the ambient temperature at which babies of different ages and sizes need to be kept if they are to maintain body temperature. It will be noticed that the temperatures are higher than those in an operating room, even if it seems very hot! In other words, an exposed baby in an operating room will get cold.

### Nervous system

At birth, myelination of the brain stem and spinal cord is incomplete and continues during the first few months of life; this is reflected in the normal milestones of development. The brain also grows rapidly in the first year of life. At birth, the lower limit of the spinal cord is at L3, and does not reach its final level of L1 until 1 year of age.

## PSYCHOLOGY

The psychological approach of children to surgery or other treatment depends on their age, maturity, emotional make-up, preadmission preparation (e.g. books, videos, ward visit, etc.), and parental attitude and support. Sympathetic explanation of events is important, preferably in the presence of a parent. Induction of anaesthesia is a major contributory factor to the psychological stress of hospitalization, and the anaesthetic team has an important role in reducing this stress. Some children are emotionally upset by their experiences in hospital and show behavioural changes such as bed-wetting, temper tantrums, nightmares, and hostility after going home. This also makes subsequent admissions to hospital more difficult.

## CONSENT

The legal age of consent is 16 years; under this age it is usual for a parent or guardian to give consent for surgery on behalf of the child. Unfortunately, the law is not quite as simple as this. In the case of unmarried parents, it is at present (in the UK) the mother who legally gives consent, not the father (although at the time of writing the Government had promised to change this).

It has also been recognized in the 'Children Act' that individuals younger than 16 years may understand the implications of proposed treatment. Thus, what has come to be referred to as a 'Gillick competent' child under the age of 16 years may consent to treatment on his or her own behalf:

> 'As a matter of law the parental right to determine whether or not their minor child below the age of 16 years will have medical treatment terminates if and when the child achieves a sufficient understanding and intelligence to understand fully what is proposed.'
> (Lord Scarman in response to Mrs Gillick's view that her daughter who was under 16 years old should not be prescribed the contraceptive pill.)

On the other hand, the legal rights of a child to refuse treatment are less clear. It would seem wise that, where there are any problems with consent, the problem should be referred to the consultants involved.

## PHARMACOLOGY

Childhood physiology contributes to differences in pharmacokinetics and pharmacodynamics compared with adults. There is a relatively increased volume of distribution and reduced protein binding, both of which influence the effective dose of drugs. The blood–brain barrier is immature and is more freely permeable, which contributes to the increased sensitivity to sedative and hypnotic drugs. Immature enzyme activity and excretory function may produce a prolonged duration of action and toxicity from delayed metabolism.

It is important to know the dose requirements of any drug given. It is wise to become familiar with a limited number of drugs and look up any others as required. Drug dosage is normally calculated according to body weight, although it might be more accurate to base it on body surface area. The appropriate dose for children of some commonly used drugs in anaesthesia are given in Table 42.3. Commercially available paracetamol elixir (Calpol) contains 120 mg in 5 ml.

**Table 42.3 Paediatric dose of drugs commonly used in anaesthesia**

| Drug | Route | Dosage |
|---|---|---|
| Atropine | i.v. | 20 μg/kg |
| Trimeprazine | Oral | 2–4 mg/kg |
| Chloral hydrate | Oral | 50 mg/kg |
| Temazepam | Oral | 0.3 mg/kg |
| Thiopentone (thiopental) | i.v. | 5–6 mg/kg (see text) |
| Propofol | i.v. | 3 mg/kg |
| Ketamine | i.v.<br>i.m. | 2 mg/kg<br>10 mg/kg |
| Suxamethonium | i.v. | 1.0–1.5 mg/kg (see text) |
| Vecuronium | i.v. | 0.1 mg/kg (use a third to half initial dose for increments) |
| Atracurium | i.v. | 0.5 mg/kg (use a third to half initial dose for increments) |
| Pancuronium | i.v. | 50–100 μg/kg (use a third to half initial dose for increments) |
| Neostigmine | i.v. | 80 μg/kg |
| Morphine | i.v. | 0.1 mg/kg (see text) |
| Pethidine | i.v. | 1 mg/kg |
| Fentanyl | i.v. | 1–2 μg/kg |
| Codeine phosphate | Oral or p.r. | 1 mg/kg |
| Paracetamol | Oral or p.r. | 15 mg/kg |
| Diclofenac | p.r. | 1.0–1.5 mg/kg |
| Ibuprofen | Oral | 5 mg/kg |
| Bupivacaine | Infiltration or epidural | up to 2 mg/kg |

### Inhalational agents

The uptake of inhalational agents is more rapid than in adults. The main reasons for this are the increased minute ventilation and reduced FRC. The increased cardiac output also increases the rate of equilibration in the tissues. Apart from neonates, the minimum alveolar concentration is inversely proportional to age (Figure 42.8).

### Induction agents

The dose of thiopentone (thiopental) required is 4–5 mg/kg for neonates, 7–8 mg/kg for infants, and 5–6 mg/kg for children. This increased requirement over that in the adult is related to the higher cardiac output. This also means that the induction agent has a shorter duration of action, and therefore the anaesthetist has to ensure a rapid transition to inhalational maintenance. Similar changes in dose requirements of other induction agents occur and are all reduced after sedative premedication.

### Analgesics

Morphine has a greater potency, longer duration of action, and causes more ventilatory depression in small babies than in older children because the blood–brain barrier is more permeable, cerebral blood flow is relatively higher, and the diffusible free fraction of morphine is higher. This is an argument for careful administration of analgesia rather than inadequate pain control. Morphine is the opioid used most commonly in children and is poorly lipid soluble; hence it penetrates the intact blood–brain barrier with difficulty. In the child aged over 6 months, a suitable loading dose of morphine is 100 μg/kg i.v. followed by infusion of 20 μg/kg per h for balanced anaesthesia. (If 1 mg/kg morphine is diluted to 50 ml in saline, 1 ml/h = 20 μg/kg per h.) For those aged under 6 months, a loading dose of 25 μg/kg is followed by maintenance of 5–10 μg/kg per h. The use of opioids in infants aged under about 6 months should be in an environment where close monitoring is possible. The use of fentanyl 1–2 μg/kg provides shorter duration of analgesia and ventilatory depression than in the adult.

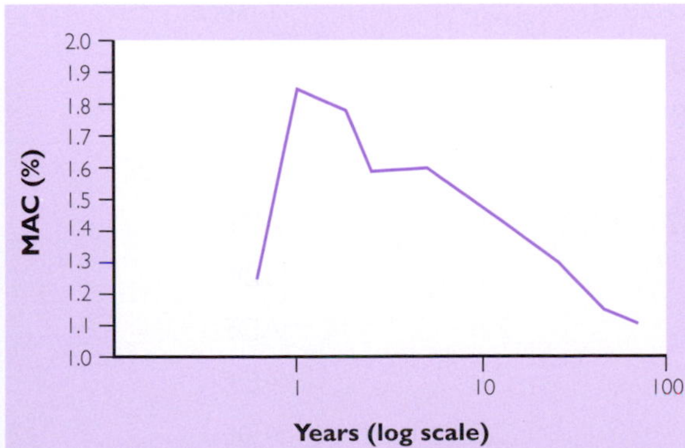


**Figure 42.8** The variation of minimum alveolar concentration (MAC) with age, illustrated with isoflurane. Anaesthetic requirements increase during the first months of life. The highest MAC values are found in infants of around 6 months of age. After this, MAC gradually decreases with age. Note that age is presented on a logarithmic scale. (From LeDez KM and Lerman J. *Anesthesiology* 1987;67:301–7.)

### Neuromuscular blockers

The volume of distribution of neuromuscular blocking drugs in infants is larger than that in children and adults. When allowance is made for these differences, infants appear to be relatively resistant to suxamethonium and sensitive to non-depolarizing relaxants. Thus, the infant may require 2–3 mg/kg of suxamethonium, but similar doses (per kilogram) of non-depolarizing agents as older children.

## PREOPERATIVE ASSESSMENT AND PREPARATION

The medical history needs to be taken from the parent and is similar to that detailed in Chapter 41. The chest and the airway need to be examined.

The predominant concurrent pathologies in children are congenital abnormalities and infections. Congenital cardiac disease is present in 8 per 1000 births. The presence of a cardiac murmur may require preliminary cardiological evaluation. The lesions found in unfamiliar syndromes will require consultation in reference texts.

Upper respiratory tract infections are common and their occurrence within the previous 6 weeks leads to increased respiratory complications in the perioperative period. There is a real dilemma because no one wishes children to be placed at increased risk and, yet, in the winter months particularly, it may be difficult to catch children between such infections! Some children seem to have a perpetually runny nose. If questioning the parents establishes that this is frequently the child's state, and there is no fever and no signs of lower respiratory tract disease, then it may be reasonable to proceed with anaesthesia for minor procedures. Children who have, for them, abnormal upper respiratory signs, who are febrile, or who have lower respiratory tract signs should have surgery postponed for a month. When surgery is urgent, a decision about the best course of action for the child has to be made and may often include proceeding with anaesthesia. Other infections such as in the chest or ear, chickenpox, measles, mumps, and rubella are contraindications to non-urgent surgery.

At the age of 5 years or so, children start to lose their primary dentition (see Chapter 6). It pays to ask the child if any teeth are loose.

There has been a dramatic change in views over the appropriate duration of preoperative starvation. Drinking of clear fluids up to 2–3 h before surgery has not shown increases in the volume or acidity of gastric contents, is less distressing to children, and is less likely to result in a hypoglycaemic, irritable child than is total fasting. It must be stressed that clear fluids do not include any milk or drinks containing particles. These and solids should be withheld for at least 6 h, although some centres are adopting more liberal times of 4 h. Hungry children need to be closely observed in the preoperative period to prevent the acquisition of food from unofficial sources!

Preparing the child for surgery takes skill, experience, and patience. The parent also requires reassurance.

Most children respond to a direct friendly explanation, in gentle terms that they can understand, of events that will occur. The child may wish to express a preference for 'gas' or 'scratch in the hand' 'way of going to sleep'. Depending on the response of the parents to hospitalization, it is usually helpful for one of them to accompany the child during induction of anaesthesia.

EMLA (eutectic mixture of local anaesthetic) cream applied on the skin over veins anaesthetizes the skin after a period of 60 min or so. Topical amethocaine has the advantage of also numbing the skin, but without causing vasoconstriction of the vein underneath. Both of these agents are effective and can make venepuncture painless. It is sensible to apply one of them 1 hour before surgery even if an inhalational induction is finally chosen.

If a sedative premedication is wanted, the oral route is preferable because of children's dislike of intramuscular injections. Unfortunately there is not a universally ideal agent. Trimeprazine is a phenothiazine derivative with antiemetic and antisialogogue properties; the degree of sedation produced is variable. Chloral hydrate is most useful in babies. Temazepam is an alternative.

An antisialogogue is somewhat less important with modern inhalational agents, which are less irritant than those formerly available. However, in infants, there is an increased risk of laryngeal spasm at induction and after extubation if excessive secretions are present. Gastric absorption of atropine is poor, so that in proximal gastrointestinal tract obstruction the effect of oral atropine is unreliable. However, in other patients, it is effective orally, although perhaps less reliably than when given intramuscularly.

## INTRAOPERATIVE CONSIDERATIONS

Before anaesthesia is induced, check that equipment suitable for the size of child is ready. This includes breathing circuits, facemasks, airways, endotracheal tubes, connectors, laryngoscopes, laryngeal mask, suction catheters, intravenous cannulae, and blood pressure cuffs (Table 42.4 gives guidelines; see Chapter 6 for photographs). Have sticky tape pre-cut to secure a cannula. Make sure that the operating room is warm.

Keep needles out of sight and prepare drugs to be used before the child arrives. It is helpful to have standard dilutions, clearly labelled, to avoid mistakes.

In general, local anaesthetic techniques as the sole anaesthetic are unsuitable, except perhaps for very young (e.g. neonatal hernia repair under spinal anaesthesia) or older children. However, local anaesthetic blocks as an adjunct to general anaesthesia can be useful in providing postoperative analgesia.

### Induction

When the child arrives, decide whether anaesthesia is going to be induced with the child sitting on a parent's lap. If so, it is helpful to look at possible veins with the child's arm behind the parent's back. Then the vein can be cannulated (22- or 24-gauge cannulae are suitable) without the child seeing. A firm grip is needed to prevent sudden withdrawal of the arm. Thiopentone is the most commonly used induction agent; among

**Table 42.4 Size of airway equipment suitable for different ages**

| Age (years) | Oral airway | Tracheal tube ID; length (cm) | LMA | Facemask[a] | Circuit |
|---|---|---|---|---|---|
| Neonate | 000 | 3.5; 10 | 1 | 0 L | T-piece |
| 6 months | 0 | 4.0; 11 | 1 (up to 5 kg) or 1.5 (5–10 kg) | 1 L | T-piece |
| 1 | 1 | 4.5; 12 | 2 (10–20 kg) | 2 L | T-piece |
| 2 | 1 | 4.5; 14 | 2 (10–20 kg) | 2 L | T-piece |
| 3 | 1 | 5.0; 14.5 | 2 (10–20 kg) | 2 L | T-piece |
| 4 | 1 | 5.0; 15 | 2 or 2.5 | 2 L | T-piece/ADE |
| 5 | 2 | 5.5; 15.5 | 2.5 (20–30 kg) | 2 B | ADE |
| 6 | 2 | 5.5; 16 | 2.5 | 2 B | ADE |
| 7 | 2 | 6.0; 16.5 | 2.5 | 2 B | ADE |
| 8 | 2 | 6.0; 17 | 2.5 | 2 B | ADE |
| 9 | 2 | 6.5; 17.5 | 2.5 | 2 B | ADE |
| 10 | 2 | 6.5; 18 | 2.5 | 2/3 B | ADE |
| 11 | 2/3 | 7.0; 18.5 | 3 (>30 kg) | 2/3 B | ADE |
| 12 | 2/3 | 7.0; 19 | 3 | 3 B | ADE |

[a]L, Laerdal; B, British Oxygen Company; LMA, laryngeal mask airway; ID, inner diameter; ADE, Mapleson A, D or E circuit (see Chapter 9).

its advantages is the lack of pain on injection. Propofol is licensed for children aged over 3 years. Lignocaine (lidocaine) mixed with the propofol helps reduce pain on injection. The rapid redistribution of induction agent because of the high cardiac output means that it is not usually possible to insert a laryngeal mask airway (LMA) immediately after propofol, as it is in the adult. Anaesthesia has to be deepened with a volatile agent and then the LMA inserted in a similar manner to in adults (see Chapter 6), although its passage is not quite as easy. Incorrect placement with obstruction by the epiglottis is encountered more frequently. Enlarged tonsils may also contribute to difficulty with placement.

An inhalational induction may be chosen, either by the child or if there are no visible veins. Some children like to blow the 'balloon' up and hear the whistle through an expiratory valve, and others are more cooperative if the gas is introduced from the circuit enclosed in the anaesthetist's hand.

Halothane has been the agent of choice because it is non-explosive and less irritant than enflurane or isoflurane. The child starts breathing 66% nitrous oxide in oxygen and halothane is gradually introduced, increasing the inspired concentration every few breaths until 2% is reached. Halothane may be contraindicated if there are repeated exposures and sevoflurane has even less irritant properties and less odour. Sevoflurane can be used in concentrations up to 8% immediately on induction and reduced to 3–4% after the child has gone to sleep. Anaesthesia is often induced quickly if leaks can be avoided. Intravenous access should then be secured.

Laryngospasm may occur during the administration of anaesthesia and intubation in children; 100% oxygen with PEEP should be used until it resolves and occasionally emergency intubation is necessary.

Infants and children are intubated with their head in the neutral position. Raising the head on a pillow does not improve the view of the larynx, because there are fewer intervertebral joints above the larynx that can be flexed. External pressure over the cricoid cartilage helps to bring the larynx into view.

Once the endotracheal tube has been passed, check that there is a slight leak when pressure of 20–25 $cmH_2O$ is applied. If the tube fits too snugly, there is a risk of postintubation croup. If there is too much leak, ventilation will be difficult. Once the position of the tube has been checked, it must be secured firmly to avoid accidental extubation or endobronchial intubation. If a nasotracheal tube is required, the same diameter as an orotracheal tube can be used up to the age of 6 years.

### Breathing circuits

These are outlined in more detail in Chapter 9. For children under 20 kg a T-piece arrangement is necessary to avoid excessive equipment dead space and also has the advantage of low resistance to expiration.

### Ventilators

Older children who are intubated with cuffed tubes may usually be ventilated with standard adult ventilators, with ventilatory parameters adjusted to allow for their smaller size.

Paediatric ventilators can be classified under various familiar headings such as cycling mechanism or flow or pressure generator (see Chapter 11).

Infants and younger children are intubated with uncuffed tubes, which are sized to allow for a small gas leak. Measurement of tidal volumes may therefore be inaccurate. Moreover, the leak may vary during the course of an anaesthetic as the patient is moved, or the compliance changes as a result of patient or surgical factors. It is usual to define paediatric ventilation in terms of inspiratory and expiratory times, which give overall rate and pressure (inspiratory, expiratory, and mean). The effectiveness of ventilation is monitored clinically and by pulse oximetry and capnometry.

In general, the total volume of the circuit should be smaller than that used for adults to reduce compliance, particularly if a humidifier is used.

### Hand ventilation

Manual ventilation using the T-piece (see Chapter 9) is frequently used, particularly during anaesthesia of infants and neonates. The 'educated thumb' of the anaesthetist can instantly detect and compensate for compliance changes, and acts as an effective disconnection alarm. It has the advantage of keeping the anaesthetist in close proximity to the patient!

### Mechanical ventilation

Ventilators such as the Penlon Nuffield with a paediatric valve, which act by effectively 'squeezing the bag' on a T-piece or Bain system, are popular. The adult version of the Penlon Nuffield is a flow generator. For paediatric use, the adult patient valve is replaced by a Newton valve, giving a rather complex picture of flow generation at low pressures and pressure generation at higher pressures. However, it is quite simple to use. The gas flow into the patient during inspiration will be the sum of the fresh gas flow set on the anaesthesia machine plus the driving gas flow from the ventilator. When first connecting the patient to such a system, it is usual first to set the inspiratory and expiratory times to give an appropriate rate. The ventilator is then turned on with the flow initially set low, gradually increasing it until the inspiratory pressure rises and tidal excursions appear clinically appropriate.

Effectiveness of ventilation is judged by clinical monitoring of the patient in conjunction with pulse oximetry and capnometry. When using a T-piece or Bain system with capnometry, it is possible to control excessive hypocapnia by reducing the ventilatory rate, and also by reducing the fresh gas flow. The reduction of fresh gas flow produces rebreathing, allowing good tidal excursions and maintaining alveolar expansion, without producing hypocapnia. The use of $CO_2$ monitoring has removed the need to calculate the fresh gas flow to produce normocapnia.

One of the potential hazards of the T-piece is that it does not incorporate a pressure-relief valve. One of these should always be used to reduce the chances of barotrauma caused by any mechanical problem. If doubt arises about the efficacy of mechanical ventilation, it is wise to switch to manual ventilation while seeking the source of the problem. It is worthwhile electively ventilating by hand in normal cases in order to practise for this scenario. Hand ventilation with an open-ended paediatric reservoir bag is a skill that needs to be learnt.

### Other ventilators

Some anaesthetists favour the type of ventilators normally used in intensive care for operating room work, such as those made by Siemens or Draeger, these providing great flexibility in use. However, those unfamiliar with them will prefer simpler ventilators attached to a T-piece or Bain system, if only because of the frequency with which the alarms are triggered in operating room use.

### Regional and other nerve blocks

It is rarely appropriate for procedures in young children to be performed solely under nerve blockade, so these blocks are normally used as an adjunct to general anaesthesia to provide analgesia during and after surgery. The exception to this rule is when caudals and spinals are used in pre-term neonates to reduce the chances of postoperative respiratory problems.

In general, regional anaesthesia in children is performed as in adults, with the same precautions. Care should be taken not to exceed the safe total drug dose (see Table 42.3 and Chapter 15).

### Caudal block

This is easy to perform in children, and is particularly suitable for penile surgery. The procedure should be sterile. A greater success is achieved with an approach to the sacral hiatus that is more parallel to the surface of the back than is usual in adults. In infants, the needle should not be introduced too far into the epidural space because the dural sac extends further caudally in this age group (see Chapter 15). Bupivacaine (0.5 ml/kg of 0.25%) is suitable, although some anaesthetists prefer to use more dilute local anaesthetic (e.g. 0.125% bupivacaine) to avoid possible complications of urine retention and leg weakness. Hypotension is very unusual and fluids rarely have to be given for this, although intravenous access is essential, as with all anaesthetics. Upward spread of the local anaesthetic through the epidural space occurs easily in children, so greater volumes of local anaesthetic may be used, for example to provide analgesia for inguinal surgery, within the limits of the safe total dose.

Penile blocks are favoured by some anaesthetists for simple circumcisions.

### Ilioinguinal block

For surgery in the inguinal region, a ilioinguinal–iliohypogastric nerve block performed with 0.25% bupivacaine is quick and easy to perform (see Chapter 15), and is as effective as caudal blockade.

### Maintenance

The same principles of anaesthesia apply as in the adult. The child's cardiovascular and respiratory parameters should be monitored by visual checks, ECG, oxygen saturation, blood pressure, and capnography. The use of a precordial or oesophageal stethoscope is favoured by some. In feeling for a pulse in a child, the carotid pulse may be difficult to feel. The brachial or axillary pulse may be easier to palpate. It can also be easily done from the head of the operating table.

Fluid requirements and the need to keep the child warm have been discussed earlier. For all but the shortest operations in older children, body temperature should be measured from an oesophageal probe. Measurement of blood loss is difficult because of the small volumes involved. Swabs can be weighed. Alternatively, they can be washed, the resulting haematocrit measured and the loss calculated from a knowledge of the preoperative haemoglobin and the volume of the washing fluid. Physiological parameters (blood pressure, heart rate, and urine output) are just as useful as they are in adults.

## POSTOPERATIVE CONSIDERATIONS

The same considerations apply as in the adult. The aim is to provide the greatest safety combined with the best possible postoperative analgesia. In general hospitals, a paediatric area in the recovery room is a good idea, providing that it is appropriately equipped for postoperative problems in the paediatric age ranges – simply sticking cartoon character posters on the wall of a cold, draughty, and ill-equipped area is useless.

Children do not always vocalize the presence of pain. Conversely, a crying child in the recovery area may just be an indication of unhappiness with the surroundings and a desire to see the mother. The idea that babies do not feel pain has long since been abandoned, but its degree may be difficult to assess. Pain may be quantified by the use of formal scales, some of which include physiological parameters (such as CHEOPS, Children's Hospital of Eastern Ontario Pain Score). Pain may also be quantified with some sort of visual analogue scale, such as selection from a series of faces (as shown in Figure 42.9; see also Chapter 5). However, the use of any formal assessment tool may be time-consuming and is often not necessary. Experienced children's nurses, and of course the parents, will be able to assist the anaesthetist in quantifying pain. Continuous morphine infusions have already been mentioned but may need supplementation with extra morphine boluses. Patient-controlled analgesia systems

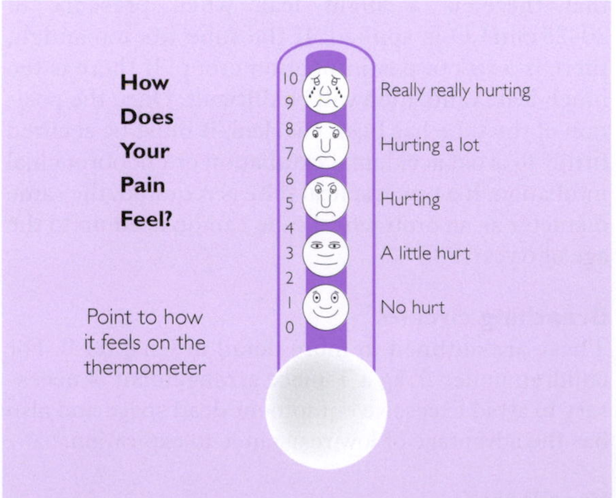


**Figure 42.9** A pain thermometer. This may help a child express how much pain is being felt. Pain 'ladders' or just a simple line analogue may be more suitable for children over 8–10 years.

can be managed by many patients over the age of 5 years.

Unless they are being transferred to an intensive care unit, patients should stay in the recovery area until they are fully awake, to recover from anaesthesia with established analgesia.

## CONGENITAL HYPERTROPHIC PYLORIC STENOSIS

This is one of the most common surgical problems of early infancy. The incidence is about 1 in 300 children with a male : female ratio of about 5 : 1. About half of these are firstborns. A thickening of the pylorus muscle causes increasing obstruction to the emptying of the stomach. The presenting symptom is vomiting, which increases in severity and becomes projectile. The infant becomes dehydrated and, as hydrochloric acid is lost from the stomach, a hypochloraemic metabolic alkalosis develops.

The diagnosis is usually confirmed by a test feed, at which the tumour may be felt (the tester taking care not to be hit by the vomit!). Sometimes confirmation by ultrasonography or radiology is needed.

The operation is not an emergency, and correction of the dehydration and replacement of sodium, chloride, and potassium must precede surgery. Before operating, the serum chloride should be above 90 mmol/L, the serum bicarbonate below 30 mmol/L, and the serum sodium and potassium within normal limits, with the baby clinically rehydrated.

Immediately before anaesthesia, the stomach is aspirated. Induction of anaesthesia is either intravenous or by inhalation, followed by a neuromuscular blocking agent. Note that cricoid pressure is effective in babies. A key aspect of anaesthesia is the maintenance of full relaxation during the splitting of the pyloric tumour, because coughing or straining could result in perforation of the mucosa, which increases postoperative morbidity. After surgery the baby is extubated awake, and can usually feed again after a few hours.

Surgical correction of pyloric stenosis is possibly the most common surgical procedure in early life performed in non-specialist centres. However, the National Confidential Enquiry into Perioperative Deaths has shown the benefits of anaesthesia and surgery being performed by those who do this on a regular basis, and this is a reason for a degree of subspecialization in larger district general hospitals.

## FURTHER READING


Cullen P. Fluid resuscitation in infants and children. *Curr Anaesth Crit Care* 1996;**7**:197–205.

Articles in: Hatch DJ, Hunter JM, eds. Postgraduate educational issue: The paediatric patient. *Br J Anaesth* 1999;**83**:1–168.

Kain ZN. Perioperative information and parental anxiety: the next generation. *Anesth Analg* 1999;**88**:237–9.

Lindahl SGE. Perioperative management of children. *Acta Anaesthesiol Scand* 1996;**40**:975–81.

Articles in: Lindahl SGE, ed. *Paediatric Anaesthesia. Baillière's Clin Anaesthesiol* 1996;**10**:605–770.

Phillips S, Daborn AK, Hatch DJ. Preoperative fasting for paediatric anaesthesia. *Br J Anaesth* 1994;**73**:529–36.

Schreiner MS, O'Hara I, Amarkakis D, Politis GD. Do children who experience laryngospasm have an increased risk of upper respiratory tract infection? *Anesthesiology* 1996;**85**:475–80.

Tatman A, Ralston C. Assessment of pain in small children. *Curr Anaesth Crit Care* 1997;**8**:19–24.

# Chapter 43 The elderly patient

G.M. Cooper

Whatever the type of surgery (excepting paediatric!), the anaesthetist cares for elderly patients. Many of the reasons for surgery are age related, e.g. cataracts, prostatic hypertrophy, degenerative changes in joints, trauma from falls, etc. More than a quarter of the surgical population is aged over 65 years, and this proportion will inevitably increase.

The normal ageing process gradually erodes all the body's safety margins, with a decreasing ability to adapt. Hence, it is not surprising that the elderly patient is at greater risk from surgery and anaesthesia than his or her younger counterpart. This is related to the increased incidence of coexisting pathology rather than any intrinsic risk. In addition, many elderly patients may attribute any physical deterioration to their age rather than to remedial pathology, and hence presentation of disease may be both occult and relatively advanced. Symptomatology is often much less florid than in the young, as shown by the 'silent infarct'. The rate of ageing is very variable and this needs to be recognized and related to a biological age rather than a chronological one.

The physiological changes of ageing are a universal and progressive degeneration of structure and function of organs and tissues. Most decrements in function start in the fourth decade of life, accelerate in the seventh decade and beyond, and are relatively irreversible. Almost all these changes affect the conduct of anaesthesia and are summarized in Tables 43.1–43.7.

The cardiovascular, pulmonary, and skeletal changes may not be inevitable, because they can be reduced in the fit and active elderly person who maintains a demand through daily exercise. However, this lifelong commitment is rare and thus the elixir of youth escapes the majority!

The importance of the decrease in renal function is often under-estimated. Acute renal failure is responsible for at least 20% of surgical deaths in elderly people.

## PREOPERATIVE ASSESSMENT

### History

Taking an adequate history can be difficult because of the problems associated with ageing. Account may need

**Table 43.1 Cardiovascular changes with age**

| Pathological change | Physiological effect | Implication |
|---|---|---|
| ↓ active myocardial fibres (size and number) | ↓ stroke volume<br>↓ resting heart rate<br>↓ maximum heart rate<br>↓ resting cardiac output | Slow arm–brain circulation<br>↓ cardiac reserve<br>↓ effect of catecholamines |
| Fibrous replacement of conducting system | Conduction disturbances | Predisposed to cardiac failure, heart block |
| Degeneration of valve ring<br>Papillary muscle dysfunction | Mitral incompetence | Avoid increasing systemic vascular resistance<br>Avoid bradycardias<br>Prophylaxis against endocarditis needed<br>Patient may be on anticoagulants |
| Aortic valve fibrosis | Aortic sclerosis | Valve function usually unaffected<br>Need to differentiate murmurs |
| Destruction of intima of vessel wall<br>↓ smooth muscle elastin loss | Fibrotic, calcified, necrotic, inelastic distributing system | Systolic hypertension<br>Blood pressure changes in response to fluid loss or gain exaggerated |
| Coronary or peripheral vessel disease | | May be asymptomatic because immobile |
| Red cell production | Haemoglobin concentration normal | Anaemia must be investigated and treated |

**Table 43.2 Pulmonary changes with age**

| Pathological change | Physiological effect | Implication |
|---|---|---|
| ↓ efficiency of lung parenchyma<br>↓ strength and mobility of muscles | ↓ vital capacity<br>↑ residual volume<br>FRC unchanged<br>↓ compliance<br>↓ $FEV_1$ | Predisposed to failure<br>Poor coughing<br>Predisposed to infection |
| Alveolar septa break | ↓ alveolar surface area | ↓ gas exchange |
| Interbronchiolar 'guy ropes' deteriorate | ↑ closing volume | Air trapping and shunting of pulmonary blood → ↓ $PaO_2$ |
| Dilatation of upper airways | ↑ anatomical dead space<br>↑ physiological dead space | Larger endotracheal tube needed<br>Inefficient gas exchange |
| ↓ reactivity | ↓ Laryngeal reflexes | Aspiration |
| ↓ reactivity | Ventilatory response to hypoxia and hypercapnia | Risk of respiratory failure |

FRC, functional residual capacity; $FEV_1$, forced expiratory volume in 1 second.

**Table 43.3 Changes in nervous system with age**

| Pathological change | Physiological effect | Implication |
|---|---|---|
| ↓ function of nerve cells | ↓ sensory abilities | ↓ appreciation of symptoms |
| Loss of myelin | ↓ motor abilities | Immobility, DVT |
| ↓ synapses and nerve fibres | ↓ intellectual function | Consent difficulties |
| ↓ neurotransmitter synthesis | Dementia | Sensitivity to anaesthetic agents (↓ MAC), opioids, neuromuscular blocking agents, and local anaesthetics<br>↓ adaptation to new surroundings |
| Above changes in sympathetic nervous system | ↓ autonomic tone | Postural hypotension<br>↓ BP in blood loss |
| Cataracts | Poor sight | Accidents |
| Presbycusis | Deafness | Communication problems |

DVT, deep vein thrombosis; MAC, minimum alveolar concentration.

**Table 43.4 Metabolic and endocrine changes with age**

| Pathological change | Physiological effect | Implication |
|---|---|---|
| ↓ lean body mass | ↓ muscle power | ↓ metabolic rate<br>Poor coughing<br>Immobility |
| Atrophy of sweat glands<br>↓ capacity to vasodilate and vasoconstrict | Poor temperature control | Slow rewarming postoperatively |
| ↓ cortisol secretion | ↓ cortisol excretion | Serum concentration unchanged |
| ↓ aldosterone secretion | | Vulnerable to sodium loss |
| Hyperthyroidism and hypothyroidism common | Presentation atypical | Often unrecognized |
| ↓ sensitivity of β cells to glucose<br>↓ insulin secretion | Glucose intolerance | Diabetes appears because of surgery<br>Care with glucose solutions |

**Table 43.5 Gastrointestinal and other changes with age**

| Pathological change | Physiological effect | Implication |
|---|---|---|
| ↓ appetite<br>Poor dentition | Malnutrition | Poor wound healing<br>Chest infection<br>Respiratory failure |
| Hiatus hernia | Oesophageal reflux | Aspiration |
| ↓ peristalsis | ↓ gastric emptying<br>Constipation | ?effect on drug absorption |
| ↓ gastric mucus | Gastritis | $H_2$-receptor antagonist therapy → drug interactions |
| ↓ muscle fibres and fibrous replacement | ↓ body height | Immobility |
| Collagen loss | Loose skin<br>Fragile veins<br>↓ ligament strength | Mobile veins<br>Haematoma formation<br>Joint dislocations |
| Osteoporosis | Fragile bones | Fractures |

**Table 43.6 Hepatic and renal changes with age**

| Pathological change | Physiological effect | Implication |
|---|---|---|
| ↓ albumin produced | ↓ serum albumin (by 20%) | ↓ drug binding |
| ↓ cardiac output | ↓ liver blood flow | Drug accumulation |
| Enzymatic activity = | Unchanged | Nil |
| ↓ protein synthesis | ↓ serum protein<br>Sufficient clotting factors | Poor healing<br>Normal coagulation |
| ↓ kidney mass | ↓ glomerular filtration rate<br>↓ tubular function | ↓ functional reserve<br>↓ water conservation<br>Dehydration<br>↓ drug excretion |
| ↓ skeletal muscle | Serum creatinine unchanged (less to excrete) | ↓ renal reserve despite normal creatinine |
| Prostatic hypertrophy | | Urinary retention |

**Table 43.7 Handling of drugs**

| Modality | Change | Example of importance |
|---|---|---|
| Renal clearance | Reduced | Digoxin, lithium, most antibiotics, curare, pancuronium |
| Hepatic clearance | Reduced | Propranolol |
| Volume of distribution | ↓ skeletal muscle mass<br>Variable ↑ fat<br>Overall variable effect | Variable effects; need to observe effects and tailor all doses |
| Pharmacodynamics | ↓ adrenoceptor density and sensitivity<br>Less ↓ in cholinergic receptors | Attenuated response to catecholamines<br>Dose of non-depolarizer unaltered, although effect may be prolonged |

to be taken of deafness. Where there is difficulty obtaining a sensible history, help must be obtained from relatives. Enquiry should be made about normal daily activities, ability to climb stairs, and general health. Ask specifically about symptoms associated with heart disease, chest disease, diabetes, anaemia, and thyroid function. Often it is very difficult to separate pathology from normal 'wear and tear'.

Frequency and nocturia secondary to prostatic hypertrophy may predict postoperative urinary retention. 'Falls' are not usually caused by external hazards, but reflect an instability associated with impaired general health. Although a remedial cause may not be found, it may alert the anaesthetist to an increased risk from surgery for the patient. Make an assessment of the patient's biological (as opposed to chronological) age.

Existing medication can both indicate the presence of underlying conditions (of which the patient may not be aware) and give warning of possible drug interactions. Of particular danger in elderly people is the combination of digoxin and diuretics. Beta-adrenoceptor blockers may attenuate an already compromised autonomic nervous system.

Multiple pathology is exceedingly common. Worsening of one pathology may hasten the deterioration of others.

### Examination

- Examine the cardiovascular and pulmonary systems and treat any abnormalities appropriately.
- Neurological deficits should be recorded in the case notes, and remember that if a stroke was recent, suxamethonium may cause a dangerous increase in serum potassium.
- Assess the ability to move all joints, especially those in the neck and jaw for intubation, and hips and knees for lithotomy position. Get the patient to put the head back to test for vertebrobasilar disease. Check the condition of the skin and review possible drip sites.
- See if the person can lie flat. If breathing is difficult, spontaneous breathing in the supine or head-down position is an unsuitable anaesthetic technique.
- Dehydration is common in sick elderly people who become disinterested in drinking. It presents with postural hypotension, dry mucosal surfaces, and oliguria. Skin turgor is often poor anyway.
- Always look at the teeth. Solitary, fragile pegs can make intubation unusually awkward.

### Investigations

Apart from those suggested by the findings of the history and examination, the following are probably satisfactory for a 'normal' elderly patient.

#### *Full blood count*

Twenty percent of 'normal patients' in this age group have anaemia, the cause of which should be elucidated.

#### *Urea and electrolytes*

Elderly people are often taking diuretics, or have occult renal disease.

**Table 43.8 Abnormal ECGs in the aged**

| Abnormality | Percentage incidence |
|---|---|
| T wave changes | 19 |
| Q/QS patterns | 10 |
| Left ventricular hypertrophy | 7 |
| Atrial fibrillation | 2–5 |
| Bundle branch block | 5 |
| Ectopic beats > 1 in 10 | 4 |
| Right ventricular hypertrophy | 1 |

#### *Blood sugar*

Occult diabetes is common.

#### *ECG*

There is a high incidence of conduction defects, signs of ischaemia, and hypertrophy (Table 43.8).

#### *Chest radiograph*

This is a useful baseline before major surgery. It not infrequently reveals occult pathology such as tuberculosis, pneumonia, tumours (primary or secondary), or an enlarged heart.

#### *Echocardiography*

This can be very useful especially where there is doubt about the quality of left ventricular function (see Chapter 48) and the proposed surgery is major.

#### *Serum thyroxine*

Up to 5% of those aged over 65 years have abnormal results.

## PREOPERATIVE PREPARATION

It is especially important for elderly people, and their relatives, to be aware of the reason for surgery as well as the anticipated period of convalescence. The need for surgery should be balanced against the risks and postoperative complications, life expectancy without surgery, and the anticipated quality of life with and without surgery. Table 43.9 highlights the increased likelihood of postoperative cardiovascular complications with older age, although this is mainly the result of the increased presence of preoperative cardiac disease. Table 43.10 illustrates the importance of older age in the development of postoperative respiratory complications. The decision whether to proceed with surgery is an important one. For elective surgery, this requires thought and discussion before admission to hospital when the pressure to continue can be inexorable.

## INTRAOPERATIVE PHASE

Pre-existing conditions should be treated appropriately. Gentleness and speed of operating with minimal exposure of tissues, and careful haemostasis are the hallmarks of a successful outcome. Therefore, be sure that

**Table 43.9 Age and postoperative cardiovascular complications**

| Source | Age group (years) | Postoperative cardiovascular complications (%) |
|---|---|---|
| Larsen *et al.* (1987)[a] | 40–59 | 1.0 |
| | 60–69 | 3.0 |
| | 70–79 | 3.8 |
| | 80+ | 4.5 |
| Seymour and Vaz (1989)[b] | 65–74 | 2.8 |
| | 75+ | 10.2 |
| Pedersen *et al.* (1990)[c] | < 49 | 2.6 |
| | 50–69 | 8.2 |
| | 70–79 | 14.3 |
| | 80+ | 16.7 |

[a]Larsen SF, Oleson KH, Jacobsen E *et al. Eur Heart J* 1987;8:179–85.
[b]Seymour DG, Vaz FG. *Age Ageing* 1989;18:316–26.
[c]Pederson T, Eliason K, Henriksen E. *Acta Anesth Scand* 1990;34:144–55.

**Table 43.10 Preoperative risk factors and postoperative respiratory complications in ageing patients**

| Preoperative risk factor | Relative risk of postoperative respiratory complication |
|---|---|
| Age > 75 years | approximately 1.5 |
| Male sex | 1.3–4 |
| Current smoker | 1.5–7 |
| > 120% of ideal weight | 2 |
| Non-elective surgery | 1.5–2.5 |
| Dyspnoea on minimal exercise | 2 |
| ASA class 3 or 4 | 2–5 |
| Incision near diaphragm | 2 |
| Past or chronic lung disease | 2 |
| Acute respiratory disease | 2–3 |
| Peak flow < 250 L/min | 1.5–2 |
| $FEV_1$/FVC < 70% | 2–3 |

$FEV_1$, forced expiratory volume in 1 second; FVC, forced vital capacity.

the surgeon is ready. Always take great care with venous cannulation as the veins are very fragile.

### Premedication

Many elderly patients are very anxious and frightened in a strange environment. Explanation of procedures is vital. It is important that the patient (and/or relative) is aware of the reason for, and the anticipated benefit of, surgery. Many elderly patients have short-term memory loss and, despite explanations on the ward, may arrive in the anaesthetic room completely unaware of what is going to happen to them.

The choice of whether to give a premedicant drug is a personal one and it is frequently best omitted. Many psychotropic drugs have unpredictable effects and both hyoscine and atropine can cause unwanted tachyarrhythmias. The effect of premedication on the dose of thiopentone (thiopental) required to induce anaesthesia is shown in Figure 43.1.

Prophylaxis against deep vein thrombosis is essential for all but the most minor surgery, because age is a major risk factor for mortality from pulmonary emboli (see Chapter 1).

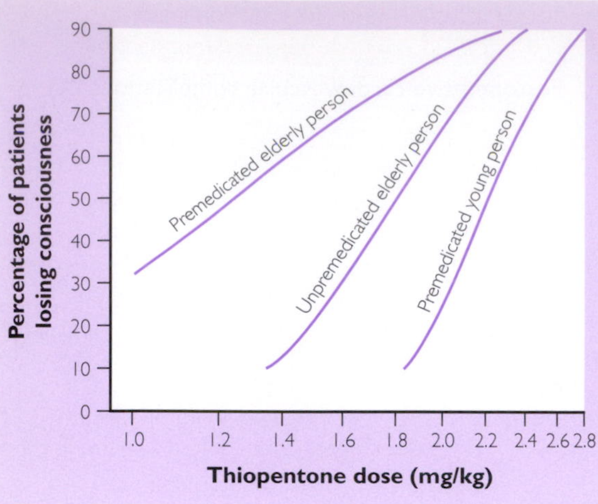


**Figure 43.1** The intravenous bolus dose of thiopentone required to produce loss of consciousness, related to age and premedication (morphine 5 mg). (Adapted from Davenport HT. *Anaesthesia in the Elderly*. London: Heinemann, 1986.)

## GENERAL OR REGIONAL?

The argument as to which is best for elderly people has continued for many years. Numerous retrospective and prospective studies have concluded that there is no significant difference in perioperative survival or major morbidity attributable directly to the choice of anaesthetic technique (Figure 43.2). In many instances it may be the postoperative care that is crucial in determining the outcome of surgery.

### Regional anaesthesia

Appropriate selection of patients is vital to success. Patients need to be mentally lucid, be able to lie flat for the duration of surgery, understand what is involved, and be able to adopt the position necessary for the block to be performed.

Often it is possible to combine a regional block with light narcosis with Entonox. Doing this, problems can arise when airway patency is lost but the patient is not deep enough to accept an airway. There are only two solutions: allow the patient to wake up or deepen anaesthesia and insert an airway.

The most common form of regional anaesthesia for operations below the umbilicus is either epidural or spinal block. An inability to flex the vertebral column and the presence of calcified ligaments may make the paramedian or full lateral approach easier (see Chapter 15) and more successful than the midline approach. To be pleasant for the patient, the lateral approach does require the liberal use of local anaesthetic around the lamina to anaesthetize the periosteum, which is often scraped by the needle.

The volume of local anaesthetic required for epidural block is reduced, as a result partly of an increased sensitivity to the drug and partly of an increased spread up and down the epidural space because of inelasticity and blocked intervertebral foramina. Whereas in young adulthood 1.5 ml local anaesthetic might block one segment, by 80 years of age only half this quantity is required (see Figure 45.2). With intrathecal block the level of anaesthesia is effectively independent of age. With both techniques, the effect of a given dose is said to last longer because of reduced tissue wash-out by the elderly spinal vessels.

The major complication of spinal and epidural block is hypotension, the degree of which increases with age for a given level of block, resulting from sympathetic blockade and loss of intrinsic homoeostatic competence. As a result of the dangers of fluid overload after the block has worn off, it is reasonable to limit intravenous fluid loading to 500 ml, and then use small incremental doses

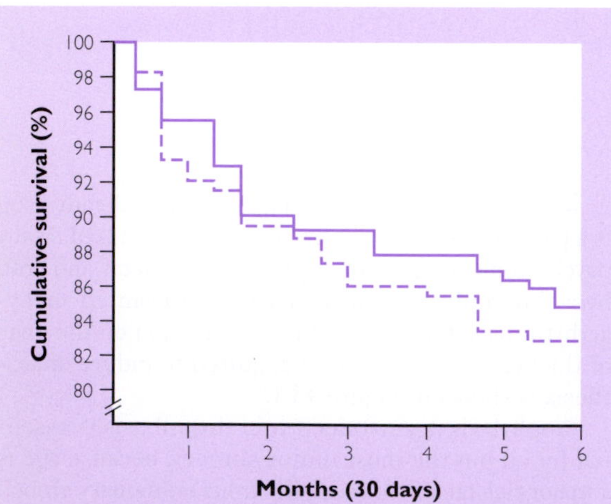


**Figure 43.2** Mortality after surgery for repair of fractured hip. Survival is compared between patients who had general anaesthesia (solid line) and those who had regional anaesthesia (dashed line). There was no difference in this nationwide (New Zealand) multicentre study. (From Davis FM *et al. Br J Anaesth* 1987;59:1080.)

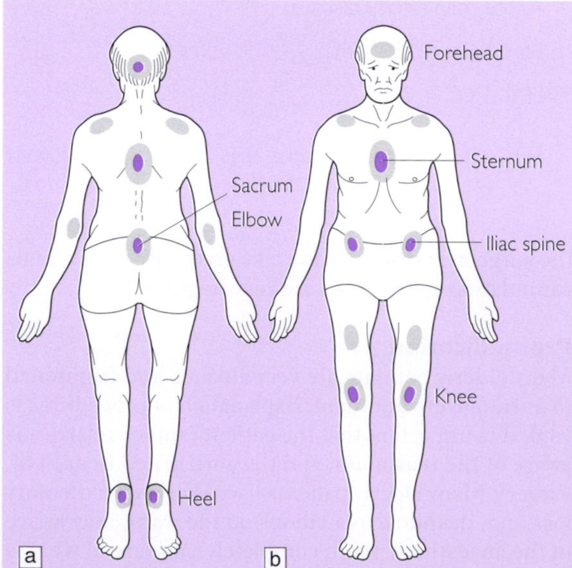


**Figure 43.3** Diagram showing the amount of pressure exerted in the supporting parts of the body in (a) the supine and (b) the prone positions. ■ < 20 mmHg; ■ > 20 mmHg. (Adapted from Davenport HT. *Anaesthesia in the Elderly*. London: Heinemann, 1986.)

of vasoconstrictors if necessary. If hypotension is associated with bradycardia, ephedrine is the drug of choice; if it is not, methoxamine is appropriate. It is important not to overshoot and produce a tachycardia associated with hypertension, thus increasing myocardial work sufficiently to cause myocardial ischaemia. The duration of action of these drugs is short and repeat doses may be required after a few minutes (see Chapter 19).

## General anaesthesia

The most important aspect is the care with which drugs are given rather than the particular choice of agent. For both regional and general anaesthesia, care is needed to protect vulnerable pressure areas, which are illustrated in Figure 43.3.

### *Induction*

Preoxygenation is important in increasing the margin of safety. Unlike the pregnant patient this is not because of a reduction in functional residual capacity which is unaltered with age (Figure 43.4). The circulation time in elderly people is much longer than in young people, and time must be allowed for incremental doses of drugs to work before others are given, otherwise gross overdosage is a real possibility. Note in Figure 43.1 the low doses of thiopentone required to induce anaesthesia, especially if the patient is premedicated. In very infirm individuals, gas induction has been favoured by some authors but others have succeeded just as well with very slow intravenous induction. Propofol does have the advantage of reducing postoperative confusion but must not be given overenthusiastically because of the dangers of hypotension.

### *Maintenance*

Spontaneous ventilation can have several problems and is only suitable for short procedures. Airway control can be very awkward in edentulous individuals with stiff necks. It can be difficult to get a good fit with a facemask and, at times, it can be advantageous to keep the dentures in (see also Chapter 6). A nasopharyngeal airway may help, but often, for spontaneously breathing patients, the best solution is to use a laryngeal mask airway. Problems related to the use of volatile agents are cardiovascular depression (with hypotension and an increased tendency to arrhythmias), ventilatory depression (increased arterial $CO_2$ tension [$Pa\text{CO}_2$] and a reduced arterial $O_2$ tension [$Pa\text{O}_2$], because of a reduced tidal volume and a high closing volume), and a delayed recovery. A bonus claimed by some is that, because the $Pa\text{CO}_2$ rises, so does cerebral blood flow, thereby offsetting the effects of a low blood pressure on cerebral perfusion.

Intubation and intermittent positive pressure ventilation is the preferred method for longer operations. Frequently, no neuromuscular block is necessary for either intubation or ventilation. If one is needed, the required dose of a non-depolarizing agent is reduced and it has an extended duration of action. Intubating those at risk of inhalation of gastric contents requires a similar rapid sequence induction as in young people. It is better to give a dose of suxamethonium, rather than 'wait and see' if it is necessary. The minimum alveolar concentration of the inhalational agents is reduced in elderly people (Figure 43.5 and see Table 43.3) and therefore lower concentrations of these drugs are required.

The low basal metabolic rate and the reduced $CO_2$ production imply that it is easy to hyperventilate elderly people and to drive their $Pa\text{CO}_2$ to very low levels. This is dangerous both from its effect on the myocardium (low contractility and hypotension) and in decreasing cerebral blood flow. Intraoperative hyperventilation also results in postoperative hypoventilation. Breath-by-breath $CO_2$ monitoring is thus invaluable. To maintain normocapnia often requires very low minute (and tidal) volumes. This can produce a lower $Pa\text{O}_2$ than expected from the fractional oxygen inspired. Airway closure occurs (see Figure 43.4 which illustrates the increased closing capacity in elderly people) and there is a danger of postoperative

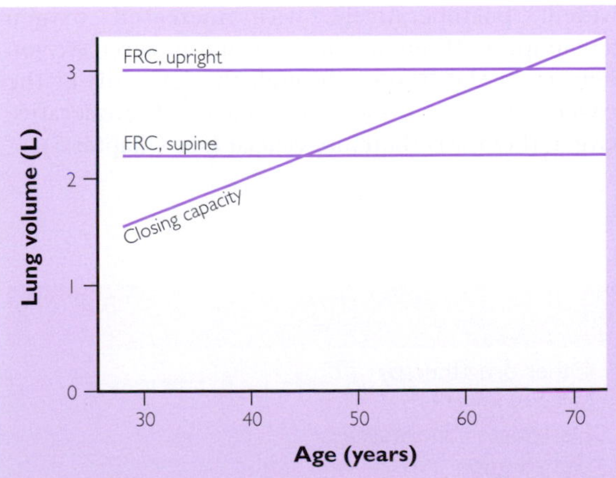


**Figure 43.4** The effect of age on closing capacity and functional residual capacity (FRC). Note that FRC does not change. (From Morgan GE. *Clinical Anesthesiology*, 1st edn. New York: Appleton & Lange: 1992.)

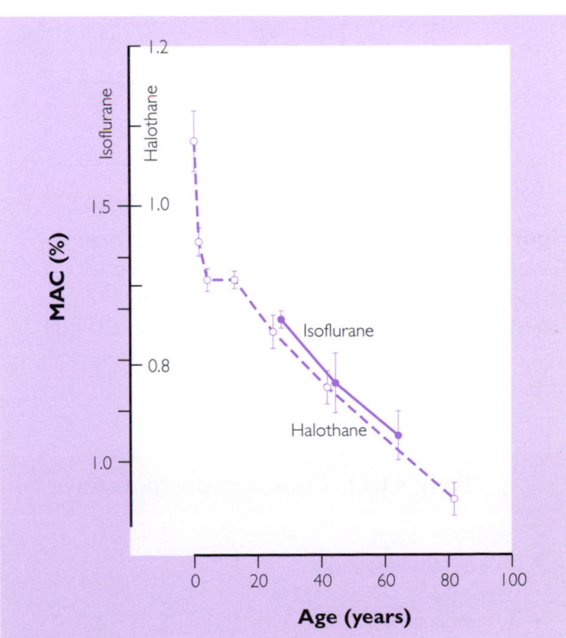


**Figure 43.5** Minimum alveolar concentration (MAC) for isoflurane and halothane decreases with increasing age. (From Quasha AL, Eger EI, Tinker JH. *Anesthesiology* 1980;53:315–34.)

pneumonia. The solution is either to add inspired $CO_2$ and increase the minute ventilation when using a minute volume divider, or to employ some sort of partial rebreathing circuit with a large tidal volume.

Elderly people are particularly at risk of becoming hypothermic during surgery; in addition to reduced heat production, absence of shivering, resetting of the thermoregulatory centre, and vasodilatation during anaesthesia, elderly people also have reduced basal metabolic rate and deficient thermoregulation (Figure 43.6 and see Table 43.4). Therefore, meticulous attention should be paid to body temperature and every effort made to keep the patient warm. This may require a warming blanket, warm intravenous fluids, humidified gases, and a temperature in the operating room that is higher than the surgeon would like it.

Induced hypotension in elderly people is a controversial subject. There are reports that it is both effective and safe as a means of reducing intraoperative blood loss. Others caution against it because of the risks of cerebral and myocardial ischaemia. With an awake patient monitored on a CM5 ECG lead, both of these problems can be detected early. Whether this allows sufficient time to reverse the detrimental effects of hypotension completely has not been recorded. In the unconscious patient, although the CM5 lead can monitor the left ventricle, there is no convenient or reliable monitor of cerebral perfusion. Therefore my practice is to maintain the intraoperative blood pressure in the preoperative range (±30 mmHg) because this is known to be both adequate and safe for the patient.

The use of opioid supplements is standard practice. The quantity of drug required to produce a pharmacodynamic effect is often surprisingly low, and much older patients usually (as a rule of thumb) need only half that required by a young adult.

Cisatracurium has the advantage of elimination that is independent of renal and hepatic function (with less laudanosine produced than with atracurium), and hence is probably the non-depolarizing neuromuscular blocking agent of choice in elderly people. Reversal of neuromuscular blockade can pose a problem because of the effect of atropine on the cardiovascular and central nervous systems, and it can be sensible to wait for spontaneous reversal, or to use glycopyrrolate.

Before reversal, if there are copious secretions, a thorough bronchial toilet can improve pulmonary function in the immediate postoperative period until the patient is able to cooperate with the physiotherapist. If the ventilatory movements are incoordinated and weak, there should be no hesitation in proceeding to a period of postoperative ventilation.

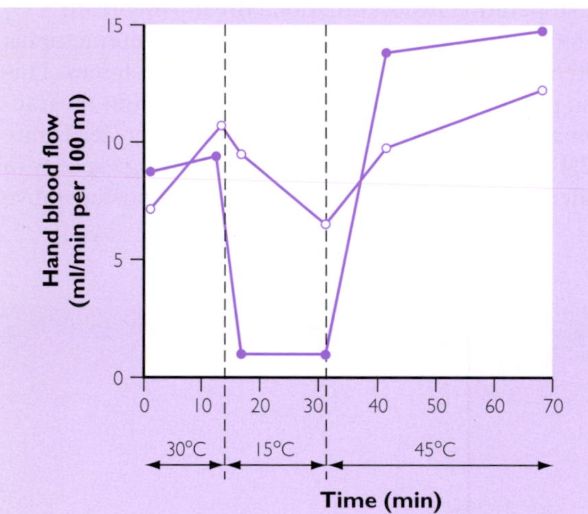


**Figure 43.6** The hand blood flow changes in an 80-year-old (○)and a 30-year-old (●) exposed to a period of cooling. (Adapted from Davenport HT. *Anaesthesia in the Elderly*. London: Heinemann, 1986.)

## POSTOPERATIVE PHASE

General principles of postoperative care are found in Chapters 4 and 5. Careful fluid balance is particularly important because the elderly patient is very susceptible to fluid overload. This, and reduced renal reserve, mean that there is much less margin for careless fluid therapy. Caution should also be exercised with the use of non-steroidal anti-inflammatory agents for postoperative analgesia, because of their effect on renal blood flow through inhibition of prostaglandins.

Postoperative confusion is common in elderly patients. This can lead to other complications such as urinary infections, pneumonia, and pressure sores and these complications can themselves cause confusion. The causes of confusion detailed in Table 43.11 should be sought and where possible corrected.

The adverse effects of hypothermia may become evident postoperatively, with increased oxygen consumption through shivering and impaired oxygen delivery to the tissues through the left shift of the oxyhaemoglobin dissociation curve. Postoperative oxygen therapy is therefore crucial (see Chapter 5).

**Table 43.11 Causes of postoperative confusion**

| | |
|---|---|
| • Sedative drugs | • Other drug therapy |
| • Pulmonary infection | • Urinary infection |
| • Hypoxia | • Electrolyte abnormalities |
| • Uraemia | • Dehydration |
| • Hypothermia | • Constipation |
| • Senile dementia | • Alcohol withdrawal |
| • Silent myocardial infarction | • Poor diabetic control |
| • Cerebrovascular accident | |

## FURTHER READING


Clarke FL, Corbitt N. Trauma and the elderly. *Curr Anaesth Crit Care* 1997;**8**:108–12.

Articles in: Dodds C, ed. *Anaesthesia and the Geriatric Patient. Baillière's Clin Anaesthesiol* 1993;**7**:1–193.

Dodds C, Allison A. Postoperative cognitive deficit in the elderly surgical patient. *Br J Anaesth* 1998;**81**:449–62.

Duey MA, McLeskey CH. Outcome after anaesthesia and surgery in the geriatric patient. In: Desmonts JM, ed. *Outcome after Anaesthesia and Surgery. Baillière's Clin Anaesthesiol* 1992;**6**:609–30.

*Geriatric Surgery: Comprehensive Care of the Elderly Patient*. Baltimore, MA: Urban & Schwarzenberg, 1990.

O'Keeffe ST, Chonchubhair AN. Postoperative delirium in the elderly. *Br J Anaesth* 1994;**73**:673–87.

Wilkins CJ. Anaesthesia and vascular surgery in the elderly. *Curr Anaesth Crit Care* 1997;**8**:113–19.

# Chapter 44 The obese patient

G.M. Cooper

Obesity, which results from excessive intake of calories, is the most common nutritional disorder in the infants, children, and adults of Western civilizations. Its incidence is increasing and it is defined as a body weight that exceeds the expected or ideal weight by more than 10%, taking into account height, age, body build, and sex. An alternative definition is that state in which more than 25% of the body weight in males or 30% in females is attributable to fat (normally 15–18% body weight is fat). Morbid obesity is defined as exceeding twice the ideal body weight. The ideal body weight in kilograms can be estimated by the patient's height in centimetres minus 100 (males) or 105 (females). Alternatively, the body mass index, which is the weight in kilograms divided by the square of the height in metres, should not exceed 25 kg/m$^2$ normally, and more than 30 kg/m$^2$ is considered obese. Grades of obesity are illustrated in Figure 44.1.

Most obese people have no other definable pathological condition apart from consuming an excess of food over need. A minority become overweight as a side effect of endocrine dysfunction (Cushing's syndrome, hypothyroidism, or hypopituitarism).

Wherever possible advice to reduce weight by dieting should be given before elective surgery. Sufficient time will have to be allowed for weight to be lost and targets should be set. Unfortunately, most patients are unsuccessful or non-compliant, despite explanations of the reduction of surgical risks, improved recovery, and life-long benefits of not being significantly overweight. This implies the necessity to anaesthetize and care for obese patients. The considerations that follow relate to the seriously fat patient, not the cuddly type! Twin examples are shown in Figure 44.2.

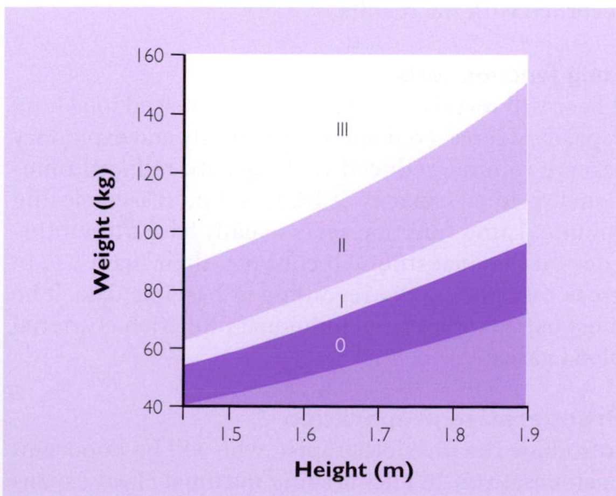


**Figure 44.1** Grades of obesity as measured using the body mass index. Grade 0 is the desirable range and grade III morbid obesity.

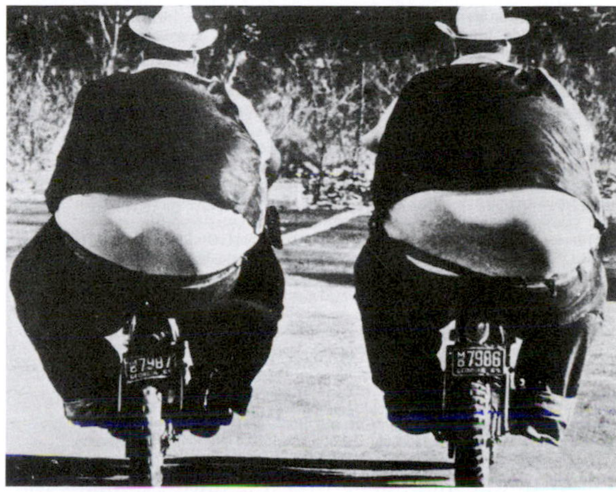

**Figure 44.2** The two-person traffic jam. (Reproduced with permission from Adams AP. Nutritional disorders. In: Vickers MD, ed. *Medicine for Anaesthetists*. Oxford: Blackwell Scientific Publications, 1977, 388.)

## PREOPERATIVE CONSIDERATIONS

### History

The effect of previous anaesthetics is particularly relevant (with knowledge of body weight at that time), because there may be information about techniques that have been either problematic or trouble free. Questioning should also try to uncover the symptoms of those diseases commonly associated with obesity that may affect anaesthesia (ischaemic heart disease, cerebrovascular disease, hypertension, hiatus hernia, and diabetes mellitus). Do not forget the possibility of an underlying anxiety neurosis because this may influence the choice of premedicant. Suspect the rare but important coexistence of endocrine dysfunction.

Enquire about somnolence as a pointer to the uncommon pickwickian syndrome. Try to get a measure of the person's normal level of activity, general mobility, and exercise tolerance. Osteoarthritis is common, and may limit exercise and also the ability to achieve the appropriate positioning for surgery or regional blocks.

Discuss the possibilities and difficulties of regional anaesthesia with both the patient and the surgeon before surgery. Endotracheal intubation can be extremely difficult. If awake intubation is anticipated, it should be fully explained in as sympathetic a manner as possible.

## Examination

Visual estimates of weight are frequently inaccurate. Ensure that the patient is weighed – if necessary double scales or the public weighbridge may be needed! Look at the patient and decide whether the standard operating table will be adequate or whether special arrangements have to be made. Take the opportunity to look for venous access points and at the condition of the skin over pressure areas.

### *Cardiovascular system*

Look for signs of cardiac failure, which can be difficult to detect in obese people. Sacral oedema is easily missed. Remember to use a large cuff to measure the blood pressure, recognizing that using a standard size cuff over-estimates the true value by as much as 20 mmHg in gross obesity.

### *Respiratory system*

Examine the extent of rib movement on deep inspiration. If it is severely restricted, ventilation will be almost totally diaphragmatic and very prone to postural deterioration. It is therefore wise to observe the breathing when supine, and check that it is both adequate and comfortable in this position. Look for sternal fat pads, which will make laryngoscopy difficult, and check the movement of the neck, the degree of mouth opening, the patency of the nostrils, and the state of the teeth. If the jaws have been wired together for weight reduction, liaise with the dentist about removal of the wires.

### *Limbs*

Arthritis is common in obese people, so examine the knees and hips for mobility, especially if the lithotomy position is anticipated.

### *Skin*

Intertrigo, boils, or vaginal candidiasis could point to occult diabetes.

## Investigations

### *Full blood count, liver function tests, and random blood sugar*

These should all be normal in uncomplicated obesity. Polycythaemia may have developed secondary to chronic hypoxia.

### *Chest radiograph*

This will assist in the detection of cardiomegaly, cardiac failure, and aortic atherosclerosis. If the last is present, it will be so throughout the body. A radiograph is an important baseline for major operations. Its necessity for minor surgery can be left to clinical judgement. (See Figure 44.3 which revealed an unsuspected paraoesophageal hernia.)

### *ECG*

Rhythm and conduction disturbances are adequately reproduced. A thick fat layer does, however, reduce the voltages recorded so that cardiac hypertrophy may remain unnoticed. There are often considerable differences in the ECG between inspiration and expiration because diaphragmatic breathing swings the cardiac vectors with respect to the electrode placements. A prolonged Q–T interval and a reduced QRS voltage are non-specific abnormalities which may be found and suggest an increased anaesthetic risk. Look for evidence of ischaemia.

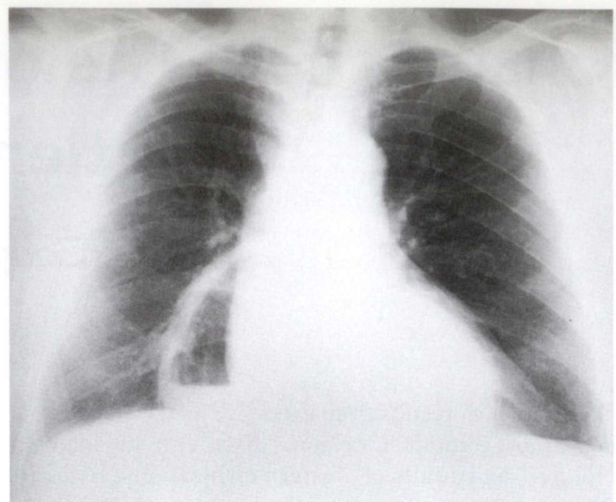

**Figure 44.3** A chest radiograph in an obese patient, showing a paraoesophageal hernia.

### *Blood gases*

These are indicated in all severely obese subjects regardless of the operation, and for major operations in less severely obese subjects. Although values may be within normal limits, the most common pattern is a normal arterial $CO_2$ tension ($P\text{a}CO_2$) with an arterial oxygen tension ($P\text{a}O_2$) reduced by up to 20% from the expected value, corrected for age, breathing air. Hypoventilation with a raised $P\text{a}CO_2$ is both rare and serious. If the need for postoperative artificial ventilation is anticipated, a preoperative baseline is invaluable. When taking an arterial sample, remember that the $P\text{a}O_2$ is dependent on posture and is lowest when supine. Hence the position of the patient should be recorded with the results.

### *Lung function tests*

These will reveal combinations of decreased total lung capacity, decreased inspiratory capacity and expiratory reserve volume, reduced vital capacity, reduced functional residual capacity (FRC), and increased closing volume. Lung function tests usually have little influence on the anaesthetic technique, their main use in gross cases being the recording of baseline data. The most useful indicator of pulmonary function is arterial blood gases.

## Preoperative preparation

Introduce the physiotherapist, who will be important postoperatively in encouraging maximal chest expansion and general mobility. Subcutaneous heparin to prevent postoperative deep vein thrombosis will be needed (see Chapter 1) where there is any doubt about immediate postoperative mobilization.

#### Premedication

The choice is personal but it is important to avoid reducing the ventilatory drive in someone with borderline pulmonary mechanics. An antisialogogue is often helpful and improves the performance of any topical local anaesthetic used subsequently. Excessive subcutaneous fat results in unreliable 'intramuscular' injections. It is sensible to reduce the volume and acidity of gastric contents by preoperative $H_2$ antagonist (e.g. ranitidine) and gastric prokinetic (e.g. metoclopramide) therapy. This needs to be started 24 hours before surgery.

## INTRAOPERATIVE PHASE

All surgical procedures, however trivial, must be taken seriously. Reference to Table 44.1 shows that the risk of death in obese subjects is increased for both surgical and non-surgical events. Anaesthetizing these patients is not a task for the novice anaesthetist. Many of the problems occur because of the sheer size of the patient. Adequate personnel must be available to transfer the patient from the ward to the operating room. It is a good idea to induce anaesthesia on the operating table (which can be tipped) in the operating room: the patient may be able to move him- or herself into position, which saves others' backs. Airway control is easier without the added difficulties of moving the patient and there need be no interruption of monitoring.

Always think carefully about the pros and cons of regional and general anaesthesia. It is often advantageous to combine them for better overall control of both the airway and the patient, and to provide analgesia and relaxation with little central depression. Peripheral nerve blocks, spinals, and epidurals can be technically difficult to perform because of the problems in locating landmarks beneath the fat (see Chapter 15). However, the distribution of fat may be such that a local anaesthetic block may not be as difficult as first envisaged. Obesity also has the reputation of making the dermatome level achieved in spinal and epidural anaesthesia unpredictable. Local anaesthetic requirements for epidural blockade are often reduced. Even if it is intended for the patient to remain fully awake during regional blockade, beware of the distress, both mental and ventilatory, that the supine or head-down position may cause.

With either local or general anaesthesia, try hard to secure a really good drip. Superficial veins may not be obvious and it can be time-consuming to cannulate that which can neither be seen nor felt easily. Watch even more carefully than usual for extravascular or intra-arterial injection. If the patient is first on the list, bring him (or more often her!) to the anaesthetic room early to get a relaxed start. Always have adequate assistance and sufficient personnel to manoeuvre the patient in an emergency. Start monitoring blood pressure, ECG, and oxygen saturation before induction.

**Table 44.1 Obese/non-obese death risk**

| Disease | Risk |
|---|---|
| Diabetes | 3.75 |
| Gallstones | 2.5 |
| Cirrhosis | 2.0 |
| Chronic nephritis | 2.0 |
| Cerebrovascular accident | 1.6 |
| Ischaemic heart disease | 1.6 |

#### Induction

Preoxygenation is essential. The reduction in FRC, increased oxygen demand (because of increased tissue mass), and ventilation/perfusion mismatch all predispose to hypoxaemia. Opinion is divided over the advantages and disadvantages of inhalational and intravenous methods of induction. The overall object is to avoid producing an unconscious patient who cannot breathe, and who cannot be ventilated or intubated. On the basis of airway assessment and clinical judgement, this can be circumvented by an awake intubation followed by induction of anaesthesia and this technique should be seriously considered.

As a result of the risk of regurgitation, there are arguments in favour of inducing anaesthesia in either the left lateral or the sitting position. A *slow* intravenous induction, converted to spontaneous ventilation with an inhalational agent, can be followed by laryngoscopy before intubation, with or without the aid of suxamethonium. Longer-acting relaxants are acceptable after the patency of the airway on a facemask has been established. Properly applied cricoid pressure, taking care not to distort the anatomy, helps avoid aspiration.

No matter how skilled the anaesthetist, induction of anaesthesia in very obese people is often harrowing and inelegant. The help of a second anaesthetist is recommended. Facemask ventilation can be exceedingly difficult and may precipitate the return of copious gastric contents to the mouth, especially if there is a hiatus hernia. Cricoid pressure should, of course, be used to prevent aspiration. The laryngeal mask may be useful to produce a clear airway in the short term, but is not a suitable management option because it does not protect against aspiration and will not permit sufficiently high inflation pressures without a leak.

#### Maintenance

Drug requirements can be difficult to estimate because of a reduction in the proportion of body water in relation to body weight. The dose of water-soluble drugs therefore needs to be reduced on a milligram per kilogram basis. Prolonged use of fat-soluble drugs such as halothane can lead to delayed recovery. There is also an association between halothane hepatotoxicity and obesity (see Chapters 1 and 33).

For all but the very shortest operations, intermittent positive pressure ventilation (IPPV) will be needed. High inflation pressures will be required because of the reduced compliance. End-tidal $CO_2$ monitoring guides the adequacy of ventilation. The dose of neuromuscular blocking drug needs to be given according to the estimated lean body weight, and further requirements guided by nerve stimulation (check that nerve stimulation is not impeded by excessive fat). Do not forget that IPPV does not necessarily require paralysis. Check that your ventilator is sufficiently powerful to ventilate the patient and monitor the inspiratory pressure.

Obesity undoubtedly creates operative difficulties for the surgeon and hence prolongs anaesthesia, even for relatively minor operations. Large abdominal packs may seriously impede venous return and cause precipitous falls in blood pressure. Indirect arterial monitoring is inaccurate in obese people and therefore, for all major operations, direct arterial monitoring is advised. This may not be technically easy but the radial artery is usually palpable.

Intraoperative fluid balance is difficult to assess. The proportion of body weight that is blood volume may be reduced from the normal 70 ml/kg to as little as 45 ml/kg. Central venous pressure monitoring is helpful with large blood losses, but again this can be technically difficult to institute and interpret. Landmarks may be hard or impossible to find. There is an increased risk of puncturing a lung and causing a pneumothorax or haemothorax with subclavian and internal jugular routes. Urine output is probably the most satisfactory measure of adequate circulating fluid volume.

Take care of the arms; do not let them fall and be careful not to cause nerve injuries through bad placement of restraints.

## POSTOPERATIVE PHASE

Beware of the operating room emptying of staff once the operation is completed. Ensure that there is adequate help to lift the patient into the bed and to tip or position him or her as necessary.

Postoperative mortality is greater in the obese patient compared with the non-obese one. In gross obesity or after major surgery, care in a high dependency unit, intensive care unit, or recovery area is mandatory. The trachea should be extubated only when the patient is fully awake. Pulmonary gas exchange is best in the sitting or semi-recumbent position (up to 45°). Oxygen therapy will be required for several days and this should be humidified. Nocturnal nasal continuous positive airway pressure can be used to prevent postoperative acute upper airway obstruction.

The dose of opioids for postoperative analgesia should be based on the ideal rather than the actual body weight. Patient-controlled intravenous administration is probably best unless regional analgesia is feasible.

Do not forget that the stress response to surgery can produce a temporary or permanent diabetic state in obese patients. The incidence of wound infection is greater and appropriate antibiotic prophylaxis will be required.

## FURTHER READING

Brodsky JB. Morbid obesity. *Curr Anaesth Crit Care* 1998;**9**:249–54.

Gray DS. Diagnosis and prevalence of obesity. *Med Clinics N Am* 1989;**73**:1–14.

Mason EE, Renquist KE, Jiang D. Perioperative risks and safety of surgery for severe obesity. *Am J Clin Nutr* 1992;**55**:516S–76S.

Oberg B, Poulsen TD. Obesity: an anaesthetic challenge. *Acta Anaesthesiol Scand* 1996;**40**:191–200.

Shenkman Z, Shir Y, Brodsky JB. Perioperative management of the obese patient. *Br J Anaesth* 1993;**70**:349–59.

Wilson AT, Reilly CS. Anaesthesia and the obese patient. *Int J Obesity* 1993;**17**:427–35.

# Chapter 45 The pregnant patient

G.M. Cooper

Apart from removal of retained products of conception, the two important areas where patients who are pregnant require anaesthesia is at the time of delivery (e.g. for caesarean section, forceps delivery, retained placenta, etc.) or for incidental surgery required during pregnancy.

Pregnancy has been described as the only physiological state where most physiological parameters are abnormal! A sound knowledge of these physiological changes is required and the reader is also referred to Chapter 30.

## USUAL OUTCOME OF PREGNANCY

Normal pregnancy is measured from the last menstrual period and is of 38 to 41 weeks' duration. Conception occurs 2 weeks after menstruation and therefore (assuming a regular 4-week menstrual cycle) there are 2 weeks before a missed period when a woman is not aware that she is pregnant.

Eighty percent of human conceptions are lost at some stage in pregnancy, of which half occur before pregnancy is discovered. Fifty percent of early abortions have chromosomal abnormalities. Congenital malformations are present in 3% of newborn babies, and one-third of these are life threatening. In most cases, the reason for abnormality is unknown: 25% have genetic or chromosomal causes and 2–3% are the result of drugs.

Implantation is completed in the second week and organogenesis occurs in weeks 4–8 after fertilization. This is the time of maximal effect of teratogens. By 20 weeks' gestation, the fetus weighs 500 g, at 30 weeks it weighs about 1 kg, and at term about 3.2 kg.

## INTERCURRENT SURGERY IN PREGNANCY

Pregnancy is the only situation where the anaesthetist is routinely caring for more than one patient simultaneously, and hence it carries additional responsibility. The particular worries of anaesthesia during early pregnancy are those of causing either fetal malformations or abortion (miscarriage). In later pregnancy the concern is about inducing premature labour.

The teratogenic risk from anaesthesia is difficult to ascertain with certainty because of:

- the high incidence of spontaneous abortion;
- the low overall incidence of birth defects;
- the low incidence of surgery in pregnancy;
- difficulty separating the effects of anaesthesia from other drugs given in pregnancy;
- the high risk of fetal loss after Shirodkar suture.

Results from epidemiological studies, however, suggest the following:

- Structural abnormalities are unlikely consequences of anaesthesia.
- The incidence of low birth weight and premature delivery are increased if women have anaesthesia at any time in pregnancy.
- The incidence of postnatal death is increased if subjected to anaesthesia and surgery in the second or third trimester of pregnancy.
- There is continued uncertainty over whether anaesthesia has any influence on the incidence of spontaneous abortion.
- There is no information about possible effects on functional abilities.

### Anaesthetic implications

Identification of pregnancy is not always easy, particularly at an early gestation. There is an argument for routine pregnancy testing in the 'at-risk' population, especially where the menstrual history is vague or a period is overdue.

In view of the information from epidemiological studies it seems wise not to perform *elective* surgery during pregnancy. Sometimes, where surgery is relatively urgent, risks have to be balanced against each other. If surgery proceeds in the first trimester of pregnancy, the patient should be informed that the risks of spontaneous abortion and behavioural deficiency are not known, but that there is no increased risk of congenital defects. With anaesthesia at any time during pregnancy, it is reasonable to inform the patient that there is an increased likelihood of a low-birth-weight baby and premature delivery.

However, despite the natural concerns that this information will cause, the most frequent and serious error is unnecessary delay of urgently required surgery. Undoubtedly, such delay increases maternal and fetal morbidity and mortality. Where surgery is necessary, the following information may help allay anxiety: the likelihood of a first-trimester miscarriage is increased from 5% to 8% because of surgery and the incidence of premature delivery is increased from 5% to 7.5%. Thus the majority of pregnancies continue as normal.

The main objectives of incidental anaesthesia in pregnancy are to:

- ensure maternal safety;
- avoid teratogenic drugs;
- avoid intrauterine asphyxia;
- prevent pre-term labour.

There is no evidence that the choice of anaesthetic agent is important, but the most relevant factor is to maintain well-oxygenated blood flow to the placenta. This is achieved by the usual good conduct of anaesthesia, which avoids hypoxia and hypotension and maintains normocapnia of pregnancy. General or regional anaesthesia may be appropriate depending on surgical site, patient preference, and the coexisting medical and surgical conditions.

At present no anaesthetic agent has been proved teratogenic in humans. As pregnancy advances, aortocaval compression, risk of regurgitation, and difficulty in intubation become increasingly relevant. The conduct of anaesthesia should then be managed as outlined for the patient at term (see below). The gestation at which endotracheal intubation (as opposed to using a facemask or laryngeal mask) is considered mandatory is controversial. Some advise that it should be from 12 weeks' gestation (especially in obese patients), whereas others suggest that it should be from 16 weeks onwards.

Ideally, the fetal heart should be monitored continuously during surgery (after 16 weeks' gestation), because it may provide an indication of abnormalities in maternal ventilation or uterine perfusion, which could be corrected. Fetal heart monitoring is not always feasible, an example being during appendicectomy.

Uterine activity should be monitored continuously during the postoperative period to detect the onset of pre-term labour. Beta-mimetic treatment, if instituted early, may prevent premature delivery.

Thought should be given to the prevention of deep venous thrombosis because of the hypercoagulability and venous stasis in pregnancy. Graduated compression stockings should be used and subcutaneous heparin is advisable after the second trimester.

Haemolytic disease of newborn babies occurs in rhesus-positive fetuses of rhesus-negative mothers. Passage of fetal blood cells into the maternal circulation (which may occur during labour, therapeutic abortion, or amniocentesis) causes formation of anti-D antibodies (the term 'rhesus positive' usually refers to the presence of D agglutinogen). These may pass into subsequent rhesus-positive fetuses, causing haemolysis that can be fatal. Thus, unless the blood group of the fetus/neonate is known to be rhesus negative, a rhesus-negative mother should be immunized with anti-D immunoglobulin after evacuation of retained products of conception, therapeutic abortion, amniocentesis, or delivery. The anaesthetist may be asked to give this during anaesthesia because intramuscular injection is painful.

## ANAESTHESIA FOR DELIVERY OR NEAR TERM

### Preoperative assessment

#### *History*

The amount of time available for assessment varies according to the urgency of surgery. Contrast the situations of a planned caesarean section known weeks in advance with those for acute prolapse of the cord, significant antepartum haemorrhage, or severe fetal distress where a speedy response can be crucial to the survival of the baby. Thus, the reason for, and urgency of, intervention are the first points to establish. Check whether it is a singleton or multiple pregnancy. Check when the mother last ate and drank (it may be quite recently!). The urgency of delivery may outweigh the need for the desired duration of starvation and must be discussed with the obstetricians.

Even when time is limited, enquire about general health, health in pregnancy, concurrent medication, and known allergies. Previous experience of general anaesthesia is important, particularly if problems have been identified. Although rare, a personal or family history of malignant hyperpyrexia is particularly relevant because general anaesthesia implies the use of both suxamethonium and a volatile anaesthetic agent, which are potent triggers of the syndrome.

Symptoms of oesophageal reflux and feeling faint when supine should be sought. Ask about excessive swelling, thinking of possible pre-eclampsia.

Obstetric patients tend to be better informed about the choices of anaesthesia available and may have already firmly decided for or against regional anaesthesia. While talking to the patient, think about possible contraindications to either form of anaesthesia (see Chapter 15) and whether particular difficulties are more likely in this patient (e.g. kyphoscoliosis may make location of cerebrospinal fluid (CSF) tricky, or severe asthma may make regional anaesthesia especially desirable).

#### *Examination*

Always look carefully at the airway, even when planning a regional technique. A block may not always be adequate and conversion to general anaesthesia may be necessary either for this reason or because of surgical complications. Alternatively, a block may extend higher than intended and intubation be necessary to control ventilation.

It is helpful to examine the back, looking at the degree of lumbar lordosis, and to feel the intervertebral spaces. If the woman has had previous back surgery, the site of the skin incision may indicate whether there will be difficulties with epidural or spinal insertion.

Venous access is normally relatively easy because of vasodilatation, but is worth checking especially in pre-eclampsia where vasoconstriction is present.

#### *Investigations*

*Full blood count*

A recent haemoglobin investigation is helpful because anaemia is common.

*Clotting screen*

This should be performed if there is a known clotting disorder, pre-eclampsia, an abruption of the placenta, or a stillbirth.

*Urea and electrolytes*

These should be available in pre-eclampsia as should a serum albumin concentration.

*Blood group*

This should always be known, in case of blood requirement and to know if anti-D immunoglobulin needs to be given (see above). Policies about having blood cross-matched vary from unit to unit, depending on the speed with which blood can be made available in an emergency. Blood should always be cross-matched where excessive blood loss can be anticipated (e.g. placenta praevia, coagulation defects, repeated caesarean sections), or if there is anaemia.

*ECG and chest radiograph*
These will rarely be required.

*Ultrasound report*
Where this is available, it is worth noting the size of the baby and the position of the placenta. This is particularly important if the placenta is overlying a previous caesarean section scar, when senior obstetric staff will be required and excessive blood loss can be anticipated.

## Preoperative preparation

Where possible, gastric acid secretion should be suppressed for the 12 hours before anaesthesia by the administration of $H_2$-receptor antagonists (e.g. ranitidine 150 mg orally on two occasions, approximately 8 h apart), in order to reduce gastric acid production and hence the likelihood of acid aspiration. Because of the delay in gastric emptying, the intravenous route will be needed for those who have received pethidine in labour. It is not always possible for an appropriate period of starvation but, for urgent cases, ensure that no further food or fluids are taken.

In the anaesthetic room, give an oral antacid such as 30 ml of 0.3 mol/L sodium citrate in order to neutralize any gastric acid remaining in the stomach. This is essential for all non-elective patients.

Sedative premedication is avoided because of adverse effects on the baby and possible oversedation of the mother.

A full explanation of the proposed method of anaesthesia, including the more common risks, should be given. With regional anaesthesia, the risks of possible dural tap and consequent headache, failure to achieve adequate block, hypotension, and consequent nausea should be identified.

## Intraoperative considerations

### Local anaesthesia

Over the last 20 years there has been a swing to perform more and more caesarean sections under regional rather than general anaesthesia. Initially the most common choice was epidural anaesthesia and this continues to be popular, especially when an epidural catheter has been successful in providing analgesia in labour. More recently, spinal anaesthesia has had a resurgence, largely as a result of the more acceptable, low incidence of postdural puncture headache associated with pencil-point needles (see Chapter 15).

The reasons for regional anaesthesia frequently being the preferred choice of both the parents and the anaesthetist are outlined in Table 45.1.

| Table 45.1 Advantages of regional anaesthesia in operative obstetrics |
|---|
| Parental participation and early bonding |
| Less depressant effect on the neonate |
| Avoids endotracheal intubation difficulties |
| Much less risk of gastric aspiration |
| Mother maintains normocapnia |
| Reduced blood loss |
| Early postoperative analgesia provided |
| Avoids 'hangover' effect of general anaesthesia |
| Reduced risk of thromboembolic problems |

Despite these advantages, there are occasions where regional anaesthesia is inappropriate. These are outlined in Table 45.2. Some would argue that a spinal block could be instituted as quickly as general anaesthesia can be induced. However, this is not always so and, in cases of extreme urgency (as in prolapsed cord where it is also difficult to position the patient appropriately!), general anaesthesia is indicated.

| Table 45.2 Contraindications to regional anaesthesia in obstetrics |
|---|
| Patient refusal |
| Significant antepartum haemorrhage |
| Coagulopathy from any cause |
| Anticoagulant therapy |
| Sepsis |
| Extreme urgency |
| Eclampsia |

The innervation of the uterus and birth canal is shown in Figure 45.1. Regional block to T10 provides good analgesia for labour, but this is not sufficient for caesarean section where a block is required from at least T6 to S5. This should be established and confirmed before surgery begins. Epidural blockade is most appropriate if this has been the method of analgesia during labour. Spinal block has the advantage of more rapid onset and denser block. Opioids (e.g. fentanyl 100 µg epidurally or fentanyl 15 µg intrathecally) added to the local anaesthetic have been used to advantage with both routes, improving the quality of analgesia.

The increase in lumbar lordosis in pregnancy can make it difficult to open up the lumbar interspaces. Also, the softening effect of progesterone on ligaments has a variable effect on the ligamentum flavum. These two factors, coupled with difficulty for some women to keep still during painful contractions, can make identification of the epidural space difficult and contribute to inadvertent dural puncture.

Increased abdominal pressure causes epidural veins to become engorged. This makes their cannulation more frequent when threading epidural cannulae, or direct intravascular injection more common in single-shot techniques.

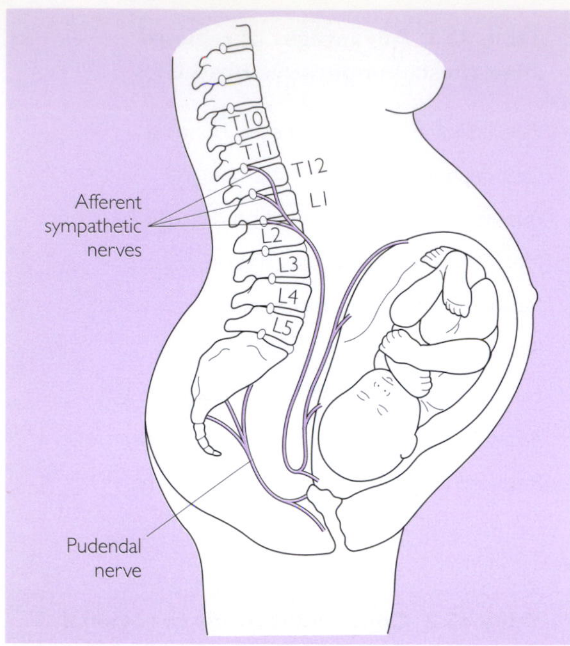


**Figure 45.1** Innervation of the birth canal. Note also the lumbar lordosis. (From Carrie LES. Regional techniques in obstetrics. In: Wildsmith JAW, Armitage EN, eds. *Principles and Practice of Regional Anaesthesia*. Edinburgh: Churchill Livingstone, 1987; 112.)

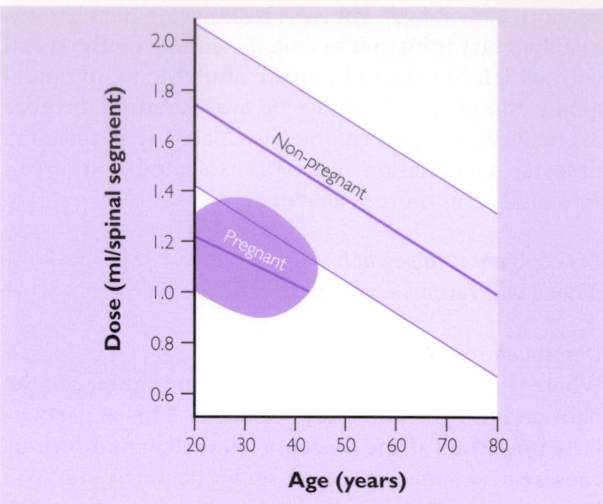


**Figure 45.2** Regression lines for dose of epidural solution and age in non-pregnant women and in pregnant women at term. The pregnant woman obviously requires much less drug: at 30 years the pregnant woman requires only 1.1 ml local anaesthetic to block each segment, compared with 1.6 ml for her non-pregnant counterpart. (From Bonica JJ. *Principles and Practices of Obstetric Analgesia and Anesthesia*, vol 1. Philadelphia: Davis, 196; 627.)

Less local anaesthetic is required in pregnancy to produce the same level of spinal or epidural block as in a non-pregnant counterpart (Figure 45.2). Previously, this has been explained by the effect of engorged veins, but recently it has been questioned whether this is the result of changes in CSF pressure during labour or of increased neurosensitivity to local anaesthetics (possibly caused by progesterone). Typically, 2.5–3.0 ml local anaesthetic (e.g. 'heavy Marcain') is needed for intrathecal block, and 20 ml of 0.5% bupivacaine for epidural block for caesarean section. The amount of local anaesthetic for epidural block is less constant than that for spinal. Incremental topping up of an epidural while monitoring the level of block is recommended.

Before inserting a block, an intravenous preload of 1 L of fluid should be given. There is no evidence that colloid is superior to crystalloid.

*The detrimental effects of aortocaval compression on uterine perfusion pressure* (see Chapter 30) *must be avoided by displacing the uterus laterally*. This is usually satisfactorily achieved by placing a wedge under the buttock to tilt the woman about 15°, although more tilt may be required where the uterus is exceptionally large, such as with multiple pregnancy or polyhydramnios. The detrimental effects of aortocaval compression are greater with regional analgesia than with general anaesthesia because more blood volume is sequestered in the legs, and the upper part of the body is already maximally vasoconstricted as a homoeostatic mechanism to maintain cardiac output.

Maternal oxygenation should be supplemented with added oxygen to breathe from a facemask or nasal prongs.

ECG, oxygen saturation, and blood pressure monitoring are just as important as they are under general anaesthesia. Any hypotension should be treated with intravenous ephedrine (e.g. 6-mg increments), as this is the vasoconstrictor with the least adverse effect on uterine blood supply. If uterine relaxation is required, this can be achieved by the mother inhaling salbutamol *before* the uterus is incised. Oxytocin, 5–10 units, is used to stimulate uterine contraction after the baby is delivered. Ergometrine is unsuitable because of the high incidence of hypertension and nausea and vomiting.

Regional anaesthesia is also preferred to general anaesthesia for forceps delivery or delivery of a retained placenta (unless there has been excessive blood loss). A block from T10 to S5 is needed for these procedures.

### *General anaesthesia*

#### *Induction*

A rapid sequence induction is mandatory. The reduced functional residual capacity and increased oxygen consumption mean that the pregnant patient becomes hypoxic much more easily than her non-pregnant counterpart. After preoxygenation followed by a period of apnoea of 1 min the arterial oxygen tension ($P\text{aO}_2$) decreases by 18.5 kPa (139 mmHg) in the pregnant woman compared with a decrease of only 7.7 kPa (58 mmHg) in the non-pregnant woman (Figure 45.3). This highlights the need for adequate preoxygenation before paralysing the pregnant patient, and the shorter time available to achieve intubation before hypoxia occurs.

Breast enlargement can cause difficulty inserting the laryngoscope (a short-handled instrument can be helpful). This, coupled with airway swelling, lateral tilt, and possible misalignment of the larynx from zealous application of cricoid pressure, makes failure to intubate the trachea 10 times more common than in the non-pregnant patient.

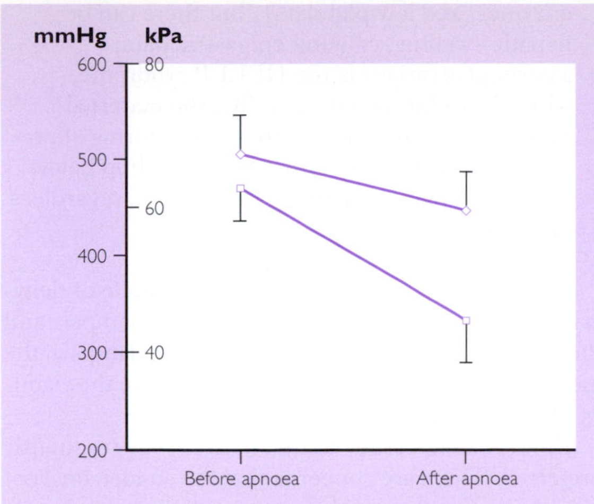


**Figure 45.3** Decrease in arterial oxygen tension after 1-min apnoea in pregnant (lower line) and non-pregnant (upper line) women. Data are mean ± SD. (Data from Archer GW and Marks GF. *Br J Anaesth* 46: 358–360.)

If a difficult intubation is encountered the drill should be followed (see Chapter 7), always remembering that failure to oxygenate is more detrimental than failure to intubate.

The lateral tilt used to avoid aortocaval compression means that the woman is precariously placed on the operating table. Induction of anaesthesia in the operating room reduces transporting accidents and allows continuous monitoring of cardiovascular and respiratory variables. It also encourages the obstetrician to start operating speedily. The duration of anaesthesia until delivery does not become important until 30 min have elapsed, which is well within the usual delivery time.

*Maintenance*

An inspired oxygen concentration of 50% allows good fetal oxygenation, although some benefits of an inspired fractional oxygen concentration of nearly 100% have been shown to be beneficial in severe fetal distress. Adequate concentrations of a volatile agent should be used to ensure unconsciousness. Ventilation to normocapnia of pregnancy provides optimal uterine blood flow. After suxamethonium has been used to achieve endotracheal intubation, a short-acting neuromuscular blocker such as atracurium, vecuronium, or rocuronium is appropriate because under normal circumstances the operation is not too lengthy.

If uterine relaxation is required (it can be particularly useful for a transverse lie or in premature delivery where the lower segment of the uterus is not well formed), this is easily achieved by increasing the inspired concentration of volatile agent before uterine incision. It is important nevertheless to ensure that there is no undue cardiovascular depression resulting in uterine hypoperfusion. Uterine contraction after delivery is aided by intravenous oxytocin.

The administration of opioid to provide intraoperative analgesia is delayed until after delivery of the baby. The exception to this is giving a short-acting opioid to prevent a hypertensive response to laryngoscopy in the pre-eclamptic patient. The person in charge of resuscitating the baby needs to know that naloxone may need to be given to the baby.

It can be difficult to assess the amount of blood loss at caesarean section because of the dilution by amniotic fluid or loss into the surgical drapes or onto the floor. Thus, one relies very much on the effect on heart rate and blood pressure. It is important to realize that large volumes of blood can be lost rapidly and unpredictably (this applies just as much when regional anaesthesia is used, although the average blood loss is less under regional block). Haemorrhage is still a leading cause of maternal death and thus blood loss should be replaced appropriately.

Thromboembolic phenomena are also leading causes of maternal mortality; thought should therefore be given to prevention by the use of graduated compression stockings and subcutaneous heparin. Guidelines have been produced by the Royal College of Obstetricians and Gynaecologists, categorizing those at high risk (this includes all emergency caesarean sections, those who have a history of thromboembolic phenomena, and obese women). Some units follow these guidelines and some administer heparin to all women who have a caesarean section on the premise that it is safe and those who need it will get it. Antibiotic prophylaxis to prevent wound infection is also commonplace.

### Postoperative considerations

Unless there are ongoing concerns about blood loss, most women, especially those who have had a regional block, are able to eat and drink in the first few hours after caesarean section, and postoperative intravenous fluids are unnecessary.

Good analgesia should be instigated in the recovery room. Once this has been achieved, in most instances further requirements for postoperative analgesia are remarkably less than for the non-pregnant counterpart with a similar incision. This is probably because of endogenous endorphins released and because the abdominal muscles have been stretched during the pregnancy. Non-steroidal analgesics are useful in combination with oral simple analgesic agents, with top-ups using opioids as required.

The return of full neurological function (motor, sensory, and bladder control) should be checked for those patients who have had a regional block. Possible postdural puncture headache should be sought and, if present, treatment options discussed (see Chapter 15).

## THE PREGNANT PATIENT WITH PRE-ECLAMPSIA

Pre-eclampsia is a multi-system disorder with many manifestations, of variable severity, which affects up to 10% pregnancies. It presents at any time after week 20 of pregnancy (if it is earlier than this, it is likely to be associated with a hydatidiform mole). It is defined by:

- hypertension (systolic > 140 mmHg, mean > 105 mmHg, diastolic > 90 mmHg or an increase of systolic blood pressure of 30 mmHg or diastolic blood pressure of 15 mmHg);
- peripheral oedema;
- proteinuria > 0.3 g/L in 24 h or > 1 g protein/L urine (+ or ++ on dipstick).

It is more common in first pregnancies, where there are twins or polyhydramnios, and in those with diabetes. The only known cure is delivery of the fetus. The cause is unknown; the initiating factor may be immunological, genetic, or simply a decrease in uterine blood flow.

One theory is that decreased placental perfusion causes trophoblasts to release a substance, causing vascular endothelial cell injury. This results in fibronectin release, which causes further damage to all vascular endothelial cells, leading to:

- loss of plasma protein which results in decreased plasma oncotic pressure;
- production of vasoconstrictors and reduced synthesis of vasorelaxing substances;
- renal damage;
- coagulation abnormalities including platelet aggregation;
- myocardial and placental endothelial damage.

There is an imbalance in the production of two prostaglandins: prostacyclin and thromboxane. Production of thromboxane, which is associated with vasoconstriction, platelet aggregation, and decreased uterine blood flow, is increased whereas the production of prostacyclin, whose effects are opposite, is decreased. This imbalance between thromboxane and prostacyclin could be related to endothelial cell injury or placental trophoblastic production of thromboxane. Substances that decrease the production of thromboxane, such as aspirin, appear to decrease the incidence and severity of pre-eclampsia in selected high-risk mothers.

The above theories illustrate the complex pathophysiology of pre-eclampsia and the multi-organ involvement. Some of the features are implied above. They may be variably prominent in an individual and aspects of presentation are listed below:

- vasoconstriction;
- increased cardiac output (although not universally);
- high blood pressure;
- low or normal central venous pressure;
- markedly reduced plasma volume;
- reduced plasma albumin;
- decreased plasma oncotic pressure;
- oedema: peripheral, pulmonary, and airway (including laryngeal);
- increased plasma renin, angiotensin, catecholamines, and atrial natriuretic peptide;
- increased blood viscosity which aggravates uteroplacental underperfusion;
- associated coagulation abnormalities, especially decreases in platelet number and function; also there is an increased bleeding time;
- cerebral irritability which may manifest as brisk reflexes, anxiety, and tremors or convulsions (eclampsia);
- decreased glomerular filtration rate and creatinine clearance; acute renal failure may ensue;
- uric acid excretion is impaired and serum urates indicate the severity of disease;
- hepatic involvement is usually mild (except in HELLP syndrome [haemolysis, elevated liver enzymes, and low platelets]) but there can be hepatic swelling, causing epigastric pain;
- a particular variant is the HELLP syndrome, which has a high fetal mortality; the maternal mortality is also higher than in other forms of pre-eclampsia. Platelet counts frequently drop below 50 000. Immediate delivery is called for, regardless of gestation.

Management, including timing and mode of delivery, depends on the severity of the pre-eclampsia and the gestation of the fetus. In severe pre-eclampsia, the mother's life may be at risk at a stage where the viability of the fetus is not assured.

Epidural anaesthesia for delivery is frequently preferred. There are concerns that the sudden onset of block with spinal anaesthesia may result in precipitate decreases in blood pressure. General anaesthesia for caesarean section will be required in the presence of coagulopathy and when the patient has eclamptic fits. Severely ill, pre-eclamptic, and eclamptic mothers require expert management in high dependency or intensive care areas. Once delivery has occurred, therapy is supportive and directed to the particular abnormalities exhibited. The mortality from this condition continues to be significant.

The treatment of choice for eclampsia is intravenous magnesium sulphate (4 g given over 20 min), although diazepam (or thiopentone [thiopental]) may be more readily available in some situations. Subsequent prophylaxis against further fits is by infusion of magnesium sulphate (approximately 2 g hourly) to maintain a plasma concentration between 2 and 3.5 mmol/L. Frequent serum estimations are often used and the infusion should be adjusted to maintain therapeutic concentrations. Overdosage can also be assessed clinically by absence of tendon reflexes (remembering to use the arms if there is a functioning epidural) and depressed ventilation. Tendon reflex response and respiratory rate should be recorded hourly. Magnesium is excreted by the kidney and toxicity is more likely if the renal output is poor. Therefore if the urine output is less than 20 ml/h, the infusion of magnesium should be decreased.

## FURTHER READING

Alahuhta S. Preanaesthetic management of the obstetric patient. *Anaesthesiol Scand* 1996;**40**:991–5.

Articles in: Bogod DG, ed. *Obstetric Anaesthesia. Baillière's Clin Anaesthesiol* 1995;**9**:591–760.

Browne DA, Morgan M. Outcome after anaesthesia for labour and operative delivery. In: Desmonts JM, ed. Outcome after Anaesthesia and Surgery. Baillière's Clin Anaesthesiol 1992;6:561–88.

Holdcroft A, Thomas TA. *Principles and Practice of Anaesthesia and Analgesia*. Oxford: Blackwell, 2000.

James MFM. Magnesium in obstetric anesthesia. *Int J Obstet Anesth* 1998;**7**:115–23.

Kumar A, Vertommen J, Van Aken H. Recent advances in epidural and spinal anaesthesia in obstetric patients. In: Van Aken H, ed. *New Developments in Epidural and Spinal Drugs Administration. Baillière's Clin Anaesthesiol* 1993;**7**:749–68.

Practice Guidelines for Obstetrical Anesthesia. *Anesthesiology* 1999;**90**:600–11.

Russell IF. Anaesthesia for emergency caesarean section. *Curr Anaesth Crit Care* 1995;**6**:202–5.

# Chapter 46 The day-stay patient

G.M. Cooper

The day-stay patient comes into hospital for a wide variety of surgical procedures so the anaesthetist will see patients from many surgical subspecialties. Apart from the individual requirements pertaining to orthopaedics, ophthalmology, gynaecology, or whatever the type of surgery, there are common elements that arise because the patient is coming in and going home on the same day as the operation. For this to be successful, one of the key features is appropriate patient selection. Some surgeons have a tendency to regard certain operations as suitable for a day-stay basis regardless of other factors. Suitability depends not only on the surgical condition but also on the general medical health and the social circumstances of the patient. It is the surgeon's responsibility to select patients, but the anaesthetist has to ensure that an appropriate choice has been made. Thus, the three key elements to be checked are: medical fitness, surgical suitability, and social circumstances.

## MEDICAL FITNESS

It is important to establish that there are not likely to be any complications resulting from a pre-existing medical condition that may be problematic after discharge from hospital – or whether the patient's medical condition would be managed better in hospital, assuming that it cannot be improved. An easy rule of thumb is to select only patients of ASA grades 1 and 2 for day-stay treatment. Nevertheless, some patients who are less fit may be allowed to go home, depending on the proposed surgery and home circumstances. It is helpful for individual borderline cases to be discussed between the surgeon and anaesthetist.

Chronological age is more important than biological age; elderly patients are more likely to have intercurrent disease but, if this is not severe, avoiding hospital admission reduces the likelihood of confusion that occurs in up to half of elderly inpatients after surgery. Children are well suited to day-stay treatment because they are well cared for by their mothers and suffer less psychological trauma than if they are admitted to hospital overnight. The exceptions to this are pre-term infants and the very young (up to 55 weeks postconceptual age) who are susceptible to postoperative apnoea for up to 12 hours after general anaesthesia; children in this age group should therefore be admitted for apnoea monitoring.

## SURGICAL SUITABILITY

The operation needs to be of relatively short duration – some authorities suggest an upper limit of 30 minutes, but there is general agreement that one hour of surgery should not be exceeded. There needs to be a low likelihood of serious complications developing after the patient has gone home. This applies particularly to situations such as occult bleeding where the patient may not notice that something is amiss. Also, it needs to be an operation where postoperative analgesia can be provided satisfactorily at home. The surgeon needs to assess the surgical condition itself, as opposed to its category, to ensure suitability. An example is that of an inguinal hernia repair, which could be simple and uncomplicated or could be an extensive procedure.

## SOCIAL CIRCUMSTANCES

On the day of surgery, there should be a responsible adult in the home who could summon help should complications occur. There needs to be easy access to a telephone. The patient needs to live near enough to hospital to make travelling to and from hospital practical. It has been suggested that a maximum of one hour's travel is a reasonable limit, although less than this may be sensible depending on the type of surgery and how well the patient feels afterwards. With sufficient notice, people who live alone may be able to make suitable arrangements at home or to stay with someone.

Financial savings that accrue through not having to staff the facilities at night have driven the increase (explosion) in day-case surgery. Nevertheless, it is generally popular with patients because there is less disruption of family routine and a preference for recovering in the comfort of home.

Another of the keys to successful day-stay treatment is good organization which ensures that suitable patients arrive, suitably prepared, to the right place at the right time. Written information is more reliably complied with than verbal: a preoperative instruction sheet should identify the following:

- Date, time, and place of admission.
- Duration of preoperative starvation required.
- Things to bring (current medication, night clothes, book, etc.).
- Need for washing before surgery.

- Area to be shaved.
- Need to be accompanied home after surgery by a responsible adult.
- Advice not to drive for at least 24 hours after surgery.
- Advice to abstain from alcohol for 24 hours after surgery.
- Need for responsible adult at home after surgery.

## PREOPERATIVE CONSIDERATIONS

### Preoperative assessment

Most patients who present are fit and healthy. The items discussed in Chapter 41 are thus all relevant: day-stay anaesthesia is not an excuse for a second-class service! For children, Chapter 42 should also be consulted. The difference between inpatients and the day-stay patient is that time for preoperative assessment is much more limited with the latter. A questionnaire, such as the one illustrated in Figure 46.1, preferably completed at the outpatient/booking clinic, which identifies any pre-existing medical conditions, drug therapy, allergies, previous surgery, dental crowns, loose teeth or dentures, etc., helps to speed up assessment. The severity of any diseases mentioned should be ascertained. Any new illnesses (e.g. coughs, colds, etc.) should be sought. The duration of preoperative starvation should be checked – it is not uncommon for patients to forget or misunderstand their instructions.

The anaesthetist should always assess the airway, whether intubation is planned or not. Body temperature, weight, resting heart rate, and blood pressure should all be noted. Relevant organ systems should be examined. The surgical site (e.g. site of lipoma, cyst, hernia, etc.) should be ascertained. In some cases, the lesion requiring surgery will have disappeared.

During this rapid assessment, the anaesthetist should always be thinking whether the patient is suitable for day-stay treatment. Be prepared to discuss any reservations with the surgeon and patient. There are always areas of controversy and although guidelines help, commonsense needs to prevail. An example is someone who is grossly obese expecting, perhaps, a laparoscopic sterilization. Although falling into the category of ASA grade 2 and listed for a suitable operation, they may be totally unsuitable because of surgical difficulties and anaesthetic hazards.

Name: ........................ Today's date is........................

Address: ........................ What is your age? ........................years

What is your approximate weight?........

1. Have you ever suffered from any of the following?
   - Heart trouble (e.g. angina, heart failure, murmurs etc.) .. Yes ❑ No ❑
   - High blood pressure........................ Yes ❑ No ❑
   - Breathing problems (e.g. asthma, bronchitis, pneumonia) Yes ❑ No ❑
   - Jaundice or liver disease ........................ Yes ❑ No ❑
   - Kidney disease........................ Yes ❑ No ❑
   - Diabetes ........................ Yes ❑ No ❑
   - Thyroid disorder........................ Yes ❑ No ❑
   - Bleeding tendency (apart from heavy periods) ................ Yes ❑ No ❑
   - Thrombosis (blood clots)........................ Yes ❑ No ❑
   - Severe arthritis (including neck and jaws) ........................ Yes ❑ No ❑
   - Severe anxiety or depression........................ Yes ❑ No ❑
   - Epilepsy, convulsions or blackouts ........................ Yes ❑ No ❑
   - Any other serious illness ........................ Yes ❑ No ❑
   
   Please give details.
2. Have you taken any medicine or tablets, used an inhaler or received any injections in the past 3 months?............. Yes ❑ No ❑
   If YES, please give details.
3. Have you had an anaesthetic previously? ........................ Yes ❑ No ❑
   If YES, please give details of operations and approximate dates below.
4. To your knowledge, have you or your family had any problems connected with anaesthesia or operations? .... Yes ❑ No ❑
   If YES, please give details.
5. Are you allergic to anything that you know of? ............... Yes ❑ No ❑
   If YES, please give details.
6. Are your parents of black African or eastern Mediterranean origin? ........................ Yes ❑ No ❑
   If YES, have you or any of your family had sickle-cell disease?........................ Yes ❑ No ❑
7. Do you smoke? If YES, how much?........................ Yes ❑ No ❑
8. Do you drink alcohol? If YES, how much?........................ Yes ❑ No ❑

**Figure 46.1** Preoperative assessment questionnaire. (Adapted from Cooper GM. Daycare anaesthesia. In: Taylor TH and Major E, eds. *Hazards and Complications of Anaesthesia*. Edinburgh; Churchill Livingston, 1993.)

### Investigations

Any investigations that are clinically indicated should be done. The usual guidelines for haemoglobin estimation (see Chapter 41) should be followed. Results of investigations should be checked to be sure that there are no abnormalities that need correction or may preclude treatment on a day-stay basis.

### Premedication

Many premedicant drugs continue to have sedative effects after anaesthesia and therefore premedication is usually avoided. Nevertheless, there are some particularly nervous patients who benefit from anxiolytic premedication, for which a suitable choice is a short-acting benzodiazepine such as temazepam. Think about giving a non-steroidal anti-inflammatory agent preoperatively, so that analgesia is effective immediately after surgery.

## INTRAOPERATIVE CONSIDERATIONS

The overall aims of anaesthesia for the day-stay patient are the safe and efficient provision of adequate operating conditions with rapid recovery and minimal complications. This can be done by a variety of techniques and with many different agents, but it is important that competent trained staff deliver anaesthesia and perform surgery to avoid unnecessary complications and admission to hospital.

### Regional anaesthesia

Many local anaesthetic techniques are particularly advantageous for day-stay surgery because of the excellent postoperative recovery, as well as being able to provide good operating conditions with minimal risk, early postoperative analgesia, and freedom from nausea and vomiting.

Regional anaesthesia is not universally applicable, however, either because of the operative site or because of its acceptance by the patient. There is a resurgence of interest in epidural and spinal anaesthesia for day stay, the speed of onset and shorter recovery times making the intrathecal route more favourable. If the dura is breached, arrangements must be made for the detection and treatment of postspinal headache, which will undoubtedly occur in some patients after returning home.

Patients and accompanying persons must be clear about the dangers of inadvertent injury to an anaesthetized limb.

### General anaesthesia

#### *Induction*

The required dose of intravenous induction agent is slightly increased in the unpremedicated patient, who may, despite preoperative explanations, continue to be apprehensive. Anxiety can make venous access more difficult to secure, but a little patience in finding a suitable vein is usually rewarded. Propofol is the induction agent that most nearly approaches ideal because of a clear-headed recovery and its antiemetic effect; nevertheless, the pain on injection is undesirable and its ventilatory and cardiovascular depressant properties may mitigate against its use in some patients. Methohexitone (methohexital) is an alternative to propofol, but has the disadvantage of causing pain on injection and excitatory phenomena, and it has a less favourable pharmacokinetic profile for recovery. Although there are misgivings about the use of thiopentone (thiopental) because full psychomotor recovery after a single induction dose has been shown to take more than 24 hours, there may be specific indications for using an induction agent that outweigh any difference in recovery. It should be remembered that the patient wakes because of redistribution of the intravenous induction agent and that sedative effects are apparent for many hours.

Excitatory phenomena such as coughing and movement are more common in the unpremedicated patient, and care is needed in airway manipulations to avoid laryngospasm. The use of propofol often aids airway management, because of the depressant effects on airway reflexes, provided manual ventilation can be effected if necessary.

#### *Maintenance*

Spontaneous or controlled ventilation can be used. Although the elimination of volatile agents favours, in order, sevoflurane, isoflurane, and enflurane over halothane, the differences in recovery after short anaesthetics are too small to be of clinical importance. Also, the incidence of nausea and vomiting is similar with all these agents and therefore the choice rests on other considerations. Maintenance with a total intravenous technique may also be equally suitable.

#### *Analgesics*

Intraoperative use of analgesics can be important where postoperative pain is anticipated, but needs to be balanced against the increased likelihood of nausea and vomiting. Local anaesthetic blocks, non-steroidal inflammatory agents, and non-opioid analgesics play an important role in postoperative analgesia.

#### *Neuromuscular blocking agents and airway management*

There has been debate about whether it is safe to send patients home after endotracheal intubation because of the potential development of laryngeal oedema. The risk of this happening several hours later is small, and must be weighed against the risks of not intubating for procedures such as those involving intraoral surgery. The laryngeal mask has enabled control of the airway without endotracheal intubation for spontaneous or controlled ventilation; it reduces the incidence of sore throat to a level comparable to that seen after the use of a facemask. It has had a significant impact on the practice of day-stay anaesthesia, but it must be remembered that it does not protect against aspiration (see Chapter 7).

The choice of neuromuscular blocking agent is influenced by the anticipated duration of surgery. The incidence of 'muscle pains' after suxamethonium is very much greater in patients who are young and ambulant, and therefore, wherever possible, other agents are preferable. Atracurium, vecuronium, cisatracurium, and rocuronium have better return of muscle power than older non-depolarizing agents (see Chapter 35). This may be important in minimizing postoperative diplopia, a distressing complication that might prejudice safety while going home and makes reading difficult.

#### *Antiemetics*

The use of routine antiemetics is debatable. The unwanted effects (sedation, extrapyramidal symptoms) need to be weighed against their effectiveness (or lack of it) and the cost. It is probably sensible to identify those most at risk (see Chapter 5) and target treatment to them. Naturally, care should be taken with administration of anaesthesia and factors such as avoiding inflation of the stomach with anaesthetic gases. Stimulation of the semicircular canals should be avoided by care with gentle manoeuvring of the patient on the trolley or bed.

#### *Monitoring*

Day-stay patients require the same quality of care as inpatients and therefore the same standard of equipment and monitoring should be used. Standard monitoring includes an ECG, non-invasive blood pressure, oxygen saturation, and capnography (see Chapter 12).

## POSTOPERATIVE CONSIDERATIONS

The need for unplanned admission after day-stay surgery should be under 1%. In large surveys the admission rate resulting from anaesthetic causes is of the order of 0.25%, and is mainly caused by nausea and vomiting or excessive drowsiness. Patients usually require only a few hours in the day unit.

Assessment of fitness to go home recognizes that recovery is incomplete but, in the absence of complications, should proceed uneventfully over a period of time. The important criteria are that the patient can stand without falling (with the eyes open and shut) and that he or she can walk satisfactorily (in a straight line without staggering or swaying). Complications such as haemorrhage should be checked for. It is helpful if the patient can eat and drink before going home because it prevents hypoglycaemia and demonstrates well-being. Many tests have been used to assess psychomotor recovery, but none is simple and reliable enough to predict safety and therefore they remain research tools.

After local anaesthesia, provided that there is no limb paralysis that makes walking difficult, it can be beneficial to allow the patient to go home while continuing to derive benefit from the analgesia. Patients should be warned to protect the affected area and to expect tingling and pain as the block wears off.

Minor complications (headache, sore throat, dizziness, etc.) are common after general anaesthesia, and the patient worries less if warned about them and informed how to alleviate them. Sufficient analgesics should be supplied before going home.

The patient needs to know what the arrangements are for follow-up, who will remove any sutures, and who to contact if things go wrong. In some units it is the family doctor and in others it is the local hospital.

Advice to refrain from driving (or operating machinery) stems from the fact that psychomotor tests reveal minor decrements in performance for 24–48 hours after anaesthetic agents. In addition to the effects of anaesthesia, it is important to bear in mind the type of surgery that has been performed. For instance, will the patient who has had his inguinal hernia repaired 3 days previously be able to apply his car brakes in an emergency? In situations such as these, it is not possible to guarantee when normality has been regained, but common sense on the part of the patient has to prevail.

Advice to refrain from alcohol ingestion relates to its synergistic effects, particularly with barbiturates, sleeping tablets, and dextropropoxyphene.

## FURTHER READING

Chung F, Mezei G. Adverse outcomes in ambulatory anaesthesia. *Can J Anesth* 1999;**46**:R18–26.

Articles in: Healy TEJ, ed. *Anaesthesia for Day Case Surgery*. *Baillière's Clin Anaesthesiol* 1990;**4**:615–818.

Heneghan C. Anaesthetics and the law. In: Klepper ID, Sanders LD, Rosen M, eds. *Ambulatory Anaesthesia and Sedation: Impairment and Recovery*. Oxford, Blackwell, 1991.

National Health Service Management Executive. *Day Surgery: Report by the Day Surgery Task Force*. Heywood, UK: Health Publications Unit. 1993.

Twersky RS. *The Ambulatory Anesthesia Handbook*. St Louis: Mosby, 1995.

Articles in: White P, ed. Mini-symposium on day-case surgery. *Curr Anaesth Crit Care* 1994;**5**:123–64.

# Chapter 47 The patient with an abnormal ECG

P. Hutton

This chapter first identifies the patients from whom an electrocardiogram (ECG) should be obtained. It then describes a systematic method of reading the ECG and correlates the components of the ECG trace with physiological changes in the heart. After this there is a consideration of the implications of abnormalities of the ECG for anaesthesia and the management of patients with pacemakers.

At the time of writing, it is difficult to be absolutely specific about the role of anticoagulants in the management of arrhythmias, both acute and chronic. Over recent years cardiological opinion has moved towards:

- long-term anticoagulant maintenance therapy;
- echocardiography before cardioversion to exclude intracardiac clots.

There is still considerable variation in opinion over the best course of action in individual cases. It is therefore important to follow locally agreed guidelines. Reasonable general principles are as follows:

- Ensure adequate anticoagulation (international normalized ratio [INR] > 2) and a clear echocardiogram for all elective cardioversions, whatever the arrhythmia, its duration, or the age of the patient.
- For acute-onset intraoperative arrhythmias which are severely affecting cardiac output and/or blood pressure and do not have a correctable non-cardiac cause (see Table 47.2), cardiovert as soon as possible (within minutes) without recourse to anticoagulants.
- For arrhythmias that have been present for hours (rather than minutes, days, or weeks), take cardiological advice.
- Only in an emergency, perform a cardioversion without first undertaking echocardiography to eliminate the presence of intracardiac clot.

All the ECG traces shown in this chapter are superimposed on paper that shows normal 'large squares' on a standard ECG, i.e. the width is 0.5 cm representing 0.2 s and the height is 0.5 cm representing 0.5 mV.

## INDICATIONS FOR A PREOPERATIVE ECG

The ECG is a basic, simple, inexpensive investigation. There are two reasons for requesting an ECG:

1. As a screening test to look for abnormalities.
2. To obtain a baseline before surgery or other events that might cause it to change.

Although it is difficult to be very specific about the indications for obtaining an ECG preoperatively, reasonable recommendations are set out in Table 47.1.

| Table 47.1 Patients who should have an ECG preoperatively |
|---|
| Patient with a history of any type of heart disease |
| Patient with a history of hypertension, even if well controlled |
| Patients taking diuretics or other cardiovascularly active drugs |
| Any patient with a diastolic BP > 95 mmHg on admission |
| Any patient who is found to have a murmur |
| Any patient with an abnormal cardiac outline on a chest radiograph |
| Patients with unexplained episodes of breathlessness |
| Smokers aged > 50 years |
| Otherwise fit people aged > 60 years |
| Patients with chronic or acute chronic pulmonary disease |
| Any patient likely to need HDU or ICU care postoperatively |

HDU, high dependency unit; ICU, intensive care unit.

## THE GENERATION OF THE ECG

Check all recordings for paper speed (25 mm/s) and sensitivity (1 mV/cm). A 12-lead ECG has three bipolar limb leads (I, II, and III), three unipolar limb leads (aVR, aVL, and aVF), and six unipolar chest leads (V1–6). The lead positions are shown in Chapter 20 (Figure 20.7). Definitions of the various named components of the ECG are shown in Figure 47.1.

### The P wave

The P wave represents atrial depolarization. It is most easily seen in leads V1 and V2, but, when abnormal, the most significant changes in shape may be best seen in leads II and V4–6. The normal P wave is less than 0.1 s in duration and less than 2.5 mm in height. An atrial repolarization wave is not seen because it is small and is obscured by the QRS complex. The following are abnormalities of the P wave:

- absent – no coordinated atrial contraction (see later, Figure 47.14);
- too tall – right atrial hypertrophy (see later, Figure 47.7a);
- too wide and/or bifid – left atrial hypertrophy delaying conduction and causing atrial asynchrony (see later, Figure 47.7b);
- inverted, too close to, or following the QRS – abnormal focus initiating atrial contraction (see later, Figure 47.15).

### The PR interval

The PR interval (see Figure 47.1) is the time taken for excitation to spread from the sinoatrial (SA) node, through the atrial muscle and the atrioventricular (AV) node, down the bundle of His, and into the ventricular conducting system. Most of the time is taken up with AV node delay (see Chapter 20, Figure 20.4). The normal PR interval is 0.12–0.2 s (three to five small squares). The following are the abnormalities:

- too short – nodal rhythm, δ wave in the QRS (see later, Figures 47.15 and 47.26);
- too long but fixed – first-degree heart block;
- variable – second- or third-degree heart block (see later, Figures 47.18–47.21).

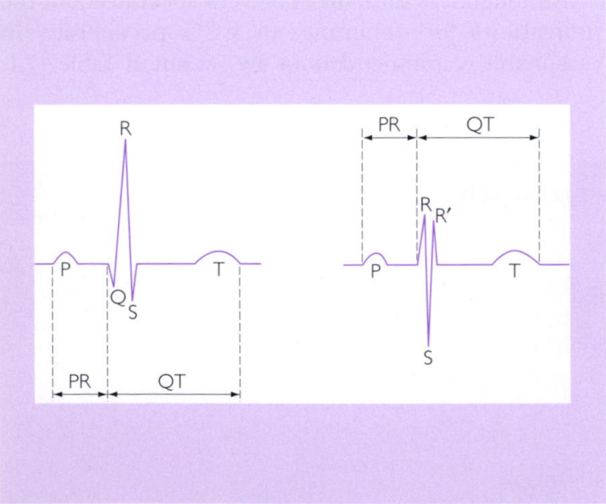

**Figure 47.1** QRS terminology: the first positive deflection is labelled R; the second R′. A negative deflection preceding an R is labelled Q. A negative deflection after an R is labelled S. The identifying letter is unrelated to the underlying event, R in a left-sided lead being equivalent to S in a right-sided lead. The QT interval varies with heart rate, the normal upper limits being 0.5 s (12.5 mm on the trace) at 40 beats/min and 0.28 s (7 mm on the trace) at 150 beats/min.

### The QRS complex

The QRS complex represents ventricular depolarization. The ventricular conducting system is shown in Figure 47.2. Depolarization should be complete within 0.12 s (three small squares) and no one lead should have a total amplitude of over 35 mm.

During normal conduction, the interventricular septum is depolarized first and activity spreads across the septum from left to right (Figure 47.3a). This simultaneously produces an upward deflection (R wave) in the right ventricular leads and a small downward deflection in the left ventricular leads (Q wave). The two ventricles then depolarize together (Figure 47.3b) and, because of the greater mass of the left ventricle, its electrical effect swamps that of the right. A downward deflection occurs in the right ventricular leads (S wave) and an upward deflection in the left ventricular leads (R wave). When the whole of the myocardium has depolarized (Figure 47.3c), the ECG returns to the baseline.

The following are the abnormalities of the QRS complex:

- too tall – hypertrophied muscle beneath the electrode;
- too short – a reduction in active muscle (infarction) or an excess of fat or lung beneath the electrode;
- deep Q wave (over 2 mm) – an absence of living myocardium beneath the electrode fails to obscure septal depolarization;
- too wide, wrong shape, wrong R : S ratio – atypical ventricular depolarization (see later, Figures 47.5, 47.6, 47.22, 47.23, and 47.28).

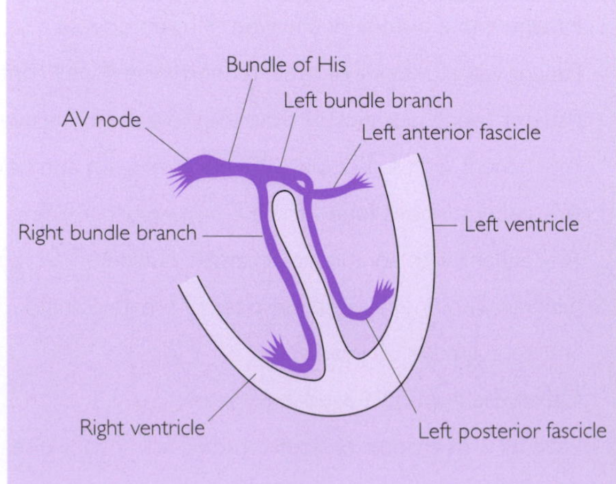


**Figure 47.2** The ventricular conducting system. AV, atrioventricular.

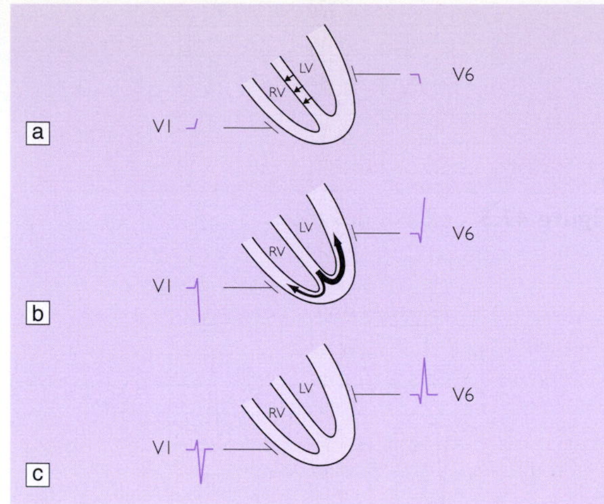


**Figure 47.3** Ventricular depolarization and the resultant ECG. See text for details.

Ventricular muscle that depolarizes in an aberrant manner also repolarizes abnormally, and there may be accompanying changes in the ST segment and T wave.

### The ST segment

The ST segment requires a period of electrical inactivity after the completion of depolarization and before the start of repolarization. It is not normally more than 0.5 mm above or below the isoelectric line in any lead. Changes in the ST segment occur when events in the myocardium and pericardium produce an electrical current secondary to injured (but not dead) or abnormal cells. By far the most common cause of marked ST changes is myocardial ischaemia (see later, Figure 48.4). Other causes are pericarditis, cardiomyopathy, ventricular aneurysm, and acid–base and electrolyte disturbances (especially severe hypokalaemia, see Figure 47.9).

The 'injury current' displaces the whole ECG up or down, except during the electrically quiescent ST segment, but the visual effect is a change in the ST segment.

### The T wave

The T wave represents ventricular repolarization, which is dependent on transmembrane ionic movement and the sodium/potassium pump. Not all myocardial cells repolarize after the same time interval or in the same electrical direction, and the wave seen represents the resultant summation of all the individual cellular repolarizations. Factors that alter the mechanism of repolarization can therefore change both the shape and the position of the T wave. These include ischaemia, infarction, ventricular hypertrophy, conduction defects, electrolyte disturbances (note potassium, see Figure 47.9), drugs (note digoxin, Figure 47.8, and see Figure 20.39), myocarditis, cardiomyopathy, pericarditis, septicaemia, hypothyroidism, and pulmonary embolism.

Repolarization in the healthy heart occurs in the same electrical sequence and along the same pathways as depolarization. The T wave is thus usually upright in those leads in which the QRS complex is upright, and vice versa. The normal T wave is always upright in leads I and II. Inversion in V1 and V2 is a normal variant.

### The QT interval

The QT interval represents the time period from the beginning of ventricular depolarization to the end of repolarization. It normally varies with heart rate (see Figure 47.1) and when abnormalities occur they are usually secondary to electrolyte changes (such as a prolonged QT in hypocalcaemia).

### Individual leads and cardiac axis

Each of the leads reflects the activity in a particular part of the heart:

- Leads I, aVL, V5, and V6 give information about the left side of the heart.
- Leads V5 and V6 are specific to the left ventricle.
- Leads V1 and V2 give information about the right ventricle.
- Leads V3 and V4 give information about the interventricular septum and the anterior wall of the left ventricle.
- Leads II, III, and aVF give information about the inferior surface of the heart.

Together, aVR, aVL, aVF, I, II, and III provide a 'clock face' view of cardiac electrical activity in the frontal plane of the body (Figure 47.4) and can be used to assess the direction of the mean frontal cardiac axis. (They say nothing about electrical vector activity at right angles to the coronal plane.) The cardiac axis is the direction of the mean electrical vector which results from all the individual cellular depolarizations during the production of the QRS. It is therefore in the approximate direction of the lead with the tallest R wave or at right angles to the lead in which the R and S waves are equal. There are only six leads available for assessment and the axis can therefore only be obtained to the nearest 30° on visual inspection. This means that firm statements can be made only when the axis deviation is considerable.

When examining an ECG, develop the habit of:

- looking at disturbances of rhythm;
- estimating the rate (divide the number of large squares between two QRS complexes into 300);

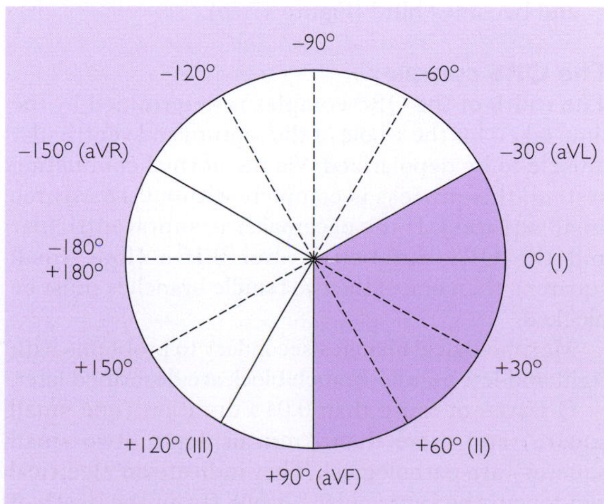


**Figure 47.4** The frontal plane cardiac axis. The range of the normal axis is shown shaded.

- sequentially assessing abnormalities in: the P wave, the PR interval, the T wave.

## CHANGES IN THE CARDIAC AXIS

In practice, axis deviation which might indicate pathology is determined by applying 'rules of thumb' to the heights of the R and S waves in leads I, II, and III.

Left axis deviation is significant when there is a deep S wave in III and the S wave is of greater amplitude than the R wave in II (Figure 47.5). It is usually caused by a conduction defect (especially left anterior hemiblock, Figure 47.5) rather than by left ventricular hypertrophy. Minor degrees of left axis deviation are found in any condition in which the heart is more horizontal than normal (e.g. short fat subjects, pregnancy, all the causes of a raised diaphragm), and rarely are associated with tricuspid atresia and ostium primum atrial septal defects.

Right axis deviation is significant when there is a deep S wave in I and the largest R wave is in III (Figure 47.6). This is associated mainly with right ventricular hypertrophy secondary to pulmonary hypertension or congenital heart disease. Minor degrees of right axis deviation occur in tall thin subjects (vertical heart), in those with left posterior hemiblock, and in ostium secundum atrial septal defects.

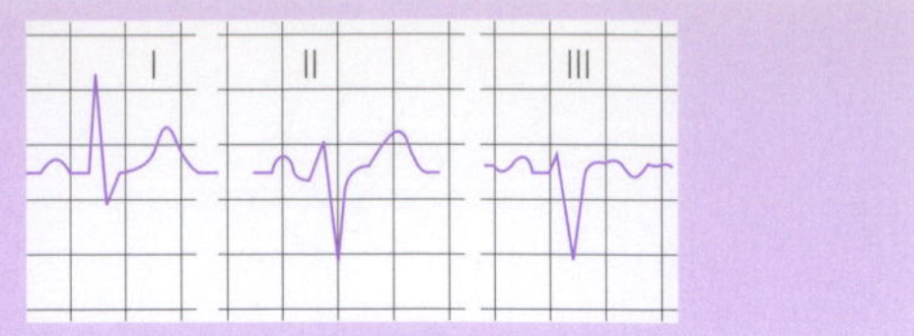


**Figure 47.5** Left axis deviation.

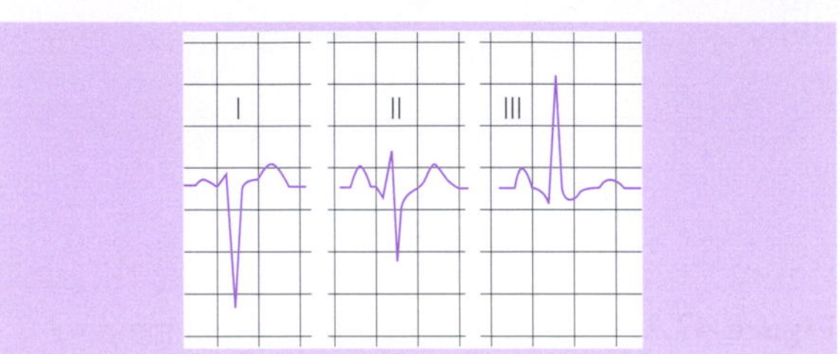


**Figure 47.6** Right axis deviation.

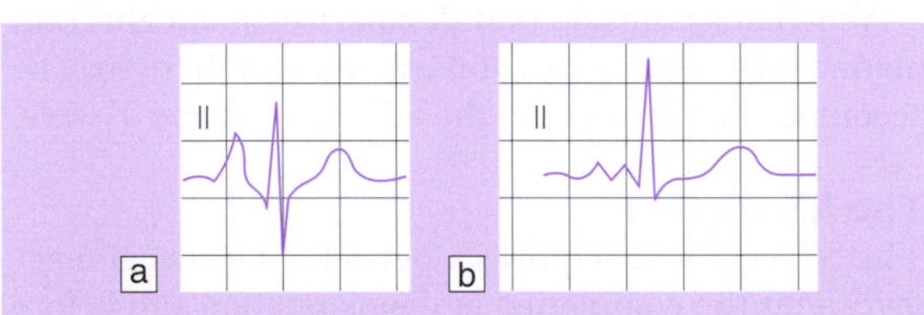


**Figure 47.7** (a) 'P' pulmonale, right atrial hypertrophy; (b) 'P' mitrale, atrial asynchrony.

## MORPHOLOGICAL CHANGES OF THE COMPONENT PARTS OF THE ECG

These have already been briefly considered above.

### The P wave

Morphological changes to the P wave are always relevant to anaesthesia and there are two well-described abnormalities:

- Any condition that causes the right atrium to become hypertrophied (pulmonary hypertension, tricuspid stenosis) causes the P wave to increase in height above the normal of 2.5 mm and become peaked (Figure 47.7a).
- Left atrial hypertrophy (usually caused by mitral stenosis) causes the left atrium to depolarize late; the P wave broadens above its upper limit of 0.1 s and becomes bifid (Figure 47.7b).

### The QRS complex

The width of the QRS complex is determined by the time taken for the whole of the septum and ventricular muscle to be depolarized. Via the normal conducting system, this process is complete within 0.12 s (three small squares). If the pacemaker is supraventricular and the QRS duration is over 0.16 s (four small squares), then one of the two bundle branches must be blocked.

Morphological changes secondary to problems with right and left bundle-branch block are described later.

Q waves of more than 0.04 s duration (one small square) and more than 2 mm in depth (two small squares) are pathological. They indicate an electrical window in the ventricular muscle (from the death of tissue) which allows a cavity potential to be recorded. They give no indication of the age of the infarction and are usually permanent. Infarction of the anterior wall of the left ventricle produces Q waves in V3, V4, and V5. Infarction of the inferior surface causes Q waves in III and aVF.

An increase in the height of the QRS complex is caused by an increase in the muscle mass of the ventricles. There are two well-defined causes:

1. Right ventricular hypertrophy is best seen in the right ventricular leads (especially V1), where the complex becomes upright. It is always abnormal if the height of the R wave exceeds the depth of the S wave in V1. This can be accompanied by a deep S in V6, right axis deviation, a peaked P wave, and (in severe cases) inversion of the T waves in V2 and V3.
2. Left ventricular hypertrophy causes a tall R wave in V5 and V6 (> 25 mm) and a deep S in V1. There are often also inverted T waves in V5, V6, aVL, and II, and there may be left axis deviation. Another commonly used guide is to say that left ventricular hypertrophy is present if the sum of the S wave in V1 and the R wave in V5 is over 40 mm.

### The ST segment

The ST segment should be on the isoelectric line but it can be elevated or depressed.

Elevation of the ST segment is an indication of acute myocardial injury (usually caused by infarction) or pericarditis. It occurs in the leads overlying the affected area, i.e. anterior damage shows in the V leads, inferior in II, III, and aVF. In infarction, the ST segment normally returns to the baseline within 24–48 hours.

Pericarditis is usually generalized and changes occur in all leads. Permanent ST segment elevation indicates a left ventricular aneurysm.

Depression of the ST segment (especially in association with an upright T wave) is usually a sign of ischaemia instead of infarction. Depression is taken to be significant when it exceeds 1 mm. It is ST depression that is looked for on an exercise ECG.

## The T wave

The most common abnormality is inversion of the T wave. This can be the result of the following.

### *Normality*

The T wave is normally inverted in aVR and sometimes in V1. In some healthy young people inversion also occurs in V2.

### *Non-specific changes*

Minor degrees of ST segment and T wave abnormality in an otherwise fit patient are usually of no great significance.

### *Bundle branch block*

The abnormal path of depolarization is usually associated with an abnormal path of repolarization (see later). Therefore, T wave abnormalities associated with QRS complexes of greater than 0.16 s duration (four small squares) have no significance in themselves.

### *Ventricular hypertrophy*

This is dealt with above.

### *Digoxin*

Digoxin is used in the management of congestive heart failure and supraventricular arrhythmias (especially atrial fibrillation and atrial flutter). It acts by inhibiting the sodium/potassium ATPase of the sarcolemma, allowing the intracellular accumulation of sodium ions. These displace bound calcium ions and make more available to take part in the contractile process. As a result of the action on the sarcolemma, digoxin produces changes of the ST segment when the patient is in sinus rhythm (Figure 47.8 and see Figure 20.39).

When used to control an excess of atrial stimuli presenting at the AV node, digoxin slows AV conduction and prolongs the AV refractory period, thus reducing the ventricular rate. When given intravenously, it has its onset of action at 30 min and peak effect at approximately 4 h. Most patients presenting with chronic atrial fibrillation will be on digoxin.

Digoxin toxicity is not rare but has become less common now that pharmaceutical preparations are more reliable, and serum levels are easy to assay. The most common side effects experienced by the patient (anorexia, nausea, vomiting, diarrhoea, and psychiatric disturbances) are unrelated to its cardiac actions. In the heart, almost any arrhythmia can be produced, the most frequent being ventricular ectopic beats, coupled beats, and ventricular tachycardia. Toxicity is more likely in the presence of hypokalaemia, hypocalcaemia, hypoxaemia, hypothyroidism, and reduced renal clearance.

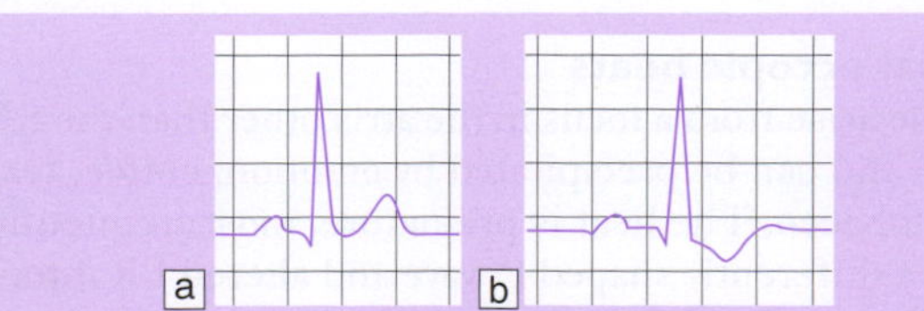


**Figure 47.8** The effect of digoxin on the lateral chest leads. (a) Before digitalization; (b) after digitalization. Note ST segment and T wave changes.

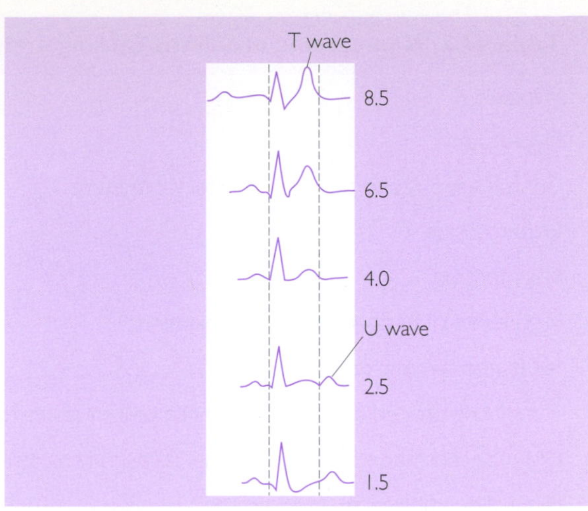


**Figure 47.9** ECG changes resulting from altered serum potassium. Note the high-voltage, peaked T wave with hyperkalaemia, and the low-voltage T wave and U wave with hypokalaemia. Values are the approximate serum potassium concentration in mmol/L.

The T wave can also be affected by electrolyte disturbances. The most significant of these are:

- hypocalcaemia which prolongs the QT interval (see above);
- potassium which has profound effects on transmembrane potential and ionic transmission, especially if the serum level changes rapidly. The ECG changes that result are shown in Figure 47.9.

## ARRHYTHMIAS AND CONDUCTION DEFECTS

Patients can either already have arrhythmias preoperatively or develop them anew in the perioperative period. It is important *always* to think of causes other than intrinsic cardiac malfunction because the proper treatment may not be the injection of an anti-arrhythmic agent, but the correction of a basic defect in anaesthesia. Non-cardiac anaesthetic problems that can produce arrhythmias are given in Table 47.2.

Hypoxia and hypotension secondary to a pneumothorax, although rare, are easily overlooked until well advanced. Arrhythmias are particularly common during dental anaesthesia, especially at a light plane of anaesthesia.

Consequently, when an arrhythmia arises, before administering anti-arrhythmic drugs, always check:

- the oxygen supply;
- the patient's colour and saturation;

| Table 47.2 Non-cardiac problems causing arrhythmias |
|---|
| Hypoxia |
| Hypercapnia |
| Central venous and pulmonary artery catheters |
| Hypertension |
| Hypotension |
| High levels of endogenous catecholamines |
| Sympathomimetic drugs |
| Stimulating procedures in the presence of light anaesthesia (e.g. traction on viscera, laryngoscopy, etc.) |
| High concentration of volatile agents (especially halothane) |
| Electrolyte imbalance |
| Acidosis |

- the adequacy of ventilation;
- the expired $CO_2$;
- the concentration of volatile agents;
- the blood pressure.

These checks take only a few moments and may be life saving. Please refer to the beginning of this chapter for notes on the role of anticoagulation in the management of arrhythmias.

### Sinus tachycardia

The normal heart rate varies from 120 beats/min in infancy to 70–80 beats/min in adults (40–50 beats/min taking trained athletes into account). Sinus tachycardia is a normal physiological event in exercise, anxiety, and light anaesthesia, and is frequently present in the postoperative period. It occurs as a compensatory mechanism in shock, anaemia, and cardiac failure, and as a toxic side effect in thyrotoxicosis and after several drugs (e.g. atropine, ephedrine). It is only important clinically when it results in myocardial ischaemia, and the treatment should first be that of the underlying cause (e.g. deeper anaesthesia, give fluids, etc.) before recourse to β-adrenoceptor blockade. It is, however, sometimes necessary to reduce the heart rate to 100 beats/min or less when reduced diastolic filling, prejudiced by a fast rate, is causing myocardial ischaemia.

Always keep in the back of your mind that onset of unexplained tachycardia during surgery could be light anaesthesia (common), awareness, or malignant hyperpyrexia (rare).

### Sinus arrhythmia

This is a normal finding in children and teenagers. Via baroreceptor control, the heart rate increases during inspiration and decreases during expiration. It is markedly attenuated during all forms of general anaesthesia.

### Sinus bradycardia

This is found in many healthy patients (particularly trained athletes), but also in hypothyroidism and hypothermia, and with raised intracranial pressure. When a bradycardia develops anew, it is often the result of excessive vagal stimulation and may resolve on stopping the stimulus (e.g. carotid sinus stimulation in carotid surgery or oculocardiac reflex in eye surgery). Although the prolonged diastole which accompanies a bradycardia aids coronary perfusion, coronary blood flow still depends on an adequate filling pressure in the aortic sinus. This, in turn, demands that the ventricle must be able to compensate for a reduction in rate by an increase in stroke volume. Although easy for a healthy ventricle, this may be impossible for one that is close to failure or that has previously been infarcted. Under these conditions, it is possible that a bradycardia (usually below 50 beats/min) will result in systemic hypotension and poor coronary filling that may be sufficient to demonstrate ischaemia on the ECG. The treatment is small incremental doses of atropine (0.1-mg steps) to return the rate to normal without overshooting to a tachycardia (unless the bradycardia occurs during carotid endarterectomy when lignocaine [lidocaine] on the carotid sinus is the treatment of choice).

The other effect of a lengthened diastole is that it allows more time for the prepotential of automatic cells to drift and reach the threshold potential, thus producing ectopic activity, most frequently from a ventricular focus. Having excluded faulty anaesthesia (particularly in small children who are very prone to bradycardia from hypoxia), treatment of sinus bradycardia is to use small doses of atropine or glycopyrrolate to increase the rate. This merely shortens diastole and prevents ectopic foci from reaching their threshold potential ('pacing them out').

### Atrial ectopic beats

These arise from a focus in the atria other than the SA node and can be precipitated by emotion, coffee, tea, and tobacco. The beat is premature, most frequently with a differently shaped P wave and altered PR interval (Figure 47.10). Usually the QRS complex is normal, but very rarely aberrant conduction can widen the QRS complex, mimicking both left and right bundle-branch block. Atrial ectopic beats predominantly occur in

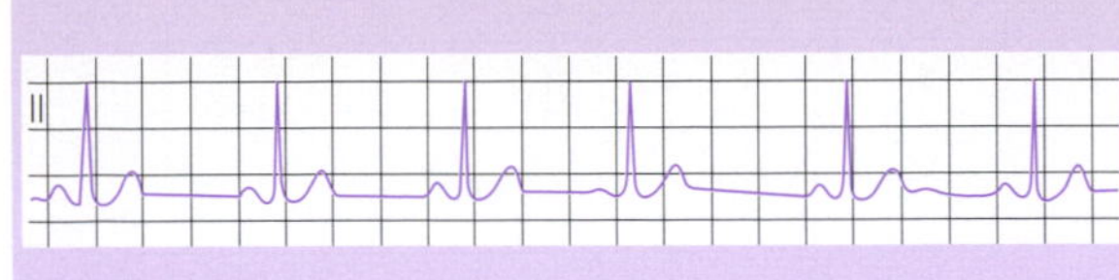


**Figure 47.10** Atrial ectopic beat. The fourth beat is premature, preceded by an abnormal P wave and followed by a compensatory pause.

normal patients and do not require treatment or pose an anaesthetic hazard.

Their only significance is in patients prone to atrial tachyarrhythmias, in whom they may herald the onset of an attack. They can usually be 'paced out' by atropine, or the excitability of atrial tissue can be reduced by β-adrenoceptor blockade or calcium antagonists.

### Wandering pacemaker

This disturbance is a form of severe atrial ectopic behaviour in which, in addition to impulses from the SA node, there are many others that originate from various foci in the atrium. As a result, there is a variation in rhythm, a changing P wave shape, and a changing PR interval. The abnormalities sometimes occur in runs and a rhythm strip may be required for the presence of other pacemakers to be seen. The QRS is usually normal (apart from rare aberrant conduction). This arrhythmia may occur in normal individuals, but is also not uncommon after myocardial infarction or digitalis therapy, and during myocarditis (especially rheumatic fever), in which case the real anaesthetic risks are those of the underlying condition.

There is little anaesthetic literature on the risks of the condition itself, but they would appear to be similar to those in the patient with atrial ectopic beats.

The term 'sinus pause' describes the failure of the atrium to depolarize at the expected time in a patient who is in sinus rhythm (Figure 47.11). Two different mechanisms may initiate it. In Figure 47.11, if $y$ is a whole-number multiple of $x$, then it is assumed that the SA node is still firing but that its effect is not transmitted throughout the atrium. This is termed 'sinoatrial block'. If there is no precise relationship between $x$ and $y$, then it is assumed that the SA node has simply ceased automatic activity, and the condition is called sinus arrest. Much debate currently exists about the exact separation of these two conditions. If the pause is sufficiently long, a subsidiary pacemaker emerges (hopefully!).

Sinus pauses can be associated with excessive vagal tone, ischaemic heart disease, digoxin, propranolol, and ageing (fibrous replacement), or be a normal variant. Whether a finding is physiological or pathological is often difficult to know. It may herald the appearance of the sick sinus syndrome (see below).

From the anaesthetist's viewpoint, a healthy SA node is one that will increase the atrial rate in response to exercise or atropine, and does not allow pauses of more than 1.5 s on the ECG. The SA node should be considered pathological when the pauses are recurrent, cause cerebral symptoms, coexist with other evidence of cardiac disease, or are in excess of 2.0 s on the ECG. Poor SA node function may prevent a physiological tachycardia, remove the atrial contribution to ventricular filling, and allow a subsidiary, slower pacemaker to emerge with a limitation on cardiac output. These cases should be treated as in sick sinus syndrome (see below).

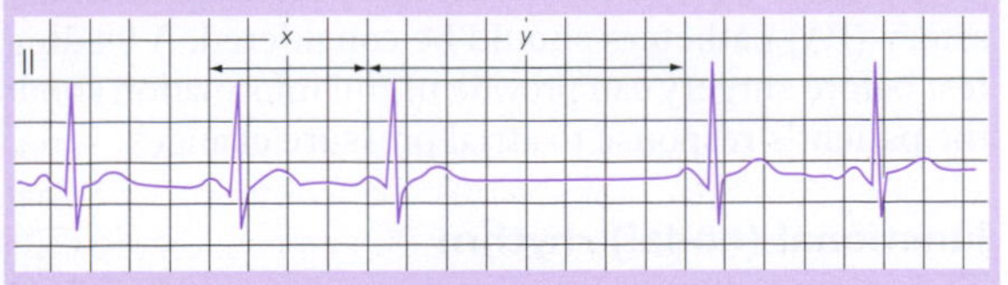


**Figure 47.11** Sinus pause; see text for details

### The sick sinus syndrome

The sick sinus syndrome is a disease of the SA node that results in unpredictable sinus pauses (see above) and inappropriate bradycardias, which at times alternate with tachycardias. It is increasingly being diagnosed in elderly people, often as a result of syncopal attacks or palpitations being investigated by a 24-hour ECG monitor. It may be associated with almost any form of heart disease or present as an isolated finding.

Many patients are asymptomatic, and sick sinus syndrome should be suspected in any elderly patient with an unexplained sinus bradycardia, particularly if direct questioning reveals evidence of cerebral symptoms. Frequently, the bradycardia (caused by degenerative changes in the SA node) is complicated by episodes of supraventricular tachycardia (SVT). The condition is treated when it is symptomatic, in which case a pacemaker is used to control the bradycardia; superimposed on this are digoxin and β-adrenoceptor blockers to suppress the tachyarrhythmias. The bradycardia may be refractory to atropine because of the disease of the SA node.

The anaesthetic implications of pacemakers are outlined later in this chapter. The anaesthetic risk for an unpaced patient, in addition to the risks of any other underlying condition, has not been quantified. A sensible approach is to use an anaesthetic technique that has little effect on cardiac conduction and excitability. The locality of equipment and personnel for pacing must be known. A wide-bore central venous cannula *in situ* facilitates emergency insertion of a temporary wire.

One unexplained feature of these patients is their propensity to pulmonary embolism, so perioperative anticoagulation (if they are not chronically anticoagulated) is sensible or should at the very least be discussed.

### Paroxysmal atrial tachycardia (PAT)

The notes on anticoagulation at the beginning of this chapter should be referred to. PAT results from the pacemaking function of the SA node being replaced by a focus somewhere else in the atrium which discharges rapidly at a rate of 130–200 beats/min. Conduction at the AV node and beyond is usually normal so the QRS complex is unaffected (Figure 47.12). In a small proportion of cases there is aberrant conduction. Each

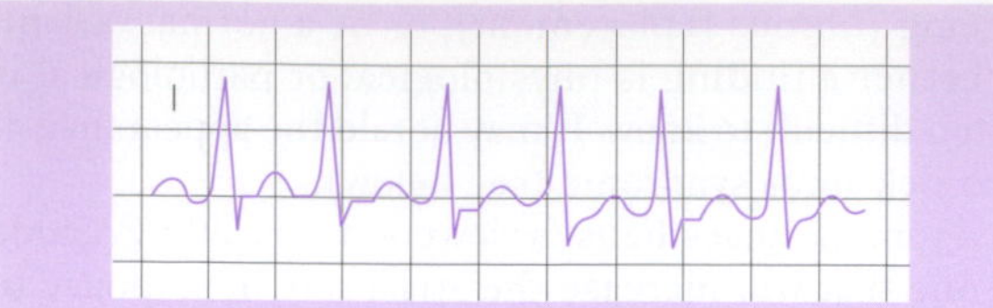


**Figure 47.12** Paroxysmal atrial tachycardia. Rate = 175 beats/min. P waves not visible.

QRS is preceded by a P wave which at rates greater than 150 beats/min is usually lost in the previous T wave.

Sixty percent of affected patients have no evidence of underlying heart disease. In others, it is associated with thyrotoxicosis, tobacco, caffeine, rheumatic mitral valve disease, coronary artery disease, and the Wolff–Parkinson– White syndrome. The tachycardia starts and ends suddenly and may last any time from seconds to days. It may precipitate angina, cardiac failure, dizziness, and syncope.

Initial treatment is by unilateral carotid sinus massage or the Valsalva manoeuvre. Verapamil or adenosine may be effective for the acute state but, if refractory, direct current (DC) countershock is usually effective. Always check the serum electrolytes as a contributory cause. Patients who have recurrences are often maintained on digoxin.

If possible, PAT should always be controlled before anaesthesia. Underlying causes should always be suspected and treated appropriately. Refractory patients requiring urgent surgery can receive DC countershock in the presence of a cardiologist immediately after induction.

### Atrial flutter

Notes on anticoagulation at the beginning of this chapter should be referred to. In atrial flutter, the atria are stimulated rapidly and regularly 250–400 times per min by an ectopic atrial pacemaker. The AV node cannot conduct at this rate and there is a varying degree of AV block, most commonly either 2:1 or 4:1. The ECG has characteristic flutter waves interspersed with normal QRS complexes (Figure 47.13).

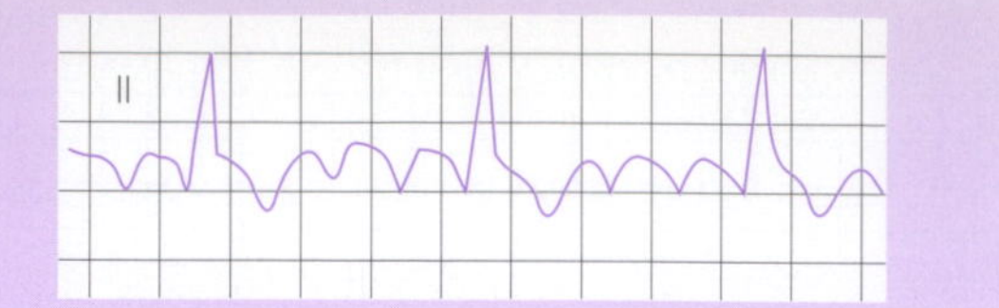


**Figure 47.13** Atrial flutter with 4:1 atrioventricular block. When identifying flutter waves, it is important to remember those coinciding with the QRS complexes and T waves.

Over 90% of cases have a basic underlying cardiac defect (rheumatic or ischaemic heart disease or atrial septal defect). Less commonly, it is associated with thyrotoxicosis, trauma to the myocardium, myocarditis, and digoxin therapy. These should be excluded before surgery. Most patients find the arrhythmia very distressing, and cardiac failure or angina is commonly precipitated early. Chronic control is by digoxin, verapamil, or β-adrenoceptor blockers. DC countershock is almost always effective in abolishing atrial flutter, and is the acute treatment of choice. This should be done as a planned procedure before elective surgery, or can be done at the induction of urgent surgery in association with a cardiologist.

### Atrial fibrillation

Notes on anticoagulation at the beginning of this chapter should be referred to. In atrial fibrillation (AF) small areas of the atrial muscle are stimulated at different times and there is no coordinated contraction (Figure 47.14). The atrial contribution to ventricular filling is lost. The ventricular rhythm is totally irregular because the majority of stimuli reaching the AV node are either too weak to stimulate it or arrive in the refractory period. The ventricular rate is usually rapid and can precipitate angina and cardiac failure. Rarely, AF in young people occurs as a congenital abnormality or is precipitated by alcohol or other drugs. Most middle-aged and elderly people have underlying acquired heart disease. Common associations are rheumatic mitral valve disease, ischaemic heart disease, and thyrotoxicosis. The last must be excluded in elderly people. Less common, acute causes of AF are pulmonary infections and infarctions, cardiothoracic surgery, cardiac trauma, and myocarditis. Two important factors affecting the onset of AF are advancing age and the presence of a large atrium. On exercise, the ventricular rate increases but the cardiac output does not and this can cause distress and possible myocardial ischaemia.

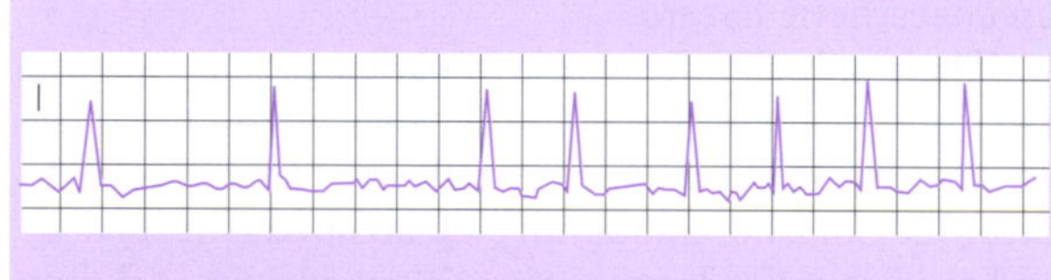


**Figure 47.14** Atrial fibrillation.

If a patient presents for surgery with AF of recent onset (it may be the cause of the admission, e.g. mesenteric infarct from an embolus), any underlying condition should be evaluated and cardiological advice taken about the wisdom of reversal of AF. It carries a high risk of embolization unless the patient is anticoagulated and, if the AF is likely to become permanent, may be an unnecessary manoeuvre.

Patients in established AF are very sensitive to changes in right and left atrial pressures because they have no atrial contractile contribution to ventricular filling and depend on the hydrostatic pressure in the atria to fill the ventricles.

Consequently, for major surgery or where large or sudden changes in circulating blood volume are anticipated, the use of central venous and possibly pulmonary artery (PA) catheters should be considered. A loading test before surgery can provide useful information about the patient's response to atrial pressure changes.

### Junctional (nodal) rhythm

This is caused by an ectopic pacemaker situated close to and either above or below the AV node. The P wave, representing atrial contraction, is therefore produced by abnormal conduction which may be retrograde. This causes the temporal relationship between atrial and ventricular contraction to be upset. Two effects follow: the P wave can precede, follow, or be buried in the QRS (Figure 47.15), and there is a diminished or absent atrial contribution to ventricular filling. Transient and permanent nodal rhythm can be found in normal people. More frequently, it follows myocardial infarction and is associated with the wide range of other organic heart diseases which produce atrial arrhythmias. Junctional rhythm is probably the most common arrhythmia seen during anaesthesia and is particularly associated with halothane.

Junctional rhythm needs treatment only when it affects the cardiac output. With rapid rates, it may be difficult to differentiate it from PAT, but both can be treated in a similar manner. If the rate is very slow, treat with atropine. During anaesthesia, in people with borderline myocardial function, the onset of junctional rhythm can cause sudden hypotension because of a reduced ejection volume. The best treatment is to remove the cause (usually halothane). If there is no response, calcium salts (calcium gluconate 250–500 mg) improve conduction and do not risk the tachycardia that is so often seen with atropine. Treatment is not always successful.

### Ventricular ectopic beats

Ventricular ectopic beats (VEs) arise because the prepotential of some automatic cells in the ventricle reaches threshold potential before the next sinus beat. Factors that increase the rate of rise of the prepotential include hypercapnia, hypoxia (global and myocardial ischaemia), catecholamines, other sympathomimetic drugs, hyperthermia (remember malignant hyperpyrexia), and hypokalaemia. More than any other arrhythmia, these may be caused by faulty anaesthesia so, when they occur, always check the adequacy of ventilation, the end-tidal $CO_2$ and other basic parameters.

Because an ectopic beat occurs prematurely, it is not preceded by a P wave. When the sinus beat does arrive, it finds the ventricles in a refractory state so there is a compensatory pause until the next one arrives. Other features are a wide and bizarre QRS complex, and abnormal ST segment and T wave (Figure 47.16). They can occur (up to 6/min) in normal people.

VEs can, however, represent underlying myocardial disease (especially after myocardial infarction) and the danger in these patients is the progression to ventricular tachycardia (VT) or ventricular fibrillation (VF). Coupled VEs are most commonly secondary to digitalis toxicity, which in the perioperative period may be precipitated by hyperkalaemia. Traditional criteria for treatment of VEs are if they are more than 6/min, multifocal, occur in runs of three or more, or show the R-on-T phenomenon (ectopic beat near the vulnerable period which can precipitate VF).

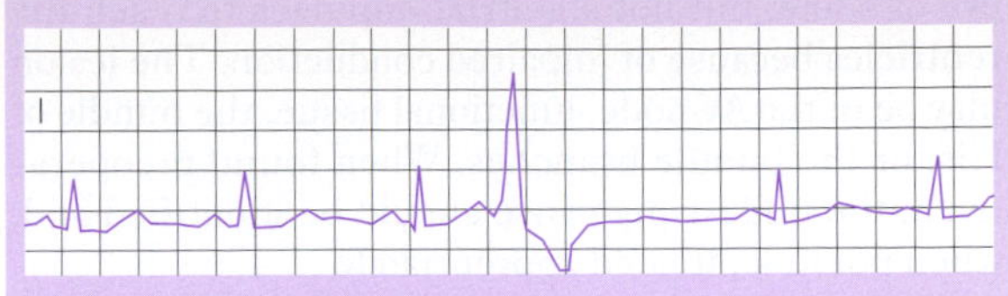


**Figure 47.16** Ventricular ectopic beat.

If treatment is commenced, then the standard regimen is intravenous lignocaine (1–1.5 mg/kg as a bolus followed by an infusion of 2–4 mg/min).

### Ventricular tachycardia

VT is always life threatening and in anaesthetic practice can be caused by anything creating ventricular ectopic behaviour. Always monitor the ECG after infiltration with epinephrine (adrenaline) in case VT is precipitated. VT is commonly associated with severe ischaemic heart disease. The pulse rate is regular and rapid (130–200 beats/min), leading to myocardial ischaemia and heart failure. The ECG (Figure 47.17) can be difficult to differentiate from PAT with aberrant conduction. DC countershock is very effective but many episodes respond to intravenous lignocaine (1–1.5 mg/kg as a bolus followed by an infusion of 2–4 mg/min).

### Atrioventricular block

#### *First-degree block*

This is an ECG definition when the PR interval is found to be above the upper limit of normal (0.2 s). It commonly occurs in the absence of any organic heart disease and implies a disturbance of conduction between the SA and AV nodes, or a delay in conduction through the AV node. It can also be caused by increased vagal tone, halothane, digitalis, ischaemia of the AV node, almost all infective diseases, cardiomyopathy, and congenital heart disease. It is of no functional significance itself, its importance being that of any underlying disease. If the prolonged PR interval is the result of excessive vagal tone and associated with a bradycardia, it responds to atropine.

#### *Second-degree block*

Clinically, this may at times be mistaken for virtually any arrhythmia and its diagnosis is by ECG. It is a fail-

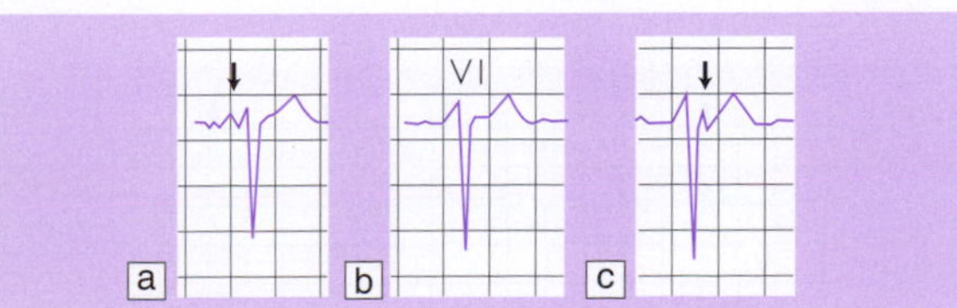


**Figure 47.15** Junctional beats: the P waves (arrowed) may (a) precede, (b) coincide with, or (c) follow the QRS complex.

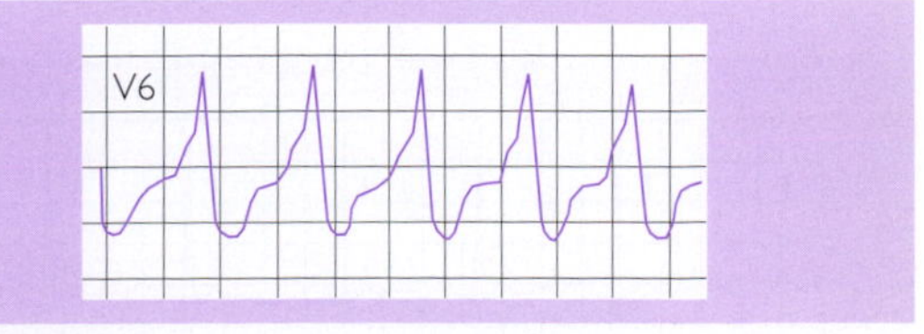


**Figure 47.17** Ventricular tachycardia. Rate = 150 beats/min.

ure of some, but not all, atrial impulses to reach the ventricles because of impaired conduction. The lesion may be in the AV node, junctional tissue, the bundle of His, or the bundle branches. When found preoperatively, the underlying cause should be identified and, when possible, treated appropriately.

The classification of second-degree block differs slightly in detail from book to book. I have described below what I think is the most logical.

*Mobitz type I block (Wenckebach)*

This has a progressive lengthening of the PR interval until there is a total failure of conduction. Then the whole cycle repeats (Figure 47.18). Type I block is usually caused by disease of the AV node (see Figure 47.2) but rarely, on occasions, results from conduction defects in the bundle of His or the bundle branches. When of nodal origin, it is benign and only very infrequently progresses to third-degree block. When it does, a reliable high-order pacemaker emerges to provide adequate ventricular rates.

*Mobitz type II block*

This is less common than type I, but carries a much graver significance. It is characterized by a sudden failure of AV conduction without previous lengthening of the PR interval (Figure 47.19). Most cases have widespread disease (fibrosis or infarction) of the bundle branches or fascicles (see Figure 47.2) so that, if third-degree block supervenes, a slow, unreliable, low-order ventricular pacemaker emerges. A small minority have a relatively well-defined lesion in the bundle of His.

*'Advanced' or 'high-grade' block*

These are terms used to describe second-degree heart block with the presence of a 2:1 or greater incidence of AV conduction failure (Figure 47.20). In this example, as there is only one PR interval to be examined, it is impossible to classify it as Mobitz type I or type II. In most cases, the underlying pathology is widespread disease of the bundles and fascicles (Mobitz type II) and it frequently progresses to total block.

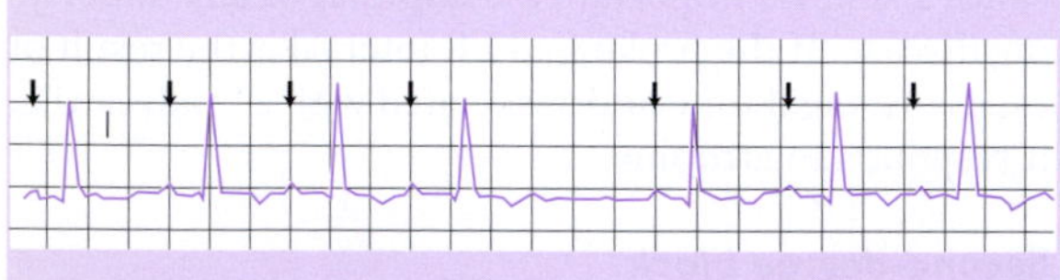


**Figure 47.18** Mobitz type I (Wenckebach) block. The P waves are arrowed.

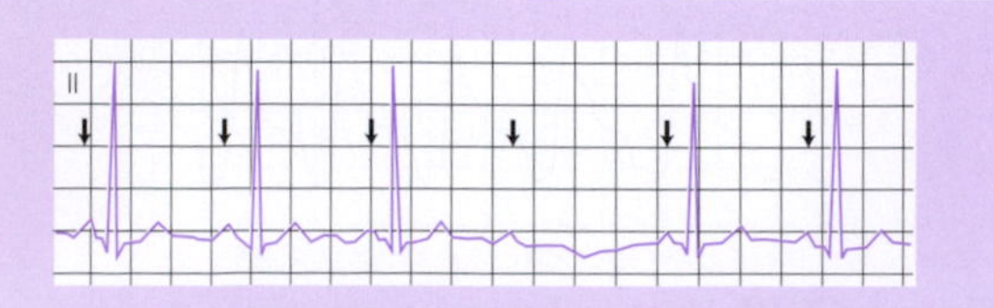


**Figure 47.19** Mobitz type II block. The P waves are arrowed.

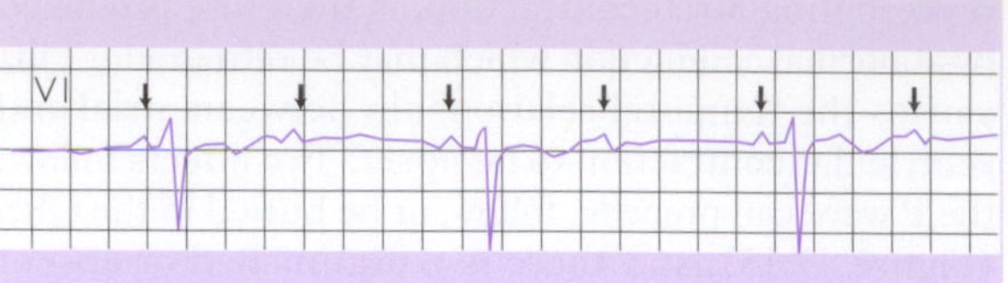


**Figure 47.20** High grade or advanced block (2:1). The P waves are arrowed

To our knowledge, there is little literature describing the effect of anaesthesia on second-degree heart block. The worry is the progression to third-degree block intra- or postoperatively. It is sensible to:

- test the effect of a very small dose of atropine before or during anaesthesia;
- have an isoprenaline (isoproterenol) infusion ready;
- know the whereabouts of pacing personnel and facilities – a wide-bore central venous cannula *in situ* facilitates the emergency insertion of a temporary wire;
- avoid drugs known to produce or intensify AV conduction defects (especially halothane);
- take care to prevent periods of postoperative hypoxia, because this may intensify the block.

## Third-degree block

All the atrial impulses are blocked in the conducting system and the ventricular rate is controlled by a subsidiary pacemaker somewhere below the block, in either the AV node or automatic tissue of the ventricles (Figure 47.21). When atrial and ventricular contractions coincide there are jugular 'cannon' waves. The most frequent causes in adults are fibrosis of the conducting tissue and infarction of the interventricular septum. The latter is ominous in that it indicates a wide area of damage.

When the ventricular pacemaker is near the AV node, the heart rate is 40–55 beats/min with a normal width QRS complex. When the pacemaker is distant to the AV node, the heart rate is 30–40 beats/min with a wide QRS complex.

Many patients are symptomatic with syncopal attacks, myocardial ischaemia, or cardiac failure. They should have a pacemaker implanted before elective surgery. Emergency pacing may be necessary in urgent cases. The same perioperative precautions should be taken as for second-degree block.

Very rarely, complete heart block is congenital in origin (1 in 20 000 live births) and one-third of these have other congenital cardiac defects. Its effect on the

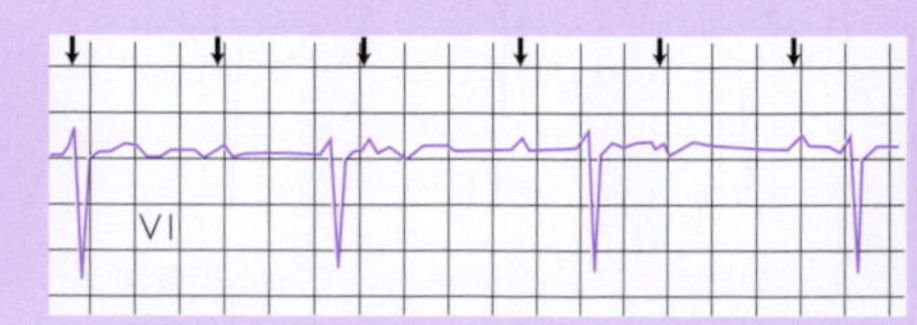


**Figure 47.21** Total (third-degree) heart block. The P waves are arrowed.

patient is very variable. Some require pacing as children, others are able to increase their cardiac output on exercise well into adult life. As the patients age, more and more need a pacemaker.

### Ventricular conduction defects

The ventricular conducting system is shown in Figure 47.2. Many texts subclassify bundle branch blocks into complete and incomplete, the latter having a normal width QRS and a less florid pattern disturbance. The distinction is arbitrary and indicates little about the potential severity of the abnormality.

#### *Right bundle branch block (RBBB)*

There is a failure of conduction of the right bundle branch (see Figure 47.2) proximally. Right ventricular depolarization is delayed because the distal right bundle branch fibres have to wait to be triggered by slow impulses passing through the septal myocardium. This results in a wide (> 0.12 s) QRS complex with an RSR′ pattern in leads V1 to V3 (Figure 47.22). Often the T wave is inverted in all these leads but right axis deviation (Figure 47.6) is usually present only when there is coexisting right ventricular hypertrophy.

As RBBB has little effect on the lateral chest leads, it is still possible to diagnose left ventricular hypertrophy and myocardial ischaemia and infarction from a 12-lead ECG or a CM5 lead.

RBBB has no underlying cause in what is variously estimated to be 1–15% of the normal adult population. Other causes are hypertensive disease, coronary artery disease, pulmonary embolism, all the causes of right ventricular hypertrophy and strain, and congenital lesions, particularly those involving the septum. The treatment and prognosis are those of the underlying condition. As an isolated finding, RBBB poses little anaesthetic risk.

#### *Left bundle branch block (LBBB)*

There is a failure of conduction of the left bundle branch (see Figure 47.2) and all impulses must pass down the right bundle branch. Septal depolarization is reversed, and the mass of the left ventricle depolarizes late and abnormally. This results in a wide (> 0.12 s) QRS complex with a notched or M shape in leads V4 to V6 (Figure 47.23). Abnormal left axis deviation is not a routine feature of LBBB. As a result of the bizarre routes of depolarization and repolarization, no further diagnostic information can be gained from examination of the QRS complex, ST segment, or T wave.

LBBB occurs almost always as a result of underlying heart disease of many types and is almost never a normal variant. It is associated with hypertension, coronary artery disease, cardiomyopathy, congenital lesions involving the septum, and valve disease. The anaesthetic management is that of the underlying condition and avoiding the induction of RBBB. This implies care in the passage of a PA catheter if it is indicated for major surgery and taking similar precautions to those listed for second-degree heart block.

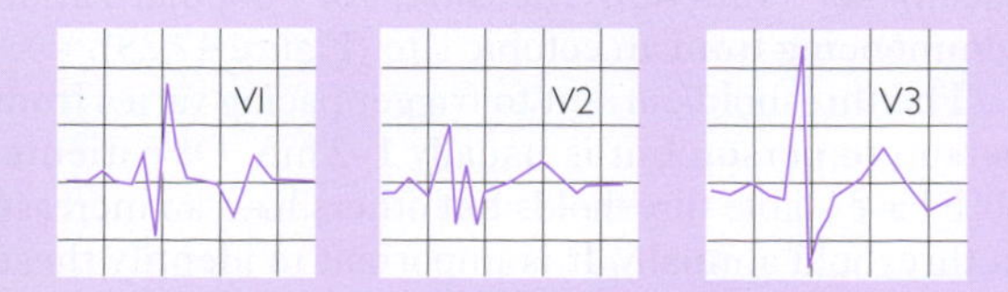


**Figure 47.22** Right bundle branch block.

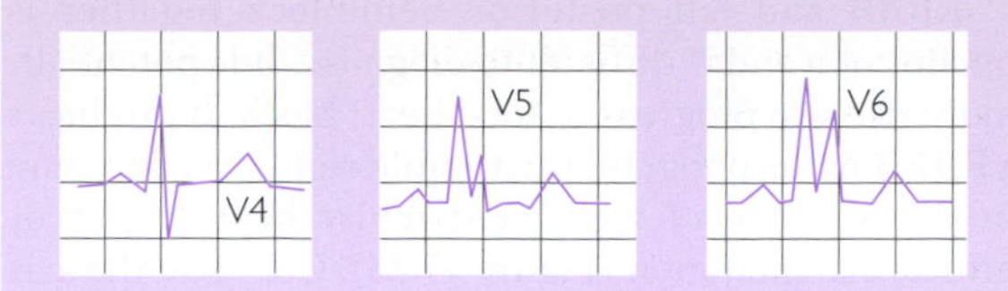


**Figure 47.23** Left bundle branch block.

#### *Hemiblock*

The left bundle branch is composed of anterior and posterior divisions (see Figure 47.2) and, if only one of them is damaged, the electrical impulse passes in an abnormal manner throughout the left ventricle, but the conduction is rapid. This causes an alteration in the cardiac axis but does *not* prolong the duration of the QRS complex.

Left anterior fascicle hemiblock causes left axis deviation and can be diagnosed if the QRS deflection is predominantly negative in lead II (see Figure 47.5) and there are no other causes of left axis deviation present. It is by far the most common form of hemiblock.

The posterior fascicle is more resistant to ischaemia because it is supplied by both the right and left coronary arteries. Hence, left posterior hemiblock is uncommon. It is manifested on the ECG only as mild right axis deviation (see Figure 47.6). It often appears as the upper limit of normal and is undiagnosable with right ventricular hypertrophy or after myocardial infarction.

#### *Bifascicular blocks*

These blocks are dangerous and imply that only a single conducting channel is available to the ventricles, and hence there is a high danger of total heart block.

RBBB and left anterior hemiblock is the most common combination. The condition is relatively stable, only 5% of patients per year progressing to total block. It produces a broad RSR′ in V1–3 with left axis deviation in the frontal plane (Figure 47.24).

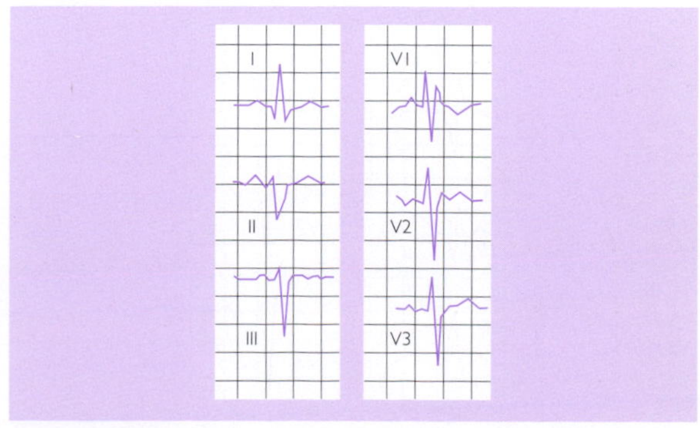


**Figure 47.24** Left anterior hemiblock with right bundle branch block.

RBBB and left posterior hemiblock together is uncommon and is difficult to diagnose. It is potentially more likely to progress to total heart block. It produces a RBBB pattern together with mild right axis deviation in the absence of right ventricular hypertrophy or myocardial infarction (Figure 47.25). Compare the axis deviation in Figure 47.25 with that normally regarded as significant in Figure 47.6.

The optimum perioperative management of bifascicular block is controversial and is patient dependent. The major concern is the onset of total block. If the patient has symptoms suggesting intermittent trifascicular block (fainting episodes, absences, etc.), seek the advice of a cardiologist about the wisdom of pacing. The asymptomatic patient can be anaesthetized with precautions taken similar to those described for second-degree heart block.

Great care is needed in the postoperative period where hypoxia may produce myocardial ischaemia and intensify the block. Patients should be monitored postoperatively in a high dependency unit.

#### *Intermittent blocks*

Various states of intermittent right and left bundle-branch and hemiblocks have been described. They have occurred in association with tachycardias, hypertension, ischaemia, hypoxia, and large tidal volumes.

### Wolff–Parkinson–White syndrome

This is the most common of the accelerated conduction syndromes, with an incidence in the population of up to 0.5%. It is usually seen in individuals who show no evidence of other organic disease, but occasionally it can be secondary to ischaemia of the AV node or myocarditis. In the otherwise normal individual, it does not alter life expectancy.

The cardiac impulse travels simultaneously down the normal conduction pathway and other anomalous fibres (the bundle of Kent bypasses the AV node). This results in a characteristically short P–R interval, wide QRS complex, and an abnormally slurred upstroke (δ wave) of the R wave (Figure 47.26).

These individuals are prone to attacks of atrial arrhythmias, usually paroxysmal atrial tachycardia and, less frequently, atrial flutter and AF.

Epicardial mapping can further define the anomalous pathways which can then be transected. If this is in the septum it may produce complete block.

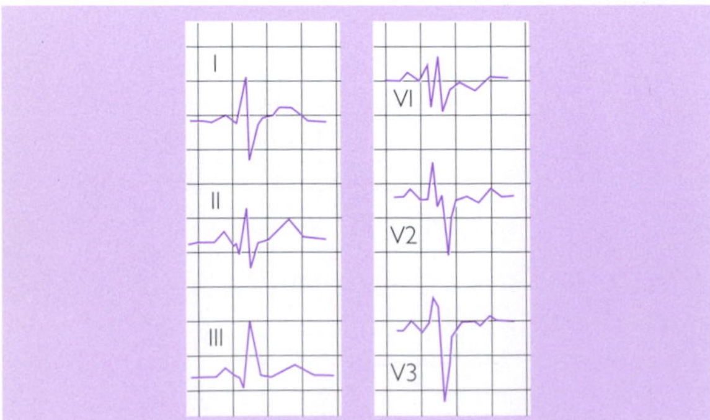


**Figure 47.25** Left posterior hemiblock with right bundle branch block.

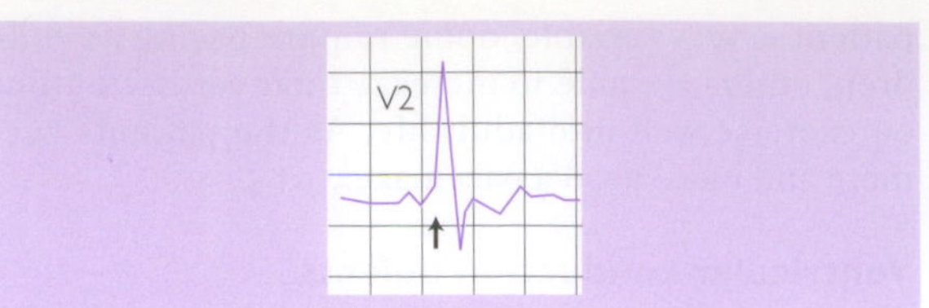


**Figure 47.26** Wolff–Parkinson–White syndrome. The δ wave is arrowed.

Medical management is now ablation of the pathway together with β-adrenoceptor blockers. These should be continued to the time of surgery. Both atropine and digitalis can precipitate and intensify the arrhythmia, as can emotional excitement.

During anaesthesia, facilities for cardioversion should be available. Light anaesthesia, catecholamines, and preoperative nervousness can all produce an attack. Therefore give a generous anxiolytic premedication and continue monitoring postoperatively.

## PACEMAKERS

Pacemakers are devices that ensure that the heart beats sufficient times per minute, irrespective of the intrinsic rhythmic activity. They are inserted for different types of conduction deficit and usually only when a patient is symptomatic. Perioperative indications are discussed under individual conditions. The criteria for insertion are continuously under review by cardiologists.

Temporary pacing wires normally use the transvenous endocardial approach and rest in the right ventricle. There are some needle electrodes which can be inserted into the myocardium via the chest wall, but these are for emergency use only, as in cardiac arrests. Oesophageal pacing is also possible.

Permanent pacemakers are usually inserted under local anaesthesia by cardiologists. The pacing wire passes via the subclavian vein and tricuspid valve to the right ventricle where it is anchored in the trabeculae by some sort of hook. A subcutaneous pocket over, or close to, the pectoralis major is constructed for the 'pacemaker box'. The typical chest-radiograph appearance of a pacemaker box and wire is shown in Figure 47.27. They are powered by various types of battery (including nuclear devices) and the power unit can usually be felt like a 'bar of soap' beneath the skin.

Less commonly, permanent pacemakers are implanted into the epicardial surface of the heart via either an epigastric incision or a mini-thoracotomy. The power unit is then placed in the rectus sheath. This approach may be preferred in children because it is easy to coil up an extra length of lead to allow for growth.

The ECG complexes are often abnormal during pacemaker function because of depolarization commencing from an ectopic site (Figure 47.28).

The threshold current to trigger pacing varies from person to person but is usually 1–2 mA. Of patients, 80% have stable thresholds but others have an increase in threshold annually. It is important to identify these (get the cardiologist to check the threshold) because it is possible that they have drifted close to the limits of

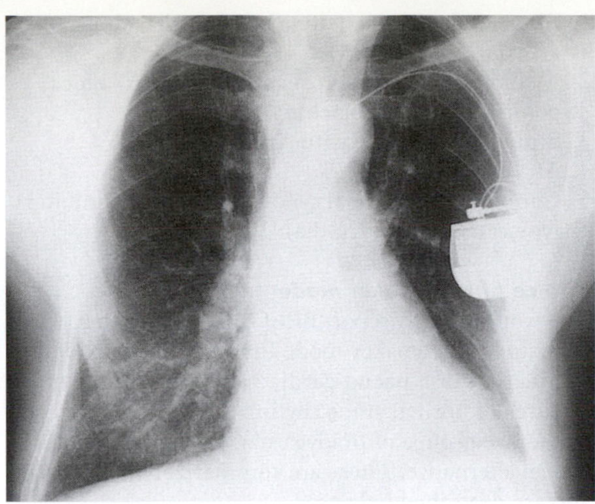

**Figure 47.27** Chest radiograph showing pacemaker box and position of pacing wire

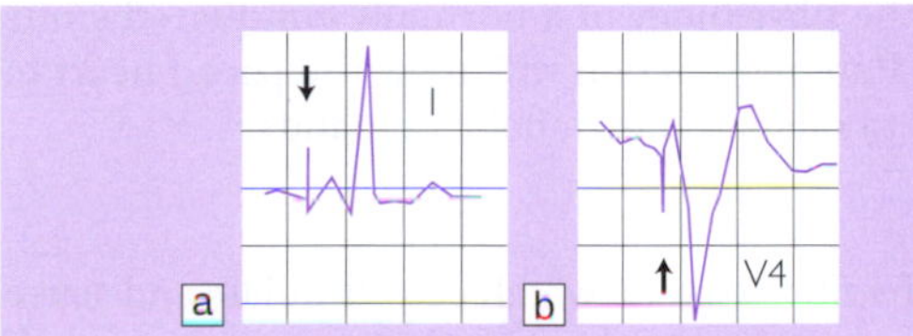


**Figure 47.28** Pacemaker ECG. (a) Atrial pacing producing a P wave and a normal QRS complex; (b) ventricular pacing from an ectopic site. The pacemaker spikes are arrowed.

safety. The threshold for triggering is increased by the extremes of acid–base disturbances and hyperkalaemia, and is decreased by hypercapnia and catecholamines.

The main functional division of types is between three modes of operation.

*Fixed rate (asynchronous)*

These produce a fixed frequency stimulus and have the advantage of simplicity. Their rate can sometimes be altered by the use of an external magnet. A theoretical disadvantage is the possibility of the pacemaker potential doing a sort of 'R-on-T' phenomenon and inducing VF. The energy required to do this is, however, much greater than that delivered by the pacemaker. Nevertheless, for this reason, a fixed-rate device is inserted only if the block is continuous. They are now rarely used.

*Demand (synchronous)*

These have an internal ability to suppress pacemaker activity if there is an adequate heart rate, but 'cut in' if the rate falls below a preset minimum. They remove any 'competition' between the heart and the electrode and, theoretically, remove the possibility of inducing VF. They are the most common type of permanent pacemaker.

*Sequential*

These are the most complex models with atrial and ventricular electrodes that try to stimulate physiological contraction and obtain the ventricular filling contribution of the atria. They are principally of the demand type (fired from P waves) and some can suppress ventricular pacing if the impulse from the atria is conducted normally. Others can be converted to fixed-rate ventricular pacemakers by an external magnet.

## Types of pacemakers

### *The NBG code*

The development of various atrial and ventricular pacing systems led to the adoption of an international identification code for the type of system. It was produced by a working party of the North American Society of Pacing and Electrophysiology (NASPE) and the British Pacing and Electrophysiology Group (BPEG), and is referred to as the NBG code. This is described in Table 47.3.

There are seven major modes of pacing:

- AAI: atrial pacing, atrial sensing, and inhibition of the pacemaker when an endogenous atrial event is sensed;
- VOO: asynchronous mode, ventricular pacing, no sensing, and no response;
- VAT: ventricular pacing, atrial sensing, and an atrial event triggers a ventricular stimulation by the pacemaker;
- VVI: most common mode of pacing to date. Ventricular pacing and ventricular sensing inhibit a pacemaker impulse;
- DVI: dual chamber sequential pacing with ventricular sensing so that a normally conducted impulse will inhibit the ventricular response. When the atrial impulse is not conducted the ventricle is paced after a preset AV delay;
- VDD: ventricular pacing with dual chamber sensing and a dual response. Atrial sensing triggers a ventricular stimulus when endogenous conduction fails and ventricular sensing inhibits a ventricular stimulus;
- DDD: dual chamber sequential pacing where both chambers are paced and both chambers are sensed. It responds to a sensed atrial beat by inhibiting the atrial pacemaker impulse and triggering a ventricular stimulus after an AV delay. When the atrial impulse is conducted normally to the ventricle, the ventricular pacing impulse is inhibited. This pacing mode shows the greatest flexibility when responding to the various changes in the patient's native rhythm.

### *Indications for pacing*

The development of more complex and more versatile pacemakers has led to a widening of indications for pacemaker implantation. Although anti-tachyarrhythmic pacemakers have been developed and are in clinical use, particularly for the treatment of atrial or supraventricular tachyarrhythmias, most pacemakers are implanted for the treatment of symptomatic bradycardias. Here they can either improve prognosis or symptomatology. There are over 30 ECG abnormalities, which can be responsible for symptomatic bradycardias and they can be summarized into five groups:

**Table 47.3 Pacemaker codes**

| First letter | Second letter | Third letter | Fourth letter | Fifth letter |
|---|---|---|---|---|
| Chamber paced | Chamber sensed | Response to sensing | Programmability | Anti-tachyarrhythmia |
| | | | Rate modulation | Function |
| O = none | O = none | O = none | O = none | O = none |
| A = atrium | A = atrium | T = triggered | P = simple programmable (up to two parameters) | P = pacing (anti-tachyarrhythmia) |
| V = ventricle | V = ventricle | I = inhibited | M = multiprogrammable | S = shock |
| D = dual (A + V) | D = dual (A + V) | D = dual (T + I) | C = communicating (telemetry) | D = dual (P + S) |
| | | | R = rate modulation | |

1. Sinus node disease (sinus bradycardia, sinus arrest, SA block): 25%.
2. AV block (intermittent second-degree AV block, complete with AV block): 42%.
3. Sinus node disease with AV block: 10%.
4. AF with AV block: 13%.
5. Carotid and vasovagal syndromes (cardioinhibitory type causing bradycardia): 10%.

### *Choice of pacemaker mode*

The working party report BPEG 1991 states that, when choosing a pacemaker mode for a patient, the ideal is production of a paced cardiac rhythm with as many features of normal sinus rhythm as possible. For each of the five groups of bradycardia, they give an optimal and an alternative. These are summarized in Table 47.4 and are described below.

#### *Sinus node disease*

In sinus node disease with normal AV conduction, pacing, and sensing, the atrium should be sufficient to restore the physiology of a normally conducted sinus rhythm. Rate modulation will allow the paced heart to respond to increased metabolic demands.

#### *AV block*

A dual chamber system, which can stimulate and sense both atrium and ventricle, will restore synchronized AV activity and therefore maintain the atrial contribution to the cardiac output.

#### *Sinus node disease with AV block*

Again a dual chamber system is needed to maintain AV synchronization. The diseased sinus node cannot be relied on to respond to metabolic challenges, therefore rate modulation is also needed.

#### *Atrial fibrillation with AV block*

Atrial tachycardia, atrial flutter, or AF might be picked up by an atrial sensing electrode and might lead to inappropriately high ventricular pacing rates. Atrial sensing is therefore contraindicated in these patients. Ventricular stimulation and sensing are recommended and adaptation to exercise might be achieved with rate modulation.

#### *Carotid sinus and vasovagal syndromes*

These patients show normal sinus rhythm with normal AV conduction at most times. Problems during exercise occur very rarely. Bradycardia attacks are accompanied by AV block in which situation both chambers need pacing.

The most common mode of pacing to date, VVI pacing, is also the cause of the most common complication of pacing – the *pacemaker syndrome*. This expresses itself as syncope or presyncope, dyspnoea, oedema, lethargy, and chest pain. The pacemaker syndrome occurs because of retrograde conduction from the ventricle through the AV node to the atrium. This retrograde conduction is intact in most patients with complete anterograde AV block. The loss of the atrial transport function, as well as the atrium contracting against a closed AV valve, results in high pulmonary pressures and a low cardiac output state. About 10% of patients suffer severe symptoms and

**Table 47.4 Recommended pacemaker modes[a]**

| Diagnosis | Optimal | Alternative |
|---|---|---|
| Sinus node disease | AAIR | AAI |
| AV block | DDD | VDD |
| Sinus node disease + AV block | DDDR<br>DDIR | DDD<br>DDI |
| Atrial fibrillation + AV block | VVIR | VVI |
| Carotid and vasovagal syndromes | DDI | DDD |

[a]definitions of pacemaker codes are given in Table 47.3.
AV, atrioventricular.

another 15% have a reduced quality of life caused by VVI pacing.

### *Malfunction*

Advancement in pacemaker technology has made modern pacemakers much more reliable but at the same time more complex. Malfunctions are infrequent in the hands of experienced pacemaker manufacturers, with an incidence of about 5%. They can be divided into malfunctions where any part of the pacemaker circuit is faulty or the pacemaker–patient interface is disturbed, and pseudomalfunctions that might be caused by inappropriate settings of the pacemaker or environmental interference with pacemaker function. Very often the patient is asymptomatic and the diagnosis can be made only via an ECG. Bradycardia and tachycardia might also be indicative of pacemaker malfunction.

The causes of pacemaker malfunction are summarized in Table 47.5.

## Anaesthetic management

Of patients with pacemakers, 50% have coronary artery disease, 20% have hypertension, and 10% have diabetes. They are often on several drugs with cardiovascular actions. For any operative procedure, underlying pathologies such as these need to be treated appropriately as described elsewhere in the book. In general, threshold changes caused by the anaesthetic agents themselves are not important.

When undertaking anaesthesia in a patient with a pacemaker, always ensure that a member of the cardiology team is aware of it and able to be contacted and respond urgently if difficulties arise with the pacing.

Remember that patients with pacemakers cannot produce a tachycardia to compensate for fluid loss or myocardial depression, which reduces stroke volume and therefore cardiac output. For the same reason avoid sudden postural changes.

The hospital environment, and in particular the operating room environment, presents a hazard for pacemaker patients in a number of ways: drugs, physiological changes with induction of anaesthesia and with surgery, and most of all electrical equipment attached to the patient.

**Table 47.5 Causes of pacemaker malfunction**

| |
|---|
| Failure to output |
| Failure to capture |
| Undersensing |
| Inappropriately high pacing rates |
| Environmental causes:<br>• electrocautery<br>• transthoracic defibrillation<br>• magnetic resonance imaging<br>• extracorporeal shock wave lithotripsy<br>• transcutaneous electrical nerve stimulation<br>• therapeutic radiation<br>• other causes |

### Preoperative pacemaker assessment

All pacemaker patients are given a European Pacemaker Identification Card which contains information about:

- make of pacemaker;
- pacemaker leads (unipolar or bipolar);
- date and place of implant;
- implanting cardiologist;
- pacing mode;
- pacing rate;
- reason for pacemaker implant and symptomatology;
- follow-up data.

The following questions should be considered:

- Is the patient pacemaker dependent? This is likely if the ECG shows that pacemaker spikes are present before each depolarization.
- Has the pacemaker been checked during the last year and found to operate without problems?
- Has the patient associated heart disease such as ischaemic heart disease or congestive heart failure? If so, is the patient's electrolyte status within normal limits? Hypokalaemia in particular can interfere with pacemaker function and cause arrhythmias.

- Is the pacemaker set in a rate-responsive mode? It is generally recommended to exclude the rate modulation function of a pacemaker by preoperative telemetric reprogramming. which can only be done by the ECG department.
- Does the patient experience any symptoms that might be the result of pacemaker malfunction? These might be syncope, dizziness, or heart failure which could be caused by true pacemaker malfunction or more commonly by the *pacemaker syndrome* in patients with VVI pacing. Palpitations and angina can indicate tachyarrhythmias resulting from either sick sinus syndrome or paced tachycardia. Any one of these symptoms should alert the anaesthetist to the possibility of intraoperative cardiovascular instability, and the patient should be referred to the cardiologists preoperatively for investigation of aetiology and for treatment.
- Do routine investigations such as an ECG or chest radiograph reveal any potential problems? As most pacemaker malfunctions are asymptomatic, careful study of the preoperative ECG is necessary to make sure that each pacemaker spike is followed by a depolarization. The ECG often provides the only indication of a potential problem. If in doubt, cardiology advice should be sought. The chest radiograph shows the position of the pulse generator, integrity of the leads, and electrode tip position, as well as heart size and pulmonary vasculature (see Figure 47.27).

Although in the past, it was recommended to apply a magnet above the pulse generator before the use of diathermy, this is potentially dangerous in some modern pacemakers. The application of a magnet can open the pacemaker for reprogramming and the additional use of diathermy can in turn induce phantom reprogramming of the pacemaker.

### Intraoperative considerations

The standards of good practice with respect to safety and monitoring (see Chapter 12) are assumed. Avoid all equipment or situations that might produce stray earth currents or microshock (see Chapters 38 and 39). Remember that a saline-filled central venous catheter can produce microshock.

Always use a means of monitoring the pulse (oesophageal stethoscope, precordial stethoscope, peripheral pulse oximeter) that is not obliterated by diathermy.

Have an isoprenaline infusion available in case the pacing fails. If there is any doubt about pacemaker function and/or if the procedure is anything but a minor procedure, insert a wide-bore central venous catheter which can accommodate a temporary pacing wire.

Induction of anaesthesia might enhance AV conduction and therefore increase the patient's heart rate or suppress AV conduction, leading to a continuously paced rhythm. Muscle contractions after suxamethonium can lead to oversensing and complete inhibition of pacemaker output. The use of suxamethonium should therefore be avoided if possible, particularly if the pacemaker is in a sensing mode with a unipolar system.

Halothane can raise the stimulation threshold and lead to a loss of capture. Its use is not recommended in pacemaker patients. The use of anaesthetic gases in the presence of hypoxia increases the potential for ectopic pacemakers within the heart and therefore the incidence of arrhythmias. They might also alter the sensing function of the pacemaker which could become competitive with the patient's spontaneous rhythm and so induce arrhythmias. Supraventricular arrhythmias should be treated with verapamil, and ventricular arrhythmias with lignocaine or amiodarone.

As described earlier, the main surgical hazard to pacemaker patients is the use of unipolar diathermy. Fixed-rate pacemakers are resistant to external interference and are usually unaffected by diathermy. Some demand pacemakers are very sensitive to interference by diathermy, which may cause VF or reprogramming. Alternatively, the diathermy signal can be interpreted as adequate myocardial complexes by the pacemaker with a resultant asystole. Be ready to treat VF. Do not apply the paddles over the pacemaker device.

The use of bipolar instead of unipolar diathermy, whenever possible, is strongly recommended. Should surgeon and anaesthetist agree that the use of unipolar diathermy is essential for a successful result of the operation, a number of precautions should be taken:

- Reprogramme the pacemaker preoperatively into an asynchronous mode.
- Place the diathermy and the ground plate as far away from the pacemaker as possible.
- Minimize diathermy to short bursts and lowest effective energy output.
- Make sure that the diathermy current from blade to plate flows at right angles to the pacemaker leads.
- Have isoprenaline available to start an infusion if the pacemaker output fails.
- Have an emergency transvenous pacing kit available and know how to use it.

### Postoperative considerations

The principles of good postoperative management should be followed as described in Chapter 5. In particular, care should be taken to minimize episodes of hypoxia for the usual reasons, but also because of its potential effect on pacemaker function.

Patients with pacemakers should be referred back postoperatively to the cardiology service for a check of their pacemaker function – settings and thresholds – especially if electrical devices have been used.

## FURTHER READING


Bennett DH. *Cardiac Arrhythmias*, 3rd edn. Bristol: Wright, 1989.

Deroy R, Graham TR. Pacemakers and anaesthesia. *Curr Anaesth Crit Care* 1995;**6**:171–179.

Feneck B, Duncan F. How to read the ECG – Parts 1 and 2. *Curr Anaesth Crit Care* 1994;**5**:223–30; 1995;**6**:29–40.

Hayashi Y, Kagawa K. Dysrhthmogenicity of anaesthetics. *Curr Anaesth Crit Care* 1998;**9**:312–17.

Nathanson MH, Gajraj NM. The peri-operative management of atrial fibrillation. *Anaesthesia* 1998;**53**:665–76.

# Chapter 48 The patient with ischaemic heart disease

G.M. Cooper and P. Hutton

This chapter describes the approach to patients with ischaemic heart disease (IHD) who are presenting for non-cardiac surgery. IHD is the most common cause of death in the developed world. It is present in a quarter of the elderly population in the UK.

## THE MANAGEMENT OF PERIOPERATIVE RISK

The numbers of interventional procedures such as coronary angioplasty and coronary artery grafting, both to treat the disease and to prevent its consequences continue to increase. Most anaesthetists will see patients who have IHD on a weekly basis, although neither of them may be aware of it because even advanced IHD can be asymptomatic. The possibility of serious but undiagnosed disease therefore makes it important to be aware of the main risk factors, even though up to half of the patients with known IHD may have no risk factors. Risk factors are listed in Table 48.1.

Patients with known IHD undergoing major non-cardiac surgery are at increased risk of cardiac complications, and those in whom ischaemia is readily inducible are at greatest risk. An infarct occurring up to 3 months before surgery carries a greater risk of reinfarction, but after 6 months the risk plateaus. The serious nature and potential cost of these complications emphasize the need for a perioperative strategy to minimize the risks. Although IHD is frequently encountered within the surgical population, surprisingly limited information is available on its optimal management and much has to be inferred from studies in other fields. Furthermore, the interventions themselves, which range from intensification of medical therapy to percutaneous transluminal coronary angioplasty and coronary artery bypass graft (CABG) surgery, carry an intrinsic risk. This risk can vary widely between patients and may exceed the risk of proceeding directly with non-cardiac surgery. Interventions will generally be appropriate only for those patients undergoing intraperitoneal, intrathoracic, vascular, or other major operations because the additional risk imparted by stable IHD is minimal after minor surgery.

Individual value judgements, taking into account the patient, his or her surgical problem, and the severity of the IHD, will need to be made. At present, there are few direct and clinical trial data upon which to base general guidelines. It is a situation in which clinical judgement remains the basis of therapy; the important thing is not to forget to consider the options. Another important point to bear in mind is that in patients who have previously undergone successful CABG surgery, perioperative mortality and long-term survival after major non-cardiac surgery approaches that of patients not known to have IHD.

Most patients with IHD awaiting major non-cardiac surgery will not have disease severe enough to warrant cardiac catheterization. Such patients have traditionally been managed in the perioperative period with increased vigilance and invasive monitoring, which has been continued postoperatively on either a high dependency or an intensive care unit. They may, however, benefit in addition from intensification of medical therapy. Of the evidence available the most compelling supports the perioperative use of β-adrenoceptor blockers. In the non-operative setting, β-adrenoceptor blockers reduce the size and mortality of myocardial infarction and atenolol increases event-free survival in patients with chronic stable angina. Given preoperatively, β-adrenoceptor blockers reduce the amount of perioperative silent myocardial ischaemia, which may be an aetiological factor in the development of perioperative infarction. Patients who suffer a perioperative infarction have a very poor long-term prognosis. Recently, atenolol administered throughout the perioperative period was shown to reduce mortality and improve cardiac event-free survival for up to 2 years after major non-cardiac surgery. Despite its relative ease of use and relatively low intrinsic risk, intensification of medical therapy has nevertheless not become a standard preoperative treatment. Beta-adrenoceptor blockade is of course negatively inotropic and must be used with great caution in patients with poor ventricular function.

Aspirin (see Table 48.1) has been clearly shown to play a major role in the primary and secondary prevention of myocardial infarction, and it also reduces mortality following infarction. Despite this, its potential role in reducing perioperative cardiac risk remains notably uninvestigated. Indeed aspirin is often withdrawn before major surgery at a time when platelet reactivity is likely to be increased. It is our current practice, in patients who are not already on low-dose therapy, to initiate its prescription (75–100 mg) in all at-risk groups, provided that it is not contraindicated. The debate with respect to local blocks is discussed in Chapter 15.

## DEFINITIONS

*Angina*

This is the pain felt when the oxygen supply to the myocardium is insufficient for its demands. In some patients, ischaemia is not accompanied by pain.

**Table 48.1 Causal and preventive risk factors for ischaemic heart disease (IHD)**

| Causal | Preventive |
|---|---|
| Family history | Low-dose aspirin |
| Cigarette smoking[a] | Oestrogen replacement therapy in women |
| Elevated cholesterol[a] | |
| Hypertension[a] | |
| Diabetes | |
| Obesity/physical inactivity | |

[a]Modification of these factors will reduce incidence of IHD.
Adapted from Hennekens CH. *Circulation* 1998;97:1095.

*Hypertrophy*

This is a physiological response of the ventricle to an increased workload. It is detectable electrocardiographically and by echocardiogram, but is not seen specifically on the chest radiograph. The increased muscle mass increases the overall oxygen demand and can thus precipitate features of coronary insufficiency.

*Ejection fraction*

This is the ratio of stroke volume to ventricular end-diastolic volume.

*Ventricular dilatation*

This occurs when the ventricle, because of intrinsic weakness or excessive workload, is unable to produce an adequate stroke volume without allowing an increase in end-diastolic volume. The ejection fraction is reduced and ventricular output depends heavily on adequate ventricular filling. It is seen by an increase in the size of the cardiac shadow on chest radiograph and is usually accompanied by the ECG changes of ventricular hypertrophy. Left ventricular failure causes breathlessness, orthopnoea, and paroxysmal nocturnal dyspnoea. Right ventricular failure produces raised central venous pressure, peripheral oedema, and ascites.

*Ventricular failure*

This is difficult to define, but can be described as that condition when ventricular output is able to match venous return only after a substantial increase in filling pressure has occurred.

## LEFT VENTRICULAR ISCHAEMIA

### Pathophysiology

The reader is also referred to Chapter 20. The distribution of the main coronary arteries is shown in Figure 48.1. They arborize on the surface of the heart to form a mass of smaller epicardial arteries, from which so-called 'B' branches perforate directly through the myocardium to reach the endocardium. The only collateral circulation exists at subendocardial level and becomes important if there is a blockage in an epicardial vessel (Figure 48.2). This arrangement has several consequences.

The intramural oxygen tension of the subendocardial muscle is normally significantly lower than that in subepicardial muscle. As a result of their length, the 'B' perforators are subject to torsion and pressure during muscular contraction. As the intravascular pressure develops during systole, there is a 'tissue' pressure, which by compression effectively halts flow in the subendocardial region. This results in most of the useful myocardial perfusion in the left ventricle occurring during diastole. Early diastolic relaxation is delayed if the myocardium is ischaemic.

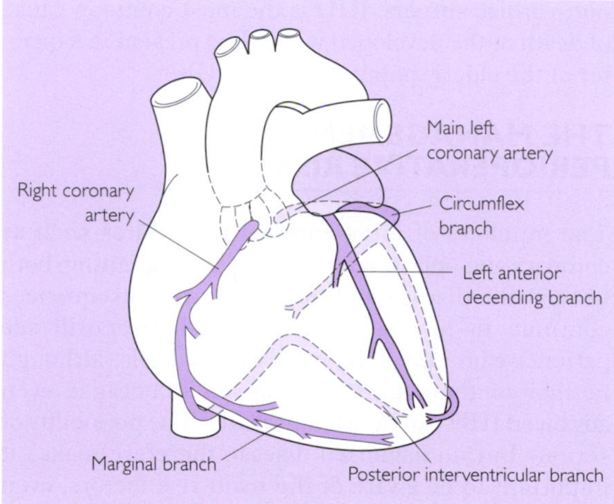


**Figure 48.1** The blood supply to the heart. (From Hutton P, Cooper G. *Guidelines in Clinical Anaesthesia*. Oxford: Blackwell Science, 1985.)

Even at low levels of activity, the heart extracts about three-quarters of the oxygen content of the blood delivered to it. Thus, an increased demand can be met only by increased supply rather than increased extraction. Although the exact mechanism of this is still debated, it is thought to be achieved in the healthy heart at the arteriolar and precapillary sphincter level. Such an increase is impossible in coronary arteries blocked by atheroma.

The main determinants of the oxygen requirement are the intraventricular systolic wall tension and compression (reflected by the systemic blood pressure), the heart rate, and myocardial contractility (influenced by the patient's own sympathetic outflow and by drugs). The effect of coronary arterial pressure on flow in health and disease is shown in Figure 48.3.

The factors that lead to relative ischaemia are summarized in Table 48.2.

A measure of myocardial oxygen demand can be approximated by the product of the systolic pressure (mmHg) and heart rate (beats/min). This is referred

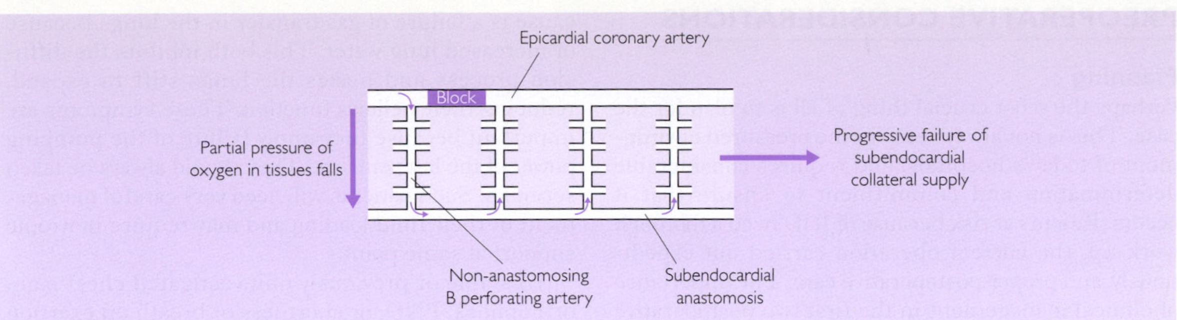


**Figure 48.2** Perfusion of the left ventricular wall. (From Hutton P, Cooper G. *Guidelines in Clinical Anaesthesia*. Oxford: Blackwell Science, 1985.)

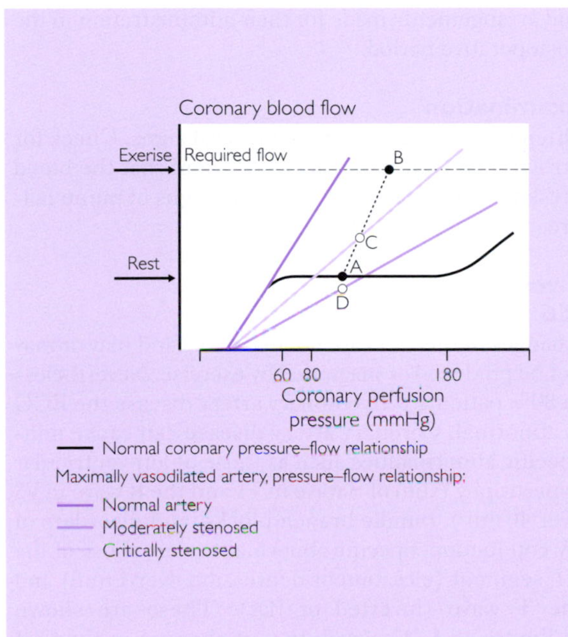


**Figure 48.3** Effect of mean coronary arterial pressure on flow. Coronary blood flow (black line) is maintained constant despite variations in perfusion pressure. At perfusion pressures below 60 mmHg coronary blood flow falls because the limit of coronary vasodilatation is reached. A maximally vasodilated coronary artery has a linear pressure–flow relationship as shown by the darkest green line. Stenoses of varying severity will alter the pressure–flow relationship of the dilated artery as shown by the green straight lines. At rest, an individual might have an artery flow at point A (perfusion pressure approximately 100 mmHg); with exercise the demand rises (dotted line) and flow increases to point B, within the capacity of a normal vessel to dilate. If the individual's coronary artery had a moderate stenosis, only point C could have been reached, which is less than the flow required, so ischaemia (angina) is produced. A critical stenosis may interfere with the delivery of the necessary resting flow (D) so ischaemia at rest ensues. (From Walker JM, Tan L-B. Cardiovascular disease. In: Souhami RL, Moxham J, eds. *Textbook of Medicine*, 3rd edn. Edinburgh: Churchill Livngstone, 1997.)

**Table 48.2 Causes of insufficient supply of oxygen to the myocardium**

| | |
|---|---|
| Low oxygen carriage per ml of blood | Hypoxia<br>Anaemia |
| Inability to perfuse main coronary arteries | Coronary artery thrombosis<br>Hypotension<br>Coronary artery spasm |
| Reduced coronary perfusion time | Tachycardia |
| Endocardial compression | Hypertension<br>Aortic stenosis |
| Increased metabolic demand | Hypertension<br>Tachycardia<br>Sympathetic drive<br>Sympathomimetic drugs<br>Catecholamines |

to as the 'rate pressure product'. Healthy adults can easily achieve levels over 20000. Its usefulness in anaesthesia is that patients known to have exercise-induced angina become symptomatic at approximately a constant value. Those who have exercise testing (ST segment depression of 0.1 mV is taken as significant) or stress echocardiography may have the figure recorded (or able to be calculated), in their notes. This can be taken as a guide to an acceptable upper limit of myocardial stress during anaesthesia.

## PREOPERATIVE CONSIDERATIONS

### Planning

Perhaps the most crucial thing of all is to plan for the case. This is not always easy in the pressured environment of today's hospitals, and requires considerable determination and commitment to ensure that it occurs. Patients at risk because of IHD need a thorough work-up, the correct operation carried out expeditiously, and proper postoperative care. The importance of clinical management in the first two postoperative days cannot be emphasized enough.

### History

IHD is usually well advanced when it declares itself clinically, and serious underlying disease (up to 70% stenosis of a major coronary artery) *may* be totally asymptomatic. Consequently, try to identify the risk factors listed in Table 48.1. Patients have two main symptoms: chest pain and breathlessness. Record the date of any known infarction and consider whether surgery is justified (see below).

Ask about the character, duration, site, and associated events of any chest pain, remembering that it may be the result of other causes. Anginal chest pain is typically central (with possible radiation to the left arm or neck), lasts between 5 and 15 min and is related to effort. More transient pain suggests oesophageal or musculoskeletal causes, whereas more prolonged pain suggests unstable angina or infarction. Anaesthetists should also distinguish between predictable angina of effort, which normally takes several minutes to come on, and that associated with emotion (anger, fear, pain), which comes on rapidly (in seconds). The latter is rare and is caused by coronary artery spasm. The differentiation is important because patients with stable angina of effort are predictable during surgery, provided that the heart rate and blood pressure are appropriately controlled, whereas those with angina of emotion are thought to be more prone to sudden episodes of ischaemia in response to sympathetic stimulation.

Unstable angina is defined as attacks that are increasingly frequent and/or prolonged, that occur at rest, or that are brought on by trivial provocation. It is a very serious finding. Such patients need immediate and intensive medical therapy and are at high risk of infarction. Other than surgery for urgent treatment of the condition itself, they should only ever be accepted for the surgery of life-threatening conditions. If anaesthesia cannot be avoided, it is best done in a hospital with facilities for cardiopulmonary bypass.

For those with stable symptoms determine the degree of exercise that invokes angina and how often it occurs. Remember that patients with peripheral vascular disease always have coronary artery disease but may not be able to exercise sufficiently to induce angina. Angina at rest, or on minimal exercise, is a bad prognostic sign. If the angina is becoming unstable and increasing in frequency and severity, myocardial infarction is a danger and any elective surgery should be delayed until the symptoms are stable.

Breathlessness not caused by intrinsic pulmonary disease is always a significant finding. It can present as orthopnoea, paroxysmal nocturnal dyspnoea (PND), or shortness of breath on (usually mild) exertion. The cause is a failure of gas transfer in the lungs because of increased lung water. This both inhibits the diffusion process and makes the lungs stiff to expand, reducing their bellows function. These symptoms are important because they imply failure of the pumping power of the left ventricle. They should always be taken seriously. Such patients will need very careful management of their fluid loading and may require inotropic support at some point.

Unstable or previously uninvestigated chest pain, orthopnoea, PND, or shortness of breath on exertion warrants a cardiological opinion before elective surgery.

The drug history is obviously of importance and hypotensives, β-adrenoceptor blockers, diuretics, and calcium antagonists should be continued until surgery, and arrangements made for their administration in the postoperative period.

### Examination

Often there are no abnormal physical signs. Check for arrhythmias, valvular heart lesions and that the blood pressure is normal, and look for any signs of pump failure.

### Investigations

*ECG*

Changes in the ECG are not invariable and may or may not be produced or magnified by exercise. Nevertheless in 80% patients with coronary artery disease the ECG is abnormal. Coronary artery disease can cause nonspecific abnormalities such as those of left ventricular hypertrophy (sum of S wave in V1 and the R wave in V5 over 40 mm), bundle branch blocks, and disorders of AV conduction. Specific abnormalities are those of the ST segment (elevation or depression over 1 mm) and the T wave (inverted or flat). These are shown in Figure 48.4. The evolution of changes in the first

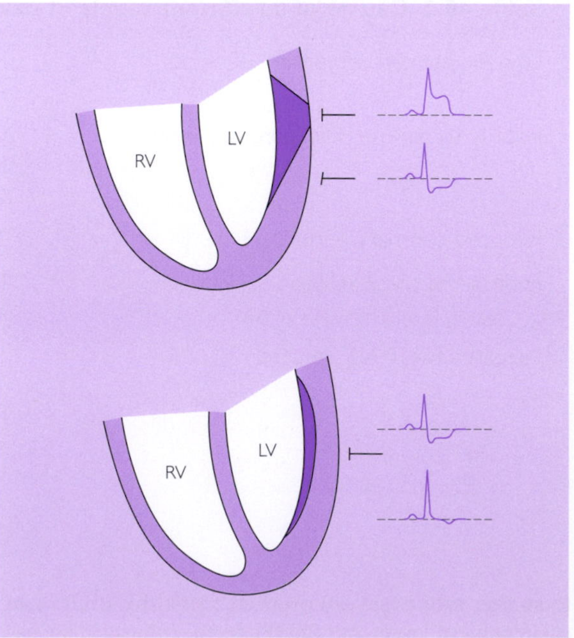


**Figure 48.4** Patterns of left ventricular ischaemia.(From Hutton P, Cooper G. *Guidelines in Clinical Anaesthesia*. Oxford: Blackwell Science, 1985.)

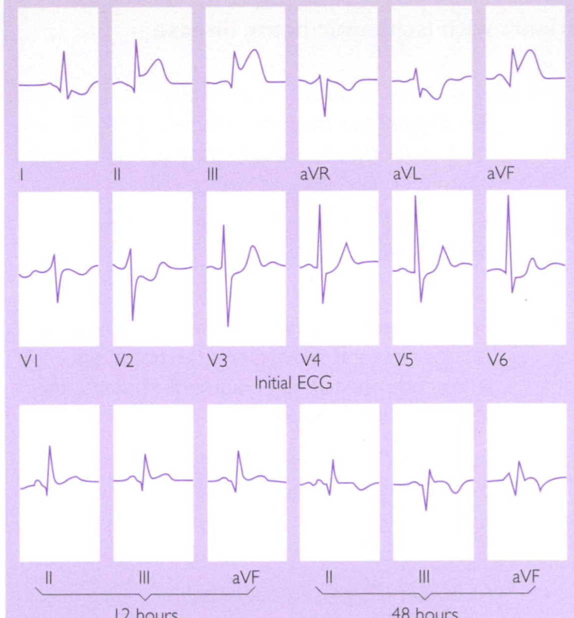


**Figure 48.5** Evolution of ECG change in an acute inferior infarction. Initially, there is marked ST segment elevation in II, III, and aVF, and reciprocal depression in V2–4. At 12 hours, a Q wave is developing in II, III, and aVF and the ST segment has returned to baseline. At 48 hours, the Q wave has deepened and broadened and there is T wave inversion. (From Walker JM, Tan L-B. Cardiovascular disease. In: Souhami RL, Moxham J, eds. *Textbook of Medicine* 3rd edn. Edinburgh: Churchill Livingstone, 1997.)

48 hours after a myocardial infarction is shown in Figure 48.5.

*Exercise ECG*

The magnitude and onset of ECG changes during exercise correlate with disease severity. ST depression that continues for a long time into the post-exercise period is associated with a poor prognosis. Some patient groups particularly at risk may not be able to exercise, e.g. those with aortic or peripheral vascular disease. In these patients, ambulatory ECG (Holter) monitoring may be useful in demonstrating ischaemic episodes.

*Chest radiograph*

This should be normal, but check for signs of an increase in the cardiothoracic ratio, pulmonary oedema, left ventricular failure, and aortic and mitral valve calcification.

*Full blood count*

The importance of the haemoglobin level is in maximizing oxygen delivery.

*Echocardiography*

This has revolutionized preoperative cardiological evaluation, because, unlike cardiac catheterization, it is non-invasive and has a very low complication rate. Right and left ventricular function can be assessed together with valve performance. Although left ventricular volumes tend to be under-estimated, they correlate well with ejection fractions. The presence of detrimental effects of myocardial ischaemia can be seen as segmental or regional abnormalities of wall motion, and are described qualitatively or quantitatively.

Although the ejection fraction depends on the amount of afterload and on the preload, in the stable patient (i.e. ordinary elective case, not suffering from fluid losses, etc.) a value of approximately 0.6 or over is normal and indicates good ventricular function. A false interpretation of a normal ejection fraction occurs if there is cardiac valvular incompetence. An ejection fraction of under 0.35 indicates a seriously compromised ventricle.

Early evaluation of stress echocardiography (performed after exercise or infusion of dipyramidole or dobutamine) suggests that it may be a particularly sensitive and specific test for predicting perioperative cardiac events. Further studies are awaited.

There is no doubt that, if IHD is picked up anew in the preoperative period, the combination of an exercise ECG and echocardiographic examination is the safest and quickest method of improving knowledge about the severity of the disease.

## PREOPERATIVE PREPARATION

A good outcome depends on team work of anaesthetists, cardiologists, and surgeons. The following questions should be considered before embarking on surgery:

- Is the operation necessary or appropriate? Would a less invasive procedure be suitable? An example would be an axillobifemoral graft instead of an aortobifemoral graft.
- Can the patient's status be improved? Examples discussed above include alterations to drug therapy for arrhythmias, heart failure or hypertension, insertion of pacemaker, coronary angioplasty, aortic valve replacement, or coronary artery grafting.
- Is it appropriate to delay surgery if there has been a recent infarct?
- Will an intensive or high dependency care bed be needed postoperatively and is there one available?

The anticipated risks should be discussed sympathetically with the patient (and relatives) and surgical colleagues.

### Premedication

The primary objective is to reduce anxiety and the consequent secretion of catecholamines. The choice of drugs is a personal one. Very anxious patients may also benefit from a benzodiazepine in the days approaching surgery. Take care to avoid excessive ventilatory depression from opioids or a tachycardia from atropine. If an opioid premedication is prescribed, ensure that the patient gets facemask oxygen at the same time.

Antianginal, antiarrhythmic, and antihypertensive medication should be continued up to and including the day of surgery. Ensure access to glyceryl trinitrate where appropriate.

Aspirin and heparin should be started before surgery to minimize the risk of coronary and deep vein thrombosis (see above and Chapter 1).

**Table 48.3 Suggested approach to monitoring patients with ischaemic heart disease**

| Patient description | Monitoring used |
|---|---|
| Stable cardiac symptoms, no signs of LVF or arrhythmias<br>Non-major surgery and major surgery lasting up to 1 h with low blood loss | Recommended minimal monitoring, (ECG, non-invasive blood pressure, capnograph and pulse oximeter)* |
| Stable cardiac symptoms; no signs of LVF or arrhythmias<br>Major surgery involving body cavities and significant fluid losses and replacement | As above (*) plus arterial line and multilumen central venous line |
| Now stable, but recent exacerbation of symptoms requiring modification to maintenance therapy for unavoidable minor surgery, e.g. setting Colles' fracture, cleaning and suturing of a deep flesh wound sustained while gardening | Recommended minimal monitoring, including capnograph and pulse oximeter but more advanced monitoring equipment immediately available. Take seriously! |
| Now stable, but recent exacerbation of cardiac symptoms requiring modification to maintenance therapy<br>Major surgery involving body cavities and significant fluid losses and replacement | As above (*) plus arterial line, multilumen central venous line and PA catheter sheath (**) |
| Patient with recent episode of cardiac instability, not fully resolved or evidence of ventricular failure<br>Major surgery involving body cavities and significant fluid losses and replacement | As above (**) plus PA catheter |

LVF, left ventricular failure; PA, pulmonary artery.

### Monitoring

The monitoring used in any particular case will almost certainly, in practice, depend on the combination of the anaesthetist, the surgeon, the patient, and the operative procedure. It is still an area where there is considerable individual variation in practice, and there are no definitive studies upon which to lay down incontrovertible rules. It is our view that monitoring needs to be applied in a balanced way, looking at the benefits and complications of each modality. There is no doubt that, on the one hand, failure to apply basic standards and, at the other extreme, to apply 'overkill' can both produce their own but different problems. A guide to the authors' current practice is given in Table 48.3. This does not cover all combinations of patient and operation, but it does indicate the philosophy of matching patients and procedures.

It would be normal practice, if an arterial line were indicated, to insert it before induction of anaesthesia. Central venous catheters would be placed only before induction if it were felt necessary to be able to inject drugs centrally during induction, or to obtain some preoperative measurements of cardiac output or pulmonary artery pressure. It is only rarely that patients are so sick that this has to be done. Details of the advantages and complications of monitoring equipment can be found in Chapter 12.

## INTRAOPERATIVE CONSIDERATIONS

There is still a widespread view, particularly held by some physicians and surgeons, that a regional or local block rather than a general anaesthetic is the technique of choice for patients with cardiovascular disease. There is no evidence to support this opinion, and it probably represents a hangover from the time when major surgery was done on spontaneously breathing subjects and patients died because they 'could not stand the anaesthetic'.

The following arguments summarize the 'pros and cons' of each technique. In some instances, it is possible to combine them and enjoy the benefits of both.

### Regional anaesthesia

#### *Advantages*

The main advantage is that profound anaesthesia is possible with a drug that is slowly absorbed into the general circulation, causing little systemic effect. Further advantages are that, if the patient is kept awake, there is no ventilatory depression in the immediate postoperative period, and complete analgesia abolishes the sympathetic response to pain. Peripheral nerve blocks or low spinal anaesthesia can be undertaken without undue risk even in the sickest cardiac patient, provided that the patient is not heavily anticoagulated.

#### *Disadvantages*

As a sole technique, regional blocks are suitable only for operations on the extremities or below the umbilicus. Spinal and epidural techniques, because of vasodilatation, drop the blood pressure and can easily provoke myocardial ischaemia. It is always important to have a dilute solution of vasopressor drawn up so that it can be titrated to just correct hypotension without overshooting. At the thoracic level, the sympathetic nerves to the heart (T2–T4) may be inactivated, resulting in a bradycardia that requires atropine or sympathomimetics. If the local anaesthetic is inadvertently administered intravenously, it can have catastrophic effects on a compromised cardiovascular system (see Chapter 15). This is particularly true of epidural, brachial plexus, and Bier's blocks where the quantity of local anaesthetic is large. Bupivacaine is more dangerous than lignocaine (lidocaine) because of its long duration of action and its affinity for the myocardium (as a result of high fat solubility).

The psychological stress of having the operation when awake may itself induce an angina attack. This is particularly likely to occur if sensitive patients are kept in an uncomfortable and embarrassing position in the presence of thoughtless operating room personnel, or if the patient has little confidence in the block.

If the anxious patient is given a sedative premedication or increments of intravenous sedatives intraoperatively, he or she may become confused and the airway can become difficult to control. Both can result partly from, or contribute to, hypoxia. This must be corrected immediately and may require general anaesthesia and intubation.

Regional blocks are no excuse for inadequate monitoring. If chosen, meticulous technique and anticipation of events are all important.

### General anaesthesia

#### *Advantages*

There is no question that monitoring and the discussion and treatment of abnormalities are easier when the patient is asleep. The surgeon is often more relaxed and, hopefully, able to work faster. The changes in heart rate and blood pressure are more easily controlled. The use of intermittent positive pressure ventilation (IPPV) ensures adequate oxygenation and allows control of the arterial $CO_2$ tension ($P\text{a}CO_2$).

#### *Disadvantages*

Induction of anaesthesia depresses the blood pressure by the direct pharmacological effect of the anaesthetic agents (both intravenous and inhalational) and by the loss of baroreflex control. Spontaneous breathing techniques with high concentrations and/or prolonged administration of a volatile agent as the main anaesthetic agent can produce marked hypercapnia and hypotension.

#### *Induction*

Preoxygenate to minimize the chance of hypoxia. Always have good intravenous access, monitor the ECG, and use a tipping trolley so that hypotension can be treated rapidly by increasing venous return. Many induction sequences are satisfactory. The key is to give the drugs slowly to minimize adverse cardiac effects. Etomidate is the induction agent that causes the least change in blood pressure and cardiac output. Thiopentone (thiopental), methohexitone (methohexital), and propofol all produce a moderate decrease in blood pressure (20–30%), but this can be lessened by using a small dose given slowly after fentanyl 4–5 μg/kg. Ketamine may produce undesirable hypertension and tachycardia.

In emergencies, suxamethonium will be necessary but may have the adverse side effect of bradycardia. Of the non-depolarizing neuromuscular blocking agents: vecuronium is particularly cardiovascularly stable; atracurium (in normal doses) and mivacurium have little effect on heart rate or blood pressure unless histamine is released; pancuronium produces a mild sympathomimetic effect; and rocuronium has a slight vagolytic effect resulting in a higher heart rate than if vecuronium was used. The truth is, however, that, used sensibly, all these agents can be satisfactory.

If intending to intubate, take over the ventilation when possible. Avoid obstructing the venous return by clumsy application of the facemask or by hand ventilation with high pressures.

Laryngoscopy and intubation under light anaesthesia stimulate the sympathetic nervous system such that hypertension and tachycardia may cause myocardial ischaemia. The main stimulus is that of laryngoscopy rather than passage of the tube into the trachea. Several techniques have been used to reduce the physiological response to this stretching of the pharynx. Local anaesthesia of the larynx and pharynx will prevent afferent neural input, but must, of course, itself be accomplished without laryngoscopy for the reflex not to occur. Laryngoscopy under deep anaesthesia, or after high-dose fentanyl, reduces the response because of central nervous depression. Beta-adrenoceptor blockade and nitroprusside do nothing to attenuate the neural or hormonal response, but prevent its peripheral actions from being apparent. Intravenous lignocaine has also been used, but its mode of action is not well defined.

By far the most convenient method of suppressing the response to laryngoscopy, if there are no contraindications, is pre-treatment with a β-adrenoceptor blocker. Those patients who are maintained on their pre-existing treatment with β-adrenoceptor blockers show markedly attenuated responses to laryngoscopy and intubation.

There is, however, no doubt that the best management is good oxygenation, careful use of drugs that one is familiar with, gentle laryngoscopy, and immediate response to adverse cardiovascular changes if they occur. Intubate gently without forcing the tube. Watch the ECG for signs of ischaemia and, if necessary, deepen anaesthesia.

Gentle insertion of a laryngeal mask does not induce marked cardiovascular responses and, hence, where there is not a risk of aspiration and, where the type of operation is suitable to manage the airway with a laryngeal mask, this has obvious advantages.

#### *Maintenance*

Spontaneous breathing using volatile agents may be suitable only for short operations because the anaesthetic dose necessary to achieve surgical anaesthesia causes an increase in $P\text{a}CO_2$ and depression of the myocardium.

Halothane primarily depresses myocardial contractility, producing a dose-dependent hypotension. As the anaesthetic progresses, some 'adaptation' or 'accommodation' occurs when the systemic vascular resistance decreases and cardiac output is maintained, thus supporting tissue oxygenation. It also depresses conduction at the sinoatrial node and may cause junctional rhythm; in addition, it precipitates ventricular ectopic activity, particularly in the presence of a high $P\text{a}CO_2$ or catecholamines.

Enflurane has similar depressant properties but a lower propensity to produce arrhythmias in the presence of hypercapnia and catecholamines.

Isoflurane reduces arterial pressure more than halothane does, but it does so by dilating resistance vessels rather than by impairing contractility. Cardiac output is well maintained and the threshold for arrhythmias in the presence of hypercapnia is higher than with halothane. Superficially, the properties of isoflurane would appear to make it the agent of choice for use with a compromised myocardium. Its ability to dilate the coronary arteries may, however, be reduced or absent in those branches whose lumina are reduced by disease. When the healthy adjacent vessels dilate, it has been suggested that there may be an inverse-steal effect shunting blood away from an area of borderline perfusion. This is, however, dependent on the amount given and is probably only significant at high levels.

Sevoflurane may have some advantages because haemodynamic control can be gained rapidly, it does not cause the 'coronary steal', and it sensitizes the myocardium less to the arrhythmic effects of catecholamines. Sound advice is to use a balanced technique with minimum alveolar concentration (MAC) values of any agent not going far above 1.0.

IPPV with a neuromuscular blocking agent, oxygen, nitrous oxide, and an opioid is the most commonly used maintenance technique. IPPV reverses the intrathoracic pressure gradients and reduces cardiac output by increasing pulmonary input impedance and causing asynchrony of the right and left ventricles. The usual acceptance of an inspiratory : expiratory ratio of 1 : 2 comes from early studies which demonstrated that, under these conditions, compensation for the inspiratory perturbations could be provided during expiration. The normal physiological response to IPPV is both peripheral and pulmonary venoconstriction, and this reduces the cyclical changes in venous return to the right ventricle and left atrium. This compensatory mechanism is reduced by poliomyelitis, polyneuritis, spinal cord transection, autonomic neuropathy, ganglion blockers, β-adrenoceptor blockers, general anaesthesia, and high spinal or epidural anaesthesia. Under general anaesthesia, the degree of vasoconstriction possible is inversely proportional to the depth of anaesthesia.

Minimize ventilator effects by adjusting to obtain low inflation pressures, a sufficient expiratory period, and an adequate circulating volume. Positive end-expiratory pressure (PEEP) should be used only to improve oxygenation in the presence of pulmonary pathology. Its action on the circulation depends on the degree to which its effect is transmitted to the blood vessels across the stiff, damaged lungs. The major acute cardiovascular effects of PEEP are to slow venous return to the right atrium and to raise the impedance to right ventricular ejection. The reduction in cardiac output can be catastrophic in the presence of hypovolaemia. Despite the improvement in oxygenation, because PEEP has such a deleterious effect on cardiac output, the concept of 'best PEEP' has arisen, which is the amount of PEEP at which the oxygen flux is maximal.

#### *Carbon dioxide*

The response to hypocapnia produced by hyperventilation is largely independent of the anaesthetic agent used. Typically, it results in a 0.5–1% reduction of cardiac output per mmHg (or per 0.13 kPa) reduction in $P\text{aCO}_2$ when the heart rate and mean arterial pressure are unchanged. There is also evidence that hypocapnia reduces coronary blood flow. The hyperdynamic response to hypercapnia under anaesthesia is strongly affected by sympathetic activity and is markedly reduced by effective β-adrenoceptor blockade. Without β-adrenoceptor blockade, cardiac output increases by approximately 1% per mmHg (or per 0.13 kPa) increase in $P\text{aCO}_2$ under halothane anaesthesia and up to 3.5% per mmHg (or per 0.13 kPa) in $P\text{aCO}_2$ with nitrous oxide and enflurane.

Consequently, it is sensible to ventilate to normocapnia or only to hyperventilate very mildly patients who have any form of cardiovascular disease because of the unpredictability and intensity of the response to changes in $P\text{aCO}_2$.

#### *Changes in blood pressure*

Treatment of intraoperative deviations of blood pressure and heart rate should be directed in a logical manner, based on the level of anaesthesia and on the changes seen in the systolic and diastolic pressure and, if measured, on the central venous pressure, the pulmonary artery wedge pressure, and the shape of the arterial pressure wave (Figure 48.6). Some guidelines are given in Table 48.4.

Many drugs are available for the management of the abnormalities listed in Table 48.4. Know the properties of a selection. A reasonable armoury would be halothane, isoflurane, sevoflurane, atropine, hydralazine, methoxamine, ephedrine, labetalol, esmolol, glyceryl trinitrate, sodium nitroprusside, dopamine, isoprenaline (isoproterenol), and calcium.

It is important to minimize heat loss during surgery because of the adverse effects of increased vascular resistance, left shift of the oxyhaemoglobin dissociation curve, and cardiac arrhythmias. There are also the added demands on the cardiovascular system during rewarming and greatly increased oxygen consumption during shivering. The importance of maintaining normothermia is described in more detail in Chapter 3.

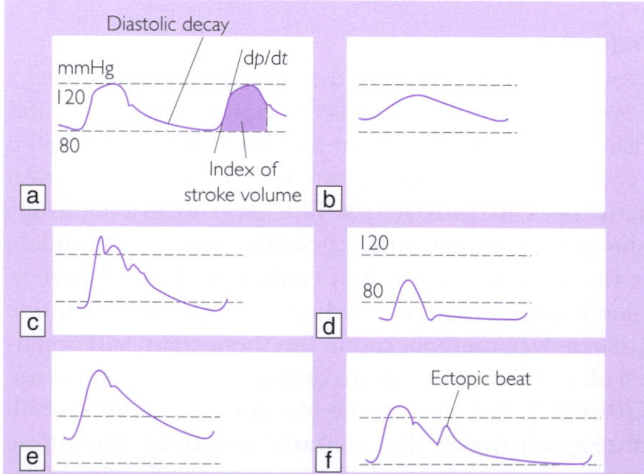


**Figure 48.6** Arterial pressure waves: (a) good trace; (b) damped trace: systolic reduced, diastolic increased, mean unchanged; (c) resonant trace: systolic increased, diastolic reduced, mean unchanged; (d) hypotension and peripheral vasodilatation; (e) hypertension and peripheral vasoconstriction; (f) beat from an ectopic focus. (From Hutton P, Cooper G. *Guidelines in Clinical Anaesthesia*. Oxford: Blackwell Science, 1985.)

**Table 48.4 Guide to logical treatment of cardiovascular abnormalities**

| Abnormality | Cause | Treatment |
|---|---|---|
| Tachycardia | Hypovolaemia | Check CVP; test infusion of fluid; give blood |
| | Light anaesthesia | Deepen anaesthesia |
| | Vasodilatation | Vasoconstrictors |
| | Above excluded, therefore sympathetic overactivity | β-Adrenoceptor blockade |
| Hypertension | Light anaesthesia | Deepen anaesthesia; increase analgesia |
| | Vasoconstriction | Vasodilate |
| | Hypercapnia | Increase ventilation |
| Hypotension | Fluid depleted | Give fluid |
| | Vasodilatation – especially epidural or spinal | Vasoconstrict |
| | Poor contractility | Inotropic support |
| | Fluid overload | Check CVP, vasodilate |
| | Hypoxia | 100% oxygen; check oxygen delivery to lungs |
| Bradycardia | Hypoxia | Correct cause. 100% oxygen |
| | Vagal stimulation | Give atropine |
| | Heart block | Give isoprenaline (isoproterenol); insert pacemaker |

CVP, central venous pressure.

## POSTOPERATIVE CONSIDERATIONS

Routine management is described in Chapter 5. Postoperatively, patients with known IHD need to go to an area where they can be cared for appropriately. A good operation is useless if followed by myocardial infarction. The proper setting can be anything from the normal healthy patient's passage first to recovery and then to the normal ward through to several days in the intensive care unit. The correct choice obviously depends on the individual situation. The important thing is that the choice is made positively and that the patient is not accommodated in what happens to be available by default at the end of the procedure.

Predictably, one of the major complications in the postoperative period is that of myocardial ischaemia. This is not surprising in view of the added myocardial work associated with stress and healing, and also the potential for hypoxaemia (see Chapter 5). Detection of ischaemia by clinical means is unreliable because postoperative myocardial ischaemia is silent in over 90% cases. The reason for the high incidence of silent ischaemia is not clear, but it may be that it is masked by factors present after surgery. These include surgical pain, residual anaesthetic agents, fluid balance abnormalities, and analgesic drugs. Postoperative patients are also approximately twice as likely to suffer painless myocardial infarction as are non-surgical patients.

The most important step in the management of postoperative ischaemia is to recognize those patients at risk and to prevent its occurrence. Twelve-lead ECG recording is of limited value in the detection of transient ischaemic episodes. Continuous ECG monitoring may be feasible only in a high dependency setting. Early treatment of haemodynamic abnormalities is vital, particularly the combination of hypertension and tachycardia. Myocardial ischaemia and infarction occur most commonly on the second and third postoperative days, which is when arterial oxygen saturation may still be low. The reason for this may be the return of rapid-eye-movement sleep and associated sleep apnoea and episodic desaturation, which had been suppressed by opioids on the first and second postoperative nights (see Chapter 5). Consequently, as a minimum, after major surgery these patients should be given supplementary oxygen for 24 hours, then overnight for two nights.

Careful analgesic regimens have been shown to reduce ischaemic episodes and help avoid hypertension and tachycardia. Equally, it is important to avoid ventilatory depression with hypercapnia and hypoxaemia.

Thought must be given to the maintenance of regular cardiovascular drug therapy, especially when the oral route is compromised. Intravenous, sublingual, and intramuscular and transdermal routes will still be available.

## FURTHER READING

Bennett DH. *Cardiac Arrhythmias*, 3rd edn. Bristol: Wright, 1989.

Deroy R, Graham TR. Pacemakers and anaesthesia. *Curr Anaesth Crit Care* 1995;**6**:171–9.

Feneck B, Duncan F. How to read the ECG – Parts 1 and 2. *Curr Anaesth Crit Care* 1994;**5**:223–30; 1995;**6**:29–40.

Hayashi Y, Kagawa K. Dysrhthmogenicity of anaesthetics. *Curr Anaesth Crit Care* 1998;**9**:312–17.

Nathanson MH, Gajraj NM. The peri-operative management of atrial fibrillation. *Anaesthesia* 1998;**53**:665–76.

# Chapter 49 The patient with hypertension

G.M. Cooper

Hypertension is an arbitrary term because there is no actual division between a normal and an abnormal blood pressure. It can be defined as an arterial blood pressure of more than 20% above baseline or increased above age-corrected limits. Most patients treated for essential hypertension are done so on the basis of a high diastolic pressure. A more flexible definition is 'the level of blood pressure above which investigation and treatment do more good than harm'. About 20% of the white adult population in Britain have blood pressures above 160/95 mmHg as measured by Korotkoff sounds. Of these, approximately 10% have a specific aetiological factor of:

- renal disease (chronic glomerulonephritis, chronic pyelonephritis, diabetic nephropathy, renal artery stenosis, polycystic kidney disease, polyarteritis nodosa);
- endocrine disease (Cushing's syndrome, Conn's syndrome, phaeochromocytoma, acromegaly);
- pregnancy (pre-eclampsia, eclampsia);
- oral contraceptive pill;
- coarctation of the aorta.

There has been debate for many years over the critical value of abnormality of blood pressure that should be treated. Guidelines are continually being updated, but the consensus now appears to be that even relatively minor degrees of hypertension are treated at younger ages. The recommendations of the British Hypertension Society at the time of writing are that specific antihypertensive treatment is indicated:

- Where the initial blood pressure is systolic ≥200 mmHg or diastolic ≥110 mmHg, treat if these values are confirmed on three separate occasions over 1–2 weeks (immediate treatment is needed if hypertension is severe or associated with heart failure).
- Where the initial blood pressure is systolic 160–199 mmHg or diastolic 90–109 mmHg (or when higher initial values fall to this range) one of the following courses of action should be taken:
  - if vascular complications or end-organ damage (e.g. left ventricular hypertrophy, renal impairment) or diabetes is present, treat if systolic ≥160 mmHg or diastolic ≥90 mmHg confirmed on at least three occasions;
  - if there are no vascular complications, no end-organ damage and no diabetes, repeat blood pressure measurements at monthly intervals for 3–6 months and treat if the average value during this period is systolic ≥ 160 mmHg or diastolic ≥ 100 mmHg;
  - if the average value is systolic < 160 mmHg and diastolic 90–99 mmHg, treatment may be withheld but continue to monitor; however, consider treatment if sustained in this range in older patients (over 60 years), and in those with a particularly high risk of cardiovascular complications (e.g. a strong family history).

The usual aim should be to reduce the systolic pressure to below 160 mmHg and the diastolic pressure to below 90 mmHg.

Malignant (or accelerated) hypertension or very severe hypertension (diastolic blood pressure > 140 mmHg) requires urgent treatment in hospital, but is not an indication for parenteral antihypertensive therapy. Normally treatment should be by mouth with a β-adrenoceptor blocker (atenolol or labetalol) or a calcium-channel blocker (nifedipine). Within the first 24 hours the diastolic blood pressure should be reduced to 100–110 mmHg. Over the next 2–3 days, blood pressure should be normalized by using β-adrenoceptor blockers, calcium-channel blockers, diuretics, vasodilators, or angiotensin-converting enzyme (ACE) inhibitors.

Patients with essential hypertension have cardiac outputs similar to those of normotensive patients. Their increased blood pressure is therefore caused by differences in vascular resistance. These are twofold:

1. The basic hypertensive lesion is a thickening of the arteriolar walls to such an extent that the luminar diameter is reduced, thereby increasing systemic vascular resistance (SVR). This also makes their SVR much more variable and sensitive to sympathetic stimulation, and produces a high diastolic pressure, because it is 'harder' for the blood in the major arteries to 'run off' peripherally during diastole.
2. Decreased vascular distensibility secondary to vessel wall degeneration causes an abrupt increase in aortic input impedance. This predominantly increases the systolic pressure.

High blood pressure does not usually cause symptoms. When a patient does present with symptoms, it indicates the presence of end-organ involvement in the nervous system, heart, or kidneys. Hypertension is the most significant risk factor in strokes and is as important as smoking in the aetiology of coronary artery disease. The level of risk has been found to correlate best with the systolic, rather than the diastolic, pressure, especially in very old people and in women, and particularly for cerebral events. Hypertension increases myocardial oxygen demand and decreases myocardial oxygen supply. The optimum functional value of blood pressure is 120/80 mmHg or less.

The complications of hypertension are:

- left ventricular failure;
- strokes and hypertensive encephalopathy;
- renal failure;
- myocardial infarction and ischaemia;
- retinopathy;
- complications of treatment (postural hypotension, hypokalaemia).

The hypertensive patient is at increased risk perioperatively of myocardial ischaemia and infarction, left ventricular failure, stroke, renal failure, and death. Greater intraoperative haemodynamic instability is also evident. These problems increase with the extent of the surgery.

## PREOPERATIVE ASSESSMENT

Only half of patients with hypertension will have been previously diagnosed as such. Most patients with hypertension are symptom-free and therefore it is often detected only by routine preoperative measurement of blood pressure. When a blood pressure is found to be elevated, several measurements should be recorded over a period of time (several hours) to determine the usual value and how much it varies.

Symptoms related to end-organ disease should be elicited, particularly myocardial ischaemia and cerebrovascular insufficiency. Unfortunately, a negative history is not always reassuring because a high proportion of hypertensive patients have silent myocardial ischaemia or infarction. The presence of any condition predisposing to hypertension should be checked for.

The nature and duration of antihypertensive therapy should be noted. It is helpful to ask whether there has been difficulty controlling the blood pressure and whether frequent changes to therapy have been necessary.

On examination any evidence of cardiomegaly or left ventricular failure should be sought. Fundoscopy revealing haemorrhages, exudates, or particularly papilloedema indicates severe hypertension.

### Investigations

#### *ECG*

One is looking particularly for evidence of left ventricular hypertrophy, conduction abnormalities, arrhythmias, and previous infarction.

#### *Echocardiography*

This is more sensitive in detecting the thickness and function of the left ventricular wall. The knowledge that this may confer may be especially helpful in managing anaesthesia and postoperative care for major surgery.

#### *Chest radiograph*

This is a useful baseline investigation before major surgery, looking for evidence of cardiomegaly or ventricular failure.

#### *Urea and electrolytes*

This is important to exclude early renal dysfunction. Hypokalaemia from diuretic therapy should be looked for.

#### *Full blood count*

The importance of this is in myocardial oxygenation, looking for anaemia or polycythaemia.

Serum glucose should be checked to exclude diabetes mellitus.

## PREOPERATIVE PREPARATION

Appropriate management of anaesthesia depends on the severity and degree of control of the hypertension, and the magnitude and urgency of surgery. There are many ways of achieving the same results, which depend on minimizing excessive hypertensive responses and any hypotension. This starts preoperatively and the approach used will almost certainly differ between individual anaesthetists. Guidelines are given here:

- *Patients with diastolic blood pressure > 110 mmHg for non-urgent surgery*: postpone surgery and refer for investigation and treatment.
- *Patients with systolic hypertension but diastolic pressure that is below normal or normal*: these patients are arteriosclerotic and are not true hypertensives. Surgery, urgent or non-urgent, can continue. Blood pressure changes during surgery will reflect the cardiac output and efforts should be directed towards keeping the blood pressure normal.
- *Patients with diastolic blood pressures of 95–110 mmHg for non-urgent surgery*: if there are no complications of hypertension, particularly left ventricular hypertrophy, surgery can probably continue safely. However, there is evidence that these patients benefit from preoperative treatment for 1–2 days with a $\beta_1$-adrenoceptor blocker (provided that there are no contraindications). Atenolol has the advantage of a long duration of action which will persist into the postoperative period. β-Adrenoceptor blockers are contraindicated in patients with asthma and chronic obstructive airway disease because even $\beta_1$-selective agents may provoke bronchospasm. A new agent, celiprolol, which has $\beta_2$-adrenoceptor agonist and $\beta_1$-and $\alpha_2$ blocking activity, may prove valuable in the perioperative period in these patients.
- *Patients with severe hypertension (diastolic pressures > 110 mmHg) or evidence of end-organ disease for urgent surgery*: here, there is little choice available to the anaesthetist. The only indications for a rapid reduction in blood pressure (over a period of less than 1 hour) are encephalopathy, acute left ventricular failure, and severe pre-eclampsia or eclampsia. Otherwise, the dangers of rapid blood pressure reduction (blindness and cerebral episodes) are outweighed by the benefits.
- *Patients with diastolic pressures of 80–95 mmHg*: proceed with care if there is no evidence of end-organ damage.

### *Premedication*

All regular antihypertensive medication *must* be continued up to the time of surgery, and thought should be given as to how these are to be given if the patient is unable to take oral medication postoperatively. An oral anxiolytic (e.g. temazepam) before elective surgery or a small dose of midazolam before emergency surgery is beneficial.

## INTRAOPERATIVE CONSIDERATIONS

The problems specific to hypertensive patients include the following:

- With all induction agents there is a greater fall in blood pressure in the hypertensive patient than there is in a normotensive patient. There is advantage in giving an opioid intravenously, in a dose appropriate to the duration of surgery, before the induction agent. This allows a reduction in the dose of induction agent required and also suppresses an exaggerated hypertensive response to laryngoscopy and intubation (and also extubation). An alternative approach to the short-lived bursts of intense adrenergic stimulation at laryngoscopy is intravenous esmolol, which has a short half-life. Thought should also be given to whether the use of a laryngeal mask, thus avoiding laryngoscopy, is appropriate for the surgical procedure.
- There is also an exaggerated response to surgical stimulation which, like that to intubation, can result in hypertension, tachycardia, arrhythmias, and myocardial ischaemia. Adequate analgesia is essential. The short-acting analgesic agent, remifentanil, may prove to have a valuable role in allowing variable and rapid control of analgesia during surgery, although care will be needed to ensure that adequate other analgesia is provided postoperatively.
- High left ventricular pressures and tachycardias increase myocardial oxygen consumption and can produce subendocardial ischaemia. This highlights the importance of continuous ECG and arterial pressure monitoring during induction, throughout surgery, and postoperatively.
- Patients receiving antihypertensive therapy that depletes norepinephrine (noradrenaline) storage in sympathetic nerve endings (e.g. guanethidine, bethanidine, debrisoquine) are very sensitive to exogenous catecholamines or direct β-adrenoceptor stimulants.
- The most common spontaneous arrhythmia during surgery is the conversion from sinus to junctional rhythm, which is associated with abrupt hypotension. This occurs most readily in the presence of hypercapnia and volatile agents.
- Atropine may cause a tachycardia leading to ischaemia. It may be preferable to use glycopyrrolate when reversing neuromuscular blockade.
- Spinal anaesthesia (except very low blocks) may result in abrupt hypotension and dangerous bradycardias in untreated or poorly controlled hypertensive patients. Epidural blockade, either alone or in conjunction with general anaesthesia, produces more gradual haemodynamic changes in well-controlled hypertensive patients. Significant hypotension from both these causes needs careful reversal by the titration of intravenous fluids and vasoconstrictors (see Chapter 15).

The approach to hypertensive episodes during and after surgery should follow logical steps (see also Table 48.4). First, check that anaesthesia is not too light, that there is no hypoxia or hypercapnia, and that the patient is not overtransfused. If pharmacological intervention is indicated, the diastolic pressure and heart rate may influence the choice of agent. In diastolic hypertension, incremental hydralazine or infusion of glyceryl trinitrate or nitroprusside may be useful. Provided that there is no evidence of conduction defects or pump failure, systolic hypertension with tachycardia may be controlled by increasing the concentration of volatile agent or by β-adrenoceptor blockade. Alternatively, combined α- and β-adrenoceptor blockade with labetalol by infusion can achieve both objectives.

## POSTOPERATIVE CARE

Adverse cardiac outcomes after non-cardiac surgery can be reduced by early detection and aggressive management of excessive myocardial oxygen demand or inadequate supply. This implies that monitoring and therapy need to be continued into the postoperative period. Oxygen therapy is always indicated. Good postoperative analgesia is important, as is the absence of ventilatory depression (see Chapter 5). Non-steroidal anti-inflammatory drugs may be best avoided because of their ability to precipitate renal failure in this vulnerable group of patients. This is especially so in patients receiving ACE inhibitors (see Chapters 5 and 20).

## FURTHER READING


Boldt J. Peri-operative hypertension and its treatment with intravenous agents. In: Skarvan K, ed. *Arterial Hypertension. Baillière's Clin Anaesthesiol* 1997;**11**:759–80.

Hansson L. The benefits of lowering elevated blood pressure: a critical review of studies of cardiovascular morbidity and mortality in hypertension. *J Hypertension* 1996;**14**:537–44.

Howell S, Foex P. Pathophysiology of arterial hypertension: implications in surgical patients. In: Skarvan K, ed. *Arterial Hypertension. Baillière's Clin Anaesthesiol* 1997;**11**:795–813.

Nahar T, Devereux RB. Hypertension, cardiac hypertrophy and the effects of anaesthesia. In: Skarvan K, ed. *Arterial Hypertension. Baillière's Clin Anaesthesiol* 1997;**11**:675–703.

Priebe H-J. Impact of systemic hypertension on peri-operative morbidity and mortality. In: Skarvan K, ed. *Arterial Hypertension. Baillière's Clin Anaesthesiol* 1997;**11**:781–94.

Prys-Roberts C. Anaesthesia and hypertension. *Br J Anaesth* 1984;**56**:711–24.

# Chapter 50 The patient with valvular heart disease

P. Hutton

For many years the most common cause of acquired valvular heart disease has been chronic rheumatic endocarditis. Its majority position is gradually being eroded (especially in mitral incompetence) as the incidence of rheumatic fever falls and the number of survivors from myocardial infarction and congenital heart disease rises. When resulting from rheumatic endocarditis, the mitral valve is affected in 80% of cases, the aortic valve in 45%, the tricuspid valve in 10%, and the pulmonary valve in 1%. Forty-five percent of cases have mitral valve disease alone. This implies that, in rheumatic heart disease, almost all aortic valve disease coexists with mitral valve disease.

It must be emphasized that the anaesthetic management of these cases can, on occasion, create unexpected intraoperative falls in cardiac output and episodes of myocardial ischaemia. For all but patients with minor degrees of dysfunction, *an experienced anaesthetist is needed.* It is always very helpful to discuss the management of patients with established disease with a cardiologist. Existing catheter studies and echocardiograms may supply important data about the resting pressures in the chambers of the heart and about the contractile nature of the myocardium.

This chapter assumes basic good standards of care as described in the first section of this book.

## PROPHYLAXIS AGAINST ENDOCARDITIS

Subacute bacterial endocarditis (SBE) occurs in people with pre-existing heart disease, especially those who have valves that are abnormal or are damaged by rheumatic fever. Prosthetic heart valves, a ventricular septal defect, and a patent ductus arteriosus also predispose to endocarditis, but an atrial septal defect does so only rarely. The bacteraemia may arise from poor dental hygiene (refer to dentist) or from the operative site (e.g. teeth, bowel, urinary tract). There is still controversy over the best prophylactic regimen but the following are guidelines.

- *Patients with valvular heart disease:* intravenous amoxycillin (1 g) at induction followed by oral amoxycillin 6 hours later; or, oral amoxycillin (3 g) 4 hours before surgery followed by oral amoxycillin (3 g) as soon as possible after the procedure; or, oral amoxycillin (3 g) plus oral probenecid (1 g) 4 hours before surgery.
- *Patients with prosthetic heart valves or who have had endocarditis:* intravenous amoxycillin (1 g) plus intravenous gentamicin (120 mg) at induction of anaesthesia followed by oral amoxycillin (500 mg) 6 hours later.
- *Patients who are penicillin sensitive or who have had penicillin in the previous month:* intravenous vancomycin (1 g) over at least 100 minutes followed by intravenous gentamicin (120 mg) at induction; or, intravenous teicoplanin (400 mg) plus gentamicin (120 mg) at induction of anaesthesia; or, clindamycin (300 mg) over at least 10 minutes at induction of anaesthesia then oral or intravenous clindamycin (150 mg) 6 hours later.

## PATIENTS WITH PROSTHETIC VALVES

Although a prosthetic valve corrects the direction and ease of blood flow, it does not immediately correct the consequent left or right ventricular hypertrophy that has occurred. Replacement of a diseased valve does, however, produce an early improvement in 90% of surviving patients and over a period of 2–5 years radiological signs of cardiomegaly and pulmonary arterial hypertension gradually decrease. Management is that of the residual ventricular condition. On auscultation, the prosthetic valve can be heard clicking. The appearance of prosthetic valves on a chest radiograph is shown in Figure 50.1.

Patients are often on anticoagulants to prevent embolization. Treat them as described for mitral stenosis. Antibiotic prophylaxis is essential. Unless there are strong indications, do not use a pulmonary artery (PA) catheter because of the increased risk of SBE.

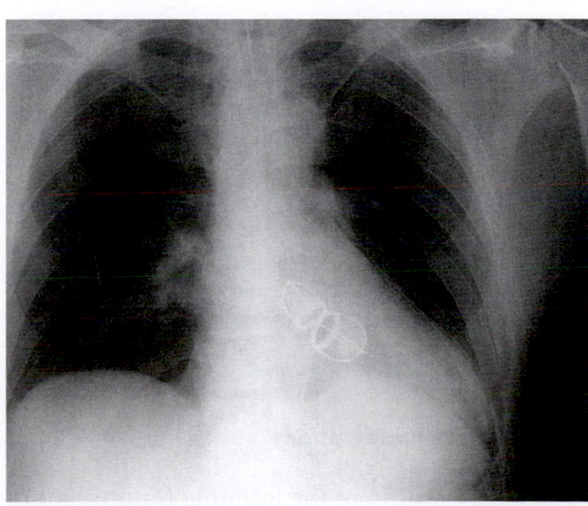

**Figure 50.1** Chest radiograph showing prosthetic aortic and mitral valves.

## MITRAL VALVE DISEASE

### Mitral stenosis

#### *Aetiology*

Over 99% of cases of mitral stenosis follow rheumatic fever, but approximately one-third of cases give no history of rheumatic fever or chorea, the acute illness being mild and escaping notice. The disease is four times more common in women than in men and the latent period from infection to presentation may be 20 years. A tiny percentage of cases are congenital, the valve being replaced by a rudimentary perforated diaphragm.

#### *Physiology*

The basic problem in pure mitral stenosis is that the left ventricle cannot fill easily during diastole because of the progressive decrease in mitral valve area. The severity of the disease parallels the reduction in orifice size. The normal cross-sectional area of the valve is over 4 $cm^2$. There are few symptoms until it has fallen to 2.5 $cm^2$, and the obstruction is severe when it is below 1.0 $cm^2$.

The narrowed mitral valve restricts flow between the left atrium and ventricle and the degree of stenosis thus limits both early diastolic ventricular filling and the contribution of atrial contraction to late diastolic ventricular filling. Increased left atrial work inevitably causes dilatation of the thin-walled left atrium. In the presence of atrial fibrillation (AF), the uncoordinated movements of the left atrium no longer contribute to the late diastolic phase, reducing end-diastolic ventricular volume by up to 30%. The sudden onset of AF may be the cause of an abrupt fall in cardiac output and rise in left atrial pressure.

In addition to the above changes, 25% of patients with severe mitral stenosis develop an active constriction of the pulmonary arterioles which eventually become hypertrophied. Pulmonary hypertension occurs, the changes become irreversible, the right ventricle hypertrophies, and there may be functional pulmonary and tricuspid valve incompetence. Congestive heart failure finally supervenes. Why only 25% of severe cases react in this way is unknown.

Some patients with severe mitral stenosis also have contraction abnormalities of the left ventricle as a result of fusion of the chordae tendinae (when measured their ejection fraction is low) and cannot increase their stroke volume even if an induced bradycardia allows greater ventricular filling time.

This account of mitral valve stenosis concentrates on the moderate or serious case. There are of course many patients with mild degrees of stenosis who live a normal life, have a good exercise tolerance, and even undertake some sporting activities. For them to undergo minor surgery, it is important not to over-react with the extent of precautions and invasive monitoring. They can be managed satisfactorily by the application of good practice using standard techniques and non-invasive monitoring.

#### *Preoperative considerations*

*History*

Symptoms result from the following features of the disease:

- Increased pulmonary venous pressure causes dyspnoea on exertion, orthopnoea, paroxysmal nocturnal dyspnoea (PND), haemoptysis, and recurrent bronchitis.
- AF (present in 40%) causes palpitations, heart failure if there is a rapid ventricular rate, and symptoms of embolization (in 10%). Patients may be on anticoagulants and/or digoxin.
- Reactive pulmonary hypertension results in a low cardiac output, causing fatigue, ankle swelling, symptoms of deep vein thrombosis, and pulmonary embolism.
- Bacterial endocarditis is uncommon in *pure* mitral stenosis.
- The patient may have angina.

The important feature of the history is to gauge the progression of the disease by the patient's exercise tolerance and the drugs needed to control symptoms. The onset of dyspnoea with exercise is the best guide to severity. Dyspnoea when walking slowly on the flat, and episodes of PND, imply a resting left atrial pressure of 15–20 mmHg and a pressure gradient between atrium and ventricle persisting throughout diastole.

*Examination*

The findings depend on whether or not there is accompanying pulmonary hypertension.

In the uncomplicated case, the facies are normal, the brachial pulse is normal or rather small in amplitude, the jugular venous pressure (JVP) is normal, and there is a tapping apex beat, sometimes with an apical diastolic thrill. The two easiest things to hear on auscultation are a loud first sound and a rumbling mid- or late diastolic murmur localized to the apex (Figure 50.2). The opening snap and presystolic crescendo (only in sinus rhythm) are heard less frequently. The murmur can be accentuated by exercising the patient and rolling him or her onto the left side. If there are any signs of left ventricular failure (LVF), suspect another added problem (mitral incompetence, aortic stenosis, or coronary artery disease).

With raised pulmonary vascular resistance, there are mitral facies, cool extremities, peripheral cyanosis, a small amplitude pulse, a large 'a' wave on the JVP if in sinus rhythm, and a parasternal heave. There may also be signs of tricuspid incompetence if the right ventricle has dilated.

*Investigations*

*ECG*

This may show 'P' pulmonale or mitrale (see Figure 47.7), AF (see Figure 47.14), right axis deviation (see

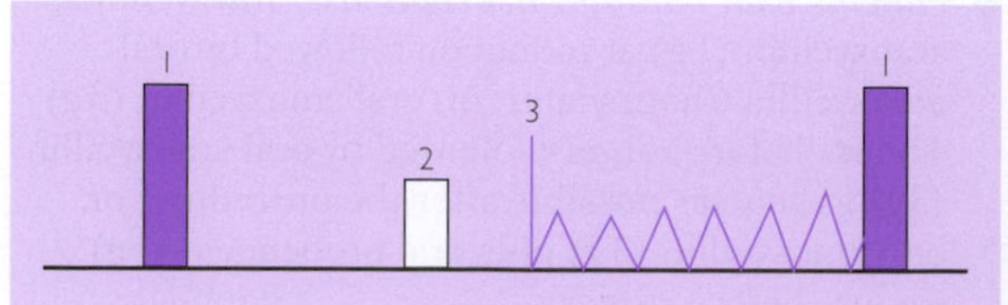


**Figure 50.2** Mitral stenosis: I, first heart sound; 2, second heart sound; 3, opening snap.

Figure 47.6), or right bundle branch block (see Figure 47.22).

*Chest radiograph*
This shows left atrial enlargement (indents the oesophagus on an oblique film), upper venous congestion, and Kerley B lines above the costophrenic angles. The mitral valve may be calcified. The aorta is small.

*Echocardiography*
This has proved to be of outstanding value in the assessment of the state of the mitral valve, by quantifying the decreased closure rate of the valve leaflets.

*Cardiac catheterization*
This records data about the normal pulmonary artery wedge pressure (PAWP) and left atrial pressure (LAP).

*Prothrombin time*
Many patients are anticoagulated and the prothrombin ratio should be approximately twice normal.

*Anaesthetic considerations*
Consider whether the patient can be improved preoperatively with drug adjustments and the merits of prophylactic digitalization. Antibiotic prophylaxis is essential.

Those patients who are on anticoagulants must be discussed with the surgeon. There is no doubt that reducing the prothrombin time to normal increases the chance of systemic embolism. It is also true that, unless it is an arterial operation or one resulting in considerable diffuse tissue damage, good surgical technique can provide perfectly adequate haemostasis when the prothrombin time is two to three times normal. Thus, a reasonable way to proceed is to keep the patient on warfarin, maintain the prothrombin time at the patient's usual level, and have fresh frozen plasma ready to return the clotting mechanism to normal if postoperative oozing or bruising becomes a problem. The half-life of warfarin is prolonged by metronidazole.

If the oral route will be unavailable postoperatively, the patient is best changed to heparin before operation.

The complications of mitral stenosis, which might occur in the perioperative period, are acute pulmonary oedema, right ventricular failure (RVF), AF, systemic embolism, SBE, and bronchitis or pneumonia. In addition, pulmonary vasoconstriction is increased by hypoxia and acidosis.

The main areas of anaesthetic consideration for these patients are heart rate, rhythm, and preload:

- Tachycardia:
  - decreases ventricular filling time and thus cardiac output;
  - increases LAP and may result in pulmonary oedema.
- Severe bradycardia:
  - causes a decrease in cardiac output as a result of a fixed stroke volume.
- AF:
  - will further decrease ventricular filling by up to 30%;
  - is often long standing and, if so, will be highly resistant to cardioversion;
  - may be induced by anaesthesia;
  - digitalis toxicity may be induced by intraoperative hypokalaemia.
- Pre-load:
  - hypovolaemia may result in reduced LAP, and thus a further reduction in left ventricular filling;
  - excessive fluid load may result in pulmonary oedema.
- After-load:
  - a large decrease in systemic vascular resistance (SVR) may cause severe hypotension as a result of a relatively fixed cardiac output.

Remember that the cardiac output cannot be effectively increased. It may be markedly decreased by reduced ventricular filling (tachycardia, reduced LAP, vasodilatation, hypovolaemia, myocardial depression), which should be avoided. A raised LAP can precipitate pulmonary oedema.

A sudden intraoperative fall in the cardiac output may be caused by the loss of the atrial contribution to ventricular filling from junctional rhythm (see Figure 47.15) or AF (see Figure 47.14). AF occurring anew intraoperatively is probably best converted immediately by direct current (DC) shock while under anaesthesia.

To prevent a tachycardia at induction, give a sympathetic explanation (to allay anxiety) and do not use atropine. Traditionally, heavy premedication is recommended but take care to avoid ventilatory depression. Continue digoxin.

Induction of anaesthesia, however it is carried out, needs to be done slowly, and time needs to be given for the drugs to act if there is a low cardiac output. Whatever type of monitoring is in place, the important principle is to observe the readings and to respond appropriately.

During maintenance of anaesthesia, high concentrations of inhalational agents such as halothane or enflurane may be dangerous in patients with a severely decreased resting cardiac output. Nitrous oxide ($N_2O$) has been shown to increase pulmonary vascular resistance and, as patients with mitral stenosis have an increased alveolar–arterial oxygen gradient, it is sensible to set the $N_2O$ : oxygen ratio at 1 : 1, and add an intravenous agent or a low concentration of a volatile anaesthetic to ensure hypnosis. It is a mistake to maintain patients at an insufficient depth of anaesthesia; adequate anaesthesia is essential to blunt the sympathetic responses to laryngoscopy and surgery, all of which result in tachycardia.

Fluid management is not easy. On the one hand, the patient requires a sufficiently high circulating fluid volume to produce the necessary right and left atrial pressures. On the other hand, there is decreased compliance of the pulmonary vasculature because of existing over-distension. Consequently, the pulmonary venous pressure and the PAWP rise more than expected with a given increase in circulating fluid volume. This pulmonary fluid overload can be delivered by exogenous fluids, a head-down posture, or peripheral vasoconstriction. The major problems occur in the spontaneously breathing patient or on the cessation of intermittent positive pressure ventilation, when pulmonary oedema may develop quickly.

The problem of fluid loading can be difficult with the use of spinal or regional anaesthesia (contraindicated if on anticoagulants) when an upper limit of 1 litre should probably be set. If peripheral vasoconstriction is necessary, methoxamine is the best choice because, despite increasing pulmonary resistance, it does not increase the heart rate.

The extent of invasive monitoring used depends on the combination of patient and operation. With mild or moderate stenosis and no reactive pulmonary hypertension, changes in the JVP will parallel changes in LAP. With severe stenosis, advanced pulmonary hypertension, and an expectation of large fluid shifts, a PA catheter is invaluable. Intraoperatively it is sensible to maintain the preoperative central venous pressure (CVP) or PAWP as the minimum for adequate left ventricular filling.

Monitoring must be continued (invasive or not) into the postoperative period and the patient nursed in a high dependency area. Postoperatively, a PA catheter may warn of impending pulmonary oedema.

Take care not to produce a tachycardia when reversing neuromuscular blockade. Glycopyrrolate is preferable to atropine or, alternatively, atracurium, vecuronium, or rocuronium could be allowed to wear off spontaneously.

Patients with mitral stenosis have decreased lung compliance, increased airway resistance, an elevated alveolar–arterial oxygen gradient, and an increased work of breathing. A period of postoperative ventilation (to normocapnia) may well be required before the patient is strong enough to sustain adequate spontaneous ventilation.

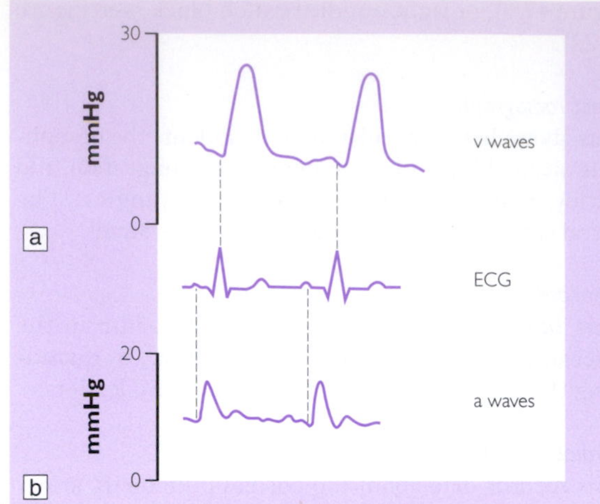


**Figure 50.3** Abnormal pulmonary artery occlusion pressure traces. (a) Giant v waves are traditionally explained as being the result of initial regurgitation but are an inconstant feature of this condition. (b) a waves result from energetic atrial systole in sinus rhythm in the presence of mitral stenosis or left ventricular hypertrophy.

## Mitral incompetence

### *Aetiology*

About half of the cases of mitral incompetence are associated with rheumatic mitral stenosis. Other causes are papillary muscle dysfunction (after infarction), ventricular dilatation from LVF (not common because the valve ring is strong), and ruptured or useless chordae tendinae. Rarer causes are congenital malformations and cardiomyopathies. Functional incompetence from a dilated valve ring may disappear after LVF is treated.

### *Physiology*

There is a regurgitant jet throughout systole and the forward flow into the aorta represents only a part of the stroke volume. This produces a large V wave on a PA-catheter trace (Figure 50.3). During diastole, there is an increased flow across the valve because the regurgitated fluid is returned with the normal pulmonary venous flow. A regurgitant fraction (RF) of 0.3 or less indicates mild mitral incompetence, and a RF of over 0.6 indicates severe regurgitation.

As the left ventricle can eject into either of two outflow paths, the impedances of each will determine the ratio of volume delivery. The volume injected into the aorta is very dependent on SVR and capable of manipulation by vasoconstricting and vasodilating drugs (e.g. methoxamine and sodium nitroprusside).

The left ventricle hypertrophies. The left atrium expands and dilates to accommodate the extra volume load. ('P' mitrale may be seen if in sinus rhythm – see Figure 47.7.) The majority of left ventricular activity is used for fibre shortening and the tension requirements for intraventricular pressure development are little different from normal. As myocardial oxygen consumption is related to left ventricular wall tension, heart rate, and contractility, and as fibre shortening itself consumes little oxygen, the energy costs of mitral incompetence are modest. Consequently, angina in patients with pure mitral incompetence is not common unless there is coexisting coronary disease.

AF is the usual end-point for severe cases. The atrial contribution to ventricular filling is, however, relatively unimportant and a deterioration from sinus rhythm to AF may cause little change in cardiac output. The mean LAP is much lower than in mitral stenosis, making pulmonary and right ventricular involvement less common. The symptom-free period is longer than in mitral stenosis, but the downhill course is rapid after the onset of LVF.

The exception to this sequence of events is those patients who develop acute mitral incompetence after myocardial infarction. They develop pulmonary oedema early because the regurgitant jet cannot be accommodated by a normally sized left atrium.

Patients who have mitral regurgitation caused by papillary muscle failure secondary to coronary artery disease, including those with recent myocardial infarction, are unlikely to be encountered outside specialist cardiac units and require extremely careful anaesthesia by experienced personnel.

'Mitral valve prolapse', which has many aetiologies, refers to a 'floppy valve' that leaks after leaflet closure because the ventricular pressure forces the edges of the valve apart and they 'prolapse' into the left atrium. Most patients are symptom-free and remain stable. Others progress chronically with a course similar to that of rheumatic valve disease.

### Preoperative considerations

#### History

There are no symptoms unless heart failure or other complications occur. The incidence of SBE is higher than with any other valve lesion, and it has been claimed that systemic embolism is no less common than in mitral stenosis. Consequently, a proportion of these patients is maintained on warfarin, especially if there is a coincident mitral stenosis.

When LVF does occur, there is usually sufficient pulmonary congestion to produce mixed symptomatology of fatigue, dyspnoea on exertion, orthopnoea, PND, haemoptysis, and recurrent bronchitis.

The progression of disease is gauged on exertional dyspnoea, and the presence and onset of LVF. The symptoms of RVF occur later. Patients are often on digoxin and diuretics.

#### Examination

The pulse wave feels normal. The apex beat is vigorous and displaced beyond the normal limits. The murmur is pansystolic and maximal at the apex (Figure 50.4) radiating to the axilla. A diastolic flow murmur in severe incompetence may be functional and does not necessarily imply stenosis. In serious disease, AF may be present. Later there are signs of first LVF and then RVF. Arterial hypertension increases regurgitant flow and may precipitate LVF.

#### Investigations

##### ECG

This can show 'P' mitrale (see Figure 47.7), AF (see Figure 47.14), or left ventricular hypertrophy (see Chapter 47).

##### Chest radiograph

This shows a large left atrium and enlarged ventricles.

##### Echocardiography

This demonstrates an increased diastolic closure rate in contrast to the reduction found in mitral stenosis. The echocardiogram also differentiates the thickened mitral cusps of chronic rheumatic endocarditis from the thin cusps of mitral incompetence, as a result of rupture of the chordae tendinae or of mitral valve prolapse.

##### Cardiac catheterization

This can give data on the normal PAWP and LAP.

#### Anaesthetic considerations

The anaesthetic aim for these patients is centred around the maintenance of forward flow through the left ventricle.

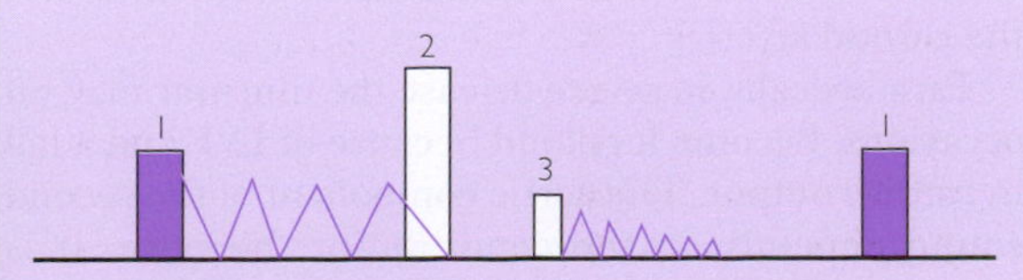


**Figure 50.4** Mitral incompetence: 1, first heart sound; 2, second heart sound; 3, third heart sound and functional mitral valve flow murmur.

- Systemic vascular resistance: an increased SVR increases the tendency for regurgitative flow, and vasoconstrictors should be avoided.
- Preload: a large increase in preload causes atrial distension and the relatively rapid onset of pulmonary oedema.
- Heart rate: bradycardia reduces ventricular filling and increases the degree of regurgitation; however, a moderate tachycardia increases forward flow and is thus preferable.

The same principles of good practice apply as for patients with mitral stenosis. As stated in that section, this account is aimed at the moderate or severe case. Minor degrees of incompetence should be taken on their merits and the anaesthetic procedure should not be made unduly complex without good reason.

*All* patients need prophylaxis against endocarditis. Those with only minor symptoms and a good exercise tolerance (e.g. can carry shopping upstairs with little discomfort) tolerate anaesthesia and surgery well. Those on anticoagulants should be treated as described in 'mitral stenosis'.

With a symptomatic patient, always consider whether or not he or she could be improved by manipulating his or her drugs, and get a cardiological opinion. Induction should be carried out slowly, applying the principles described in Chapter 2.

Maintenance using high concentrations of volatile agents is contraindicated. Patients with symptomatic mitral incompetence already have depressed contractility and the negative inotropic effects of these agents more than offsets the mild decrease in SVR, and there is a fall in stroke volume and cardiac output.

Although bradycardias are to be avoided because there is no reserve stroke volume to compensate for the reduced heart rate, mild tachycardias are tolerated well because there is no obstruction to diastolic left ventricular filling. It is important to sustain an adequately high LAP by careful fluid management, otherwise the left ventricular end-diastolic pressure (LVEDP) falls to below the 'knee' of the ventricular performance curve, causing a sudden drop in stroke work. The dilated, hypertrophied ventricle of mitral incompetence is very sensitive to this mechanism and must be maintained at a sufficient degree of 'stretch' for its optimum contractile performance.

Anything that increases SVR (sympathetic vasoconstriction, drugs) leads to an increased portion of stroke volume returning through the mitral valve, and a consequent fall in cardiac output. This problem (outside cardiac units) potentially occurs chiefly with light anaesthesia and the excessive use of vasoconstrictors during regional block. The solutions are to deepen anaesthesia, to give a generous fluid load during regional block, and to give vasoconstrictors only in tiny incremental doses. If the cardiac output is low because of unexplained peripheral vasoconstriction (this can occur in the postoperative period), the afterload can be reduced by sodium nitroprusside in doses that do not produce a marked tachycardia.

The atrial contribution to ventricular filling is less important in patients with mitral regurgitation, and loss of sinus rhythm does not have the catastrophic effect seen in mitral stenosis. Atrial tachyarrhythmias form part of the natural history of the disease and it is worthwhile, before anaesthesia, discussing with a cardiologist the wisdom of attempting reversal.

As usual, the extent of invasive monitoring depends on the particular combination of patient and operation. As a result of the propensity to SBE, catheters should not be placed in the major vessels without very good reason. The features of the PA trace in mitral incompetence have already been described (see Figure 50.3). The advantages that a PA catheter gives are the ability to maintain the PAWP at any desired level, and an indication of whether a fall in PAWP is caused by hypovolaemia or RVF. It can also be used to measure the effectiveness of treatments to increase the cardiac output by inducing falls in peripheral vascular resistance. The major advantages are obviously found in those patients with moderate or severe disease who experience large fluid shifts.

If the patient has disease that is sufficiently severe and chronic to induce pulmonary vascular changes, then refer to the relevant sections in the anaesthetic management of mitral stenosis.

### Mixed mitral valve disease

Optimum management is by a compromise of the above, depending on whether stenosis or incompetence is the dominant feature. This is ultimately decided by catheterization but, if the pulse volume is small and there is no left ventricular hypertrophy (in the absence of failure), stenosis is more likely to be dominant.

## AORTIC VALVE DISEASE

### Aortic stenosis

#### *Aetiology*

If the valvular stenosis is of rheumatic origin (presents at < 60 years of age), almost all cases are accompanied by mitral valve disease. Other causes are a congenital bicuspid valve (presents at about 60 years) and degenerative calcification (presents at > 70 years). Functional, but not true, valvular stenoses at either the supravalvular or subvalvular level are very rare.

#### *Physiology*

The progressive resistance to flow through the aortic valve causes the pressure during systole to be higher in the left ventricle than in the aorta. The valve must be narrowed to about 25% of its normal area (approximately 3 cm$^2$) before there is a significant obstruction to flow across it. This results in massive hypertrophy of the left ventricle, which becomes stiff and increasingly dependent on the contribution from left atrial contraction for adequate filling. Ventricular dilatation occurs when there is associated regurgitation or when the ventricle fails. Angina may occur without significant coronary artery disease because of the precarious balance of oxygen supply and demand.

Several factors conspire to attenuate the delivery of oxygen to the subendocardium. The stiff hypertrophied ventricle has impaired relaxation during early diastole, and the metabolic demands of the muscle are increased because of the high intraventricular pressures. The thickness of the ventricular wall may itself hinder an adequate oxygen flux from the distributing epicardial arteries to the subendocardial capillaries (see Figure 48.2). It is thought that the relative failure of nitroglycerin to relieve the angina of aortic stenosis is because the coronary vessels are already maximally dilated under 'resting' conditions. Any reduction in the duration of diastole (e.g. from exercise, emotion) quickly induces angina and, on some occasions, acute LVF or ventricular fibrillation (VF), which results in sudden death. Coronary filling is further impeded because the diseased valve distorts the aortic architecture and reduces the back flow of blood from the mainstream into the coronary sinuses. The coronary ostia can also be narrowed by calcification.

Optimum performance of the left ventricle becomes very dependent on the correct heart rate. The rate must be low enough to allow adequate time for filling and ejection, but not so slow that the end-diastolic volume is excessive. Gradually, higher filling pressures are needed to maintain cardiac output and the ventricle becomes increasingly dependent on atrial contraction to ensure diastolic filling, and the atrium (in sinus rhythm) contributes up to 40% of left ventricular end-diastolic volume (LVEDV) in aortic stenosis, compared with 10–15% in normal individuals. This can produce 'a' waves on a PA catheter trace (see Figure 50.3). The sudden onset of AF (which suggests a rheumatic aetiology) can precipitate a major fall in cardiac output. For obvious reasons, coincident coronary artery disease is a serious added risk factor for these patients.

With aortic stenosis there is usually a long (can be up to 30–50 years or more) asymptomatic period, and sudden death may be the first presenting feature. The most common symptoms are angina, syncope, dyspnoea, and arrhythmias. When symptoms finally occur, the stenosis is severe, their significance is ominous, and if the stenosis is not surgically corrected death occurs within a few years.

#### *Preoperative considerations*

##### *History*

There may be no symptoms or there can be angina (see above), dizziness and syncope on effort (low cardiac output), and dyspnoea (LVF). Once diagnosed, the patient is usually on digoxin and diuretics. Nitroglycerin is not as effective in relieving ischaemic pain as usual (see above) and may be harmful in reducing diastolic pressure. A sudden deterioration in exercise tolerance is often the result of the onset of AF.

##### *Examination*

There is a slow rising, slow falling, regular, low-amplitude plateau pulse. AF usually indicates associated mitral valve disease. There is a sustained and heaving apex beat. Signs of LVF may be present. There may be a thrill over the aortic area (Figure 50.5) which radiates to the neck. A loud midsystolic ejection murmur is heard in the aortic area which may be transmitted to the carotid arteries.

Paradoxically, in severe disease the murmur may, on occasions, become less loud because of LVF and a fall in cardiac output. The aortic component of the second sound depends on the condition of the valve. It is normal or increased in some cases of congenital origin and soft or absent with a rigid calcified valve. The ejection click has a similar variable presence. In severe stenosis, left ventricular systole is considerably prolonged and, in expiration, the aortic sound falls well behind the pulmonary sound – the so-called reversed split (Figure 50.5).

*Investigations*

*ECG*

This may show signs of left ventricular hypertrophy (see Chapter 47). If not present, the stenosis is not severe.

*Chest radiograph*

There is no increase in transverse cardiac diameter unless ventricular dilatation has occurred. The aorta is small but there can be post-stenotic dilatation and a calcified valve.

*Echocardiography*

This demonstrates the restricted movements of the aortic valve, and indicates calcification to a sufficient degree of accuracy for an accurate diagnosis of the severity to be made.

*Cardiac catheterization*

This is used to determine the true severity of the condition.

*Anaesthetic considerations*

In severe cases requiring major elective surgery, discuss the possibility of a valve replacement with cardiology colleagues. If this is not decided on, the physiological objective is to maintain the basic haemodynamic state by carefully managing heart rate, filling pressure, and systemic blood pressure.

*Hypotension*

This is very dangerous. It may be caused by low cardiac output, hypovolaemia, or vasodilatation. It implies that a ventricle generating high intracavity pressures is being perfused by a low-pressure arterial system. Immediate correction with an α-adrenoceptor agonist is needed, while the underlying cause is remedied.

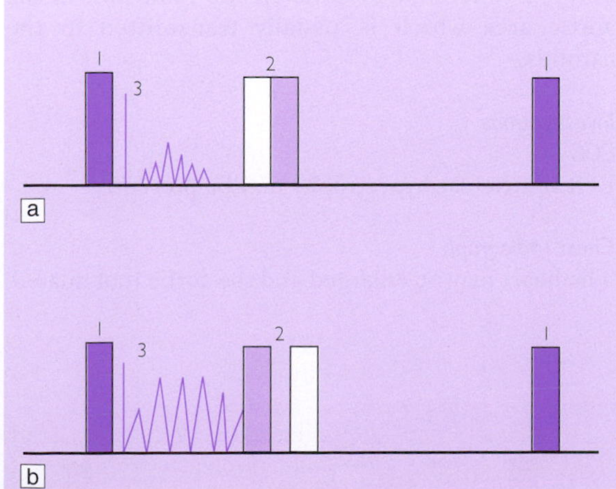


**Figure 50.5** Aortic stenosis: I, first heart sound; 2, second heart sound; 3, ejection click. (a) In mild stenosis the pulmonary component of the second sound follows the aortic component. (b) In moderate-to-severe stenosis the aortic sound follows the pulmonary sound in expiration.

*Tachycardia*

This too is dangerous. It produces myocardial ischaemia (sometimes acute LVF) and reduces cardiac output by increasing dynamic impedance of stenosis. Treat the cause (light anaesthesia, hypovolaemia, etc.). *Do not* give β-adrenoceptor blockers. Persistent arrhythmias affecting cardiac output may need DC countershock.

*Bradycardia*

Moderate degrees are tolerated. It reduces the dynamic impedance of stenosis. If severe with very low diastolic pressures, use tiny doses of glycopyrrolate and avoid over-correction at all costs.

*Preload on left ventricle*

This must be maintained to ensure filling of the hypertrophied ventricle.

*Afterload on left ventricle*

Changes have little effect on valve pressure gradient and hence LV load, but the effect on systemic blood pressure in the aortic root significantly changes coronary perfusion.

Always prescribe prophylaxis against SBE.

Patients with a symptomatic aortic stenosis are *always serious anaesthetic risks* because the disease is advanced at presentation. If discovered incidentally during the preoperative assessment for elective surgery, it is *essential* to involve a cardiologist. Valve replacement may be recommended and if so should be done before elective surgery for other conditions.

Possible complications during the operative and postoperative period include spontaneous VF, acute LVF, and myocardial ischaemia.

The single most important variable to monitor until well into the recovery period is probably the direct arterial pressure. Not only does it give beat-by-beat information about the diastolic pressure (which is critical for coronary perfusion), but the diastolic decay also indicates how fast the stroke volume 'runs off' peripherally.

*Hypotension is the greatest danger* to adequate coronary perfusion and may be caused by peripheral vasodilatation, fluid loss, an inadequate stroke volume against a high peripheral resistance, or LVF. Combined readings from arterial and PA catheters are invaluable in identifying the cause in severe cases.

The need for a PA catheter depends on the severity of aortic valve disease, the magnitude of surgery, and the expected changes in fluid balance. A PA catheter should not be inserted without good reason because its passage through the right ventricle can induce ventricular tachycardia. The problems of interpretation of the trace have already been discussed (see Figure 50.3).

Induction of anaesthesia must follow preoxygenation and must be accomplished slowly. Hypotension after induction must be treated promptly with vasoconstrictors (e.g. metaraminol in 0.5-mg increments) to ensure minimum reduction in coronary artery flow.

High concentrations of volatile agents such as halothane and enflurane not only depress contractility (with little reduction in SVR) with consequent systemic hypotension, but also depress the sinoatrial node automatically and may cause a junctional rhythm to emerge.

In patients with severe aortic stenosis, the maintenance of sinus rhythm is paramount because the left ventricle is dependent on a properly timed atrial systole to achieve an adequate end-diastolic volume. Disturbances of rhythm should first be avoided (check the serum electrolytes and the dose of drugs, especially digoxin) and then treated by removal of the cause (e.g. switch off halothane, withdraw the CVP line), before resorting to drug therapy or DC shock. Calcium is probably the drug of choice for persistent junctional rhythm. Sinus tachycardia frequently produces myocardial ischaemia and can be caused by an insufficient depth of anaesthesia or insufficient circulating fluid volume. If there is no response after correction of these, then use *small* incremental doses of a β-adrenoceptor blocker. This is potentially dangerous, however, because the patient may be depending on endogenous β-adrenoceptor stimulation to maintain myocardial contractility.

Severe bradycardia can also be detrimental because, if the ventricle is working to its maximum possible pressure before the bradycardia, no increase in cardiac output is possible. Heart rates of less than 45–50 beats/min associated with a low diastolic blood pressure and myocardial ischaemia can be treated by tiny doses of atropine, but at all costs avoid the 'overshoot' to a tachycardia.

More complex arrhythmias, unresponsive to simple measures, are probably best managed by DC shock.

At the end of surgery either allow time for the neuromuscular blocking drugs to be metabolized or use glycopyrrolate (*not* atropine) to prevent the bradycardia of neostigmine.

If cardiac arrest occurs, rapid resolution is essential because only *internal* cardiac massage is really effective as a result of the valvular stenosis.

## Aortic regurgitation

### Aetiology

The most common causes are rheumatic valve disease (chronic) and infective endocarditis (acute). It may also be associated with chest trauma, connective tissue disorders (Marfan's syndrome), congenital lesions, (bicuspid valve), and aneurysms of the ascending aorta. Syphilis as a cause is now rare. The importance of hypertensive dilatation of the aortic root is disputed.

### Physiology

During diastole, the left ventricle is filled by blood leaking back through the aortic valve, in addition to that received from the left atrium. Consequently, only a proportion of that blood ejected into the aorta actually reaches the periphery. Patients with an RF over 0.6 of the stroke volume have severe disease. The left ventricle dilates and hypertrophies to accommodate the increased diastolic volume. The duration of ventricular systole is normal and hence there is rapid forward flow, causing a functional systolic murmur.

The determinants of the regurgitant volume are the valve area available for back flow, the diastolic pressure gradient from aorta to left ventricle, and the time available. Thus, the regurgitant fraction is increased by a high SVR, a compliant left ventricle, and a bradycardia. The influence of heart rate on controlling regurgitation is said to explain the clinical observation that patients with aortic regurgitation often tolerate exercise well but may develop symptoms of pulmonary congestion at rest.

Mild or moderate degrees of back flow are tolerated well and are compatible with a normal life. The life expectancy of patients with significant aortic regurgitation is about 9 years. Sudden death is rare. If the disease progresses, LVF or ischaemic heart disease occurs which leads to death in 1–3 years. In acute aortic regurgitation (secondary to dissection or acute SBE), which is rare outside specialist units, there is a sudden volume overload of the left ventricle with a dramatic rise in the LVEDP. Ventricular dilatation enlarges the mitral valve annulus, resulting in functional mitral regurgitation. Pulmonary oedema is marked and refractory. This is a very serious condition.

### Preoperative considerations

#### History

The patient may be completely symptom-free until features of LVF (dyspnoea on exertion, orthopnoea, PND) or angina occur. Sudden death is rare. They are often on digoxin and diuretics. RVF secondary to LVF is a late event.

#### Examination

The pulse is regular, of large amplitude (high systolic, low diastolic), and collapsing. If AF is present, suspect mitral involvement. The left ventricle is large, and the apex beat hyperdynamic and displaced beyond the normal limits.

There is abrupt distension and collapse of the carotid arteries (Corrigan's sign), and there is said to be capillary pulsation in the nail beds.

Aortic regurgitation may be difficult to detect on auscultation. Classically, there is a blowing, high-pitched murmur beginning immediately after the second sound, loudest at the third and fourth left intercostal spaces close to the sternum (Figure 50.6). Sometimes it can be elicited only at the end of expiration when the patient leans forward. There is almost always a functional systolic ejection murmur in the aortic area which is usually transmitted to the carotids.

#### Investigations

##### ECG

Left ventricular hypertrophy may be present.

##### Chest radiograph

The heart may be enlarged and the aortic root dilated.

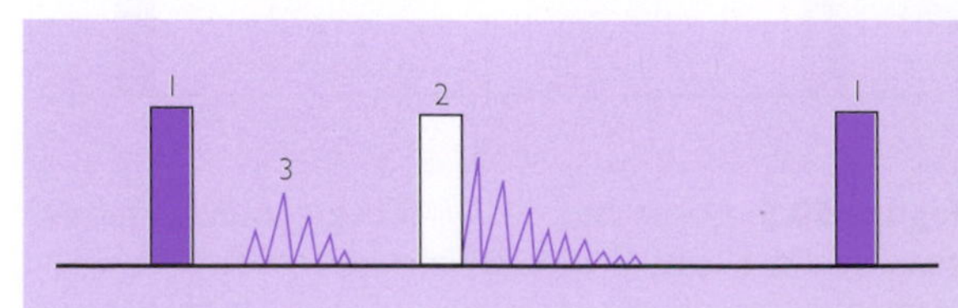


**Figure 50.6** Aortic regurgitation: 1, first heart sound; 2, second heart sound; 3, added functional flow murmur.

*Echocardiography*
This will detect the movement of the aortic valve leaflets and eliminate or confirm coexistent mitral involvement.

*Anaesthetic considerations*
Optimal management implies maintenance of acceptable physiological parameters.

*Tachycardia*
If mild, it is well tolerated, because it increases dynamic impedance of reverse flow through the valve.

*Preload*
This needs to be maintained to keep the dilated ventricle full.

*Afterload*
This needs to be kept low to enhance forward flow. A balance has to be found between good cardiac output and an aortic perfusion pressure adequate to perfuse the coronary arteries of the dilated ventricle.

*Bradycardia*
This allows time for back flow into the ventricle and increases the regurgitant fraction. Treat carefully with glycopyrrolate or very small doses of epinephrine (adrenaline) or isoprenaline (isoproterenol).

All patients need prophylaxis against SBE. Those with minor degrees of regurgitation and a good exercise tolerance tolerate anaesthesia and surgery well.

The management of a more serious case should always be discussed with a cardiologist. It may be possible to improve the medication or valve replacement might be offered before elective major surgery.

Induction of anaesthesia must be accomplished slowly and follow the principles of good practice described in Chapter 2. Maintenance using high concentrations of volatile agents is contraindicated. The dilated, hypertrophied myocardium already has depressed contractility, and the negative inotropic effects of these agents can produce a marked drop in stroke volume and cardiac output.

As in mitral regurgitation, the atrial contribution to left ventricular filling is relatively unimportant, provided that the LVEDV is maintained. The dilated left ventricle is very sensitive to fibre length and, if it falls below the 'knee' of the ventricular performance curve, there may be a sudden drop in stroke work. Some patients are exquisitely sensitive to venodilatation because of this mechanism. In cases in which large fluid shifts are expected, a PA catheter can be invaluable in maintaining the optimal PAWP.

When adverse changes in cardiac output occur, the combination of direct arterial monitoring and PA catheter can be required to evaluate the cause. Cardiac output is a balance of heart rate, stroke volume, contractility, and SVR. Anything that increases SVR (sympathetic vasoconstriction, drugs) leads to an increased portion of the stroke volume returning through the aortic valve and a consequent fall in cardiac output. This potential problem (outside cardiac units) occurs chiefly with light anaesthesia and the excessive use of vasoconstrictors during regional block. The solutions are to deepen anaesthesia, to give a generous fluid load during regional block, and to give vasoconstrictors only in tiny incremental doses.

Although a fall in SVR reduces regurgitant flow, it also induces hypotension and may lead to an inadequate coronary artery filling pressure. Vasodilators, when employed to reduce left ventricular afterload, must be used carefully to prevent this happening.

A mild tachycardia is permissible, provided that it does not prejudice left ventricular filling. Bradycardia is poorly tolerated because of the increased regurgitant flow (see above) and should be corrected by small doses of atropine or prevented by the use of a vagolytic neuromuscular blocking agent such as pancuronium.

### Mixed aortic valve disease

The dominance of stenosis or incompetence is indicated clinically by the deviation of a normal pulse to either plateau or collapsing. The true contribution of each is possible only by catheterization.

## TRICUSPID VALVE DISEASE

### Tricuspid stenosis

Organic tricuspid valve disease only very rarely occurs in isolation and *the cardiac picture is usually dominated by other associated abnormalities*.

Almost all cases of tricuspid stenosis are of rheumatic origin with mitral involvement. Very rare isolated lesions occur in the carcinoid syndrome, systemic lupus erythematosus, and as congenital abnormalities. There is invariably a regurgitant component.

Tricuspid stenosis produces a low cardiac output state with a high right atrial pressure. This, in turn, may lead to throbbing headaches and a pulsating liver which can progress to mild chronic jaundice and cirrhosis. There is fatigue and peripheral oedema. Large 'a' waves are seen in the JVP. The murmur of tricuspid stenosis is similar in timing to that of mitral stenosis, maximal in the tricuspid area, and accentuated during inspiration. A pansystolic murmur of tricuspid incompetence is usually also present. 'P' pulmonale may be seen on the ECG (see Figure 47.7). The enlarged right atrium is prominent on the right heart border of the chest radiograph. Management is by diuretic therapy and low physical exertion. Anaesthetic considerations are analogous to those for mitral stenosis, with left atrial changes being equivalent to right atrial changes, left ventricular changes mirroring those of the right ventricle, and changes in systemic vascular resistance being equivalent to changes in pulmonary vascular resistance (PVR) (i.e. LA = RA, LV = RV and SVR = PVR). Fluid overload in tricuspid stenosis does not lead to early pulmonary oedema.

### Tricuspid incompetence

The majority of cases are rheumatic in origin with coexistent mitral involvement. Congenital lesions are Ebstein's anomaly and endocardial cushion defects. An increasing, but still rare, cause is acute bacterial endocarditis in mainlining drug addicts. Dilatation of the relatively weak valve ring in RVF may produce a serious regurgitant state. This usually responds well to medical treatment. Symptoms are similar to those of tricuspid stenosis, but there are jugular 'v' waves and signs of right ventricular hypertrophy. A pansystolic murmur louder in inspiration is heard at the lower end of the sternum. The ECG shows right ventricular hypertrophy, and the chest radiograph has an enlarged cardiac shadow.

The physiological consequences of tricuspid incompetence itself are very well tolerated because of the highly distensible systemic venous system, and even complete removal of the valve is possible. However, this equilibrium is easily upset by an increased right ventricular load secondary to pulmonary hypertension or LVF. In extreme cases, low right ventricular output and massive regurgitation can result in a CVP that is higher than the LAP.

Anaesthetic considerations are as for valve disease in general. The optimum care of the right ventricle is produced by meticulous attention to left ventricular function and by avoiding drugs that appreciably increase pulmonary vascular resistance.

## PULMONARY VALVE DISEASE

Most cases are congenital stenotic lesions and account for 10% of all cases of congenital heart disease; 90% are valvular and 10% infundibular. Ten percent of cases have an associated atrial septal defect, and infundibular lesions are usually accompanied by a ventricular septal defect. Rheumatic and carcinoid causes are very rare.

Symptoms may be absent but severe stenoses produce fatigue, angina (ischaemic right ventricle), and syncope. There is usually a thrill in the pulmonary area with a systolic or continuous murmur. The other physical signs and positive findings on investigation are those secondary to right ventricular hypertrophy and/or failure. The most important haemodynamic disturbance of marked stenosis is a low cardiac output. Anaesthetic considerations are analogous to those for aortic stenosis. There is, in severe cases, a sufficient gradient across the pulmonary valve such that changes in pulmonary vascular resistance have little effect on cardiac output.

Pulmonary stenosis is rare in general anaesthetic practice. When symptomatic it needs to be managed by those with experience. Two major problems are the intrinsic 'low power' of the right ventricle, which responds poorly to inotropes, and the (almost) inevitable abnormal pulmonary circulation and mechanics.

## FURTHER READING

Fisher DM, Lynch III C, Neerhut RK, Hanson EW. Mitral valve prolapse. *Anesthesiology* 1996;**85**:178–95.

Hultman J. Pre-anaesthetic evaluation and management of patients with cardiovascular disease. *Acta Anaesthesiol Scand* 1996;**40**:996–1003.

Mangano DT. Perioperative cardiac morbidity. *Anesthesiology* 1990;**72**:153–84.

Souhami RL, Moxham J, eds. *Textbook of Medicine*, 3rd edn. Edinburgh: Churchill Livingstone, 1997.

Walker JM, Cooper J. Modern methods for assessing cardiac function. In: Kaufman L, ed. *Anaesthesia Review 10*. Edinburgh: Churchill Livingstone, 1993: 1–14.

# Chapter 51 The patient with congenital heart disease

P. Hutton

The overall incidence of congenital heart disease is approximately one case per 200 live births. An increasing percentage now survive to adulthood because of improved methods of treatment. Most are discovered at birth because of routine physical examination. Diagnosis and treatment recommendations are a specialist's prerogative. In addition to corrective procedures involving open-heart surgery, there are recent advances where some corrections can be performed, without the need for bypass, by cardiac catheterization. Almost all cases have been well investigated before being seen by the anaesthetist for non-cardiac surgery, although some still present as a new finding on admission.

Congenital heart disease may present as an isolated cardiac abnormality or as part of a more generalized systemic syndrome. The cardiac abnormality can be single or a combination of lesions. Well over 100 conditions have been described but less than 10 occur commonly. These can be divided into left-to-right shunts, right-to-left shunts, and outflow obstructions. The management of these will be discussed in general terms so that the conclusions can be applied to other, rarer syndromes. It must be emphasized that *it is an area in which things can go unpredictably wrong* and that, for all but the simplest cases, *experienced help is needed.*

All patients need antibiotic prophylaxis to protect against subacute bacterial endocarditis (see Chapter 50). If anomalous murmurs and signs are discovered anew during the preoperative visit, it is always best to get a cardiological opinion.

## LEFT-TO-RIGHT SHUNTS

Irrespective of their exact site, these lesions all produce an increased pulmonary blood flow. The magnitude of this is a function of both the size of the hole and the pressures on either side of it. These pressures are themselves partly dependent on systemic and pulmonary vascular resistances. Thus, variations in these resistances indirectly influence the magnitude of the shunt. Theoretically, drugs that decrease pulmonary vascular resistance or increase systemic resistance will increase the shunt.

If the flow is high enough, some patients will develop reactive pulmonary hypertension with right ventricular hypertrophy. Ultimately, this progresses to a reversal of the shunt (Eisenmenger's syndrome) and to right and left ventricular failure. The philosophy of treatment is to prevent pulmonary hypertension occurring by closure of the defect at a sufficiently early stage. Eisenmenger's syndrome is rare, difficult to manage, and not considered further.

### Atrial septal defects

Atrial septal defects (ASDs) comprise 15% of all congenital heart disease; 95% of these are ostium secundum and 5% ostium primum defects.

#### *Ostium secundum*

This defect is usually well tolerated by the child and, untreated, it often does not present until the second or third decade, when there is irreversible pulmonary hypertension. It is often discovered incidentally or because of repeated chest infections.

#### *Ostium primum*

This defect is embryologically different and often involves the atrioventricular valves. Symptoms present more floridly and earlier than in the secundum defect, reflecting a bigger and more complex lesion.

#### ***Examination***

The pulse volume is normal and, when the pulmonary blood flow exceeds the aortic blood flow by approximately 3 : 1, there is a loss of sinus arrhythmia. The defect itself produces no murmur but, because of the increased blood flow through the lungs, there is a pulmonary ejection systolic murmur in the pulmonary area and there may on occasions be a diastolic tricuspid murmur (Figure 51.1). The murmurs are louder on inspiration and the second sound has a fixed split. There are often signs of a hypertrophied, hyperkinetic, right ventricle.

#### ***Investigations***

*ECG*

Right bundle branch block and right axis deviation are common (see Figures 47.22 and 47.6).

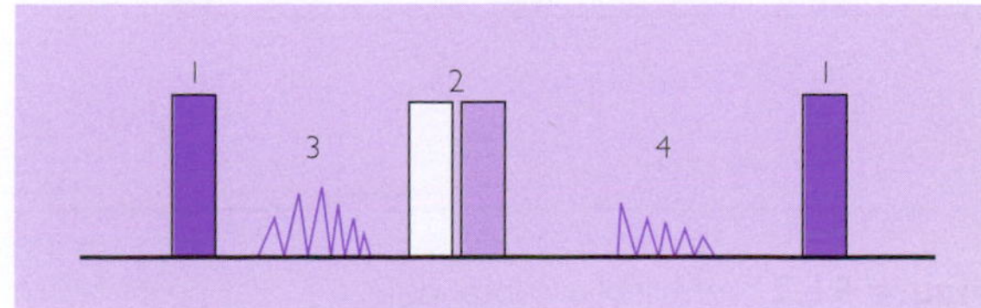


**Figure 51.1** Atrial septal defect: 1, first heart sound; 2, second heart sound with fixed split, pulmonary valve closure coming late; 3, pulmonary valve flow murmur; 4, tricuspid valve flow murmur.

*Chest radiograph*
This may be normal or may show large pulmonary vessels and an enlarged right atrium.

***Anaesthesia***
Defects with left-to-right shunts and no evidence of ventricular failure pose few problems. Theoretically, because of increased pulmonary blood flow, the uptake of gaseous agents is rapid and the effect of intravenous agents is slow in onset. Although systemic air embolism is theoretically unlikely from a left-to-right shunt, it is good practice to be meticulous in removing air from syringes and cannulae before use. By effects on the pulmonary and systemic vascular beds, intermittent positive pressure ventilation (IPPV) and volatile agents tend to reduce the shunt. Postoperative chest infections are common, so vigorous physiotherapy and early mobilization are vital.

## Ventricular septal defects

Ventricular septal defects (VSDs) comprise 30% of congenital heart disease. The presentation and clinical manifestations depend on the size of the lesion. Small defects are haemodynamically unimportant, but may have a loud murmur and 20–30% close spontaneously. They are compatible with a normal life. Large defects can present with failure to thrive, tachypnoea, and heart failure within a month of birth. Between these extremes, the magnitude of the shunt is assessed by ECG evidence of left ventricular hypertrophy, increased cardiac diameter on chest radiograph, signs of pulmonary hypertension, and ultimately cardiac catheterization.

***Examination***
Often the patient is symptom-free but if symptoms occur they are those of any significant left-to-right shunt (frequent bronchitis, dyspnoea). The pulse is of normal volume and with significant lesions there is an abrupt and forceful apex beat (volume overload of the left and to a lesser extent the right ventricles).

The murmur of the defect is a harsh pansystolic murmur in the third or fourth intercostal space at the left sternal edge, which intensifies on expiration. Superimposed on this are the flow murmurs of the pulmonary and mitral valves (Figure 51.2).

***Investigations***
*ECG*
This may be normal or show the voltage changes of left ventricular hypertrophy (see Chapter 47).

*Chest radiograph*
This may be normal or show large pulmonary vessels, a large left atrium, and biventricular enlargement.

*Anaesthetic considerations*
These are similar to those of an ASD.

## Patent ductus arteriosus

Patient ductus arteriosus (PDA) comprises 10% of congenital heart lesions. In a PDA, the shunt is from the aorta into the pulmonary artery. The majority are asymptomatic and discovered incidentally. It may be part of the rubella syndrome. If there is a large shunt, recurrent bronchitis and dyspnoea on exertion occur. Untreated, heart failure and pulmonary hypertension appear in the teens.

***Examination***
The pulse volume is normal when the defect is small but becomes high volume and collapsing as it increases in size. There is an abrupt forceful apex beat from a dilated and hypertrophied left ventricle which has an abnormally large stroke volume. Blood flows through the ductus throughout the cardiac cycle and produces a continuous murmur, maximal at the first left intercostal space, which is loudest towards the end of systole and on expiration (Figure 51.3). In addition, there may be superimposed aortic and mitral flow murmurs (but these are usually obscured) from the excessive flow of blood through these valves.

***Investigations***
*ECG*
This may be normal or show changes of left ventricular hypertrophy (see Chapter 47).

*Chest radiograph*
This may be normal or may show enlargement of pulmonary vessels, ascending aorta, aortic knuckle, left atrium, and ventricles.

*Anaesthetic considerations*
These are similar to those for an ASD.

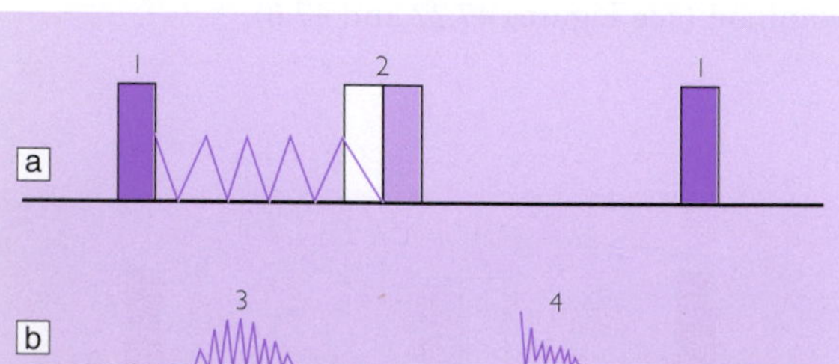


**Figure 51.2** Ventricular septal defect: 1, first heart sound; 2, second heart sound, pulmonary valve closes later than aortic. (a) Sounds of the defect; (b) added sounds. 3, Pulmonary flow murmur; 4, mitral flow murmur.

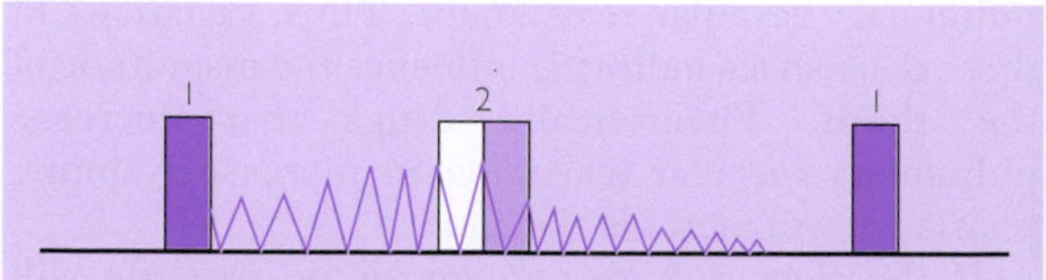


**Figure 51.3** Patent ductus arteriosus: 1, first heart sound; 2, second heart sound. Normally the pulmonary valve closes last but with a large defect there is a reversed split with aortic closure falling appreciably after pulmonary-valve closure during expiration.

## RIGHT-TO-LEFT SHUNTS

A right-to-left shunt needs a communication between the systemic and pulmonary circulations and an imbalance in ventricular pressures (there may be a common ventricle), such that venous blood can enter the aorta by bypassing the lungs. There is usually reduced pulmonary blood flow. *Air embolism from intravenous injection is a great danger.*

The only commonly occuring defect is Fallot's tetralogy which comprises 10% of all congenital heart disease and 65% of cyanotic heart disease.

### Fallot's tetralogy

#### Physiology

There is a large VSD (functionally a common ventricle) in which the shunt is from right to left because of pulmonary stenosis (infundibular and/or valvular and/or in the pulmonary artery). There is an accompanying over-riding of the aorta, which sits over the septal defect. The load on the right ventricle results in right ventricular hypertrophy completing the tetralogy.

Alteration of the relative resistance of the pulmonary and aortic outflow tracts changes the magnitude of the shunt. Although the resistance of a pulmonary artery or valve defect is effectively fixed, that of the infundibulum, which is dependent on tone, can be increased by emotional crises, catecholamines, or sympathetic activity from light anaesthesia, and reduced by halothane, β-adrenoceptor blockers, and deep anaesthesia. There is no resistance to flow into the aorta and the aortic impedance is controlled by the systemic vascular resistance, a fall in this increasing the right-to-left shunt and the cyanosis.

#### History

Failure to thrive, growth retardation, dyspnoea, syncope, and squatting (thought to increase systemic vascular resistance by kinking major blood vessels) are common.

#### Examination

Cyanosis and finger clubbing (over 6 months) are obvious. Considering the gravity of the defect, auscultation is disappointing. The murmur of pulmonary stenosis is heard in the pulmonary area but there is no VSD murmur because it is so large (Figure 51.4). Heart failure is rare in infancy.

Complications include emboli, strokes, epilepsy, endocarditis, cerebral abscesses and, most important of all, cyanotic and syncopal attacks (which can be fatal).

#### Investigations

*Full blood count*

Polycythaemia is usual.

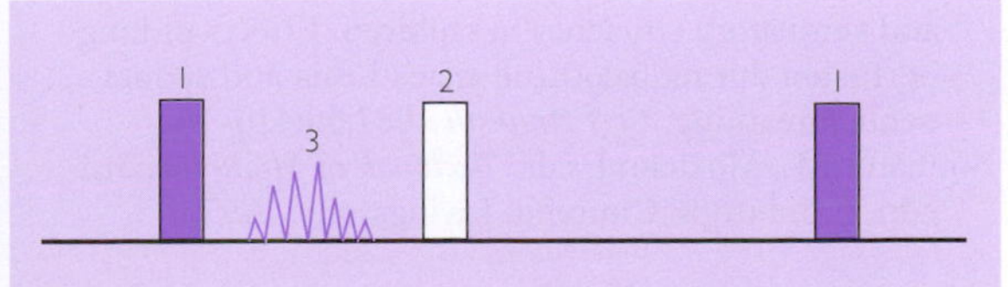


**Figure 51.4** Fallot's tetralogy: 1, first heart sound; 2, second heart sound; 3, pulmonary stenosis.

*ECG*

Right axis deviation is usual (see Figures 47.6 and 51.5).

*Chest radiograph*

The aorta is large (right sided in 25% of cases) and the pulmonary vasculature shows only faintly (Figure 51.5).

*Blood gases*

The arterial carbon dioxide tension is normal or low, and hypoxia and metabolic acidosis are evident.

#### Treatment

This is now definitive total correction at 4–6 years of age, which may or may not be preceded by a palliative

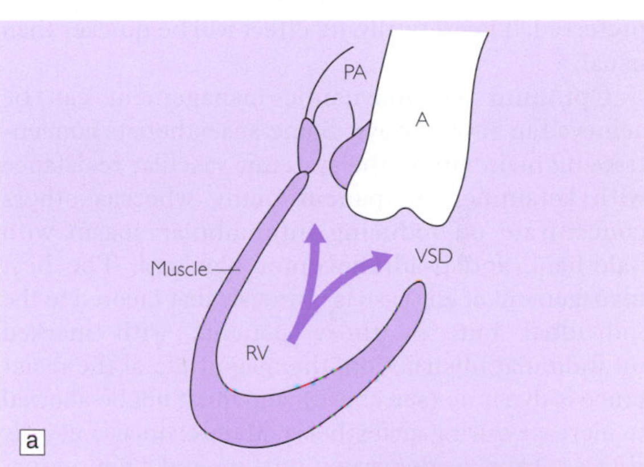


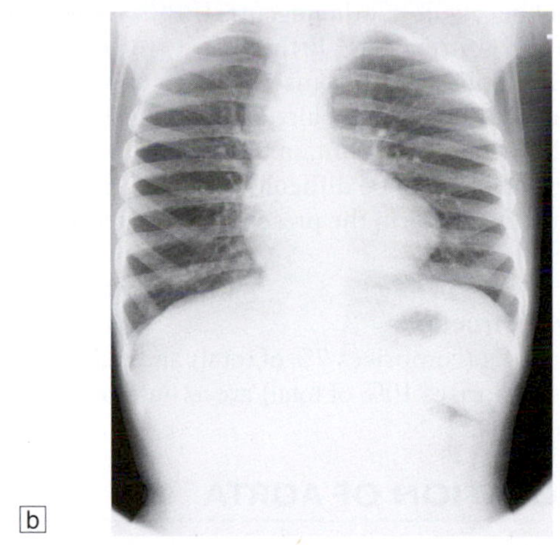


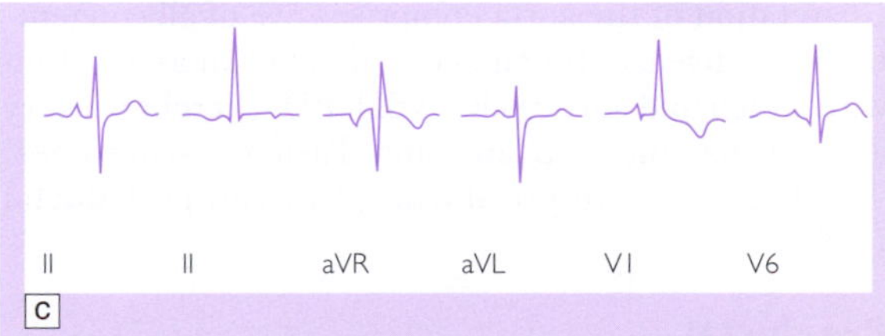


**Figure 51.5** Features of Fallot's tetralogy: (a) diagram of abnormality: PA, pulmonary artery; A, aorta; VSD, ventricular septal defect; RV, right ventricle; (b) chest radiograph showing characteristic cardiac silhouette of severe right ventricular hypertrophy which lifts the cardiac apex, oligaemic lung fields and a prominent aortic shadow; (c) ECG showing right atrial and ventricular hypertrophy and right-axis deviation. (From Walker JM and Tan LP. Cardiovascular disease. In: Souhami RL and Moxham J, eds. *Textbook of Medicine,* 3rd edn. Edinburgh: Churchill Livingstone, 1997.)

operation to increase pulmonary blood flow. Many children with cyanotic attacks are now on propranolol to control infundibular obstruction.

### Anaesthesia

Often the children dislike hospitals. Do not allow them to become dehydrated through prolonged withholding of fluids. A generous premedication (oral followed by intramuscular) should ensure a sedated child at induction. Crying and fighting at induction can lead to a cyanotic attack.

The overall principle in the uncorrected case is to prevent the complications of the condition, and not to increase the shunt and thereby intensify the hypoxia. Venous access is usually easy and intravenous (or intramuscular) induction with a small dose of the agent is preferred. Theoretically, its effect will be quicker than usual.

Optimum haemodynamic management can be achieved in several ways. Some anaesthetists concentrate on maintaining the systemic vascular resistance with ketamine and pancuronium, whereas others concentrate on reducing infundibular spasm with halothane and β-adrenoceptor blockers. The best management of any case is obviously that tailored to the individual but, in those patients with marked infundibular obstruction, the magnitude of the resistance is dynamic (see above), and must not be allowed to increase during anaesthesia. Maintenance is usually with a nitrous oxide/oxygen mixture and a neuromuscular blocking agent ± other agents. IPPV with normal inflation pressures has little effect in reducing pulmonary blood flow because the resistance of the pulmonary outflow tract is already so great. Keep the child well hydrated to maintain the blood pressure.

These patients can be difficult to handle and should be anaesthetized only in the presence of an experienced anaesthetist.

### Outflow obstructions

Aortic stenosis (comprises 7% of total) and pulmonary stenosis (comprises 10% of total) are as outlined under valvular disease.

## COARCTATION OF AORTA

Coarctation of the aorta comprises 5% of all congenital heart disease. It can occur alone or in association with a bicuspid aortic valve, VSD, PDA, cerebral artery aneurysms, and Marfan's and Turner's syndromes. The two types are pre-ductal (2%) and post-ductal (98%).

### Pre-ductal

This is the most florid form, presenting within the first weeks of life and is frequently associated with other cardiac defects and severe biventricular failure. Medical treatment is with digoxin and diuretics, and early (often semi-emergency) surgical correction. They rarely present untreated for any other operation than correction itself.

### Post-ductal

This is a much less severe form which may not present until adulthood when it may only be a chance finding. It is less frequently associated with other major defects but 20–50% have a bicuspid aortic valve. Untreated the majority die in the third or fourth decade from endocarditis, cerebrovascular accident, or left ventricular failure (LVF).

### History

Sixty percent are asymptomatic, and 40% have symptoms of hypertension, cerebrovascular accidents, endocarditis, or intermittent claudication.

### Examination

Proximal hypertension is common. The blood pressure (BP) is higher in the arms than in the legs and there is frequently a difference in BP between the right and left arms. The radial pulse is felt before the femoral one. Occasionally, there are visible, palpable, or audible scapular collaterals. A loud, rough, systolic murmur is heard at the apex of the left lung. There is a forceful apex beat often displaced beyond the normal limits.

### Investigations

*ECG*

This shows signs of left ventricular hypertrophy (see Chapter 47).

*Chest radiograph*

This may reveal a double aortic knuckle, a small descending aorta, rib notching, and increased cardiac size.

### Anaesthesia

If not in LVF (which should be treated), these patients are effectively normal, except that those parts of the body supplied by the collateral circulation are at risk of ischaemia. This can produce damage to both the spinal cord and kidneys, and is disastrous when it happens.

A good plan is to measure the BP in *both arms and legs* preoperatively, and to maintain these values throughout surgery. This requires careful attention to fluid balance and may necessitate the use of vasoactive drugs. Some texts suggest that the mean BP in the legs should not fall below 50 mmHg. A good, convenient, non-invasive measurement of leg BP is obtained from an oscillometric or oscillotonometric cuff applied to the calf. It is, however, desirable to use the same cuff and measuring system preoperatively and intraoperatively because there is considerable variation between instruments, particularly if the cuff size is different.

## FURTHER READING

Hoffman JE, Rudolph AM, Heymann MA. Pulmonary vascular disease with congenital heart lesions: pathologic features and causes. *Circulation* 1981;**64**:873–7.

Lindahl SGE, Olsson A-K. Congenital heart malformations and ventilatory efficiency in children. Effects of lung perfusion during halothane anaesthesia and spontaneous breathing. *Br J Anaesth* 1987;**59**:410–18.

Souhami RL, Moxham J, eds. *Textbook of Medicine*, 3rd edn. Edinburgh: Churchill Livingstone, 1997.

# Chapter 52 The patient with anaemia

G.M. Cooper

Anaemia is a feature of many underlying conditions which may, or may not, be related to the necessity for surgery. It can be defined as a diminished oxygen-carrying capacity of the blood as a result of a reduction in the number of red cells, or in their haemoglobin (Hb) content, in the presence of a normal blood volume. Anaemias are usually classified according to their aetiology which is summarized in Figure 52.1:

- Blood loss: in Western societies this is the most common cause and results from conditions that can remembered because they begin with 'p' (piles, peptic ulcer, periods, pain-killers, parturition, polyps). The two common routes of blood loss are gastrointestinal and vaginal. In chronic form, the net loss of blood induces an iron-deficient state.
- Decreased red cell survival (increased haemolysis):
  - red cell abnormalities (spherocytosis, haemoglobinopathies);
  - splenomegaly;
  - toxins.
- Red cell production failure:
  - reduced number of stem cells (aplastic anaemia);
  - reduced manufacturing capacity (marrow infiltrates);
  - shortage of manufacturing components (vitamin B12, folate, iron);
  - bone marrow 'depression' (anaemia of chronic diseases, e.g. rheumatoid arthritis, infection);
  - reduced erythropoietin secretion (e.g. in renal failure).

Alternative classifications are based on red cell morphology and appearance, which give a guide to causation:

- Hypochromic/microcytic: iron deficiency including chronic haemorrhage, thalassaemia.
- Normochromic/normocytic: chronic disease, e.g. infection, malignancy, renal failure, aplastic anaemia, bone marrow disease, or infiltration.
- Normochromic/macrocytic: vitamin B12 or folate deficiency.

## PHYSIOLOGY

The oxygen tensions and carrying capacities of normal arterial and mixed venous blood are given in Table 52.1. The Hb concentration is assumed to be 15 g/dl.

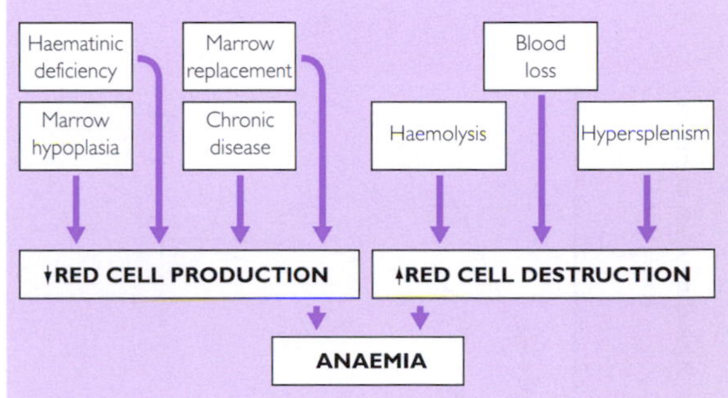


**Figure 52.1** The aetiology of anaemia. (Adapted from Linch DC. Haematological disorders. In: Souhami RL and Moxham J, eds. *Textbook of Medicine*, 3rd edn. Edinburgh: Churchill Livingstone, 1997.)

Figure 52.2 shows a comparison of the oxyhaemoglobin dissociation curve in a normal person whose Hb concentration is 15 g/dl and in one who is made acutely anaemic by loss of blood and transfusion of clear fluid so that his Hb is 7.5 g/dl. To deliver 5 ml $O_2$/100 ml blood, a normal person moves from A (arterial point) to B (mixed venous point) and still has 15 ml $O_2$/100 ml blood remaining. The anaemic person, despite full oxygenation to an arterial oxygen tension ($Pa\text{O}_2$) of 13.3 kPa (100 mmHg) starts with only 10 ml $O_2$/100 ml blood at C (arterial point) and moves to D (mixed venous point) with a mixed venous $P\text{O}_2$ of 3.5 kPa (26 mmHg) and a reserve of only 5 ml/100 ml of blood. The partial pressure of oxygen ($P\text{O}_2$) in tissue is closely related to the mixed venous $P\text{O}_2$ and hence anaemia can produce tissue hypoxia, an effect that is intensified if there are high oxygen requirements (e.g. shivering, pyrexia, hypermetabolism, sepsis). To prevent tissue hypoxia, the body decreases the amount of oxygen released per 100 ml of blood and effectively moves the mixed venous point to E. This is achieved by reducing the transit time through the capillaries by increasing tissue blood flow. Hence anaemic patients often have a high cardiac output. The ability to compensate with an increased cardiac output depends on the health of the underlying cardiovascular system.

A corollary of the above arguments is that decreases of cardiac output should be avoided in the anaemic patient, and that those techniques known to reduce cardiac output are positively contraindicated. In addition, although the $Pa\text{O}_2$ confirms the adequacy of lung oxygenation, the mixed venous $P\text{O}_2$ is a valuable measure of the adequacy of cardiac output and tissue oxygenation. It is therefore not unreasonable to measure the mixed venous $P\text{O}_2$ preoperatively, and to

**Table 52.1 The oxygen-carrying characteristics of normal arterial and mixed venous blood**

| | Arterial blood | Mixed venous blood |
|---|---|---|
| $Po_2$[a] | 13.3 (100) | 5.3 (40) |
| Oxygen attached to haemoglobin per 100 ml blood (ml) | 20 | 15 |
| Oxygen in solution per 100 ml of blood (ml) | 0.3 | 0.15 |

[a]$Po_2$, partial pressure of oxygen. Values are kPa; mmHg in parentheses.

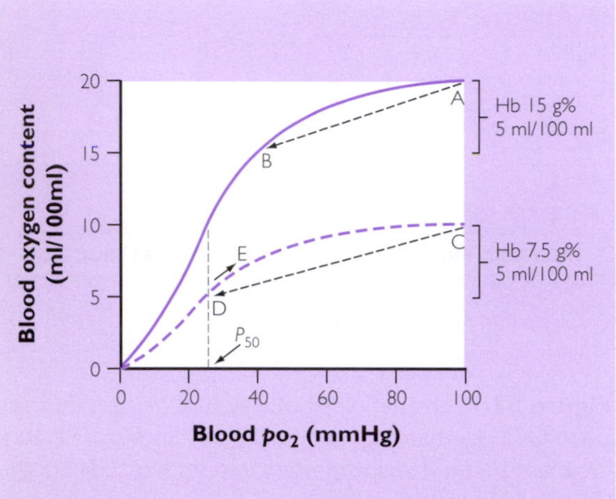


**Figure 52.2** The oxyhaemoglobin dissociation curve in a normal man and in one who is acutely anaemic. (See text.)

use it as a guide during major operations. The lowest mixed venous $Po_2$ compatible with life is approximately 2.7 kPa (20 mmHg).

The quantity of oxygen released to the tissues is also affected by the shape and position of the oxyhaemoglobin dissociation curve, which can be moved to the right or the left (Figure 52.3). Shifts in this curve are described by changes in the $P_{50}$ (the $Po_2$ at 50% saturation). Regardless of any change in left or right shift of the oxyhaemoglobin dissociation curve, if lung function is normal, when blood leaves the lungs it always carries approximately the same quantity of oxygen at a $Pao_2$ of 13.3 kPa (100 mmHg). This can be described as point F. However, to release 5 ml oxygen/100 ml blood, the curve with the right shift has accomplished it at point G when the mixed venous $Po_2$ is 6.7 kPa (50 mmHg), whereas the curve with the left shift has had to fall to a mixed venous $Po_2$ of 3.3 kPa (25 mmHg) at point H. Thus right shifts allow oxygen delivery to the tissues to occur more easily and at a higher tissue $Po_2$ (decreased Hb affinity for oxygen). Left shifts do the reverse.

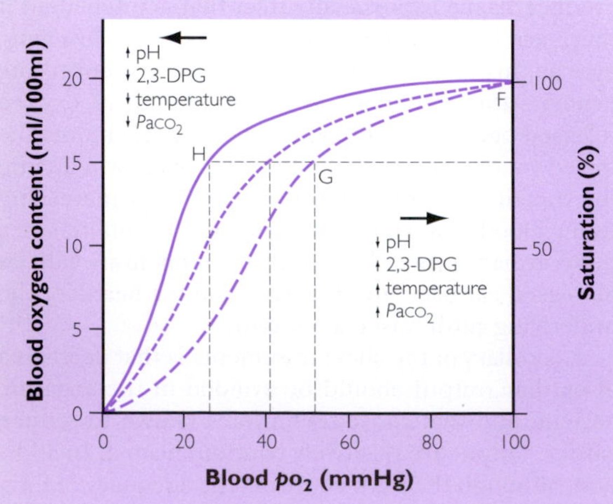


**Figure 52.3** Factors affecting the lateral position of the oxyhaemoglobin dissociation curve. 2,3-DPG, 2,3-diphosphoglycerate. (See text.)

As the venous point is on the steep part of the oxygen dissociation curve, even moderate changes in the $P_{50}$ have a considerable effect on the amount of oxygen that can be released to the tissues. If the $Pao_2$ is 13.3 kPa (100 mmHg) and the mixed venous $Po_2$ is 5.3 kPa (40 mmHg), with a $P_{50}$ of 3.5 kPa (26 mmHg), 25% of the oxygen carried is released to the tissues. If the $P_{50}$ increases to 4.7 kPa (35 mmHg), 40% of the oxygen carried will be released.

Factors that affect the $P_{50}$ are physiological alterations such as changes in temperature, hydrogen ion concentration (the arterial $CO_2$ tension [$Paco_2$] exerts an effect by altering pH), and intracellular enzyme abnormalities (these are rare) or abnormal haemoglobins. These are summarized in Table 52.2. The detrimental effects of the excessive use of bicarbonate, hyperventilation, and hypothermia can be estimated.

Within the erythrocyte, apart from the concentration of Hb, it is the intracellular concentration of 2,3-diphosphoglycerate (2,3-DPG) that has the greatest effect on the delivery of oxygen to the tissues via the changes it induces in the $P_{50}$. The levels of 2,3-DPG are increased in all forms of anaemia, and this shifts the oxyhaemoglobin dissociation curve to the right, enhancing oxygen delivery to the tissues. In chronic anaemia, there is little increase in cardiac output until the Hb has fallen to less than 9 g/dl. Below this level, any increase in oxygen demand can be met only by an increased tissue flow. The effect of changes of pH and temperature have an immediate effect on the $P_{50}$, whereas the 2,3-DPG level takes hours or days to exert its effect.

A useful summary is to think of the equation:

$$\text{Delivery of } O_2 = \text{Cardiac output} \times \text{Volume of } O_2 \text{ carried} \times \text{Fraction of } O_2$$

where the delivery is to tissues per unit time, the volume (ml) is per unit volume of arterial blood and depends on $Pao_2$ and Hb concentration (height of oxyhaemoglobin dissociation curve) and the fraction of

| Table 52.2 Typical values of $P_{50}$[a] | |
|---|---|
| | $P_{50}$[a] |
| Normal | 3.5 (26) |
| Pyrexia (temperature 40°C) | 3.9 (29) |
| Hypothermia (temperature 34°C) | 2.8 (21) |
| Alkalosis (pH 7.7; [H+] 20 nmol/L) | 2.4 (18) |
| Acidosis (pH 7.1; [H+] 80 nmol/L) | 5.0 (38) |
| ≠ 2,3-DPG in anaemia | 4.4 (33) |
| Pyruvate kinase deficiency (↑ 2,3-DPG) | 5.1 (38) |
| Hexokinase deficiency (↓ 2,3-DPG) | 2.5 (19) |
| Sickle-cell anaemia (HbSS) | 6.1 (46) |

[a]$P_{50}$ is the partial pressure of oxygen at 50% saturation; values are in kPa; mmHg in parentheses.
$[H^+]$, hydrogen ion concentration; 2,3-DPG 2,3-diphosphoglycerate.

$O_2$ is the content released to tissues, which depends on $P_{50}$ (lateral position of oxygen dissociation curve).

## CLINICAL SETTING

### History

The anaesthetist is often presented with a patient who is known to be anaemic, because of either the pathology requiring surgery or routine preoperative screening (see Chapter 41). However, the anaesthetist should be alert to the non-specific symptoms common to all anaemias, which are tiredness, lassitude, dyspnoea (especially on exertion), dizziness, fainting, irritability, and difficulty in concentrating. With severe anaemia (Hb < 8 g/dl), the compensatory increase in cardiac output may be sensed by the patient and described as palpitations. Angina and heart failure can be induced by anaemia.

The cause of anaemia should be identified. Questioning is necessary about the following.

#### *Blood loss*

This may be from menstruation, haemorrhoids, or peptic ulcer, or be associated with pregnancy. Ask about indigestion and melaena.

#### *Drugs*

Salicylates cause occult blood loss, anticonvulsants may cause folate deficiency, and cytotoxic agents and chloramphenicol cause bone marrow depression.

#### *Previous surgery*

Malabsorption, colitis, or absence of intrinsic factor may be the cause.

#### *Diet*

People with alcohol problems can have folate deficiency. Insufficient dietary iron, folate, or vitamin C is not uncommon among elderly or poor people. Vegans may have vitamin B12 deficiency. Do not overlook the possibility of carcinoma causing anorexia and weight loss.

### Examination

The characteristic finding is pallor, which is a poor guide to the Hb concentration. When the palmar creases are as pale as the surrounding skin, the Hb is usually less than 7 g/dl. Clinical signs of an increased cardiac output (tachycardia with a wide pulse pressure and a systolic ejection murmur) or cardiac failure may be present. Glossitis and stomatitis are found in several anaemias. Koilonychia occurs in iron deficiency. Mild jaundice can indicate excessive red cell destruction.

Neck lymph nodes might be enlarged in leukaemia, in reticuloses, or in those with secondary deposits. The abdomen may reveal splenomegaly, hepatomegaly, or neoplasms of the stomach, colon, or uterus.

Vitamin B12 deficiency is occasionally associated with mental disturbances and subacute combined degeneration of the cord (symmetrical paraesthesia with loss of proprioceptive and vibration senses).

Look for signs of associated chronic diseases (e.g. chronic renal failure, connective tissue disorders).

### Investigations

A full blood count is necessary to confirm the diagnosis and define the type of anaemia. Normal adult reference values are shown in Table 52.3. If further tests are required by the haematologist (bone marrow, serum folate, vitamin B12, iron, iron-binding capacity, ferritin) these should be done before transfusion or other treatment.

All black patients must be screened for sickle-cell disease. A sickledex test takes only a few minutes to perform. A positive test indicates the presence of HbS, but does not distinguish between the homozygous and the heterozygous state. This requires Hb electrophoresis, which takes 24 hours. Often, a black patient will know his or her own sickle status because of previous screening, and may carry a card stating which haemoglobins are present. The anaesthetic implications of HbS are discussed at the end of this chapter.

A normal Hb concentration is 20 g/dl at birth, which decreases to 15 g/dl by 1 month of age and reaches a low

**Table 52.3 Normal haematological values**

| | Males | Females |
|---|---|---|
| Haemoglobin (g/dl) | 14–18 | 12–16 |
| Packed cell volume (ratio) | 0.42–0.55 | 0.36–0.48 |
| Red cell count ( × $10^{12}$/L) | 4.8–6.5 | 4.1–5.5 |
| Mean corpuscular haemoglobin (pg) | 27–32 | 27–32 |
| Mean corpuscular volume (fl) | 76–96 | 76–96 |
| Mean corpuscular haemoglobin concentration (g/dl) | 30–35 | 30–35 |
| Reticulocytes (%) | 0.2–2.0 | 0.2–2.0 |
| White cell count ( × $10^9$/L) | 4.0–11.0 | 4.0–11.0 |
| Platelets (× $10^9$/L) | 150–400 | 150–400 |

of 10 g/dl at 3 months. Adult values are gained by 2–5 years and differences between the sexes are seen during the years of menstruation.

Features of common anaemias are outlined in Tables 52.4–52.7.

## PREOPERATIVE PREPARATION

Having detected the presence of anaemia and its causation, it is necessary to decide whether the anaemia should be corrected and by what means. There is a tendency to transfuse blood less frequently than previously because of possible complications, which are outlined in Chapter 14. The rationale of the traditionally accepted minimum Hb concentration of 10 g/dl for *elective* surgery is based on the benefits of reduced viscosity, which reduces myocardial work and yet oxygen flux is maintained (see Chapter 14). However, below this Hb concentration, myocardial work has to increase substantially to maintain oxygen flux. The decision to transfuse blood to correct anaemia needs to take into account the following:

- Is the circulating volume reduced? If bleeding is acute and continuing, surgery should take place to stop the bleeding at the same time as giving blood.
- Is surgery urgent or is there time for correction of anaemia by correction of deficiency states (e.g. oral iron)?
- Does the patient have a coexisting condition that might impair oxygen transport or be particularly jeopardized by reduced oxygen delivery, such as inadequate cardiac, pulmonary, or renal function, or cerebrovascular disease?
- How complex is the proposed surgery and what is the likelihood of blood loss, and especially is bleeding likely to be sudden and torrential?
- Has the patient compensated well for the anaemia and are they only undergoing minor surgery unlikely to incur blood loss?
- Is there increased oxygen consumption such as seen in shock, sepsis, trauma, or infective processes?

**Table 52.4 Hypochromic anaemia**

| |
|---|
| Shortage of iron for cell manufacture |
| Most common cause is chronic blood loss |
| Low mean corpuscular volume |
| Red cells appear small and pale on blood film |
| Low or low–normal serum iron (normal = 9–29 μmol/L) |
| High iron-binding capacity (normal = 45–72 μmol/L) |
| Treatment with oral iron (ferrous sulphate 200 mg three times daily) increases the haemoglobin concentration by 2 g/dl in 3 weeks |
| Failure to respond to oral iron indicates failure to take tablets, continued bleeding, connective tissue disorders, chronic infection, chronic renal failure, malabsorption, or sideroblastic anaemia (marrow stores full of iron that cannot be used) |
| Intravenous iron (1 g) can be used for the poorly compliant |

If the decision is taken to transfuse blood it is best done at least 2 days before surgery. This allows sufficient time to excrete any excess fluid load and to correct the deficiency in 2,3-DPG present in stored blood.

### Pulmonary disease

Cyanosis may not be seen in anaemia (or only when severely hypoxic) because it is detected only when 5 g/dl or more of Hb is deoxygenated. Thus, in the presence of compromised pulmonary function, baseline arterial blood gases should be established. Smokers can have up to 15% of their Hb in the form of carboxyhaemoglobin, which is then unavailable for oxygen transport.

### Premedication

This is a personal choice but should avoid causing ventilatory depression.

| Table 52.5 Macrocytic anaemia |
|---|
| Caused by impaired DNA synthesis required for maturation and reducing size of the reticulocyte as it is changed to erythrocyte |
| Most commonly caused by vitamin B12 or folic acid deficiency |
| In vitamin B12 deficiency serum level is low (normal = 103–517 pmol/L) |
| Body stores of vitamin B12 sufficient for 3–6 years |
| Causes of vitamin B12 deficiency are poor diet, increased needs (e.g. in pregnancy, neoplastic disease, hyperthyroidism), or impaired absorption (caused by lack of intrinsic factor in stomach, ileal resection, coeliac disease, intestinal lymphoma, or parasitic disease) |
| Folic acid is most common dietary vitamin deficiency |
| Folic acid stores sufficient only for 3 months |
| Folic acid deficiency shows as decreased serum value (normal 4–20 nmol/L) and low red cell folate (normal 340–1020 nmol/L) |
| Folic acid deficiency found where intestinal absorption impaired |
| Megaloblastic changes in bone marrow disappear within 24 hours of starting treatment |
| Care is needed with transfusion because macrocytic anaemia is associated with an increased circulating blood volume |
| Anaemia usually corrected within 1–2 months of starting treatment |
| If folic acid is given in the presence of a vitamin B12 deficiency, mental disturbances and symptoms of subacute combined degeneration of the cord may be precipitated or intensified |

| Table 52.6 Normocytic/normochromic anaemias |
|---|
| Most are secondary to other chronic diseases such as connective tissue disorders, carcinoma, chronic infection, and renal failure |
| Mild anaemia may accompany endocrine deficiency (e.g. hypothyroidism, Addison's disease, and panhypopituitarism) |
| Serum iron-binding capacity is low (normal 45–72 μmol/L) |
| Serum iron, folate, and vitamin B12 usually normal |
| Unusual to have haemoglobin < 10 g/dl unless the cause is renal failure in this type of anaemia |
| Rarely, a normocytic/normochromic anaemia is the result of primary bone marrow failure when the anaemia can be severe and other cell lines are usually affected, e.g. aplastic anaemia, leukaemia, etc. |
| Treatment is that of the underlying cause |

## INTRAOPERATIVE PHASE

The usual considerations relating to the patient, surgeon, and site of operation apply when a choice is being made between a regional technique and general anaesthesia. Although there may be important factors governing the choice, which are related to the condition causing the anaemia, there are two specific problems of regional block related to anaemia itself:

- If hypotension secondary to vascular dilatation is treated with clear fluid, the fall in Hb concentration (e.g. by 20% if 2 L of physiological [0.9%] saline is given to a 70-kg man) can temporarily exacerbate the anaemia. In those with a macrocytosis, it might precipitate heart failure when the vascular tone returns to normal. Consequently, after infusing 500 ml of crystalloid fluid, it is logical to use vasoconstrictors to sustain the blood pressure and replace only blood loss intravenously.
- Patients with vitamin B12 deficiency may develop neurological symptoms postoperatively anyway. Thus, it is probably advisable not to offer regional anaesthesia lest it be blamed as the cause.

When general anaesthesia is employed, the aims are to avoid hypoxia, maintain cardiovascular stability, and minimize those factors that produce an adverse shift in the oxygen dissociation curve (see Figure 52.3).

| Table 52.7 Haemolytic anaemias |
|---|
| Anaemia caused by premature destruction of red blood cells |
| Compensatory increase in erythrocyte production with increased reticulocyte count |
| Intravascular haemolysis results in haemoglobinuria and jaundice whereas destruction in the reticuloendothelial system produces only jaundice |
| Jaundice is mild and liver function is normal |
| Gallstones common in chronic cases |
| Inherited causes are haemoglobinopathies (most common are sickle-cell disease and thalassaemia) |
| Acquired causes are erythrocyte defects (spur cell anaemia or paroxysmal nocturnal haemoglobinuria), physical damage from an artificial or stenotic heart valve, extracorpuscular effects (e.g. direct or immunologically mediated cell damage from drugs, infections, burns, radiation damage, venoms, malignancy, connective tissue disorders, and mismatched blood transfusions) |
| The rare presence of a 'cold antibody' has maximal haemolytic effect at 20°C. If it is detected on routine screening, blood transfusion should be avoided because the cold agglutinin reacts with an antigen that is present on almost all stored red cells. If transfusion is vital, blood should be given at 37°C. The patient must be kept warm to avoid intravascular agglutination. |

### Induction

This should be preceded by preoxygenation and the induction agent should be given slowly to minimize cardiovascular disturbances. If a rapid sequence induction is essential, for frail patients an arterial line inserted before induction will allow the most rapid detection and correction of blood pressure and heart rate changes.

### Maintenance

Never forget that cyanosis is a very late sign of hypoxia in the anaemic patient, and that its absence does not imply adequate oxygenation. Arterial samples for blood gas analysis are advisable in lengthy procedures. Beware the possibility of awareness if the inspired oxygen concentration is raised to 50% in nitrous oxide. In theory, nitrous oxide is a bad choice of anaesthetic in macrocytic anaemia because of its effect on the bone marrow.

Spontaneous ventilation with its high physiological dead space is suitable only for short procedures. To overcome hypoxia secondary to hypoventilation, the inspired oxygen concentration should be increased to 50% (see Chapter 5). High concentrations of volatile agents depress ventilation and myocardial performance, both of which are necessary for the maintenance of oxygen flux. The resultant change to mild respiratory acidosis does not, however, impair oxygen delivery to the tissues. Pay particular attention to airway control and, if there are difficulties, intubate earlier rather than later.

Controlled ventilation is preferred for longer operations. Ventilate to normocapnia; alkalosis impairs oxygen delivery (see Figure 52.3 and Table 52.2), and hypocapnia reduces cardiac output.

Remember that a mild tachycardia and a wide pulse pressure may be physiological rather than a sign of light anaesthesia. On the other hand, these compensatory mechanisms may be obtunded by anaesthetic agents. Adequate tissue perfusion can be judged clinically by blanching the ear lobes, nose, or forehead with pressure and watching the pallor disappear, and quantitatively by measuring the mixed venous $P\text{O}_2$.

Keep the patient as warm as possible by using a warming blanket, maintaining a high operating-room temperature, and heating all intravenous fluids. Blood loss intraoperatively should be replaced promptly by packed cells or whole blood. Falls in systemic blood pressure and cardiac output produced by venous pooling secondary to adverse posturing can be a problem. Positioning of the patient in such instances needs prior discussion with the surgeon so that postural effects can be minimized.

## POSTOPERATIVE PHASE

Extubate the patient only when there are signs of powerful ventilatory effort. The first 12–24 hours should be spent in a recovery or high dependency area where the patient's ventilation can be monitored and oxygen-enriched air given from a facemask. Anaemic patients are put at great risk by the factors producing postoperative hypoxia. If shivering occurs, give 100% oxygen over the acute period because the oxygen requirement may increase to over five times the resting level. It should be emphasized to the nursing staff that hypoxia may not manifest itself as cyanosis, but is likely to result in confusion and drowsiness.

Elderly people are at an increased risk of developing pulmonary oedema in the postoperative period if they have been transfused. Check the Hb postoperatively and adjust the intravenous fluid regimen appropriately.

## SICKLE-CELL SYNDROMES

The structure of haemoglobin and abnormal haemoglobins is described in Chapter 31. HbS is of particular importance to the anaesthetist. HbS is thought to confer a biological advantage against malaria and is most common in black populations. It is occasionally found (especially as the sickle trait – HbAS) in southern Italians, Greeks, Indians, and mixed-race people. HbAS is found in 10% of the UK black population. Sickle-cell anaemia (HbSS) is found in 0.25% of the UK black population and double heterozygous states (HbSC or HbS thalassaemia) are found in 0.04% of the UK black population.

In the deoxygenated state, HbS crystallizes to form tactoids. These distort the cell membrane and produce a characteristic sickle shape. These altered cells initiate capillary and venous thrombosis which can progress to infarction. They are also removed prematurely from the circulation by the spleen. This results in anaemia (see Table 52.7) and a high reticulocyte count. The ease with which sickling occurs depends on the percentage of deoxygenated HbS in the red cell, the blood pH, the presence of other abnormal haemoglobins, and coincident infection. Sickling may therefore be precipitated during anaesthesia or as a result of surgery.

### Preoperative considerations

It is vital to establish whether the patient is at risk of sickling. This is done by routine sickledex testing of the population at risk (i.e. Afro-Caribbean/American blacks). The risks of sickling with different genotypes are summarized in Table 52.8. Note that those with a *high* risk of sickling are usually also anaemic. The important exception is HbSC where the Hb concentration is normal and yet the risk of sickling is high.

History and examination findings are not helpful in detecting the presence of HbS because patients with both HbAS and HbSC are asymptomatic and have no abnormal physical findings. Thus, it is important to determine the genotype by Hb electrophoresis in all patients who are sickledex positive. Figure 52.4 illustrates electrophoresis patterns seen with different haemoglobins. Patients may have been screened already and know the result or carry a card identifying their genotype. In urgent situations, where electrophoresis results are unavailable, it is essential to treat all patients who are sickledex positive (even with a high Hb) as being at risk of sickling.

If the sickle trait is found, it does not incur a high anaesthetic risk but sickling might occur under extreme conditions. Knowledge of the sickle state may also affect the surgical procedure undertaken, influence decisions on day-case surgery, help in the diagnosis of postoperative complications, reassure the anaesthetist, have medicolegal implications, and determine the need for management in a high dependency area.

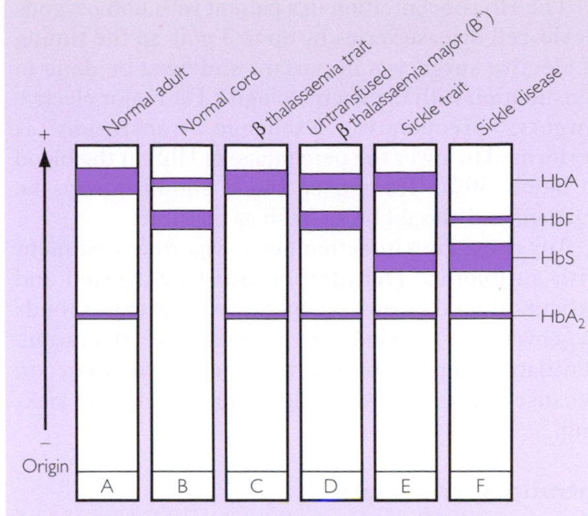


**Figure 52.4** Diagrammatic representation of haemoglobin electrophoresis at pH 8.9 to demonstrate the constituent haemoglobins present in normal blood, cord blood and haemoglobinopathies. (Adapted from Walker JM, and Tan LP. Haematological disorders. In: Souhami RL and Moxham J, eds. *Textbook of Medicine*, 3rd edn. Edinburgh: Churchill Livingstone, 1997).

Patients who are homozygous for HbS have sickle-cell anaemia and will have been symptomatic since childhood with 'crises' of bone and joint pains. There may be neurological damage from cerebral infarction. Vascular occlusions in the spleen can mimic an acute abdomen. There is often lymphadenopathy with an enlarged liver and spleen, jaundice, and the clinical signs of anaemia. The heart may be enlarged. Infarction of the renal medulla with haematuria is common, as are gallstones. Life expectancy is severely reduced.

The crises that occur are principally of two types:

1. Sequestration crises are caused when there is a sudden increase in the number of sickled red cells. These may be provoked by hypoxia, acidaemia, cold peripheries, infection, trauma (including surgery), pyrexia, and pregnancy.
2. Aplastic crises occur when the bone marrow is unable to keep pace with the high rate of red cell destruction, usually during a viral infection.

The clinical picture of patients with HbS thalassaemia is similar to homozygous sickle-cell disease.

**Table 52.8 Sickling risk and haemoglobinopathies**

| Genotype | Sickledex result | Haemoglobin content | Haemoglobin concentration | Risk of sickling |
|---|---|---|---|---|
| HbAA | Negative | 98% HbA, 2% $HbA_2$ | Normal | Absent |
| HbAS | Positive | 40% HbS, 58% HbA, 2% $HbA_2$ | Normal or mild anaemia | Low |
| HbSS | Positive | 95% HbS, 5% HbF | 5–8 g/dl | High |
| HbSC | Positive | 50% HbS, 50% HbC | Normal | High |
| HbS thalassaemia | Positive | 75% HbS, 20% HbF, 5% $HbA_2$ | 5–8 g/dl | High |

The Hb concentration in a patient with homozygous sickle-cell disease varies by up to 3 g/dl, so the timing of elective surgery is important and *must* be done in consultation with the haematologist. For major elective surgery, preoperative exchange transfusion is performed to lower the percentage of HbS in the blood to below 30%. Transfused blood should always be warmed and should be as fresh as possible.

Any coexisting infection needs vigorous treatment with antibiotics. Dehydration must be averted and patients should receive preoperative intravenous fluids to cover the period of preoperative starvation. Ventilatory depression must not be allowed to occur, because hypoxia and/or acidosis may precipitate sickling.

### Intraoperative phase

Many specific treatments have been suggested to prevent sickling. These include sodium bicarbonate, urea, promazine, megestrol acetate, warfarin, cyanate, carbamyl phosphate, dextran, and aspirin. None of these is of proven value and the mainstay of prevention of crises is avoidance of all the factors that predispose to sickling (hypoxia, hypotension, dehydration, acidosis, hypothermia), and taking the precautions essential to any case of anaemia (see above).

Although patients with HbAS are much less likely to sickle than those with HbSS, HbSC, or HbS thalassaemia, it is sensible to treat them with the same care during the perioperative period. Whatever anaesthetic technique is chosen, it is essential to keep the patient well hydrated, well oxygenated, and warm. Check the operating room temperature, warm all intravenous fluids, and actively warm the patient. Humidify the inspired gases. Monitor the patient's temperature. Transfuse blood to replace losses, aiming for a Hb concentration of approximately 10 g/dl.

Whether regional or general anaesthesia is chosen, factors predisposing to sickling must be avoided. Tourniquets with resultant stasis, acidaemia, and hypoxia are contraindicated. Local anaesthetic field blocks with epinephrine-containing solutions should not be done.

Sympathetic blockade secondary to regional anaesthesia can produce falls in blood pressure, cardiac output, and tissue perfusion. In the areas not affected by the blockade there is a compensatory vasoconstriction. The first-line treatment is the infusion of warm intravenous fluids, augmented by atropine if there is a bradycardia. Vasoconstrictors, although raising central blood pressure, can reduce peripheral tissue blood flow. Supplementary oxygen from a facemask is sensible.

Before general anaesthesia, always preoxygenate the patient. Give the induction agent slowly and never tolerate a poor airway. Maintain the fractional oxygen inspiration ($F\text{IO}_2$) at 50%. Cyanosis is doubly difficult to detect in a black person who is also anaemic, so oxygen saturation must always be measured. When ventilating, make sure that normocapnia is maintained. Acidosis predisposes to sickling and alkalosis reduces oxygen delivery to the tissues. In long operations, as well as maintaining the $P\text{aO}_2$, it is valuable to monitor the mixed venous $P\text{O}_2$ because this is a better index of cardiac output and tissue oxygenation. The preoperative baseline mixed venous $P\text{O}_2$, with an $F\text{IO}_2$ of 21%, is the minimum acceptable intraoperatively. Lower values require an appropriate correction to the cardiac output.

### Postoperative phase

This is the most hazardous period for patients with sickle-cell disease. All those who are at high risk of sickling need nursing in a high dependency area for at least 24–48 hours, and should receive oxygen supplementation for the first 24 hours. They must be kept warm and well hydrated with a good circulating blood volume. Encourage early mobilization to promote tissue circulation and prevent thrombosis. Adequate analgesia is required to prevent the vasoconstrictive reaction to pain (and impaired diaphragmatic movement with an upper abdominal incision) but guard against excessive ventilatory depression.

After major abdominal incisions, prophylactic antibiotic cover is also important to prevent pulmonary infections.

Crises can occur in the postoperative period and may be heralded by odd, unexpected aches and pains. These are obviously difficult to detect after major surgery and a high index of suspicion is required. Close cooperation must be maintained with the haematologist because the treatment of a crisis in a postoperative patient is complex. If severe bone pains occur, patients are anticoagulated to try to prevent pulmonary embolization.

## FURTHER READING

Carson JL, Poses RM, Spence RK, Bonavita G. Severity of anaemia and operative mortality and morbidity. *Lancet* 1988;**i**:727–9.

Articles in: Drummond GB, Hall GM, eds. Perioperative anaemia: Risk and treatment. *Br J Anaesth* 1998;**81**:S1–82.

Huisman THJ. The structure and functions of normal and abnormal haemoglobins. *Baillière's Clin Haematol* 1993;**6**:1–25.

Levack ID, Gillon J. Intraoperative conservation of red cell mass: controlled hypotension or haemodilution – not necessarily mutually exclusive? *Br J Anaesth* 1999;**82**:161–3.

Souhami RL, Moxham J, eds. *Textbook of Medicine*, 3rd edn. Edinburgh: Churchill Livingstone, 1997.

Vijay V, Cavenagh JD, Yate P. The anaesthetist's role in acute sickle cell crisis. *Br J Anaesth* 1998;**80**:820–8.

# Chapter 53 The patient with asthma

G.M. Cooper

Asthma is an inflammatory condition of the tracheobronchial tree that is associated with hyper-reactivity of the airways. It affects 5% of adults and up to 15% of children in the UK. The predominant symptoms are dyspnoea and wheeze of fluctuating severity. Narrowing of the airways as a result of inflammation may lead to irreversible airflow obstruction.

The prevalence of asthma is increasing. Genetic factors may determine an individual's relative risk of developing asthma, but the major determinants and reasons for the recent increases are likely to be environmental. House-dust mite and animal hair are probably important factors, possibly because of changes in housing, but dietary changes may enhance the effects of these environmental influences. Pollution and smoking are less important than previously assumed, although maternal smoking may have particular importance in childhood asthma.

The importance of the inflammatory element of asthma has been recognized only relatively recently. Pathological changes in the submucosa of the airways include inflammatory cell infiltration, oedema of the bronchial mucosa, secretion of mucus, and epithelial desquamation. The most active chemical mediators are thought to be histamine, the leukotrienes, and platelet-activating factor, although neural mechanisms also contribute to the bronchial responses. Asthma cannot be cured. However, good care and optimum drug treatment can convert asthma from a major handicap to a minor inconvenience. In the long-term treatment of asthma, emphasis is currently placed on the administration of regular inhaled anti-inflammatory drugs such as corticosteroids (beclomethasone, budesonide, or fluticasone), sodium cromoglycate and nedocromil sodium, and long-acting β-adrenoceptor agonists. Large controlled studies of treatment have now shown that the regular use of short-acting β-adrenoceptor agonists three or four times daily results in no discernible clinical benefit compared with their use 'as needed'. The leukotriene antagonists and 5-lipoxygenase inhibitors are available in some countries, and their place in relation to other drugs is currently being assessed.

Asthma should always be treated with respect by anaesthetists because aspects of airway management and the administration of drugs that cause histamine release can result in acute and catastrophic deterioration of gas exchange. It is very frightening for the anaesthetist (and the patient if he or she is awake) to be unable to get air either in or out of the lungs, which is the situation in severe asthma.

## PREOPERATIVE ASSESSMENT

### History

Ask about the frequency and severity of asthmatic attacks, what drugs the patient takes, and what has successfully aborted attacks in the past. Enquire whether admission to hospital or to an intensive care unit has ever been necessary. Elective surgery should be performed only when bronchospasm is optimally controlled and in the absence of infection.

### Examination

The lung fields should be auscultated for the presence of bronchospasm. In the presence of long-standing disease, there will be a barrel chest, with hyperinflated lungs. The ease of exhalation can be estimated visually by asking the patient to breathe out quickly after maximal inhalation.

### Investigations

The most sensitive indices of bronchial tone are the peak expiratory flow rate (PEFR) and the forced expiratory volume in 1 s ($FEV_1$). In severe asthma, the likelihood of needing postoperative ventilation can be anticipated in the presence of an $FEV_1$ of less than 1 litre, an $FEV_1$/VC ratio of less than 40% (VC is vital capacity), or a PEFR of less than 120 L/min. Arterial blood gases will also be needed in severe cases as a baseline: a raised arterial $CO_2$ tension ($Pa\text{CO}_2$) is serious and indicates the probable need for postoperative ventilation. A chest radiograph will show hyperinflated lungs with a narrow heart shadow; bullae may also be evident. However, because of underlying lung tissue, bullae may be visible only by computed tomography or from an oblique chest film. Figure 53.1 shows a chest radiograph of a child with asthma, where a mucus plug has blocked the left main bronchus.

## PREOPERATIVE PREPARATION

The inhaled, and other, medication usually used by the patient should be continued until surgery, and be brought to the operating room so that it is available in recovery. Physiotherapy and prophylactic antibiotic therapy should be started preoperatively before major surgery. Corticosteroid cover will be required if these drugs have been used in the previous 13 months (see Chapter 56), and a short course of steroids will also be indicated if inflammation is present.

Adequate premedication is important because an attack can be precipitated by fear. An antihistamine

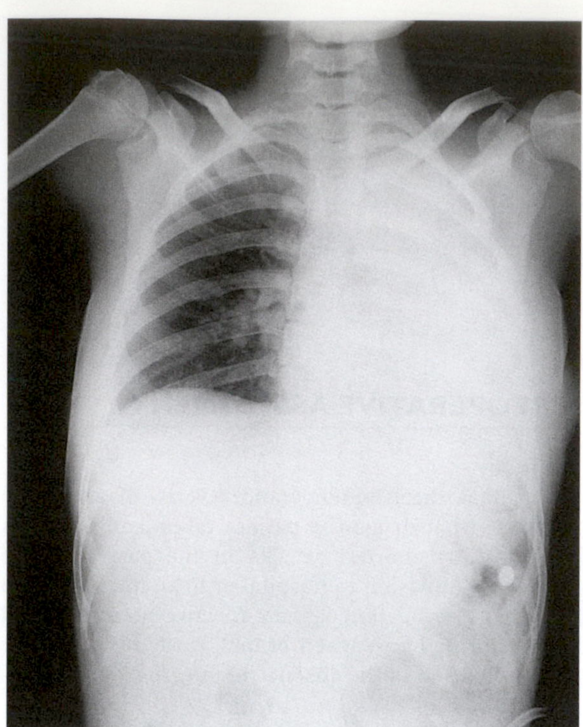

**Figure 53.1** Chest radiograph of a child with asthma who has a mucus plug blocking the left main bronchus.

such as promethazine can be particularly useful in both preventing bronchospasm and producing general sedation. Alternatively, benzodiazepines are satisfactory. The importance of avoiding drugs that release histamine peripherally (such as morphine) is unclear. Until proved safe, it seems sensible to choose a drug such as pethidine that does not release histamine if analgesia is desired as part of the premedicant.

## INTRAOPERATIVE CONSIDERATIONS

Regional analgesia is very advantageous when the surgical site is suitable. Local blocks that may cause a pneumothorax should be avoided.

Bronchospasm on induction of anaesthesia may be caused by histamine release from drugs used or by instrumentation of the airway, the carina being particularly sensitive to stimulation. Propofol, etomidate, methohexitone (methohexital), and ketamine are all suitable induction agents. Ketamine is the only intravenous induction agent with bronchodilator properties. It is important not to instrument the airway during light anaesthesia. During intubation, only sufficient endotracheal tube should be passed for the upper part of the cuff to be just below, not touching, the cords. Thiopentone (thiopental) has been implicated as causing severe bronchospasm; it is not clear whether the mechanism is histamine release or insufficient depression of airway reflexes. Although its implication is controversial, the ready availability of alternatives without this reputation render thiopentone a less suitable choice.

Rapid sequence induction can be difficult. Adequate depth of anaesthesia is important. Suxamethonium releases histamine, but the response of people with asthma to all histamine-releasing drugs is unpredictable. Aspiration of acid into the lungs is a potent bronchoconstrictor with adverse longer-term consequences, therefore the need for a rapidly acting neuromuscular blocker and the predicted ease of intubation need to be weighed up in each individual situation. Atracurium and tubocurare release histamine, and therefore vecuronium, rocuronium, or pancuronium are the neuromuscular blocking agents of choice.

Fentanyl and its analogues are free from bronchoconstrictor properties and are ideal intraoperative analgesics. As discussed earlier, morphine is probably best avoided.

Halothane, enflurane, isoflurane, desflurane, sevoflurane, and ether are all bronchodilators. However, halothane sensitizes the heart to the effects of exogenous and endogenous catecholamines. Halothane also interacts with aminophylline to produce serious ventricular arrhythmias, even when theophylline levels are within the therapeutic range. Therefore halothane is best avoided. By reducing hypoxic pulmonary vasoconstriction, inhalational agents may worsen ventilation–perfusion inequalities and increase hypoxia. Total intravenous anaesthesia with propofol is a satisfactory alternative method for maintaining anaesthesia.

When setting the ventilator, ensure that the expiratory phase is sufficiently long. The inspiratory flow rate should be adjusted to achieve the lowest inflation pressures. Changes in ventilatory parameters may herald the onset of bronchospasm or the occurrence of a pneumothorax, and hence they should be monitored closely.

Hypotensive anaesthesia can pose problems. There is no evidence, if there is normal preoperative lung function, that it is in any way harmful. However, bronchospasm under hypotensive anaesthesia (which invariably increases physiological dead space) can be disastrous, so β-adrenoceptor blockers, ganglion blockers, and trimetaphan should never be used as part of the technique. Safer methods include regional blockade, sodium nitroprusside, and inhaled volatile agents.

Intraoperative arrhythmias, if they need treating (and are not the result of hypoxia or a raised $P\text{aCO}_2$), are better treated with lignocaine (lidocaine), verapamil, or disopyramide rather than β-adrenoceptor blockers.

### Treatment of acute bronchospasm

During anaesthesia bronchospasm is recognized by increased inflation pressures (the bag may be very difficult to squeeze, or inflation pressures even in excess of 60 mmHg noted) and the presence of wheezing. With very severe bronchospasm, the audible wheeze may be absent. The position of the endotracheal tube should be checked and, if necessary, pulled back from the carina. There are then four possible therapeutic approaches (see Chapter 21 for further detail of mechanisms of action):

1. Probably the easiest manoeuvre is to try to deepen anaesthesia with a volatile agent. It is best to choose an agent other than halothane because of the potential arrhythmic effect if sympathomimetic bronchodilators are subsequently used.
2. The use of a sympathomimetic agent. The standard drug is salbutamol (2–4 μg/kg i.v. over

15 min or an infusion of 3–20 µg/min). Alternatively, terbutaline (250 µg i.v. or an infusion of 3–20 µg/min) can be given. Although much smaller doses can be effective when the drug is inhaled by a conscious person experiencing an asthmatic attack, aerosols are extremely difficult to use effectively on an unconscious person.
3. The use of a theophylline derivative. By inhibition of phosphodiesterase, this prevents the breakdown of cyclic AMP and thereby increases its intracellular concentration. This results in relaxation of the bronchial muscle. Aminophylline (up to 7 mg/kg i.v. over 15 min) is commonly used and may be the drug of choice for use during anaesthesia because it does not have the same degree of generalized sympathomimetic activity that $\beta_2$-adrenoceptor agonists possess.
4. The prophylactic use of corticosteroids at this stage is controversial.

If these measures fail and hypoxia persists with high inflation pressures, always suspect a pneumothorax (see Chapter 54). Preferential ventilation or air trapping can cause an emphysematous bulla to burst and a large pneumothorax quickly develops. This may well become a tension pneumothorax, and on time- and volume-cycled ventilators the inflation pressure will continue to rise. Urgent action is required to prevent a fatality. Examination of the chest reveals mediastinal displacement away from the pneumothorax, hyperresonance on percussion, absent breath sounds, reduced chest movement on the side of the pneumothorax, and hypotension. At the least suspicion, insert a wide-bore cannula (a large intravenous cannula will do in emergencies) and immediately follow it with a chest drain. In a ventilated patient, this should always be put onto free drainage to an underwater seal because suction pumps cannot deal with the gas transmission into the pneumothorax during intermittent positive pressure ventilation (IPPV).

## POSTOPERATIVE CONSIDERATIONS

There is no problem reversing neuromuscular blockade because the bronchoconstrictor effects of anticholinesterases are blocked by muscarinic receptor antagonists. Non-steroidal anti-inflammatory agents are contraindicated in people with asthma, although some patients know that they are not susceptible to bronchospasm from them. Pethidine, fentanyl, or alfentanil are the preferred opioids because they do not stimulate histamine release. Regional analgesia is beneficial. Postoperative oxygen should be humidified. There is no need to limit the inspired oxygen concentration because carbon dioxide responsiveness is retained in all those apart from the rare patients on hypoxic drive, who will have been identified earlier as respiratory cripples (see Chapter 54).

## THE TREATMENT OF SEVERE ASTHMA

The changes in lung volumes during an asthmatic attack are shown in Figure 53.2b. Note the greatly increased residual volume and functional residual capacity, the prolonged inspiratory and expiratory time, and the reduced VC and inspiratory reserve volume. Apart from the degree of ventilatory distress and inability to speak, the following clinical features suggest that the attack is severe, and that treatment will be required in a high dependency area:

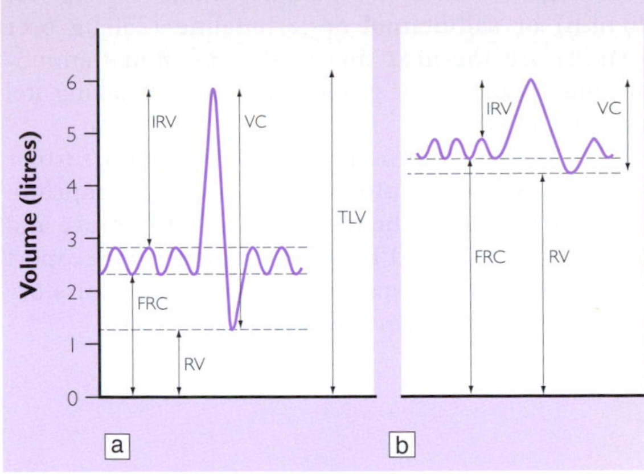


**Figure 53.2** Lung volumes: (a) normal; (b) during a severe asthma attack. FRC, functional residual capacity; IRV, inspirational reserve volume; RV, residual volume; TLV, total lung volume; VC, vital capacity.

- Tachycardia over 120 beats/min. The heart rate will slow in profound hypoxia.
- Marked pulsus paradoxus (systolic blood pressure at least 20 mmHg lower in inspiration than in expiration). Later, hypotension occurs from hypoxia.
- Indrawing of the intercostal muscles as well as the use of accessory muscles.
- Mental and physical tiredness.
- Life-threatening features are confusion, drowsiness, central cyanosis, and so little air entry that there is a 'silent chest'.

Inability to talk implies inability to drink and patients usually require aggressive rehydration.

### Investigations

An erect inspiratory chest radiograph should always be performed to exclude a pneumothorax, pneumomediastinum, atelectasis, or infiltration. Arterial blood gases are essential and a low arterial oxygen tension combined with a rising $Pa\text{CO}_2$ is evidence that the patient's ventilation is failing. It may not be possible to perform pulmonary function tests in a severe attack. A PEFR of less than 50% of predicted normal indicates a severe attack, and one of less than 30% of predicted normal is a life-threatening feature.

### Management

Oxygen (60–100%) must be given immediately. Salbutamol (5 mg) or terbutaline (10 mg) should be given by an oxygen-driven nebulizer. Hydrocortisone (200 mg i.v. or 30–60 mg prednisolone if able to drink) is then administered. *All sedative drugs must be avoided.* When life-threatening features are present, ipratropium (0.5 mg) (an antimuscarinic bronchodilator) should be added to the nebulized β-adrenoceptor agonist. Intravenous aminophylline (250 mg over 20 min) or salbutamol or terbutaline (250 μg over 10 min) are the next line of therapy. Bolus aminophylline should not be given to those already taking oral theophyllines.

If there is no improvement after 15–30 min, further steroid, β-adrenoceptor agonist, and ipratroprium should be given. If the patient does not improve and exhaustion ensues, IPPV will be required with expert help to adjust the inspiratory flow rate and expiratory pause to maximize gas exchange.

## FURTHER READING

Bishop MJ. Anesthesia for patients with asthma. Low risk but not no risk. *Anesthesiology* 1996;**85**:455–6.

The British Guidelines on Asthma Management 1995. Review and position statement. *Thorax* 1997;**52**:S1–21.

Flood-page PT, Partridge MR. Asthma: a changing perspective on management. *Curr Anaesth Crit Care* 1996;**7**:260–5.

Stoelting RK. Asthma. *Curr Anaesth Crit Care* 1989;**1**:47–53.

Warner DO, Warner MA, Barnes RD, Offord KP, Schroeder DP, Gray DT, Yunginger JW. Perioperative respiratory complications in patients with asthma. *Anesthesiology* 1996;**85**:460–7.

# Chapter 54 The patient with poor pulmonary function

G.M. Cooper

Respiratory diseases are responsible for a large proportion of premature mortality and serious morbidity among the population and, at the same time, for a large amount of minor illness. They are the second most common cause of death after cardiovascular disease. Chronic airflow limitation is particularly common in urban communities.

The relationship between lack of pulmonary reserve before surgery and postoperative morbidity and mortality is well recognized. When compared with healthy adults, patients with chronic lung disease have a 20-fold increase in postoperative pulmonary complications. After major surgery, smokers have a sixfold increase in pulmonary complications when compared with non-smokers. The highest incidence of complications (and about double the mortality) occurs after major thoracic and upper abdominal procedures. The intraoperative management is usually straightforward.

For patients with any form of pulmonary dysfunction, the key to successful anaesthesia lies in preoperative assessment and preparation, and in postoperative management.

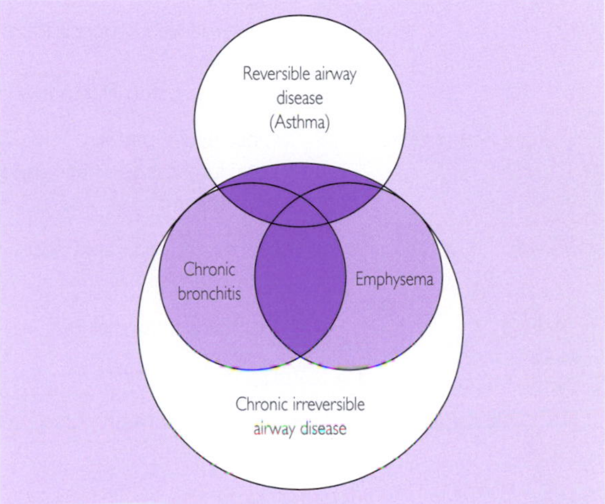

**Figure 54.1** The interrelationships between reversible airway disease, chronic bronchitis, and emphysema.

## CHRONIC OBSTRUCTIVE AIRWAY DISEASE

Chronic obstructive airway disease (COAD) is caused by the narrowing of the peripheral parts of the bronchial tree by muscular activity, oedema, or mucus, and presents as chronic bronchitis, emphysema, or asthma. The inter-relationship between the three conditions is shown in the Venn diagram of Figure 54.1. They may occur singly or in combination in any patient. The airway narrowing associated with chronic bronchitis and emphysema is largely irreversible. There is, however, a degree of overlap with asthma because some people with asthma have a productive cough and patients with chronic bronchitis and emphysema may have a component of reversible airway constriction.

### Chronic bronchitis and emphysema

Chronic bronchitis is defined clinically as a persistent cough with sputum production for more than 3 months of each year, for 3 consecutive years. Emphysema is defined purely pathologically as dilatation of air spaces distal to the terminal bronchioles, with destruction of their walls. Its extent can only be determined *post mortem*. A tiny minority of patients have pure emphysema. The rest have mixed disease which is related to cigarette smoking, urban pollution, and low social class. Chronic bronchitis causes airway obstruction by mucus in the lumen and inflammation in the walls of the bronchioles. Emphysema causes obstruction by loss of elastic tissue and airway collapse on expiration.

Patients present with any degree of ventilatory disablement. Exacerbations are often the result of superimposed infection by *Haemophilus influenzae* and *Streptococcus pneumoniae*, and these should be treated before surgery. Even at their best, these patients have excess bronchial mucus, predisposing to infection and distal collapse from blocked airways. Clinically, they are represented by a continuous spectrum, ranging from the 'pink puffer' to the 'blue bloater'. The underlying cause for these two distinct entities is not known. Although, at postmortem examination the 'pink puffer' always has extensive emphysema, it can also be found to a similar extent in 'blue bloaters', so the exact underlying physiological and pathological processes are still unclear. The two syndromes are contrasted in Table 54.1.

The degree of reversible airway obstruction is assessed by a trial of the effects of bronchodilators and/or steroids on the results of lung function tests (usually the peak expiratory flow rate [PEFR] and the forced expiratory volume in 1 s [$FEV_1$]).

### Preoperative considerations

The main objectives are to identify and minimize risk factors and to predict postoperative problems. Elective surgery needs to be delayed only if the patient's condition can be improved. In emergencies, even those with severe pulmonary disease will, with appropriate

| Table 54.1 The clinical and investigative findings in the 'pink puffer' and the 'blue bloater' | | |
|---|---|---|
| | 'Pink puffer' | 'Blue bloater' |
| Clinical features | Pink, breathless<br>Not cyanosed<br>Thin, wasted<br>Signs of cardiac failure and fluid retention rare | Warm blue hands<br>Central cyanosis<br>Obese<br>No dyspnoea<br>Signs of cor pulmonale common |
| ECG | Normal | Changes of cor pulmonale |
| Full blood count | Haemoglobin normal | Polycythaemia |
| Chest radiograph | Normal in mild–moderate<br>Later, marked hyperinflation, with long small heart<br>Large retrosternal window on lateral view | Normal in mild–moderate disease<br>Later, normal sized lung fields with cardiomegaly and upper-lobe blood diversion |
| Lung function tests | Obstructive pattern<br>Total lung capacity increased<br>VC reduced | Obstructive pattern<br>Normal lung capacity<br>VC reduced |
| Gases | Normal at rest, rapid onset of hypoxia with exercise | Hypoxaemic with raised $Paco_2$ |
| Asleep | Maintains a normal $Pao_2$ | May have frequent spells of oxygen desaturation |

VC, vital capacity; $Pao_2$, arterial oxygen tension; $Paco_2$, arterial carbon dioxide tension.

management, survive the operation. The greatest danger is in the postoperative period.

### *History*

Frequently, people with chronic lung disease, because of its insidious onset, come to regard their own state as 'normal', so it is essential to ask leading questions about coughing, sputum, breathlessness, smoking, and the limitations of physical activity. If there are positive replies to any of these questions, determine whether or not this is an acute exacerbation, which could be improved with treatment before surgery, or whether this is his or her normal condition, making a delay unnecessary. Although patients are not always good predictors of their own state, do not ignore complaints of being worse than usual.

Dyspnoea is an undue awareness of breathing or awareness of difficulty in breathing and can be caused by:

- an increase in the work of breathing (all the causes of airway obstruction, decreased pulmonary compliance, restricted chest expansion);
- increased pulmonary ventilation (compensatory for any cause of increased physiological dead space);
- hysteria;
- hyperventilation to reduce the arterial $CO_2$ tension ($Paco_2$) in compensation for a metabolic acidosis;
- a weakness of the muscles of ventilation (neuromuscular defects);
- chest expansion being limited by pain.

The variability of symptoms and the severity of exertional dyspnoea are particularly important. Variable symptoms tend to be caused by reversible airway disease (see Chapter 53).

The degree of exertional dyspnoea gives an index of the patient's compromised pulmonary function. It is graded according to Roizen's classification (Table 54.2).

Ask about coughing and whether it is productive. A dry cough indicates bronchial irritation, pulmonary congestion, or, rarely, distortion of the trachea or bronchi. Establish whether the sputum is purulent or mucoid and what volume is produced daily. These

| Table 54.2 Roizen's classification of dyspnoea | |
|---|---|
| Grade 0 | No dyspnoea while walking on the level at a normal pace |
| Grade I | Able to walk long distances at own pace |
| Grade II | Exercise limited after specific distance (e.g. 100–200 m) |
| Grade III | Dyspnoea on mild exertion (e.g. a few metres) |
| Grade IV | Dyspnoea at rest |

factors are particularly important in deciding the optimum condition likely to be attained.

Check on the amount and duration of smoking. Assess the patient's mental state. Mild confusion is not uncommon in sick elderly people who have pulmonary disease, resulting from $CO_2$ retention, hypoxia, electrolyte imbalance, or hypoglycaemia, or who have had a cerebrovascular accident secondary to the primary pathology. It is important to identify the cause of confusion because it may well be reversible. Initially, $CO_2$ retention gives rise to disturbed sleep and early morning headaches, but as the $Pa\text{CO}_2$ rises further it causes poor concentration, drowsiness, and confusion.

Note the patient's medication, especially bronchodilators, antibiotics, and steroids. Determine the effects of previous anaesthetics, and, where possible, look at the anaesthetic record for clues as to the best management.

If the patient is on intermittent oxygen therapy, record the fractional inspired oxygen concentration ($F\text{IO}_2$) that does not suppress the ventilatory drive.

### Examination

#### General

Get a good view of the chest from the end of the bed and observe any asymmetry of movement. Diminished movement means pathology on that side of the chest. Note the use of the accessory muscles of respiration. The patient may be unable to finish a sentence without taking a breath, and may be leaning forward propped up on a pillow or on his or her hands. Facial anxiety, pursed lips (providing a physiological positive end-expiratory pressure to prevent airway closure), and clubbed, warm, blue hands (central cyanosis) complete the picture of severe pulmonary disease. A tracheal tug may be present.

Restrictive lung disease tends to produce rapid, shallow breathing. Always look for tobacco-stained fingers and the ominous signs of weight loss.

#### Chest

Inspection, palpation, percussion, and auscultation will reveal localizing signs, the significance of which are outlined in Table 54.3. Think whether this will influence intraoperative positioning or the use of endobronchial tubes.

The three clinical signs of COAD are hyperinflation, prolongation of the expiratory phase, and expiratory rhonchi. Hyperinflation causes the chest wall to be held permanently in the almost inflated position, the ventilatory excursion being provided by the diaphragm and the accessory muscles of respiration (which lift the whole rib cage vertically). There may be sufficient hyperinflated lung between the heart and the chest wall to cause loss of cardiac dullness to percussion, and to make the heart sounds difficult to hear.

Prolongation of the expiratory phase may be obvious. In borderline cases, problems of expiration can be unmasked by asking the patient to breathe out from a maximal inspiration. In patients without COAD, the expiration should be complete within 5 s, and the patient should be capable of extinguishing a lighted match with an open mouth from 15 cm (Snider match test).

In severe cases, expiratory rhonchi are audible from the end of the bed. In mild cases, they can be produced if the patient does a series of deep breaths and forced expirations.

The presence of sputum is usually obvious from a productive cough. Sputum is retained when the expulsive movements of coughing are so compromised by expiratory resistance or lack of muscle power that the airways are not cleared by the rapid exhalation of dead space and alveolar air. If there are coarse moist sounds at the lung bases, which clear on deliberate coughing, it is likely that there is no serious inability to expel sputum. The only rider to this is that very severe sputum retention may cause a silent area on auscultation, because there is insufficient movement in the small air passages to produce either crepitations or rhonchi.

#### Cardiovascular system

Look for signs of cor pulmonale. Chronic hypercapnia is associated with poor handling of salt and water, so there is often peripheral oedema and a raised jugular venous pressure (JVP). The dilated vascular bed results in a rapid, high-volume, bounding pulse and, because the cardiac output is frequently increased, the blood pressure may be raised. Pulsus paradoxus (see Table 54.3) is seen in COAD, and its degree is a reflection of the severity of obstruction. A difference between the systolic blood pressure in inspiration and expiration of 40 mmHg may be reached in severe disease.

#### Abdomen

There may be excessively strenuous movements to aid expiration in both obstructive and restrictive lung disease. Look to see if the patient is obese, which would augur badly for postoperative breathing difficulties.

#### Nervous system

Hypercapnia may be revealed by a coarse tremor or irregular twitching of the outstretched dorsiflexed hands.

### Investigations

#### Urea and electrolytes, and liver function tests

These should all be normal. If the urea is elevated, check the nephrotoxicity of antibiotics and the dose of diuretics. Abnormalities of serum potassium are usually the result of diuretics or steroids. Persistent cor pulmonale with a raised JVP can produce altered liver function tests.

#### Full blood count

If polycythaemia is present suspect chronic hypoxia. An increased white cell count may indicate a chest infection.

#### Arterial blood gases

The physical signs of hypoxia and $CO_2$ retention are variable and need to be quantified by arterial blood gas estimations. They may be indicated if abnormalities are found on physical examination, and are essential in patients with severely compromised ventilatory reserve. Baseline values can be invaluable in diagnosing and predicting postoperative problems. The following are some points to remember in their interpretation:

- The arterial $O_2$ tension ($Pa\text{O}_2$) varies throughout life, decreasing from a peak in young adulthood.

**Table 54.3 Clinical findings in chest disease**

| Pathology | Chest wall movement | Mediastinal displacement | Tactile vocal fremitus | Percussion note | Breath sounds | Added sounds |
|---|---|---|---|---|---|---|
| Consolidation (e.g. lobar pneumonia, extensive pulmonary infarction, pneumonic tuberculosis) | Reduced on affected side | None | Increased | Dull | Bronchial | Fine crepitations early, coarse later |
| Massive collapse (e.g. obstruction by carcinoma, foreign body) | Reduced on affected side | Towards lesion | Absent | Dull | Decreased | None |
| Large pleural effusion | Reduced on affected side | Towards opposite side | Absent | Stony dull | Absent | Absent or pleural rub |
| Large pneumothorax | Reduced on affected side | Towards opposite side | Decreased | Hyper-resonant | Decreased | None |
| Fibrosis | Reduced slightly on affected side | Towards lesion | Increased | Dull | Bronchial | Coarse crepitations |
| Emphysema | Reduced bilaterally (barrel chest) | None | Decreased | Hyper-resonant | Decreased | Absent |
| Bronchitis | Reduced bilaterally | None | Normal | Normal | Prolonged expiration | Rhonchi, coarse crepitations |
| Asthma | Reduced bilaterally | None | Normal or decreased | Normal | Prolonged expiration | High-pitched expiratory rhonchi |

Several regression equations are available but none has an upper limit of over 75 years. Consequently, $PaO_2$ values for ages above this are all reached by unreliable extrapolation.

- The increased pulmonary venous admixture, secondary to airway closure in dependent lung zones (an effect that increases with age), causes a reduction in $PaO_2$ of over 1 kPa (7.5 mmHg) from the sitting to the supine position. Hence, the position of the patient should always be recorded with the results. A useful regression equation predicting the $PaO_2$ between the ages of 15 and 75 years for a patient sitting propped to 70° with the legs horizontal is that of Mellemgaard:

$$PaO_2\ (\text{kPa}) = 13.8 - (0.036 \times \text{age in years})$$
$$PaO_2\ (\text{mmHg}) = 104 - (0.27 \times \text{age in years})$$

- The marked effect that venous admixture has on the $PaO_2$ occurs because of the non-linearity of the oxygen dissociation curve. It causes little change in the $PaCO_2$, which remains constant throughout life.
- It is essential to relate the blood gas results to the inspired oxygen concentration. Unless breathing air or intubated, a fixed performance device such as a Ventimask should be used.

The patterns of blood gas derangement fall into three main subdivisions: hyperventilation, alveolar hypoventilation, and a shunt or gas transfer defect. Often the last two categories are mixed:

- In hyperventilation, the $PaCO_2$ is normal or elevated and the $PaO_2$ is reduced. It is almost invariably the result of anxious overventilation on the part of the patient and merely indicates healthy lungs. It is usually of no clinical importance. Exceptions are the hyperventilation of cerebral origin and the low $PaCO_2$ that is compensating for a metabolic acidosis.
- Alveolar hypoventilation can result from COAD, impaired mechanical ventilation (acute airway obstruction, stiff lungs, flail chest, pneumothorax), muscular weakness (myopathy, neuropathy), or central depression from drugs. In essence, there is insufficient alveolar ventilation both to oxygenate the blood and to wash out the $CO_2$ so the $PaCO_2$ is elevated and the $PaO_2$ is reduced. It is important to recognize the presence of alveolar hypoventilation because the $PaO_2$ (but not the $PaCO_2$) can be greatly improved by increasing the $FIO_2$. If the failure of alveolar ventilation is secondary to chronic abnormal neuromuscular function, the patient often shows little clinical distress, but if it is secondary to a mechanical problem, he or she will make vigorous efforts to increase the tidal and minute volumes.
- Shunt or gas transfer defects describe those situations in which there is no airway obstruction and the lungs are expanded normally, but there is imperfect interfacing of pulmonary blood and alveolar air. This can arise from both generalized parenchymal conditions (sarcoidosis, fibrosing alveolitis, shock lung) and localized problems (pulmonary embolus, lobar collapse, lobar pneumonia). This collection of circumstances results in a situation where the $PaCO_2$ is normal (because hyperventilation can wash out the $CO_2$ adequately from the normal lung tissue) but, because of the necessary mixing of blood with varying oxygen tensions in the pulmonary veins and because of the shape of the oxygen dissociation curve, the $PaO_2$ is reduced. In the presence of a shunt of 50% of the cardiac output, there is very little to be gained from increasing the $FIO_2$ to very high levels. This merely increases the risk of pulmonary oxygen toxicity without improving the $PaO_2$.

### *Chest radiograph*

The systematic interpretation of a chest radiograph is outlined in Chapter 6. The following are indications for a preoperative chest radiograph:

- symptoms or signs of active lung disease;
- patients with possible bronchogenic carcinoma (Figure 54.2) or pulmonary metastases;
- symptoms and signs of heart disease;
- recent immigrants from countries where tuberculosis is endemic and who have not had a chest radiograph in the previous year.

It is important to realize that the chest radiograph gives little indication of the efficiency of the lungs as gas exchangers. Figure 54.3 shows that of a patient with severe kyphoscoliosis and the results of her arterial blood gases and pulmonary function tests.

A chest radiograph is often most useful as a baseline before major surgery. Any subsequent postoperative findings can then be compared. Figure 54.4 illustrates a right phrenic nerve palsy found on preoperative chest radiograph.

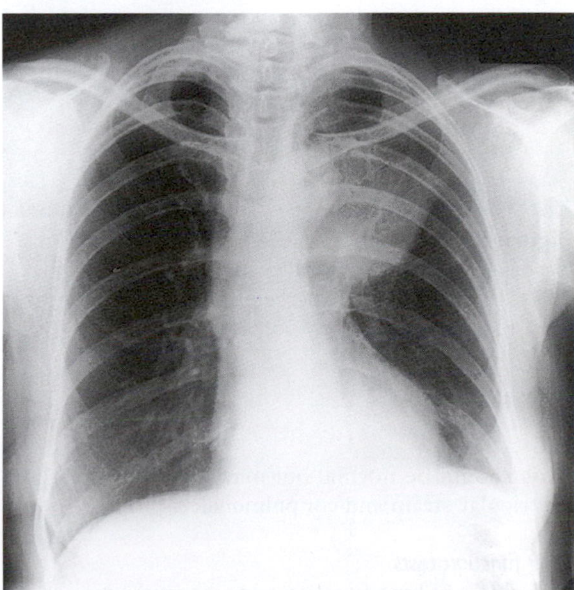

**Figure 54.2** Preoperative chest radiograph showing a left bronchogenic carcinoma in a heavy smoker. Lung function tests were normal.

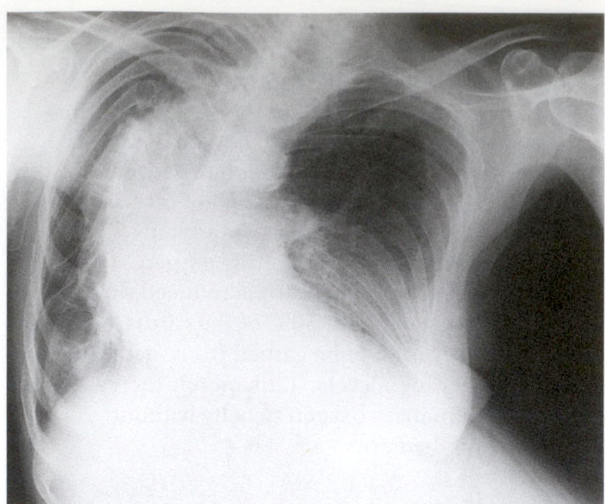

**Figure 54.3** Preoperative chest radiograph of a 67-year-old ex-smoker who was scheduled for vaginal repair. Severe kyphoscoliosis was evident clinically. Arterial blood gases taken breathing air were pH 7.39, $P\text{CO}_2$ = 5.3 kPa (40 mmHg), $P\text{O}_2$ = 7.6 kPa (57 mmHg), base deficit = 0.7. Her $\text{FEV}_1$ and FVC were reduced, being 0.62 and 0.92 L respectively (predicted values being 1.57 and 1.92 L), with no improvement after bronchodilators. This confirmed the restrictive pattern of disease as a result of kyphoscoliosis. The repair was successfully performed under spinal anaesthesia.

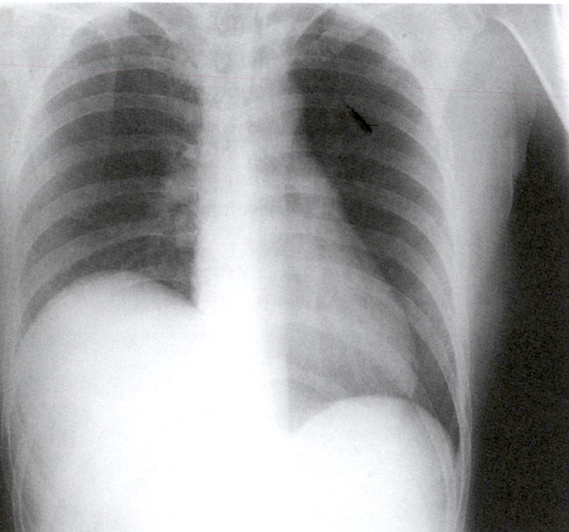

**Figure 54.4** Preoperative chest radiograph. The film was taken during full inspiration and demonstrates the effects of a right phrenic nerve palsy. This predicted the need for postoperative physiotherapy.

*ECG*

This should be normal but may show signs of right ventricular strain and cor pulmonale.

*Lung function tests*

The object of lung function tests is to put a numerical index on a given physiological variable, so that the patient can be compared with a normal peer, the effect of treatment can be monitored, or the progress of disease or recovery from anaesthesia and other insults can be assessed. Lung function tests need to be related to age, sex, and height in standard tables. There is a wide range of normal values, the 95% confidence limits being approximately 20% on either side of the mean.

The three most useful and commonly measured variables are the vital capacity (VC or forced vital capacity, FVC), $\text{FEV}_1$, and PEFR. They can all be measured at the bedside and depend on the patient's cooperation. All lung function tests should be repeated at least three times and the best values taken. They can be done before and after bronchodilator treatment to assess the influence of reversible airway obstruction. Causes of a reduced VC are given in Table 54.4.

The PEFR (normal range in healthy adults is 450–650 L/min) is a reproducible estimate of airway obstruction, but it is extremely effort dependent and the value is low whenever the VC is reduced (Table 54.4). It is useful for following the progress of asthma and neuromuscular disorders. One of its most important uses is serial measurements in the same patient to assess the response to the treatment of airway obstruction. A genuine PEFR of less than 120 L/min indicates severe obstruction. An artificially high PEFR can be obtained by the patient doing a sort of trick cough. An artificially low PEFR can be obtained from failure to expire from a maximal inspiration.

Another function sometimes recorded is the maximum breathing capacity (MBC) which is the amount of air that can be breathed in 1 min. It can be measured directly as an expired volume during exercise (e.g. on a treadmill). It is dependent on expiratory effort and reflects total cardiorespiratory function. Its particular value may be that it also depends on intangible variables of cooperation, motivation, and stamina. The MBC can also be calculated from $\text{FEV}_1 \times 35$ or peak flow × 0.25 but this does not reflect the less tangible variables. MBC greater than 60 L/min is normal and less than 25 L/min indicates severe pulmonary impairment.

Most studies relating pulmonary function to postoperative complications have concentrated on those undergoing lung resections. Nevertheless, some general observations about pulmonary function are useful in understanding postoperative breathing difficulties:

- If the tidal volume ($V_{\text{T}}$) is close to the VC, then there is little 'ventilatory reserve', and the adequacy of postoperative ventilation easily deteriorates with opioids and residual neuromuscular block (including that provided by a thoracic epidural).
- Irrespective of the cause, perhaps the most important feature of low values of $\text{FEV}_1$ and PEFR is an indication that the patient cannot expel air rapidly. Although these tests are not a direct measure of the 'power' of a cough, they are closely related to the ability to expel sputum. An $\text{FEV}_1$ of less than 2 litres and/or an $\text{FEV}_1$/VC ratio of less than 50% are sometimes quoted as values that define serious disease. The lower the value recorded, the more important it is to optimize the patients' state preoperatively, to monitor them closely in the postoperative period, and to subject them to vigorous and frequent physiotherapy.

**Table 54.4 Some causes of reduced vital capacity**

| | |
|---|---|
| Reduced lung volume | Pulmonary fibrosis and infiltrations<br>Large pleural effusions<br>Collapsed or absent lobes or lung<br>Pulmonary oedema<br>Skeletal abnormalities |
| Inability to expand lungs | Limitation by pain<br>Obesity<br>Splinted diaphragm |
| Severe airway obstruction (because of premature airway closure) | Asthma<br>Emphysema<br>Chronic bronchitis |
| Muscular weakness | Neuromuscular blocking drugs<br>Myopathies<br>Neuropathies<br>Myasthenia gravis |

- When lung function tests reveal abnormal results, it is obviously important to combine them with a blood gas estimation. It is only this that demonstrates the effect that the ventilatory defect has on the efficacy of gas exchange. A $P\text{aO}_2$ of less than 7.1 kPa (53 mmHg) or less than 70% of normal for age, in combination with dyspnoea at rest, has been shown to predict dependence on postoperative respiratory support in patients undergoing upper abdominal surgery. The $P\text{aCO}_2$ is of little predictive value of the need for postoperative ventilation. However, it may be useful for the detection of those with a hypoxic respiratory drive in whom postoperative administration of oxygen will need careful monitoring.

Other pulmonary function tests must be carried out in a specialized laboratory and tend to be done only on selected patients. They are used primarily to follow the progress of chronic disease and are not usually helpful in preoperative assessment. For absolute lung volumes, a measurement involving residual volume must be done, usually by helium dilution. The single-breath carbon monoxide test is used for measuring the barrier to the diffusion of gases, and tests of regional lung function require the use of radioisotopes. A single-breath nitrogen test estimates the closing capacity, and more recently the response to rebreathing $CO_2$ has been used as an index of the sensitivity of the respiratory centre to a change in the $P\text{aCO}_2$.

## Preoperative preparation

The degree of pulmonary incapacity will be apparent from the preoperative assessment. The objective is to optimize pulmonary function before surgery. In emergencies this may be impossible. Patients for elective operations who have chronic lung disorders need to be admitted several days before surgery and at a time of year when their condition is not exacerbated. Six aspects need to be considered.

### *Smoking*

The adverse effects of smoking are spasm and collapse of small airways, hypersecretion of mucus, and impairment of tracheobronchial tree clearance. Improved mucociliary transport and small airway function, and a decrease in airway secretions and reactivity, occur after several weeks' cessation of smoking. At least 6–8 weeks of abstinence are required and this is rewarded with a decreased incidence of postoperative respiratory complications. Even though as few as 20% smokers are successful at giving up well in advance of elective surgery, encouragement to do so is essential.

If this has been unsuccessful, as a bare minimum try to prevent smoking in the 24 hours before surgery, in order to reduce the carboxyhaemoglobin content of the blood and hence improve oxygen transport. There are, however, some badly addicted patients who, if they have coexisting heart disease, may have angina induced in the stressful preoperative period because they are unable to experience the relaxing effects of a pipe or cigarette. With them, discretion must be exercised. One solution is to allow smoking to continue; another is to prescribe an anxiolytic.

### *Dilating the airways*

Patients who have increased airway responsiveness and who are therefore candidates for preoperative bronchodilatation are smokers, atopic individuals, patients with COAD, and people with asthma (see Chapter 53). Some sources recommend inhaled β-adrenoceptor agonists and/or anticholinergics as first-line therapy and inhaled steroids as back-up, whereas other sources recommend inhaled steroids as first-line therapy.

### *Loosening the secretions*

The most efficacious method of loosening secretions is by hydration. The most common method is by use of a jet humidifier or ultrasonic nebulizer (see Chapter 8). A heated sterile water aerosol is produced and delivered from a close-fitting mask for 20 min. The patient is instructed to breathe deeply. Good systemic hydration must also be ensured, either orally or intravenously. Mucolytic agents (such as acetylcysteine) are of only limited benefit.

#### *Removing the secretions*

The physiotherapist and patient should meet as early as possible to establish rapport. This enables postural drainage, percussion, coughing, and breathing exercises to be practised preoperatively. Incentive spirometry has also been used with success in patients with COAD, but its exact position and benefits are as yet undetermined. Sputum should be collected and antibiotics prescribed according to the results of culture and sensitivity.

#### *General measures*

Weight loss should be encouraged in obese patients. Malnutrition may require preoperative treatment by nasogastric or intravenous feeding. Any other concurrent medical problems (e.g. diabetes or angina) should be stabilized.

#### *Motivation, education, and facilitation of postoperative care*

Outline the problems of postoperative analgesia to the patient and discuss the acceptability of various techniques. Make sure that a member of the acute pain team comes to see the patient and ask for his or her help with psychological preparation. Orientation to the high dependency or intensive care environment may be advantageous, encouraging a positive but realistic approach.

It is important during this period to assess the patient's ability to breathe when lying flat, especially if local, regional, or facemask techniques are envisaged.

For premedication, it is sensible to avoid ventilatory depressant drugs. If an anxiolytic is required, a small dose of a short-acting benzodiazepine is suitable (e.g. temazepam 10–20 mg).

### Intraoperative phase

Opinions differ widely as to the best method of anaesthetizing patients with pulmonary disease. Views vary from those who would use a local or regional technique at all costs, to those who recommend intermittent positive-pressure ventilation (IPPV) on all occasions. The pros and cons of each technique are described below. In practice, the optimum management is a reasoned decision based on the site and length of operation, and the wishes of the patient, anaesthetist, and surgeon.

#### *Minimal interference techniques*

The logic of this philosophy is to use local or regional blocks to provide adequate anaesthesia and to keep the patient conscious or only mildly sedated, while breathing spontaneously and retaining the ability to cough. It is most applicable to fairly short operations on the limbs and lower abdomen.

Advantages are that it avoids upsetting the patient's ventilatory control and the problems of weaning from the ventilator. If the patient's ventilation is barely adequate, it does not reduce the patient's functional residual capacity (FRC) or increase the physiological dead space ($V_D$) as does a general anaesthetic. There is no reversal of physiological intrathoracic pressure swings, which might put emphysematous bullae at risk. It also avoids residual neuromuscular block. Another advantage is that the patient can use his or her nebulizer if bronchodilatation proves necessary.

Disadvantages are that an awake patient must be acceptable to the surgeon, and the operating room staff must be careful with their comments. The patient may have to lie still for long periods in an embarrassing position, resulting in both mental and physical discomfort. The postural change may worsen compromised ventilatory function to a distressing level, but this can often be overcome by operating with the patient semirecumbent. Long procedures are likely to be punctuated by coughing, making the operation longer if not impossible (e.g. tendon suturing, hernia repair, prostatic resection). The patient needs to have a robust personality because the treatment of intraoperative anxiety with intravenous sedatives, although often successful, can be harmful. Sedatives can reduce the conscious level, suppress ventilation, cause confusion, and create problems with the airway. Similar problems surround the use of sedative premedications. Nitrous oxide/oxygen/air mixtures given through a lightly applied facemask are often well tolerated. With patients who rely on a hypoxic drive, the $F_{IO_2}$ must not be allowed to rise to the level that suppresses ventilation.

It is important not to minimize the potential dangers of regional techniques. A pneumothorax from a supraclavicular block or an intravenous injection during a brachial plexus block can be disastrous in the presence of a compromised cardiopulmonary system. When using spinal or epidural blockade, beware of fluid overload which may later cause pulmonary oedema. A reasonable upper limit of fluid load is 500 ml of 0.9% saline in addition to the intraoperative losses. Hypotension caused through sympathetic blockade not responding to this is best treated with vasconstrictors.

An awake patient is no excuse for inadequate monitoring but the extent will depend on the individual case. If it is felt necessary to have an arterial line purely for sampling intraoperative blood gases, then minimal interference is probably the wrong technique to choose because the blood gas status can be corrected only by manual manoeuvres.

#### *Maximal support techniques*

In fit, healthy, anaesthetized patients breathing spontaneously, there is a reduction in the FRC. The $V_D : V_T$ ratio (including apparatus dead space) is approximately 0.5 when intubated and 0.65 when breathing from a mask. It is not uncommon for the alveolar ventilation to fall to below 2 L/min and for the $P_{aCO_2}$ to rise to 9.3 kPa (70 mmHg) after 1 h. Consequently, in patients with pulmonary disease, spontaneously breathing techniques are really suitable only for short procedures (e.g. check cystoscopy).

For longer operations, particularly those on the upper abdomen, there is an increasing tendency to use a balanced technique with paralysis, analgesia, and ventilation. Once this decision has been made, there is usually no intraoperative problem in maintaining the $P_{aO_2}$ and $P_{aCO_2}$ at any desired level, and the anaesthetist has effectively transferred most of his or her difficulties to the postoperative period. A combination of general and local anaesthesia can have the advantage of minimizing the dose of neuromuscular blocking agent needed (and hence the likelihood of postoperative muscle weakness) and avoiding ventilatory depression from opioids.

The extent of invasive monitoring is an individual decision and may be determined by the type of surgery; however, in most of the severe 'respiratory cripples', an arterial line for the measurement of blood gases proves invaluable.

In the fit, healthy patient having a general anaesthetic, there is a virtual shunt of 10% of the cardiac output producing an alveolar–arterial $P_{CO_2}$ gradient of only 0.08 kPa (0.6 mmHg). There is also a well-defined alveolar plateau when the expired $CO_2$ is recorded (see Figure 3.3a), which therefore represents an accurate measure of $P_{aCO_2}$. In the patient with pulmonary disease, there is frequently not only an increased virtual shunt, but also a wide variation in the efficiency of alveolar gas exchange causing a slope in the expired $CO_2$ trace (see Figure 3.3b). Under these conditions, the $P_{aCO_2}$ cannot be estimated accurately from the end-tidal $P_{CO_2}$ and arterial blood samples are needed.

There are good theoretical reasons for maintaining the intraoperative $P_{aCO_2}$ at the preoperative level. This continues the previous steady-state acid–base homoeostasis and prevents shifts in cerebrospinal fluid bicarbonate which would take time to recover later. With high tidal and minute volumes, this often necessitates the addition of $CO_2$ to the fresh gas flow or the use of a partial rebreathing circuit. An alternative is to ventilate to a $P_{aCO_2}$ of 5.3 kPa (40 mmHg), and allow the $P_{aCO_2}$ to rise at the end of the operation. Doing this, spontaneous ventilation, if it resumes, is usually triggered at a $P_{aCO_2}$ below the preoperative level. A prolonged period of intraoperative hyperventilation inevitably produces a net loss of $CO_2$ from the body. In the postoperative period, this implies that there will be an obligatory period of hypoventilation while the deficit is repaid.

There is little hard evidence available that certain ventilatory patterns are preferable to others. However, it is logical to supply large tidal volumes (12–15 ml/kg) and a sufficient inspiratory time (either with a slow rate or an inspiratory hold) to maximize the equality of ventilation between fast and slow alveoli. Similarly, the expiratory phase should be long enough for a full exhalation. Avoid excessively high inflation pressures because of the dangers of bursting an emphysematous bulla.

Patients with copious secretions or focal sepsis may benefit from appropriate positioning to keep the affected lung dependent, or endobronchial intubation to isolate the good lung from the bad lung. Frequent aspiration should be carried out to prevent soiling of the good lung.

Intraoperative fluid balance is important. Dehydration makes secretions more viscous and difficult to suck out, and over-hydration risks postoperative pulmonary oedema. In the presence of normal renal function, the latter can, provided that it is recognized, be treated effectively with diuretics.

Two classes of drug to prescribe with great care are sedatives and β-adrenoceptor blockers. Over-sedation can precipitate ventilatory failure. β-Adrenoceptor blockers cause bronchoconstriction via $\beta_2$-adrenoceptors. Thus, if they are needed, a cardioselective type (e.g. acebutalol, atenolol, metoprolol) should be used, but only in very small doses. Even then, it may cause a rapid deterioration in effective ventilation.

All patients with chronic airflow limitation, and especially those with over-distended lungs, are at risk of developing a pneumothorax. This should always be suspected if there is a sudden onset of breathlessness (especially if it is associated with sudden pleuritic chest pain) in the perioperative period. It is a particular risk during anaesthesia when high ventilation pressures are required, and the location of a chest drain should always be known.

Hypotension in these patients can be dangerous for three reasons. First, collapsed lung segments are often poorly perfused because of compensation by hypoxic pulmonary vasoconstriction. The use of sodium nitroprusside and other vasodilating agents reduces this compensation, thus increasing the shunt and reducing the $P_{aO_2}$. Second, hypotension always causes an increase in the physiological dead space with consequent deterioration in $CO_2$ removal and the $P_{aO_2}$. Third, the use of ganglion and β-adrenoceptor blockers as part of the technique may precipitate or intensify the bronchoconstrictive component of airway obstruction. Posturing and subcutaneous injections of local anaesthetics with epinephrine (adrenaline) are really the only safe methods of assisting haemostasis.

## Postoperative phase

### *The normal response to anaesthesia*

In all patients who have been anaesthetized with nitrous oxide, there is an unimportant, transient decrease in the $P_{aO_2}$ of up to 1.3 kPa (10 mmHg) which lasts for 10 min, when they resume breathing air. It can be prevented by giving 100% oxygen for 2 min at the end of the operation.

The major effects of anaesthesia on pulmonary gas exchange in the postoperative period depend on the site of surgery. In the operative and immediate postoperative period, the FRC is reduced with alveolar gas trapping and there is an increased right-to-left shunt. The cause is unknown, but it can produce falls in $P_{aO_2}$ of up to 4.0 kPa (30 mmHg) when breathing air and compared with the preoperative level. It is easily corrected by giving 30–40% oxygen on a facemask. After the first hour or two, those patients who have undergone limb or superficial body surgery reverse these changes and effectively return to their normal preoperative state. However, when patients with previously healthy lungs undergo abdominal or thoracic surgery, this reduction in oxygenation continues for at least 48 hours and may extend for up to 5 days. This effect is worst with upper abdominal, thoracic, and paramedian incisions, and least with lower abdominal incisions. Factors known to exacerbate these effects are wound pain (prevents deep breathing, can reduce VC by up to 50%, reduces expiratory force), abdominal distension (splints the diaphragm), the supine position (when the relationship of FRC to closing volume is least favourable), and over-transfusion (tendency to pulmonary oedema).

All the above changes are intensified in patients with poor preoperative lung function, cigarette smokers, obese individuals, and very old people. They are also the groups most at risk from infection and segmental collapse secondary to sputum retention.

### Assessment and initial management

After reversal of neuromuscular block some patients will make ventilatory movements that are obviously adequate on clinical grounds alone, and they can be extubated immediately. In others, it is preferable to make a more formal assessment of the ventilatory state before extubation. Some anaesthetists do this purely on clinical grounds, principally by assessing distress, ventilatory rate, tachycardia, and adequacy of tissue oxygenation. Others apply numerical values such as a ventilation rate below 30 breaths/min, a $Pa\text{O}_2$ over 9.3 kPa (70 mmHg) on 40% $F\text{IO}_2$, a VC of over 12–15 ml/kg, and an inspiratory force of over 30 cm$H_2O$.

Once the patient is extubated, it can be very difficult to make an accurate visual assessment of the adequacy of ventilation, or to measure tidal or minute volumes. Other measurements such as VC and PEFR are dependent on the cooperation of the patient and may indicate low values because of sedation, pain, or residual neuromuscular block, and may not reflect the adequacy or otherwise of ventilation. *If there is any doubt, it is best to measure the blood gases on a known* $F\text{IO}_2$.

If ventilation is absent or obviously inadequate, continue IPPV while the cause is being identified. Once muscular weakness has been excluded by peripheral nerve stimulation, the major factors influencing apnoea are the $Pa\text{CO}_2$, the level of sedation, and drug-induced ventilatory depression. Gradually let the $Pa\text{CO}_2$ rise to the preoperative value and allow sufficient time for the elimination of volatile agents. If the pupils are small, consider opioid reversal with naloxone, the dose being titrated so as not to aggravate postoperative pain. Once spontaneous ventilation recommences, keep the endotracheal tube in place. This allows accurate control of the inspired gas mixture and ease of aspiration of secretions until ventilation is established as satisfactory.

Further measures that can improve borderline ventilation are continuous positive airway pressure and nursing the patient in the sitting or semi-recumbent position. Both of these measures improve the FRC. Another possibility is to 'drive' ventilation with the stimulant drug doxapram. There is a wide variation in the infusion rate required, and it must be adjusted to give adequate ventilation without an unpleasant level of nausea, mental anxiety, or peripheral tremor.

Occasionally, in that minority of patients who are on hypoxic drive (they normally have a preoperative $Pa\text{O}_2$ of below 6.7 kPa [50 mmHg]), it will be necessary to lower the $F\text{IO}_2$ to stimulate ventilation. It is pertinent here to stress the dangers of uncontrolled oxygen therapy to these patients. Initially, the $Pa\text{O}_2$ is maintained but the $Pa\text{CO}_2$ rises and ultimately leads to coma, cessation of breathing, and hypoxia. Once they are extubated, use fixed performance masks (such as a Ventimask) with either 24% or 28% $O_2$.

If there is still clinical and objective evidence of ventilatory failure, IPPV must be continued. This may only be a short-term requirement to allow for further metabolism of drugs and return of full muscle power.

### Management after extubation

After extubation, the patient should ideally go to a high dependency unit. If this is not available, in borderline cases, an overnight stay on an intensive care unit is the safest recourse, despite the possibly unnecessary use of expensive resources.

#### Posture

Provided that the surgical procedure allows it, minimize the factors reducing the FRC by sitting the patient up.

#### Oxygen therapy

Hypoxia persists for several days after upper abdominal and thoracic operations. Oxygen therapy is universally advocated, but the desirable amount and duration are poorly established. A sensible approach is to supply $F\text{IO}_2$ (by mask or nasal prongs) sufficient to maintain adequate oxygenation, usually for 24 hours. At this time reassess if it needs to be continued. Always identify and treat any cause of alveolar hypoventilation (opioids, pneumothorax, pain, sputum retention).

#### Analgesia

Good pain relief allows maximal ventilatory activity. When using opioids, this represents a balance between pain reduction and the depression of ventilation and conscious level. There is enormous individual variation in the response to opioids, and it is often better to give the initial dose gradually intravenously and titrate it against ventilatory depression (this is usually maximal from 5 to 10 min after injection). Patient-controlled analgesia can be excellent with a cooperative patient.

The reduction of pain of upper abdominal incisions by regional blockade has frequently been quoted as optimizing postoperative lung function. Thoracic epidurals have the facility for easy top-ups and can certainly provide excellent analgesia. Epidural analgesia can be with a local anaesthetic or opioid, given intermittently, or by continuous infusion. Remind the nursing staff of the dangers of hypotension, especially in the sitting position. A problem occasionally encountered in severe restrictive lung disease is a deterioration in gas exchange as a result of paralysis of intercostal and abdominal musculature. Intercostal blockade, although effective, is not easy to repeat and can cause a pneumothorax.

#### Secretions

The ability to cough and remove secretions is paramount and a 'fruity' cough with no sputum production is a bad prognostic sign. Try to remove secretions by postural drainage and physiotherapy. This is not always possible because of the surgical procedure. The best results are obtained if the peak actions of both the analgesia and the physiotherapist coincide.

A portable chest radiograph will help to identify any localized problems such as lobar collapse. Fibreoptic bronchoscopy under local anaesthesia by a skilled user can sometimes remove a plug of mucus without recourse to intubation.

#### Obstructive apnoea

Although the magnitude of the problem is not yet defined, sleep apnoea has, over the past few years, been regarded with increasing suspicion as a cause of postoperative hypoxia. It has been shown that sleep, and most probably anaesthesia, causes a reduction in the muscle tone of the tongue and pharynx, thus allowing these structures to collapse inwards and occlude the airway. These changes may possibly persist up to 12 hours after anaesthesia and are more common when parenteral opioids are used.

Apnoeic periods occur almost entirely during sleep and are associated with oxygen desaturation. When patients with obstructive airway disease fall asleep they may develop severe hypoxia associated with obstructive apnoea.

The loss of muscular tone is also apparent in the intercostal muscles (but not the diaphragm which has little spindle control), and these have a poor compensatory response to partial or complete obstruction of the airway.

## FURTHER READING


Craig DB. Postoperative recovery of pulmonary function. *Anesth Analg* 1981;**60**:46–52.

Gal TJ. Anaesthesia for patients with lung disease. In: Pearl RG, ed. *The Lung in Anaesthesia and Intensive Care. Baillière's Clin Anaesthesiol* 1996;**10**:63–76.

Leeman M. The pulmonary circulation in lung diseases. In: Pearl RG, ed. *The Lung in Anaesthesia and Intensive Care. Baillière's Clin Anaesthesiol* 1996;**10**:215–30.

Kafer ER. Respiratory and cardiovascular functions in scoliosis and the principles of anesthetic management. *Anesthesiology* 1980;**52**:339–51.

Nunn JF, Milledge JS, Chen D, Dore C. Respiratory criteria of fitness for surgery and anaesthesia. *Anaesthesia* 1988;**43**:543–51.

Selsby DS, Jones JG. Some physiological and clinical aspects of chest physiotherapy. *Br J Anaesth* 1990;**64**:621–31.

Sykes MK. *Respiratory Support. Principles and Practice Series*. London: BMJ Publishing Group, 1995.

Tarhan S, Moffit EA, Sessler AD. Risk of anesthesia and surgery in patients with chronic bronchitis and chronic obstructive pulmonary disease. *Surgery* 1973;**74**:720–6.

# Chapter 55 The patient with diabetes

G.M. Cooper

Diabetes mellitus is the most common endocrine disorder that the anaesthetist encounters, affecting about 2% of the population in the UK. It is a disorder of glucose metabolism characterized by a relative or complete lack of insulin.

Normally, approximately 50 units (a quarter of the store) of insulin are released daily in response to carbohydrate foods. Insulin enhances the entry of glucose into muscle and fat cells by facilitated diffusion across the cell membrane. It stimulates glycogen formation (in liver and muscle), inhibits glycogenolysis and gluconeogenesis, and encourages fat deposition, both by inhibiting lipase and by the transport of glucose into fat cells. Insulin also facilitates potassium transport into cells. Feedback mechanisms maintain the blood glucose in normal individuals between 3.5 and 7.0 mmol/L. Peak values after meals rarely exceed 8 mmol/L and hence glycosuria never occurs unless the renal threshold for glucose reabsorption is below the normal value of 10 mmol/L.

Patients with diabetes are divided into type 1 (insulin dependent) and type 2 (non-insulin dependent). Although this stemmed from their prior classification into juvenile onset, who were insulin dependent, and maturity onset, who were non-insulin dependent, this distinction has become blurred; this is because those type 2 patients who were previously treated with diet and/or oral hypoglycaemic agents are sometimes now treated with insulin in order to gain better control of serum glucose.

Diabetes mellitus may be primary or secondary. It is now accepted that type 1 diabetes results from autoimmune destruction of the β cells in the pancreatic islets, the propensity to which is partly determined by heredity (Figure 55.1). The genetic markers for diabetes susceptibility are much more common than the disease, which suggests that an additional, probably environmental, factor is superimposed. Only 5% of cases of diabetes result from a recognizable pathological process, or are secondary to some other condition. Such causes include:

- pancreatic insufficiency from chronic pancreatitis, haemochromatosis, pancreatectomy, or carcinoma of the pancreas;
- secretion or ingestion of substances that antagonize insulin at the cellular level, e.g. steroids (Cushing's syndrome), growth hormone (acromegaly), epinephrine (adrenaline) (phaeochromocytoma), hyperthyroidism, glucagonoma;
- pregnancy (increased insulin requirements);
- liver disease;
- drugs, especially steroids, but also the oral contraceptive pill, and thiazide diuretics;
- major injuries, especially burns.

People with type 2 diabetes have been noted to have amylin (a peptide similar to amyloid, also known as islet-associated polypeptide) deposition near the β-cell membrane. It is thought that amylin may be responsible for the secretory defect in people with type 2 diabetes; in animal models pharmacological doses of amylin have been shown to cause a decrease in insulin sensitivity.

The aim of treatment in diabetes is to prevent the acute consequences of hyperglycaemia and hypoglycaemia, and to reduce, or prevent, long-term complications. The long-term complications are significant causes of morbidity and mortality, and frequently lead to the need for surgery. Indeed, 50% of people with

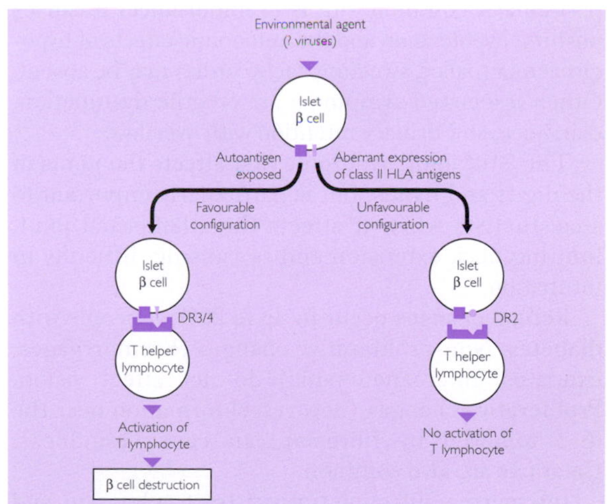


**Figure 55.1** Hypothetical scheme for the autoimmune β-cell destruction in type 1 diabetes mellitus. Viruses or other agents could induce islet β cells to express class II antigens and to 'expose' autoantigens (viral antigens could be expressed on β cells, or a normal β-cell antigen could mimic viral antigens). The autoantigen (shown in pale green), when co-expressed with HLA-DR3 and/or -DR4, has a 'favourable' configuration, which activates T-helper lymphocytes and triggers autoimmune damage. By contrast, HLA-DR2 has an 'unfavourable' configuration, which prevents this from happening. (Adapted from Williams G and Monson JP. Diabetes mellitus and lipid metabolism. In: Souhami RL and Moxham J, eds. *Textbook of Medicine*, 3rd edn. Edinburgh: Churchill Livingstone, 1997.)

**Table 55.1 The long-term complications of diabetes**

| | |
|---|---|
| Vascular (large vessels) | Ischaemic heart disease<br>Peripheral vascular disease<br>Cerebrovascular disease |
| Vascular (small vessels) | Renal impairment<br>Retinopathy |
| Neurological | Peripheral neuropathy, mainly sensory<br>Autonomic neuropathy |
| Joints | Stiffness |
| Infection | Increased susceptibility |

diabetes require surgery at some time. Tight glycaemic control has now been shown to reduce retinopathy and nephropathy. The complications of diabetes are summarized in Table 55.1. It must be appreciated that, although type 2 is often described as 'mild' diabetes, these patients are nevertheless susceptible to chronic diabetic complications.

Vascular complications are responsible for 75% of all deaths from diabetes. Both large and small vessels are affected. Ischaemic heart disease is five times more frequent than in people who do not have diabetes, and atheromatous disease in peripheral vessels is 50-fold more common than in normal individuals. Hypertension and cerebrovascular disease are also common in people with diabetes.

Severe cases of sensory neuropathy result in chronic painless ulcers, which frequently become infected and may progress to gangrene. Autonomic neuropathy is not particularly common, but is of importance. It causes postural hypotension and the autonomic effects of hypoglycaemia (pallor, sweating, tachycardia) may be absent. Other associated symptoms are erectile dysfunction, diarrhoea, and urinary retention with overflow.

The 'stiff joint' syndrome first affects the joints of the digits and hands, but is particularly important to anaesthetists when it affects the atlantoaxial joint, limiting neck extension and so causing difficulty in intubation.

Retinal changes occur in up to 20% of people with diabetes. Non-proliferative changes (haemorrhages, exudates, microaneurysms) do not affect vision. Proliferative changes (new vessel formation near the disc followed by fibrosis) can cause blindness. Cataracts are also common.

Intercurrent infection (urinary tract, vulva, skin, and chest) is common in people with diabetes, and can worsen control of blood sugar. Tuberculosis is not unusual, especially in elderly people.

It will be appreciated that some of the complications of diabetes pose a threat to the safety of surgery; historically, people with diabetes had a greatly increased mortality. With better overall control of diabetes, and newer antibiotics, operative morbidity and mortality are now nearer those of the non-diabetic population.

## PREOPERATIVE ASSESSMENT

Most people with diabetes will already be diagnosed, but always be alert to the common presenting features (polyuria, fatigue, pruritus vulvae, thirst), whether there is a family history, if female whether she has had babies weighing over 4.5 kg, maintenance therapies (corticosteroids, thiazides), and obesity.

It is important to assess the degree of control of the diabetes. Poor control is indicated by frequent hospital admissions with either hyperglycaemia or hypoglycaemia. An indication of good control is frequent self-measured blood glucose within normal limits charted in a booklet. In between these extremes is a chart showing blood glucose estimations varying between normal and erratically high. The annual review by a diabetologist records the level of glycosylated haemoglobin ($HbA_{1c}$) which reflects the exposure of adult haemoglobin (HbA) to glucose over the preceding 6–8 weeks. Non-diabetic values of $HbA_{1c}$ are about 5–8% of total HbA; well-controlled diabetic values are 8–10% and poorly controlled diabetes is reflected by values over 12%.

### Drug history

It is important to be aware of the type of insulin and/or oral hypoglycaemic drugs being taken. Short-acting oral drugs include glipizide, tolbutamide, and tolazamide. Glibenclamide has a medium half-life but is concentrated in the islet cells and is effective for over 24 hours. Chlorpropamide has a very long half-life and may still be acting after 50 hours.

Since the 1980s, insulin has been manufactured with the human amino acid sequence by recombinant DNA technology, using genetically programmed yeast or bacteria. About 80% of insulin used in the UK is 'human' insulin, although highly purified pork and beef preparations are still available and are preferred by some patients. There is a perception that an insulin that is exactly the same as the one produced endogenously is intrinsically better, although the highly purified porcine insulin has similar immunogenicity and is available at a similar price. The availability of insulin 'pens', which are pre-filled multi-dose portable syringes, has facilitated the more intensive management regimens and improved the lifestyle of many patients.

Insulin analogues have recently become available for clinical use. They are 'designer' insulins with a similar action to human insulin. The rapidly acting analogue, insulin lispro, is now marketed and other analogues, including long-acting ones, are under study. Insulin lispro is produced by interchanging amino acids at positions 28 and 29 in the human B chain to make

**Table 55.2 Characteristics of some insulin preparations**

| | Example | Onset (h) | Peak effect (h) | Duration (h) |
|---|---|---|---|---|
| Rapid acting | Insulin lispro | 0.25 | Approx. 2 | 2–5 |
| Short acting | Actrapid<br>Velosulin<br>Humulin S | 0.5–2 | 2–6 | 8 |
| Intermediate acting | Insulatard<br>Protophane<br>Isophane<br>Humulin I | 2–4 | 4–11 | 24 |
| Long acting | Monotard<br>Ultratard<br>Lente | 2–8 | 8–12 | 30 |

an insulin whose monomeric molecules are more rapidly absorbed. This means that an injection given before a meal mimics more closely the normal peripheral insulin profile seen in people who don't have diabetes, and hypoglycaemia may be less common. Insulin lispro is given immediately before a meal rather than 30 min before eating as with soluble insulin.

The characteristics of some of the more common insulin preparations are summarized in Table 55.2. The time of administration should be noted and cognisance made of the relationship to ingested food. The importance of this is highlighted when insulin has been given but an accident or sudden illness occurs and food intake is omitted.

Look for evidence of any of the complications of diabetes.

*Cardiovascular system*

Evidence of angina, myocardial infarction, intermittent claudication, gangrene, and postural hypotension (systolic fall of > 30 mmHg on standing) should be sought.

*Nervous system*

Involvement may show as numbness, pain, paraesthesia, leg ulcers, strokes, transient ischaemic attacks, erectile dysfunction, or gustatory sweating. Postural hypotension is a late sign of autonomic neuropathy; loss of heart rate variability during deep breathing is the most reliable early sign.

*Kidney*

Symptoms may include polyuria (from glycosuria or renal failure), frequency, dysuria, and pruritus, or the secondary symptoms of anaemia or hypertension.

*Skin*

Look for boils and at the pressure areas.

*Joints*

Look at the hands and neck movements.

**Investigations**

*Full blood count, and urea and electrolytes*

These should be normal.

*Blood glucose*

This is an essential investigation in all people with diabetes. The desired value is between 5 and 10 mmol/L. Test strips (e.g. BM-stix and Glucostix), which contain glucose oxidase and a dye that reacts with the hydrogen peroxide generated by the oxidation of glucose in the blood sample, allow measurements to be made on the ward (or in the operating room) without the delay of a laboratory result. The colour change on the strip can be read either visually, or electronically by a reflectance meter.

*Urine analysis*

Look for glucose (hyperglycaemia), ketones (poor control), protein (renal complications), and at the bacteriology (infection).

*ECG*

This should be normal. Look for evidence of ischaemic heart disease.

*Chest radiograph*

This should be normal. Check for tuberculosis.

## PREOPERATIVE PREPARATION

Hypoglycaemia leads to permanent neuronal death and hyperglycaemia increases the likelihood of infection, as well as accelerating catabolism and delaying wound healing. Thus, the aim is to maintain the blood glucose within the normal range throughout the perioperative period. The constraints on this are:

- the need for preoperative starvation to prevent gastric aspiration;
- the metabolic response to surgery leading to hyperglycaemia; the extent and duration of the response are reflected by the magnitude of surgery;
- an inability to eat and drink normally after surgery;
- any hypoglycaemic agent already given.

There are several ways that normoglycaemia can be maintained. It is not important *how* it is achieved. Whatever method is chosen, it has been shown that the most important factor in good glycaemic control perioperatively is frequent measurement of blood glucose and appropriate interpretation and intervention. It is normal for insulin requirements to increase in the postoperative period. Putting the patient first (or early) on the morning list aids management. Guidelines are offered here.

### Person with diabetes controlled by diet

Treat as a normal patient but monitor the blood glucose in case insulin is required in the early postoperative phase. This is likely after major surgery.

### Person with diabetes controlled by oral drugs

#### *Minor surgery*

Ensure that chlorpropamide is withheld for 48 hours before surgery and other oral hypoglycaemic drugs are omitted on the day of surgery. Careful monitoring of blood sugar is usually all that is required. Hypoglycaemic drugs can be started postoperatively when food is taken.

#### *Major surgery*

Oral hypoglycaemic drugs should be stopped. Insulin and glucose infusions are started on the day of surgery (see below).

### Person with insulin-controlled diabetes

#### *Elective minor surgery*

If:

- the patient will be able to eat very soon after surgery,
- an early morning operation is arranged,
- the blood sugar is 5–10 mmol/L,
- there is no long-acting insulin circulating,

it is quite appropriate to omit food and insulin on the morning of surgery ('no food/no insulin' regimen) and take lunch with an appropriately reduced soluble insulin based on previous requirements.

#### *Elective intermediate/major surgery*

In the few days before surgery switch the patient to purely short-acting insulins. Doing this means that any long-acting insulin preparation is no longer present. There are then two main alternative methods of approach:

1. On the day of surgery, whatever time the operation is scheduled, stop the regular subcutaneous insulin, omit breakfast, and set up a continuous intravenous infusion of balanced amounts of glucose, potassium, and insulin (Table 55.3). This scheme (adapted from that of Alberti) has the advantage that any alteration of infusion rate (inadvertent or otherwise) changes the infusion of glucose and insulin simultaneously. A disadvantage is that the whole bag has to be changed if the glucose strays outside the desired 5–10 mmol/L.
2. Separate infusions of insulin and dextrose (with potassium) allow the insulin dosage to be altered more easily in response to blood glucose values. It must be emphasized that when using this technique, regular measurements of blood glucose (hourly) must be made. There is sometimes, even with short-acting insulins, a lag phase before the response to insulin is seen. This can then be followed by continued insulin action from that already infused, and thus glucose may need to be given to prevent hypoglycaemia. This method has increased in popularity recently, partly because of the ready availability of 'bedside' blood glucose monitoring kits.

For patients who are already on insulin preoperatively, determine an appropriate baseline infusion rate by dividing their daily dose by 24 and run this in, in units per hour. For patients not receiving insulin who become diabetic in the perioperative period, if the blood glucose is more than 10 mmol/L, begin the infusion at 5 units/h. Subsequent management of both groups is then guided by a sliding scale. There is no universal set of sliding scale figures that will apply to all patients. Tables 55.4 and 55.5 give two examples of sliding scales: one is for a 'sensitive' patient and the other for a more 'resistant' patient. Both of these have been used recently in the author's practice. It cannot be emphasized too strongly that, although sliding scales can give excellent control:

- the blood glucose must be measured at least hourly;
- the possibility of a lag in response should not be forgotten;
- 50% glucose must be readily available to give intravenously both to prevent and to treat hypoglycaemia;
- the prescribed scale may need changing in the light of the patient's response.

#### *Emergency surgery, previously well controlled*

The only additional problem is the presence of any long-acting insulin already given, which may result in

| Table 55.3 Glucose–potassium–insulin regimen for surgery |
|---|
| 15 units soluble insulin + 10 mmol KCl in 500 ml 10% dextrose |
| Infuse 100 ml hourly |
| Check blood glucose hourly:<br>if glucose < 5 mmol/L: replace bag with one containing 10 units insulin + KCl<br>if glucose > 10 mmol/L: replace bag with one containing 20 units insulin + KCl |

KCl, potassium chloride.
Adapted from Alberti KGMM. Thomas DJB. *Br J Anaesth* 1979;51:693–710.

| Table 55.4 Insulin dose according to blood glucose: an example for a relatively 'sensitive' patient | |
|---|---|
| Blood glucose (mmol/L) | Insulin dose (units/h) |
| 0–4 | 0 |
| 4–8 | 0.5 |
| 8–12 | 1.0 |
| 12–16 | 1.5 |
| 16–20 | 2.0 |
| > 20 | 3.0 |

| Table 55.5 Insulin dose according to blood glucose: an example for a relatively 'resistant' patient | |
|---|---|
| Blood glucose (mmol/L) | Insulin dose (units/h) |
| < 3 | 0 |
| 3–5 | 1 |
| 6–8 | 2 |
| 8–10 | 3 |
| 10–15 | 5 |
| 15–20 | 10 |
| >20 | 15 |

hypoglycaemia. This can be countered with intravenous infusion of dextrose and careful monitoring of the blood glucose.

#### *Emergency surgery, poorly controlled*

In general, all surgery should be avoided in those with uncontrolled diabetes but, occasionally, it is necessary to operate on a patient who is ketoacidotic. This is usually for an intra-abdominal problem. There are two diagnostic difficulties:

1. Severe abdominal pain may be caused by ketoacidosis.
2. Severe peritonitis may present with minimal pain because of neuropathy.

Once surgery is decided on, each case must be managed individually. It is a serious undertaking. The object of management is not to try to correct everything as quickly as possible, achieving in an hour what normally takes 1–2 days. Rapid changes produce dangerous swings in serum osmolality (which can result in cerebral oedema) and imbalances the serum and cerebrospinal fluid pH (which disturbs the ventilatory compensation of acidosis). It is sufficient, before urgent surgery, to correct acute hypovolaemia and produce a falling blood glucose. The likely abnormalities are highlighted in Table 55.6. The biochemical basis and pathophysiological disturbances of diabetic ketoacidosis are summarized in Figure 55.2.

| Table 55.6 Probable abnormalities to be corrected before emergency surgery in ketoacidosis |
|---|
| Fluid losses – 100 ml/kg |
| Electrolyte losses:<br>sodium – 8 mmol/kg<br>potassium – 4 mmol/kg |
| Hyperglycaemia and hyperosmotic plasma<br>Osmolarity = [glucose] + [urea] + 2[$Na^+$ + $K^+$] |
| Metabolic acidosis, compensated by hyperventilation and a low $PaCO_2$ |
| Hypotension if severely hypovolaemic and acidotic |

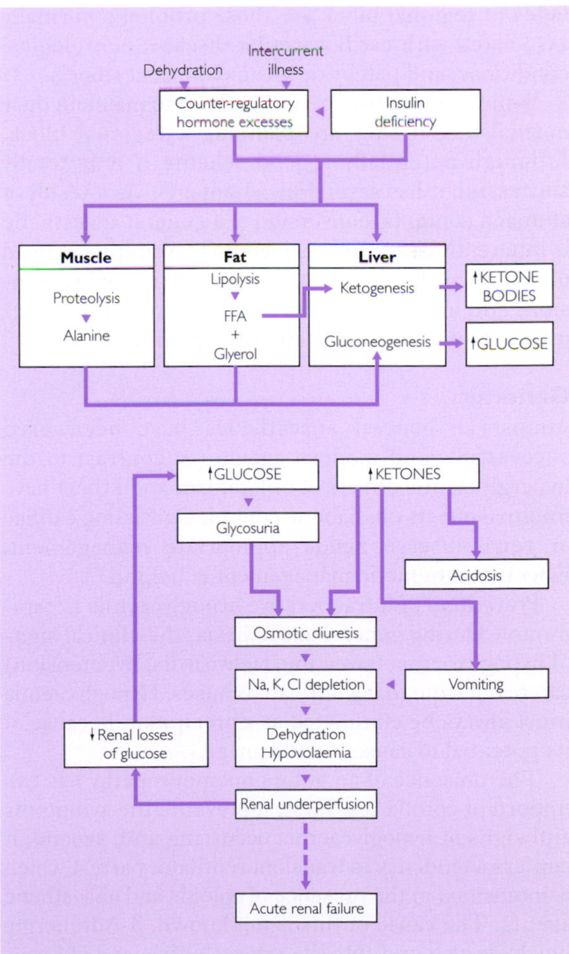


**Figure 55.2** (a) The biochemical basis and (b) pathophysiological disturbances of diabetic ketoacidosis. FFA, free fatty acid. (Adapted from Williams G and Monson JP. Diabetes mellitus and lipid metabolism. In: Souhami RL and Moxham J, eds. *Textbook of Medicine*, 3rd edn. Edinburgh: Churchill Livingstone, 1997.)

It is important to remember that ketoacidosis delays gastric emptying and therefore cricoid pressure will always be required.

These patients must be managed in an intensive care area where facilities for resuscitation and ventilation are available. The details of treatment are beyond the remit of this book but in brief: intravenous fluids (saline), insulin (20 units i.v. stat) followed by 10 units/h should be given, with continuous ECG monitoring. Regular blood glucose, potassium, and arterial gases guide therapy.

For all people with diabetes, the need for antibiotic prophylaxis must be considered.

## INTRAOPERATIVE PHASE

There is no evidence that, with appropriate management, either general or local anaesthesia is better. For some operations, general anaesthesia is the only possibility.

### Local

The advantages of regional anaesthesia are reduction of the stress response, early detection of hypoglycaemia in the awake patient, less postoperative nausea, and easy postoperative control of diabetes. The disadvantages of regional block are those problems normally associated with cardiovascular disease, neurological conditions, and patchy or incomplete anaesthesia.

Some anaesthetists permit patients to maintain their normal diet if they are planning a regional block. Although potentially a good scheme if it is totally successful, it has several disadvantages. As a result of stomach contents, conversion to a general anaesthetic is inherently risky, there is likely to be vomiting instead of nausea in response to a transient period of hypotension, and any convulsion secondary to intravascular injection of local anaesthetic risks aspiration.

### General

Almost all general anaesthetics have been used successfully and modern agents (in contrast to the hyperglycaemic effects of chloroform and ether) have minimal effects on diabetic control. Coexisting cardiac or renal disease needs appropriate management. Effective antiemetic management is helpful.

Prevention of intraoperative hypoglycaemia is paramount. During general anaesthesia, the clinical signs of hypoglycaemia (sweating, tachycardia, hypotension) can result from many unrelated causes. Hypoglycaemia must always be eliminated as a precipitant because of its potential to cause brain damage.

The presence of an autonomic neuropathy has two important corollaries. First, it prevents the symptoms and signs of hypoglycaemia occurring and, second, it confers a tendency to transient ventilatory arrest which is intensified in the presence of opioids and anaesthetic agents. The cause of this is not known. β-Adrenergic blockade also prevents the sympathetic signs of hypoglycaemia. Patients with autonomic neuropathy are also at risk during changes of intraoperative posture and may develop hypotension on institution of intermittent positive pressure ventilation.

Intraoperative fluid replacement can be as normal, although lactate (Hartmann's solution) and fructose-containing solutions should probably be avoided. Concentrated solutions of dextrose are irritant to veins and if needed should be given into a central vein.

#### *In ketoacidosis*

On the rare occasion that a ketoacidotic patient requires general anaesthesia, it is important to appreciate that the arterial $CO_2$ tension ($P\text{a}CO_2$) must be controlled to the level at which the patient is compensating for the metabolic acidosis. Otherwise, ventilation to normocapnia may produce an acute and dangerous fall in blood pH. However, if the $P\text{a}CO_2$ is very low, there can be a serious fall in cardiac output during anaesthesia. Under these conditions, it may be preferable to infuse bicarbonate and allow the $P\text{a}CO_2$ to rise by reducing the ventilation. It must be stressed that great care is needed to prevent dangerous swings in pH and serum potassium (which can be sufficient to produce cardiac arrest).

Blood gases will need to be done frequently (every 15 min) throughout the operation, and the ventilation adjusted accordingly. Reversal of neuromuscular blocking agents may be impaired in the presence of acidosis. In serious cases, a period of postoperative ventilation may be required until the diabetes is under better control.

## POSTOPERATIVE PHASE

Aim to get the patient back to a normal diet and insulin (or oral hypoglycaemics) as soon as possible. There is some evidence that better control is attained if an insulin infusion is maintained for 72 hours after surgery. This is relevant to the more major operations and is important because better diabetic control improves wound healing. Insulin requirements are increased postoperatively because of the stress response and if infection is present.

Write clear instructions to the nursing staff about the frequency of glucose estimations (e.g. hourly) and what to do, or who to call, if it falls outside prescribed limits (e.g. 5–10 mmol/L).

Remember that people with diabetes are prone to infection (examine the chest regularly) and arrange physiotherapy and antibiotics as necessary. Always suspect an occult infection if diabetic control worsens unexpectedly. Increased insulin requirement usually precedes the symptoms of infection.

## FURTHER READING


Alberti KGMM. Diabetes and surgery. *Anesthesiology* 1991;**74**:209–11.

Hirsch IB, McGill JB, Cryer PE, White PF. Perioperative management of surgical patients with diabetes mellitus. *Anesthesiology* 1991;**74**:346–359.

Libowitz HE. Diabetic ketoacidosis. *Lancet* 1995;**345**:767–71.

McKenzie CR, Charlson ME. Assessment of perioperative risk in the patient with diabetes mellitus. *Surg Gynecol Obstet* 1988;**167**:293–9.

Milaskiewicz RM, Hall GM. Diabetes mellitus and anaesthesia. *Curr Anaesth Crit Care* 1992;**3**:30–6.

Milaskiewicz RM, Hall GM. Diabetes and anaesthesia: the past decade. *Br J Anaesth* 1992;**68**:198–206.

Williams G. Management of non-insulin dependent diabetes mellitus. *Lancet* 1994;**343**:95–100

# Chapter 56 The patient with a thyroid, pituitary, or adrenal disorder

P. Hutton

## THE THYROID GLAND

### Physiology

The detailed physiology of the thyroid gland and its hormones is given in Chapter 29. In summary, the thyroid gland, located immediately below the larynx, secretes the hormones thyroxine ($T_4$) and triiodothyronine ($T_3$), whose functions are the regulation of tissue metabolism. Ninety percent of the hormonal release is $T_4$ of which some is subsequently deiodinated to $T_3$. Both hormones have quantitatively similar effects but $T_3$ is more potent and is shorter acting. Iodine (about 1 mg weekly) is essential for the formation of thyroid hormones. Iodine deficiency in the first 2 years of life results in irreversible mental handicap (cretinism).

To maintain a normal basal metabolic rate, thyroid hormone secretion is regulated by a specific feedback mechanism. Thyrotrophin-releasing hormone (TRH) from the hypothalamus directly increases output of thyroid-stimulating hormone (TSH) by the anterior pituitary gland. TSH in turn increases both the secretion and formation of $T_3$ and $T_4$. These are both stored bound to thyroglobulin in thyroid follicles but are released from the gland in the free form. They are then bound to thyroxine-binding globulin and thyroxine-binding prealbumin, and a small proportion to albumin. The unbound fraction, which can now be measured, increases the overall metabolic rate and, in children, stimulates growth.

The clinical problems associated with the thyroid result from excessive or deficient hormone secretion (hyperthyroidism or hypothyroidism) or, alternatively, from physical enlargement of the gland which may, or may not, be associated with hormonal dysfunction.

### Hypothyroidism

Hypothyroidism affects 1.4% of women and 0.1% of men. It is also referred to as myxoedema which, strictly, is the non-pitting oedema caused by mucopolysaccharide accumulation in subcutaneous tissues. The causes are:

- autoimmune destruction;
- iatrogenic (surgery and radioiodine);
- failure of adequate replacement therapy;
- drugs (lithium, amiodarone);
- iodine deficiency (rare because of iodized table salt);
- secondary hypothyroidism (pituitary disease, TRH deficiency);
- congenital.

#### *Anaesthetic considerations*

*History*

You should always have a high index of suspicion because this disease is one of the 'great imitators'. Common symptoms are weakness, fatigue, lethargy, dry coarse skin, voice change, intolerance of cold, moderate weight gain despite anorexia, poor memory and hearing, arthralgia, constipation, and swelling of the hands, face, and extremities. Be careful not to confuse the poor memory of hypothyroidism ('myxoedema madness') with that of cerebrovascular insufficiency of senile dementia. Check that those patients already treated with thyroxine are no longer clinically hypothyroid. Observe later if there are symptoms or signs of an enlarged gland.

*Examination*

*General*

Body and scalp hair are reduced and the skin is coarse, cool, and sallow.

*Cardiovascular system*

Bradycardia is common, with a low stroke volume. The heart sounds may be distant and the heart enlarged. A pericardial effusion is common but rarely leads to clinical problems.

*Nervous system*

Cerebellar ataxia may be present. Delayed relaxation of deep tendon reflexes, peripheral neuropathy, and carpal tunnel syndrome all resolve with hormone replacement.

*Respiratory system*

The ventilatory sensitivity to both hypoxia and hypercapnia is greatly decreased while hypothyroid. Ventilatory depressant drugs may precipitate myxoedema coma. History of hoarseness is important, indicating vocal cord involvement. Assessment of goitre should be thorough, as for hyperthyroidism.

*Investigations*

*Serum thyroxine*

A reduced free $T_4$ index is diagnostic of hypothyroidism unless the patient is on large doses of salicylates or phenytoin.

*Full blood count*

This should be normal or show only mild normochromic/normocytic anaemia.

*Urea and electrolytes*
The glomerular filtration rate is reduced and the ability to excrete free water is reduced. Inappropriate antidiuretic hormone (ADH; vasopressin) secretion may lead to a low serum sodium.

*ECG*
This may indicate bradycardia, cardiomegaly, and ischaemia.

*Chest radiograph*
This may reveal cardiomegaly or a pericardial effusion. Check that there is no retrosternal extension of the thyroid gland.

*Preoperative preparation*
The patient who is on replacement hormone treatment and who is clinically euthyroid does not present any particular anaesthetic problem and can be treated as normal. Patients found to be hypothyroid on admission should be rendered euthyroid before surgery with $T_4$ (50–200 μg daily) over a week or 10 days. For urgent cases, the previously undiagnosed patient can be given $T_3$ intravenously over a few hours. This must be done in a high dependency unit (HDU), with full monitoring in case myocardial ischaemia develops in response to enhanced metabolism.

*Intraoperative and postoperative management*
For the treated euthyroid patient, this should progress satisfactorily. It is, however, sensible to be alert to the fact that the patient may be hypothyroid and start with reduced dosages of all sedatives, induction agents, analgesics, and volatile agents. The presence of hypothyroidism makes the patients:

- sensitive to all sedatives and opioids;
- sensitive to all intravenous and volatile anaesthetics;
- easy to hyperventilate to hypocapnia because the low metabolic rate is producing less $CO_2$ than usual;
- prone to episodes of hypotension;
- prone to hypothermia;
- prone to hyponatraemia from reduced water excretion.

## Hyperthyroidism

Like hypothyroidism, hyperthyroidism is more common in females: 1.9% of the female and 0.2% of the male population are affected, the peak incidence being between 20 and 40 years. The major symptoms reflect the hypermetabolic state (the basal metabolic rate is increased 30–60%), which is produced by excess circulating thyroid hormone. There can be a familial incidence. The following are the causes:

- Common: Grave's disease; multinodular diffuse enlargement;
- Rarer: thyroid adenoma; choriocarcinoma; thyroiditis; pituitary adenoma.

Diagnosis is confirmed by elevated serum concentrations of free and total $T_4$ and $T_3$ and undetectable serum TSH. The most reliable clinical sign is a sleeping heart rate of more than 80 beats/min.

### Preoperative considerations

*History*
Agitated fatigue, palpitations, muscle weakness, and heat intolerance are frequent complaints. Weight loss is common, despite an increased appetite. Bowel habit may be increased infrequency and, rarely, there is diarrhoea. In premenopausal women, amenorrhoea may occur and, in older patients, angina or heart failure may be worsened. Hyperthyroidism *is often asymptomatic in elderly people*.

*Examination*
*General*
Thyroid enlargement is common (refer to later section for assessment and management). Thyroid bruits are sometimes heard because of the increased blood flow. The ocular signs of hyperthyroidism include stare, lid lag, lid retraction, and proptosis. Look for raised, thickened skin on the legs or feet (pretibial myxoedema – rare). The hair is usually fine and silky.

*Cardiovascular system*
Tachycardia, atrial arrhythmias, widened pulse pressure, systolic flow murmurs, and increased intensity of the first heart sound are classic signs. Check that the thyrotoxic state has not precipitated heart failure, which, along with atrial arrhythmias, may be the only presenting symptoms and findings (especially atrial fibrillation in elderly people).

*Nervous system*
A fine tremor of the fingers and tongue, together with hyper-reflexia, is characteristic.

*Investigations*
*Full blood count*
Leukopenia may occur as a side effect of antithyroid drugs.

*ECG and chest radiograph*
These may show evidence of the cardiac effects and the presence of a retrosternal goitre.

*Serum $T_4$*
Confirm euthyroid state by a free $T_4$ index.

### Preoperative preparation

If surgery is being performed on the thyroid gland, the antithyroid drugs can be modified with oral iodine (e.g. potassium iodide 60 mg three times daily) for the week preceding surgery, in order to reduce the vascularity of the gland. Check that the drugs have been taken. When premedicating, sedate the patient well, especially if nervous. Continue β-adrenoceptor blockade on the day of surgery.

### Intraoperative phase

There is no contraindication to the usual anaesthetic agents or techniques, although it is wise to avoid drugs that stimulate the sympathetic nervous system (e.g. ketamine, ether, cyclopropane, and possibly pancuronium). This is because exaggerated adrenergic effects may result. For the same reason, avoid hypercapnia. Similarly, use a direct-acting sympathomimetic amine (e.g. methoxamine or phenylephrine) in reduced dosage if vasoconstriction is required.

The usual principles of good practice are assumed. Make sure that any epinephrine (adrenaline) administered to reduce bleeding is within safe limits and, if a volatile agent is used, select one that is an ether (e.g. isoflurane) and not one that predisposes to cardiac arrhythmias (e.g. halothane). If undertaking thyroid surgery, a head-up tilt is common. Do not forget that venous air embolism is possible in this position.

#### Postoperative phase

The considerations relating to the operation of thyroidectomy are referred to later (and in Chapter 16). The important complication of hyperthyroidism itself is thyroid crisis. With adequate preoperative preparation, it should not occur. However, if there is an excessive release of thyroid hormones, they cause exaggerated symptoms of thyrotoxicosis, either during the operation or, more commonly, in the early postoperative period. A true thyroid crisis in a well-prepared patient is now very rare.

Such a crisis is characterized by a rapidly rising pulse rate, abdominal pain, pyrexia, sweating, diarrhoea, restlessness, and ultimately arrhythmias and cardiac failure. It has a mortality rate of 20–40%. A thyroid crisis must be distinguished from the postoperative complications of sepsis, septicaemia, haemorrhage, and transfusion or drug reactions. The aims of treatment are:

- to reduce tachycardia by β-adrenoceptor blockade;
- to inhibit further release of thyroid hormone by intravenous iodine (e.g. sodium iodide, 250 mg 6-hourly);
- to cool the patient externally (the use of salicylates is inappropriate because they increase the release of thyroid hormones);
- to treat with hydrocortisone any acute adrenal insufficiency resulting from the increased biotransformation and utilization of corticosteroids;
- to inhibit further thyroid hormone synthesis with propylthiouracil, 400 mg 6-hourly by mouth.

### The enlarged thyroid

The enlarged gland may or may not have an associated abnormal hormone secretion, and the possibility of hypo- or hyperthyroidism should always be considered. (Refer to earlier sections for the relevant clinical findings.)

Thyroid swelling can be benign or malignant; it may be diffuse, a single nodule or multinodular, and can extend retrosternally into the thorax. Surgery is indicated when there are pressure symptoms, if there is a suspicion of malignancy, and for selected thyrotoxic cases.

#### Preoperative considerations

##### History

Probably the most common complaint is that of the adverse effect on appearance. Pressure symptoms may cause difficulty in swallowing or in breathing. Rarely, a bleed into the gland can cause acute enlargement and severe ventilatory obstruction, which needs relieving urgently. Stridor may be noticed, particularly on the alteration of neck posture. A change of voice ideally requires indirect laryngoscopy before surgery to evaluate recurrent laryngeal nerve function, and may be indicative of malignancy.

##### Examination

Thyroid swelling is best demonstrated by inspecting the anterior neck and asking the patient to swallow with the neck moderately extended. Feel for the position of the trachea, remembering that it can be grossly deviated. This, and tracheal compression, are important factors in anticipating a difficult intubation. Retrosternal extension can be demonstrated by jugular venous distension and suffusion of the face in extending the patient's arms over his head (Pemberton's sign). Note the position (often sitting up) in which the patient has least difficulty breathing and plan the conduct of anaesthesia accordingly. A very enlarged goitre is shown in Figure 56.1, and see Figure 7.25.

##### Investigations

Thyroid function tests. These should always be performed in order to confirm that the patient is euthyroid.

##### Chest radiograph

This is helpful in revealing a retrosternal extension and will also demonstrate any tracheal deviation.

##### Lateral neck radiographs

A view of the thoracic inlet is particularly helpful to see tracheal narrowing and to anticipate the size of endotracheal tube required.

##### Tomograms and computed tomography scan

These identify tracheal deviation and extent of the goitre best of all.

#### Intraoperative phase

Do not over-sedate the patient if the gland is large enough to cause severe ventilatory embarrassment. Otherwise, there are no contraindications to usual premedicants.

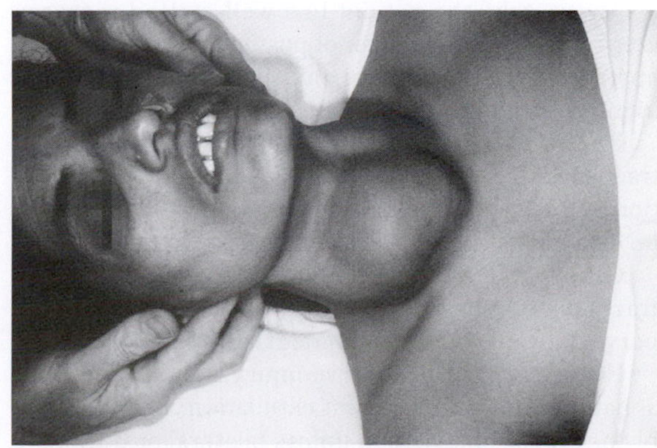

**Figure 56.1** A patient with an obviously enlarged thyroid gland. This led to difficulties with intubation.

Laryngoscopy is usually satisfactory; the problem can be the passage of the tube down the trachea after it has passed the vocal cords. If the gland is only moderately large, and the trachea is undeviated, there is unlikely to be any problem in intubation. An armoured tube is preferred in order to reduce the likelihood of kinking of the tube with movement of the head. A smaller than normal orotracheal tube may be required to negotiate tracheal compression. This is often most easily achieved over a long gum elastic bougie (see Figure 6.46). If there is compression of the trachea, intraoperatively, this is usually overcome by inflation of the cuff.

When a difficult intubation is anticipated, the pros and cons of awake intubation should be considered and a range of endotracheal tube sizes and types, as well as introducers, should be available. With a cooperative patient, a good compromise is gas induction. If the patient is only able to breathe satisfactorily while sitting, retain this position until control of the airway is achieved. Skilled efforts to intubate are essential as tracheostomy is not an attractive alternative. Paralyse the patient only if the airway can be managed safely.

Take all the usual precautions of head and neck surgery (i.e. check that all connections are secure, protect the eyes, secure the endotracheal tube with sticky tape rather than bandage, and provide moderate head up-tilt). There are protagonists for both spontaneous ventilation and intermittent positive pressure ventilation (IPPV); if the operation is likely to be long and difficult, IPPV is certainly preferred. As a result of head-up tilt, remember the possibility of air embolism in the spontaneously breathing patient.

With thyroid carcinoma especially, be aware of the possibility of tracheal damage and have tracheostomy tubes available. At the end of surgery, on extubation, look at the cords to ensure that both sides are moving fully, in case of recurrent laryngeal nerve damage. Suck out the pharynx carefully to remove any blood or mucus, but try not to cause too much coughing, which increases the likelihood of reactionary haemorrhage.

#### *Postoperative phase*

On the return of spontaneous ventilation, tracheal collapse can occur. This is a particular problem after the removal of large goitres which have eroded tracheal cartilages or, after thyroidectomy for malignancy, when a tracheal cartilage may have been removed inadvertently during a difficult dissection. Reintubate the patient immediately and consider tracheostomy.

Always take the patient to a well-staffed recovery area because of the danger of postoperative ventilatory obstruction. The cause of any obstruction should be identified and the appropriate action taken promptly.

Reactionary haemorrhage causes pressure on the trachea and, if it is severe, requires immediate evacuation of the haematoma. Stitch cutters and/or clips must be immediately available at the bedside for 24 hours.

Other uncommon problems that can occur are tracheo-oesophageal fistula, pneumothorax, phrenic nerve damage, and pneumomediastinum

Recurrent laryngeal nerve injury should have been apparent on laryngoscopy at extubation. It will probably not cause obstruction unless bilateral or if there is concomitant oedema. If the nerve injury does not resolve, tracheostomy may have to be done.

Stridor caused by laryngeal oedema does not usually present until 2 or 3 days after the operation and may require reintubation.

If the parathyroid glands have also been inadvertently removed, tetany may occur (8 h to 8 days after the operation). This needs treatment with up to 20 ml 10% calcium gluconate, given slowly intravenously and repeated as necessary.

## PITUITARY GLAND

The detailed physiology of the pituitary gland and its hormones is outlined in Chapter 29. In summary, this small gland (0.5–1.0 g, 1 cm in diameter) is located in the sella turcica at the base of the brain. Together, the hypothalamus and the pituitary form a control unit that regulates growth (growth hormone), lactation (prolactin), thyroid (TRH and TSH), adrenal (corticotrophin-releasing factor [CRF], and adrenocorticotrophin hormone [ACTH]), and gonadal (follicle-stimulating hormone, and luteinizing hormone) function from the anterior pituitary and the state of hydration (ADH) from the posterior pituitary.

The three most common pituitary tumours release excess hormones that cause acromegaly (growth hormone), Cushing's syndrome (ACTH), and lactation (prolactin). Tumours releasing gonadotrophins and thyrotrophins are exceedingly rare. All tumours may cause neurological symptoms or signs, particularly visual field defects, because of pressure on the optic chiasma. Prolactin-secreting tumours, apart from their space-occupying effect, should not pose much problem to the anaesthetist. Acromegaly is discussed under pituitary gland disorders and Cushing's syndrome under adrenal gland disorders. Abnormally low release of hormones may be caused by tumours, surgical hypophysectomy, or radiation. This results in a hypopituitary state which may affect all hormones (panhypopituitarism), ADH (diabetes insipidus), ACTH (Addison's disease), TSH (hypothyroidism), or growth hormone.

### Acromegaly

Acromegaly should always be treated with respect by the anaesthetist. This account assumes that the patient is being treated for an intercurrent problem. It does not consider the problems associated with hypophysectomy. Acromegaly is a chronic disease of middle life characterized by over-growth of bone, connective tissue and viscera as a result of prolonged excessive release of growth hormone. If this defect occurs before puberty, the long bones continue to grow and gigantism results. Acromegaly affects both sexes equally. Once diagnosed it is treated by pituitary ablation. The associated features of importance to the anaesthetist are the following.

#### *Airway and respiratory system*

- Large lips, jaw, tongue and epiglottis. Facemask ventilation may be very difficult or impossible.
- Hypertrophy of pharyngeal and laryngeal structures may make the anatomy difficult to interpret, the cords may not be seen, and the larynx may be resistant to external manipulation, all resulting in a difficult intubation.

- Voice changes may indicate vocal cord involvement (glottic stenosis, calcification).
- Nasal airways obstructed by polypoid growth and mucosal hyperplasia.
- Somnolence, obstructed breathing, and sleep apnoea.

*Other symptoms*

- Hypertension.
- Diabetes mellitus and its complications.
- Cardiomyopathy.
- Proximal myopathy and nerve entrapment.
- Rarely, hypopituitarism, diabetes insipidus, goitre, and hypercalaemia.

### Preoperative considerations

*History*

The onset of symptoms is insidious, but the person with advanced acromegaly is easily recognized. Common complaints are needing larger hats, gloves, rings, and shoes, and headaches, visual disturbances, amenorrhoea, loss of libido, and arthralgia. A third of patients originally seek medical advice for an unrelated illness. Ask about the symptoms of diabetes mellitus (see Chapter 55) and hypertension (see Chapter 49). When diabetes is present it is usually easily controlled. Drug therapy frequently includes a diuretic and antihypertensive agents.

In the treated patient, gauge the arrest of the disease by the progress of symptoms since treatment. Look for signs of hypopituitarism. Any previous anaesthetic record may indicate the degree of difficulty with airway management.

*Examination*

*General*

Note the characteristic enlarged hands, feet, nose, and jaw and the coarseness of facial features. Examine the mobility of any joints affected by osteoarthritis. Look for kyphoscoliosis and degenerative signs in the back if an epidural or spinal block is envisaged.

*Respiratory system*

Examine the airway, note the size of the jaw, and check neck movements carefully. Ask to see the patient's tongue, which is often enlarged. Listen for a hoarse voice, indicating thickening of the vocal cords or soft tissue obstruction of the pharynx. See if the patient can breathe through the nose. In the light of these findings, carefully consider the options for endotracheal intubation.

*Cardiovascular system*

Hypertension occurs in 25%. Check that cardiac failure is not present. If anticipating arterial cannulation, test the ulnar collateral supply to the hand because it may be compromised.

*Nervous system*

Look for peripheral neuropathy resulting from nerve trapping, especially if anticipating local anaesthetic blocks.

*Investigations*

*Full blood count, and urea and electrolytes*

These should be normal.

*Chest radiograph*

Look at the heart size, for the presence of cardiac failure or kyphoscoliosis, and at the position of the trachea.

*ECG*

Look for left ventricular hypertrophy.

*Echocardiograph*

Invaluable for assessing ventricular performance.

*Urinalysis*

Check for glucose.

*Blood glucose*

Do a random blood sugar to uncover occult diabetes.

*Skull radiograph*

There is no need for this to be done routinely. If it is done, the sella turcica will be seen to be enlarged. These films may also predict the difficult intubation already anticipated clinically.

### Anaesthetic management

First consider whether local or regional anaesthesia is possible or advisable. Whether a local or a general anaesthetic is chosen, *always be prepared for a difficult intubation*. Have available a long-bladed laryngoscope, long endotracheal tubes of varying sizes (a smaller diameter tube than predicted may be needed if there is a supra- or subglottic stenosis), and any other aids or introducers likely to help. Consider awake fibreoptic intubation. This may be the best and safest option. Always make sure that your assistant is experienced and well prepared.

Management of the airway on a facemask is likely to be difficult and is only suitable for short operations. Use a large facemask and make sure that the large tongue does not cause obstruction. A size 4 oral airway is usually necessary. A nasopharyngeal airway can be successful, but often there is considerable haemorrhage and difficulty in passing one because of hypertrophied nasal mucosa.

If intubating asleep, the best technique depends on the individual patient and anaesthetist. Although theoretically correct, deepening anaesthesia by spontaneous ventilation with volatile agents (and assessing the problem at laryngoscopy before attempting intubation or giving a neuromuscular blocking agent) is often very difficult to do smoothly. If the intubation on preoperative assessment, or from a previous anaesthetic record, appears relatively straightforward, preoxygenation, intravenous induction, and suxamethonium are probably the sequence of choice. Handle all tissues gently: blood in the larynx can make things much worse. Facilities for performing a tracheostomy must be readily available.

Manage hypertension, diabetes, and kyphoscoliosis as outlined in other chapters.

Postoperatively, do not extubate until there is good muscle power and the patient is awake. There is a tendency to postoperative hyperglycaemia. As a result of the associated problems of acromegaly for all but the most minor procedures, postoperative care should be on an HDU or specially identified bed in a normal ward. On some occasions a period of ventilation on an intensive care unit may be necessary.

**Table 56.1 The causes of diabetes insipidus (DI)**

| Neurogenic DI | Nephrogenic DI |
|---|---|
| Primary | Primary |
| Secondary<br>Trauma<br>Tumour (primary or secondary)<br>Infection<br>Vascular causes | Secondary<br>Hypercalcaemia<br>Hypokalaemia<br>Drugs (lithium, demeclocycline, glibenclamide, amphotericin B, methoxyflurane) |

### Diabetes insipidus

Diabetes insipidus (DI) is a disorder resulting from impaired renal conservation of water because there is either a failure of production of arginine vasopressin (AVP) (neurogenic DI) or a failure of the kidneys to respond to AVP (nephrogenic DI). The causes are summarized in Table 56.1.

If not unconscious from a head injury, the patient notices polyuria and polydipsia. The urine has a low specific gravity (< 1.010) and the volume can be up to 24 litres daily in extreme cases. Plasma osmolality rises. Normal function of the thirst centre ensures that polydipsia closely matches polyuria so that, unless fluid is withheld (e.g. preoperative starvation), dehydration does not normally occur. Diagnosis is by failure to concentrate urine (> 800 mosmol/L) after fluid deprivation. For elective surgery, no patient should be anaesthetized if the DI is uncontrolled.

Routine management of neurogenic DI is with desmopression (DDAVP), 10–20 μg twice daily nasally. It can also be given intramuscularly or intravenously. If the patient has some residual ADH function, this can be enhanced by chlorpropamide, clofibrate, or carbamazepine.

Preoperatively, look for the signs of dehydration (see Chapter 14) and correct appropriately. The patient should not undergo prolonged preoperative fasting without intravenous fluids. Do not hesitate to insert a catheter during surgery if you need to check that there is adequate urine production.

In practice, intraoperative and postoperative fluid management is not difficult. Monitor urine output and serum osmolality. The serum osmolality can be estimated from the sum of the concentrations of the serum glucose and urea, and twice those of sodium and potassium (normal range 283–285 mosmol/L). If the osmolality reaches over 290 mosmol/L, hypotonic fluids should be given and desmopressin given intramuscularly or intravenously.

Probably the most common group of patients with DI seen by the general anaesthetist is organ donors who have died from intracranial trauma or some other physiological insult.

## THE ADRENAL GLANDS

### The adrenal medulla

The detailed physiology of adrenal gland hormones is given in Chapter 29. In summary, the adrenal medulla is functionally part of the sympathetic nervous system and is derived from neural crest tissue. Under normal conditions, it secretes epinephrine (80%) and norepinephrine (noradrenaline) (20%) into the circulation. Here they have a similar effect to direct sympathetic stimulation. The half-lives of epinephrine and norepinephrine in the circulation are only a few minutes. The adrenal medulla is not essential for life, and its ablation has little apparent effect.

In the doses secreted by the medulla, epinephrine has α- and β-adrenoceptor-stimulating activity with the β effects predominating. The net result is an increase in heart rate, cardiac contractility, cardiac output, and systolic blood pressure. The vessels to skeletal muscle are dilated and those to skin, mucosae, and the kidneys are constricted. Overall, this results in a lowering of peripheral vascular resistance and diastolic blood pressure.

Norepinephrine is predominantly an α stimulant and the peripheral resistance rises in almost all vascular beds. There is an increase in both systolic and diastolic pressures with a reflex reduction in heart rate.

Management of a secreting tumour of the medulla (phaeochromocytoma) is not considered further here. They almost never present for intercurrent surgery, and details of the management of this can be found in more specialized texts.

If, however, an unexpectedly high blood pressure is recorded on admission in a patient who has had an adrenalectomy, or if the patient complains of a recurrence of symptoms, they must be taken seriously. It could indicate a recurrence of a secreting tumour at an ectopic site. This needs prompt referral to an endocrinologist and appropriate investigation.

### The adrenal cortex

The adrenal cortex is a true endocrine gland derived from embryonic mesothelium. It is essential for life. All its products are based on the cholesterol skeleton and daily it produces on average 20 mg hydrocortisone (glucocorticoid), 0.15 mg aldosterone (mineralocorticoid), and 20 mg androgenic hormones.

The release of hydrocortisone is directly controlled by ACTH (from the anterior pituitary), which in turn is controlled by CRF (from the hypothalamus). The serum level of hydrocortisone produces negative feedback inhibition at both anterior pituitary and hypothalamic levels. There is a diurnal variation with a 'low' at midnight and a 'high' just after breakfast. Its role is principally in the control of intermediary metabolism with an overall catabolic effect. Protein breakdown, nitrogen excretion, and gluconeogenesis are all increased and the peripheral utilization of glucose is decreased. Hydrocortisone has an anti-insulin action.

The secretion of glucocorticoids is increased during periods of stress (serum levels rise only minutes after the start of surgery) and is essential for survival. The exact reason for this is as yet undefined, but is thought to be a result of the fact that circulating glucocorticoids may be necessary for the maintenance of vascular reactivity to catecholamines. In addition, glucocorticoids are necessary for catecholamines to exert their full free fatty acid mobilizing action.

Aldosterone has its most important effect on the renal tubules, conserving sodium and excreting potassium, hydrogen, and magnesium ions. The control of its secretion is complex. It is secreted in response to stress (via ACTH), a high extracellular potassium, and as the final end-point in the renin–angiotensin system.

Only four clinical syndromes resulting from malfunction of the adrenal cortex are of importance in anaesthesia: over- and under-production of glucocorticoids, iatrogenic suppression of the adrenal cortex, and over-production of aldosterone.

### Cushing's syndrome

This results from a chronic excess of glucorticoids, the causes of which are summarized in Table 56.2. If affects three times as many females as males, and usually presents between the ages of 30 and 50 years. Demonstrating increased plasma and urine concentrations of cortisol makes the diagnosis. Treatment is by surgical removal of the source of excess ACTH or glucocorticoid.

The glucocorticoids are present in such large amounts that they exert a significant mineralocorticoid action, and there may be potassium depletion, and weakness. Protein catabolism reduces the muscle bulk, the skin becomes thin and striae form, wounds heal poorly, minor injuries cause ecchymoses, and there is a reduction in the bone matrix, causing osteoporosis. The decreased peripheral utilization of glucose may produce diabetes (in up to 20% of cases), and the immune response and fibroblastic activity are inhibited.

Conditions associated with the disease are diabetes mellitus, hypertension, chronic infections (chest and urinary), muscular weakness, obesity, bone pain, and vertebral collapse. Indigestion may be caused by peptic ulceration. Aggressive behaviour or euphoria can result from 'steroid psychosis'. Patients may be immunosuppressed.

Few patients with Cushing's disease present for incidental surgery. If they do, management is that of the complications described above. Be prepared for difficult intubation. The involvement of an endocrinologist is important to optimize perioperative drug regimens.

Postoperative ventilatory function is often poor because of muscular weakness. The first postoperative day should be spent in a high dependency area with oxygen-enriched air to breathe and regular physiotherapy. Treat infections early with antibiotics.

Glucocorticoid insufficiency (vomiting, weakness, tachycardia, low-grade fever, hypotension) and electrolyte abnormalities can occur. This requires treatment with hydrocortisone and electrolyte replacement, and a change in the weaning regimen. This frequently involves an adjustment in the ratio of hydrocortisone and fludrocortisone given. Physiotherapy and early mobilization are very important. Curative operations to remove the adenoma are a specialized area of practice and for this reference should be made to specialist texts.

**Table 56.2 Causes of Cushing's syndrome**

| ACTH-dependent disease (60–70%) |
|---|
| Pituitary-dependent (Cushing's disease) producing bilateral adrenal hyperplasia |
| Ectopic ACTH-producing tumours (bronchial, pancreatic carcinoma) |
| ACTH administration |
| **Non-ACTH-dependent causes** |
| Adrenal adenomas |
| Adrenal carcinomas |
| Glucocorticoid administration |
| **Other** |
| Alcohol-induced pseudo-Cushing's syndrome |

ACTH, adrenocorticotrophin hormone.

### Adrenocortical insufficiency

The incidence of primary adrenocortical insufficiency (Addison's disease) is about 1 per 100 000. It affects both sexes and all ages. When it is caused by destruction of the cortex by granulomatous disease (most commonly tuberculosis), meningococcal septicaemia, fungal infections, cancer, haemorrhage, infiltrations (amyloid, haemochromatosis, leukaemia), or autoimmune processes, both cortisol and aldosterone are lacking. When the deficiency is secondary to a lack of pituitary ACTH, aldosterone secretion remains normal. Adrenocortical insufficiency occurs after bilateral adrenalectomy.

These states tend to be chronic and may have superimposed (addisonian) 'crises' when the adrenal gland is unable to meet the demands of stress for increased glucocorticoids.

The onset of chronic disease is insidious. The patient feels generally unwell and weak, and has anorexia, nausea, vomiting, or abdominal pain with weight loss. Pigmentation (resulting from melanocyte-stimulating hormone secretion) occurs particularly in exposed portions of the body (resembling a suntan), at points of pressure and friction, and in the palmar creases. The most notable finding is hypotension (usually with a postural drop) and tachycardia. If the cause is autoimmune, there may be coexistent diabetes mellitus, hypothyroidism, or hypoparathyroidism. Hyperkalaemia may be present.

The diagnosis is made by a reduced plasma cortisol response to ACTH. Maintenance therapy is cortisone acetate and fludrocortisone.

The known chronic case who is stable on maintenance therapy presents few problems and should be treated similarly to patients on steroid therapy (see later and Chapter 5). Problems arise when the patient presents for the first time, because of the stress of an acute illness requiring surgical correction. This is very rare. The picture is indistinguishable from oligaemic shock. The patient is usually apathetic and may be suffering from hypoglycaemia. Diagnosis is made by thinking of the possibility of hypoadrenalism and as a result of investigations, especially those of serum electrolytes. The author has never seen an acute case but has suspected several. In all cases, hypotension and electrolyte abnormalities have been secondary to fluid depletion from dehydration or blood loss.

### Iatrogenic adrenocortical suppression

Patients present on steroid therapy for a variety of reasons. The reason for steroids being prescribed (e.g. rheumatoid arthritis, asthma) may itself have a significant impact on the optimal management of anaesthesia.

Until recently it was common to prescribe supraphysiological doses of steroids to mimic the stress response to surgery. It is now thought, however, that using the minimum amount of steroid replacement aids postoperative recovery and avoids the adverse effects on would healing, of glucose intolerance, peptic ulceration, bowel perforation and adverse cardiovascular effects, which include arrhythmias and myocardial infarction. Adequate replacement therapy is essential to avoid peri-operative haemodynamic instability. Guidelines for different situations are given in Table 56.3.

### Conn's syndrome

This is the result of an adrenal adenoma secreting aldosterone. It is rare, accounting for less than 1% of people with hypertension. It is twice as common in women as in men.

The clinical features reflect the physiological effect of aldosterone.

#### *Sodium conservation*

The patient becomes hypertensive and the blood volume is expanded.

#### *Potassium depletion*

Muscle weakness, areflexia, tetany, and paraesthesiae occur. The ECG abnormalities of hypokalaemia (ST depression, flattened T waves, and the appearance of U waves, see Figure 47.9) and idioventricular arrhythmias may be present. Metabolic alkalosis follows together with hyperkalaemia because of the excess excretion of hydrogen ions.

The diagnosis should always be suspected when hypertension and unprovoked hypokalaemia coexist. Treatment is surgical removal of the adrenal gland containing the adenoma. If they are bilateral, medical therapy with the mineralocorticoid antagonist, spironolactone, is preferred.

The main anaesthetic implications in the well patient presenting for intercurrent surgery are:

- the effects of previous hypertension, associated with cardiomegaly and renal and retinal damage;
- 50% of patients have an abnormal glucose tolerance test;
- adjustment of perioperative mineralocorticoid and glucocorticoid therapy (usually relevant only if both adrenal glands removed).

No specific anaesthetic technique is necessary as long as the principles of good practice are adhered to.

## FURTHER READING

Breivik H. Perianaesthetic management of patients with endocrine disease. *Acta Anaesthesiol Scand* 1996;**40**:1004–15.

Ladenson PW, Levin AA, Ridgway EC, Daniels GH. Complications of surgery in hypothyroid patients. *Am J Med* 1984;**77**:261–6.

Murkin JM. Anesthesia and hypothyroidism: a review of throxine physiology, pharmacology, and anesthesia. *Anesth Analg* 1982;**61**:371–83.

**Table 56.3 Guidelines for steroid cover in the peri-operative period**

| Usual steroid therapy | Type of surgery | Peri-operative steroid cover |
|---|---|---|
| < 10 mg/day | All | No additional cover required |
| > 10 mg/day | Minor | 25 mg hydrocortisone at induction |
| | Moderate | Usual preoperative steroids<br>+ 25 mg hydrocortisone at induction<br>+ 100 mg hydrocortisone/day for 24 h |
| | Major | Usual preoperative steroids<br>+ 25 mg hydrocortisone at induction<br>+ 100 mg hydrocortisone/day for 48–72 h |
| High dose for immunosuppression | All | Continue immunosuppressive dose in peri-operative period |
| Stopped < 3 months ago | All | As if currently on steroid therapy |
| Stopped > 3 months ago | All | No peri-operative steroids required |

Adapted from Nicholson G, Burrin JM, Hall GM. *Anaesthesia* 1998;53:1091–1104.

Nicholson G, Burrin JM, Hall GM. Peri-operative steroid supplementation. *Anaesthesia* 1998:**53**:1091–104.
Roizen MF. Diseases of the endocrine system. In: Katz J, Benumof J, Kadis L, eds. *Anesthesia and Uncommon Diseases*, 3rd edn. Philadelphia: WB Saunders. 1990: 245–92.
Schlaghecke R, Kornley E, Sante R, Ridderskamp P. The effect of long-term glucocorticoid therapy on pituitary-adrenal responses to exogenous corticotropin-releasing hormone. *N Engl J Med* 1992;**326**:226–30.
Sebel PS. Thyroid and parathyroid disease. *Curr Anaesth Crit Care* 1992;**3**:23–9.

# Chapter 57 The patient with arthritis

G.M. Cooper

At least half a million people in the UK have rheumatoid arthritis; nearly as many have gout and ankylosing spondylitis, and 5 million are affected by osteoarthritis. These conditions often lead to the need for surgery (e.g. joint replacement, arthrodesis, osteotomy, tendon repair) but are sufficiently common that they will regularly be seen coincidentally.

## PREOPERATIVE ASSESSMENT

### History

The level of mobility and exercise tolerance should be assessed. Many patients are so immobile that angina or breathlessness is not generated in the presence of myocardial disease. Ask the patient which joints are worst affected, functionally and from the point of view of deformities or causing pain. Always specifically ask about neck movement. Symptoms of cervical spine instability can include aching over the occiput, the nape of the neck, and the shoulders, and dizzy spells related to head movement (vertebrobasilar insufficiency). Ask if a neck collar is worn.

Enquire of any other neurological symptoms. These usually have mechanical causes (carpal tunnel, ulnar nerve entrapment, spinal root compression [usually cervical]), but rarely there is a neuropathy secondary to vasculitis of the vasa nervorum.

Listen for hoarseness or stridor which may indicate laryngeal involvement in rheumatoid disease.

A drug history is vital because many drugs used in the treatment of arthritis cause gastrointestinal blood loss, affect platelet function, can depress the bone marrow, can cause proteinuria, and can affect the carriage of other drugs. Patients may be on steroids and/or antidepressants.

### Examination

Make sure the patient is weighed; those with rheumatoid disease may be deceptively light and those with osteoarthritis heavier than average.

#### *Musculoskeletal*

Look at the affected joints and their range of movement, bearing in mind the operative positioning and the best choice of sites for cannulation. Assess the knee and hip joints, especially if the lithotomy position is anticipated. It is vital to check the movement of the neck and the ability to adopt the intubating position, especially in rheumatoid disease and in ankylosing spondylitis. Temporomandibular involvement may reduce mouth opening in rheumatoid disease. Figure 57.1 shows the differences between rheumatoid arthritis and osteoarthritis in their involvement of joints in the hand.

#### *Respiratory system*

Look for restricted rib movement, especially in rheumatoid arthritis and ankylosing spondylitis. Small pleural effusions are present in up to 20% patients with rheumatoid arthritis.

#### *Cardiovascular system*

Pericarditis is relatively common in rheumatoid arthritis, but rarely becomes constrictive or leads to tamponade. Left-sided valvular incompetence caused by rheumatoid granulomas is rare.

Aortic regurgitation is present in about 4% of those with ankylosing spondylitis, and therefore signs of cardiac failure, collapsing pulse, low diastolic blood pressure, and an aortic diastolic murmur should be sought in these patients.

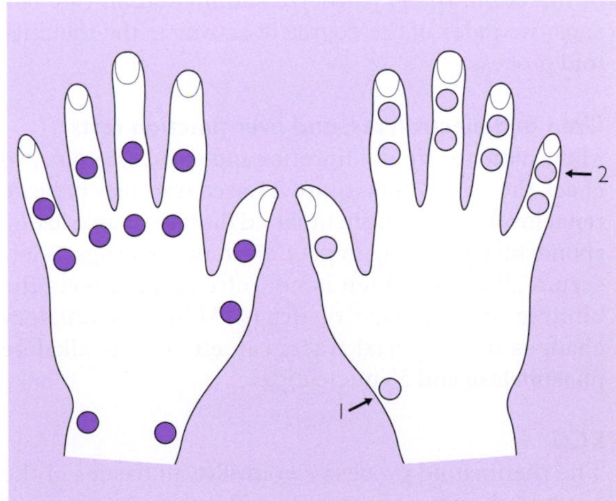


**Figure 57.1** Joints of the hands involved in rheumatoid arthritis (left) and osteoarthritis (right). Note how osteoarthritis affects the carpometacarpal joint of the thumb, and how rheumatoid arthritis affects the wrist. 1, Osteoarthritis of the first carpometacarpal joint gives an appearance of a 'square hand' as a result of enlargement of the joint and adductive deformity of the metacarpal joint. 2, Osteophytes of the terminal interphalangeal joints are called 'Heberden's nodes'. (Adapted from Hazleman B. Musculoskeletal and connective tissue disease. In: Souhami RL and Moxham J, eds. *Textbook of Medicine,* 3rd edn. Edinburgh: Churchill Livingstone, 1997.)

*Nervous system*

Any neurological deficit should be recorded and is more likely in rheumatoid arthritis. Paraesthesia and weakness in the hands and arms can be secondary to cervical root compression. Peripheral neuropathies secondary to vasculitis of the vasa vasorum are usually sensory. The most frequent peripheral nerve entrapment is median nerve compression in the carpal tunnel.

*Gastrointestinal tract*

A large spleen indicates possible thrombocytopenia (Felty's syndrome) and rectal examination can reveal gastrointestinal bleeding.

*Skin*

Examine the state of pressure areas, look for the presence of skin fragility, and feel for subcutaneous nodules, thinking of any problems that they may cause in intraoperative positioning.

### Investigations

*Full blood count*

In inflammatory joint disease, a moderate normocytic/normochromic anaemia is common and its severity reflects disease activity. However, if the haemoglobin is below 10 g/dl, then suspect a superimposed cause such as drug-induced gastrointestinal bleeding (common) or more rarely a coexisting pernicious or haemolytic anaemia. Impaired release of folate from erythrocytes causing a macrocytic anaemia is five times more common than in the general population.

A raised white cell count of $12–20 \times 10^3$, with a neutrophilia, occurs in infective arthritis, acute gout, and juvenile chronic polyarthritis, and in patients with rheumatitis who receive corticosteroids. In the absence of infection, the erythrocyte sedimentation rate is a sensitive index of the degree of activity in the rheumatoid process.

*Urea and electrolytes, and liver function tests*

Many patients are on diuretics and corticosteroids, so check the serum potassium. A raised urea may indicate renal involvement in rheumatoid disease or ankylosing spondylitis, resulting in poor clearance of drugs. A low serum albumin, which is not infrequent, affects the binding and carriage of drugs. Mild inflammatory changes in the portal tracts can elevate the alkaline phosphatase and 5′-nucleotidase.

*ECG*

The rheumatoid process can involve all tissues of the heart leading to arrhythmias and ischaemic changes. Ten percent of patients with ankylosing spondylitis have cardiac conduction disturbances, the most frequent being atrioventricular block.

*Radiographs*

*Chest*

Small pleural effusions are found occasionally in rheumatoid disease, but are usually of little significance. Less often there are rheumatoid nodules which can occur throughout the lung fields and resemble neoplasms. They can be accompanied by a massive fibrotic reaction (Caplan's syndrome). Rarely, there is a true diffuse pulmonary fibrosis. Look for vertebral flexion deformities and evidence of rib cage joint fixation. Figure 57.2 shows the head in a fixed flexed position which obliterates much of the lung fields on the chest radiograph!

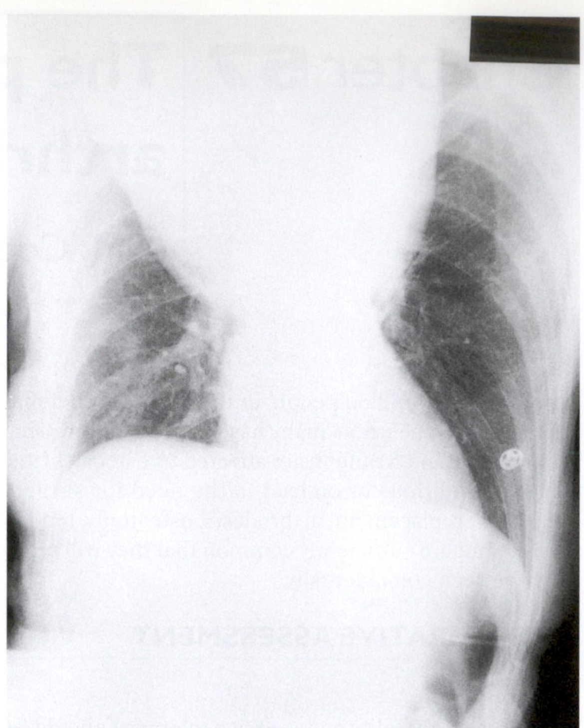

**Figure 57.2** A chest radiograph of a woman with ankylosing spondylitis. The opacity obliterating the upper lung fields is her head which is fixed in flexion. Incidentally a button is also apparent.

In ankylosing spondylitis, the edges of the vertebral bodies become eroded and in severe disease anterior longitudinal ligaments and apophyseal joints are ossified resulting in the 'bamboo spine'. Also seen in severe disease are chronic fibrotic changes in the upper lung, which resemble tuberculosis. A large left ventricle may indicate decompensation secondary to aortic incompetence.

*Cervical spine*

In all but the most trivial cases of rheumatoid arthritis and ankylosing spondylitis, it is mandatory to take a radiograph of the cervical spine. Radiographs should be taken in flexion and extension, and on flexion may show posterior displacement beyond the normal limit of 3 mm. If radiographs of the feet are as in Figure 57.3, it is important to look at the cervical spine.

*Lung function tests*

These are indicated in severe disease to assess functional disability and to provide baseline data. They assume greater importance when the disease is severe and an upper abdominal incision is required for surgery. Arterial blood gas measurement is also helpful.

## PREOPERATIVE PREPARATION

With the help of physiotherapy, encourage maximum mobility. Consider the use of splints to minimize defor-

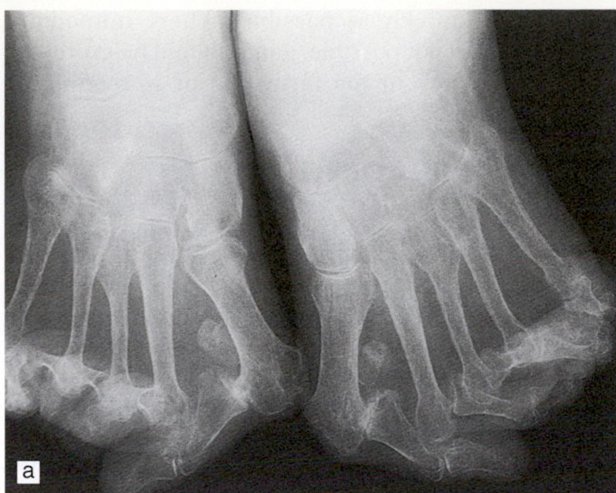

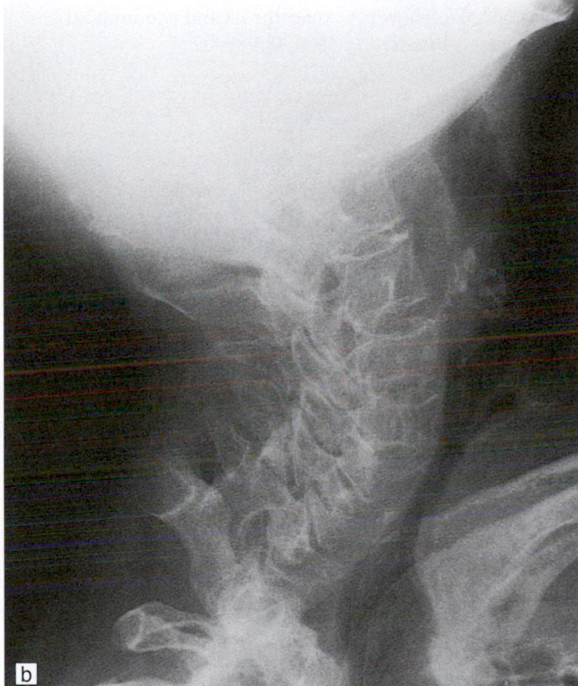

**Figure 57.3** Radiograph of the feet of a woman with rheumatoid arthritis. A lateral view of her cervical spine shows subluxation.

mities. Discuss the use of regional blockade with the patient and the surgeon, bearing in mind whether the patient can adopt the position necessary to perform the block. Treat any cardiac failure or chest infection.

## INTRAOPERATIVE PHASE

### Premedication

There is a wide range of possibilities but beware of ventilatory depression and remember steroid cover where appropriate (see Chapter 56).

### Regional techniques

Consider the use of nerve blocks. Be sure that the patient is comfortable before surgery starts, because it may be difficult to adjust position once the operation is under way. Joint contractures can make it necessary to adopt odd postures. Immobile joints can become very painful during even moderately lengthy operations, and pressure areas are at great risk.

In ankylosing spondylitis, spinals, caudals, or epidurals are at best difficult and often impossible. If attempted, a lateral approach is recommended to minimize the passage through calcified ligaments.

### General anaesthesia

Site the cannula carefully so that the patient is at minimum disadvantage postoperatively. The cannula needs to be secured meticulously because of the danger of cutting through fragile veins.

Position the patient carefully for intubation before induction. Cervical vertebrae may easily become subluxated during the usual extension of the neck required for laryngoscopy, resulting in serious neurological dysfunction by pressure on the cord, or vertebrobasilar insufficiency. Those at risk in rheumatoid arthritis are the upper cervical discs, in contrast to the lower ones in osteoarthritis. Therefore always give good support to the head and neck and be very gentle with cervical manipulation. Consider the use of a vacuum head mould or judiciously placed sandbags. If the patient normally wears a cervical collar, it may be best to keep it on. Let the patient position his own head to his limit while awake. It is often best to do this on the operating table to minimize movement. When an unconscious patient has to be moved, ensure that there are sufficient helpers to protect arthritic joints, especially those of the neck. Always be careful not to strain any affected joint when the patient is unconscious.

If a facemask is to be used, a nasopharyngeal airway can be superior to an oral airway in terms of neck position. Topical local anaesthesia given preoperatively can usefully shrink the nasal mucosa to minimize bleeding. Where intubation is not mandatory, a laryngeal mask airway inserted carefully can avoid neck manipulations, and eases management of a difficult airway.

Equipment should always be available for a difficult intubation. In severe arthritis involving the neck, awake nasal or oral intubation may be essential. The alternative of awake tracheostomy will not be viable if the neck is in fixed flexion, as seen sometimes in ankylosing spondylitis. Even in less severe cases, it is wise not to use a neuromuscular blocking agent until the ability to ventilate the lungs from a facemask has been checked.

In ankylosing spondylitis, neck and thoracic spine rigidity can make internal jugular or subclavian approaches for central venous access difficult. Where this is required, a long line from the antecubital fossa may be preferable.

Where there is any question about respiratory inadequacy, intermittent positive pressure ventilation will be indicated. A reduced dose of non-depolarizing neuromuscular blocking agent will suffice or can often be omitted altogether, mild hyperventilation in the presence of opioids permitting mechanical ventilation.

For patients taking non-steroidal anti-inflammatory drugs, it is important that sufficient intravenous fluids are given in order to prevent renal failure developing.

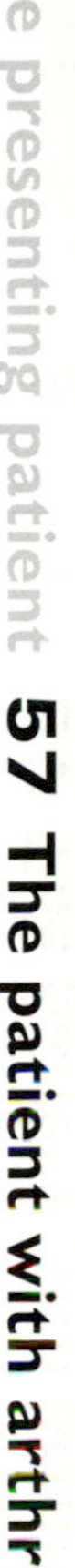

## POSTOPERATIVE PHASE

After IPPV, it is particularly important to be sure that resumed spontaneous ventilation is adequate before extubation; reintubation may not be easy. In addition to relying on physical signs (see Chapter 4), it is wise to test the adequacy of reversal of neuromuscular blocking agent by nerve stimulation (see Chapter 4), before awakening, which should show a well-sustained tetanus and minimally decrementing train of four. Control of the airway before the patient is fully awake should never be left to an inexperienced person.

Consider the use of regional blockade for postoperative analgesia. This may reduce the need for drugs that reduce ventilation. Many patients already take NSAIDs and it is sensible to continue their preferred one. Alternative routes of administration need to be considered when the gastrointestinal tract is temporarily out of action. Remember to continue steroids where appropriate. Organize early chest physiotherapy and mobilize as quickly as possible. Where immediate mobilization is not possible, joints should be exercised passively to prevent the formation or worsening of contractures.

## FURTHER READING


Benumof JL. Management of the difficult adult airway. With special emphasis on awake tracheal intubation. *Anesthesiology* 1991;**75**:1087–100.

Latto IP. Management of difficult intubation. In: Latto IP, Vaughan RS, eds. *Difficulties in Tracheal Intubation*, 2nd edn. Philadelphia: WB Saunders, 1997: 107–61.

Nicholson G, Burrin JM, Hall GM. Peri-operative steroid supplementation. *Anaesthesia* 1998;**53**:1091–104.

Salathe M, Johr. Unsuspected cervical fractures: a common problem in ankylosing spondylitis. *Anesthesiology* 1989;**70**:869–70.

Sinclair JR, Mason RA. Ankylosing spondylitis. The case for awake intubation. *Anaesthesia* 1984;**39**:3–11.

Skues MA, Welchew EA. Anaesthesia and rheumatoid arthritis. *Anaesthesia* 1993;**48**:989–97.

# Chapter 58 The patient with jaundice

G.M. Cooper

Four broad categories of disease cause jaundice:

- prehepatic (unconjugated hyperbilirubinaemia);
- hepatitis;
- intra- or extrahepatic obstructive jaundice;
- chronic liver disease.

The jaundiced patient must always be taken seriously, and an accurate preoperative diagnosis of the cause is exceedingly important. Although an experienced clinician can expect to achieve a correct diagnosis in approximately 66% of cases on the basis of history and examination alone, this is increased to over 95% by the use of special investigations. An unnecessary laparotomy in a patient with severe hepatocellular failure may well prove fatal, whereas posthepatic biliary obstruction should be relieved at the earliest opportunity. In addition, any operative procedure on a jaundiced patient carries a risk of renal failure which may be intensified if the anaesthetic is badly managed.

One prehepatic cause of jaundice is haemolysis where there is unconjugated hyperbilirubinaemia. Features of haemolytic anaemias are discussed further in Chapter 52. Another prehepatic cause of jaundice is defective uptake of bilirubin into hepatocytes as found in Gilbert's syndrome. A much more serious congenital defect in bilirubin conjugation, as found in the Crigler–Najjer syndrome, results in deep jaundice. This syndrome is rare and is unlikely to be encountered by the anaesthetist. The infective problems of hepatitis are discussed in Chapter 60.

It is important to distinguish between the jaundiced patient who has abnormal liver function and the one whose liver function is unaffected. For this reason the assessment of liver function is discussed first. The chapter then concentrates on the anaesthetic management of jaundice itself, such as might be necessary for the removal of gallstones causing severe obstructive jaundice. If the jaundice is complicated by cirrhosis or severe parenchymal failure, the additional material later in the chapter should be taken into account.

## ASSESSMENT OF LIVER FUNCTION

In terms of its biochemical capabilities, the liver has a large margin of safety with considerable cellular reserves available for use in abnormal conditions. Coupled with its ability to regenerate hepatocytes, this implies two important facts: first, liver disease may not become clinically apparent until it is well advanced and, second, liver function tests (LFTs), which reflect the spilling of intracellular contents into the circulation (e.g. aspartate transaminase, alanine transaminase), may be abnormal in the presence of relatively normal synthetic function (as in mild cirrhosis). Consequently, LFTs in many cases are only crude indicators of the real hepatic state and must always be related to the clinical condition of the patient. If, however, serial tests are abnormal over a long period, it is an indication that considerable cellular damage is occurring. Conversely, one isolated biochemical abnormality may be of little significance.

After acute episodes (e.g. viral hepatitis, drug-induced cholestasis, stone in the common bile duct) the return of LFTs to normal gives good evidence of recovery but, in chronic disease (e.g. cirrhosis), abnormal levels give little guide to the severity of disease activity.

It is also important to remember that abnormal LFTs may be related to the effect of systemic diseases on the liver (e.g. congestive cardiac failure, connective tissue disorders, cystic fibrosis, granulomatous and malignant infiltrations, and poisoning) which must be taken into account in the overall anaesthetic management.

A summary of LFTs and what abnormalities might indicate is given in Table 58.1 The normal ranges given for LFTs differ from laboratory to laboratory.

*Bilirubin (normal range ≤17 μmol/L)*

When the serum concentration rises above 20 μmol/L, there is usually sufficient bilirubin sequestered in the tissues to cause jaundice. This is best seen in the sclera under white light – it can easily be missed on the artificially illuminated ward.

The serum bilirubin can be divided into conjugated and unconjugated fractions. These are not normally assayed separately by the laboratory. An increase in the unconjugated fraction (which cannot enter the urine and produces acholuric jaundice) results from an abnormal bilirubin load (haemolysis) or from a biochemical defect at, or proximal to, the site of conjugation on the smooth endoplasmic reticulum of the hepatocyte. The latter is typified by Gilbert's syndrome, a benign condition of intermittent jaundice affecting 5% of the population.

An elevation of the serum conjugated bilirubin is always evidence of liver pathology and indicates defective excretion via the normal route into the biliary tree. Once conjugated, bilirubin is water soluble and can enter the urine.

Traditional teaching suggests that disordered LFTs, interpreted with the conjugated to unconjugated bilirubin ratio, can specify whether the problem is pre-,

**Table 58.1 Liver function tests**

| Test | Normal range | If abnormal, may indicate |
|---|---|---|
| Aspartate aminotransferase | 10–40 units/L | Hepatocellular damage/necrosis |
| Alanine aminotransferase | 10–37 units/L | Hepatocellular damage/ necrosis |
| Alkaline phosphatase | 35–100 units/L | Cholestasis |
| γ-Glutamyl transpeptidase | 11–64 units/L | Alcohol- or drug-related damage |
| Serum albumin | 30–44 g/L | Decreased synthetic function |
| Prothrombin time | 1–1.3 INR | Decreased synthetic function |
| Serum bilirubin | | |
| Total | 4–17 μmol/L | Assessment of jaundice/primary biliary cirrhosis |
| Unconjugated | < 0.3 μmol/L | Gilbert's syndrome |
| 5′-Nucleotidase | 1–18 units/L | Cholestasis |
| Total serum bile acids | 0–6 μmol/L | Cholestasis/portosystemic shunt |
| Serum iron | 8–31 μmol/L | Increased ferritin and transferrin suggests haemochromatosis |
| Transferrin saturation | < 50% | |
| Ferritin | 10–250 μg/L | |
| Ceruloplasmin | 1.1–2.9 μmol/L | Low with low copper suggests Wilson's disease |
| Serum copper | 11–24 μmol/L | – |
| $\alpha_1$-Antitrypsin | 25–64 μmol/L | Low in deficiency disease |
| α-Fetoprotein | < 0.29 nmol/L | Increased in hepatoma |

INR, international normalized ratio.
After Strunin L. *Baillière's Clinical Anaesthesiology* 1992;6:781–93.

intra-, or posthepatic. Although neat in theory, this can rarely be done in practice because parenchymal disease ultimately possesses an obstructive component and obstructive disease produces cellular dysfunction. A more definitive diagnosis may be made with the aid of investigations such as serum virology, transhepatic cholangiography, ultrasonography, liver biopsy, and endoscopic retrograde cholangiopancreatography (ERCP).

*Aspartate transaminase (normal serum value 10–50 units/L)*
This is an enzyme that facilitates transamination in the heart, skeletal muscle, and the kidney as well as in the liver. Consequently, it may be raised not only in the liver disease but also after myocardial infarction and in the active phase of a myopathy. Therefore, the clinical presentation is important in its interpretation.

*Alanine aminotransferase (normal serum value 10–37 units/L)*
This is more specific to the liver but this enzyme is less stable than other enzymes in stored serum.

*Alkaline phosphatase (normal serum value 30–100 units/L)*
This is found in high concentrations in bile canaliculi, osteoblasts, small intestine, and the placenta, each tissue containing different isoenzymes. Accordingly, the levels are high in liver disease (especially with cholestasis), bone disease, and pregnancy. Isoenzyme determinations are not widely available and the coexistence of an elevated 5′-nucleotidase (found in the kidney, liver, pancreas, and prostate) is often used to confirm the hepatic origin of an abnormal alkaline phosphatase.

*γ-Glutamyl transpeptidase (normal < 60 units/L)*
This is found in the liver, kidney, pancreas, and prostate and is a non-specific marker. It is less sensitive than other enzymes to biliary obstruction. It is, however, sensitive to enzyme-inducing drugs such as phenytoin and alcohol, both of which can cause quite marked elevation in serum levels in the absence of significant liver damage.

*Remember* that all hepatic enzyme changes are indicative of cellular damage and give no guide to the functional ability of the residual cells.

*Serum proteins*
Serum albumin (normal 30–44 g/L) is an indicator of the synthetic power of the liver. A level below 25 g/L indicates extensive liver damage (provided the nephrotic syndrome and excessive protein losses in gastrointestinal disease have been excluded). $\alpha_1$-Globulins (normal 1–5 g/L) are also low in hepatocellular disease. Other globulin levels (normal serum

globulin 25–30 g/L) may increase but these changes are not diagnostic.

*Prothrombin time (1–1.3 international normalized ratio)*
Most clotting factors are synthesized in the liver and the synthesis of factors II, VII, IX, and X is dependent on vitamin K. Deficiency of these factors prolongs the prothrombin time. In obstructive jaundice, vitamin K is not absorbed from the intestine because bile salts are absent. Parenteral vitamin K begins to act within a few hours and will usually return the prothrombin time to normal within 24 hours. If it remains elevated ('vitamin K resistant'), this indicates cellular damage, the hepatocytes being unable to synthesize the clotting factors in the presence of active substrate.

## PREOPERATIVE CONSIDERATIONS IN JAUNDICE

### History
Most patients will have been accurately diagnosed before the anaesthetist's visit and most of those outside specialist units will have biliary obstruction. Mistakes are occasionally made, so it is always valuable to consider other causes (hereditary, haemolytic, cirrhotic, infective, toxic). Ask about any family history of jaundice, contact with jaundiced individuals, blood transfusions, tattooing, acupuncture, drug addiction, sexual orientation and contacts, foreign travel, immigration, alcohol intake, recent drug ingestion, general health, and occupational hazards. If the answer to any of these questions is positive, it should be brought to the attention of the clinician in charge of the patient. Unexplained jaundice of 4 weeks' duration or longer will prove to be caused by obstruction in about 75% of patients.

Gallstones in the common bile duct are usually accompanied by pain and pyrexia, and may present as pancreatitis, with or without jaundice. Weight loss suggests an underlying neoplasm of the bile ducts or the pancreas, and weight gain should raise the possibility of ascites secondary to cirrhosis.

Malaise, lethargy, nausea, and pruritus are common and related to obstructive jaundice. Personality and mental changes are rare, unless there is severe hepatocellular failure. The symptoms of anaemia may be secondary to occult or frank (haematemesis or melaena) blood loss. In the cirrhotic patient the most common site of blood loss is oesophageal varices.

Always enquire about bruising or bleeding after minimal trauma such as at venepuncture sites (coagulation defects), oedema (cardiac failure, hypoproteinaemia with ascites), breathing difficulties (restricted diaphragm, pulmonary effusions), and recent anaesthetics (drug effects). If the patient takes medication regularly, note the dose and the effect on the patient: it may give a measure of the liver's metabolic capacity.

### Examination
In a mildly jaundiced patient with simple biliary obstruction, there are few additional physical signs and the object of the preoperative assessment is to look for features that point to hepatocellular failure (see later).

Hepatomegaly, although important to elicit, is not helpful in the differential diagnosis of jaundice. A palpable gallbladder normally indicates obstruction of the common bile duct.

### Investigations
These are to confirm the type of jaundice and then to find its cause.

*Liver function tests*
See above.

*Full blood count*
A low haemoglobin may be the result of concealed blood loss or haemolysis. A raised white cell count is present in cholecystitis and cholangitis.

*Urea and electrolytes*
These should be normal. An elevated and rising urea is important and requires urgent treatment (see below).

*Urine testing*
Once biliary obstruction is complete, bilirubin appears in the urine. Otherwise a raised bilirubin is reflected by excess urobilinogen in the urine.

*Clotting studies*
The prothrombin time may be prolonged.

*Virology*
Hepatitis B may need to be excluded.

*Radiographs*
*Chest*
Both cholecystitis and hepatomegaly inhibit right-sided diaphragmatic movement, thus giving a propensity for lower right chest infections and pulmonary effusions.

*Abdominal*
Only in a minority of cases does the radiograph show gallstones. It may have the 'ground glass' appearance of ascites.

*Barium meal or endoscopy*
This radiograph will reveal oesophageal varices. Distortion and fixation of the duodenum occurs in carcinoma of the pancreas.

*Cholangiography*
The percutaneous approach to cholangiography is the most effective once the jaundice has resolved. ERCP has a low complication rate and is effective at demonstrating the site of obstruction, even when the obstruction is complete. The choice of approach depends on the personnel available, the presence of abnormal clotting, and the presence of infection.

*Ultrasonography and computed tomography*
These investigations will demonstrate grossly dilated ducts. In experienced hands, they also give information about the liver parenchyma, gallbladder, and even the site of an obstruction.

*Liver biopsy*
Percutaneous needle biopsy is now accepted as a routine investigation in liver disease. It allows histo-

logical differentiation between intrinsic parenchymal disease and that secondary to biliary obstruction. Although it should be approached with care, especially where there are clotting abnormalities in experienced centres, it is very safe.

## PREOPERATIVE PREPARATION

It is imperative to make the maximum effort to avoid renal damage during surgery on jaundiced patients. Renal failure may complicate any form of jaundice but does so most commonly with obstructive jaundice and, the higher the serum bilirubin, the higher the risk. This risk is greatly increased if there is an endotoxaemia from infected bile. If there is a rising urea preoperatively, it is imperative that the biliary obstruction is relieved immediately, however ill the patient. If it is untreated, the progression to irreversible renal failure approaches 100%. In extreme cases, haemodialysis has been recommended before surgery, but this is not without problems because a period of hypotension during dialysis can intensify the renal failure. Its value is as yet unproven.

More frequently, the jaundiced patient presents for surgery with normal renal function and the object is to prevent postoperative renal failure. One of the dangerous factors predisposing to renal failure in the presence of bilirubinaemia is hypovolaemia, which reduces urine production. Consequently, the patient must not be allowed to present for surgery relatively dehydrated because of the preoperative fast. A young fit patient can be given intravenous fluids liberally; 2 L of dextrose saline (0.18% saline in 4% dextrose) in the 4 h before surgery is reasonable. Those with borderline cardiac function need more careful handling with a fluid load titrated against a moderate-to-high central venous pressure (CVP). This is best done in a high dependency area. In the pre-, intra-, and postoperative periods, there should be a diuresis of at least 1.0 ml/kg per h. Urine flow needs to be monitored accurately by catheter collection, but its insertion is often delayed (perhaps unwisely) until the patient is in the operating room.

If, *despite adequate hydration*, the urine flow is too low, or if the serum bilirubin is over 140 μmol/L, 10% mannitol is the treatment of choice, 500 ml being given over approximately 1 h. Some authors have also used frusemide (furosemide) to maintain a diuresis. It is strongly emphasized that it is potentially disastrous to use mannitol or loop diuretics to maintain a high urine flow in the presence of a low circulating fluid volume – this combination can lead to a deterioration in renal function.

As stated earlier, renal damage is more likely to occur if there is an endotoxaemia, and this can be produced during surgical manipulation of the biliary tree. Consequently, an adequate serum concentration of a suitable antibiotic (usually gentamicin or a cephalosporin) should be attained before surgery by administering it with the premedication or at induction.

Clotting studies are mandatory and, if the prothrombin time is prolonged, parenteral vitamin K is required. This takes up to 24 hours for the maximal effect to be reached and, if liver function is sufficiently compromised, it may make little difference to the prothrombin time (vitamin K resistant, see earlier). In this case it is necessary to use fresh frozen plasma (FFP), the amount being titrated against the improvement in prothrombin time.

Postoperative chest infections are common, so preoperative physiotherapy to optimize pulmonary function and familiarize the patient with his or her postoperative treatment is important.

### Premedication

The derangement of drug metabolism is not usually severe in obstructive jaundice, so a wide choice of oral or parenteral drugs is available, but a lower than normal dosage is advised for safety. For an opioid, pethidine has a theoretical advantage in that it is said to constrict the sphincter of Oddi less than other agents. Whether this has any relevance to a diseased biliary tree subjected to surgical instrumentation has not been established. Avoid intramuscular injections if the prothrombin time is prolonged.

## INTRAOPERATIVE PHASE

Contrary to what is required, all anaesthetic techniques, both general and regional, reduce splanchnic blood flow, as do β-adrenoceptor blockers and ganglion blockers. Consequently, the anaesthetic technique used should aim to reduce liver and kidney blood flow as little as possible, and to maintain a good urine production. Therefore, *avoid hypoxia, hypovolaemia, and hypotension, maintain normocapnia, hydrate well,* and if necessary give a repeat dose of mannitol to ensure a urine output of over 1.0 ml/kg per h.

Virtually all operations on people with obstructive jaundice are for the relief of jaundice, and hence the incision is an upper abdominal one. This, and the possibility of clotting disorders, mitigates against regional blockade as the sole anaesthetic technique. If clotting is satisfactory, think about epidural blockade for analgesia during and after the operation. Be careful to avoid hypotension with its associated reduction in liver blood flow.

The degree of monitoring above the basic requirements (ECG, blood pressure [BP], pulse, urine production) depends on the magnitude of the procedure and the anaesthetist's preferences. For a Whipple's operation on a sick patient, an arterial line, CVP, and pulmonary artery catheter may be appropriate; for the removal of a single stone in the common bile duct of a fit patient, they are unnecessary.

### Induction

Apart from unavoidable situations such as rapid sequence induction, preoxygenation should be followed with the induction agent given slowly for its effects to be manifest. The choice of induction agent does not appear to be important. Hypotension during induction requires the prompt infusion of fluid and/or a head-down tilt.

### Maintenance

Except for very short procedures, spontaneous breathing techniques using volatile agents are unsatisfactory because of the falls in blood pressure, cardiac output, and splanchnic blood flow, which occur if surgical anaesthesia is to be achieved.

Ventilation to normocapnia with end-tidal $CO_2$ monitoring or arterial blood gas sampling is the ideal. Atracurium, with its spontaneous breakdown by Hofmann elimination, has great advantages. Nitrous oxide is not contraindicated. Provided that liver function is satisfactory, there is no reason not to use parenteral analgesics (pethidine, fentanyl) and, if they were given as premedication, their effects can be judged when the patient arrives in the anaesthetic room. Halothane and other volatile agents are not automatically contraindicated, but should be used only in low concentrations that do not cause cardiovascular depression.

Theoretically, the presence of hyperbilirubinaemia can augment the intrapulmonary shunt, so it is often recommended to increase the inspired oxygen concentration to 40% or above. The necessity for this can easily be checked by intraoperative blood gas analysis.

The importance of fluid balance and urine flow has been emphasized above. Unless liver failure is present, the choice of maintenance fluids is not important. There are good arguments for letting the haematocrit fall because this increases renal plasma flow (which is beneficial to a compromised kidney), provided that there are healthy pulmonary and cardiovascular systems to maintain a high oxygen flux. The postoperative haemoglobin should not, however, fall below 10 g/dl. FFP may be needed if clotting is defective.

## POSTOPERATIVE PHASE

Take the patient to a good recovery area with sufficient staff and monitoring facilities. Good reversal of neuromuscular block and adequate ventilation before extubation are essential. Once extubated, give oxygen-enriched air.

Analgesia is important in the prophylaxis of lower lobe atelectasis and can be achieved satisfactorily by intravenous or epidural opioids, or by intercostal blockade with local anaesthetic. Beware of undue ventilatory depression with opioid analgesia. Intercostal blocks are good but need to be repeated every few hours. Ventilatory function often improves if the patient is sat up, but it is vital to monitor the BP assiduously after topping up an epidural with local anaesthetic because of the danger of a 'sitting faint' and cerebral hypoxia. Optimum analgesia is probably obtained using a weak concentration of local anaesthetic (e.g. 0.1% bupivacaine) combined with an opioid (e.g. fentanyl 1–2 μg/ml).

Continue to monitor the urine output and treat accordingly. Ensure that physiotherapy has been arranged. Postoperative chest infections are common, usually originating from a focus in the right lower lobe.

The use of postoperative antibiotics is important, especially if infected bile was found at operation. Care must be exercised with the aminoglycosides because of their nephrotoxic effects.

## THE PATIENT WITH CHRONIC LIVER DISEASE

The response of the liver to disease is strictly limited, such that many diverse conditions have the final common pathway of cirrhosis. Cirrhosis is a pathological definition describing the end-point of the sequence cellular necrosis, fibrosis, and nodular regeneration with distortion of architecture. Histologically, there are further subdivisions based on the nodule size and the location of the fibrosis, but the functional result is the same. The causes of cirrhosis are summarized in Table 58.2. The activity of the cirrhotic process is assessed by clinical, biochemical, and histological observations, and subsequently classified as progressive, stationary, or regressive.

In many cases cirrhosis is compatible with good health and completely normal biochemical tests, the patient being totally unaware of his or her condition. About one-third of the cases of cirrhosis seen at necropsy have been unsuspected in life. This end of the clinical spectrum is termed 'latent and well compensated'. When severe, cirrhosis can run an aggressive course, culminating in liver failure and death, and is then termed 'active and decompensated'.

The well-compensated patient can almost be regarded as normal. The following discussion of the management of cirrhosis describes the treatment of patients with serious decompensation. The optimum

| Table 58.2 The causes of cirrhosis |
|---|
| Unknown or cryptogenic (30% in UK) |
| Alcoholic (30% in UK and rising) |
| Viral hepatitis, types A, B, C, D, and E; also Epstein–Barr, cytomegalovirus, and herpes simplex and zoster |
| Prolonged cholestasis, intra-, or extrahepatic obstruction |
| Hepatic venous outflow obstruction |
| Metabolic disease, e.g. haemochromatosis, Wilson's disease, $\alpha_1$-antitrypsin deficiency, storage diseases |
| Autoimmune<br>• primary biliary cirrhosis<br>• chronic active hepatitis<br>• 'lupoid hepatitis' |
| Drugs e.g. methotrexate, isoniazid, methyldopa |
| Intestinal bypass surgery for obesity |

conduct of anaesthesia for any given patient requires a skilful clinical decision based on where he or she falls between these two extremes.

Some patients admitted with apparent decompensation may previously have been well compensated and have subsequently deteriorated because of some added stress. In addition, the brain of the patient with chronic liver disease is unduly sensitive to a number of insults that would not affect normal individuals. Factors that may precipitate decompensation are diarrhoea, vomiting, haemorrhage, hypotension, paracentesis, infection, alcohol excess, portosystemic shunting, intestinal obstruction, previous surgery, myocardial infarction, or drugs (antidepressants, diuretics, sedatives, opioids).

The clinical presentation of cirrhosis is related to either hepatocellular failure or portal hypertension.

## Hepatocellular failure

Hepatocellular failure is indicated by the presence of jaundice, ascites, and encephalopathy. The anaesthetic implications of jaundice have already been discussed.

### *Jaundice*

In hepatocellular failure, this is the result of failure of the liver cells to metabolize a normal bilirubin load and so the serum bilirubin concentration is some guide to the severity of liver cell failure.

### *Ascites*

The two most important factors in the development of ascites are a lowered plasma oncotic pressure (because of the failure of albumin synthesis) and portal venous hypertension. When more fluid enters the peritoneal cavity than leaves it, ascites develops. This results in depletion of the effective intravascular volume, which causes the renal tubules to retain sodium and water. This in turn encourages further formation of ascites. Ascites may develop suddenly or insidiously over a period of months.

### *Encephalopathy*

This neuropsychiatric syndrome may complicate liver disease of almost all types. The cause is not fully understood but is in part the result of the passage of toxic substances of intestinal origin to the brain. Other metabolic events of liver failure contribute. Early clinical signs are disturbed consciousness with sleep disorders, reduced spontaneous movement, a fixed stare, and apathy. Personality changes, intellectual deterioration, slurred speech, and a 'flapping' tremor also occur. The clinical course fluctuates but a guide to the severity is shown in Table 58.3.

## Portal hypertension

In cirrhosis, the portal vascular bed is distorted and diminished, and the portal blood flow is mechanically obstructed. Some of the portal venous blood is diverted into collateral venous channels and some bypasses the liver cells and is shunted directly into the hepatic vein. The normal portal venous pressure is 7 mmHg. In cirrhosis it can be raised up to 50 mmHg. The clinical features of portal hypertension are oesophageal varices, prominent collateral veins radiating from the umbilicus, dilated rectal veins, and splenomegaly. Surgical treatment may sometimes be indicated.

**Table 58.3 Severity of encephalopathy**

| | |
|---|---|
| Grade 1 | Confused<br>Altered mood or behaviour |
| Grade 2 | Drowsy<br>Inappropriate behaviour |
| Grade 3 | Stuporous but speaking and obeying simple commands<br>Inarticulate speech<br>Marked confusion |
| Grade 4 | Coma |
| Grade 5 | Deep coma with no response to painful stimuli |

## Preoperative considerations

### *History*

Establish the likely aetiology of the cirrhosis, and check that the patient is hepatitis B negative. Usual general complaints are weight loss, weakness, lethargy, anorexia, and loss of libido. Weight gain and swelling of the abdomen and legs suggest fluid retention and ascites. Dyspnoea may result. Details of jaundice, hepatitis, medications, and alcohol intake are important. Bleeding, and personality and mental changes are suggestive of encephalopathy.

Note the effects of any recent anaesthetics, and ask about the symptoms of diabetes mellitus, which frequently coexists with cirrhosis.

### *Examination*

#### *General*

Look for signs of liver malfunction: jaundice, gynaecomastia (may be secondary to spironolactone), spider naevi in the drainage area of the superior vena cava, white nails, paper money skin, palmar erythema, Dupuytren's contracture, bruising, parotid swelling, testicular atrophy, and loss of secondary sexual hair.

#### *Cardiovascular system*

Hepatocellular failure produces a hyperkinetic circulatory state with a high cardiac output, tachycardia, flushed extremities, bounding pulses, capillary pulsation, and an ejection systolic murmur. The BP may be low, and it is vital to differentiate between this state and that secondary to occult blood loss. Cyanosis is often present and hypoxia, acidosis, and electrolyte disturbances may cause arrhythmias.

#### *Respiratory system*

About one-third of patients with a decompensated cirrhosis have a reduced arterial oxygen tension and are cyanosed. This is secondary to intrapulmonary shunting and pulmonary vasodilatation. Chest infections are common, and ascites can impair diaphragmatic movement.

#### *Gastrointestinal tract*

Examine carefully for ascites and hepatosplenomegaly. Melaena may indicate bleeding oesophageal varices, and dilated veins suggest portal hypertension.

*Central nervous system*
Look for signs of encephalopathy and grade it accordingly. Cerebellar ataxia and peripheral neuropathy may occur in alcoholics without encephalopathy.

### Investigations

*Full blood count*
If the haemoglobin concentration is low look for a cause of occult blood loss. Exclude haemolysis.

*Urea and electrolytes*
These should be normal. The serum potassium may be high from spironolactone therapy or low from potassium-losing diuretic treatment. A low serum potassium can produce a metabolic alkalosis because of hydrogen ion excretion by the kidney, which attempts to preserve potassium. If possible, correct the hypokalaemia before surgery. An elevated and rising urea, and a low and falling plasma sodium, indicate a poor prognosis and require urgent treatment to prevent the hepatorenal syndrome.

*Glucose*
Chronic cirrhosis has an association with diabetes mellitus.

*Liver function tests*
See pages 885–887.

*ECG*
This should be normal. Arrhythmias occur in seriously decompensated states. Check that electrolyte and acid–base disturbances are not the cause.

*Clotting studies*
See the section on the jaundiced patient above.

*Chest radiograph*
Look for pleural effusions, pulmonary oedema, and a dilated heart.

*Blood gases*
These are indicated in severe disease or if there is cyanosis. Usually there is a hypoxic picture with compensatory hyperventilation and a low arterial $CO_2$ tension. There may be a metabolic alkalosis secondary to chronic potassium loss or a metabolic acidosis secondary to poor tissue perfusion.

*Endoscopy*
If there is evidence of gastrointestinal blood loss, endoscopy is useful in identifying oesophageal varices, both for controlling it with sclerotherapy and for establishing the presence or absence of the commonly coexisting peptic ulcer or gastric erosions.

*EEG*
The changes are non-specific but occur early in hepatic encephalopathy. There is a slowing from the normal $\alpha$ range of 8–13 cycles/s to the $\delta$ range of less than 4 cycles/s.

*Cerebrospinal fluid*
No abnormality is expected.

### Risks of surgery

The principles of management are essentially the same whether the patient is well compensated or decompensated, but the latter has a greatly reduced margin of safety. It can be helpful to grade the severity of liver disease according to a modification of Child's grouping, outlined in Table 58.4. For each of the variables listed, points are awarded as shown and the total calculated. A score of 5 or 6 points is considered to indicate a low operative risk (group A); a score of 7, 8, or 9 points indicates a moderate risk (group B); a score of 10–15 points indicates high operative risk (group C). Although this grouping was introduced to estimate the risk from portosystemic shunting, it can be helpful in deciding the risks of other surgery.

Where possible only patients in group A should be considered for elective surgery; those in group C should be considered for surgery only in life-threatening conditions.

### Preoperative preparation

If the patient with cirrhosis is jaundiced, this indicates an excess of liver cell necrosis over regeneration and carries a bad prognosis. This section assumes that, where relevant, the problem of jaundice and a prolonged prothrombin time are managed as described earlier.

The problems of ascites, cirrhosis, fluid retention, and the kidney are inextricably connected. About 80% of patients seriously ill with cirrhosis, who may or may not be jaundiced, have some element of renal failure,

**Table 58.4 Modified Child's grouping of the severity of liver disease (the grading of encephalopathy is outlined in Table 58.3)**

| Clinical and biochemical measurement | 1 point | 2 points | 3 points |
|---|---|---|---|
| Grade of encephalopathy | Absent | 1 and 2 | 3, 4 and 5 |
| Bilirubin (μmol/L) | < 25 | 25–40 | > 40 |
| Albumin (g/L) | 35 | 28–35 | < 28 |
| Prothrombin time (seconds prolonged) | 1–4 | 4–6 | > 6 |
| Ascites | Absent | Slight | Moderate |

the exact aetiology of which is not understood. The degree of renal failure is often worsened by sepsis, haemorrhage, hypotension, hypoxia, and surgery.

For the anaesthetist, the presence of ascites implies abnormal binding and metabolism of drugs, abnormal excretion of electrolytes, possible poor renal function, and compromised diaphragmatic movement. If the ascites is very tense and causes breathing problems, enough ascitic fluid should be removed to alleviate the symptoms and allow an adequate tidal volume and vital capacity. Do not forget that ventilatory function is worse when supine. Complete paracentesis carries a high risk of precipitating both renal and hepatic failure and encephalopathy, but this total drainage is sometimes inevitable in the course of an abdominal operation.

The preoperative treatment of ascites by bed rest and diuretics to increase the sodium loss (combined with a low-salt diet) must be done very gradually with careful observation of the clinical condition of the patient. Time is required to allow the fluid to shift from the ascitic to the central compartment, and weight loss should not exceed 0.5 kg/day. If it does, the central circulating volume is reduced by the action of the diuretic on the kidney faster than it is replaced from the ascitic fluid, and there is a high risk of developing a diuretic-induced uraemia. The organization of diuretic therapy is best done by hepatologists who will select the appropriate drugs and balance the dose against the patient's glomerular filtration rate. Occasionally, it is useful to expand the circulating fluid volume by the use of salt-poor albumin. In specialist units, refractory ascites can be treated by ultrafiltration. The ascitic fluid is drained via a peritoneal dialysis cannula, passed through a dialyser with a molecular sieve (passes molecules up to a molecular weight of 50 000) and the protein-concentrated fluid is returned to the patient intravenously. Weight loss is both direct and via increased urine output. Although large volumes of fluid can be lost quickly, it is a complex procedure with complications of infection, pulmonary oedema, heart failure, and haemorrhage.

If the patient has signs of encephalopathy, the absorption of the products of bacterial degradation of protein should be reduced. Magnesium sulphate enemas, oral lactulose, and/or oral neomycin are given to alter and reduce chronic bacterial flora.

For all but the most minor procedures, always have blood cross-matched (as fresh as possible) and check that FFP is available.

The effect of drugs in the patient with cirrhosis is unpredictable. Changes in albumin and globulin levels affect binding, alterations in the response at cellular level make the patient more 'sensitive', and a reduction in metabolic degradation prolongs the action of the active drug and its breakdown products.

#### *Premedication*

Many premedicant drugs will themselves precipitate encephalopathy. Morphine has a particularly bad reputation for this, although it is the dose, rather than the type of opioid, that is important. A well-tried combination is a small dose of intramuscular promethazine combined with a *small* dose of pethidine (e.g. 0.1–0.3 mg/kg). For sedation alone, oxazepam is probably best. In some cases, if the patient is agreeable, premedication can be avoided.

If a premedication is given, observing its effects when the patient arrives in the anaesthetic room may help in assessing the response to drugs. If the patient is on steroids increase the dose appropriately for the operation (see Chapter 56).

### Intraoperative phase

The maintenance of an adequate arterial blood pressure is vital in cirrhosis because the cirrhotic liver receives most of its blood supply from the hepatic artery. Hence, even a patient with well-compensated cirrhosis should not be offered hypotensive anaesthesia for an elective operation (e.g. plastic or middle-ear surgery). Other factors that minimize any disturbance of liver and kidney perfusion are the avoidance of hypoxia and hypovolaemia. If necessary, inotropes (at low doses) can be used to maintain the arterial blood pressure once a high CVP is established.

Invasive monitoring, if it is to be used, is best put in under local anaesthetic at the outset so that the haemodynamic effects of induction can be monitored. This is especially useful during rapid sequence induction. The necessity of arterial, central venous, and pulmonary artery catheters must be judged in individual cases, and their benefits balanced against the risks in patients with a potential coagulation problem. They are indicated most in those patients with preoperative arrhythmias, hypoxia, and hypotension. Patients presenting with a tachycardia and a peripherally dilated vascular bed tolerate blood loss and decreases of cardiac output badly.

When dealing with patients with hepatitis, take care with blood and bodily fluids in order to avoid cross-infection to yourself or other operating room personnel (see Chapter 60).

#### *Induction*

After preoxygenation, induction agents should be given slowly to minimize reductions in cardiac output and to allow time for their effects to become apparent. In the sick patient, only very small doses will be required, but, in the patient with compensated cirrhosis, increased binding to globulins, or enzyme induction, may lead to an increase in requirements. Barbiturates may worsen encephalopathy. Etomidate has the theoretical advantage of cardiovascular stability.

If there has been acute gastrointestinal bleeding, a rapid sequence induction (or awake intubation) will be necessary, with the usual precautions (preoxygenation, spare laryngoscope, cuff checked on the endotracheal tube, and large capacity sucker). In extreme cases with bleeding oesophageal varices, an oesophageal tamponade tube (e.g. Sengstaken) will be in place. They have up to four lumina: oesophageal and gastric balloons, a tube in the stomach, and a fourth lumen for aspiration above the oesophageal balloon. Suck on the last before induction. Do not remove the tamponade tube (intubation is quite possible with it *in situ*) and do not deflate the balloons. It should be left in place to minimize blood loss until the surgeon is ready for either injection sclerotherapy or oesophageal trans-section.

It has been suggested that in patients with cirrhosis low serum pseudocholinesterase prolongs the action of suxamethonium, but there is little evidence of this being a practical problem.

#### *Maintenance*

The importance of avoiding hypotension has already been emphasized. Careful cardiovascular monitoring is essential (pulse, BP, CVP, ECG) and you should always be ready to give warmed blood early, thus allowing a relatively slow transfusion and time for the adequate metabolism of citrate. This is a particular problem in patients with bleeding oesophageal varices, in whom very high levels of serum citrate have been found during multiple transfusions. With normal liver function, the risk of lowering the serum ionized calcium is small, unless blood is transfused at a rate greater than 1 unit/5 min or more than 4 units are given in total. These limits are eroded in hepatocellular failure, and calcium supplements may need to be given earlier, especially if the QT segment on the ECG indicates hypocalcaemia.

If non-surgical blood loss is a problem, repeat the clotting screen and give fresh blood and/or FFP and platelets according to the results.

For routine maintenance fluids (apart from the replacement of a loss of circulating volume), avoid giving solutions with a high sodium content: 5% dextrose is probably the fluid of choice unless the patient is hyponatraemic. Human plasma protein fraction has a high sodium content: 140–160 mmol/L.

Normocapnia should be maintained because of the beneficial effect on liver blood flow. The fractional inspired oxygen concentration is best set initially at 50% to offset the possible effects of intrapulmonary shunting. Infusion of alfentanil at 30–50 μg/kg per h provides analgesia satisfactorily. Low concentrations of volatile agents are acceptable, provided that they do not depress BP and cardiac output.

Patients with cirrhosis have low reserves of glycogen, so their blood glucose needs checking half-hourly.

The response to non-depolarizing neuromuscular blocking agents is not always predictable, because of abnormal protein binding and possible increased sequestration in the liver. Normally this is not a problem if the patient has adequate renal function, because the kidney is the major route of excretion. Nevertheless, it is advantageous to monitor the level of neuromuscular block in prolonged procedures, to ensure that only the minimum total dose is administered. Atracurium is the most appropriate neuromuscular blocking agent because its metabolism is independent of liver function.

Nasogastric tubes, when required, should be passed carefully if there are any oesophageal varices.

Respectfully remind the surgeon, if he or she is working abdominally, not to put packs on the hepatic artery or portal vein! Similar pressure on the inferior vena cava is probably the most common cause of episodic intraoperative hypotension

#### Postoperative phase

Patients require a good recovery area with adequate staff and monitoring facilities. They need oxygen-enriched air and their BP should be measured every few minutes. Adequate oxygenation may prevent unwanted metabolites occurring because of reductive pathway metabolism. Often patients take a long time to recover from anaesthetic drugs and can require intermittent positive pressure ventilation to ensure good oxygenation until they are conscious.

Do not forget that the operation itself might cause confusion. Always eliminate hypoglycaemia as a cause of this. Conversely, remember that a diabetic state may be precipitated. Allow time for the effects of the anaesthetic drugs to wear off before giving postoperative analgesia. This can be provided with epidural local anaesthetics combined with opioid, provided that there is no coagulopathy. Do not allow hypotension to occur. In the presence of portal hypertension, the epidural veins are often engorged and bloody taps are not infrequent.

If using parenteral analgesics, give only very small incremental does (e.g. 0.01 mg/kg morphine i.v.) until the effect has been determined. Large or 'normal' doses of any opioid can be fatal. If postoperative sedatives are required, it is best to use those that are excreted renally (e.g. sodium barbitone, phenobarbitone [phenobarbital], or oxazepam).

Other problems that occur during the first few postoperative days are frequent chest infections (prescribe early and regular physiotherapy), and a deterioration in hepatic and renal function. This is especially likely if the ascites has been totally drained because of the surgical procedure. If the ascites remains, postoperative ventilatory insufficiency is common.

### FURTHER READING


Browne DRG. Anaesthesia in impaired liver function. *Curr Anaesth Crit Care* 1990;**1**:220–7.

Eagle CJ, Strunin L. Drug metabolism in liver disease. *Curr Anaesth Crit Care* 1990;**1**:204–12.

Sear JW. Effect of renal and hepatic disease on pharmacokinetics of anaesthetic agents. In: Prys-Roberts C, Hug CC Jr, eds. *Pharmacokinetics of Anaesthesia*. Oxford: Blackwell Scientific Publications, 1984: 64–88.

Souhami RL, Moxham J, eds. *Textbook of Medicine*, 3rd edn. Edinburgh: Churchill Livingstone, 1997.

Strunin L. Preoperative assessment of hepatic function. *Baillière's Clinical Anaesthesiology*. 1992;**6**:781–93

# Chapter 59 The patient with impaired renal function

G.M. Cooper

The function of the kidney in health falls into three main areas:

- excretion of waste products;
- maintenance of the constancy of the internal environment;
- biosynthesis of hormones.

These functions are discussed in detail in Chapter 25. Their importance is vividly demonstrated in renal disease, in which a wide variety of symptoms and signs is associated with disordered metabolism. The sophistication of the various functions of the kidney is evident from the striking contrast between the limited efficacy of the various forms of artificial dialysis treatment, and the virtual normalization of body function that attends reversal of kidney dysfunction or successful transplantation. The anaesthetist will be involved with patients with acute and chronic renal failure.

## ACUTE RENAL FAILURE

The anaesthetist meets acute renal failure in two ways. First, he or she becomes involved with the avoidance, recognition, and treatment of acute renal failure in the 'at-risk' patient both during surgery and on the intensive care unit (ICU). Second, he or she has to anaesthetize patients who are in established acute renal failure. The latter present either for the investigation of renal outflow obstruction or for surgical treatment of the precipitating cause (e.g. major trauma, burns, drainage of infections, vascular repair).

Acute renal failure occurs when there is a rapid deterioration in the ability of the kidney to perform its task of excretion, metabolism and acid–base homoeostasis. Irrespective of the exact aetiology, waste products of protein metabolism, such as urea and creatinine, accumulate in the blood and there is inadequate excretion of hydrogen ions. Sodium and water balance is disturbed and hyperkalaemia may occur.

Established acute renal failure in the perioperative period is a serious condition associated with an overall mortality rate of about 50%. A high incidence is found after open-heart, major vascular, and trauma surgery.

Traditionally, acute renal failure is defined as a sudden reduction in urine output to below 400 ml/day. Although this is the most common presentation, it is an imperfect definition because up to 30% of cases (especially those resulting from loop diuretic or antibiotic toxicity) are polyuric, and acute renal failure develops with the production of normal or increased volumes of isotonic urine.

Those patients who are at risk of developing acute renal failure should be identified. The predisposing factors are listed in Table 59.1. These patients should be monitored carefully, looking for the first signs of renal failure. This is important because, with correct and vigorous treatment, the progression to established renal failure may, at times, be averted.

### Prevention and detection in the perioperative period

The cornerstone of prophylaxis is to keep the patient well hydrated with a satisfactory blood pressure. He or she should never be allowed to become hypovolaemic, hypotensive, or hypoxic. Aim for a moderately high central venous pressure (CVP $> 6$ mmHg) and if necessary use inotropic agents at a *low* dosage level to maintain renal perfusion. Pushing these to moderate or high levels is counterproductive because of the resultant vasoconstriction. Measure the urea and electrolytes, and serum creatinine at least daily in the perioperative period, and chart the urine volume every 2 h (or hourly). Urinary catheterization is therefore mandatory, but is usually required anyway to aid the management of other pathologies. Take great care to ensure accurate collections. Directly nephrotoxic drugs to be avoided are listed in Table 59.2.

When a person is managed as described above, any sustained fall in the urine output (always check for a blocked catheter) in the presence of a constant fluid load must be investigated. It is wrong to wait until some arbitrary figure of daily urine output has been reached (e.g. 400 ml/day) before taking the situation seriously.

A reduction in urine flow can precede the rapid rise in blood urea and creatinine levels by 24–72 h. Once renal failure has occurred, in the untreated patient the serum potassium rises at 0.5–3.0 mmol/day (this may be intensified by excessive tissue damage) and acidosis occurs from the production of approximately 1 mmol hydrogen ions per kg per day. All these changes are intensified by catabolism. Later, hypertension, anaemia, and clotting abnormalities may occur.

#### *Management of oliguria*

Some patients are not brought to the attention of the anaesthetist until the blood urea is already elevated. In those who have not had effective circulatory support, uraemia may be still be reversible, provided that restoration of circulating fluid volume and improvement of renal blood flow occur at a stage when renal excretory, concentrating, and reabsorptive mechanisms are still adequate. Established acute renal failure will

**Table 59.1 Factors associated with acute renal failure**

| Patient factors | Perioperative factors |
|---|---|
| Advanced age | Hypotension |
| Aortic surgery | Hypovolaemia: |
| Atherosclerosis (especially aortic) | • diuretic therapy |
| Cardiac surgery | • preoperative starvation |
| Chronic renal disease | • gastric aspiration/vomiting |
| Cirrhosis | • ileus/obstruction |
| Diabetes | • diarrhoea/bowel preparation |
| Heart failure | • surgical oedema |
| Hypertension | • prolonged tissue exposure |
| Jaundice | • blood loss |
| Myeloma | Hypoxia |
| Nephrotoxic drugs | Tissue damage/inflammation |
| Outflow blockage (note: prostate) | Ischaemia and reperfusion |
| Pre-eclampsia/eclampsia | Major burns |
| Sepsis | Pancreatitis |
| Systemic disease involving kidneys (e.g. connective tissue disorders) | Multiple fractures |
| | Muscle damage |
| Undernourishment | Transfusion reactions |

inevitably supervene if the factors causing the low urine output are not corrected promptly.

The concentrating power of the kidney may be assessed by the urinary specific gravity or osmolality. The colour of the urine, which is caused by urochromes, is totally unrelated to its quality in terms of excretion and acid–base homoeostasis.

Measurement of urine and plasma osmolality and creatinine can help distinguish between renal underperfusion and intrinsic renal failure (Table 59.3). However, the fractional excretion of sodium ($FE_{Na}$) is a more accurate guide to renal integrity:

$$FE_{Na} = \frac{(U_{Na}/P_{Na})}{(U_{Cr}/P_{Cr})}$$

where $U_{Na}$ and $U_{Cr}$ are the urinary sodium and creatinine concentrations and $P_{Na}$ and $P_{Cr}$ are plasma sodium and creatinine concentrations, respectively.

When first encountering a patient with a low (about 0.5 ml/min) or deteriorating urine flow, it is important to differentiate between true renal failure and an exaggerated physiological response to hypovolaemia. This differentiation is important because, depending on the cause of the oliguria, the correct treatment is either to increase fluids or to restrict them. The renal response of a healthy kidney to poor perfusion is the excretion of small volumes of highly concentrated urine (> 500 mosmol/L), which is low in sodium content (< 10–20 mmol/L) because of maximum tubular reabsorption. Once acute renal failure is established, the urine excreted (usually of small volume) is iso-osmotic with plasma (about 290 mosmol/L) with a high concentration of sodium (> 40 mmol/L).

All oliguric patients require catheterization so that the urine output can be measured accurately. Initial management should be directed to the primary cause and to the correction of any *hypoxia and haemodynamic abnormalities* that may be present.

If oliguria persists despite adequate resuscitation, and there is a satisfactory blood pressure and a moderately high CVP (> 6 mmHg), it is appropriate to give an intravenous diuretic challenge. A suitable regimen is mannitol (up to 0.7 g/kg) followed by frusemide (furosemide) in increasing doses of 40 mg, 80 mg, 160 mg, and 250 mg. Between each prescription, allow at least 1–2 h to assess the response. Note that giving frusemide to patients who are hypovolaemic can itself produce acute renal failure. There are two possible responses to the diuretic challenge:

**Table 59.2 Nephrotoxic drugs**

| Drug group | Examples |
|---|---|
| Aminoglycosides | Amikacin<br>Gentamicin<br>Kanamycin<br>Neomycin<br>Tobramycin |
| Chemotherapeutic agents | Amphotericin<br>Cephaloridine<br>Colistin<br>Tetracycline<br>Vancomycin |
| NSAIDs | Diclofenac<br>Ketorolac<br>Tenoxicam |
| Radiocontrast media | |
| Volatile agents that release fluoride | Enflurane<br>(methoxyflurane) |

NSAIDs, non-steroidal anti-inflammatory agents.

**Table 59.3 Common urinary indices**

| | Underperfusion | Intrinsic renal failure |
|---|---|---|
| *U/P* osmolality | > 1.5 | < 1.1 |
| *U/P* creatinine | > 40 | < 20 |
| $U_{Na}$ (mmol/L) | < 20 | > 40 |
| $FE_{Na}$ (%) | < 1 | > 3 |

U, urine; P, plasma; $FE_{Na}$, fractional excretion of sodium.

1. No effect: this confirms renal failure with the possible need for dialysis and fluid restriction.
2. An increased output of hypotonic urine: this means that acute renal failure has been aborted or that oliguric failure has been converted to polyuric failure. If the latter has occurred, the patient's biochemistry will still deteriorate quickly. Careful monitoring of the U&Es and acid–base status must continue in order to differentiate these two conditions.

Once acute renal failure has been diagnosed it should be managed as outlined below.

### *Management of acute renal failure*

The overall philosophy of management is to keep the patient alive by whatever means are required, until spontaneous recovery of renal function occurs. Simultaneously, the basic cause of the renal failure should be treated aggressively. The ease of management depends greatly on the precipitating cause. Patients with extensive soft tissue trauma, septicaemia, multiple fractures, or burns are the most difficult. They readily become catabolic, and thus have increased metabolic activity and protein breakdown superimposed on grossly inadequate or temporarily non-existent renal function. Once renal failure is established, measure all daily fluid losses from vomit, urine, faeces, etc.

Hyperkalaemia develops early in the course of acute renal failure and is completely asymptomatic. The ECG (see Figure 47.9) and serum potassium must be monitored for changes, and wide QRS complexes and peaked T waves treated urgently. These are usually evident with a serum potassium of about 6 mmol/L but, if the development of hyperkalaemia is very gradual, the ECG can remain unaffected until the serum potassium is much higher. The terminal cardiac event is ventricular tachycardia progressing to ventricular fibrillation. The first-line emergency treatment is calcium chloride (to stabilize the myocardium) and sodium bicarbonate (to reduce the acidosis). Never give these together in the same intravenous line because calcium bicarbonate will precipitate out. These measures can be followed by glucose and insulin, but this serves only to transfer potassium ions to the intracellular space. To remove excess potassium from the body, which is ultimately required, ion exchange resins, dialysis, or haemofiltration is necessary.

The optimum management for an individual patient is often difficult to decide on, and is usually undertaken by specialist renal physicians. The choices are conservative management, peritoneal dialysis, haemodialysis, or haemofiltration.

The problem with conservative management is that, while awaiting spontaneous recovery, the biochemistry of the body continues to deteriorate, and this does not provide the optimum setting for renal function to improve. Consequently, many centres limit their trial of conservative therapy to only 24–48 h before active steps are taken. This has the important effect of allowing adequate nutrition, which is now thought to be crucial in early recovery. Whenever possible, use the enteral route, otherwise commence intravenous feeding. Parenteral nutrition presents considerable problems because of the inevitable fluid load, the use of hypertonic glucose, and the potassium content of some amino acid solutions. Skilful dialysis and adjustment of the regimen are required to minimize disturbances.

Peritoneal dialysis is better for the safe removal of excess fluid, is technically simpler, and is better tolerated in children and elderly people. Its disadvantages are that it can splint the diaphragm, thus encouraging pulmonary infection, it corrects uraemia only slowly, and it may be contraindicated after abdominal surgery or trauma. With the recent improvements in filter technology and the increased familiarity with intravenous techniques, peritoneal dialysis is now less frequently used than in the past. It is, however, still effective, simple, and safe.

Haemodialysis is far more efficient in removing the waste products of metabolism, but can potentiate cardiac irregularities and requires the patient to be heparinized. Emergency dialysis used to be done with arteriovenous (AV) shunts, but now single-cannula dialysis via the subclavian vein is increasing in popularity.

Haemofiltration employs the use of an extracorporeal circulation which is usually perfused from an AV shunt. A semipermeable membrane allows an ultrafiltrate of plasma to be produced and the losses are replaced from new solutions via a separate intravenous line. Continuous AV haemofiltration (CAVH) is a slow, continuous (24 h/day) treatment that has advantages in very sick patients because it produces haemodynamic changes to a lesser degree. Continuous AV haemodiafiltration also has these advantages. These two techniques are compared in Table 59.4. As seen, CAVH is more suitable for hypercatabolic patients. Haemodialysis, haemofiltration, and haemodiafiltration are shown diagrammatically in Figure 59.1.

**Table 59.4 Comparison of continuous arteriovenous haemofiltration (CAVH) and haemodiafiltration (CAVHD)**

| | CAVH | CAVHD |
|---|---|---|
| Clearance | Convection | Diffusion + convection |
| Urea clearance (ml/min) | 10 | 30 |
| Creatinine clearance | 10<br>(UFR 600 ml/h)<br>($Q_B$ 200 ml/min) | 30<br>($Q_D$ 35 ml/min)<br>($Q_B$ 200 ml/min) |
| Hypercatabolic patient | Inadequate | Adequate |
| Drug pharmacokinetics | Known | Uncertain |
| Total parenteral nutrition, e.g. amino acids | Up to 25% lost | Uncertain |
| Replacement fluids | High volumes (complex intravenous replacement) | Low volumes (simpler) |
| Hyperkalaemia | Poor control | Good control |
| Hypotensive patients | Falling UFR and clearance | Dialysis maintained at ≥ 60 mmHg systolic blood pressure |

UFR, urinary filtration rate; $Q_D$, dialysate outflow rate; $Q_B$, blood blow. From Sweny P. *Curr Anaesth Crit Care* 1991;2:39.

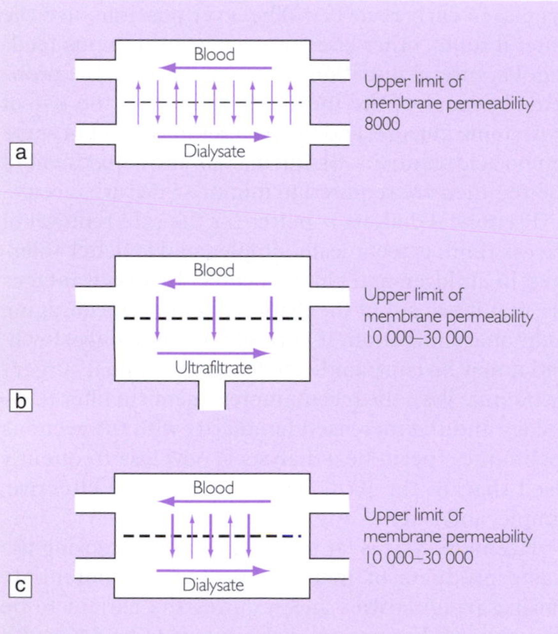


**Figure 59.1** Diagrammatic representation of (a) haemodialysis, (b) haemofiltration, and (c) haemodiafiltration. (Adapted from Sweny P. *Curr Anaesth Crit Care*. 1991; 2: 37–43.)

The ventilatory response to metabolic acidosis reduces the arterial $CO_2$ tension ($P$aCO$_2$) and thus minimizes the pH change. If the patient has insufficient ventilatory reserve to make this compensation, there will be a rapid rise in the serum hydrogen ion concentration. Consequently, ventilatory support with intermittent positive pressure ventilation (IPPV) is not infrequently required, especially if there is coexisting pulmonary trauma, chest infection, pulmonary oedema, or septicaemia. Haemodialysis itself increases the pulmonary shunt by the sequestration of white blood cells in the lung and the activation of complement. A problem associated with ventilation, and especially the use of positive end-expiratory pressure, is the inappropriate secretion of antidiuretic hormone (ADH; vasopressin), which further suppresses urine formation.

Infection is a major risk and can occur in any body system or organ. If unchecked, it rapidly progresses to septicaemia. Routine cultures of blood, sputum, urine, and drainage fluids are required.

Stress ulcers in the stomach and duodenum occur in up to 25% of patients with acute renal failure. Combined with the bleeding tendency of these patients, intestinal blood loss may be brisk and massive. Prophylactic $H_2$-receptor blockade is indicated. Magnesium salts should be avoided in acute renal failure. Anaemia and hypertension tend to be later complications. It is important to remember that the doses of any drugs prescribed must be adjusted if their excretion depends on good renal function.

#### *Anaesthetic management of patients with acute renal failure*

The background presentation, physiology, and management of acute renal failure have already been described. Many patients presenting for surgery have other major surgical or medical problems around which any anaesthetic must be tailored. For the management of these individual problems themselves, the reader should refer to the appropriate chapters.

The philosophy of any anaesthetic procedure must be, first, to optimize the patient's condition within the time available (this is usually undertaken by a renal physician) and, second, to give an anaesthetic that least jeopardizes existing renal function.

### Preoperative considerations

#### *History*

Establish the cause of acute renal failure, time of onset, progress of symptoms, prognosis, and mode of treatment. Ask the staff about the patient's morale and record the patient's mental state. Be suspicious that any bloody nasogastric aspirate or melaena might be from a stress ulcer or caused by a blood dyscrasia. In patients with multiple problems, consider whether or not a tracheostomy could usefully be fashioned during the same anaesthetic. If the patient is ventilated or sedated, see how long drug dosages have lasted, because the duration is often markedly altered by renal function. Note especially whether, on the one hand, inotropes and a high CVP are necessary to maintain cardiac output or, on the other, antihypertensives are needed for reducing the blood pressure.

If the patient has had haemodialysis, record any problems encountered, especially postdialysis hypotension or pulmonary oedema, both of which occur most easily in patients who are very sensitive to changes in circulating fluid volume. Check the daily allowance of intravenous fluids. Before surgery, contact renal physicians and ask their advice on intraoperative fluids and whether or not transfused blood needs special treatment (e.g. washed cells).

If the patient is fit enough, discuss the possibility of regional or local anaesthetic techniques.

### Examination

Examine the significance of precipitating factors in relation to the proposed procedure (e.g. fractured spine, crush injuries, etc.). Look at the condition of the skin and check the quality of the drip sites. If a new or additional one is required, it can often best be established in a relaxed atmosphere on the ICU before moving to the operating room. If a shunt is present, make a mental note to protect it intraoperatively.

#### *Respiratory system*

If the patient is breathing spontaneously, look for cyanosis (may be masked by anaemia) and assess the ventilatory rate, the chest expansion, and the use of the accessory muscles of respiration. Note the presence of air hunger and any anxious facial expressions. The patient will probably be hyperventilating to normalize the blood pH.

Borderline ventilation when sitting may become inadequate when supine. If the patient is able to cooperate, the preoperative vital capacity and tidal volume are sensible measurements to take. The comparison between them gives an indication of the ventilatory reserve. Auscultate carefully for equal air entry and crepitations. Ventilation may deteriorate with both haemodialysis and peritoneal dialysis. Check the ability to breathe deeply and cough, and examine a specimen of sputum for macroscopic evidence of infection or blood.

If the patient is on a ventilator, note the settings required to maintain adequate arterial blood gases. This will affect the anaesthetic technique and great care may be necessary to prevent hypoxia and/or hypercapnia while transporting the patient to the operating room.

#### *Cardiovascular system*

Check the stability of the blood pressure (BP) under the treatment regimen. Examine for signs of anaemia (pale, tachycardic, bounding pulse). Auscultate for murmurs (usually flow murmurs in the aortic region and at the left sternal edge, but rarely can be endocarditis), or added sounds (left ventricular failure [LVF]). Check the postural fall in BP. Examine the neck veins or measure the CVP. Look for sacral and ankle oedema, and listen for the crepitations of pulmonary oedema. Note any petechiae or ecchymoses secondary to a blood dyscrasia (often best seen under the BP cuff).

#### *Gastrointestinal tract*

Examine the nasogastric aspirate and faeces for the presence of blood. Regular nasogastric tube aspiration or vomiting can reduce the rate of rise of serum potassium. In patients on peritoneal dialysis, an opalescence in the dialysis fluid often indicates infection.

#### *Nervous system*

From a conversation (if this is possible), make a crude estimate of the mental state. Record any preoperative neurological symptoms, signs, or injuries. The muscular twitchings of uraemia usually occur late with a very high blood urea, and do not occur in dialysed patients. Therefore, if odd neuromuscular movements are present, or there is blunted consciousness, always suspect an occult cause (e.g. cerebral oedema).

### Investigations

#### *Urea and electrolytes*

These are obviously very important, particularly the serum potassium shortly before surgery.

#### *Full blood count*

Anaemia in acute renal failure is measurable after 1 week and is maximal by 1 month. If the haemoglobin is unexpectedly low, taking into account all the features of the case, look for other occult sites of blood loss, especially from the gastrointestinal tract. The presence of a raised white cell count should suggest infection.

#### *Clotting studies*

Acute renal failure often produces clotting abnormalities, which might require the use of fresh frozen plasma or platelet concentrate. Remember that patients are heparinized during haemodialysis.

#### *Chest radiograph*

Look at the heart size, and for the presence of pulmonary oedema or pleural effusions.

#### *ECG*

Look for signs of potassium toxicity (see Figure 47.9) and for arrhythmias. A sinus tachycardia is common.

#### *Sputum*

Do regular cultures.

#### *Blood gases*

These are useful as a baseline and to give a guide to the extent of the ventilatory compensation necessary to counter the metabolic acidosis. Avoid causing any unnecessary trauma to an artery which may be needed subsequently for an AV shunt or fistula.

#### *Preoperative preparation*

The basic preparation is as in 'management of acute renal failure'. For urgent operations with a normal ECG and a serum potassium of 6.0 mmol/L or less, the operation can probably proceed immediately.

#### *Premedication*

This may not be required. If it is, try to avoid intramuscular injections, which cause bruising. Beware of ventilatory depressant drugs in a patient who is hyperventilating to compensate for acidosis.

### Intraoperative phase

Always remember that a patient with acute renal failure may require haemodialysis in the future. Therefore, it is vital to avoid potential shunt and fistula sites with intravenous and arterial cannulae.

#### *The effect of anaesthesia*

The only two anaesthetic agents that have not been implicated in reducing urine production are nitrous oxide and droperidol. Volatile anaesthetics, opioids, sympathomimetic drugs, endogenous catecholamines, and surgery itself all reduce urine flow by a variety of mechanisms, including hypotension, vasoconstriction, and the release of ADH. Free fluoride ions from the breakdown of enflurane are directly nephrotoxic.

The most important factors of all in protecting the kidney are unrelated to the choice of the anaesthetic drugs. *The features that must be avoided at all costs are hypoxia, hypovolaemia, and hypotension.* There are obviously several ways of achieving this.

#### *Monitoring*

It is essential to monitor the BP and ECG from before the induction of anaesthesia through to the postoperative period. The need for an invasive measurement of BP obviously differs from case to case, but an arterial cannula should be used only if it is going to play a vital role. Whenever possible, avoid the radial and brachial arteries. The dorsalis pedis is probably the artery of choice.

A central venous catheter also has the potential for damaging potential fistula sites. Although it is useful for assessing fluid balance and for testing the response of a compromised cardiovascular system to a fluid load, do not use one without good reason. The best sites are the internal jugular or subclavian veins. The subclavian route is less preferable after recent haemodialysis because there is no facility for applying pressure if the patient bleeds.

The acid–base status can be followed either by repeated arterial blood sampling or from measurement of the end-tidal $CO_2$. The latter is preferable from the non-invasive viewpoint, but the former also confirms the adequacy of oxygenation. As a result of the increased pulmonary shunt present in many of these patients, a good case can be made for the placement of an arterial line during major surgical procedures. It is likely to be needed afterwards anyway because the majority require postoperative ventilation on the ICU.

A nerve stimulator can be used to follow the progress of neuromuscular blockade. It is most useful in confirming the presence of a significant residual block at a time when 'top-up' doses would normally be given. Atracurium is the most sensible choice of neuromuscular blocker. Any prolonged procedure is an indication for the use of a warming blanket and body temperature measurement.

Fentanyl and alfentanil are appropriate choices of intraoperative analgesic. The metabolites of morphine accumulate with poor renal function. One of these, morphine 6-glucuronide, is a potent analgesic, and is thought to be responsible for the prolonged clinical effects that have been reported. Morphine should therefore be used with care, and not as a continuous infusion. The action of pethidine is also altered and one of its metabolites, norpethidine, accumulates. Although it has only weak analgesic activity, it can cause excitatory phenomena and convulsions. Non-steroidal anti-inflammatory drugs should be avoided.

#### *Fluid balance*

Optimal fluid balance is difficult to achieve. The major problem is that of fluid overload resulting in postoperative pulmonary oedema. Those patients on conservative management are at the greatest risk, and often it must be accepted that postoperative dialysis will be necessary. It is almost inevitable after major surgery.

Many anaesthetic agents produce arteriolar and venous dilatation. This results in a fall in BP which responds to an infusion of fluid. Fluid has to be given because hypotension and hypovolaemia might further jeopardize the kidneys. Use physiological (0.9%) saline because dextrose solutions produce acute hyponatraemia.

Dextrose 5% is satisfactory for 'keeping a line open' when it is required for injecting drugs. It can be given up to the daily allowance plus estimated evaporative losses.

Frank blood losses obviously need replacement by physiological saline, blood, blood products, or a plasma expander (but not dextran, which is nephrotoxic). When giving blood, always watch the T wave closely on the ECG. The high serum potassium of stored blood is not always rapidly reabsorbed by the red cells as it is in the 'normal' patient, and hyperkalaemia can occur. Do not over-transfuse. A high haematocrit reduces renal plasma flow. A postoperative haemoglobin of over 11g/dl is almost certainly contraindicated unless required for other purposes (e.g. to maintain oxygen flux in severe adult respiratory distress syndrome). If the haemoglobin had already fallen preoperatively because of the renal disease alone, treat as a case of chronic renal failure.

#### *Regional anaesthesia*

The normal indications for and contraindications to this type of anaesthesia apply. Problems can arise during the spinal or epidural anaesthesia if a large fluid load is given to maintain BP. As vascular tone returns, pulmonary oedema may occur.

#### *General anaesthesia*

*Induction*

Always preoxygenate. If the patient is starved give the drugs slowly to minimize haemodynamic disturbances. Even doing this, BP can still fall dramatically. If a rapid sequence induction is necessary be ready to infuse physiological saline to restore BP.

Potassium release after suxamethonium is not exaggerated in people who are only moderately uraemic with a normal serum potassium. There are, however, many patients in acute renal failure who have a serum potassium that is high initially and/or associated tissue or neurological damage. In these patients, the succeeding rise is more likely to reach dangerous levels.

#### *Maintenance*

Spontaneous ventilation is usually suitable only for short procedures such as diagnostic radiology, the reason being that most patients in acute renal failure have some degree of ventilatory compensation for their metabolic acidosis. This compensation is suppressed by volatile agents that cause the $Pa\text{CO}_2$ to rise and the alveolar ventilation to fall (see Chapter 54). There are consequent rapid changes in the pH and, if there is a large pulmonary shunt, unexpected falls in the arterial oxygen tension. Therefore, meticulous airway control is essential and the fractional inspired oxygen ($F\text{IO}_2$) should be set to 50%. If there is any doubt about the adequacy of the airway, always intubate. End-tidal $CO_2$ measurement is very helpful and, if it rises appreciably (> 1%), manual assistance of the ventilation is often sufficient to return it to the preoperative value.

Measure BP at least every 5 min. Hypotension secondary to a volatile agent may necessitate a change in technique.

Controlled ventilation is preferred for any long procedure and particularly for those where blood and/or insensible fluid losses will be appreciable. The necessity for maintaining the $Pa\text{CO}_2$ and the possibility of unexpected hypoxia have already been discussed. Many patients with acute renal failure are already being ventilated on the ICU before surgery. If so, and they have been stable, their $F\text{IO}_2$ and minute ventilation can be maintained intraoperatively. Otherwise, they should be ventilated with a large tidal volume, a minute volume sufficient to achieve their preoperative $Pa\text{CO}_2$, and an $F\text{IO}_2$ that prevents hypoxia.

Patients with renal failure often need only small doses of a non-depolarizing neuromuscular blocking agent, if any at all, to maintain IPPV. When they are required, atracurium has the advantage of non-renal excretion. Vecuronium and rocuronium are partially renally excreted, and, although they can be used successfully in renal failure, they will accumulate after multiple doses or infusions. Mivacurium is metabolized by plasma and tissue esterases. Plasma cholinesterase activity is reduced in renal failure but the increase in duration of effect of mivacurium is minimal. Gallamine is contraindicated because the kidney is the sole route of its excretion. Pancuronium, alcuronium, and curare have an extended duration of action in renal failure. It is, however, often possible after intubation to ventilate the patient without the need for further neuromuscular blocking agent. Supplementation with a volatile agent combined with an opioid can usually augment the neuromuscular block sufficiently to prevent any troublesome movement, but care must be taken to avoid hypotension.

Despite careful anaesthesia and meticulous attention to fluid balance, the BP may start to fall gradually. Provided that it is certain that the patient is not hypovolaemic, this is best treated by low-dose inotropes (dopamine or dobutamine) to increase cardiac contractility and cardiac output. Moderate or high dosages of these agents are contraindicated because of possible vasoconstrictor actions. It is difficult to give exact figures for when to treat hypotension, but it is not unreasonable in patients with renal failure to aim never to allow the systolic BP to fall below 100 mmHg.

### Postoperative phase

Reversal of neuromuscular block should be attempted only if there is evidence that recovery has commenced spontaneously (e.g. by nerve stimulation or by ventilatory efforts). If not, have no hesitation in deciding to continue ventilation. Recurarization is a real danger. A low body temperature combined with a prolonged action of non-depolarizing neuromuscular blocking agents can produce an extended paralysis. If the body temperature is low (< 35°C) at the end of the operation, reversal may be impossible until the body is rewarmed.

Return the patient to a high dependency area and maintain a high $F\text{IO}_2$. If he or she is breathing spontaneously, instruct staff to be alert to the possibilities of pulmonary oedema and recurarization. On rare occasions, pulmonary oedema needs acute treatment by IPPV. Dialysis or haemofiltration is then required for the bulk removal of excess fluid.

The BP, ECG, and breathing need to be monitored closely for several hours, and any irregularities must be treated early. The most frequent causes of abnormalities after careful anaesthesia are those common to any operation, such as hypoxia, a high $Pa\text{CO}_2$, pain, and the excessive use of analgesics.

Postoperatively, chest infections are common. Early physiotherapy is very important and, if antibiotics are required, thought must be given to their potential nephrotoxicity.

## CHRONIC RENAL FAILURE

In contrast to acute renal failure, most cases of chronic renal failure are totally unavoidable. The annual rate of incidence of end-stage renal disease in the UK is about 150/million population. Of these, about 50% are suitable for renal replacement therapy, although in practice only about 70% of those suitable receive it. The remaining 30% die untreated.

The several forms of glomerulonephritis continue to provide the largest group treated in renal units. Other causes are pyelonephritis, polycystic disease, diabetic nephropathy, hypertensive nephropathy, gout, analgesic abuse (paracetamol [acetaminophen]), the collagen diseases, hypercalcaemia, obstruction from an enlarged prostate gland, retroperitoneal fibrosis, and, very rarely, incompletely resolved acute renal failure. Patients with diabetic nephrosclerosis account for a steadily increasing number of those receiving treatment.

The choice of treatment depends on the patient's age, intelligence, social resources, employment, associated diseases, geographical situation, and motivation.

### The features relevant to the anaesthetist

#### *Presentation*

Chronic renal failure has a variable presentation because it can, indirectly, cause any organ system to be affected. Most commonly, there is a non-specific history of lethargy, anorexia, polyuria, nocturia, and general ill-health. Nausea, vomiting, bruising, pruritus, and weight loss follow. There are few physical findings except the signs of anaemia, hyperventilation, hypertension, and a pallid complexion. Mental confusion, pericarditis, and neuropathy are late features.

Sometimes renal failure is discovered because significant albuminuria or hypertension is found at a routine medical examination. Renal impairment may progress to a relatively advanced stage without any symptoms but, as yet, most renal disease can be neither prevented nor treated. Its detection is aided by routine screening of urine samples from every patient admitted for surgery. Significant proteinuria (> 150 mg in 24 h) should make one think, not only of renal disease, but also of the consequences of the resultant hypoalbuminaemia. Proteinuria in patients with healthy kidneys may disappear on lying supine or may be associated with congestive cardiac failure, fever, or exercise. A specific gravity of 1.023 or more in a random urine sample implies normal renal concentrating power. A more accurate, but less readily available, measurement is urine osmolality. Maximal dilution and concentration produces urine osmolalities from 50 mosmol/L to 1400 mosmol/L.

Never test the concentrating power of the kidneys by fluid restriction if you suspect chronic renal failure. It may precipitate an irreversible deterioration in function.

### *Physiology and management*

Once chronic renal failure has been discovered, the first line of attack is to search for any treatable cause (e.g. post-renal obstruction), and to treat complicating factors that may accelerate the deterioration in renal function.

The advanced stage of all types of chronic renal failure is characterized by uraemia and the production of urine with a fixed specific gravity of 1.010. Under these conditions, because of the failure of the kidney to handle variations in water and salt intake, on the one hand, the patient faces possible dehydration, hypoperfusion, and volume contraction and, on the other, crystalloid overload may precipitate peripheral oedema, pulmonary oedema, and hypertension.

Reduction of dietary protein to 40 g/day is usually adequate to keep the urea below 25 mmol/L. A high calorie intake is nevertheless necessary to suppress breakdown of endogenous protein.

Fortunately, various compensatory mechanisms enable the patient in chronic renal failure to retain some regulating ability, the most important being an increase in the excretory power of the surviving nephrons (intact nephron hypothesis). A large intake of water (3 L/day) results in an increased urine flow and, hence, increases the daily losses of urea, potassium, and other toxins. Large doses of frusemide are sometimes prescribed to assist diuresis (rarely up to 1.5 g/day).

When the patient is producing large volumes of dilute urine, serum potassium is not a problem, but the inability to excrete hydrogen ions and other fixed acids leads to a metabolic acidosis. This is partly alleviated by oral bicarbonate. However, if arterial blood gases are measured, they always show a metabolic acidosis with ventilatory compensation. The level of $Pa\text{CO}_2$ is very important because it indicates the degree of hyperventilation. Mild-to-moderate hyperventilation is difficult to detect from clinical observation. Its presence is important because of the effects of anaesthetic agents and opioids on ventilatory drive. By increasing the $Pa\text{CO}_2$, they may produce dangerous swings in pH and serum potassium. Another effect of the acidosis is to shift the oxygen dissociation curve of haemoglobin to the right, thus increasing oxygen delivery to the tissues. This mechanism is further enhanced by the increase of 2,3-diphosphoglycerate in chronic anaemia (see Chapter 52).

Anaemia in chronic renal failure results from marrow suppression secondary to a failure of production of erythropoietin. Red cell survival is also reduced. In addition, there is a qualitative platelet defect and, frequently, occult blood loss from the gut that exacerbates the condition. Adequate oxygen flux is maintained by a compensatory tachycardia and increased cardiac output. This can produce premature symptoms of angina and LVF.

Hypertension is almost invariable but the exact role of renin and aldosterone is uncertain. It should be treated vigorously, and commonly needs several drugs for good control. A reduction in dietary sodium, which is sometimes useful in essential hypertension, is inappropriate because of the inevitable reduction in renal blood flow that follows. In very severe and terminal renal failure, salt and water retention worsen the hypertension, but it may respond to a reduction in the extracellular fluid volume. This can be accomplished either by high-dose diuretic therapy (if the kidney will respond) or by dialysis.

Thyroid function tests are often abnormal with low serum thyroxine ($T_4$) and triiodothyronine ($T_3$) levels. These figures reflect abnormal binding characteristics and the free $T_4$, $T_3$, and thyroid-stimulating hormone assays are normal.

Chronic renal failure affects calcium metabolism in two ways: phosphate is retained and patients can no longer hydroxylate 25-hydroxycholecaliferol to 1,25-dihyroxycholecalciferol (1,25-DHCC). Phosphate retention produces a reciprocal fall in serum calcium, which can nevertheless create conditions that precipitate ionic calcium because of chemical instability. There may thus be paradoxical ectopic calcium deposition in the presence of a low serum calcium.

Overall, the ionic hypocalcaemia produces a state of chronic, but appropriate, hypersecretion in the parathyroid glands. This secondary hyperparathyroidism results in a permanently high level of parathyroid hormone (PTH), which acts directly on bone osteoclasts, increasing their numbers and activity. This results in accelerated bone resorption, increased osteoblastic activity, high bone turnover and variable degrees of peritrabecular fibrosis. The clinical picture is one of bone pains, generalized decalcification, and pseudofractures, although bony swellings, subperiosteal erosions, and bone cysts are rare.

There is evidence that the early control of rising phosphate levels may delay the onset of renal osteodystrophy. Calcium supplements and restriction of dietary phosphorus helps. Aluminium hydroxide is used to bind phosphorus to the gut, but there is increasing concern that ingestion of aluminium hydroxide may lead to its accumulation in the brain, causing 'dialysis dementia'. 1,25-DHCC is now available commercially and can be successful in preventing demineralization.

Tetany from hypocalcaemia is most unusual, but the maintenance of the unbound calcium fraction depends heavily on hypoproteinaemia and metabolic acidosis, and corrective changes in these two variables can precipitate tetany.

People with diabetes who develop renal failure often have a change in their insulin requirements. On the one hand, insulin requirement can decrease because poor renal function reduces insulin degradation in the kidney; on the other, insulin requirement can increase because of the effect of acidosis and uraemia at the cellular level where insulin acts.

Renal and other intercurrent infections need prompt antibiotic therapy. This, in itself, may cause problems from drug nephrotoxicity and ideally, although this is not always possible, antibiotics should be administered only after the results of culture and sensitivity are available. In general, ampicillin is safe, gentamicin needs dose reduction and measurement of serum levels, the cephalosporins should be used only with great care as a reserve, and nitrofurantoin and the tetracyclines are contraindicated (see Table 59.2).

The renal physicians who take an overall view and decide on a long-term plan, follow up the patient for life. Dialysis or transplantation is usually considered when the renal function is approximately 10% of the norm.

***Prescribing drugs***

Patients with chronic renal failure often react unpredictably to a normal drug dosage, implying that the initial dose of any drug should err on the low side. There are many reasons for this erratic response.

Although gastrointestinal absorption of drugs itself is essentially normal, antacids hinder the absorption of antibiotics, warfarin, and fat-soluble vitamins. Poor renal function reduces the protein binding of drugs for reasons that are unclear. If the patient also has hypoalbuminaemia, the free drug fraction can be greatly in excess of normal. This is a problem with sulphonylureas, warfarin, frussemide, and sulphonamides. The distribution volume of many drugs is markedly altered. The most frequently quoted example is digoxin whose distribution volume is halved compared with normal.

As yet few hard data are available to demonstrate the effects of chronic renal failure on drug metabolism. It is, however, well established that the reduction of hydrocortisone and the hydrolysis of procaine and suxamethonium are slowed.

The total clearance of an active drug and its active metabolites is the sum of the renal and non-renal clearances. The renal clearance of any drug, irrespective of the exact mechanism, is broadly proportional to the creatinine clearance. Consequently, those drugs relying heavily on renal clearance have a greatly prolonged and exaggerated action (Figure 59.2). The two classic examples are a non-depolarizing neuromuscular blocker (especially gallamine) and digoxin. The β-adrenoceptor blockers, atenolol, pindolol, and sotalol, are all excreted unchanged through the kidney.

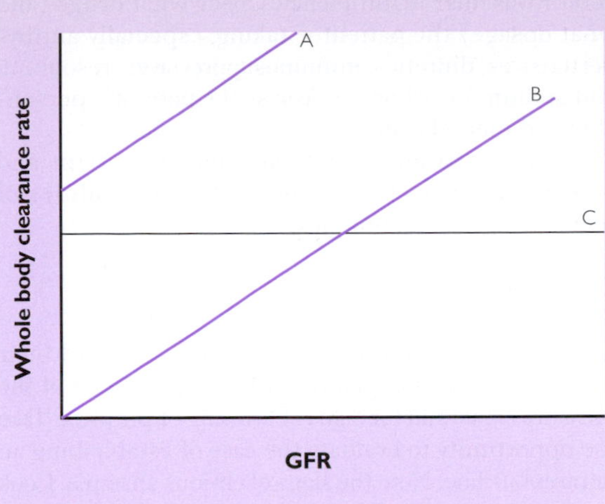


**Figure 59.2** Effect of changes of the glomerular filtration rate (GFR) on the elimination of different drugs. Drug A is cleared by both the kidney and the liver; Drug B is cleared by the kidney alone; Drug C is cleared by the liver alone – its clearance rate is unaffected by changes in the GFR. (From Cunningam J. Renal and urinary disease. In: Souhami RL, Moxham J, eds. *Textbook of Medicine*, 3rd edn. Edinburgh: Churchill Livingstone 1997, 894.)

In addition to these problems, patients with chronic renal failure appear to be more sensitive than normal individuals to a given serum level of a drug. This is particularly so with opioids, barbiturates, phenothiazines, and sedatives. It has been suggested that the chronically high serum urea in some way affects the uptake across the cell walls and the blood–brain barrier.

## Anaesthetic management of non-dialysed patients with chronic renal failure

The background presentation, physiology and management are as described above. Any anaesthetic given should jeopardize existing renal function as little as possible. This revolves around maintaining the normal flow of oxygenated blood to the kidney by *avoiding hypoxia, hypovolaemia, and hypotension*.

***Preoperative considerations***

*History*

Establish the original cause of the renal failure, the duration of treatment, and the limitations and quality of everyday life. Be clear what the outlook and long-term plans for therapy are, particularly with regard to possible future haemodialysis or transplantation. Discuss the patient's morale with the nursing staff; it is important to establish good rapport. Once these patients are accepted for haemodialysis, they tend to be regular customers. Note the usual fluid allowance and the daily urine output.

If the renal failure was caused by a generalized systemic disease, enquire about the associated anaesthetic problems of the background condition (e.g. connective tissue disorders, diabetes mellitus). Polycystic disease of the kidneys may be associated with pulmonary cysts and 14% of affected patients have intracerebral aneurysms.

Ask about exercise tolerance and the symptoms of anaemia, myocardial ischaemia, LVF, pericarditis, and cerebrovascular insufficiency. Check what drugs (and what dosage) the patient is taking, especially antihypertensives, diuretics, immunosuppressives, resonium, and sodium bicarbonate. Assess the patient's personality and mental state.

If the operation is suitable, and the patient and surgeon are cooperative, discuss the possibilities of regional or local techniques.

*Examination*

*General*

The patients tend to be underweight, so record their weight. Look at the quality of the skin, the state of the pressure areas, and for signs of bruising or purpura. Take the opportunity to evaluate the ease of establishing an intravenous line. Note the signs of obvious anaemia. Look for pyrexia because of the susceptibility to infection.

*Cardiovascular system*

Measure the BP with the patient supine and standing, looking for both absolute levels and any postural drop. A tachycardia is usual and is necessary to maintain the oxygen flux in anaemia. Auscultate for murmurs (a high cardiac output may cause flow murmurs in the aortic region and down the left sternal edge), added sounds (LVF), or rubs (pericarditis occurs late in uraemia). Quiet heart sounds in a person of normal build might suggest a pericardial effusion if there is severe uraemia. Listen for pulmonary crepitations and look for sacral and ankle oedema. Peripheral oedema can result from both right ventricular failure and a low serum albumin. The important differentiator is the jugular venous pressure.

*Respiratory system*

Mild hyperventilation can often best be noticed by the inability to coordinate speech and breathing perfectly, extra breaths being taken from time to time. Small pleural effusions present on a chest radiograph are rarely detectable clinically. Basal crepitations are always significant and indicate a degree of LVF. Examine any sputum for possible infection and send it for culture.

*Investigations*

*Full blood count*

If the anaemia is not normochromic and normocytic, with a haemoglobin of 7–8 g/dl, suspect an additional occult blood loss.

*Clotting studies*

These are normal unless the uraemia is severe.

*Urea and electrolytes*

These are mandatory within a few hours of surgery. Treat a high serum potassium as outlined in acute renal failure. Figure 59.3 shows that, at low levels of renal function, the serum creatinine concentration is a sensitive indicator of the glomerular filtration rate (GFR).

*ECG*

A sinus tachycardia is almost invariable. Check for arrhythmias and the signs of potassium toxicity (see Figure 47.9).

*Chest radiograph*

Look for the signs of pulmonary oedema, cardiomegaly, and pleural effusions. The last are most common in the nephrotic syndrome.

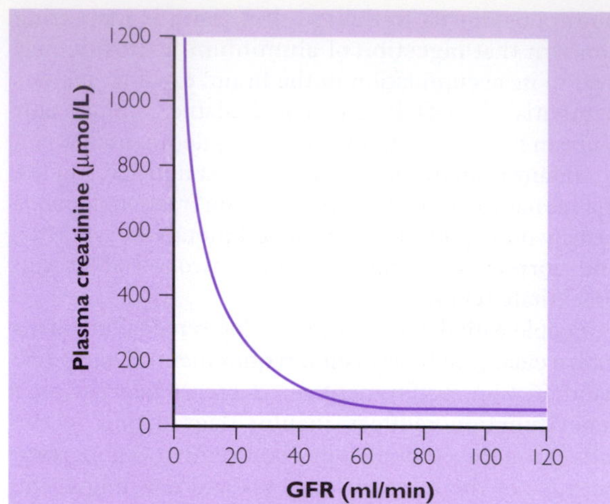


**Figure 59.3** Relationship between the glomerular filtration rate (GFR) and plasma creatinine concentration. The normal range of plasma creatinine is shaded. At high GFR, changes are associated with relatively small changes of plasma creatinine, which remains within the 'normal' range until the GFR falls to about 45 ml/min. At low levels of renal function, plasma creatinine becomes a more sensitive indicator of the GFR. (From Cunningham J. Renal and urinary disease. In: Souhami RL, Moxham J, eds. *Textbook of Medicine*, 3rd edn. Edinburgh: Churchill Livingstone, 1997, 849.)

*Preoperative preparation*

Optimize the person's BP, serum potassium, and metabolic state within the limits of the time available and in conjunction with his or her physician. Treat infections vigorously with antibiotics and physiotherapy.

Never transfuse blood preoperatively without first consulting a renal physician, even if blood loss is anticipated at operation. Most patients with chronic renal failure depend on a low haematocrit to provide a high renal plasma flow, and hence maximize the GFR. If the haematocrit is artificially raised to a normal level, renal function may suddenly deteriorate and never recover. There is also a risk of precipitating pulmonary oedema. If it is anticipated that blood *will* be required, check with the renal physician whether washed cells are advisable (to avoid sensitizing the patient because of future transplantation).

***Intraoperative phase***

The important considerations are almost identical to those of patients in acute renal failure and to those who are anaemic. Please refer to these sections. Only extra points specific to chronic renal failure are given here.

Continue antihypertensive therapy up to the time of surgery. Intraoperatively, these drugs react synergistically with volatile agents and there may be unexpected falls in blood pressure. This is most easily corrected by switching off the offending agent or avoided altogether by using a total intravenous technique.

For all but the shortest procedures, a urethral catheter should be passed to monitor intraoperative urine production. With good hydration, an adequate

CVP and BP, urine flow should be maintained at 1 ml/kg per h. If it is not, despite good hydration, etc., mannitol (25 g over 10–15 min) is the first line of treatment. A small dose of frusemide may then be tried.

Intraoperative fluid and blood replacement requires considerable skill in judgement. The object of blood replacement should be to maintain the final haemoglobin to within 1 g/dl of the initial level. Over-transfusion not only reduces the renal plasma flow (see above), but also creates a higher load of products that are toxic to the kidney.

If a patient has been maintained for a long period on conservative management, it is reasonable to assume that his or her $P\text{aCO}_2$, pH oxygen dissociation curve characteristics, and cardiac output have compensated to give maximum oxygen delivery to the tissues. To maintain this state, his or her intraoperative end-tidal $CO_2$ or $P\text{aCO}_2$ should be monitored, and the ventilation adjusted to achieve the preoperative level.

#### Postoperative phase

The postoperative course obviously depends on the nature and extent of surgery. After minor surgery, the patient should return as soon as possible to his or her preoperative regimen. After major surgery, it may be necessary to dialyse or haemofiltrate the patient temporarily (for the first week or so). Depending on the site and extent of the operation, peritoneal dialysis or haemodialysis can be used. The best modern technique is probably haemodialysis via a two-way subclavian cannula inserted at the time of the operation.

### Patients on long-term dialysis

The patient is assumed to have *no* effective renal function and that recovery is impossible. It is therefore *unnecessary* to take extreme and complex measures to maintain intraoperative renal blood flow to prevent further damage.

#### Haemodialysis

Chronic renal failure patients being followed up by a renal physician, are, if considered suitable, prepared for haemodialysis when their creatinine clearance is approximately 10 ml/min. Under local anaesthesia, an AV fistula is created, usually at the wrist of the non-dominant hand. This takes 4–8 weeks to develop fully and to dilate the veins of the forearm sufficiently to allow easy access.

Most patients are started on dialysis when uraemic symptoms develop that are not corrected by a protein-restricted diet. The most common regimen is to dialyse for 5 h three times per week. After starting dialysis, urine flow falls off and patients are limited to a fluid intake of 600 ml/day plus the urine loss. Not adhering to this results in hypertension and pulmonary oedema. Dialysis does nothing to correct the anaemia and many patients require transfusions to keep the haemoglobin above 6 g/dl. The anaemia can intensify when on dialysis: first, because the necessary heparinization aggravates any occult blood loss (e.g. from a duodenal ulcer) and, second, because red cells are sequestered in the extracorporeal system.

Renal osteodystrophy is a frequent finding and patients may be treated with 1,25-DHCC or present for a parathyroidectomy.

Tiredness, breathlessness, malaise, emotional instability, depression, angina, and claudication occur all too frequently. It is tempting to think that haemodialysis restores the internal environment to normal; it is vital to remember that this is not so. These patients are severely abnormal and, for instance, commence dialysis with a serum creatinine of anything from 700 to 2000 mmol/L.

The two major problems of fistulae are aneurysmal dilatation and LVF. The latter can occur when the fistula flow is above about 1 L/min. The most common causes of death in people on haemodialysis are premature myocardial infarction, LVF, and strokes. After these is infection which is often from opportunist organisms.

*Anaesthetic considerations*

Essentially the preparation and management are as for chronic renal failure. There are a few additional details.

Before the operation, discuss intraoperative fluids with the renal physician. Over-transfusion of red cells is less important than in people who are not on dialysis because the GFR no longer needs to be maximized. However, which pack of cells is transfused is important because of future transplantation. Rapid transfusion in haemodialysis patients carries a high risk of producing hyperkalaemia, because the red cells do not act as ‘potassium sponges’ as they do in normal patients.

It is important to coordinate the times of dialysis and surgery. Ideally, dialysis should finish 3–6 hours preoperatively and, after coming off the machine, full blood count, urea and electrolytes and a clotting screen *must* be done. The patient should also be weighed. Many units give a calcium resonium enema routinely. Shortly after dialysis, the patient is relatively hypovolaemic and his or her BP is very sensitive to most intravenous and volatile anaesthetic agents. Hypotension should be corrected promptly by physiological saline. Dextrose solutions produce a dilutional hyponatraemia and are to be avoided.

If the patient receives excess fluid intraoperatively, postoperative pulmonary oedema is a very real risk and requires further dialysis.

The site of the AV fistula should be noted and that limb must be carefully protected. It should never have a BP cuff applied to it, every effort must be made to establish the intravenous drip site in another arm or leg, and intraoperatively it should be wrapped in warm Gamgee. Some units use a stellate ganglion block or brachial block to dilate the blood vessels of the relevant arm. There is a theoretical objection, in that the major effect of the dilatation is on the small vessels and this may produce a ‘steal’ from the fistula. Probably, the major factor in ensuring fistula patency is the maintenance of cardiac output and BP. Some centres measure fistula flow intraoperatively with an ultrasonic flowmeter.

Patients with fistulae can be very difficult to handle psychologically. They know their outlook and many are young with family responsibilities. Often a brash exterior hides chronic anxiety. A sedative oral premedication is probably the best choice and, as they usually present for surgery on several occasions for a variety of procedures, there is frequently a previous anaesthetic record to guide prescription.

There is no contraindication to local or regional techniques provided that the clotting screen is normal and a high level of sterility is observed. Care must be taken not to allow the BP to fall, and vasoconstrictors should be used at an earlier stage than in normal people to avoid an excessive fluid load. A block may wear off more quickly than expected, especially if it is in the arm with a fistula where there is a tremendous 'wash-out' potential.

#### *Peritoneal dialysis*

Until recently, peritoneal dialysis was used only as a semi-emergency technique to cover a period of acute renal failure. Now, many centres in the UK have up to 30% of patients on chronic ambulatory peritoneal dialysis. The most common complication is infection (usually in the peritoneum), which can be detected by eye because the dialysate on the return to the bag is opalescent. Failure to empty the peritoneum properly can result in congestive cardiac failure, basal atelectasis, and chest infection from a splinted diaphragm.

The advantage of the technique to the patient is that it is good at removing excess fluid and allows much greater dietary freedom than does haemodialysis.

##### *Anaesthetic considerations*

Patients present for a variety of operations (genitourinary surgery, surgery for congenital urinary tract abnormalities or blocked cannulae, renal transplantation). Their management is essentially the same as for patients with chronic renal failure. It is best to spigot the peritoneal cannula during surgery because the dialysis bags are a nuisance. Always check that the patient can breathe adequately when lying flat, and that he or she is not in cardiac failure and does not have an underlying chest infection.

## FURTHER READING


Bennett WM, Aronoff GR, Gloper TA *et al. Drug Prescribing in Renal Failure*, 2nd edn. Philadelphia, PA: American College of Physicians, 1991.

Bevan DR. Renal function and the safety of anaesthesia. In: Taylor TH, Major E, eds. *Hazards and Complications of Anaesthesia*, 2nd edn. Edinburgh: Churchill Livingstone, 1993: 103–11.

Cottam S, Eason J. Anaesthesia for renal transplantation. In: Kaufman L, ed. *Anaesthesia Review 8*. Edinburgh: Churchill Livingstone, 1991: 159–78.

Hunter JM. Recent advances in the management of renal disease: their relevance to the anaesthetist. *Curr Opin Anaesthesiol* 1990;**3**:452–6.

Lote CJ. Renal physiology and acute renal failure. *Curr Anaesth Crit Care* 1992;**3**:124–32.

Novis BK, Roizen F, Aronson S, Thisted RA. Association of preoperative risk factors with postoperative renal failure. *Anesth Analg* 1994;**78**:143.

Souhami RL, Moxham J, eds. *Textbook of Medicine*, 3rd edn. Edinburgh: Churchill Livingstone, 1997.

Sweny P. Haemofiltration and haemodiafiltration – theoretical and practical aspects. *Curr Anaesth Crit Care* 1991;**2**:37–43.

# Chapter 60 The patient with an infection

M.J. Wilson

The horror of the 'Black Death' caused it to be considered an agent of God's punishment. In *Corialanus*, Volumina refers to it as 'th' hoarded plague o' th' gods'.

The fact that *Yersinia pestis* may now be treated successfully with antibiotics has done little to dispel our lingering dread of communicable disease; indeed there are those who point to a similar divine retributive hand in the origin of acquired immune deficiency syndrome (AIDS), a currently incurable modern plague!

Anaesthetists are rarely involved in the primary diagnosis and management of infectious disease; however, there are areas of this medical field that are directly relevant to anaesthetic practice:

- The decision to proceed with or delay an anaesthetic as a result of an incidental infection is one that a trainee is likely to be called upon to make at an early stage in his or her career, yet it is rarely taught or considered systematically.
- Anaesthetic procedures in the presence of systemic infection are associated with specific hazards, which require aggressive techniques of monitoring and management.
- New chemotherapeutic regimens and treatment modalities have resulted in a significant increase in longevity and reduced morbidity in sufferers of chronic systemic communicable infections such as the human immunodeficiency virus (HIV) or the hepatitis viruses. Surgical procedures in this population related or incidental to their primary pathology will become more commonplace.

## THE PATIENT WITH AN INCIDENTAL RESPIRATORY INFECTION

> 'I've had a bit of a cough recently doctor, will it matter for the surgery?'

An infective disorder discovered by the anaesthetist during routine preoperative assessment is a complex situation to manage well. Cancellation of a surgical procedure is an inconvenience to all and the decision to do so should be treated with gravity.

Upper respiratory tract infections (URTIs) represent the most common anaesthetic dilemma. Evidence-based conclusions are scant in this area. Central to the assessment of a patient with an URTI is the question of whether they are at optimum fitness to undergo anaesthesia and whether the intercurrent infection will increase operative morbidity.

The presence of a cough productive of purulent sputum which is associated with systemic manifestations of infection such as a pyrexia or rigors, suggestive of a bacterial chest infection, represents an unequivocal situation. Unless the procedure is urgent or life saving, the risk of sputum retention, desaturation, and collapse/consolidation of lung parenchyma outweighs the potential benefit of operating early. However, the patient must be assessed in the context of his or her pattern of health – it makes little sense to cancel an urgent procedure for a productive cough in a patient with chronic bronchitis!

The pattern of morbidity associated with anaesthesia in the presence of a viral URTI is strongly age related. This results from the relatively larger effect of mucosal inflammation on airway calibre and reactivity in children.

As resistance to airflow is inversely proportional to the fourth power of the airway radius in laminar gas flow (Hagen–Poiseuille equation), any reduction in airway size results in an exponential increase in resistance to airflow and work of breathing. In conditions of turbulent flow, e.g. crying, the effect of reduced airway calibre is further exaggerated.

The clinical manifestation of these physical laws is an increase in morbidity associated with general anaesthesia in small children, including laryngospasm, bronchospasm, and associated hypoxaemia.

The population at greatest risk is children aged 1 year or younger, and there is good evidence to suggest that elective surgery should be postponed for a minimum period of 6 weeks for children of this age who have a URTI.

For older children up to the age of 6 years, there is an excess of morbidity associated with general anaesthesia; however, it is not as significant. This group is problematic because, as any parent knows, in children of this age there is a high 'turnover' of respiratory infection and one may wait indefinitely for a symptom-free 6 weeks! Unless symptoms are particularly severe or there is an associated history of asthma, postponement of anaesthesia is unlikely to offer significant benefit.

There is little evidence to suggest that delaying anaesthesia in fit adults with a viral URTI has any impact on anaesthetic morbidity. These cases should be judged in the light of their medical history and individual symptomatology.

Once the decision to proceed in the presence of infection has been taken, there are measures that can reduce the chance of respiratory complications. The simplest is to avoid general anaesthesia entirely and to choose a regional or local anaesthetic technique. If general anaesthesia is required, a spontaneously breathing technique employing the laryngeal mask airway to avoid endotracheal intubation may reduce the risk of airway hyper-reactivity. Ultimately, there is no substitute for a smooth anaesthetic and a heightened sense of awareness for potential problems.

## THE PATIENT WITH SYSTEMIC SEPSIS

'Sepsis' implies blood-borne infection or its systemic manifestations. The nomenclature of sepsis has undergone significant change in response to the recognition that a common pathophysiological syndrome results from a spectrum of aetiologies. Systemic inflammatory response syndrome (SIRS) is a multisystem disorder, which can result from an infective process or other causes such as trauma, burns, pancreatitis, or indeed any major physiological insult.

The central 'lesion' of SIRS is an abnormal activation of the acute phase response, producing a characteristic haemodynamic picture. Peripheral vasodilatation with subnormal systemic vascular resistance (SVR) is associated with hypotension and a hyperdynamic circulation. A reduction in mean arterial blood pressure, coupled with peripheral shunting of oxygenated blood, results in inadequate tissue oxygenation and dysfunction of vital body systems.

The activation of the acute phase cascade at a tissue level also results in a capillary endothelial leak. Extravasation of fluid into the extravascular space produces relative intravascular hypovolaemia.

The search for the mediator responsible for SIRS continues apace. Many potential culprits have been implicated, including endotoxin, interleukins IL1 and IL6, tumour necrosis factor, and the ubiquitous nitric oxide. It is more likely that SIRS is not the manifestation of the release of a single substance, but a complex interaction or imbalance of many mediators at cellular level.

### Preoperative assessment

The first task of the anaesthetist is to recognize the patient at risk of, or suffering from, SIRS so that appropriate steps can be taken to manage the situation. The signs of a systemic inflammatory response include pyrexia, a hyperdynamic cardiovascular system with tachycardia, bounding pulses, and warm peripheries associated with hypotension, hypovolaemia, and oliguria. Tissue oxygenation is compromised, despite an increase in oxygen demand, resulting in organ dysfunction and a metabolic acidaemia.

It is important to note that, if this situation persists, it may progress to cardiovascular decompensation and collapse.

### Preoperative preparation

The principle of preoperative resuscitation is paramount in these patients. This is often best undertaken in an intensive care unit (ICU) environment because the resuscitative process is optimally guided by invasive monitoring techniques.

#### *Fluid resuscitation*

Intravascular hypovolaemia is almost uniform and fluid replacement should be aggressive in early management to re-establish circulating volume. Loss of fluid into the extravascular space as a result of capillary endothelial leak makes the assessment of fluid depletion and requirements notoriously difficult. It is common practice to use central venous pressure or pulmonary capillary wedge pressure monitoring to guide optimal filling.

The colloid versus crystalloid debate over which fluid is ideal for initial fluid resuscitation continues without resolution. Colloid solutions would seem to offer significant advantages in the face of potential continuing capillary leak. However, it can be argued that colloids are more likely to become fixed in extravascular sites and cause further tissue damage in the post-resuscitative phase. In practice, gelatin- or starch-based colloid solutions represent a good first-line approach.

Basic clinical signs, such as an improvement in blood pressure or urine output, also provide a valuable guide to fluid therapy.

#### *Oxygenation*

The combination of impaired tissue oxygen delivery and increased requirement associated with SIRS means that supplemental oxygen therapy should be uniform. It is sometimes necessary to use mechanical ventilation preoperatively in pursuit of optimal oxygenation if the patient is unable to sustain an adequate respiratory pattern.

#### *Correction of hypotension*

Systemic hypotension often persists even in the face of adequate intravascular filling as a result of the peripheral vasoplegia, which is a cardinal feature of SIRS. In these circumstances, invasive monitoring of arterial pressure should be used because it is often necessary to intervene with inotropic support. Norepinephrine (noradrenaline) administered by infusion is the agent most commonly used to increase peripheral vascular resistance by $\alpha$-adrenoceptor-mediated vasoconstriction.

Vasoconstrictor therapy is best directed by monitoring derived haemodynamic variables such as cardiac output/index and SVR, using a pulmonary artery occlusion catheter. The goal is to achieve an adequate perfusion pressure to ensure vital organ function and reversal of metabolic acidaemia.

#### *Treatment of underlying cause*

Once haemodynamic stability has been achieved, attention can be directed to the specific aetiology of the SIRS and its appropriate treatment, which may include antimicrobial therapy or surgical intervention.

### Intraoperative considerations

Much of the preceding discussion is relevant to the intraoperative management of these patients. Surgical intervention can often refuel the inflammatory process anew and further destabilize the situation. Senior experienced anaesthetic personnel should be present and the operation should be performed by a senior surgeon.

The technique of choice in these circumstances is a balanced anaesthetic using an inhalational agent, intermittent positive pressure ventilation with short-acting neuromuscular blockade, and systemic opioid analgesia. This provides the best environment for maintaining cardiovascular stability. Regional anaesthesia/analgesia by epidural or spinal blockade is contraindicated because blood-borne bacteria may provide a focus for epidural abscess formation. Further vasodilatation of a septic patient is also undesirable.

Invasive monitoring should be employed to facilitate the rapid identification and correction of suboptimal vital indices, and to prevent any exacerbation of organ dysfunction.

Management of the patient postoperatively should be continued in an ICU environment and consideration given to electively continuing ventilation into the postoperative phase to optimize oxygenation and allow for a staged, controlled withdrawal of respiratory support.

The challenge of safe anaesthetic management of these patients requires the integration of acute physiology with the principles of intensive care.

## THE PATIENT WITH AN ABSCESS

Incision and drainage of peripheral abscesses comprises a significant proportion of the emergency work undertaken by junior anaesthetists. It is easy to trivialize such cases. There are, however, specific concerns relevant to their management.

There is often little consideration given to factors that may predispose to peripheral infection. Recurrent abscess formation or the involvement of multiple sites should alert the anaesthetist to seek specific causes. Diabetes may present with recurrent infection. Enquiry about associated symptomatology such as polydipsia and polyuria is simple to include in a preoperative assessment, while urinalysis and blood sugar estimation are easy tests to perform at the bedside. Evidence of any associated systemic sepsis should be sought such as pyrexia, rigors, or tachycardia. The gravity of staphlycoccal septicaemia is not to be underestimated!

The site of the abscess may not immediately appear relevant; however, there are often implications for positioning the patient intraoperatively. It is not uncommon for drainage of perineal lesions to be performed in lateral or prone positions.

These lesions are often very painful. This is relevant intraoperatively in that incision of an abscess is often profoundly stimulating. Inadequate depth of anaesthesia at this point can precipitate coughing or laryngospasm. Analgesia for these procedures is often poorly prescribed. Systemic opioids are probably required in the immediate postoperative phase and their efficacy may be enhanced by combination with non-steroidal anti-inflammatory drugs. Regional anaesthesia/analgesia is worth considering in the absence of systemic sepsis and is probably under-utilized.

## THE PATIENT WITH A COMMUNICABLE INFECTION

Although many potentially transmissible infections are encountered in routine medical practice, there are only a handful that represent a significant risk to anaesthetic/operating room staff or other patients. HIV, hepatitis B and C, and pulmonary tuberculosis will be considered in this chapter.

### HIV and hepatitis

These viral infections can be usefully considered together because they are both transmissible by contact with infected body fluids, and the anaesthetic management of infected patients shares many of the same principles.

AIDS was first recognized as a clinical entity in the early 1980s; since then there has been an exponential increase in the number of seropositive individuals. Two major patterns of transmission of the retrovirus responsible have emerged. In developing countries, the predominant mechanisms of spread are heterosexual intercourse and vertical transmission from infected mothers to infants. In developed countries, the major routes of transmission are homosexual intercourse between men and the sharing of contaminated equipment for intravenous drug abuse. HIV infection preferentially affects T-helper cells, eventually resulting in both the loss and impaired function of CD4 lymphocytes. The inevitable consequences for host immunity result in opportunistic infection, e.g. pneumocystis pneumonia, malignancies such as Kaposi's sarcoma, and neurological manifestations.

Hepatitis B is a small, enveloped DNA virus, which is responsible for much morbidity and mortality worldwide. Transmission occurs vertically, by sexual contact, or by inoculation with infected material. The pathological significance of the virus results from the high incidence of chronic carriage resulting from infection, leading to cirrhosis and hepatic malignancy. The existence of hepatitis C was long predicted on epidemiological grounds as a cause of post-transfusion hepatitis. The disease is transmitted by exposure to infected blood and blood products and, although most cases recover, 20–40% suffer persisting hepatitis with the risk of late cirrhosis or hepatocellular carcinoma.

#### *Patient assessment*

Patients may present for surgery related to their primary infective pathology, e.g. tumour excision or drainage of an infected focus, or operations incidental to their condition.

Preoperative assessment should include a review of systems potentially compromised by the disease process. This implies clinical and laboratory assessment of hepatic function in patients with hepatitis and a review of respiratory, gastrointestinal and neurological systems in HIV.

Establishing a rapport with these patients and careful explanation of procedures are important in the context of the psychological impact of these diseases and being treated as an infective risk

#### *Conduct of anaesthesia*

The tripod of immunization, communication, and universal precaution provides a useful *aide-memoire* when planning the anaesthetic management of an infected case.

##### *Immunization*

Both active and passive immunization against hepatitis B is possible. Hepatitis B vaccines contain hepatitis B surface antigen derived from human plasma or recombinant DNA technology. A course of three injections provides active protection which lasts 3–5 years.

A recipient's antibody response can be easily monitored and immunization provides the basis for protection of operating room staff exposed to infected patients. There is currently no equivalent vaccine for the HIV.

*Communication*

The effective management of an infected patient depends on the dissemination of accurate, relevant information to the operating room team. Informing the operating room nurse in charge early allows all professionals involved to plan well in advance.

It is often sensible to schedule such a patient last on a routine operating list, to allow adequate time for cleaning the operating room and equipment without disrupting the progress of other procedures.

*Universal precautions*

These procedures are designed to protect operating room staff from body-fluid-borne infection and should be employed in cases of hepatitis and HIV. The recommendations include the use of gloves if there is any risk of contact with infected fluids. Protective goggles or visors and gowns should be worn to protect against exposure to splashed fluids. Facemasks are employed to reduce the risk from aerosolized infected matter. If contact with body fluids occurs, the affected part should be washed immediately. Open or exudative wounds should be covered or, better still, the individual with such wounds should not take part in the procedure. Needles should not be resheathed or passed between individuals and must be disposed of immediately after use.

Specific anaesthetic precautions include the use of disposable airway equipment or its sterilization between cases. Breathing systems outside the patient do not constitute a risk unless they become contaminated with blood. Bacterial filters should still be routinely employed.

#### *Invasive monitoring*

The use of invasive monitoring in infected individuals represents a dilemma worth considering. Percutaneous cannulation of peripheral arteries or central veins not only increases the risk of needle-stick injury to the clinician, but, in the case of HIV infection, exposes an immunocompromised patient to the risk of line-related sepsis.

These risks must be balanced against the potential benefit of the procedure proposed.

#### *Exposure to infection*

If exposure does occur, despite precautions, it is the responsibility of the anaesthetist to coordinate the appropriate response. The site of an inoculation injury should be encouraged to bleed. Splashes into the eye or face should be washed with copious volumes of clean water.

Further therapy should be led by an identified expert, e.g. a microbiologist or occupational health physician. This ordinarily involves investigation of the HIV/hepatitis status of the patient concerned and estimation of the potential risk of the exposure. It is important that these measures are carried out quickly because protective measures such as the administration of hepatitis B-specific immunoglobulin, zidovudine (AZT), or other specific therapy may be required.

Such an incident also requires meticulous record keeping.

Further guidelines to the treatment of these patients can be found in *HIV and other blood borne viruses – guidance for anaesthetists* published by the Association of Anaesthetists.

### Pulmonary tuberculosis

Tuberculosis is a granulomatous disease caused by infection with some species of *Mycobacterium*. It can be a multisystemic disorder; however, the most common sites of infection are the lungs and lymph nodes. The pulmonary form of the disease is highly infectious and tuberculosis can cause severe morbidity and high mortality in all age groups.

It is uncommon for patients with active, untreated tuberculosis to undergo anaesthesia; however, it is not unusual to undertake surgical procedures in individuals receiving antimicrobial chemotherapy and who are still considered an infective risk or for patients to require diagnostic surgery when mycobacterial infection is suspected.

#### *Patient assessment*

A systematic review of these patients is required before anaesthesia. It is easy to focus on pulmonary pathology; however, other important sites that may be affected include the bowel, peritoneum, meninges, kidneys, bones, and joints.

Primary pulmonary tuberculosis characteristically manifests as a persistent, dry cough in addition to generalized symptoms of pyrexia, night sweats, anorexia, and weight loss. Pulmonary tuberculosis may be endobronchial, with granulomas causing partial airway obstruction. There is often a fixed wheeze on auscultation over the affected airway and signs of bronchial occlusion should be sought on a chest radiograph.

Some thought should be given to the possibility that tuberculosis may represent an opportunistic infection in an immunocompromised patient, e.g. in undiagnosed AIDS.

#### *Conduct of anaesthesia*

Again, the basis of the protection of operating room staff and other patients is the immunization programme, which is undertaken nationally in the UK in secondary-school-age children. However, specific measures in the operating room can reduce the likelihood of transmission from one patient to another by inhalation of infected material.

In the case of diagnostic lymph node biopsy, it may be possible to avoid general anaesthesia by employing a local or regional technique. If general anaesthesia is required, there is a risk of contamination of the anaesthesia machine and breathing system with infected material and transmission to subsequent patients.

To reduce this risk, disposable breathing systems should be employed in conjunction with a bacterial filter between anaesthetic machine and circuit. Circle systems with low gas flows should not be employed, and expired gases should be scavenged effectively. Breathing systems should be discarded after use and disposed of as biohazardous material.

A final point relevant to the management of all infected cases is that a detailed, accurate description of the precautions employed should form an integral part of the anaesthetic record to provide medicolegal protection to both anaesthetist and patient.

## FURTHER READING


Association of Anaesthetists of Great Britain and Ireland. *HIV and Other Blood Borne Viruses – Guidance for Anaesthetists*. London: AAGBI, 1992.

Batai I, Kerenyi M, Tekeres M. The impact of drugs used in anaesthesia on bacteria. *Eur J Anaesthesiol* 1999;**16**:425–40.

Baxter F. Septic shock. *Can J Anaesth* 1997;**44**:59–72

Bowring D. History of infection control in anaesthesia. *Anaesth Intensive Care* 1996;**24**:150–3.

Breslin ABX. Tuberculosis – the threat re-emerges. *Anaesth Intensive Care* 1996;**24**:176–9.

Dwyer DE. Anaesthesia and emerging infectious diseases. *Anaesth Intensive Care* 1996;**24**:184–90.

Hogarth I. Anaesthesia machine and breathing system contamination and the efficacy of bacterial/viral filters. *Anaesth Intensive Care* 1996;**24**:154–63.

Jones ME. Screening for HIV: ratios, risks and rationality. *Anaesth Intensive Care* 1996;**24**:191–6.

Komesaroff D. Disposable and autoclavable anaesthetic circuits: the future is now. *Anaesth Intensive Care* 1996;**24**:173–5.

Knoblanche GK. Revision of the anaesthetic aspects of an infection control policy following reporting of hepatitis C nosocomial infection. *Anaesth Intensive Care* 1996;**24**:169–72.

Liddle C. Hepatitis C. *Anaesth Intensive Care* 1996;**24**:180–3.

Tomkins DP, Van der Walt JH. Needleless and sharp free anaesthesia. *Anaesth Intensive Care* 1996;**24**:164–8.

# Chapter 61 The patient with an acute abdomen

M.J. Wilson

The 47th aphorism of Hippocrates, section 6, states that 'persons who are benefited by venesection or purging should be bled or purged in spring'. His conviction that certain seasons provided the optimum conditions for therapeutic success resounds with contemporary poignancy for those practising the art of anaesthesia for the acute abdomen –'timing is everything!'

'The acute abdomen' is a blanket term applied to a heterogeneous group of patients and pathologies that reside on a spectrum of anaesthetic risk. At one end sits the 'previously fit-and-well' young adult suffering from appendicitis, at the other the multi-system devastation in an elderly patient precipitated by faecal peritonitis.

The practice of relegating emergency abdominal surgery to junior surgeons and the next available slot in the operating room has largely been consigned to history. There is now a recognition that these procedures should be performed by experienced surgeons only after adequate resuscitation of the patient.

The purpose of this chapter is not to provide an exhaustive list of all potential abdominal surgical emergencies, but to equip the 'front-line' anaesthetist with a system for assessing and managing these patients.

## BLACK BOXES AND THIRD SPACES

The abdomen has remained stubbornly resistant to the advance of diagnostic technologies and, even in the age of ultrasonography and computed tomography, is still something of a 'black box', requiring a greater measure of clinical judgement than other surgical fields of endeavour. As such it retains some of the mystique that was uniform to medicine in less enlightened times. The very language used to describe the processes of the acute abdomen is haunted by this lingering cadence. We still refer to extravascular fluid sequestration at the site of pathology or surgical trauma as loss into the 'third space', endowing it with the cosmic significance of a dimension-warping 'black hole'.

## PREOPERATIVE ASSESSMENT

### Patient history

In addition to the routine questions of any preoperative interview (see Chapter 41), there are specific areas of enquiry that are pertinent to emergency anaesthesia for an abdominal procedure. The mandatory use of rapid sequence induction means that meticulous assessment of the airway for the history or signs of a difficult intubation is essential.

The duration and severity of presenting symptoms such as pain, vomiting, diarrhoea, or other evidence of hollow viscus obstruction, can be extremely helpful in anticipating the fluid deficit and degree of physiological disturbance that is present.

The presence of thirst is important. The site and character of pain may help in diagnosis. Enquiry should be made for any history of blood loss from the gastrointestinal tract. A history of fever or rigors suggests infective pathology such as cholecystitis or intra-abdominal abscess.

A detailed drug history is also of particular relevance. The time of ingestion in relation to onset of abdominal symptoms is important because routine medications may not have been absorbed. Special consideration should be given to those patients taking cardiovascular drugs with a short half-life requiring multiple daily doses, e.g. antihypertensive/antiarrhythmic agents.

People with diabetes present special problems. Acute illness disrupts diabetic control with a hyperglycaemic stress response. Patients may omit oral hypoglycaemic agents if they are unable to eat food, further exacerbating the situation. Conversely, insulin or long-acting oral hypoglycaemics (particularly chlorpropamide) may be given to a starved patient with consequent hypoglycaemia. Evidence of ketosis and hypoglycaemia should be specifically sought.

Other important causes of acute abdominal pain should also be considered. In women the date of the last menstrual period should be established and ectopic pregnancy actively excluded. An elderly patient admitted with acute back and abdominal pain may be suffering from a dissecting abdominal aortic aneurysm.

Rapid diagnosis and expeditious therapy in these, potentially life-threatening, intra-abdominal emergencies depends on a high index of suspicion.

Thought should be given to non-surgical cases of abdominal pain such as myocardial infarction, endometriosis, diabetic ketoacidosis, or porphyria. Anaesthesia in these circumstances could be unnecessary or disastrous.

### Examination

Patients with acute abdominal pathology are subject to profound changes in their internal milieu from concealed dehydration and the metabolic consequences of their illness.

Fluid depletion occurs as a result of:

- overt losses such as vomiting and diarrhoea;

- covert losses through fluid sequestration in the gut lumen or wall;
- insensible losses from the body surface and lungs; these are exacerbated by pyrexia and hyperventilation.

Clinical assessment of fluid status is fundamental to resuscitation in anticipation of surgery. The same principles of clinical examination and interpretation of vital signs apply to homoeostatic disturbance from any source. The conventional classification of dehydration according to water loss relative to body weight is shown in Table 61.1.

Unfortunately, changes in total body weight are not a reliable indication of the amount of fluid lost from the circulation as a result of sequestration in tissues. Furthermore, there is rarely an accurate record of the patient's normal weight and patients may be too sick to be weighed at presentation.

The clinical signs are therefore important in estimation of fluid depletion. Skin turgor and capillary refill should be assessed and the mucous membranes examined. Heart rate and blood pressure should be measured and recorded at regular (e.g. half-hourly) intervals. It may not always be practical to look for orthostatic hypotension. Urine output needs to be measured accurately.

The metabolic consequences of an acute abdomen are myriad and range from metabolic acidosis to metabolic alkalosis with associated electrolyte disturbances. A moderate metabolic acidaemia is very common in dehydrated patients. This results from a combination of tissue under-perfusion and hypercatabolism. The patient may be avidly fluid retaining, haemoconcentrated, and hypernatraemic.

This contrasts with the patient who has a history of intractable vomiting, e.g. in gastric outflow obstruction (pyloric stenosis), who presents with a hypokalaemic, hypochloraemic, metabolic alkalosis with paradoxically acid urine (if fluid depletion is sufficiently advanced).

### Investigations

#### *Full blood count*

This is essential and helps to assess haemoconcentration, the potential for systemic sepsis, anaemia, and transfusion requirement.

#### *Urea and electrolytes, and creatinine*

These help to elucidate the extent of metabolic disturbance, estimate the magnitude of any renal dysfunction, and guide fluid resuscitation.

#### *Blood group and save*

This is mandatory for abdominal surgery. In cases with the potential for blood loss, a minimum cross-match of four units of packed cells is recommended.

#### *Chest radiograph*

This may demonstrate or exclude perforation and pneumoperitoneum (Figure 61.1).

#### *Plain abdominal films*

Erect and supine films determine whether there is an abdominal obstruction and the presence of calculi. Peritoneal fluid and gas under the diaphragm may also be evident.

#### *ECG*

This is mandatory for all patients with cardiac histories or acute electrolyte disturbances, and in elderly patients (see Chapter 43). The diagnosis of acute myocardial infarction may need to be excluded as a cause of abdominal pain.

#### *Arterial blood gas analysis*

This provides an objective insight into metabolic status and oxygenation and yet is a sadly under-utilized investigation. It can be repeated during the course of resuscitation to follow the effectiveness (or otherwise) of therapy.

#### *Liver function tests and serum amylase*

Although of limited help, these may indicate hepatobiliary dysfunction and exclude acute pancreatitis.

#### *Abdominal and pelvic ultrasonography*

This may assist in the diagnosis by detection of tumours, localized abscesses, and free peritoneal fluid or ascites. Ruptured aortic aneurysm or ectopic pregnancy may also be evident.

#### *Urinalysis and urine microscopy and culture*

These are important to exclude urinary tract infection.

**Table 61.1 Classification of dehydration**

| Severity | Weight loss (% body weight) | Fluid volume lost (in 70-kg man) (litres) | Clinical signs |
|---|---|---|---|
| Mild | 4 | 3 | Severe thirst<br>Dry mucous membranes<br>Capillary refill > 2 s<br>Reduced skin turgor |
| Moderate | 5–8 | 4–6 | As above plus:<br>Tachycardia<br>Oliguria (< 0.5 ml/kg per h)<br>Orthostatic hypotension |
| Severe | 8–10 | ≥ 7 | As above plus:<br>Hypotension<br>Cardiovascular collapse |

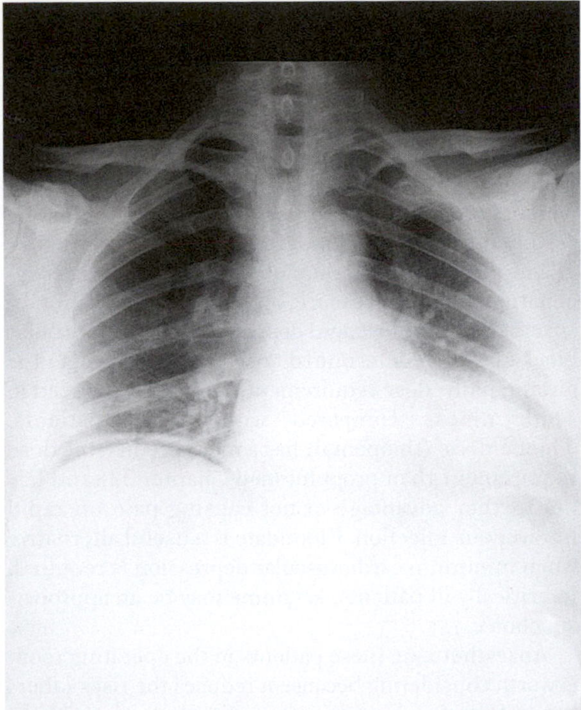

**Figure 61.1** An erect chest radiograph of a man with a left lower lobe pneumonia whose condition deteriorated. He had developed a stress ulcer which perforated. Note the air under the right hemidiaphragm

## PREOPERATIVE PREPARATION

The focus of anaesthetic management is often misplaced exclusively to the intraoperative period. Effective preoperative resuscitation can often be achieved with simple bedside measures. At a minimum it should address the following issues.

### Oxygenation

Abdominal distension and peritoneal pain with associated splinting of the abdominal musculature result in a reduced functional residual capacity and tidal volumes. Decompression with a large-bore (14 or 16 French gauge) nasogastric tube is a simple therapeutic measure which may dramatically improve oxygenation. It has the further advantage of emptying the patient's stomach, ensuring safer conditions at intubation.

Supplemental oxygen therapy delivered through a high-airflow oxygen entrainment (HAFOE) device, combined with attention to patient position, ideally sitting up, should be uniformly applied to these patients to optimize oxygen delivery to all tissues.

### Fluid resuscitation

Based on an assessment of the patient's fluid status, this should aim to correct any deficit from the underlying pathology and make some provision for replacing the maintenance requirements invariably 'lost to follow-up' on admission to hospital. Rules regarding fluid replacement are widespread, complicated, and, on the whole, unhelpful. In practice, the following may be used as a guide:

- Fluid depletion is almost uniform in these patients.
- Any significant intravascular depletion is best corrected with rapid infusion of isotonic crystalloid, blood, colloid, or starch-based solutions with 'physiological saline'-equivalent osmolar contents (e.g. Gelofusin or Pentaspan) through a wide-bore intravenous cannula (14 or 16 gauge).
- Losses into the gut, although difficult to estimate in volume and composition, should be replaced with 0.9% (physiological) saline over the hours before surgery. It must be noted that all infused sodium ions remain in the extracellular fluid.
- Total body water deficits, including lost maintenance requirements, should be replaced with 5% dextrose. After cellular glucose metabolism, the free water remaining distributes itself across both intracellular and extracellular fluid compartments.
- Potassium replacement remains problematic. The best pragmatic approach is to titrate replacement to requirement by adding 20–40 mmol potassium chloride to each litre of 0.9% saline and re-estimating the serum potassium frequently. Profound hypokalaemia should be treated with central replacement and continuous ECG monitoring.

The 'Holy Grail' of fluid resuscitation is to establish normovolaemia and an adequate urine output before induction. In the presence of a normal heart and unimpaired renal function, 0.5 ml/kg per h in the catheter bag implies adequate renal perfusion.

It is worth noting here that a critically ill patient will benefit from a period of aggressive preoperative resuscitation on the intensive care unit (ICU), guided by invasive monitoring, before surgery.

### Resuscitation of major intra-abdominal bleeding

Some surgical emergencies do not allow time for staged resuscitation. Dissecting abdominal aortic aneurysms and ruptured ectopic pregnancy can present with catastrophic hypovolaemia. Haemorrhage progresses to produce cardiovascular decompensation and neurological compromise or frank unconsciousness. Anaesthetic response must be modified to deal with different priorities:

- **A**: secure a patent, protected airway.
- **B**: ensure adequate ventilation with 100% oxygen.
- **C**: establish intravenous access. Two wide-bore intravenous cannulae (minimum 14 gauge) should be inserted. Intraosseous needles (see Chapter 78) and 'cut-down' access are acceptable alternatives if peripheral access is difficult.
- Commence fluid replacement to re-establish circulating volume.
- Send relevant investigations and start planning definitive therapy simultaneously with resuscitation.

#### *Fluid therapy*

Hypotension resulting from hypovolaemia implies loss of 30–40% of circulating volume and must be treated with the utmost urgency. Crystalloid infusion may be life saving by re-establishing an adequate cardiac output; however, blood loss of this magnitude should be treated with prompt transfusion of blood or packed cells to optimize tissue oxygen delivery and avert organ damage.

Although fluid resuscitation to restore circulating volume is extremely important, these lesions must be rapidly corrected surgically and transfer to the operating room should not be delayed in an attempt to attain 'normal' physiological parameters. Partial resuscitation of such patients before definitive surgical control of haemorrhage is therefore acceptable. Indeed there is some evidence to suggest that vigorous resuscitation of dissecting aortic aneurysm before cross-clamping is detrimental to long-term outcome. It is suggested that so-called 'permissive hypotension' reduces clotting factor dilution, tissue oedema, and disruption of newly formed clot, reducing peri-operative morbidity and mortality.

#### *Investigations*

Only investigations directly relevant to managing the resuscitation process should be performed. Blood should be sent for full blood count and clotting screen to establish a baseline for resuscitation and to look for evidence of a coagulopathy (this is likely to worsen with the effects of a massive blood transfusion). Cross-match at this stage should take into account immediate and intraoperative requirements. A minimum of six units of blood and four units of fresh frozen plasma is a reasonable starting point.

The continued intraoperative management of such major haemorrhage requires the early involvement of senior, experienced anaesthetic and surgical personnel.

##### *Analgesia*

Patients with acute abdominal pathology are often in significant pain. Apart from a humanitarian duty, the control of acute pain offers significant advantages in subsequent management. Intravenous systemic opioids titrated at the bedside to the patient's individual analgesic requirement remain difficult to beat. Absorption from intramuscular injection is unpredictable in states of fluid depletion and this route of administration should be avoided. Non-steroidal anti-inflammatory drugs are relatively contraindicated because of their effects on renal perfusion.

For those patients suffering from major haemorrhage discussed above, effective analgesia presents further challenges. Reduced cardiac output and central nervous system dysfunction make the effects of systemic opioids difficult to predict and increase the risk of significant respiratory depression. A practical compromise is to use small intravenous increments of a potent short-acting opioid such as fentanyl to achieve 'bridging' analgesia before definitive operative intervention. Ketamine is a useful alternative analgesic in such circumstances.

Prophylaxis against deep vein thrombosis and infection is particularly important in this group of patients.

## INTRAOPERATIVE CONSIDERATIONS

The anticipation of problems allows for their early recognition and treatment. A structured approach to the task of anaesthetizing a patient with an acute abdomen gives one the framework from which to respond to acute intraoperative events.

### Induction

The risk of regurgitation and aspiration of gastric contents in the presence of an ileus means that all patients anaesthetized for an acute abdomen must be assumed to have a full stomach. This implies the use of a rapid sequence induction technique with preoxygenation, cricoid pressure, and the administration of suxamethonium for rapid depolarizing neuromuscular blockade. A predetermined dose of induction agent is given rapidly; dose requirement is normally reduced in acute illness compared with in fit patients. Thiopentone (thiopental) has a more predictable dose requirement than propofol (see Chapter 32) and has the further advantage of not causing pain on rapid intravenous injection. Etomidate is a useful alternative when minimum cardiovascular depression is required. In critically ill patients, ketamine may be an appropriate choice.

Anaesthetizing these patients in the operating room is worth considering because it reduces the risks inherent to transfer. Monitoring facilities are also almost uniformly better in the operating room than in anaesthetic rooms.

### Monitoring

Monitoring at induction should include oxygen saturation, continuous ECG, and non-invasive blood pressure estimation as a minimum. Capnography to establish correct placement of the endotracheal tube is also essential.

For any patient at high risk of adverse events as a result of pre-existing disease processes or the surgical pathology requiring operative intervention, invasive arterial blood pressure recording and central venous pressure estimation should be employed to direct intraoperative fluid therapy.

Insertion of an arterial line 'awake' under local anaesthesia and continuous invasive blood pressure monitoring during induction is an under-used technique. It provides valuable information at a time when cardiovascular stability and tissue oxygenation may be significantly compromised. It also allows for convenient intraoperative blood sampling for blood gases or estimation of transfusion requirements.

Intraoperative urine output should be closely monitored because it provides a sensitive guide to renal perfusion. The much quoted axiom 'if you don't get oliguric, you don't get anuric' retains considerable wisdom.

### Maintenance

Generations of stressed FRCA candidates have dutifully rolled out the 'balanced anaesthetic technique' as the panacea to their examiners' probing enquiries. What do we mean by this? It implies a general anaesthetic technique combining an inhalational anaesthetic agent with non-depolarizing neuromuscular blockade and systemic opioids titrated to the patient's needs. It is difficult to improve on for an ideal combination of cardiovascular stability and analgesia, hence its unassailable position.

The duration of emergency surgery can be unpredictable, so short-acting non-depolarizing neuromuscular blocking agents such as atracurium, vecuronium, or rocuronium should be used. Nitrous oxide can cause unwanted bowel distension and is probably best avoided.

Heat loss is frequently excessive during laparotomy because latent heat of vaporization is absorbed during evaporation from exposed abdominal contents. Temperature should be monitored, ideally with a nasopharyngeal probe, and techniques to reduce heat loss employed, i.e. warming intravenous fluids, humidification of inspired gases, and the use of a warming blanket.

Emergency abdominal surgery performed under regional anaesthesia alone is still rare outside delivery suites! However, the combination of regional analgesia with thoracic or lumbar epidural and an inhalational anaesthetic has attractive properties, provided that there is no residual hypovolaemia or systemic sepsis.

Reversal of neuromuscular blockade and emergence from anaesthesia/extubation requires active management because the patient must still be considered at risk of aspiration. Extubation should be performed in the operating room only after a full return of airway reflexes, in a lateral position with monitoring still *in situ*. Return of spontaneous respiratory activity and adequate ventilatory function should be established before the patient is discharged to recovery.

## POSTOPERATIVE CONSIDERATIONS

### Environment

The decision about where the patient is cared for postoperatively should be based on preoperative status, intraoperative stability, and surgical findings.

Clearly, any patient requiring mechanical ventilation or inotropic support can be adequately cared for only in an ICU. For the patient who is breathing spontaneously, surgical factors exert a significant influence. Any evidence of peritonitis from hollow viscus contents, e.g. small bowel leak or faecal peritonitis, puts the patient at risk of developing systemic inflammatory response syndrome (SIRS; see Chapter 60). Invasive postoperative monitoring and aggressive interventional management of problems such as oliguria, hypotension, or hypoxaemia are required even if the patient appears stable immediately after the operation.

Any patient who has undergone a primary anastomosis in a peritoneal field should be closely monitored because this practice carries a risk of anastomotic breakdown or leak. Intravenous antibiotic therapy should also be continued into the postoperative phase in this subgroup.

### Analgesia

If analgesia has been established with systemic opioids, it is reasonable to continue these into the postoperative phase. Patient-controlled analgesia safely balances pain relief with analgesic requirements, provided that the patient understands what is required (see Chapter 5). Unpredictable absorption and peaks and troughs of analgesia make intermittent intramuscular administration of opioids for major abdominal surgery unsatisfactory.

Regional analgesia combined with a general anaesthetic technique arguably provides ideal intraoperative conditions and postoperative pain relief for laparotomy. Thoracic epidural analgesia with a combination of local anaesthetic and opioid delivered by infusion preserves the functional residual capacity and respiratory excursion. The preservation of adequate ventilation and coughing permitted by good analgesia prevents basal atelectasis and retention of secretions. The environment to which the patient returns after surgery is a significant consideration when contemplating this form of analgesia. Safe management of thoracic epidural analgesia usually implies care in a high dependency unit or ICU.

Peripheral nerve blockade is seldom used for abdominal emergencies; however, field block of the right ilioinguinal and iliohypogastric nerve can provide effective analgesia for appendicectomy.

### Fluids

Fluid prescriptions should include baseline requirements and a supplement for any predictable losses, e.g. continued fluid sequestration at the operative site or SIRS with an associated capillary endothelial leak. None of us has a crystal ball for spying into the near future! There is no substitute for going back to the patient, reassessing vital signs, and adjusting therapy accordingly.

### Oxygen

The simple postoperative considerations are often the most important. Supplemental oxygen therapy should be almost uniform after abdominal surgery and goes some way towards compensating for the compromise of respiratory function. Ideally this should be humidified to prevent further dehydration and cooling, and delivered with a fixed performance HAFOE device.

## FURTHER READING

Gallagher CJ, Lubarsky DA. *Board Stiff: Preparing for the Anesthesia Orals*. Boston: Butterworth-Heinemann, 1990.

Reed AP, ed. *Clinical Cases in Anesthesia*, 2nd edn. New York: Churchill Livingstone, 1995.

# Chapter 62 The patient needing transport

M. Manji

## OVERVIEW

Organization of collection and transportation of severely injured people developed in the eighteenth century under the influence of Barron Dominique-Jean Larrey, Napoleon's chief military surgeon. Specially adapted horse-drawn carts *(ambulances volantes)* were used for primary transport of the injured to a place of safety, where they received immediate treatment, débridement, cleansing, and primary suturing. Over the years, our understanding of the pathophysiology of critical illness has expanded, together with the recognition of the need for safe and efficient transport systems.

Transport of critically ill people can be divided into two independent but complementary systems: primary (from the site of initial injury or illness) and secondary (between hospitals). This chapter examines mainly secondary interhospital transport and provides an overview of the underlying principle governing the safe and efficient transfer of critically ill patients.

It has been estimated that over 11 000 interhospital transfers take place in the UK each year. Proposed centralization of intensive care provision and other major specialities in tertiary centres, compounded by bed restrictions on intensive care units (ICUs), will undoubtedly increase transfer numbers. Despite the large number of interhospital transfers, mounting evidence suggests that transport systems are deficient in many situations. Regretfully, there still remains an urgent need for a coordinated approach to safe interhospital transfer in the UK. In the US, Australia, and other European countries, dedicated transfer teams have been established, properly coordinated, and audited. For example, in France the law requires public provision of an Emergency Medical Assistance Service (Service d'Aide Medicale Urgente). Several bodies are now addressing the issue of interhospital transfer in Britain. Guidelines have been published by the British Trauma Society, the Neuroanaesthesia Society of Great Britain and Ireland, the Intensive Care Society, and the Paediatric Intensive Care Society. A Department of Health Working Party has issued guidelines on admission to and discharge from ICUs and high dependency units (HDUs).

A few centres have developed their own transport teams, and evidence suggests that, when transfers are conducted by these specialist groups, outcomes are better than for non-specialist transfers. Although having a specialized mobile intensive care team might be the ideal, limited resources prevent its widespread adoption. Although monetary factors should not determine standard of care, the reality is that most ICUs in the UK will have to continue to perform transfers of critically ill patients without the benefit of such specialized teams. It is therefore essential that those responsible for the transfer possess the appropriate skills and are sufficiently experienced to ensure that critically ill patients separated from the secure environment of the ICU or HDU are cared for adequately.

## THE TRANSFER

The decision for suitability of transfer should be made by a senior doctor experienced in intensive care. The sole purpose of the transfer is to provide the patient with a higher level of care than that available at the base hospital, with the expectation that outcome will be improved. The indications for transfer outlined in Table 62.1 show that many of the reasons revolve around the fact that the provision of special facilities and expertise needs to be concentrated in a few centres to provide optimum care. The increased numbers of patients who are recognized as benefiting from intensive care (which has not been paralleled by appropriate increase in resources) means that transfer because of lack of a staffed bed locally is relatively frequent compared with a few years ago. The heterogeneity of case mix emphasizes the need to employ staff with experience in all aspects of intensive care management and diagnosis, and with advanced life-support skills to care for the patients during transport. Such specialized teams should be able to respond to all clinical categories encountered, enabling the ICU environment to be moved with the patient.

The Association of Anaesthetists of Great Britain and Ireland, the Intensive Care Society, and the Joint Commission on Accreditation of Hospitals in the USA suggest that the responsibility of transfer should lie with the receiving hospital as soon as acceptance of the patient is confirmed. Unfortunately, this practice is rarely observed in health care systems with limited resources.

## ASSESSMENT AND STABILIZATION

Table 62.2 identifies the essentials of transport assessment and management. It is important to pay meticulous attention to resuscitation and stabilization of the patients to avoid complications during the journey. Transfer must not take place until the patient is physiologically stable. Avoidable factors identified as contributing to death in children after head injury include failure of diagnosis of intracranial lesion,

**Table 62.1 Reasons for transfer: case mix and some special problems**

| |
|---|
| Regional paediatric intensive care expertise. Care of neonates, pre-term babies, and infants especially for problems associated with congenital abnormalities (e.g. cardiac, tracheo-oesphageal fistula, gastroschisis) |
| Regional adult specialty expertise – thermal injury, head and spinal injury |
| Advanced organ support – fulminant hepatic failure, critical oxygenation for extracorporeal monitoring oxygen |
| Surgical intervention: neurosurgical, cardiac, major vascular – emergencies often unstable |
| Clinical investigations: computed tomography scan, magnetic resonance imaging – therapy and monitoring facilities often suboptimal |
| Insufficient local resources; never transfer for cost-shifting strategies |

inadequate management of airway, and poor management of transfer between hospitals. Active airway management is particularly important. Another audit published in 1990 revealed a 32% incidence of untoward events in patients transferred to a neurosurgical unit, with the airway compromised in 25% of cases.

The decision to transfer should be made by the senior medical staff (usually the consultant) after full assessment of the patient and a careful evaluation of the benefits to be gained against the possible risks. A thorough, disciplined, and methodical approach is required. Immediate attention may have to be directed to correcting life-threatening physiological aberration before more detailed systematic evaluation of other organ systems.

The assessment should start with a thorough history and physical examination, supplemented by details from nursing staff, relatives, and other medical staff. Careful documentation is essential, particularly of neurological status in patients with head injury or those who require sedation and paralysis for transfer. Physical examination should be systematic and begin with the ABC of resuscitation. Critical illness implies unstable physiology that will be adversely affected by movement. Unstable variables should be identified, stabilized, and corrected. Assessment should also include anticipation of potential complications that might occur during transfer, particularly cardiorespiratory variables, which may influence tissue oxygenation.

## MEDICAL CONSIDERATIONS

### Airway and ventilation

Airway obstruction, hypoxia, and hypercapnia are major causes of physiological deterioration and all are poten-

**Table 62.2 Transport: questions, systematic assessment, and management**

| | |
|---|---|
| Is transfer absolutely necessary and will it alter patient management or outcome? | |
| Is the patient deteriorating or likely to deteriorate? | |
| What critical incidents could occur during transfer? | |
| What action should be taken before transfer to prevent them? | |
| Airway | Airway management and protection; intubate if in doubt |
| Ventilation | Mechanical if intubated<br>Prevention of hypoxia or hypercapnia<br>Need for positive end-expiratory pressure facilities<br>Need for complex ventilatory facilities, e.g. inverse ratio |
| Cardiovascular | Circulating volume, blood loss<br>Inotropic requirement<br>Identification and treatment of arrhythmias |
| General | Sedation, analgesia, need for paralysis |
| Metabolic | Blood glucose, acid–base status, serum potassium<br>Renal function, circulating volume, and bladder catheterization |
| Fractures | Fixation and immobilization |
| Drugs | Adequate to patient's anticipated need, including oxygen (see Table 62.3) |
| Monitoring | Comprehensive facility and tailored to patient's condition (see Table 62.4) |
| Personnel | Senior staff, adequate numbers, training |

tially avoidable. They result from inadequate assessment and management of the airway. Potential airway compromise must be identified, with measures to correct this receiving the highest priority. The adequacy of gas exchange must be assessed by blood gas analysis before transfer and, other than in exceptional cases, the aim is to maintain the arterial oxygen tension at at least 13 kPa (98 mmHg) and normal arterial $CO_2$ tension unless otherwise specifically indicated. Airway management, protection, and reliable oxygenation may be achieved only by tracheal intubation and mechanical ventilation, and the attending physician must possess the necessary skills and knowledge of technique and equipment. Intubation and mechanical ventilation are mandatory for unconscious patients. It is easier to extubate a patient in a controlled stable environment if this is deemed necessary, than to try to intubate an hypoxic, unstable patient during transfer. The latter is more hazardous and suggests failure of adequate assessment and preparation.

### Cardiovascular

An appropriate haemoglobin, circulating volume, and perfusion pressure must be achieved to maintain stability and function of major organ systems. This may require intravenous volume loading with colloid and/or crystalloid initially. Whether colloids or crystalloids are used is a long-standing controversy; whatever the choice, enough quantities must be used because hypovolaemic patients tolerate transfer poorly. Blood loss must be controlled and replaced with packed cells. A patient who remains hypotensive despite resuscitation must not be transferred until the cause is determined and corrected. When massive transfusion of intravenous fluid is required, due consideration must be given to warming of fluids. Good intravascular access is necessary and is usually secured via two large-bore cannulae (smaller in children). In children, when intravascular access may be very difficult, the intraosseous route for infusion of resuscitative fluids is very valuable (see Chapter 78). In general, intubated patients should also have a central venous cannula. This is a particularly useful route for vasoactive drug therapy. Inotropic therapy is probably best guided in unstable patients by detailed intravascular monitoring with the use of a pulmonary artery catheter.

### Fractures

Fractures must be immobilized and stabilized to provide neurovascular protection. In trauma patients, intracranial and spinal cord injuries must be excluded or stabilized, and treatment optimized so that the potential for further secondary insult is eliminated. Cervical spine instability should be considered and control must be maintained during intubation. This usually requires the presence of an experienced assistant and usually takes the form of manual inline traction and immobilization.

### Sedation and analgesia

It is inappropriate to allow an intubated, critically ill patient to breathe spontaneously during the transfer. These patients should be paralysed and meticulous attention must be given to analgesia and sedation appropriate to the individual patient's need. Undersedation and inadequate analgesia can have serious pathophysiological effects. Even those who are unconscious require an induction agent for laryngoscopy and intubation with continuing sedation and analgesia.

### Others

Urinary bladder catheterization should be performed unless specifically unwarranted, along with the passage of an oral or nasogastric tube. Both must be allowed free drainage. The latter will facilitate ventilation by decompressing the stomach, especially in paediatric patients.

Recent radiographs and other results should be reviewed along with current therapies, which should be continued during transfer. A chest drain should be inserted if a pneumothorax is present or likely as a result of thoracic trauma.

Neurological function must be evaluated as part of the initial assessment. The Glasgow Coma Scale should be used as the minimum, not the sole, measure to evaluate orientation and cognitive function. Pupillary size and responsiveness to light as well as motor function and reflexes in all limbs are examined. Metabolic parameters are often ignored – particular attention should be paid to blood glucose, serum potassium levels, and acid–base status.

## ACCOMPANYING PERSONNEL AND EQUIPMENT

The safety of the patient and accompanying staff takes precedence over all other considerations. Inadequate and unsupervised care during transfer is dangerous. The transfer team should consist of at least two attendants: a physician and an experienced nurse familiar with the patient's clinical condition, intensive care procedures, and with all the transport equipment. Patients who are critically ill must be attended by a physician skilled in resuscitation, airway management, ventilation, and other organ support. This will usually be an anaesthetist or critical care specialist, but the precise specialty label is less important than the skills implied. Safety of the patient is not secured merely by the presence of a physician, and training courses are essential. Even for the shortest journey, the transfer team should be capable of initiating a response to a patient's deterioration to the same degree and rapidity as would occur in the ICU. In this context, involvement of additional specialists may also be necessary according to patients' needs, for example, transfers involving neonates or those with spinal trauma.

Ideally, critically ill patients requiring interhospital transfer should be attended by a dedicated specially trained transport team from the receiving hospital. Such a team should have clear management structure and responsibilities, be familiar with transport equipment, and have the authority to determine suitability for transfer and its timing. Alternatively, a central retrieval team specializing in interhospital transfer, as in some neonatal units or with international air transfers, may be available. However, with current financial constraints, this may not be feasible. It is important that all critical care personnel are trained in transport skills because the proposed regional transfer teams cannot always respond with the urgency that may be required. Delay in treatment is a substantial risk factor for multiple organ failure and intensive care mortality, and a balance must be maintained between waiting for a specialist team and providing prompt transfer of a stabilized patient to a specialized centre for definitive treatment. In the absence of such a specialized team, the responsibility of transfer of a critically ill patient is often wrongly delegated to a junior trainee. This is unacceptable and must be avoided at all times.

### Communication

Good and clear record-keeping is essential at all stages of the transfer. Not only does this reflect good medical practice, but medicolegal requirements dictate that the purpose of the transfer should be explained to the patient, if competent, and/or relatives. Indications, risks, and alternatives must be clearly documented. The history, examination findings, diagnosis, resuscitative measures, and response to such treatment must be recorded. Detailed discussion with senior medical staff at the receiving hospital must take place before transfer. Documentation of the clinical condition throughout the transfer must continue. This type of information can also be used for the purpose of audit and training to maintain and improve standards. The receiving unit should be informed of the departure and estimated time of arrival.

The transfer team should be equipped with a method of communicating with their base and the receiving hospital. Despite the risk of interference with electronic equipment, a portable telephone can be useful in these circumstances.

### Monitoring equipment

The dimly lit, noisy, and crowded environment of an ambulance is hostile to the monitoring of critically ill patients. Ideally, monitoring during transfer should be as comprehensive as that in an ICU to ensure physiological stability. The guidelines for monitoring patients for administration of a general anaesthetic, as published by the Association of Anaesthetists of Great Britain and Ireland, should serve as the minimum standard and includes the following: continuous ECG monitoring; intermittent, frequent, automated non-invasive blood pressure measurement; respiratory rate; and continuous pulse oximetry.

Continuous intra-arterial pressure monitoring is the preferred standard and is the only reliable method in transit; this should be the method of choice whenever possible. Non-invasive oscillotonometric measurement is sensitive to motion artefact and tends to over-estimate low pressure and under-estimate high pressure. This inaccuracy may be increased at extremes of pressure and is subject to further increases in the presence of arrhythmias. Hypotension can be significant in poorly conducted transfer and can severely affect outcome. The Finapress is a constant-volume finger plethysmograph designed for continuous non-invasive blood-pressure measurement. Although potentially very attractive for transport, there are still concerns regarding its accuracy.

Central venous access and pressure transduction should be used if this is necessary for clinical management. Monitoring of pulmonary artery pressure and cardiac output measurements may be needed for long journeys, but are generally more important for pre-transfer stabilization.

Pulse oximetry provides a simple and reliable means of detecting hypoxaemia, provided its limitations are appreciated. In selected patients, it may be necessary to measure airway pressure and continuous end-tidal $CO_2$, but current portable capnometry is of limited use and at best provides only a crude guide to actual values. Advancements in technology have allowed the development of miniature, continuous, intravascular blood gas electrodes (e.g. Paratrend 7), but at present these are not sufficiently well developed or available for routine use during transfer. Body temperature (particularly in children) and urine output should generally be measured in all critically ill patients requiring transport.

Audible alarms are essential on all monitoring devices, infusion equipment, and the mechanical ventilator during transfer, because the attendant's attention is often distracted. All equipment should be small, lightweight, robust, resistant to movement/vibrational artefacts, easy to operate, battery powered with a battery life of at least 2 hours for the average transfer, and able to function from the power supply of the transport vehicle for longer journeys. There are several multi-channel monitors now available which satisfy most of these requirements. Additional requirement might include the facility to store and download data for research and audit.

### Ventilator and gas supply

Mechanical ventilation is mandatory in intubated patients because manual or spontaneous ventilation is unreliable and unsatisfactory during transfer. Ideally, portable ventilators should be gas-powered, time-cycled, pressure-limited, and provide a positive end-expiratory pressure facility, a range of tidal volumes, respiratory rates, and oxygen concentration to accommodate differing clinical circumstances. They should be armed with a disconnection alarm. However, most of the transport ventilators do not provide full ICU-type support. It is important that emergency means of manual ventilation are available in the unlikely event of ventilator failure.

Oxygen supplies should be sufficient to meet at least twice the total anticipated period of transfer to compensate for possible delays: a size F cylinder (1360 L) will provide approximately 30 min of ventilation using 100% oxygen for the average adult. This includes the patient's consumption as well as that which may be used to operate the ventilator. This will usually be secured by carrying two size G (3400 L) oxygen cylinders or their equivalent. Liquid-oxygen containers, of capacity up to 34 000 L, have been developed which can be used with portable ventilators during prolonged interhospital transport.

### Other supplies

The requirement of monitoring equipment and ventilator has already been highlighted. Drugs and small items should be available in basic packs with extra room to add a limited number of items specific for individual patients need. The list of drugs and other equipment required should be kept as simple as possible.

Tables 62.3 and 62.4 show some of the items that should be considered. A designated person should be responsible for the regular maintenance and restocking of the pack. Particular attention should be paid to controlled drugs, out-of-date drugs, drugs that need to be kept in a refrigerator, and battery-operated equipment.

Heat loss can be a problem, especially for transfers of children. Measures to minimize this include raising ambient temperature, foil wrapping, warming blankets, and heat and moisture exchange units in the breathing circuit. Incubators are essential for neonatal transfer. Fluid administration may require the use of pressure bags because gravity-dependent devices are often unreliable, especially in the crowded environment. Syringe drivers are preferable to volumetric devices for continuous administration of drugs.

| Table 62.4 Examples of small equipment required for interhospital transfer |
|---|
| Comprehensive airway management (e.g. masks, oral airway, endotracheal tubes, bougies, tracheostomy tubes) |
| Spare batteries |
| Self-inflating bag with reservoir and connectors, mask |
| Direct-current defibrillator |
| Suction and catheters |
| Intravenous cannulae and giving sets |
| Syringes and needles |
| Chest drain, Heimlich valve |
| Gloves, scissors, pens, torch |

### Modes of transfer

Transport could be carried out by ground, air, or sea. Proper coordination and audit are required for the success of any transport service. The factors determining choice of mode of transport include severity of illness, distance and transport time, weather, traffic conditions, availability, and cost. Limited space is a problem common to all modes of transport, but the method chosen ideally should accommodate the full transfer team and allow them to perform emergency procedures such as endotracheal reintubation and cardiopulmonary resuscitation. Safety and comfort are important for the attendants and vehicle operator, as well as the patient. The problems relating to inertial forces, speed, and altitude are discussed below.

Transport stretchers generally should be lightweight, portable, and flexible, with an undercarriage to mount securely other essential equipment such as monitors, infusion equipment, intravenous pumps, transducers, and oxygen tanks. Due regard to the presence of possible spinal injury must be given.

Land transport is met by paramedic ambulance, is relatively cheap, and is readily available. It is the most common form of patient transport employed in cities when distances and transport times are relatively short. Adequate preparation before the journey allows subsequent transport at normal road speeds; hurried transfers are dangerous and usually reflect poor preparation. Traffic police may be of great value, but the emphasis remains on a smooth and controlled ride rather than on speed.

Many of the inherent problems of transport were realized by those transporting the wounded from battle fields. The features of early designs of transport are illustrated in Figure 62.1. Modern transport is illustrated in Figures 62.2 and 62.3.

Some of the problems associated with air transfer are shown in Table 62.5. Helicopters are useful in primary transport, especially in rural areas, but there is very little difference in outcome between air and ground transport over short distances. They are practical for intermediate distances to avoid traffic congestion and complex routing, and have the added advantage of being able to operate from urban centres.

**Table 62.3 Classes and examples of stock drugs required for interhospital transfer**

| | |
|---|---|
| Anticonvulsants | Phenytoin, diazepam, thiopentone (thiopental) |
| Analgesics | Controlled drugs (to be prepared and booked out for individual patient) |
| Antiarrhythmics | Lignocaine (lidocaine), amiodarone, adenosine |
| Anaesthetic/hypnotics | Midazolam, propofol |
| Bronchodilators | |
| Cardiovascular/resuscitation drugs | Hospital resuscitation boxes, nitrates, isoprenaline (isoproterenol), norepinephrine, ephedrine |
| Diuretics | |
| Fluids | Cross-matched blood, physiological saline, colloids |
| Neuromuscular blocking agents | Suxamethonium, atracurium |
| Miscellaneous | Hydrocortisone, bicarbonate, naloxone, antiemetics |

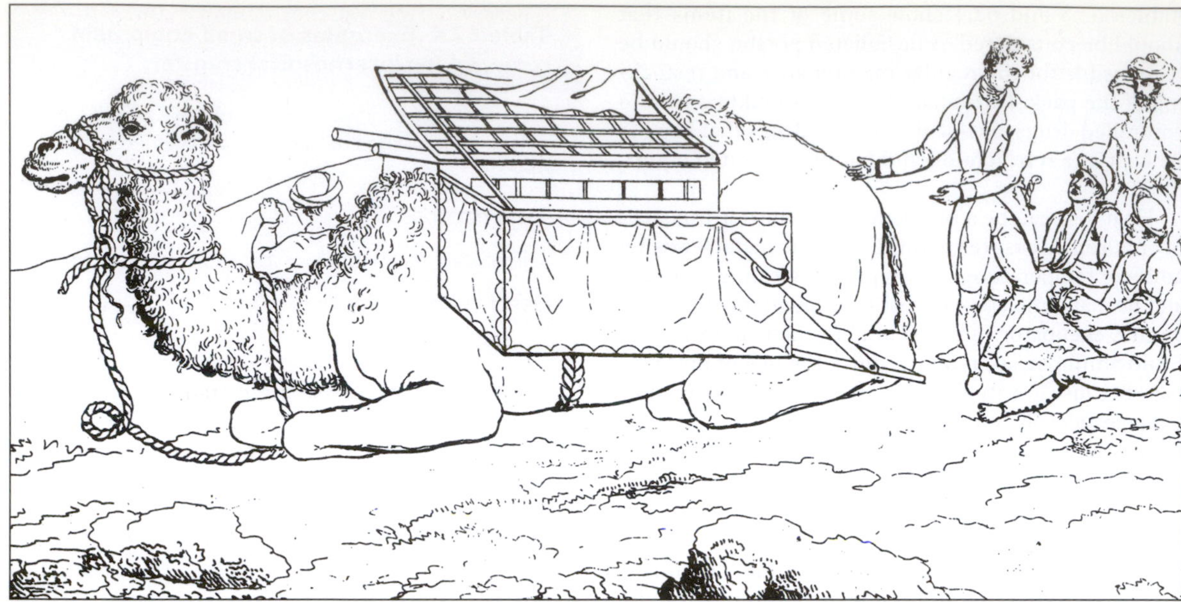

**Figure 62.1** Transport for the wounded from the campaign in Syria (1798): '. . . it was necessary to employ camels, the only means of conveyance which the country afforded, and to render the transportation convenient to the wounded, and to the animal. For this purpose I caused a hundred panniers to be made, two for each camel, disposed in the form of a cradle, which the animal carried on each side of his dorsal projection, suspended by elastick straps. Their construction was such as neither to impede the progress of nor motion of the animal: they were, however, made of sufficient length, by means of a moveable foot-board, to carry a man while lying at full length.' (From Larrey DJ. *Memoirs of Military Surgery.* Baltimore: Joseph Cushing, 1987.)

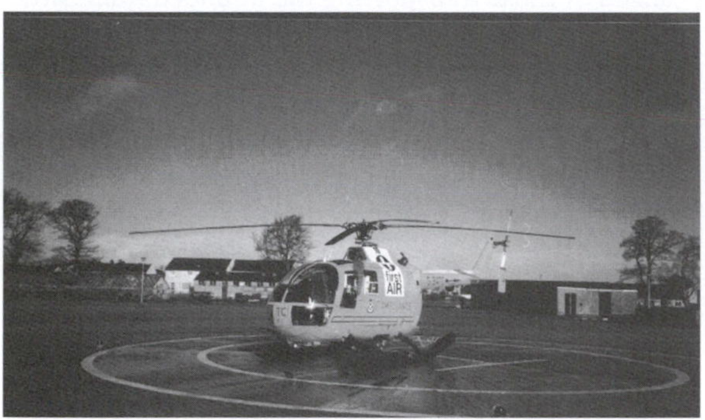

**Figure 62.2** A transport helicopter on the landing pad.

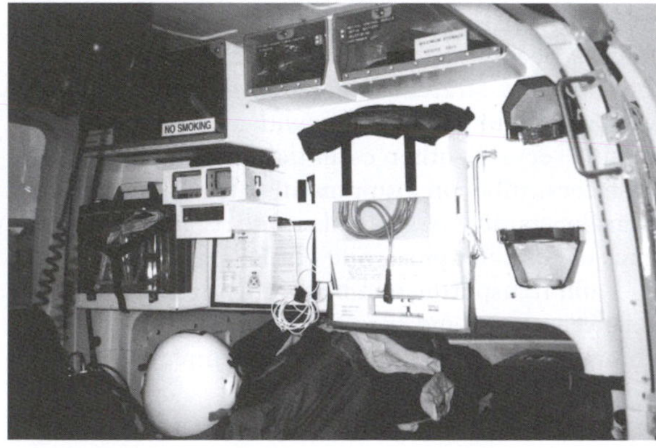


**Figure 62.3** Conditions inside a transport helicopter are very cramped.

Fixed-wing aircraft are especially useful for very long distance transport. Unlike a helicopter, a proper airfield is necessary, which means that supplementary ground transport is always required. This adds further to the total transit time, as well as increasing the costs and the need for more personnel.

### Movements and altitude/barometric pressure

Critically ill patients tolerate transfer poorly. Physiological instability is often compounded by disturbance and moving the patient. The mechanisms of this are not entirely understood but may be related to failure of autonomic reflexes and homoeostatic mechanisms. Sudden acceleration and deceleration must be avoided and, if possible, patients should be positioned transversely. Large shifts of body fluids can take place as a result of acceleration forces, with deterioration in both cardiovascular and central nervous systems. This is particularly marked in the presence of hypovolaemia.

The hazards associated with air transport depend largely on whether it is a fixed-wing aircraft or a helicopter. Altitude effects (pressure and temperature) may be a problem with non-pressurized aircraft. Although some air ambulance and military transport planes such as Hercules and VC 10 can achieve sea-level cabin pressure, the pressure in most aircraft is equivalent to that at an altitude of 2500 metres. This will reduce the ambient partial pressure of oxygen from 150 mmHg (20 kPa) to about 110 mmHg (15.5 kPa). In healthy individuals, this will cause a decrease in arterial $P\text{O}_2$ tension, reducing the oxygen saturation to 93%, and

| Table 62.5 Common problems with transport |
|---|
| Heating and temperature loss |
| Poor lighting |
| Limited space and supplies |
| Insubstantial power source |
| Noise and motion |
| Communication |
| **Specific problems with air transport** |
| Unavailable at short notice |
| Landing facilities – necessitating further transport by road |
| Increased cost and personnel |
| Helicopters – dangerous in severe weather conditions, mountainous terrain, night flying |
| Increased noise and vibration |
| Communication |
| Very limited cabin space |
| Barometric/altitude effects |

may result in a more serious desaturation in patients with acute or chronic cardiopulmonary disease. Enclosed gas-containing cavities, such as pneumothorax, lung cysts, sinuses, the gut, and the endotracheal tube cuff, will enlarge as the ambient pressure decreases. A pneumothorax will expand by 20% by a change in altitude of 6000 feet. Middle-ear air cavity expansion may increase the likelihood of vomiting and aspiration. Intravenous infusion rates may also alter unless controlled by infusion devices.

The risk to which the transfer team is exposed must not be dismissed, especially with air transport. This includes the effect of altitude, dysbarisms, hypoxia, environmental temperature, gas expansion, motion sickness, and fatigue. Attending staff who cannot equalize pressure in the middle ear or suffer from severe motion sickness should not fly.

## SPECIAL CONSIDERATIONS

Some clinical conditions pose particular specific transport difficulties, e.g. burn injuries, head and spinal injuries, fulminant hepatic failure, neonates, high-risk pregnant women, and obese patients. Patients with fulminant acute hepatic failure may appear relatively stable before transfer, but develop progressive multiple organ failure rapidly, and may suffer fatal brain herniation during the journey. Burned patients present the additional problems of progressive airway and lung injury, fluid losses, vascular access, and rapid hypothermia. Head- and spinal cord-injured patients are at obvious risk of secondary injury if there are deficiencies in elementary standards of preparation and management for transfer.

There is strong evidence demonstrating a significant decrease in mortality for low-birth-weight infants born in or transported to a tertiary specialized centre. There is also a need for transport of high-risk maternal cases for optimal outcome. The success of these programmes depends on the direct involvement of other specialists such as paediatricians/neonatologists and obstetricians who should form an essential part of the transfer team.

## AUDIT, EDUCATION, AND TRAINING

There is an urgent need for a national coordinated effort to provide efficient and safe transport of critically ill patients on a 24-hour basis. A centralized effort to help each hospital to establish clear guidelines and communication channels to initiate interhospital transfer of the critically ill needs to be established.

There should be planning of transport at local, regional, and national levels. Appropriate resources must be identified and made available to meet demands, as well as fund audit and training. Hospitals that provide transfer retrieval teams should not be penalized by the lack of regional or national funding. The key to the effectiveness of transport programme is not only training but adequate funding. To address limitations with funding, regional services may consider establishing transport teams funded by contributions from individual trusts and/or direct contribution from the purchasing authorities.

Data collection is paramount for the purpose of audit and assessment of quality assurance and risk management. It is essential to improve training and to maintain standards. All staff involved in transfer of patients should be competent in the care of the critically ill patient and should be familiar with equipment. Resources are required to achieve this and joint training courses covering all aspects of transport medicine need to be established.

The transport staff as well as the patient are vulnerable to accidents and/or disability during the transfer. Individuals need to be insured against such events and a written confirmation of medical indemnity must be provided by the employing body.

## FURTHER READING


Association of Anaesthetists of Great Britain and Ireland. *Recommendation for the Transfer of Patients with Acute Head Injuries to Neurosurgical Units*. London: AAGBI, 1996.

Association of Anaesthetists of Great Britain and Ireland. *Intensive Care Services: Provision for the Future*. London: AAGBI, 1998.

Bion JF, Wilson IH, Taylor PA. Transporting critically ill patients by ambulance: audit by sickness scoring. *BMJ* 1988;**296**:170.

Davies MJ. Crystalloid or colloid: does it matter? *J Clin Anesthesiol* 1989;**1**:464–71.

Gentleman D, Jennett B. Audit of transfer of the unconscious head injured patients to a neurosurgical unit. *Lancet* 1990;**335**:330–4.

Gentleman D, Jennett B. Hazards of interhospital transfer of comatose head injured patients. *Lancet* 1981;**ii**:853–5.

Gilligan JE. Stabilisation, transport and the critically ill. *Clin Anaesthesiol* 1995;**3**:789–811.

Guidelines Committee of The American College of Critical Care Medicine. Guidelines for the Transfer of Critically Ill Patients. *Crit Care Med* 1993;**6**:931–7.

Intensive Care Society. *Guidelines for the Transport of the Critically Ill Adult.* London: Intensive Care Society, November 1997.

Paneth N, Kiely JL, Phil M, *et al*. Newborn intensive care and neonatal mortality in low-birth-weight infants: A population study. *N Engl J Med* 1982;**307**:149–55.

Purdie JM, Ridley SA, Wallace PM. Effective use of regional intensive care units. *BMJ* 1990;**300**:79–81.

Ramage CMH, Kee SS, Bristow A. A new portable oxygen system using liquid oxygen. *Anaesthesia* 1991;**46**:395–7.

Saule H, Riegel K, Beltinger C. Effectiveness of neonatal transport systems. *J Perinatal Med* 1988;**72**:515–21.

Sharples PM, Storey A, Aynsley-Green A, Eyre JA. Avoidable factors contributing to death of children with head injury. *BMJ* 1990;**300**:87–91.

Stack CG. Stabilization and transport of the critically ill child. *Curr Anaesth Crit Care* 1997;**8**:25–30.

Webb A, Shapiro MJ, Singer M, Suter P, eds. *Oxford Textbook of Critical Care*. Oxford: Oxford University Press, 1999.

# Chapter 63 The patient with neurological disease

P. Hutton

## DISORDERS OF THE CENTRAL NERVOUS SYSTEM

### Epilepsy

This term represents a group of disorders (incidence of 1 in 200 people) characterized by local or general seizure activity, or temporary absences. The following are the causes:

- Unknown (idiopathic epilepsy).
- Intrinsic brain disease: tumour, abscess, post-trauma, malaria.
- An abnormality external to, but affecting brain cell function:
  - faints (vasovagal, micturition, emotion);
  - intra- and extracerebral vascular disease;
  - insufficient cardiac output (Stokes–Adams attacks, heart block);
  - hypotension (often postural) as a result of drugs (especially in elderly people);
  - metabolic insults (hypoglycaemia, renal failure, hepatic failure, water intoxication, drug overdose);
  - eclampsia of pregnancy.

The age of onset may give a clue to the underlying aetiology. Young children are prone to febrile convulsions, which they usually grow out of. Fits in adolescence are usually idiopathic or follow trauma. Onset between 30 and 50 years is caused by brain tumours in 30%. Over the age of 50 years, cerebrovascular disease is the most frequent cause.

#### Clinical manifestations

*Petit mal epilepsy*

Brief absences (up to 30 s) may be accompanied by muscular jerks. This almost always disappears at adolescence, but can be succeeded by grand mal fits.

*Temporal lobe epilepsy*

Altered consciousness is accompanied by déjà vu or visual, gustatory, or olfactory hallucinations. There is often a sense of oppression or depersonalization. On occasions automatism follows the aura.

*Jacksonian or focal epilepsy*

These fits commence in a localized part of the body and gradually increase to involve more of that side. Ultimately, they may spread to the whole body and be followed by Todd's paralysis (lasts from several minutes to hours).

*Grand mal epilepsy*

The fit is often preceded by an aura. Tonic and clonic phases are followed by a deep sleep. During the fit, cyanosis usually occurs as a result of combined high oxygen consumption and brief ventilatory arrest. Tongue biting and incontinence of urine and faeces can occur. Bilateral upgoing plantar reflexes may be elicited.

#### Preoperative considerations

Assess the severity of epilepsy by the frequency of fits. Ask if they are increasing or decreasing in frequency. Find out when the patient last had a fit. Enquire whether there are any precipitating factors, e.g. fever, hypoglycaemia, flashing lights.

Ask about drug therapy and whether the dosage has been modified because of increasing fits. Check when serum levels were last measured and if they were satisfactory.

There are no abnormal findings on examination in idiopathic epilepsy. Any abnormalities may indicate another underlying cause.

#### Investigations

Although the electroencephalogram (EEG) is the most important test in evaluation and follow-up, it is unnecessary in the routine preparation for surgery.

*Full blood count, and urea and electrolytes*

These are indicated because a number of anticonvulsant drugs have an effect on blood cells and serum. These are listed in Table 63.1.

#### Anaesthetic considerations

Unless other diseases are present, the main problems are those of the effects of maintenance therapy and the prevention of a fit in the perioperative period. This is important, not only because of potential airway problems, but also because people with epilepsy are allowed to hold a driving licence only if they have not had a daytime fit for 3 years. Phenobarbitone (phenobarbital) and phenytoin are both enzyme inducers. This often makes the effective half-lives of drugs shorter and the concentration of metabolites (which may be toxic) higher. There is likely to be an increased danger from repeated halothane administration in patients on phenobarbitone, especially if breakdown occurs via a reductive pathway (see Chapter 28).

*Premedication*

Continue anticonvulsant medication on the day of surgery to prevent a withdrawal fit. Fits can be

**Table 63.1 Blood abnormalities that may be caused by anticonvulsant drugs**

| Effect | Drug |
|---|---|
| Haemoglobin level reduced | Phenytoin<br>Phenobarbitone<br>Vigabatrin |
| Thromobocytopenia | Sodium valproate<br>Carbamazepine<br>Ethosuximide<br>Primidone |
| Leukopenia | Carbamazepine<br>Primidone |
| Low serum sodium | Carbamazepine |
| Abnormal liver function tests | Sodium valproate<br>Carbamazepine |

induced by extreme nervousness, so a sedative premedication is advisable. Diazepam has the same metabolic pathway as phenytoin and may precipitate phenytoin toxicity (dizziness, diplopia, nystagmus, ataxia, confusion, and coma). Cholinergic drugs and phenothiazines can also invoke convulsions and are best avoided.

#### *Induction and maintenance*

There is no special technique that is preferred, but it is sensible to avoid those drugs and situations that are known to provoke, or reduce the threshold for, a fit. These are listed in Tables 63.2 and 63.3.

#### *Postoperative care*

This should follow the guidelines of good practice outlined in Chapter 5, taking into account the procedure undertaken and the clinical condition of the patient. Especially during emergence from general anaesthesia, avoid photic or auditory stimulation. This might produce a seizure. Do not misinterpret the shivering of 'halothane shakes' as a fit, and ensure that they are not recorded as such on the chart because of the legal implications for the patient. Continue anticonvulsant therapy, if necessary parenterally.

When prescribing drugs for reasons unrelated to epilepsy, use alternatives to those agents that interact with phenytoin and phenobarbitone and compete for plasma-protein binding sites (e.g. salicylates, warfarin, sulphonamides).

It is essential to continue anticonvulsant therapy into the postoperative period, and anticonvulsant levels must be checked postoperatively. Some anticonvulsants (e.g. carbamazepine) have no parenteral preparation and, in a sedated patient, should be administered via a nasogastric tube or as a suppository.

Recurrent seizures, sometimes leading to status epilepticus, can occur in the postoperative period. They may be precipitated by any of the factors in Table 63.2.

Seizure activity invokes a high cerebral oxygen consumption and risks brain damage. The mortality rate for untreated status epilepticus is over 10% and a further 10–30% have permanent neurological damage.

Treatment must therefore be rapid and aggressive, and any precipitating factors must be corrected. The drugs of choice for terminating seizures are thiopentone (thiopental), diazepam, and phenytoin, except for an eclamptic fit where magnesium is indicated (see Chapter 45). Check the serum level of the maintenance therapy.

Recurrent seizures or status epilepticus should be treated with infusion of chlormethiazole and the patient monitored in a high dependency unit (HDU). Ventilatory support may be required. Neuromuscular blocking agents, ventilation, and a good cardiac output prevent acidosis from the intense muscle activity associated with seizures. Continuous electroencephalographic monitoring is mandatory in such circumstances.

### Cerebrovascular disease

Transient ischaemic attacks are brief episodes of focal neurological disturbance with an abrupt onset and, usually, full recovery within a few minutes. Most authors accept 'transient' as a duration of symptoms and signs for up to a maximum of 24 hours. They are often associated with amaurosis fugax, and are caused by small emboli from the carotid (listen for a bruit) or vertebral arteries. The patients are sometimes maintained on antiplatelet therapy (e.g. aspirin). If the frequency of attacks increases it can indicate a prestroke syndrome.

A stroke or cerebrovascular accident (CVA) implies an area of permanent brain damage resulting from a circulatory disturbance. As symptoms develop, it is called a 'stroke in evolution' and once they are stationary it is called a 'completed stroke'. CVA can result from thrombosis, embolism, or haemorrhage. Clinical differentiation between these causes is impossible, except that embolism is more likely if there is atrial fibrillation, after myocardial infarction, or in endocarditis. Haemorrhage is more common in people with hypertension, and thrombotic episodes tend to have a slower, more protracted evolution. Definitive diagnosis is now usually made by computed tomography. In Britain over 100 000 people are living with the permanent effects of CVA.

**Table 63.2 Agents and other factors that might cause a seizure in the perioperative period**

| Patient related | Serum related | Drug related | Technique related |
|---|---|---|---|
| Poor existing control | Hypoglycaemia | Omission of anticonvulsant therapy | Hypoxia |
| Pre-eclampsia | Hyponatraemia | Proconvulsant drugs | Hypercapnia |
| Pyrexia | Uraemia | | Hypocapnia |

| Table 63.3 Use of anaesthetic drugs in people with epilepsy | | |
|---|---|---|
| Indicated | Probably safe | Contraindicated |
| Thiopentone | Propofol | Methohexitone |
| Benzodiazepines | Lignocaine | Ketamine |
| Isoflurane | | Etomidate |
| Halothane | | Enflurane |
| Opioids | | |
| Nitrous oxide | | |

***Preoperative considerations***

Look for a cause for the CVA (hypertension, excess anticoagulation, heart disease) and treat it appropriately. Otherwise, the extent of the stroke must be recorded carefully, both for baseline data and for medicolegal reasons. If there has been an accurate diagnosis of thromboembolic disease, the patient may be on anticoagulant or antiplatelet drugs. This therapy must be continued unless there are serious indications to the contrary.

Many patients have expressive rather than receptive problems, so ask questions in a manner that allows the patient to answer 'yes' or 'no' rather than with a full sentence. Emotional lability is common and dementia may occur. Taking a history can be impossible or unreliable. In long-standing cases, look for drip sites on the non-spastic limb and position them carefully to give maximum freedom of the wrist.

***Intraoperative phase***

Apart from careful positioning of the affected limbs, which often have poor quality skin, the main aim is to maintain cerebral haemodynamics at their preoperative level by controlling the blood pressure and cerebral blood flow. Remember that much of the work on cerebral blood flow quoted for healthy brains does not apply to diseased brains in which there is a loss of autoregulation.

The patient should be maintained normotensive and normocapnic. Hypotension may cause ischaemic infarction whereas hypertension may cause a cerebral haemorrhage. Intubation is an obvious time of danger and a smooth technique must be the aim.

In the acute phase after a CVA, there is an area of luxury perfusion to recoverable tissue around the lesion where there is maximum vasodilatation. If the arterial $CO_2$ tension ($Paco_2$) rises (or high concentrations of volatile agents are used), blood flow to other healthy areas of the brain increases and the luxury perfusion may fall, causing an increase in neuronal death (steal syndrome). Alternatively, if the $Paco_2$ falls, blood flow to the healthy areas falls, but flow to the area around the lesions is maintained (inverse steal). It has been postulated that this may lead to further infarction of 'healthy' brain. Consequently, normocapnia is essential. For all but the shortest operations, this implies intermittent positive pressure ventilation (IPPV).

Suxamethonium can produce changes in potassium flux after an upper motor neuron injury, similar to those secondary to a lower motor neuron injury. The mechanism for this is unclear because the motor endplate is unaffected.

***Postoperative phase***

The patient requires good recovery facilities and facemask oxygen. The blood pressure is often labile. Avoid ventilatory depression with consequent hypercapnia and hypoxia. Postoperative confusion is frequent. Treat the cause (hypoxia, hypotension, pain, full bladder, hypoglycaemia, etc.). Sedation may make matters worse. Good physiotherapy reduces atelectasis and pneumonia, and prevents contractures.

## Parkinson's disease

Parkinson's disease is predominantly a disease of elderly people, affecting over 1% of the population over 65 years old. It is probably under-diagnosed. It presents as a disturbance of voluntary motor function with:

- rigidity of the limb and trunk muscles (lead-pipe or cogwheel rigidity of the elbows and knees);
- a shuffling gait, bradykinesia;
- an expressionless, unblinking face;
- monotonous slurred speech;
- a 'pill-rolling' tremor (5/second) of the hands;
- autonomic instability.

Often the symptoms are asymmetrical, and there is emotional lability and depression. Eventually the patient may become wheelchair bound and have difficulty swallowing.

Most cases are idiopathic; some are ascribed to previous encephalitis, some are associated with widespread cerebrovascular disease, and some are secondary to phenothiazine or butyrophenone therapy. This last group is represented mainly by people with schizophrenia or manic depression. All cases result from the depletion of dopamine in the basal ganglia.

The main anaesthetic problems, which are worse if treatment is suboptimal, are:

- taking an adequate history;
- poor motivation to assist in their own recovery postoperatively;
- muscular weakness and rigidity.

Muscle weakness can result in hypoventilation. Aspiration pneumonia may also occur. Phenothiazines or butyrophenones should not be included in the anaesthetic or be used to treat postoperative confusion.

Most patients are maintained on levodopa, which is decarboxylated to dopamine in the brain. It is effective in reducing most symptoms in 75% of all patients, but especially so in those with bradykinesia. Decarboxylase is widespread throughout the body, and hence using levodopa is equivalent to giving a dopamine infusion. Side effects are common; those that affect the patient most are anorexia, nausea, and vomiting. Those that affect the anaesthetist are the cardiovascular effects (arrhythmias, tachycardia, hypertension, postural hypotension, peripheral vasconstriction, and dilatation of mesenteric and renal vessels). Levodopa is often combined with carbidopa, an extracerebral decarboxylase inhibitor. This, by reducing the peripheral breakdown of levodopa, enables the effective dose of levodopa to be lowered and the peripheral side effects of nausea, vomiting, and the cardiac disturbances to be minimized. Unfortunately, there is occasionally an increased incidence of abnormal involuntary movements.

#### *Factors relevant to anaesthetic management*

The principles of good practice outlined in section 1 of the book are assumed:

- The half-life of levodopa is only 4 hours. Cessation may cause rebound parkinsonism with the difficulties of excessive salivation and chest rigidity. This can be severe enough to interfere with adequate ventilation. It should therefore be continued on the day of surgery. Sudden withdrawal of levodopa or use of antidopaminergic drugs may result in life-threatening, centrally mediated pyrexia (neuroleptic malignant syndrome) and may impair the patient's postoperative mobility.
- There have been reports of suxamethonium producing hyperkalaemia, and of pethidine worsening rigidity.
- There may be excessive salivation and oesophageal reflux.
- There may be autonomic neuropathy and postural hypotension.
- Postoperatively, there may be a high incidence of obstructive and central sleep apnoea.
- If an antiemetic is required, ondansetron is the agent of choice. Metoclopramide and phenothiazines are contraindicated.

Note that well-planned postoperative care is required because of the factors listed above. Physiotherapy is particularly important.

### Multiple sclerosis

This is a disease of the central nervous system (CNS) in which acute episodes of neurological deficit appear irregularly in both time and site. It is principally a disorder of young adults, with an onset between 15 and 40 years and an average expectation of life of 20–30 years after the first symptoms. The incidence is high in temperate latitudes (1 per 1700 population) and low in the Tropics. Certain inbred groups (e.g. Orkney Islanders) appear to have an inherited predisposition.

Pathologically, the lesions are areas of demyelination, occurring most commonly in the optic nerves, brain stem, cerebellum, and dorsal and pyramidal tracts. Initially, symptoms disappear completely after the acute episode has passed, but eventually with subsequent attacks residual deficits increase. The most common deficits are optic atrophy, diplopia, nystagmus, vertigo, cerebellar signs, paraesthesia, loss of proprioception, upper motor neuron lesions, and disordered bladder function. There may be euphoria or depression. The disease process often culminates in an incontinent, wheelchair-bound, spastic individual suffering from flexor spasms and bed sores. Diagnosis can be confirmed by a magnetic resonance imaging scan of the brain and spinal cord. There is no specific treatment. Immunosuppressive therapies (e.g. beta-interferon and low-dose methotrexate) modify the disease process in a minority of patients; however, their place in routine treatment has yet to be determined. Despite the relatively high prevalence of multiple sclerosis there is surprisingly little literature giving clear-cut advice with respect to anaesthetic management.

#### *Anaesthetic considerations*

During the preoperative visit, assess the patient's mental state, look for contractures and bed sores (think of positioning during the operation), and check the drug therapy (some are on adrenocorticotrophic hormone or steroids). Of particular relevance are the presence of a bulbar palsy (making gastric reflux and inhalational pneumonia probable complications) and autonomic hyper-reflexia (see Chapter 64). Assess the ventilatory reserve.

All elective surgery should be performed only if the patient is free from infection (pulmonary or other). Record the patient's preoperative disability on the anaesthetic sheet.

It has frequently been said that pregnancy or any form of stress, emotional or surgical, can lead to a relapse of intensification of symptomatology. These effects usually abate after 10–14 days and are thought to be the result of a rise in body temperature (as small as 0.5–1°C) producing a conduction block in demyelinated nerves. It is therefore logical to use sedative premedication, prophylactic antibiotics, and a mild antipyretic (e.g. aspirin) postoperatively.

##### *General anaesthesia*

There is no hard evidence that any one particular technique or combination of drugs has advantages over any other. Monitor the temperature in long operations and do not allow it to rise by the over-enthusiastic use of humidified gases or warming blankets. Neuromuscular blocking agents should be used sparingly. During a period of active upper motor neuron demyelination, there may be a rise in serum potassium after giving suxamethonium. Suxamethonium is therefore contraindicated unless the disease is quiescent and there is a specific reason to use it (e.g. expected difficult intubation). In those with bulbar palsy, endotracheal intubation is indicated for most operations, and especially if the patient is likely to be put in the head-down position.

##### *Regional anaesthesia*

There is reluctance to use local anaesthetics because the patient may attribute any subsequent relapse to the anaesthetic if a limb has been therapeutically paralysed. There is, however, no evidence that surgery under regional blockade is any more, or less, likely to precipitate a relapse. Despite this, most anaesthetists avoid it for medicolegal reasons.

The most common request for regional blockade is that of epidural analgesia for childbirth. In this situation, the pros and cons of the procedure should be fully explained to the mother. Some anaesthetists would suggest that she ought to sign a consent form for medicolegal protection. If used, the wording should indicate that no relapse of the multiple sclerosis will be attributed to the epidural. Postoperatively, well planned physiotherapy is important for two reasons:

1. It aids removal of pulmonary secretions which are a problem in those with poor ventilatory function and/or bulbar palsy.
2. It prevents contractures and bed sores in affected limbs.

### Motor neuron disease

Motor neuron disease is characterized by a selective degeneration of the motor neurons of the corticospinal pathways, the brain stem, and the anterior horns of the spinal cord. There are, therefore, a mixture of upper and lower motor neuronal signs. The onset is usually insidious and death occurs within 2–3 years. There are three main clinical varieties, which overlap:

1. Progressive muscular atrophy presents with the symptoms of a lower motor neuron lesion, most commonly in the hands and arms. Fasciculation, wasting, weakness, stiffness, clumsiness, and cramp-like pains occur. Gradually, all muscles in the body may be affected.
2. Progressive bulbar palsy presents with a wasted, strawberry, fibrillating tongue. Control of the tongue is poor; the muscles of the larynx and pharynx become involved. Speech suffers because of paresis of the lips, tongue, and palate. Swallowing becomes increasingly difficult, food regurgitates, and inhalational pneumonia is common. Emaciation characterizes the later stages. A pseudobulbar palsy (upper motor neuron lesion) is frequently superimposed with its attendant emotional lability.
3. Amyotrophic lateral sclerosis describes a degeneration of the upper motor neurons in the corticospinal tracts. This adds a further element of weakness, spasticity, and exaggerated tendon jerks. Spasticity is usually more prominent in the legs than in the arms.

#### *Anaesthetic considerations*

- There is usually poor airway control and a high risk of inhalational pneumonia.
- Suxamethonium may induce hyperkalaemia.
- There may be a myasthenic-like response to non-depolarizing neuromuscular blocking agents.
- Patients are often emaciated with poor ventilatory reserve. They need intensive postoperative physiotherapy.

This is no literature to suggest that any particular anaesthetic technique is the best.

### Hereditary ataxias

This term covers a group of closely related disorders, usually hereditary or familial, which are characterized by degeneration of some or all of the following parts of the nervous system: the optic nerves, the cerebellum, the olives, and the long ascending tracts of the spinal cord. The most common (which is still rare) is Friedreich's ataxia.

Cerebellar ataxia is noted first in the legs and then in the hands, between the ages of 5 and 15 years. Pyramidal tract disease produces upper motor neuron lesions of the legs with muscle weakness and spasticity. Dorsal column involvement results in absent tendon jerks. Proprioceptive changes are inconsistent. There may be a mild dementia and optic atrophy. Nystagmus and diplopia are common. There is an associated cardiomyopathy with arrhythmias and heart failure which is usually the cause of death at the age of 40–50 years.

There are few published data on the anaesthetic management of these patients. The considerations are those of suxamethonium during or after a demyelinating episode, the sparing use of non-depolarizing neuromuscular blocking agents in people with muscular weakness, and the management of cardiomyopathy and arrhythmias. These patients present principally for elective orthopaedic procedures on the feet.

### Neurofibromatosis (von Recklinghausen's disease)

Neurofibromatosis is inherited as a mendelian dominant condition, with an incidence of approximately 1 in 3000. Its severity varies enormously and it has an equal sex incidence. It is usually characterized by cutaneous pigmentation and tumours on the peripheral nerves (neurofibroma) and skin (cutaneous fibroma). Blood loss from lesions in the gastrointestinal tract can be a problem. Less commonly, neurofibromas also form on the spinal nerve roots within the CNS (acoustic neuroma), in the autonomic nervous system, and in the pharynx and larynx. Epilepsy may occur. Other rare but associated abnormalities are kyphoscoliosis, interstitial pulmonary fibrosis, phaeochromocytoma ($<1\%$), medullary carcinoma of the thyroid, and hyperthyroidism.

Most patients live a normal span and neurofibromatosis is an unimportant condition unless symptoms arise as a result of the size and position of the tumour or because an associated disease develops.

Anaesthetic management is that of the individual symptoms that the patient presents with (e.g. effective cord transection from large fibroma), and screening for and dealing with any associated disorder, especially phaeochromocytoma. Caution is required when deciding to perform spinal and epidural techniques. Intrancranial pressure may be raised – dural puncture or trauma to a neurofibroma could be disastrous. Lumbar neurofibromas can be large but asymptomatic, making entry to the epidural or subarachnoid space difficult. Apart from this, there are no specific anaesthetic recommendations.

### Spina bifida

Spina bifida is a congenital condition caused by a failure of the neural tube to fuse posteriorly, usually in the lumbar region. It has a presentation that is variable in severity. The incidence varies widely across the world but is typically 2 per 1000 live births. Improved prenatal diagnosis has resulted in many being aborted, so the current incidence is difficult to estimate.

There are, however, now many people with spina bifida who have survived earlier surgery and are now teenagers and young adults. For these survivors who have had the defect closed, their life is often characterized by recurrent hospital admission for a variety of complications of their condition. They present for urological, bowel, orthopaedic, and neurological procedures and are encountered at some time by most anaesthetists. The spectrum of problems and presentations is very variable, and each patient must be assessed and dealt with individually. Always try to get the patient weighed: their weight is difficult to estimate because of the under-growth of the lower body. The complications for anaesthesia are given below.

*Mental state*

Their level of intelligence can vary from learning disabled to highly intelligent. The level of cerebral performance may not be apparent on an initial meeting, because their appearance and often distorted, slow speech can give a false impression. Some also have hearing and vision difficulties. Care, sympathy, and respect for the individual's intelligence are obviously important in communication. It is not infrequent also to have to deal with other members of the family, social workers, or a local support group. Some patients are understandably unhappy and are on antidepressants.

*Central nervous system*

There are often associated abnormalities of the whole of the spinal cord and sometimes the brain. Many have ventriculoperitoneal shunts inserted and they can present with the complications of these in both the brain and peritoneum. Disinterest, disorientation, and, most importantly, reduced conscious level may, on occasion, be the result of a blocked shunt.

*Cardiovascular system*

As a result of the restricted lifestyle, usually in a wheelchair, angina of effort or shortness of breath on exertion may not present as symptoms. They are, however, as likely as any other members of the public to develop ischaemic heart disease.

*Respiratory system*

The upper airways can be either normal or, on occasions, very abnormal. Abnormalities result from malformation of the spinal column, surgical fusions, and contractions of the cervical musculature. A number of people with spina bifida have severe kyphoscoliosis, with a restrictive pattern of breathing and poor respiratory reserve. Some have a bulbar palsy and swallowing difficulties with repeated pulmonary aspiration.

*Kidney*

Almost all these patients are catheterized, and if not they will have had ureteric reimplantation with consequent effects on serum electrolytes. Others have anatomical and structural abnormalities of the urinary tract, which results in stones and renal impairment.

*Locomotor system*

Spina bifida patients are often crippled in appearance, especially from the waist downwards. The cervical spine may be abnormal, and the combination of this and kyphosis may mean the use of a number of pillows to make them comfortable. A number have symptoms of cervical nerve compression in the shoulders and anus. Contractures of joints, particularly the hips and knees, may be present.

#### *Anaesthetic considerations*

*Preoperative*

A full work-up taking account of the features listed above is essential. It is vital to be absolutely clear what the surgical procedure is going to be, and, very importantly, what position the patient will have to adopt.

No particular anaesthetic technique is preferred.

*Induction and intubation*

If this is anticipated to be difficult, the counsel of perfection may be to establish endotracheal intubation with the patient awake. However, the mental state of some of these patients is such that it may be distressing for them, or they may be unable to understand what is involved. What is required is for an experienced anaesthetist to decide on balance and clinical judgement what is best for that individual patient. This may range, as suggested above, from an awake intubation to more imaginative approaches such as a sitting inhalational technique. In part, the position that the patient is able to adopt may determine the method chosen.

*Maintenance*

Positioning (see Chapter 3) is very important and can be very time-consuming. The patient may not have lain flat for years, and careful padding with foam and pillows may be necessary to support the back, limbs, and head in unusual positions. Positioning can be even more of a problem if the prone position is required.

*Recovery*

This needs to be carried out with considerable care:

- Before consciousness returns, place the patient in a position that they are known to be comfortable adopting. This may require them to be semi-recumbent or even sitting. When moving from the horizontal to such a position, monitor the pulse and blood pressure (BP) carefully.
- Do not extubate until the patient is fully awake.
- Make proper arrangements for them to be cared for appropriately on the ward, HDU, or intensive care unit (ICU), depending on their needs and circumstances.

## PERIPHERAL NERVOUS SYSTEM DISORDERS

### Guillain–Barré syndrome

The anaesthetist meets patients with the Guillain–Barré syndrome on the ICU and for anaesthesia for tracheostomy. The condition has a mortality rate of up to 10% depending on its severity.

It is defined as a subacute polyneuritis of unknown aetiology, which is thought to be secondary to an allergic phenomenon affecting the peripheral nerves. In 60% of cases, in the month preceding onset, there has been an infection (viral or bacterial), an injury (traumatic or surgical), or an immunization.

Symptoms, characterized by weakness, pain, and sensory abnormalities, develop over days or weeks, with 50% of patients having a maximal disability by 2 weeks, and 90% by 4 weeks. Weakness is symmetrical and more pronounced proximally. Areflexia occurs early and the cranial nerves (especially the facial) may be affected.

There is then a stationary phase of days or weeks followed by a slow recovery. Only a minority have residual neurological defects. Most patients resume their occupation by 6 months, but full recovery may take up to 2 years. In addition to the characteristic peripheral sensory and motor nerve changes, autonomic nerves may be affected with bladder and cardiovascular instability.

The cornerstone of therapy is to keep the patient as well as possible until spontaneous recovery occurs. This implies good nursing (to avoid pressure sores), intensive physiotherapy (to prevent chest infection or limb contractures), some sort of urinary collection if necessary (e.g. Paul's tubing, catheterization), a cheerful, friendly, forward-looking environment (to prevent depression), and an assiduous check on ventilatory and pharyngeal musculature.

The greatest danger for these patients is ventilatory failure. Serial blood gases are useless. Abnormal results indicate only that corrective measures are being taken too late. The best way of monitoring ventilatory function is to monitor the vital capacity at least twice daily, and to plot it on a chart. If there is an inexorable downward trend, once the vital capacity is less than twice the tidal volume, artificial ventilation needs to be considered. Elective tracheostomy should be done early. If there are weak respiratory muscles, there are usually problems with swallowing and inhalational pneumonia is a very real danger. It is then best to insert a nasogastric tube for feeding and commence a standard regimen. The patient seriously ill with the Guillain–Barré syndrome may not reveal his or her anxiety because of facial weakness. There is a high risk of deep venous thrombosis and pulmonary embolus, and some authorities recommend routine anticoagulation.

From the patient's viewpoint, this is a frightening disease because the obvious paralysis and danger to life occur in full consciousness. Therefore, constant sympathetic reassurance is vital for morale and, if possible, the patient should have some means of attracting the attention of staff when he or she wants to. This often requires improvisation with the positioning of a buzzer or bell pull.

Monitor the ECG and BP routinely. Abnormalities may result from a pulmonary embolus or from an autonomic neuropathy. Treat cardiovascular changes if these are symptomatic or dangerous.

Approximately three out of every four patients show a persistent tachycardia with one having postural hypotension. Other cardiac arrhythmias such as bradycardia and sinus arrest have been reported. One-third of patients have excessive episodic sweating. In those affected sufficiently to be on an ICU, a common finding is severe postural hypotension. It is important to look for this positively and to alert nurses and physiotherapists to its dangers. The patient at particular risk is the one who is 'sat out for a few minutes' while the bed is changed. The use of steroids in this condition is controversial.

#### *Anaesthetic considerations*

A patient with the Guillain–Barré syndrome may require anaesthesia for tracheostomy.

The major problem is the instability of the cardiovascular system. Large falls in BP can be produced by induction agents, changes in posture, blood loss, or IPPV. The patient should therefore be preoxygenated, a large-bore intravenous cannula inserted, and the induction drugs given slowly. Fluid loading may be necessary to maintain the blood pressure. Exercise care in the use of α- and β-adrenoceptor agonists to produce peripheral vasconstriction. These patients are exquisitely sensitive to their actions.

Measures to prevent thromboembolism (see Chapter 1) are mandatory. Suxamethonium should be avoided in the active stages of the condition because widespread denervation may result in hyperkalaemia.

## NEUROMUSCULAR JUNCTION DISORDERS

### Denervation hypersensitivity

The lower motor neuron exerts a trophic influence on the myoneural junction and any disease affecting it results in a loss of organization of the end-plate. This degeneration starts at about 24 hours, is maximal at 2–4 weeks, and lasts for up to 9 months. Its effect is to make the whole muscle membrane (not just the end-plate region) sensitive to acetylcholine and its analogues (this applies to suxamethonium but not to non-depolarizing neuromuscular blocking agents, which are structurally dissimilar). When depolarization occurs, it does so throughout the whole muscle membrane surface, with the potential for massive ionic swings. Most of the work on this effect has been done in animal models. Evidence in humans is limited to isolated case reports, but these are sufficient in number to be certain that rises in serum potassium of up to 6 mmol/L are possible after suxamethonium is given, especially if repeat doses are used. Pre-treatment with a non-depolarizing neuromuscular blocking agent is unpredictable in reducing the level of the potassium efflux, and the best method of prevention is the avoidance of suxamethonium in the crucial period.

Although the mechanism has never been explained, similar changes in potassium flux after suxamethonium administration have been described in patients with hemiplegia (upper motor neuron), tetanus, and encephalitis.

Acute rises in serum potassium after suxamethonium administration also occur frequently in patients with burns and massive tissue damage, and rarely in patients with myopathy and myositis. The mechanism here is not, however, the result of disorganization of the motor end-plate and its loss of trophic ability, but is an abnormality of the muscle membrane itself which 'leaks' during fasciculation.

### Myasthenia gravis

'True' myasthenia is an autoimmune disease with antibodies to acetylcholine receptors, which affects the post-junctional membrane. It can occur in association with other conditions:

- thymoma;
- thyroid disorders;
- rheumatoid arthritis;
- other autoimmune conditions (e.g. systemic lupus erythematosus).

Myasthenia is rare with an incidence of 1 in 20 000 adults and a 2 : 1 female : male ratio.

The clinical onset is usually slow and progressive over 5 years or more, but it can occasionally follow a fulminant course. There can be periods of remission of up to 3 years. Clinically, it presents as a muscular weakness characterized by fatiguability after repetitive or sustained contraction. It is most marked in the face and eyes, producing diplopia and ptosis. Speech and swallowing become affected and there may be a proximal upper limb weakness. The lower limbs are affected last. The greatest danger is the involvement of the ventilatory muscles (this may be very insidious) and bulbar palsy. In myasthenia crisis, ventilatory function should be monitored as in the Guillain–Barré syndrome (see page 932). Rarely, there is a cardiomyopathy.

Treatment of the neuromuscular weakness is by a long-acting anticholinesterase (e.g. pyridostigmine). This merely presents more acetylcholine to the postsynaptic membrane. Atropine may occasionally be required to prevent bradycardia and to reduce abdominal cramps. Many patients also take ephedrine. An overdose of anticholinesterase can result in a depolarizing block (cholinergic crisis), which is difficult to distinguish clinically from a myasthenic crisis. The two can usually be separated by the lack of response to edrophonium in a cholinergic crisis. The management of both is similar to that of the Guillain–Barré syndrome (see above): control of the airway, suction, and, if necessary, artificial ventilation until medical management is effective. A change in an individual's requirements for anticholinesterase can be the result of progression of the disease or of intercurrent infection.

In addition to anticholinesterase, long-term drug treatment is by steroids and/or azathioprine and/or thymectomy, in an effort to control the progress of the autoimmune process. Also, plasmapheresis is becoming increasingly employed, particularly in the more fulminant cases.

#### *Preoperative considerations*

Assess the patient carefully. Warn of the likelihood of postoperative ventilation. Put the patient where he or she can be closely observed on the day before the operation. In the past, the accepted procedure was to omit the dose of anticholinesterase immediately before surgery if intraoperative IPPV was planned, but continue it if spontaneous ventilation was to be used. Nowadays, opinion has swung towards giving maintenance therapy as usual, together with any other relevant drugs (e.g. steroids, azathioprine, cyclosporin).

A benzodiazepine premedication is usually safe, and prophylaxis against acid aspiration should be routine.

#### *Intraoperative phase*

Regional or general anaesthesia may be used. Lignocaine (lidocaine) is the preferred local anaesthetic. After its use, the patient requires close observation until the drug has been absorbed and metabolized. For operations on the arms, legs, lower abdomen, and perineum, regional block is often the method of choice.

For general anaesthesia, only short cases in those patients with good ventilatory function (measure vital capacity) ought to be done on a facemask or laryngeal mask airway. All others require intubation and IPPV. Thiopentone or propofol is suitable for induction. If intubation is required, care needs to be taken with the use of neuromuscular blocking agents.

Resistance to suxamethonium occurs as a result of blockade of acetylcholine receptors, so increased doses are often needed for rapid sequence induction. Even so, the dose required is unpredictable, both 'resistance' and 'sensitivity' having been recorded. (If the patient has had a plasma exchange for a myasthenic crisis, it takes several days for the pseudocholinesterase to be replaced unless fresh frozen plasma is given.)

Patients with myasthenia have an exaggerated response to non-depolarizing neuromuscular blocking agents, and these should be used with great care. Sensitivity to these agents occurs as a result of reduced numbers of acetylcholine receptors; one-tenth the normal dose will often provide adequate relaxation. Atracurium and vecuronium have both been used safely in patients with myasthenia and can be completely reversed. Neuromuscular monitoring is mandatory for titration of neuromuscular blocking agents.

Reversal of residual block with neostigmine and atropine is safe, but excessive doses above those that the patient is taking orally may precipitate a cholinergic crisis; 1 mg neostigmine i.v. is equivalent to 30 mg orally because of its poor bioavailability. Another approach that has been satisfactorily used by the author is to avoid the use of neuromuscular blocking agents altogether. Anaesthesia is deepened after induction by ventilating on a facemask with a volatile agent. Intubation is achieved after spraying the vocal cords with local anaesthetic. As a result of the possibility of postoperative ventilation, it may be best to intubate nasally with an endotracheal tube that has a low-pressure cuff. Maintenance is by nitrous oxide, oxygen, and an opioid, with or without a volatile agent.

Any cardiomyopathy should be treated appropriately.

#### *Postoperative phase*

Most patients with well-controlled or mild myasthenia will tolerate anaesthesia as described above with relatively few problems. After satisfactory extubation, they need careful monitoring for at least 24 hours on an HDU or in an environment used to caring for such patients.

However, some patients, especially if they have had major surgery, who were difficult to control preoperatively and have continuing infection, may have increased anticholinesterase requirements. It is, therefore, often best in these cases to continue IPPV on the

ICU and gradually increase the dose of anticholinesterase (given intravenously or via the nasogastric tube) until respiratory muscle power is satisfactory. Typical criteria for extubation are a forced vital capacity of more than 15 ml/kg and a peak occlusion pressure of more than 30 $cmH_2O$. Only extubate when the vital capacity and tidal and minute volumes are adequate and have been stable for 12–24 hours in the presence of effective analgesia. This whole process can take up to 10 days in difficult cases. Problems also occur in the postoperative period because of the concomitant administration of potassium-depleting diuretics and the 'micin' group of antibiotics.

### The myasthenic syndrome (Eaton–Lambert syndrome)

This is a myasthenic-like condition associated with an underlying carcinoma (usually oat cell of the bronchus). It is rare, even within thoracic units. The fundamental lesion is unlike that of true myasthenia. It is caused by a prejunctional failure to release acetylcholine. This results in a poor response to anticholinesterase (negative edrophonium test), a transient increase in strength before fatigue, and a sensitivity to all neuromuscular blocking agents.

Management is as for myasthenia gravis. It should be thought of as a possibility in all patients having investigations and surgery for presumed carcinoma of the bronchus, particularly in the presence of non-specific, unexplained, muscular weakness.

## DISORDERS OF MUSCLES

### The muscular dystrophies

These are a group of related disorders which are familial, primary, degenerative myopathies. They are usually progressive and all are rare.

The most common is Duchenne (pseudohypertrophic) dystrophy which occurs exclusively in males. It presents before the age of 5 years with lower limb weakness and hypertrophied calves, but some cases are undiagnosed when they present for anaesthesia. The serum creatine phosphokinase is elevated. Associated problems are cardiomyopathy, which can be life threatening under anaesthesia (they usually have ECG changes), a restrictive pattern of pulmonary disease (see Chapter 54), and an inability to cough well.

#### *Anaesthetic considerations*

Apart from anticholinesterase therapy, the principles of management of all muscular dystrophies is similar to that of myasthenia gravis and the Guillain–Barré syndrome, with special attention being paid to the cardiac and ventilatory complications. Suxamethonium is contraindicated because it releases both potassium and myoglobin from the muscles. Patients are very sensitive to non-depolarizing neuromuscular blocking agents and the myocardial depressant effects of volatile agents. In advanced cases, a period of postoperative ventilation is almost inevitable after major surgery.

### Myotonia

Myotonia is the inability of the muscle to relax normally after contraction. It is associated with a very rare group of diseases.

The most common of these diseases is dystrophia myotonica. This is a hereditary disorder producing increasingly more severe symptoms and signs with time. Presenting in the second decade, there is progressive involvement of skeletal, cardiac, and smooth muscle. The 'classic' case has frontal balding, ptosis, an expressionless face, cataracts, wasting of the shoulder and thigh muscles, and testicular or ovarian failure. There may be a severe cardiomyopathy (with sudden death from an arrhythmia) and diabetes mellitus. Mental deficiency is sometimes evident. The respiratory muscles may be affected with a restrictive pattern of breathing (see Chapter 54) and recurrent chest infections. Myotonia increases with cold, fatigue, and excitement.

#### *Anaesthetic considerations*

Apart from anticholinesterase therapy, management is as for myasthenia gravis and the Guillain–Barré syndrome, with the additional problems of cardiomyopathy, diabetes mellitus, and restrictive lung disease. Even in the absence of any evidence of cardiomyopathy, arrhythmias must be anticipated. The following are important aspects of care:

- Suxamethonium is totally contraindicated. As well as releasing potassium, it may cause a prolonged (up to 3 min), generalized, muscular contraction, clamping the jaw shut and making ventilation difficult or impossible. The response to non-depolarizing neuromuscular blocking agents is prolonged.
- Sensitivity to thiopentone, opioids, and benzodiazepines has been reported, so give small, incremental doses and observe the effect.
- As cold can intensify the myotonia, the operating room should be warm, there should be a warming blanket on the table, the inspired gases may be heated and humidified, and the patient's temperature should be monitored.
- High-quality postoperative care is essential.

## INFECTIONS

### Tetanus

As a result of widespread immunization, tetanus is now rare. When it does occur, it is more common in very young children and elderly people who have not been immunized. It has an incubation period of 4–10 days and may follow surgery, burns, otitis media, dental infection, or abortion; the practice of 'skin popping' among narcotic addicts accounts for a proportion of cases in urban centres.

The clinical features are given in Table 63.4. A poor outlook is associated with:

- short incubation period;
- rapid progress from local to general spasms;
- injury site close to the head;
- extremes of age;
- frequency and intensity of convulsions.

Severe cases have a mortality rate of 50%.

Anaesthetists become involved with the established case in transporting patients to regional centres, anaes-

| Table 63.4 Clinical features of tetanus |
| --- |
| **Early manifestations** |
| Muscle stiffness |
| Spasm of masseter muscle (trismus or lockjaw) |
| **Later manifestations** |
| Tetanospasms occur causing:<br>• clenching of the jaw (risus sardonicus)<br>• arching of the back (opisthotonos)<br>• flexion of arms, extension of legs |
| Autonomic involvement: hypo-/hypertension, arrhythmias |
| Respiratory failure, aspiration pneumonia |
| Fractures, especially of thoracic vertebrae |

thetizing them for wound debridement, and ventilating them on the ICU.

*Prophylaxis*

When anaesthetizing any patient with a dirty wound, it is the duty of all medical staff to ensure that the patient is immunized and receives either antibiotics (benzylpenicillin) or antitetanus immunoglobulin (Humotet).

*The established case*

The causative organism is *Clostridium tetani*, a spore-bearing anaerobe which enters via a wound contaminated by infected material (e.g. soil). The bacilli produce a potent toxin which is absorbed by the motor end-plate and moves centrally to the nerve cell bodies. Prediction of the severity of the attack is difficult, except that the sooner the onset of symptoms from injury (2 days is short, 3 weeks is long), the more likely that the attack is severe. All infected patients require antibiotics, passive and active immunization, and wound cleaning.

After the diagnosis, treatment is essentially supportive with close observation for the onset of complications.

*Muscular problems*

Traditionally, patients are moved into a dark room to suppress spasms. Modern thinking supports a quiet, but well-lit, room to aid the early detection of laryngeal and other muscular spasms. Mild muscle spasms respond well to diazepam. Those that do not respond need treatment with dantrolene (1 mg/kg over 2–3 hours). This, by controlling the spasms, may avoid tracheal intubation. Autonomic overactivity (with tachycardia and increased BP) can be treated by β-adrenoceptor blockade (e.g. propranolol, labetolol). Prophylactic use of these drugs is advised if intubation is planned.

Protection of the airway is vital and, if there are signs of laryngospasm, it is better to intubate early. Severe laryngospasm can sometimes be induced by swallowing saliva or attempting to pass a nasogastric tube. If there are sustained contractions of peripheral and trunk muscles, despite diazepam and dantrolene, therapeutic paralysis and IPPV are required.

*Fluid balance*

Patients with tetanus often have a profuse production of saliva and sweat. If this happens, give enough fluid to maintain a urine output of 1–2 L/day as the means of controlling fluid balance.

*Cardiovascular*

Autonomic disturbances are common. They usually appear as episodes of hypertension, tachycardia, arrhythmias, and peripheral vasoconstriction. Hypotension occasionally occurs, but if persistent it is usually pre-terminal. There are grossly exaggerated responses to intubation and tracheal suction.

***Anaesthetic considerations***

As a result of the exaggerated responses to intubation, it should be preceded by β-adrenoceptor blockade. Despite disturbances of the motor end-plate, many publications recommend a thiopentone and suxamethonium induction sequence. There have been isolated incidents of hyperkalaemia. Maintenance is best done with a nitrous oxide/oxygen/neuromuscular blocking agent/analgesic technique. Ensure a sufficient depth of anaesthesia to prevent over-reaction to visceral stimuli. Careful monitoring of the BP and ECG is essential.

All patients need to receive thromboembolic prophylaxis, and feeding (preferably enteral) should be established early. When speaking to relatives, if recovery is likely, warn them that it may take 2–4 weeks.

If called on to accompany an affected patient to another hospital, unless he or she is *very* well controlled, it is best to intubate before departure: there are many stimuli during an ambulance journey that might provoke a seizure (see Chapter 62).

## FURTHER READING


Azaar I. The response of patients with neuromuscular disorders to muscle relaxants: a review. *Anesthesiology* 1984;**61**:173–87.

Cucchiara RF, MichenfelderJD. *Clinical Neuroanaesthesia*. Edinburgh: Churchill Livingstone, 1990.

Hambly PR, Martin B. Anaesthesia for chronic spinal cord lesions. *Anaesthesia* 1998;**53**:273–89.

Haywood T, Divekar N, Karalliedde LD. Concurrent medication and the neuromuscular junction. *Eur J Anaesthesiol* 1999;**16**:77–91.

Jones RM, Healy TEJ. Anaesthesia and demyelinating disease. *Anaesthesia* 1980;**35**:879–84.

Russell SH, Hirsch NP. Anaesthesia and myotonia. *Br J Anaesth* 1994;**72**:210–16.

Van Aken H. *Neuro-anaesthetic Practice*. London: BMJ Publishing Group, 1995.

# Chapter 64 The injured patient

A.J. Sutcliffe

Patients involved in accidents vary widely with regard to the number of injuries sustained, the physiological and anatomical complexity of the injury, and the relevance of each injury to resuscitation, anaesthesia, and the eventual outcome. Each patient requires detailed assessment and an individually planned and carefully executed anaesthetic. Advanced Trauma Life Support (ATLS) guidelines provide a comprehensive method of preoperative assessment which, for most patients, will ensure that all significant injuries are diagnosed, that resuscitation is prompt and effective, and that a structured management plan can be implemented.

## ATLS: RESUSCITATION, ASSESSMENT, INVESTIGATION, AND DIAGNOSIS

### The primary survey: rapid assessment and management of life-threatening injuries

The assessment and management of the injured patient is divided into three phases. The first phase is the primary survey when **a**irway, **b**reathing, **c**irculation, and **d**isability are rapidly assessed, the patient's clothes are removed so that he or she is **e**xposed, and treatment is begun. Oxygen via a facemask may be all that is required, but inability to maintain the airway, loss of protective reflexes with the risk of pulmonary aspiration of stomach contents, and significant oropharyngeal haemorrhage or injury are indications for endotracheal intubation. Breathing difficulty is an indication for controlled mechanical ventilation if simple measures such as analgesia or drainage of a pneumothorax do not help. Ventilation is also indicated for head-injured patients with a Glasgow Coma Score of 8 or less (Table 64.1) who are at risk of raised intracranial pressure (ICP).

Before endotracheal intubation, it is important to recognize the risk of cervical spine instability, particularly in unconscious patients and those with blunt injury above the clavicle. A plain lateral radiograph showing all seven cervical vertebrae is essential, and other views may be required to demonstrate injury. If a cervical spine injury cannot be excluded, the neck must be immobilized using a spinal board, sandbags, and tape or a rigid, well-fitting collar.

Hypovolaemia should be suspected in the presence of either injuries known to cause significant blood loss (Table 64.2) or hypotension and tachycardia. Although severe brain-stem injury may cause hypotension, this is usually associated with bradycardia. Head injury should never be assumed to be the cause of hypotension until all causes of haemorrhage have been excluded. In the presence of hypovolaemia, fluid should be given through

**Table 64.1 Glasgow Coma Score**

| Scoring criteria | Response |
|---|---|
| **Eye opening** | |
| 4 | Spontaneous |
| 3 | To speech |
| 2 | To pain |
| 1 | None |
| **Verbal** | |
| 5 | Orientated |
| 4 | Confused conversation |
| 3 | Inappropriate words |
| 2 | Incomprehensible sounds |
| 1 | None |
| **Best motor response** | |
| 6 | Moves limb to command |
| 5 | Localizes painful stimulus |
| 4 | Withdraws from painful stimulus |
| 3 | Abnormal flexion |
| 2 | Extension, decerebrate posturing |
| 1 | None |

**Table 64.2 Blood loss after injury**

| Injury | Blood loss (litres) |
|---|---|
| Fractured humerus | 0.5–1.0 |
| Foot or ankle fracture | 0.5–1.0 |
| Lower leg fracture | 1.0–2.0 |
| Femoral fracture | 1.5–3.0 |
| Pelvic fracture | 1.0–4.0+ |
| Rib fractures | 0.5–3.0 |
| Intracavity injury | 1.0–6.0+ |

Note that losses are a guide only and are based on the total losses measured in the first 24 hours after injury.

two large-bore cannulae positioned above and below the diaphragm. Up to 2 L of crystalloid should be given, followed by colloid and blood. Although prompt and accurate replacement of fluid loss is recommended for most injured patients, recent evidence suggests that patients with penetrating thoracic injury do better if fluid resuscitation is delayed until surgery has started. There is a trend towards delayed fluid resuscitation or restricted, hypotensive (i.e. systolic blood pressure of 80 mmHg) resuscitation for other injuries causing major blood loss. The success of this approach depends on early surgical control of haemorrhage. Its precise place in the management of the injured patient has yet to be fully evaluated.

### Secondary survey: history, examination, investigation, and treatment planning

During the primary survey, assessment and life-saving treatment occur simultaneously. They may continue during the second phase known as the secondary survey. This phase is divided quite distinctly into assessment and investigation, followed by definitive treatment, which should be planned in an orderly manner appropriate to the number and type of injuries. A detailed history obtained from relatives, witnesses, or paramedics may give clues to the type and severity of injuries sustained. A mnemonic – AMPLE – helps to remind the anaesthetist to identify **a**llergies, **m**edication, **p**ast illnesses, **l**ast meal, and **e**vents/**e**nvironment. The last may indicate additional problems for the anaesthetist, such as hypothermia caused by prolonged entrapment, or hazards such as chemical spills. A past history of diabetes or ischaemic heart disease may suggest a medical incident as the cause of the accident. After a full history has been obtained, the patient is examined from head to toe using:

- the eyes to detect anatomical deformities, bruising, or bleeding from wounds and orifices;
- touch to detect boggy swellings, tenderness, and crepitus or steps indicating fractures;
- ears to listen for abnormalities of airway control, breathing, and gastrointestinal function.

It is important to examine the patient's back. Log-rolling is essential if there could be a spinal injury.

The physical examination will usually identify which body compartments are injured and confirmation of the diagnosis is made by radiological and laboratory tests. Blood for cross-match and arterial blood gas analysis should be taken as soon as possible after admission, usually at the time that the cannulae are placed. The presence of a metabolic acidosis is important and indicates tissue hypoxia secondary to respiratory insufficiency and/or hypovolaemia. It is customary to measure haemoglobin, but the result will be misleadingly normal if the blood sample is drawn before fluid resuscitation has been given and haemodilution has occurred. Biochemical testing frequently reveals hypokalaemia and hyperglycaemia. These abnormalities are a manifestation of the humoral stress response to injury, and usually return to normal without specific treatment as resuscitation progresses.

The treatment plan will include ongoing resuscitative measures, initiation of appropriate monitoring of the respiratory, cardiovascular, renal, and nervous systems, provision of analgesia, and, if necessary, planned surgical intervention and a period in intensive care.

### Reassessment

The last phase of ATLS is reassessment. Knowledge of the patient's injuries will enable the anaesthetist to make a judgement regarding the level of respiratory and cardiovascular support that should be required. If there is a discrepancy between the support actually needed and that expected, an occult injury should be suspected. Re-examination of the patient may reveal an undiagnosed injury in the chest or abdomen. Stab wounds to the upper abdomen may have penetrated the diaphragm, leading to cardiac tamponade or tension pneumothorax. Occasionally, severe soft tissue injury, a large scalp laceration, or a heavy nose bleed causes unexpectedly large blood losses. Reassessment should occur at repeated intervals for at least the first 48 hours after injury. Fractures, particularly those that are not surgically immobilized, and soft tissue injuries continue to ooze for many hours. Furthermore, vasoconstriction in response to haemorrhage resolves slowly, unless reversed pharmacologically as part of planned treatment or during anaesthesia. Both situations require continued blood replacement. Rarely, a small laceration of the liver, spleen, or diaphragm may remain undetected for several days.

### Anaesthetic considerations relating to the timing of surgery

The ATLS system provides a method by which the anaesthetist and surgeon may assess, monitor, and plan definitive treatment of the injured patient in a structured way. Detailed discussion may be necessary to decide the optimum time for surgery, which should occur when the risks of early intervention outweigh the benefits of delay to permit completion of resuscitation and optimization of pre-existing medical diseases. Emergency anaesthesia, when resuscitation occurs in tandem with definitive treatment, may be indicated for injuries to the major airways or chest and abdominal injuries causing uncontrollable haemorrhage. In the past, emergency procedures were performed, first to overcome the immediate threat to life and, second, to complete the definitive repair. There has been a recent trend towards a new method known as damage-control surgery. During damage-control surgery, the life-saving and repair components of surgery are staged, with the patient being nursed in intensive care between each surgical procedure. The philosophy is that each surgical procedure is limited to that which causes the minimum physiological derangement. The interim period in intensive care is used to restore circulating blood volume, optimize oxygenation, correct clotting abnormalities, and restore normothermia.

Urgent anaesthesia in the first 24 hours after injury is common. It may be required for the evacuation of intracerebral haematomas, the control of intrathoracic or intra-abdominal haemorrhage, the repair of damaged intrathoracic or intra-abdominal organs, or surgical fixation of fractures. There is a widespread belief that early surgical fixation of fractures reduces the incidence of pulmonary complications, facilitates nursing care, and promotes a more rapid recovery from injury. Outcome is, however, more dependent on the severity of concurrent head and chest injuries and the quality of their management than on the timing and method of treating fractures. Each patient should be considered as an individual when decisions are made regarding the timing of surgery.

## ANAESTHESIA FOR THE INJURED PATIENT: GENERAL CONSIDERATIONS

From the anaesthetist's perspective, the timing of surgical treatment will depend on the need for resuscitation, the need for optimization of concurrent medical conditions, and the need to empty the stomach.

### The full stomach

Stomach emptying is delayed or may cease completely from the time of injury for up to 24 hours afterwards. This is true even for minor injuries such as Colles' fracture. The effect of injury on stomach emptying is compounded by pain, fear, and opioid analgesics. It is prudent to assume, therefore, that all injured patients have a full stomach for a prolonged period after injury. Consideration should be given to active removal of liquid stomach contents using a large-bore nasogastric tube, enhancing stomach emptying using metoclopramide, and neutralizing acidity with antacids. Continued acid secretion can be reduced with $H_2$-receptor antagonists. The traditional delay of 4–6 hours between injury and induction of anaesthesia is rarely appropriate. Rationally, the period of starvation should be sufficient to allow the measures described to become effective. Even then, the anaesthetist should assume that the stomach is full and employ a rapid sequence induction with preoxygenation and cricoid pressure. Caution is necessary for patients with penetrating eye injuries when suxamethonium is contraindicated.

### Resuscitation and treatment of concurrent medical conditions

Resuscitation for haemorrhage has already been described. It is important to remember also that elderly patients with fractures, who have been unable to summon help, may be dehydrated and require preoperative treatment with crystalloid solutions. Medical conditions that are amenable to a brief period of optimization before anaesthesia and surgery include hypertension, arrhythmia, cardiac failure, chest infection, and diabetes mellitus.

The causes of unconsciousness may be broadly divided into four primary groups: intracranial events, alcohol and drugs, metabolic and endocrine, and critical illness (Table 64.3). It is important to remember that more than one primary cause of unconsciousness may be present. For example, a head-injured patient may have consumed sufficient alcohol to affect assessment of his or her conscious level. Furthermore, the primary cause of unconsciousness may have other

**Table 64.3 Causes of unconsciousness**

| Intracranial events | Alcohol and drugs | Metabolic and endocrine | Critical illness |
|---|---|---|---|
| **Primary causes** | | | |
| Direct head trauma | Alcohol | Diabetes mellitus | Sepsis |
| Extradural haematoma | Amphetamines | Addison's disease | Post-cardiac arrest; hypoxic brain injury |
| Subdural haematoma | Cocaine | Hyponatraemia | Hypoxia |
| Stroke | LSD | Hypernatraemia | Hypovolaemia |
| Subarachnoid haemorrhage | Overdose of sedative, opiate, anticonvulsant or antidepressant | Hypothyroidism | |
| Intracerebral haemorrhage | Carbon monoxide poisoning | Hypothermia | |
| Epilepsy | | Hyperthermia | |
| | | Uraemia | |
| | | Hepatic failure | |
| **Secondary causes** | | | |
| Epilepsy | Subarachnoid haemorrhage | Raised ICP | |
| Raised ICP | Intracerebral haematoma | | |
| Fat embolism | | | |

ICP, intracranial pressure; LSD, lysergic acid diethylamide.

effects that also cause unconsciousness. A common example is that fitting can occur after head injury, so that the depressed conscious level may be a combined effect of cerebral contusion and the postictal state. As for all patients, a detailed history and careful examination, followed by appropriate investigations, will assist with making the correct diagnosis and hence aid anaesthetic management.

Metabolic and endocrine disorders require correction of biochemical abnormalities or specific therapy such as insulin or hydrocortisone. Patients with epilepsy who are treated with phenytoin may have a megaloblastic anaemia, making them intolerant of haemoglobin loss. Sodium valproate is reported to impair blood clotting. Recreational drugs, particularly amphetamines and cocaine, cause fever, hypertension, and tachycardia, which may confuse the diagnosis and mask the signs of hypovolaemia (see also Chapter 65). Acute alcohol intoxication not only causes sedation and increases the depth of coma, it also induces a diuresis, which may cause dehydration and render urine output an unreliable measure of adequate volume replacement. Reduced doses of anaesthetic agents are often required, although chronic alcohol abusers have an increased requirement (see also Chapter 65). LSD inhibits cholinesterase activity and increases the toxicity of esterase local anaesthetics.

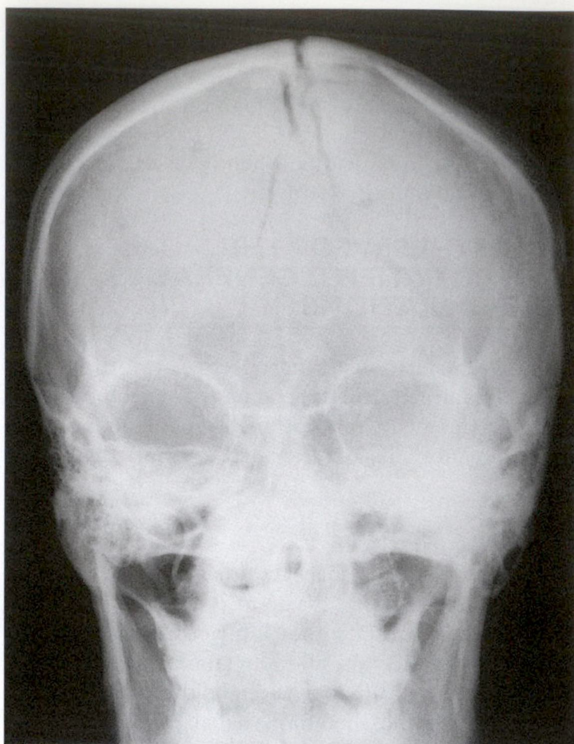

**Figure 64.1** Sagittal fracture following compression of the skull in a motorcyclist who was wearing a crash helmet.

## ANAESTHESIA FOR SPECIFIC TYPES OF INJURY

The principles described above are applicable to all injured patients. Specific injuries, described below, have special problems that influence anaesthetic management.

### Head injury

Primary brain damage may be caused by a depressed skull fracture, haematoma, or brain contusion. Skull radiographs (Figure 64.1) and computed tomography (Figures 64.2–64.4) help in diagnosis and subsequent management. Damaged brain tissue cannot recover and it is important to prevent secondary brain injury caused by hypotension, hypoxia, seizures, infection, and raised ICP resulting from a haematoma, hypercapnia, and oedema. All these secondary insults are amenable to correction. All head-injured patients should be treated according to ATLS guidelines; other injuries should be excluded.

Head-injured patients may be hypoxic as a result of airway obstruction, pulmonary aspiration of stomach contents, chest injury, or neurogenic pulmonary oedema caused by a massive sympathetic discharge at the time of injury. If the patient is hypoxic, ventilation is indicated and, as a general rule, arterial oxygen tension should be maintained above 8 kPa (60 mmHg).

Hypotension reduces cerebral perfusion and causes tissue hypoxia. The systolic blood pressure should be maintained above 100 mmHg. Combined hypoxia and hypotension has a cumulative effect, and the incidence of comatose patients who either die or survive in a vegetative state is around 70% if the target values described are not met.

Measures to reduce raised ICP include evacuation of haematomas, control of arterial carbon dioxide tension ($Pa\text{CO}_2$) to around 4 kPa (32 mmHg), 40° head-up tilt, moderate hypothermia and analgesia, sedation (including barbiturate coma), and paralysis. Hypocapnia is no longer recommended except for the emergency control of raised ICP when other measures have failed, because severe vasoconstriction may reduce cerebral blood flow and cause brain ischaemia. Mannitol, an osmotic diuretic, in a dose of 0.5 mg/kg, is a useful emergency measure to buy time until definitive surgery can be performed to remove an intracranial blood clot. Dexamethasone is useful to reduce swelling associated with tumours, but not for cerebral swelling caused by head injury.

If ICP is being measured, the anaesthetist should aim to maintain the cerebral perfusion pressure, defined as mean arterial blood pressure (MAP) minus ICP, at 70 mmHg because autonomic regulation of cerebral blood flow is lost when the brain is injured. Crystalloids, colloids, and blood may be used, but care should be taken to avoid circulatory overload. Dextrose solutions are best avoided because glucose is metabolized to lactate in the ischaemic brain, and high lactate levels are thought to be associated with a poor outcome. If restoration of the circulating blood volume does not raise the MAP sufficiently, inotropes are indicated. Prophylactic anticonvulsants and antibiotics should be given.

The anaesthetic technique should accommodate all of the above measures. The technique chosen should permit a smooth induction without coughing or a hypertensive response to intubation. With the exception of ketamine, all induction agents are safe. Short-acting analgesics such as alfentanil or fentanyl are acceptable. Muscle paralysis to allow ventilation, with

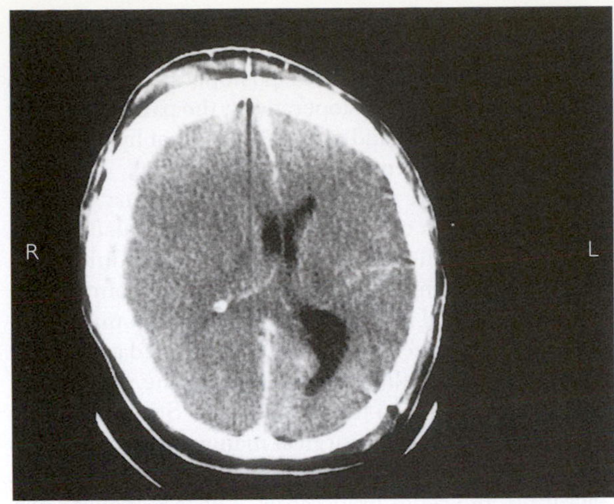


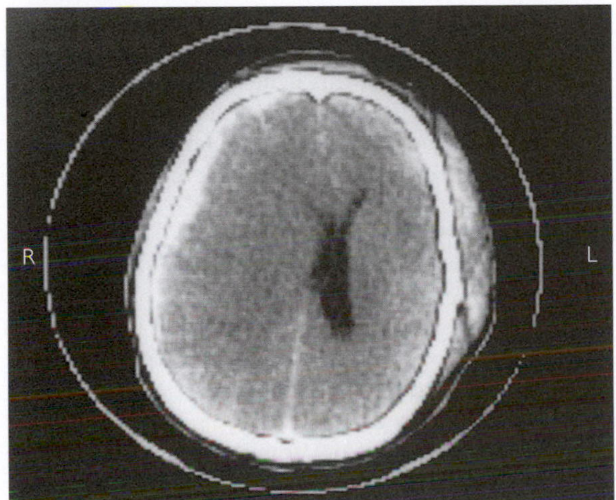


**Figure 64.2** These two computed tomography scans show a right-sided subdural haematoma with underlying cerebral oedema obliterating the ventricle on the right side. It is identified as a subdural (rather than an extradural) haematoma because of the diffuse nature without clear angulation at the dura.

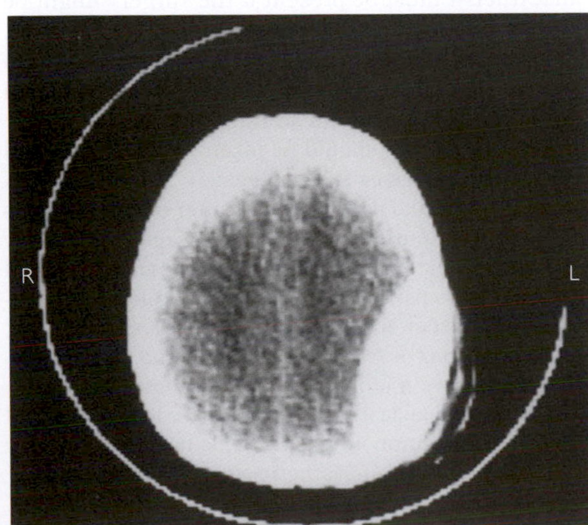


**Figure 64.3** Computed tomography scan showing an extradural haematoma. Note the acute angle at which the haemorrhage is bounded by the dura.

control of arterial oxygen tension ($Pa\text{O}_2$) and $Pa\text{CO}_2$, is indicated. Anaesthesia may be maintained with isoflurane in concentrations of less than 1 MAC (minimum alveolar concentration), which do not cause vasodilatation, or a propofol infusion. Postoperatively, neurological monitoring must continue. If the patient is not sedated and paralysed, codeine phosphate is an appropriate analgesic because it does not cause sedation or mask other neurological signs. If the patient has other painful injuries, local anaesthetic techniques can be helpful. If there is evidence of cerebral oedema, the anaesthetist and surgeon may elect to ventilate the patient postoperatively. As the associated sedative and paralysing drugs will reduce the availability of clinical neurological signs, it is advisable to place an ICP monitoring device while the patient is still in the operating room.

## Spinal injury

Spinal injury may be conveniently divided into two groups of patients: those with and those without neurological deficit. In the latter group, it is particularly important to avoid any movement of the spine because this may cause spinal cord damage. In the former group, movement is also avoided to minimize the risk of further spinal cord damage. The clinical signs depend on the level of the lesion. Visceral and somatic sensation is lost for up to 6 weeks, and is accompanied by loss of autonomic reflexes, and flaccid paralysis. Vasodilatation and hypotension are common and assume greater significance when the lesion is above T1 because the cardiac ganglion is involved. Bradycardia occurs as a result of unopposed vagal activity, and the patient loses his or her reflex ability to compensate for blood loss caused by other injuries. Lesions below C5 spare the diaphragm and, depending on the level, some intercostal nerves. Breathing will be adequate but paradoxical. Patients with lesions at C4–C5 are able to breathe but their vital capacity is reduced to around 25% of normal. They cough weakly and may require ventilatory support. Intercostal and diaphragmatic paralysis occurs with lesions above C4 and ventilatory support is always required. Other complications of spinal cord injury include acute gastric dilatation, paralytic ileus, impaired thermoregulation, urinary retention, and pressure sores.

ATLS guidelines should be followed during resuscitation. Fluids should be given with caution and monitoring with a central venous pressure (CVP) line or thermodilution catheter is advisable. Fluid overload can cause pulmonary oedema and the risk is increased if the injury was associated with a sympathetic surge and neurogenic pulmonary oedema. If fluid is insufficient to restore the blood pressure, a vasoconstrictor such as norepinephrine (noradrenaline) can be used. Bradycardia that compromises the blood pressure should be treated with atropine. $Pa\text{O}_2$ and $Pa\text{CO}_2$ should be monitored and supplemental oxygen with or without ventilatory support provided to maintain the arterial blood gases within the normal range. There is good evidence that methylprednisolone, administered in a dose of 30 mg/kg within 8 hours of injury, aids the recovery of motor, but not sensory, function.

During anaesthesia, movement of the injured spine and hypotension must be avoided. The latter can be

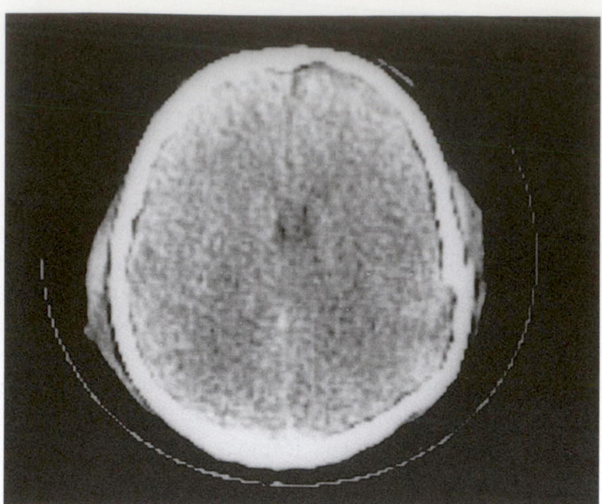

**Figure 64.4** Computed tomography scan showing severe cerebral oedema. There are no skull fractures but the lateral ventricles are obliterated.

achieved by adequate volume replacement and the judicious use of drugs and volatile agents, combined with low peak ventilatory pressures. The former is often the anaesthetist's prime concern, particularly if the cervical spine is injured. The requirement to avoid movement of the cervical spine outside the neutral position causes several problems:

- airway obstruction resulting from hard collars or fixation devices;
- inability to extend the neck, making intubation more difficult;
- the risk that cricoid pressure will cause spinal subluxation.

Furthermore, cervical spine injuries are often associated with facial and head injuries, and the likelihood of regurgitation is increased by gastric dilatation and a paralytic ileus. Endotracheal intubation can be extremely difficult. The use of suxamethonium in the acute phase is controversial because of its association with hyperkalaemia and life-threatening arrhythmias. Some authors state that its use is acceptable in the first 3 days after injury whereas others say that it is safe only in the first 3 hours after injury. Ideally, suxamethonium should not be used at all. Atropine should be given to prevent bradycardia and dry secretions. Options for intubation include:

- fibreoptic awake intubation using local anaesthesia;
- oral or nasal intubation under local or general anaesthesia;
- elective tracheostomy.

There is no hard evidence that one method is better than another. What is clear is that the neck must not be moved. It is preferable to have a colleague maintaining manual inline traction until the neck can be immobilized by the surgeon. Provided that the blood pressure is maintained, specific anaesthetic agents are not preferred for maintenance of anaesthesia. Meticulous monitoring and the use of somatosensory evoked potentials are important. It is also necessary to avoid hypothermia, to pad pressure areas, and to use intermittent calf compression to reduce the likelihood of postoperative deep vein thrombosis (DVT). Postoperatively, the patient must be carefully monitored and steps taken to treat hypotension, bradycardia, and ventilatory insufficiency.

After the acute phase of spinal cord injury, there is a gradual return of sympathetic activity, muscle tone, and reflexes. There is a loss of descending inhibition and the development of abnormal synaptic connections within the spinal cord. After 8 weeks, autonomic dysreflexia, characterized by a massive disordered autonomic response to stimuli below the level of the injury, is of major importance to the anaesthetist. Stimuli such as bladder distension or surgical manipulation of viscera may provoke the response, which causes hypertension, sweating, and reflex bradycardia. These responses may cause intracerebral haemorrhage, seizures, myocardial ischaemia, and death. Autonomic dysreflexia is most common in patients with a spinal lesion above T7. During anaesthesia, the most effective treatment is to remove the trigger. If this is not possible, pharmacological control of hypertension with glyceryl trinitrate, hydralazine, clonidine, or phentolamine is indicated. Other anaesthetic considerations include:

- chronic hypovolaemia;
- an exaggerated hypotensive response to raised intrathoracic pressure;
- respiratory insufficiency;
- risk of bony injury as a result of osteoporosis;
- skin injury caused by pressure;
- loss of thermoregulation;
- anaemia resulting from persistent low-grade infection;
- increased risk of DVT;
- urinary retention;
- delayed gastric emptying;
- muscular spasms;
- chronic pain.

As a result of the loss of sensation, many procedures can be performed without anaesthesia, although an anaesthetist must be present if the surgery might be compromised by autonomic dysreflexia or spasms. Many patients with chronic spinal cord injury prefer to receive general anaesthesia. The use of deep general anaesthesia may obtund the autonomic dysreflexic response, but care should be taken with all drugs and volatile agents that cause hypotension. Suxamethonium is contraindicated until 9 months after injury and non-depolarizing neuromuscular blocking agents are rarely required after intubation has been achieved. Spinal anaesthesia is particularly helpful for urological procedures because it obtunds the hyper-reflexic response, although it may be technically difficult and some anaesthetists believe that hypotension is a significant problem. Epidural anaesthesia is said to be less successful in preventing autonomic dysreflexia because of patchy spread of the local anaesthetic agent.

### Pulmonary contusion and intrathoracic injuries

Injury to the lung parenchyma is characterized by hypoxia, although radiological evidence of injury may not be visible for the first 24 hours. Physical examination may reveal localizing signs of pneumothorax or haemothorax (see also Table 54.3). If the patient is deteriorating rapidly, there will not be time to take a chest radiograph (Figure 64.5) before inserting a chest drain.

All patients with evidence of injury to the chest wall, such as bruising, seat-belt marks, or fractured ribs, should be presumed to have underlying pulmonary contusion. Contused lung is characterized by a zone of parenchymal damage surrounded by a zone of oedema and atelectasis. Fluid overload increases the area of oedema, delays resolution of the lung injury, and reduces the ability of the lung to combat infection. The anaesthetic technique and monitoring used must be chosen to permit meticulous fluid balance.

Where there is lung contusion, myocardial contusion must also be suspected and an ECG performed. Patients with pre-existing myocardial compromise or myocardial contusion often benefit from monitoring with a pulmonary artery catheter. Enflurane may be the volatile agent of choice because there is some evidence to suggest that it does not impede hypoxic vasoconstriction, which facilitates maintenance of the lung's normal ventilation–perfusion characteristics.

If surgery on an intrathoracic organ is planned, the anaesthetist may wish to assist the surgeon by using a double-lumen tube and providing the facility to collapse one lung to assist surgical access. The decision to use a double-lumen tube depends on the type of injury and the extent of the pulmonary injury. If the 'good' lung is collapsed, it may be impossible to maintain adequate oxygenation. Alternatively, if the injured lung is to be collapsed or removed, ventilation–perfusion relationships in the remaining lung tissue may be improved.

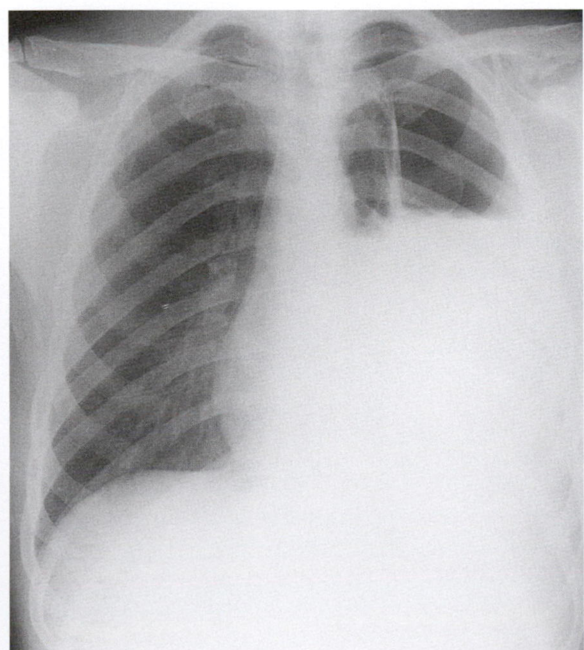

**Figure 64.5** A chest radiograph showing a large left-sided haemopneumothorax. Note the collapsed lung on the left showing the presence of pneumothorax.

### Multiple injuries

The patient with multiple injuries presents the greatest challenge to the anaesthetist. It may be necessary to balance the conflicting requirements of diverse injuries and the anaesthetist may find him- or herself the arbiter in planning which surgical interventions take priority. It is helpful to remember the order of priority used during resuscitation – namely, airway, breathing, circulation, and neurological disability.

The key to success is careful preoperative preparation of the patient and meticulous planning of the anaesthetic technique, monitoring, and order of precedence for surgical intervention. By far the greatest challenge is the patient with major haemorrhage. If there are no contraindications, less popular drugs such as ketamine and pancuronium can be extremely useful because they cause an increase in blood pressure. Adequate venous access in the form of short, large-bore, intravenous cannulae is essential. Rapid infusion devices capable of adequate warming should be used if they are available. Large transfusions of cold fluid can cause hypothermia, which is an independent variable associated with increased mortality after injury. Other methods of maintaining core temperature such as heated blankets and humidified gases should be used, if appropriate. The ability to transfuse fluid rapidly carries the risk of circulatory overload. Monitoring of cardiovascular parameters is, therefore, mandatory. This may be difficult in a crisis, but is facilitated by the use of alarmed monitors displaying trends. If such a monitor is not available, an assistant with responsibility for monitoring is helpful. The assistant must receive clear instructions to inform the lead anaesthetist of significant and potentially detrimental changes in monitoring parameters.

### Fractured neck of femur

A large number of elderly patients undergo surgery for hip fractures. Often surgery is undertaken within the first 24 hours after injury, in order to facilitate early mobilization and to reduce the incidence of complications associated with prolonged bed rest. Elderly patients are frequently dehydrated and suffer from concurrent medical illnesses. The anaesthetist must balance the risks of early anaesthesia combined with suboptimally treated respiratory or cardiovascular abnormalities against the delays incurred when patients are treated for acute chest infection, hypertension, arrhythmias, or hypovolaemia. It appears that those patients anaesthetized between 2 and 4 days after hip fracture have the best outcome, probably because they are optimally prepared but have not yet developed bronchopneumonia or pressure sores. It is not important to survival whether general or regional anaesthesia is used (see Figure 43.2).

## CONCLUSION

Anaesthesia for the injured patient is challenging because of the vast interpatient variations that are encountered. The anaesthetist's involvement begins, ideally, at the time of admission and continues until discharge from intensive care. Many injured patients are young and a successful outcome depends on the ability of the surgeon and anaesthetist to coordinate resuscitation, surgery, and postoperative care in a way that provides the optimum conditions for recovery of every injured organ.

## FURTHER READING


Alderson JD, Frost EAM. *Spinal Cord Injuries*. London: Butterworths, 1990.

Baker AJ. Management of the severely head injured patient. *Can J Anaesth* 1999;**46**:R35–40.

Bickell WH, Wall MJ, Pepe PE, *et al*. Immediate versus delayed fluid resuscitation for hypotensive patients with penetrating torso injuries. *N Engl J Med* 1994;**331**:1105–9.

Bracken MB, Shepard MJ, Collins WF, *et al*. Methyl-prednisolone or naloxone treatment after acute spinal cord injury: 1-year follow-up data. *J Neurosurgery* 1992;**76**:23–31.

Bullock R, Chesnut RM, Clifton G, *et al*. *Guidelines for the Management of Severe Head Injury*. New York: Brain Trauma Foundation, 1995.

Chesnut RM, Marshall LF, Klauber MR, *et al*. The role of secondary brain injury in determining outcome from severe head injury. *J Trauma* 1993;**34**:216–22.

Gupta KG, Nolan JP. Emergency general anaesthesia for hypovolaemic trauma patients. *Curr Anaesth Crit Care* 1998;**9**:66–73.

Kenzora JE, McCarthy RE, Lowell JD, Sledge CB. Hip fracture mortality. *Clin Orthop Rel Res* 1984;**186**:45–56.

Lindsay KW, Bone I, Callander R. *Neurology and Neurosurgery Illustrated*, 3rd edn. Edinburgh: Churchill Livingstone, 1994.

Rose EF. Factors influencing gastric emptying. *J Forens Sci* 1979;**24**:200–6.

Skinner D, Driscoll P, Earlam R, eds. *ABC of Major Trauma*, 2nd edn. London: BMJ Publishing Group, 1996.

# Chapter 65 Consent, psychiatric disease, and drug abuse

P. Hutton and G.M. Cooper

## CONSENT

Obtaining consent is a fundamental part of medical practice. Failure to obtain consent from a patient before the most minor examination may theoretically lead to a civil action for trespass, assault, or battery, or to a criminal trial for common, aggravated, or indecent assault, depending on the circumstances.

Consent may be 'implied' or 'express'. Implied consent assumes that when the patient presents him- or herself to a doctor, he or she has already tacitly agreed to some sort of limited examination. This is normally taken to mean nothing more advanced than inspection, palpation, percussion, and auscultation. Any other procedure (e.g. blood tests, endoscopy, radiology, and rectal and vaginal examinations) requires express consent. The anaesthetist should always obtain express consent for any procedure that causes a material risk. This includes the provision of local anaesthetic blocks. The patient's agreement should be noted on the anaesthetic chart.

Express consent means exactly what it says. The patient gives his or her consent expressly for a well-defined procedure to be undertaken after a full explanation of its objectives. This consent may be oral or written; both are of equal validity if adequately witnessed. Written consent has the advantage of permanence and easy proof, which may be important in subsequent litigation.

Patients have the right to refuse treatment, with or without good reason. If a patient refuses to consent to the anaesthetic technique that the anaesthetist believes to be the most appropriate, then reasonable attempts should be made to persuade the patient that the proposed technique is associated with the least risk of adverse sequelae. Coercion is not acceptable, but advantages and disadvantages of the proposed procedure and reasons for the advice should be explained clearly.

Until recently, consent for any medical or dental procedure could be given only by conscious, mentally sound adults. This implies that it must have been obtained before premedicant drugs were given. An adult, for these purposes, was anyone over 16 years of age and, below this age, consent was obtained from the parent or guardian. This approach, although still used in most cases, has now been modified by extending the rights of children to determine their own treatment. Since the results of a number of test cases, in Britain, if a minor is able to understand what is involved in a procedure they have the right to determine whether or not to permit it. If a child who is able to understand what is involved in a given operation therefore refuses consent, in the first instance his or her wishes should be respected and the situation reviewed later with the involvement of other doctors and the parents.

No other person can consent to treatment on behalf of an adult, including incompetent adults. Difficulties therefore arise because of psychiatric illness when an adult of unsound mind is unable to give consent for surgery on either him- or herself or a dependant under the age of consent. The doctor is therefore in the position that he or she has to judge whether a treatment or investigation in a mentally incapacitated adult is in the patient's best interest, bearing in mind knowledge about the patient's background. Views about the patient's preferences given by the patient's family, carer, legal representative, or other third party properly authorized to act on the patient's behalf should nevertheless be taken into account. Wherever possible, however, any patient (whether detained under the provisions of mental health legislation or not) should be given the appropriate information to try to obtain his or her informed consent, and be given the opportunity to make a voluntary decision about his or her health care. Where a patient's capacity to consent is in doubt, or where differences of opinion about his or her best interest cannot be resolved satisfactorily, experienced colleagues should be consulted and, if necessary, you should apply to the court for a ruling. The court's approval should be sought where a patient lacks the capacity to consent to a medical intervention that is non-therapeutic or controversial, for example, sterilization, or organ or tissue donation.

Another potentially difficult situation arises where a patient who has become of unsound mind (e.g. as in presenile or senile dementia) has indicated preferences in an advance statement ('advance directive' or 'living will'). Provided that the decision in the advance statement is clearly applicable to the present circumstances, and there is no reason to believe the patient would have changed his or her mind in the intervening period, a refusal of treatment should be respected.

When a minor is prevented from receiving treatment considered to be of benefit to him or her, or because the adult guardian holds peculiar beliefs or is mentally handicapped, there are two courses of action for the doctor. He or she can seek the assistance of the Children's Officer of the Local Authority who may, with a magistrate, convene an emergency court at the bedside. The magistrate may then authorize the removal of the child's custody from the parent to a 'fit person' (usually the Children's Officer), who is then able to authorize the operation or treatment. This procedure is very rarely used and a directive from the Minister of Health in 1961 advised its abandonment. Instead, he recommended that the doctor involved should get a written supporting opinion from a colleague that the patient's life is in danger without the proposed line of treatment, and he or she should then go ahead provided that he or she is competent to accomplish the task.

Another recent change in the approach to consent in the UK relates to the pregnant woman at term and her unborn child. A recent judgement on a woman who was forced to have a caesarean section in the interests of both herself and the fetus decided that the doctors were indeed guilty of trespass. If the appeal on this fails, it will effectively mean that, unless a pregnant women can be certified mentally ill, she can, herself alone, determine what will happen to her and the fetus. The father and unborn child apparently have no rights until the child is born. In such circumstances, it is therefore vital that proper procedures are followed so that subsequent litigation cannot be pursued on the back of a procedural error.

At present, in the UK and most European nations, surgical consent forms include consent to anaesthesia. This implies that the surgeon taking consent is capable of discussing the anaesthetic technique adequately with the patient. This is obviously not so in many cases but, nevertheless, is the situation that currently exists.

Consequently, every effort should be made by anaesthetists to see all patients preoperatively so that the patient knows what to expect and can ask questions about what is going to happen. It is possible that patients may wish to express their choice about such things as local anaesthetic blocks, remaining awake during surgery, and methods of postoperative analgesia. If patients do not wish to know such detail or become involved in making choices about their care, they usually make this very clear early in the conversation. When difficulties arise, or choices are made, they should be documented briefly in the anaesthetic record.

In true emergency life-threatening situations the treatment of the unconscious, previously normal person, and the mentally handicapped one, is the same. If rapid consent cannot be obtained from a relative, guardian, or medical officer, the operating team act as 'agents of necessity', and proceed as they think fit. In so doing, it is assumed that a normal, adult patient finding him- or herself in this situation would give willing consent.

Consent is currently a 'hot topic' in the medicolegal world and case law is continuing to develop precedent. It is an area that needs constant monitoring to ensure that one's personal practice is in line with current guidelines. Help can readily be obtained from the medical defence societies.The key to success is to provide unbiased information. All patients should be given the opportunity to ask questions, and honest answers should be provided.

## PSYCHIATRIC DISORDERS

### Affective disorders

These are all characterized by a primary disturbance of mood, with altered behaviour and changes in energy, sleep, appetite, and weight. The extremes are intense excitement and elation (mania and hypomania) and severe depression. Depression can arise by itself with no apparent cause (endogenous), be secondary to psychic trauma (reactive), or follow physical illnesses, surgery, and the prescription of certain drugs (reserpine, methyldopa, sulphonamides, barbiturates, the contraceptive pill). The overall incidence is about 2%. The patient always has a depressed mood and may have retarded physical activity and learning disorders. Occasionally, delusional ideas, altered perception, and a lack of insight are prominent. History-taking can be tedious and unreliable. If the depression is chronic, there may be cachexia, obesity, or evidence of alcohol or drug abuse. The anaesthetist mainly encounters depressed patients when they are scheduled for electroconvulsive therapy.

There are several physical illnesses that may present as, or are particularly associated with, depression. These include hypothyroidism, Parkinson's disease, pernicious anaemia, and carcinoma of the lung or prostate. Consequently, it is reasonable for all depressed people, especially those in middle age or older, to have their drug therapy reviewed and to have some investigations (e.g. full blood count [FBC], urea and electrolytes [U&Es], liver function tests [LFTs], thyroid function tests, acid phosphate, and a chest radiograph) performed.

The major implication for the anaesthetist is that of the prescribed antidepressant drugs (see later). The patient is usually passive, accepting whatever treatment is recommended, but is not prepared to contribute to his or her own recovery. A firm hand is often required with regard to physiotherapy and mobilization. Encouragement from relatives may help.

Mania and hypomania are much less common than depression and are only rarely attributable to an organic cause. The major differential diagnosis is that of drug abuse with amphetamines and hallucinogens such as LSD. The anaesthetic problems are related to the patient's drugs (e.g. lithium).

### People with learning disorders

Most patients with learning disorders are normal variants, but some have the condition as part of a broader syndrome, the features of which may affect anaesthetic management. Consequently, all such patients need a thorough examination of the cardiovascular and respiratory systems. Usually such patients have been investigated at length by paediatricians. If they have been diagnosed with a named syndrome, then check on the implications of this.

Communication difficulties are very similar to those of paediatric anaesthesia. If the patient is an adult, he or she is much stronger than a child and interpersonal skills play a vital role in dealing with these patients.

The preoperative visit is best made when the parent or guardian is with the patient. This enables the relevant history to be obtained (both medical and psychological), the consent for surgery to be signed, advice to be taken regarding fears or phobias (e.g. masks, needles, trolleys), and the most likely way to gain cooperation to be discussed. The patient will also recognize the anaesthetist and form some sort of trust.

Make an estimate of the mental age of the patient and explain what is going to happen in language appropriate to that age. The patient may ask very direct questions, which ought not to be evaded but answered according to the patient's understanding. If the mental age is below 4 years explanations are not likely to help.

Heavy oral or intramuscular premedication may be of benefit, but each patient needs individual assessment. Time the arrival in the anaesthetic room so that the patient has minimal waiting. Sensible parents or a 'helper' can provide invaluable assistance at induction by reassurance, but their presence can be detrimental if they are frightened. Concessions may have to be made regarding the donning or removing of clothing (remember false teeth) and posture (e.g. sitting, or even standing) for induction of anaesthesia. Ensure that there is adequate help with lifting. Whether anaesthesia is induced by gas or an intravenous technique must be determined individually, but both may call for exceptional skills and expert firm assistants for successful management. On occasion, forceful restraint or intramuscular ketamine is required. Always be prepared for a possible difficult intubation.

The presence of parents, guardian, or a familiar comfort object can help to avoid disturbances in the postoperative period. Always remember that the patient may not vocalize pain.

### Down's syndrome

Down's syndrome is a chromosome abnormality (trisomy 21) that is more likely to occur with older maternal age. Although it only accounts for 1% of mental retardation, its associated medical conditions (particularly congenital heart disease, especially atrial and ventricular septal defects, Fallot's tetralogy and patent ductus arteriosus; [see Chapter 51]) mean that they frequently present for anaesthesia. Dental care often requires general anaesthesia. There is a high mortality from the disorder in early childhood, but many now survive to adulthood.

Patients with Down's syndrome have characteristic abnormalities in the anatomy of the face and skull. The midfacial structures are crowded, the tongue is large, and the jaw is small. Nasal passages are constricted, and excessive secretions are common. All these features predispose to difficult intubation and airway management. They are affected more than usual by ventilatory depressant drugs. Their eyes are very sensitive to atropine but this is not a problem with the normal systemic doses. Extubation stridor occurs frequently and may require nursing in a humidified atmosphere.

### Neurosis

Neuroses are the most common psychiatric disorders seen, and represent up to 20% of all general practitioner consultations. They are diseases in which the personality remains intact and contact with reality is preserved. The symptoms are subjective, persistent, and troublesome, and are associated with malaise, an inability to cope, and feelings of anxiety. Neurosis is frequently seen in surgical patients simply because it is so common in the general public.

Many patients are on anxiolytics (usually benzodiazepines) or antidepressant drugs. Normally, they are very anxious and a heavy sedative premedication and reassurance are advisable. Anaesthetically, they cause few problems. Occasionally, those obsessed with regular purgations have chronic electrolyte alterations. Phobias (e.g. claustrophobia, agoraphobia, needle phobia) need sympathetic and imaginative but *firm* management.

### Schizophrenia

The incidence of schizophrenia in the general population is 0.8% and does not vary between countries and cultures. It is best seen as a developmental disorder of the brain to which genetic and perinatal factors (birth trauma or maternal viral infection) contribute; it manifests itself in late adolescence when brain maturation is finally completed. It is a syndrome of personality change and other symptoms that can lead to a dramatic disintegration of the personality. Some symptoms are cardinal (e.g. primary delusions, thought disorders, hallucinations) and others are less specific (loss of drive, blunted emotions, lack of interpersonal contact, stereotypical movements). The presentation and progress of the disease are classically divided into simple, hebephrenic, paranoid, and catatonic. Acute schizophrenic symptoms respond well to phenothiazines, with 30% of patients having only one episode. Longer-term management is more difficult and involves prevention of relapse and coping with chronic disability. Antipsychotic drugs used (e.g. chlorpromazine, thioridazine, trifluoperazine, haloperidol, flupenthixol) have sedative, antimuscarinic, and extrapyramidal effects in varying degrees. Of importance is the rare but potentially fatal neuroleptic malignant syndrome. Treatment for this condition is bromocriptine and dantrolene. Newer treatments for schizophrenia are clozapine and risperidone, both of which have fewer side-effects than previously used drugs.

The anaesthetist's problems are those of the underlying disease requiring surgery, difficult history-taking, obtaining consent, drug therapy, and the patient's loss of contact with reality.

### Organic cerebral syndromes

These are of considerable importance to the anaesthetist and should always be suspected when there is an abnormal mental state. Their aetiology may affect anaesthesia and they may be curable.

Organic cerebral syndromes are caused by dysfunction at the cellular level, resulting from ischaemia, toxins, inflammation, tumour, or trauma. The lesion may be reversible, permanent but stationary, or progressive. They present with a mixture of intellectual impairment, memory loss, change in personality, and confusion. Focal neurological signs may be present. The causes are listed in Table 65.1. They are frequently seen in elderly people on an intensive care unit.

It is therefore essential, if an organic cerebral syndrome is suspected, to have a thorough preoperative work-up. Its presence, especially in elderly people, is easily missed.

The history is usually difficult to obtain and may have to come from relatives. On examination, look for the presence of right and left ventricular failure, cyanosis, hepatomegaly, and chest infection.

Direct investigations towards abnormalities elicited in the history and examination. Tests that may be indi-

**Table 65.1 Causes of organic cerebral syndromes**

| Broad group | Examples and notes |
|---|---|
| Drugs | Alcohol, barbiturates, steroids, any psychotropic medication |
| Infections | Meningitis, encephalitis, any systemic infection causing a fever<br>Neurosyphilis is now rare |
| Electrolyte disturbances | GI tract disturbances in elderly people<br>After GI and GU surgery |
| Hypoxia | Especially in elderly people, e.g. from chest infections, LVF |
| Intracerebral | Abscess, tumour, trauma (especially subdural haematoma in elderly people) |
| Cardiovascular | Intracerebral arteriosclerosis, low cardiac output, severe anaemia |
| System failure | Renal or hepatic failure, hypothyroidism, Cushing's syndrome, Addison's disease, non-ketoacidotic diabetic coma |
| Recognized dementia | Senile dementia, Alzheimer's disease, Pick's disease, Huntingdon's disease, Parkinson's disease, etc. |
| Toxic | Carbon monoxide, heavy metals (all are rare) |
| Microemboli, ischaemia | After repeated TIAs, prolonged hypotension, cardiac bypass surgery |

GI, gastrointestinal; GU, genitourinary; LVF, left ventricular failure; TIAs, transient ischaemic attacks.

cated are FBC, U&Es, LFTs, thyroid function tests, arterial blood gases, ECG, chest radiograph, urine and serum screening for the presence of drugs, and computed tomography scanning. If there are no signs of raised intracranial pressure, a lumbar puncture may be done. In an emergency, LFTs and thyroid function tests will not be available because they are assayed in batches.

Anaesthetic management is that of any underlying disease found. Both before, and especially after, surgery these patients can pose major ward problems. Frequently, because of their antisocial activities, they tend to be ignored by the ward staff, who request sedation to keep them quiet. Patients cannot grasp what is happening and the environment appears strange and frightening to them. They often misinterpret events around them, and may suffer both delusions and hallucinations that leave them tearful and terrified. This leads to overactivity, objectionable behaviour, and episodes such as attempts to leave the ward or refuse medication. Drips and catheters are pulled out and oxygen masks thrown away. The clouding of consciousness is always worse at night when the visual cues are less clear.

Sometimes calm nurses and doctors are all that is required. On other occasions, there is so much activity on the ward that constant stimuli unsettle the patient. At times it may become essential to sedate such patients for their own benefit. This should never be done without first ensuring that they are not hypoglycaemic or hypoxic, that they are not hypotensive or in heart failure, that they have no electrolyte imbalance, and that they have not had a pulmonary embolus.

### Eating disorders

Eating disorders occur predominantly in teenage and young adult females (male : female = 1 : 10). Their incidence is increasing.

#### *Anorexia nervosa*

This is a state of self-induced weight loss far beyond that accepted as normal dieting. Some investigators require a loss of 25% of the original body weight to confirm the diagnosis. The current incidence is up to 1% of the schoolgirl population aged 16–18 years. Amenorrhoea is a constant feature.

The main differential diagnoses are organic causes of weight loss, such as malabsorption, thyrotoxicosis, or an occult neoplasm. Severe cases, in general, have the same anaesthetic problems as those with malnutrition. Vomiting or purging can produce electrolyte abnormalities. Iron-deficiency anaemia is common. A chest radiograph is helpful because there is an increased incidence of tuberculosis secondary to reduced immune competence.

#### *Bulimia nervosa*

This is more common than anorexia and is characterized by episodic gluttony followed by self-induced purgation and vomiting. The physical consequences of this include erosion of dental enamel from exposure to gastric acid, Mallory–Weiss oesophageal tears, and even oesophageal rupture. Repeated vomiting causes hypokalaemia and metabolic alkalosis, which are the main anaesthetic hazards. The patients are usually of normal weight, but in a minority the condition can overlap with (and may be regarded as an unusual form of) anorexia nervosa.

## PSYCHIATRIC DRUGS

Many of the drugs used in psychiatric illness have implications for anaesthesia. These are listed in Table 65.2.

**Table 65.2 Implications for anaesthesia of drugs used in psychiatric illness**

| Drug | Action | Comments |
|---|---|---|
| Tricyclic antidepressants | • Block uptake of norepinephrine and serotonin at sympathetic nerve endings<br>• Strong anti-muscarinic actions | • Take 2–3 weeks to act; when stopped serum level falls 50% in 2–3 days<br>• Sympathomimetic drugs produce enhanced effects with hypertension, tachycardia, hyperthermia, and sweating<br>• If vasoconstrictor required, methoxamine is drug of choice<br>• Anticholinergic agents may cause confusion<br>• In animal models potentiate CNS depressants, barbiturates, and opioids<br>• In overdosage, produce cardiac arrhythmias (mainly ventricular ectopics) which may be fatal; require ECG monitoring and may need treatment with intravenous lignocaine |
| Tetracyclics | • As above | • As above, but fewer side effects and interactions than with the tricyclic antidepressants |
| Monoamine oxidase inhibitors | • Prevent breakdown of norepinephrine, serotonin, and dopamine throughout body<br>• Increased norepinephrine available in peripheral nerve endings | • Can be discontinued 2–3 weeks before surgery and medication changed, or continued and drug interactions avoided<br>• Patients very sensitive to indirectly acting sympathomimetic drugs (ephedrine, metaraminol) which produce hypertension and adrenergic crises; direct-acting sympathomimetics are still dangerous but less so than indirectly acting agents<br>• Pethidine interacts to produce hypertension, rigidity, convulsions, restlessness, and hyperpyrexia<br>• Morphine and dihydrocodeine are safe<br>• Potentiation of effects of barbiturates, hypnotics, and other opioids; titrate these drugs carefully |
| Phenothiazines Butyrophenones | • Main therapeutic effect is antidopaminergic<br>• Action also elevates serum prolactin<br>• Some anticholinergic and anti-adrenergic actions<br>• Antiemetic<br>• Peripheral α-blockade | • Can cause dysphoria in normal people<br>• Dermatological reaction in 5%<br>• Rarely, obstructive jaundice and blood dyscrasias<br>• Rarely, neuroleptic malignant syndrome<br>• Potentiate opioids, hypnotics, benzodiazepines (note ventilatory effects)<br>• Can have additive effects with atropine or hyoscine<br>• Main side effects: hypotension, sedation, and extrapyramidal symptoms<br>• Also adynamic ileus, glaucoma, urinary retention, agitation, confusion<br>• Synergistic with other anticholinergics |
| Benzodiazepines | • Via benzodiazepine receptors | • Potentiation of all opioid and hypnotic drugs<br>• Additive effect with competitive neuromuscular blocking agents |

cont.

**Table 65.2 Implications for anaesthesia of drugs used in psychiatric illness (cont.)**

| Drug | Action | Comments |
|---|---|---|
| Lithium | • Inhibits release and increases uptake of norepinephrine<br>• Increases serotonin synthesis in CNS<br>• Main route of excretion via kidney where it interacts with sodium | • Therapeutic level (0.4–1.0 mmol/L) close to toxic level<br>• Plasma concentrations should be monitored<br>• Potentiates effect of depolarizing and non-depolarizing neuromuscular blocking agents<br>• Potentiates all anaesthetic agents<br>• Sodium balance important. If sodium intake is lowered (preoperative fast), or sodium excretion enhanced (loop diuretics), intoxication can occur; put up saline infusion before surgery<br>• Acute toxicity characterized by vomiting, profuse diarrhoea, ataxia, dysarthria, focal neurological signs, convulsions, coma<br>• Chronic toxicity causes nephrogenic diabetes insipidus with polyuria and polydypsia (responds to stopping lithium), low free thyroxine (but most patients euthyroid), and depression of T wave.<br>• Also leukocytosis, dermatitis, and vasculitis<br>• Check serum level before surgery and omit last two doses |

## DRUG AND SUBSTANCE ABUSE

Drug abuse is a world-wide problem and a multi-billion dollar illicit industry. People who are drug and substance abusers pose a number of problems for anaesthetists related to

- the effects of the drugs;
- attendant infections (HIV, hepatitis B);
- medicolegal considerations.

Drug abuse means taking a drug in a way that exceeds its proper medical or social use. Drug dependence is the development of a state in which people have to continue taking the drug because they need its mental effects (psychological dependence) or because they become ill if they stop (physical dependence). The opioids, alcohol, and barbiturates produce a strong psychological dependence and can have severe (often not dose-related) physical dependence.

Physical dependence has developed when the presence of the drug in the body is required for normal cellular metabolism. Therefore withdrawal of necessity produces physiological symptoms (anxiety, irritability, sweating, lacrimation, mydriasis, tremors, piloerection, nausea, vomiting, abdominal cramps, diarrhoea, muscle spasms) which may be so severe as to be life threatening (e.g. fits after barbiturate or alcohol withdrawal).

Those drugs that do not produce physical dependence do not precipitate physical withdrawal symptoms when stopped, but they can produce a desperate craving. There is, however, no physiological risk in their sudden cessation.

There are many reasons why the person who is a substance abuser may present for anaesthesia or intensive care. Apart from the 'normal' reasons of intercurrent illness, there are hazards related to their habit, unclean techniques, overdose, trauma, and violence from the society in which they live. The signs and symptoms of substance abuse are given in Table 65.3. Possible reasons for emergency or inpatient care related to their habit are given in Table 65.4. In the case of Ecstasy, the complications can occur as a result of a single tablet and may be an idiosyncratic response. Dantrolene has been used successfully in the treatment of the associated hyperthermia.

The fact that a substance abuser is often unrecognized highlights the need for always wearing gloves when in contact with any body fluids. A high index of suspicion should alert the anaesthetist to ensure that all staff take proper precautions (as recommended in the publication of the Association of Anaesthetists of Great Britain and Ireland; see Further reading), such as wearing extra gowns, goggles, and overshoes in the operating room in case the patient is HIV or hepatitis B positive.

### History

*Known* addicts are usually frank and cooperative about their drug problem. Take a thorough drug history, ascertaining the type of drug, the usual dosage (tolerance occurs to many drugs), when they had their last dose, and what drugs they have had since being in hospital. Check whether they are registered with an addiction centre or psychiatrist. Contact the centre/psychiatrist to verify the story because extreme cases may fake physical illness so as to obtain drugs. If they are 'new addicts', engage the help of a doctor working with addicts at an early stage.

Drug addiction is most common in young adults, so have a high index of suspicion in 15–40 year olds who behave oddly, and particularly if there is evidence of venepuncture.

### Examination

Always look carefully for signs of infection (as a result of general debility or infected needles), especially those of

**Table 65.3 Signs and symptoms of substance abuse**

| Substance | Signs and symptoms |
|---|---|
| Narcotics | • Euphoria (most marked with heroin)<br>• Conscious level ↓ → coma<br>• Pinpoint pupils with overdose<br>• Respiratory depression<br>• Hypotension<br>• Constipation<br>• Chronic respiratory dysfunction (see Table 65.4) |
| Cocaine and amphetamines | • Sympathetic stimulation, excitement, delirium, hyper-reflexia, tremors, convulsions, mydriasis, sweating, hyperpyrexia<br>• Labile blood pressure; hypertension<br>• Hallucinations (tactile = 'cocaine bugs', visual = 'snow lights') → psychosis<br>• Exhaustion and coma with overdose |
| Hypnotics, benzodiazepines, and barbiturates | • CNS depression<br>• Mood calming<br>• Overdose → respiratory depression and coma<br>• Hypothermia and cardiovascular depression |
| Hallucinogens: phencyclidine derivatives; LSD | • Altered perception and judgement<br>• High doses may progress to toxic psychosis<br>• Sympathomimetic and feeble analgesic effects<br>• Phencyclidine produces dissociative anaesthesia with increasing doses |
| Volatile solvents | • Altered perception<br>• Euphoria<br>• Overdose produces coma with progression similar to effects of general anaesthesia<br>• Respiratory and cardiovascular depression<br>• Ventricular arrhythmias from halogenated hydrocarbons |
| Cannabis | • Effects variable but dose related<br>• Euphoria<br>• Occasional anxiety and panic reactions<br>• Rarely psychosis<br>• Pulse rate ↑<br>• Blood pressure ↑↓<br>• Chronic use may induce poor memory and decreased motivation |
| Ecstasy (3,4-methylenedioxy-methamphetamine, MDMA) | • Agitation, muscle spasms, disseminated intravascular coagulation, renal failure, sympathomimetic effects, convulsions, coma, hyperthermia |

From Wood PR, Soni N. *Anaesthesia* 1989;44:672–80.

endocarditis and pulmonary infection. Look for jaundice. The high incidence (> 80%) of hepatitis B in those who use injected drugs means that all patients should be assumed to be carriers until proven otherwise.

Assess the patient neurologically. Rarely, with narcotic addicts, a transverse myelitis occurs that would contraindicate spinal anaesthesia.

## Investigations

### *Full blood count*

There may be a mild anaemia resulting from general debility.

### *Chest radiograph*

Look for signs of infection.

### *Liver function tests*

The hepatitis carrier state must be identified. Liver function is frequently deranged.

## Preoperative preparation

It is generally agreed that the perioperative period is not the time to withdraw drugs that cause physical dependence. For elective operations, the possibility of deferring surgery until withdrawal is complete should be discussed. The patient may welcome this help and should be referred to a suitable psychiatrist. If the patient declines this offer, or if surgery is urgent, the maintenance dose of the drugs that cause physical dependence (e.g. opioids, barbiturates) should be continued.

## Anaesthetic technique

Local and general anaesthesia can be used with the usual indications and contraindications (e.g. no local blocks in sepsis). The main problems occur postoperatively and are related to withdrawal symptoms and analgesia.

**Table 65.4 Pathology related to substance abuse**

| Pathology | Presentation | Comments |
|---|---|---|
| Results of acute intoxication or overdose | • Primary = CNS stimulation or depression: fitting, coma<br>• Hyperthermia from stimulant abuse<br>• Arrhythmias, BP crises (hyper-/ hypotension)<br>• Respiratory depression: hypoxic fits | Overdose most common cause of death in heroin addicts (diagnosis = coma, miotic pupils, and respiratory rate 2–6 breaths/min) |
| | • Pulmonary oedema with heroin intoxication | Common postmortem finding |
| | • Secondary = trauma, including head injuries<br>• Pancreatitis | Localizing signs important in assessment |
| Acute medical and surgical problems associated with abuse habits | • As venous injection sites lost intra-arterial injections initiated → spasm, mycotic, and false aneurysms, vessel rupture<br>• Extravasation of intravenous injections (lymphatic and venous obliteration = 'puffy hand' syndrome) | |
| | • Subcutaneous injections (abscesses + necrotizing fasciitis; 'skin popping' intravenous injections ('mainlining') → circulatory complications, including acute and subacute endocarditis (right or left sided)<br>• Systemic emboli from left-sided disease valve destruction → cardiac failure (high mortality)<br>• Candida septicaemia | Tricuspid valve pathology + pulmonary infarcts with positive blood cultures in absence of pre-existing venous disease is highly suggestive of narcotic addiction |
| | • Heroin addicts have recurrent chest problems – asthma common<br>• Aspiration is likely when acutely intoxicated<br>• Tuberculosis occurs in heroin addicts<br>• Respiratory disease (especially pneumocystis pneumonia) most common presentation of HIV disease | Often asthmatic since childhood |
| | • Heroin addicts may present with pseudo-obstruction<br>• Mechanical obstruction from swallowed cocaine or heroin: 'body packers', 'stuffers and swallowers' | May have signs of acute intoxication<br>Massive overdose may result |
| | • Septic techniques may produce tetanus<br>• Psychiatric illness, mood disorders<br>• Cerebral emboli/abscess from endocarditis | Differential diagnosis of tetanus = Parkinson's disease from 'designer drugs' |
| Related surgical and obstetric | • Dental caries common in narcotic addicts<br>• Old trauma may require orthopaedic or plastic correction<br>• Obstetric care: late presentation<br>• Pre-eclampsia ↑ in heroin addicts | |

From Wood PR, Soni N. *Anaesthesia* 1989;44:672–80.

### Pain relief

Pain relief is principally a problem in opioid addicts. The advice given by Wood and Soni is as follows (see Further reading).

Opioid addicts may present with a background of illicit street use, or more rarely they may be under supervision on a methadone-maintenance programme. The following principles are important in perioperative management:

- The addict's usual total daily dose should be discovered. This must then be considered a 'physiological requirement' and it (or an equipotent dose of another narcotic) becomes the minimal daily requirement irrespective of additional considerations of acute pain relief, background analgesic, or sedation. Analgesic requirements will be excessive and withdrawal precipitated if the principle is not observed. This principle must not be neglected if regional techniques are employed.
- Street addicts are notorious for exaggeration about their doses, in the hope of obtaining increased quantities of the drug. Overdose can easily result if their true tolerance is exceeded. Therefore, when acute analgesia is necessary, the time of the addict's own last dose may be important (the half-life of heroin is normally 4–6 hours).
- Narcotic addicts should be offered the assistance of specialists in drug dependency and their narcotic doses stabilized before the operation if surgery is not urgent.
- The normal daily dose can be given intramuscularly early on the day of elective operation in methadone-stabilized addicts. Premedication and perioperative analgesia is then given in addition.
- The late postoperative period (48 hours) is a suitable time to convert the total daily narcotic dose to oral methadone after uncomplicated emergency surgery on a street addict. This requires supervision by a drug-dependence specialist and assumes a compliant patient.
- Postoperative analgesia may be a problem. The use of intermittent injections is likely to produce peaks and troughs with consequent demands for both increased frequency and size of dosage. Infusions are therefore better, but have the risk of increased self-administration. They should be used only in high dependency areas.

### Withdrawal features and treatment

This has again been described well and summarized by Wood and Soni (see Further reading).

Symptoms of opioid withdrawal appear 8–12 hours after the last dose and include fatigue, weakness, restless sleep ('yen'), yawning, lacrimation, rhinorrhea, perspiration, fever, diarrhoea, and dehydration. Piloerection produces gooseflesh ('cold turkey'). Symptoms peak at 48–72 hours and continue for 7–10 days if untreated. Acute withdrawal is rarely fatal unless precipitated by the injection of an opioid antagonist in an addict who has not overdosed.

The symptoms are a result of sympathetic hyperactivity and are modified by the $\alpha_2$ agonist clonidine. This drug is now established in the clinical treatment of heroin withdrawal. Cramps, sweating, and abdominal symptoms are particularly relieved, but postural hypotension can be a problem.

Acute withdrawal is usually treated with methadone alone; 10 mg is given orally and, after a delay of 20 min, a further 10 mg is given and every 10 min thereafter. A favourable response is judged by a decrease in pulse rate and a return to a normal blood pressure. The same dose of methadone may be given intramuscularly or subcutaneously, or diluted and given intravenously in small boluses.

Barbiturate withdrawal is potentially life threatening if abrupt or misdiagnosed. The sequence of anxiety, weakness, insomnia, headache, and tremors progresses after 24 hours to hypotension, vomiting, and grand mal fits. Management using a pentobarbitone substitution technique is described, but benzodiazepines are equally effective. Abuse of benzodiazepines is also associated with a barbiturate-type withdrawal response. Abrupt withdrawal can result in major convulsions and, if completed, prolonged psychological problems may result. Treatment involves the reintroduction of the drug with a slow reduction in dose over a period of days to weeks.

Withdrawal from the stimulants cocaine and amphetamine can be difficult to recognize. Some abusers enter a prolonged sleep phase ('crash') (up to 24–48 hours) at the end of a period of chronic heavy usage, followed by hunger, depression, delirium, delusions, and hallucinations. This is thought to represent catecholamine depletion, the opposite mechanism to that of acute intoxication. The syndrome should be left to run its course, but severe depression may warrant expert psychiatric help.

Abstinence from hallucinogenic drugs is rarely a problem. Classically, 'trips' are separated by a period of days because tachyphylaxis occurs to the CNS effects. Psychotic episodes occur on rare occasions in susceptible individuals, days or months after ingestion. Benzodiazepines are appropriate treatment if abstinence from cannabis produces symptoms in a chronic user. The importance of correct identification and treatment of delirium tremens is such that this condition must be a differential diagnosis in any withdrawal of uncertain aetiology.

## ALCOHOL DEPENDENCE

Alcoholism is an increasingly serious social problem. It is defined by the World Health Organization (WHO) as drinking that causes emotional, social, or physical damage to the individual. There is no accurate way to establish the total number of alcohol-dependent people because alcohol is freely available for purchase. However, about 10% of the adult population are teetotal, and 66% of women and 75% of men drink regularly. As an example, the number of heavy drinkers (> 80 g alcohol/day in men and > 40 g day in women) in the 55 million population of the UK, at the last estimation in the late 1970s, was two million. About one-third of these are problem drinkers, of whom 10% are so dependent on alcohol that they suffer withdrawal symptoms when they stop drinking. In 1995, the British Government issued guidelines to sensible drinking. These are up to

28 units weekly for men and up to 14 units weekly for women. A unit of alcohol is that contained in half a pint of beer, one glass of wine, or a single measure of spirits.

About 20% of admissions to medical wards are the result of alcohol or alcohol-related diseases. Of males attending at accident and emergency departments, 40% have drink-related problems. Furthermore, up to 50% of all trauma on the roads is alcohol related. The potential for patients having withdrawal symptoms in the perioperative period is therefore considerable.

### Preoperative assessment

The key to success is a high index of suspicion, but even then detection can be difficult. Relatively few people are honest about their alcohol intake. A heavy drinker may appear anywhere in the range from normal to that of a person with a bloated face, telangectasia, acne, blood-shot eyes, tophi, awful gums, gynaecomastia, pot belly with striae, tremulous fingers, Dupuytren's contracture, bruises, an odd history of faints, mental symptoms and signs, and peripheral vasodilatation with a bounding pulse. Oesophagitis, gastritis, pancreatitis, cirrhosis, cardiomyopathy, pneumonia, tuberculosis, gout, and bone demineralization all have a high associated incidence.

Although there are many abnormal investigations and tests in patients with alcoholism, they are all the result of secondary organ damage and are therefore non-specific. Diagnosis can be confirmed by a random sample (e.g. in outpatients) for blood alcohol. With no signs of inebriation, a blood alcohol level of over 80 mg/dl is suggestive, and that of over 150 mg/dl is diagnostic, of alcohol dependence.

The following are the anaesthetic considerations:

- Those of associated disorders secondary to alcoholism (see above).
- Those caused by the effect of alcohol itself. This depends on whether or not the patient is intoxicated.
- Management of withdrawal symptoms.

### Anaesthetic management

The known alcohol-dependent patient should continue his or her usual daily consumption throughout the period in hospital. Preoperative assessment should be directed at finding any of the associated disorders outlined above, with reference to appropriate chapters. In particular, signs of cardiomyopathy, peripheral neuropathy, and cirrhosis must be looked for. The patient who does not admit, or is not aware of, his or her dependence is likely to take alcohol normally before surgery, but may develop withdrawal symptoms in the postoperative period.

The chronic alcohol abuser who is sober (but continuing his or her usual alcohol intake) and whose cellular machinery is, for him or her, working normally, exhibits cross-tolerance to many sedative, hypnotic, and anaesthetic agents. Larger doses of induction and maintenance agents are therefore likely to be required, but care must be taken in the presence of cardiomyopathy. Induction of anaesthesia can be stormy, particularly if a gaseous technique is chosen. There is no cross-tolerance to opioids, whose actions are potentiated, thereby increasing the risk of ventilatory depression. Opioids with short duration of action are preferable. If there is a history of alcohol-induced seizures, ketamine and enflurane should be avoided.

The presence of chronic liver disease will infer management according to Chapter 58.

### Acute intoxication

In people who are not alcohol dependent, blood alcohol levels of 30–70 mg/dl affect coordination, sensory perception, and intellectual functions. Drunkenness is associated with levels of between 50 and 150 mg/dl. In chronic alcoholism, tolerance to alcohol occurs so that there may be no apparent impairment of intellectual or motor function at levels of 100 mg/dl. Disorientation and stupor are more common than alcoholic coma, which is likely with blood levels above 400 mg/dl. Measuring the blood alcohol level may therefore help distinguish whether unconsciousness is the result of intoxication or whether another contributory cause should be suspected (e.g. head injury, epilepsy, diabetes, or other drugs taken with alcohol).

Although it is always preferable not to anaesthetize patients who are acutely intoxicated, the need to treat acute injuries may not allow delay. The patient must always be assumed to have a full stomach and be at risk of aspiration. In the period before and after surgery, whenever the conscious level is blunted, the patient must be placed in the lateral position. A rapid sequence induction of anaesthesia will be required. This may be made difficult by an obstreperous, confused, or even violent patient. Additional help may therefore be needed.

Acutely intoxicated patients (whether alcohol dependent or not) are sensitive to, and require reduced dosages of, opioids, sedatives, and hypnotics. The danger with normal doses is severe ventilatory depression.

Hypoglycaemia can occur so blood glucose levels should be monitored regularly, especially while unconscious. The administration of 5% dextrose intravenously is a sensible precaution.

#### *Withdrawal symptoms*

The first suspicion of alcohol dependence may occur only in the postoperative period. Withdrawal symptoms vary from mild irritability and uncooperative behaviour to the fully developed unmistakable delirium tremens. In particular, it should be suspected if there is confusion, disorientation, nausea, anxiety, or sweating. Withdrawal can be fatal because of cardiac arrhythmias and convulsions. Convulsions occur 12–48 hours after alcohol withdrawal, and can be either isolated events or last for up to 7 days. Hallucinations can be so vivid that the person, if not physically robust, can develop nervous and physical exhaustion and cardiovascular collapse. The withdrawal syndrome can be treated with alcohol, diazepam, chlormethiazole, or chlordiazepoxide. It is best done in conjunction with the help of a psychiatrist.

## FURTHER READING


Association of Anaesthetists of Great Britain and Ireland. *HIV and Other Blood Borne Viruses – Guidance for Anaesthetists*. London: AAGBI, 1992.

Association of Anaesthetists of Great Britain and Ireland. *Information and Consent for Anaesthesia*. London: AAGBI, 1999.

Eklund J. Alcohol abuse and postoperative complications. Do we ask the right questions? *Acta Anaesthesiol Scand* 1996;**40**:647–8.

Holder KJ, Weller RM. Alcohol consumption and anaesthesia. *Curr Anaesth Crit Care* 1997:**8**:231–6.

Mason D, Peters K. Consent: how to get it and what to do if you cannot. *Curr Anaesth Crit Care* 1998;**9**:274–7.

Waisel DB, Truog RD. Informed consent. *Anesthesiology* 1997;**87**:968

Wood PR, Soni N. Anaesthesia and substance abuse. *Anaesthesia* 1989;**44**:672–80.

# Chapter 66 The patient with a transplanted organ

G.M. Cooper

## GENERAL FEATURES

There are steadily increasing numbers of people who have transplanted organs, some of whom present for incidental surgery. Such transplantations are performed at regional centres, which may be some distance from the patient's home. Thus, the need for unrelated surgery may arise in hospitals that are not familiar with transplant management. For the purposes of this chapter, the principles of anaesthetic implications that are discussed are those in which the transplanted organ is functioning normally. Nevertheless, whatever the organ transplanted, the adequacy of its function must be checked.

Successful transplantation often offers a transformation of lifestyle to patients with major organ failure. Patient and graft survival are steadily improving. The current graft survival rates are shown in Table 66.1.

The function of the transplanted organ is under constant review by the relevant transplant team. Transplant recipients usually have a record book with the latest information obtained at the last hospital visit. Thus the function of the transplanted organ can be readily confirmed. Effective communication about patients who have received transplants is usually well developed, and patients have 'help-line' telephone contact numbers which may be useful if there is any doubt.

A number of aspects are common to all transplanted patients because of immunosuppressant agents used to prevent graft rejection.

### Neoplasia

There is a greater incidence of malignant neoplasms and lymphoma among transplant recipients than in the general population. The risk appears to be related to the intensity of the immunosuppressive regimen and the time from transplantation. Those who have had a heart transplantation are at greater risk in this respect than those who have had a renal transplantation. Surgery may be required for treatment of such tumours.

### Infection

Infection presents a major risk to immunosuppressed patients and is a significant cause of morbidity and mortality. Infections appear to be most common in the early months after transplantation. Viral (e.g. cytomegalovirus, herpes simplex), bacterial, protozoal, and fungal infections all occur. It is paramount that aseptic techniques are practised and that patients are protected from cross-infection. Reverse-barrier nursing may be appropriate in some instances. Antibiotic prophylaxis is important. In addition to the agents indicated by the nature of the surgery, it may be appropriate to give a single dose of an anti-staphylococcal agent (e.g. flucloxacillin) to cover the insertion of all percutaneous cannulae. This obviously needs to be given when the first peripheral cannula is inserted. Extra vigilance should be exercised to detect infection, which should be investigated early and treated accordingly.

### Drug effects

The mainstay of anti-rejection therapies are cyclosporin, azathioprine, and corticosteroids. These are all potent immunosuppressants with toxic side effects. The introduction of cyclosporin has been significant in improving survival. It is a fungal metabolite which causes a dose-dependent increase in serum creatinine and urea and is markedly nephrotoxic. The predominant toxic effect of azathioprine is myelosuppression, although hepatic toxicity is also well recog-

**Table 66.1 First cadaveric graft transplant survival (UK and Republic of Ireland)**

| Organ | No. at risk on day 0 | At 1 year (%) | At 5 years (%) | At 10 years (%) |
|---|---|---|---|---|
| Heart (1985–1994) | 2182 | 75 | 64 | – |
| Lung (1989–1994) | 351 | 65 | 42 | – |
| Heart–lung (1985–1994) | 586 | 63 | 39 | – |
| Liver (1985–1994) | 2801 | 65 | 55 | – |
| Kidney (1985–1993) | 10 856 | 84 | 70 | 58 |

Statistics prepared by the UK Transplant Support Service Authority from the National Transplant Database maintained on behalf of the UK transplant community.

nized. Thus the results of full blood count, urea and electrolytes, and liver function tests need to be reviewed preoperatively. High doses of steroids are used and the patient becomes cushingoid (see Chapter 56). Perioperatively, the dose of steroids must be maintained.

Cyclosporin, azathioprine, and steroids can all be given intravenously if the oral route is compromised because of surgery. It is vital to ensure continued therapy to prevent rejection.

Drug therapy may also include antifungal and antiviral agents in addition to $H_2$-receptor blockers.

### Psychological effects

Patients who have received transplants are only too aware of the fragility of life and have justified fears about possible rejection of their donated organ. It may be helpful to reassure them that contact has been made with their transplant centre about their need for treatment. Anxiolytic premedication may also be advisable. Organic mental disorders also occur, particularly depression and anxiety. These may lead to non-compliance with drug therapy, which can be a significant factor in many cases of organ rejection.

### Graft protection

Whatever the organ in question, it is paramount to maintain it with a well-oxygenated blood supply by the application of the principles of good anaesthetic management outlined in Section 1. Points relevant to particular organs are outlined below.

## FEATURES OF INDIVIDUAL TRANSPLANTED ORGANS

### Renal transplantation

Reference to Table 66.1 shows that the non-specialist anaesthetist is most likely to encounter a successful kidney transplantation. Rejection, although usually heralded by pain in the graft, malaise, oedema, and arthropathy, may be completely asymptomatic, so knowledge of the preoperative electrolytes is important.

Many patients with a healthy transplant still have a functioning fistula, which should be protected as described in Chapter 59.

### Cardiac transplantation

A transplanted heart is denervated. It has a faster resting heart rate (generally 90–100 beats/min) because of the absence of vagal tone. No autonomic reinnvervation takes place after transplantation, so the normal sympathetic responses to laryngoscopy and intubation are absent. The heart does, however, respond to circulating catecholamines, but the response time may be up to 5 min from an intravenous dose. It is therefore important to wait for a response, otherwise an effective overdose can easily occur. The normal baroreceptor reflexes are absent, and carotid sinus massage and Valsalva manoeuvre have no effect on heart rate. There is no pain felt as a result of myocardial ischaemia, so the warning sign to rest from exercise is absent.

Thus, there is no tachycardia in response to light anaesthesia or hypovolaemia. Increases in cardiac output are achieved by increasing stroke volume rather than heart rate. The patient with a heart transplant may show exaggerated blood pressure changes to alterations in posture, hypovolaemia, or decreases in systemic vascular resistance. Care therefore needs to be taken to avoid excessive volume of fluid loss, dehydration, or significant peripheral vasodilatation. The reflex tachycardia in response to vasodilating drugs such as hydralazine, sodium nitroprusside, or glyceryl trinitrate is absent and hypotension may be exaggerated.

Drugs with autonomic activity, such as atropine, neostigmine, suxamethonium, and pancuronium, have little effect on heart rate. Digoxin has inotropic effects but no significant effect on heart rate or atrioventricular nodal conduction. The transplanted heart responds in a normal manner to exogenous epinephrine (adrenaline), isoprenaline (isoproterenol), dopamine, and dobutamine. The development of an intraoperative bradycardia is of great concern, and therefore an infusion of isoprenaline should be readily available.

In isolated heart transplantations (as opposed to heart–lung transplantations), the diseased heart is removed during bypass, leaving right and left atrial remnants. Consequently, the postoperative ECG may exhibit two P waves. Some patients have an indwelling pacemaker fitted at the time of transplantation. The function of this should be checked as outlined in Chapter 47.

Because of the risk of infection, invasive monitoring should be used only when it is absolutely essential. During the course of routine follow-up, cardiac biopsies are taken via the right internal jugular vein, and so the antecubital fossa or left internal jugular routes should be used where central venous pressure monitoring is needed.

Fluid balance needs to be meticulous, all infusions should be fitted with bacterial filters, and injection ports should be kept capped and sterile.

### Lung transplantation

The transplanted lung is denervated distal to the bronchial anastomosis and there is no functional reinnervation. Modulation of the mechanics of breathing is regarded as being under brain-stem control. In the early postoperative period after lung transplantation there are sometimes rhythmic disturbances of breathing, but the normal pattern appears to return quickly. The lung responds normally to exercise and carbon dioxide.

Of particular importance to the anaesthetist is the fact that the stimulation of any airway distal to the bronchial anastomosis does not elicit a cough reflex. Expectoration from the transplanted lung has to be encouraged by postural drainage and physiotherapy. Despite denervation, bronchoconstriction can still occur. One complication of lung transplantation is bronchial stenosis at the anastomosis. This can result in distal collapse and accumulation of secretions. When this occurs, bronchoscopy is usually necessary and if it is recurrent a stent may be needed.

In patients with isolated lung allografts, care should be taken to avoid excessive airway pressures, which may stress the bronchial anastomosis. A transplanted lung is deprived of lymphatic drainage and great care should be taken to avoid fluid overload in these patients. It has been postulated that prolonged increased oxygen concentrations may be deleterious to the graft, and therefore it seems sensible to administer oxygen according to need rather than as a routine.

## Liver transplantation

With a successful liver transplantation, there are no special precautions other than those for transplantations in general. It is worth noting the reason for the transplantation in case there are associated congenital abnormalities.

## Corneal transplantation

Although a corneal transplantation does not have the same high profile of the solid organs mentioned above, it can similarly revolutionize life for the recipient. The point of anaesthetic relevance is that specific care should be taken in airway management, so as not to damage the cornea with clumsy application of the facemask or corneal abrasions.

## Xenotransplantation

The shortage of human organs available for transplantation is unlikely to be rectified, because of medical, sociopolitical and religious reasons. This implies that either artificial organs or living organs procured from other species (xenotransplantation) are needed. Successful xenotransplantation presents formidable scientific problems, as well as logistic and ethical ones. Animal size, functional characteristics of the potential xenograft, availability in sufficient numbers, and ethical acceptability constrain the choice of species. Although primates might seem the obvious choice, they breed slowly and are already endangered species. It is estimated that up to 40 000 animals per year would be required to sustain the world's current transplant programme.

Interest has therefore turned to the pig. Pigs grow quickly and are slaughtered for food already, and are likely to give rise to fewer ethical concerns than using organs from primates.

Rejection of discordant xenografted tissue is hyperacute, occurring within minutes. Current efforts to circumvent this problem centre on manipulation of the donor. Transgenic pigs have been produced which have had regulators of complement activation inserted into their genome. It is hoped that this will prevent hyperacute rejection. The results of experiments in which organs from these pigs have been transplanted into monkeys are encouraging – hyperacute rejection of hearts did not occur, and 20% functioned for more than 60 days. It therefore seems possible that transplantation of organs from pigs to man may be on the horizon.

# FURTHER READING


Bricker SR, Sugden JC. Anaesthesia for surgery in a patient with a transplanted heart. *Br J Anaesth* 1985;**57**:634–7.

Bowman H, Lennard TWJ. Immunosuppressive drugs. *Br J Hosp Med* 1992;**48**:570–7.

House RM, Thompson TL. Psychiatric aspects of organ transplantation. *JAMA* 1988;**260**:535–9.

Shaw IH, Kirk AJB, Conacher ID. Anaesthesia for patients with transplanted hearts and lungs undergoing non-cardiac surgery. *Br J Anaesth* 1991;**67**:772–8.

# Section 4

# Special subjects: physiology and pharmacology

# Chapter 67 Properties of the endothelium

D.G. Ririe

## THE ROLE OF THE ENDOTHELIUM IN ANAESTHESIA

A single layer of confluent cells known as the endothelium lines the cardiovascular system, including blood vessels and myocardium. Historically, the endothelium was considered a simple physical barrier between the blood and other tissues. However, the diverse and complex physiological function of the endothelial cells is now well recognized (Table 67.1). Functions of the endothelium can be divided into four distinct areas:

- a structural barrier;
- the regulation of vascular tone;
- the regulation of coagulation;
- inflammation.

## STRUCTURAL BARRIER

The endothelial cells provide a heterogeneous gatekeeping function by regulating flow of nutrient substances, diverse biologically active molecules, and blood cells from the circulating blood to the various tissues and organs of the body. In the intestine, endocrine glands, and kidneys, the fenestrated endothelial cell layer facilitates permeability for absorption, secretion, and filtering. In other areas, a discontinuous endothelial layer permits efficient cell movement through intercellular gaps.

| **Table 67.1 Physiological roles of the endothelium** |
|---|
| Maintenance of permeability barrier |
| Maintenance of basement membranes and arterial wall |
| Regulation of vascular tone |
| Provision of non-adherent, non-thrombogenic surface |
| Haemostasis and vascular repair |
| Synthesis and secretion of cytokines and growth factors |
| Adhesion and activation of leukocytes |
| Angiogenesis and vasculogenesis |
| Secretory, synthetic, metabolic and immunological functions |

A specific adaptation exists in the brain and retina where the endothelium has continuous tight junctions between adjacent cells, forming the less permeable and protective blood–brain barrier (BBB). Solutes with a high lipid solubility can readily penetrate the BBB. As most anaesthetic drugs are highly lipid soluble, they frequently produce a rapid central effect (e.g. fentanyl, volatile anaesthetics, etc.). In contrast, the relatively lipid-insoluble, charged molecules such as glycopyrrolate and neuromuscular blockers cannot readily cross the intact BBB.

Various insults can disrupt the tight junctions forming the BBB (trauma, infection, tumour, etc.). Drugs may pass freely into the central nervous system after disruption of the normal protective function of this specialized endothelium.

## REGULATION OF VASCULAR TONE

The endothelial cells modulate vascular tone through production and secretion of vasoactive molecules. Among many vasoactive factors released from the endothelium, the principal mediators of vascular tone include:

- nitric oxide (NO);
- endothelin (ET);
- prostacyclin ($PGI_2$);
- to a lesser extent, platelet-activating factor (PAF).

### Nitric oxide

NO synthase produces NO in the endothelial cell (Figure 67.1). NO decreases vascular tone through activation of the enzyme guanylyl cyclase in the vascular smooth muscle cell. NO regulates vascular tone through both basal production and stimulated production. Although NO plays a significant role in regulating basal vascular tone, it has many other actions on the endothelial cell (Table 67.2).

Volatile anaesthetics at low concentrations appear initially to increase vascular tone, probably through decreased production, inhibition of action, or increased destruction of NO. However, higher concentrations of volatile anaesthetics produce direct effects on vascular smooth muscle, overwhelming the NO effect, and producing vascular relaxation and decreased blood pressure. NO and its effects are discussed more thoroughly in Chapter 71.

### Prostacyclin

$PGI_2$ is an eicosanoid produced from arachidonic acid at sites of vascular injury. It directly relaxes smooth

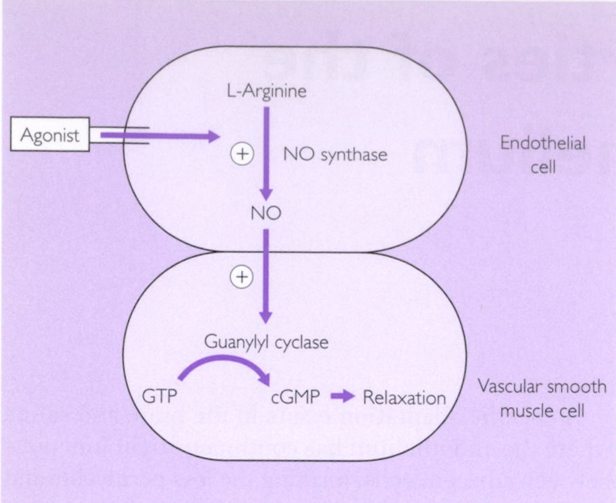


**Figure 67.1** Nitric oxide (NO) production in endothelial cells, and in vascular relaxation.

muscle, causing vascular dilatation. Unlike NO, $PGI_2$ is not produced under basal conditions and does not regulate basal vascular tone. In addition to its role in vascular tone, $PGI_2$ also has other important physiological effects (Table 67.3).

### Endothelin

ET, a very potent vasoconstrictor peptide synthesized by endothelial cells, binds to G protein coupled to receptors on the smooth muscle cells. ET stimulates an increase in the intracellular calcium concentration, which increases smooth muscle tone. As a result of the increase in intracellular calcium, ET increases the sensitivity of the vessel to the vasoconstrictive effects of catecholamines. Hypoxia, ischaemia, and shear stress on the vessel wall stimulate the production of an inactive ET precursor, which is cleaved to the active peptide.

| **Table 67.2 Effects of nitric oxide at the endothelial cell** |
|---|
| Regulation of basal vascular tone |
| Inhibition of smooth muscle cell proliferation/ migration |
| Inhibition of leukocyte adhesion |
| Inhibition of platelet adhesion and aggregation |

| **Table 67.3 Physiological effects of prostacyclin** |
|---|
| Retards platelet aggregation and adhesion |
| Relaxes vascular smooth muscle |
| Modulates local inflammatory response |

### Platelet-activating factor

PAF is a phospholipid which, in pathological states such as shock or sepsis, may cause vasoconstriction or vasodilatation, depending on the vascular bed and concentration of PAF. Although playing only a minor role in regulation of vascular tone, PAF plays an important role in inflammation.

## REGULATION OF COAGULATION

The intact endothelium serves as a natural inhibitor of coagulation; damaged endothelium promotes coagulation (Table 67.4). Our understanding of the interplay between these fascinating and complex opposing functions continues to evolve. The coagulation cascade is also discussed in Chapter 31.

### Inhibition of coagulation

The enzyme thrombin activates platelets, coagulation enzymes, and inflammation. Under normal circumstances, the endothelium must control thrombin activity to prevent clot formation. The endothelium contains heparin sulphate which promotes the activity of the associated antithrombin III to inhibit thrombin activity. The endothelial cell expresses thrombomodulin which binds and activates thrombin to catalyse activation of protein C and trigger synthesis of protein S; thrombomodulin also promotes inactivation of factors V and VIII and plasminogen activator inhibitor (PAI).

Endothelial cells also regulate coagulation through the production of plasminogen activators (PAs). The prototype, tissue plasminogen activator (t-PA), is a profibrinolytic molecule which causes plasminogen to be converted to plasmin. Plasmin catalyses conversion of fibrinogen and fibrin to fibrin monomer, producing clot lysis. Plasmin also degrades factors V, VII, IX, and X. PAIs modulate the PA. The clinical use of t-PA is for clot lysis in acute thrombolytic processes (e.g. stroke, myocardial infarction, and pulmonary embolism). A relative imbalance of PAI and PA may underlie pathological thrombus formation. In the future, manipulation of the balance between endogenous PAI and PA may be used to prevent undesirable thrombus formation, particularly after coronary artery bypass grafting and major orthopaedic surgery.

| **Table 67.4 Functions of endothelial cells in coagulation** |
|---|
| Produce and express tissue factor |
| Produce and bind von Willebrand's factor |
| Receptors for thrombin, fibrin, and other coagulation factors |
| Production of tissue plasminogen and fibrinolysis |
| Thrombomodulin expression |
| Production of protein S |
| Receptors for protein S and activation of protein C |

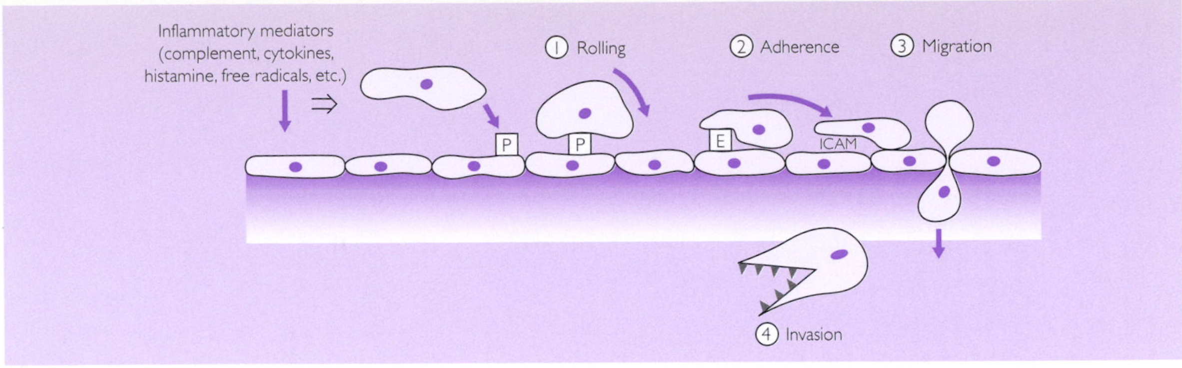


**Figure 67.2** Endothelial/leukocyte interaction in inflammation. P, P-selectin; E, E-selectin; ICAM, intercellular adhesion molecule.

In addition, endothelial production of NO and $PGI_2$ is important in inhibiting coagulation through inhibition of platelet aggregation.

### Promotion of coagulation

Inflammation and coagulation are closely related through endothelial damage or stimulation. The endothelium promotes coagulation by the expression of tissue factor, the initiator of the extrinsic coagulation pathway. Thrombin, endotoxin, cytokines, hypoxia, and mechanical injury stimulate production of tissue factor. The presence of tissue factor activates the coagulation cascade and produces fibrin on the endothelial cell surface. In addition, endothelial cells have numerous receptors for various coagulation factors, including, but not limited to, thrombin and fibrin, which are important in endothelial cell proliferation, migration, and retraction. These factors play a role in thrombus formation in the artery and may promote further narrowing or blockage of stenotic vessels.

Endothelial cells also produce and bind von Willebrand's factor. This is an important cofactor for haemostasis, functioning as a cofactor for factor VIII and the binding of platelets through glycoprotein Ib on the platelet surface. Deficiency of von Willebrand's factor results in von Willebrand's disease, and manifests as an autosomal dominant characteristic with impaired aggregation of platelets and decreased factor VIII activity.

Platelet adhesion to endothelium represents an early event in inflammation. Platelets contribute to spread of inflammation and form important links between coagulation and inflammation. One such link produced by vascular injury or inflammation is stimulation of endothelium production of PAF, which induces leukocyte and platelet adhesion and forms another link between coagulation and inflammation.

## INFLAMMATION

Normally, the endothelium provides a consistent barrier to the flow of white blood cells into tissues. However, when activated or injured, the endothelium enhances leukocyte activity in a series of actions (Figure 67.2) initiated by expression of cell surface receptors.

Injury to the endothelium causes P-selectin expression. P-selectin initiates the rolling phase in margination of leukocytes. E-selectin then maintains leukocyte adherence to the endothelial cell while P-selectin is rapidly internalized. Subsequently, the activated leukocyte binds to intercellular adhesion molecules 1 or 2 (ICAM-1 or ICAM-2). Activation of the leukocyte or the endothelium causes local endothelial damage and allows migration and invasion of leukocytes, with further localized tissue damage. Expression of certain ICAMs may be involved in tissue rejection, reperfusion injury, and sepsis.

## CONCLUSION

The endothelium regulates a vast number of physiological processes throughout the body, particularly in relation to the cardiovascular system. Understanding of the role of the endothelium in normal physiological processes and in pathophysiological states may underlie future treatments for hypertension, and coronary artery and peripheral vascular disease.

For the anaesthetist, the importance of the endothelium relates primarily to pharmacology. In particular, an understanding of how anaesthesia and specific anaesthetics regulate endothelial function may allow more appropriate selection of anaesthetic and vasoactive drugs.

## FURTHER READING

Cicala C, Cirino G. Linkage between inflammation and coagulation: an update on the molecular basis of the crosstalk. *Life Sci* 1998;**62**:1817–24.

Cines DB, Pollak ES, Buck CA, *et al*. Endothelial cells in physiology and in the pathophysiology of vascular disorders. *Blood* 1998;**91**:3527–61.

Johns RA. Endothelium, anesthetics, and vascular control. *Anesthesiology* 1993;**79**:1381–91.

Rapaport SI, Rao LV. The tissue factor pathway: how it has become a 'prima ballerina'. *Thromb Haemost* 1995;**74**:7–17.

Simonson MS, Dunn MJ. Cellular signaling by peptides of the endothelin gene family. *FASEB J* 1990;**4**:2989–3000.

Verrier E. The microvascular cell and ischemia–reperfusion injury. *J Cardiovasc Pharmacol* 1996;**27**(suppl 1):S26–30.

# Chapter 68 Adhesion molecules

J.J. McCloskey

Adhesion molecules facilitate the cell-to-cell contact that is necessary for diverse biological processes such as differentiation and inflammation. Many adhesion molecules have been described; however, the majority can be classified into four groups: integrins, members of the immunoglobulin superfamily, selectins, and cadherins (Table 68.1). The first three groups are primarily involved in inflammatory responses, whereas cadherins mediate cell growth and differentiation. The cadherin group will be discussed briefly, but this review will focus on the integrins, selectins, and members of the immunoglobulin superfamily because anaesthetists frequently encounter patients with inflammatory conditions.

## CADHERINS

Cadherins are cell surface adhesion molecules that interact with the intracellular actin cytoskeleton via plakoglobulin and catenin molecules. Intercalation of extracellular adhesion molecules into 'zipper-like' structures leads to stability of cell-to-cell junctions. To date, four cadherin molecules have been described: neural, epithelial, and placental cadherins, and liver cell adhesion molecule.

Malignant tumours demonstrate significant evidence of their biological role. Decreased production and function of cadherin molecules lead to detachment and metastasis of cancerous cells.

## INTEGRINS

The integrins are glycoproteins composed of two subunits, $\alpha$ and $\beta$, which mediate cell-to-cell and cell-to-cellular-matrix interactions. Sixteen $\alpha$ and eight $\beta$ units are known, and combinations of these units give rise to the various integrins. Classification of the integrins is defined by the $\beta$ units.

$\beta_1$-Integrins, also known as the very late antigen (VLA) superfamily, are primarily involved in tissue organization. $VLA_4$, however, also serves as a receptor for vascular adhesion molecule-1 (VCAM-1).

$\beta_2$-Integrins, or leukocyte integrins, are uniquely expressed on leukocytes. Individual binding of four various $\alpha$ chains to the specific $\beta_2$ chain, CD18, gives rise to four common integrin molecules: lymphocyte function-associated antigen (LFA-1), complement receptor 3 (Mac-1), gp 150 and 95, and $\alpha_d/\beta_2$. These $\beta_2$-integrins on leukocytes bind specifically to intercellular adhesion molecules (ICAM-1, -2, and -3).

The integrin molecules are characterized by having two-way signal transduction at the level of the cell membrane. Binding of a specific ligand to an integrin can elicit such responses as gene expression and apoptosis. However, an activated cell, such as a neutrophil stimulated by a bacterial peptide, can transmit a signal to the cell surface integrin, increasing the affinity of the integrin for binding of immunoglobulins.

**Table 68.1 Cell adhesion molecules**

| Integrins | Immunoglobulin superfamily | Selectins | Cadherins |
|---|---|---|---|
| **$\beta_1$ integrins** | ICAM-1, -2, -3 | Endothelial (E-) | Neural |
| VLA-4 | VCAM-1 | Platelet (P-) | Epithelial |
| **$\beta_2$ integrins** | PECAM-1 | Leukocyte (L-) | LCAM |
| LFA-1 | | | |
| Mac-1 (complement receptor 3) | | | |
| gp 150, gp95 | | | |
| $\alpha_d/\beta_2$ | | | |

ICAM, intercellular adhesion molecule; LCAM, liver cell adhesion molecule; LFA, lymphocyte function-associated antigen; PECAM, platelet–endothelial cellular adhesion molecule; VCAM, vascular cellular adhesion molecule; VLA, very late antigen.

## SELECTINS

Of the adhesion molecules considered here, the selectins probably have the greatest relevance to anaesthetic practice because of their role in inflammation. These molecules, including endothelial (E-), platelet (P-), and leukocyte (L-) selectin, are involved in the adhesive interactions of leukocytes, platelets, and endothelial cells. The name selectin is derived from the lectin portion of the molecule. All the selectins also share other common structural elements such as an epidermal growth factor-like domain, a variable number of complement regulatory domains, and a transmembrane sequence. Unlike the other classes of adhesion molecules, which bind proteins, the selectins bind to sialylated, fucosylated carbohydrate moieties.

E-selectin is expressed on the surface of activated endothelial cells. Activators include such agents as endotoxin, interleukin-1 (IL-1), and tumour necrosis factor (TNF). The expression of this selectin peaks at 4–6 hours and returns to basal levels in 24–48 hours.

P-selectin is constitutively synthesized and is stored intracellularly in platelets and endothelial cells. Agents such as thrombin, histamine, terminal complement components, and hydrogen peroxide activate platelets and endothelium which produces a rapid surface expression of the molecule.

Compared with the other selectins, L-selectin is constitutively expressed only by leukocytes. Activation of leukocytes leads to a shedding of L-selectin in minutes.

## IMMUNOGLOBULIN SUPERFAMILY

The immunoglobulin superfamily of adhesion molecules consists of cell surface proteins whose structure is characterized by a variable number of extracellular domains similar to those found in immunoglobulins. The most important members of this family include ICAM-1, ICAM-2, ICAM-3, VCAM-1, and platelet–endothelial cellular adhesion molecule-1 (PECAM-1).

ICAM-1 and ICAM-2 are predominately found on endothelium, but are also constitutively expressed on a variety of other cells. Both molecules bind to the leukocyte integrin, LFA-1, and Mac-1. VCAM-1, however, binds to the leukocyte integrin, VFA-4. Like E-selectin, expression of ICAM-1 and VCAM-1 on endothelial cells increases after stimulation with TNF or IL-1. ICAM-2 expression is not, however, increased by cytokines.

Unlike the selectins, molecules of the immunoglobulin superfamily require protein synthesis anew, so the onset of expression is slower and more prolonged. These adhesion molecules may mediate a more chronic role in inflammation.

## IMPLICATIONS OF CELL ADHESION MOLECULES IN ANAESTHESIA

To understand the potential involvement of adhesion molecules in anaesthesia, either directly or indirectly, one must have an understanding of the role of these molecules in inflammatory processes.

The adhesion molecules play a critical role in the recruitment of leukocytes, including neutrophils, monocytes, and lymphocytes, from the bloodstream to areas of inflammation (Figure 68.1). Initiation of an inflammatory process leads to the release of mediators, specifically cytokines, which in turn leads to the increased expression of adhesion molecules on a variety of cell surfaces and signalling of cellular recruitment. This action of recruitment can be broken down into three steps: initial attachment (tethering, rolling), adhesion, and migration. Expression of selectins leads to a slowing or rolling of leukocytes on endothelial surfaces. Up-regulation of integrins on leukocytes, and members of the immunoglobulin superfamily lead to the adhesion of the leukocytes to endothelium. Activation of two-way signal transduction by integrins

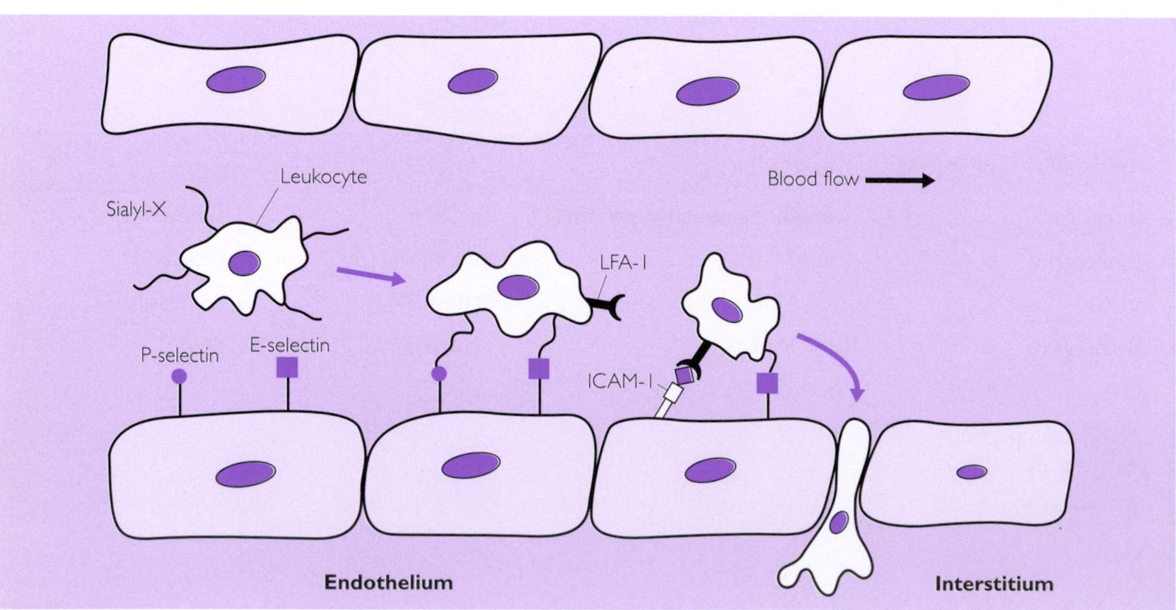


**Figure 68.1** Adhesion molecule interactions. ICAM, intercellular adhesion molecule; LFA, lymphocyte function-associated antigen.

then leads to migration of the leukocytes across the endothelial barrier into inflamed tissue.

As anaesthetists are presented with patients with inflammatory conditions (sepsis, inflammatory bowel disease, or connective tissue disorders) and those who will develop an inflammatory condition secondary to surgery (sepsis, cardiopulmonary bypass, or organ transplantation), in the future they may need to administer agents that modulate the expression or effects of adhesion molecules during surgery. Steroids, non-steroidal anti-inflammatory drugs, and a new class of agents, leumidins, can also be used perioperatively to modulate adhesion molecule expression.

Although little research has been done on the direct effects of anaesthetic agents on adhesion molecule expression, there is some evidence in a rat model that halothane can evoke ICAM-1-dependent leukocyte adhesion whereas sevoflurane up-regulates P-selectin expression in the mesenteric circulation.

Although cadherins, integrins, selectins, and members of the immunoglobulin superfamily are not yet daily concerns for anaesthetists, further research into the roles of these molecules and time course in inflammation may, in the future, require anaesthetists to tailor their anaesthetic plan according to the inflammatory process.

## FURTHER READING


Bevilacqua MP, Nelson RM. Selectins. *J Clin Invest* 1993;**91**:379–87.

Frenette PS, Wagner DD. Adhesion molecules: part I. *N Engl J Med* 1996;**334**:1526–9.

Frenette PS, Wagner DD. Adhesion molecules – part II: blood vessels and blood cells. *N Engl J Med* 1996;**335**:43–5.

Henricks PA, Nijkamp FP. Pharmacological modulation of cell adhesion molecules. *Eur J Pharmacol* 1998;**344**:1–13.

Morisaki H, Suematsu M, Wakabayashi Y, *et al.* Leukocyte–endothelium interaction in the rat mesenteric microcirculation during halothane or sevoflurane anesthesia. *Anesthesiology* 1997;**87**:591–8.

# Chapter 69 G proteins

P.P. McCaslin

Most signalling molecules bind to specific receptor proteins on the membrane of the target cell and cause changes in the intracellular environment of the cell that are relayed by secondary molecules. Of the three major classes of cell surface receptors, GTP-protein-linked (G-protein-linked) receptors represent a primary class, and the intermediary proteins involved in the signal transduction of the G-protein-linked receptors, the G proteins, will be the focus of this chapter. Many protein hormones, peptides, lipids, biogenic amines, proteases (thrombin), and sensory stimuli (vision and smell) mediate their effects via G proteins. Many of the agents used during anaesthesia to augment the patient's blood pressure, heart rate, and myocardial contractility, such as epinephrine (adrenaline), atropine, adenosine, and esmolol, produce effects that are amplified and mediated by G proteins. Important G-protein-linked receptors and the specific G proteins associated with these receptors are listed in Table 69.1.

G proteins are attached to the intracellular surface of the plasma membrane adjacent to the surface membrane receptor (Figure 69.1). When a hormone or other signalling molecule binds to its receptor, a conformational change occurs in the receptor and it transmitted intracellularly to the G protein. The G protein, comprising three polypeptides ($\alpha\beta\lambda$), dissociates into an $\alpha$ fragment and $\beta\lambda$ dimer when GTP displaces GDP from the $\alpha$ fragment. The GTP $\alpha$ fragment and $\beta\lambda$ dimer then diffuse to various enzymes or ionic channels where they serve as molecular switches. Proteins activated or inactivated by the G-protein subunits are called effectors and include enzymes such as adenylyl cyclase, phospholipases A, C, and D, and various membrane channels specific for calcium or potassium ions. There are multiple classes of G proteins, and a single cell often expresses many different classes. Moreover, several receptors on a cell may activate the same G protein, and a G protein may

**Table 69.1 G-protein-linked receptors and their effects**

| G proteins[a] | G-protein-linked receptors (usually named after signalling molecule) | G-$\alpha$ effects | G-$\beta\lambda$ effects |
|---|---|---|---|
| $G_i$ | Acetylcholine muscarinic ($M_2$, $M_4$), adenosine ($A_1$, $A_3$), adrenoceptor ($\alpha_2$), angiotensin ($AT_1$, $AT_2$), cannabinoid, dopamine ($D_{2-4}$), metabotrophic glutamate ($mGlu_{2-4, 6-8}$), $GABA_B$, 5HT (serotonin) ($5HT_{1a-f}$), melatonin, neuropeptide Y, opioid, prostanoid, protease-activated, somatostatin | Inhibits adenylyl cyclase → ↓ cAMP | stimulates $PLA_2$ or PLC → ↑ arachidonic acid or $IP_3$ |
| $G_{olf}$ | Sensory olfactory | Stimulates adenylyl cyclase → ↑ cAMP; stimulates PLC → ↑ $IP_3$ | |
| $G_q$ | Acetylcholine muscarinic ($M_1$, $M_3$, $M_5$), angiotensin ($AT_1$), bombesin, bradykinin, cholecystokinin, endothelin, metabotrophic glutamate ($mGlu_{1,5}$), histamine ($H_1$), $5HT_{2-c+}$, leukotriene, prostanoid, protease-activated, $P2Y_{1,2,4,6}$, tachykinins (substance P), vasopressin | Stimulates PLC and/or PLD → ↑ $IP_3$ and/or ↑ PA | Stimulates PLC → ↑ $IP_3$ |
| $G_s$ | Adenosine ($A_2$), adrenoceptor: $\alpha_1$, $\beta_{1,2,3}$, dopamine ($D_1$, $D_5$), histamine ($H_2$), $5HT_{4-7}$, prostaglandin, vasoactive intestinal peptide, vasopressin | Stimulates adenylyl cyclase → ↑ cAMP | Stimulates PLC → ↑ $IP_3$ |
| $G_t$ | Rhodopsin (activated by photons) | Stimulates PDE → ↓ cGMP | |

[a]heterotrimeric (i.e. $\alpha\beta\lambda$) G-protein subfamilies (subscript is often arbitrarily assigned); cAMP, cyclic adenosine monophosphate; cGMP, cyclic guanosine monophosphate; 5HT, 5-hydroxytryptamine; GABA, $\gamma$-aminobutyric acid; $IP_3$, inositol trisphosphate; PA, phosphatidic acid; PDE, phosphodiesterase; PLC, phospholipase C; PLD, phospholipase D; PKC, protein kinase C.

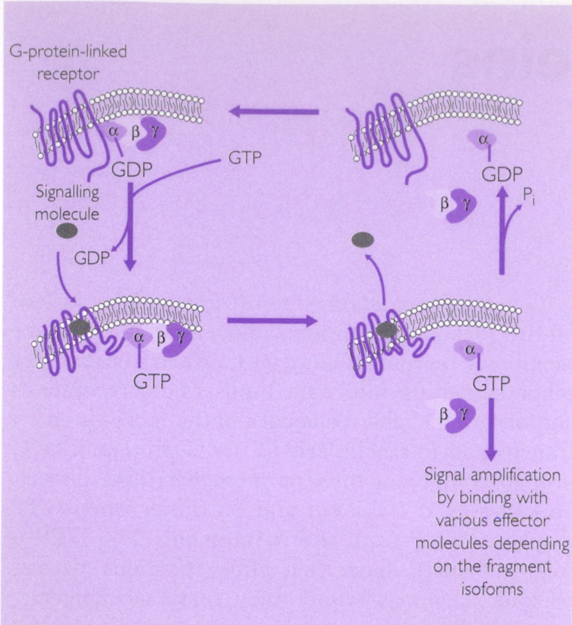


**Figure 69.1** G-protein regulatory cycle. In the first phase of the cycle, the receptor is not associated with the signalling molecule and GDP is bound to the α subunit of the G-protein complex. A conformational change occurs in the receptor upon binding of the signalling molecule, which is relayed to the G protein. This causes the α subunit to bind GTP and to split from the βλ dimer, both of which diffuse to various effector molecules where the second messenger is generated. The cycle is completed when GTP is hydrolysed and the G protein reassociates with the membrane-bound receptor.

activate more than one effector. The unique response of a cell to the signalling molecule arises from these different combinations.

As is the case for the G-protein-linked receptors, the G proteins themselves constitute a superfamily of proteins whose genomic repertoire numbers up to 100 forms in each individual. Adenylyl cyclase, the enzyme responsible for synthesizing cAMP, is inhibited by $G_i\alpha$ and stimulated by $G_s\alpha$. The $G_q\alpha$ subfamily stimulates phospholipase C, the enzyme that synthesizes inositol trisphosphate ($IP_3$), and the $G_t\alpha$ subfamily stimulates cGMP-dependent phosphodiesterase. The opening of various potassium and calcium channels is inhibited by the $G_i\alpha$ and $G_o\alpha$ subfamilies. Figure 69.2 illustrates these interactions. In each case, when the α-bound GDP is replaced with a GTP, the fragment dissociates from the trimeric molecule, enabling it to interact with the effector. Although less is known about the βλ dimer, it activates effector molecules as well. Most notably, this leads to the activation of the potassium channel ($G_i\beta\lambda$ subfamily) and P/Q- and L-type calcium channels ($G_s\beta\lambda$ subfamily), and the inhibition of the N- and P/Q-type calcium channels ($G_i\beta\lambda$ and $G_o\beta\lambda$ subfamilies).

Figure 69.3 illustrates how different autonomic receptors produce physiological effects depending on the presence of the receptors in selective tissues. In the heart, stimulation of muscarinic and adrenergic receptors produces opposite effects which can largely be explained by their opposing effects on adenylyl cyclase. Vagal stimulation results in the release of acetylcholine which activates the muscarinic receptor ($M_2$) found on cardiac cells (via $G_i$) whereas sympathetically mediated norepinephrine (noradrenaline) stimulates the $\beta_1$-adrenoceptors with the activation of adenylyl cyclase (via $G_s$) producing respective decreases and increases in cAMP.

However, the effects of acetylcholine and norepinephrine on the myocardium represent only one component of blood pressure control. Sympathetic input from the central nervous system (CNS) and G-protein activity in vascular smooth muscle are additional components that must be considered (Figure 69.3). Fenoldopam, a selective $D_1$-dopamine receptor agonist, is linked with $G_s$ and causes an elevation of cAMP in vascular smooth muscle, which leads to vasodilatation in smooth muscle. This is opposed to the effects of norepinephrine on smooth muscle, which causes vasoconstriction by activating a different adrenoceptor than that found on myocardium, the $\alpha_1$ receptor, in which case the elevation of $IP_3$ results from the actions of $G_q\alpha$ on phospholipase C. The control of blood pressure is further complicated by the CNS effects of clonidine, an $\alpha_2$-adrenoceptor agonist, which is linked to $G_i$ and produces a decrease in cAMP levels. As a result of the presynaptic location of these receptors in the CNS and peripheral vasculature, the sympathetic outflow is decreased, and clonidine produces effects opposite to those of norepinephrine.

Changes in G-protein expression have recently been found to occur in several pathological conditions. Hypertension, a major risk factor for myocardial infarction and stroke, has been linked to a G-protein isotype displaying a 41-amino-acid in-frame deletion from the $G_s\beta$. Idiopathic ventricular tachycardia is another condition that has been linked to a G protein, at least in one patient. Brief episodes of short runs of ventricular tachycardia followed by sinus rhythm characterize the condition. A single point mutation was found in the $G_i\alpha$ subunit which rendered focal areas of the heart unresponsive to normal suppression by adenosine. Normally, adenosine plays an important regulatory role by lowering cAMP levels, effects that are the opposite to those of epinephrine and norepinephrine. The $G_i$ family has also been linked to ischaemic preconditioning, where exposure of the myocardium to brief ischaemic episodes affords protection during a much longer ischaemic period that follows. A direct interaction of the $G_i\beta\lambda$ dimer with the ATP-activated potassium channel may be the mechanism of preconditioning. The $G_i$ family has also been linked to end-stage heart failure and various cardiomyopathies. The down-regulation of the $\beta_1$-adrenoceptor occurs simultaneously with the up-regulation of the $G_i\alpha$. Angiotensin-converting enzyme inhibitors and β-adrenoceptor antagonists owe part of their therapeutic effects to reversing the up-regulation of the $G_i$ subunit.

In summary, G proteins amplify the primary signal through the stimulation or inhibition of enzymes that synthesize second messengers such as cAMP and $IP_3$. G-protein subunits also directly bind to and regulate membrane channels. A large variety of pharmaceuticals and pathological conditions are mediated by G proteins.

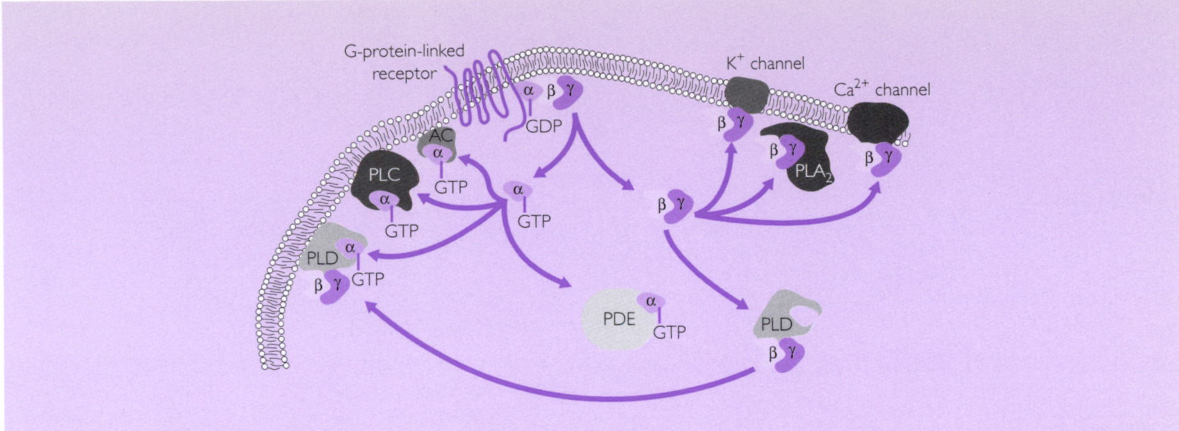


**Figure 69.2** Effector molecules activated by the α fragment and βλ dimer. After the ligand binds to the receptor, both the Gα and Gβλ dissociate from the receptor and diffuse to effector proteins, depending on the G protein subfamily. For example, $G_i\alpha$ and $G_s\alpha$ inhibit and activate, respectively, adenylyl cyclase (AC). $G_q\alpha$ stimulates phospholipase C (PLC) whereas $G_t\alpha$ inhibits phosphodiesterase (PDE). More recently, the βλ dimer associated with $G_i\alpha$ and $G_s\alpha$ has been shown to activate phospholipase $A_2$ ($PLA_2$)and PLC, respectively, and the βλ dimer of several subfamilies activates both potassium and calcium channels. Both the βλ and α subunits of $G_q$ have been linked with activation of phospholipase D (PLD).

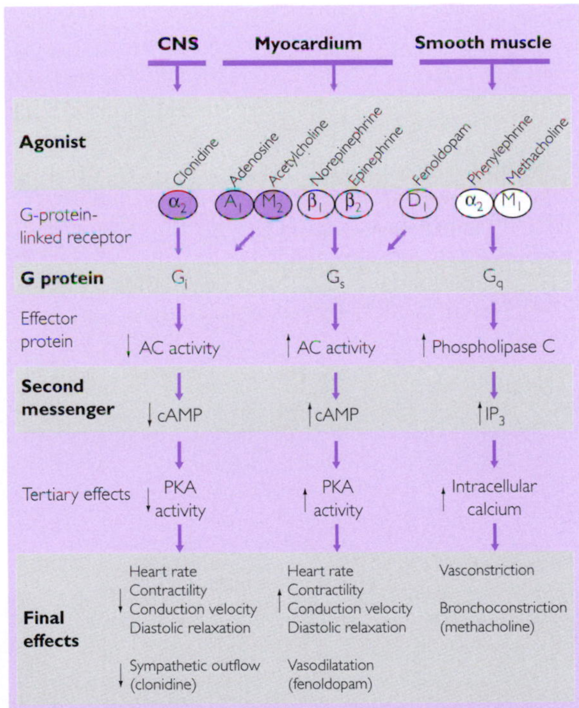


**Figure 69.3** Interaction of autonomic agonists on G proteins from three organ systems. The effect of G-protein-linked receptor activation depends on the presence or absence of the receptor in a particular organ system, as well as on the specific G protein associated with the receptor. For example, muscarinic and β-adrenergic activation in the heart have opposing effects. Even though fenoldopam's effects are mediated via $G_S$, receptors are located only on the vasculature smooth muscle and not in the heart, partially explaining why it produces a decrease in blood pressure. AC, adenylyl cyclase; cAMP, cyclic adenosine monophosphate; $\alpha_1$, $\alpha_2$ and $\beta_1$, $\beta_2$ represent adrenoreceptor subtypes; $D_1$, dopamine receptor; $IP_3$, inositol trisphosphate; $M_{1,2}$, cholinergic muscarinic receptors; PKA, protein kinase A.

## FURTHER READING


Alexander SPH, Peters JA. Receptor and ion channel nomenclature. *Trends Pharmacol Sci* 1997(suppl).

Cason BA, Gordon HJ, Avery IV EG, Hickey RF. The role of ATP sensitive potassium channels in myocardial protection. *J Cardiovas Surg* 1995:**10**:441–4.

Ford CE, Skiba NP, Bae H, *et al.* Molecular basis for interactions of G protein β-λ subunits with effectors. *Science* 1998;**280**:1271–4.

Lerman BB, Dong B, Stein KM, Markowitz SM, Linden J, Catanzaro DF. Right ventricular outflow tract tachycardia due to a somatic cell mutation in G protein subunit $\alpha_{i2}$. *J Clin Invest* 1998;**101**:2862–8.

Rodbell M. G proteins: out of the cytoskeletal closet. *Mt Sinai J Med* 1996;**63**:381–6.

Schmitz W, Boknik P, Linck B, Muller FU. Adrenergic and muscarinic receptor regulation and therapeutic implications in heart failure. *Mol Cell Biochem* 1996;**157**:251–8.

Schneider T, Igelmund P, Hescheler J. G protein interaction with K$^+$ and Ca$^{2+}$ channels. *Trends Pharmacol Sci* 1997;**18**:8–11.

Selbie LA, Hill SJ. G protein-coupled-receptor cross-talk: The fine-tuning of multiple receptor-signalling pathways. *Trends Pharmacol Sci* 1998;**19**:87–93.

Siffert W, Rosskopf D, Siffert G, *et al.* Association of a human G-protein (3 subunit variant with hypertension. *Nature Gen* 1998;**18**:45–8.

Wickman K, Clapham DE. Ion channel regulation by G protein. *Physiol Rev* 1995;**75**:865–85.

# Chapter 70 Cellular ageing

D.M. Colonna

In 1961, Hayflick and Moorehead (see Further reading) reported that human tissue cultures would predictably stop dividing after a certain number of divisions (approximately 50 divisions in human fibroblast cells). When cells reach their replicative limit (the Hayflick limit), they express particular gene products typical of cellular senescence and cease dividing. Do ageing cells simply have a clock that determines their lifespan? How well do cell cultures model ageing in the human? Through focusing on five main topics, this chapter attempts to answer these questions and provides the reader with some of the basic tenets of cellular ageing:

- the cell cycle;
- the role of telomeres in cell replication limits, ageing, and cancer formation;
- the roles of mitochondria and nucleoli in cellular ageing;
- the relationships between these mechanisms and novel treatments of chronic degenerative diseases;
- the perspective on human ageing provided by this analysis.

## THE CELL CYCLE

As an organism matures, cells divide during normal growth and differentiation, sorting into functionally different tissues. Cells divide to replace those damaged or lost: shed skin cells, cells of the gut mucosa, and blood cells lost from wear and tear. Germ cells undergo a specialized form of cell division, meiosis, producing ova or spermatozoa (see also Chapter 18).

Cells pass through predictable phases during the cell cycle, with specific replication processes occurring during each phase. For taxonomic purposes, the cell cycle includes two phases: (1) M phase (mitosis), the process of nuclear division and actual cell division (cytokinesis); and (2) interphase, everything that happens between M phases. Rather than a period of quiescence, interphase represents active portions of a cell's lifespan, and is functionally divided into three phases. Immediately following M phase is $G_1$, where the cell grows and performs its function within the organism. If cell signals do not stimulate further cell divisions, the cell can enter $G_0$, a specialized resting state, and remain there for months or years. If the cell reaches a critical size threshold, it enters S phase, where its DNA is replicated. After DNA replication is complete, structures needed for mitosis to occur, the centrioles and mitotic spindle, are created and organized during $G_2$ phase. At the completion of $G_2$, and when all is in readiness, mitosis (nuclear splitting) begins and subsequently complete cellular division (cytokinesis) follows.

A complex formed by a family of different cyclins plus cyclin-dependent kinase (CDK) regulates cell cycle processes. CDKs are activated when bound by cyclin, and deactivated when cyclin concentrations drop, shifting the equilibrium towards unbound CDK. Thus, when conditions during $G_1$ favour cell division, levels of $G_1$ cyclin increase, bind to CDK and initiate entry into S phase. Activated CDKs phosphorylate cellular proteins (at serine and threonine), initiating coordinated cell cycle processes (Figure 70.1).

## TELOMERES AND CELLULAR AGEING

During S phase, higher-order animals with linear chromosomes (excluding bacteria and many viruses with circular DNA) replicate their DNA in anticipation of mitosis. This presents a minor logistical problem, however. DNA is synthesized only in the $5' \rightarrow 3'$ direction, and the enzyme DNA polymerase requires a short section of RNA to attach to before initiating synthesis of the new DNA strand. At the end of the parent DNA segment, the RNA primer is released after DNA replication is complete, but *that* segment of parent DNA is not replicated. In short, the DNA sequence to which RNA polymerase attaches is not copied. Thus, each time a cell divides, a portion of DNA is 'lost' (Figure 70.2). A solution used by protozoa, fungi, plants, and mammals is provided by the DNA sequences found at the ends of chromosomes, consisting of repeating G nucleotides. In humans, this end portion of the chromosome is known as the telomere and has repeating TTAGGG sequences (Figure 70.3). These repeating sequences are the loci for DNA polymerase binding

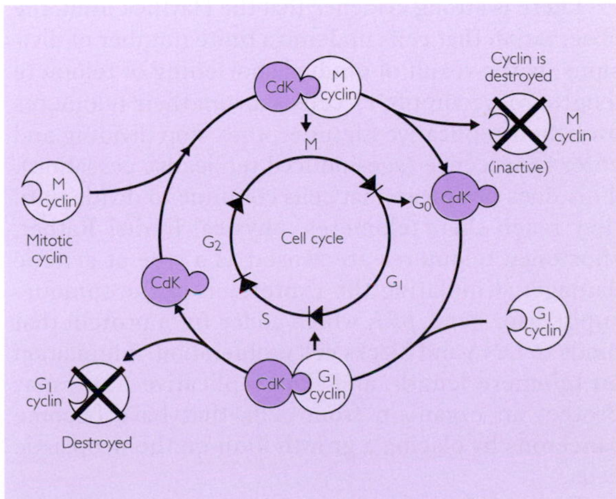


**Figure 70.1** Cyclin: cyclin-dependent kinase (Cdk) controls the cell cycle. The $G_1$ cyclin–Cdk complex stimulates the cell to enter the S phase and begin replication. The M cyclin–Cdk complex stimulates the cell to undergo mitosis and cytokinesis.

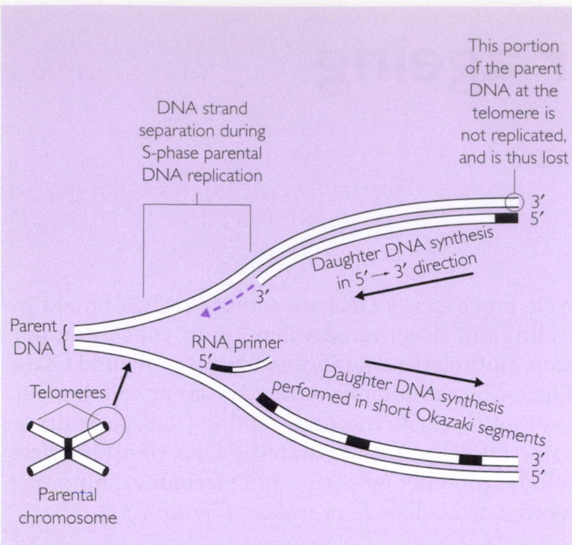


**Figure 70.2** Loss of parental DNA at the telomeres during S-phase DNA replication.

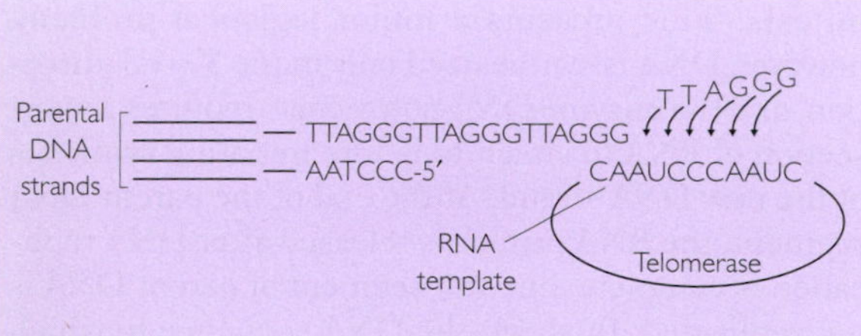


**Figure 70.3** Action of telomerase to lengthen telomeres. Human telomerase is a reverse transcriptase, adding TTAGGG bases to the chromosomes. Telomerase incorporates a portion of RNA to encode the repeating TTAGGG bases within the telomere.

and do not code for any gene products. Therefore, cell replications result in gradual shortening of the telomere.

There is strong evidence that the Hayflick limit, the observation that cells undergo a finite number of divisions, is the result of gradual shortening of telomere length. More simply, as cells shorten their telomeres over their replicative lifetimes, they stop dividing and enter senescence (age-induced replicative cessation). This does not mean that cells continue to divide until they reach their telomeres' physical limits. Rather, shortened telomeres are sensed as a type of genetic damage, stimulating the expression of the tumour-suppressor gene, *p53*, which codes for a protein that binds to DNA and blocks cell proliferation. A limitation on telomere length, and thus replicative limit, may protect an organism from cells that have become cancerous by placing a growth limit on the neoplastic cells.

Telomere length probably correlates inversely with cellular senescence and ageing of the organism. Globally speaking, having a replicative limit on cells with high turnover rates could be viewed as a problem. Such cells include haemopoietic stem cells, endometrial cells, cells lining the gut, and hair follicles. Nature does provide a solution to this conundrum: the enzyme telomerase, which lengthens telomeres. The above-mentioned cells with high replicative rates periodically express telomerase. There is a consensus that telomeres fulfil the requirement of a biological clock within an organism, determining the limits of organism viability (thought to be about 120 years in humans). In a recent report by Bodnar and colleagues (see Further reading), transfecting senescent human cell cultures with a gene for the catalytic component of telomerase reversed senescence and extended the Hayflick limit. Does this represent an elixir for eternal youth? Read further.

Interesting implications concerning telomeres and telomerase activity arise in cancer biology. Telomerase activation does not cause cancer but it does allow a cancer to grow if telomerase is expressed within that tumour. Indeed, telomerase is detected in the majority of malignant tumours. The relationship between telomerase and a cell's lifespan suggests an interesting strategy for cancer treatment – administration of telomerase inhibitors, or gene therapy aimed at inhibiting telomerase expression.

## MITOCHONDRIA, THE NUCLEOLUS, AND CELLULAR AGEING

The relationship between telomere length and the Hayflick limit is well established, producing a functional biological clock. This relationship does not explain many of the additional findings observed in ageing cells. The age-related decline in mitochondrial function proves of particular importance. Mitochondria, as the site of cellular respiration, are at high risk for oxygen-radical damage, especially to mitochondrial DNA. This phenomenon could explain, in part, the increased longevity associated with energy restriction in rats. A diet lower in calories reduces cellular metabolism, mitochondrial respiration, and free-radical-mediated damage. In the presence of the antioxidant ascorbate, ageing of human fibroblast cultures is delayed as mitochondrial respiration systems are preserved. Further evidence of ageing-induced changes in mitochondria includes the observation that nuclear transcription factors OXBOX–REBOX, which stimulate the synthesis of mitochondrial proteins, exhibit decreased nuclear binding in senescent human fibroblasts.

The yeast *Saccharomyces cerevisiae* has yielded important knowledge about cellular ageing in humans. A mutant of the *SGS1* gene in *S. cerevisiae* produces a 60% reduction in the yeast's lifespan. The *SGS1* gene has a homologue in humans found to be defective in people with Werner's syndrome, which includes premature ageing as well as other polyglandular disorders. Immunolocalization studies in *S. cerevisiae* demonstrate that *SGS1* resides in the nucleolus. In addition, senescent yeast cells with mutant *SGS1* genes have enlarged and fragmented nucleoli.

## CELLULAR AGEING MECHANISMS AND CHRONIC DISEASE

Clinical ageing represents a multifactorial set of processes, subject to environmental influences (air pollution, ionizing radiation), diet (either rich or poor in antioxidants, total energy intake), coexisting diseases (diabetes, hypertension), and personal habits (smoking, alcohol consumption). Nevertheless, cellular ageing and replicative limits probably play a role in the course of different age-related disease states, e.g. atherosclerosis. Aged and senescent cells exhibit altered patterns of gene expression, affecting both cellular and organism function. For example, age-related changes in skin include loss of collagen, increased collagenase, and decreased elastin. These dermal changes *in vivo* parallel alterations in gene expression observed in cultured human dermal fibroblasts *in vitro*.

Vascular endothelial cells are exposed to increased shear stress at arterial bifurcations, the site of early atherosclerotic changes. Such stress stimulates greater cell turnover and age-related changes. If vascular endothelial cells harvested from these sites are examined, telomere lengths are found to be shortened. This provides additional evidence that cellular senescence plays an important role in human atherosclerosis.

## CONCLUSION

This chapter presents only a portion of the ample evidence linking cellular replicative senescence with age-related telomere shortening. Additional evidence links cellular senescence with many chronic diseases, including atherosclerosis, ultraviolet-induced skin damage, osteoarthritis, failed bone marrow transplantation, and AIDS-induced loss of CD4 lymphocytes. Telomere biology is only a piece of the human ageing puzzle. Other cellular age-related changes have been discussed, including oxygen-radical mitochondrial damage, and nucleolar degeneration resulting from ribosomal DNA mutations. Many more mysteries must be solved before the human lifespan potential will change.

## FURTHER READING


Alberts B, Bray D, Lewis J, *et al*. The cell-division cycle. In: *Molecular Biology of the Cell*, 3rd edn. New York: Garland Publishing, Inc., 1994: 863–910.

Bodnar AG, Ouellette M, Frolkis M, *et al*. Extension of life-span by introduction of telomerase into normal human cells. *Science* 1998;**279**:349–52.

Fossel M. Telomerase and the aging cell: implications for human health. *JAMA* 1998;**279**:1732–5.

Hayflick L. The cell biology of human aging. *Sci Am* 1980;**242**:58–65.

Hayflick L, Moorehead PS. The limited *in vitro* lifetime of human diploid cell strains. *Exp Aging Res* 1961;**25**:585–621.

Johnson FB, Marciniak RA, Guarente L. Telomeres, the nucleolus and aging. *Curr Opin Cell Biol* 1998;**10**:332–8.

Shay JW, Bacchetti S. A survey of telomerase activity in human cancer. *Eur J Cancer* 1997;**33**:787–91.

# Chapter 71 Nitric oxide and anaesthesia

J.R. Tobin

The ubiquitous presence of nitric oxide (NO) in living systems has only been recognized over the past three decades. A free-radical gas with a half-life of only a few seconds (being inactivated when complexed with haemoglobin and other molecules), NO has wide ranging physiological importance, which resulted in its designation by *Science* as 'Molecule of the Year' in 1992. The discovery of NO and early work describing its physiology were recognized by awarding of the Nobel prize in 1998.

NO has critical physiological actions including cardiovascular regulation (as endothelial-dependent relaxing factor), neurotransmission (the first of many gaseous neurotransmitters that have been described), and immunological function (bactericidal and antineoplastic activities). Contemporary work reveals that alterations in the NO system may cause serious, even life-threatening, pathophysiology.

Multiple nitric oxide synthases (NOSs) utilize arginine as the substrate from which to produce NO and citrulline (Figure 71.1). Differing enzyme isoforms reside specifically in certain tissues, but may be cross-expressed under certain conditions. Neuronal and endothelial NOS (both of which are constitutive NOSs) require calcium, whereas the inducible NOS isoform (found predominantly in activated white blood cells, Kupffer cells, and vascular smooth muscle) does not require calcium, and, when induced by cytokines or endotoxins, will produce nanomolar quantities of NO. NOS function requires multiple other cofactors, including reduced nicotinamide adenine dinucleotide phosphate (NADPH), flavin mononucleotide (FMN), flavin adenine dinucleotide (FAD), calmodulin, and oxygen. Differences between enzyme isoforms may permit selective inhibition by newly developed compounds. NO stimulates multiple second-messenger systems, has retrograde messenger activity, and demonstrates autocrine-type activity on some of its generator cells. The second-messengers include cGMP (formed by activation of guanylyl cyclase), activation of multiple DNA- and RNA-binding factors, and poly(ADP-ribose) synthetase. NO also inactivates some enzyme systems and may produce toxicity through free-radical chemical interactions with cellular organelles. In high concentrations, NO can disrupt aerobic energy production by injuring mitochondrial electron-transport mechanisms.

The discovery of the NO–guanylyl cyclase system revealed how the nitrovasodilators (nitroglycerin and sodium nitroprusside) work. Nitrovasodilators represent precursor molecules that generate NO, the active vasodilator. Endogenous endothelial NO or NO produced by exogenous nitrovasodilators crosses the endothelium into vascular smooth muscle, activating guanylyl cyclase and increasing cGMP, which subsequently induces vasorelaxation. Furthermore, regulation of organ blood flow is critically linked to local microcirculatory NO generation. Deficiencies in NO production may contribute to hypertension or organ ischaemia, whereas excess NO formation produces hypotension and diminishes cardiac performance.

Significant work on the NO system has relevance to anaesthetic mechanisms and actions, as well as to the clinical practice of the anaesthetist. Volatile

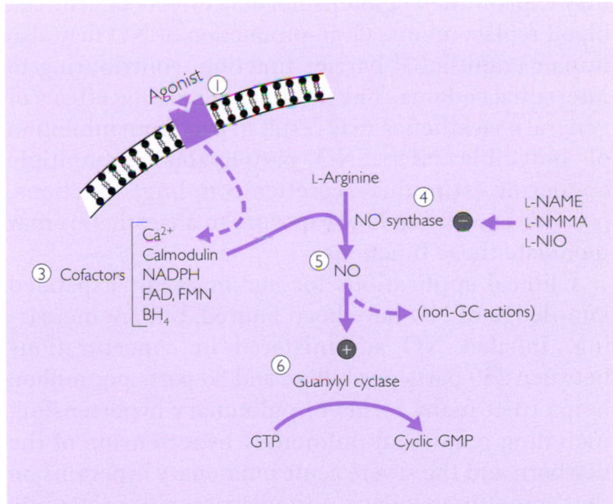


**Figure 71.1** The nitric oxide (NO) signalling pathway. In the brain and endothelium, NO is produced from L-arginine by similar consititutive enzymes called NO synthase(s). These enzymes are activated by the binding of calcium ($Ca^{2+}$) and calmodulin, often in response to agonist–receptor interaction, leading to increased cytosolic calcium. They are homologous to cytochrome P450 reductase enzymes, having recognition sites for reduced nicotinamide adenine dinucleotide phosphate (NADPH), flavin mononucleotide (FMN), and flavin adenine dinucleotide (FAD). Tetrahydrobiopterin ($BH_4$) is another cofactor. After its production, NO binds to the haem moiety of guanylyl cyclase (GC) which catalyses the production of cyclic GMP (cGMP) from GTP. Specific analogues of L-arginine, including nitro-L-arginine methyl ester (L-NAME), $N^G$-monomethyl-L-arginine (L-NMMA), and *N*-imino-ornithine (L-NIO), are competitive inhibitors of NOS. The numbers 1–6 represent potential sites of inhalational anaesthetic interaction, as discussed in the text. (Adapted from Johns RA. *Anesthesiology* 1993;79:1381–91.)

anaesthetics inhibit NO production from endothelial cells. NOS inhibition may reduce the minimum anaesthetic concentration (MAC) of volatile anaesthetics (although these results are controversial), suggesting a role of NO in consciousness and as an important neurotransmitter involved in the mechanism of general anaesthesia. Even though volatile general anaesthetics inhibit endothelial NO release (which should result in vasoconstriction), vasodilatation and negative inotropy represent the predominant haemodynamic responses and they are produced by other direct mechanisms (inhibition of calcium channel activity) in these tissues, as well as indirectly through reduced sympathetic activity.

Atherosclerosis interferes with basal NO production, which may contribute to hypertension associated with atherosclerosis. NO inhibits platelet aggregation and adhesion. The impaired endothelial function of atherosclerotic vessels, including impaired local vasodilatation, may predispose to local platelet adhesion and aggregation. NO plays a significant role in normal vascular autoregulation and in the balance of coagulation. These actions may be important in the acute and chronic administration of nitrates, and must be considered as significant potential side effects to inhaled NO. NO may actually have a haemodynamic hormonal function, albeit brief, while carried on haemoglobin, which may explain the angiotensinogenic effects of artificial blood replacements. Over-production of NO may also impair endothelial barrier function, contributing to interstitial oedema. The immunomodulating effects of general anaesthetics may result in part from inhibition of inducible NOS. NO participates in multiple endocrine (stimulus–secretion coupling) functions, possibly explaining how exposure to anaesthetics may modulate these functions.

Clinical applications for our markedly expanded knowledge of NO have been limited, but are increasing. Inhaled NO administered in concentrations between 250 parts per billion and 80 parts per million helps treat many forms of pulmonary hypertension, including persistent pulmonary hypertension of the newborn and the severe acute pulmonary hypertension that sometimes follows administration of protamine sulphate. Some authors advocate a trial of NO inhalation to determine recruitability of pulmonary vascular dilatation in the algorithm of decision-making regarding heart versus heart–lung transplantation. As inhaled NO would 'selectively' vasodilate well-ventilated lung regions, inhaled NO might improve $\dot{V}/\dot{Q}$ matching in acute respiratory distress syndrome (ARDS), permitting less aggressive positive pressure ventilation and oxygen exposure. However, results regarding use of NO in ARDS have been mixed. Many centres are currently conducting intraoperative and critical care clinical trials of inhaled NO either for acute therapy of pulmonary hypertension or to reduce right ventricular afterload (impedance). Inhaled NO must be used with caution in the patient with coagulopathy or thrombocytopenia because pulmonary haemorrhage may result.

Many investigators are determining whether inhibition of endothelial (constitutive) and inducible NOS is an appropriate therapy for shock. Overproduction of NO may cause severe vasodilatation and cardiac depression in septic shock. Although investigators have successfully restored vascular tone and augmented cardiac performance with inhibitors of NOS (arginine derivatives and other agents), overall survival in animal models and early human studies has not been encouraging. Furthermore, NOS inhibitors may evoke pulmonary hypertension, necessitating use of inhaled NO to prevent right ventricular failure or severe hypoxaemia. With the synthesis of more selective inhibitors of NOS isoforms, better targeted therapy of the NOS systems may evolve.

Neuronal NOS is expressed in many areas of the brain, spinal cord, and peripheral nerves. Many investigators have inhibited NOS with arginine analogues to determine the results of decreased NO production. Others have developed gene knock-out models to study the implications of the absence of one NOS isoform. Controversy exists about whether inhibition of NOS reduces the MAC of volatile anaesthetics, and whether the NO pathway might be involved in general anaesthetic mechanisms. It remains unclear whether volatile agents inhibit neuronal NOS activity directly or inhibit the NO–cGMP cascade at a different site. NO plays an important role in long-term potentiation and memory formation in the brain. Neuronal and endothelial NOSs are involved in cerebrovascular autoregulation. The cerebral vasculature responds to NO; thus, nitrovasodilators may increase cerebral blood volume and this must be considered carefully in patients with increased intracranial pressure. NO may underlie glutamate-induced neurotoxicity.

Spinal nitroxidergic neurons are involved in both spinal nociceptive transmission and descending antinociceptive pathways. Selective manipulation of NO pathways in the spinal cord may offer new analgesic developments. However, inhibition of NOS in the spinal cord may result in ischaemia. Dorsal root ganglion, dorsal horn and intermediolateral tract foci of nitroxidergic neurons respond differently to acute and chronic pain. Insights into the control of signal transduction mechanisms for these responses may offer more promise than direct inhibition of NOS itself.

Nitroxidergic neurons represent one of many of the non-cholinergic, non-adrenergic neuron groups responsible for smooth muscle dilatation in the gastrointestinal tract and for the vasodilatation necessary for penile erection. Opioid- and volatile anaesthetic-induced reduction in gastrointestinal peristalsis may involve diminished NO production. In the kidney, NO affects the microcirculatory perfusion pressure gradients necessary for filtering functions, and has a paracrine function in regulation of renin production. As a proinflammatory molecule, NO may be important in transplant rejection. NO also regulates adrenal steroidogenesis and adrenal function in response to stress and shock.

Future directions in NO research will include further identification of its role in developmental physiology, neurotoxicity and plasticity, cardiovascular homoeostasis, cancer, transplantation biology, inflammation, and immunology. Whether systemic administration of NOS inhibitors will improve survival in shock states remains unclear. The efficacy of inhaled NO for multiple disease states is being studied. The interactions of different classes of anaesthetic agents with the NO system may help elucidate the central mechanism(s) of consciousness/sedation or general anaesthesia. In addition, future analgesics and advances in pain research may exploit the nitroxidergic signalling system in the central, autonomic, and peripheral nervous systems.

## FURTHER READING


Adachi T, Kurata J, Nakao S, *et al*. Nitric oxide synthase inhibitor does not reduce minimum alveolar anesthetic concentration of halothane in rats. *Anesth Analg* 1994;**78**:1154–7.

Galley HF, Nelson LR, Webster NR. Anaesthetic agents decrease the activity of nitric oxide synthase from human polymorphonuclear leucocytes. *Br J Anaesth* 1995;**75**:326–9.

Ignarro LJ. Signal transduction mechanisms involving nitric oxide. *Biochem Pharmacol* 1991;**41**:485–90.

Jia L, Bonaventura C, Bonaventura J, Stamler JS. S-Nitrosohaemoglobin: a dynamic activity of blood involved in vascular control. *Nature* 1996;**380**:221–6.

Johns RA. The nitric oxide–guanylyl cyclase signally pathway. In: Yaksh TL, Lynch C, Zapol WM, *et al*., eds. *Anesthesia Biologic Foundations*. Philadelphia: Lippincott-Raven, 1998: 131–44.

Johns RA, Moscicki JC, DiFazio CA. Nitric oxide synthase inhibitor dose-dependently and reversibly reduces the threshold for halothane anesthesia. A role for nitric oxide in mediating consciousness? *Anesthesiology* 1992;**77**:779–84.

Meller ST, Gebhart GF. Nitric oxide (NO) and nociceptive processing in the spinal cord. *Pain* 1993;**52**:127–36.

Moncada S, Palmer RM, Higgs EA. Nitric oxide: physiology, pathophysiology, and pharmacology. *Pharmacol Rev* 1991;**43**:109–42.

Mullner M. Nobel prize for medicine awarded for work on nitric oxide. *BMJ* 1998;**317**:1031.

Palmer RM, Ferrige AG, Moncada S. Nitric oxide release accounts for the biological activity of endothelium-derived relaxing factor. *Nature* 1987;**327**:524–6.

Parker TA, Kinsella JP, Abman SH. Response to inhaled nitric oxide in persistent pulmonary hypertension of the newborn: relationship to baseline oxygenation. *J Perinatol* 1998;**18**:221–5.

Petros A, Lamb G, Leone A, *et al*. Effects of a nitric oxide synthase inhibitor in human with septic shock. *Cardiovasc Res* 1994;**28**:34–9.

Rossaint R, Falke KJ, Lopéz F, *et al*. Inhaled nitric oxide for the adult respiratory distress syndrome. *N Engl J Med* 1993;**328**:399–405.

Rossaint R, Gerlach H, Schmidt-Ruhnke H, *et al*. Efficacy of inhaled nitric oxide in patients with severe ARDS. *Chest* 1995;**107**:1107–15.

Szabo C. Alterations in nitric oxide production in various forms of circulatory shock. *New Horiz* 1995;**3**:2–32.

Todd MM, Wu B, Warner DS, Maktabi M. The dose-related effects of nitric oxide synthase inhibition on cerebral blood flow during isoflurane and pentobarbital anesthesia. *Anesthesiology* 1994;**80**:1128–36.

Zuo Z, Tichotsky A, Johns RA. Halothane and isoflurane inhibit vasodilation due to constitutive but not inducible nitric oxide synthase. Implications for the site of anesthetic inhibition of the nitric oxide/guanylyl cyclase signaling pathway. *Anesthesiology* 1996;**84**:1156–65.

Moncada S, Palmer RM, Higgs EA. Nitric oxide: physiology, pathophysiology and pharmacology. *Pharmacol Rev* 1991;43:109–42.

[illegible] Nobel prize for medicine awarded for work on nitric oxide. *BMJ* 1998;317:1031.

Palmer RM, Ferrige AG, Moncada S. Nitric oxide release accounts for the biological activity of endothelium-derived relaxing factor. *Nature* 1987;327:524–6.

[illegible] JJ, Kinsella JP, Abman SH. Response to inhaled nitric oxide in persistent pulmonary hypertension of the newborn: relationship to baseline oxygenation. *J Perinatol* 1998;18:221–5.

Petros A, Lamb G, Leone A, *et al.* [illegible] nitric oxide synthase inhibitor in humans with septic shock. *Cardiovasc Res* 1994;28:34–9.

[illegible]

[illegible] 1996;[illegible]

[illegible] Alterations in nitric oxide production in various forms of circulatory shock. *New Horiz* 1995;3:[illegible]

Todd MM, Wu B, Warner DS, Maktabi M. The dose-related effects of nitric oxide synthase inhibition upon basal cerebral blood flow during halothane and pentobarbital anesthesia. *Am J Physiol* 1994;[illegible]

[illegible] Johns RA. [illegible] anesthetics, and [illegible] nitric oxide synthase, implications for the [illegible] the inhibition of the nitric oxide/cyclic GMP signaling pathway. *Anesthesiology* 199[illegible]

[illegible] of general anaesthesia. In addition, inhalational [illegible] in [illegible] the nitric oxide signalling system in the central, autonomic, and peripheral nervous systems.

## FURTHER READING

Adachi T, Kurata J, Nakao S, *et al.* Nitric oxide synthase inhibitor does not reduce minimum alveolar anesthetic concentration of halothane in rats. *Anesth Analg* 1994;78:1154–7.

Galley HF, Nelson LR, Webster NR. Anaesthetic agents decrease the activity of nitric oxide synthase from human polymorphonuclear leucocytes. *Br J Anaesth* 1995;75:326–9.

[illegible]

[illegible]

Johns RA. The nitric oxide/cyclic GMP signaling pathway. In: [illegible] (eds) *Anesthesia: Biologic Foundations.* Philadelphia: Lippincott-Raven, 1998, 123–44.

Johns RA, Moscicki JC, DiFazio CA. Nitric oxide synthase inhibitor dose-dependently and reversibly reduces the threshold for halothane anesthesia. A role for nitric oxide in mediating consciousness? *Anesthesiology* 1992;77:779–84.

Malmberg AB, Yaksh TL. Spinal nitric oxide [illegible] processing in the spinal cord. *Pain* 1993;[illegible]

# Chapter 72 Mechanisms of general anaesthesia

S.J. Mihic

The use of general anaesthetics to prevent pain perception during surgery forms a cornerstone of modern medicine, and began in the 1840s with demonstrations by Long and Morton of the therapeutic utility of ether anaesthesia. A number of general anaesthetic agents have since been introduced into clinical practice, but without any definitive knowledge of their mechanisms of action. Chemicals with diverse structures can produce anaesthesia, including gases such as xenon and nitrous oxide, and a variety of alkanes, alkanols, ethers, and cycloalkanes. Larger molecules such as barbiturates, steroid anaesthetics, and the dissociative anaesthetic ketamine also produce general anaesthesia. This structural diversity in chemicals all producing the same desired clinical end-point has long interested pharmacologists and has led to considerable speculation about the mechanisms of action of general anaesthetics.

At the turn of the twentieth century, H.H. Meyer and E. Overton independently formulated their now famous hypothesis that anaesthetics with greater solubility in lipophilic solvents such as olive oil possess greater potency *in vivo*. As available evidence suggested the importance of cell membranes in regulating neuronal excitability, and because they have a high lipid content, cell membranes were studied intensively in an attempt to determine the mechanism of action of general anaesthetics. In cell membranes, anaesthetics could conceivably act on lipids, on membrane-bound proteins, or at the interfaces between lipids and proteins. Initially, most research focused on the disordering effects of anaesthetics on membrane structure. Anaesthetic molecules, by dissolving into the lipid portions of cell membranes and affecting membrane properties such as volume or order, were believed to then indirectly affect the function of membrane-bound proteins. Volatile anaesthetics disorder lipid bilayers and cell membranes at concentrations achieved therapeutically; however, these effects are small and can be mimicked by small increases in temperature which themselves do not produce anaesthesia. More recently, Eger and colleagues (see Further reading) identified compounds chemically related to general anaesthetics that appear to violate the Meyer–Overton hypothesis by not producing immobilization, despite their having high oil : gas partition coefficients. Difficulties with lipid-based theories of volatile anaesthetic action eventually led to a shift in research emphasis to other potential molecular targets.

By the early 1980s, protein sites of action of general anaesthetics gained increasing attention. Pharmacologically relevant concentrations of a variety of anaesthetics were found to inhibit the function of the lipid-free firefly enzyme luciferase. Based on this work, and that performed using other model proteins, it was reasoned that proteins found in cell membranes might be possible targets for anaesthetic agents. The voltage-gated ion channels, which rapidly alter cellular excitability, were among the first to be studied. Voltage-gated sodium, potassium, and calcium ion channels, important in mediating axonal signal conduction and neurotransmitter release, are all affected by volatile anaesthetics but, with a few exceptions, only at supratherapeutic concentrations.

The actions of volatile anaesthetics on the function of neurotransmitter-activated ion channels have been extensively studied in the past decade, with some of the most promising candidates being the γ-aminobutyrate ($GABA_A$), glycine, and glutamate receptors. Most of these receptors are located at synapses and thus are crucial to neurotransmission. As with the voltage-gated ion channels, modifying the function of these membrane-bound proteins would be expected to alter neuronal excitability rapidly. $GABA_A$ and glycine receptors contain integral anion-conducting channels and, with the related serotonin-3 ($5HT_3$) and nicotinic acetylcholine receptors, form a receptor superfamily. A number of classes of modulatory agents allosterically affect the functioning of these receptors.

The $GABA_A$ receptor is the major inhibitory neurotransmitter receptor system in the mammalian central nervous system, and a current forerunner among candidate sites for general anaesthetic action. Many sedative/hypnotic/anaesthetic agents, possessing diverse chemical structures, affect $GABA_A$ receptor function, including the benzodiazepines, alcohols, barbiturates, some steroids such as alphaxalone, and volatile anaesthetics. Administration of GABA analogues to rats and mice produces analgesia, sedation, and loss of the righting reflex. Studies by a number of investigators using biochemical and electrophysiological techniques demonstrate enhancement of $GABA_A$ receptor function by volatile and non-volatile anaesthetics, including: enflurane, halothane, isoflurane, propofol, alphaxalone, and a variety of alcohols. Importantly, all these compounds enhance $GABA_A$ receptor function at general anaesthetic concentrations. Furthermore, *in vivo* differences between the potencies of isomers of isoflurane match the differences in their potencies in enhancing GABA-mediated responses. These *in vivo* differences are very difficult to explain using lipid-based theories of anaesthetic action, and partially contributed to the shift in research interest to protein-based theories. In summary, the extensive literature describing anaesthetic effects on the $GABA_A$ receptor makes it one of the most likely molecular sites of action. In fact, most general anaesthetics, with the exceptions of ketamine and xenon, affect the $GABA_A$ receptor at therapeutically relevant concentrations.

Although the $GABA_A$ receptor is primarily responsible for inhibitory neurotransmission in the brain, the glycine receptor performs that role in the spinal cord and brain stem. Like the $GABA_A$ receptor, it contains an integral chloride channel and, because of the significant amino acid sequence homology of $GABA_A$ and glycine receptors, it is not surprising that glycine receptors are also sensitive to general anaesthetics (Figure 72.1). Although fewer studies have examined general anaesthetic effects on glycine receptors, enflurane, halothane, isoflurane, chloroform, and propofol, as well as a variety of alcohols, all potentiate glycine-mediated currents. Recent studies suggesting that anaesthesia may involve a significant spinal cord component also underscore the potential importance of glycine receptors in anaesthesia.

General anaesthetics also affect cationic currents through nicotinic acetylcholine and $5HT_3$ receptor-associated channels. However, because the function of nicotinic acetylcholine receptors in the brain is not well understood, the physiological relevance of anaesthetic-mediated current inhibition remains unknown. The scarcity of $5HT_3$ receptors in the brain probably limits their importance in producing anaesthesia, although their presence in the area postrema suggests an involvement in anaesthetic-induced nausea. Therapeutic concentrations of volatile anaesthetics enhance $5HT_3$ receptor responses, but even extremely high concentrations of propofol are without effect, perhaps explaining the decreased incidence of nausea accompanying its use.

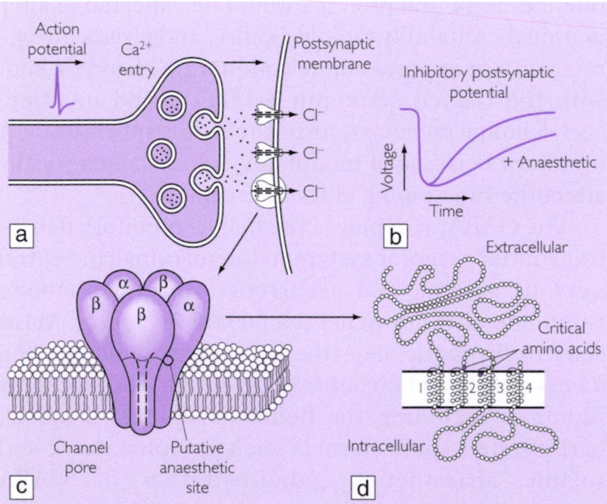


**Figure 72.1** My research group has found that single amino acid substitutions at two positions remove the potentiating effects of volatile anaesthetics and ethanol on $GABA_A$ (γ-aminobutyric acid) and glycine receptors. (a) $GABA_A$ and glycine receptors bind the neurotransmitters that are released at inhibitory chemical synapses, and open to allow chloride ions ($Cl^-$) to diffuse across the postsynaptic membrane. (b) The main effect of volatile anaesthetics is to prolong channel opening and, hence, to increase postsynaptic inhibition. (c) The receptor channels consist of pentamers of closely related subunits, and the structure of a single subunit is shown in (d). The two critical amino acids may form a binding site for general anaesthetics and ethanol. (Adapted from Mihic SJ *et al. Nature* 1997;389:385–9.)

Glutamate receptors are divided into the *N*-methyl-D-aspartate (NMDA) and non-NMDA receptor classes. Both types of receptor are linked to integral cation channels and share amino acid sequence homology between themselves, but not with the $GABA_A$ receptor class. Glutamate receptors comprise the primary excitatory neurotransmitter system in the brain, and inhibition of their function would be consistent with the production of an anaesthetized state. NMDA receptors are sensitive to the inhibitory effects of the dissociative anaesthetic ketamine, but not pentobarbitone (phenobarbital). Ethanol inhibits the function of neuronal NMDA receptors and receptors composed of defined combinations of subunits, but the inhibitory effects of volatile anaesthetics and propofol are generally weak. Inhibition of glutamate release may explain the strong effect of volatile anaesthetics on NMDA receptor function reported in the spinal cord.

Non-NMDA glutamate receptors are subdivided into the α-amino-3-hydroxy-5-methyl-4-isoxazole proprionate (AMPA) and kainate subclasses. Both are generally weakly sensitive to clinically relevant concentrations of volatile anaesthetics in both neuronal and recombinant receptor preparations. Furthermore, the intravenous anaesthetic propofol has no effect on AMPA receptors, even at concentrations greatly exceeding those that produce anaesthesia. However, as for NMDA receptors, AMPA and kainate receptors are strongly inhibited by subanaesthetic-to-anaesthetic concentrations of ethanol and other small alcohols. In summary, for both the NMDA and non-NMDA receptors, justifications can be made for their involvement in the behavioural actions of ethanol and ketamine, but the situation is less clear with the volatile anaesthetics. The minor effects produced by pharmacologically relevant concentrations may be important *in vivo*, but this has yet to be ascertained.

General anaesthesia is not a single clinical entity, but instead represents a spectrum of physiological states that include loss of consciousness, amnesia, and the failure to respond reflexively to a noxious stimulus. Although significant progress has been made in understanding the actions of general anaesthetics *in vitro*, it is not yet possible to ascribe the clinically observed signs of anaesthesia to the result of specific changes in any of the biochemical sites detailed above. Different sites probably mediate the effects of volatile anaesthetics on amnesia and the suppression of movement by a noxious stimulus; some non-immobilizing lipophilic compounds that deviate from the Meyer–Overton hypothesis still possess amnestic properties. Recently, specific amino acids of $GABA_A$, glycine, and glutamate receptors were identified as being responsible for the effects of volatile anaesthetics on receptor function. Anaesthetic-insensitive receptors have been constructed and tested *in vitro*, and it is now feasible to contemplate the genetic engineering of mice bearing these insensitive receptors. This will allow the various *in vivo* aspects of general anaesthetic actions to be associated with the receptors mentioned above, which may lead to a more complete understanding of the molecular mechanisms of general anaesthesia.

## FURTHER READING

Eger EI II, Koblin DD, Harris RA, *et al*. Hypothesis: inhaled anesthetics produce immobility and amnesia by different mechanisms at different sites. *Anesth Analg* 1997;**84**:915–18.

Franks NP, Lieb WR. Do general anaesthetics act by competitive binding to specific receptors? *Nature* 1984;**310**:599–601.

Franks NP, Lieb WR. Molecular and cellular mechanisms of general anaesthesia. *Nature* 1994;**367**:607–14.

Harris RA, Mihic SJ, Dildy Mayfield JE, *et al*. Actions of anesthetics on ligandgated ion channels: role of receptor subunit composition. *FASEB J* 1995;**9**:1454–62.

Janoff AS, Pringle MJ, Miller KW. Correlation of general anesthetic potency with solubility in membranes. *Biochim Biophys Acta* 1981;**649**:125–8.

Koblin DD, Chortkoff BS, Laster MJ, *et al*. Polyhalogenated and perfluorinated compounds that disobey the Meyer–Overton hypothesis. *Anesth Analg* 1994;**79**:1043–8.

Mihic SJ, Sanna E, Whiting PJ, *et al*. Pharmacology of recombinant $GABA_A$ receptors. *Adv Biochem Psychopharmacol* 1995;**48**:17–40.

Mihic SJ, Ye Q, Wick MJ, *et al*. Sites of alcohol and volatile anaesthetic action on GABA(A) and glycine receptors. *Nature* 1997;**389**:385–9.

Minami K, Wick MJ, SternBach Y, *et al*. Sites of volatile anesthetic action on kainate (Glutamate receptor 6) receptors. *J Biol Chem* 1998;**273**:8248–55.

Moody EJ, Harris BD, Skolnick P. The potential for safer anaesthesia using stereoselective anaesthetics. *Trends Pharmacol Sci* 1994;**15**:387–91.

Rampil IJ, Mason P, Singh H. Anesthetic potency (MAC) is independent of forebrain structures in the rat. *Anesthesiology* 1993;**78**:707–12.

# Chapter 73 Thermoregulation during anaesthesia

K. Leslie

During general and major regional anaesthesia, loss of central thermoregulation and exposure to the cold operating room environment lead to core hypothermia. Recently, hypothermia has been established as a major contributor to perioperative morbidity and mortality. Understanding how hypothermia develops will help anaesthetists choose appropriate means of prevention and treatment.

## TEMPERATURE REGULATION IN UNANAESTHETIZED PATIENTS

Temperature-sensitive nerve endings in deep tissues, the central nervous system, and the skin contribute thermal information to the hypothalamic nuclei. An integrated input temperature of less than the threshold temperature for 'cold' responses triggers autonomic responses aimed at increasing core temperature. Conversely, an input temperature exceeding the threshold temperature for 'warm' responses triggers autonomic responses aimed at decreasing core temperature (Table 73.1). Behavioural responses are also very important in awake humans. In this way, the hypothalamus keeps very tight control over core temperature: only a temperature range of 0.2°C (36.9–37.1°C) is tolerated without producing a response.

## TEMPERATURE REGULATION IN ANAESTHETIZED PATIENTS

During general anaesthesia, the hypothalamus allows core temperature to vary by up to 4°C without initiating a response. The core temperature triggering arteriovenous shunt vasoconstriction is decreased by about 3°C, and the core temperature triggering vasodilatation and sweating is increased by about 1°C. Shivering is profoundly impaired and non-shivering thermogenesis is abolished completely. Most anaesthetics, including volatile agents, propofol, opioids, and $\alpha_2$ agonists, cause a similar degree of impairment, regardless of their direct effects on the peripheral circulation, emphasizing the crucial role of the hypothalamus in thermoregulation.

Epidural and spinal anaesthesia also impair thermoregulation. Sympathetic nervous system blockade prevents sweating, vasoconstriction, and shivering in the area of the block. In addition, thermoregulatory responses are impaired in the area *not* affected by the block. The hypothalamus misinterprets loss of thermal input from the lower body as an increase in skin temperature. This *apparent* increase in lower body skin temperature results in increased tolerance of hypothermia. As a result, vasoconstriction and shivering thresholds in the upper body decrease by about 0.6°C during spinal and epidural blockade.

## HEAT BALANCE IN ANAESTHETIZED PATIENTS

Most patients are vasoconstricted when they arrive in the operating room. When either general or major regional anaesthesia is induced, a core temperature that formerly triggered vasoconstriction no longer does, and arteriovenous shunts dilate. This allows core-to-peripheral redistribution of body heat, and results in a precipitous decrease in core temperature. Redistribution of body heat represents the most important cause of hypothermia throughout general and major regional anaesthesia.

In addition, anaesthesia disturbs the balance between heat loss and heat production. The surgical

**Table 73.1 Autonomic and behavioural responses to changes in core temperature**

| 'Cold' responses | 'Warm' responses |
|---|---|
| Arteriovenous shunt vasoconstriction | Arteriovenous shunt vasodilatation |
| Non-shivering thermogenesis | Sweating |
| Shivering | |
| Behavioural responses:<br>↑ activity<br>↑ coverings<br>↑ ambient temperature | Behavioural responses:<br>↓ activity<br>↓ coverings<br>↓ ambient temperature |

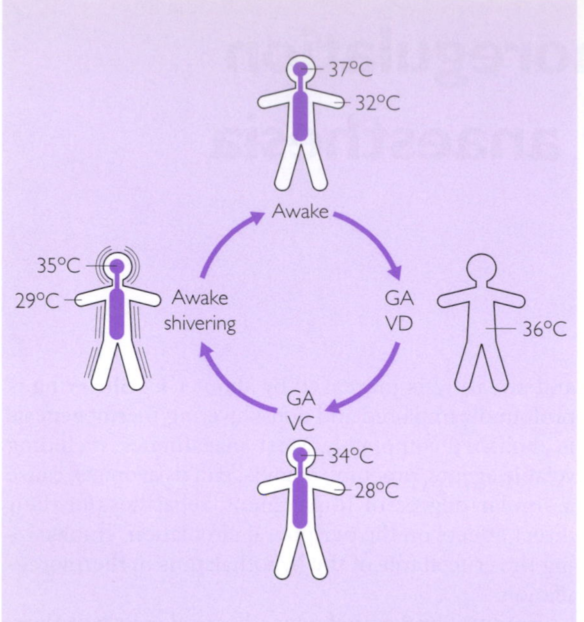


**Figure 73.1** Patients usually come to the operating room vasoconstricted. Vasodilatation (VD) after induction of anaesthesia results in redistribution of body heat. The core-to-peripheral temperature gradient is restored when vasoconstriction (VC) is triggered. Heat loss incurred during general anaesthesia (GA) must be restored by shivering.

wound and cold intravenous fluid administration increase heat loss across the skin. Heat production decreases during general anaesthesia by 5% per °C. Heat production does not decrease during regional anaesthesia, and may actually increase if shivering occurs.

In the absence of active warming, core temperature eventually stabilizes during general anaesthesia at 34°C. Triggering of vasoconstriction and re-establishment of the core-to-peripheral temperature gradient produce this plateau, protecting the core from further heat loss, but the peripheral compartment continues to lose heat to the environment. A significant heat debt may develop (Figure 73.1). An effective core-temperature plateau usually fails to develop during central axial regional anaesthesia because the legs remain vasodilated.

## PREVENTION AND TREATMENT OF HYPOTHERMIA DURING ANAESTHESIA

Unintended perioperative hypothermia represents a major cause of perioperative morbidity (Table 73.2). In addition, shivering triggered by hypothermia can be very uncomfortable for patients. Normothermia should therefore be maintained unless a specific indication for hypothermia exists.

Pre-warming with a forced-air warmer or pre-treatment with vasodilators can prevent redistribution hypothermia. Infusing warmed fluids, covering or warming exposed skin, and maintaining a high ambient temperature can counteract heat loss during surgery. Shivering during epidural or spinal anaesthesia can be abolished by warming skin *not* affected by the block. Intravenous or epidural opioids (especially pethidine), clonidine, and ketanserin, are also effective. These strategies can also be used to treat shivering after general anaesthesia. Oxygen consumption is increased during rewarming and hence postoperative oxygen therapy is essential.

## CONCLUSIONS

General and major regional anaesthesia impair thermoregulation. Hypothermia develops as a result of redistribution of body heat and augmented heat loss. Because perioperative hypothermia adversely affects outcome from surgery, normothermia should be maintained unless hypothermia is indicated for organ protection.

**Table 73.2 Risks and benefits of mild perioperative hypothermia**

| Risks | Benefits |
|---|---|
| Increased duration of hospital stay | Organ protection (e.g. brain, heart) |
| Increased surgical wound infections | Augmented anaesthetic effects |
| Increased oxygen consumption with rewarming | Decreased triggering of malignant hyperthermia |
| Decreased wound healing | |
| Increased morbid cardiac events and | |
| Ventricular tachycardia | |
| Increased operative blood loss | |
| Prolonged drug effects | |
| Prolonged recovery from general anaesthesia | |
| Increased nitrogen loss | |
| Shivering | |

## FURTHER READING

Frank SM, Fleisher LA, Breslow MJ, *et al*. Perioperative maintenance of normothermia reduces the incidence of morbid cardiac events: a randomized clinical trial. *JAMA* 1997;**277**:1127–34.

Kurz A, Sessler DI, Lenhardt R. Perioperative normothermia to reduce the incidence of surgical wound infection and shorten hospitalization. *N Engl J Med* 1996;**334**:1209–15.

Schmied H, Kurz A, Sessler DI, *et al*. Mild hypothermia increases blood loss and transfusion requirements during total hip arthroplasty. *Lancet* 1996;**347**:289–92.

Sessler DI. Consequences and treatment of perioperative hypothermia. *Anesthesiol Clin North Am* 1994;**12**:425–56.

Sessler DI. Mild perioperative hypothermia. *N Engl J Med* 1997;**336**:1730–7.

# Chapter 74 Performing an arterial cannulation

L. Groban and J. Butterworth

Measurement of blood pressure is fundamental to cardiovascular monitoring in the anaesthetized or critically ill patient. Although there are numerous non-invasive methods for measuring arterial blood pressure, direct intra-arterial monitoring remains the most accurate and reliable measurement technique. This chapter focuses on the site selection, equipment and the technique for arterial cannulation. Tables 74.1 and 74.2 list the indications and risks of arterial cannulation.

## SITE

Ideally, the arterial pressure waveform should be measured in the ascending aorta. As this is impractical, several alternative peripheral sites have been used for arterial cannulation, including the radial, dorsalis pedis, femoral, axillary, brachial, and ulnar arteries. Nevertheless, the pressure measured in peripheral arteries does not usually correspond exactly with the aortic pressure; the more distal the site for measuring arterial pressure, the greater the systolic pressure and the lower the diastolic pressure (Figure 74.1). The mean arterial blood pressure remains nearly constant at all sites. Waveform distortion by the addition of reflected waves as the arterial waveform travels distally in the arterial tree causes the changing arterial pressure. With ageing, reflected waves occur at progressively more proximal cannulation sites.

| Table 74.2 Site-specific risks |
|---|
| Ischaemia/necrosis (all) |
| Thrombosis (all) |
| Cerebral embolism (R, B, A) |
| Haemorrhage/haematoma (all) |
| Infection (all) |
| Nerve injury (F, B, A) |
| Pseudoaneurysm (R, F, B) |

R, radial; F, femoral; B, brachial; A, axillary; D, dorsalis pedis.

The site selected for arterial cannulation depends on:

- the operative site (e.g. during head and neck surgery, the dorsalis pedis artery may be preferred because the anaesthetist is closer to the patient's feet than to the head);
- the possibility of arterial compromise resulting from surgical manipulation (e.g. during repair of thoracic aortic aneurysms, the right radial artery is

| Table 74.1 Indications for invasive arterial pressure monitoring in surgical patients |
|---|
| **Medical** |
| • Continuing haemodynamic instability<br>• Recent myocardial infarction (< 3 months), severe coronary artery disease, heart failure, pulmonary hypertension, significant valvular heart disease with haemodynamic instability<br>• Need for inotropic/vasoactive drugs (e.g. epinephrine [adrenaline], norepinephrine [noradrenaline], dobutamine)<br>• An intra-aortic balloon pump<br>• Circulatory shock |
| **Surgical** |
| • Surgery involving large fluid shifts and/or blood loss<br>• Surgery involving the use of deliberate hypotension or deliberate hypothermia<br>• Surgery involving aortic clamping (e.g. thoracic/abdominal aortic aneurysmal repair, renal artery revascularization)<br>• Surgery requiring cardiopulmonary bypass<br>• Surgery requiring one-lung ventilation for lung resection |
| **Convenience** |
| • Frequent arterial blood gases<br>• Frequent blood sampling (e.g. for electrolyte and metabolic disturbances) |

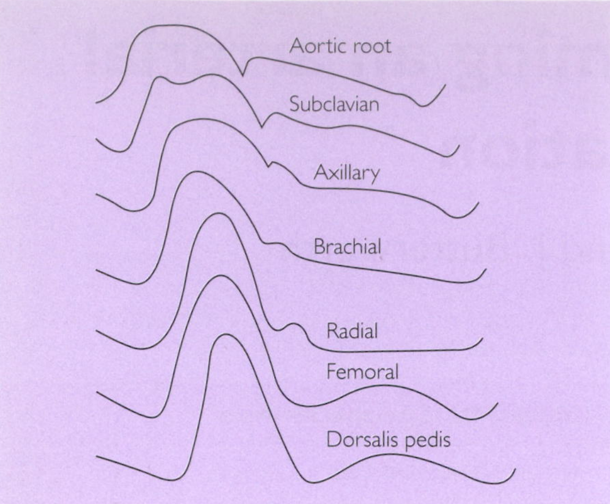


**Figure 74.1** Comparison of arterial pressure waveform configurations from various sites in the arterial tree. (Adapted from Bedford RF. Invasive blood pressure monitoring. In: Blitt CD, ed. *Monitoring in Anesthesia and Critical Care Medicine*, 3rd edn. New York: Churchill Livingstone, 1985:41–85.)

**Figure 74.2** Schematic drawing of a Wheatstone bridge. The bridge consists of three fixed resistances and one resistance that varies with the applied pressure. A change in resistance changes the electrical output current. (Adapted from Saidman LJ, Smith NT. *Monitoring in Anesthesia*, 3rd edn. Woburn, MA: Butterworth–Heinemann, 1993.)

preferred because flow in the left radial artery ceases upon aortic clamping near the left subclavian artery);

- concerns about the safety or accuracy of the recorded blood pressure (e.g. cannulation of the dorsalis pedis artery is not recommended in patients with femoral arteriosclerosis).

## COMPONENTS OF PRESSURE MONITORING

Arterial pressure waves represent the transmission of forces generated in the cardiac chambers. Measurement of these forces needs a device, called a transducer, that converts mechanical energy into electrical energy. This electrical energy then travels through an amplifier which enlarges and filters the signal before its display on an oscilloscope. The most common type of pressure transducer is the strain gauge, which senses pressure through a Wheatstone bridge. A Wheatstone bridge consists of four resistance wires, or silicone crystals, connected to one another to form a square (Figure 74.2). This square of wires lies directly beneath the surface of the transducer diaphragm. Pressure applied to the diaphragm distorts its shape and lengthens the wires or crystals beneath the diaphragm. This change in length alters the electrical resistance. A change in resistance changes the electrical current. Therefore, changes in transducer current are proportional to changes in pressure.

## TECHNIQUE

### Radial artery cannulation

The radial artery, a branch of the brachial artery, extends down the anterior radial aspect of the forearm before entering the hand beneath the flexor retinaculum, where it forms the palmar arch. In most individuals, the radial artery is not the dominant vessel of the hand, and is preferred over the ulnar artery for cannulation. Although the Allen test is widely performed to determine adequacy of collateral blood flow to the hand, evidence fails to show that avoiding radial artery cannulation in the presence of an abnormal Allen test increases safety. Table 74.3 lists the equipment needed for radial artery cannulation.

With the patient's hand and wrist dorsiflexed over a rolled towel and loosely secured to an arm board with adhesive tape, identify the radial artery by palpation proximal to the wrist creases, lateral to the tendon of

| Table 74.3 Equipment required for radial artery cannulation |
|---|
| Sterile gloves |
| Antiseptic solution |
| 2-ml syringe of 1% lignocaine (lidocaine) (25- or 27-gauge needle) |
| 10-ml syringe of heparinized saline (2 units heparin/ml 0.9% saline) |
| Arterial extension tubing with stopcock |
| Arm board |
| Towel roll |
| 20-gauge 5-cm catheter (for adults) |
| 18-gauge needle (optional) |
| Tincture of benzoin |
| Sterile dressing |

flexor carpi radialis (Figure 74.3). After washing the skin with antiseptic solution (iodophor or alcohol), infiltrate the site of the intended puncture (Figure 74.4a) with 0.5 ml lignocaine (lidocaine) (or a comparable local anaesthetic). Advance the 20-gauge intravenous cannula through the skin to the point of palpation at a 30–40° angle from the wrist (Figure 74.4b). When arterial blood flashes back into the hub of the needle, lower the angle of the catheter (Figure 74.4c) and advance the entire catheter-over-the-needle system 1–2 mm into the artery (Figure 74.4d). Then slide the catheter over the needle into the artery (Figure 74.4e). Apply pressure to the radial artery proximal to the cannula to reduce blood loss, while connecting an extension tubing with a stopcock (Figure 74.4e). Secure the catheter with adhesive tape and, if desired, suture it to the skin. This technique is referred to as direct cannulation.

The transfixation method represents another technique commonly used for arterial cannulation. When blood flashes back into the needle hub, insert the catheter through both walls of the artery to transfix the artery from front to back (Figure 74.5a). Then remove the needle completely from the catheter, and slowly withdraw the catheter until pulsatile blood emerges from the catheter end, indicating that its tip has entered the arterial lumen (Figure 75.5b) and the catheter should be advanced into the artery (Figure 74.5c). If the catheter cannot be advanced into the arterial lumen, pass a sterile guidewire through the catheter into the artery and advance the catheter over the wire. Monitor the adequacy of perfusion distal to the site of cannulation during the residence of a radial artery catheter by placing a pulse oximeter on the ipsilateral index finger.

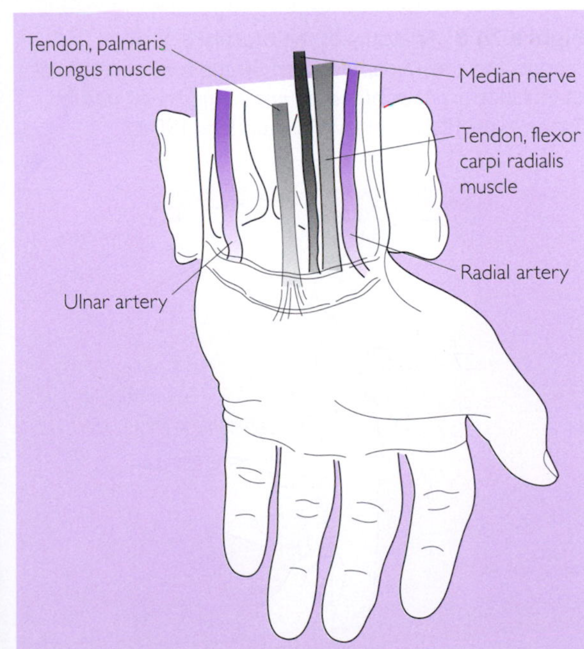


**Figure 74.3** Anatomy of the radial artery cannulation site. (Adapted from Butterworth JF. Arterial cannulation. In: *Atlas of Procedures in Anesthesia and Critical Care*. Philadelphia: WB Saunders 1992.)

## Femoral artery cannulation

The femoral artery, a continuation of the external iliac artery, traverses beneath the inguinal ligament in the leg. It can be located at the midpoint of an imaginary line drawn between the anterosuperior iliac crest and the symphysis pubis. The femoral vein lies medial to the artery, and the femoral nerve lies lateral to the artery in the femoral sheath (Figure 74.6). The femoral artery is usually cannulated using a Seldinger technique. Advance a 20- or 21-gauge needle (6–7 cm in length) 2–4 cm through the skin overlying the point of maximal pulsation into the artery. Next advance a 0.035-cm sterile guidewire through the needle and, subsequently, an 18-gauge catheter (16 cm) over the wire. Finally, suture the catheter to the skin and apply a sterile dressing. The femoral artery can also be cannulated using the direct method with an appropriate length angiocath.

Figures 74.7, 74.8, and 74.9 depict the approaches used for cannulation of the dorsalis pedis, brachial, and axillary arteries.

## Dorsalis pedis artery cannulation

The dorsalis pedis artery extends subcutaneously as a continuation of the anterior tibial artery down the

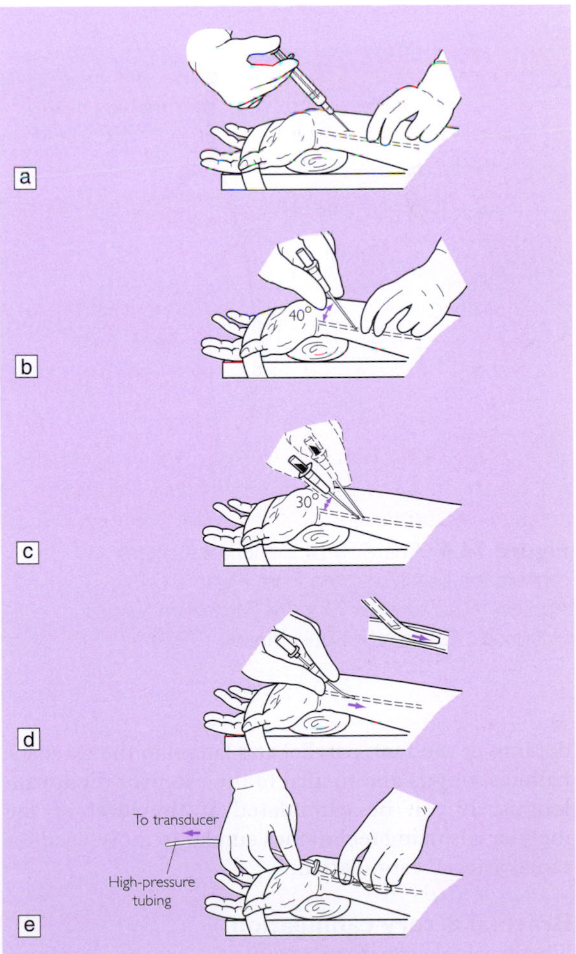


**Figure 74.4** Cannulation of the radial artery using the direct technique. See text for details. (Adapted from Morgan GE Jr, Mikhail MS. *Clinical Anesthesiology*, 2nd edn. Stamford, CT: Appleton & Lange, 1996.)

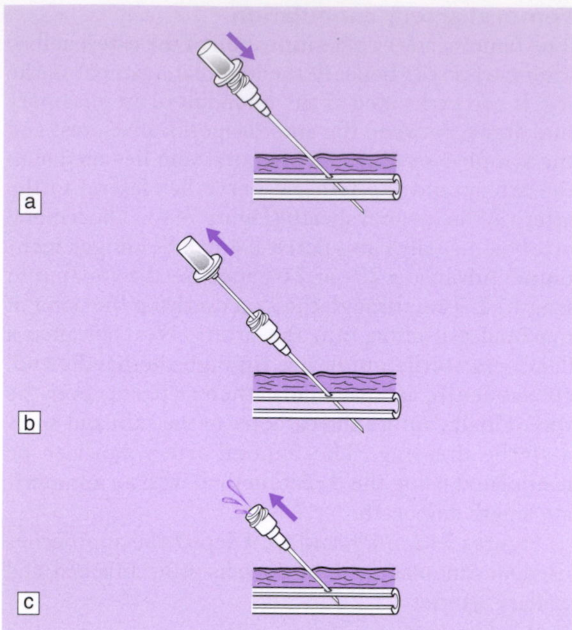


**Figure 74.5** Cannulation of the radial artery using the transfixation technique. See text for details. (Adapted from Butterworth JF. Arterial cannulation. In: *Atlas of Procedures in Anesthesia and Critical Care*. Philadelphia: WB Saunders, 1992.)

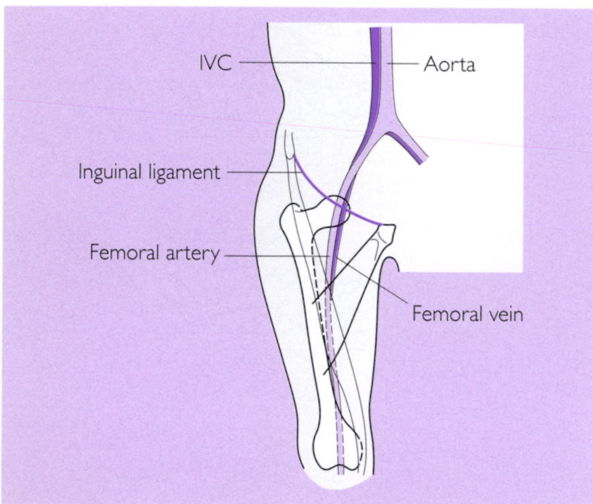


**Figure 74.6** Anatomy of the femoral artery cannulation site. (Adapted from Hiyama DT, Appleby TC, Daneker GW. *The Mont Reid Surgical Handbook*, 4th edn. St Louis: Mosby, 1997.)

dorsum of the foot, parallel and lateral to the extensor hallucis longus and medial to the extensor digitorum longus. It can be cannulated at the level of the metatarsals using techniques similar to those used for radial arterial cannulation.

### Brachial artery cannulation

The brachial artery extends into the arm as a continuation of the axillary artery, emerging from under the medial edge of the biceps muscle. It can be palpated medial to the biceps tendon and lateral to the median nerve and pronator teres in the antecubital fossa. The

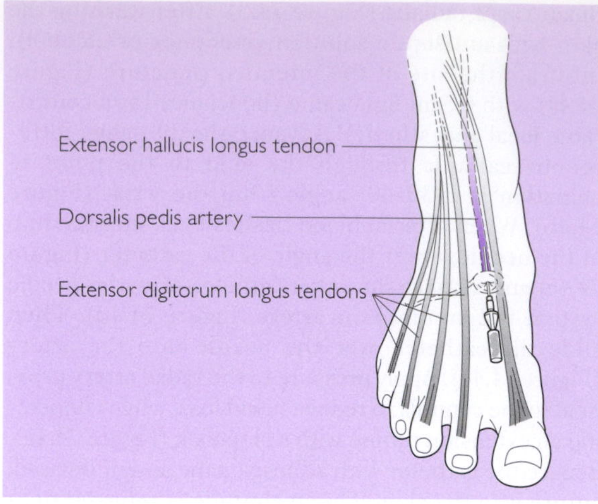


**Figure 74.7** Anatomy of the dorsalis pedis cannulation site. (Adapted from Butterworth JF. Arterial cannulation. In: *Atlas of Procedures in Anesthesia and Critical Care*. Philadelphia: WB Saunders, 1992.)

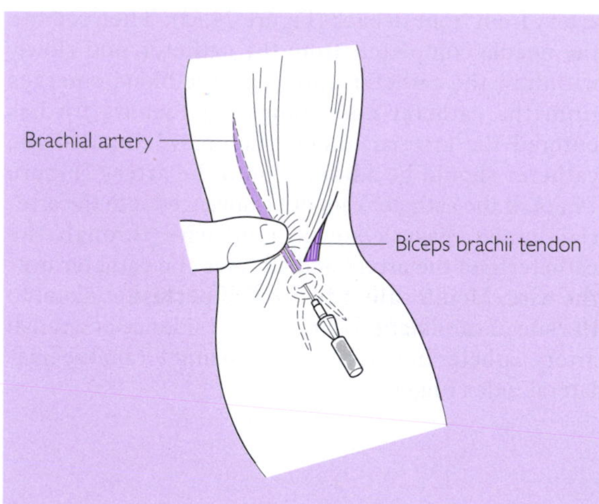


**Figure 74.8** Anatomy of the brachial artery cannulation site. (Adapted from Butterworth JF. Arterial cannulation. In: *Atlas of Procedures in Anesthesia and Critical Care*. Philadelphia: WB Saunders, 1992.)

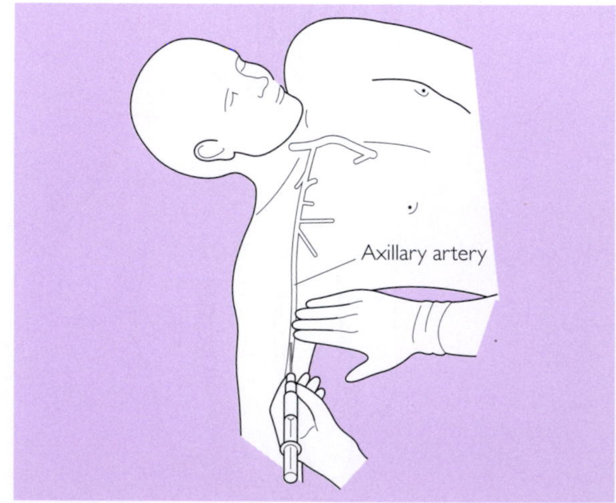


**Figure 74.9** Schematic of axillary artery cannulation. (Adapted from Hiyama DT, Appleby TC, Daneker GW. *The Mont Reid Surgical Handbook*, 4th edn. St Louis: Mosby, 1997.)

brachial artery can be cannulated just proximal to the skin crease of the antecubital fossa (Figure 74.8). With the arm extended at the elbow, the technique used for radial artery cannulation may be employed. The brachial artery is a more proximal artery and, thus, pressures recorded at this site are less likely to be altered by reflected waves. Therefore, the brachial artery provides a more accurate blood pressure (relative to the aorta) than the radial artery after cardiopulmonary bypass. Median nerve damage and distal vascular ischaemia occur infrequently with brachial artery cannulation.

### Axillary artery cannulation

The axillary artery, the continuation of the subclavian artery within the axillary sheath, forms a neurovascular bundle with the axillary vein and the three cords of the brachial plexus. With the arm abducted and externally rotated, palpate the axillary arterial pulse just below the biceps muscle. Insert a 20-gauge, 5-cm long, thin-walled arteriotomy needle within the axilla at a 35° angle to the skin. Then employ the Seldinger technique to place a 16-cm catheter over a guidewire. As with both radial and brachial artery cannulae, take particular care during flushing of the axillary arterial cannula to prevent embolic matter from entering the cerebral circulation. Damage to the brachial plexus represents another potential risk associated with axillary artery cannulation owing to its location within the neurovascular sheath.

## ACCURACY OF THE PRESSURE MEASUREMENT

Following catheter insertion, flush the arterial tubing to eliminate air bubbles and attach it to the cannula. For accurate monitoring, zero the transducer at the level of the heart. The transducer must be moved in parallel with the patient when altering the height of the bed. During neurosurgery, monitor cerebral arterial pressure by placing the transducer at the level of the ear (which approximates the circle of Willis).

## USES OF THE INTRA-ARTERIAL CANNULA

Intra-arterial monitoring provides information about beat-to-beat variations in arterial pressure, a means to obtain multiple blood samples for electrolyte and blood gas analyses, and an indication of organ perfusion as determined by mean arterial pressure (MAP). The MAP can be measured directly by integrating the area under the arterial waveform trace over time, or can be estimated using the formula:

$$\text{MAP} = (\text{SAP} - \text{DAP}) + \frac{\text{DAP}}{3}$$

where SAP is the systolic arterial pressure, and DAP the diastolic arterial pressure. Besides continuous blood pressure measurements, the arterial waveform provides useful information about the patient's haemodynamic status, including:

- the large respiratory variations and a narrow pulse pressure (SAP –DAP) suggestive of hypovolaemia or excessive tidal volumes;
- a visual estimate of the immediate blood pressure consequences of various arrhythmias;
- heart rate determination during electrocautery interference;
- verification of electrical–mechanical coupling associated with pacemaker initiation.

## FURTHER READING


Bedford RF, Shah NK. Blood pressure monitoring: invasive and non-invasive. In: Blitt CD, Hines RL, eds. *Monitoring in Anesthesia and Critical Medicine*. New York: Churchill Livingstone, 1995: 95–117.

Butterworth JF. Arterial cannulation. In: *Atlas of Procedures in Anesthesia and Critical Care*. Philadelphia, WB Saunders, 1992: 115–24.

Mangano DT, Hickey RF. Ischemic injury following uncomplicated radial artery catheterization. *Anesth Analg* 1979;**58**:55–7.

Slogoff S, Keats AS, Arlund C. On the safety of radial artery cannulation. *Anesthesiology* 1983;**59**:42–7.

Thys DM, Reich DL. Invasive cardiovascular monitoring. In: Saidman LJ, Smith NT, eds. *Monitoring in Anesthesia*, 3rd edn. Woburn, MA: Butterworth-Heinemann, 1993: 51–62.

# Chapter 75 Establishing central venous access

L. Groban and J. Butterworth

Central venous catheterization provides secure access to the venous circulation and permits quantitative assessment of right ventricular filling pressure. This chapter discusses the normal central venous pressure (CVP) waveform along with pathological waveforms seen with abnormalities of right heart function. The indications (Table 75.1), complications (Table 75.2), and the method of obtaining central venous access are also described.

**Table 75.1 The perioperative indications for obtaining central venous access**

| |
|---|
| Monitoring of volume status/guide for fluid replacement |
| Evaluation of cardiac function (normal heart) |
| Provision of access for:<br>• vasoactive infusions<br>• blood/fluid replacement<br>• blood sampling<br>• air emboli aspiration<br>• introduction of a pulmonary artery catheter |

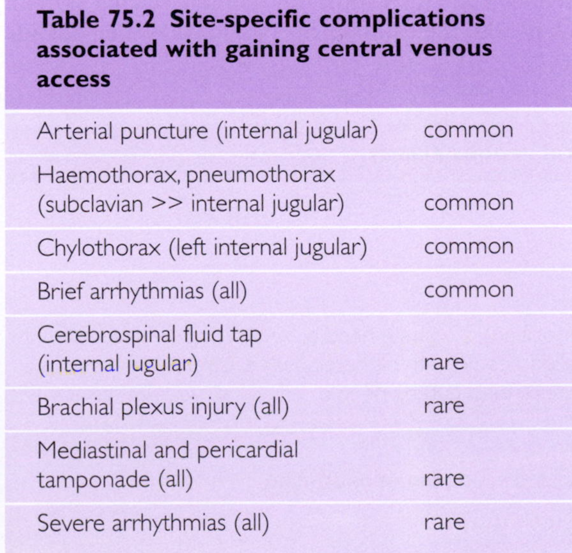

**Table 75.2 Site-specific complications associated with gaining central venous access**

| | |
|---|---|
| Arterial puncture (internal jugular) | common |
| Haemothorax, pneumothorax (subclavian >> internal jugular) | common |
| Chylothorax (left internal jugular) | common |
| Brief arrhythmias (all) | common |
| Cerebrospinal fluid tap (internal jugular) | rare |
| Brachial plexus injury (all) | rare |
| Mediastinal and pericardial tamponade (all) | rare |
| Severe arrhythmias (all) | rare |

## CENTRAL VENOUS PRESSURE WAVEFORM

Figure 75.1 depicts the normal CVP waveform as it corresponds to the ECG. Right atrial contraction produces the A wave which disappears during atrial fibrillation. Giant or 'cannon' A waves are observed with atrial contraction against a closed tricuspid valve (tricuspid stenosis), or with concurrent contraction of the right atrium and right ventricle (junctional rhythm). The C wave results from bulging of the tricuspid valve into the right atrium with the onset of ventricular systole. The *x* descent follows the C wave. The atrium relaxes and the tricuspid valve is pulled downwards, reducing atrial pressure. The positive V wave corresponds to diastolic filling of the right atrium while the tricuspid valve is closed. Large V waves indicate tricuspid regurgitation. The *y* descent corresponds to right ventricular relaxation and early filling of the right ventricle while the tricuspid valve is open.

## TECHNIQUE

A Seldinger technique (catheter-over-guidewire) is most commonly used for central venous cannulation and is described here (Figure 75.2). Table 75.3 lists the necessary equipment.

Place the patient in the Trendelenburg position. After antiseptic cleansing of the skin, position a fenestrated drape (or several sterile towels) to reveal the anticipated puncture site. Identify the central vein by

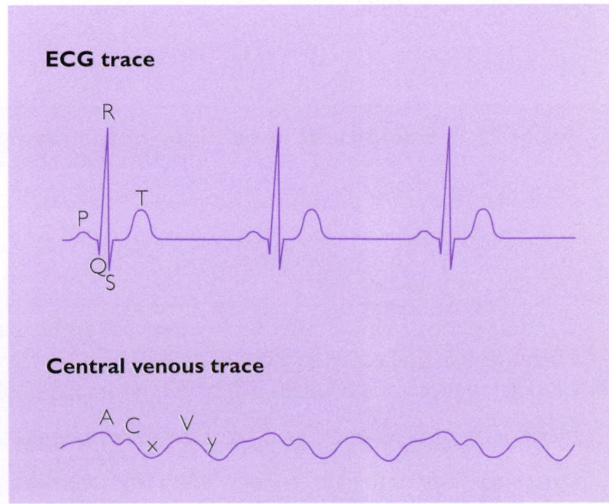


**Figure 75.1** Schematic of normal and central venous pressure waveform, as it corresponds to the ECG.

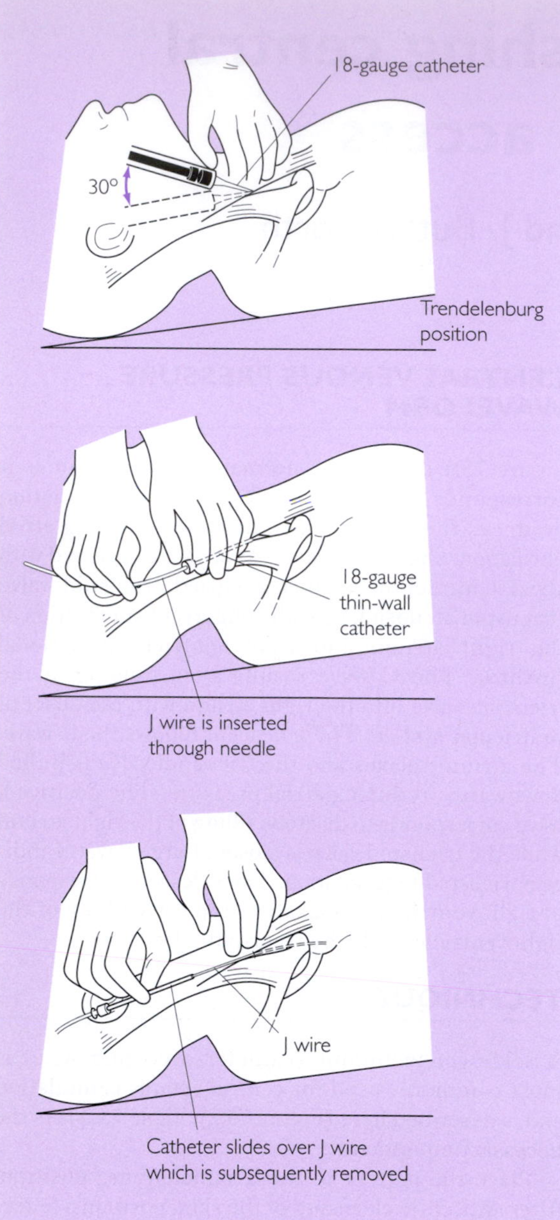


**Figure 75.2** Central venous cannulation using the Seldinger technique. (Adapted from Morgan GE Jr, Mikhail MS. *Clinical Anesthesiology*, 2nd edn. Stamford, CT: Appleton & Lange, 1996.)

the aspiration of venous blood through an 'exploring' 22-gauge 4-cm needle attached to a 3-ml syringe. Remove the 'exploring' needle before attaching a 5-ml syringe to an 18-gauge intravenous catheter or thin-wall arteriotomy needle, and insert it through the skin in an identical manner. After aspirating venous blood into the syringe, advance the entire assembly an additional 1 mm to ensure placement of the tip of the catheter fully within the vein. Before proceeding with the guidewire, verify that the catheter (from which the needle has been withdrawn) or arteriotomy needle is within the vein by comparing the colour of a sample of blood aspirated from the cannula with a contemporaneous arterial sample.

If the two samples are of similar colour, do not proceed further because an artery may have been cannulated. If a firm decision cannot be made as to whether an artery or vein has been cannulated, or an arterial blood sample is not available, transduce the cannula (while maintaining sterility) with an electrical transducer or a venous manometer. A venous manometer requires only that sterile venous tubing be attached to the cannula. After passively filling the tubing with blood, hold the tubing upright while still attached to the cannula. The height of the blood defines the CVP. If the catheter lies within the carotid artery, pulsatile blood will emerge from the end of the tubing and the column of blood will not fall. Arterial puncture does not usually present a serious problem, except when a large catheter or introducer sheath has been accidentally passed into the artery. Such instances may necessitate surgical exploration and repair.

After confirmation of venous puncture, insert the guidewire through the catheter (or arteriotomy needle) into the central venous circulation, leaving about half its length outside the patient. Next, remove the catheter. Premature beats often occur during wire insertion, particularly when the wire is advanced further than necessary. Make a small skin incision at the puncture site. A plastic dilator passed over the wire previously can facilitate placement of the central venous catheter over the guidewire. After withdrawing the guidewire, suture the correctly sited catheter to the skin.

In most cases, a chest radiograph should be obtained to confirm correct location of the central venous catheter within the thoracic venous system. Generally, the catheter tip should be located outside

| **Table 75.3 Equipment needed for obtaining central venous access** |
|---|
| Sterile gloves |
| Antiseptic solution |
| Intravenous fluid and tubing |
| Central venous cannula tray (3-ml syringe, 1% lignocaine (lidocaine), 22-gauge needle, 5-ml syringe, J-wire, 18-gauge thin-walled arteriotomy needle, 18-gauge thin-walled needle with catheter over it, central venous cannula of appropriate length, 3/0 or 4/0 non-absorbable suture on a cutting needle |
| Monitoring of ECG and blood pressure (recommended) |
| Means to place patient in Trendelenburg (for internal jugular and subclavian vein) position |
| Resuscitation drugs/equipment |

the heart but near the cavoatrial junction. When the catheter has been placed specifically for aspiration of air emboli (e.g. during neurosurgical procedures performed with the patient in the sitting position), the catheter can be transformed into an extension of an ECG lead 'V' for intravascular ECG. Alternatively, the catheter can be positioned at the cavoatrial junction using fluoroscopy as a guide.

Although there are multiple potential access sites for central venous catheterization, the internal jugular and subclavian veins represent the most popular in anaesthesia and critical care medicine. Approaches to these central veins are discussed separately.

## INTERNAL JUGULAR VEIN

The right internal jugular vein is preferred over the left because of its straight, valveless course through the superior vena cava to the right atrium, and because the thoracic duct is on the opposite side. Cannulation of the internal jugular vein may not be possible in patients with previous neck surgery, neck tumours, or obstruction of the superior vena cava. With the patient in the Trendelenburg position, the right internal jugular vein can be approached using the low anterior (or middle), high anterior, or posterior approaches.

### Low anterior (middle) approach

Introduce the needle at the apex of the triangle formed by the two heads of the sternocleidomastoid muscle, and direct it towards the ipsilateral nipple at a 30° angle to the skin (Figure 75.3).

### High anterior approach

Introduce the needle at the medial border of the sternocleidomastoid muscle just lateral to the carotid pulse. Direct the needle towards the ipsilateral nipple at a 30° angle to the skin (Figure 75.4).

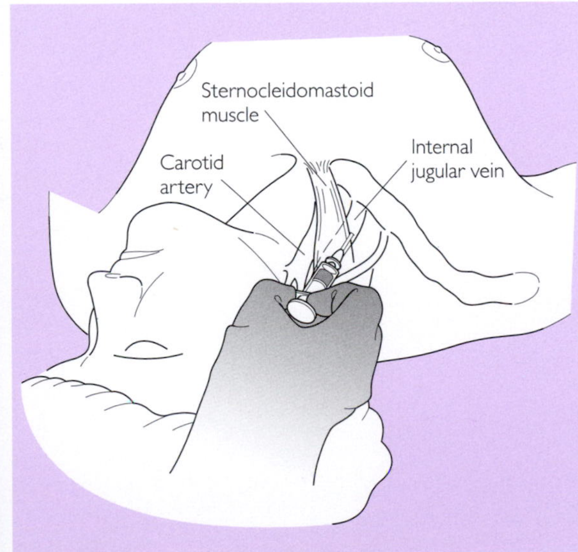


**Figure 75.3** Low anterior (middle) approach to cannulation of the right internal jugular vein. (Adapted from Butterworth JF. Arterial cannulation. In: *Atlas of Procedures in Anesthesia and Critical Care*. Philadelphia: WB Saunders, 1992.)

### Posterior approach

Introduce the needle at the junction of the posterior border of the sternocleidomastoid muscle and the external jugular vein. Then direct the needle towards the ipsilateral corner of the sternal notch (Figure 75.5).

## SUBCLAVIAN VEIN

Although subclavian vein cannulation results in a higher incidence of complications (pneumothorax, haemothorax) than internal jugular vein cannulation,

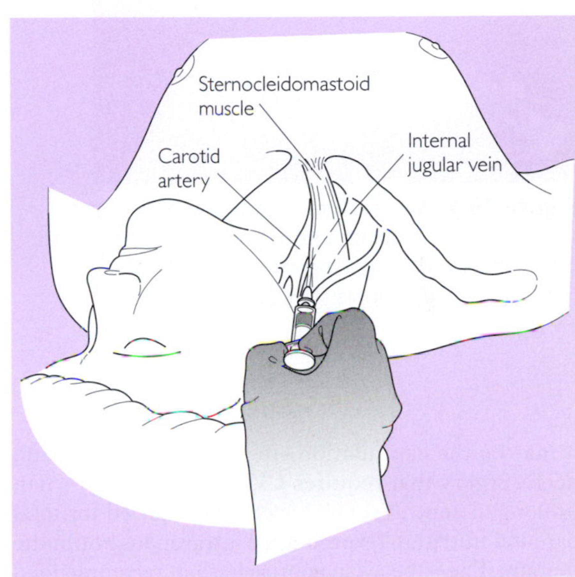


**Figure 75.4** High anterior approach to cannulation of the right internal jugular vein. (Adapted from Butterworth JF. Arterial cannulation. In: *Atlas of Procedures in Anesthesia and Critical Care*. Philadelphia: WB Saunders, 1992.)

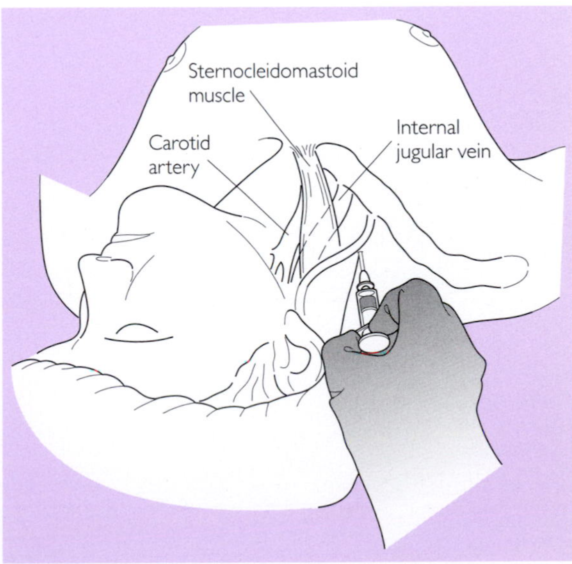


**Figure 75.5** Posterior approach to cannulation of the right internal jugular vein. (Adapted from Butterworth JF. Arterial cannulation. In: *Atlas of Procedures in Anesthesia and Critical Care*. Philadelphia: WB Saunders, 1992.)

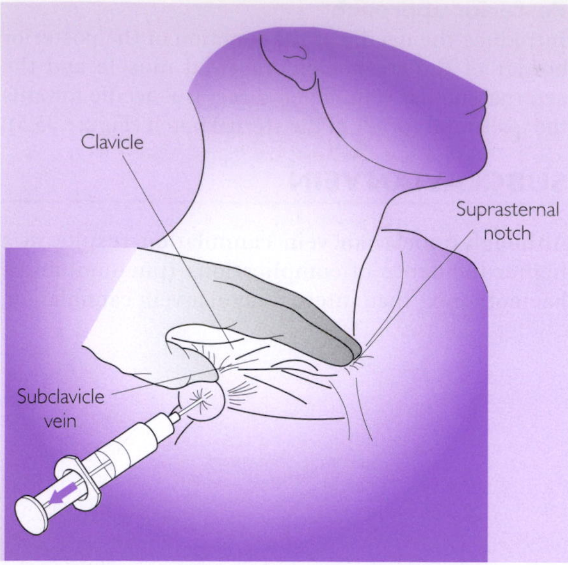


**Figure 75.6** Approach to cannulation of the right subclavian vein. (Adapted from Butterworth JF. Arterial cannulation. In: *Atlas of Procedures in Anesthesia and Critical Care*. Philadelphia: WB Saunders, 1992.)

it may be the cannulation site of choice in head and neck surgery that requires CVP monitoring, or when prolonged central venous access is required for total parental nutrition or prolonged intravenous antibiotic therapy. The subclavian approach is not recommended for patients with a bleeding diathesis or for those receiving anticoagulants, because of the risk of haematoma formation in the rare instance of subclavian artery puncture. The Trendelenburg position, with the arms by the side and the head turned slightly away from the side of venepuncture, offers optimal positioning for insertion of a subclavian catheter. Place a rolled towel along the thoracic spine between the scapulae, extending to the shoulders. Unlike internal jugular vein cannulation, an exploring needle is not routinely used before subclavian vein cannulation. Insert the 18-gauge, thin-walled needle a fingerbreadth inferior to the midpoint of the clavicle and direct the needle just beneath the bone, towards the sternal notch, until it enters the subclavian vein and blood is aspirated (Figure 75.6). Verify that the needle is within the vein before proceeding with insertion of the guidewire, by comparing the colour of a sample of blood aspirated with that of a simultaneously drawn arterial sample, as described for internal jugular vein access.

## FURTHER READING

Bedford RF, Shah NK. Central venous pressure monitoring. In: Blitt CD, Hines RL, eds. *Monitoring in Anesthesia and Critical Medicine*. New York: Churchill Livingstone, 1995: 173–213.

Butterworth JF. Central venous cannulation. In: *Atlas of Procedures in Anesthesia and Critical Care*. Philadelphia: WB Saunders, 1992: 75–100.

Butterworth JF. Intravascular electrocardiography. In: *Atlas of Procedures in Anesthesia and Critical Care*. Philadelphia: WB Saunders, 1992: 101–4.

Mark JB. Getting the most from your CVP catheter. ASA Refresher Course Lectures 1995.

Thys DM, Reich DL. Invasive cardiovascular monitoring. In: Saidman LJ, Smith NT, eds. *Monitoring in Anesthesia*, 3rd edn. Boston: Butterworth-Heinemann, 1993: 63–7.

# Chapter 76 Pulmonary artery catheter introduction and interpretation

L. Groban and J. Butterworth

Pulmonary artery (PA) catheterization is commonly used to assess intravascular volume status (left ventricular preload), vascular resistance, and cardiac output, and in particular to assess responses to therapy. It is potentially useful during major surgical procedures associated with a high risk of haemodynamic complications (e.g. complex cardiac and vascular surgery) and in unstable intensive care patients. Although PA catheterization has been used for more than 20 years, debate continues as to the appropriate indications for its use. In individual patients, whether to use a PA is a judgement based on the likelihood of haemodynamic stability, combined with the condition of the patient and the proposed operation. Patient factors might include a low ejection fraction (< 40%), severe left or right ventricular failure or hypertrophy, conduction defects, or pulmonary hypertension. Many institutions now have guidelines, and trainees are advised to follow those pertaining at the time. The following chapter includes a description of the catheter, the technique for its insertion, how to interpret the data obtained, and the risks associated with its use (Table 76.1).

## DESCRIPTION OF THE PA CATHETER

The standard adult PA catheter is a 7.0–7.5 French gauge, polyvinyl chloride, radio-opaque, balloon-tipped, flow-directed, multi-lumen catheter, as shown in Figure 76.1. It is 110 cm long and marked with black rings at 10-cm intervals from the distal tip. A thick black ring indicates 50 cm. It contains three lumina, a thermistor, and a balloon. The distal lumen terminates at the tip of the catheter, and is used for measuring PA pressures, and blood sampling. The right ventricular lumen is 20 cm from the tip and can be used for fluid and drug administration, and in some catheters as a conduit for a right ventricular pacing electrode. The proximal lumen opens 30 cm from the tip and it is used for measuring central venous pressure, for fluid and drug administration, and for injecting the fluid bolus for cardiac output determination; 3–5 cm from the distal tip a thermistor bead connects, via a wire, to the cardiac output monitor. Also, at the distal end, there is a 1.5-ml capacity latex balloon which facilitates advancement of the catheter tip through the right heart and into the PA. Specially designed catheters with capabilities for monitoring continuous cardiac output, mixed venous oxygen saturation, right ventricular ejection fraction, and for right atrial and ventricular pacing are available. A smaller PA catheter is available for use in children.

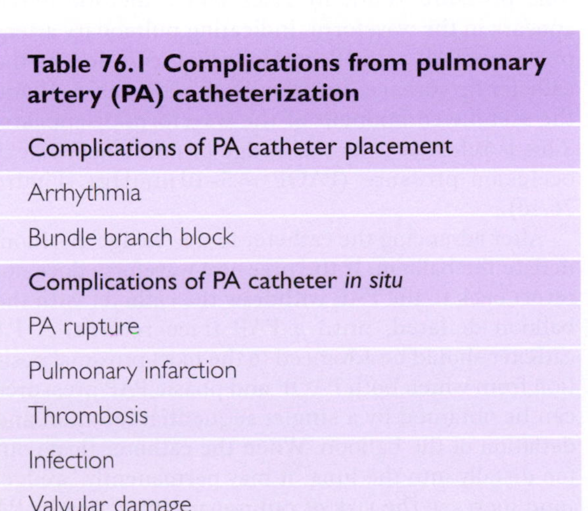

| Table 76.1 Complications from pulmonary artery (PA) catheterization |
|---|
| **Complications of PA catheter placement** |
| Arrhythmia |
| Bundle branch block |
| **Complications of PA catheter *in situ*** |
| PA rupture |
| Pulmonary infarction |
| Thrombosis |
| Infection |
| Valvular damage |

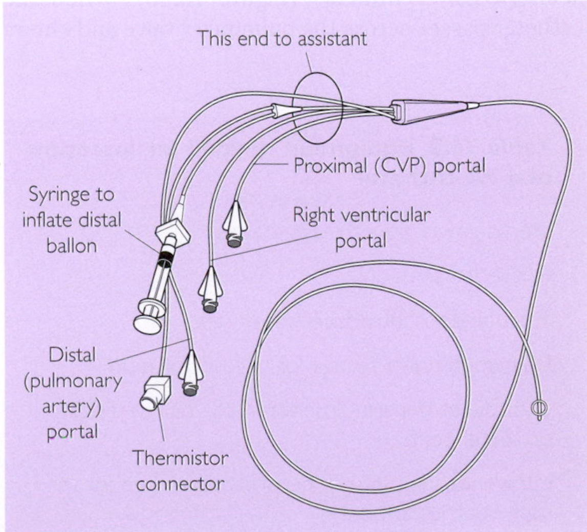



**Figure 76.1** Schematic of adult pulmonary artery catheter. (Reproduced with permission from Butterworth JF. Arterial cannulation. In: *Atlas of Procedures in Anesthesia and Critical Care*. Philadelphia: WB Saunders, 1992.)

## PREPARATION

Table 76.2 lists the equipment needed for insertion of a PA catheter. The clinician, gowned and gloved, prepares the skin overlying the area of insertion with antiseptic solution. Next, a wide area is draped to minimize the chance of catheter contamination. The PA catheter is nearly always introduced through a sheath previously inserted in a central vein. Sheaths can also be inserted via the basilic vein. In anaesthetic practice, the right internal jugular vein is most popular. The method for insertion of the introducer/sheath apparatus into the right internal jugular vein is identical to that discussed in Chapter 75, except that the dilator is inserted through the sheath/introducer before advancing the entire unit (dilator/introducer) over the J-wire into the vein (Figure 76.2). Pull the wire and dilator out together to create a closed system, reducing the risk of air embolization.

After placing the introducer, flush the PA catheter channels with saline to remove the air. With the aid of an assistant, attach the proximal ends of the central venous and distal (PA) ports to pre-zeroed transducers. Attach the right ventricular port to a saline-filled syringe or an infusion line. Place a sterility guard over the catheter (Figure 76.3). 'Test' inflate the balloon using a 3-ml syringe, preset to a 1.5-ml limit.

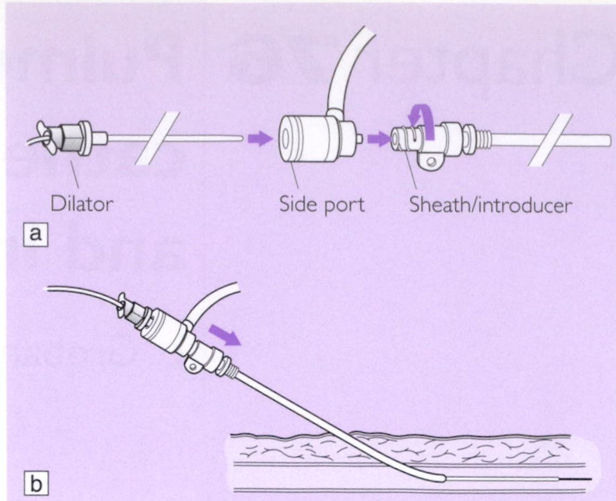


**Figure 76.2** Schematic of dilator, side port, sheath/introducer apparatus (a) and insertion over the J-wire (b) into the vein. (Adapted from Butterworth JF. Arterial cannulation. In: *Atlas of Procedures in Anesthesia and Critical Care*. Philadelphia: WB Saunders, 1992.)

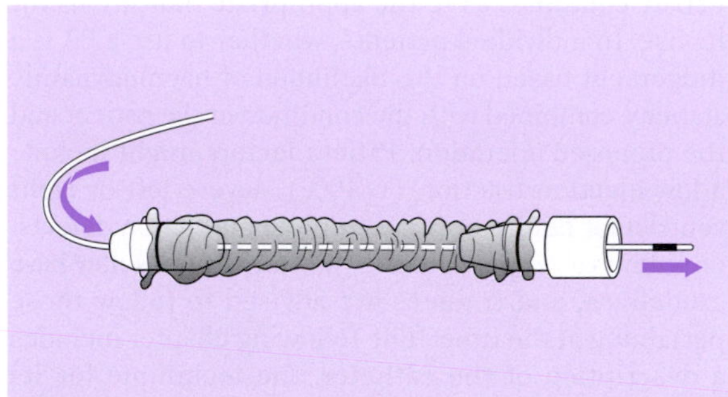

**Figure 76.3** Schematic of sterility guard placed over pulmonary artery catheter. (Adapted from Butterworth JF. Arterial cannulation. In: *Atlas of Procedures in Anesthesia and Critical Care*. Philadelphia: WB Saunders, 1992.)

## FLOTATION

Insert the PA catheter, with the balloon deflated, into the introducer sheath and advance until the catheter reaches the vena cava, approximately 20 cm beyond the skin insertion site. Then inflate the balloon and gently advance the catheter while monitoring the pressure waveform from the distal lumen (Figure 76.4). On entrance into the right atrium, a central venous pressure tracing appears on the oscilloscope (right atrial pressure ≃ 0–8 mmHg) (Figure 76.4a). Once the tip crosses the tricuspid valve and enters the ventricle at approximately 30–35 cm, right ventricular pressures are seen (≃ 25/0–5 mmHg) (Figure 76.4b). When the catheter passes across the pulmonary valve and enters the PA, approximately 5–10 cm further along, the diastolic pressure suddenly rises and a dicrotic notch appears in the waveform, indicating pulmonary artery pressure (PAP ≃ 25/10 mmHg) (Figure 76.4c). As the catheter tip advances into the PA an additional 5–10 cm, the systolic component of the waveform disappears. This is referred to as the wedge or pulmonary artery occlusion pressure (PAOP ≃ 5–10 mmHg) (Figure 76.4d).

After advancing the catheter to the 'wedge' position, deflate the balloon. If the pressure waveform does not revert back to the PAP, withdraw the catheter with the balloon deflated, until a PAP trace returns. A PA catheter should be advanced to the most proximal position from which both PAOP and phasic PAP pressures can be obtained by a single, sequential inflation and deflation of the balloon. When the catheter floats out too distally into the lung, it may permanently 'wedge' (and increase the risk of pulmonary infarction or PA rupture). If the catheter tip remains too proximal in the

| Table 76.2 Equipment needed for insertion of a PA catheter |
|---|
| Sterile gown, gloves, mask, drapes |
| Antiseptic solution |
| Percutaneous introducer/sheath tray |
| PA catheter and syringe for balloon inflation |
| Transducer/heparin-flush assembly for the distal and proximal ports |
| Intravenous infusion or heparinized syringe for the right ventricular port |
| Transducer/oscilloscope equipment |
| Monitoring devices (ECG, blood pressure) |
| Resuscitation drugs and equipment |

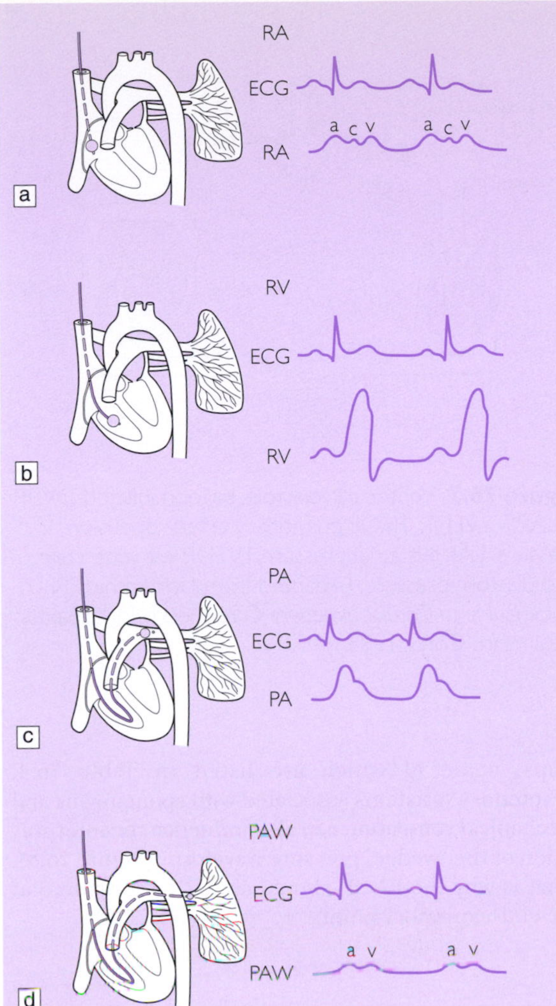


**Figure 76.4** Normal pressures and waveform tracings during PA catheter flotation. See text for details. RA, right atrial pressure; RV, right ventricular pressure; PA, pulmonary artery pressure; PAW, pulmonary artery wedge pressure; a, atrial systole; c, backward bulging from tricuspid valve closure; v, ventricular systole. (Adapted from Lichtenthal PR. *Quick Guide to Cardiopulmonary Care*. Deerfield, IL: Baxter Healthcare Corp., 1998.)

main PA, the catheter tip may whip into and out of the right ventricle. Under these circumstances, the diastolic pressure will be misinterpreted as being too low. Once the catheter is in the proper position, advance the sterile sheath over the catheter and attach it to the introducer. Table 76.3 describes the difference in catheter insertion distances (e.g. internal jugular versus the subclavian vein) to the PA.

The pattern of traces seen during an easy and uncomplicated passage is shown in Figure 76.4e.

## INTERPRETATION

The accurate interpretation of the data obtained from the PA catheter requires an understanding of the relationship between the PAOP and the cardiac chamber pressures and volumes. Ideally, when advanced into the 'wedge' position, the PA catheter resides in a region of the lung where the PAP exceeds pulmonary venous and alveolar pressures. This represents zone 3 of the lung (Figure 76.5). It is assumed that, in this position, a static column of fluid exists between the distal tip of the PA catheter and the left ventricle (Figure 76.6). In the absence of valvular disease, airway pressure changes, or ventricular compliance alterations, the PAOP will track left atrial pressure, which represents left ventricular end-diastolic pressure (LVEDP) (Figure 76.7). The LVEDP directly reflects left ventricular end-diastolic volume (Frank–Starling). Therefore, under

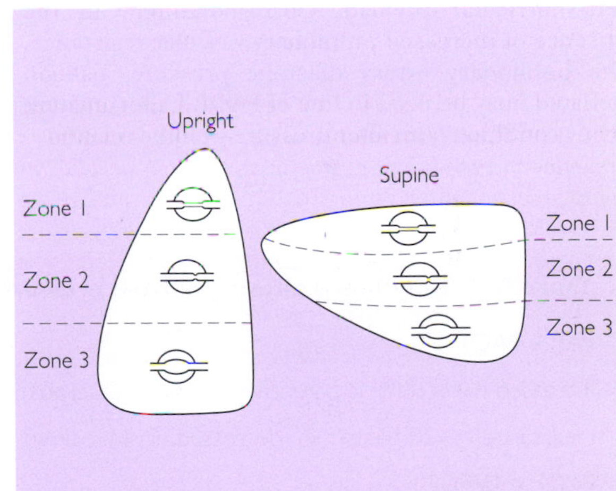


**Figure 76.5** Lung zones in upright and supine position. Zone 1: PAP < $PA_LP$ > PvP. Zone 2: PAP > $PA_LP$ > PvP. Zone 3: PAP > $PA_LP$ < PvP. PAP, pulmonary artery pressure; $PA_LP$, pulmonary alveolar pressure; PvP; pulmonary venous pressure. (Adapted from Lichtenthal PR. *Quick Guide to Cardiopulmonary Care*. Deerfield, IL: Baxter Healthcare Corp., 1998.)

**Table 76.3 Catheter insertion distances**

| | Right atrium (cm) | Right ventricle (cm) | Pulmonary artery (cm) |
|---|---|---|---|
| Internal jugular vein: | | | |
| Right | 20 | 30 | 45 |
| Left | 25 | 35 | 50 |
| Subclavian vein | 10–15 | 25 | 40 |
| Femoral vein | 40 | 50 | 65 |

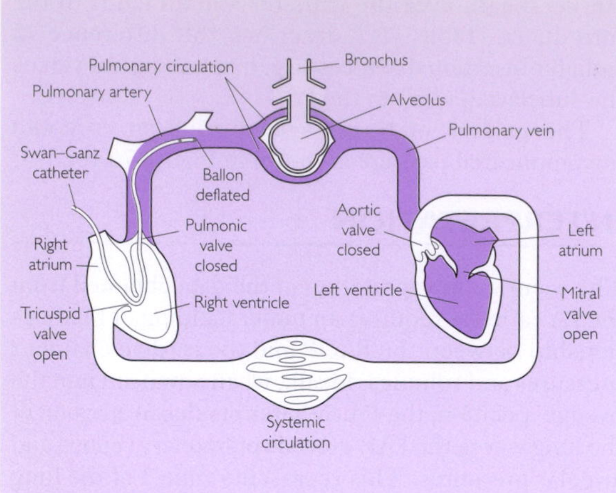


**Figure 76.6** Ventricular diastole, balloon deflated: PADP ≈ LAP ≈ LVEDP. PADP, pulmonary artery diastolic pressure; LAP, left atrial pressure; LVEDP, left ventricular end-diastolic pressure. (Adapted from Lichtenthal PR. *Quick Guide to Cardiopulmonary Care*. Deerfield, IL: Baxter Healthcare Corp., 1998.)

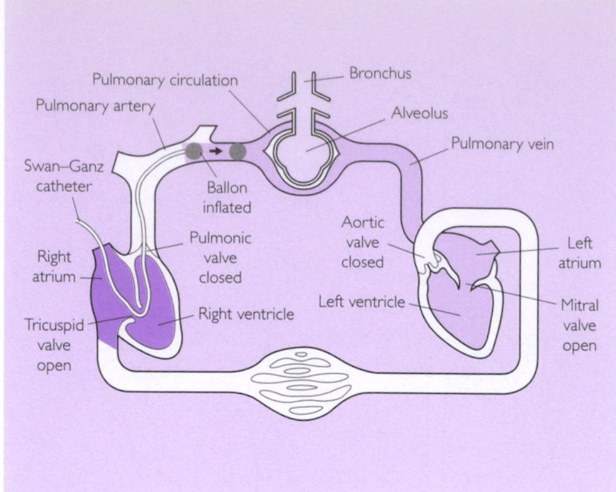


**Figure 76.7** Ventricular diastole, balloon inflated: PAOP ≈ LAP ≈ LVEDP. PAOP, pulmonary artery occlusion pressure; LAP, left atrial pressure; LVEDP, left ventricular end-diastolic pressure. (Adapted from Lichtenthal PR. *Quick Guide to Cardiopulmonary Care*. Deerfield, IL: Baxter Healthcare Corp., 1998.)

normal conditions, the PAOP can be used to estimate left-ventricular preload. Correspondingly, in the absence of increased pulmonary vascular resistance, the pulmonary artery diastolic pressure, balloon deflated, may be used in lieu of PAOP. Unfortunately, many conditions can alter pressure–volume relationships, some of which are listed in Table 76.4. Respiratory variations associated with spontaneous and mechanical ventilation can also influence the interpretation of the 'wedge' pressure waveform (Figure 76.8). That is why the PAOP should always be measured at the end-expiratory point.

| **Table 76.4 Conditions altering normal pressure–volume relationships** |
|---|
| **PAP > PAOP** |
| Increased PVR (chronic parenchymal lung disease, pulmonary embolism, alveolar hypoxia, vasoactive drugs) |
| Heart rate > 120 beats/min (decreased diastolic time) |
| **PAOP > LVEDP** |
| Positive pressure ventilation |
| PEEP |
| Increased intrathoracic pressure |
| Chronic obstructive airway disease |
| Increased pulmonary vascular resistance |
| Mitral valve disease (stenosis, regurgitation) |
| Left atrial myxoma |
| **PAOP < LVEDP** |
| Non-compliant left ventricle (ischaemia, hypertrophied LV) |
| Aortic regurgitation |

PAP, pulmonary artery pressure; PVR, pulmonary vascular resistance; PAOP, pulmonary artery occlusion pressure; LVEDP, left ventricular end-diastolic pressure; PEEP, positive end-expiratory pressure; LV, left ventricle.

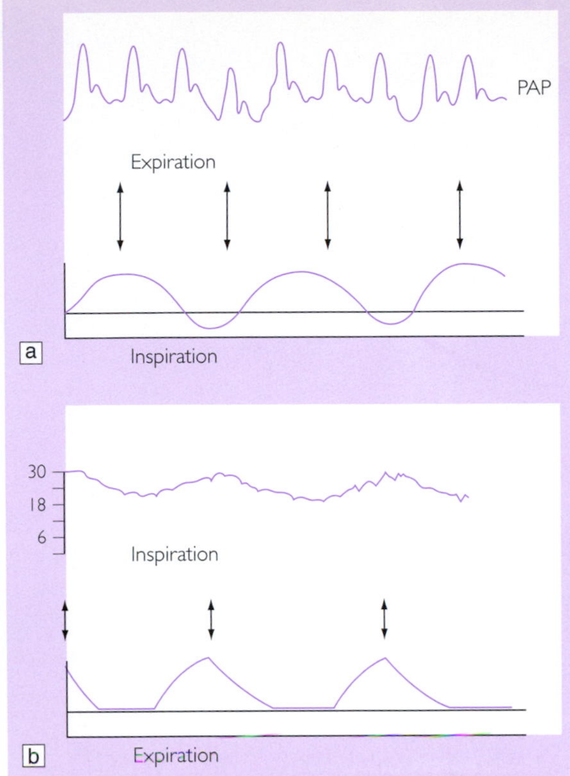


**Figure 76.8** Pulmonary artery pressure waveform variations associated with spontaneous breathing (a) and controlled mechanical ventilation (b). The values recorded should be obtained at end-expiration when the influence of intrathoracic pressure is minimal. (Adapted from Lichtenthal PR. *Quick Guide to Cardiopulmonary Care*. Deerfield, IL: Baxter Healthcare Corp., 1998.)

## FURTHER READING


American College of Cardiology Expert Consensus Document. Present use of bedside right heart catheterization in patients with cardiac disease. *J Am Coll Cardiol* 1998;**32**:840–64.

American Society of Anesthesiologists. Practice Guidelines for Pulmonary Artery Catheterization. A Report by the American Society of Anesthesiologists Task Force on Pulmonary Artery Catheterization. *Anesthesiology* 1993;**78**:380–94.

Butterworth JF IV. Pulmonary artery catheterization. *Atlas of Procedures in Anesthesia and Critical Care*. Philadelphia: WB Saunders, 1992: 105–10.

Gomez CMH, Palazzo MGA. Pulmonary artery catheterization in anaesthesia and intensive care. *Br J Anaesth* 1998;**81**:945–56.

Hines, RL, Barash PG. Pulmonary artery catheterization. In: Blitt CD, Hines RL, eds. *Monitoring in Anesthesia and Critical Care Medicine*, 3rd edn. New York: Churchill Livingstone, 1995: 213–59.

Sprung CL: *The Pulmonary Artery Catheter: Methodology and Clinical Applications*. Rockville, MA: Aspen Systems Corporation, 1983.

Thys DM, Reich DL. Invasive cardiovascular monitoring. In: Saidman LJ, Smith NT, eds. *Monitoring in Anesthesia*, 3rd edn. Stoneham, MA: Butterworth-Heinemann, 1993: 67–71.

Vender JS. Pulmonary artery catheter monitoring: an update. *ASA Refresher Course* 1993;**21**:189–204.

# Chapter 77 Methods of measuring cardiac output

M.H. Wall

Since Fick first described his technique in 1870, numerous methods have been proposed for measuring cardiac output (CO). These methods include both invasive (Fick, dye dilution, thermodilution) and non-invasive (Doppler, bioimpedance, and pulse waveform analysis) techniques. This chapter describes these methods and their use in clinical practice. The Fick principle and the technique of integration of dye dilution curves are described in Chapter 37 (Figures 37.68 and 37.23, respectively).

## FICK METHOD

Adolph Fick proposed that CO (L/min) could be calculated based on the principle of conservation of mass, by measuring oxygen consumption ($\dot{V}O_2$, ml $O_2$/min) and the difference in arterial and mixed venous oxygen content, where:

$$\frac{\text{Total arterial}}{O_2\text{ content}} = \frac{\text{Total venous}}{O_2\text{ content}} + O_2\text{ uptake}$$

$$\text{CO} \times CaO_2 \times 10 = \text{CO} \times C\bar{v}O_2 \times 10 + \dot{V}O_2 \qquad (1)$$

Solving for CO:

$$\text{CO} = \frac{\dot{V}O_2}{CaO_2 - C\bar{v}O_2} \times 10 \qquad (2)$$

where $CaO_2$ is the arterial oxygen content (ml/100 ml), and $C\bar{v}O_2$ is the mixed venous oxygen content (ml/100 ml).

From equation (2), $CaO_2$ and $C\bar{v}O_2$ can be directly measured in arterial and mixed venous blood samples using co-oximetry. $\dot{V}O_2$ is measured by collecting all exhaled gases and measuring the amount of oxygen that was inhaled and exhaled, the difference representing oxygen consumption.

Measurement of CO using the Fick technique is standard in physiological laboratories with controlled conditions and stable haemodynamics. However, in the clinical environment, this technique presents many problems, including: the assumption that $\dot{V}O_2$ and CO remain constant during the inspired and expired gas analysis; the difficult and time-consuming task of performing the expired gas collection; the need for a ventilator circuit free of leaks; the inability to measure high COs with accuracy as a result of a small $CaO_2 - C\bar{v}O_2$ difference. Finally, the technique provides only a single, discontinuous measurement.

The availability of continuous arterial pulse and mixed venous oximetry, continuous intra-arterial blood gas analysis, and continuous inspiratory and expiratory gas analysers has made the almost continuous Fick CO determination possible. Preliminary reports in small numbers of patients show the potential for continuous non-invasive Fick-derived monitoring of CO in the future; however, none of these techniques is currently in widespread clinical use.

## DYE DILUTION

This technique is based on the principle that, if a known mass is placed in an unknown volume and the concentration can be measured, the volume can be calculated:

$$\text{Volume} = \frac{\text{Mass}}{\text{Concentration}} \qquad (3)$$

This same principle can be used to calculate flow if a known mass is added, and the concentration can be measured downstream over time. The flow ($V/t$) will equal the mass divided by the area under the concentration versus time curve or:

$$\text{Flow} = \int_0^\infty \frac{\text{Mass}}{\text{Concentration } dt} \qquad (4)$$

This is the Stewart–Hamilton equation for measuring CO, in which a known amount of dye (often indocyanine green [ICG]) or lithium is injected intravenously, then the downstream arterial concentration is measured by a densitometer. The area under the concentration versus time curve is calculated and equation (4) can be solved for CO. This technique is accurate; however, multiple arterial samples must be analysed to produce the concentration versus time curve, and dye can accumulate, making subsequent concentration measurements more difficult. Thus, thermodilution methods (see below) have largely replaced dye dilution.

## THERMODILUTION

Thermodilution CO uses the principle of conservation of heat to calculate CO. The change in temperature measured is analogous to change in dye concentration during dye dilution. The expression used to calculate CO is the Stewart–Hamilton equation modified for thermodilution, where $V_{inj}(T_b - T_t)$ is the 'mass of cold' and $\int \Delta T_{blood}(t)\,dt$ is the 'concentration of cold'. This can be written (see Appendix 77.1) as:

$$CO = \frac{V_{inj}(T_b - T_t)}{\int_0^{t3} \Delta T_{blood}(t)dt + A} \times K$$

A typical thermodilution curve is shown in Figure 77.1.

Accurate and precise thermodilution requires the following:

- the correct volume of injectate;
- stable CO during measurement;
- stable baseline pulmonary artery temperature;
- complete mixing of the injectate;
- no loss or gain of injectate volume before measurement by detector (no shunts);
- correct detection and calculation of temperature versus time curve;
- correct use of constants (computation constant [$k$] and correction factor [$F$] entered into CO computer).

However, with spontaneous or mechanical ventilation, pulmonary artery temperature can vary by 0.01–0.05°C, and true CO (blood flow) also varies (by more than 10%), and the magnitude and direction of the changes are unpredictable. Furthermore, animal and human studies that have compared thermodilution CO at various phases of respiration have come to different conclusions regarding optimal timing.

Theoretically, larger volumes of colder solutions should cause larger temperature changes in the blood and minimize some of the impact of baseline pulmonary artery temperature variation. However, larger volumes of colder solutions may increase the possibility of measurement errors and loss of indicator (cold) before mixing with blood. Studies examining the effect of volume and temperature have found no differences in the accuracy or reproducibility in patients between iced or room temperature, and between 5- or 10-ml bolus injections. Multiple factors can cause errors in the integration of the temperature versus time curve (Table 77.1). Nevertheless, bolus thermodilution has shown correlation coefficients ($r$ values) of 0.90–0.94 with Fick, dye dilution, and electromagnetic flow probes in multiple *in vivo* and *in vitro* studies.

To summarize, the measurement of thermodilution CO has many potential errors; however, measurement in triplicate using 5 or 10 ml iced or room temperature solution given at the same phase in respiration (end expiration) will optimize reproducibility while having minimal effect on accuracy, and should allow for more reliable comparisons of CO over time.

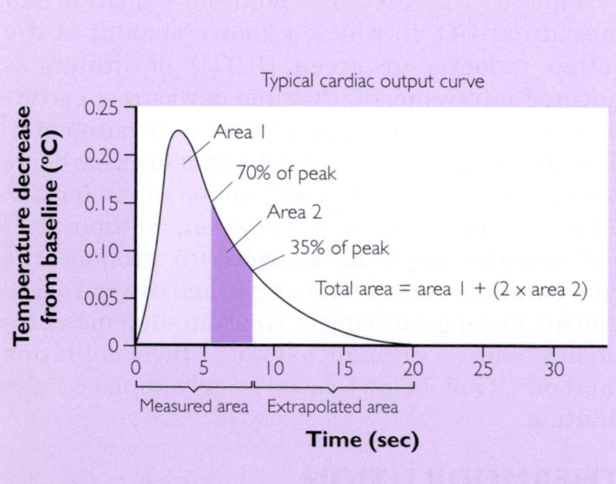


**Figure 77.1** An example of an algorithm for calculating the area under the temperature versus time curve. Area 1 is the area under the curve until the temperature decrease reaches 70% of the peak. Area 2 is the area between 70% and 35% decrease. The extrapolated area is defined as being equal to area 2. (Adapted from Bazaral MG, Petre J, Novoa R. *Anesthesiology* 1992;77:31–7.)

## CONTINUOUS THERMODILUTION

The intermittent performance of most CO measurement techniques represents their major drawback. Yelderman developed a technique in which multiple small boluses of heat, delivered by a thermal filament on a pulmonary artery catheter, cause temperature

| **Table 77.1 Factors affecting the integration of the temperature versus time curve** |
|---|
| Inadequate injectate mixing |
| Patient movement or shivering |
| Haemodynamic instability |
| Rapidly changing CO, HR, or BP |
| Arrhythmias |
| Shunting |
| Valvular regurgitation – tricuspid or pulmonary regurgitation |
| Recirculation |
| Inadequate change in blood temperature |
| Small injectate volume |
| Small patient/injectate temperature gradient (i.e. hypothermic patient) |
| High CO |
| Electrocautery interference |
| PA temperature baseline drift |
| Post-hypothermic cardiopulmonary bypass |
| Respiratory variation |
| Intravenous fluid administration |
| Poor thermistor response |
| Improper catheter position |
| Catheter thrombus |
| Catheter contact with vessel wall |

CO, cardiac output; HR, heart rate; BP, blood pressure; PA, pulmonary artery. Modified, with permission from Mantin R, Ramsay JG. *Int Anesthesiol Clin* 1996;34:79–107.

changes of 0.007°C. The distal thermistor senses these small heat boluses, resulting in a temperature versus time concentration curve similar to that seen with bolus thermodilution. CO data are generated every 30–90 s, and the CO displayed represents an average over the last 5–10 min. Several studies have verified the accuracy and safety of this technology, but the failure to produce 'real-time' measurement rather than an average CO over the sampling period represents a major disadvantage.

## DOPPLER-DERIVED CARDIAC OUTPUT

The Doppler principle describes a shift in sound frequency that occurs when a sound emitted from a stationary transducer reflects off a moving object and returns to the transducer. The shift in frequency is proportional to the velocity ($V$), which is calculated from the Doppler equation (described in Chapter 37):

$$V = \frac{C \times F_d}{2F_0 \times \cos\theta} \qquad (5)$$

where $C$ is the speed of sound in blood, $F_d$ is the frequency shift, $F_0$ is the frequency of sound emitted, and $\theta$ is the angle between emitted sound and the moving object.

This velocity is displayed as velocity versus time (Figure 77.2; see also Chapter 37, Figure 37.67). The area under this curve $\int_0^{VET} V(t)\,dt$ (where VET is the ventricular ejection time) is the velocity–time integral. Stroke volume (SV) can be calculated by SV = CSA × VTI, where CSA is the cross-sectional area, and finally CO = SV × HR (heart rate).

For accurate measurement of CO by Doppler, the following must be true:

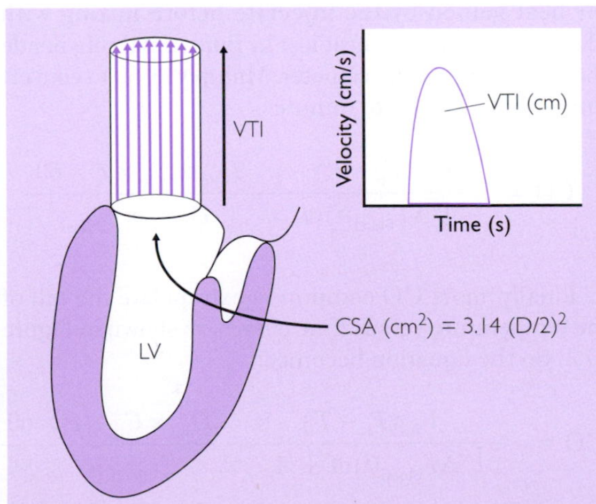


**Figure 77.2** Calculation of stroke volume. The cross-sectional area (CSA) is calculated as a circle based on a two-dimensional echo diameter D measurement. The length of the cylinder of blood ejected through this CSA on a single beat is the velocity time integral (VTI) of the Doppler curve – the area under the velocity–time curve. Stroke volume is calculated as CSA × VTI. (Adapted from Otto CM, Pearlman AS. *Textbook of Clinical Echocardiography*. Philadelphia: WB Saunders, 1995.)

- accurate measurement of CSA;
- laminar flow;
- parallel angle (θ) between Doppler beam and blood flow;
- velocity and blood flow measurements made at the same site.

Major problems are the estimation of CSA and the necessary assumption of a square velocity profile (see Chapter 37).

### Suprasternal Doppler

Studies of suprasternal Doppler evaluation of blood flow through the ascending aorta have had success in critically ill patients. However, training and experience are required to get consistent results. The probe requires frequent repositioning, preventing continuous evaluation, and in many patients an adequate signal cannot be obtained.

### Transoesophageal Doppler

A Doppler probe attached to an oesophageal stethoscope can be used to determine flow velocity in the descending aorta. Problems with this technique include:

- a correction must be made to calculate the total CO because the measurement takes place in the descending aorta;
- unless the descending aorta is directly measured, a nomogram is used to determine CSA;
- the Doppler beam is at an approximately 45° angle to the aortic blood flow, so a correction must be made for this angle;
- optimum positioning requires training;
- the probe needs to be adjusted.

Despite these limitations, this technique has been widely studied and continues to improve with modifications to the probe, new nomograms, and correction factors. The transoesophageal location has the greatest potential of the Doppler techniques.

### Transtracheal

A Doppler probe has been mounted on an endotracheal tube and used to measure aortic diameter and Doppler flow. So far, this has not found a routine place in CO measurement.

### Intrapulmonary artery Doppler

A pulmonary artery catheter with an array of four Doppler probes has been used to measure main pulmonary artery CSA and flow velocity directly, to generate continuous CO data. Preliminary studies showed a fair correlation with CO measured by electromagnetic flow probes, even though it may be difficult to site the Doppler array appropriately in the main pulmonary artery.

Overall, the suprasternal, transoesophageal, transtracheal, and intrapulmonary techniques require advanced training, frequent repositioning to optimize the Doppler signal, and thus far the absolute accuracy when compared with bolus thermodilution or electromagnetic flow probes is low. With continued refinement of algorithms and nomograms, the transoesophageal approach seems most promising.

## TRANSOESOPHAGEAL ECHOCARDIOGRAPHY

Transoesophageal echocardiography (TEE) has been used to calculate CO using Doppler and two-dimensional imaging at the mitral, aortic, tricuspid, and pulmonic valves, the ascending and descending aortas, and pulmonary artery. These methods and thermodilution closely agree.

Problems with TEE include expensive technology and the requirement of advanced training for placement, acquisition, and interpretation of Doppler and two-dimensional images.

Recently, three-dimensional TEE, with the ability to calculate left ventricular volumes, has been investigated.

## BIOIMPEDANCE

In 1966, Kubicek *et al.* presented an empirical equation for the calculation of SV based on changes in thoracic impedance (measured by introducing a low-amplitude, high-frequency alternating current, and sensing the impedance change with electrodes placed around the thorax). Ventilation and pulsatile blood flow produce these changes in impedance. The original formula was:

$$SV = [pL^2/Z_0{}^2] \times VET \times Max\ (dZ/dt)$$

where $p$ is the resistivity of blood ($\Omega \times$ cm), $L$ is the thoracic length (cm), $Z_0$ is the basal thoracic impedance ($\Omega$), VET is the ventricular ejection time (s), and Max $dZ/dt$ is the maximum rate of impedance change during systolic upstroke.

Bernstein modified this equation, and its place in clinical practice has recently been revised. Some studies have demonstrated the accuracy of bioimpedance whereas others have shown poor correlation with thermodilution CO.

Clearly, more research will be needed before bioimpedance can replace other methods of CO determination.

## PULSE CONTOUR ANALYSIS OR PULSE WAVEFORM

For more than 30 years, many different algorithms have tried to predict SV from an analysis of the peripheral arterial waveform. Unfortunately, despite multiple attempts, no algorithm has proved successful in a wide range of patient populations.

## CONCLUSION

The quest for an accurate, precise, continuous, non-invasive CO device that is simple to operate and inexpensive continues. Several methods (Doppler, bioimpedance) appear promising, but for now thermodilution remains the standard clinical technique.

## APPENDIX 77.1: THERMODILUTION

Thermodilution CO uses the principle of conservation of heat to calculate CO, where the amount of heat lost by blood must equal the amount of heat gained by a cold injectate. Mathematically, heat gained equals heat lost or:

$$D_{inj} \times C_{inj} \int_{t_1}^{t_2} Q(f)\ [T_{blood}(t) - T_{inj}(t)]dt = D_{blood} \times C_{blood} \int_{t_1}^{t_2} \Delta T_h(t)(CO_{blood})dt$$

where $D_{inj}$ is the density of injectate = 1.018 g/ml for dextrose 5% in water, 1.005 g/ml for physiological saline; $C_{inj}$ is the specific heat of injectate = 0.965 cal/g per °C for dextrose 5% in water, 0.997 cal/g per °C for physiological saline; $t_1$ is the time of injection; $t_2$ is the end of integration where all cold blood passed the detector site; $Q(f)$ is the input flow of the indicator; $T_{blood}$ is the baseline temperature of blood; $T_{inj}$ is the temperature of injectate (°C); $D_{blood}$ is the density of blood = 1.045 g/ml; $C_{blood}$ is the specific heat of blood = 0.87 cal/g per °C; $\int_{t_1}^{t_2}\Delta T_h(t)dt$ is the area under temperature versus time curve (°C · s); $CO_{blood}$ is the cardiac output.

If the injection of cold is a bolus then $\int_{t_1}^{t_2} Q(t)\ dt$ = volume injected = $V_i$, and $T_b$ and $T_i$ remain constant, the equation may be rewritten as:

$$D_{inj} \times C_{inj} \times V_{inj}(T_b - T_i) = D_{blood} \times C_{blood} \int_{t_1}^{t_2} \Delta T_{blood}(t)(CO_{blood})dt$$

If CO is constant, the equation becomes the Stewart–Hamilton equation modified for thermodilution where $V_{inj}(T_b - T_i)$ is the 'mass of cold', and $\int_{t_1}^{t_2}\Delta T_{blood}(t)dt$ represents the 'concentration' of cold':

$$CO = \frac{V_{inj}(T_b - T_i) \quad \times \quad D_{inj} \times C_{in}}{\int_{t_1}^{t_2}\Delta T_{blood}(t)dt \ \times \ D_{blood} \times C_{blood}}$$

An empirical correction factor $F$ is added to account for heat gained by the injectate before mixing with blood, and additional heat lost by fluid remaining inside the dead space of the catheter. Multiply by 60 to convert units from seconds to minutes.

$$CO = \frac{V_{inj}(T_b - T_i) \quad \times \quad D_{inj} \times C_{in} \times F \times 60}{\int_{t_1}^{t_2}\Delta T_{blood}(t)dt \ \times \quad D_{blood} \times C_{blood}}$$

Finally, most CO computers extrapolate the tail of the temperature versus time curves, as shown in Figure 77.1. So the equation becomes:

$$CO = \frac{V_{inj}(T_b - T_i) \quad \times \quad D_{inj} \times C_{in} \times F \times 60}{\int_0^{t_3}\Delta T_{blood}(t)dt + A \quad \times \quad D_{blood} \times C_{blood}}$$

where $t_3$ represents the time set by the algorithm and $A$ is the area of the extrapolated tail of the curve. Finally, the constants $D_{inj}$, $C_{inj}$, $F$, 60, $D_{blood}$, and $C_{blood}$ are all combined to form the computation constant ($K$), which is specific for each catheter, volume, temperature, and type of injectate resulting in the equation:

$$CO = \frac{V_{inj}(T_b - T_t)}{\int_0^{t_3}\Delta T_{blood}(t)dt + A} \times K$$

## FURTHER READING


Bashein G. Cardiac output: measurement and clinical significance. 41st Annual Refresher Course Lectures. Park Ridge (IL): American Society of Anesthesiologists, 1990: 216.

Critchley LA. Impedance cardiography: the impact of new technology. *Anaesthesia* 1998;**53**:677–84

Heerdt PM, Pond CG, Blessios GA, Rosenbloom M. Comparison of cardiac output measured by intrapulmonary artery Doppler, thermodilution, and electromagnetometry. *Ann Thorac Surg* 1992;**54**:959–66.

Hirschl MM, Binder M, Gwechenberger M *et al.* Noinvasive assessment of cardiac output in critically ill patients by analysis of the finger blood pressure waveform. *Crit Care Med* 1997;**25**:1909–14.

Jansen JR. The thermodilution method for the clinical assessment of cardiac output. *Intensive Care Med* 1995;**21**:691–7.

Krishnamurthy B, McMurray TJ, McClean E. The perioperative use of oesophageal Doppler monitor in patients undergoing coronary revascularization. A comparison with the continuous cardiac output monitor. *Anaesthesia* 1997;**52**:624–9.

Linton R, Band D, O'Brien T *et al.* Lithium dilution cardiac output measurment: a comparison with thermodilution. *Crit Care Med* 1997;**25**;1796–1800.

Mantin R, Ramsay JG. Cardiac output technologies. *Int Anesthesiol Clin* 1996;**34**:79–107.

Mihm FG, Gettinger A, Hanson CW 3rd *et al.* A multicenter evaluation of a new continuous cardiac output pulmonary artery catheter system. *Crit Care Med* 1998;**26**:1346–50.

Miller DM, Wessels JA. A simple method for the continuous noninvasive estimate of cardiac output using the Maxima breathing system. A pilot study. Anaesth Intensive Care 1997;**25**:23–8.

Perrino AC Jr, Harris SN, Luther MA. Intraoperative determination of cardiac ouput using multiplane transesophageal echocardiography: a comparison to thermodlution. *Anesthesiology* 1998;**89**:350–7.

Singer M. Esophageal Doppler monitoring of aortic blood flow: beat-by-beat cardiac output monitoring. *Int Anesthesiol Clin* 1993;**31**:99–125.

Yelderman M. Continuous measurement of cardiac output with the use of stochastic system identification techniques. *J Clin Monit* 1990;**6**:322–32.

# Chapter 78 Intraosseous access and infusion

M.L. Cannon

In any emergency, vascular access for resuscitative fluid and drug administration is crucial. However, in the critically ill neonatal or paediatric patient, obtaining adequate venous access is often difficult and time-consuming. By placing an intraosseous needle, venous access can usually be obtained rapidly, permitting immediate delivery of resuscitative fluids and medications to the central circulation.

Josefson published one of the earliest descriptions of intraosseous infusion in humans in 1934. Recent animal studies have shown that intraosseous drug infusions have pharmacokinetics and efficacy comparable to peripheral intravenous infusions. To date, all standard medications and fluids used for resuscitation have been given successfully by intraosseous injection. One report describes an infant being resuscitated and anaesthetized via the intraosseous route. Intraosseous injection has provided regional anaesthesia in adult patients. Finally, other non-resuscitative medications may be administered via the intraosseous route (Table 78.1).

Intraosseous injection is generally under-utilized. Guidelines published by Kanter *et al.* state that intravenous access should be accomplished within 5 min of a paediatric cardiopulmonary arrest (see Further reading). The guidelines for Pediatric Advanced Life Support published by the American Heart Association and the American Academy of Pediatrics state that no more than three attempts at intravenous cannulation or 90 s should occur before inserting an intraosseous needle into an unstable, critically ill child.

Intraosseous injection can also be used in adults. With a bone injection gun, an intraosseous needle can easily be inserted, and emergency fluids and medications effectively administered.

**Table 78.1 Other medications acceptable for intraosseous infusion**

| |
|---|
| Ampicillin |
| Cefotaxime |
| Ceftriaxone |
| Dexamethasone |
| Diazoxide |
| Digitalis |
| Ephedrine |
| Gentamicin |
| Heparin |
| Insulin |
| Levarterenol |
| Local anaesthetics |
| Morphine |
| Penicillin |
| Phenobarbitone (phenobarbital) |
| Phenytoin |
| Propranolol |
| Sulphonamides |

Adapted with permission from Fiser DH. Intraosseous infusion. In: Dieckmann RA, Fiser DH, Selbst, eds. Illustrated *Textbook of Pediatric Emergency and Critical Care Procedures*. St Louis: Mosby-Year Book, 1997: 220–4.

## COMPLICATIONS AND CONTRAINDICATIONS

Intraosseous needle placement and infusion have some complications, including the potential of infection, which is minimized by use of the correct technique. Growth plate injury and growth disturbance in the cannulated bone may also occur. However, a study of 10 patients who had undergone intraosseous infusion one year earlier failed to detect significant tibial length discrepancy. Other reported complications include tibial fracture, compartment syndrome, osteomyelitis, and tissue/skin necrosis. Microscopic pulmonary embolism of bone marrow and fat has been reported; however, a recent animal study found no difference in the numbers of emboli between animals receiving cardiopulmonary resuscitation alone and those receiving cardiopulmonary resuscitation with intraosseous infusion.

Contraindications to intraosseous needle placement and infusion include disruption of the cortex of the bone in the ipsilateral extremity from fracture, or a previous failed intraosseous needle placement. Patients with osteopetrosis and osteogenesis imperfecta represent contraindications to intraosseus infusion. Avoid insertion through infected tissue to prevent osteomyelitis.

## SITE SELECTION AND TECHNIQUE

The medullary sinusoids of the long bones drain into medullary venous channels, which then flow into the systemic venous circulation via nutrient and emissary veins. In children less than 6 years of age, the most frequently recommended and utilized site for intraosseous cannulation is the medial aspect of the tibia, approximately 1–3 cm below the proximal tibial tuberosity (Figure 78.1). This site is ideal because of the virtual absence of overlying muscle, nerves, and vascular structures. Tibial cannulation does not interfere with airway management or chest compressions. Other potential sites include the distal femur, distal tibia, and anterosuperior iliac spine (Figures 78.2–78.4). Note that differing angles of approach are used to cannulate the various sites.

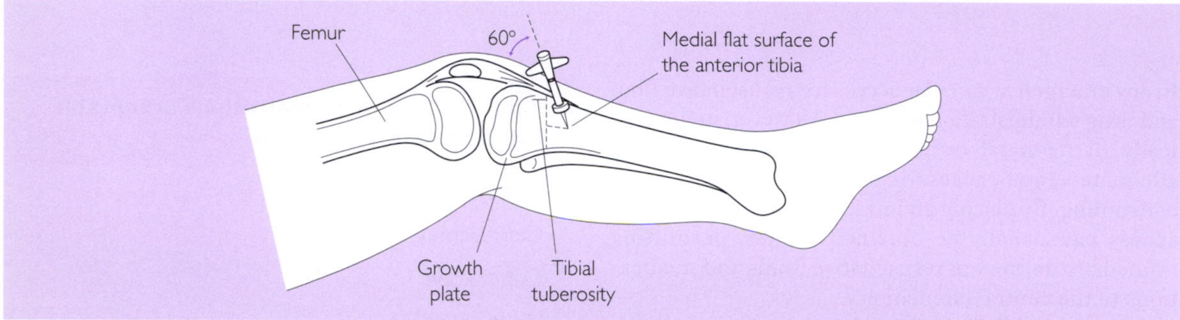


**Figure 78.1** Standard anterior tibial approach: the insertion point is in the midline on the medial flat surface of the anterior tibia, 1–3 cm (2 finger-breadth) below the tibial tuberosity. (Adapted from Dieckmann RA, Fiser DH, Selbst, eds. Illustrated *Textbook of Pediatric Emergency and Critical Care Procedures*. St Louis: Mosby, 1997: 220–4.)

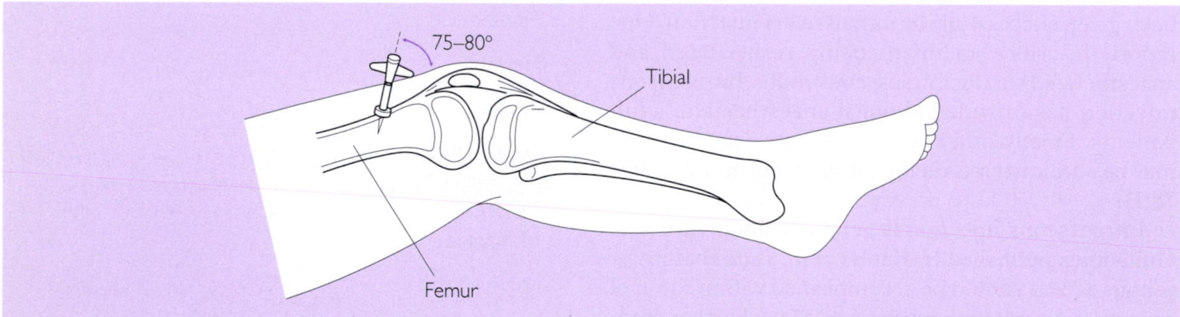


**Figure 78.2** Distal femur approach: insert the needle prodromal to the external condyle in the midline, and superiorly at an angle of 75–80°. (Adapted from Dieckmann RA, Fiser DH, Selbst, eds. Illustrated *Textbook of Pediatric Emergency and Critical Care Procedures*. St Louis: Mosby, 1997: 220–4.)

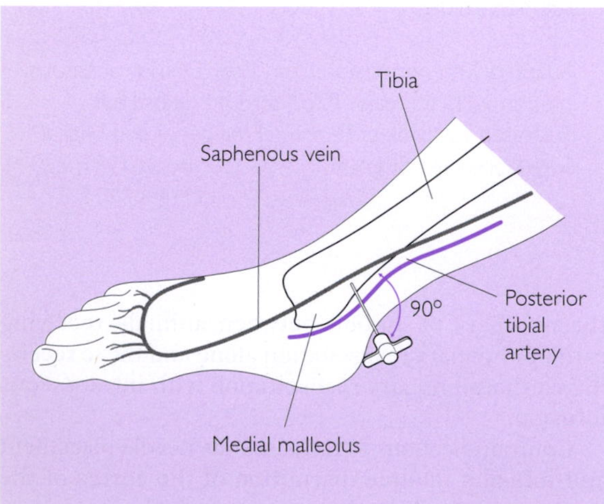


**Figure 78.3** Distal tibia approach: insert the needle perpendicularly just proximal to the middle malleolus and posterior to the saphenous vein. (Adapted from Dieckmann RA, Fiser DH, Selbst, eds. Illustrated *Textbook of Pediatric Emergency and Critical Care Procedures*. St Louis: Mosby, 1997: 220–4.)

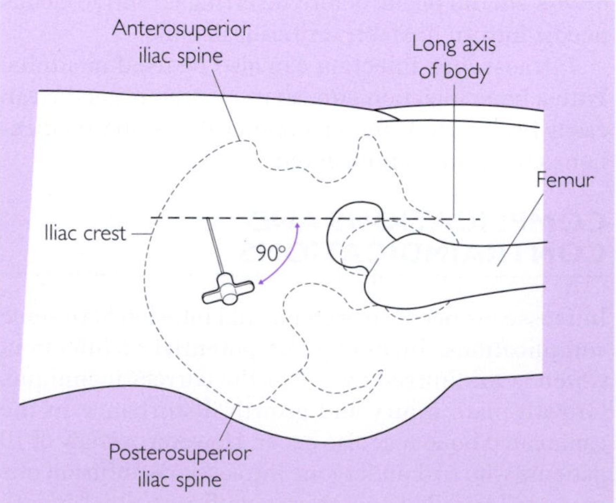


**Figure 78.4** Anterosuperior iliac spine approach: insert the needle at an angle of 90° to the long axis of the body. (Adapted from Dieckmann RA, Fiser DH, Selbst, eds. Illustrated *Textbook of Pediatric Emergency and Critical Care Procedures*. St Louis: Mosby, 1997: 220–4.)

**Table 78.2 Method for intraosseous access**

| | |
|---|---|
| 1. | Locate the site of cannulation. Palpate the site of intraosseous cannulation 1–3 cm below and medial to the tibial tuberosity. |
| 2. | Wash hands and put on gloves. |
| 3. | Clean the cannulation site with antiseptic solution. |
| 4. | Assure that the intraosseous needle's outer bevel and internal stylet bevel are properly aligned. |
| 5. | Grasp the thigh and knee above the proposed insertion site with the non-dominant hand. Do not place any portion of your hand posterior to the insertion site. Support the patient's leg on a firm surface. |
| 6. | In conscious patients, inject 1% lignocaine (lidocaine) (or equivalent) in skin and periosteum of cannulation site. |
| 7. | Insert the needle through the skin and through the bony cortex perpendicular to the medial surface of the tibia and slightly caudad. Avoid the epiphyseal plate. Use steady, firm pressure and twisting motion to advance the needle until a sudden decrease in resistance is noted. |
| 8. | Remove the cap and stylet and confirm that bone marrow can be aspirated. Flush the needle after aspirating bone marrow to prevent clogging. Nevertheless, marrow cannot always be aspirated through a correctly placed needle. |
| 9. | Stabilize the needle and slowly inject 10 ml saline. There should be little resistance to injection if the needle is properly placed. Closely observe the site and surrounding tissue for signs of infiltration. |
| 10. | If the test injection is uneventful, begin infusing resuscitation fluids and medications. |
| 11. | If the needle placement is unsatisfactory, remove the needle and attempt placement with another needle in the opposite extremity. |

Adapted from the American Heart Association. *Pediatric Advanced Life Support*, 1997.

A bone marrow needle (Jamshidi-type) or a specially designed intraosseous infusion needle should be used. Short large-bore spinal needles with an internal stylette may be used in an emergency if no better alternative is available.

Intraosseous cannulation should be done using an aseptic technique. Table 78.2 outlines the steps for intraosseous cannulation of the proximal tibia.

## CONCLUSION

Intraosseous needle placement and infusion represent relatively simple life-saving procedures. The complication rate is low when standard techniques are employed. All physicians and paramedical personnel who are involved in the acute care of children should be prepared to place intraosseous needles and infuse drugs and fluids through this route.

## FURTHER READING


American Heart Association. *Pediatric Advanced Life Support*. Dallas TX: American Heart Association, 1997.

Fiser DH. Intraosseous infusion. In: Dieckmann RA, Fiser DH, Selbst S, eds. *Illustrated Textbook of Pediatric Emergency and Critical Care Procedures*. St Louis: Mosby, 1997: 220–24.

Fiser RT, Walker WM, Seibert JJ, *et al*. Tibial length following intraosseous infusion: a prospective, radiographic analysis. *Pediatr Emerg Care* 1997;**13**:186–8.

Hodge D III. Intraosseous infusions: a review. *Pediatr Emerg Care* 1985;**1**:215–18.

Josefson LM. A new method of treatment – intraossal injections. *Acta Med Scand* 1934;**81**:550–64.

Kanter RK, Zimmerman JJ, Strauss RH, Stoeckel KA. Pediatric emergency intravenous access: evaluation of a protocol. *Am J Dis Child* 1986;**140**:132–4.

Miner WF, Corneli HM, Bolte RG, *et al*. Prehospital use of intraosseous infusion by paramedics. *Pediatr Emerg Care* 1989;**5**:5–7.

Orlowski JP, Julius CJ, Petras RE, *et al*. The safety of intraosseous infusions: risks of fat and bone marrow emboli to the lungs. *Ann Emerg Med* 1989;**18**:1062–7.

Schleien, CL, Kuluz JW, Shaffner DH, Rogers MC. Cardiopulmonary resuscitation. In: Rogers MC, ed. *Textbook of Pediatric Intensive Care*, 3rd edn. Baltimore: Williams & Wilkins, 1996: 3–49.

Waisman M, Waisman D. Bone marrow infusion in adults. *J Trauma* 1997;**42**:288–93.

# Chapter 79 Diagnostic peritoneal lavage

J.S. Kelly and J.F. Butterworth

Intra-abdominal blood loss and/or hollow viscus perforation with peritoneal contamination remains the leading cause of preventable morbidity and mortality in the trauma patient. The specific mechanism of injury coupled with abnormal physical findings (such as guarding, rebound tenderness, ileus, and abdominal distension) may suggest a high likelihood of intra-abdominal injury, and the need for emergency laparotomy in the awake, cooperative patient. However, many trauma patients present with confounding factors which render the abdominal physical examination unreliable (Table 79.1). Consequently, additional diagnostic studies are often required to rule out significant intra-abdominal injuries in this patient population. Diagnostic peritoneal lavage (DPL) continues to be extensively used for this purpose.

## PROCEDURE DESCRIPTION

The technique for performing DPL has changed little since its original description and is well characterized in standard textbooks. After decompression of the stomach and bladder by nasogastric and urinary catheter drainage, the abdomen is surgically prepared with topical antiseptic between each anterior axillary line from the xiphoid to the symphysis pubis, and draped in a sterile fashion. Local anaesthetic containing epinephrine (adrenaline) is then injected in the midline, approximately one-third of the distance between the umbilicus and pubic symphysis. A midline supraumbilical site is used in the setting of advanced pregnancy or pelvic fracture to avoid violating the gravid uterus or a developing pelvic haematoma. A vertical skin incision of 3–5 mm is made through the anaesthetized area, followed by passage of a peritoneal dialysis catheter at approximately a 45° angle caudad and posteriorly into the peritoneal cavity. This may be accomplished by using an open technique (vertically incising the underlying fascia and peritoneum, with catheter passage under direct visualization), a closed technique (Seldinger approach using a hollow 18- to 21-gauge needle, guidewire, and blunt dilator), or a semi-open technique (skin and fascia incised, followed by the Seldinger approach described above).

Most centres use either the open or closed technique, with proponents of the latter advocating it as a much quicker but equally safe approach. An initial aspirate is then attempted and, if negative for gross blood or intestinal contents, followed by infusion of 1 L (10 ml/kg in children) of warmed isotonic crystalloid through the catheter. The abdomen is gently agitated for 5 min, followed by fluid return to its original container by gravity. All fluid collected is subsequently sent to the laboratory for microscopic analysis. Table 79.2 summarizes the gross and microscopic criteria defining a positive DPL. Note that the red blood cell count is based on the expected dilution of 20–30 ml of gross blood into 1000 ml of isotonic crystalloid. This over-sensitivity to detect small amounts of bleeding from clinically insignificant injuries may subject occasional patients to unnecessary emergency laparotomy.

## DISCUSSION

DPL was first introduced as a diagnostic adjunct to the physical examination over 30 years ago by Root and colleagues (see Further reading), and remains the gold standard against which more recent diagnostic studies (ultrasonography and double-contrast computerized tomography [CT]) are compared. The indications, contraindications, advantages, disadvantages, and complications of each are summarized in Tables 79.3–79.5. Although the accuracy and sensitivity of the three techniques are similar in experienced hands

| Table 79.1 Factors contributing to an unreliable abdominal examination in the trauma patient |
|---|
| Alterations in mentation (head injury, alcohol, illicit drugs, shock) |
| Alterations in sensation, i.e. spinal cord injury |
| Painful extra-abdominal injuries (particularly to adjacent areas such as the lower ribcage, lower thoracic spine/lumbar spine, and pelvis) |
| Inability to communicate (language barriers, sensorineural hearing deficits, pre-hospital intubation, maxillofacial trauma) |
| Fright, anxiety, fear, etc. (as seen in the paediatric trauma victim) |

**Table 79.2 Criteria defining a positive peritoneal lavage**

| |
|---|
| Grossly positive aspiration for any of the following:<br>• > 10–20 ml of blood<br>• vegetable matter/digested food<br>• bile |
| Lavage fluid positive for either of the following:<br>• RBC count > 100 000/mm$^3$<br>• WBC count > 500/mm$^3$ |

RBC, red blood cell; WBC, whole blood cell

(consistently > 90% in most series), ultrasonography and, particularly, CT have the potential to yield additional information regarding specific organ injuries.

The superior ability of CT scanning to identify and quantitate injuries to the liver, spleen, diaphragm, and retroperitoneum (kidney, great vessels) overcomes one of DPL's main shortcomings, and has led many trauma centres to use it as their initial diagnostic procedure in haemodynamically stable, blunt-trauma patients. However, a CT scan may miss perforations of hollow viscera. Some clinicians thus advocate performing DPL in haemodynamically stable patients when CT scanning demonstrates intra-abdominal fluid accumulation, a stable or insignificant injury to the liver or spleen, a high-risk mechanism for bowel injury (e.g. lap belt over the abdomen), or abnormal physical findings out of proportion to injuries demonstrated by CT. An elevation of the lavage fluid white blood cell (WBC) count may identify hollow visceral injury if performed a minimum of 2–3 h after the time of injury. As such, DPL

**Table 79.3 Advantages and disadvantages of diagnostic options in abdominal trauma**

| Option | Advantages | Disadvantages |
|---|---|---|
| Diagnostic peritoneal lavage | Quick and simple<br>Familiar and time-honoured<br>Low complication rate<br>Low cost<br>Can be simultaneously performed during resuscitation, non-abdominal emergency surgery, or while obtaining other diagnostic studies | Invasive<br>Alters serial physical examinations<br>Lacks specificity<br>Over-sensitivity<br>Misses retroperitoneal and diaphragmatic injuries |
| Ultrasonography | Non-invasive<br>Quick<br>Can be serially repeated<br>Potentially useful where DPL contraindicated (e.g. pregnancy)<br>Less expensive than CT<br>Can be simultaneously performed during resuscitation, non-abdominal emergency surgery, or while obtaining other diagnostic studies | Requires technology/interpretation expertise<br>Requires patient immobility<br>Lacks specificity/poorer organ definition compared with CT<br>Misses diaphragm, bowel, and retroperitoneal injuries<br>Misses some injuries to solid organs (liver, spleen, pancreas) |
| Computed tomography | Most specific for individual organ injuries (especially liver, spleen, retroperitoneum, and diaphragm)<br>Ability to scan for other injuries (head, spine, chest, pelvis) | Requires technology/interpretation expertise<br>Requires patient immobility<br>Most expensive<br>Requires intravenous and oral contrast media<br>Time-consuming<br>Limited patient access/remote geographical site<br>Increased aspiration risk (oral contrast media)<br>May miss some diaphragm, bowel, and pancreas injuries |

DPL, diagnostic peritoneal lavage; CT, computed tomography.

| **Table 79.4 Indications and contraindications of diagnostic options in abdominal trauma** | | |
|---|---|---|
| Option | Indications | Contraindications |
| Diagnostic peritoneal lavage | Haemodynamically unstable blunt-trauma patient with one or more of the following:<br>• confounding variables (as per Table 79.1)<br>• equivocal physical examination<br>• ultrasonographic expertise unavailable<br>• extended loss of patient contact anticipated (emergency anaesthetic for other injuries, arteriography)<br>Anterior abdominal stab wounds demonstrated to violate the peritoneum on local wound exploration | Absolute:<br>• obvious indication for emergency laparotomy<br>Relative<br>• prior abdominal surgeries<br>• pregnancy<br>• morbid obesity<br>• cirrhosis/ascites<br>• coagulopathy |
| Ultrasonography | Haemodynamically unstable blunt-trauma patient with one or more of the following:<br>• confounding variables (as per Table 79.1)<br>• equivocal physical examination<br>• extended loss of patient contact anticipated (emergency anaesthetic for other injuries, arteriography) | Absolute:<br>• obvious indication for emergency laparotomy<br>Relative:<br>• prior abdominal surgery<br>• morbid obesity<br>• subcutaneous emphysema<br>• excess bowel gas<br>• lack of interpretation expertise |
| Computed tomography | Haemodynamically stable trauma patient without physical findings mandating emergency laparotomy and one or more of the following:<br>• confounding variables (as per Table 79.1)<br>• contraindications to DPL or ultrasonography<br>• gross haematuria<br>• pelvic fracture<br>• delayed patient presentation<br>• urgent anaesthesia required for associated injuries<br>• penetrating trauma to back or flank | Absolute:<br>• obvious indication for emergency laparotomy<br>• haemodynamic instability<br>Relative:<br>• significant time delay<br>• poor patient cooperation<br>• history of contrast allergy<br>• lack of interpretation expertise |

DPL, diagnostic peritoneal lavage; CT, computed tomography.

| **Table 79.5 Complications of diagnostic options in abdominal trauma** | | |
|---|---|---|
| Diagnostic peritoneal lavage (< 1%) | Ultrasonography | Computed tomography |
| Haemorrhage (incision-related, vascular perforation) | None | Contrast allergy (~0.1%) |
| Hollow viscus or bladder perforation | | |
| Injury to retroperitoneal structures | | |
| Wound infection | | |

and CT scanning complement each other in blunt-trauma victims and overcome some inherent limitations of each modality in this population. DPL may also prove useful in diagnosing hollow viscus injury in patients sustaining anterior abdominal stab wounds that have proved under local wound exploration to violate the peritoneum. DPL's accuracy rate under these circumstances is approximately 90%. Lavage fluid WBC counts of more than 3000/mm$^3$ (rather the standard 500/mm$^3$) are more likely to yield positive laparotomy results in this setting.

In patients with marginal or unstable haemodynamics, CT scanning is impractical and DPL or bedside ultrasonography is more appropriate. Given that the latter two have comparable sensitivity, specificity, and accuracy, the choice between them depends on which technique rapidly yields the most accurate information, given the expertise and technology available within a given institution. Ultrasonography may also miss some hollow visceral perforations, and selective use of DPL after ultrasonography in high-risk patients may detect such injuries. Most American centres continue to rely primarily on DPL, whereas bedside ultrasonography is becoming increasingly popular in some European centres.

## FURTHER READING


American College of Surgeons. *Advanced Trauma Life Support for Doctors*, 6th edn. Chicago: American College of Surgeons, 1997: 193–211, 217–18.

Cue JI, Miller FB, Cryer HM III, *et al*. A prospective, randomized comparison between open and closed peritoneal lavage techniques. *J Trauma* 1990;**30**:880–3.

Fabian TC, Croce MA. Abdominal trauma, including indications for celiotomy. In: Feliciano DV, Moore EE, Mattox KL,eds. *Trauma*, 3rd edn. Stamford, CT: Appleton & Lange, 1996: 441–59.

Feliciano DV. Diagnostic modalities in abdominal trauma. Peritoneal lavage, ultrasonography, computed tomography scanning, and arteriography. *Surg Clin North Am* 1991;**71**:241–56.

Feliciano DV, Bitondo-Dyer CG. Vagaries of the lavage white blood cell count in evaluating abdominal stab wounds. *Am J Surg* 1994;**168**:680–3.

Kearney PA Jr, Vahey T, Burney RE, Glazer G. Computed tomography and diagnostic peritoneal lavage in blunt abdominal trauma. Their combined role. *Arch Surg* 1989;**124**:344–7.

Liu M, Lee CH, P'eng FK. Prospective comparison of diagnostic peritoneal lavage, computed tomographic scanning, and ultrasonography for the diagnosis of blunt abdominal trauma. *J Trauma* 1993;**35**:267–70.

Meyer DM, Thal ER, Weigelt JA, Redman HC. Evaluation of computed tomography and diagnostic peritoneal lavage in blunt abdominal trauma. *J Trauma* 1989;**29**:1168–70.

Root HD. Abdominal trauma and diagnostic peritoneal lavage revisited. *Am J Surg* 1990;**159**:363–4.

Root HD, Hauser CW, McKinley CR *et al*. Diagnostic peritoneal lavage. *Surgery* 1965;**57**:633–7.

# Chapter 80 Antibiotics for surgical prophylaxis and infection

D.A. MacGregor and R.J. Sherertz

Antimicrobial prophylaxis for surgery serves to prevent perioperative infections, which rank among the most common (and costly) nosocomial infections in hospitals. The well-recognized benefit of using antibiotics to prevent perioperative infections must be weighed against the potential risks of allergic and toxic reactions, adverse drug interactions, and development of antimicrobial resistance. Unfortunately, personal experiences, anecdotal successes or failures, or habit, rather than scientific data, form the basis of perioperative antibiotic selection. This chapter focuses on three important considerations in the selection of antibiotics for surgical prophylaxis and treatment: the timing of peak plasma or tissue concentrations, the location and nature of the surgery, and the hospital-specific considerations for antimicrobial therapy. Prophylaxis against subacute bacterial endocarditis for at-risk patients is discussed in Chapter 50.

## TIMING OF INITIAL DOSE, AND SUBSEQUENT DOSING SCHEDULE

Ideally, antibiotics should reach peak concentrations in the at-risk tissues at the moment of surgical incision, and maintain bactericidal concentrations beyond the time of wound closure. Laboratory and clinical studies have demonstrated that antibiotics are optimally administered approximately 30 min before surgical incision. Prophylaxis proves significantly less effective when given more than 2 h before the incision or after the incision is made. The anaesthetist often has the responsibility for administering antibiotics in the operating room, and must be cognisant of the short- and long-term complications, including potentiation of neuromuscular blocking agents, allergic reactions, and end-organ toxicity.

The antibiotics commonly used for surgical prophylaxis have therapeutic effects that exceed the duration of most operations (2–3 h), thus usually obviating intraoperative redosing. Although it is common practice to continue antibiotics for up to 24 h after the surgery, there is *no* conclusive evidence that any postoperative doses of antibiotics are required. Indeed, excessive duration of antibiotic therapy represents the most common error in the use of perioperative antibiotics. Potential exceptions to this 'single-dose' philosophy include circumstances where the surgical procedure leads to prolonged exposure of contaminated mucosa (e.g. open wounds with draining fistulae), or placement of foreign devices into infected fluids (e.g. continuous ventriculostomy or biliary drains). Although the relevant data are conflicting, postoperative antibiotics may reduce morbidity or mortality during ongoing exposure of sterile body fluids or tissues to grossly infected or contaminated material. The clinician must distinguish among bacterial contamination, wound colonization, and true infection, because only the last warrants antimicrobial therapy in most instances. Interventional educational programmes that include surgeons, anaesthetists, and nurses can dramatically reduce inappropriate perioperative antibiotic use. Table 80.1 summarizes the recommendations of a consensus conference concerning risk stratification and the use of perioperative antibiotics.

**Table 80.1 Risk stratification for the use of perioperative antibiotics**

| Type of surgical procedure | Recommended antibiotic regimen |
|---|---|
| Abdominal contamination by recent (< 12 h) perforation, whether traumatic or surgical | Single-dose prophylaxis |
| Resectable intra-abdominal infections, such as gangrenous cholecystitis/appendicitis or ischaemic bowel without frank perforation | 24 h of perioperative antibiotics |
| Advanced intra-abdominal infections at the time of surgery | 2–5-day course of antibiotics dictated by the patient's clinical course |

**Table 80.2 Likely pathogens and therapeutic options by type of operation**

| Type of surgery | Potential pathogens | Comments | Recommended regimen |
|---|---|---|---|
| Cardiac<br>Thoracic (non-cardiac) | *Staphylococcus epidermidis, S. aureus*, enteric Gram-negative bacilli | Single-dose first- or second-generation cephalosporin or vancomycin[a] | Cefuroxime: single dose pre-incision |
| Neuro<br>Orthopaedic<br>Vascular, including amputation<br>Traumatic, without perforation of viscus | *S. aureus, S. epidermidis*<br>Less likely to have Gram-negative organisms | Single-dose first-generation cephalosporin or vancomycin[a] | Cefazolin: single dose pre-incision |
| Gastrointestinal<br>• Upper tract (oesophagus, stomach, small bowel) | Enteric Gram-negative bacilli, Gram-positive cocci | High risk (advanced age, morbid obesity, oesophageal obstruction, or reduced gastric motility) defines need for expanded coverage | Low risk: cefazolin<br>High risk: cefuroxime, cefoxitin, Cefotetan, or ampicillin + sulbactam |
| • Biliary tract | Enteric Gram-negative bacilli, clostridia, *Enterococcus* sp. | High risk (advanced age, acute cholecystitis, common duct stones or obstructed/non-functioning gallbladder) defines need for expanded coverage | Low risk: cefazolin<br>High risk: cefuroxime, cefotetan, or ampicillin + sulbactam |
| • Colorectal, including non-perforated appendix | Enteric Gram-negative bacilli, anaerobes, *Enterococcus* sp. | Anaerobic coverage should be included | Cefoxitin, cefotetan, or ampicillin + sulbactam |
| Contaminated abdominal surgery: ruptured appendiceal or biliary abscess, ruptured viscus, penetrating traumatic injuries | Enteric Gram-negative bacilli, anaerobes, *Enterococcus* sp. | Frequently requires drainage tubes or devices, potentially warranting coverage beyond the operative period | Cefoxitin, cefotetan, or clindamycin + aminoglycoside |

[a]When methicillin-resistant *Staphylococcus aureus* (MRSA) is known to be a problem within the hospital or surgical centre.

## LOCATION AND NATURE OF THE SURGERY

Virtually all surgical operations involve disruption of the cutaneous barrier, which exposes the patient to *Staphylococcus* and *Streptococcus* species. For most operations, a single dose of a first-generation cephalosporin such as cefazolin provides adequate coverage to prevent infection by these bacteria at the surgical site. Disruption of the intestinal mucosa during surgery necessitates broader antibiotic coverage for aerobic Gram-negative bacilli and anaerobic bacteria. Cephalosporins such as cefoxitin or cefotetan are often recommended because of their activity against both enteric aerobes and anaerobes, including *Bacteroides fragilis*. Clindamycin or metronidazole, combined with an aminoglycoside, have also been used for this purpose. 'Expanded spectrum' cephalosporins (e.g. ceftriaxone, ceftazidime, and others) and penicillins, (e.g. piperacillin–tazobactam, ticarcillin, and others) are generally not recommended for surgical prophylaxis because they are more expensive, have less efficient coverage for *Staphylococcus*, and maintain higher activity against pathogens not commonly encountered in elective surgery. Although broader-spectrum antibiotics may reduce the incidence of postoperative bacterial infections, the risk of antimicrobial resistance and development of serious fungal infections increases. Table 80.2 displays the type of surgery with the most likely pathogens and recommendations for perioperative antimicrobial therapy.

## HOSPITAL-SPECIFIC CONSIDERATIONS

When hospitalized patients undergo an operation, the bacteria that cause perioperative infections tend to correlate with the bacteria colonizing the hospital. For example, if most of the staphylococcus isolates are resistant to methicillin, then patients within that hospital who develop staphylococcal infections have a much higher likelihood of having staphylococci that are also resistant to methicillin. In hospitals where methicillin-resistant *Staphylococcus* prevails as a postoperative pathogen, the use of vancomycin may be justified for prophylactic use. Routine use of vancomycin for prophylaxis is strongly discouraged, however, because its overuse promotes the development and spread of vancomycin-resistant *Enterococcus* species.

Infection control programmes in many hospitals monitor the relative frequency of certain bacteria recovered from patients. Through these programmes, the hospital can monitor for outbreaks of unusual bacteria, such as *Legionella* or *Acinetobacter* species which can be isolated from contaminated water or ventilation systems, or *Serratia* species which have contaminated equipment in operating rooms and intensive care unit (ICU) areas. Outbreaks in a given operating suite or ICU location often implicate nurse- or physician-associated transference of bacteria. In addition, infection control surveillance can uncover changes in antimicrobial resistance patterns, and result in changes in antimicrobial therapy. Anaesthetists must remain aware of these hospital-specific considerations to ensure adequate prophylaxis, as well as to understand the changes in antimicrobial resistance that may result from overuse of a single antibiotic regimen.

## CONCLUSIONS

Antibiotics can effectively reduce the incidence of perioperative infections, but may also cause complications such as drug interactions, allergic reactions, and organ toxicity. To be effective, antibiotics must be present at the time of incision in bactericidal concentrations, and must be effective against the organisms likely to be encountered. Although prophylactic antibiotics prove extremely effective, they cannot substitute for adequate sterile technique.

## FURTHER READING


Abramowicz M. Antimicrobial prophylaxis in surgery. *Med Lett Drugs Ther* 1989;**31**:105–8.

Brown EM. Antimicrobial prophylaxis in neurosurgery. *J Antimicrob Chemother* 1993;**31**(suppl B):49–63.

Burke JF. The effective period of preventive antibiotic action in experimental incisions and dermal lesions. *Surgery* 1961;**50**:161–8.

Cheng EY, Nimphius N, Hennen CR. Antibiotic therapy and the anesthesiologist. *J Clin Anesth* 1995;**7**:425–39.

D'Amelio LF, Wagner B, Azimuddin S, Sutyak JP, Hammond JS. Antibiotic patterns associated with fungal colonization in critically ill surgical patients. *Am Surg* 1995;**61**:1049–53.

DiPiro JT, Vallner JJ, Bowden TA Jr, Clark B, Sisley JF. Intraoperative serum concentrations of cefazolin and cefoxitin administered preoperatively at different times. *Clin Pharm* 1984;**3**:64–7.

Evans RS, Pestotnik SL, Classen DC, Clemmer TP, Weaver LK, Orme JF Jr, Lloyd JF, Burke JP. A computer-assisted management program for antibiotics and other antiinfective agents. *N Engl J Med* 1998;**338**:232–8.

Gyssens IC, Geerligs IE, Nannini-Bergman MG, Knape JT, Hekster YA, van der Meer JW. Optimizing the timing of antimicrobial prophylaxis in surgery: an intervention study. *J Antimicrob Chemother* 1996;**38**:301–8.

Schein M, Wittmann DH, Lorenz W. Duration of antibiotic treatment in surgical infections of the abdomen. Forum statement: a plea for selective and controlled postoperative antibiotic administration. *Eur J Surg* 1996;**576**(suppl):66–9.

Stone HH, Hooper CA, Kolb LD, Geheber CE, Dawkins EJ. Antibiotic prophylaxis in gastric, biliary and colonic surgery. *Ann Surg* 1976;**184**:443–52.

# Chapter 81 Enteral and parenteral nutrition

S. Nath, S.L. Hack,
P.H. Roberts, and
T.H. Clutton-Brock

In the 1960s, the ability to feed patients intravenously instead of via the gastrointestinal tract was developed. Dudrick and colleagues (see Further reading) reported growth and development with total parenteral nutrition (TPN), initially with beagle puppies and then later in infants. At that time TPN referred only to intravenous dextrose and amino acids. Today's TPN includes the ability to provide all nutrients that patients require, and represents an alternative method of feeding patients when the gastrointestinal tract is not accessible or functional.

Current indications for TPN include: small bowel fistulae, malabsorption secondary to extensive bowel resections, severe diarrhoea, radiation enteritis, recent bone marrow transplantation, complications of chemotherapy or radiotherapy, severe pancreatitis, chylothorax, hyperemesis gravidarum, stressed patients unable to receive enteral nutrition for more than 5–7 days, and perioperative nutrition in severely malnourished patients to decrease postoperative complications.

More recently, the emphasis has shifted with the realization that many critically ill patients are in fact able to absorb from their gastrointestinal tract, and the early introduction of enteral nutrition is now an important part of modern intensive care management. Ideally, in many of the above situations, enteral feeding can be successfully administered in time. However, TPN can supply vital nutrients until the patient can tolerate enteral feeding. Enteral feeding is preferred over TPN whenever possible.

## NORMAL NUTRITIONAL REQUIREMENTS

Normal cellular function relies on an adequate nutritional intake. There are a series of equilibria that need to be maintained in order to prevent an imbalance in the metabolic function of cells. Thus, a normal nutritional requirement takes account of energy balance, nitrogen balance, fluid balance, electrolyte balance, and the requirement for micronutrients. These are dependent on age, sex, height and weight, level of physical activity, presence of concurrent stresses or illness, and pre-existing nutritional state. The normal *daily* requirements for a healthy 70-kilogram man are shown in Table 81.1. Of the total energy requirement, carbohydrate makes up 47% and fat 33%.

### Energy balance

All cells require energy in the form of adenine triphosphate (ATP) to preserve normal metabolic function. ATP is generated through a series of complex biochemical pathways from carbohydrate, protein and fat. This is discussed further in Chapter 18.

*Anabolism* is the predominant metabolic process when there is an excess of nutrition. This allows energy to be stored as glycogen, muscle (protein), and adipose tissue. Conversely, *catabolism* is the break down of these nutrients to supply energy. This is seen when nutritional demand exceeds supply. Such conditions are not uncommon and can arise as a result of a combination of: reduced nutritional intake, increased loss of nutrients, and/or increased demand for nutrients.

Basal metabolic rate (BMR) is defined as the energy required by the body at rest. It is described by the Harris–Benedict equations, which take account of age, sex, height, and weight:

$$\text{Male: BMR} = 66 + (13.7 \times \text{body weight in kg}) + (5 \times \text{height in cm}) - (6.8 \times \text{age})$$

$$\text{Female: BMR} = 655 + (9.6 \times \text{body weight in kg}) + (1.7 \times \text{height in cm}) - (4.7 \times \text{age}).$$

Alternatively, a more accurate reflection of energy requirement is the resting energy expenditure which may be assessed by measuring energy production using direct or indirect calorimetry. It takes account of the additional factors of physical activity, presence of concurrent stresses or illness, and pre-existing nutritional state.

### Nitrogen balance

The assessment of nitrogen balance is of prime importance because this represents the total body protein mass. Each gram of nitrogen is equivalent to 6.25 g of protein or 30 g of muscle tissue. Nitrogen balance is defined as the difference between input of nitrogen and nitrogen loss, and in catabolic states there is an overall *negative* nitrogen balance. Nitrogen losses may be estimated:

$$\text{Nitrogen loss in g per 24 h} = (\text{Urinary urea in mmol per 24 h} \times 0.028) + 4.$$

Loss is predominantly in the urine as urea, but in addition there is loss in the faeces, skin, and hair. In the equation above, 0.028 is a factor to convert urea in millimoles to grams of nitrogen. Loss of protein (nitro-

**Table 81.1 The normal daily nutritional requirements of a 70-kg man**

| | | |
|---|---|---|
| Energy | Calories | 2000–2500 kcal (8400–10 500 kJ) |
| | Glucose | 230–285 g |
| | Fat | 70–90 g |
| Nitrogen | Protein | 55–70 g (equivalent to 9–11 g nitrogen) |
| Fluid | Water | 2000–2500 ml |
| Electrolytes (macronutrients) | Sodium | 70 mmol |
| | Potassium | 90 mmol |
| | Calcium | 18 mmol |
| | Magnesium | 12 mmol |
| | Chloride | 70 mmol |
| | Phosphate | 18 mmol |
| Trace elements/vitamins (micronutrients) | Iron | 160 μmol |
| | Zinc | 145 μmol |
| | Manganese | 26 μmol |
| | Copper | 19 μmol |
| | Selenium | 0.9 μmol |
| | Chromium | 0.5 μmol |
| | Iodide | 1.0 μmol |
| | Vitamin A (retinol) | 0.6 mg |
| | Vitamin D (calciferol) | 7.5 μg |
| | Vitamin E (tocopherol) | 4.0 mg |
| | Vitamin K (phylloquinone) | 70 μg |
| | Vitamin B1 (thiamine) | 1.0 mg |
| | Vitamin B6 (pyridoxine) | 1.3 mg |
| | Vitamin B12 (cyanocobalamin) | 1.4 mg |
| | Vitamin C (ascorbic acid) | 37 mg |
| | Folate | 0.2 mg |

gen) in the hair, faeces, skin, and urine (as non-urea nitrogen) is estimated at 4 g per day.

### Fluid and electrolyte balance

Normal daily requirements for water account for losses in the urine and faeces and insensible losses through the skin as sweat (and also fistulae and drains if present). When patients are catabolic, their water requirement increases primarily as a result of increased insensible losses. Total body water is distributed across three major body compartments: intracellular, interstitial, and vascular compartments. In stress or starvation, these compartments alter in their composition.

Electrolyte distribution also changes in disease. There are many disorders of electrolytes but primarily they relate to renal or gastrointestinal abnormalities. Fluid and electrolyte balance is more fully explained in Chapters 14 and 19.

### Micronutrients

*Trace elements* are inorganic elements that have a concentration in the body of less than 50 mg/kg. They have functions as cofactors or coenzymes for normal metabolic function, and allow optimal use of nutrients. *Vitamins* are complex organic compounds, which are essential for normal metabolic functions. They are classed as either fat soluble (vitamins A, D, E, K) or water soluble. Deficiency of micronutrients can lead to well-recognized diseases such as anaemia in iron deficiency and hypothyroidism in iodine deficiency, or rarer conditions such as scurvy in vitamin C deficiency or beri-beri in vitamin B1 deficiency. Chapter 18 has a fuller account of the function of these elements and compounds.

### Children and elderly people

At the extremes of age, nutritional requirements are different, primarily in terms of energy and fluid balance. In children, energy requirements are relatively increased when corrected for surface area. This occurs because the predominant metabolic process in growth is anabolism, and because their surface area : volume ratio is large, leading to increased losses of energy as heat. Fluid is also lost at an increased rate, making children prone to dehydration in times of stress or starvation. However, they are also sensitive to fluid overload because of the smaller circulating blood volume.

Several important metabolic changes occur in elderly people. There is a reduction in muscle mass which accounts for a reduced BMR and reduced physical activity. Energy requirements are therefore relatively reduced. Food intake is not reduced in parallel, resulting in an increased body fat content. However, there is an increased incidence of chronic illness among elderly people, and so they are prone to malnutrition. This then leads to increased incidence of infection, immobility, increased risk of trauma, and ultimately increased frequency of hospital admission. Table 81.2 summarizes the changes seen in children and elderly people.

**Table 81.2 Nutritional requirements for children and elderly people**

| | | | |
|---|---|---|---|
| **Children** | | | |
| Energy | Calories | 0–3 years | 120–95 kcal/kg |
| | | 3–6 years | 95–90 kcal/kg |
| | | 6–10 years | 90–65 kcal/kg |
| | | 10–15 years | 65–45 kcal/kg |
| | Glucose | 13.8–5.4 g/kg | |
| | Fat | 4.25–1.7 g/kg | |
| Nitrogen | Protein | 3.1–0.72 g/kg (equivalent to 0.5–0.1 g nitrogen/kg) | |
| Fluid | Water | 1500–2000 ml | |
| **Elderly people** | | | |
| Energy | Calories | 2300–2500 kcal (9660–10 500 kJ) | |
| | Glucose | 257–280 g | |
| | Fat | 81–88 g | |
| Nitrogen | Protein | 53–60 g (equivalent to 8.5–9.6 g nitrogen) | |
| Fluid | Water | 1750–2500 ml | |

## STRESS AND STARVATION

Stress and starvation represent opposite extremes of energy metabolism and are clinically relevant in the hospital setting. In the metabolic response to stress or illness, there are two phases: the ebb phase and the flow phase. The ebb phase is usually a short period lasting 1–2 days and is characterized by a depression in the physiological functions of the body (fall in blood pressure, body temperature, and oxygen use). The flow phase is itself divided into two stages. The first and most important stage is the catabolic period, characterized by an inflammatory response, where there are marked energy and protein losses; this is commonly seen in patients in the intensive care setting. This is followed by the anabolic period where the stores are re-established, and this heralds patient recovery. By contrast, in the starved state energy is derived from endogenous stores, and there is an attempt to minimize losses of glucose, fat, and in particular protein. Many patients in hospital are fasted either intentionally in preparation for a surgical or medical procedure, or as a result of a disease process that does not allow ingestion or absorption of food.

Nutritional requirements increase in times of stress or illness as a result of development of an overall catabolic state (Table 81.3). In particular, with major catabolic insults, there is a marked loss of nitrogen in the urine as a result of increased amino acid turnover and overall proteolysis (muscle breakdown), and this accounts for the increase in energy requirement. In addition, there is an increase in carbohydrate and fat turnover with increased glycogenolysis and lipolysis.

In starvation the predominant processes are a reduction in energy expenditure and the minimization of protein loss. It may be regarded in terms of *early* and *prolonged* starvation. Energy is generated primarily from the stores of carbohydrate (glycogen) in the first 24 hours, and then from the fat in adipose tissue thereafter. Certain cells (erythrocytes and renal medulla) are obligate glucose utilizers and so, in states of prolonged starvation, glucose can be derived only from gluconeo-

**Table 81.3 Nutritional requirements in catabolic states**

| | | Minor catabolism, e.g. uncomplicated surgery, mild fever, exercise | Major catabolism, e.g. major surgery, trauma, sepsis, burns, adult respiratory distress syndrome |
|---|---|---|---|
| Energy | Calories | 1750–2100 kcal[a] (25–30 kcal/kg) | 2100–2800 kcal[a] (30–40 kcal/kg) |
| | Glucose | 165–242 g | 246–301 g |
| | Fat | 58–89 g | 47–57 g |
| Nitrogen | Protein | 83–105 g (equivalent to 14–17 g nitrogen) | 110–140 g (equivalent to 18–22 g nitrogen) |
| Fluid | Water | 2500–3000 ml | 2700–3200 ml |

[a]70-kg patient

genesis with amino acids as the substrate. There is therefore an obligatory loss of protein of at least 20 g/day after a 3-week fast. The central nervous system is usually an obligatory glucose utilizer, but with prolonged fasting ketone bodies become the substrates for energy production. Ketone bodies are derivatives of fatty acid metabolism formed in the liver, and they may be utilized by most other cells early in the fasted state.

Several surveys have shown that many patients in hospital are malnourished. This may be as a result of chronic illness where a marasmus-like picture is seen; alternatively, it may be as a result of severe protein–energy malnutrition as seen in patients in intensive care who are in a state of major catabolism (Table 81.4). During critical illness, cellular demand for some non-essential amino acids (e.g. arginine, glutamine, cysteine) may exceed the body's synthetic capabilities; in this case the amino acid becomes 'conditionally essential'. No current parenteral amino acid formulation contains glutamine because of problems with stability. Some formulations lack cysteine.

The importance of nutritional therapy has long been recognized. There is increased morbidity and mortality associated with malnutrition, where patients are at an increased risk of developing postoperative complications and acquiring infections, and are likely to be hospitalized for longer periods. Nutritional therapy is therefore aimed at restoring the balance.

Nutrition may be administered by one of several routes. Introduction of food into the gastrointestinal tract is the *enteral* route. This relies on a functional gut, and is the usual and preferred method of feeding patients. The *parenteral* route bypasses the gastrointestinal tract, nutrition being administered intravenously.

## ENTERAL NUTRITION

Most patients will ingest food via the oral route. Alternatively, food may be introduced directly into the stomach or jejunum via a polyurethane or polyvinyl chloride tube inserted intranasally; this is the nasogastric or nasojejunal route. More recently, other techniques have been developed to place a tube either directly into the stomach from the anterior abdominal wall as a percutaneous endoscopic gastrostomy (PEG) (Figure 81.1) or into the jejunum as a percutaneous jejunostomy at the time of laparotomy. The nasogastric or nasojejunal route is preferred for short-term nutritional support and placement is relatively simple and inexpensive. Use of a PEG or jejunostomy tube may be considered for longer-term needs. However, insertion of these is more invasive and in some cases requires a general anaesthetic. They are expensive and are prone to complications both at the time of insertion and thereafter.

### Indications for PEG or jejunostomyenteral nutrition

Indications for PEG or jejunostomy feeding fall into two categories (Table 81.5):

- patients with a neuromuscular deficit where airway protection cannot be guaranteed;
- patients with the upper gastrointestinal tract pathology.

### Composition of enteral feeding regimens

Enteral feed is prepared under sterile conditions to prevent infection because it provides an optimal growth medium for micro-organisms. Generally feeds are polymeric (containing intact proteins) and provide energy (1–2 kcal/ml), protein (0.04–0.06 g/ml), and the recommended allowances for minerals and vitamins. They are milk based (lactose free) and free of gluten. A vari-

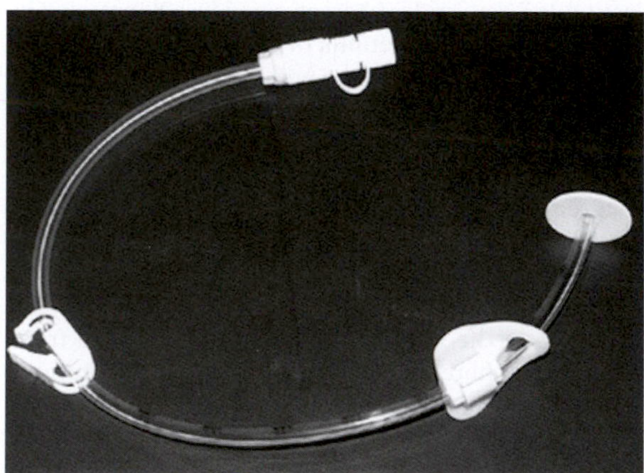

**Figure 81.1** A PEG tube.

**Table 81.4 Summary of metabolic changes in the fed, fasted, and stressed states**

| Fed state | Fasted (marasmus-like) state | Stressed (kwashiorkor-like) state |
|---|---|---|
| Major hormone: Insulin | | Major hormones: counter-regulatory hormones (glucagon, catecholamines, adrenocorticotrophic hormone, glucocorticoids) |
| Glycogenesis<br>Protein synthesis<br>Lipogenesis | Glycogenolysis (initially)<br>Lipolysis<br>Ketogenesis<br>Gluconeogenesis | Glycogenolysis<br>Lipolysis<br>Gluconeogenesis<br>Proteolysis |
| Anabolism predominant | Energy conservation<br>Minimal catabolism | Catabolism predominant |

| Table 81.5 Indications for PEG/jejunostomy enteral nutrition | |
|---|---|
| Central nervous system | Coma/unconsciousness<br>Cerebrovascular disease (e.g. cerebrovascular accident, bulbar palsy)<br>Brain-stem lesions (e.g. tumour, trauma, haemorrhage)<br>Head injury<br>Multiple sclerosis<br>Neuropathy (e.g. Guillain–Barré syndrome, vitamin deficiencies)<br>Myasthenia gravis<br>Myopathy<br>Psychological (eating disorder) |
| Gastrointestinal system | Obstructive lesions of the mouth (e.g. pharyngeal tumour)<br>Obstructive upper gastrointestinal lesions (e.g. oesophageal or gastric tumour)<br>Pancreatitis<br>Inflammatory bowel disease<br>Catabolic states (e.g. trauma, sepsis, etc.)<br>To supplement oral intake |

**Table 81.6 Typical constituents of a *standard* 500-ml bottle of enteral feed (Nutrison)**

| Energy | 500 kcal | Electrolytes | | Trace elements | | Vitamins | |
|---|---|---|---|---|---|---|---|
| Protein | 20 g | Sodium | 18 mmol | Iron | 5.0 mg | A | 0.3 mg |
| Nitrogen | 3.2 g | Potassium | 18 mmol | Zinc | 5.0 mg | D | 2.5 μg |
| Carbohydrate | 62 g | Calcium | 6.3 mmol | Copper | 0.8 mg | E | 5.5 μg |
| Sugars | 5.0 g | Magnesium | 4.1 mmol | Manganese | 0.3 mg | K | 20 μg |
| Polysaccharides | 56 g | Chloride | 18 mmol | Selenium | 4.2 μg | B1 | 0.5 mg |
| Fat | 20 g | Phosphate | 8.0 mmol | Chromium | 3.3 μg | B6 | 0.7 mg |
| Saturates | 1.5 g | | | Fluoride | 0.1 mg | B12 | 1.0 μg |
| Polyunsaturates | 6.2 g | | | Iodide | 10 μg | C | 25 mg |
| | | | | | | Folate | 66 μg |
| Water | 425 ml | | | | | | |
| Energy ratio (protein : carbohydrate : fat) 1:3:2 | | | | | | | |

ety of formulations is commercially available. A *standard* formulation (Table 81.6) delivers the average daily nutritional requirements. *Specialized* formulations are modified to treat specific nutritional abnormalities. Examples of these may be: feeds with an increased calorific content, reduced concentration of electrolytes, reduced fluid volume, increased fibre content, or increased fat : carbohydrate ratio (for patients with carbon dioxide retention).

### Monitoring of enteral feeding

Patients are monitored to assess their tolerance to and effectiveness of feeding, and to reduce the risk of complications associated with enteral feeding. Tolerance to food is measured by regular aspiration of the nasogastric tube to check for a gastric residual, the presence of which suggests malabsorption or gastric stasis. The latter is a common cause of failure to establish enteral feeding in critically ill patients. It occurs after abdominal surgery, where there is early return of small bowel function but delayed return of gastric function. This is also seen with heavily sedated patients, after head injury, with opioid use, and is associated with metabolic conditions such as diabetic ketoacidosis. It may be treated with prokinetic agents such as metoclopramide or erythromycin. The effectiveness of feeding is assessed by regular measurement of weight, anthropometric measurements, biochemical testing (e.g. urea, albumin), and measurement of energy/fluid requirements. Adjustments are then made to the regimen to meet the changing nutritional needs. Complications associated with enteral feeding are shown in Table 81.7.

## PARENTERAL NUTRITION

### Types of admixtures

There are two main methods of administering the nutritional components. One method is with all of the above nutrients mixed into one container. This is often

**Table 81.7 Complications of enteral nutrition**

| | |
|---|---|
| Gastrointestinal system | Diarrhoea<br>Nausea and vomiting<br>Abdominal pain and distension |
| Respiratory system | Aspiration pneumonia |
| Metabolic | Hyperglycaemia<br>Hypo- or hyperkalaemia<br>Hypocalcaemia<br>Hypomagnesaemia<br>Hypophosphataemia |
| Mechanical | Tube perforation<br>Tube blockage<br>Tube migration<br>Nasal or oesophageal perforation |

referred to as a total nutrient admixture (TNA). Another method blends all of the ingredients together in one container *except* lipids, which are infused separately. Both types of admixture are very complex, and component compatibility and stability issues are a primary concern.

In April 1994, the US Food and Drug Administration (FDA) released an alert after two deaths and at least two cases of respiratory distress were reported secondary to formation of precipitates of calcium phosphate in TPN (see McKinnon in Further reading). These precipitants can result in intravenous line occlusion and pulmonary emboli. There are now established guidelines regarding the proper mixing order for TPN ingredients to limit the risk of precipitation.

### Methods of administration

Intravenous nutrition may be delivered via peripheral or central veins. Osmolality limits peripheral TPN administration because peripheral venous access sites poorly tolerate osmolalities of more than 900 mosmol/L. Both dextrose and amino acids contribute to the osmolality of TPN; however, lipids are iso-osmotic. Peripheral formulae usually supply more calories from lipids than from central formulations; nevertheless, the overall amount of lipids should not exceed 50–60% of total calorific intake via TPN. As lipids may decrease risk of phlebitis, TNA formulations are preferred. The patient's ability to tolerate larger water volumes may also limit peripheral administration. As formulations must be dilute for venous tolerance, larger volumes are usually required in order to meet complete nutritional needs. On the other hand, more concentrated formulations can be administered via a central venous catheter. Appropriate catheter location must be confirmed before initiation of TPN to minimize complications.

Most commonly, TPN flows at a continuous rate over 24 hours, but central formulations may be administered by a 'cyclic regimen' in which the patient receives the full day's supply of nutrition over 10–18 hours. Most cyclic regimens are given to outpatients over 12 hours, thus allowing patients to be mobile for part of each day.

### Composition of parenteral feeding regimens

There are several commercially available regimens, which provide average nutritional requirements, but feed of this type should be tailored to the need of the individual (Figure 81.2). A dietitian therefore assesses the dietary requirements of each patient in order to devise an individual TPN regimen. Considerations are as for enteral nutrition in terms of: energy, nitrogen, fluid and vitamins, and minerals.

The components of TPN are provided in a predigested state because they bypass the gastrointestinal tract. Glucose-rich parenteral regimens cause many problems, for example: hyperglycaemia leading to fatty infiltration of the liver; hyperosmolar dehydration; excess carbon dioxide formation; hypophosphataemia causing reduced tissue oxygenation; fluid retention secondary to hyperinsulinaemia; and decreased immune function. Therefore the energy must be provided by carbohydrate *and* fat. This prevents the problems primarily by avoiding overload of the metabolic pathways. Fat in PN regimens is provided in the form of emulsions that contain a triglyceride core, surrounded by phospholipid from soya, sunflower oil, or egg. In this way, the fat is more soluble and therefore more easily metabolized. Fat is also included to prevent essential fatty acid deficiency (of linoleic and α-linolenic acid). A typical regimen is shown in Table 81.8.

### Complications of parenteral nutrition

The most important risk with TPN is the development of infection. As with enteral feeds, the composition of the TPN provides an optimal medium for the growth of micro-organisms. The feed is therefore made up

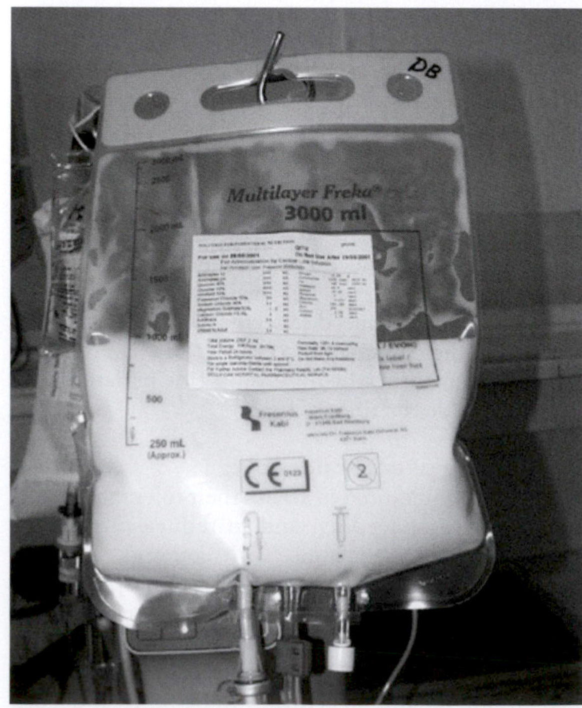


**Figure 81.2** A 3-litre bag of TPN.

**Table 81.8 Typical constituents of a parenteral nutrition regimen**

| | | | |
|---|---|---|---|
| Aminoplex 12 | 1000 ml | Potassium | 60 mmol |
| Glucose 24% | 1000 ml | Sodium | 85 mmol |
| Intralipid 20% | 500 ml | Calcium | 4.6 mmol |
| Calcium chloride 13.4% | 5 ml | Magnesium | 5 mmol |
| Additrace | 10 ml | Zinc | 146 μmol |
| Solivito N | 1 ml | Chloride | 143 mmol |
| Vitlipid Adult | 10 ml | Phosphate | 18 mmol |
| | | Acetate | 5 mmol |
| Protein : carbohydrate : fat | 1:3:3 | | |

into bags under sterile conditions by the pharmacy department to minimize the risk of infection, and the bags are changed every 24 hours. The feed is administered via a *dedicated* central venous catheter, which may be tunnelled to further reduce the risk of infection.

Complications of the use of TPN relate to the TPN itself, and also to catheter-related problems (Table 81.9).

Other complications include: acid–base disorders, fatty liver, cholestasis, cholelithiasis, trace element deficiencies, and even toxicity if a patient were to develop hepatic or renal failure with metabolite accumulation. The liver abnormalities are usually reversible when they present early in therapy. Patients on long-term TPN should have their liver enzymes checked regularly.

**Table 81.9 Complications of parenteral nutrition**

| | |
|---|---|
| **TPN** | |
| Immediate | Hyperglycaemia |
| Long term | Sepsis<br>Liver dysfunction<br>Hypo- or hyperkalaemia<br>Hypercalcaemia<br>Hypomagnesaemia<br>Hypo- or hyperphosphataemia<br>Dyslipidaemias<br>Essential fatty acid deficiency |
| **Catheter** | |
| Immediate | Haemorrhage<br>Pneumothorax or haemothorax<br>Arrhythmias<br>Cardiac tamponade |
| Long term | Chylothorax<br>Thrombosis and pulmonary embolism<br>Pleural effusion or pericardial effusion<br>Subacute bacterial endocarditis<br>Venopulmonary fistula |

### Monitoring of parenteral nutrition

To determine whether a patient is tolerating TPN and responding to it, a multitude of factors need to be considered. Weight, total fluid intake and output, electrolytes, and blood glucose levels should be monitored frequently to minimize complications, particularly in the critical care setting. Visceral protein concentrations (i.e. albumin, prealbumin or transthyretin, and transferrin) can be useful in assessing adequacy of the nutritional support administered. Liver function studies such as alkaline phosphatase, aspartate transaminase, and alanine transaminase, and bilirubin concentrations should be checked weekly, until the clinical status of the patient justifies reduced surveillance.

## CURRENT ISSUES

Recently, there has been much interest in the area of *immunonutrition*. This is the suggestion that certain nutrients have the potential to modulate immune function. In particular these include glutamine, arginine, and ω-3 fatty acids. There is increasing evidence that glutamine may enhance gut immunity and lymphocyte function. Arginine may also have positive effects on lymphocyte function and wound healing. ω-3 fatty acids are *essential* polyunsaturated fatty acids found in fish oils, and their role may be to modulate the immuno-inflammatory response to sepsis and trauma.

Certainly the evidence is by no means conclusive, and ongoing studies are required to clarify the effects of these compounds.

## CONCLUSIONS

For numerous reasons, including lower costs and risks of complications, enteral feeding is the preferred route of nutritional support. TPN offers an alternative when oral/enteral feeding is not an option. Patients receiving TPN require extensive monitoring, particularly at initiation of therapy, and must be diligently assessed for signs of infection or other complications. TPN formulations are complex and require expertise and specific education regarding compatibility issues and compounding of the mixtures. Although TPN has been significantly improved over the past 30 years, it remains a far from perfect substitute for the alimentary tract.

## FURTHER READING

American Society of Parenteral and Enteral Nutrition. Guidelines for the use of parenteral and enteral nutrition in adult and paediatric patients. *J Parenter Enteral Nutr* 1993;**17**(4 suppl):1SA–52SA.

Civetta JM, Taylor RW, Kirby RR, eds. Enteral and parenteral nutrition. In: *Critical Care*, 2nd edn. Philadelphia: JB Lippincott, 1992.

Committee on Medical Aspects of Food Policy. *Dietary reference values for food energy and nutrients for the United Kingdom*. 41 DOH, 4th edn. *Report of the Panel on Dietary Reference Values.* London: HMSO, 1991.

Daly JM, Masser E, Hansen L, *et al*. Peripheral vein infusion of dextrose/amino acid solutions ± 20% fat emulsion. *J Parenter Enteral Nutr* 1985;**9**:296–9.

Dudrick SJ, Wilmore DW, Vars HM, *et al*. Long term total parenteral nutrition with growth, development, and positive nitrogen balance. *Surgery* 1968;**64**:134–42.

Klein CJ, Stanek GS, Wiles III CE. Overfeeding macronutrients to critically ill adults: Metabolic complications. *J Am Diet Assoc* 1998;**98**:795–806.

Kumar PJ, Clark ML, eds. Nutrition. In: *Clinical Medicine*, 3rd edn. Glasgow: Baillière Tindall, 1994: 153–74.

McKinnon BT. FDA safety alert: hazards of precipitation associated with parenteral nutrition. *Nutr Clin Pract* 1996;**11**:59–65.

Mainous MR, Deitch EA. Nutrition and infection. *Surg Clinics North Am* 1994;**74**:659–76.

Nussbaum MS, Fischer JE. Parenteral nutrition. In: Zaloga GP, ed. *Nutrition in Critical Care.* St Louis: Mosby, 1994: 371–97.

Roberts PR, Zaloga GP. Enteral nutrition in the critically ill patient. In: Shoemaker WC, Grenvik AN, Ayres SM, *et al*., eds. *Textbook of Critical Care*, 4th edn. Philadelphia: WB Saunders, 2000: 875–98.

Rolandelli RH, Ullrich JR. Nutritional support in the frail elderly surgical patient. *Surg Clinics North Am* 1994;**74**:79–92.

Wilmore DW, Dudrick SJ. Growth and development of an infant receiving all nutrients exclusively by vein. *JAMA* 1968;**208**:860–4.

# Chapter 82 Carbon monoxide poisoning

M.A. Cannon and R.C. Prielipp

During the past decade, carbon monoxide (CO) has represented the leading cause of both intentional and unintentional poisoning in the US. The incomplete combustion of fossil fuels creates this colourless and odourless gas. In the USA, approximately 4000 deaths per year occur from CO poisoning. Exposure to CO usually occurs secondary to smoke inhalation during fires, or the use of poorly functioning furnaces or combustion engines in poorly ventilated areas. Less commonly, CO poisoning may follow exposure to methylene chloride (paint strippers), which is converted to CO *in vivo*.

## DIAGNOSIS

Physicians must maintain a high index of suspicion to diagnose CO poisoning. The variability of symptoms often obscures the diagnosis, making it difficult to document the actual number of afflicted patients. Non-specific symptoms – most commonly resembling viral influenza – often lead to misdiagnosis (Tables 82.1 and 82.2). Any history of working in a closed space (e.g. garage, basement, ship), or around a fire in an enclosed space, requires an evaluation for CO exposure. Similarly, when multiple family members present with common non-specific symptoms during winter months, environmental exposure to CO should be considered. Fire victims must be evaluated for poisoning caused by multiple agents because the burning of industrial and household items releases many toxic chemicals (i.e. hydrogen cyanide, nitrogen oxide, acrolein).

The initial evaluation of patients exposed to CO must be thorough and thoughtful. However, the presence of metabolic acidosis in the absence of hypotension, sepsis, cardiogenic shock, or diabetic ketoacidosis may offer a clue to CO poisoning. Pulse oximetry is grossly inaccurate in estimating actual arterial haemoglobin saturation in the presence of CO. Carboxyhaemoglobin cannot be differentiated by the infrared light used in standard pulse oximetry. The resulting arterial oxygen saturation ($Sa\text{O}_2$) calculated by the sum of carboxyhaemoglobin and oxyhaemoglobin is erroneously high. In contrast, percutaneous partial oxygen pressure analysers, which measure current resulting from oxygen transport across two electrodes, retain accuracy in the presence of CO. Arterial blood gas analysis, like pulse oximetry, provides little useful information. The arterial oxygen tension quantifies the partial pressure of oxygen dissolved in the plasma. This does not correlate with saturated haemoglobin in the presence of CO. Co-oximetry represents the *definitive* test for carboxyhaemoglobin. During co-oximetry, a blood sample is exposed to six different wavelengths of light to quantify the fractions of reduced haemoglobin, oxyhaemoglobin, methaemoglobin, and carboxyhaemoglobin. Any value of carboxyhaemoglobin above 5% in non-smokers and 10% in smokers indicates an acute exposure.

**Table 82.1 Common misdiagnoses of patients with isolated carbon monoxide poisoning**

| |
|---|
| Viral influenza |
| Myocardial infarction |
| Gastroenteritis |
| Drug abuse |
| Psychiatric disorders |

**Table 82.2 Clinical features of carbon monoxide poisoning**

| Carboxyhaemoglobin level (%) | Clinical signs |
|---|---|
| 10–20 | Mild headache<br>Slight shortness of breath |
| 20–30 | Moderate headache<br>Weakness<br>Difficulty with concentration |
| 30–40 | Irritability<br>Nausea/vomiting<br>Dizziness<br>Visual changes |
| 40–50 | Tachycardia, tachypnoea, arrhythmias<br>Ataxia, confusion |
| 50–60 | Stupor, convulsions<br>Often fatal |
| 60–70 | Coma, cardiac depression |

## PATHOPHYSIOLOGY

Absorption of CO depends on environmental concentration and minute ventilation. Tissue injury results from hypoxia and tissue ischaemia. CO has a 240 times greater affinity for haemoglobin than has oxygen. The high affinity of CO competitively inhibits oxygen binding to haemoglobin during gas exchange in the lung. In addition, carboxyhaemoglobin changes the configuration of the protein itself, preventing the release of any bound oxygen. Thus, the oxygen dissociation curve is shifted to the left, further decreasing oxygen delivery to the tissue. Lastly, it appears that CO inhibits cellular respiration, possibly through cytochrome $A_3$, but that has yet to be proved.

CO poisoning ultimately affects all organ systems. Those with the greatest oxygen demand, i.e. the heart and brain, are most immediately affected. Premature ventricular contractions occur commonly with CO poisoning, and patients with pre-existing cardiovascular disease have a significantly increased risk for cardiac mortality after CO poisoning. Cardiac arrhythmias represent the most common cause of death in fatal CO poisoning. The central nervous system exhibits acute and chronic effects. Acute symptoms include headache, confusion, lethargy, stupor, etc. Chronic symptoms, including impulsiveness, mood changes, perceptual deficits, and cognitive abnormalities, occur in 10–60% of patients treated, usually 10–40 days after exposure. Magnetic resonance imaging commonly shows hyperintensive areas in the thalamus and globus pallidus, consistent with progressive demyelination.

## TREATMENT

The initial treatment of CO poisoning should include 100% oxygen by facemask or an endotracheal tube. Hyperbaric oxygen, when available, is considered optimal; however, no prospective randomized trial has compared outcome after treatment with hyperbaric oxygen with that after treatment with normobaric oxygen. At present, most patients never receive hyperbaric oxygen. The average elimination half-life of CO for a patient breathing room air is 300 min. With 100% normobaric oxygen, the half-life falls to 80 min. The elimination half-life is further reduced to 23 min during treatment with hyperbaric oxygen at 3 atmospheres. In the conscious patient, no improvement in clinical outcome has been shown with hyperbaric oxygen compared with normobaric oxygen therapy. The use of carboxyhaemoglobin concentrations to dictate treatment has been shown to correlate poorly with clinical outcome. However, severity of clinical symptoms can vary dramatically in patients with similar carboxyhaemoglobin concentrations. Thus, symptoms, not carboxyhaemoglobin concentrations, should direct choice of treatment modalities (see Table 82.2). The only exception is that any pregnant patient presenting with a carboxyhaemoglobin level above 20% should be treated with hyperbaric oxygen (Table 82.3). The risk of fetal mortality increases significantly when the concentration increases above 20% (Figures 82.1 and 82.2).

| **Table 82.3 Indications for hyperbaric oxygen treatment** |
|---|
| Severe central nervous system impairment |
| Pregnant patients with carboxyhaemoglobin levels > 20% |
| Unconscious patients |
| Ischaemic chest pain or clinical signs of acute cardiac ischaemia |

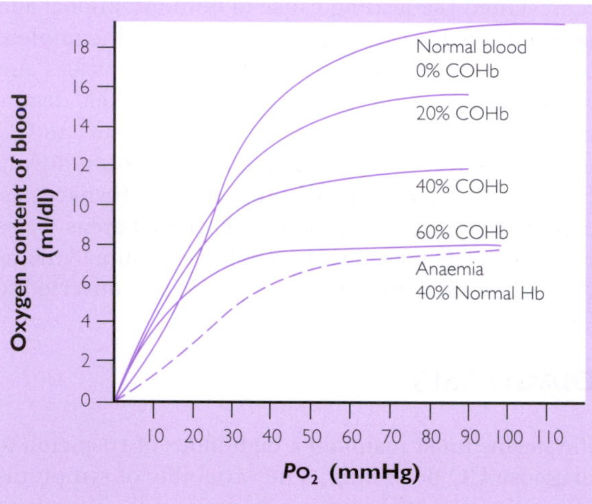


**Figure 82.1** Blood oxygen content with increasing percentages of carbon monoxide (CO). Oxygen content and oxygen delivery both decrease with increasing CO levels. 1 mmHg = 133 Pa.

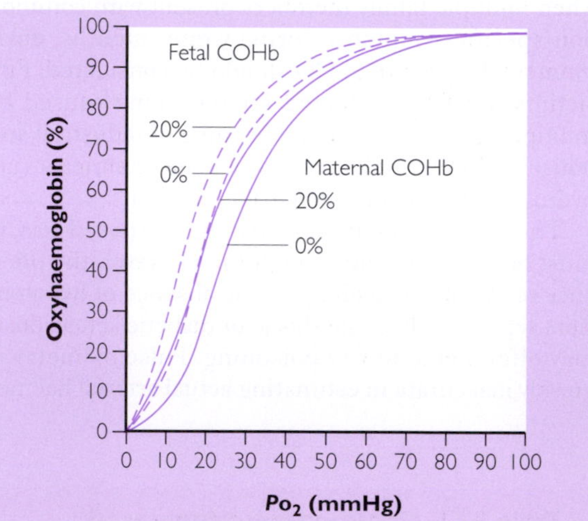


**Figure 82.2** Fetal (dashed lines) and maternal (solid lines) oxyhaemoglobin saturation curves demonstrating effect of carbon monoxide (CO). Fetal curve normally lies to the left of the maternal curve. In the presence of CO, both curves are further shifted to the left. COHb indicates carboxyhaemglobin, and $Po_2$ the partial oxygen pressure. (Adapted from Van Hoessen KB *et al. JAMA* 1989;261:1039–43.)

## FURTHER READING


Barker SJ, Tremper KK. The effect of carbon monoxide inhalation on pulse oximetry and transcutaneous $pO_2$. *Anesthesiology* 1987;**66**:677–9.

Dolan MC. Carbon monoxide poisoning. *Can Med Assoc J* 1985;**133**:392–9.

Ginsburg ME. Carbon monoxide intoxication: clinical features, neuropathy and mechanism of injury. *J Toxicol Clin Toxicol* 1985;**23**:281–8.

Joels N, Pugh LG. The carbon monoxide dissociation curve of human blood. *J Physiol (Lond)* 1958;**142**:63–77.

Kaplan H, Grand A, Hartzell G. *Combustion Toxicology: Principles and Test Methods.* Lancaster, PA: Technomic, 1983.

Kovac AL. Diagnosis and treatment of smoke inhalation injuries. *Anesthesiol Rev* 1994;**21**:93–100.

Lacey DJ. Neurologic sequelae of acute carbon monoxide intoxication. *Am J Dis Child* 1981;**135**:145–7.

Raphael JC, Elkharrat D, Jars-Guincestre MC, *et al.* Trial of normobaric and hyperbaric oxygen for acute carbon monoxide intoxication. *Lancet* 1989;**ii**:414–19.

Siesjo BK. Carbon monoxide poisoning: mechanism of damage, late sequelae and therapy. *Clin Toxicol* 1985;**23**:247–8.

Van Hoesen KB, Camporesi EM, Moon RE, *et al.* Should hyperbaric oxygen be used to treat the pregnant patient for acute carbon monoxide poisoning. *JAMA* 1989;**261**:1039–43.

Vegfors M, Lennmarken C. Carboxyhaemoglobinaemia and pulse oximetry. *Br J Anaesth* 1991;**66**:625–626.

# Chapter 83 Techniques and considerations in the diagnosis of cerebral death

K.D. Rorie, T.J. Jones, and D.A. Stump

The diagnosis of cerebral death has become increasingly important as a result of public awareness about 'quality of life' in terminal illnesses. Thus, the diagnosis must be precise and expedient, particularly when organ procurement for transplantation is under consideration.

Improved technology has removed some of the uncertainty from the diagnosis of cerebral death. However, the technology has also made the diagnosis of cerebral death much more complicated.

## HISTORY

The concept of brain death was first formally proposed in a Special Communication to the *Journal of the American Medical Association* in 1968 by the Ad Hoc Committee of the Harvard Medical School to Examine the Definition of Brain Death. This publication contained the first peer-reviewed criteria for brain death: coma, apnoea, lack of spontaneous or purposeful movements, absence of elicitable reflexes, and normothermia without evidence of pharmacological depression for at least 24 hours. The Committee also recommended that two electroencephalograms (EEGs) be performed at least 24 hours apart; when both were isoelectric, the diagnosis was supported.

More than a decade later, the National Institute of Neurologic and Communicative Disorders and Stroke (NINCDS) sponsored a fixed protocol study of brain death at eight clinical centres throughout the US. As a result of this collaborative research programme, the criteria for cerebral death were revised. In 503 (primarily adult) patients, the NINCDS study confirmed that the loss of pupillary, oculovestibular, oculocephalic, and corneal reflexes was necessary before the pronouncement of brain death. Moreover, the research group concluded that a drug screen (specifically confirming the absence of barbiturates) and an EEG were mandatory before the diagnosis of brain death. Based, in part, on these findings, one year after the publication of the NINCDS study, a US Presidential Commission published consensus guidelines for the diagnosis of brain death. These guidelines specified two criteria for determining death:

1. Irreversible cessation of circulatory and respiratory functions;
2. Irreversible cessation of all functions of the entire brain, including the brain stem.

In addition, this report also questioned the applicability of these guidelines in children because of developmental factors, a possible greater tolerance to asphyxia, and the ability of infants and children to demonstrate significant recovery despite prolonged coma.

The conceptual and diagnostic difficulties created by the term 'brain death' are universal. In the UK, the first clinical guidelines for the diagnosis of brain death were published in 1976. As a result of the increase in organ transplantation, by 1983 the Health Departments issued a code of practice with set criteria to be followed when making the diagnosis of brain death. At the request of the Health Departments, the Royal College of Physicians, on behalf of the Academy of Royal Colleges, published a revised and updated *Code of Practice for the Diagnosis Of Brain Stem Death* in 1998. They suggested the term 'brain death' be replaced by 'brain-stem death,' stating that it is not the entire death of the brain, but rather death of the brain stem, that must be established before changes in treatment priorities should be addressed. The diagnosis of brain-stem death may be made only after demonstrating the absence of all brain-stem reflexes with no motor response to appropriate stimulation, and no respiratory movements occurring when exceeding the threshold for respiratory stimulation. Two senior clinicians who are not members of a transplantation team must make the diagnosis. The tests must be repeated at a time interval dictated by clinical judgement.

These guidelines are not universally practised throughout Europe. French law similarly requires the diagnosis to be established by two senior clinicians neither of whom may be involved in transplantation activity. However, two isoelectric EEGs or the demonstration of cessation of cerebral perfusion by arteriography should confirm the diagnosis. This resembles protocols followed in many Western countries based on satisfying predetermined conditions, demonstration of loss of cerebral function and brain-stem reflexes, with confirmation by either EEG or angiography. In 1997, Germany passed a law recognizing brain-stem death as being equivalent in law to death. Before this, death was recognized only as the time when the heart stopped beating. The Australia and New Zealand Intensive Care Society defined brain death as 'when there is irreversible loss of consciousness and irreversible loss of brain-stem reflex responses and respiratory centre function, or irreversible cessation of intracranial blood flow'. The diagnosis may be made after clinical testing of brain-stem function with established preconditions satisfied, but if this is not possible cerebral angiography is required.

## DIAGNOSTIC CRITERIA

The diagnosis of brain death requires that many criteria be met, and the exclusion of reversible causes of coma before its pronouncement. Therefore, the original cause of the coma must be established in order to confirm that a catastrophic brain injury has occurred. Causes of catastrophic injuries include trauma, hypoxia, hypotension, hydrocephalus, haemorrhage, infarction, infection, tumour, metabolic disorders, seizures, and intoxication. The absence of a known brain injury should cast doubt on the diagnosis of brain death and prompt further investigation. Some primary brain-stem lesions or drug intoxications may surreptitiously satisfy the criteria of brain death.

Clinical examination provides additional criteria for proving the absence of cortical and brain-stem function. Requisite criteria include an unresponsive coma, absence of motor and brain-stem reflexes, and apnoea. When prerequisite criteria cannot be met (e.g. therapeutic barbiturate coma) or when brain death diagnosis proves uncertain, neuroradiological and neurophysiological tests should be employed to confirm cerebral death. Arteriography or intravenous digital subtraction angiography, transcranial Doppler (TCD), magnetic resonance imaging and angiography, or radionuclide cerebral angiography may confirm the absence of cerebral blood flow. Angiography has been regarded as definitive for diagnosing the absence of cerebral blood flow. Brain death results in vascular stasis, or the absence of progression of contrast medium during a prolonged series (of 1 min duration). Although cerebral angiography yields a sensitivity of 100%, it has several disadvantages:

- it is expensive, requiring specialized personnel and technology;
- it requires the transportation of critically ill patients from the intensive care unit;
- it is invasive and uses contrast media that may be detrimental to the patient's already compromised organs, such as the kidneys.

TCD can effectively assess cerebral circulation. However, in one series, the sensitivity of TCD as a one-time test was low (60%) and was related to the inability to obtain a TCD signal, either unilaterally or bilaterally in many patients. This may have resulted from displacement of the cerebral vessels, lack of a temporal window, or interference from other equipment connected to the patient. Subsequently, the authors argue that the 'no signal' may be artefactual and not necessarily indicate circulatory arrest. False-negative findings do not question the clinical diagnosis of cerebral death. Rather, they stress that it is possible to find a TCD spectra inconsistent with brain death by insonating the area of the middle cerebral artery. Therefore, a 'no signal' detection via TCD calls for confirmation by cerebral angiography.

Radionuclide angiography (RA) represents a first-pass technique and does not depend on subsequent localization of the radiopharmaceutical. An important feature of RA is its ability to detect blood flow in patients comatose from drug intoxication. RA can also be done safely and effectively at the patient's bedside. However, RA has several shortcomings including:

- sporadic technical failures;
- inadequate visualization of the vertebrobasilar system;
- false-negative studies caused by severely reduced, but not absent, cerebral blood flow.

Moreover, at least 12 hours must pass before repeating a radionuclide study, to allow dissipation of the radiopharmaceutical from the circulation.

The EEG is one of the most widely used tests for the confirmation of brain death. At the time of death, the EEG usually, but not always, depicts a flat line. Data suggest that, in patients suspected of having brain death, there is about a 64% chance that, if the first EEG shows activity, a second EEG would be isoelectric and presumably confirm the diagnosis of brain death. However, the presence of some activity in the second EEG warrants continued observation for a period of at least 2 days. The return of EEG activity does not predict potential recovery, but only demonstrates a change in central nervous system (CNS) function which has to be considered in conjunction with, but not in isolation from, other clinical data to assist the clinician.

Factors that may depress the EEG include hypothermia, CNS-depressant drugs, and isolated destruction of the cerebral cortex with sparing of the brain stem. In a series of 2650 patients presenting with isoelectric EEG of up to 24 hours' duration, the only three patients who recovered cerebral function were those in coma resulting from overdose of CNS-depressant drugs. Similarly, methaqualone, diazepam, meprobamate, and trichloroethylene may produce reversible isoelectric EEGs.

## CONCLUSION

The need for transplantable organs forms the most compelling reason for objective, instrument-based criteria for brain death. Accurate diagnosis of brain death relies on the medical history (the original cause of coma and the circumstances, which should be inconsistent with recovery), on clinical criteria (an irreversible coma, loss of brain-stem reflexes, apnoea), and on confirmatory tests showing an absence of cerebral blood flow (e.g. TCD, radionuclide uptake, and cerebral angiography), and an absence of spontaneous brain electrical activity on an EEG. The presence of potential confounding factors (CNS-depressant drugs, hypothermia, or metabolic disturbances) mandates confirmatory tests. In reaching the diagnosis of brain death, the physician must consider the emotional impact that confirmatory diagnostic procedures will have on the patient's family and medical staff. Therefore, diagnosis of brain death should not supersede consideration for the patient and the patient's family.

## FURTHER READING


Ashwal S. Brain death in the newborn: Current perspectives. *Clin Perinatol* 1997;**24**:859–82.

Department of Health. Cadaveric organs for transplantation. *A Code of Practice including the Diagnosis of Brain Death*. London: HMSO, 1983.

Diagnosis of brain death. Statement issued by the honorary secretary of the Conference of Medical Royal Colleges and their Faculties in the United Kingdom on 11 October 1976. *BMJ* 1976;**ii**:1187–8.

NINCDS. *The NINCDS Collaborative Study of Brain Death: Monograph No. 24.* NIH Publication No. 81-2286, 1980: 1–203.

Paolin A, Manuali A, Di Paola F, *et al*. Reliability in diagnosis of brain death. *Intensive Care Med* 1995;**21**:657–62.

President's Commission. *Guidelines for the Determination of Death*. Report of the medical consultants on the diagnosis of death to the President's Commission for the Study of Ethical Problems in Medicine and Biomedical and Behavioral Research. *JAMA* 1981;**246**:2184–6.

Rouse MO. Remarks of the AMA president. *JAMA* 1968;**205**:85–8.

Royal College of Physicians. *A Code of Practice for the Diagnosis of Brain Stem Death including Guidelines for the Identification and Management of Potential Organ and Tissue Donors*. London: HMSO, 1998.

Williams MA, Suarez JI. Brain death determination in adults: more than meets the eye. *Crit Care Med* 1997;**25**:1787–8.

# Chapter 84 Hazards of laparoscopy

T.N. Harwood

Ever since the description of laparoscopy in 1902 by Kelling, the procedure has been increasingly accepted for diagnostic and therapeutic indications by gynaecologists, general surgeons, and urologists. With the current trend towards 'minimally invasive' surgery, a further increase in the number of laparoscopic procedures can be expected.

Although laparoscopy is a relatively safe procedure, complications such as haemorrhage, gas embolism, cardiovascular collapse, pneumopericardium, pneumothorax, pneumomediastinum, perforation of the viscera, and peritonitis occur with a reported incidence between 0.6% and 2.5% (Table 84.1). The published mortality rate from laparoscopy ranges from 0.03% to 0.49%.

Although anaesthetic options for patients undergoing laparoscopy include general, regional, and local anaesthesia, by far the most commonly used method is general anaesthesia with an endotracheal tube. Insufflation of the abdomen and use of the Trendelenburg position indicate controlled ventilation in most patients. Surgeons most commonly insufflate the abdomen with carbon dioxide ($CO_2$), chosen because it is soluble and does not support combustion. If an insoluble gas were to be used, any gas remaining in the peritoneal cavity at the end of the procedure would be irritant, causing shoulder pain. Furthermore, in the event of accidental intravenous administration, the insoluble gas collects in the right ventricle and is resistant to absorption. Nevertheless, carbon dioxide insufflation under pressure is a major aetiological factor for complications. Raised intra-abdominal pressure and $CO_2$ absorption produce the pathophysiological changes associated with adverse events reported in laparoscopy. During prolonged procedures, absorption of $CO_2$ can be sufficient to cause hypercapnia. Minute ventilation may need to be increased by 50–75% in order to maintain normocapnia.

| Table 84.1 Complications reported during and after laparoscopic surgery |
|---|
| Pulmonary complications |
| Hypercapnia |
| Hypoxaemia |
| Aspiration |
| Pneumothorax |
| Pneumomediastinum/pericardium |
| Cardiovascular complications |
| Hypertension |
| Hypotension |
| Reduced cardiac output |
| Arrhythmias |
| Gas embolism |
| Miscellaneous complications |
| Subcutaneous emphysema |
| Vascular injury |
| Perforation of gastrointestinal or genitourinary structure |

Intra-abdominal pressures, commonly increased to 15–20 mmHg during $CO_2$ insufflation, may reduce diaphragmatic excursion or compliance and thus decrease intrapulmonary compliance. During volume-controlled ventilation with low inspiratory flow rates or pressure-controlled ventilation, alveolar ventilation may decline to levels less than those required for normocapnia. The use of the Trendelenburg position frequently exacerbates this reduced compliance. Trendelenburg postioning and increased intra-abdominal pressure can also reduce functional residual capacity, potentially leading to ventilation–perfusion mismatching and hypoxaemia in patients with lung disease. Moving the patient to a reverse Trendelenburg position may reduce this problem. The Trendelenburg position also encourages gastro-oesophageal reflux (see Chapter 16).

Insufflation, through stretching of the peritoneum, may increase vagal tone and trigger bradycardia. This is usually temporary but may require acute desufflation or intravenous atropine. Insertion of the insufflating trocar may result in direct trauma to a variety of intra-abdominal structures. In a review, Nordestgaard *et al.* (see Further reading) identified 20 cases of major vascular injuries during laparoscopic procedures. Of the reported vascular injuries, most involved the distal aorta and its major branches, or the inferior vena cava and its tributaries. Penfield (see Further reading) concluded that factors such as failure to place the patient in the Trendelenburg position, failure to elevate or stabilize the abdominal wall, lateral insertion of the needle or trocar, inadequate pneumoperitoneum, and failure to rotate the trocar during insertion could also lead to large-vessel injury during pelvic laparoscopy.

Almost any intra-abdominal organ can be damaged. This includes the bladder, bowel, stomach (especially if distended through poorly administered ventilation from a facemask before intubation), uterus, liver, spleen, and even the ureters. The bladder should always be emptied before the trocar is inserted. It is important to have a high index of suspicion for bowel injury when there is more postoperative pain than usual. Unrecognized bowel perforation can be fatal.

Increased intra-abdominal pressure has effects on the cardiovascular system. Small increases in intra-abdominal pressure may have no effect or increase venous return, and may decrease, increase, or have no impact on cardiac output. With increases in intra-abdominal pressure up to 20 mmHg, venous return and cardiac output diminish. Concurrently, systemic vascular resistance may increase as a result of increased pressure on the abdominal aorta, further reducing cardiac output. Joris (see Further reading) examined the cardiovascular changes that occurred in healthy patients undergoing laparoscopic cholecystectomy. With an intra-abdominal pressure of 14 mmHg and normocapnia, systemic vascular resistance increased by 65% and cardiac output decreased by 20%. With the addition of general anaesthetic agents and the reverse Trendelenburg position, cardiac output decreased by 50%. Clearly, patients with compromised ventricular function might not tolerate changes of this magnitude.

With continued insufflation, $CO_2$ may dissect into the mediastinum, pleural cavity, or subcutaneous tissue. Although the latter may not cause pathophysiological consequences, pneumomediastinum or pneumothorax can lead to cardiac and/or pulmonary compromise. Fatal $CO_2$ embolism can occur from initial insufflation. Just as occurs with venous air emboli, amounts of gas injected into the venous system may be large enough to impede blood flow through the right heart and pulmonary vasculature, leading to hypoxaemia and shock. This is an important reason for limiting the initial gas flow to 500 ml/min until one is certain that the gas is entering the peritoneal cavity. Detection of $CO_2$ embolism is by ECG changes (as $CO_2$ encounters the right bundle branch, causing bizarre broad complexes) and *decreasing* end-tidal $CO_2$ values.

Raised intracranial pressure (ICP) is also a reported effect of laparoscopy. Bloomfield and others studied pigs undergoing laparoscopy with an intra-abdominal pressure of 25 mmHg. The ICP rose from a mean of 8 to 21 mmHg, and the cerebral perfusion pressure decreased from 82 to 62 mmHg. Thus, laparoscopy should be used cautiously in patients with known or suspected increased ICP.

Laparoscopy for diagnostic and therapeutic purposes is a safe procedure that only rarely causes any complication. However, major abdominal arterial and venous injury may occur and requires prompt recognition and treatment. Anaesthetists and laparoscopists must be vigilant for these rare and potentially lethal complications, which mandate immediate laparotomy and application of appropriate vascular surgical techniques to re-establish arterial and venous continuity.

## FURTHER READING


Bloomfield GL, Ridings PC, Blocher CR, Marmarou A, Sugerman HJ. Effects of increased intra-abdominal pressure upon intracranial and cerebral perfusion pressure before and after volume expansion. *J Trauma* 1996;**40**:936–43.

Bradfield ST. Gas embolism during laparoscopy (letter). *Anaesth Intensive Care* 1991;**19**:474.

Joris JL, Noirot DP, Legrand MJ, Jacquet NJ, Lamy ML. Hemodynamic changes during laparoscopic cholecystectomy. *Anesth Analg* 1993;**76**:1067–71.

Kalhan SB, Reaney JA, Collins RL. Pneumomediastinum and subcutaneous emphysema during laparoscopy. *Cleve Clin J Med* 1990;**57**:639–42.

Kane MG, Krejs GJ. Complications of diagnostic laparoscopy in Dallas: a 7-year prospective study. *Gastrointest Endosc* 1984;**30**:237–40.

Kashtan J, Green JF, Parsons EQ, Holcroft JW. Hemodynamic effect of increased abdominal pressure. *J Surg Res* 1981;**30**:249–55.

Liu SY, Leighton T, Davis I, Klein S, Lippmann M, Bongard F. Prospective analysis of cardiopulmonary responses to laparoscopic cholecystectomy. *J Laparoendosc Surg* 1991;**1**:241–6.

Nordestgaard AG, Bodily KC, Osborne RW Jr, Buttorff JD. Major vascular injuries during laparoscopic procedures. *Am J Surg* 1995;**169**:543–5.

Penfield AJ. Trocar and needle injury. In: Phillips JM, ed. *Laparoscopy*. Baltimore, MA: Williams & Wilkins, 1977: 236–41.

# Chapter 85 Analgesia for labour

L.S. Dean

The severity of pain associated with childbirth varies from woman to woman (and from pregnancy to pregnancy, although subsequent labours tend to be less painful than the first), but it is universally acknowledged as potentially one of the most painful of life's experiences. The ideal labour analgesic would cause neither maternal nor fetal side effects, nor impair the progress of labour. The mother must know what techniques are available to her and keep an open mind about her requirements (which may change during the course of labour). Early first-stage labour pain is visceral and is transmitted via T10–L1 nerve roots. During late first stage and throughout the second stage, the labour pain becomes somatic in nature and is transmitted through the pudendal nerve (S2–S4) (Figure 85.1). The goal of obstetric analgesia is to interfere with pain transmission or its perception.

Multiple approaches have been used successfully, including a number of non-pharmacological techniques, which are summarized briefly.

## NON-PHARMACOLOGICAL TECHNIQUES

### Psychoprophylaxis

The importance of this is in the education of the mother about the process of childbirth. By knowing what is happening, fear is removed, anxiety is lessened, and the pain seems less intense. Conditioned pain reflexes associated with uterine contractions can be replaced with 'positive' conditioned reflexes by concentrating on breathing and the release of muscle tension. This can help the woman to cope with the pain but does not remove it. There are no neonatal adverse effects.

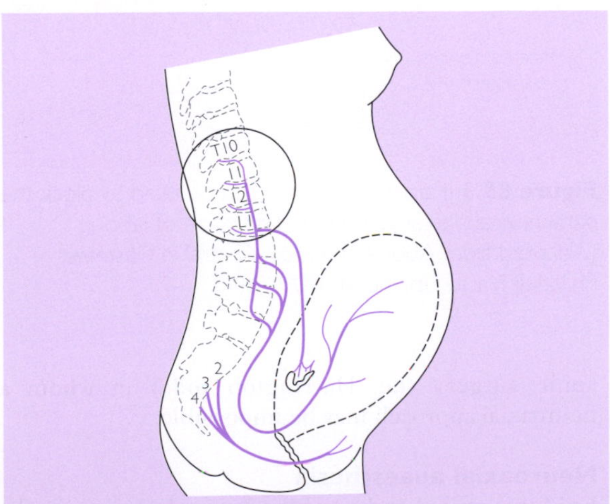


**Figure 85.1** Somatic and visceral pain pathways of labour. Afferent impulses from the cervix and uterus are transmitted via sympathetic fibres that enter the spinal cord at T10–L1. The pudendal nerve S2–4, carries pain pathways from the perineum. (Adapted from Bonica JJ. *Clin Obstet Gynaecol* 1975;2:511.)

### Hypnosis

This is only possible in susceptible candidates and requires a series of conditioning sessions. At these the mother achieves progressively greater degrees of trance until analgesia is achieved, usually in a hand. The mother is then conditioned to transfer the analgesia from the hand to the abdomen and perineum. This technique is time-consuming, not always effective even in susceptible subjects, and can induce acute anxiety states in the mother.

### Acupuncture

There are no traditional acupuncture points for vaginal delivery because Chinese women have not expected to use analgesia for childbirth. Although the acupuncture points for vaginal hysterectomy and dysmenorrhoea have been used, results have been inconsistent. There are no deleterious effects on the neonate.

### Transcutaneous electrical nerve stimulation (TENS)

This is the application of pulsed current through surface electrodes placed on the skin at the appropriate dermatomes (T10–L1 for the first stage of labour; S2–S4 for the second stage). It is thought to work by low-frequency stimulation increasing endorphin production and by high-frequency stimulation closing the 'gate' (see Chapter 34) in the spinal cord to the transmission of pain information. About 20% of selected patients gain useful help from TENS, although it can take up to 40 min to become effective. TENS is non-invasive, does not interfere with fetal heart monitoring, and does not harm the mother or neonate.

## INHALATIONAL ANALGESIA

Historically, trichloroethylene and methoxyflurane were used, but are no longer available. Although enflurane and isoflurane have been used occasionally, only nitrous oxide has widespread acceptance. The basis of inhalational analgesia is that uterine contractions have to be anticipated and the agent starts to be inhaled some 30 seconds before each contraction, so that there is sufficient gas tension in the brain by the time the contraction reaches its painful phase.

Nitrous oxide is suitable because of its analgesic properties and because it can be used in concentrations that do not cause unconsciousness. It is available as a 50% mixture of nitrous oxide in oxygen known as Entonox. It can be self-administered via a low-resistance breathing system from cylinders after pressure reduction. Deep and slow breathing should be encouraged and it should not be used between contractions. Satisfactory pain relief is obtained in approximately 50% of mothers who choose this form of analgesia.

## SYSTEMIC ANALGESIA

The μ-opioid receptor agonists, pethidine and morphine, have long been administered intravenously or intramuscularly to diminish pain perception. Morphine has lost favour because of its prolonged duration of action and the unpredictable duration of labour. Pethidine remains popular among obstetricians. Opioid agonist–antagonists, butorphanol and nalbuphine, are often chosen because of their ceiling effect on respiratory depression. Opioid patient-controlled analgesia (PCA) is also gaining in popularity, and may lead to reduced total drug doses and increased patient satisfaction compared with intermittent bolus techniques. All opioids may cause decreased fetal heart rate variability. Ketamine in 0.25 mg/kg doses can rapidly provide analgesia for the second and third stages of labour without dissociative side effects. In single doses greater than 1 mg/kg, ketamine can cause neonatal depression and muscle rigidity.

## REGIONAL ANALGESIA

### Pudendal nerve block

Pudendal (S2–S4) nerve block provides the perineal analgesia needed during the second stage of labour for low outlet forceps delivery, for vacuum extraction, or for episiotomy repair. Local anaesthetic in 7–10 ml volumes is injected on each side as described in Figure 85.2.

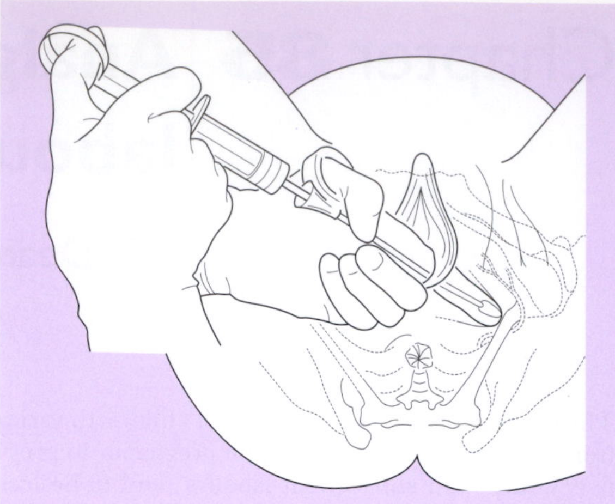

**Figure 85.2** Pudendal nerve block. The index and middle fingers of the operator's hand are inserted through the vagina to rest on the ischial spine. A needle guide is inserted between the fingers until its tip is against the vaginal wall just proximal to the ischial spine. A 20-gauge needle is inserted through the guide, the vaginal wall is pierced, and the needle is advanced into and through the sacrospinous ligament, just posterior to the ischial spine. Local anaesthetic is injected after careful aspiration. (Adapted from Pritchard JA, MacDonald PC, Gant NF. *Williams obstetrics*. Stamford, CT: Appleton & Lange, 1997: 359.)

### Paracervical nerve block

Paracervical plexus (T10–L1) block (Figure 85.3) effectively relieves pain during the first stage of labour, but reports of sustained fetal bradycardia, acidosis, and death resulting from systemic absorption of local anaesthetic and increased uterine arterial and myometrial tone have essentially precluded its use.

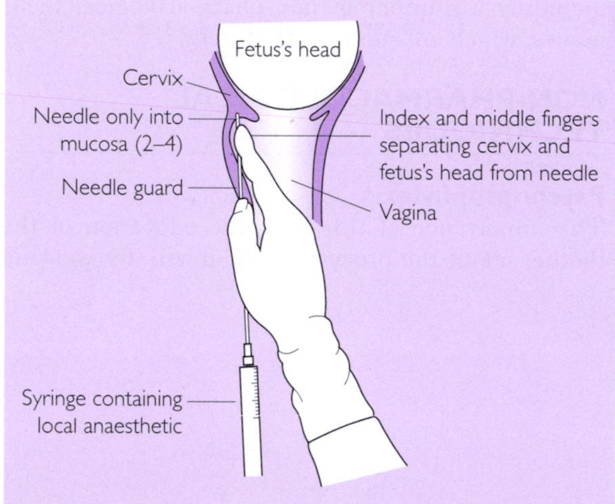


**Figure 85.3** Paracervical block can be used to block the paracervical plexus during the first stage of labour. (Adapted from Abouleish E. *Pain Control in Obstetrics*. Philadelphia: JB Lippincott, 1977: 344.)

### Lumbar sympathetic blocks

Paravertebral lumbar sympathetic block (T10–L1) interrupts transmission of pain during the first stage of labour. With the patient in the sitting position, use a 22-gauge needle to identify the transverse process of L2 and then redirect it so that the tip lies just anterior to the vertebral body. After careful aspiration, slowly inject 10 ml of local anaesthetic and repeat the block on the other side. Risks include hypotension, total spinal block, postdural puncture headache, local anaesthetic toxicity, and retroperitoneal haematoma. This technique proves useful in the patient who has had prior spine surgery (i.e. Harrington rods) in whom a neuroaxial approach may be impossible.

### Neuroaxial anaesthesia

Epidural, spinal and combined spinal/epidural techniques efficiently provide labour analgesia (Figure 85.4). Caudal anaesthesia has been used in labour, but difficulty in positioning the patient and maintenance of sterility in labour have decreased its use. Table 85.1 lists the contraindications to neuroaxial anaesthesia. Emergency resuscitation equipment (see Chapter 15)

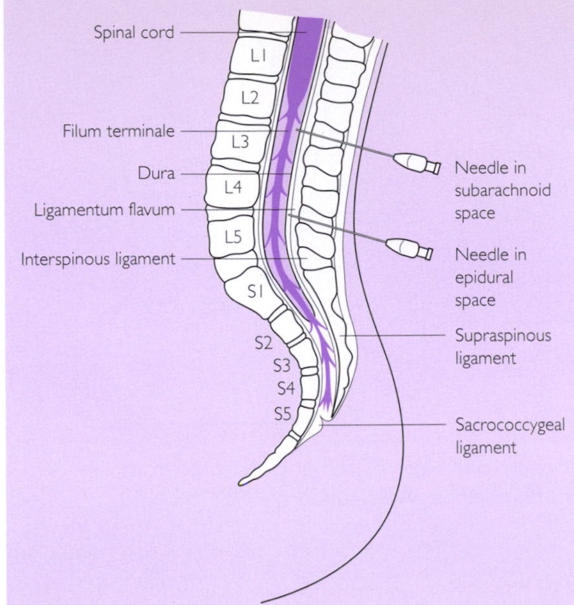


**Figure 85.4** Lumbosacral anatomy depicting placement of subarachnoid and epidural needles. (From Shnider SM, Levinson G, Ralston DH. Regional anesthesia for labor and delivery. In: Shnider SM, Levinson G, eds. *Anesthesia for Obstetrics*, 3rd edn. Baltimore, MA: Williams & Wilkins, 1993: 135–55.)

| **Table 85.1 Contraindications to neuroaxial anaesthesia** |
|---|
| Patient refusal or inability to cooperate |
| Coagulation defect |
| Infection at site of placement |
| Hypovolaemia/hypotension |
| Known intracranial mass |

should be readily available in case of intravascular injection or total spinal block. Continuous fetal heart rate monitoring should be employed.

## Epidural anaesthesia

Epidural anaesthesia remains the most commonly used neuroaxial method of pain relief in labour. Advantages include continuous analgesia for an indefinite time period and the ability to convert a labour epidural to a surgical anaesthetic for a caesarean section. Table 85.2 shows the disadvantages and complications of epidural anaesthesia. Correct positioning is crucial for neuroaxial block placement (Figure 85.5). Table 85.3 depicts one protocol for epidural placement. Various test doses facilitate the recognition of subarachnoid or intravascular catheter placement (Table 85.4). Some practitioners question the necessity of test dosing. With each redose, one must recognize the possibility that the epidural catheter may have migrated to an intravenous or subarachnoid location. Any dysfunctional epidural

| **Table 85.2 Complications of epidural analgesia** |
|---|
| High failure rate requiring replacement (10%) |
| Hypotension with resultant nausea and vomiting and potential fetal bradycardia |
| High/total spinal block |
| Accidental intravascular injection of local anaesthetic |
| Accidental placement of subarachnoid or subdural catheter |
| Urinary retention |
| Postdural puncture headache |

signifies intravascular placement unless proved otherwise. Table 85.5 provides dosing guidelines for continuous epidural infusion of local anaesthetic. The absence of sensory block, or an unexpectedly high block identifies catheter migration to an intravenous or subarachnoid location, respectively. Opioids may be added to lower concentrations of local anaesthetics to achieve less motor block, in the hope of retaining analgesic efficacy comparable to more concentrated solutions of local anaesthetics.

If an unintentional dural puncture occurs during attempted epidural placement, consider a continuous spinal catheter technique, particularly for a patient at high risk for repeat dural puncture (e.g. obesity or scoliosis). Alternatively, attempt epidural placement at a different interspace. I prefer the latter unless I anticipates difficult replacement or imminent delivery.

Debate continues as to whether regional anaesthesia delays the progress of labour, but there is general agreement that, when cervical dilatation exceeds 4 cm, epidural analgesia will not alter the course of labour.

## Spinal anaesthesia

Intrathecal local anaesthetics, opioids, or combinations in single or repeated doses provide effective analgesia for labour. Proposed advantages over epidural anaesthesia include more rapid onset, more reliable analgesia, and reduced motor block. The technique can allow ambulation in early labour and proves more practical than epidural techniques for providing analgesia in late labour when delivery appears imminent. Intrathecal administration of opioids without local anaesthetics allows normal motor function. Table 85.6 shows the side effects of intrathecal opioids and their treatment. Possible drug choices include fentanyl (20 μg), sufentanil (10 μg), and pethidine (20 mg) with or without bupivacaine (1–2.5 mg). Drawbacks of single-shot spinal techniques include finite duration of action, hypotension, pruritus, and nausea. The incidence of postdural puncture headache relates to the size and tip design of the spinal needle. The use of 27- and 29-gauge needles can reduce the risk to less than 1.5%.

## Combined spinal/epidural analgesia

Combined spinal/epidural (CSE) analgesia has recently become popular in obstetric anaesthesia. Using loss-

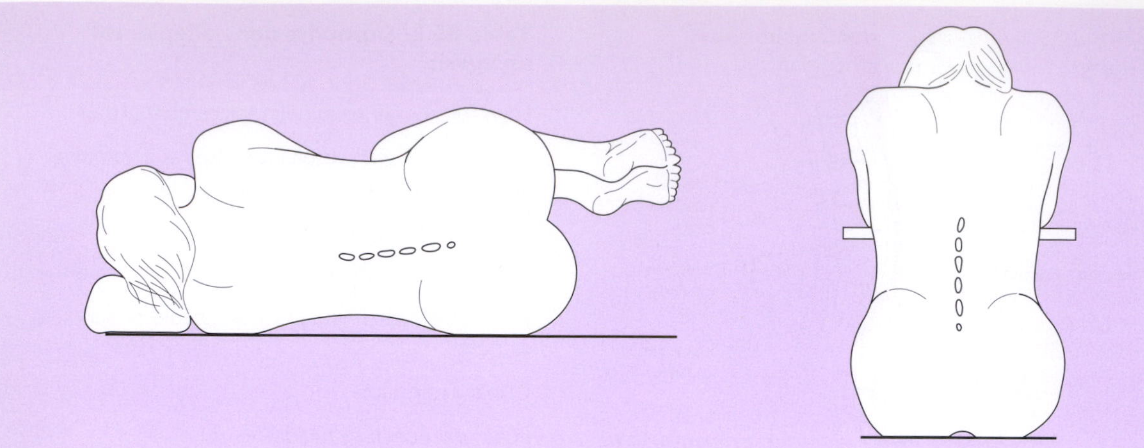

**Figure 85.5** Correct lateral decubitus and sitting position for neuroaxial block placement. (Adapted from Butterworth JF. *Atlas of Procedures in Anesthesia and Critical Care*. Philadelphia: WB Saunders, 1992: 184.)

| **Table 85.3 One technique for epidural catheter placement** |
|---|
| Patient position: lateral or sitting |
| Sterile prep and drape |
| 1% lignocaine (lidocaine) skin weal at L3–L4 or L4–L5 interspace |
| 17-gauge Tuohy–Schiff needle to locate epidural space using loss of resistance to air or saline |
| Thead 18-gauge catheter 4–6 cm in epidural space |
| 2 ml 2% lignocaine for subarachnoid test dose |
| Wait 5 min then inject 5 ml 2% lignocaine for intravenous test dose |
| Confirm bilateral sensory block to pinprick |
| If additional analgesia required give 5 ml 0.25% bupivacaine |
| Start 0.125% bupivacaine infusion with or without fentanyl at 10–14 ml/h |
| Give patient-controlled epidural analgesia with 5-ml bolus and 10-min lockout period |

From D'Angelo R, Berkebile BL, Gerancher JC. *Anesthesiology* 1996;84:88–93.

| **Table 85.4 Test dose to detect intravascular or subarachnoid (SA) catheter** |
|---|
| **Characteristics of an ideal test dose** |
| 1. Amount of local anaesthetic sufficient to allow easy identification of an intrathecal catheter without causing a total spinal or haemodynamic compromise |
| 2. Amount of local anaesthetic sufficient to produce reliable intravascular symptoms if given intravenously without being detrimental to mother or fetus |
| 3. The test dose should be readily available and have relatively high sensitivity and specificity |
| **Examples of commonly used test doses** |
| Lignocaine 40–60 mg for SA test followed by lignocaine 80–100 mg for intravenous test |
| Chloroprocaine 40 mg for SA test followed by chloroprocaine 80–100 mg for intravenous test |
| Bupivacaine 5–10 mg SA test |
| Lignocaine 45 mg with 1 : 200 000 epinephrine (adrenaline) for both SA and intravenous test (monitor for increase in heart rate and blood pressure and fetal stress with intravenous injection of epinephrine) |

| **Table 85.5 Guidelines for continuous epidural infusions for labour analgesia** | |
|---|---|
| Bupivacaine | 0.0625–0.25% at 8–15 ml/h |
| Lignocaine | 0.5–1.0% at 8–15 ml/h |
| 2-Chloroprocaine | 0.75% at 27 ml/h |

Adapted with permission from Glosten B. Local anesthetic techniques. In: Chestnut DH. *Obstetric Anesthesia: Principles and Practice*. St Louis: Mosby, 1994: 363.

| **Table 85.6 Side effects of intrathecal opioids and their treatment** | |
|---|---|
| Itching | Diphenhydramine 25 mg i.v.<br>Nalbuphine 5–10 mg i.v.<br>Propofol 10 mg i.v.<br>Naloxone 40 mg i.v. |
| Nausea and vomiting | Metoclopramide 5–10 mg i.v.<br>Nalbuphine 5–10 mg i.v.<br>Propofol 10 mg i.v.<br>Naloxone 40 mg i.v. |
| Hypotension | Intravenous fluids<br>Ephedrine 5–10 mg i.v. increments |
| Urinary retention | Naloxone 400–800 mg i.v.<br>Bladder catheterization |

Adapted with permission from Cheek TG, Gutsche BB. Analgesia for labor. In: Dewan D, Hood D. *Practical Obstetric Anesthesia*. Philadelphia: WB Saunders, 1997: 114.

of-resistance-to-air technique, an epidural needle identifies the epidural space and then a 25- or 27-gauge needle is inserted through the epidural needle to puncture the dura. Intrathecal opioid or a combination of local anaesthetic and opioid is administered. The spinal component provides rapid onset, reduced motor block, and initial reliability. The epidural then provides an indefinite duration of analgesia and can be utilized for surgical delivery. This procedure proves particularly useful for the multiparous patient who requests analgesia in the late active phase of labour. Alternatively, it may allow ambulation in the latent phase of labour. Unfortunately, a failure rate as high as 13% may occur with the needle-through-needle technique for the reasons depicted in Figure 85.6. In addition, it is difficult to predict which patients are likely to deliver during the spinal portion of the therapy, and the success of the epidural component of CSE is probably no greater than a traditional epidural. The side-effect profile of CSE includes pruritus, nausea, vomiting, hypotension, and postdural puncture headache.

The results of a national study of the use of analgesia during childbirth in the UK shows that few women having their first baby use no analgesia at all (Figure 85.7). It is apparent that most women rely on a combination of methods of analgesia. The most commonly used method is Entonox followed by pethidine. It can be seen that relaxation and massage are important components of analgesia. Although epidural analgesia may not be available on a 24-hour basis in all units, it is striking that the use of this method increases with increasing duration of labour, reflecting its undoubted effectiveness, allowing rest and the ready possibility of sufficient analgesia for caesarean section when required. The low use of TENS may have been affected by its availability being restricted to certain units.

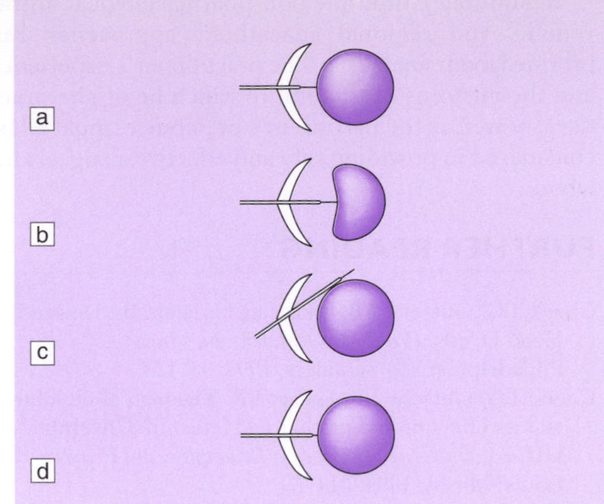


**Figure 85.6** Various possible reasons for combined spinal/epidural failure as a result of incorrect positioning of epidural or spinal needle. (a) The length of the spinal needle protruding from the tip of the epidural needle is too short. (b) The tip of the spinal needle 'tents' the dura without piercing it. (c) The epidural needle is malpositioned. (d) Correct placement of both epidural and spinal needles. (From Rawal N, Van Zundert A, Holmstrom B, Crowhurst JA. *Reg Anesth* 1997;22:406–23.)

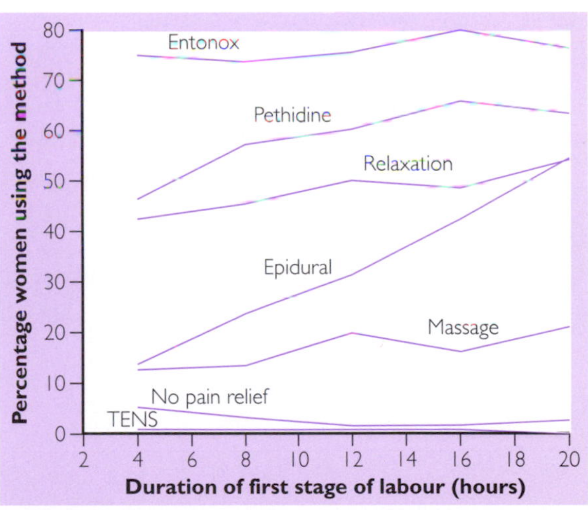


**Figure 85.7** Percentage of first-time mothers using different types of analgesia, according to duration of labour. Note that some mothers used more than one type of analgesia. (From Chamberlain G, Wraight A, Steer P, eds. *Pain and its Relief in Childbirth. The results of a national survey by the National Birthday Trust*. Edinburgh: Churchill Livingstone, 1993.)

In summary, multiple non-pharmacological, intravenous, and regional anaesthetic approaches can provide labour analgesia. The practitioner's experience and the customs of the unit in which he or she practises, as well as the parturient's preference, must all be considered in providing safe and effective analgesia for labour.

## FURTHER READING


Cheek TG, Gutsche BB. Analgesia for labor. In: Dewan D, Hood D, eds. *Practical Obstetric Anesthesia.* Philadelphia: WB Saunders, 1997: 95–124.

Cheek TG, Gutsche BB, Gaiser RR. The pain of childbirth and its effect on the mother and fetus. In: Chestnut DH, ed. *Obstetric Anesthesia Principles and Practice.* St Louis: Mosby, 1994: 314–29.

Hawkins JL. New techniques for labor analgesia. *Anesth Analg* 1998;(suppl):57–60.

Practice guidelines for obstetrical anesthesia: a report by the American Society of Anesthesiologists Task Force on Obstetrical Anesthesia. *Anesthesiology* 1999;**90**:600–11.

Rawal N, Van Zundert A, Holmstrom B, Crowhurst JA. Combined spinal–epidural technique. *Reg Anesth* 1997;**22**:406–23.

Reynolds F, Russel R. Central neural blockade for labour. *Curr Opin Anaesthesiol* 1997;**10**:345–9.

Shnider SM, Levinson G. Anesthesia for cesarean section. In: Shnider SM, Levinson G, eds. *Anesthesia for Obstetrics*, 3rd edn. Baltimore, MA: Williams & Wilkins, 1993: 211–45.

Wakefield ML. Systemic analgesia: opioids, ketamine and inhalational agents. In: Chestnut DH, ed. *Obstetric Anesthesia Principles and Practice.* St Louis: Mosby, 1994: 340–78.

# Chapter 86 Safety precautions when using lasers

A.G. Pashayan and
M.A. Polkinghorne

The word 'laser' is an acronym for **l**ight **a**mplification of the **s**timulated **e**mission of **r**adiation and refers to a wide variety of devices that produce coherent light used for commercial, scientific, and medical applications. Laser light is being applied to an ever-increasing number of medical and surgical interventions that require anaesthesia care, so the anaesthetist must understand the hazards and safety procedures associated with this form of electromagnetic radiation.

Sunlight consists of waves of varying frequencies and wavelengths, which travel in a diffuse, spreading pattern. Laser light, on the other hand, is coherent, meaning that waves are of uniform length, travel in phase with each other, and are non-divergent (Table 86.1).

Stimulation of a homogeneous population of molecules, known as the lasing medium, to emit photons (Figure 86.1) produces coherent light in the optical cavity of the laser device. The photons are focused into spots of extremely high-energy density which are applied clinically for their thermal effects, to cut, coagulate, or vaporize tissues.

The exact effect of a particular laser on tissue depends on the wavelength of the beam, the tissue being irradiated, and the beam's power density. Table 86.2 lists commonly used wavelengths, their respective lasing media, and their general characteristics. Note that the carbon dioxide ($CO_2$) laser produces light in the far-infrared range, which is readily absorbed by all types and colours of tissues, hence the $CO_2$ laser beam exerts its effect on whatever surface it strikes first. In contrast, the green beam of the potassium titanyl phosphate (KTP) laser passes through clear tissues without interaction but is highly absorbed by tissues pigmented by haemoglobin and melanin.

The same tissue thermal effects that provide the clinical applications of laser light also present hazards to the patient being treated and to nearby health care workers. Accidental exposure to a direct or reflected laser beam can cause burns to normal tissues or ignition of flammable materials. Should the eye be exposed, visual impairment may result from corneal injury (e.g. $CO_2$ lasers) or retinal damage (e.g. argon, KTP, Nd:YAG [neodymium : yttrium–aluminium–garnet] lasers). Vaporized tissue produces a smoke known as the 'laser plume' which may contain infectious particles, irritate the respiratory tract or induce nausea. Lasers are classified by their potential to cause tissue injury, such that the higher the class of laser, the greater the potential hazard (Table 86.3). Most lasers used in medical and surgical interventions are in class 4, so that a formal laser safety programme must be implemented by health care facilities operating these devices.

Assurance that their surgeons and physicians are trained and qualified for the specific wavelength of the lasers that they are operating represents a key issue in the laser safety programme of any health care facility. Personnel other than the operating surgeon who work around the laser should also learn the potential risks of the laser, and the appropriate management of complications. During medical use of a laser, warning signs

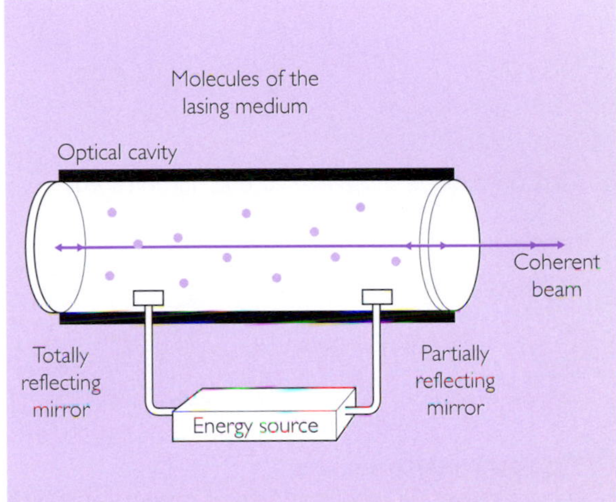


**Figure 86.1** The three principal parts of a laser: the energy source; the lasing medium; and the optical cavity. (Adapted from Pashayan AG. Lasers and laser safety. In: Kirby RR, Gravenstein N, eds. *Clinical Anesthesia Practice*. Philadelphia: WB Saunders, 1994: 1370–9.)

| **Table 86. Characteristics of coherent radiation** |
|---|
| Monochromaticity: all waves are of the same wavelength or colour |
| Collimation: all waves are parallel to each other and do not diverge |
| Coherence: all waves travel in phase in the same direction |

**Table 86.2 Lasers commonly used in the operating room**

| Laser | Wavelength (nm) | General considerations |
|---|---|---|
| Argon | 488–515 (blue/green) | Absorbed selectively by haemoglobin and melanin or other similar pigments<br>Transmitted through clear substances<br>Tissue penetration: 0.5–2 mm |
| KTP[a] (frequency-doubled YAG) | 532 (green) | Strongly absorbed by haemoglobin, melanin, and similar pigments<br>Transmitted through clear substances<br>Tissue penetration: 0.5–2 mm |
| Dye laser | Variable with dyes | Wavelength can be tuned to suit application, e.g. 585 nm (yellow) for haemoglobin absorption and 630 nm (red) for photodynamic therapy |
| Nd :YAG[b] | 1064 (near infrared) | More readily absorbed by dark tissue<br>Transmitted through clear fluids<br>Tissue penetration: 2–6 mm |
| Carbon dioxide ($CO_2$) | 10 600 (far infrared) | Strongly absorbed by water and thus by all tissue, pigmented or not<br>Tissue penetration: < 0.5 mm |
| He–Ne[c] | 633 (red) | Used as a low-power coaxial aiming beam for non-visible laser ($CO_2$ and Nd :YAG)<br>Has no significant tissue interaction |
| Holium YAG | 650 (green) | Vaporizes and coagulates tissue |

[a]Potassium titanyl phosphate.
[b]Neodymium (Nd)-doped yttrium–aluminum–garnet (YAG).
[c]Helium–neon.

**Table 86.3 Classification established by the American National Standards Institute for Lasers and Laser Hazards**

| Class | Description | Examples | Control measures |
|---|---|---|---|
| 1 | Beam is totally contained and device cannot emit accessible laser radiation | Lasers used in laboratories for diagnostic work | No |
| 2 | Low-power visible lasers that are not intended for prolonged viewing; the normal blink reflex will protect the eye | He–Ne aiming beam for $CO_2$ and Nd :YAG lasers | Yes |
| 3a<br>3b | Normally would not pose a hazard if viewed momentarily with the unaided eye<br>May produce a hazard if viewed directly (intra-beam viewing and specular reflection) | Some ophthalmological lasers are higher class 3 | Yes |
| 4 | Hazardous if viewed directly or from diffuse reflection. Also produces fire hazards and skin hazards | Most medical lasers including $CO_2$, Nd :YAG, argon, and KTP | Yes |

Abbreviations as Table 86.2. Reproduced with permission from the *American National Standard for the Safe Use of Lasers*. Orlando: Laser Institute of America, 1993.

that specify the class and wavelength of laser should clearly mark all entrances to the operating room or treatment room. Protective goggles should be provided for all people in the treatment area; such goggles must be able to filter out the specific wavelength of the laser in use. The patient's eyes should be lubricated with a water-based, non-flammable solution and then closed and covered with wet gauze. Normal tissues in and around the operative site may also be protected with wet drapes and gauze. Metallic instruments in and around the operative field should have a matte rather than a glossy finish, so as to diffuse the reflection of the beam. Flame-retardant drapes should be used to impede the spread of a fire.

Laser-ignited airway fires are of particular concern to the anaesthetist. Many laryngologists favour lasers because the resection of airway tumours or other obstructions can be very precise and produces minimal oedema when compared with traditional excisional techniques. $CO_2$ lasers prove particularly useful in airway surgery as a result of the shallow depth of burn and extreme precision. However, the oxygen-rich environment and the presence of flammable materials, such as polyvinyl chloride (PVC) tracheal tubes in the airway during general anaesthesia, increase the risk of fire. Severe, life-threatening burns of the larynx and trachea have occurred in such situations, and airway fires have extended up the anaesthesia circuit throughout the operating room, risking the safety of health care personnel as well.

Airway endoscopy can be divided into upper airway procedures (operations at or above the larynx) and lower airway procedures (operations on the trachea and bronchi). Elimination of the tracheal tube, either with jet or spontaneous ventilation, during laser surgery on the upper airway lowers the risk of airway fire. A metal, blunt-tipped needle mounted in the operating laryngoscope can be used to direct a high-velocity jet of oxygen down the airway lumen; the risk of fire is low because there are no flammable objects in the path of the laser beam. However, jet ventilation may not provide adequate gas exchange in patients with decreased pulmonary compliance or increased airway resistance, such as morbidly obese or bronchospastic patients; jet ventilation also risks pneumothorax and other forms of barotrauma. Spontaneous ventilation of potent inhaled agents in oxygen through the operating laryngoscope offers yet another means of avoiding tracheal intubation. However, the spontaneously breathing patient cannot receive neuromuscular blockers and could move during surgery, potentially mistargeting the laser beam. Non-intubation techniques make capnography and spirometry difficult, if not impossible, compounding the risk of hypoventilation by obfuscating its detection. Other risks in the non-intubated airway include aspiration of gastric contents, aspiration of laser plume, and accidental laser perforation of the trachea distal to the surgical site.

Tracheal intubation secures the airway and provides for optimal ventilatory monitoring. However, conventional tracheal tube materials are readily ignitable and flammable (Table 86.4). During traditional, non-laser surgery, PVC represents the tracheal-tube material of choice because it is clear and soft, and it maintains a patent lumen while conforming to the natural curves of the airway anatomy. PVC tubes have a higher oxygen index of flammability than other traditional tracheal tube materials (Table 86.4), and thus require a higher concentration of oxygen to sustain a flame than either red rubber or silicone. However, PVC tubes can ignite as a result of either high oxygen concentration or excess laser exposure and, once ignited, can sustain a torch-like flame, which propagates down the lumen of the tube into the patient's trachea. For these reasons, unprotected PVC tracheal tubes are not recommended for airway laser surgery.

Alternative tracheal tube materials include red rubber and silicone. Red rubber can sustain combustion in room air (Table 86.4), so that it is susceptible to extraluminal fires. However, because red rubber resists penetration by the laser, making the deadly intraluminal fire unlikely, many practitioners prefer it. Silicone, much like red rubber, can ignite in room air (Table 86.4). When ignited, silicone rapidly oxidizes to a brittle, crumbling ash which could result in the retention of tube segments and debris in the airway.

To protect flammable materials, the anaesthetist may wrap tracheal tubes in metallic tapes or metallic-based sponges. The use of one of the commercially available laser-resistant tracheal tubes (Table 86.5) offers an alternative to wrapping tubes. Although these products greatly reduce the risk of airway fire, they all contain flammable material that a laser can ignite. Flammable material in the airway necessitates measures to reduce the risk of fire, such as limiting the fractional inspired oxygen concentration ($F\text{IO}_2$) and using helium in the gas mixture if tracheal intubation is used during airway laser surgery (Table 86.6).

During laser operations on the trachea and bronchi, a metal bronchoscope is typically used to access the lower airway, and ventilation may be maintained through the side arm of the bronchoscope. The risk of

**Table 86.4 Combustion properties of materials composing conventional tracheal tubes**

| Material | Oxygen index of flammability[a] | Penetration time (s)[b,c] | Mean time to ignition (s)[b] |
|---|---|---|---|
| Polyvinylchloride | 0.263 | 0.77 | 3.06 |
| Silicone | 0.189 | Not tested | Not tested |
| Red rubber | 0.176 | 41.48 | 33 |

[a]Fractional concentration of oxygen that sustains a candle-like flame. From Wolf GL, Simpson JI. Flammability of tracheal tubes in oxygen and nitrous oxide enriched atmosphere. *Anesthesiology* 1987;67:236–9.
[b]Times with a 10-W laser beam and 50% oxygen and 50% nitrogen.
[c]Ossoff RG. *Laryngoscope* 1989;99(suppl 48):1–26.
Pashayan AG. Lasers and laser safety. In: Kirby RR, Gravenstein N, eds. *Clinical Anesthesia Practice*. Philadelphia: WB Saunders, 1994: 1370–9.

fire is low with a metal bronchoscope, although desiccated tissue can sustain combustion. Should a flammable fibreoptic cable or a fibreoptic bronchoscope be used to deliver the laser beam, the risk of fire increases, and $F\text{IO}_2$ must be limited.

The team of surgeon, anaesthetist, and operating room nurse should be vigilant for the signs of airway fire during airway laser surgery, and should be trained in how to manage such a catastrophe (Table 86.7).

**Table 86.5 Advantages and disadvantages of commercially available laser-resistant tracheal tubes**

| Description of resistant tube | Applicable laser | Advantages | Disadvantages |
|---|---|---|---|
| Aluminum/silicone spiral with self-inflating foam cuff (Fome-Cuf, Bivona, Inc., Gary, IN, US) | $CO_2$ | Atraumatic external surface; cuff maintains seal even if punctured by laser; non-flammable inner surface | Contains flammable material (silicone); cuff difficult to deflate if punctured |
| Airtight, stainless steel, corrugated spiral with polyvinyl chloride tip and double cuff (Laser Flex, Mallinckrodt, St Louis, MO, US) | $CO_2$, KTP | Tube maintains shape well, double cuff maintains seal after proximal cuff puncture; body of tube is non-flammable; non-cuffed version available | Cuffed version contains flammable material polyvinyl chloride; tubes are thick walled; metal may reflect beam onto non-targeted tissue |
| Silicone tubes wrapped with aluminum and Teflon, with methylene blue in cuff (Laser-Shield, Xomed, Inc., Jacksonville, FL, US) | $CO_2$, KTP | Wrapping protects flammable material and is smoother than manual tape wrapping; methylene blue aids in detection of cuff perforation | Contains flammable material (silicone); single cuff is vulnerable to laser damage |

$CO_2$, carbon dioxide; KTP, potassium titanyl phosphate.

Reproduced with permission from Pashayan AG, Ehrenwerth J. Lasers and electrical safety in the operating room. In: Ehrenwerth J, Eisenkraft JB, eds. *Anesthesia Equipment: Principles and Applications*. Philadelphia: Mosby, 1993: 436–69.

**Table 86.6 Measures to reduce the risk of airway fire during laser endoscopy**

| Measurement | Considerations |
|---|---|
| $F\text{IO}_2$ | The lowest $F\text{IO}_2$ compatible with $Sp\text{O}_2 \geq 95\%$ should be employed. Only nitrogen or helium should be used as oxygen diluents. Nitrous oxide can serve as an oxidizer and will promote flames |
| Helium | Helium with its high thermal diffusiveness, lowers heat at the site of laser contact, thus decreasing the risk of ignition |
| Positive airway pressure (PEEP) | Application of low levels of PEEP (5 cm) sustains gas flow across laser-induced holes, thus cooling the site of laser contact |
| Power density | Limitation of laser to the lowest clinically acceptable power density |
| Tracheal tube cuff | Fill the tracheal tube cuff with saline instead of air to decrease risk of cuff ignition |

$F\text{IO}_2$, fractional inspired oxygen concentration; PEEP, positive end-expiratory pressure; $Sp\text{O}_2$, blood oxygen saturation measured with a pulse oximeter.

**Table 86.7 Response to fires during laser operations on the airway**

| Steps | Measure |
|---|---|
| **Immediate** | |
| First | Disconnect oxygen source at Y piece and remove burning objects from the airway |
| Second | Irrigate site with water if fire is still smouldering |
| Third | Ventilate the patient by mask or reintubate the trachea and ventilate with as low an $FiO_2$ as possible |
| **Secondary** | |
| Fourth | Evaluate extent of injury by bronchoscopy and laryngoscopy |
| Fifth | Reintubate the trachea or perform a tracheostomy if needed |
| Sixth | Monitor with oximetry, arterial blood gas analysis, or both, and chest radiographs |
| | for at least 24 hours |
| Seventh | Use ventilatory support, steroids, and antibiotics as needed |

$FiO_2$, fractional inspired oxygen concentration.
Reproduced with permission from Pashayan AG, Ehrenwerth J. Lasers and electrical safety in the operating room. In: Ehrenwerth J, Eisenkraft JB, eds. *Anesthesia Equipment: Principles and Applications*. Philadelphia: Mosby, 1993: 436–69.

## FURTHER READING


American National Standard for the Safe Use of Lasers. Orlando: Laser Institute of America, 1993.

ASTM Subcommittee F29.02.10: Pashayan AG *et al*. Upper airway management guide provided for laser airway surgery. Park Ridge, IL: Anesthesia Patient Safety Foundation Newsletter 1993; 2:13–6.

International Organization for Standardization (ISO). ISO TR 11991: Guidance on airway management during laser surgery of upper airway. Geneva, Switzerland: ISO; 1995. 10

International Organization for Standardization (ISO). ISO 14408: Tracheal tubes designed for laser surgery – requirements for marking and accompanying information. Geneva, Switzerland: ISO; 1998.

International Organization for Standardization (ISO). ISO TR 11990: Optics and optical instruments – lasers and laser-related equipment – determination of laser resistance of tracheal tube shafts. Geneva, Switzerland: ISO; 1999.

Pashayan AG, Ehrenwerth J. Lasers and electrical safety in the operating room. In: Ehrenwerth J, Eisenkraft JB, eds. *Anesthesia Equipment: Principles and Applications*. Philadelphia: Mosby, 1993: 436–69.

# Chapter 87 Management of porphyria

S.Y. Dolinski

## PATHOPHYSIOLOGY

Porphyria is a disease resulting from a partially inherited or acquired enzyme defect in haem biosynthesis. Porphyrias are classified as either hepatic or erythropoietic, depending on the site of the haem production defect (Table 87.1). There are multiple specific enzyme defects; nevertheless, all porphyrias result in excesses of haem precursor, a porphyrinogen, which when oxidized becomes a porphyrin (Figure 87.1). Porphyrin accumulates in tissues and, as a highly reactive oxidant, leads to tissue injury and the clinical disturbances associated with the disease. It seems that neurological tissue takes up δ-aminolaevulinic acid (δ-ALA) which inhibits sodium/potassium ATPase, which in turn results in inhibition of nerve conduction.

**Table 87.1 Classification of porphyrias**

| |
|---|
| **Hepatic porphyrias** |
| Acute intermittent porphyria |
| Hereditary coproporphyria |
| Variegate porphyria |
| Plumboporphyria |
| **Hepatic non-acute porphyrias** |
| Porphyria cutanea tarda |
| **Erythropoietic porphyrias** |
| Erythropoietic uroporphyria |
| Erythropoietic protoporphyria |

Adapted from Moore MR. *Disorders of Porphyrin Metabolism*. New York: Plenum, 1987.

Normally δ-ALA synthase catalyses the rate-limiting step in haem production. Intermediates are rapidly metabolized and haem itself acts as an inhibitor of further haem synthesis. The various enzyme defects result in less mitochondrial haem synthesis, less negative feedback of δ-ALA synthase activity, and accumulation of intermediate species.

Of the five types of hepatic porphyria, four have importance for the anaesthetist: acute intermittent porphyria (AIP), hereditary coproporphyria (HCP), and variegate porphyria (VP); plumboporphyria represents a very rare hepatic porphyria which, unlike the others, is inherited in an autosomal recessive fashion. These four types prove indistinguishable in regard to the presentation of a neurovisceral crisis (central nervous system [CNS] and gastrointestinal symptomatology) and management. However, HCP and VP also demonstrate photosensitivity and skin fragility which AIP does not. Only the porphyrias producing neurovisceral symptoms are called acute. Porphyria cutanea tarda is

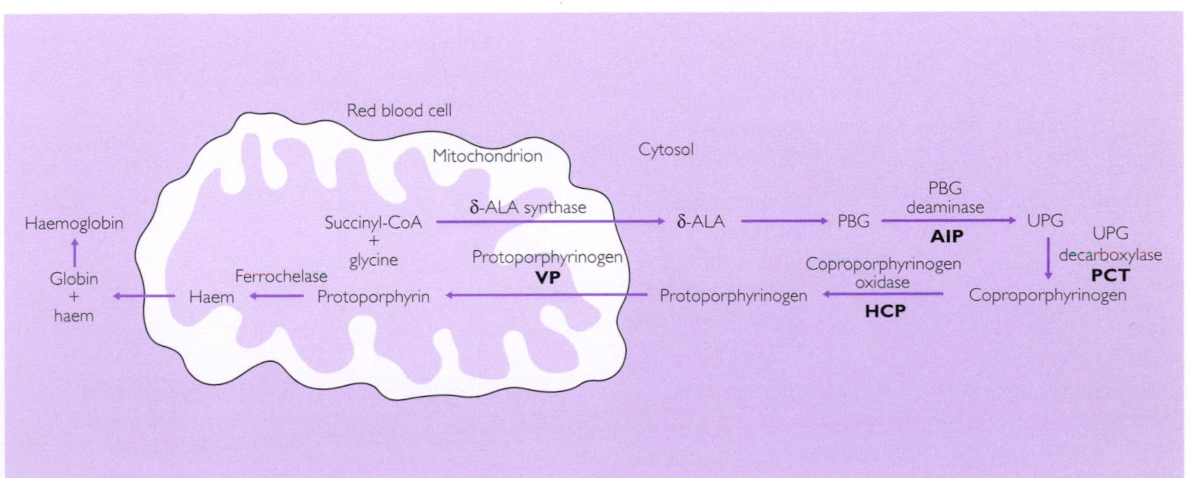


**Figure 87.1** Porphyrin pathway to haem biosynthesis. δ-ALA, δ-aminolaevulinic acid; PGB, porphobilinogen; UPG, uroporphyrinogen. Abbreviations in bold indicate the type of porphyria that results from the enzyme defect: AIP, acute intermittent porphyria; PCT, porphyria cutanea tarda; HCP, hereditary coproporphyria; VP, variegate porphyria.

associated with liver disease but not with drug-induced crises. Likewise, drug-induced crises do not occur in the red-blood-cell-derived porphyrias.

Acute attacks occur more commonly in women than in men and rarely before puberty. Acute attacks include abdominal pains (see Chapter 61), peripheral neuropathies, and changes in mental status that can be triggered by drugs, most notoriously the barbiturates. An unrecognized attack can be fatal (Table 87.2). In addition to drugs, fasting, infection, alcohol intake, psychological stress, menstruation, and pregnancy can precipitate attacks. Most porphyria-inducing drugs decrease haem levels by three possible mechanisms. First, they can stimulate cytochrome P450 synthesis, which leads to greater incorporation of haem. Second, they can destroy cytochromes, requiring more haem to be utilized in cytochrome production and thereby preventing haem from acting as the enzyme inhibitor. Last of all, they can alter the haem molecule such that it cannot negatively influence δ-ALA synthase.

## CLINICAL FEATURES

Patients with porphyria normally remain asymptomatic, but can develop occasional acute attacks featuring abdominal, neurological, and laboratory test alterations. An autonomic neuropathy resulting from neurotoxic metabolite deposition causes the colicky abdominal pain. Other common symptoms and signs include nausea, vomiting, constipation, diarrhoea, and dehydration. Further evidence of autonomic dysfunction includes tachycardia, hypertension, and orthostatic hypotension. During severe sympathetic discharge, sudden death can ensue secondary to cardiac arrhythmias. Besides autonomic neuropathy, these patients can develop peripheral motor neuropathies resulting in paresis or paralysis of the proximal extremities. They can be asymmetrical and focal or involve cranial nerves. Bulbar neuropathies cause dysphonia, dysphagia, and, rarely, diaphragmatic paralysis and respiratory compromise. Sensory involvement tends to be patchy, leading to paraesthesias and numbness.

**Table 87.2 Anesthetic drug interactions with porphyria**

| Drug class | Safe drugs | Unsafe drugs | Safety unclear |
|---|---|---|---|
| Benzodiazepines | Midazolam<br>Lorazepam | Flunitrazepam<br>Nitrazepam<br>Chlordiazepoxide | Diazepam |
| Induction agents | Propofol | Barbiturates<br>Etomidate | Ketamine |
| Opioids | Morphine<br>Fentanyl | Pentazocine | Sufentanil |
| Neuromuscular blocking agents | Succinylcholine<br>Vecuronium<br>*d*-Tubocurarine | | Pancuronium<br>Atracurium |
| Anticholinesterases | Neostigmine | | |
| Local anaesthetics | Bupivacaine<br>Procaine | | Lignocaine |
| Cardiovascular | Atenolol<br>Labetalol<br>Phentolamine<br>Reserpine<br>Guanethidine | α-Methyldopa<br>Hydralazine<br>Phenoxybenzamine | |
| Premedicants | Scopolamine<br>Atropine<br>Droperidol<br>Chloral hydrate<br>Diphenhydramine<br>Cimetidine | | |
| Inhalational agents | Nitrous oxide | Enflurane | Sevoflurane<br>Desflurane<br>Isoflurane<br>Halothane |
| Other | Glucose loading<br>Anticonvulsants | Oral contraceptives<br>Griseofulvin<br>Endogenous steroids | |

Dysfunction of hypothalamic supraoptic and paraventricular nuclei can manifest as the syndrome of inappropriate antidiuretic hormone secretion and pyrexia. These can lead to or contribute to other CNS disturbances, including psychosis, confusion, seizures, and coma. Porphobilinogen (PBG) and δ-ALA, probable neurotoxins, may inhibit neurotransmitter release. Altered neural haem synthesis may contribute to CNS findings. Decreases in haem synthesis impair tryptophan metabolism, which inhibits gluconeogenesis with concomitant hypoglycaemia. Altered laboratory findings include hypochloraemia, hyponatraemia, hypokalaemia, and hypomagnesaemia from vomiting, diarrhoea, and dehydration. Tachycardia presents a sensitive indicator of worsening disease. As the patient improves, the tachycardia resolves. Paresis and the emotional/psychological disturbances often persist.

## DIAGNOSIS

The diagnosis can be confirmed only when laboratory studies are available, because the symptomatology is non-specific. Patients experiencing an acute attack will have elevated concentrations of δ-ALA and PBG in their urine. The specific type of porphyria can be identified by detection of porphyrins in urine and/or faeces. Other diseases are associated with haem biosynthesis abnormalities such as lead poisoning and hereditary tyrosinosis. (For a summary of tests see Further reading: Sumner, and McCarroll). Any patient with known porphyria or one who has a family history of porphyria should be considered potentially at risk for developing an acute porphyric attack.

## PREOPERATIVE EVALUATION

Any patient presenting with acute abdominal pain, changes in mental status, and peripheral neuropathy should be considered possibly to have porphyria, and anaesthetic drugs known to trigger a porphyric attack should be avoided. When symptoms are present in a patient known to have porphyria, one should perform and document the neurological examination. Preoperatively, this may sway the anaesthetist from performing regional anaesthesia and enhance the anaesthetist's awareness of any new postoperative peripheral nervous system findings. Porphyric patients should receive ample premedication to avoid psychological stress. In addition, the patient should receive liberal intravenous fluids containing dextrose and the time of preoperative fasting should be minimized.

## INTRAOPERATIVE MANAGEMENT

### Induction

As patients with porphyria can have an attack precipitated by mechanisms other than drugs, any drug concurrently administered while the patient develops an attack could be implicated. Numerous case reports demonstrate that barbiturates have been given to patients with acute porphyria who are not in crisis, without leading to an attack. Two studies showed that patients with latent porphyria received barbiturates with no symptomatic consequences. However, as barbiturates have been shown to be porphyrinogenic in animals and in many case reports, they are contraindicated. In one fatal case involving the use of barbiturates, δ-ALA synthase activity was increased 40-fold.

Propofol has not been implicated in animal models as contributing to or causing an attack. One report showed a trend in increased δ-ALA synthase activity in rats, but it was not statistically significant. Many case reports show successful use of propofol in humans. However, there are case reports of patients who remained symptomatic with increased urinary porphyrins after continuous infusions of propofol. Only recently has there been a case report of porphyric symptoms exhibited after a 16-hour propofol infusion. The benzodiazepines, midazolam and lorazepam, are considered safe. Diazepam, in particular, has been associated with AIP attacks. Etomidate can be porphyrinogenic and should be avoided. Ketamine has been used clinically without precipitating any porphyric symptoms, although one induced porphyric crisis has been reported. In animal research the results are conflicting. ALA synthase activity increases in chick embryos injected with ketamine whereas no change in enzyme activity occurs after high concentrations of ketamine.

### Maintenance

Enflurane represents the only inhalational agent classified as unsafe based on animal experiments. Neither of the two newer inhalational anaesthetics sevoflurane or desflurane has been reported to be porphyrinogenic. Opioid and nitrous oxide combinations can also be used. Suxamethonium, *d*-tubocurarine, and vecuronium are deemed safe. Pancuronium has been labelled porphyrinogenic based on animal data. Rocuronium and cisatracurium have not been associated with porphyria.

### Monitoring

Haemodynamic variability from autonomic neuropathy, potential hypovolaemia, and hypertension requires careful monitoring of arterial blood pressure. Invasive monitoring may be indicated, depending on the extent of surgery.

### Postoperative management

Postoperative nausea and vomiting can be treated with droperidol, chlorpromazine, or promethazine. Metoclopramide should be avoided. The safety of the anti-serotonin agents such as ondansetron has not been determined.

## REGIONAL ANAESTHESIA

As porphyric patients often develop peripheral neuropathies, some clinicians avoid regional techniques in these patients. Lignocaine (lidocaine) is often cited as being porphyrinogenic on the basis of animal experiments; nevertheless, it has been used in porphyric patients without precipitating attacks. Procaine and bupivacaine have been widely used and recommended. Some proponents of regional anaesthesia favour spinal over epidural anaesthesia because of the lower blood concentrations of local anaesthetics.

## ACUTE SYMPTOM MANAGEMENT

Tachycardia and hypertension can be treated with propranolol or atenolol. The other β-adrenoceptor have not been adequately studied. α-Methyldopa and hydralazine are considered unsafe antihypertensives. For the treatment of seizures, the use of phenytoin and valproic acid remains controversial. Lorazepam or midazolam represent the best initial drugs. Any drug implicated as a potential trigger of the attack should be discontinued. Intravenous glucose solutions should be initiated because they will suppress porphyrin synthesis. Haematin (3–4 mg/kg per day) offers the most effective therapy in an acute attack. It suppresses δ-ALA synthase activity. Acute attacks should be closely monitored in the intensive care unit and the above treatment measures undertaken. Without treatment, the symptoms tend to subside within 5 days.

## PSEUDOPORPHYRIA

Tetracycline, dapsone, naproxen, frusemide (furosemide), and pyridoxine are associated with pseudoporphyria, a drug-induced bullous photosensitivity. Up to 16% of haemodialysis patients can develop bullous dermatosis of haemodialysis. In this condition porphyrins remain normal and no modification in anaesthetic agents is required.

## CONCLUSION

As new drugs are constantly being introduced without having been tested for porphyria-inducing characteristics, one should preferentially use those with a history of safety.

## FURTHER READING


Asirvatham SJ, Johnson TW, Oberoi MP, Jackman WM. Prolonged loss of consciousness and elevated porphyrins following propofol administrations. *Anesthesiology* 1998;**89**:1029–31.

Bolognia JL, Braverman IM. Skin manifestations of internal disease. In: Fauci AS, *et al*., eds. *Harrison's Principles of Internal Medicine*, 14th edn. New York: McGraw-Hill, 1998: 310–28.

Harrison GG, Meissner PN, Hift RJ. Anaesthesia for the porphyric patient. *Anaesthesia* 1993;48:417–421.

Kappas A, Sassa S, Galbraith RA, Nordmann Y. The porphyrias. In: Scriver CR, Beaudet AL, Sly WS, Valle D, eds. *The Metabolic and Molecular Bases of Inherited Disease*. New York: McGraw-Hill, 1995: 2103–59.

McCarroll NA. Diseases of metabolism (porphyrias). *Anal Chem* 1995;**67**(suppl):425R–8R.

Meissner PN, Harrison GG, Hift RJ. Propofol as an i.v. anaesthetic induction agent in variegate porphyria. *Br J Anaesth* 1991;**66**:60–5.

Mustajoki P, Heinonen J. General anesthesia in 'inducible' porphyrias. *Anesthesiology* 1980;53:15–20.

Stone DR, Munson ES. Anaesthetics and porphyria. *Br J Anaesth* 1979;**51**:809.

Sumner E. Porphyria in relation to surgery and anaesthesia. *Ann R Coll Surg Engl* 1975;**56**:81–8.

# Index

Page numbers in *italic* denote figure legends where there is no textual reference on the same page.
GI = gastrointestinal  IV = intravenous